John C. Young, M.D.

Primary Care *for* Women

Primary Care *for* Women

Edited by

Phyllis C. Leppert, MD, PhD
Chair
Department of Obstetrics and Gynecology
State University of New York at Buffalo
Buffalo, New York

Formerly Professor of Obstetrics and Gynecology
University of Rochester School of Medicine and Dentistry
Chair, Department of Obstetrics and Gynecology
Rochester General Hospital
Rochester, New York

Fred M. Howard, MD
Assistant Professor of Obstetrics and Gynecology
University of Rochester School of Medicine and Dentistry
Associate Chief
Department of Obstetrics and Gynecology
University of Rochester School of Medicine and Dentistry
Rochester General Hospital
Rochester, New York

with 106 contributing authors

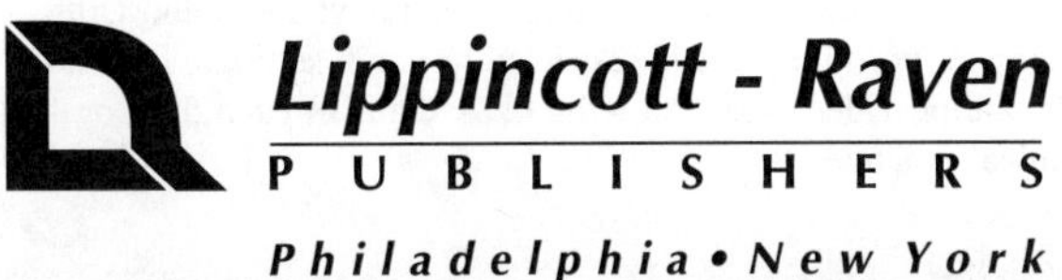
Lippincott - Raven
PUBLISHERS
Philadelphia • New York

Acquisitions Editor: Lisa McAllister
Developmental Editor: Emilie Linkins
Associate Managing Editor: Elizabeth A. Durand
Production Manager: Caren Erlichman
Production Coordinator: MaryClare Malady
Design Coordinator: Melissa Olson
Indexer: Maria Coughlin
Printer: Quebecor/Kingsport

Primary care for women / edited by Phyllis C. Leppert, Fred M. Howard; with 106 contributing authors.
p. cm
Includes bibliographical references and index.
ISBN 0-397-51523-5
1. Women—Diseases. 2. Women—Health and hygiene. 3. Primary care (Medicine)
I. Leppert, Phyllis Carolyn. II. Howard, Fred M.
[DNLM: 1. Women's Health. 2. Primary Health Care. WA 309 P9521 1997]
RC48.6.P75. 1997
616′.0082—dc20
DNLM/DLC 96-30176
for Library of Congress CIP

9 8 7 6 5 4 3 2 1

To our patients,
who have taught us what is primary and essential in caring for women,
and to our students and residents,
who, as learners, also taught us that medicine is a profession
where learning is lifelong.

Contributors

J. Gary Abuelo, MD
Associate Professor of Medicine
Department of Medicine
Brown University School of Medicine
Rhode Island Hospital
593 Eddy St.
Providence, RI 02903

Carol Achilles, MA
Adjunct Faculty
School of Nursing
University of Rochester
Nurse Practitioner
Department of Obstetrics and Gynecology
Rochester General Hospital
Medical Office Bldg., Suite 445
1445 Portland Avenue
Rochester, NY 14621

C. Douglas Angevine, MD
Clinical Associate Professor of Medicine
Division of Rheumatology
University of Rochester School of Medicine
Rochester General Hospital, Rheumatology Unit
1415 Portland Avenue, Suite 100
Rochester, NY 14621

Marie E. Aydelotte, MD
Clinical Assistant Professor of Medicine
University of Rochester School of Medicine
St. John's Home
150 Highland Avenue
Rochester, NY 14620

Cesar Barada, MD
Clinical Instructor
University of Rochester School of Medicine
Department of Obstetrics and Gynecology
Perinatal Division, Suite 585
1415 Portland Avenue
Rochester, NY 14621

David Baram, MD
Associate Professor of Obstetrics & Gynecology and Psychiatry
Department of Obstetrics and Gynecology
University of Rochester School of Medicine and Dentistry
Strong Memorial Hospital
601 Elmwood Avenue
Box 668
Rochester, NY 14642

Michael W. Barrett, MD
Chief Resident in General Surgery
University of Rochester School of Medicine and Dentistry
Department of Surgery
601 Elmwood Avenue
Rochester, NY 14642

G. William Bates, MD
Professor, Obstetrics and Gynecology
University of South Carolina School of Medicine
Vice President, Medical Education
Greenville Hospital System
701 Grove Road
Greenville, SC 29605

Eric L. Berman, MD
Clinical Assistant Professor
Ophthalmology and Neurology
University of Louisville
100 East Liberty Street
Suite 800
Louisville, KY 40202

Karl R. Beutner, MD, PhD
Associate Clinical Professor
Department of Dermatology
University of California, San Francisco
Sutter Solano Dermatology Associates
127 Hospital Drive
Suite 204
Vallejo, CA 94589-2500

Janet Kay Bobo, PhD
Associate Professor
Section on Epidemology
Department of Preventive and Societal Medicine
University of Nebraska Medical Center
Student Life Center 3033
600 South 42nd Street
Omaha, NE 68198-4350

Marjorie A. Boeck, MD, PhD
6012 Twin Coves
Dallas, TX 75248

Donald R. Bordley, MD, FACP
Associate Professor of Medicine
Associate Chief of General Medicine
University of Rochester School of Medicine
Strong Memorial Hospital
Department of Medicine
601 Elmwood Avenue
Rochester, NY 14642

Martin Brower, MD
Associate Professor of Oncology in Medicine
Division of Oncology
Department of Medicine
Rochester General Hospital
University of Rochester
1425 Portland Avenue
Rochester, NY 14621

Marc D. Brown, MD
Associate Professor of Dermatology and Otolaryngology
Department of Dermatology and Otolaryngology
University of Rochester
Strong Memorial Hospital
601 Elmwood Ave, Box 697
Rochester, NY 14624

Joanna M. Cain, MD
Professor and Chair
Department of Obstetrics and Gynecology
Pennsylvania State University
M. S. Hershey Medical Center
500 University Drive
Hershey, PA 17033

Michelle Carpenter-Bradley, MD
Department of Medicine
Rochester General Hospital
Independent Living for Seniors
695 Bay Road
Rochester, NY 14580

David A. Carrier, MD
Associate Attending Physician
Orthopaedics Department
Rochester General Hospital
1415 Portland Avenue
Rochester, NY 14621

Robert H. Carrier, MD
Chief
Orthopedics Department
Rochester General Hospital
1425 Portland Avenue
Rochester, NY 14621

Steven S. T. Ching, MD
Associate Professor
Department of Ophthalmology
University of Rochester School of Medicine and Dentistry
Strong Memorial Hospital
Rochester, NY 14642

Edward C. Clark, MD
Assistant Professor of Medicine
Department of Medicine
University of Rochester School of Medicine
Rochester General Hospital
1425 Portland Avenue
Rochester, NY 14621

Richard S. Constantino, MD
Chief, Division of Ambulatory Services
Department of Medicine
Vice President
Rochester General Hospital
1445 Portland Avenue, Suite 302
Rochester, NY 14621

Patricia Coury-Doniger, RN, FNPC
STD Clinical Services Manager
Infectious Disease Unit
Department of Medicine
University of Rochester
601 Elmwood Avenue
Rochester, NY 14642

David L. Crosby, MD
Associate Professor of Dermatology
Medical College of Wisconsin
MCW Clinic at Froodtert
Department of Dermatology
9200 West Wisconsin Avenue
Milwaukee, WI 53226

Elizabeth A. deLahunta, MD
Assistant Professor
Department of Emergency Medicine
University of Rochester School of Medicine and Dentistry
Strong Memorial Hospital
601 Elmwood Avenue, Box 655
Rochester, NY 14642

Giuseppe Del Priore, MD, MPH
Assistant Professor of Gynecologic Oncology
New York University School of Medicine
Chief, Gynecologic Oncology
Bellevue Hospital
550 First Avenue
New York, NY 10016

Brent DuBeshter, MD
125 Lattimore Road
Rochester, NY 14620

Karin Dunnigan, MD
Clinical Associate Professor
Gastroenterology Unit
Department of Medicine
Rochester General Hospital
1425 Portland Avenue
Rochester, NY 14621

Paul S. Dziwis, MD
Associate Attending in Medicine
Gastroenterology Division
Department of Medicine
Rochester General Hospital
1425 Portland Avenue
Rochester, NY 14621

Ann R. Falsey, MD
Assistant Professor of Medicine
Department of Medicine
University of Rochester School of Medicine and Dentistry
Attending Physician
Rochester General Hospital
1425 Portland Avenue
Rochester, NY 14621

Howard A. Farrell, MD
Clinical Assistant Professor of Otolaryngology
University of Rochester School of Medicine
Rochester Otolaryngology Group, P.C.
Rochester General Hospital
1425 Portland Avenue
Rochester, NY 14621

Anthony J. Fedullo, MD
Professor of Medicine
Division of Pulmonary Medicine
Department of Medicine
University of Rochester School of Medicine and Dentistry
Rochester General Hospital
1425 Portland Avenue
Rochester, NY 14621

James V. Fiorica, MD
Associate Professor
Department of Obstetrics and Gynecology
Division of Gynecologic Oncology
University of South Florida College of Medicine
H. Lee Moffitt Cancer Center
12902 Magnolia Drive
Tampa, FL 33612

Patricia G. Fitzpatrick, MD
Associate Professor of Medicine
Department of Medicine
University of Rochester School of Medicine
and Dentistry
Director, Cardiac Catherization Laboratories
Associate Chief of Cardiology
Rochester General Hospital
1415 Portland Avenue, Suite 210
Rochester, NY 14621

Edward G. Flickinger, MD
Professor of Surgery
Department of Surgery
University of Rochester School of Medicine and Dentistry
Chief of Surgery
Rochester General Hospital
1425 Portland Avenue
Rochester, NY 14621

Charles W. Francis, MD
Hematology Unit
Department of Medicine
University of Rochester School of Medicine and Dentistry
P.O. Box 610
University of Rochester Medical Center
601 Elmwood Avenue
Rochester, NY 14642

James Frank, MD
Chief Resident
Department of Ophthalmology
Strong Memorial Hospital
601 Elmwood Avenue
Rochester, NY 14642

Aasha S. Gopal, MD
Assistant Professor of Medicine
Associate Director, Echocardiography
Department of Cardiology
Mt. Sinai Medical Center
1 Gustave Levy Place, Box 1030
New York, NY 10029

Catherine F. Gracey, MD
Senior Instructor in Medicine
Department of Medicine
University of Rochester
University Health Service
250 Crittenden Blvd.
Rochester, NY 14642

Jeanne E. Grove, DO, FACOG
Clinical Instructor
Department of Obstetrics and Gynecology
Rochester General Hospital
1425 Portland Avenue
Rochester, NY 14621

James A. Hadley, MD, FACS
Clinical Associate Professor of Surgery (Otolaryngology)
University of Rochester
Rochester General Hospital
1425 Portland Avenue
Rochester, NY 14621

Rosalind Hayes, MD
Clinical Faculty
Obstetrics and Gynecology Residency Program
Rochester General Hospital
Institute for Reproductive Health and Infertility
1561 Long Pond Road
Suite 410
Rochester, NY 14626

Joshua Hollander, MD
Associate Professor of Neurology
Department of Neurology
University of Rochester School of Medicine and Dentistry
Rochester General Hospital
1425 Portland Avenue
Rochester, NY 14621

Allison Holm, MD
30 N. Union Street
Rochester, NY 14607

Gerald W. Honch, MD
Associate Professor of Neurology
University of Rochester School of Medicine and Dentistry
Attending Neurologist
Rochester General Hospital
1425 Portland Avenue
Rochester, NY 14621

Maria K. Hordinsky, MD
Associate Professor
Department of Dermatology
University of Minnesota Health System
Box 98
420 Delaware Street, SE
Minneapolis, MN 55455

Cynthia R. Howard, MD, FAAP
Assistant Professor
University of Rochester School of Medicine & Dentistry
Pediatric Director, Mother-Baby Unit
Department of Pediatrics
Rochester General Hospital
1425 Portland Avenue
Rochester, NY 14621

Fred M. Howard, MD
Assistant Professor of Obstetrics and Gynecology
University of Rochester School of Medicine and Dentistry
Associate Chief
Department of Obstetrics and Gynecology
University of Rochester
Rochester General Hospital Division
1425 Portland Avenue
Rochester, NY 14621

Brenda L. Johnson, MD
Suburban Medical Group PC
Reading, Massachusetts

Jonathan D. Klein, MD, MPH
Assistant Professor of Pediatrics and of Community & Preventive Medicine
Division of Adolescent Medicine
Department of Pediatrics
University of Rochester School of Medicine
601 Elmwood Avenue, Box 690
Rochester, NY 14642

Tarun Kothari, MD, FACG, FACP
Clinical Assistant Professor of Medicine
University of Rochester School of Medicine and Dentistry
Attending Gastroenterologist
Rochester General Hospital
1425 Portland Avenue
Rochester, NY 14621

Peter A. Kouides, MD
Assistant Professor of Medicine
Department of Medicine
University of Rochester School of Medicine & Dentistry
Attending Physician
Department of Medicine
Rochester General Hospital
1425 Portland Avenue
Rochester, NY 14621

Joseph Kozlowski, RPA-C
Department of Obstetrics and Gynecology
Rochester General Hospital
1425 Portland Avenue
Rochester, NY 14621
Phone: 716-336-3784

Richard E. Kreipe, MD
Associate Professor of Pediatrics
Division of Adolescent Medicine
Department of Pediatrics
University of Rochester
Strong Memorial Hospital, Box 690
601 Elmwood Avenue
Rochester, NY 14642

John S. Lambert, MD
Assistant Professor
Department of International Health, Medicine, and Pediatrics
Johns Hopkins Medical Institution
Johns Hopkins Hospital
600 North Wolfe Street
Baltimore, MD 21205

Raymond Lanzafame, MD, FACS
Associate Professor of Surgery
University of Rochester School of Medicine and Dentistry
Director, Laser Center
Department of Surgery
Rochester General Hospital
1425 Portland Avenue
Rochester, NY 14621

Dr. Rahul Laroia
Department of Obstetrics and Gynecology
Rochester General Hospital
1425 Portland Avenue
Rochester, NY 14625

Ruth A. Lawrence, MD
Department of Pediatrics
Professor of Pediatrics and Obstetrics & Gynecology
University of Rochester School of Medicine & Dentistry
601 Elmwood Avenue
Rochester, NY 14642

Adrian Leibovici, MD
Clinical Assistant Professor
Department of Psychiatry
University of Rochester
Associate Chief
Department of Psychiatry
Rochester General Hospital
1425 Portland Avenue
Rochester, NY 14621

Phyllis C. Leppert, MD, PhD
Chair
Department of Obstetrics and Gynecology
State University of New York at Buffalo
Buffalo, New York

Harold Lesser, MD, PhD
Senior Instructor in Neurology
Department of Neurology
Rochester General Hospital
1425 Portland Avenue
Rochester, NY 14621

Richard Allan Lewis, MD
Assistant Professor of Orthopaedics
Department of Orthopaedics
University of Rochester School of Medicine and Dentistry
Attending, Orthopedics Department
Strong Memorial Hospital
601 Elmwood Ave, Box 665
Rochester, NY 14642

Kathleen Louise Martin, MD
Clinical Instructor
Department of Obstetrics and Gynecology
University of Rochester
Director of Urogynecology
Rochester General Hospital
1415 Portland Avenue, Suite 445
Rochester, NY 14621

Henry S. Metz, MD
Professor of Ophthalmology
University of Rochester School of Medicine
Department of Ophthalmology
Rochester General Hospital
1425 Portland Avenue
Rochester, NY 14621

Matthew R. Moog, MD
Department of Medicine
University of Rochester Medical Center
Strong Memorial Hospital
601 Elmwood Avenue
Rochester, NY 14642

Eberhard Karl Muechler, MD
Clinical Associate Professor of Obstetrics and Gynecology
University of Rochester School of Medicine and Dentistry
Attending Physician
Department of Obstetrics and Gynecology
Rochester General Hospital
Director, Department of Gynecology
Park Ridge Hospital
1561 Long Pond Road
Suite 410
Rochester, NY 14626

Peter Mulbury, MD
Chair, ENT
Rochester Otolaryngology Group
1415 Portland Avenue, Suite 200
Rochester, NY 14621

Ajai K. Nemani, MD
Pain and Symptom Management Center
Rochester General Hospital
1415 Portland Avenue, Suite 580
Rochester, NY 14621

Paul Nyirjesy, MD
Assistant Professor of Obstetrics and Gynecology and of Medicine
Department of Obstetrics and Gynecology
Temple University Hospital
3401 North Broad Street
Philadelphia, PA 19140

Christopher W. Olcott, MD
Chief Resident
Department of Orthopaedics
Strong Memorial Hospital
601 Elmwood Avenue, Box 665
Rochester, NY 14642

John P. Olson, MD
Professor of Medicine
University of Rochester School of Medicine and Dentistry
Attending Hematologist
Department of Medicine - Hematology Unit
Rochester General Hospital
1425 Portland Avenue
Rochester, NY 14621

Anita S. Pakula, MD
Clinical Instructor
Division of Dermatology
University of California, Los Angeles
10833 LeConte
Los Angeles, CA 90024

Pradyumna D. Phatak, MBBS, FACP
Associate Professor of Medicine
University of Rochester School of Medicine
Chief, Hematology Unit
Rochester General Hospital
1425 Portland Avenue
Rochester, NY 14621

Ronald D. Plotnik, MD
Assistant Professor of Ophthalmology
Department of Ophthalmology
University of Rochester School of Medicine and Dentistry
Strong Memorial Hospital
601 Elmwood Avenue, Box 659
Rochester, NY 14642

Douglas L. Powell, MD
Resident
University of Rochester
Department of Dermatology
Strong Memorial Hospital
601 Elmwood Avenue, Box 697
Rochester, NY 14642

Thomas M. Price, MD
Greenville Hospital System
701 Grove Road
Greenville, SC 29605

Gilbert P. Proper, MD
Associate Clinical Instructor
Department of Anesthesiology
University of Rochester
Pain and Symptom Management Center
Department of Anesthesiology
Rochester General Hospital
1425 Portland Avenue
Rochester, NY 14621

Stephen M. Rauh, MD
Assistant Clinical Professor of Surgery
University of Rochester College of Medicine & Dentistry
Attending Surgeon
Rochester General Hospital
1650 Elmwood Avenue
Rochester, NY 14620

Cynthia A. Reddeck, MD
Clinical Assistant Professor in Medicine
University of Rochester Medical School
Attending Cardiologist
Rochester General Hospital
1425 Portland Avenue
Rochester, NY 14621

Geoffrey P. Redmond, MD
President
Foundation for Developmental Endocrinology, Inc.
Five Commerce Park Square
23200 Chagrin Boulevard, Suite 325
Beachwood, OH 44122

Janet R. Reiser, MD
Clinical Assistant Professor of Medicine
Gastroenterology Unit
Department of Medicine
Rochester General Hospital
1425 Portland Avenue
Rochester, NY 14621

Ann T. Riggs, MD
Senior Instructor of Medicine
Department of Medicine
University of Rochester
Monroe Community Hospital
Department of Medicine
435 E. Henrietta Road
Rochester, NY 14620

Christopher T. Ritchlin, MD
Assistant Professor of Medicine
University of Rochester School of Medicine & Dentistry
Chief, Rheumatology Unit
Rheumatology Unit
Rochester General Hospital
1415 Portland Avenue, Suite 100
Rochester, NY 14621

Jay K. Roberts, MD, MS, FACS
Clinical Assistant Professor
Division of Otolaryngology
University of Rochester School of Medicine and Dentistry
The Rochester Otolaryngology Group, PC
1641 East Avenue
Rochester, NY 14610

Steven J. Rose, MD
Clinical Assistant Professor
Department of Ophthalmology
University of Rochester Medical Center
890 Westfall Road
Rochester, NY 14618

Reinaldo Sanchez, MD
Clinical Instructor
Department of Obstetrics and Gynecology
Rochester General Hospital
1425 Portland Avenue
Rochester, NY 14621

Beth Schorr-Lesnick, MD, FACP, FACG
Assistant Professor
Department of Medicine
Albert Einstein College of Medicine
Assistant Attending
Department of Medicine
Beth Israel Medical Center
Suite 1B-20
First Avenue at 16th Street
New York, NY 10003

Ashok N. Shah, MD, FRCP(C), FACS
Clinical Professor of Medicine
Center for Digestive and Liver Diseases
Department of Gastroenterology
University of Rochester Medical Center
Department of Medicine, Gastroenterology
Strong Memorial Hospital
601 Elmwood Avenue
Rochester, NY 14642

Ronald Sham, MD
Assistant Professor of Medicine
Department of Medicine, Hematology Unit
Rochester General Hospital
1425 Portland Avenue
Rochester, NY 14621

William V. R. Shellow, MD
Associate Professor of Medicine (Dermatology)
UCLA School of Medicine
Chief, Inpatient and Consultation Dermatology
VA Medical Center West Los Angeles
11301 Wilshire Boulevard
Los Angeles, CA 90073

Cynthia Shortell, MD
Clinical Assistant Professor
Vascular Surgery
Rochester General Hospital
1425 Portland Avenue, Suite 125
Rochester, NY 14621

Timothy R. Siegel, MD
Attending Surgeon
Department of Surgery
Salem Hospital
55 Highland Avenue
Suite 202
Salem, MA 01970

Stephen M. Silver, MD
Assistant Professor of Medicine
Nephrology Unit
Rochester General Hospital
1425 Portland Avenue
Rochester, NY 14621

Aaron Spital, MD
Associate Professor of Medicine
University of Rochester School of Medicine
Genesee Hospital
Nephrology Unit
224 Alexander Street
Rochester, NY 14607

Gwen K. Sterns, MD
Clinical Professor of Ophthalmology
Department of Ophthalmology
University of Rochester
Rochester General Hospital
1425 Portland Avenue
Rochester, NY 14621

Richard H. Sterns, MD
Professor of Medicine
Chief, Department of Medicine
University of Rochester School of Medicine and Dentistry
Rochester General Hospital
1425 Portland Avenue
Rochester, NY 14621

Derek J. tenHoopen, MD
Clinical Instructor
Department of Obstetrics and Gynecology
University of Rochester School of Medicine and Dentistry
Associate Attending and Clinical Faculty
Department of Obstetrics and Gynecology
Rochester General Hospital
3101 Ridge Road West
Rochester, NY 14626

Paul Topf, MD
Clinical Assistant Professor of Otolaryngology
Department of Surgery
University of Rochester School of Medicine and Dentistry
Rochester General Hospital
1425 Portland Avenue
Rochester, NY 14621

Charlene Varnis, MD
Senior Instructor
University of Rochester
Division of Rheumatology
Rochester General Hospital
1415 Portland Avenue. Suite 100
Rochester, NY 14621

Maggie Vill, MD
Clinical Instructor
Perinatology Division
Department of Obstetrics and Gynecology
Rochester General Hospital
Medical Office Building
1425 Portland Avenue
Rochester, NY 14621

Laura J. von Doenhoff, MD, FACC
Clinical Instructor in Medicine
Department of Medicine/Cardiology
University of Rochester School of Medicine
Attending Physician in Medicine
Rochester General Hospital
1415 Portland Avenue, #555
Rochester, NY 14621

Gary W. Wahl, MD
Associate Professor of Medicine
University of Rochester School of Medicine and Dentistry
Pulmonary and Critical Care Unit
Rochester General Hospital
1425 Portland Avenue
Rochester, NY 14621

David P. Warshal, MD
Clinical Assistant Professor
Temple University School of Medicine
Department of Gynecologic Oncology
Abington Memorial Hospital
Division of Gynecologic Oncology
1200 Old York Road
Suite 311, Rorer Building
Abington, PA 19001-3788

Barbara E. Weber, MD, MPH
Assistant Professor of Medicine
University of Rochester School of Medicine & Dentistry
Chief, General Medicine Unit
St. Mary's Hospital
89 Genesee Street
Rochester, NY 14611

Roy S. Wiener, MD
Cardiologist
Department of Medicine
Rochester General Hospital
1415 Portland Avenue, Suite 210
Rochester, NY 14621

Robert A. Wild, MD
Professor and Chief
Section of Research and Education in Women's Health
Department of Obstetrics and Gynecology
University of Oklahoma
PO Box 26901
801 NE 13th, CHB RM. 215
Oklahoma City, OK 73190

Sophie M. Worobec, MD
Assistant Professor of Dermatology
Department of Dermatology
University of Rochester
601 Elmwood Avenue, Box 697
Rochester, NY 14642
2180 S. Clinton Avenue
Suite D
Rochester, NY 14618

Morris Wortman, MD
Clinical Associate Professor
Department of Obstetrics and Gynecology
University of Rochester School of Medicine and Dentistry
601 Elmwood Avenue
Rochester, NY 14642
200 White Spruce Blvd.
Rochester, NY 14623

Preface

Primary care for women, as currently practiced, is not provided solely by a specific subspecialty of medicine. Only obstetrician–gynecologists limit their practice exclusively to the care of women. However, others also deliver primary care to women, among them family practitioners, internists, and pediatricians. Increasingly, nonphysician providers such as physician assistants, professional midwives, and nurse practitioners give primary care to women as well within their scope of practice. There are unique aspects of primary care for women, just as there are for children or for men. This book is written to address the unique aspects of such care and to address possible approaches to women's health care.

The chapters in this text are written to allow primary care practitioners of varying backgrounds to supplement their knowledge beyond that traditionally covered in their education and training. For example, the internist can use this book to gain knowledge about family planning, menstrual abnormalities, and orthopedic injuries, or the gynecologist may use it to supplement knowledge about hypertension, renal disease, and dermatologic disorders. No one provider can be all things to all patients, so the chapters suggest when referral to a subspecialist is appropriate. In our view, primary care is not synonymous with ambulatory care, nor is it to be equated with a concept of a single provider treating an individual woman completely throughout her lifetime from the cradle to the grave for all medical and health problems she encounters. Although referrals are indicated, the primary care physician needs a level of basic knowledge that allows him or her to continue to coordinate the woman's care and to serve as her medical advisor and counselor.

This text discusses age specific issues in women's primary care. Because reproductive health is paramount to women's health at all ages, specific information regarding reproductive tract health and disease is included in this text. As an example, ambiguous genitalia is included, because many such children are raised as females and primary care providers need to be cognizant of this problem. Likewise, we include basic mechanisms of labor and delivery not because we expect all primary care providers to practice obstetrics, but because childbirth is an important event in the lives of the majority of women and their primary care providers need to appreciate the basic physiology of this event. The text also includes specific information regarding the effects of pregnancy on various medical conditions as well as the effects of various diseases on pregnancy. Finally, we promote and emphasize the concept that primary care for women is comprehensive care that is much broader than reproductive health.

This text is based on the premise that there is a core of medical knowledge that all providers of primary care for women must comprehend and understand irrespective of the practice organizational patterns or, to use a current term, the integrated delivery system, in which they function. In a very fundamental sense the primary care physician needs a wider range of care knowledge than a subspecialist and a sharper diagnostic ability to truly serve the primary care needs of women. This text attempts to cover the basic requisite knowledge of a variety of problems in an accessible and concise format. As is the case with all textbooks, the editors anticipate and hope that the core knowledge presented will stimulate further inquiry and pursuit of greater depths of knowledge when appropriate. It is a truism that the practice of medicine and the provision of primary preventive care demand lifelong learning. Primary care places great demands on its practitioners to honestly accept and admit what is not known or understood, either by themselves as individual practitioners, or by medical and health sciences in general. Then they must have the integrity to admit a lack of knowledge and to seek to expand that knowledge in order to help women.

It is only by practicing their art and science with complete integrity that providers of primary care for women will be able to give comprehensive, continuous, and coordinated care to those in need.

It has been a major and exciting challenge to bring together fundamental knowledge from various medical disciplines that care for women in the publication of this textbook, *Primary Care for Women*. From the moment of the inception of the idea to the reading of the final page proofs, it has been exceedingly apparent that specialty groups approach many of the same diseases and physiological conditions from different perspectives. As the text is a multispecialty-authored book, each author contributed to the final manuscript the point of view of his or her individual specialty. What may seem at first glance to be redundant and repetitious is the result of a conscious decision to have each chapter as complete as possible and able to stand on its own point of view. Thus, discussion of estrogen replacement therapy is a theme in many chapters. Venous thromboembolism is currently treated by hematologists as well as cardiovascular specialists and others in medicine and is thus included in two sections. Every effort has been made to be consistent, however, so as not to confuse the student.

Textbooks are often used as references rather than being read in one sitting. Therefore, the volume is organized by age groups and then organ systems, and each section is complete in itself.

Phyllis C. Leppert, MD, PhD
Fred M. Howard, MD

Acknowledgments

We wish to thank Drs. Anthony Fedullo, John Olson, Robert Carrier, Joshua Hollander, Peter Mulbury, and Sophie Worobec for their diligent editorial assistance generously given.

Contents

Primary Care *for* Women

Primary Care for Women, edited by Phyllis C. Leppert and Fred M. Howard. Lippincott-Raven Publishers, Philadelphia © 1997.

I
Principles of Primary Care of Women

1
Uniqueness of Women's Health

PHYLLIS C. LEPPERT

The constitution of the World Health Organization defines health as a state of complete physical, mental, and social well-being. For women, this concept has far-reaching implications, and the impact of these implications on the health professions is only now beginning to be realized.

Women's health is related to far more than health during childbirth and means more than the absence of gynecologic disease. Women's health encompasses the total well-being of each individual woman. Every physiologic system in the human female is influenced by XX chromosomes and by a lifetime of variations in reproductive hormones. Therefore, women's health incorporates the combined knowledge of all the traditional specialties of medicine, public health, nursing, midwifery, social work, and other health professions.

At the same time, women's health has a much broader perspective than that of these traditional health professions. Epidemiology has helped in the understanding that the social and political climate in which a woman finds herself may be the most important determinant of that woman's health. In societies where women are undervalued, the necessary human, economic, and scientific resources are seldom allocated to women's health. Thus, in these circumstances the health needs of women are not met. This fact holds true in all countries, and it is true in the United States. The status of women's health, whether it be the shockingly high maternal mortality rate of 1 in 20 in some parts of Africa, or the unacceptably high prevalence of domestic violence and trauma in the United States, reflects the lack of value placed on women's lives.

In nations that allocate economic resources to maternal and child health, all too often most of the money is used for child health, with the effect that the maternal component is neglected. Although the health and well-being of children are essential to the survival of the human species and our multitude of cultures, too many nations do not adequately address the compelling health needs of women. Women contribute to the nurture, development, and success of nations and to the world culture, whether or not they are mothers. Nations that value women educate all women to their full intellectual potential. Education of women is a vital element in reducing infant mortality, improving the overall well-being of the family, ensuring optimal health for all women, encouraging women's economic stability, and preparing women for community, national, and world leadership. There is substantial evidence that women are not valued for their full potential, because educational barriers and hurdles exist for women worldwide.

Women's health is unique as well because of the plain fact that the female reproductive system is an anatomically and physiologically complex system. This system is subject to a large number of disease processes. The signs and symptoms of female reproductive tract disease are more varied and often more subtle than those of the male reproductive tract. Women are subject to diseases and dysfunctions of the reproductive tract throughout life, not only in the reproductive years: they may occur at any age, from intrauterine life to old age. These pathologic conditions occur whether or not an individual has borne children; furthermore, the fact that she has borne children may alter her risk for a particular disease.

The female reproductive tract is a common site for the formation of neoplasms, both benign and malignant. Most of these tumors occur at the end of the reproductive years or in the menopausal period. The multiplicity of the pathologic classification of female reproductive tract neoplasms attests to the wide variety of tumors affecting women at any stage of life. Gynecologic and mammary gland malignancies are so common that all providers of women's primary care must be cognizant of the natural history, signs, symptoms, and methods of diagnosis of these neoplasms. There is no parallel in males to uterine leiomyomata in females. These benign tumors today account for 25% to 30% of the hysterectomies performed in the United States.

Sexually transmitted diseases occur in both men and women, but in women the consequences of these diseases are more serious. For biologic and social reasons, women are more likely to become infected, are less likely to seek care, and are often more difficult to diagnose. Women with sexually transmitted diseases suffer serious sequelae, including chronic pelvic pain, ectopic pregnancies, and infertility. Women infected with sexually transmitted disease are more often subjected to social discrimination. Prevention is difficult for women because the most effective method of prevention, the condom, is controlled by men. There is no current method that a woman may use for herself without her partner's cooperation to prevent sexually transmitted disease. The female condom is still not widely accepted by many people.

Women's health care providers must always be cognizant of the fact that a woman's reproductive role means that she faces health risks, including complications and death, from causes related to pregnancy. Too many and too closely spaced pregnancies are health risks for women. A woman's ability to control fertility so that all pregnancies are wanted and occur at the appropriate time is fundamental to her health and well-being.

Pregnancy can be prevented by methods controlled by an individual woman. Many of these methods, however, pose potential health risks. Abstinence is the only certain and sure way to prevent both unwanted pregnancy and sexually transmitted disease. However, abstinence as the only strategy to prevent both pregnancy and sexually transmitted disease in the age of AIDS is unrealistic. Abstinence as the only strategy is exceedingly unrealistic when health care providers consider the fact that most women worldwide live in social situations where they are compelled by custom or physical force to have sexual intercourse not desired by them. Abstinence as the only strategy is also unfair to women, because women bear a heavier health and social burden for pregnancy and for sexually transmitted disease when this method is the only health strategy available.

There is increasing recognition that research conducted on men does not necessarily apply to women as well. This is another way in which women's health care is unique. Recently, the National Institutes of Health (NIH) has begun many initiatives to study problems of women's health.

HISTORY OF WOMEN'S HEALTH IN THE UNITED STATES

In the United States, a unique history has affected women's health and women's status in society. This history plays a role in the current health care of women of all ages.

Throughout all of world history, women have cared for women during their time of greatest need—childbearing. As humans developed the slender hip configuration essential for an upright posture, and as, correspondingly, the human infant developed a large brain, childbirth became more difficult for humans than for other primates. In humans, a fetus must pass through a tight, curved space, and the infant is usually born facing away from the mother. Thus, women have needed assistance in childbirth, not only for themselves but for their offspring. The very survival of the infant and mother demands the help of another human, and universally that woman has been a midwife. Midwifery has been appropriately called the oldest profession. In fact, "midwife" in Old English means "with woman."

In colonial times and until the middle part of the 19th century, midwifery in the United States and Canada was a respected profession. In the mid-1800s, as education for medicine became more organized and elitist, midwifery became the province of male obstetricians who considered midwives ignorant and unskilled. In many states, especially in the North, the medical establishment of that time convinced public health authorities that midwifery as a profession should be abandoned. This attitude contrasted markedly with that of European and Asian countries, where midwives were accepted by the medical community and considered worthy and essential members of the health care professions. At the turn of the century in the United States, especially in New York City, the medical profession attacked the European-born immigrant midwife for the maternal and infant mortality of the time. These attacks were unjustified in view of the poor sanitary conditions in many urban centers during the early part of the century. The effect of the nonacceptance of the midwife was to deny women access to a large body of midwifery knowledge affecting many aspects of women's reproductive health and women's health in general.

In the intervening years, scientific medicine advanced the safety of childbirth for all women. Finally, after a long struggle, nurse-midwifery has become accepted by physicians, bringing midwifery knowledge into the mainstream of health care.

This historical trend to diminish the influence of midwifery was paralleled by the birth of the women's movement and the movement toward women's suffrage. Women became social workers and trained nurses, as well as physicians. Unfortunately, many women physicians received their training in schools that did not survive the changes in medical education that occurred in the early 20th century. Medical schools, largely because of the Flexner report, began to emphasize the science of medicine. The admission standards of these scientifically oriented schools made it difficult for women to enter the medical profession. Although women did become physicians, they were not encouraged to do so. The result was that women were denied access to the profession. It was not until the 1970s that women entered medicine in fairly large numbers, and it was not until the 1990s that women entered medical school in proportion to the number of women in the general population.

The effect of these historical trends was that women's health was not studied in a broad sense, because the male-dominated profession tended to focus on illnesses that affected men. Women's health was taught in fragmented and incomplete ways. Young physicians did not understand that symptoms of certain diseases in women might differ from symptoms of the same diseases in men. This knowledge was simply not understood.

Currently, women physicians are not represented at the higher levels of medical education and professional organizations, although this is changing. This lack of women's input has had a direct impact on the content, organization, and delivery of health care for women.

The rise of scientific medicine at the turn of the 20th century has contributed to tremendous health gains for women. For example, in the United States and other developed countries, maternal mortality has decreased dramatically, contraception has allowed women to control fertility, and screening for cervical cancer has eliminated considerable mortality from that disease. All these advances have been remarkable and should be celebrated. The problem is that while medicine was improving women's health by improving reproductive health, women felt excluded in decisions affecting their health and well-being. This was compounded in the United States by the fact that the medical profession was predominantly male.

Unfortunately, as this history unfolded, some women took the extreme position that only women providers were appropriate as women's health workers. It is hoped that we are in an era where it is realized that women respond positively to competent, compassionate care given by health professionals of both sexes. Both women and men are capable of being nurturing individuals. Those responsible for health care policy and education are realizing that women's health involves an interdisciplinary effort by health care providers and researchers. Providers of women's health must drive researchers so that all women reach optimal health.

In the final analysis, all women, no matter how poor or uneducated, respond positively to compassionate, competent care. This compassion and competence should pervade the complete knowledge that leads to the physical, mental, and social well-being of women.

SOME TRENDS IN WOMEN'S HEALTH TODAY IN THE UNITED STATES

Birth and death rates and life expectancy are the parameters usually evaluated in determining the nation's health in comparison to other countries. These rates are also used as the basis for observing trends.

Birth Rates

In 1991, in the United States, 4,110,907 births were recorded, for a birth rate of 16.3 live births per 1000 population. This was a decrease of 1% from 1990. However, between 1986 and 1990, there had been an 11% increase in births. In that same year, the fertility rate, as determined by the number of births to the number of women of childbearing years (15 to 44 years of age), was 70.9 live births per 1000 population.

A significant trend over the past decade has been an increase in the birth rate for women aged 30 to 34 years. In 1980, this was 61.9 per 1000. In 1990, it was 80.8 per 1000, but by 1991 the birth rate of this age group declined slightly. Similarly, in the 1980s, the birth rate for women aged 35 to 39 years increased from 19.8 per 1000 to 31.7 per 1000. The number of births in this age group continued to rise in 1991. Women aged 40 to 44 years had a 14.5% increase in their birth rate from 1988 to 1990. The rate increased from 4.8 per 1000 in 1988 to 5.5 per 1000 in 1990. The rate remained stable in 1991.

The birth rate for adolescents aged 15 to 17 years in 1989 was 8% higher than in 1988, or 36.5 per 1000, and in 1991 the rate climbed to 38.7 per 1000. The rate for young women aged 18 to 19 years was 86.4 per 1000, the highest since the 1970s, and it was 94.4 per 1000 in 1991, a 7% increase. This rise reflects the number of teens who are sexually active. In 1988, the number of teens sexually active rose to 38% among those aged 15 to 17 years; among those aged 18 to 19 years, three out of four were sexually active (Table 1-1). A 1990 survey by the Centers for Disease Control found that 32% to 67% of these students were sexually active.

In 1990, fertility rates were higher (91.9 per 1000) for black women than for white women. Birth rates for Hispanic women have also increased and are consistently higher. In 1992, the fertility rate for Hispanic women in the United States was 95 per 1000. These rates are higher than for non-Hispanic women at all ages, but the greatest differences between Hispanic and non-Hispanic are seen among teenagers and among women 40 and older.

Among black women 18 to 34 years of age, the fertility rate increase was higher than among whites, but the increase in fertility among white females aged 17 years and under and among ages 35 to 44 was higher than that of blacks. There has been a dramatic rise in the number of births to unmarried women aged 20 years and older, due to the fact that the number of teens in the population declined during the 1980s. During this decade, the increase in birth rates for white unmarried women was greater than the increase for blacks or Hispanics.

The birth rate for married women has decreased. This has resulted in a noticeable increase in the proportion of births to unmarried women, from 18.4% in 1980 to 28.0% in 1990. Some of these changes are due to women's ability to control their own fertility because of the general availability of contraception. Data from studies of unwanted births suggest that unmarried women accept single motherhood and plan for it.

The perinatal mortality and morbidity rates in the United States are not decreasing as rapidly as those in other countries. The trends in the United States of increasing births to single women, to teens, and to older women do not parallel those of countries with excellent perinatal morbidity and mortality statistics—notably Japan, where most births are to married women between ages 25 and 34 years. In most analyses of factors affecting perinatal mortality and morbidity, marital status and age are contributors to outcome, with ages 25 to 34 and married status traditionally associated with the lowest perinatal mortality rates.

Chronic Conditions

Data from three national health surveys and vital statistics in the United States demonstrate the impact of seven chronic conditions by age and sex: arthritis, visual impairment, hearing impairment, ischemic heart disease, chronic obstructive pulmonary disease, diabetes mellitus, and malignant neoplasms. Impact is divided into three categories: activity limitations, visits to physicians, and hospital stays.

Data indicate that limitation impact, or the likelihood of reduction in daily functioning, in all conditions increases for both sexes from young to middle adulthood, ages 18 to 44 and ages 45 to 64. It increases only slightly more for women at age 65 and over, except for visual impairment, where both sexes are affected. Heart disease has its greatest impact on limitation of both sexes at ages

Table 1-1. Percentage of Women Aged 15 to 19 Years Who Had Ever Had Sexual Intercourse, 1982 and 1988

	15–19 YEARS		15–17 YEARS		18–19 YEARS	
Race/Ethnicity	***1982***	***1988***	***1982***	***1988***	***1982***	***1988***
Total	47.1	53.2	32.6	38.4	64.1	74.4
Non-Hispanic white*	44.5	52.4	29.8	36.2	60.8	74.3
Non-Hispanic black	59.0	60.8	44.4	50.5	79.1	78.0
Hispanic	50.6	48.5	35.6	36.1	70.1	70.0

*Includes Asians and others who are not black or Hispanic.

(Data from the National Survey of Family Growth, Alan Guttmacher Institute, from Forrest JD, Singh S. The sexual and reproductive behavior of American women, 1982–1988. Fam Plan Perspect 1990;22:208. Reprinted with permission from Horton JA [ed]. The women's health data book: a profile of women's health in the United States. Jacobs Institute of Women's Health. New York: Elsevier, 1992:139.)

45 to 64, but this is true for men only at ages 18 to 44. There is a somewhat lesser impact of chronic obstructive pulmonary disease for women and a greater impact of visual impairment for women than for men at all ages. For instance, cataracts are ranked fourth in prevalence for women but tenth for men.

In analyzing the impact on physician visits, or the likelihood that a person with a particular condition will visit a physician, medical contacts are similar for men and women with the same condition, except for more care among young men with heart disease and more care among women with visual impairment at all ages. Cancer and diabetes have a higher visit impact among middle-aged women than among middle-aged men.

The impact on hospitalization, or the likelihood that a person with a given condition will be hospitalized, is similar for both sexes for all conditions except ischemic heart disease, where greater hospitalization is seen for young men than for young women. It has been suggested that men are likely to receive more aggressive treatment at that age, rather than that men's conditions are more severe. In people of middle and older ages, no differences by sex are seen for hospital impact for ischemic heart disease.

Leading causes, or principal diagnosis, of hospital stays per 10,000 population are also revealed by analysis of the surveys. Among women aged 18 to 44 years, the leading causes are complications of pregnancy (97.4), other female genital tract problems (63.2), and diseases of female pelvic organs (62.8). Major causes for hospitalization are related to reproductive health. Among men in this age range, the major causes are fractures, alcohol dependence syndrome, and laceration and open wound.

In people aged 45 to 64 years, both women and men are hospitalized primarily with the principal diagnosis of malignant neoplasms, with the rate for women (179.2 per 10,000) slightly higher than that for men (144.4 per 10,000). Among women, the next ranked conditions are diseases of the urinary system and benign neoplasms, whereas men show ischemic heart disease and acute myocardial infarction. In people aged 65 years and over, both men and women show malignant neoplasms and cerebrovascular disease as the leading causes of hospitalizations. The third-ranked condition leading to hospitalization differs in this age group, with fractures among women and prostate and other genital disorders among men. It is only in this age category that a condition related to reproductive health appears among the three main causes of hospital stays for men. However, among women, conditions related to reproductive health appear as major causes throughout the three age ranges.

Data relating to the principal diagnosis for visits to office-based physicians differ between the sexes. For example, diseases of the reproductive system ranked prominently in women aged 18 to 44 years. These included diseases of pelvic organs (ranked second), other female genital tract problems (ranked fourth), diseases of the urinary system (ranked fifth), complications of pregnancy (ranked sixth), and menstruation disorders (ranked ninth). In contrast, men showed few reproductive system conditions, with the top listing being prostate and other genital problems, ranked eighth in the age group 18 to 44 years.

Diagnoses become more similar in patients aged 45 to 64 years. The three leading reasons for office-based physician visits for both men and women are essential hypertension, ischemic heart disease, and diabetes. In the group aged 65 years and over, men and women are again more similar and make office-based visits for essential hypertension and chronic eye conditions. The third-ranked condition differs, with diabetes for women and malignant neoplasms for men.

Death Rates

The number of people who died in 1990 totaled 2,148,500. The crude death rate was 863.8 per 100,000 population. Age-adjusted death rates were higher for men than for women, and higher for blacks than for whites. Heart disease and cancer were the leading causes of death in women of all races.

For both men and women, heart disease is the leading cause of death. Heart disease accounts for more than a third of all deaths among women, and the rate is higher among black women than among white women. In 1988, three times more women died from heart disease than from breast and lung cancer together.

Women tend to develop the symptoms of heart disease 10 years later than men. The rate of coronary heart disease is 10-fold higher among women over 55 years of age than it is among younger women. The risk of coronary heart disease for younger women is less than for men, but as women age the mortality from heart disease increases. By age 75, the incidence of heart disease is essentially the same in both sexes. Because women aged 55 and over are at higher risk for coronary artery disease, it is hypothesized that the increased risk is associated with the changes of menopause. The ongoing Women's Health Initiative planned by the National Institutes of Health is designed in part to understand the effect of menopause and hormonal replacement therapy on the risk of heart disease.

Research efforts aimed at understanding heart disease have predominantly included men, due to the fact that women typically develop symptoms of heart disease at later stages of life. Therefore, women are not included in studies because they have other medical conditions and diseases that are thought to be confounding factors for study research design. Treatment studies, furthermore, tend to include the high-risk group of middle-aged men for the simple reason that conclusions of studies can be reached fairly quickly with a smaller sample size.

Cancer is the second leading cause of death among women in the United States, with black women having a higher incidence of death from cancer than white women. Five-year survival from cancer is considered a potential cure. The 5-year survival rate, which includes a calculation of normal age-adjusted life expectancy, is used as a measure for the detection and treatment of early-stage cancer. Although some cancers, such as breast cancer, may recur 5 years after the diagnosis of the primary cancer, a 5-year survivor is usually considered cured. Table 1-2 lists incidence and mortality rates and 5-year relative survival rates by cancer sites and time period for women.

In 1990, more women died from lung cancer than from breast cancer, and an estimated 51,000 women died of lung cancer in 1991. Because symptoms of lung cancer appear at advanced stages of the disease, it is difficult to detect in its earliest stages. Lung cancer is a preventable disease: if cigarette smoking were stopped, most lung cancer cases would be eliminated.

The risk of breast cancer increases as women age, and the disease occurs more frequently among white women 45 years of age and over than among black women of the same age. Screening for breast cancer through mammography, self-examination, and clinical examination is an essential element in health care for women. To date, not all women are obtaining necessary screening examinations and mammograms to detect early breast cancer. Over the past decades, breast cancer has been treated successfully with less aggressive surgical intervention, thus increasing the quality of life and self-image of women with this disease.

Table 1-2. Age-adjusted Incidence and Mortality Rates and 5-year Relative Survival Rates by Cancer Site and Time Period for Women

	INCIDENCE 1983–1987*		MORTALITY 1983–1987*		SURVIVAL 1981–1986†	
SITE	*White*	*Black*	*White*	*Black*	*White*	*Black*
Lung and bronchus	36.3	39.2	26.6	29.0	16.2	13.7
Breast	105.0	89.7	27.9	31.7	77.5	64.3
Female genital system	48.3	43.7	14.9	18.7	67.0	52.4
Cervix uteri	7.8	15.8	2.3	6.4	67.3	57.1
Corpus uteri	23.0	13.9	2.0	2.8	84.0	55.0
Uterus (NOS‡)	0.3	0.6	1.8	2.7	25.2	25.3
Ovary	14.3	10.0	8.2	5.8	38.7	37.6
All sites	334.5	332.5	138.7	164.6	57.0	44.4

*Incidence and mortality rates are per 100,000 and are age-adjusted to the 1970 U.S. standard population.
†Survival rates are expressed as percentages.
‡Not otherwise specified.
(Adapted from NCI cancer statistics review 1973–87. Bethesda, Md.: NCI, NIH Pub. No. 90-2789, 1990:I-54-9. Reprinted with permission from Horton JA [ed]. The women's health data book: a profile of women's health in the United States. Jacobs Institute of Women's Health. New York: Elsevier, 1992.)

Cervical cancer is prevented by the use of the Pap smear, which identifies very early cancer and its precursors. Despite this usage, an estimated 13,000 new cases of invasive cervical cancer were diagnosed in 1991. Among black women, the incidence of cervical cancer is twice as high as that of white women. Hispanic and Native American women have a higher incidence of cervical cancer as well. Sexual behavior plays a part in risks for cervical cancer, as multiple sexual partners and first intercourse at an early age increase the risk for development of cervical cancer.

Endometrial cancer is more common among white women than among black women, and more common among older women than among younger women, both black and white. The incidence increased quickly in the decade when unopposed estrogen was used in postmenopausal women to prevent the complications of menopause. Estrogen replacement therapy was more common among white women, which may explain the fact that endometrial cancer is more common among white women.

Ovarian cancer is rare. However, it is particularly worrisome because it often does not cause symptoms until the disease is in a late stage. Furthermore, the risk of ovarian cancer increases with age. The use of oral contraceptives and increased parity decrease the risk of this disease. The 5-year survival rate for ovarian cancer is a low 38%.

Primary prevention of cancer in women includes smoking reduction and cessation, reduction of promiscuous sexual behavior, and the screening strategies of Pap smears, mammograms, and regular gynecologic and general checkups. Basic, clinical, and epidemiologic research must focus on the multiple unanswered questions involving the etiology, prevention, and treatment of cancers in women.

Deaths in women due to acquired immunodeficiency syndrome (AIDS) have increased since the beginning of the epidemic in the United States. Half of the women with AIDS were exposed to human immunodeficiency virus (HIV) by injecting drugs. Of those exposed through heterosexual contact, almost two thirds indicated that their sexual partners were intravenous drug users. See Table 1-3 for a summary of exposure categories.

TABLE 1-3. Female Adult and Adolescent AIDS Cases Reported October 1992Tthrough September 1993* and Cumulative Totals Through September 1993, United States

	ETHNICITY					CUMULATIVE TOTALS	
EXPOSURE CATEGORY	*White non Hispanic (%)*	*Black non Hispanic (%)*	*Hispanic (%)*	*Asian/Pacific Islander (%)*	*American Indian/Alaskan Native (%)*	*Oct. 1992–Sept. 1993 total‡ (%)*	CUMULATIVE TOTAL (%)
Injecting drugs	1718 (46)	3861 (48)	1265 (44)	15 (15)	17 (37)	6891 (47)	19,878 (49)
Heterosexual contact	1387 (37)	2884 (36)	1192 (41)	57 (58)	20 (43)	5545 (37)	14,997 (37)
Hemophilia/coagulation disorder	14 (0)	7 (0)	5 (0)	1 (1)	— —	27 (0)	73 (0)
Transfusion or tissue recipient	223 (6)	167 (2)	88 (3)	16 (16)	2 (4)	496 (3)	2388 (6)
Risk not identified§	398 (11)	1089 (14)	327 (11)	10 (10)	7 (15)	1833 (12)	3366 (8)
Total	3740	8008	2877	99	46	14,792	40,702

*Includes 9 months of data collected under the 1993 AIDS surveillance case definition for adults and adolescents.
†Some percentages do not add up to 100 due to rounding.
‡Includes 75 females whose race/ethnicity is unknown.
§"Risk not identified" refers to persons whose mode of exposure to HIV is unknown. This includes persons under investigation; persons who died, were lost to follow-up, or declined to be interviewed; and persons whose mode of exposure remains unidentified after investigation.
(Centers for Disease Control and Prevention. HIV/AIDS surveillance report 1993;5:8.)

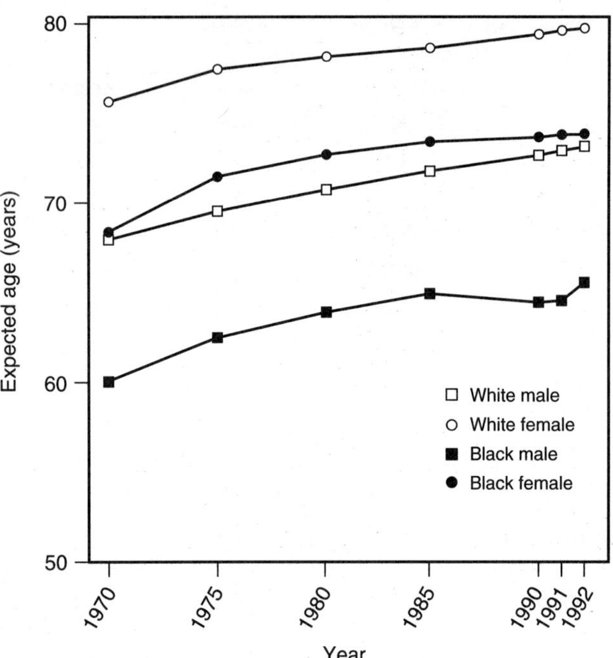

Figure 1-1. Life expectancy at birth according to race and sex, United States, 1970–1992. Data from 1992 are provisional. (National Center for Health Statistics. Health, United States, 1993. Hyattsville, Maryland: Public Health Service, 1994:91.)

Major depressive disorders are more common among women than among men. The consensus among health care professionals is that the observed differences between women and men are real. Depression occurs most frequently among women under age 24. Suicide and suicide attempts indicate depression, and many in our society who attempt suicide are depressed. Again, further research is needed to determine the biologic and psychosocial parameters leading to depression.

Life Expectancy

In 1988, infants born had a life expectancy of 74.9 years (Fig. 1-1). The life expectancy for white females was 78.9 years and for black females was 73.4 years. Women are living longer than in previous generations, a major reason why their health care needs now encompass more than reproductive health. Menopausal and postmenopausal health has become an essential component of health care.

Women are more likely than men to suffer many debilitating diseases, such as osteoporosis, lupus, and rheumatoid arthritis. These lead to restrictions in independent living. Women are also more likely than men to be the objects of violence and rape, and this leads to psychosocial difficulties. It has been estimated that violence against women accounts for about 5% of the disease and incapacitation in women worldwide.

Over the last 20 years, women have become more articulate in stating their health needs. All women must have universal access to quality health care, including reproductive health care, and they must have respect for their individual rights. These are goals all health care providers must strive to achieve.

BIBLIOGRAPHY

Fathalla M (ed). World report on women's health. Special issue. Int J Gynecol Obstet 1994;1:258.

Fletcher SW. Commentary: summing up epidemiology's effect on women's health—and vice versa. Ann Epidemiol 1994;4:174.

Horton JA (ed). The women's health data book: a profile of women's health in the United States, 2d ed. Jacobs Institute of Women's Health. New York: Elsevier, 1995.

Leigh WA. The health status of women of color. Washington DC: Women's Research and Educational Institute, 1994.

National Institutes of Health. Opportunities for research on women's health. Hunt Valley, Md., Sept. 4–6, 1991.

Verbrugge LM, Patrick DL. Seven chronic conditions: their impact on U.S. adults' activity levels and use of medical services. Am J Public Health 1995;85:173.

Voelker R. A new agenda for women's health. JAMA 1994;272:7.

Primary Care for Women, edited by Phyllis C. Leppert and Fred M. Howard. Lippincott-Raven Publishers, Philadelphia © 1997.

2

Primary Care Concept

PHYLLIS C. LEPPERT

Temporis ars medicina fere est (The art of medicine is usually a matter of time).

Ovid

It is the sick who need medicine and not the well.

Thomas Jefferson

Listen to women.

The American College of Nurse-Midwives

The word "primary" in English means "the first in time or development" and also connotes "that from which something is derived." In this sense, the word "primary" means fundamental, basic, or essential. Primary care, then, is the bedrock on which all health care is grounded. By defining primary care by considering the meaning of "primary" in its true sense, it becomes evident that the content of primary care is care that is fundamental and basic to the health of all persons. For providers of health care, it encompasses the total and complete knowledge base that is fundamental for the provision of competent care to all persons and their families. The concept of primary care implies that the core content is the shared basis of practice for all practitioners. Primary care is in the necessary province of all medical practitioners and is within the scope of practice of other health care professionals. This concept of primary care cuts across all disciplines within the medical profession and across other professions, such as nursing, midwifery, and social work. Health care providers must articulate what the shared content of primary care is so that they can meet their obligation to society: improving the health of all persons.

It has been customary to define primary care in narrow terms. Medical specialists and subspecialists argue about which specialty is truly practicing primary care, or if nurse-practitioners and physician assistants really can practice primary care. This approach misses the mark because it begins to fragment the health profession and creates unnecessary territorial battles that in the end do not contribute to society's needs. Each professional discipline has knowledge that is fundamental to the total health of populations and individuals and must become part of the core of primary care for women.

Just as "primary" is defined as "fundamental," "preventive" is defined as "providing effectual hindrance." It implies that actions are taken to keep something from occurring. In health care, "preventive" implies prophylactic measures, as opposed to remedial interventions. Preventive is not synonymous with primary. Not all primary care in the sense of fundamental care is preventive, and not all preventive care is primary. In the course of caring for a woman during her first pregnancy, much of the care given is preventive and is aimed at avoiding the complications of gestational diabetes or preeclampsia and pregnancy hypertension. If this same woman develops a urinary tract infection, remedial and therapeutic care is essential. The treatment prescribed by the provider is fundamental and, thus, primary care. It also has a preventive function in that it prevents further pregnancy complications and poor outcomes. Conversely, a woman with ovarian cancer who undergoes radical surgery performed by a highly qualified gynecologic oncologist needs preventive care to avoid serious complications, such as thromboembolus. If, after surgery, this patient develops a urinary tract infection, the same oncologist treating her would prescribe therapy in the same fundamental or primary manner as the physician prescribing medication for the pregnant woman. This, then, is also primary care. The point is that primary care and preventive care are defined in terms of the basic knowledge needed to provide for both women.

Primary care is not defined in terms of who the provider happens to be. For instance, a woman with acute onset of lower abdominal pain who is diagnosed with an ectopic pregnancy has a fundamental need for surgery. Thus, some surgical procedures must be considered to be primary care. There is a danger in labeling certain procedures as primary or not primary, as health care is dynamic and ever-changing. Thus, primary care is the care that encompasses the fundamental knowledge necessary for the health of all persons.

In terms of women's health, these concepts are important because women's fundamental health needs are met by providers in many disciplines. The health needs of women extend from infancy to advanced age and include both the social and biologic dimensions of health. Because of their reproductive role, women have a biologic advantage: at all stages of life, from intrauterine life to old age, females are better survivors than men. However, societies all too often do not reward women. Women are discriminated against and subordinated, and these gender discriminations adversely affect women's health. Therefore, practitioners of fundamental health of women draw on basic, primary knowledge gleaned from obstetrics and gynecology, pediatrics, medicine, surgery, family practice, education, and anthropology. Many other disciplines also contribute to the essential knowledge of primary care for women. The challenge of the next few decades will be for all these diverse disciplines and for women themselves to define what is primary care for women. This care must not be fragmented by territorialization on the part of professionals.

Two trends are emerging. One trend has been for physicians trained by education and experience in internal medicine and primary care to expand their knowledge and practice base to include aspects of reproductive health. The other trend has been for obstetricians and gynecologists to move beyond a narrow focus of treating only the female genital tract and to assume the role of physician for women. Obstetrics and gynecology is a multifaceted brand of medicine that encompasses virtually the entire span of a woman's adult life. Obstetrician-gynecologists offer a wide range of care to women, including preventive and primary care, medical care during pregnancy and childbirth, and medical and surgical management of reproductive tract disorders and diseases. The obstetrician-gynecologist, therefore, is also a primary physician who is mainly responsible for the patient's welfare, whether the need is for primary, secondary, or tertiary care, or for a consultant specialist. This concept is distinct from the concept of the primary care physician currently in use, in which the physician or provider deals with problems of self-limiting disease and is a "gatekeeper." Clearly, the roles of primary care and preventive care are encompassed within the obstetrician-gynecologist's practice as a primary physician. Thus, most obstetrician-gynecologists act as both specialists and primary physicians.

Other specialties, such as internal medicine, family practice, general surgery, pediatrics, and psychiatry, also play roles in the primary care of women. Physicians in these specialties, especially female physicians, have proposed a new specialty in women's health, largely because internists, family practitioners, psychiatrists, and others have realized that the biology, psychology, and sociology of women's health, wellness, and illness are distinct from those of men. These physicians have advocated increased research in women's health issues as well as a separate specialty for women. The other reason behind this trend has been that in the not-so-distant past, obstetrics and gynecology was dominated by male physicians and by an approach to the field that was mostly surgical. Only in the past 2 to 3 years has the leadership in obstetrics and gynecology adopted the concept of primary care for women. In the future, these two trends will merge, a prospect that will truly enhance the health care of women.

In the United States, there may well be too few primary physicians relative to specialists. The American Association of Medical Colleges and other professional and educational associations are taking steps to increase the number of primary physicians practicing in the United States.

Many women view their obstetrician-gynecologist as their primary physician. Health maintenance organizations in Rochester, New York, have enabled women enrolled in their programs to choose obstetrician-gynecologists as primary care providers. Studies confirm that obstetrician-gynecologists spend up to 78% of their practice in primary care roles. Defining primary care by the "gatekeeper" concept ignores the fact that health care is complex and that primary, secondary, and tertiary care may overlap. The American College of Obstetricians and Gynecologists has adopted this working definition of the primary care physician:

> A primary care physician is a physician directly accessible to patients for their initial contact. This physician will see patients who have a specific or an undifferentiated complaint or patients who desire health maintenance through periodic health checkups. The primary care physician also provides continuity of care and is readily available to the patient when he or she has either a specific or nonspecific complaint. Such physicians perform initial evaluation and management within their expertise. The primary care physician advises when referral to another physician is indicated, coordinating subsequent and continuing care to assure the patient of appropriate comprehensive care.

One way to overcome this complexity is to develop health care teams that include physician and nonphysician providers, such as nurse-midwives, physician assistants, and nurse practitioners. Each member of the team would function fully according to his or her scope of practice, and each member would also practice preventive care. Only by opening the boundaries of professional territories can complete health care for women be realized. Health care of the future will be given by teams, and for this team concept to work, all members must be highly confident and trusting. No one member can "own" the patient. No one can be the "captain," because leadership is dynamic and is based on expertise. For example, in the case of a pregnant woman with class C diabetes, the maternal-fetal medicine specialist would be the team leader. In a case of straightforward mild preeclampsia, the leader might be a family practitioner. In the case of term twin delivery, the team would be led by an obstetrician, but in a normal birth the team leader could be the nurse-midwife. Different geographic regions of the United States could and should develop unique care teams.

Finally, a multidisciplinary approach to health care for women, including the need for research in all areas of women's health at the basic science and clinical levels, must be fully integrated into medical school curricula. All physicians should be educated in the complete range of women's health care. This educational program for all medical students would include the unique sex differences in health and disease issues and the recent results of women's health research.

The medical profession is at a crossroads. Women's health care can no longer be considered solely care of the reproductive organs. As Egyptian obstetrician-gynecologist M.F. Fathalla has written:

Our profession should evolve into a profession for women's health. We can no longer play the ostrich, bury our head in the sands of biology, and turn our back to social realities that adversely impact on women's health. We have only one place to stand: with women, beside women, and behind women, and when the moment of truth is called, we will stand up and be counted.

BIBLIOGRAPHY

American College of Obstetrician-Gynecologists. Obstetrician-gynecologists: specialists in reproductive health care and primary physicians for women. Statement of policy as issued by the executive board of ACOG. Washington DC: ACOG, 1986.

American Medical Association. The graduate education of physicians. Chicago: AMA, 1986.

Clancy CM, Massion CT. Commentary: American women's health care—a patchwork quilt with gaps. JAMA 1992;268:1918.

Educational objectives: core curriculum for residents in obstetrics and gynecology, 4th ed. Washington DC: Council on Resident Education in Obstetrics and Gynecology, 1992.

Fathalla M. Women's health: an overview. Int J Gynecol Obstet 1994;46:105.

Leppert PC. Developing sound interpersonal relationships among maternity care professionals. A presentation at the 75th anniversary of Maternity Center Association, New York, November 1993.

Lowey NM. National policy perspectives: Women's health and medical school curricula. Acad Med 1994;69:280.

Primary Care for Women, edited by Phyllis C. Leppert and Fred M. Howard. Lippincott-Raven Publishers, Philadelphia © 1997.

3

The Well Woman Visit: Prevention and Screening

BARBARA E. WEBER

Preventive health-care services are increasingly being incorporated into patient care. Clinical preventive services include screening tests, counseling, immunizations, and chemoprophylaxis. Several organizations, including the American College of Physicians (ACP), the Canadian Task Force (CTF), and the U.S. Preventive Services Task Force (USPSTF), have developed practice guidelines, emphasizing critical appraisal of the evidence rather than relying on expert opinion to recommend specific interventions. This chapter will review the theory behind these guidelines, discuss several approaches to disease prevention, and provide summary tables of preventive services.

THEORY

Screening is defined as disease detection at an asymptomatic or preclinical stage. The purpose of screening is to improve patient outcomes, often evaluated as decreased morbidity or mortality. The following major principles of screening should be assessed:

- Burden of suffering from the target condition. To be appropriate for screening, the target condition or disease should be prevalent and a significant cause of mortality, and there must be a preclinical phase that can be detected.
- Efficacy of screening test. The screening test should be inexpensive, harmless, accurate, and reliable. The test should detect the target condition earlier than without screening and with sufficient accuracy to avoid producing large numbers of false-positive and false-negative results.
- Effectiveness of early detection. There should be an effective intervention for patients with a positive screening test, and it should favorably influence outcome. Patients with disease who are detected early should have a better clinical outcome than those who are detected without screening. Early detection should also be cost-effective.
- Population benefit. The total number of deaths prevented due to the screening test should be considered, not simply the relative reduction in risk. Cost, both direct (the screening test) and indirect (false-positives and false-negatives), should be considered.

Screening always advances the diagnosis (lead time bias) and thereby improves survival from the time of diagnosis, but not necessarily from the time when the patient would have presented clinically. This is crucial in assessing the effectiveness of a screening intervention (Fig. 3-1).

Although a test may be accurate (high sensitivity and specificity), the true usefulness of a test is best determined by the positive predictive value (true-positive results divided by the sum of true-positive and false-positive results). The predictive value of a positive screening test increases as the prevalence of the target condition increases. Screening for some target conditions is best performed for the entire population (eg, blood-pressure determination for hypertension), but other screening tests should be performed

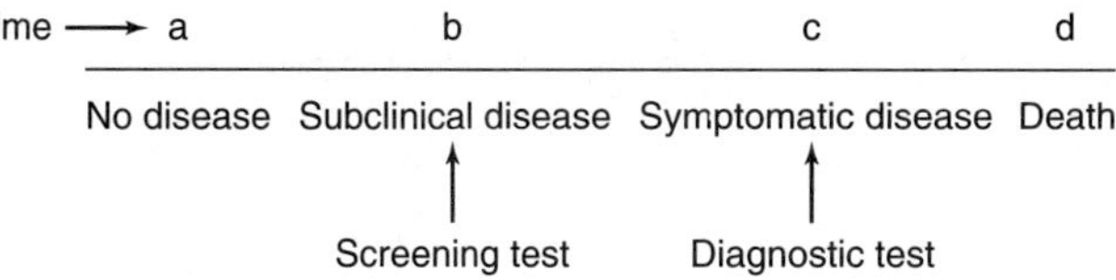

FIGURE 3-1. If *d* occurs at the same time whether the disease is detected at time *b* or *c*, the screening test is not effective. If the time until *d* occurs is extended, or if the disease is detected at time *b* rather than *c*, the screening test is effective.

only for selected high-risk populations (eg, thyroid palpation for thyroid cancer in patients exposed to upper-body radiation).

The need for evidence of effectiveness is especially important when cost is considered. Ensuring that benefits outweigh risks is critical, especially when interventions are recommended to healthy, asymptomatic patients.

Recommendations for preventive care occasionally conflict. This may be related to differences in the intended target population, in the objectives of the intervention, or in the interpretation of the evidence of the intervention's effectiveness.

The periodic health assessment should be seen as more than a traditional history (current symptoms, past medical history, medications, allergies, past surgical history, family history, and review of systems) and physical examination. It should focus on risk-factor assessment, disease screening, immunization, and health education needs. Equally important is the establishment of the clinician-patient relationship. Acquiring a complete database (eg, tobacco use, family history of cancer) allows the clinician to stratify patients into average or high risk for certain diseases.

BARRIERS

Both patient and clinician barriers must be overcome to ensure compliance with preventive care guidelines. Patient barriers include lack of knowledge about the role of preventive health care, fear of screening tests (eg, discomfort, anxiety generated by a false-positive test in a healthy patient), and cost. Clinician barriers include concern over conflicting recommendations, cost, uncertainty that patient outcomes will be improved, and inadequate tracking systems that identify patients eligible for screening. Methods for surmounting these barriers include education for both patient and clinician, cautious selection of highly accurate screening tests, minimizing cost to patients, improving the identification of patients due for preventive services, and improving patient access, especially for the elderly.

DISEASE-FOCUSED APPROACH

Prevention can be thought of in terms of the target condition (eg, cervical cancer, accidental injury, influenza) or the intervention (eg, Pap smear, seatbelt counseling, immunization). The next two sections and Tables 3-1 and 3-2 describe the epidemiology of the leading causes of death (burden of suffering) and provide an overview of the effectiveness of interventions to decrease morbidity and mortality from these diseases. Subsequent chapters address each specific disease.

Mortality

The most common causes of death for women of all ages are heart disease, cancer, cerebrovascular disease, pneumonia and influenza, and chronic obstructive lung disease. The number of deaths due to each of the diseases varies with age (see Table 3-1). Risk factor modification and disease prevention are keys to decreasing mortality from the most common causes of death.

Table 3-1. Reported Deaths for the 10 Leading Causes of Death for Females by Age, United States, 1991

ALL AGES	15–34	35–54	55–74	75+
All causes 1,047,853	All causes 24,822	All causes 72,218	All causes 299,422	All causes 629,118
Heart disease 361,048	Accidents 6944	Cancer 29,302	Cancer 111,419	Heart disease 263,041
Cancer 242,277	Cancer 3434	Heart diseases 84,865	Heart disease 97,388	Cancer 97,388
Cerebrovascular diseases 86,767	Homicide 2838	Accidents 4695	COLD 17,049	Cerebrovascular diseases 65,870
Pneumonia and influenza 42,646	Suicide 1831	Cerebrovascular diseases 3321	Cerebrovascular diseases 16,889	Pneumonia and influenza 33,971
Chronic obstructive lung disease (COLD) 40,165	Heart diseases 1491	Suicide 2296	Diabetes mellitus 10,995	COLD 21,272
Accidents 29,617	HIV infection 1440	Cirrhosis 2274	Pneumonia and influenza 5699	Diabetes mellitus 14,485
Diabetes 27,855	Cerebrovascular diseases 540	Diabetes 2009	Accidents 5221	Accidents 10,073
Septicemia 11,081	Congenital anomalies 408	HIV infection 1615	Cirrhosis 4442	Atherosclerosis 9566
Nephritis 10,942	Pneumonia and influenza 375	COLD 1502	Diseases of arteries 3104	Alzheimer's disease 7908
Atherosclerosis 10,784	Diabetes 342	Homicide 1498	Nephritis 2812	Septicemia 7622

(Wingo PA, Tong T, Bolden S. Cancer statistics, 1995. CA 1995;45:8.)

Table 3-2. Reported Deaths for the Five Leading Cancer Sites for Females by Age, United States 1991

ALL AGES	15–34	35–54	55–74	75+
All cancer 242,277	All cancer 3434	All cancer 29,302	All cancer 111,419	All cancer 97,388
Lung 52,068	Breast 660	Breast 9188	Lung 30,154	Lung 16,400
Breast 43,583	Leukemia 432	Lung 5372	Breast 19,900	Colon & rectum 15,727
Colon & rectum 29,017	Uterus 343	Colon & rectum 1999	Colon & rectum 11,117	Breast 13,834
Ovary 13,247	Brain & CNS 328	Uterus 1978	Ovary 6720	Pancreas 6637
Pancreas 13,161	Non-Hodgkin's lymphoma 209	Ovary 1779	Pancreas 5669	Ovary 4601

(Wingo PA, Tong T, Bolden S. Cancer Statistics, 1995. CA 1995;45:8.)

Risk factors for ischemic heart disease include hypertension, smoking, tobacco use, hypercholesterolemia, diabetes, obesity, sedentary lifestyle, and deprivation of estrogen after menopause. Most research to date on the primary prevention of ischemic heart disease has been performed in men, and it is unclear if the results can be generalized to women. Table 3-3 gives an overview of interventions for the primary prevention of myocardial infarction.

Treatment for a risk factor may be recommended, but the clinician must also consider the efficacy of screening for that risk factor. Screening for hypertension is recommended for all women, but screening for hypercholesterolemia is not, especially in women over age 70. Mathematical models suggest a mortality benefit from lowering blood pressure and cholesterol and tobacco cessation for women at high risk for ischemic heart disease. Women must be educated about their risk for ischemic heart disease and counseled to avoid smoking, follow a diet low in saturated fat, and maintain a moderate level of physical activity to help control weight. If these behaviors do not also control hypertension or diabetes, pharmacologic intervention is often necessary.

Risk factors for stroke include hypertension, age, diabetes, tobacco use, oral contraceptive use, heart disease, transient ischemic attacks (TIAs), and atrial fibrillation. Hypertension is the most prevalent risk factor and has the strongest association with stroke (relative risk about 4). Treatment of hypertension, including

Table 3-3. Quality of Available Data, Achievable Reductions in Risk, and Efficacy of Modification Strategies for Interventions in the Primary Prevention of Myocardial Infarction.

INTERVENTION	SOURCE OF DATA	ESTIMATED MEAN REDUCTION IN RISK OF MYOCARDIAL INFARCTION*	EFFICACY OF CURRENT STRATEGIES TO MODIFY RISK FACTOR
Smoking cessation	Observational studies	50–70% lower risk in former as compared with current smokers, within 5 years of cessation	Fair
Reduction in serum cholesterol	Metanalysis of randomized trials	2–3% decline in risk for each 1% reduction in serum cholesterol. Reductions in total cholesterol average 10% with diet therapy and often exceed 20% with drug therapy.	Fair to good
Treatment of hypertension	Metanalysis of randomized trials	2–3% decline in risk for each reduction of 1 mm Hg in diastolic blood pressure. Reductions in diastolic blood pressure average 5–6 mm Hg with combination dietary and drug therapy, although decreases of at least 20 mm Hg are frequently achieved in clinical practice.	Good
Exercise	Metanalysis of observational studies	45% lower risk for those who maintain an active as compared with a sedentary lifestyle	Fair
Maintenance of ideal body weight	Observational studies	35–55% lower risk for those who maintain ideal body weight as compared with those who are obese (≥20% above desirable weight)	Poor
Maintenance of normoglycemia in diabetic patients	Randomized trials (in progress)	Data insufficient to provide estimates	Fair to poor
Postmenopausal estrogen-replacement therapy	Metanalysis of observational studies	44% lower risk in users as compared with nonusers, although no estimates for combined estrogen-progestin therapy are available	Data not available.
Mild to moderate alcohol consumption	Observational studies	25–45% lower risk for those who consume small to moderate amounts of alcohol as compared with nondrinkers	Data not available
Prophylactic low-dose aspirin	Metanalysis of randomized trials	33% lower risk in users as compared with nonusers	Data not available

*Estimated reductions in risk refer to the independent contribution of each risk factor to myocardial infarction and do not address the wide range of known or hypothesized interactions between them. As Rothman notes, given the numerous interrelated causal mechanisms associated with any chronic disease process, "the total of the proportion of the disease attributable to various causes is not 100 percent but infinity."

(Manson JE, Tosteson H, Ridker PM, et al. The primary prevention of myocardial infarction. N Engl J Med 1992;326:1406.)

isolated systolic hypertension, reduces the risk of stroke by as much as 36%. There is still limited information on the best treatment for women, given the preponderance of men in antihypertensive trials. Primary prevention of stroke with aspirin is not recommended for all women, but certain high-risk patients (eg, those with nonvalvular atrial fibrillation or prior TIA or cerebrovascular accident [CVA]) may benefit from aspirin. Concerns about the efficacy of aspirin in women are not supported by the data; therefore, women should be considered for secondary stroke prevention. Smoking cessation decreases the frequency of stroke.

Immunization with pneumococcal and influenza vaccines has been shown to be safe and cost-effective in preventing pneumococcal pneumonia and influenza, in addition to reducing serious complications from these diseases.

Cigarette smoking accounts for 82% of the deaths from chronic obstructive lung disease. With cessation of smoking, the rate of ventilatory function loss declines, but lost function cannot be regained.

Cancer

The five most common sites causing death from cancer for women of all ages are the lung, breast, colon and rectum, ovary, and pancreas. The number of deaths due to each of the cancer sites varies with age (see Table 3-2). Subsequent chapters address specific details regarding screening for some of the more common cancers. This section discusses recommendations for the woman at average risk for each of the cancers mentioned.

Lung cancer screening with chest radiography or sputum cytology has not been proven to be an effective intervention. Primary prevention may be more effective than screening, as cigarette smoking is responsible for over 90% of all lung cancers.

Breast cancer screening can be performed with clinical breast examination (physical examination), mammography (test), or self-breast examination (counseling). Tables 3-4 through 3-6 provide recommendations for each of these interventions. Breast palpation accounts for 50% to 67% of the value of breast examination and mammography. The three expert panels (ACP, CTF, USPSTF) recommend an annual clinical breast examination for women over age 40. Mammography has been the best-studied intervention. Eight randomized controlled trials have been conducted since the 1963 HIP trial. A recent metanalysis of the efficacy of screening mammography showed a relative risk for breast cancer mortality of 0.74 in women aged 50 to 74 (95% confidence interval, 0.66 to 0.83) and 0.93 in women aged 40 to 49 (95% confidence interval, 0.73 to 1.13). The results for women younger than 50 are controversial. Some trials have shown benefit and others have not, but most have not had the power to show a statistical benefit. The controversy emanates from differences in study design, the quality and type of mammography, the length of follow-up, and the performance of mammography in the control arm. The evidence also suggests that mammography is less effective in women over age 70. The three expert panels agree on the need for annual mammography beginning at age 50, recognizing that 75% of all breast cancers occur in women over age 50. Some organizations recommend mammography for women aged 40 to 49. Self-breast examination is not recommended by any of the three panels because of low accuracy.

Colorectal cancer screening can be performed with the digital rectal examination, fecal occult blood testing, barium enema, or sigmoidoscopy. The effectiveness of each of these interventions is controversial. Since the last recommendation of the three panels, published reports show a decrease in mortality from colon cancer after screening with fecal occult blood testing (33%) or sigmoidoscopy (70%). Because fecal occult blood testing assumes that tumors bleed, relies on a second test of visualization of the colon in a patient with a positive test, has poor sensitivity, and is associated with poor patient compliance, some experts have advised waiting for more conclusive evidence to support routine use of this screening intervention. Because there are barriers to the use of sigmoidoscopy (eg, cost, patient discomfort and fear), the quality of the evidence is inferior, and prospective data are unlikely to be available for years, some experts advise cautiously proceeding with the ACP guidelines of regular (every 3 to 10 years) sigmoidoscopy after age 50.

Ovarian cancer screening with bimanual rectovaginal pelvic examination, CA-125 testing, or transvaginal ultrasonography has not been proven to be effective in women with one or no first-degree relatives with ovarian cancer. Because ovarian cancer has a low prevalence, even if a screening test had 99% specificity and 100% sensitivity, the positive predictive value would still be less than 5%. Thus, the National Institutes of Health (NIH) consensus panel concluded that average-risk women should not be screened for ovarian cancer. The NIH and the ACP concur that screening should be individualized for women at increased risk, although the evidence does not support a mortality benefit.

Pancreatic cancer screening with abdominal palpation or ultrasonography has not been proven to be an effective intervention.

Morbidity

Although principles of effective screening emphasize a mortality benefit, prevention of acute illness and symptoms should not be neglected. Significant morbidity is associated with alcohol and substance abuse, sexually transmitted diseases, low back pain, sexual abuse, upper respiratory tract infection, urinary tract infection, incontinence, osteoporotic fractures, and impaired vision and hearing. Counseling to prevent such morbidity is addressed in Table 3-6.

In the elderly, health should be defined by the absence of disease, the maintenance of optimal function, and the presence of an adequate support system. The USPSTF major principles of screening are less applicable to the elderly, for whom the concept of compression of morbidity is especially important. There is inadequate evidence to support the effect of many preventive services on morbidity or mortality in the elderly.

INTERVENTION-FOCUSED APPROACH

Three expert panels (ACP, CTF, USPSTF) have evaluated the evidence for the effectiveness of a broad range of preventive services. Each recommendation is linked to the strength of the evidence. Tables 3-4 through 3-8 review each preventive service and the recommended policy for implementation in general and selected populations. They are organized by intervention: history and physical examination, testing, counseling, immunization, and chemoprophylaxis. Evidence-based recommendations and expert opinions are represented. The tables were adapted from preventive care guidelines published in 1991 and 1994 and are updated with current data:

(text continues on page 23)

Table 3-4. History and Physical Examination Recommendations

AREA	AMERICAN COLLEGE OF PHYSICIANS (ACP)	CANADIAN TASK FORCE ON PERIODIC HEALTH EXAMINATION (CTF)	U.S. PREVENTIVE SERVICES TASK FORCE (USPSTF)	OTHER
Height and Weight				
General	Not considered	[C] No recommendation	[B] 18+ every 1–3 y†	**Frame:** 18+ every 4 y **Oboler & LaForce:** 20+ every 4 y **IOM:** 18+ every 5 y **AHA:** 18+ every 5 y
Selective	Not considered	[B] 18+ if one or more: woman of low socioeconomic status, food faddist, adolescent woman, native Indian or Inuit		
Blood Pressure Measurement				
General	18+ y every 1–2 y and at every visit for other reasons	[A] 25–64 at least every 5 y and at every visit for other reasons‡ [A] 65+ every 2 y	[A] 18+ every 2 y and at every visit for other reasons	**Frame:** 18+ every 2 y **IOM:** 18+ every 5 y **JNC, AHA:** 18+ every 2 y **Oboler & LaForce:** 20+ every 2 y
Selective	18+ every 1 y if diastolic BP is 85–89 mm Hg 18+ at least every 1 y if one or more: previous HTN, DM, known cardiovascular disease, moderate or extreme obesity, black race, history of HTN in parents or siblings	No recommendation	18+ every 1 y if diastolic BP is 85–89 mm Hg	**JNC, AHA:** 18+ every 1 y if diastolic BP is 80–89 mm Hg; measure BP more frequently if diastolic BP > 89 mm Hg
Assessment of Cognitive Impairment				
General	"Elderly," functional assessment screening, including measures of cognitive status	[C] No recommendation	No recommendation§	NIH: clinical evaluation
Selective	No recommendation	No recommendation	No recommendation	
Assessment of Depression and Suicidal Intent				
General	"Elderly," functional assessment screening, including measures of emotional status	[D] Recommendation against	No recommendation[1]	**Frame:** recommendation against
Selective	No recommendation	[C] 18+ for suicide risk if one or more: evidence of a psychiatric disorder, substance abuse, family history of suicide attempt	18+ for suicide risk if one or more: adolescent, young adult, personal or family history of depression, chronic illness, living alone, recent bereavement or separation or unemployment, sleep disturbance, multiple somatic complaints, drug or alcohol abuse	
Assessment of Visual Impairment				
General	Not considered	[C] No recommendation	No recommendation [B] 65+ every 1 year	**Oboler & LaForce:** 60+ every 1 y by Snellen chart or similar test **AAO:** 40-64 every 2–4 y 65+ every 1–2 y
Selective	Not considered	No recommendation	No recommendation	**AAO:** 20–39 every 3–5 y if black race
Assessment of Hearing Impairment				
General	Not considered	[B] 18+ by history	[B] 65+ by history	**IOM:** 40+ every 5 y **Oboler & LaForce:** 60+ every 1 y by audioscope
Selective	Not considered	18+ by history if one or more: exposure to jet engines or other noisy machinery, farm equipment, amplified music, gunfire, snowmobiles, or model airplanes for more than 2 hours several times per week	[C] 19–64 if regularly exposed to excessive noise	

(continued)

Table 3-4. History and Physical Examination Recommendations *(Continued)*

AREA	AMERICAN COLLEGE OF PHYSICIANS (ACP)	CANADIAN TASK FORCE ON PERIODIC HEALTH EXAMINATION (CTF)	U.S. PREVENTIVE SERVICES TASK FORCE (USPSTF)	OTHER
Examination of Oral Cavity to Detect Oral Cancer				
General	Not considered	[C] 65+ every 1 y	[C] Recommendation against	**Frame:** recommendation against¶ **ACS, NCI:** 20–39 every 3 y **Oboler & LaForce:** recommendation against
Selective	Not considered	[C] 18+ if tobacco use	18+ if one or more: tobacco use, excessive alcohol exposure, suspicious lesions detected through self-examination	
Carotid Auscultation for Cervical Bruit				
General	Not considered	[C] No recommendation	No recommendation	**Frame:** recommendation against **Oboler & LaForce:** recommendation against
Selective	No recommendation	40+ if one or more TIA symptoms, previous stroke, HTN, smoking, CAD, atrial fibrillation, DM		
Thyroid Palpation				
General	Not considered	Not considered	[D] Recommendation against	**Oboler & LaForce:** recommendation against
Selective	Not considered	Not considered	[C] 18+ if personal history of upper body radiation	**Oboler & LaForce:** 18+ every 1 y if irradiation to head, neck, or mediastinum during childhood
Complete Skin Examination				
General	Not considered	[D] Recommendation against	Recommendation against**	**Frame:** recommendation against **ACS, NCI:** 20–39 every 3 y 40+ every 1 y **Oboler & LaForce:** 20+ once **IOM:** 18+ once
Selective	Not considered	[B] 18+ if one or more: outdoor occupation, contact with polycyclic aromatic hydrocarbons [C] 18+ if personal or family history of dysplastic nevi	18+ if one or more: increased sun exposure, personal or family history of skin cancer, dysplastic nevi, or congenital nevi	**Oboler:** 20+ every 1 y if one or more: dysplastic mole, six or more moles larger than 5 mm in diameter, previous skin cancer, family history of melanoma
Breast Examination by Clinician				
General	40+ every 1 y	[C] 40–49 every 1 y [A] 50–59 every 1 y [B] 60+ every 1 y	[C] 40–49 every 1 y [C] 50–60 every 1 y	**Frame:** 18–49 every 2 y 50+ every 1 y **ACS, NCI:** 20–40 every 3 y 40+ every 1 y **ACOG:** 18+ every 1 y **IOM:** 18+ every 2 y **Oboler & LaForce:** 40+ every 1 y **AGS:** 65+ every 1 y
Selective	18+ every 1 y if personal history of breast cancer	35+ every 1 y if family history of premenopausal breast cancer in a first-degree relative or otherwise at "high risk"	[C] 35+ every 1 y if family history of premenopausal breast cancer in a first-degree relative	**ACS:** 20+, more frequently if family history of breast cancer

(continued)

Table 3-4. History and Physical Examination Recommendations *(Continued)*

AREA	AMERICAN COLLEGE OF PHYSICIANS (ACP)	CANADIAN TASK FORCE ON PERIODIC HEALTH EXAMINATION (CTF)	U.S. PREVENTIVE SERVICES TASK FORCE (USPSTF)	OTHER
Pelvic Examination by Bimanual Palpation				
General	Recommendation against	Not considered	[D] Recommendation against††	**Frame:** recommendation against **Oboler & LaForce:** recommendation against **ACS, NCI:** 20–40 every 1 to 3 y 40+ every 1 y **ACOG:** 18+ every 1 y **NIH:** recommendation against
Selective	Recommendation against‡‡	Not considered	No recommendation	**NIH:** if 1 or more first-degree relatives with ovarian cancer, consult MD if hereditary ovarian cancer syndrome, every 1 year‡‡

†The USPSTF recommends routine evaluation of height and weight using a table of desirable weights or a body mass index of more than 27.3 in women as a basis for further intervention.

‡If diastolic BP is <90 mm Hg, blood pressure should be measured at least every 5 y and at every visit made for other reasons.

§Clinicians should periodically inquire about the functional status of elderly patients at home and at work.

‖Refers to use of formal instruments to screen for depression.

¶All patients should be taught self-examination of the oral cavity for malignancy.

**Although routine screening for skin cancer by complete skin examination is not recommended, clinicians should be alert to skin lesions with malignant features when examining patients for other reasons.

††Although the USPSTF states that screening of asymptomatic women for ovarian cancer is not recommended, they advise examination of the adnexa when doing gynecologic examinations for other reasons.

‡‡ACP and NIH recommend against screening asymptomatic women for ovarian cancer with CA-125 or pelvic ultrasound. For women at increased risk of ovarian cancer (more than one first-degree relative with ovarian cancer), the decision to screen should be individualized after discussing the lack of evidence that mortality from ovarian cancer is decreased by screening. For women from a family with the rare hereditary ovarian cancer syndrome, referral for specialist care is recommended.

AAO, American Academy of Ophthalmology; *ACOG,* American College of Obstetrics and Gynecology, *ACS,* American Cancer Society, *AGS,* American Geriatrics Society; *AHA,* American Heart Association; *BP,* blood pressure; *CAD,* coronary artery disease; *DM,* diabetes mellitus; *HTN,* hypertension; *IOM,* Institute of Medicine; *JNC,* Joint National Committee; *NCI,* National Cancer Institute; *NIH,* National Institutes of Health; *TIA,* transient ischemic attack.

Tables 3–4 through 3–8, recommended intervention is listed in the first column. "General" screening refers to routine testing of asymptomatic persons who have no risk factors, other than age or gender, associated with the target condition. "Selective" screening refers to testing of asymptomatic persons who are at increased risk for the target condition.

Square brackets enclose a one-letter "strength of recommendation" code, if available. Indicated next is the age range to which the recommendation applies and the frequency with which the test should be done (in years), if specified by the health organization. For selective screening strategies, risk factors are listed. Not all panels graded recommendations for all topics.

[A] denotes a favorable recommendation based on strong evidence.

[B] denotes a favorable recommendation based on weak evidence.

[C] denotes an intermediate recommendation in which the evidence is too weak to support a positive or a negative recommendation despite grade C evidence ("Yes [C]" or "No [C]"), but the usual recommendation with grade C evidence is "no recommendation."

[D] denotes an unfavorable recommendation (exclude the intervention) based on fair evidence.

[E] denotes an unfavorable recommendation based on good evidence.

"Not considered" indicates that the health organization has not published a practice guideline about the preventive care intervention.

"Recommendation against" means that the intervention should be excluded from routine preventive care for the age, sex, and risk status indicated.

"No recommendation" indicates that an authority considered the intervention, but, for lack of convincing evidence, refrained from making a specific recommendation either for or against it.

(Adapted from Hayward RSA, Steinberg EP, Ford DE, Roizen MF, Roach KW. Preventive care guidelines, 1991. Ann Intern Med 1991;114:758 and Sox HC. Preventive health services in adults. N Engl J Med 1994;330:1589.)

Table 3-5. Laboratory Test Recommendations

TEST	ACP	CTF	USPSTF	OTHER
Hemoglobin Measurement for Iron-Deficiency Anemia				
General	Recommendation against	[C] Recommendation against	No recommendation	**IOM:** 40+ every 20 y
Selective	18+ if one or more: recent immigrant from underdeveloped country, institutionalized elderly	[C] 18–64 if of low socioeconomic status	[B] Pregnant women at first prenatal visit	
Urinalysis				
General	Recommendation against screening for bacteriuria	[D] Recommendation against screening for bacteriuria or for bladder cancer	[C] 60+ screening for bacteriuria, hematuria, proteinuria	**IOM:** 40+
Selective	Recommendation against	[B] 18+ urine cytology to screen for bladder cancer in smokers and persons occupationally exposed to bladder carcinogens	[C] 18+ to screen for bacteriuria if diabetic	
Fasting Plasma Glucose				
General	Recommendation against	[D] Recommendation against	Recommendation against	**Frame:** recommendation against **IOM:** 40+ every 5 y
Selective	18+ if intends to become pregnant and has risk factors for DM as listed below; 18+ if one or more: DM in first-degree relative, age >50 y, weight >25% over ideal weight, personal history of gestational DM, membership in ethnic group with high prevalence of DM. 40+ once if obese and a diagnosis of DM would motivate weight loss.	[B] 18+ if one or more: family history of DM, hyperglycemia associated with pregnancy, evidence of early occlusive vascular disease	18+ if one or more: family history of DM, marked obesity, personal history of gestational DM	**ADA:** 18+ every 3 y if one or more: family history of DM in first-degree relative; >20% over ideal body weight; American Indian, Hispanic, or black race; age ≥40; previously identified impaired glucose tolerance; HTN, hypercholesterolemia or hyperlipidemia; personal history of gestational DM or birthweight of babies >9 lb
Nonfasting Cholesterol†				
General	18–70 every 5 y	[C] No recommendation	[C] 18+ every 5 y‡	**Frame:** 18–70 every 4 y **AHA:** 20–60 every 5 y **NCEP:** 20+ every 5 y
Selective	18+ more frequently if one or more: smoker, family history of hypercholesterolemia or premature cardiovascular disease in a parent or sibling, use of lipid-altering drugs, HTN, CAD, or secondary cause of hyperlipidemia such as DM	[C] No recommendation	18+ more frequently if one or more: previous abnormal cholesterol, male, early CAD in a first-degree relative, smoker, HTN, HDL < 35 mg/dL (0.91 mmol/L), DM, previous stroke or PVD, severe obesity	
Thyroid FunctionTesting§				
General	Recommendation against	[D] Recommendation against screening for hyperthyroidism [C] Recommendation against screening for hypothyroidism	[D] Recommendation against	**Frame:** recommendation against
Selective	50+ if one or more general symptoms that could be caused by thyroid disease	[C] 40+ no recommendation if postmenopausal	[C] 60+ may be clinically prudent for populations at increased risk for hypothyroidism, such as older women	
HIV Serology				
General	Recommendation against	[C] No recommendation	[C] Recommendation against	**CDC:** recommendation against
Selective	18+ if one or more: member of a high-risk population by virtue of sexual or drug-taking behavior, woman of childbearing age with any risks of HIV infection, received a blood transfusion between 1978 and 1985, person planning marriage who may be at increased risk	[A] Recommend if member of high-risk population [C] No recommendation if pregnant and living in low-prevalence area	[A] 18–64 if one or more: recently acquired STD, homosexual or bisexual man or partner of same, IV drug abuser or partner of same, prostitute, has multiple sexual contacts or partner of same, received blood transfusion between 1978 and 1985, long-term resident of high-prevalence area	**CDC:** 18+ if one or more: treated for STD, IV drug abuser or partner of same, prostitute, HIV-infected sexual partner, received blood transfusion between 1978 and 1985, resident of high-prevalence area, considers self at risk **New York State Department of Health:** pregnant women

(continued)

Table 3-5. Laboratory Test Recommendations *(Continued)*

TEST		ACP	CTF	USPSTF	OTHER
Syphilis Serology					
	General	Recommendation against	[D] Recommendation against	Recommendation against	**Frame:** recommendation against
	Selective	18+ if one or more: sexual contact of known case, member of high-risk group, resident of area of high prevalence	[A] 18–64 if multiple sexual partners	[A] 18–64 if one of more: sexual contact of proved case, prostitute, multiple sexual partners, resident of area of high prevalence, pregnant	**Frame:** 18+ if member of high-risk group
Resting Electrocardiogram					
	General	18–65 recommendation against	[C] Recommendation against	Recommendation against	**Frame:** recommendation against **IOM:** 40–45 once **AHA:** 20+ every 20 y **ACC:** adults every 5 y
	Selective	65+ no recommendation 18+ no recommendation if one or more cardiac risk factors are present (risk factors include DM, HTN, tobacco use, hypercholesterolemia)¶	[C] No recommendation	No recommendations for women; doubtful that recommendations for men are applicable to women given the lower prevalence of CAD: ie, 18+ if a cardiac event would endanger public safety, 40+ if sedentary and planning to begin vigorous exercise program; 40+ if two or more: hypercholesterolemia, smoker, DM, first-degree family history of early-onset CAD**	
Exercise Stress Test					
	General	[C] Recommendation against	[C] Recommendation against	Recommendation against	**Frame:** recommendation against
	Selective	No recommendation if one or more: occupation that puts others at risk, sedentary and about to begin a program of physical conditioning No recommendation if of "increased age" and one or more: family history of CAD, smoker, systolic BP > 140 mm Hg, DM, hypercholesterolemia, total: HDL cholesterol ratio > 6	No recommendation	No recommendations for women; doubtful that recommendations for men are applicable to women given the lower prevalence of CAD: ie, 18+ if a cardiac event would endanger public safety, 40+ if sedentary and planning to begin vigorous exercise program; 40+ if two or more: hypercholesterolemia, smoker, DM, first-degree family history of early-onset CAD	**Frame:** once for high-risk groups, especially if planning exercise program A**CSM:** 46+ once if planning exercise program **ACC, AHA:** no recommendation for women
Assessment of Intraocular Pressure by Clinician‡					
	General	Not considered	[C] Recommendation against	18–64 recommendation against 65+ by eye specialist	**Frame:** recommendation against **AAO:** 20–39 every 2–4 y 65+ every 1–2 y
	Selective	Not considered	No recommendation	No recommendation	**AAO:** 20–39 every 3–5 y if black race

(continued)

Table 3-5. Laboratory Test Recommendations *(Continued)*

TEST	ACP	CTF	USPSTF	OTHER
Tuberculin Skin Testing (PPD)				
General	No considered	[E] Recommendation against	Recommendation against	**Frame:** recommendation against
Selective	Not considered	[A] 18+ if exposed to TB at home or work or living in community with high infection rate	[A] 18+ if one or more: exposed to TB case in the home, clinics or shelters for the homeless, nursing homes, substance abuse treatment centers, dialysis units, correctional institutions, recent immigrants or refugees from high-prevalence areas; migrant workers; HIV or renal failure, immunosuppressive drugs, including steroids	**Frame:** 18+ for high-risk groups, including immigrants, alcoholics, contacts of TB cases, health-care personnel, persons with a family history of TB, and persons living in institutions **CDC:** 18+ if one or more: close contact with persons suspected to have TB; medical risks such as HIV infection, silicosis, previous gastrectomy, renal failure, DM, malignancy, prolonged corticosteroid use; foreign-born from area of high TB prevalence; member of high-risk racial, ethnic, or low-income population; alcoholic or IV drug user, resident of long-term care facility
Chest Radiograph to Detect Lung Cancer				
General	Recommendation against	[D] Recommendation against	Recommendation against	**Frame:** recommendation against **ACS:** recommendation against **Oboler & LaForce:** recommendation against
Selective	Recommendation against if smoker	[D] Recommendation against if smoker	Recommendation against if smoker	
Bone Mineral Content Testing[‡‡]				
General	Perimenopausal, recommendation against	[D] Recommendation against	No recommendation	**Frame:** recommendation against
Selective	18+ no recommendation; risk factors: postmenopausal, white race, low body weight; roles of calcium intake and exercise in prevention are controversial; consider if decision to start long-term estrogen therapy will be based on knowledge of bone mass and related fracture risk	[C] 40+ no recommendation if one or more: Caucasian, surgical menopause, early natural menopause, low body weight for height, immobile; uncertain roles for smoking, calcium intake, alcohol use, falls	40–64 if one or more: perimenopausal, Caucasian, bilateral oophorectomy before menopause, slender build; and if estrogen therapy is being considered for prophylaxis against osteoporosis but would not otherwise be indicated	**Frame:** 18+ no recommendation if one or more: Caucasian, early menopause, small body frame, family history of osteoporosis, sedentary lifestyle, low dietary calcium, steroid use
Mammography				
General	50+ every 1 y	[A] 50–59 every 1 y [B] 60+ every 1 y	[A] 50–69 every 1–2 y [C] 40-49 every 1–2 y [C] ≥70 every 1-2 y	**Frame (1986):** 50+ every 1 y **ACS,NCI, AMA, AAFP (1989):** 40–50 every 1–2 y; 50+ every 1 y **ACOG (1989):** 35–40 once; 40–50 every 1–2 y; 50+ every 1 y **AGS (1989):** 65–85 every 2–3 y **Oboler & LaForce (1989):** 40+ every 1 y
Selective	18+ every 1 y if personal history of breast cancer 40+ every 1 y if family history of breast cancer or at increased risk after consideration of marital status, multiparity, late first pregnancy, early menarche, late menopause, history of benign breast conditions, high-fat diet (1989)	35+ every 1 y if "at high risk," especially if family history of premenopausal breast cancer in a first-degree relative (1986)	35+ every 1 y if family history of premenopausal breast cancer in a first-degree relative (1989)	See text for discussion of controversy

(continued)

Table 3-5. Laboratory Test Recommendations *(Continued)*

TEST	ACP	CTF	USPSTF	OTHER
Papanicolaou Smear (Cervical Cytology)[§§]				
General	20–65 every 3 y	[B] 18–35 every 3 y [B] 36–74 every 5 y	18–65 every 1–3	**Frame:** 18–69 every 2 y **ACS, NCI, ACOG, AAFP:** 18+ every 1–3 y[‖‖] **Oboler & LaForce:** 20+ every 3 y **IOM:** 18+ every 5 y **AGS:** 60–70 every 3 y **ACS:** 18+ more frequently if one or more: early age at first intercourse, multiple sexual partners, other risk factors
Selective	20–65 every 2 y if at increased risk after consideration of main risk factors (multiple sexual partners, early onset of sexual activity, smoking) and additional risk factors (black, Hispanic, Native American ethnic origins; certain partner characteristics, history of STD, oral contraceptive use) 66–75 every 3 y if not screened in the 10 years before age 66	[B] 18–74 every 1 y if one or both: early onset of sexual activity, multiple sexual partners	[A] 18+ more frequently if one or more: early onset of sexual activity, multiple sexual partners, low socioeconomic status 65+ every 1–3 y if no documentation of consistently normal cervical cytology in the previous 10 years	
Gonorrhea Culture[¶¶]				
General	Not considered	[D] Recommendation against	Recommendation against	**Frame:** recommendation against **Oboler & LaForce:** recommendation against **IOM:** 18–24 once
Selective	Not considered	[A] 18–64 if multiple sexual partners	[A] 18–64 if one or more; prostitute, multiple sexual partners, sexual contact with proved cases, history of repeated STDs	**Oboler & LaForce:** 18+ if one or more; prostitute, sexual contact with proved cases, history of repeated gonorrhea
Chlamydia Testing[***]				
General	Not considered	[D] Recommendation against	Recommendation against	**Frame:** recommendation against **Oboler & LaForce:** recommendation against
Selective	Not considered	[C] 18+ if in high-risk group such as partners of persons with nongonoccocal urethritis	18–64 if one or more: attending STD clinic or other health-care setting that sees high-risk patients, multiple sexual contacts, partner of persons with positive cultures	**CDC:** 18+ if one or more: attending STD clinic or other health-care setting that sees high-risk patients, low socioeconomic status, multiple sexual partners, partner with multiple sexual contacts, partner of persons with positive cultures
Endometrial Aspirate or Biopsy				
General	Not considered	[D] Recommendation against	Not considered	**Frame:** recommendation against[†††]
Selective	Not considered	No recommendation	Not considered	**ACS:** at menopause, if one or more: history of infertility, obesity, anovulation, uterine bleeding, estrogen therapy **ACOG:** perimenopausal, if unexpected break-through bleeding during estrogen replacement therapy
Stool Examination for Occult Blood				
General	50+ every 1 y	18–39 recommendation against [C] 40+ no recommendation	[C] No recommendation	**Frame:** 40–50 every 2 y 50+ every 1 y **ACS, NCI, ACOG:** 50+ every 1 y **IOM:** 40+ every 1 y
Selective	40+ every 1 y if one or more: personal history of inflammatory bowel disease, familial polyposis coli, family history of colon cancer in first-degree relative	[C] 45+ no recommendation if family history of colorectal cancer detected after age 40 in a first-degree relative [D] recommend against if kindred of cancer family syndrome	[C] 50+ every 1 y if one or more: personal history of adenomatous polyps or colorectal cancer or inflammatory bowel disease, first-degree relative with colorectal cancer [C] 50+ every 1 y if personal history of one or more: endometrial, ovarian, breast cancer	See text for discussion of controversy

(continued)

Table 3-5. Laboratory Test Recommendations *(Continued)*

TEST	ACP	CTF	USPSTF	OTHER
Sigmoidoscopy				
General	50+ every 3–5 y‡‡‡	[C] 40+ no recommendation	[C] 40+ no recommendation [D] 18–39 recommendation against	**Frame:** recommendation against **ACS, NCI, ACOG:** 50+ every 3–5 y
Selective	No recommendation	18–29 if family history of familial polyposis [C] 40+ no recommendation if family history of colorectal cancer detected after age 40 in one or more first-degree relatives [C] 40+ if personal history of one or more: endometrial, ovarian, breast cancer [D] recommend against if kindred of cancer family syndrome	[C] 50+ every 3–5 y if one or more: personal history of adenomatous polyps or colorectal cancer or inflammatory bowel disease, first-degree relative with colorectal cancer after age 40 [C] 50+ every 3–5 y if personal history of one or more: endometrial, ovarian, breast cancer	**ACS:** 18–49 more frequently if one or more: personal history of familial polyposis, Gardner syndrome, ulcerative colitis, previous polyps or colon cancer; family history of colorectal cancer See text for discussion of controversy
Colonoscopy				
General	Recommendation against	[C] 40+ no recommendation	Recommendation against	
Selective	40+ every 3–5 y if one or more: personal history of inflammatory bowel disease, familial polyposis coli, family history of colon cancer in first-degree relative§§§	[C] 18+ if personal history of one or both: ulcerative colitis or adenomatous polyps of 10 years' duration, previous colorectal cancer [C] 30+ if family history of familial polyposis [C] 40+ no recommendation if two or more first-degree relatives with colorectal cancer [B] 40+ recommend if kindred of cancer family syndrome	[A] 18+ if family history of hereditary polyposis syndromes [B] 18+ if personal history of 10 or more years of ulcerative colitis [B] 18+ if personal history of colorectal cancer or adenomatous polyps [B] 40+ if two or more first-degree relatives with coloretal cancer, particularly if age of onset is before 40	

†Measurement of nonfasting total serum cholesterol level by venipuncture. All authorities stress the importance of submitting samples to an accredited laboratory with good quality control. Abnormal results should be confirmed by a repeat nonfasting cholesterol level, and the mean of the two results should be used for decision making.

‡Periodic total cholesterol screening is most important for middle-aged men and may be clinically prudent for others.

§Sensitive thyrotropin (TSH) immumoradiometric assay or free thyroxin index.

||Most groups recommend testing with a Western blot test after repeatedly reactive results on enzyme immunoassay tests.

¶Although no specific advice is given for the use of a resting electrocardiogram to screen for coronary artery disease in persons with risk factors for such disease, the ACP background paper states that general screening recommendations do not apply to persons with the characteristics listed.

**The USPSTF lists the same high-risk groups as possible candidates for exercise and rating electrocardiography, but observes that there is insufficient evidence to determine which is the better screening test for these persons.

††Tonometry and ophthalmoscopy done by primary-care provider.

‡‡Methods for assessing the risk for osteoporosis-related fractures with bone mineral content testing include single-photon absorptiometry, dual-photon absorptiometry, and quantitative computed tomography.

§§ ACP, ACS, CTF, Frame, Oboler and LaForce, and USPSTF suggest initiating screening with two or three annual smears at the onset of sexual activity. Recommendations pertain to women who are sexually active.

|| ||After three normal annual examination results, the Papanicolaou test may be done less frequently at the discretion of the physician.

¶¶Culture from urethral, rectal, throat, or endocervical swabs.

***Culture or immunofluorescent assay of endocervical or urethral swabs.

††† All women should be taught to report postmenopausal bleeding.

‡‡‡ Air-contrast barium enema every 5 years may be substituted for sigmoidoscopy.

§§§ Air-contrast barium enema may be substituted for colonoscopy.

AAFP, American Academy of Family Physicians; *AAO,* American Academy of Ophthalmology; *ACC,* American College of Cardiology; *ACOG,* American College of Obstetrics and Gynecology; *ACS,* American Cancer Society; *ADA,* American Diabetes Association; *AGS,* American Geriatrics Society; *AHA,* American Heart Association; *AMA,* American Medical Association; *CAD,* coronary artery disease; *CDC,* Centers for Disease Control and Prevention; *DM,* diabetes mellitus; *HDL,* high-density lipoprotein; *HTN,* hypertension; *IOM,* Institutes of Medicine; *NCI,* National Cancer Institute; *NCEP,* National Cholesterol Education Project; *PVD,* peripheral vascular disease; *STD,* sexually transmitted disease.

(Adapted from Hayward RSA, Steinberg EP, Ford, DE, Roizen MF, Roach KW. Preventive care guidelines, 1991. Ann Intern Med 1991;114:758 and Sox HC. Preventive health services in adults. N Engl J Med 1994;330:1589.)

Table 3-6. Counseling Recommendations

TOPIC	ACP	CTF	USPSTF	OTHER
Dietary Assessment and Nutritional Counseling				
Caloric balance	18+ provide guidelines for a healthful, well-balanced diet and encourage behavior modification to reduce and prevent obesity	Not considered	18+ provide diet and exercise advice to all persons to achieve and maintain desirable weight by keeping caloric intake balanced with energy expenditures	**NAS:** 18+ advise to balance food intake and physical activity to maintain appropriate body weight
Fat, cholesterol		[C] No recommendation	[A] 18+ give dietary guidance on how to reduce total fat intake to <30% of total calories, saturated fat consumption to <10% of total calories, and dietary cholesterol to <300 mg/d [B] 18–59 advise to adopt low-fat diet for CAD prevention [C] 60+ advise to adopt low-fat diet for CAD prevention [A] 18+ repeated dietary change messages from multiple sources to effect decrease in fat content of diet	**NAS:** 18+ advise to reduce total fat intake to 30% or less of calories, saturated fatty acid intake to <10% of calories, and cholesterol intake to <300 mg/d **ACS:** 18+ advise to reduce intake of calories from fat to 25% to 30% or less of total calorie intake
Fiber		Not considered	[B] 18+ encourage patients to eat a variety of foods with emphasis on whole-grain products, cereals, vegetables, fruits	**NAS:** 18+ advise to eat five or more servings of vegetables and fruits daily and increase intake of complex carbohydrates **ACS:** 18+ advise to eat more high-fiber foods such as whole-grain cereals, legumes, vegetables, fruits
Sodium		Not considered	[C] 18+ advise patients to eat foods low in sodium and to limit salt added to food in preparation or consumption	**NAS:** 18+ advise to limit total intake of salt to 6 g/d or less by avoiding salty foods and limiting salt added to foods **ACS:** 18+ advise to limit consumption of salt-cured, smoked, and nitrite-preserved foods
Calcium		[C] 18+ maintain liberal intake of natural and supplemental calcium	[B] 18+ counsel about methods to ensure adequate calcium intake	**NAS:** 18+ advise maintaining adequate calcium intake
Iron		[C] 18–44 selective counseling for women of low socioeconomic status, food faddists	[C] 18–64 all menstruating women, counsel about adequate iron intake	
Physical Activity and Exercise				
Physical activity		[C] 40+ teach effect of immobility on bone mass	[A] 18+ provide all patients with information on the role of regular physical activity in disease prevention and assist in selecting an appropriate type of exercise [C] 18+ for primary prevention of CAD [A] 18+ for primary prevention of HTN, obesity, or bone loss	**Frame:** 18+ encourage exercise
Cancer Surveillance				
Skin self-examination		Not considered	[C] No recommendation (1989)	**Frame:** 18+ teach skin self-examination
Breast self-examination		[C] 18–40 no recommendation (1986)	[C] No recommendation (1996)	**Frame:** 18+ every month (1986) **ACS, NCI:** 20+ every month (1988) **IOM:** 25+ every month (1978) **AGS:** 65+ every month (1989) **Oboler and LaForce:** no recommendation (1989) **WHO:** no recommendation (1984)

(continued)

Table 3-6. Counseling Recommendations *(Continued)*

TOPIC	ACP	CTF	USPSTF	OTHER
Sexual Practices				
STD		Not considered	[B] 18+ use of barrier methods to reduce risk for STD [C] 18–64 counsel STD transmission, partner selection, condom use, avoiding anal intercourse	**CDC:** Education of those at risk on the means for reducing the risk for transmission (1993)
HIV		Not considered	[A] 18+ teach blood, needle, sexual behavior precautions for same high-risk groups for whom HIV testing is indicated	**CDC:** Education of those at risk on the means for reducing the risk for transmission (1993)
Unintended pregnancy		[B] 18+ prevent unwanted pregnancy by asking teenagers about sexual activity and recommending appropriate contraception	18–64 counsel about unintended pregnancy and contraceptive options	
Substance Abuse				
Tobacco	18+ actively counsel patients to quit smoking	[A] 18+ counsel to prevent tobacco use; emphasize if one or more: oral contraceptive use, DM, HTN, high cholesterol level; asbestos, uranium, silica, grain exposure	[A] 18+ repeated smoking cessation messages from multiple sources over an extended period of time; primary prevention messages to nonsmoking adolescents	**Frame:** 18+ every 10 y screen for tobacco use
Alcohol	18+ patient education and counseling about the appropriate use of alcohol	[B] 18–64 case finding to identify problem drinking, followed by counseling	18+ counsel to limit alcohol consumption, to stop alcohol consumption during pregnancy, not to drive after drinking	**Frame:** recommendation against screening for alcoholism **NAS:** 18+ advise patients to limit alcohol consumption to < 1 ounce of pure alcohol per day
Intravenous street drugs	18+ patient education and counseling about licit and illicit drugs	Not considered	18–64 counsel IV drug users about dangers of psychoactive drug use, encourage cessation of drug use, alert to risks of using unsterilized needles	
Injury Prevention				
Motor vehicle accidents	18+ counsel patients to use seatbelts	[C] 18–64 ask and teach about seatbelt safety; control underlying medical conditions that increase risks associated with driving	[C] 18+ advise about seatbelt use, alcohol- or drug-related risks with driving, general road safety, motorcycle helmet use	**Frame:** 18+ encourage use of seatbelts
Back injuries		Not considered	18–64 teach injury prevention if one or more: previous back injury, high-risk body configuration, current or planned high-risk activities	**Oboler and LaForce:** 18+ if high-risk occupation: nursing, manual labor, driving
Falls among the elderly		[C] Encourage safety in home and community	18+ teach domestic safety to elderly adults and persons with elderly adults in the home	
Fire injuries		[C] Encourage safety in home and community	18+ encourage smoke detector installation and maintenance and discuss danger of smoking near bed or upholstery	
Violence and firearm injuries		Not considered	19–39 teach dangers of hand weapons, violent behavior; keep firearms in child-resistant containers	
Promoting Dental Health				
Dental hygiene teaching		[A] 18–74 every 1 y, encourage daily oral hygiene, dental visits	[A] 18+ every 1 y (plaque) [C] 18+ every 1 y (caries), encourage regular tooth brushing, flossing, dental visits	**Oboler and LaForce:** 20+ every 1 y, teach about dental hygiene and importance of regular dental visits
Stress and Bereavement				
Functional assessment	Elderly, functional assessment screening including measures of emotional status and domestic adaptation	[C] 18–64 elicit history of marital and sexual problems [C] 46–64 preretirement counseling [B] 65+ every 1–2 y, assess physical, social, and psychological function	18+ remain alert for symptoms of abnormal bereavement, depression, physical abuse, and suicide risk in persons with recent bereavement, divorce, separation, unemployment, alcohol or other substance abuse, depression, living alone, serious medical illness	

ACS, American Cancer Society; *AGS,* American Geriatrics Society; *CAD,* coronary artery disease; *CDC,* Centers for Disease Control; *DM,* diabetes mellitus; *HTN,* hypertension; *IOM,* Institutes of Medicine; *NAS,* National Academy of the Sciences; *NCI,* National Cancer Institute; *STD,* sexually transmitted disease; *WHO,* World Health Organization.

(Adapted from Hayward RSA, Steinberg EP, Ford, DE, Roizen MF, Roach KW. Preventive care guidelines, 1991. Ann Intern Med 1991;114:758 and Sox HC. Preventive health services in adults. N Engl J Med 1994;330:1589.)

Table 3-7. Adult Immunization Recommendations

VACCINE		ACP	CTF	USPSTF	OTHERS
Hepatitis B-Inactivated Virus Vaccine					
	General	Sexually active young adult (1994)	Recommendation against	Recommendation against	
	Selective	18+ initial series if at increased risk for occupational, environmental, social, or family exposure; intimate family contact with infected persons, resident of institutions for the mentally retarded, prison inmate, homeless person, person with multiple sexual partners, person with multiple STDs or partner of same, intimate contact with persons from endemic areas, early renal disease or hemophilia, health-care worker, IV drug abuser	[A] 18+ initial series if one or more: dialysis, blood product exposure, health-care personnel, institutionalized mentally retarded person, IV drug abuser, contact with patients with disease or carriers	[A] 18+ initial series if one or more: IV drug user, blood product recipient, health-care worker with blood product exposure	**CDC:** 18+ initial series if one or more: health-care worker with blood product exposure, client or staff of institution for the developmentally disabled, staff of nonresidential day-care programs, hemodialysis patient, person with multiple sexual partners or recent STD, prostitute, user of illicit injectable drugs in household or sexual contact with HBV carriers, inmate of long-term correctional facilities, recipient of certain blood products
Inactivated Influenza Vaccine					
	General	65+ every 1 y	[E] 18–64 recommendation against [A] 65+ every 1 y	[A] 65+ every 1 y	**Frame:** recommendation against **IOM:** 60+ every 1 y **CDC:** 65+ every 1 y
	Selective	18–64 every 1 y if one or more: resident of nursing home or chronic-care facility, health-care occupation, chronic cardiopulmonary disorder or other chronic disease requiring regular medical care, HIV-infected patient, organ transplant recipient, alcoholic, cancer patient, person providing care to high-risk persons, or resident of area with increased risk for exposure (eg, dormitories, military barracks)	[A] 18+ every 1 y if chronic debilitating disease	[A] 18+ every 1 y if one or more: resident of chronic-care facility, chronic cardiopulmonary disease, hemoglobinopathy, DM, metabolic disease, renal dysfunction, immunosuppression; health-care provider for high-risk patients	**Frame:** 18+ every 1 y if at high risk for lower respiratory tract infection **CDC:** 18+ every 1 y if one or more: resident of nursing home or chronic-care facility, chronic cardiovascular or pulmonary disease, person who has required regular medical care because of chronic metabolic or renal disease, person with hemoglobinopathy or immunosuppression; health-care worker, home care provider, household member of high-risk persons
Measles Live Virus Vaccine†					
	General	No recommendation	Not considered	No recommendation	
	Selective	18+ two doses if born after 1956 and without proof of immunity or documentation of receipt of live vaccine; revaccinate if college student or health-care worker and previously given only one dose of vaccine or killed measles vaccine	Not considered	[A] 18+ once if born after 1956 and no proof of immunity, documentation of receipt of live vaccine or physician-documented measles [B] 2nd MMR if adolescent/young adult in settings where such individuals congregate	**CDC:** 18+ if medical personnel or student born after 1956 and lacking evidence of two live measles vaccination, physician-diagnosed measles disease, or laboratory evidence of measles immunity
Pneumococcal Polysaccharide 23-Valent Vaccine					
	General	65+ once; consider revaccination after 6 years	[C] 55+ no recommendation	[B] 65+ once; consider revaccination after 6 years	**Frame:** recommendation against **CDC:** 65+ once
	Selective	18–64 once if one or more: chronic cardiac or pulmonary disease, asplenia, chronic liver disease, alcoholism, DM, chronic renal failure, hematologic malignancy, undergoing chemotherapy, organ transplant recipient, HIV infection, CSF leak, nursing home resident	[A] 18+ once if one or both sickle-cell anemia; asplenia [A] 55+ once if living in an institution [D] recommendation against if immunocompromised	[C] 18+ once if one or more: chronic cardiopulmonary disease, sickle-cell disease, nephrotic syndrome, Hodgkin's disease, asplenia, DM, alcoholism, cirrhosis, multiple myeloma, renal disease, immunosuppression, HIV infection	**Frame:** 18+ once if sickle-cell disease or asplenia **CDC:** 18+ once; consider revaccination after 6 years if one or more: chronic illness such as cardiopulmonary disease, DM, alcoholism, cirrhosis, CSF leak; immunosuppression, such as splenic dysfunction, hematologic malignancy, renal failure, organ transplantation, HIV infection
Rubella Live Virus Vaccine*					
	General	Recommendation against	Recommendation against	Recommendation against	
	Selective	18+ once if lacking documentation of receipt of live vaccine or after first birthday, particularly women of child-bearing age and young adults studying or working in educational, health-care, or military institutions	[A] 18–44 once if lacking proof of immunity and agreeing not to become pregnant for 3 months	[A] 18 to menopause once if lacking proof of vaccination or serologic evidence of immunity and agreeing not to become pregnant for 3 months	**Frame:** 18+ once if not pregnant and has had lack of immunity determined **CDC:** 18+ once if not pregnant and lacking adequate documentation of immunity, serologic laboratory evidence, or record of immunization on or after first birthday

(continued)

Table 3-7 Adult Immunization Recommendations *(Continued)*

VACCINE	ACP	CTF	USPSTF	OTHERS
Tetanus-Diphtheria Toxoid (Td booster)				
General	18+ every 10 y or 1 booster at age 50 for persons who have completed the full pediatric series, including the teenage/young adult booster (1994)	[A] 18+ every 10 y	[A] 18+ every 10 y	**Frame:** 18+ every 10 y
Selective	No recommendation (1990)	No recommendation	No recommendation	

*Most authorities advise using a combined mumps, measles, and rubella vaccine.

CDC, Centers for Disease Control and Prevention, *CSF,* cerebrospinal fluid; *DM,* diabetes mellitus; *IOM,* Institutes of Medicine; *STD,* sexually transmitted disease.

(Adapted from Hayward RSA, Steinberg EP, Ford, DE, Roizen MF, Roach KW. Preventive care guidelines, 1991. Ann Intern Med 1991;114:758 and Sox HC. Preventive health services in adults. N Engl J Med 1994;330:1589.)

1. *History and physical examination.* A complete history and physical examination should be performed to assess risk factors and document baseline abnormalities. Emphasis should be placed on maneuvers that will assess risk and influence recommendations for further testing, counseling, immunizations, and chemoprophylaxis. It is clearly the most cost-effective aspect of preventive care.
2. *Laboratory testing.* Performance should be based on explicit goals and documented efficacy of the test.
3. *Counseling.* Although "talk is cheap," clinicians should consider the cost and inconvenience of recommendations for behavior modification. Tobacco cessation must be emphasized, as it is responsible for more than one of every six deaths in the United States and is the most important single preventable cause of death and disease in our society. Cigarette smoking accounts for 21% of coronary heart disease deaths, 87% of lung cancer deaths, and 30% of all cancer deaths. Tobacco use is a major risk factor for chronic bronchitis and obstructive lung disease; cancer of the lung, larynx, pharynx, oral cavity, esophagus, pancreas, and bladder; respiratory infections; and peptic ulcers. Because ischemic heart disease is the number-one cause of death in women, it is practical for clinicians to focus counseling efforts on modifying the risk factors for cardiovascular disease (see Table 3-3). This paradigm addresses many features of a healthy lifestyle.
4. *Vaccinations.* True primary prevention can be accomplished, but the efficacy of vaccines in the groups most at risk for disease is controversial.
5. *Chemoprophylaxis.* This section is limited to advice about heart disease and osteoporosis prevention. The ACP has published a detailed review of hormone replacement therapy in postmenopausal women.

Table 3-8. Adult Chemoprophylaxis Recommendations

DRUG	ACP	CTF	USPSTF	OTHERS
Aspirin				
General	Not considered	[C] No recommendation	No recommendation	See text for discussion of controversy
Selective	[A] Nonvalvular atrial fibrillation: first choice, warfarin; second choice, ASA 325 mg/day [C] ASA may not be useful >75 y [A] Prior TIA, CVA; [C] Any dose	Women not considered	No recommendations for women; unclear if recommendations for men are applicable to women given the lower prevalence of CAD: ie, M 40+ if risk factors for myocardial infarction such as high cholesterol, smoking, DM, family history of early onset of CAD, and no history of GI or other bleeding problems, other risks for bleeding, or cerebrovascular hemorrhage (1989)	
Hormone Replacement Therapy				
General	Consider in all postmenopausal women	Recommendation against	Recommendation against	
Selective	Consider if surgical menopause, with or at increased risk for CAD	[C] 40+ consider if white race, peri-menopausal, surgical or early menopause, low body weight for height, smoking, medication, alcohol use, inadequate dietary calcium	[B] 40+ at menopause; consider if peri-menopausal and at risk because of white or Asian race, bilateral oophorectomy before menopause, early menopause, slender build and no abnormal vaginal bleeding, active liver disease, thromboembolic disorders, hormone-dependent cancer	Frame: 40+ assess risk for osteoporosis at menopause and individualize therapy with estrogen and calcium

CAD, coronary artery disease; *CVA,* cerebrovascular accident; *DM,* diabetes mellitus; *TIA,* transient ischemic attack.

(Adapted from Hayward RSA, Steinberg EP, Ford, DE, Roizen MF, Roach KW. Preventive care guidelines, 1991. Ann Intern Med 1991;114:758 and Sox HC. Preventive health services in adults. N Engl J Med 1994;330:1589.)

This chapter has emphasized disease prevention and screening (testing in asymptomatic women). Interventions should be considered for general implementation after considering the four major principles of screening. Women at average risk for disease differ considerably from those at high risk. Care must always be individualized and patient preferences should be considered.

BIBLIOGRAPHY

Ahlquist DA, Weiand HS, Moertel CG, et al. Accuracy of fecal occult blood screening for colorectal neoplasia. JAMA 1993;269:1262.

American Cancer Society. Summary of current guidelines for the cancer-related checkup: recommendations. Atlanta: American Cancer Society, 1988.

American College of Physicians, Medical Practice Committee. Periodic health examination: a guide for designing individualized preventive health care in the asymptomatic patient. Ann Intern Med 1981;95:729.

American College of Physicians. Guidelines for counseling postmenopausal women about preventive hormone therapy. Ann Intern Med 1992;117:1038.

American College of Physicians. Guidelines for medical treatment for stroke prevention. Ann Intern Med 1994;121:54.

American College of Physicians. Screening for ovarian cancer: recommendations and rationale. Ann Intern Med 1994;121:141.

American College of Physicians. Guide for adult immunization, 3d ed. Philadelphia: American College of Physicians, 1994.

Anastos K, Charney P, Charon RA, et al. Hypertension in women: what is really known? Ann Intern Med 1991;115:287.

Canadian Task Force on the Periodic Health Examination. The periodic health examination. Can Med Assoc J 1979;121:1193.

Canadian Task Force on the Periodic Health Examination. The periodic health examination: 1984 update. Can Med Assoc J 1984;130:1278.

Canadian Task Force on the Periodic Health Examination. The periodic health examination: 1985 update. Can Med Assoc J 1986;134:724.

Canadian Task Force on the Periodic Health Examination. The periodic health examination: 1987 update. Can Med Assoc J 1988;138:618.

Canadian Task Force on the Periodic Health Examination. Periodic health examination: 1989 update. Can Med Assoc J 1989;141:209.

Canadian Task Force on the Periodic Health Examination. Periodic health examination, 1990 update: 1. Early detection of hyperthyroidism and hypothyroidism in adults and screening of newborns for congenital hypothyroidism. Can Med Assoc J 1990;142:955.

Canadian Task Force on the Periodic Health Examination. Periodic health examination, 1990 update: 2. Early detection of depression and prevention of suicide. Can Med Assoc J 1990;142:1233.

Canadian Task Force on the Periodic Health Examination. Periodic health examination, 1990 update: 3. Interventions to prevent lung cancer other than smoking cessation. Can Med Assoc J 1990;143:269.

Canadian Task Force on the Periodic Health Examination. Periodic health examination, 1991 update: 1. Screening for cognitive impairment in the elderly. Can Med Assoc J 1991;144:425.

Canadian Task Force on the Periodic Health Examination. Periodic health examination, 1991 update: 2. Administration of pneumococcal vaccine. Can Med Assoc J 1991;144:665.

Canadian Task Force on the Periodic Health Examination. Periodic health examination, 1991 update: 5. Screening for abdominal aortic aneurysm. Can Med Assoc J 1991;145:783.

Canadian Task Force on the Periodic Health Examination. Periodic health examination, 1991 update: 6. Acetylsalicylic acid and the primary prevention of cardiovascular disease. Can Med Assoc J 1991; -145:1091.

Canadian Task Force on the Periodic Health Examination. Periodic health examination, 1993 update: 2. Lowering blood cholesterol to prevent coronary heart disease. Can Med Assoc J 1993;148:521.

Canadian Task Force on the Periodic Health Examination. Periodic health examination, 1993 update: 3. Periodontal diseases: classification, diagnosis, risk factors and prevention. Can Med Assoc J 1993;149: 1409.

Canadian Task Force on the Periodic Health Examination. Periodic health examination, 1994 update: 2. Screening strategies for colorectal cancer. Can Med Assoc J 1994;150:1961.

Canadian Task Force on the Periodic Health Examination. Periodic health examination, 1994 update: 4. Secondary prevention of elder abuse and mistreatment. Can Med Assoc J 1994;151:1413.

Carlson KJ, Skates SJ, Singer DE. Screening for ovarian cancer. Ann Intern Med 1994;121:124.

Colditz GA, Bonita R, Stampfer MJ, et al. Cigarette smoking and the risk of stroke in middle-aged women. N Engl J Med 1988;318:937.

Eaker ED, Chesebro JH, Sacks FM, et al. Cardiovascular disease in women. Circulation 1993;88:1999.

Eddy D. ACS report on the cancer-related health checkup. CA 1980;30:194.

Eddy DM. Clinical decision making: from theory to practice. Resolving conflicts in practice policies. JAMA 1990;264:389.

Eddy DM (ed). Common screening tests. Philadelphia: American College of Physicians, 1991.

Fiebach N, Beckett W. Prevention of respiratory infections in adults. Influenza and pneumococcal vaccines. Arch Intern Med 1994; 154:2545.

Frame PS, Carlson SJ. A critical review of periodic health screening using specific screening criteria. Part 1: Selected diseases of respiratory, cardiovascular, and central nervous systems. J Fam Pract. 1975;2:29.

Garber AM, Sox HC Jr, Littenberg B. Screening asymptomatic adults for cardiac risk factors: the serum cholesterol level. Ann Intern Med 1989;110:622.

Grady D, Rubin SM, Petitti DB, et al. Hormone therapy to prevent disease and prolong life in postmenopausal women. Ann Intern Med 1992; 117:1016.

Hayward RSA, Steinberg EP, Ford DE, Roizen MF, Roach KW. Preventive care guidelines, 1991. Ann Intern Med 1991;114:758. (Erratum, Ann Intern Med 1991;115:332.)

Kerlikowske K, Grady D, Rubin SM, Sandrock C, Ernster VL. Efficacy of screening mammography: a meta-analysis. JAMA 1995;273:149.

Klinkman MS, Zazove P, Mehr DR, Ruffin MT IV. A criterion-based review of preventive health care in the elderly. Part 1: Theoretical framework and development of criteria. J Fam Pract 1992;34:205.

Krumholz HM, Seeman TE, Merrill SS, et al. Lack of association between cholesterol and coronary heart disease mortality and morbidity and all-cause mortality in persons older than 70 years. JAMA 1994;272:1335.

Littenberg B, Garber AM, Sox HC Jr. Screening for hypertension. Ann Intern Med 1990;112:192.

Mandel JS, Bond JH, Church TR, et al. Reducing mortality from colorectal cancer by screening for fecal occult blood. N Engl J Med 1993;328:1365. (Erratum, N Engl J Med 1993;329:672.)

Manson JE, Tosteson H, Ridker PM, et al. The primary prevention of myocardial infarction. N Engl J Med 1992;326:1406.

Matchar DB, McCrory DC, Barnett HJM, Feussner JR. Medical treatment for stroke prevention. Ann Intern Med 1994;121:41. (Erratum, Ann Intern Med 1994;121:470.)

National Academy of Sciences Institute of Medicine. Preventive services for the well population. Washington, DC: National Academy of Sciences, 1978.

NIH Consensus Development Panel on Ovarian Cancer. Ovarian cancer: screening, treatment, and follow-up. JAMA 1995;273:491.

Nystrom L, Rutqvist LE, Wall S, et al. Breast cancer screening with mammography: overview of Swedish randomised trials. Lancet 1993; 341:973.

Oboler SK, LaForce FM. The periodic physical examination in asymptomatic adults. Ann Intern Med 1989;110:214.

Ransohoff DF, Lang CA. Sigmoidoscopic screening in the 1990s. JAMA 1993;269:1278.
Selby JV, Friedman GD, Quesenberry CP Jr, Weiss NS. A case-control study of screening sigmoidoscopy and mortality from colorectal cancer. N Engl J Med 1992;326:653.
Selby JV, Friedman GD, Quesenberry CP Jr, Weiss NS. Effect of fecal occult blood testing on mortality from colorectal cancer: a case control study. Ann Intern Med 1993;118:1.
Shapiro S. Periodic screening for breast cancer: the health insurance plan project and its sequelae, 1963–1986. Baltimore: Johns Hopkins University Press, 1988.
SHEP Cooperative Research Group. Prevention of stoke by antihypertensive treatment in older persons with isolated systolic hypertension: final results of the Systolic Hypertension in the Elderly Program. JAMA 1991;265:3255.
Sox HC. Preventive health services in adults. N Engl J Med 1994;330:1589.
Taylor WC, Pass TM, Shepard DS, Komaroff AL. Cholesterol reduction and life expectancy: a model incorporating multiple risk factors. Ann Intern Med 1987;106:605.
U.S. Department of Health and Human Services, Public Health Service. Healthy people 2000: national health promotion and disease prevention objectives. Washington DC: DHHS, 1990.
U.S. Preventive Services Task Force. Guide to clinical preventive services: an assessment of the effectiveness of 169 interventions. Baltimore: Williams & Wilkins, 1996.
Wingo PA, Tong T, Bolden S. Cancer statistics, 1995. CA 1995;45:8.
Wolf PA, D'Agostino RB, Kannel WB, Bonita R, Belanger AJ. Cigarette smoking as a risk factor for stroke: the Framingham study. JAMA 1988;259:1025.
Zazove P, Mehr DR, Ruffin MT IV, et al. A criterion-based review of preventive health care in the elderly. Part 2: A geriatric health maintenance program. J Fam Pract 1992;34:320.

Primary Care for Women, edited by Phyllis C. Leppert and Fred M. Howard. Lippincott-Raven Publishers, Philadelphia © 1997.

4

The Importance of the Gynecologic Examination

PHYLLIS C. LEPPERT

Because a woman's reproductive tract health from birth to death is essential for her total health, the gynecologic examination is especially important. Unfortunately, this examination often is not performed as part of the complete physical examination, or, if it is carried out, it may not be done adequately. The gynecologic history is distressing for many women, because very personal questions need to be asked to understand the woman's problem or to prevent disease. A history and examination includes an assessment of the total woman and her physical, psychological, and cultural well-being. Many women avoid a gynecologic examination for fear of discomfort or embarrassment; many more avoid it because they fear an abnormality will be found.

ATTITUDES TOWARD HEALTH PROVIDERS

A physician or provider of either sex is an authority figure; thus, women will relate to individual providers based on their own experience with authority. Women with less money or less education than the physician may view the physician in an unfavorable light because of past negative experiences with persons in authority. Although nonphysician health care providers such as midwives and physician assistants are perceived as having less power than physicians, the same dynamics may apply, especially among medically underserved women in poor communities. When women in focus groups in a medically underserved neighborhood were asked why they did not keep regular appointments for gynecologic examinations, they stated that they thought the doctor might report them for legal transgressions (eg, to the county government about welfare issues). In this case, the women's image of the physician was of a person with power over them. Those who are sick are in a dependent situation, especially if they are seriously ill. This extreme dependency further distances them from the physician. A woman may then subconsciously see the physician as a father or mother figure. This subconscious thought is especially apt to interfere with adequate pelvic examinations unless physicians conducting pelvic examinations understand how to accept and deal with the feelings of the women they treat.

Both male and female physicians must understand the fact that a totally professional, caring attitude is essential to ease any psychological distress connected with the pelvic examination, due to cultural attitudes toward sexuality and the reproductive tract. The United States includes many diverse cultural groups. Some of these groups believe that the only male a woman should reveal her genital organs to is her mate. Other women may be uncomfortable with a woman physician because of culturally derived attitudes toward sexuality.

GYNECOLOGIC TEACHING ASSOCIATES

In the mid-1970s, departments of obstetrics and gynecology (or in some instances departments of medicine) in U.S. medical schools began to use gynecologic teaching associates (GTAs) to educate students in the art of the gynecologic examination. However, GTAs are not only surrogate patients: in well-organized departments, these well-versed women are teachers too, and teach students in teams without the presence of a physician. The use of GTAs, more than any other recent innovation in medical education, has had a great impact on the sensitive performance of a thorough gynecologic examination.

Medical students are taught that the problem solving essential to making an accurate diagnosis demands a completely open and nonjudgmental attitude. A woman must have confidence in her health care provider.

WHEN A GYNECOLOGIC EXAMINATION SHOULD BE DONE

A gynecologic examination is mandatory in these circumstances:

- A general physical examination
- A prenatal examination
- A premarital examination, or an examination before prescribing any method of contraception

- In women taking hormones, such as hormone replacement therapy, or in those exposed to hormones, such as diethylstilbestrol
- In women with any abdominal or genital complaint.

There are four essential parts to a complete gynecologic examination: (1) the initial contact; (2) a detailed history; (3) the physical examination; and (4) the postexamination interview.

INITIAL CONTACT

As in all physician-patient relationships, the initial contact begins well before the woman seeking care actually meets the doctor. An impression of the sort of caring or noncaring provider the physician is begins with the first phone call to the office. The receptionist is a key part of the establishment of trust. He or she must be kind, courteous, and well-mannered. The receptionist must be skilled in distinguishing acute or emergency problems from chronic situations and must be able to ask enough questions to delineate the problem at hand. After the physician-patient relationship is established, the receptionist is a vital person in maintaining this professional alliance. A woman with vaginal bleeding should be scheduled in a more urgent manner than a woman requesting an annual examination. Routine examinations are not usually scheduled when a patient is menstruating. It is helpful for the receptionist to ask a patient to bring valuable medical records and a carefully written menstrual calendar. The patient should be advised about routine laboratory procedures included in the examination, such as a Pap smear. Women should know that they should not douche for at least 2 days before a gynecologic examination. A woman who has pain at a particular point in her menstrual cycle should be scheduled at that same approximate time in her cycle, and infertility patients should be scheduled a few days before their anticipated menses.

The first meeting between the physician and a woman patient should occur in a consultation room or other suitable place. The patient should be dressed and sitting face to face with the physician. It is inappropriate and leads to discomfort to have the patient lying on an examination table the first time she meets a provider. On the surface, this might appear to be the most efficient way to initiate contact and proceed with the examination, but it is not. It is impossible to perform an adequate examination on an uncomfortable, tense patient, so important history and physical findings are missed. This scenario is inefficiency at its worst.

TAKING A DETAILED HISTORY

A gynecologic examination cannot be performed without a careful history. Although a nurse or other person may obtain a preliminary screening history, a physician should personally obtain the medical history from the patient. It is only by obtaining a careful history that a differential diagnosis can be made and then narrowed. Thus, a physician who takes an unhurried, accurate history in a relaxed setting ultimately is a more efficient health care provider than one who is hurried; in the latter case, inadequate care and misdiagnosis result. It is important for all health care providers to emphasize this to the administrators of managed care plans.

All health care providers must appreciate and respect the patient's temperament. Initially, some personal conversation develops the physician-patient relationship. A good beginning is "What brings you to the office?" Open-ended questions can be asked regarding the history of the presenting problem. In this type of questioning, no particular response is suggested. At times, some questions need to be directed to avoid irrelevancies. These questions should be used only as necessary. The historical interview is one of the most important skills a health care provider must master. The physician should have the attitude that the physical findings confirm a careful history.

After elucidating the precise history of the problem at hand, a review of systems should be carried out. The purpose of the systematic review is to uncover problems or diseases that might be missed in obtaining the history of the present problem. It is obtained by asking questions in a logical sequence regarding anatomic areas, beginning with the head and neck and proceeding down to the feet. Clues to gynecologic illness may be obtained in this fashion. Information may point to a systemic problem as a cause of the gynecologic problem. At an initial visit to a physician giving primary care to a woman, a complete history includes a past history, family history, and social history. Information pertinent to the gynecologic examination is asked in an interested but matter-of-fact professional manner. Information to be elicited is the patient's age at menarche, the type of menstrual cycle normal for her, her last menstrual period, and the previous menstrual period. An inexperienced practitioner may believe a woman's periods are heavy when in fact the menstrual flow is normal for her. Therefore, information regarding the number of perineal pads or tampons usually worn, how often they are usually changed, and the use of double pads should be ascertained. A history of menstrual changes that interfere with work or other activities is significant. If a woman complains of pelvic pain, this must be related to the timing of the menstrual period. Without this information, ovulatory pain, a ruptured corpus luteal cyst, ectopic pregnancy, or endometriosis cannot be diagnosed with accuracy. Equally important are the number of pregnancies and the amount and type of sexual activity and experience. Careful, gentle questioning regarding contraception usage and history of sexually transmitted disease is mandatory.

The physician who explains to the woman the reasons for these very personal questions will obtain a more accurate and useful history than the one who is rushed and judgmental. Exceptional skill in framing questions yields the most accurate diagnosis. This area of expanded diagnosis separates the professional approach from the nonprofessional "cookbook" approach to the history. A woman's personal and social history offers a portrait of her lifestyle and gives an idea of how her environment may be contributing to her presenting problem. Information on smoking, consumption of alcoholic beverages, and use of illicit drugs is essential. It is necessary to inquire about a history of sexual assault or possible domestic violence. Questions of this nature may well be asked during the physical examination, especially if findings suggest possible abuse. A sensitive provider is attuned to the possibility that a woman may initially deny the existence of sexual abuse by a partner.

The actual symptoms elicited, placed in sequence in the course of a gynecologic history, usually identify a problem; the physical examination provides the correct diagnosis. The three most common symptoms described by women are abnormal vaginal bleeding, vaginal discharge, and pelvic pain. Abnormal bleeding suggests pregnancy or malignancy, but other conditions can cause abnormal bleeding as well. A good history determines the quality and quantity of the blood loss and determines if hormones or other medications are being taken. Abnormal bleeding may indicate malignant disease, leiomyomata, pelvic inflammatory disease, or endometriosis. In young women of childbearing age, bleeding or spotting at the time of a normal period may indicate unruptured ectopic pregnancy or an early intrauterine pregnancy. A history of spotting or bleeding after several missed menstrual periods suggests a threatened abortion. Irregular bleeding suggests carcinoma of the cervix, endometrial or cervical polyps, dysfunctional uterine bleeding due to hormonal abnormalities, or endometrial cancer.

When evaluating vaginal discharge, the physician must appreciate that not all discharges are pathologic. Some women may have excessive vaginal discharge and not have a single symptom, but others with slight discharge may have many symptoms. A heavy discharge associated with normal vaginal flora often makes the proper diagnosis difficult. A cheesy white discharge is a classic symptom of moniliasis and needs to be confirmed by a wet smear. A chronic, irritating moniliasis is difficult to eradicate and is often associated with diabetes or HIV infection. An irritating, foul-smelling, frothy, yellow-green discharge of trichomoniasis may be worse after a menstrual period. The diagnosis is made by a hanging drop smear. Bacterial vaginosis is also irritating and often has a fishy smell. A discharge may mean a gonococcal infection. The physician must ask when the discharge began, the amount of discharge, the nature of the odor, and if blood is seen in the discharge. Knowledge of whether or not the patient has been taking antibiotics is helpful. Finally, questions determining the relation of the discharge to sexual intercourse and the menstrual cycle are essential.

Pain is probably the most difficult symptom to deal with, from the point of view of both the women and the practitioner. In the case of dysmenorrhea, it is important to ascertain if the problem is primary or secondary. The type of pain needs to be elicited. Is it sharp? Aching? Dragging? Burning? Cramping? Colicky? Is it bearing-down pressure-type pain? Is it steady or intermittent? Is it present before, during, or after menses? At what point in the cycle is the pain most intense? What is its location, and does it radiate? Does position change the pain?

Ovarian and fallopian tube pain may be referred to the lower abdomen just above the groin. It may radiate down the medial aspect of the thigh. Pain in the lower rectum may radiate to one or both legs. The physician should ask if the pain interferes with work or sleep. A backache of pelvic origin is never higher than S1. Uterine pain can be diffuse: it can be hypogastric in location, or it may be transmitted to the inner aspect of the thigh, but it is never below the knee.

PHYSICAL EXAMINATION

A gynecologic examination is not merely an examination of the genitalia and the pelvic organs. A general physical examination should be completed first to look for signs that might explain the presenting symptomatology. For instance, the condition and texture of the patient's hair should be observed and noted, because her hormonal status can be reflected in hair texture and its pattern of growth. Careful attention should be paid to the thyroid, as abnormalities in its function often cause disturbances in the menstrual cycle.

Breast Examination

The breast examination must include inspection, palpation, and examination of any secretions. When examining the breasts, a careful physician instructs the patient how to carry out a breast self-examination. This is also an opportune moment to educate the patient about the appropriate timing of mammography.

Both breasts should be carefully palpated as a part of every complete physical examination. This should be done as a routine measure, and not only for women who have particular signs and symptoms. Breast cancer can be cured if it is detected early in its course. Early detection depends on accurate physical examination and appropriate use of mammography.

A systematic approach to the examination is most important. The patient should disrobe so that adequate observation can be made. A towel or gown can cover her breast, except for the time of the actual examination. The patient should first be sitting up when the breasts are examined, and then asked to lie flat with the opposite arm elevated above her head.

The first part of the examination is inspection. This cannot be overlooked or rushed, as important information is acquired. The physician must remember that breasts look and feel different earlier in the menstrual cycle than they do later in the same cycle. All women have a degree of asymmetry of the breasts. However, an increase in size of one breast over the other may indicate the development of a tumor, cyst, or inflammation. Observation of the size and symmetry of the breasts is done with the patient in a sitting position. The skin overlying the breasts is carefully observed. Edema may be associated with certain carcinomas. An ulceration of the nipple is seen in Paget's disease. Skin retraction usually indicates carcinoma. For the physician to see this sign best, the patient should sit erect and raise her arms overhead. This position exerts a pull on the suspensory ligaments of the breasts, and any lesion producing a shortening of these ligaments will result in skin retraction as well as deviation of the nipple. Alternative methods of eliciting this information are by asking the patient to put both palms of her hands together and push against them, or by asking her to place her hands on her hips and push against them. Another way is to ask the patient to lean forward at the waist with her hands on the back of a chair. These procedures are helpful in detecting early lesions. Lastly, the nipples should be inspected carefully for evidence of bleeding, discharge, retraction, or ulceration, and the axillary and supraclavicular regions must be observed for evidence of bulging, edema, and retraction.

Next, palpation is done. The consistency of normal breast tissue varies widely from one woman to another, and it also varies according to age, weight, stage of the menstrual cycle, and pregnancy. Palpation of the breast should be done systematically so that all areas of the breasts and their lymphatic drainage can be evaluated. Most providers usually begin with the left breast. Palpation is done with the fingertips, lightly at first. It is carried out in a clockwise fashion until the complete breast is examined. The nipple is palpated and the presence of discharge determined; this can be done by a gentle stripping motion of the nipple. The right breast is then examined in a similar fashion. Palpation is done with the patient sitting, then lying, and next with her arms at her sides and then overhead. The axillary and supraclavicular areas are also palpated.

At the completion of the examination, any abnormalities found should be described accurately. Location should be described by quadrant. Note should be made of whether the lesion is multiple or solitary. The consistency and extent of the mass should be noted, as well as its tenderness. The examiner should record whether the mass is movable or fixed to the wall, whether the nipple is displaced or retracted, and if regional lymph nodes are palpable.

The breast examination must be conducted in a complete manner. Mammograms have an important place in the screening of women for breast cancer, but they are an adjunctive measure and do not replace a thorough manual and visual examination.

Pelvic Examination

The pelvic examination is an essential part of any complete physical examination of a woman and is considered a basic skill for all providers, just as an examination of the heart and lungs is a basic skill for all. For the nonspecialist, the examination is carried out to ascertain that the reproductive organs are normal and to identify women who need referral to a specialist.

Because women have a different sense of the pelvic examination than they do for examination of other parts of the body, many women are embarrassed. They may be less embarrassed with a female provider, but this is not always the situation.

The patient must be comfortable. She should be helped into the lithotomy position and draped adequately for the examination. Gentleness is essential: not only is it reassuring, but it also is essential for the accurate completion of the examination and prevents the involuntary contraction of the anal sphincter, which makes the examination uncomfortable. Roughness interferes with the accuracy of the examination. Thus, movements of the examiner's hands must be light at first and deliberate. Quick, darting, or jabbing motions hurt the patient and make the examination impossible. Beginning the examination in a careful way is essential to the rest of the examination.

First, the external genitalia are inspected. This inspection usually takes 2 minutes. Abnormalities to be noted are erythema, skin lesions of the perineum, and evidence of vaginal discharge. Palpation is conducted to determine if there are Bartholin cysts or abscesses, or if the Skene glands are enlarged or inflamed. This is determined by gently stripping the areas upward and observing for purulent discharge from the urethral meatus. The strength of the perineal support is ascertained by asking the patient to bear down. Cystoceles and rectoceles are observed by this method.

The cervix and upper vagina are next inspected by using a vaginal speculum. One of the most important considerations in this examination is choosing the right-sized speculum. This minimizes patient discomfort and allows adequate observation. Vaginal specula are nondisposable metal or disposable plastic. If the disposable speculum is used, great care must be taken not to pinch the skin as the bills are being opened. A disadvantage of these specula is that they tend to be all one size and thus are not tailored to the patient. Metal specula are either the Graves or duckbill type, or the Pedersen type. The bills of the Graves speculum are wide and spoon-shaped; those of the Pedersen speculum are narrowed. Both speculum types come in various sizes from large to small. Except for very obese women, a medium-sized Pedersen speculum is adequate and more comfortable. The vaginal speculum has a movable anterior blade and a fixed posterior blade. A metal speculum can be warmed beforehand, and most modern examination tables have a warming tray at the foot in which the speculum may be kept. If lubrication is needed, warm water can be used.

The technique of inserting the speculum is most important. The speculum is held firmly by the blades between the index and middle fingers. When the speculum is inserted, the blades should be held obliquely and pressure placed against the posterior fourchette. The angle of insertion should be downward toward the sacrum. The blades should not be inserted in a horizontal manner, as this stretches the introitus and causes pain. When the blades are vertical, the suburethral area is touched, causing pain. When the blades are almost past the introitus, they should be rotated to a horizontal position and the handle elevated. When the speculum is fully inserted, the blades should be separated. The examiner's thumb presses the thumbpiece on the side to elevate the top blade and the hand lifts the handle to lower the fixed posterior blade.

The cervix can then be inspected. The Pap smear is obtained. The most important part of this examination is to obtain an adequate endocervical sample. A cytobrush is inserted into the endocervical canal and turned several times. The material obtained is spread immediately on a slide. (A cytobrush is not used for pregnant patients.) The cervical face and vaginal pool samples are next obtained by using the hand of the wooden Ayres spatula and spreading the sample on the slide. Because the cellular specimen must be fixed immediately, the slide and the bottle of fixative or spray should be prepared and labeled in advance to ensure prompt fixing of the cells.

Cervical cytology does not replace a biopsy. If an apparent lesion or suspicious area is noted, it should be biopsied. In fact, any lesion noted by the naked eye should be biopsied. Abnormal cytology should be evaluated by colposcopy, and abnormal areas of the cervix noted in this examination should be biopsied. If an abnormality is noted, a negative cytologic report does not remove the need for a biopsy.

As the speculum is removed, the walls of the vagina should be inspected for lesions. After the speculum is removed, a bimanual examination is conducted. The abdominal hand brings the pelvic structures to the intravaginal fingers for palpation. The abdominal hand must be positioned to hold the pelvic organs between it and the intravaginal hand. If the abdominal hand is placed too low on the abdomen, the pelvic organs will be missed. This hand should be placed at least three quarters of the way to the umbilicus. The fingers examining intravaginally must be well lubricated and gently inserted into the vagina over the posterior fourchette. The elbow of the intrapelvic hand can rest on the examiner's knee if the physician places a foot on a stool or footrest.

The cervix is easily palpated. It usually points away from the fundus—in other words, if the cervix points posteriorly, the fundus is found anteriorly. Movement of the cervix should be painless. Pain due to pathologic conditions such as an ectopic pregnancy or pelvic inflammatory disease is indicated by the patient without the need for questioning.

The uterus should be held between the examining hands and its size, contour, and mobility noted. The cul-de-sac should be examined for masses, tenderness, and irregularities. The broad ligament and fallopian tubes are usually not palpable. The intravaginal fingers should go posteriorly under the broad ligament while the abdominal fingers on the sides of the uterus can approach the broad ligament. Next, the intravaginal fingers should move down and toward the lateral wall on one side, and the abdominal hand should move to just inside the anterior-superior spine of the ilium. This process should be repeated on the opposite side. In this manner, the size, shape, and mobility of the ovaries are noted. In postmenopausal women, the ovaries should not be palpable.

A vaginal probe ultrasound replacing the vaginal fingers can accurately determine abnormalities of the reproductive tract. This method of the gynecologic examination is so accurate that many authorities recommend its routine use in the proper conduct of the vaginal examination. To ease patient discomfort, the woman is instructed to insert the probe herself under guidance. After its insertion, the provider manipulates the probe to facilitate examination of the reproductive organs. Used in this manner, the vaginal probe ultrasound is considered an essential part of the examination, just as a sphygmomanometer is essential for the observation of blood pressure. Some argue that this ultrasound examination should be considered a part of the gynecologic examination and included in the fee for the examination. With ultrasound examination, ectopic pregnancies can be diagnosed before rupture, and ovarian masses can be discovered at an earlier stage, with great benefit for health and well-being. Some authorities feel that physicians who charge extra for the vaginal ultrasound and thus increase costs have done a disservice to women.

The bimanual pelvic examination is completed by rectovaginal abdominal palpation. The middle finger should be inserted into the rectum and the index finger into the vagina. The examiner palpates the adnexal areas, the posterior surface of the broad ligament, and the rectum.

The health care provider must explain to the woman the steps of the physical examination as it is conducted. Honest discussion of possible discomfort must be expressed in an open manner.

Postexamination Interview

On completion of the physical examination, brief comments should be given regarding the findings of the examination so that the woman is not left to imagine them. Either reassurance or a brief discussion of abnormal findings is in order. The woman is then asked to get dressed. After this, a postexamination discussion of the physical findings is held in a separate consultation room or in the examination room. Good health habits and preventive measures should be discussed. If necessary, specific procedures or tests indicated for diagnostic purposes should be described and the reasons for them discussed. Time must be allotted to answer the patient's questions. Therapeutic measures, prescriptions, and side effects should be explained.

Communication between the health care provider and the patient is best when the patient's anxiety is lessened—hence the need for a brief summation of the findings before the more detailed postexamination conference. The postexamination conference is conducted after the patient is fully clothed because this allows the discussion to be held on a more equal footing. The patient is more comfortable and thus is more likely to hear the discussion and to be compliant with a health care program or specific therapeutic measures.

It is fashionable in the name of efficiency to "move female patients through a system." The woman sees the physician quickly and then is seen by a nurse or other worker for the postexamination conference. Although there is a place for a nursing or dietitian conference to extend health or specific illness teaching, it is false economy to leave all teaching to other professionals. First, it interferes with the trust necessary to the relationship between the primary provider and the patient. Second, compliance is improved if the provider and other health care professionals spend time with the patient. Third, it is an opportunity for the provider to obtain important feedback.

The Picker-Commonwealth survey conducted at Rochester General Hospital demonstrated that patients wanted and needed advice and information regarding prescription drugs from the person prescribing the medication, not from the pharmacist. Focus groups conducted in the neighborhoods surrounding the hospital pointed out that patients wanted and needed time from their primary care provider, not from a nurse, to review laboratory and diagnostic tests. Taking time to educate a female patient saves time in the long run.

In summary, careful examination of the reproductive system is an essential part of a complete physical examination for women. Its skillful performance should be in the armamentarium of every primary care practitioner.

BIBLIOGRAPHY

Bishop FM, Forelich RE. Interviewing techniques. In: Rakel RE, ed. Essentials of family practice. Philadelphia: WB Saunders, 1992:103.

Female genitalia. In: Barkauskas VH, Stoltenberg-Allen K, Baumann LC, Darling-Fisher C, eds. Health and physical assessment. St. Louis: Mosby, 1994:661.

Female genitalia. In: Bates B, ed. A guide to physical examination and history taking, 5th ed. Philadelphia: JB Lippincott, 1991:385.

King GD. Female pelvic examination. In: Judge RD, Zuidema GD, eds. Clinical diagnosis: a physiologic approach. Boston: Little, Brown, 1989:389.

Timor-Tritsch I, Greenidge S, Admon D, Reuss ML. Emergency room use of transvaginal ultrasonography by obstetrics and gynecology residents. Am J Obstet Gynecol 1992;166:866.

Timor-Tritsch IE, Monteagudo A. Transvaginal sonography. In: Nichols DH, Sweeney PJ, eds. Ambulatory gynecology, 2d ed. Philadelphia: JB Lippincott, 1995:350.

Zuidema GD. Breast. In: Judge RD, Zuidema GD, eds. Clinical diagnosis: a physiologic approach, 5th ed. Boston: Little, Brown, 1989:311.

Primary Care for Women, edited by Phyllis C. Leppert and Fred M. Howard. Lippincott-Raven Publishers, Philadelphia © 1997.

5

Primary Care of the Cancer Patient

JOANNA M. CAIN

A woman with cancer enters a complex world of specialists and a bewildering array of possible treatments, and has the entire basis of her life view challenged. In the midst of this maelstrom, the primary care provider can be called on for complex supportive therapy, such as treatment of neutropenic sepsis, or for guidance and support during this confusing process. To be an adequate guide, the primary care provider must have a current understanding of the genetic nature of cancer and the implications for future therapy, a basic understanding of the terminology of cancer staging and therapy, a clear view of the psychosocial sequelae from the diagnosis and treatment of cancer, and the ability to be aware of the particular complications or side effects of cancer therapy that may come their way in the primary care of such patients.

THE NATURE OF CANCER

A complex interaction of genetic inheritance, environmental influences, and chance ultimately results in a genetic alteration that leads to cancer. The understanding of oncogenes and their functions is rapidly expanding, along with the potential for treatments based on this knowledge. These advances also may allow presymptomatic testing for genetic tendencies toward cancer; this in turn raises several issues for the primary care of patients. All these discoveries have been dependent on the laboratory tools developed along with the genome project and sequencing initiative. Most of these changes are too small to be seen by cytogenetic analysis, which, for example, shows more gross triploidy or polymorphisms. Instead, restriction enzymes are used that generate sequences or clipped bits of DNA that have different sizes than normal sequences. Southern blot analysis detects these restriction fragment length polymorphisms; however, this takes several days and detects only 1% to 5% of altered DNA. It also requires fresh tissue. More recently, polymerase chain reaction using primers and short sequences of DNA that stick to certain areas but are too far apart to yield a product in normal tissue has been used to fingerprint cancers. PCR is ten times as sensitive and can be used on fixed tissues. These techniques are merely ways of identifying commonalities among cancers; the actual sequencing of these defects and the identification of the genetic sequence of interest, such as in breast cancer, are far more elegant and far from complete.

The underlying biology of cancer is being understood at a much more complex level than before. Most somatic cell mutations are phenotypically silent, especially if they are in nonessential or redundant genes. If they are in essential genes, they more often result in death of the affected cells, but sometimes result in changes in the growth patterns of cells by either directly stimulating growth or attracting growth factors to stimulate growth and avoid the normal cell death (apoptosis). This altered growth is propelled by oncogenes, altered genes whose presence leads to cancer. Their normal counterparts are known as proto-oncogenes (sometimes termed "wild-type") that have a normal gene sequence and produce the proteins that control cellular growth and function.

Oncogenes are uncovered in three ways. The number of copies of a gene can be increased; this is called amplification (eg, the HER-2/neu or C-erb B 2 proto-oncogene). This gene determines the number of receptors for epidermal growth factor and is of particular interest in ovarian and breast cancers. The number of copies per cell in cancer cells is amplified. Therefore, the upstream decrease or modulation of the number of receptors is lost, and the cell is stimulated by epidermal growth factor (EGF) to grow inappropriately.

The second way an oncogene is uncovered is by a change in the sequence of the DNA (eg, the ras oncogene). The change of a single 3-base codon is enough to make an oncogene. The third type of event requires the loss of a matching gene (loss of heterozygosity [LOS]), which destroys function. Most oncogenes are heterozygous and are affected by the loss of matching normal alleles as well as by transpositions that change the upstream control of the gene. The best example is the Philadelphia chromosome of chronic myelocytic luekemia (CML), in which the ABL gene transfers from chromosome 9 to 22 and forms BCR-ABL, which is oncogenic. This is also how Burkitt lymphoma works, with transpositions from chromosomes 8 to 14.

The loss of heterozygosity is particularly important for tumor suppressor genes. These genes cause cancer by their absence, such as in retinoblastoma, where Knudson's two-hit (or loss) theory has been proved. One allele is missing in the germ cell line, so it takes only the loss of the second tumor suppressor gene in the somatic cell lines for the cancer to occur. Other important tumor suppressor genes code for proteins p-53 and p-16, or multiple tumor suppressor I, a cell cycle regulator.

p-53 is a nuclear phosphoprotein that arrests cells in G-1. To progress to synthesis, p-53 must be inactivated. This gene should be at p13 on the short arm of 17. Often, the remaining p-53 allele harbors point mutations and the mutant allele remains after the normal p-53 allele is lost. Normal functioning of p-53 is closely tied to programmed cell death (apoptosis); this may also provide new therapeutic opportunities.

Extension of Genetic Findings to New Directions in Cancer Therapy

Identifying genes that encode for recognizable antigens or cytokines that might be put in cells to attract the attention of the immune system is of active interest. As an example of how this research might be of use for treatment, genes that encode for antibiotic sensitivity, tumor necrosis factor (TNF), or interleukin-2 (IL-2) could be placed specifically in tumor cells. Treatment is then targeted to the presence of a gene—for example, ganciclovir is given to tumor cells, which are then differentially destroyed by the presence of genes that confer ganciclovir sensitivity.

Immunotherapies will also be affected by new genetic information. Those subjected to trials in the past relied on passive or adoptive immunotherapy. T cells can recognize single amino acid substitutions that differentiate a tumor antigen from a self-antigen. They then attract other cells by secreting cytokines such as IL-2 that cause inflammation so that leukocyte (tumor-infiltrating leukocytes and activated killer cells) and macrophage infiltration can occur, potentially eradicating solid tumors. Early attempts to use the immune system stimulated the whole system, but this was not as successful as had been hoped. These therapies have been subject to trials in ovarian cancer, often with intraperitoneal infusions, but probably because of a lack of specificity have not been particularly successful. Tumor cells have a remarkable ability to use growth factors and other antigenic markers to evade this system.

More than 50 gene therapy protocols have been approved by the National Institutes of Health. The efficacy of gene therapy depends on the following factors:

- An ability to insert a "normal" gene physically into the target cell and have it remain long enough to exert an effect. Adenoviruses are gaining as a vector because they are more efficient at getting the gene in even quiescent cells, whereas retroviruses require active division.
- Ensuring that the new gene will be expressed in the cell at the appropriate level
- The new gene or the vector should not harm the cell or the person.

Presymptomatic Testing

Presymptomatic testing for oncogenes will require the identification of genes associated with different cancers and a far better understanding of the variability of their expression. Major difficulties will continue to be the sensitivity and specificity of these tests and the fact that environmental factors continue to play a major role in the ultimate development of cancer. The area of presymptomatic testing is fraught with ethical, psychological, and economic pitfalls. Even for patients for whom no present presymptomatic test is available, genetic counseling can be offered, but this is beset with issues such as unwarranted life changes, depression, and suicide if it is not undertaken with adequate training in the vagaries of genetic counseling. Furthermore, the inclusion in a medical record of a "family history of" may end up as an exclusion in the patient's insurance for all ovarian or colon cancer therapy, even when the risk may be only minimally increased over the baseline.

When presymptomatic testing is available, the impact on the patient of such information is only one of the features that must be considered. The current concept of informed consent and autonomy is challenged by this genetic diagnostic technique that inherently requires the consent and involvement of other genetically related family members. The potential for insurance discrimination and job discrimination based on an inherited tendency for a particular cancer or a susceptibility to environmental toxins is real. The physician who includes such testing in the primary care of patients must give careful consideration to the medical and societal consequences, making sure that appropriate safeguards and education have been provided.

STAGING

Once cancer has been diagnosed, the therapy chosen is closely tied to the stage of the malignancy. Staging is done by various measures, depending on the tumor site and type. A stage is assigned at the time of the original diagnosis and never changes after that, despite the presence of recurrent disease. For instance, a recurrent cancer would be described as the original stage, with recurrent disease. An erroneous description might lead a consultant to a different conclusion regarding the need for referral, further evaluation, or therapy. Describing someone with, for example, a stage I carcinoma of the cervix with a central recurrence implies entirely different therapeutic options and evaluation needs than does a stage III cancer of the cervix. Clear communication between providers is essential to optimize therapy and to advance knowledge about cancer, and staging is one way to do so.

Most cancers are staged by the TNM system, which assigns stages according to tumor size (T), the presence of suspicious or positive nodes (N), and the presence or absence of metastatic disease (M). For some cancers unique to women, staging follows guidelines set by the International Federation of Gynecologists and Obstetricians. Staging systems for common cancers in women and cancers unique to women are outlined in Table 5-1.

PSYCHOSOCIAL CONTEXT OF CANCER

Women undergoing surgery, radiation, and chemotherapy for malignancies present particular challenges for primary care providers. Familiarity with the psychological and physical side effects of such treatment can clarify appropriate treatment and can help support the patient during her oncology treatment. The process of helping a

Table 5-1. Staging of Common Cancers

SITE	MOST COMMON SITE OF METASTASIS	T DEFINITION	METHODS FOR STAGING
Lung	Depends on cell type	AJC* T1 = <3 cm T2 = >3 cm or pleural atelectasis, pneumonitis, or hilar involvement T3 = Direct extension beyond T2	Bronchoscopy Chest roentgenogram Biopsy, other radionuclide or CT scans as appropriate
Colon	Liver	Dukes by extension from mucosa T1 = Mucosa T2 = Serosa or peritoneal fat T3 = Adjacent structures	Resection required for staging
Breast	Regional lymph nodes	AJC/UICC† T1 = <2 cm T2 = >2 cm, <5 cm T3 = >5 cm T4 = direct extension	Physical examination Biopsy Bone scan
Cervix	Regional lymph nodes	FIGO‡ I = confined to cervix II = in parametrium III = to sidewall IV = direct extension or distant	Physical examination Biopsy Other radiographic tests as appropriate
Ovary	Abdominal cavity	FIGO‡ I = Ovaries only II = Ovaries plus pelvis III = Abdomen IV = Outside abdominal cavity	Surgically staged Chest x-ray
Uterus	Regional nodes	FIGO‡ I = Uterine cavity II = Uterine cavity plus cervix III = Plus pelvic area IV = Distant	Surgically staged Chest x-ray

*American Joint Commission
†International Union Against Cancer
‡International Federation of Gynecologists and Obstetricians

patient live with a diagnosis of cancer often begins with informing her of the results of a biopsy and the diagnosis. This is the start of an intense period of personal challenge for the patient, and gentle truthfulness from caregivers supports the patient's ability to make choices and trust her caregivers. Withholding information from a patient rarely serves her best interests and does not respect her right to make choices, ranging from whether referral is appropriate to whether a particular proposed therapy is acceptable.

Early identification of social and psychological adjustment problems, a close watch of the patient's use and the availability of support systems, and clear communication that the primary care provider is available for consultation for any reason can help assuage the terrible isolation and loneliness raised by a diagnosis of cancer.

Psychological Effects

A diagnosis of cancer profoundly affects fundamental assumptions of daily life, particularly the human frailty of assuming that we have control of our destiny, as well as raising the specter of death. In addition, the woman's ability to carry on her various roles, particularly that of caregiver in her relationships, is altered, adding to her distress. Finally, many aspects of the treatment of cancer affect self-image, from loss of hair to loss of body parts integral to a patient's identity as a woman. Thus, the psychological context of cancer care should be the first consideration in the primary care of women with cancer.

Adjustment to Diagnosis

A woman's reaction to a diagnosis of cancer depends on three major factors: the psychological background of her prior adjustment, her societal or cultural context, and the medical factors of the particular diagnosis. There is a clear difference in the morbidity and mortality of women with cancer between different racial or ethnic and socioeconomic groups. The legacy of poverty for women includes unemployment with lack of health coverage, malnutrition, higher smoking rates, lack of basic health education, and a cognitive fatalism; all these affect choices in seeking health care. Attention to improving women's social and economic status, particularly for minority women, will improve medical and psychological outcomes with cancer and is a proper concern for the primary caregiver.

The coping abilities the woman had before the cancer diagnosis are brought into the spotlight by the diagnosis. If her coping was poor, it will still be poor in response to this challenge. Her emotional maturity, her ability to modify plans, and the availability of emotional support are also the same as before the diagnosis. A major role of the primary care provider can be to identify support systems and coping patterns to sustain the patient through this turbulent time. However, it is unreasonable to assume that her ability to deal with this stress will improve miraculously because of a diagnosis of cancer. Patients who are stoic remain so, and those who lose all ability to function in crises tend to do so. The two axioms of support for primary caregivers are these:

1. Do not expect the patient to change her coping mechanisms. Accept her approach and suggest more successful strategies.
2. If the woman is well known to the primary caregiver, and pretest (eg, prebiopsy) counseling can be done before the diagnosis, this should be offered if possible.

Sexual Dysfunction

One of the factors in a woman's response to certain types of cancer is the inextricable cultural link between the breasts, ovaries, and uterus and womanhood. Although much has been made of the connection and the ultimate impact of those cancers on a woman's sexuality and body image, the link is actually stronger to her previous sexual satisfaction and psychological health. According to Schover's 1991 article, which includes a review of multiple authors' work, the breast-conserving strategies for the treatment of breast cancer clearly resulted in better body image but had little or no impact on marital satisfaction, psychological adjustment, frequency of sex, and sexual dysfunction. For gynecologic cancers, the extent of sexual disruption is overshadowed by the overall coping skills of individual patients, making it difficult to assess the sequelae independently. There is a strong suggestion in the available data, however, that the number of sexually active women drops during and after treatments, that the frequency of intercourse declines, and that arousal deficits emerge. As Anderson (1989) notes, "the cancer-related sexual difficulties for couples may provide a sufficient, added vulnerability if sexual intercourse is already problematic for other reasons." Also, pelvic surgery may affect sensation or increase dyspareunia.

Chemotherapy and hormonal therapies can have significant effects on the vaginal mucosa, along with other side effects, with resultant dyspareunia and sexual dysfunction. Schover and colleagues (1995) found that chemotherapy was a major predictor of greater psychosocial distress and sexual dysfunction.

Of particular concern to primary caregivers should be the finding by Thranov and Klee (1994) that although 74% of gynecologic cancer patients expressed little or no desire for sexual relations, 54% had had sexual relations within the past month, primarily patients under age 55. This suggests that these women are trying to fulfill their normal roles and retain normal sexual function but are not getting concomitant support and attention for their sexual dysfunction.

Given the general lack of attention to this area of life in medicine overall, it is important to initiate such inquiries and support with all patients. Caregivers must not assume that older women are less concerned with sexual dysfunction following diagnosis and therapy for cancer. The discrepancy between sexual desire and actual sexual relations reported for younger women does not seem to be as strong in women over age 55, but this seems to be due to a concomitant finding that many of the elderly patients' partners also had no desire for a sexual relationship. Thus, although sexual function for the older group of women did not seem to be as discordant and problematic as for younger women, individual patients may still desire a better evaluation and support for these issues, regardless of age. This is another area where the primary caregiver can be of particular assistance and support.

Quality of Life

Much has been said about quality-of-life issues in cancer therapy, but the measurement of such factors and our ability to affect the various domains of psychological and functional adaptation to cancer remain in the early stages. It is important for medical caregivers to note that estimates of a patient's quality of life by others, including medical caregivers, correlate poorly with the patient's own assessment. Listening to the individual patient about whatever part of her quality of life is the most troublesome during the diagnosis and treatment of cancer is the approach most likely to allow primary caregivers the opportunity of adequately addressing these issues. For some patients, spirituality or sexuality rather than physical function is the biggest concern, and failure to pay attention to that concern will result in a poorer outcome.

The entire family's experience is often important for women with cancer. The partner's or family's quality of life has an impact on the perceived quality of life of the woman with cancer, so it may be appropriate to assess more than just the patient. Some suggest that because spouses have different coping styles, assessment of quality of life should be done separately.

PHYSICAL CHANGES RELATED TO CANCER THERAPY

Surgical changes related to cancer care encompass many organ systems and have varying sequelae. It is important for the caregiver to understand the possible complications in the general care of women with cancer. A few selected problems are outlined here.

Venous Access Devices

Patients receiving chemotherapy often have a subcutaneous port (arm or chest wall) or a transcutaneous catheter. These are used for the frequent blood draws that chemotherapy entails, and maintenance of skin integrity and avoidance of infection are critical. Transcutaneous catheters may have a Dacron cuff portion to stabilize the catheter in the subcutaneous tissue. If the transcutaneous catheter does not have such a cuff, fixation to the skin with sutures must be maintained, and loss of a stabilizing suture must be replaced. The primary caregiver should be able to draw blood through various catheter systems and to evaluate these devices for infection. Breakdown of the skin over a port or extension of erythema and purulent drainage above the Dacron cuff (or down the catheter channel in those without cuffs) of a transcutaneous catheter warrants expert evaluation. Upper extremity deep venous thrombosis, evidenced by arm or neck edema, also requires immediate attention, because pulmonary embolism can occur.

Limb Edema With Cancer Surgery

Removal of regional lymph nodes, particularly axillary and groin dissections, can lead to lymphedema of the limb. Multiple systems for diminishing lymphedema exist; passive compression and sequential compression are the major functional elements in these strategies. The use of sleeves or socks with varied pressure (Jobst) often prevents accumulation of fluid in the limb. The major complication of this lymphedema is lymphangitis or local skin cellulitis because of the poor drainage of the tissues. Often the only change is a slightly greater redness or heat in one extremity. The usual agents are skin flora, and antibiotic therapy should be instituted as soon as lymphangitis or cellulitis is suspected. Avoidance of blood draws, intravenous sites, and trauma to the arms post–axillary dissection is based on this risk of infection.

Radical Pelvic Surgery

Radical pelvic surgery for malignancies in women is never undertaken lightly. The physical changes from these surgeries affect self-image and sexual function and create a new set of problems.

Urinary Reconstruction

Urinary reconstructions range from bladder augmentation to ileal urinary conduits. The health-related quality of life seems to be better with bladder substitution (continent) than ileal conduit because of the decreased risk of leaks and the ability to avoid ostomy appliances. However, all reconstructive surgery on the urinary tract increases the risk of pyelonephritis and stone formation with entrapment at anastomotic strictures, and the development of partial or complete ureteral obstruction with strictures. Infections can be particularly difficult to assess because reconstructions with ostomies are chronically colonized. Fever, back pain, or ureteral symptoms should alert the practitioner to the need for careful evaluation for one of the sequelae of these surgeries.

Pelvic Exenteration and Reconstruction

The development of new surgical techniques allows the preservation of bowel and bladder function as well as pelvic and vaginal reconstruction after exenterative surgery for recurrent cervical or colon cancers. One of the major advances has been the development of multiple graft techniques to restore normal anatomy.

Skin and Muscle Grafts

When an area has received significant radiation therapy, the microvascular blood supply is often inadequate for normal healing. The use of myocutaneous and other flaps has allowed for reconstruction of a neovagina after such surgery. These flaps can be plumper than the original vaginal and surrounding tissue and can cause discomfort from compression. In addition, the cutaneous sensation remains transmitted to the brain, at least initially, as though it were originating from the donor site—for instance, if a gracilis myocutaneous graft is used, sensation is referred to the medial thigh. This is normal for such grafts. Anesthesia of a graft site can also occur if there is significant damage to the graft nerves or, in the use of free flaps, if the original neural bundle is not maintained. Because grafts are placed in the original tumor bed, examination of these areas for abnormalities is important in the detection of recurrent disease.

SIDE EFFECTS OF CANCER TREATMENT AND THEIR MANAGEMENT

Hair Loss

Hair loss with chemotherapy is common. It is also a visible sign of cancer therapy to the patient and others and a visible change in appearance. A proactive approach to hair loss (eg, teaching about alternative head wraps, selection of wigs or hairpieces made with the patient's own hair) should be done before or shortly after the first chemotherapy session. Women must be reminded that they are likely to lose more heat and be more susceptible to sunburn with thinner hair or a bald scalp. The hair follicles can also become quite sensitive early in hair loss, and the use of loosely fitted, 100% cotton scarves or turbans can help treat this sensitivity.

Pain

The pain associated with cancer treatment, whether the anticipated outcome is death or cure, is woefully undertreated. The etiology of pain may be multiple. Cancer itself and the surrounding nerve pressure and inflammation can cause pain. The procedures (even diagnostic) and therapies can cause their own varying types of pain and anxiety. It is important to differentiate neuropathic pain from tissue damage pain, as therapy for each differs markedly. Anticonvulsants and antidepressants are appropriate for neuropathic pain, whereas the more traditional pain medications, from nonsteroidal antiinflammatory drugs (NSAIDs) through the opiates, are appropriate for tissue damage pain. Therapy of osseous pain may require corticosteroids and local radiation therapy.

The routine assessment of pain, using a scale that the practitioner is comfortable with, substantially improves pain control. The most important aspect of cancer pain management, however, is believing the patient's perspective and reassuring her regarding the "addictive" properties of opioids. There is a common misunderstanding regarding the difference between addiction and drug-seeking behavior and the habituation that occurs when patients take substantial doses of narcotics over a long period of time. Although this habituation means that these patients cannot stop their pain medicine abruptly without suffering withdrawal symptoms, appropriate withdrawal from narcotics when the need has resolved is successful. This usually requires patient and family education regarding pain therapy with narcotic medications, as well as encouragement from the health care team to report pain. No patient with cancer should have to suffer untreated pain.

Futile Care

The concept of quality of life is also used to address ethical issues in cancer therapy. For example, when is further curative therapy of no further benefit to the patient? What constitutes a "life not worth living" to individual patients? These are often difficult decisions for patients and their caregivers. The need to treat and offer assistance is integral to the practice of medicine, but treatment can be given with palliative as well as curative intent. It is important for the caregiver to make an honest assessment of the likelihood of cure with additional treatment and with what side effects, to identify when further curative therapy is unlikely to meet that goal, and to transmit this information in a supportive setting. Such actions respect the patient's right to make choices about what the benefits and harms of particular treatments mean to her quality of life.

Of course, the information given must be correct. Some patients with metastatic disease are told that no further therapy is of benefit. It may be quite true that there is no curative therapy, but there still are therapies with relatively tolerable side effects that can both prolong life and delay or change the emergence of pain, bowel obstruction, and other difficult terminal symptoms. To ignore this information is clearly not in the best interests of the patient. The choice should be hers, based on her evaluation of how the side effects will affect her life. Telling the truth and eliciting the patient's goals and wishes in a respectful way allow the patient and caregiver to make the best decision about terminal therapy.

REFERENCES

Andersen BL, Anderson B, deProsse C. Controlled prospective longitudinal study of women with cancer: I. Sexual functioning outcomes. J Consult Clin Psychol 1989;57:683.

Anderson B. Yes, there are sexual problems. Now what can we do about them? Gyn Oncol 1994;52:10.

Baquet CR, Horm JW, Gibs T, Greenwald P. Socioeconomic factors and cancer incidence among blacks and whites. J Natl Cancer Inst 1991; 83:551.

Bertelsen K. Sexual dysfunction after treatment of cervical cancer. Dan Med Bull 1983;30:31.

Bjerre BD, Johansen C, Steven K. Health-related quality of life after cystectomy: bladder substitution compared with ileal conduit diversion. A questionnaire survey. Br J Urol 1995;75:200.

Blitzer PH. Reanalysis of the RTOG study of the palliation of symptomatic osseous metastasis. Cancer 1985;55:1468.

Bonica JJ. Cancer pain. In: Bonica JJ, ed. The management of pain, 2d ed., Vol. 1. Philadelphia: Lea & Febiger, 1990:400.

Brennan SC, Redd WH, Jacobsen PB, et al. Anxiety and panic during magnetic resonance scans. Lancet 1988;2:512.

Cain J, Stacey L, Jusenius K, Figge D. The quality of dying: financial, psychological, and ethical dilemmas. Obstet Gynecol 1990;76:149.

Cleeland CS. Barriers to the management of cancer pain. Oncology 1987;1:19.

Cleeland CS, Cleeland LH, Dar R, Rinehardt LC. Factors influencing physician management of cancer pain. Cancer 1986;58:796.

Ehmann JL, Sheehan A, Decker G. Intervening with alopecia: exploring an entrepreneurial role for oncology nurses. Oncol Nurs Forum 1991;18:769.

Farncombe M, Daniels G, Cross L. Lymphedema: the seemingly forgotten complication. J Pain Symptom Manag 1994;9:269.

Gleeson N, Baile W, Roberts WS, et al. Surgical and psychosexual outcome following vaginal reconstruction with pelvic exenteration. Eur J Gyn Oncol 1994;15:89.

Goluboff ET, McKiernan JM, Todd G, Nowygrod R, Smith D, Olsson CA. Reconstruction of urinary and gastrointestinal tracts in total pelvic exenterations. Urology 1994;44:666.

Holland JC. Fears and abnormal reactions to cancer in physically healthy individuals. In: Holland JC, Rowland JH, eds. Handbook of psychooncology: psychological care of the patient with cancer. New York: Oxford University Press, 1989:13.

Hunter T. Cooperation between oncogenes. Cell 1991;64:249.

Kagawa-Singer M. Socioeconomic and cultural influences on cancer care of women. Semin Oncol Nursing 1995;11:109.

Keung YK, Watkins K, Chen SC, Groshen S, Silberman H, Douer D. Comparative study of infectious complications of different types of chronic central venous access devices. Cancer 1994;73:2832.

Korf B. Molecular medicine: molecular diagnosis. N Engl J Med 1995;332:1218.

Lerman C, Rimer BK, Engstrom PF. Cancer risk notification: psychosocial and ethical implications. J Clin Oncol 1991;9:1275.

Management of cancer pain: clinical practice guidelines. Agency for Health Care Policy and Research, Rockville, Md., Publication No. 94-0592, March 1994.

Massie MJ, Holland JC. Psychological reactions to breast cancer in the pre- and postsurgical treatment period. Semin Surg Oncol 1991;7:320.

Presant CA. Quality of life in cancer patients: who measures what? Am J Clin Oncol 1984;7:571.

Quaid KA. Psychological and ethical considerations in screening for disease. Am J Cardiol 1993;72:64D.

Rosenthal N. Regulation of gene expression. N Engl J Med 1994;331:931.

Rosenthal N. Fine structure of a gene—DNA sequencing. N Engl J Med 1995;332:589.

Sachs BP, Korf B. The Human Genome Project: Implications for the practicing obstetrician. Obstet Gynecol 1993;81:458.

Schneiderman LJ, Jecker NS, Jonsen AR. Medical futility: its meaning and ethical implications. Ann Intern Med 1990;112:949.

Schover LR. Sexuality and chronic illness: an integrative model. In: Schover LR, Jensen SB, eds. Sexuality and chronic illness: a comprehensive approach. New York: Guilford Press, 1988:6.

Schover LR. The impact of breast cancer on sexuality, body image, and intimate relationships. CA 1991;41:112.

Schover LR, Yetman RJ, Tuason LJ, et al. Partial mastectomy and breast reconstruction: a comparison of their effects on psychosocial adjustment, body image, and sexuality. Cancer 1995;75:54.

Thranov I, Klee M. Sexuality among gynecologic cancer patients: a cross-sectional study. Gynecol Oncol 1994;52:14.

Varmus H. A historical overview of oncogenes. In: Weinberg RA, ed. Oncogenes and the molecular origins of cancer. New York: Cold Spring Harbor Laboratory Press, 1989:12.

Yunis JJ. The chromosomal basis of human neoplasia. Science 1983;221:227.

Zacharias DR, Gilg CA, Foxall MJ. Quality of life and coping in patients with gynecologic cancer and their spouses. Oncol Nurs Forum 1994;21:1699.

Primary Care for Women, edited by Phyllis C. Leppert and Fred M. Howard. Lippincott-Raven Publishers, Philadelphia © 1997.

6

Smoking, Alcohol Use, and Cessation Techniques

JANET KAY BOBO

Smoking and problems with alcohol often present as comorbidities in primary care settings. Smokers are much more likely to drink, and drink heavily, than nonsmokers, and heavy drinkers are much more likely to smoke than nondrinkers. Alcohol and tobacco also share a unique legal status: they are the only recreational mood-altering drugs legally produced and sold to age-eligible adults, even though the economic consequences of their use substantially exceed that of all illegal drugs combined.

Despite these commonalities, there are important distinctions. Therefore, this chapter mirrors the frequent comorbidity of alcohol and tobacco problems by reviewing the two topics in tandem and digressing as necessary to highlight significant differences in epidemiology, diagnosis, and treatment. *Smoking* here refers only to the consumption of tobacco as packaged in cigarettes; less than 1% of U.S. women consume other forms of tobacco, such as chew or snuff. *Alcohol problems* is an umbrella term encompassing both alcoholics and the broader population of problem drinkers/alcohol abusers, who lack the classic signs and symptoms of chemical dependence.

EPIDEMIOLOGY

Smoking is gradually decreasing among women of all ages, but the rate of decline is slower than the corresponding drop among men. National Health Interview Survey (NHIS) data from 1991 found male and female prevalence rates for current smoking of 28.1% and 23.5%, respectively. Corresponding rates by gender from the 1974 NHIS survey were 43.4% and 31.2%. Female rates are steadily approaching male rates, in part because recent quit ratios—the proportions of ever smokers who have become former smokers—for women are lower than those observed for men, and in part because girls are no longer less likely than boys to take up smoking. Quit ratios were markedly higher in 1991 for men (51.6%) than for women (44.7%), but tobacco use rates among males and females ages 18 to 24 were essentially comparable at 23.5% and 22.4%, respectively. Statistical models based on nationwide surveys of tobacco use suggest that by the year 2000, 23% of all adult women but only 20% of all adult men will be current smokers.

At least five different studies have reported tobacco use rates in samples of women receiving treatment for alcohol problems. The lowest observed prevalence was 82%, and three studies found rates that exceeded 90%. Problems with alcohol are also much more common among smokers. NHIS data on a representative sample of women in the general population found that binge drinking, defined in that survey as five or more drinks per day on 10 or more days in the past year, was four times more likely in current smokers than in never smokers (8.5% versus 2.2%).

In contrast to the epidemiology of smoking, which considers only smokers and nonsmokers, the epidemiology of alcohol problems considers a continuum of use. A 1984 U.S. survey found that 36% of women were abstainers, 50% averaged one drink a day or less, 9% had one or two drinks a day, and 5% averaged more than two drinks per day and had consumed five or more drinks on at least one occasion during the prior year. The 1992 National Longitudinal Alcohol Epidemiologic Survey (NLAES) data similarly showed a 1-year prevalence of 4.1% for alcohol dependence and abuse in women; the corresponding male value was 11%. These data suggest that about one in 20 women drink heavily enough to compromise their health, and more than one in ten exceed conservative guidelines for moderate drinking.

When all ages are considered together, the rates of alcohol use, alcohol problems, and alcohol-related deaths have remained relatively stable for at least 30 years. However, some evidence of increasing rates among women age 21 to 34 has been reported.

Pregnant women are less likely to drink and smoke than nonpregnant women, but their use of alcohol and tobacco continues to be a major public health concern. In a series of studies by the Centers for Disease Control, the prevalence of smoking during pregnancy ranged from 19% to 30%, the prevalence of drinking from 4% to 13%. The Pregnancy Risk Assessment Monitoring System (PRAMS) collected data on the use of alcohol and tobacco from over 6000 randomly selected births in four states in 1988–89. Among women who drank at all during the 3 months before pregnancy, 14% drank an equal or greater amount during the final trimester, 10% drank less, and 76% stopped drinking entirely. Among women who smoked before their pregnancy, 29% quit, 39% smoked less per day, and 32% smoked as much or more. In 1995, the Smoking Cessation in Pregnancy study reported that among over 5000 women attending public clinics for prenatal care, nearly 50% reported smoking at study enrollment, and only 11% of all smokers reported having quit by the eighth month of pregnancy. The proportion of women who continue to smoke and drink throughout pregnancy is unknown.

Rates of problem drinking and smoking among pregnant and nonpregnant women vary markedly when age, ethnicity, and social status indicators such as education are considered. Most studies have found age to be inversely related to the prevalence of alcohol problems. In the 1992 NLAES data, rates of alcohol dependence and abuse ranged from 9.8% in women age 18 to 29 to 0.3% in women 65 and older. A similar relation with smoking was reported for the 1991 NHIS data, although the highest rate of 28% was observed in women age 25 to 44. About 15% of women between 65 and 74 were current smokers, as were nearly 8% of those 75 or older.

Ethnicity may be associated with both behaviors. Among adults, problems with alcohol are somewhat more likely in white than in nonwhite women. In a sample of pregnant adolescents in Pittsburgh, heavy drinking was more common initially among white women, but white and nonwhite rates were comparable near the end of the pregnancy. Most studies have found higher rates of smoking among white women.

Level of education is positively correlated with the probability of regular drinking, but negatively correlated with the prevalence of alcoholism, according to at least one population-based survey. Smoking consistently shows a pronounced negative correlation with education. In a 1991 survey, 32% of women with 12 years of education (high school only) were current smokers compared to 12% of those with 16 years or more. Similarly, a large national sample of pregnant women indicated that at least 35% of those with less than a high school education but only 17% of those with some post-high school education were current smokers.

In the PRAMS study, the source of prenatal care, another surrogate for socioeconomic status, predicted tobacco use. Women who received publicly funded care accounted for 43% of all prepregnancy smokers but only 27% of the total sample.

ETIOLOGY

Much remains unknown about the etiology of problem drinking and smoking among women. A review of the neurobiologic consequences of ethanol exposure concluded that the cellular effects of alcohol extend far beyond the changes in cell membrane fluidity postulated previously. Although no specific receptor sites for ethanol have been identified, alcohol consumption clearly triggers various behavioral and neurochemical CNS changes. The strength of these changes depends on the amount of alcohol consumed and on the relative sensitivities of the various CNS components to ethanol. Adaptation occurs with chronic alcohol use, making the effects of such changes on the molecular, neurochemical, and behavioral levels hard to predict. The reinforcing and addicting properties of ethanol probably result from its effect on neurotransmitters such as GABA, dopamine, and serotonin, which affect mood.

The addictive component of tobacco is nicotine. Nicotine, unlike ethanol, has specific receptor sites in both the central and peripheral nervous systems. These account, in part, for the wide-ranging effects of smoking, including mood elevation via changes in dopamine levels, pressor responses, changes in cardiac acceleration, and appetite suppression.

Social factors also contribute to the onset of smoking and alcohol problems. Several studies have found higher rates of a history of childhood sexual abuse among problem drinkers and alcoholics. Most problem drinkers report experimentation with alcohol, and often progression to regular use, during the teenage years. Almost all smokers began smoking in adolescence, typically before entering high school. In a sample of 1400 female high school students in California, 50% reported some use of tobacco by age 13.5 years. Studies of alcohol and tobacco use in adolescence have identified four important predictors of early use: peer pressure, peer modeling, parent modeling, and exposure to product advertising.

There may be a genetic component to the propensity to smoke or develop problems with alcohol. A U.S. study of over 1000 female twin pairs estimated the heritability of liability to alcoholism in women as ranging from 50% to 61%, depending on the restrictiveness of the diagnostic criteria used. A large Australian study reported a similar range for married twins but a higher rate of 76% for unmarried twins, suggesting a strong role for the moderating effect of spousal drinking.

The U.S. twin study also found a genetic link with smoking, which was consistent with data from a study of over 13,000 male twins identified through World War II military service records. The latter study reported an adjusted heritability estimate for smoking of 35%. No specific gene, or combination of genes, has been found that consistently mediates susceptibility to alcoholism or smoking.

CLINICAL COURSE

The clinical course for smoking is typically characterized by early onset, almost always in adolescence or young adulthood, repeated attempts to quit smoking before eventual success or death, and increased likelihood of quitting by age 65. Occasional smokers are rare: fewer than 10% of all smokers consume five cigarettes or fewer per day. In a nationwide survey of women who currently or formerly smoked, only 9% of current smokers said they had never thought about trying to quit. Among all those who had tried to quit in the past year, 58% had gone back to smoking. The corresponding relapse rate among women over 65 was substantially less, at 28%.

Despite the use of the disease label in many discussions of alcoholism, the clinical path women with alcohol problems follow, if not treated, is largely unpredictable. Drinking levels tend to decline spontaneously with age, and natural recoveries are common. Wilsnack and colleagues conducted a national survey to identify 178 women who met their criteria for problem drinking. When these women were reinterviewed 5 years later, 33% were completely free of alcohol problems. Another study found that heavy drinking among college women was not a good predictor of later problem drinking or alcoholism. Early signs of problems with alcohol should not be ignored, however, because in women who continue to drink heavily, progression to the advanced stages of alcoholism often occurs much more rapidly than in men.

Women, on average, are older than men when they start drinking heavily, but both genders tend to enter drug treatment programs at about the same age. Several studies have suggested that women are also more likely to relapse to alcoholism or problem drinking after completing alcohol treatment. One explanation for these disparities is that a given dose of ethanol results in higher blood-alcohol levels in women, because they tend to have more body fat per unit of weight and less body water. Another is that the enzyme alcohol dehydrogenase is less active in women, which results in more alcohol passing through the digestive system and into the bloodstream.

Women also may be more likely than men to develop alcoholic liver disease. The link between liver disease and hormones is difficult to study, given the potential for reciprocal effects, but there is some evidence that the effects of alcohol on the liver are compounded by female hormones. In one study of postmenopausal women, estradiol levels were significantly elevated in those with alcohol-induced liver disease.

MORBIDITY AND MORTALITY

The full impact of smoking on women's health is often underestimated. The 1990 Surgeon General's report on the health benefits of smoking cessation presented 4-year mortality data on 658,748 women enrolled in the second American Cancer Society Cancer Prevention Study. After controlling for age and excluding participants who at enrollment reported a history of cancer, heart disease, or stroke or said they were "sick," women smoking one to 19 cigarettes per day were 82% more likely to die during follow-up than women who had never smoked (relative risk = 1.82). Women smoking a pack a day or more were more than twice as likely to die during follow-up (relative risk = 2.46).

Data from this study added further scientific validity to the old adage, "It's never too late to quit." There was a strong inverse association between the length of time off cigarettes and the risk of death among former smokers, even among women age 50 to 74. After 16 or more years of nonsmoking, overall mortality rates for former smokers were comparable to those of women who had never smoked.

U.S. death certificate data have been used to compare cause-specific mortality risks in smokers and nonsmokers. Women who smoke are nearly 18 times more likely to die of larynx cancer, almost 12 times more likely to die from a cancer of the trachea, lung, or bronchus, and over 10 times as likely to die from esophageal cancer (Table 6-1). There are also substantial increases in risk associated with cerebrovascular diseases, particularly in women age 35 to 64, and with bronchitis and emphysema.

Lung cancer has surpassed breast cancer as the leading cause of death among women (Fig. 6-1). In contrast to the paucity of knowledge about effective primary prevention strategies for breast cancer, enough is known about the etiology of lung cancer to prevent the overwhelming majority of cases in women. Several studies have found that the causal link between smoking and lung cancer appears to be even stronger in women than it is in men. When men and women are considered together, the relative risk for lung cancer in smokers is around 10, and tobacco use accounts for at least 85% of all such cancers. Data from a study by Risch and colleagues of lung cancer suggest that almost all lung cancer cases in women can be attributed to smoking.

The risk of cervical cancer is substantially increased among regular smokers. Some studies have also reported an association between benign breast disease and smoking, but tobacco use does not appear to increase the risk of developing breast cancer.

The cardiovascular disease burden of smoking exceeds that of all tobacco-related cancers combined. Willett and colleagues followed 119,404 female registered nurses for 6 years and found that the relative risks for smokers compared to nonsmokers were 5.5 for fatal coronary heart disease, 5.8 for nonfatal myocardial infarction, and 2.6 for angina pectoris. Even women smoking as few as one to four cigarettes per day were at increased risk. Subsequent follow-up of the cohort documented similar significant increases in the risk of subarachnoid hemorrhage, ischemic stroke, and cerebral hemorrhage. Other studies have shown a significant increase in the risk of stroke and subarachnoid hemorrhage among smokers who use oral contraceptives.

Table 6-1. Relative Risk for Death Attributed to Smoking in Women Aged 35 Years and Older

CAUSE OF DEATH	RELATIVE RISK
Neoplasms	
Lip, oral cavity, pharynx	5.6
Esophagus	10.3
Pancreas	2.3
Larynx	17.8
Trachea, lung, bronchus	11.9
Cervix uteri	2.1
Urinary bladder	2.6
Cardiovascular diseases	
Hypertension	1.7
Ischemic heart disease	
Persons age 35–64 yrs	3.0
Persons age ≥65 yrs	1.6
Cerebrovascular diseases	
Persons age 35–64 yrs	4.8
Persons age ≥65 yrs	1.5
Atherosclerosis	**3.0**
Aortic aneurysm	3.0
Other arterial disease	3.0
Respiratory diseases	
Pneumonia and influenza	2.2
Bronchitis, emphysema	10.5
Chronic airway obstruction	10.5
Other respiratory diseases	2.2

*Current smokers related to women who have never smoked
(Adapted from MMWR August 27, 1993, p. 646.)

An increased risk of developing duodenal and gastric ulcers, a significant loss in bone density, premature wrinkling, and an earlier onset of menopause are other common consequences of smoking. Studies of cigarettes and ulcer disease have shown that smoking increases the risk and that smoking cessation may be a necessary component of effective treatment. Bone density data suggest that women smoking a pack or more of cigarettes per day from early adulthood to menopause have a 5% to 10% deficit in bone density, an amount sufficient to increase the risk of fracture. Current smoking has also been shown to negate the protective effects of oral estrogen replacement therapy on the risk of hip fractures among older women. Premature skin wrinkling is typically limited to skin exposed to the sun but may be prominent, especially among white women. Menopause occurs, on average, 1 to 2 years earlier in smokers than nonsmokers, accounting in part for the increased risk of cardiovascular disease among smokers.

Other important hormonal consequences of tobacco use relate to pregnancy and fertility. Smoking significantly depresses birthweight and is thus an important contributor to peri- and neonatal mortality. In a 1981 study, perinatal mortality rose from 22 deaths

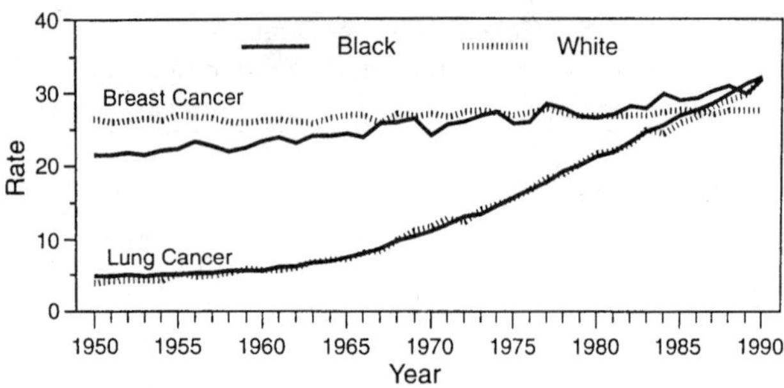

FIGURE 6-1. Age-adjusted lung and breast cancer death rates for women by race, United States, 1950–1990. Rates per 100,000 women, standardized to the 1970 age distribution of the U.S. population. (MMWR 1993;42;865.)

per 1000 live births in nonsmokers to 28.2 deaths per 1000 in smokers. Another study found that infants of smokers had higher perinatal mortality at every level of birthweight evaluated. The effect of smoking on birthweight has been found to be most pronounced among older women. Smoking has also been shown to decrease fertility and substantially increase the risk of sudden infant death syndrome.

Some investigators have reported a beneficial effect of nicotine treatment on ulcerative colitis, Parkinson disease, and major depressive disorder, but cigarettes are not the recommended route of drug administration. There is no minimal level of tobacco use that can safely be recommended for the general population.

The effects of alcohol on morbidity and mortality are more complex than the corresponding effects of smoking. U.S. death certificate data suggest that alcohol use accounted for 5% of all deaths in 1990, ranking alcohol behind only tobacco at 19% and diet/activity patterns at 14%. An 11-year follow-up study of 100 women who had been hospitalized for treatment of alcoholism found a mortality rate of 31%, a value four times higher than that observed in the general population. The leading cause of death in the 11-year study was disease of the digestive system, including cirrhosis and pancreatitis, which accounted for 29% of all deaths. Unintentional injuries and violence ranked second at 26%, followed by cancers at 19%, circulatory diseases at 16%, and respiratory diseases at 10%.

On the other hand, moderate drinking has repeatedly been linked with important reductions in cardiovascular disease risk. A longitudinal study of over 72,000 women in the Kaiser Permanente Medical Care Program reported a 20% reduction in the risk of cardiovascular death among moderate drinkers (one or two drinks per day) compared to lifelong abstainers (relative risk = 0.80). Daily drinkers in the Nurses Health Study were significantly less likely than nondrinkers to develop severe heart disease, including nonfatal myocardial infarctions. The risk of ischemic stroke was also reduced. However, the risk of subarachnoid hemorrhage was increased, even at low levels of consumption.

Despite these cardiovascular benefits, most experts do not recommend advising initiation or resumption of alcohol use among nondrinkers. There is no minimal level of use that is categorically safe for all women, and it is impossible to predict which occasional drinkers will progress to heavy drinking or alcoholism. Even moderate drinking in the Kaiser sample significantly increased the risk of other adverse outcomes, including death due to cirrhosis or other "unnatural" causes. At higher levels of drinking, the overall mortality risk increased substantially. Women consuming three to five drinks per day were 20% more likely to die during the follow-up period (relative risk = 1.2); the relative risk associated with six or more drinks per day was 2.2.

Breast cancer may be weakly associated with alcohol use, although findings from many epidemiologic studies are inconclusive. Other consequences of problem drinking include effects on bone density, menstruation, and pregnancy. Osteoporosis, osteomalacia, secondary hyperparathyroidism, fractures, and avascular necrosis have all been associated with alcoholism. Compounding the presence of these disorders is the increased risk of falling or experiencing other forms of trauma commonly observed among alcoholics and binge drinkers. The effects of moderate or minimal levels of alcohol consumption on bone mass remain unclear.

Problem drinking and alcoholism have been associated with a broad spectrum of reproductive problems, including amenorrhea, anovulation, luteal-phase dysfunction, and ovarian pathology. In Wilsnack and colleagues' study of female problem drinkers, sexual dysfunction was common and was a consistent predictor of continued binge drinking and alcohol dependence.

Alcohol has been firmly established as a human teratogen, but most women who drink occasionally during pregnancy are not at risk for delivering an infant with fetal alcohol syndrome (FAS). Conservative estimates of the rate of FAS in the general population range from 0.33 to 1.9 cases per 1,000 births. One study of infants born to women who averaged four or more drinks per day during pregnancy found only 5% to 10% who scored abnormally low on tests of mental and psychomotor development. These data offer important reassurances to women who become alarmed by the fact that they had a few drinks before they knew they were pregnant. Although FAS and the less severe syndrome of fetal alcohol effects occur infrequently, prenatal alcohol exposure is one of the leading causes of mental retardation in the Western world. Afflicted children often have severe problems that persist throughout the early school-age years.

Efforts to establish safe levels of minimal drinking in pregnancy have not been successful. Data clearly support the hazards of binge drinking (three or more drinks on any given day), but the risks associated with having an occasional beer or glass of wine remain unclear. Conservative practice thus advises all pregnant women to abstain from alcohol entirely or to drink moderately on only rare occasions.

When daily smoking is combined with heavy drinking, the adverse health effects are compounded. Blot and colleagues documented a synergistic increase in risk for women smoking 20 to 40 cigarettes per day and having five to 14 drinks per week. Women who both smoked and drank at these amounts were almost seven times more likely to develop an oropharyngeal cancer than those who neither drank nor smoked. Women who smoked at that level but rarely or never drank were about twice as likely to develop a cancer as nonsmokers. Among women who had five to 14 drinks per week but did not smoke, a 30% increase in risk was observed. Other researchers have found evidence of similar additive or multiplicative effects for cirrhosis, cardiovascular disease, and adverse pregnancy outcomes.

DIAGNOSIS

Diagnosing tobacco use is easy: just ask. The use of cotinine, a sensitive biomarker for nicotine, is rarely required. Most smokers also readily provide the other two pieces of data needed to guide treatment planning.

The first piece of information is the patient's stage of readiness to change with respect to quitting smoking. Assessing a smoker's current stage of readiness to change and then matching treatment counseling to that stage has been found to more than double the odds the smoker will quit within 12 to 18 months. Determining which stage the smoker is in can be accomplished with three questions. First ask, "Are you thinking about trying to quit smoking in the next 6 months?" If she answers yes, ask "Are you thinking about trying to quit in the next month?" If she answers yes again, ask "Have you taken any preliminary steps already, such as trying to quit for 24 hours or reading some brochures on tips to help you quit?"

The five stages of readiness to change are precontemplation, contemplation, preparation, action, and maintenance. Precontemplators are patients who are not seriously thinking about quitting within the next 6 months. Smokers who have tried to quit repeatedly without success sometimes become stuck in this stage if they have decided they cannot possibly succeed at quitting. Contemplators are more optimistic and more interested in quitting. They are thinking about quitting in the next 6 months, but not in the next 30 days. People in the preparation stage are ready to quit. They have also recently taken one or more concrete steps toward quitting, such as talking with friends or relatives who used to smoke, reading literature on the nicotine patch, trying to go without cigarettes for at least 1 day, or conscientiously delaying smoking the first cigarette each morning for as long as possible. If a smoker tells you she is planning to quit in the next month but has not taken any preliminary steps, assume she is still in the contemplation stage.

People in the action stage have already quit, but only recently. For example, a woman in for her first prenatal care visit may tell you she quit smoking last week, just as soon as she found out she was pregnant. Because relapsing is very common, it is wise to assume a smoker is still in the action stage until she has been completely off cigarettes for at least 6 months. At that point, you can begin to think of her as a former smoker, in maintenance. Women who relapse reenter the cycle at one of the first three stages.

The second piece of information concerns the patient's degree of physical dependence on nicotine. Most smokers are psychologically dependent on smoking, but some are not physically addicted and can quit without much difficulty. Highly addicted smokers are more likely to need pharmacologic support. The easiest way to assess dependence is to inquire about prior cessation attempts. Smokers who report substantial problems with irritability, frustration, anger, anxiety, difficulty concentrating, restlessness, appetite changes, weight gain, or craving during the early days and weeks after quitting were probably experiencing nicotine withdrawal symptoms and may be nicotine dependent. Alternately, smokers who have never tried to quit can be asked to complete the six-question Fagerstrom Test for Nicotine Dependence (Table 6-2). Women who report needing a cigarette as soon as they wake up each morning and those with scores of 7 or more are likely to be physically dependent.

Many opportunities to diagnose alcoholism arise in primary care settings. Heavy drinkers tend to make frequent office visits with complaints of stomach or abdominal pain, hypertension, chronic headaches, insomnia, sexually transmitted diseases, fatigue, depression, chronic diarrhea, and memory loss. Even when other explanations are apparent, assessing alcohol use as a possible cause is often worthwhile. Adding screening questions to intake procedures for new patients is also appropriate, given the high prevalence of problem drinkers in the general population. One or two questions about alcohol use should be included in most annual examinations, because drinking patterns can vary markedly from year to year.

Despite its high prevalence, accurate diagnosis can be difficult. Women are less likely than men to drink in public settings and rarely present with obvious signs of intoxication. Denial of excessive alcohol use can be flagrant, and even gentle attempts to probe may threaten dependent drinkers. Use of other mood-altering substances in addition to alcohol often complicates the picture. Many polydrug users admit to a problem with marijuana or cocaine but deny alcohol abuse or dependence despite a long history of heavy

Table 6-2. Fagerstrom Test for Nicotine Dependence

ITEMS	RESPONSES	SCORE
1. How soon after you wake up do you smoke your first cigarette?	≤5 min	3
	6–30 min	2
	31–60 min	1
	>60 min	0
2. Do you find it difficult to refrain from smoking in places where it is forbidden (eg, in church, at the library, in the cinema)?	Yes	1
	No	0
3. Which cigarette would you hate most to give up?	The first one in the morning	1
	All others	0
4. How many cigarettes per day do you smoke?	≤10	0
	11–20	1
	21–30	2
	≥31	3
5. Do you smoke more frequently during the first hours after waking than during the rest of the day?	Yes	1
	No	0
6. Do you smoke if you are so ill that you are in bed most of the day?	Yes	1
	No	0

Scoring: 0–4, low; 5, medium; 6 or 7, high; 8–10, very high level of nicotine dependence.

(Adapted from Fagerstrom KO, Heatherton TF, Kozlowski LT. Nicotine addiction and its assessment. Ear Nose Throat J 1992;69(11):763–767.)

drinking. Very recent heavy drinking is detectable with laboratory testing, but many problem drinkers do not show abnormal values using current biomarkers.

Accurate diagnosis is thus part art and part science. The social stigma of alcoholism continues to be much greater for women than men, so considerable care must be taken to avoid provoking major problems with denial. A nonjudgmental demeanor and attentive listening are critical. The science of assessment uses a sequential process that starts with a simple screen to assess the consequences of prior drinking and then moves to a review of recent alcohol use patterns. If there is any sign of adverse consequences or if quantity and frequency indicators of use exceed recommended levels for moderate drinking, further evaluation is warranted. Figure 6-2 shows a screening and assessment algorithm developed by the National Institute of Alcohol Abuse and Alcoholism.

Patients who responded affirmatively to a neutral lead-in query about occasional drinking should be given the extensively validated one-minute CAGE screening test, which consists of four questions: "Have you ever felt you ought to **C**ut down on your drinking?" "Have people **A**nnoyed you by criticizing your drinking?" "Have you ever felt **G**uilty about your drinking?" "Have you ever had a drink first thing in the morning to steady your nerves or get rid of a hangover (an **E**ye-opener)?" Assign one point for each "yes" response. Patients with scores of 0 or 1 are experiencing few adverse consequences of drinking.

To assess patterns of alcohol use, first ask about the average number of days per week during the past month when any alcohol was consumed (frequency). The frame of reference must be broad enough to exclude recent illnesses that might have temporarily altered drinking behavior. Then ask about the average number of drinks per day on a typical day when alcohol was consumed (quantity). A standard drink is 12 ounces of beer, 5 ounces of table wine, 4 ounces of fortified wine, or a shot of liquor (80 proof). Some experts also recommend asking about binge drinking: "During the past year, have you ever had more than three drinks on any one day?"

Several guidelines for moderate drinking have been proposed. The most conservative set recommends no more than one drink per day, with several alcohol-free days each week. More liberal guidelines permit one to two drinks per day, or a maximum of 14 drinks per week. The risk with the latter guideline is that it can obscure significant binge drinking: having one drink per day on Monday through Thursday and then five drinks each on Friday and Saturday is not equivalent to two drinks per day over a 7-day interval. Parallel standards for men are typically higher to allow for gender differences in alcohol metabolism and in the rate of progression from problem drinking to frank alcoholism.

All women with CAGE scores of 2 or more and most with lower scores but more than moderate levels of drinking should undergo further assessment to distinguish abusive or harmful, but not chemically dependent, drinkers from those who have advanced to overt alcoholism. The distinction is crucial, because many nondependent drinkers are good candidates for treatment in the primary care setting. In most outpatient settings, the ratio of problem drinkers to alcoholics is about 4:1. Several definitions of alcoholism are popular. A succinct version used in the 1990 Institute of Medicine report is: "A chronic, progressive, and potentially fatal biogenetic and psychosocial disease characterized by tolerance and physical dependence manifested by a loss of control, as well as diverse personality changes and social consequences."

Table 6-3 shows the DSM-IV criteria for alcohol abuse and dependence. These guidelines, which replaced the DSM-IIIR crite-

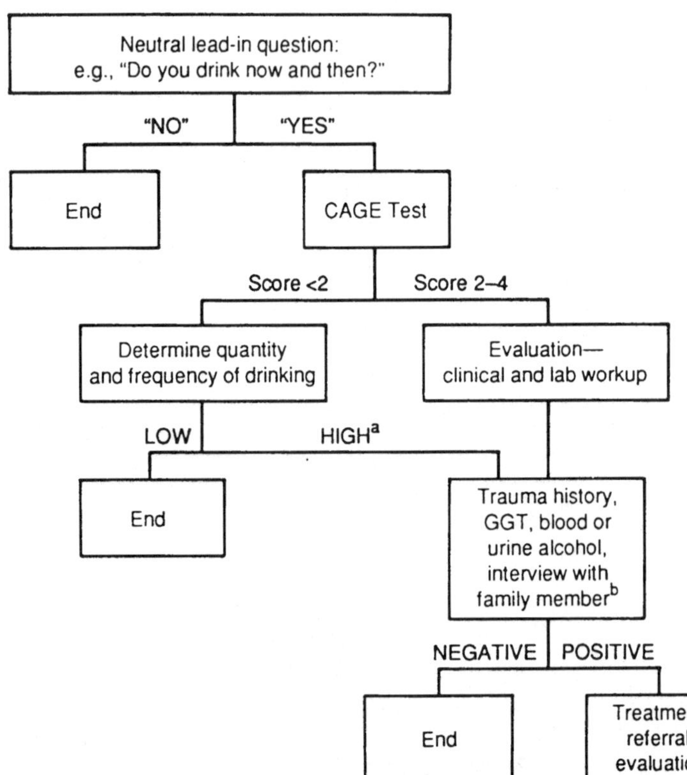

FIGURE 6-2. Decision algorithm for assessment of alcohol problems in primary care settings. [a]See text for consumption levels that exceed moderate drinking. [b]See text for details. (Adapted from U.S. Department of Health & Human Services PH. Alcohol & health—7th special report to U.S. Congress. Rockville, MD: National Institute of Alcohol Abuse and Alcoholism, 1990.)

Table 6-3. Abuse/Harmful Use and Dependence Criteria in DSM-IV

Abuse

A. A maladaptive pattern of alcohol use, leading to clinically significant impairment or distress, as manifested by one (or more) of the following:
   1. Recurrent alcohol use resulting in a failure to fulfill major role obligations at work, school or home
   2. Recurrent alcohol use in situations in which it is physically hazardous
   3. Recurrent alcohol-related legal problems
   4. Continued alcohol use despite having persistent or recurrent social or interpersonal problems caused or exacerbated by the effects of alcohol

B. Never meets the criteria for alcohol dependence

Dependence

A maladaptive pattern of alcohol use, leading to clinically significant impairment or distress, as manifested by three (or more) of the following occurring at any time in the same 12-month period:

1. Tolerance as defined by either of the following:
   (a) Need for markedly increased amounts of alcohol to achieve intoxication or desired effect
   (b) Markedly diminished effect with continued use of the same amount of alcohol
2. Withdrawal as manifested by either of the following:
   (a) characteristic withdrawal syndrome for alcohol
   (b) use of alcohol to relieve or avoid withdrawal symptoms
3. Alcohol is often taken in larger amounts or over a longer period than was intended
4. Persistent desire or unsuccessful efforts to cut down or control alcohol use
5. A great deal of time spent in activities necessary to obtain alcohol, use alcohol, or recover from its effects
6. Important social, occupational or recreational activities are given up or reduced because of alcohol use
7. Continued alcohol use despite knowledge of having had a persistent or recurrent physical or psychological problem that is likely to be caused or exacerbated by alcohol

(Adapted from Schuckit MA, Hesselbrock V, Tipp J, Anthenelli R, Bucholz K, Radziminski S. A comparison of DSM-III-R, DSM-IV and ICD-10 substance use disorders diagnoses in 1922 men and women subjects in the COGA Study. Addiction 1994;89:1629–1638.)

ria in 1994, contain more restrictive criteria for alcohol dependence but more liberal criteria for alcohol abuse.

Withdrawal symptoms are a major indicator of dependence. Major alcohol withdrawal signs are acute delirium, with confusion and disorientation; agitation, often with belligerence; marked elevation of vital signs; pronounced tremens, diaphoresis, and flushing; hallucinations with an inability to test reality; and seizure. More minor withdrawal symptoms include tremors, sweats, flushing, anxiety, insomnia, anorexia, tendon hyperreflexia, nightmares, dysphoria, diarrhea, nausea and vomiting, aches and pains, restlessness, and abdominal cramps.

To assess withdrawal, tolerance, and harmful use, ask additional questions, interview a family member or friend if the woman is agreeable, and consider obtaining laboratory data. Women should be asked about their history of trauma since age 18, including fractures, dislocations, and head injuries stemming from fights; assaults, or motor vehicle injuries. If responses are positive to any of these queries, ask if alcohol use contributed to the injury in any way. Alternately, have the patient complete the 10-minute Self-Administered Alcoholism Screening Test (Table 6-4). Responses to these questions provide a clearer picture of the nature and extent of alcohol problems and are a powerful tool for motivating women into treatment when warranted.

Several types of laboratory data can be informative. The first includes blood-, urine-, and breath-alcohol levels. In nontolerant drinkers, a blood-alcohol concentration of 0.02 to 0.05 g/dL generally produces euphoria and reduces anxiety. At 0.06 to 0.10 g/dL, judgment and motor coordination become impaired; 0.10 g/dL is the standard for driving while intoxicated in most states. At 0.20 to 0.25 g/dL, signs of sedation appear, with anesthetic effects and loss of consciousness likely at 0.30 g/dL. Higher levels can induce coma and then death through loss of adequate respiration. An elevated value in a woman who appears sober strongly suggests the development of alcohol tolerance. Other tests of more limited value in primary care settings include the gamma-glutamyl transferase test, which measures cellular injury to the liver; the mean corpuscular volume test, which assesses injury to cells that manufacture red blood cells; and the plasma carbohydrate-deficient transferrin test, which measures nonspecific alcohol-related changes. Individually, these tests tend to have low sensitivity and specificity, but combining the results from two or more measures has been shown to improve the predictive value.

Diagnosing alcohol problems often unmasks serious problems with depression, anxiety, and the use of other illicit drugs. In one study of over 20,000 men and women, comorbid disorders were common. Among the 13.5% of the sample with a lifetime history of any alcohol disorder, 45% also had some other mental health or drug abuse disorder. Specifically, 19% also had evidence of an anxiety disorder and 13% reported a history of depression. Hesselbrock and colleagues collected data on 90 female hospitalized alcoholics and found 52% with a history of major depression. In a recent midwestern study of over 200 women undergoing intensive alcohol treatment, 84% met enrollment criteria for depression and 64% reported use of one or more illicit drugs in the year before treatment admission.

TREATMENT

The importance and effectiveness of treating cigarette smoking in the primary care environment was demonstrated in the 1980s when the National Cancer Institute (NCI) funded five randomized controlled trials of brief cessation interventions in physician practices. These studies involved over 30,000 patients and 1000 physicians in a wide variety of outpatient settings. In most settings, the intervention required about 3 minutes per smoker, more if follow-up visits were arranged. Patients from these practices were followed for 12 months and biologic samples were obtained to verify smoking cessation. In practices where physicians consistently followed a protocol similar to the one presented here, patient smoking cessation rates were up to six times higher than quit rates in control practices where the usual care protocols prevailed.

The NCI protocol to help patients quit smoking is based on the four-step **A**sk, **A**dvise, **A**ssist, and then **A**rrange (for follow-up) process. *Asking* consists of assessing current use, nicotine dependence, and stage of readiness to change. Office systems can be structured to increase the likelihood that all new patients are

TABLE 6-4. Self-Administered Alcoholism Screening Test

1. Do you enjoy a drink now and then?	YES	NO
2. Do you feel you are a normal drinker (that is, drink no more than average)?	YES	NO
3. Have you ever awakened in the morning after drinking the night before and found that you could not remember a part of the evening?	YES	NO
4. Do close relatives ever worry or complain about your drinking?	YES	NO
5. Can you stop drinking without a struggle after one or two drinks?	YES	NO
6. Do you ever feel guilty about your drinking?	YES	NO
7. Do friends or relatives think you are a normal drinker?	YES	NO
8. Are you always able to stop drinking when you want to?	YES	NO
9. Have you ever attended Alcoholics Anonymous (AA) because of your drinking?	YES	NO
10. Have you gotten into physical fights when drinking?	YES	NO
11. Has your drinking ever created problems between you and your partner, wife, husband, parents, or a near relative?	YES	NO
12. Has your partner, wife, husband, or other family member ever gone to anyone for help about your drinking?	YES	NO
13. Have you ever lost friendships because of your drinking?	YES	NO
14. Have you ever gotten into trouble at work because of drinking?	YES	NO
15. Have you ever lost a job because of drinking?	YES	NO
16. Have you ever neglected your obligations, your family, or your work for 2 or more days in a row because of drinking?	YES	NO
17. Do you ever drink in the morning?	YES	NO
18. Have you ever felt the need to cut down on your drinking?	YES	NO
19. Have there been times in your adult life when you found it necessary to avoid alcohol completely?	YES	NO
20. Have you ever been told you have liver trouble? Cirrhosis?	YES	NO
21. Have you ever had delirium tremens (DTs)?	YES	NO
22. Have you ever had severe shaking, heard voices, or seen things that were not there after heavy drinking?	YES	NO
23. Have you ever gone to anyone for help about your drinking?	YES	NO
24. Have you ever been in a hospital because of drinking?	YES	NO
25. Have you ever been told by a doctor to stop drinking?	YES	NO
26. A. Have you ever been a patient in a psychiatric hospital or on a psychiatric ward of a general hospital?	YES	NO
B. Was drinking part of the problem that resulted in your hospitalization?	YES	NO
27. A. Have you ever been a patient at a psychiatric or mental health clinic or gone to any doctor, social worker, or member of the clergy for help with any emotional problem?	YES	NO
B. Was drinking part of the problem?	YES	NO
28. Have you ever been arrested, even for a few hours, because of:		
A. Drunken behavior (not driving)?	YES	NO
How many times? _____		
B. Driving while intoxicated?	YES	NO
How many times? _____		
29. Have any of the following relatives ever had problems with alcohol?		
A. Parents.	YES	NO
B. Brothers or sisters.	YES	NO
C. Husband or wife.	YES	NO
D. Children.	YES	NO

Scoring: For questions 2, 5, 7, and 8, code is no = 1, yes = 0. For *all* other questions, code no = 0, yes = 1. Totals less than 7 suggest an absence of serious problems with alcohol. Totals of 7, 8, or 9 suggest possible alcoholism. Scores of 10 or higher suggest probable alcoholism.

(Adapted from Hurt RD, Morse RM, Swenson WM. Diagnosis of alcoholism with a self-administered alcoholism screening test. Mayo Clinic Proc 1980:55:365–370.)

asked about smoking and that the topic is revisited periodically with established patients who are current or former smokers. Relapses can occur even after many years of nonsmoking. NCI recommends including questions about tobacco use on patient enrollment forms and having a receptionist or a nurse flag medical records of smokers.

Advising consists of telling the patient in a clear, direct way that smoking is compromising her health and that she needs to quit. The message is most effective if it is tailored to specific aspects of her medical history and also reflects what you know about her current stage of change. For example, "I understand you're not planning to quit smoking any time soon. Nevertheless, I want to be sure you know that continuing to smoke puts you at high risk for developing the kind of heart problems that led to your mother's death. I think it is very important that you start thinking about when you will be able to quit."

The physician's actions in the *assisting* step depend on what she or he has learned about the patient's stage of readiness for quitting and whether or not she is nicotine dependent. The goal is to move each patient one stage closer to quitting. If the woman is in precontemplation, the physician can help her advance to the contemplation stage. Rather than pushing her to agree to quit within the next week or two, the physician should try to get her to agree to think seriously about quitting in the next 6 months. This can often be done by providing more personalized information on the health effects of smoking, either through direct education or by providing pamphlets and brochures. The local American Cancer Society office can help locate appropriate low-cost materials developed specifically for women.

Women in the contemplation stage need to be encouraged to start making concrete preparations for quitting. The physician can help by underscoring their growing conviction that they need to quit and are capable of doing so and by reminding them of the substantial health and social benefits of quitting. Patients should be assured that even if they have tried and failed before, there is a good chance that their next attempt will be successful. A few anticipatory tasks can be assigned to the patient, such as finding a buddy for moral support, going without cigarettes for 24 hours just for practice, making a list of the pros and cons of smoking, or reading literature on nicotine replacement methods. Asking her to consider setting a definite quit date may accelerate this process.

Many women in the preparation stage have already set a target date and are willing to commit to a specific plan for quitting. Often the best plan is the simplest. A nationwide survey of over 2000 former smokers found that nearly 90% used the "cold turkey" approach. They abruptly just quit, without participating in a structured cessation program or relying on any sort of pharmacologic assistance. However, opinions differ on how much support should be offered to patients ready to make their first serious attempt at quitting.

Hughes and others recommend a stepped-care approach. Only after a woman has tried to quit without chemical assistance and failed should she be considered for drug therapy. Other experts regard nicotine replacement methods as a first-line strategy and argue for the advantages of maximizing the likelihood of successful quitting from the beginning. An interim position would offer pharmacologic support during the early months of nicotine withdrawal for women with Fagerstrom nicotine dependence scores in the high or very high range, but would also encourage less dependent smokers who have never tried to quit to use the cold turkey approach.

Women who have tried to quit with pharmacologic assistance but relapsed should be encouraged to try another round of treatment in conjunction with behavioral therapy or counseling. Most studies have found that behavioral therapy enhances quit rates among patients concurrently treated with nicotine replacement methods or other nonspecific pharmacotherapies. Information on smoking cessation programs in the community is often available at local hospitals and public health departments. Women with substantial tobacco-related morbidity who fail to quit after intensive outpatient treatment may benefit from referral to a residential drug-treatment program that specializes in nicotine dependence. Such programs are becoming increasingly common across the United States.

Arranging for follow-up, the fourth step, underscores the seriousness of the patient's need to quit, enhances compliance with treatment recommendations, and provides an opportunity for further problem solving. Follow-up is essential with pharmacotherapy.

Four types of medications have theoretical or demonstrated effectiveness for smoking cessation: deterrent therapies, blockade therapies, nonspecific pharmacotherapies, and nicotine replacement or substitution therapies.

Deterrent medications produce aversive side effects when used with tobacco. Silver acetate formulations combine with tobacco to create an unpleasant metallic taste, but they may also induce argyria and are not recommended. Blockade therapies have demonstrated effectiveness for several illicit drugs but have not proved useful for nicotine. Nonspecific therapies use drugs such as clonidine to counter nicotine withdrawal symptoms, especially depression and anxiety. Nicotine dependence is not an approved indication for clonidine, a centrally acting alpha-agonist licensed as an antihypertensive drug, but at least five studies have suggested that it can modestly enhance long-term quit rates in women. Glassman and colleagues randomly assigned 168 female smokers to clonidine or placebo. After 12 months, 16% of the treatment group but only 7% of the control group had quit smoking. Almost all studies, including Glassman's, have failed to find a corresponding effect for men. In addition to showing some efficacy as an adjunct to smoking cessation, clonidine has previously demonstrated effectiveness in reducing alcohol and opioid withdrawal symptoms.

A wide array of nicotine substitution and replacement therapies has been developed. Nicotine substitution products such as the various lobeline-containing OTC formulations (eg, CigArrest, Bantron, Nicoban) have not demonstrated their utility in clinical trials and have been removed from the market. Nicotine replacement products have shown substantial promise and include nicotine polacrilex, transdermal patches, and nasal sprays, which are still undergoing research and development.

Nicotine polacrilex has been on the market for nearly two decades. In 1994, Silagy and colleagues reported that use of the gum increased the likelihood of success by about 61%. Package instructions on proper chewing procedures must be followed precisely for effective buccal administration. The 2-mg dose may not be sufficient for more heavily addicted smokers and should be replaced by the 4-mg dose or by simultaneous use of two 2-mg pieces, one in each cheek. Studies assessing use of the gum as a stand-alone therapy without any sort of accompanying behavioral adjunct have found little or no evidence of long-term effectiveness.

Transdermal nicotine offers several important advantages over nicotine gum. The most important is that it appears to be more effective. Two independent metanalyses of patch-versus-placebo studies found that use of the patch more than doubled the odds of success. Fiore and associates reported 6-month success rates of 22% in patch users versus 9% in controls. Few studies have provided gender-specific quit rates, so the applicability of these findings to women must be inferred. Unlike nicotine gum, the patch has been shown to improve quit rates even in primary care settings where counseling and supportive follow-up were limited. Other benefits are enhanced ease of use, greater patient compliance, and more stable blood-nicotine levels.

Table 6-5 summarizes the patch formulations. Higher doses may be necessary for more heavily addicted smokers. Sleep disturbances have been reported in some 24-hour users, but women with strong early-morning cravings may benefit from higher blood-nicotine levels on awakening. Research studies have failed to demonstrate any significant benefit in extending patch use beyond 8 weeks or in gradually weaning patients to lower doses. Occasional use of nicotine polacrilex in conjunction with the patch during the first few weeks off cigarettes may provide a means of coping with intense urges to smoke in high-stress situations. However, the importance of not smoking while on the patch, or while using nicotine gum, must be emphasized to avoid potentially toxic blood-nicotine levels.

Other issues that warrant discussion with many smokers are the effects of nicotine withdrawal on mood and on caffeine blood levels, fears about weight gain after quitting, timing of the quit attempt with respect to the menstrual cycle, the potential impact of quitting on the risk of relapse to alcohol among problem drinkers and recovering alcoholics, and ways of responding to occasional slips back to smoking and to complete relapses.

Although one study of smoking cessation in women age 65 or older suggested that depression symptoms increased the likelihood of successfully quitting, most studies have found that depressed smokers who try to quit experience more withdrawal symptoms, are less likely to succeed initially, and are more likely to relapse than nondepressed smokers. Perhaps more worrisome are case report data suggesting that efforts to quit smoking can precipitate a significant relapse in depressive symptomatology among women with a history of major depression. Frequent monitoring in the primary care setting or psychiatric referral should be considered for all women who report becoming seriously depressed during prior attempts to quit smoking and for many women with a chronic history of dysphoria. Limited clinical trial data suggest that transdermal nicotine and clonidine may reduce the risk in vulnerable patients.

The link between nicotine and caffeine is important because some smokers routinely drink large quantities of coffee, tea, and other caffeine-rich beverages. Human laboratory data suggest that even when caffeine consumption is held constant, plasma caffeine concentrations increase, on average, by a factor of 2.5 and remained elevated for at least 6 months after quitting smoking. In coffee drinkers, this is equivalent to nearly tripling the average number of cups per day. These data suggest that some women may be able to limit withdrawal symptoms of anxiety, irritability, and restlessness by concurrently reducing their customary level of caffeine consumption when they quit smoking.

Concerns about gaining weight are a major barrier to quitting among some women. Most smokers do put on weight when they quit, but most add less than 10 pounds. Several investigators have documented lower average body weights in smokers than nonsmokers and concluded that the weight gain associated with quitting is corrective. It is not clear why quitters gain weight, as few studies have been able to document decreases in activity levels with smoking cessation and several have found no evidence of higher caloric intake. A popular theory is that nicotine has a direct effect on metabolism, resulting in an increase in energy expenditure. Several studies have found that the extra weight is rarely deposited in areas previously associated with an increased risk of cardiovascular problems. In any case, the adverse health effects of a 5- to 10-pound weight gain are usually more than offset by the overall benefits of quitting smoking.

Table 6-5. Comparison of Selected Features of Nicotine Patch Brands

	PRODUCT NAME (MANUFACTURER)			
FEATURE	*Habitrol (CIBA-GEIGY)*	*Nicoderm (Marion Merrell Dow)*	*Nicotrol (Parke-Davis)*	PROSTEP (Lederle Laboratories)
Delivered dose	21 mg/24 h	21 mg/24 h	15 mg/16 h	22 mg/24 h
	14 mg/24 h	14 mg/24 h	10 mg/16 h	11 mg/24 h
	7 mg/24 h	7 mg/24 h	5 mg/16 h	—
Patches per box	30	14	14	7
Adjuvant treatments provided with patches	Stop smoking contract: social support guide; self-help guide; motivational/relaxation audiotape from American Lung Association; toll-free telephone hotline	Self-help guide	Smoke Stoppers self-help kit: Smoke Stoppers social support guide: Dentyne chewing gum; motivational/relaxation audiotape: smoking self-monitoring form; toll-free Smoke Stoppers telephone counseling	Toll-free telephone number for smoking counseling and local smoking cessation program referrals; rebates for those who relapse within 1 y; self-help guide; squeeze ball; pay pharmacists to counsel patients on patch use

(Fiore MC, Jorenby DE, Baker TB, Kenford SL. Tobacco dependence and the nicotine patch—clinical guidelines for effective use. JAMA 1994;268:2692.)

Research on dieting to limit weight gain during the early weeks of smoking cessation have generally found such efforts to be counterproductive. Few quitters successfully maintain their initial weight, and relapse rates back to smoking tend to be higher among dieters. The latter is consistent with animal work documenting predictable increases in drug-seeking behavior during caloric deprivation. Some studies have found that use of either nicotine polacrilex or one of the transdermal patches restricts weight gain temporarily, but others have observed little or no effect. Without dismissing cosmetic and social concerns about weight as unimportant, clinicians can best help female smokers by emphasizing the health benefits of quitting and by suggesting that weight-reduction efforts can follow at a later date.

The popular notion that smoking cessation attempts may be more likely to succeed during certain phases of the menstrual cycle is appealing, but research data are too inconsistent to justify blanket recommendations. Women who ask about this should be encouraged to monitor their smoking for a month or two and then consider timing their quit attempt to coincide with an interval when their desire to smoke seems likely to be less intense.

Many smokers also have a history of problems with alcohol. When can recovering alcoholics and problem drinkers safely try to quit smoking? Is the stress of trying to quit likely to increase the risk of a relapse to drinking? Traditional wisdom in alcohol-treatment centers has tended to discourage efforts to quit during the first 1 to 2 years of sobriety. However, several thorough reviews of the literature have failed to uncover a single study in which quitting smoking had any adverse effect whatsoever on the alcohol recovery process. Three retrospective studies have reported data suggesting that quitting may prove beneficial. Unfortunately, each of these had limitations that restricted the general application of their findings. Small-scale prospective studies in Minnesota and Nebraska have found lower alcohol relapse rates among drinkers who were encouraged to quit smoking, but results from definitive trials have not yet been reported.

Quitting smoking could benefit alcohol control for at least three reasons: a reduction in environmental cues for drinking, a lessening of internal cues or alcohol cravings (if nicotine does, in fact, activate similar neurobiologic pathways), and an enhancement of overall self-esteem and well-being. These possibilities, together with the health benefits of quitting, suggest that the issue of tobacco use in women with alcohol problems should be treated exactly as it is with women who have no history of such problems. In addition, recovering alcoholics who are active in Alcoholics Anonymous (AA) should be encouraged to seek smoke-free AA meetings and to try applying the principles of AA to their smoking. Several studies of smoking cessation attempts among recovering alcoholics have found that those who quit cold turkey and relied on the principles of AA were more likely to remain off cigarettes than those who used other methods.

Despite extensive research on relapse prevention strategies, there are no known methods for reliably reducing the odds of returning to smoking. Three low-cost approaches that have shown some efficacy in clinical trials are encouraging the smoker to identify factors that contributed to prior relapses; encouraging her to regard an occasional cigarette as a slip, not a complete relapse; and providing brief in-person or telephone follow-up. Encouraging smokers to learn from their prior experiences is consistent with the stages-of-change approach to quitting. The patient should spend some time before the target quit date on creative problem solving, identifying the three or four situations in which she is most likely to want to go back to smoking and then developing a list of alternative behaviors (eg, chewing gum, going for a walk, asking for moral support from a friend).

The "abstinence violation effect" theory suggests that when smokers or drinkers view an isolated instance of use as an indication of a major relapse or failure, they are more likely to engage in negative thinking and then fall back into a pattern of regular use. Sometimes this downward spiral can be prevented if smokers learn to regard the occasional cigarette as just a slip that is very common even among successful quitters. The AA slogan of "progress, not perfection" is an appropriate philosophy.

Brief follow-up can be especially helpful. To limit the time devoted to this task, a staff member can become the office expert on smoking and can assume responsibility for all in-person or telephone follow-up. Women who quit smoking during pregnancy are likely to relapse in the early postpartum months and may particularly benefit from additional encouragement during this period.

Clinical judgment is essential to planning treatment for women with drinking problems. As with smoking, there is no one-size-fits-all approach. Issues include the appropriate level of treatment intensity, the need for management of withdrawal symptoms, the possible influence of related social and mental health factors, and, if necessary, denial or ambivalence.

The continuum of treatment options mirrors the broad spectrum of alcohol problems. The least intensive level of treatment consists of supportive counseling within the primary care environment. Good candidates are the many problem drinkers who show no signs of alcohol dependency and who have no history of prior alcohol treatment. A few brief (10 to 15 minutes) weekly or monthly visits with a gradual tapering of follow-up are sufficient for many patients. The content of these visits varies but should include some emphasis on positive reinforcement, anticipatory guidance, and social support. Miller and Rollnick's text on motivational interviewing provides practical guidelines for interventions in outpatient settings. Most patients need reassurance that the psychological and physical stresses of making a major lifestyle change eventually abate. Encouraging the recovering alcoholic or problem drinker to find as many sources of social support during the difficult transition process is almost always worthwhile.

Research data have supported the effectiveness of brief therapy, particularly when coupled with use of self-help materials. Appropriate patient brochures can be obtained from the national Office for Substance Abuse Prevention or the Hazelden publication office in Minnesota. A strong faith in the physician's knowledge and a well-established patient–physician relationship are also helpful. If heavy drinking persists despite this extended show of concern, referral to a well-established alcohol-treatment program is warranted.

The American Society of Addiction Medicine uses a four-level topology to classify treatment options that include care provided by addiction specialists. Level I consists of outpatient care with less than 9 contact-hours per week. Many community mental health centers offer individualized or group therapy programs that fall within this category. Level II is more intensive outpatient care, with at least 9 contact-hours per week, and may include partial hospitalization. Some level II programs provide evening and weekend treatment to accommodate employed patients.

Level III is medically monitored inpatient or residential therapy, with care provided by a multidisciplinary team. Much of the counseling is provided by staff who are themselves recovering alcoholics or problem drinkers. Residential facilities typically have on-call access to physicians but rely on nursing staff for day-to-day medical supervision. Most Level III programs follow the Minnesota model of treatment, which combines professional diagnostic and intervention activities with the 12-step recovery program advocated by AA. The length of stay in these programs traditionally has been 28 days, but in many communities insurance companies and managed care programs are forcing significant reductions in the maximum amount of care allowed.

Many communities have treatment programs tailored to female patients. Some women are more likely to comply with a referral to women-focused or women-only programs. Such programs typically bolster standard alcohol-treatment protocols with additional attention to female socialization patterns, communication styles, and coping responses, as well as the special issues of reproductive health and sexuality. The long-term benefits of these gender-specific treatment components are still being debated.

Level IV, medically managed intensive inpatient care, is reserved for patients whose acute or complex problems warrant primary medical and nursing care with access to the full resources of a general hospital.

Appropriate candidates for intensive level III and IV care should have one or more of the following characteristics: a history of relapsing back to drinking despite completion of one or more rounds of treatment at a less intensive level; the presence of a concurrent medical condition such as pregnancy that makes immediate cessation of heavy drinking imperative; evidence of significant comorbid depression, anxiety, or other cognitive-behavioral dysfunction that could limit their participation in an outpatient setting; concurrent use of other psychoactive substances to the extent that detoxification requires close medical supervision; or residence in a community where less intensive options are unavailable.

Research data have failed to support the popular belief that inpatient treatment consistently achieves better results than outpatient treatment. Outpatient care offers important advantages for many patients in terms of cost and convenience and should not be viewed or presented as a less desirable option in most instances.

Alcohol withdrawal in many patients is unpleasant but uncomplicated and can be managed in an outpatient setting. Tremulousness is the most common symptom and usually begins within hours of the last drink. Nausea and vomiting may occur. Protracted withdrawal signs such as unstable blood pressure, tension, anxiety, depression, and insomnia occur in some patients and may persist for several weeks. The few patients who develop signs of withdrawal delirium (eg, clouding of consciousness, disorientation, autonomic hyperactivity, difficulty in sustaining concentration) should be considered for hospitalization.

Acute withdrawal symptoms are more likely in patients who have had problems during prior withdrawals, have a recent history of very heavy drinking, or have also been using other addictive drugs. The importance of taking a careful history to identify such patients cannot be overemphasized. When acute withdrawal problems are likely, patients should be referred for management of detoxification to addiction specialists.

Except for the administration of the B-complex vitamins, there is no consensus on the need for pharmacotherapy during mild withdrawal. Some experts recommend the use of a long-acting benzodiazepine (eg, diazepam 10 to 20 mg t.i.d. or chlordiazepoxide 50 to 100 mg t.i.d.) to increase patient comfort. Oxazepam may be preferable in patients with liver damage. Other formulations that have shown promise in some settings are clonidine, propranolol, and atenolol.

The only FDA-approved medications for reducing the risk of drinking relapses are disulfiram and naltrexone. Disulfiram (Antabuse) is an alcohol-sensitizing agent that interrupts the metabolism of alcohol. The resulting accumulation of acetaldehyde leads to pronounced nausea and hypotension. The most common dose is 250 mg/day. Evidence of its effectiveness on long-term drinking patterns is mixed, in part because compliance is often a major problem. Few trials have reported gender-specific results. Highly motivated patients who specifically request disulfiram and are willing to let someone else monitor their use of it may find it helpful. Naltrexone is an opioid antagonist that has shown considerable promise in clinical trials. Results reported in the literature have either been pooled by gender or are limited to men, so its utility with women remains unknown. Most experts recommend prescription only by physicians familiar with addiction treatment and then only in conjunction with psychosoical interventions.

Social and mental health factors that should be considered during treatment planning include the nature and composition of the patient's family, her ability to find social support while making significant behavioral changes, and her overall outlook on life. Women with ongoing parenting responsibilities may not see inpatient or residential treatment as an option, unless they can be referred to a program with a child-care component. Some resist entering treatment because they fear the social stigma of being labeled as an alcoholic mother. The presence of other alcoholics or problem drinkers in the patient's home can be an additional barrier.

Many of these problems are best addressed with the assistance of an addiction treatment specialist. Referral to a self-help group can also be useful. AA has been criticized for its rigid insistence on total abstinence and its strong emphasis on spirituality, but millions of people worldwide credit the 12-step model as the key to their alcohol recovery. AA meetings differ markedly in terms of gender and social status composition. Many communities have a central referral office that can direct the patient to a suitable group. Smoke-free meetings are available in most areas.

When signs of depression are seen concurrently with problem drinking or alcoholism, decisions about simultaneous treatment with antidepressants should rest on the severity of symptoms and the patient's most recent consumption of alcohol. Clinical data on women undergoing intensive alcohol treatment have shown that depression symptoms often remit spontaneously after 3 to 4 weeks of continuous abstinence. However, some women continue to remain depressed, and psychiatric referral or treatment with standard antidepressants may be necessary. Findings from follow-up studies of female alcohol-treatment patients with a concurrent history of depression have yielded mixed results, suggesting that the long-term effects of depression on drinking are complex and difficult to predict.

How can the physician help a woman who is obviously drinking too much, but actively denies problems with alcohol? If the situation is not acute, an approach with the stages of readiness to change can be used. The physician should reemphasize his or her concern about the health consequences of heavy drinking and should urge the patient to start cutting down, or at least to start thinking about cutting down, as soon as possible. Although abstinence is the only long-term solution for women who alternate periods of heavy and then more controlled drinking, moderate drinking may be a more realistic and less threatening goal than abstinence for many problem drinkers. Arranging for follow-up visits to discuss progress underscores the seriousness of the physician's concern.

If the current level of drinking is high enough to put her at risk of harming herself or others, the physician should try to schedule a follow-up visit that includes several family members or close friends. *Gentle* confrontation in a caring environment is often sufficient to motivate a patient into treatment. Alternatively, she can be encouraged to seek care for a problem that may be related to her drinking (eg, depression or anxiety) and then referred to a therapist who is also experienced with the diagnosis and treatment of alcohol problems.

PREVENTION

Despite the tools now available to help patients stop smoking and resolve their problems with alcohol, prevention remains the most humane and cost-efficient option. Primary care practitioners are in an ideal position to intervene proactively, as they often provide primary care for adolescents and often have established long-term relationships with many of their patients. An emphasis on prevention can be shoehorned into even the busiest of offices. Revising clinic forms to prompt screening and intervention activities and encouraging staff to see prevention as an important practice goal are critical first steps. At well-child checks, the physician can reinforce the importance of making healthy choices and taking good care of their bodies. At sports physicals, the physician should ask about the use of tobacco and alcohol. Adolescents know that smoking is harmful, but they tend to underestimate the addictive potential of nicotine. When adolescent or adult patients are grieving or experiencing other acute situational stress, their coping processes should be noted. The office environment should be monitored as well: adolescents are particularly quick to spot mixed messages and are likely to notice if smoking is permitted on the premises or if clinic personnel smell of tobacco.

Finally, physicians may want to show their concern for the health consequences of smoking and alcohol problems by getting involved in community medicine. Physicians and other health care professionals are well positioned to influence local policies on adolescent access to alcohol and tobacco. There are many opportunities for cost-effective prevention efforts in most neighborhoods, such as lecturing in elementary and junior-high classrooms, working to ban cigarette vending machines, persuading owners of small grocery stores to forbid sales to minors, supporting higher taxes on tobacco and alcohol, and pushing for restrictions on product advertisements near schools and at local sporting events.

Acknowledgement

This work was supported in part by NIH grant AA09233 from the National Institute of Alcohol Abuse and Alcoholism to Dr. Bobo.

BIBLIOGRAPHY

Adams MM, Brogan DJ, Kendrick JS, Shulman HB, Zahniser SC, Bruce FC. Smoking, pregnancy, and source of prenatal care. Obstet Gynecol 1992;80:738.

American Psychiatric Association. Diagnostic and statistical manual of mental disorders, 4th ed. Washington DC: American Psychiatric Association, 1994.

Blot WJ, McLaughlin JK, Winn DM, et al. Smoking and drinking in relation to oral and pharyngeal cancer. Cancer Res 1988;48:3282.

Cornelius MD, Day NL, Cornelius JR, Geva D, Taylor PM, Richardson GA. Drinking patterns and correlates of drinking among pregnant teenagers. Alcohol Clin Exp Res 1993;17:290.

Fertig JB, Allen JP (eds). Alcohol and tobacco—from basic science to policy. NIAAA Monograph Series. DHHS: National Institute on Alcohol Abuse and Alcoholism, 1995.

Fiore MC, Jorenby DE, Baker TB, Kenford SL. Tobacco dependence and the nicotine patch. JAMA 1992;268:2687.

Fiore MC, Smith SS, Jorenby DE, Baker TB. The effectiveness of the nicotine patch for smoking cessation: a meta-analysis. JAMA 1994;271:1940.

Fiore MC, Wetter DW, Bailey WC, Bennet G, Cohen SJ. The Agency for Health Care Policy and Research Smoking Cessation Clinical Practice Guidelines. JAMA 1996;275:1270.

Glassman AH, Covey LS, Dalack GW, et al. Smoking cessation, clonidine, and vulnerability to nicotine among dependent smokers. Clin Pharmacol Ther 1993;54:670.

Glassman AH, Helzer JE, Corey LS, et al. Smoking, smoking cessation, and major depression. JAMA 1990;264:1546.

Hesselbrock MN, Meyer RE, Keener JJ. Psychopathology in hospitalized alcoholics. Arch Gen Psychiatry 1985;42:1050.

Hoffmann NG, Halikas JA, Mee-Lee D, Weedman RD. Patient placement criteria for the treatment of psychoactive substance use disorders. Am Soc Addic Med 1993;8:1.

Hughes JR. An algorithm for smoking cessation. Arch Fam Med 1994;3:280.

Lowinson JH, Ruiz P, Millman RB, Langrod JG (eds). Substance abuse: a comprehensive textbook. Baltimore: Williams & Wilkins, 1992.

Kendler KS, Heath AC, Neale MC, Kessler RC, Eaves LJ. A population-based twin study of alcoholism in women. JAMA 1992;268:1877.

Klatsky AL, Armstrong MA, Friedman GD. Alcohol and mortality. Ann Intern Med 1992;117:646.

MacKenzie TD, Bartecchi CE, Schrier RW. The human costs of tobacco use. N Engl J Med 1994;975.

Manley MW, Epps RP, Glynn TJ. The clinician's role in promoting smoking cessation among clinic patients. Med Clin North Am 1992;76:477.

Miller WR, Rollnick S. Motivational interviewing—preparing people to change addictive behavior. New York: Guilford Press, 1991.

Orleans CT, Slade J (eds). Nicotine addiction—principles and management. New York: Oxford University Press, 1993.

Pierce JP, Lee L, Gilpin EA. Smoking initiation by adolescent girls, 1944 through 1988; an association with targeted advertising. JAMA 1994;271:608.

Prochaska JO, Goldstein MG. Process of smoking cessation; implications for clinicians. Clin Chest Med 1991;12:727.

Risch HA, Howe GR, Jain M, Burch JD, Holowaty EJ, Miller AB. Are female smokers at higher risk for lung cancer than male smokers? A case-control analysis by histologic type. Am J Epidemiol 1993; 138:281.

Rosenberg L, Metzger LS, Palmer JR. Alcohol consumption and risk of breast cancer: a review of the epidemiologic evidence. Epidemiol Rev 1993;15:133.

Silagy C, Mant D, Fowler G, Lodge M. Meta-analysis on efficacy of nicotine replacement therapies in smoking cessation. Lancet 1994;343:139.

Smith EM, Cloninger CR, Bradford S. Predictors of mortality in alcoholic women: a prospective follow-up study. Alcohol Clin Exp Res 1983;7:237.

U.S. DHHS. Special issue on women and alcohol. Alcohol Health and Research World 1994;18:169.

U.S. DHHS. The health benefits of smoking cessation: a report of the Surgeon General. Rockville, Md.: Centers for Disease Control, Center for Chronic Disease Prevention and Health Promotion, Office of Smoking and Health, 1990.

U.S. DHHS. Special report to the US Congress on alcohol and health from the Secretary of Human Services. Rockville, Md.: National Institute on Alcohol Abuse and Alcoholism, 1993.

U.S. Institute of Medicine. Broadening the base of treatment for alcohol problems. Washington DC: National Academy Press, 1990.

Wilcox AJ. Birth weight and perinatal mortality: the effect of maternal smoking. Am J Epidemiol 1993;137:1098.

Willett WC, Green A, Stampfer MJ, et al. Relative and absolute excess risks of coronary heart disease among women who smoke cigarettes. N Engl J Med 1987;317:1303.

Wilsnack SC, Klassen AD, Schur BE, Wilsnack RW. Predicting onset and chronicity of women's problem drinking: a five-year longitudinal analysis. Am J Public Health 1991;81:305.

Primary Care for Women, edited by Phyllis C. Leppert and Fred M. Howard. Lippincott-Raven Publishers, Philadelphia © 1997.

II

Age Specific Issues in Women's Health Care

7

Newborns and Children

PHYLLIS C. LEPPERT

"It's a girl!" With these words, new parents immediately begin to dream of their daughter's future. The new mother will imagine her life to come: how she will learn to be a woman; what a future husband might be like; and whether or not she will become a scientist, or perhaps a successful businesswoman. The new father might imagine that she will succeed in soccer, or rowing, or basketball. But both parents will probably give a baby girl a different style of mothering and fathering than they would give to a boy. This different style is based on the feelings of the young parents toward their relationship as a couple, their relationship to their own mothers, and the customs of their society. Perhaps the new mother will be very gentle with her baby girl.

Every culture, through individual families, has its own rituals of teaching the ways of society to children, beginning with the manner in which each child is received. In some families, the arrival of a girl is treated differently from the arrival of a boy. If the new parents wanted a boy, the adjustment to parenthood may be more prolonged than usual. All the routines of newborn care—feeding, bathing, dressing, sleeping, diaper changing, holding, and rocking—tend to give an infant security. These routines are not exactly the same for girls as they are for boys. The rearing of a baby girl tends to be gentle, and girls are usually raised in an environment where they may express emotions. Thus, not only is the newborn girl physically different from a boy, she is also socially different from the moment of birth. Now that parents may learn the sex of the fetus in early pregnancy, perhaps this difference is noted then. How a baby girl's society views her role will determine her future health and well-being, just as critically as her anatomy and physiology do.

This chapter will focus on the basic health issues unique to female infants and young girls. More definitive pediatric textbooks discuss in depth all aspects of newborn and childhood care.

EMBRYOLOGY OF THE FEMALE

Figure 7-1 illustrates differentiation of male and female internal genitalia. In the early embryo, the gonads of males and females are indistinguishable. The external genitalia are female-like and undifferentiated. Müllerian and wolffian ducts exist side by side at the sixth and seventh week of embryonic development. By 8 or 9 weeks gestation, the gonads are distinguishable by sex. Ovarian differentiation occurs slightly later than testicular differentiation, both under the control of genetics. Genes also control the differentiation of the müllerian and wolffian ducts. Genes code for a testicular determining factor on the Y chromosome. However, autosomal genes are also necessary for the development of the normal ovary and normal testes. Autosomal genes act at a site common to early germ cell development.

In the absence of a Y chromosome, the undifferentiated gonad develops into an ovary. 45,X human fetuses have germ cells, but by birth the ovarian follicles have degenerated. In XY gonadal dysgenesis, oocytes are seen. Ovarian maintenance genes exist on both the short and long arm of the X chromosome.

In the absence of testosterone and the absence of the antimüllerian hormone, the müllerian ducts develop into a uterus and fallopian tubes and the external genitalia develop female characteristics. Hormones, such as androgens taken during pregnancy, also affect the appearance of the external genitalia.

NORMAL NEWBORN AND CHILDHOOD GROWTH AND DEVELOPMENT

The genitalia of a normal newborn respond to hormones. Maternal estrogen passively crosses the placenta. In newborn girls, this can cause vulvar edema, vaginal discharge, and a prominent hymen. The newborn vaginal epithelium contains glycogen-rich cells due to estrogen stimulation, and the physiologic vaginal discharge is similar to that of a woman of reproductive age. Ten percent of female newborns experience some estrogen withdrawal bleeding. Enlargement of breast tissue in both sexes may be noted in the newborn period, and two thirds of these babies secrete colostrum-like fluid followed by a small amount of milk. These hormonal effects of estrogen resolve in the first 6 to 8 weeks of life, but the hymen may remain thick and redundant-appearing up to age 2

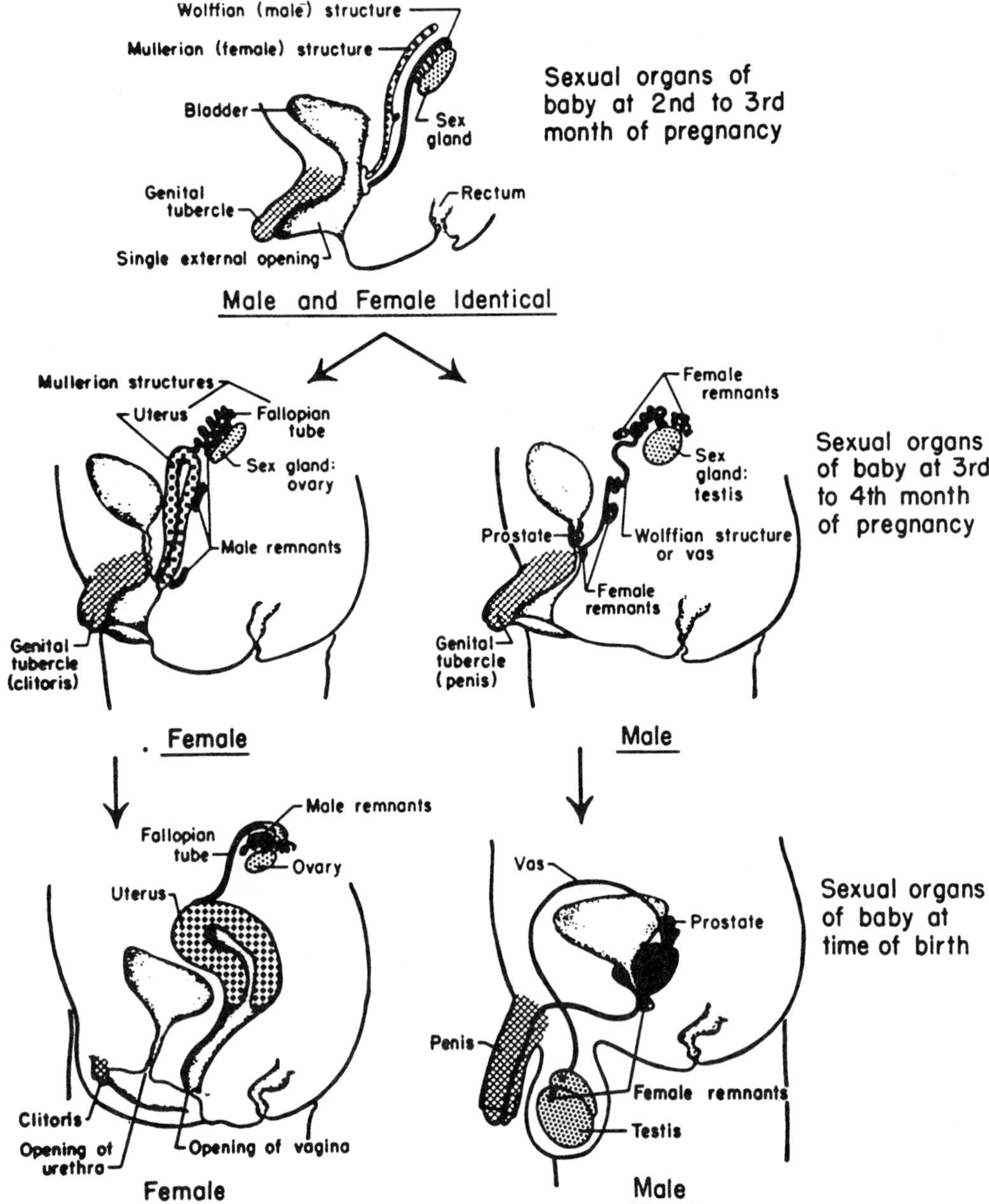

Figure 7-1. Teaching diagram: differentiation of the internal genitalia. (Money J. Psychological aspects of disorders of sexual differentiation. In: Carpenter SE, Rock JA, eds. Pediatric and adolescent gynecology. New York: Raven Press, 1992:109. Reproduced by permission.)

years. A preterm female infant appears to have a relatively large clitoris; this is normal. Once out of the neonatal period, a time of quiescence is noted until puberty is reached. The infant uterus, stimulated by maternal estrogens prior to birth, decreases in size; not until age 5 does the uterus regains its newborn size.

Infants and children grow rapidly and pass through incredible developmental periods, affected by both heredity and the environment. This ever-changing aspect of the child's development makes the evaluation of her situation challenging because the physician must be alert to reevaluation of these elements. Because infants and young girls are fragile physically and emotionally, the pediatric practitioner must understand their social environment and help the family and society to enable them to reach their potential. Infants and young children have a collection of personal characteristics called temperament. This collection includes (1) activity level; (2) rhythmicity; (3) approach or withdrawal from new stimuli; (4) adaptability; (5) intensity of reaction; (6) responsiveness threshold; (7) mood; (8) distractibility; and (9) attention span and persistence. Gender and birth order have been associated with certain behaviors. In general, infant girls are less irritable and become calm more readily than infant boys. First-born boys are thought to be more irritable than second-born boys. Girls are thought to be more neurologically mature at birth and, thus, may have less random activity and distractibility. Parents may reinforce these traits in girls over time.

Intelligence, defined in Western societies as a series of traits, includes the use of language, use of numbers, discrimination of objects in space, separation of an element from its background, problem solving, reasoning, and mastery of concepts. Not all of these skills are present at birth, nor are they all learned in childhood: they are acquired throughout childhood, adolescence, and young adulthood. The sex differences in some areas begin in adolescence. Females score higher on verbal ability, and males score, in general, higher in spatial and mathematic abilities. However, boys raised in father-absent families have a reversal of these abilities, and girls in mother-absent families have more "male" abilities, indicating that environmental factors may modify what was previously considered due to heredity.

A girl's family, school, and peer groups greatly influence her social, psychological, physical, and intellectual development. Proposed reasons for lower achievement in science by girls in grade school and high school include low expectations by families, educators, and peers. The National Assessment of Educational Progress shows gaps in science achievement scores between girls and boys as early as age 9. Studies show that self-confidence in math is an important determinant of success in science. Therefore, with family support, supportive learning environments, and highly qualified, caring teachers and mentors, girls can achieve their potential. Practitioners caring for girls must encourage parents to help develop their daughters' intelligence. Girls also need to be encouraged to be active physically in sports and athletic events, as active exercise is essential for health and well-being.

All children pass through psychosocial, cognitive, and social learning stages. In terms of psychosocial growth and development, female infants and children must learn to develop basic trust in others and in themselves. They then must learn to develop autonomy, which implies self-control, self-esteem, and a sense of pride. Finally, young girls develop initiative and a sense of goals to be achieved. Cognitive skills in infancy focus on progressing from reflex to purposeful activity and rudimentary thought. In early childhood, prelogical thought progresses into the development of language and the use of symbols. Young girls develop socially from being centered on themselves and their own behavior at first, to a stage in which learning is family-centered.

PHYSICAL EXAMINATION OF NEWBORNS AND CHILDREN

The most important aspect of the physical examination of newborns and young girls is the physician's gentleness and patience. These qualities are essential for all aspects of the pediatric examination, but the genital examination of a prepubescent female demands the most gentleness and patience. Any lack of rapport with the infant girl or older child prevents an adequate examination. Furthermore, roughness or lack of patience might pose a risk of inadvertent nosocomial sexual abuse. Before the examination, the physician must explain the process of the examination to the mother and child in terms they understand. Any instruments used, such as a Cameron-Miller vaginoscope, must be explained. The mother must understand that the hymen will not be "broken," because normally a virginal introitus is not completely covered by the hymen.

An initial evaluation of the hormonally sensitive tissue gives the physician information as to the girl's endocrine status. Information about sex steroid production can be determined by breast development, vaginal mucosal maturation index, pattern of hair growth, and apocrine gland activity. The abdomen must be carefully examined as well, because an ovarian mass would be palpated as an abdominal mass rather than as a pelvic mass. An inguinal hernia could represent an undescended testis in a child with undiagnosed male pseudohermaphroditism. Inspection of the external genitalia, including the clitoris, labia, perineal body, and hymen should be carried out carefully. In newborns, this is easily accomplished with the infant supine. For examination of the vaginal vault and cervix, the knee-chest position is superior (Fig. 7-2).

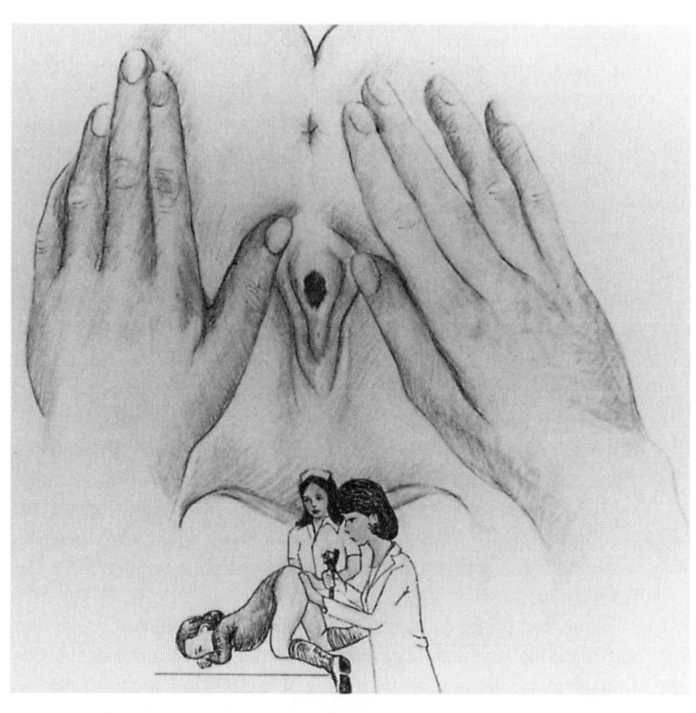

Figure 7-2. Examination of the prepubertal child in the knee-chest position. (Emans SJ, Goldstein DP, eds. Pediatric and adolescent gynecology. Boston: Little Brown, 1982.)

The ovaries and uterus may be palpated on rectal examination. Ovaries are not completely quiescent in the prepubertal period, so functional cysts may be present. Ovarian cysts are considered abnormal in girls under age 12 years if the cysts are greater than 9 mm in diameter. Any ovarian cyst that does not resolve in 6 to 8 weeks, or any cyst with sonographic findings suggesting a malignancy, must be evaluated by surgical exploration. In young girls, ovarian cysts more commonly become subject to torsion than do cysts in adult women.

Occasionally, a young girl must be examined under anesthesia to complete an adequate examination. An examination under anesthesia is mandatory in cases of undiagnosed vaginal bleeding, especially with a history of trauma.

CHILDHOOD VULVAR DISEASE, VAGINAL DISCHARGE, AND VAGINAL BLEEDING

Labial adhesions are probably due to the hypoestrogenic state of a prepubescent girl. They are often asymptomatic and do not require therapy, as they spontaneously resolve at puberty. Parents may mistake labial adhesions as vaginal agenesis, so reassurance of the family is paramount. If treatment of labial lesions is required because of interference with urination or drainage of vaginal secretions, the parent should apply an estrogen cream twice a day for 2 weeks, then once a day, usually at bedtime, for 1 or 2 more weeks. At that time, there should be complete resolution of the problem. When the cream is applied, gentle traction on the line of the adhesion is necessary. Some authorities recommend further application of Vaseline for a few weeks to a month with the goal of preventing re-formation of the adhesions.

Sexually transmitted diseases are not uncommon in prepubescent girls. They may be due to sexual molestation or transmission from the mother. Gonococci infect the thin vaginal epithelium and produce a vaginal discharge that can cause vulvar irritation. The infection should be treated with soothing lotions or cool sitz baths. If the urethra is irritated by the vaginal discharge, voiding may be uncomfortable. Cool sitz baths or soothing lotions are again helpful. In children, the gonococcus does not usually cause cystitis. Because the gonococcus does not infect the vaginal epithelium after the menarche, an older method of treatment was to use intravaginal estrogen suppositories to produce a thickening of the vaginal epithelium. This treatment is no longer current. Modern treatment is one dose of ceftriaxone, 125 mg intramuscularly, for children under 40 kg, or 250 mg for those above 45 kg. Alternatively, streptomycin 40 mg/kg intramuscularly can be used if one dose is given. A child over age 8 should also receive 100 mg doxycycline every 12 hours for 7 days.

Congenital syphilis is a serious disease transmitted to the infant by an infected mother. It is diagnosed by tests of the blood serum and must be treated with adequate doses of penicillin to prevent systemic sequelae. It is customary to test the mother's blood or cord blood obtained at delivery, or both, to screen for congenital syphilis. Syphilis acquired in childhood is difficult to diagnose. In children, the chancre is usually seen as a superficial ulceration with marked edema. Lymphadenitis is common as well, but is usually not tender. The condition is diagnosed by appropriate blood tests and is treated with penicillin, or erythromycin in the case of penicillin allergy. Retreatment is necessary if there is a sustained fourfold increase in titer, or if clinical signs and symptoms recur. After adequate treatment, there should be a fourfold decrease in the original titers.

Herpes simplex can be transmitted to an infant from an infected mother at the time of birth. Most pregnant women are followed carefully for evidence of herpes simplex because it is a serious disease in infancy. However, herpetic lesions may not have been apparent during pregnancy, although the mother was infected. Therefore, herpetic lesions seen in the first week of life point to maternal transmission. The most serious form of the disease in newborns is herpetic encephalitis. Herpes simplex may be acquired in childhood by sexual contact. The lesions have a classic appearance and the diagnosis is usually easily made: herpes culture, immunofluorescence test, and the Tzank reaction are confirmatory. Acyclovir orally four times a day for 5 days has been given to children age 3 years and older without complications or adverse effects. For infections in the first year of life, 30 mg/kg of acyclovir daily in divided doses every 8 hours is suggested. Other sexually transmitted diseases need to be searched for, as they may also be present.

Condyloma acuminata may be transmitted to the infant at the time of birth or from sexual contact. The incubation period of the human papillomavirus (HPV) may be as long as 3 to 6 months, so the lesions acquired at birth may not be apparent until 6 months later. HPV may infect the larynx, causing serious respiratory difficulties. The HPV should be typed if possible. The lesions should be treated using a fine-wire cautery tip. In children, the procedure should be done under general anesthesia. Condyloma has been seen in the vagina, urethra, and perianal area as well as the vulva.

Molluscum contagiosum may affect the vulva of young girls. It must be diagnosed by biopsy using a small key punch under local anesthesia. Spontaneous remission usually occurs in 3 months.

Candidiasis of the vulva is common in children. The pruritus may cause the child to scratch the infected area. A topical antifungal cream such as miconazole or terconazole is effective. Some authorities recommend a 1% to 2% hydrocortisone cream for intense pruritus.

Eczema, vitiligo, and lichen sclerosus may occur. Dermatitis of the vulva may be produced by irritation from a vaginal infection. A foreign body in the vagina may cause dermatitis due to a discharge; therefore, vulvar dermatitis should alert the physician to consider a foreign body as an etiology. Dermatitis may be a major problem, as the local irritation is difficult to treat. Thus, all efforts should be made to identify the cause of the irritation and to eliminate it.

In infants, diaper rash can be treated with zinc oxide or, in serious cases, with 1% hydrocortisone cream.

Tumors of the vulva include hemangioma, the initial treatment for which is observation and reassurance. Malignant tumors, such as carcinoma and embryonal rhabdomyosarcoma, are extremely rare.

The vagina at birth is stimulated from estrogen and has, therefore, thickened epithelium, but by a few weeks this epithelium has become smooth, thin, and atrophic. The vagina in a young girl is a good environment for bacterial growth because of its neutral pH and because it lacks the antibodies found later in life. In addition, the prepubertal girl has no labial fat pads, no pubic hair, small labia minora, and a rectum in close proximity to the vagina, which contribute to the tendency to acquire vulvovaginitis. Poor hygiene, including incorrectly cleaning the perineum from the rectal area to the vulva, contributes to the problem as well. Young girls must be instructed that proper perineal hygiene includes wiping from the front to the back.

Specific causes of vaginal discharge are pinworm infestation and chemical irritants. The classic symptoms of pinworm infestation are perianal and vulvar itching at night. The diagnosis can be made by parents who are instructed to inspect the vulva at night, as pinworms can be observed at that time. Alternatively, the pinworm eggs can be recovered on cellophane tape applied to the rectum. The treatment is one 100-mg dose of oral mebendazole given to the child and all members of the household over age 2 years. Some young girls are especially sensitive to bubble baths, perfumes, or soaps, which can act as irritants and cause vulvar vaginitis. The chemical irritant should be discontinued and the girl should be taught to practice good perineal hygiene.

Any girl who develops vaginal bleeding before puberty must be examined carefully. Causes include urethral prolapse; hemangioma; neoplasms; precocious puberty; the presence of a foreign body, most commonly toilet paper; and genital trauma, due to sexual abuse or bicycle or straddle injuries. It is rare for a blood dyscrasia to present as vaginal bleeding in a prepubescent female, although this finding is a common cause of excessive bleeding at menarche.

TRAUMA TO THE VULVA AND VAGINA AND SEXUAL ABUSE OF FEMALE CHILDREN

Trauma to the vulva and vagina may occur accidentally or as the result of sexual abuse. One study reported that about 90% of perineal injuries to girls were due to sexual abuse. However, the trauma might be the result of an accidental injury. With vulvar or vaginal injury in a young girl, a seemingly minor injury can in actuality be very extensive. Therefore, vaginal bleeding in a child age 4 to 12 years must be investigated by an examination under anesthesia for possible extension of a laceration into the peritoneum, broad ligament, bladder, or rectum. Vulvar and perineal trauma followed by microscopic hematuria must be evaluated by a computed tomography (CT) scan. If there is gross hematuria, then both a CT scan and a voiding cystourethrogram are necessary.

The examination of a young girl with trauma begins with the classic primary survey. First, the airway must be evaluated and maintained. Breathing, circulation, and neurologic status are quickly and accurately assessed, followed by an assessment for gross bleeding. Accurate and complete written documentation is necessary. Only if these parameters are stable can a further examination be done. Sedation is recommended before the examination of the perineum. The labia are gently retracted and the examiner looks closely for hematomas, blood, and feces. In a prepubertal girl, rectal and abdominal examination should be performed. A small hematoma of the vulva may be treated conservatively, but any hematoma of the vulva that appears to be extensive or expanding must be opened under general anesthesia and bleeding points ligated appropriately. A vaginal inspection using small vaginoscopes or small nasal specula must be conducted. If a bladder injury is suspected, a cystoscopic examination should be carried out. A rectoscopic examination should be conducted for suspected anorectal trauma. Penetration of the wound to the peritoneum requires an exploratory laparotomy.

The vulva and vagina of young girls may be accidentally injured in several ways. Straddle injuries, thought to account for 75% of all accidental genital injuries, occur commonly as the result of straddling playground or gym equipment or the center bar of a boy's bicycle. These injuries usually involve the mons pubis, clitoris, urethra, and anterior labia minora and labia majora. They usually do not extend to the vagina. These lesions may be treated conservatively by moist compresses and careful observation. Antibiotics and analgesics should be prescribed. Accidental penetration by foreign bodies is another way in which a young girl's vulva and vagina may be injured. A girl may fall accidentally on a sharp object, or pens, pencils, crayons, or other foreign bodies may be placed in the vagina as a result of curiosity or self-manipulation. These accidents are common among 2- to 4-year-old girls. Sometimes ecchymosis or an obvious puncture wound is observed, but it is not unusual for a child to present with hematuria, vaginal discharge, or bleeding. As mentioned previously, small pieces of toilet tissue can be lodged in the vagina and cause bleeding as well as discharge. Buttons, coins, and toys have all been recovered from the vagina. Any persistent vaginal discharge in a young girl or toddler requires a vaginal examination for detection of a foreign body. Removal of a foreign body that has been in the vaginal vault for a prolonged time should be preceded by the initiation of antibiotic therapy. The vagina can also be injured when a young girl is held directly over a swimming pool fountain, as the high-pressure force of the water causes trauma. The perineum and vagina can be injured in water skiing and motor vehicle accidents in which lacerations occur because of sudden abduction of the lower extremities.

The incidence of sexual abuse of children is difficult to estimate. It has been reported to occur in 7% of reported cases of maltreatment of children. However, many authorities believe that the true incidence is higher than the actual reported cases. Victims may repress sexual abuse. Surveys have suggested that as many as 20% of women reported unwanted sexual experiences during childhood, although these studies may be biased. Child sexual abuse is often overlooked by medical personnel.

The legal definition of child sexual abuse includes sexual contact, fondling, intrusion into body orifices, or forcing a child to fondle or perform fellatio on the abuser. It also includes other acts such as exhibitionism, involvement in child pornography, and deliberate exposure of a child to sexually explicit photographs or materials. Such abuse usually begins with acts that confuse a child but do not harm her; then they slowly increase in intensity.

Because the young child is especially dependent and therefore vulnerable, sexual abuse begins in many victims in the first few years of life. This child feels misled and fearful. The physical examination of such a child is carried out with respect for the child's family and their privacy. The examination must be gentle and care must be taken so that the examiner does not reinforce the child's sense of victimization. The examination must be thorough from head to toe. This gives the examiner an opportunity to gain the child's trust and to allow the child to become accustomed to the physician's touch. The provider should also examine for evidence of sexual abuse in other parts of the body, such as mouth, breasts, and abdomen. Careful documentation must be performed. Time and patience are vital. The primary care clinician would then refer a child and family to the appropriate facility for further multidisciplinary care.

Female circumcision is practiced in 26 African countries and occurs among many immigrants to the United States and Canada. Girls are usually circumcised during ages 4 to 10, but some cultures perform the procedure on infants. Toubia classified female circumcision into four types. Type I, or Sunna circumcision, involves the removal of part or all of the clitoris. Type II involves the excision of the clitoris and part of the labia minora. Bleeding from the clitoral artery and raw surfaces is stemmed by sutures of catgut or thorn, or by the application of poultices. Type III is a modified or intermediate infibulation and involves the removal of the clitoris and labia minora, and incision into the labia majora. This creates raw surfaces that are stretched together. The anterior two thirds of the labia majora are stretched together in this manner. Type IV is total infibulation: the clitoris is removed, the labia minora is removed, and the labia majora is incised and stretched together to cover the entrance of the vagina with a hood of skin: only a very small posterior opening is left for the passage of urine and menstrual blood. Complications of these procedures are hemorrhage, severe pain, and shock and death in some cases. Severe anemia and local and systemic infections also can occur. Long-term complications include chronic pelvic infections, chronic urinary tract infections, and renal damage. Dermoid cysts may form along the scar, and severe dyspareunia may occur. Childbirth represents other risks. Severe perineal tears may occur, and fetal death and vesicovaginal fistula formation also have been reported. Women who have undergone infibulation need not be delivered by cesarean section; a deinfibulation procedure should be done to allow a vaginal birth.

In 1992, the International Federation of Gynecology and Obstetrics and the World Health Organization published a joint statement condemning female circumcision, and in 1993 the World Health Assembly issued a similar statement. As Toubia stated, no ethical defense can be made for preserving a cultural practice that damages a woman's health. But it is important to become familiar with the cause and meanings of cultural practices, and realize that it may take time and new information for people to abandon a traditional practice. In this case, the practice ensures a good marriage in a culture where marriage is essential in a woman's life and where she has no other options.

CONGENITAL DEFECTS OF THE GENITALIA, INCLUDING AMBIGUOUS GENITALIA

The parents' first look at their newborn infant establishes in a few brief seconds the sex of that person for a lifetime. Usually, a rapid glance at the external genitalia is sufficient. This is so innate an event that an infant born with ambiguous genitalia is a difficult event for all present at the birth. The birth of any infant with this condition is an emergency. The midwife or obstetrician must explain immediately that the sex of the child cannot be determined by a simple examination. The parents must be told that a number of examinations are needed before deciding the sex of the child. Help must be obtained from a team consisting of a pediatrician, an endocrinologist, a gynecologist, a urologist, and a psychologist experienced in the difficulties of the diagnosis of sex differentiation. The family is told that laboratory tests will take several days to be determined. Initially, the physicians treating the infant and the family must keep a neutral opinion regarding the sex, using words such as *baby*, *gonads*, and *phallus* (rather than penis or clitoris). When the appropriate sex is decided, the baby must be given a first name that is unequivocally masculine or feminine.

The birth of an infant with ambiguous genitalia is sometimes a medical emergency as well. This occurs when the genetic mutation that produced the ambiguous genitalia produces life-threatening symptoms. Thus, once a day the levels of serum electrolytes and glucose must be checked. The baby needs to be weighed daily. In the case of the salt-losing forms of congenital adrenal hyperplasia (21-hydroxylase, 3-B hydroxy steroid dehydrogenase, isomerase deficiencies), acute adrenal crisis of hyponatremia, hyperkalemia, and hypoglycemia develop between days 2 and 6 of life. This is accompanied by dehydration and marked weight loss of the baby in acute adrenal crisis. Without therapy, death occurs.

It is important early in life to establish the preferred sex for rearing of the child. This decision is best made during the first month of life. It seems to be difficult to make a sex change after age 1 or 2. Assignment of sex is complex and is best handled by an expert medical team; therefore, prompt referral to a tertiary care facility is mandatory. Figure 7-3 shows the pathology related to ambiguous genitalia based on the karyotype.

The primary care provider must also be alert for symptoms and observations that suggest a congenital anomaly of the uterus. These symptoms become evident in adolescence and young adulthood and include difficulty using tampons, dysmenorrhea, menorrhagia, difficulty with intercourse, and a palpable mass. The congenital uterine anomaly may first be noted on an intravenous pyelogram, at the time of dilatation and curettage, or on a pelvic ultrasound. During pregnancy, fetal malpresentation, abnormal uterine contour, or a pregnancy despite the presence of an intrauterine device suggests the possibility of a uterine anomaly.

PRECOCIOUS PUBERTY

Puberty is usually considered precocious if it occurs before age 8. Precocious puberty is classified as central or true precocious puberty, or as independent of pituitary gonadotropin. Most situations in girls are deemed central puberty in origin. In early development of precocious puberty, no organic lesion is found, but the onset is at an early age. CNS tumors, such as hypothalamic

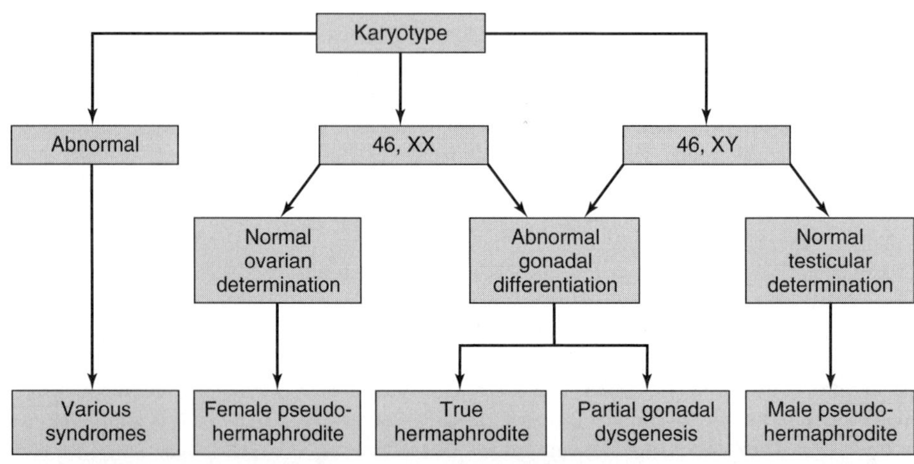

Figure 7-3. Scheme for the determination of the pathology related to ambiguous genitalia based on the karyotype. In 46,XY infants with normal testicular formation, the condition is termed male pseudohermaphroditism. In 46,XX infants with normal ovarian formation, the condition is termed female pseudohermaphroditism. In 46,XX or 46,XY infants with abnormal gonadal differentiation, the condition may be true hermaphroditism or partial gonadal dysgenesis. (Carpenter SE, Rock JA, eds. Pediatric and adolescent gynecology. New York: Raven Press, 1992. Reproduced by permission.)

hematomas, may cause precocious puberty. Other tumors, gliomas, neurofibromas, and hydrocephalus also cause precocious puberty. Other causes are head trauma, encephalitis, meningitis, and CNS irradiation.

Central precocious puberty is associated with a linear growth velocity, advanced skeletal age, and luteinizing hormone (LH) and follicle-stimulating hormone (FSH) in the pubertal range. Multiple samples of LH and FSH are needed, particularly at night. The infusion of gonadotropin-releasing hormone (GnRH) causes the levels of LH and FSH to fluctuate, so sampling should be done at regular intervals.

Treatment with GnRH agonists is the treatment of choice, although it is not approved by the FDA. Factors that determine if this treatment is desirable are the girl's age, her psychosocial adjustment, and the rapidity of the progression of the precocious puberty. For instance, a 2-year-old clearly would benefit from treatment, but it might not be desirable to treat a 7-year-old.

The second type of precocious puberty is due to a source of estrogen independent of the pituitary excretion of gonadotropin. Examples are ovarian or adrenal estrogen-producing tumors and severe and prolonged hypothyroidism (associated with the formation of multicystic ovaries). One form of primary hypothyroidism is associated with pituitary enlargement, galactorrhea, and precocious puberty.

A child with McCune-Albright syndrome has café-au-lait spots, polyostotic fibrous dysplasia, and precocious puberty. Breast development and vaginal bleeding are sometimes associated with increased estradiol levels in conjunction with one or more ovarian cysts. The treatment of McCune-Albright syndrome is with medroxyprogesterone acetate and testolactone.

A thorough search for a source of exogenous estrogen must be made. A young girl may ingest oral contraceptives or use skin creams containing estrogen. One authority cites eating of meat of an estrogen-treated animal as a cause of precocious puberty.

Isolated abnormal breast development can occur, usually between ages 1 and 4, for various reasons. Although no treatment is usually given, close follow-up is indicated.

Premature adrenarche or the appearance of pubic hair before age 8 can also be noted. This is often due to adrenal androgen secretion. Late-onset adrenal hyperplasia may present as premature adrenarche.

A young girl with any abnormality of premature sexual development must be referred to a physician with an interest and expertise in pediatric endocrinology.

HIRSUTISM

Virilization is caused by excessive androgen from adrenal gland tumors, congenital adrenal hyperplasia, or ovarian tumors. Masculinization occurs in girls with extremely elevated androgen levels. It is demonstrated by upper body obesity, temporal and frontal baldness, clitoromegaly, hirsutism, prevention or absence of breast development, and an increase in muscle mass. The physician must be alert to an androgen-producing tumor or congenital adrenal hyperplasia as a cause.

However, hirsutism may be seen in some situations without androgen excess, including acromegaly and chronic skin irritation. Phenytoin and oxandrolone cause hypertrichosis, not hirsutism. Hypertrichosis is increased vellus hair, giving a "fuzzy" look. Androgenic causes are androgenic drugs: occasionally a young girl ingests danazol, methyltestosterone, or stanozolol. Young girls with incomplete testicular feminization or XY gonadal dysgenesis develop hirsutism, clitoromegaly, and breast development in the peripubertal period.

Congenital adrenal hyperplasia, discussed previously, is a syndrome representing several different enzyme deficiencies in the adrenocortical synthesis of cortisol. This leads to masculinization and hirsutism. Late-onset adrenal hyperplasia is a disease all primary care providers should be aware of, as 1% to 6% of girls or women with various degrees of hirsutism have this problem. Treatment is with corticosteroid replacement. Hirsutism is seen in hyperandrogenism, insulin resistance, acanthosis nigricans syndrome, Cushing syndrome, androgenic tumors, and hyperthecosis (islands of hyperplastic luteinized theca cells seen in polycystic ovarian syndrome). Occasionally, a girl with hirsutism has normal free and total androgen levels, and after repeated studies her hirsutism is labeled idiopathic.

A workup for hirsutism includes a careful history of drug use, the progression of pubertal development, any history of vaginal bleeding, and the onset and progression of the hirsutism. Often, acne is noted along with the condition. A physical examination should be carefully conducted to observe for other signs of androgen excess, such as Tanner staging, clitoromegaly, and cushingoid features. Attention should be paid to other endocrine glands, such as the thyroid gland. Appropriate laboratory evaluations should be carried out to determine total and free serum testosterone, sex hormone-binding globules, dehydroepiandrosterone sulfate (DHEAS), and 17-hydroxyprogesterone.

TUMORS OF THE VULVA, VAGINA, CERVIX, UTERINE CORPUS, AND OVARY

Tumors of the reproductive tract in the newborn and young girl are very uncommon. Because of their rarity, neoplasms may be confused with other conditions, leading to serious delays in diagnosis and treatment.

Vulvar lesions must be carefully evaluated. The most common neoplasm of the lower genital tract in infants and young girls is embryonal rhabdomyosarcoma of the botryoid type. Endodermal sinus tumors may be seen in the infant vagina. Clear cell adenocarcinoma has been seen in the vagina and cervix of infants and young girls exposed to diethylstilbestrol (DES) in utero. The use of DES decreased in the mid-1950s, so these tumors should be rare today. In children, the most common clinical symptom of uterine tumors is vaginal bleeding, so a genital neoplasm must be seriously entertained as a cause. Only 5% of all ovarian malignancies occur in children and adolescents. Almost two thirds of these tumors are germ cell tumors.

BIBLIOGRAPHY

Carpenter SE, Rock JA, eds. Pediatric and adolescent gynecology. New York: Raven Press, 1992.

Emans SJH, Goldstein DP, eds. Pediatric and adolescent gynecology. Boston: Little, Brown & Co., 1982.

Hoekelman R, Friedman SB, Nelson NM, Seidil HM. Primary pediatric care, 2d ed. St. Louis: Mosby Year Book, 1992.

Money J, Lamacz M. Genital examination and exposure experience as nosocomial sexual abuse in childhood. J Nerv Ment Dis 1987;175:713.

Toubia N. Female circumcision as a public health issue. N Eng J Med 1994;331:11.

Primary Care for Women, edited by Phyllis C. Leppert and Fred M. Howard. Lippincott-Raven Publishers, Philadelphia © 1997.

8
Adolescent Health Care Issues

JONATHAN D. KLEIN
RICHARD E. KREIPE

Adolescents receive care from many different types of primary care providers. In this chapter, we review the biologic, psychological, and social developmental issues characteristic of adolescents, issues in communicating with adolescents and their families, and the effect that these issues may have on some of the major health problems affecting young women. We review the major causes of morbidity and mortality of young women, preventable health problems amenable to primary care interventions, and the special health care needs and issues of greatest concern to practitioners. Finally, special issues affecting the accessibility and availability of primary care services to adolescents are discussed.

THE BIOPSYCHOSOCIAL MODEL APPLIED TO ADOLESCENT DEVELOPMENT

The biopsychosocial model is an appropriate paradigm for the primary care of adolescent females because it recognizes the complex interaction of the biologic, psychological, and social phenomena that influence individuals during this stage of development. In many situations in primary health care for adolescent females, a biopsychosocial approach, although time-consuming, is essential. For instance, a biologic problem such as diabetes mellitus in a 14-year-old girl will affect, and will be influenced by, her psychological development and social interactions with family and peers. A psychological problem such as depression in a 15-year-old girl may result, or begin, in loss of friends and social isolation, but it may also be associated with a biologic deficiency of CNS neurotransmitters, such as serotonin; depression resulting from either cause could lead to a suicide attempt. A social problem such as recurrent runaway behavior in a 16-year-old may be associated with numerous other high-risk behaviors, including substance abuse, exposure to sexually transmitted diseases or unintended pregnancy, and violence.

Thus, the "psychosocial" aspects of primary care adolescent medicine are best incorporated into the overall care of the adolescent, not just after specific behavioral problems arise. The physician must be observant and must become acquainted with the adolescent, as well as the adolescent's family, peers, and school. He or she must interview in a style that resembles conversation more than interrogation and must take a developmentally oriented approach to the patient and a systems-oriented approach to the family.

Physical Growth and Development

Adolescent growth and development during puberty are characterized by the biologic changes that accompany puberty. The most visible changes of puberty, beginning for girls between ages 8 and 14, result from the gonadal hormones affecting the maturation of the musculoskeletal and reproductive systems. Equally significant but less obvious changes occur in the adolescent's cognitive abilities, with the onset of a young woman's abilities to engage in formal operational thought. Additionally, adolescents undergo a predictable process of psychosocial development. Each of these developmental processes may affect the health of young women.

Clinicians may find it useful to consider four tasks of adolescence that relate to these pubertal, cognitive, and psychosocial developmental processes. The tasks necessary to enter adulthood are (1) acceptance of the physical changes resulting in an adult body and reproductive capability, (2) attainment of independence and autonomy from the family of origin, (3) emergence of a stable identity, and (4) development of adult thinking patterns.

Key concepts with respect to adolescent female pubertal growth and development include secular trend, sequencing, tempo, and variability. *Secular trend* is the reduction in the age of pubertal development from the middle of the 19th to the middle of the 20th centuries in industrialized countries. Although this was thought to have plateaued over the last few decades, recent evidence indicates that many girls are demonstrating pubertal changes by age 8. This suggests that standards for normal growth and pubertal development used in primary care may need to be reconsidered. *Sequencing* is the progression of secondary sex characteristics, which follows a predictable sequence. *Tempo* refers to the timing of the onset and the velocity of changes in secondary sex characteristics. The interindividual *variability* of sequencing is small, but that for tempo is great.

Pubertal maturation occurs as a result of activation of the hypothalamic-pituitary-gonadal system. Puberty in females begins when the hypothalamus becomes decreasingly sensitive to the negative feedback of estrogen, resulting in the cyclic release of gonadotropins during sleep. The exact triggering mechanism for puberty is unknown. Hypothalamic gonadotropin-releasing hormone acts on the anterior pituitary gland to produce follicle-stimulating hormone (FSH) and luteinizing hormone (LH). FSH stimulates the production of estrogen and stimulates the growth of the ovarian follicle. LH stimulates and initiates ovulation, the corpus luteum, and the production of progesterone.

The physical changes associated with puberty and the average time course for these events are shown in Figure 8-1. As noted, the events of puberty progress in a relatively fixed and predictable sequence, but the timing of these events is quite variable. Thus, chronologic age varies widely within any given maturational stage. Determination of sexual maturation by examining breast and pubic hair development, using Tanner's maturational stages as a reference standard, is an important part of routine care delivery to young women. Plotting and monitoring growth and development are critical to helping young women and their families understand the normal nature of changes that are happening. Staging pubertal

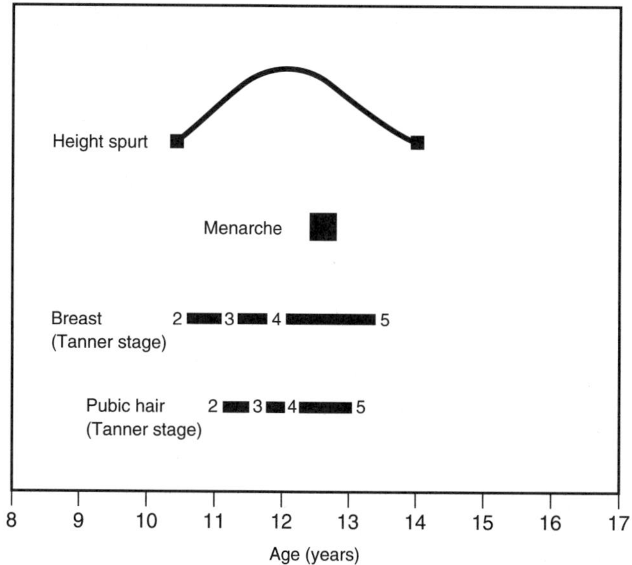

Figure 8-1. Pubertal events in females. (Copeland KC, Brookman RR, Rauth JL. Assessment of pubertal development. Ross Laboratories PREP Series. Columbus, OH: Ross Laboratories, 1986:6, with permission.)

changes has substantial value for predicting the likely course of developmental events, as most women complete their pubertal growth within 4 years of its onset. Additionally, sexual maturity rating (SMR) has implications for assessment of pubertal delay, short stature or other growth failure, and amenorrhea.

One of the earliest visible changes resulting from increasing estrogen levels due to activation of the hypothalamic-pituitary-gonadal axis is breast budding (thelarche). The appearance of dark, straight pubic hair over the mons veneris (adrenarche or pubarche) indicates activation of the hypothalamic-pituitary-adrenal axis. These mark SMR (also called Tanner stage) II of pubertal development and generally occur around 11 years of age. Breast development proceeds to SMR V (adult) over the next 4 years; completion of breast development may occur as quickly as 18 months or take as long as 9 years (Fig. 8-2). Pubic hair development generally takes about 18 to 40 months to complete (Fig. 8-3). About 1 year after the initiation of breast development, during SMR III, females experience a very rapid increase in their height. The peak of this growth spurt (peak height velocity) precedes the onset of menstruation (menarche) by about 6 months (Figs. 8-4 and 8-5). Menarche is regularly preceded by the peak growth spurt, but may occur normally as early as age 10 or as late as age 16 years. Thus, menarche is a relatively late pubertal event, occurring during or just before the SMR IV stage of breast development.

Pubertal females experience a gain in lean body mass, but also gain body fat. The average fat-to-lean ratio changes from 1 : 5 at the start of the growth spurt to 1 : 3 at the time of menarche. Weight velocity and weight gain standards are shown in Figures 8-6 and 8-7. As the external appearance changes, the internal organs also are developing. For example, as they develop, the mucus-secreting cells lining the uterus may produce a scant, thin, acidic, odorless physiologic vaginal discharge before menarche, called physiologic leukorrhea.

Psychological and Cognitive Development During Adolescence

Piaget first described the transition from concrete to formal operational thought as occurring in the early and midteen years. Although there is great variation, most young people develop this ability to think abstractly between ages 12 and 16. Before acquiring this ability, young people have difficulty applying general principles to different situations and realistically appraising and planning for the future. In contrast, formal operational thought includes the capacity to think about abstractions, such as ideas and thoughts. This developmental task is usually marked by a gradual transition from primarily egocentric or concrete thinking. Formal operational thought facilitates adolescents' thinking about independence, interdependence, career and life choices, or personal moral choices. However, some people successfully function as independent adults without ever developing formal operational thinking.

The development of formal operational thinking is also a crucial milestone with regard to planning the care of adolescents. For example, youths who are concrete operational are probably not capable of true emancipation or informed consent. Adolescents capable of formal operational thought can consider the consequences and the risks and benefits of immediate decisions with a realistic future orientation. However, this ability may be inconsistently applied when dealing with emotionally charged situations, such as those that may arise within families or around sexuality issues.

Finally, the psychosocial tasks of adolescence should be considered. The Eriksonian task of adolescence is identity formation, allowing development of independence from parents and intimacy with other individuals as adults. In contrast, Baumrind and other recent developmental theorists have defined the goals of adolescent social development as interdependence, reflecting the continuing relationships and importance of the connections between adult children and their families.

It is useful to divide adolescence into three stages: early (10 to 14 years old), middle (15 to 16 years old), and late (17 to 21 years old). Each stage can be understood with regard to adolescents' changing relationships with family, school, and peers. The developmental changes of adolescents also affect their risks, evaluation, management, and outcome. The early onset of puberty in girls (and also the later onset of puberty in boys) is associated with increased levels of risky behavior. Under stress, the ability to think and solve problems in formal operational ways may regress. For early adolescents, concrete thought processes make motivation for behav-

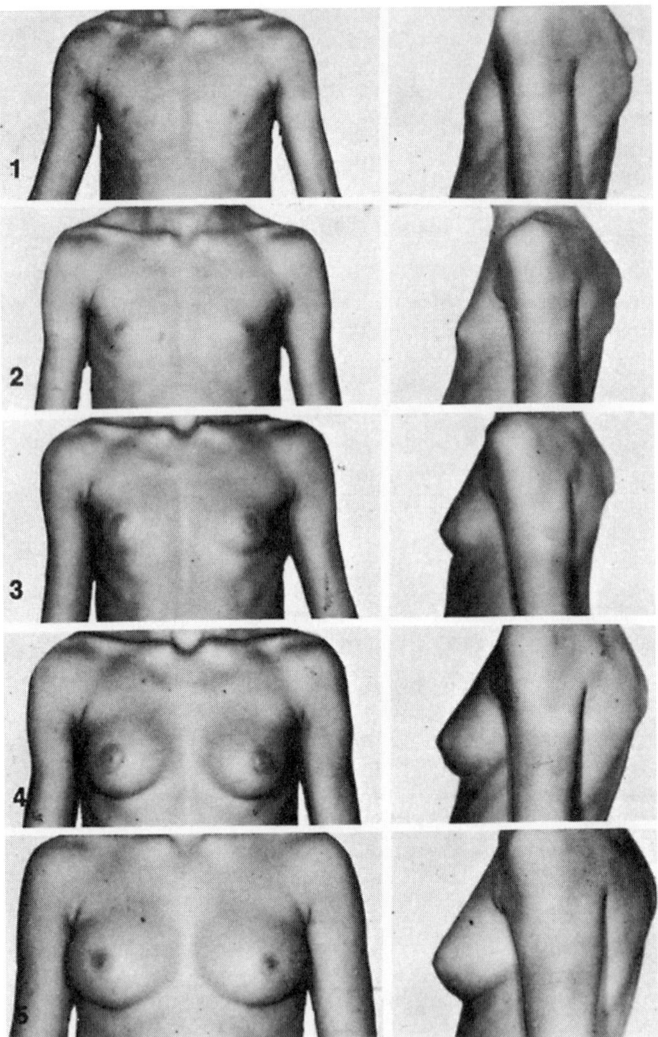

Figure 8-2. Sexual maturity ratings—pubertal development of the female breast. Stage 1: Preadolescent—elevation of the papillae only. Stage 2: Breast bud—elevation of the breast and papilla forms a small mound. Stage 3: Continuing enlargement of the breast and areola without separation of their contours. Stage 4: The areola and papilla project to form a secondary mound above the level of the breast. Stage 5: Mature adult—the areola has recessed to the countour of the breast. (Tanner JM. Growth at adolescence, 2nd ed. Oxford: Blackwell Scientific, 1962.)

ioral change dependent on short-range goals (eg, don't smoke because it may make you smell bad, run slower, or stain your teeth, rather than because of the risk of lung cancer or heart disease).

Early Adolescence (10 to 14 Years Old)

The early adolescent years are marked by rapid physical growth, both somatically and sexually. Increases in sex hormones are partly responsible for these changes, preparing the girl for womanhood and reproduction. Physical and sexual changes lead the girl in early adolescence to question her identity in terms of "Am I normal?" As she begins to identify more with her peer group, she gradually seeks autonomy or independence. Insecurity and self-consciousness characterize this stage. Although some 13-year-old girls are sexually active, it is usually for nonsexual reasons, such as seeking peer approval or independence, rather than a true seeking for intimacy, which is developmentally impossible to achieve until late adolescence or young adulthood. Furthermore, even though a girl may strive for independence from her family, when challenged by a crisis she will most often retreat to them. For girls, relationships generally have greater value than the achievement and domination implied in the term "independence." Thus, dependency in childhood tends to give way to interdependence in adolescence and young adulthood for girls. Even the cognitive structure of the early adolescent is fluctuating and highly variable, primarily limited to the present (concrete operational) and occasionally expanding to consider abstractions, things as they might be, or the future (formal operational).

Middle Adolescence (15 to 16 Years Old)

The middle adolescent has already experienced most of her physical growth and development. Most middle adolescents accept their adult body and reproductive capacity, but adolescents with chronic illness may have delayed growth and development. Autonomy, conflict with authority, testing of limits, and experimentation characterize middle adolescent behavior. "Who am I?" is the critical question of the emerging identity during middle adolescence. Sexuality usually is directed toward opposite-sex partners and individual dating is often initiated, even for women who will be lesbian as adults. Formal operational cognition also allows considering the feelings of others and the development of insight and a future orientation.

Although middle adolescents do not bring the same egocentricism to concrete objects that younger children do, they remain quite narcissistic and egocentric, and often believe that others share their thoughts. This gives rise to what has been called the "imaginary audience," through which an adolescent believes everyone is

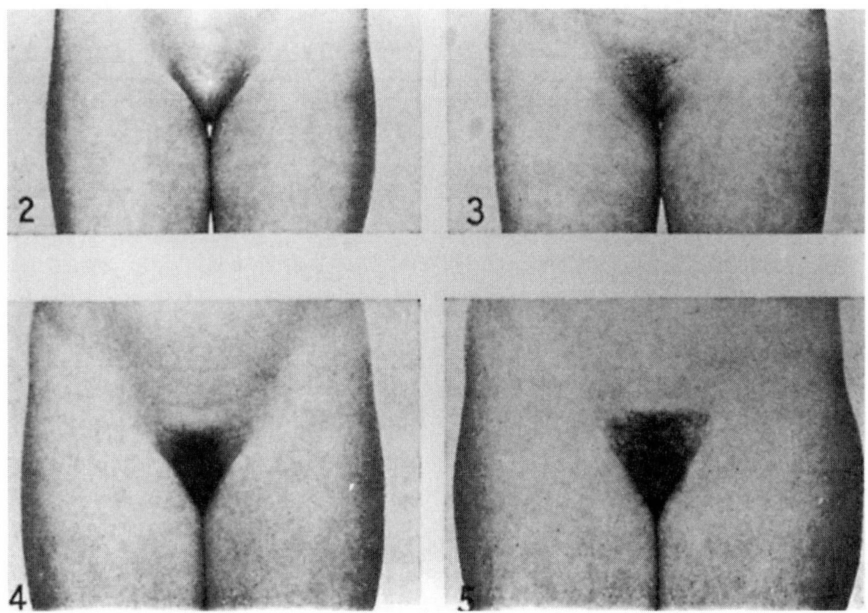

Figure 8-3. Sexual maturity ratings—pubertal development of pubic hair. Stage 1: Preadolescent—no pubic hair. Stage 2: Sparse growth of long, slightly pigmented straight or slightly curly pubic hair along labia only. Stage 3: Darker, coarser, and more curled hair spreading upward over the pubic area. Stage 4: Adult type and pattern of hair, without extension onto the thighs. Stage 5: Adult type, quantity, and pattern of hair, with extension onto the thighs. (Tanner JM. Growth at adolescence, 2nd ed. Oxford: Blackwell Scientific, 1962.)

concerned about and attentive to her unique, special actions. It also results in the "personal fable," in which adolescents see themselves as invulnerable to harm.

Late Adolescence (17 to 21 Years Old)

The late adolescent is even more concerned about the future than are middle adolescents. Adult habitus has usually been achieved. Issues concerning future education, vocation, individuation, and sexuality assume primacy in her developmental scheme. Her emerging identity question at this stage is "Who am I in relation to other people and to the future?" Late adolescents and young adults often physically or emotionally move away from their families and face the responsibilities of economic and physical independence, marriage, working, and the reality of an uncertain future. Thus, although the patient may appear as an adult physically, it is important for the primary care provider to recognize her developmental vulnerability due to a lack of adult experiences or skills. The late adolescent female may have the thinking skills and body of a woman, but may still be vulnerable and not yet ready for adulthood because of unresolved issues relating to her experiences, skills, autonomy, and identity.

HEALTH RISK BEHAVIOR AND PREVENTIVE CARE OF YOUNG WOMEN

Many adolescents engage in risky behaviors that can affect their health. The leading cause of death among all adolescents is unintentional injury, with 80% of all injury deaths due to motor vehicle accidents. Suicide and homicide are the second and third leading causes of death for all adolescents, followed by neoplasm, cardiovascular diseases, and congenital anomalies. Many of these causes of death are associated with preventable behavioral choices that place young people at risk for these adverse outcomes. As many as one in four adolescents are also at high risk for substance abuse, sexually transmitted diseases, early unintended pregnancy, interpersonal violence, and school failure. These choices, along with choices about diet, exercise, and other issues (eg, safety, such as through using seatbelts), have profound implications for the prevention of adult chronic disease. The lifestyles and behaviors adopted by teens often persist, resulting in excess adult morbidity and mortality.

Tobacco, alcohol, and marijuana use remain epidemic among adolescents, with as many as one in three adolescents smoking cigarettes. Nearly 90% of adolescents have drunk alcohol; of greater concern, nearly 25% of high school seniors report engaging in binge drinking (more than five drinks at one sitting) within a 2-week period.

One million adolescents in the United States become pregnant each year. By age 15, 25% of girls have had sexual intercourse. By age 19, 83% of black females and 76% of white females have had intercourse. Only about half of all adolescents report using contraceptives at their last intercourse. Although the proportion reporting regular condom use continues to increase each year, nearly half of all young people who are sexually active do not take adequate precautions against HIV, other sexually transmitted diseases, or pregnancy.

Much of the morbidity and mortality among our nation's adolescents is preventable; thus, effective health promotion and disease prevention for adolescents is a critical part of primary care (Tables 8-1 and 8-2). In addition to school- and community-based strategies, clinical preventive services delivered by primary care providers have an important role in health promotion and disease prevention efforts. Most adolescents see a physician or other provider each year, but only 15% of all visits are for preventive care. Additionally, most providers perform recommended preventive services at relatively low rates.

In 1992, an American Medical Association interdisciplinary expert panel developed the *Guidelines for Adolescent Preventive Services*, or GAPS, included as an appendix to this chapter. The GAPS guidelines are a set of recommendations to help primary care providers organize and deliver comprehensive preventive services to adolescents. GAPS recommendations address the organization of services, the promotion of healthy lifestyles, screening for physical, emotional, and behavioral problems, and immunizations. The goals of GAPS are to make the entire clinical visit part of a health-promoting experience.

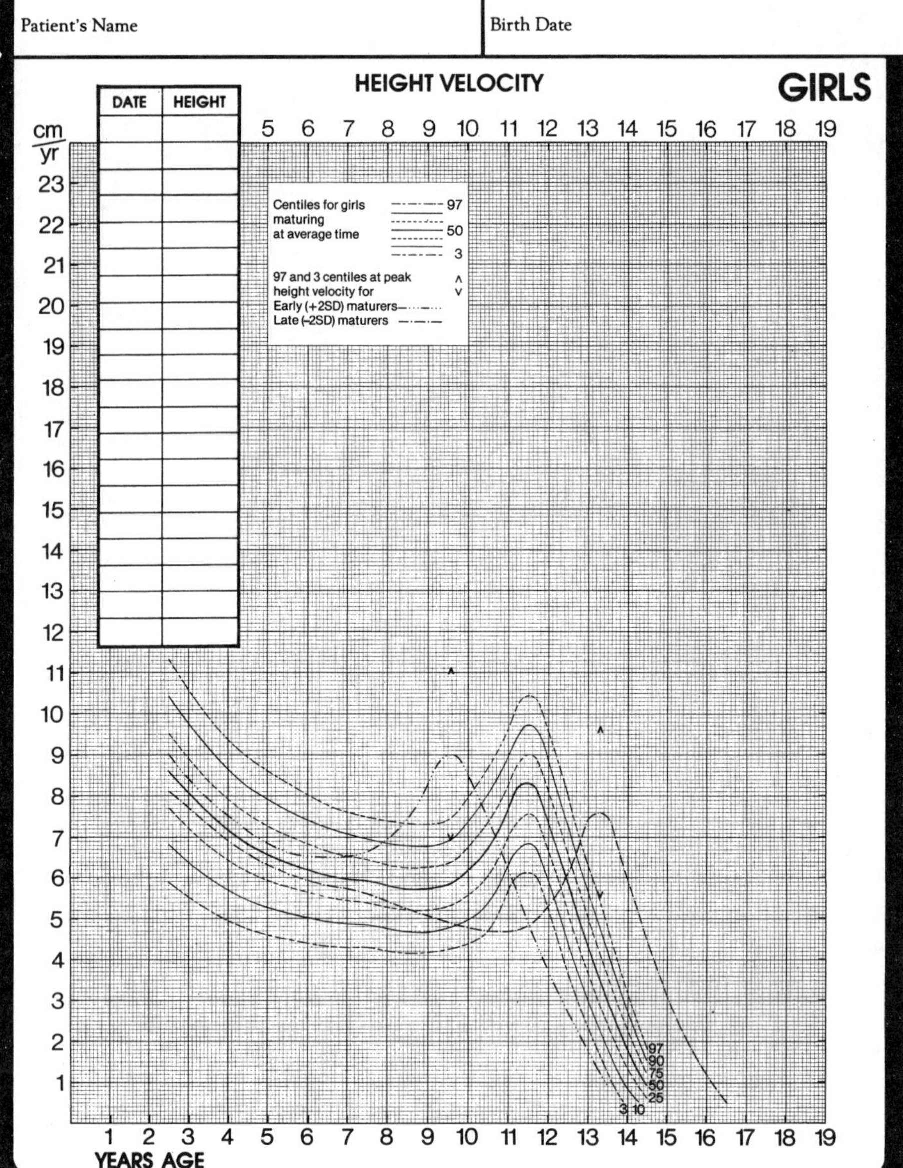

Figure 8-4. Height attained for adolescent females. (Modified with permission from Tanner JM, Davies PW. Clinical longitudinal standards for height and height velocity for North American children. J Pediatr 1985; 107:317.)

MEDICAL CONDITIONS AFFECTING ADOLESCENTS

Medical conditions affecting adolescents can be the residual effects of childhood illnesses, the start of adult disease processes, or conditions unique to adolescence. Additionally, a few conditions have different manifestations in adolescence than in either adults or children. In the following sections, conditions characteristically found in adolescents are reviewed briefly, with attention focused on diagnosis and management in primary care settings.

Acne

Acne occurs in more than 85% of adolescents and is identified as a major health concern by nearly all teenagers. Acne pimples, or comedones, are formed by thickening, occlusion, and inflammation of hair follicles on the face, forehead, back, and chest. Androgens stimulate increased secretion and estrogens inhibit secretion of the pilosebaceous glands. Thus, most adolescent girls report acne flares, often just before menarche. The increased growth of *Propionibacterium acnes* during puberty also contributes to the increasing number of comedones and the increase in symptomatic acne during adolescence. Although most adolescents outgrow acne, 5% to 10% of young adults continue to report significant numbers of acne lesions into their twenties.

To evaluate acne, the type, number, and severity of lesions should be documented. Unless an androgen or corticosteroid excess is suspected, laboratory studies are not indicated. Use of oral contraceptives may improve or exacerbate acne; the use of progestational contraceptive agents is usually associated with increased acne. Several other drugs, including corticosteroids, anabolic steroids, isoniazid, lithium, and phenytoin can cause papular and pustular acneiform lesions. Similarly, cosmetics and hair-care products can cause or exacerbate acne, although fatty foods and chocolate do not cause acne exacerbation.

Recognition and treatment of acne is an important part of adolescent practice. Therapy goals are to prevent scarring, improve self-esteem, and reduce the number and severity of comedones.

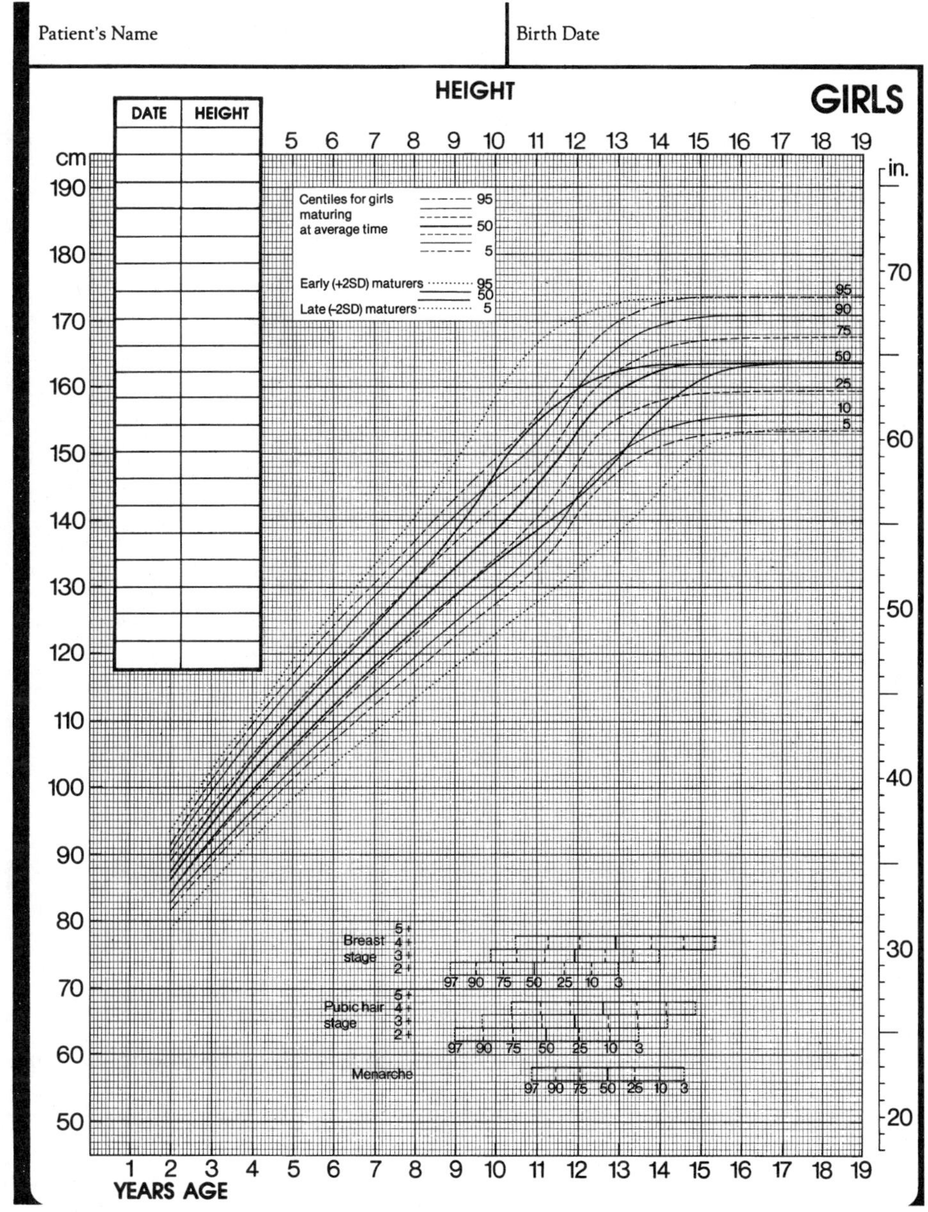

Figure 8-5. Height velocity for adolescent females. (Modified with permission from Tanner JM, Davies PW. Clinical longitudinal standards for height and height velocity for North American children. J Pediatr 1985; 107:317.)

Picking and squeezing lesions should be avoided, as scarring is more likely to occur. Routine skin care should be limited to a mild soap, and the use of cosmetics or cover-ups should be discouraged; if used, they should be nonacnegenic.

Topical treatment is usually the first line of therapy. Over-the-counter 5% topical benzoyl peroxide cream applied once or twice daily is recommended as initial therapy. Tretinoin cream 0.025% may also be used, both to prevent new lesions and to treat existing ones. The use of gel preparations, as well as stronger strengths, of both of these medications often causes dryness and irritation of the skin. Topical erythromycin or clindamycin are often added to benzoyl peroxide or tretinoin. Systemic erythromycin or tetracyclines are also used effectively, especially in cases of moderate to severe inflammatory acne. If oral tetracyclines are used, pregnancy status must be carefully monitored, as these drugs are teratogenic. Additionally, oral antibiotics may alter the metabolism of estrogens in oral contraceptives; thus, barrier contraceptives are an important adjuvant to systemic antibiotic treatment in sexually active women with acne. Additionally, both topical and systemic acne treatments can increase sensitivity to ultraviolet radiation, so adequate sunscreen use should be recommended.

A period of 4 to 6 weeks is generally required to assess the efficacy of any particular treatment, and sufficient time should be allowed before adding additional therapies or abandoning the current regimen. Combination regimens often result in increasingly effective treatment. Many adolescents with severe, resistant, and cystic acne also benefit from systemic isotretinoin (retinoic acid). Adolescents with severe acne or with significant scarring, and candidates for retinoic acid therapy should be referred to dermatologists or others familiar with the use of these drugs. The initial course is generally 16 to 20 weeks long and may be associated with significant side effects. As retinoic acid is highly teratogenic, intensive counseling, serial pregnancy testing, and the use of two effective methods of birth control are recommended.

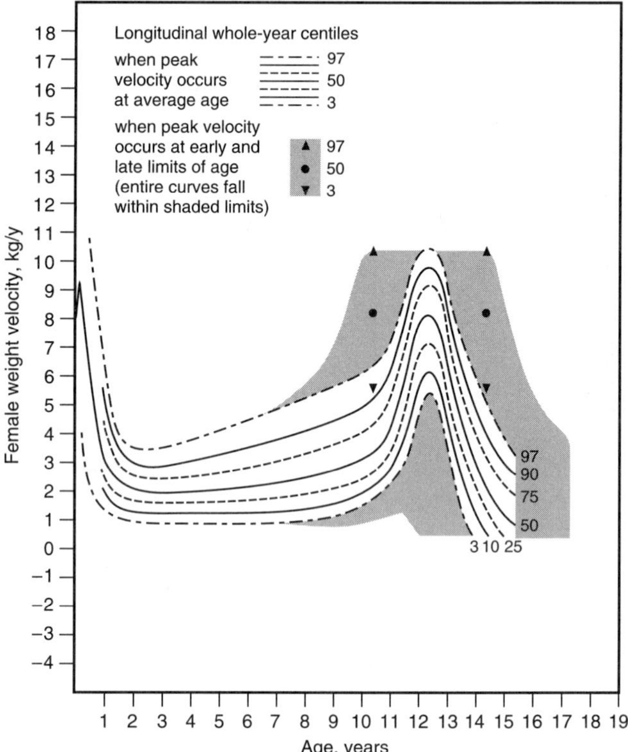

Figure 8-6. Weight attained for adolescent females. (Modified with permission from Tanner JM, Whitehouse RH. Clinical longitudinal standards for height, weight, height velocity, weight velocity and stages of puberty. Arch Dis Child 1976; 51:170.)

Vision and Hearing

The onset of myopia is most common between ages 11 and 13. Adolescence is also often a time when preexisting nearsightedness undergoes rapid change. Additionally, adolescents are at relatively high risk for traumatic eye injuries from sports or motor vehicle accidents. Hyphema, or hemorrhage into the anterior chamber of the eye, is a common form of injury; baseball, tennis, and soccer are the leading causes. Corneal abrasion is also a common result of trauma to the eye.

Protective eyeguards should be used by adolescents who have only one functioning eye, and for those who engage in sports involving projectiles (eg, baseball). Patients with significant eye trauma should be referred for ophthalmologic evaluation without delay.

During adolescence, the differential diagnosis of bacterial conjunctivitis must be broadened to include infections with gonorrhea, chlamydia, and herpes simplex virus in addition to other bacterial, viral, mechanical, and allergic causes. These conditions, which are easily treated by the primary care provider, must be differentiated from acute glaucoma, corneal abrasion or inflammation, acute iritis, and acute scleritis, all of which present with varying degrees of pain in the affected eye and require prompt referral to an ophthalmologist.

Hearing loss is one of the most common chronic health disorders, affecting 16 of every 1000 adolescents. Although the most common cause of hearing loss in adolescents is meningitis, the development of the *Haemophilus influenzae* vaccine should significantly reduce this cause in the future. Irreversible acoustic trauma may result from single and recurrent noise exposures louder than 80 decibels, either from loud music or from occupational exposures. In general, adolescents should be counseled to limit such noise exposures, to allow recovery time between episodes, and to use protective earplugs. Those with a significant exposure history should be screened for hearing loss on a regular basis and counseled accordingly.

Pharyngitis and Oral Conditions

Pharyngitis, one of the most common presenting complaints among children, remains common among adolescents. Viral infections and streptococcal pharyngitis remain the leading causes of disease in adolescents; however, the spectrum of viral and bacterial etiologies changes compared to younger children. For example, in 1% to 4% of adolescents with *Neisseria gonorrhoeae* infection, the pharynx is the only site of infection. Other sexually transmitted pathogens can also cause pharyngitis; however, oropharyngeal involvement with sexually transmitted conditions is usually seen in conjunction with genitourinary symptoms, rather than alone. Additionally, although infectious mononucleosis may present with pharyngitis in adolescents, there is at least a 30% incidence of concurrent infection with Epstein-Barr virus and streptococcal disease. Streptococcal pharyngitis, in particular, requires accurate diagnosis and treatment with antimicrobials, as poststreptococcal systemic disease remains a significant and preventable cause of morbidity. Rheumatic heart disease accounts for 25% to 45% of cardiovascular disease in all age groups.

Sexually transmitted diseases are also a major cause of oral ulcerative disease in adolescents. Primary herpes simplex viral infection may cause extensive and painful oral lesions. Treatment with oral acyclovir, if initiated early in the course of herpes infection (whether oral or genital), shortens the duration and decreases the extent of symptoms. Acyclovir may also be effective in the sup-

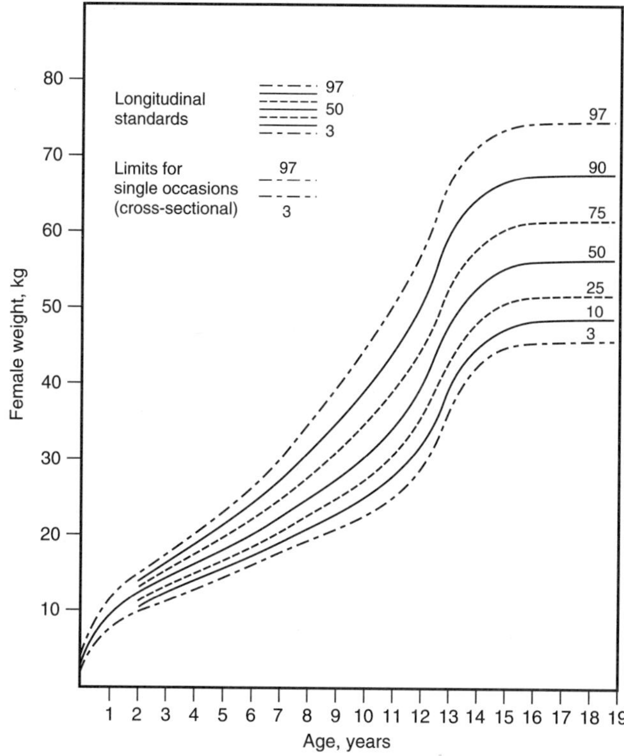

Figure 8-7. Weight velocity for adolescent females. (Modified with permission from Tanner JM, Whitehouse RH: Clinical longitudinal standards for height, weight, height velocity, weight velocity and stages of puberty. Arch Dis Child 1976; 51:170.)

pression of frequently recurring lesions, although persistence or spread of herpes simplex lesions should prompt investigation of the patient's ability to mount an immune response.

In addition to herpes, syphilis must also be considered in the differential diagnosis of ulcerative lesions. Aphthous oral ulcers may be a sign of extraintestinal inflammatory bowel disease or rheumatologic diseases such as Behçet or Reiter syndrome. Adolescence is a time when systemic manifestations of these chronic conditions often present. Because these signs may be the first manifestations of these chronic diseases, clinicians must remain open to the possibility of these diagnoses, especially when faced with atypical or persistent (> 2 weeks in duration) ulcerative disease.

Adolescents' dental and oral care concerns include traumatic injury to the teeth, adequate dental hygiene and prophylaxis, use of smokeless tobacco products, and onset of periodontal disease. Thus, the primary care provider has an important role to play in promoting appropriate dental hygiene, including brushing and use of preventive dental services. As with other preventive health behaviors, the importance of this counseling is magnified by the fact that health habits adopted during the teenage years are likely to persist throughout adulthood. Screening for injury and tobacco exposure risks, and counseling about the appropriate use of protective helmets and mouthguards during sports and about tobacco prevention and cessation are important in primary care practice. Adolescents with bulimia nervosa and some patients with anorexia nervosa who vomit risk dental erosion, as regurgitation of gastric acid may dissolve tooth enamel and dentin on the lingual surface of the teeth.

During adolescence, the third molars ("wisdom teeth") erupt, and these may require extraction. Additionally, female adolescents occasionally develop gingivitis and gum hypertrophy, similar to the gingivitis seen during pregnancy. This inflammation, which may occur in response to oral contraceptives, is believed to be due to a combination of local and hormonal influences. Although the spontaneous condition may persist for years, cases due to oral contraceptive use generally resolve when the additional hormone is withdrawn. Therapy consists of frequent oral hygiene and removal of plaque.

Respiratory and Environmental Conditions

The lung volume increases and alveoli grow throughout adolescence, corresponding to increases in the height and growth of the thorax. Asthma remains a highly prevalent disease, affecting nearly 10% of children and adolescents; nearly half of these patients have some functional impairment in their ability to perform normal daily activities. Although many school-age children with asthma become symptom-free during adolescence, 60% to 70% of these adolescents have airway hyperreactivity when challenged, and many adults with reactive airway disease first became symptomatic during adolescence. The incidence of asthma and the incidence of death from asthma have risen in recent decades. Exercise-induced asthma, which also often starts in adolescence, may present with cough or shortness of breath in addition to wheezing. Girls are less likely to improve during their adolescent years, and the sex ratio for asthma changes from 1 : 3 to 1 : 1 female : male between childhood and adulthood.

Exposure to particulate and chemical toxins, including cigarette and marijuana smoke, pollution, and occupational dust and chemical fumes, may increase during adolescence. All of these exposures cause lung irritation and may cause the destruction of lung tissue. Passive environmental smoke exposures and the

Table 8-1. Death Rates per 100,000 Due to Seven Leading Causes of Death for Adolescents and Young Adults by Age and Gender, 1991

	MALES			FEMALES		
CAUSE	*10–14*	*15–19*	*20–24*	*10–14*	*15–19*	*20–24*
Motor vehicle accident	7.9	41.4	49.2	4.2	20.5	15.7
Other accidents	7.2	15.1	17.7	2.2	2.8	3.4
Suicide	2.3	18.0	25.4	0.7	3.7	3.9
Homicide	2.9	32.8	41.1	1.3	5.5	8.2
Malignant neoplasms	3.6	5.0	6.5	2.4	3.5	4.6
Cardiovascular disease	1.3	3.3	5.1	1.2	2.1	3.4
Congenital anomalies	1.3	1.5	—	1.1	1.2	—
Infectious disease (including HIV)	—	—	4.7	—	—	1.9

National Center for Health Statistics. Vital Statistics of the United States, 1991. Vol II. Mortality. Part A. USPHS Publication No. 96-1101. Washington, DC: US Government Printing Office, 1996.

sniffing of glue or other inhalants may also exacerbate reactive airway disease. Thus, appropriate screening and history taking and counseling for protective measures should be part of routine primary care screening. Similar consideration should also be given to dermatologic and systemic manifestations of occupationally or environmentally mediated diseases. Some chemical exposures (eg, petrochemicals, solvents) can lead to pneumonias, aspiration, pulmonary edema, and death. Occupational medicine and toxicology consultations, available in many centers, may be appropriately used by primary care providers to evaluate harmful vocational or recreational exposures and to act to reduce them.

Inhaled beta-adrenergic agents, corticosteroids, and anticholinergic medications are the current mainstay of acute asthma management. Cromolyn sodium also has a major role, especially in the prevention of exacerbations due to known precipitants. Theophyllines are no longer considered first-line or routine drugs for asthma management.

Because of the increasing rates of death due to asthma in recent years, current therapeutic interventions for asthma should include explicit algorithms for home nebulizer use so that patients do not overestimate their margin of safety with regard to respiratory failure. Understanding compliance with chronic medication use and adolescent adaptation to a chronic illness is also a key part of successful asthma management during adolescence.

In adolescents with cystic fibrosis, several issues are affected by puberty. First, these young people are often delayed in their pubertal development and menarche by several years. Second, their appearance (clubbed fingers, barrel-shaped chest, cachexia) and their behaviors (coughing, sputum production, foul-smelling stools, frequent hospitalizations) may make social integration with peers difficult. Third, up to 20% of girls with cystic fibrosis are fertile, and the average life expectancy is now well into the third decade. Contraception must be addressed in sexually active girls with cystic fibrosis, as pregnancy is likely to worsen pulmonary function. Information about the effect of other risky health behaviors on the adolescent's pulmonary status should also be provided, along with routine preventive health counseling.

Cardiovascular Diseases

The growth and sexual maturation of puberty result in a variety of changes in the cardiovascular system. Adolescents' heart rates slow and their stroke volume, cardiac output, and blood pressure gradually increase to adult levels. Because physical size is important to these physiologic measurements, it is necessary to use age- and gender-referenced norms (Fig. 8-8).

The risk of coronary artery disease is well established by adolescence, and the first visible lesions of atherosclerosis often appear

Table 8-2. Death Rates per 100,000 Due to Seven Leading Causes of Death for Adolescents and Young Adults by Age and Race,* 1991

	BLACK			WHITE			OTHER		
CAUSE	*10–14*	*15–19*	*20–24*	*10–14*	*15–19*	*20–24*	*10–14*	*15–19*	*20–24*
Motor vehicle accident	6.1	19.4	25.5	6.1	34.1	34.6	5.9	19.8	24.7
Other accidents	7.8	12.2	13.1	4.3	8.7	10.4	6.6	10.7	11.7
Suicide	1.1	6.9	11.1	1.6	11.8	15.7	1.0	7.8	11.3
Homicide	6.5	75.8	104.0	1.4	9.2	12.2	5.2	60.8	81.2
Malignant neoplasms	2.8	4.3	6.3	3.1	4.4	5.6	2.6	4.1	5.7
Cardiovascular disease	2.1	4.4	9.3	1.1	2.4	3.5	1.8	3.8	7.8
Congenital anomalies	1.2	1.4	—	1.2	1.4	—	1.2	1.2	—
Infectious disease (including HIV)	—	—	10.9	—	—	2.2	—	—	8.4

*Hispanics may be of any race.

National Center for Health Statistics. Vital Statistics of the United States, 1991. Vol II. Mortality. Part A. USPHS Publication No. 96-1101. Washington, DC: US Government Printing Office, 1996.

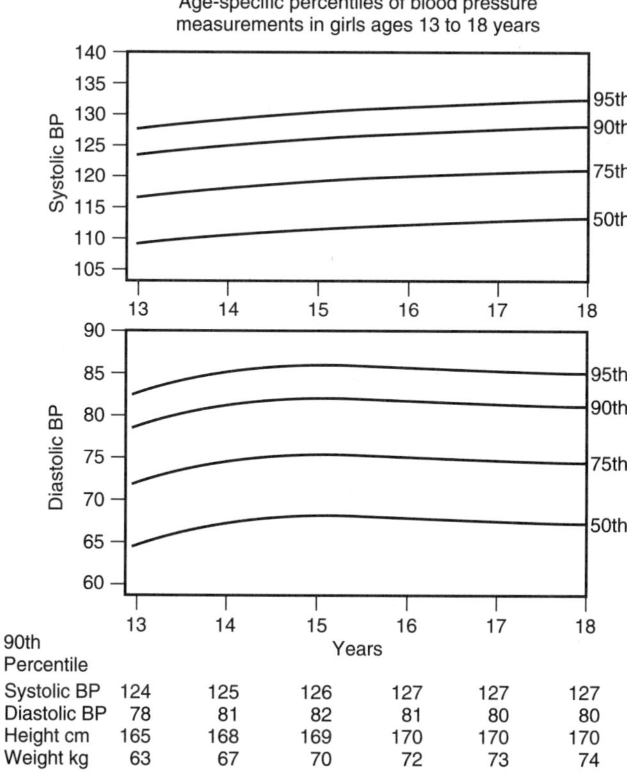

90th Percentile						
Systolic BP	124	125	126	127	127	127
Diastolic BP	78	81	82	81	80	80
Height cm	165	168	169	170	170	170
Weight kg	63	67	70	72	73	74

Figure 8-8. Blood pressure by age for girls, ages 13–18 years. (With permission from the Task Force on Blood Pressure Control in Children. Pediatrics 1987; 79:1.)

during the second decade of life. High-fat diets, inactivity, and smoking are the major causes of preventable cardiovascular mortality in the United States. Other risk factors include obesity, hyperlipidemia, hypertension, and diabetes mellitus. These risk factors are primarily genetically rather than behaviorally determined; however, risk factor modification has clear benefits to adolescents, with regard to both immediate health effects (eg, smoking cessation or weight reduction) and long-term cardiovascular risk reduction. Many providers manage adolescents with high cholesterol and triglyceride levels with the help of a nutritionist to promote lifestyles that include heart-healthy dietary and exercise habits.

Sudden cardiac death, although rare, is of concern to families and schools, in part because it tends to happen during vigorous exercise. Most of these cases are due to hypertrophic cardiomyopathy. Less commonly, these deaths are due to congenital coronary artery anomaly, arrhythmias (most often prolonged QT syndrome), or preexisting structural cardiac disease. Screening by history and physical examination is recommended. Adolescents with a prior history of cardiovascular disease or syncope, or with a family history of cardiac or unexplained sudden death, should be referred to a pediatric cardiologist for a comprehensive evaluation. Similarly, adolescents with potentially pathologic murmurs should be referred for evaluation.

Relatively few congenital or acquired cardiac defects are first detected during puberty. However, primary care providers increasingly share in caring for adolescents and young adults who have repaired congenital cardiac lesions. Management of endocarditis prophylaxis, exercise restrictions, family planning, and psychosocial adjustment should be coordinated with the patient's cardiologist.

Heart murmurs are caused by turbulent blood flow. The timing, location, and other characteristics of heart murmurs are determined by their anatomy. Most heart murmurs in adolescent females arise from turbulent flow in anatomically normal hearts. However, there are no normal diastolic murmurs. Normal systolic murmurs include pulmonary ejection murmurs (heard best during midsystole at the second left intracostal space, with radiation to the axilla); pulmonary souffle murmurs (also heard best at the second left intracostal space, especially in high-cardiac-output states, as a soft, midsystolic murmur, without radiation); venous hums (heard above the clavicle with patients in upright position only); and Still murmurs, soft, short, musical or vibratory ejection murmurs heard over the precordium. Adolescents with murmurs that do not fall into one of these categories should be evaluated by a cardiologist.

Mitral valve prolapse is one of the cardiac conditions that is often detected during adolescence. The mid-late systolic click of mitral valve prolapse is common in normal adolescents and young adults, increasing from less than 2% among children to 20% or so by the third decade of life. The high-pitched or honking murmur of mitral valve regurgitation is also relatively common. Mitral valve prolapse is three times more common in women than in men, and is most often diagnosed in tall, slender women. It is associated with Marfan syndrome and with connective tissue disorders. Thus, adolescents with murmurs consistent with mitral valve prolapse must be evaluated for these conditions. The other major differential diagnosis causing a midsystolic click is normal splitting of the first heart sound.

Cardiology referral is indicated, as is echocardiography, to assess the extent of mitral regurgitation. Electrocardiograms are normal in over 80% of patients and are significant only for nonspecific T-wave changes in those that are positive. As the risk of bacterial endocarditis increases ten times for individuals with mitral regurgitation, endocarditis prophylaxis is indicated for adolescents with mitral valve prolapse. Additionally, arrhythmias are somewhat more common in adolescents with mitral valve prolapse, although they remain relatively rare overall. In controlled studies, chest pain and panic and anxiety attacks were not found to be more often associated with mitral valve prolapse than with controls.

Hematologic Conditions

Puberty causes an increase in hemoglobin and red cell volume, especially in males, as testosterone directly stimulates erythropoiesis. Boys aged 12 to 14 have an average hemoglobin of 14 g/dL, with an increase of 1 g/dL through age 18 and another 1 g/dL after age 18. Although hemoglobin does not increase dramatically in girls, both males and females increase their MCV from 84 fL to the adult value of 90. During puberty, menstrual blood loss also initiates an increase in dietary iron requirements for women.

Some mild bleeding disorders escape detection until adolescence. As many as 20% of adolescent girls with severe menorrhagia presenting at menarche have a primary coagulation disorder (most often von Willebrand disease).

Iron-deficiency anemia is not uncommon among adolescents, especially among menstruating females. Total body iron is balanced between dietary intake and GI absorption and excretion. Iron is lost through the skin and stool at approximately 0.75 mg/day. Girls also lose an average of 0.6 mg/day through menstrual blood loss. In contrast, the average intake of dietary iron is 10 to 12 mg/day, of which approximately 10% is absorbed. Because many adolescent girls do not consume a diet rich in heme iron (eg, meat), they may develop iron-deficiency anemia. Athletes are at particular risk because they have increased losses from sweating, and from physical red cell damage and hematuria resulting from exercise.

As many as 20% to 30% of adolescent girls are thought to suffer from iron deficiency without frank anemia. Fewer become symptomatic, with lethargy or decreased exercise tolerance. Mild iron deficiency generally presents with a normocytic anemia and a reduced serum ferritin level. Later, a more typical microcytic anemia develops, with elevated free erythrocyte protoporphyrin, increased iron-binding capacity, and decreased serum iron. The differential diagnosis of iron-deficiency anemia includes hemoglobinopathies and the anemia of chronic disease.

Treatment of iron-deficiency anemia includes replacing body iron stores and treating any abnormal source or rate of ongoing blood loss. Ferrous sulfate in a dose that provides 6 mg/kg/day of elemental iron is generally recommended for symptomatic iron deficiency. Absorption is facilitated by taking the iron with orange juice. Although the reticulocyte count rises within days and the hemoglobin level rises by 0.5 to 1.0 g/dL per week, therapeutic doses are recommended for 2 to 3 months to replenish the body's iron stores. Doses of 2 mg/kg/day are recommended for prevention among patients with known blood loss or low iron intake.

Megaloblastic anemias are uncommon among adolescents, although adolescents occasionally take medications (eg, oral contraceptives, anticonvulsants) that can interfere with folate absorption. However, because folate deficiency has been associated with congenital anomalies (including neural tube defects), folate supplementation is recommended before conception and during early pregnancy for adolescents or young adults. Because many pregnancies during adolescence are unplanned, some authorities are recommending routine multivitamin use by women. Vitamin B_{12} deficiency is rare except among people maintaining strict vegetarian diets.

Endocrine Conditions

Graves' disease and autoimmune (chronic lymphocytic, or Hashimoto) thyroiditis are the most common causes of hyper- and hypothyroidism, respectively, during adolescence. Behavioral changes may be part of the initial manifestation of thyroid disease. Similarly, growth failure, weight loss or gain, and amenorrhea or menorrhagia may be part of the presentation of young women with thyroid dysfunction. Hypothyroidism may also present as depression in adolescents and as precocious puberty or precocious thelarche in younger women. Providers should consider thyroid hormone problems when approaching patients with generalized problems, should examine patients for thyroid bruits or goiter, and should obtain thyroid hormone and thyroid-stimulating hormone levels as indicated in the evaluation of adolescents with most systemic complaints.

Most cases of complete congenital adrenal hyperplasia are diagnosed in early childhood. However, the diagnosis of partial enzyme deficiencies causing milder endocrine disturbances is often delayed until adolescence. The most common of these disorders is 21-hydroxylase deficiency, which results in excess levels of 17-OH progesterone. Some patients are asymptomatic; more typically, signs of androgen excess are seen, including hirsutism, premature pubic hair growth, advanced bone age, and growth acceleration. These symptoms may be difficult to differentiate from those of polycystic ovaries, or Stein-Leventhal syndrome.

Delayed puberty in women is generally defined as the absence of breast development by age 13 or the absence of menstrual periods by age 15 (Table 8-3). However, these statistical norms mean that about 2.5% of girls start their maturation outside of these ages. In constitutional delay, the woman is delayed but otherwise normal. The most common cause of hypergonadotropic hypogonadism is gonadal dysgenesis. Thus, a karyotype, as well as FSH and LH levels (and, in younger women, a bone age), often should be part of an initial evaluation for pubertal delay. Carefully reviewing the growth history, plotting and assessing height and weight and growth velocity, and examining anatomic structures are also important. Nutritional compromise, chronic illness, malignancies and their treatment, and infectious disease are also relatively common causes of pubertal delay. For example, 30% to 40% of all cases of inflammatory bowel disease present during adolescence. Although prepubertal onset of this condition may result in suppression of total linear growth, all adolescent girls with inflammatory bowel disease eventually reach full sexual maturation. In one study, the average age of menarche among girls with inflammatory bowel disease was 14.6 ± 1.9 years (compared to 12.8 years among white and 11.8 years among black girls in the United States).

Diabetes

Although diabetes is not unique to adolescents, several challenges occur during adolescence that can make diabetes control difficult. (Many of these issues are true for all youths with chronic disease.) For example, dietary compliance may become more difficult when medical regimens conflict with peer group behaviors, especially as young people begin to take responsibility for their

Table 8-3. Causes of Delayed Adolescence in the Phenotypic Male and Female

Hypergonadotropic Conditions
Variants of ovarian and testicular dysgenesis
Gonadal toxins (antimetabolite and radiation treatment)
Enzyme defects (17α-hydroxylase deficiency in the genetic male or female and 17-ketosteroid reductase deficiency in the genetic male)
Androgen insensitivity (testicular feminization)
Other miscellaneous disorders
Hypogonadotropic Conditions
Multiple tropic hormone deficiency
Isolated growth hormone deficiency
Isolated gonadotropia deficiency
Miscellaneous syndrome-complexes (eg, Prader-Willi syndrome)
Systemic conditions, nutritional and psychogenic disorders: increased energy expenditure
Other endocrine causes: hypothyroidism, glucocorticoid excess, hyperprolactinemia
Constitutional delay in growth and development
Eugonadotropic Conditions: Delayed Menarche
Gonadal dysgenesis variants with residually functioning ovarian tissue
Abnormalities of müllerian duct development
Polycystic ovary disease
Hyperprolactinemia

McAnarney ER, Kreipe RE, Orr D, Comerci G. Textbook of adolescent medicine. Philadelphia: WB Saunders, 1992.

own management, independent of their parents' or family's role. Thus, adolescents must learn to think ahead and adjust their insulin appropriately for dietary and exercise changes. Additionally, as young people become capable of formal operational thought and assume direct control for management of their diabetes, they may realize in a new way that their condition is permanent. This may result in denial, anger, and other stages of mourning for their normalcy. Although this adjustment to chronic disease is normal, adolescents, their families, and their health care providers should anticipate these conflicts and may need help in managing this period of adjustment.

In addition to adjusting as a developing adult to the presence of chronic disease, pregnancy and alcohol use pose special risks for diabetics. Diabetic women in poor control are more likely to develop nephropathy and retinopathy during pregnancy. Additionally, congenital anomalies are much more common among infants of diabetic mothers whose sugars are poorly controlled. Alcohol use can affect glucose metabolism, causing an initial rise in blood glucose levels, followed by a drop. Alcohol also enhances the glucose-lowering effects of insulin and prolongs its effect for up to 8 to 36 hours after consumption, increasing the risk of hypoglycemia. Because of these serious potential effects, adolescents should be counseled about the effects of drinking alcohol on their blood sugar. The American Diabetes Association recommends that alcohol should be used only if diabetes is well controlled, that drinking should be in moderation (no more than two drinks once or twice a week), and that insulin doses do not need to be changed. Others recommend that adolescents should avoid high-carbohydrate beverages (ie, beer) and should eat foods with complex carbohydrates, protein, and fat while drinking; this provides excess glucose over the period during which their glucose-regulatory mechanisms may be impaired.

Eating Disorders

Eating disorders (see Chap. 157) affect up to 5% of adolescent and young adult females, resulting in medical, psychological, and social dysfunction. Because the symptoms of an eating disorder may cause a young woman to visit (or be brought by her parents to) a primary care provider, practitioners must be able to recognize, evaluate, and initiate appropriate treatment, and when necessary make a referral for more intensive treatment.

Anorexia nervosa is a syndrome in which caloric intake insufficient to maintain weight is associated with a delusion of being fat and an obsession to be thinner, neither of which diminishes with weight loss. Patients with anorexia nervosa truly believe they are fat, even when emaciated (delusion). Likewise, they are driven to lose weight (obsession) through a variety of means (compulsions), including dieting and enhancing caloric output. The primary method of increasing caloric output is exercise, used by more than 75% of patients; vomiting and cathartics are less common means. A feature that differentiates simple dieting from anorexia nervosa is the difficulty that an affected person has in identifying, or being satisfied with, a healthy weight goal. Affected persons have a relentless pursuit of becoming thinner; thus, they repeatedly lower their goal weight as weight loss persists. Anorexia also may result in severe malnutrition.

The key clinical feature of bulimia nervosa is binge eating (not, as is often assumed, vomiting). Awareness that the binge eating pattern (ingesting large amounts of food over a short interval) is abnormal leads to depressed moods and self-deprecating thoughts. Temporary relief of the distress precipitated by a binge is sought through means intended to rid the body of the effects of calories; more than 80% of patients with bulimia nervosa engage in self-induced vomiting or laxative or diuretic abuse for this purpose. Fasting or exercise also may be used to avoid weight gain, but many patients with bulimia nervosa remain at normal to slightly above normal weight. Patients with bulimia are more likely than patients with anorexia nervosa to be impulsive, not only in eating behavior but also in their use of drugs and alcohol, self-mutilation or self-harm, sexual promiscuity, lying, stealing, and other manifestations of personality disturbance.

Anorexia nervosa and bulimia nervosa are not mutually exclusive diagnoses. Approximately 40% of patients with anorexia nervosa have a bulimic phase in the course of their illness or recovery. Binge eating disorder is also common in young adult females and is not associated with significant medical morbidity other than weight gain, but it is associated with emotional distress.

Regardless of how well a patient may appear, a detailed physical examination is indicated whenever there is concern about eating problems. For example, due to the recent availability of low-fat or nonfat foods and new food-labeling laws, some adolescents limit their fat intake to unhealthy levels, often to less than 10 g/day. Signs found on physical examination can be used as evidence that the patient is unhealthy. The presence of an organic condition, such as inflammatory bowel disease, thyroid disease, or a CNS lesion, must also be ruled out.

In patients with eating disorders, serum protein and albumin levels are generally normal. Liver function tests may reveal mildly elevated (up to two times normal) enzyme levels. Cholesterol levels are often elevated, sometimes dramatically, in starvation states. Some practitioners also routinely obtain thyroid screening; if abnormal, the T_3 level is usually low, a means of reducing the metabolic rate in association with low caloric intake. Patients typically have a clinical picture that suggests both hypothyroidism (fatigue, constipation, bradycardia, hypothermia) and hyperthyroidism (weight loss, excessive activity, anxiety), but the treatment for these symptoms is healthy nutrition and weight gain. The other endocrinopathy that is suggested by the constellation of weight loss, fatigue, and a small heart is Addison disease; the serum cortisol level tends to be high in anorexia nervosa, however. An electrocardiogram may be useful to determine the nature of profound bradycardia.

Obesity

An increasing proportion of adolescents in the United States are physically unfit and obese. Obesity is defined as having an increased amount of body fat (usually > 30% of body weight). Morbid obesity is defined as weight two times normal or 100 pounds above normal. Obesity is also associated with an increase in body weight or skinfold thickness, or by a body mass index above 30 (body mass index = weight in kg/[height in m]^2).

Normal puberty in females is associated with at least a doubling of the percentage of body weight that is fat. Thus, increases in weight in adolescent females must be interpreted in light of pubertal development, exercise patterns, and body composition. However, obesity tends to occur at least three times more commonly among girls than boys, especially in lower socioeconomic groups, and is more likely to persist into adulthood if it is present in childhood and adolescence.

The primary cause of most adolescent female obesity is a combination of excessive caloric intake and inadequate expenditure of energy in exercise. Ready access to high-fat, calorically dense fast foods and snacks, together with an increasingly sedentary lifestyle, accounts for numerous cases of adolescent obesity. Furthermore, there is growing evidence that pregnancy among some adolescents may be associated with weight gain that is not lost postpartum. Depressed moods, low self-esteem, and feelings of inadequacy are also often found in obese adolescent females, although the cause-and-effect relation is unclear.

When evaluating weight gain in early adolescents, it is important also to chart changes in height. Exogenous obesity, in which excessive calories account for the increase in weight, is characterized by an increase in height; endocrine causes of obesity are marked by growth retardation rather than acceleration. Recent evidence underscores the importance of genetic influences; however, environmental influences also play a role in obesity. Thus, even if there is a strong family history of obesity, there is still reason to institute effective weight-management practices.

Successful treatment of obesity in adolescent females is difficult (Table 8-4). Early adolescents may be especially difficult to treat due to lack of motivation. Food is often used as a source of comfort or as a reward; its ready availability ensures immediate gratification. Diets may be seen as restrictive, punitive, or controlling. If a parent institutes limitations in caloric intake without the active participation of the adolescent, she may interpret this as rejection by the parent. Such circumstances often lead to surreptitious eating, acting out adolescent rebellion in a way that only she can control. On the other hand, permissive parents often find it onerous to restrict their daughter's intake, perceiving such behavior as uncaring, even when the adolescent herself wants to lose weight. Thus, even though a primary care provider may recognize the value of losing weight for medical or psychosocial reasons (Table 8-5), it is best not to institute definitive therapy until the younger adolescent and at least one of her parents are interested in change. For older adolescents, individual motivation may be sufficient. Regardless, it is best to provide information regarding ways to control weight in a nonthreatening and nonjudgmental manner.

Obesity treatment is often viewed as futile, but there are many effective strategies primary care providers can use to help overweight adolescents adopt healthy lifestyles. "Dieting: the best way to gain weight" is a popular aphorism that underscores the importance of changing eating habits and patterns instead of dieting, which may be viewed as restraining and limiting. Unfortunately, adolescents and young adults are bombarded by advertisements that promise quick, effortless weight loss through dieting programs of dubious value. There is no scientific evidence to substantiate most of the claims of these diets or formulas. Diets alone rarely lead to healthy, sustained weight loss.

Rather than prescribing a diet, the primary care provider should help the adolescent learn to make nutritional choices that are balanced, healthy, sustainable, and enjoyable (Table 8-6). Thus, preprinted diets have less value than an exchange system of meal planning, in which she can choose from a wide variety of foods that will meet her daily preferences and requirements while also allowing her to control her weight in a healthy manner.

Table 8-4. Evaluation of the Obese Adolescent Patient

History

Family history: obesity and stature, endocrine problems, psychiatric problems

Past medical history: serious illnesses, surgery, menstrual history

History of obesity: abrupt onset vs. chronic history, physical problems or development at time of rapid weight gain, etc.

Dietary history: 24-hour diet recall, review of eating habits including timing and circumstances surrounding mealtimes and snacks, history of previous weight-loss attempts

Social history: family, school, and individual stressors, especially at times of rapid weight gain

Physical Examination

Anthropometrics: height, weight, triceps skinfolds

Sexual maturity rating

Vital signs, including blood pressure taken with appropriate-size cuff

Complete physical examination for causes of secondary obesity and complications of obesity

Laboratory Tests

Routine screening with cholesterol and triglyceride levels

Endocrine studies *only* if suggested by history or physical examination

Estimate of basal metabolic rate may be helpful

(McAnarney ER, Kreipe RE, Orr D, Comerci G. Textbook of adolescent medicine. Philadelphia: WB Saunders, 1992.)

TABLE 8-5. Complications of Obesity

During Adolescence

Psychosocial

Disturbed body image

Poor self-image/self-esteem

Poor family relations: scapegoat and source of embarrassment

Poor peer relations and social isolation

Exclusion from activities, especially dating

Acting out and depression

Medical

Potentially lethal:

Obstructive sleep apnea, pickwickian syndrome

Pancreatitis

Heart failure from cardiomyopathy

Less severe:

Orthopedic: slipped capital femoral epiphysis, coxa vara, Perthes disease, ankle fracture, genu valgum

Metabolic: gallstones, hypercholesterolemia

Skin problems: candidal infections, breakdown

Pseudogynecomastia

Neurologic: pseudotumor cerebri

Increased risk of adult obesity

During Adulthood

Psychosocial

Job discrimination

Others as during adolescence

Medical

Cardiovascular disease: hypertension, hypercholesterolemia, diabetes mellitus, coronary artery disease, cerebrovascular disease (increased with "android" fat distribution)

Cancer: endometrial, breast, prostate, colon

Orthopedic: gouty and degenerative arthritis

Genitourinary incontinence, male sexual dysfunction

Surgical: increased operative morbidity and mortality

(McAnarney ER, Kreipe RE, Orr D, Comerci G. Textbook of Adolescent medicine. Philadelphia; WB Saunders, 1992.)

Weight-reduction programs that do not include an increase in physical activity are doomed to failure. School buses, escalators, elevators, and remote-control devices are all conveniences that reduce physical activity. Adolescents trying to lose weight should be encouraged to seek ways to burn calories in their activities of daily living. In addition, they should be involved in a regular exercise program for at least 20 minutes a day, 3 to 5 days a week.

Adolescents can also benefit from participation in group weight-loss programs (eg, Take Off Pounds Sensibly [TOPS], Overeaters Anonymous [OA], Weight Watchers). Shapedown is a successful comprehensive program that is highly structured and focuses on changing behavior patterns related to eating, emotional conflicts, and family life. It is targeted at adolescents and requires at least one parent to be an active participant along with the adolescent.

Several drugs that induce anorexia have recently been approved. However, there is little evidence for their use in the treatment of adolescent obesity.

Menstrual Cycle Disorders

Menstrual periods begin relatively late in puberty, usually during Tanner stage 4 (see Figs. 8-2 and 8-3). The normal menstrual cycle averages 28 days, with a range from 21 to 35 days. Adolescents often have even longer cycles, especially during their first 2 years of menstruation (see Chap. 9). Negative feedback of estradiol on the hypothalamus and pituitary is present throughout infancy and childhood. However, the positive feedback of estrogens on the pituitary, with the resulting LH surge, develops in middle to late puberty. Increasing positive feedback occurs as the hypothalamus becomes decreasingly sensitive to negative feedback during early puberty. However, without positive feedback, ovulation does not occur. Thus, regular ovulation often does not occur for several years after menarche, and most young women have a mixture of ovulatory and anovulatory cycles. Many early adolescent cycles are due to negative feedback and cyclic production of gonadotropin and estrogen, and many of these cycles may be anovulatory. In fact, 28- to 42-day cyclic FSH and LH hormone levels are present in pubertal girls even before menarche. During these anovulatory periods, stimulation of ovarian hormonal activity may result in physiologically normal ovarian enlargement and multiple cyst formation. Dysmenorrhea may become significantly worse after a few years of menstrual cycles, as young women develop predominantly ovulatory cycles.

Menstrual irregularity in young women may present anywhere along the spectrum of frequent, prolonged bleeding to complete amenorrhea. Although the most common cause of amenorrhea or abnormal uterine bleeding is pregnancy, this can usually be diagnosed easily. Primary care providers should be aware of the high likelihood of anovulatory cycles during puberty and should be

Table 8-6. Principles of Healthy Eating

Use the food pyramid (6–11 servings of bread, cereal, rice, or pasta; 3–5 servings of vegetables; 2–4 servings of fruit; 2–3 servings of milk, yogurt, or cheese; 2–3 servings of meat, dry beans, eggs, or nuts as sources of protein; and sparse use of oils, fats, and sweets) to plan the daily intake.

Avoid "good food"/"bad food" dichotomies that can lead to unhealthy, monotonous choices and guilt feelings when a "bad" food is ingested.

Spread daily intake evenly over three well-balanced meals plus one or two snacks.

Recognize breakfast as the most important meal of the day.

Reduce intake of calories gradually and not excessively.

Consider how foods are prepared, as well as their intrinsic caloric content and density.

Combine reduction of caloric intake with increase in caloric expenditure through regular, moderate exercise.

Accept small weight losses.

A number of these goals can be more easily achieved within a behavior-modification system that increases motivation and rewards appropriate actions.

familiar with the diagnosis and management of menstrual disorders.

Persistent stimulation of the endometrium by estrogen, in the face of inadequate LH to produce ovulation, may present as short cycles, excessive bleeding, oligomenorrhea, or amenorrhea. In contrast, low-estrogen states, due to lack of gonadotropin stimulation or to end-organ unresponsiveness (ovarian failure), results in an atretic uterine lining and amenorrhea. Amenorrhea in young women may also be due to severe underweight or abnormal body composition, due to chronic illness, poor nutrition, or excessive exercise. These conditions probably act by suppression of gonadotropin-releasing hormones from the hypothalamus; thus, amenorrhea may also be seen with high levels of stress and in response to drugs. When presenting with galactorrhea, amenorrhea is likely to be due to a prolactinoma, to elevated prolactin levels due to drugs (including phenothiazines, cocaine, and marijuana), or to pregnancy.

Another common pattern of menstrual irregularity is associated with androgen excess. Generally, estrogen levels are normal or high, but gonadotropin levels do not fluctuate normally, LH levels are quite high, and LH : FSH ratios exceed 3 : 1. These patients appear hirsute and obese. Some present with premature pubic hair and acne development, occasionally due to mild 21-OH deficiency or another adrenal etiology for androgen excess. However, most present with hirsutism, acne, and accelerated weight gain during puberty, without any enzymatic deficiency. When present with oligomenorrhea, these symptoms characterize Stein-Leventhal syndrome, or polycystic ovary syndrome. The differential diagnosis of amenorrhea and obesity in adolescents also includes adrenocorticoid excess (both endogenous and exogenous) and hypothyroidism. However, hypothyroidism may also present as excessive periods, especially in women presenting later in puberty.

Management of irregular menses in adolescents requires accurate history taking and a careful physical examination. Menstrual calendars may help with regard to bleeding, hormonally related cyclic changes, and other symptoms. For example, anovulatory bleeding is usually painless and is not accompanied by the breast soreness or cramps often associated with ovulatory cycles. A review of the patient's history for sexual activity; chronic illness; congenital anomalies; herniorrhaphy (suggesting an XY karyotype); hormonal, radiation, or CNS insult; or drug exposure and a developmental and sexual developmental history should also be obtained.

Examination should include careful evaluation for developmental stage, hirsutism, galactorrhea, and genital anatomy. Estrogenization of the vaginal introitus should be assessed; this can be quantified by Pap fixation of a vaginal smear. Enlargement of the clitoris suggests androgen excess. The vagina should be examined either by a digital examination or with a cotton-tipped applicator probe, and a bimanual vaginal or rectal examination should be performed to assess uterine size and adnexae. Laboratory examinations should include a urine beta-HCG to rule out pregnancy, thyroid function tests, and serum LH, FSH, and prolactin levels. Often a progestin challenge with medroxyprogesterone (Provera), 10 mg/day for 10 days, is sufficient to induce menses and diagnose anovulatory cycles in nonpregnant amenorrheic patients. If an LH:FSH ratio greater than 3 : 1, hirsutism, or other signs of androgen excess are present, androgen levels should also be obtained. In patients with polycystic ovaries, low-progestin oral contraceptives allow regular cycles and also lower androgen levels. Weight control is also an important component of therapy. Oral contraceptives are often the treatment of choice for excessive bleeding due to dysfunctional uterine bleeding (see Chap. 9), for dysmenorrhea (as a first-line therapy for sexually active teens, and as a second choice after nonsteroidal antiinflammatory drugs in women who are not sexually active), and for premenstrual syndrome.

Orthopedic Conditions and Sports-Related Injuries

Scoliosis, or lateral curvature of the spine, is a common problem during adolescence. Due to its low specificity, screening examination for scoliosis in school settings generates many unnecessary referrals. However, screening in primary care practice is indicated.

A scoliosis screening examination is performed by first observing the young woman from behind, looking for asymmetric shoulder height, prominent scapula, unequal arm-to-trunk length, or palpable lateral curves of the spine. She should next be asked to bend forward from the waist with her palms opposed and her elbows straight. Elevation of one scapula is characteristic of scoliosis; the right scapula is elevated in 95% of cases. Patients should also be observed closely for asymmetry of the chest wall or lumbar area.

Scoliosis is usually idiopathic, or it may be due to neuromuscular disease, congenital anomaly, congenital injury, or intraspinous processes. The significance of scoliosis depends on the location and degree of the curvature. The severity of scoliosis is determined by radiologic evaluation. In general, nonprogressive and painless curves less than 25° do not require active treatment. Those greater than 25°, as well as all curves accompanied by pain or neurologic symptoms, should be referred to an orthopedic surgeon for further evaluation. Scoliosis tends to progress most rapidly during the growth spurt, during SMR 2 and 3 in girls, and adolescents should be monitored as frequently as every 3 months during this period of rapid growth. Bracing prevents curves greater than 30° from progressing but does not eliminate any preexisting curvature. Those greater than 40° often continue to progress into adulthood and often require surgery to halt progression of the curvature.

Although relatively rare, slipped capital femoral epiphysis almost always occurs during the adolescent growth spurt. Rapid growth, obesity, trauma, inflammatory diseases, and genetic factors all play a role in this condition. Most symptoms and cases are subacute, with limping and mild intermittent pain as the most common presenting symptoms. Physical examination findings include pain on motion and limited internal rotation and abduction of the affected hip; the leg is held flexed and externally rotated. The limp is typically a Trendelenburg gait due to weak hip abductors on the affected side. A high index of suspicion, accurate radiographic diagnosis (including lateral views), and rapid fixation to prevent further slipping and, if needed, to realign the trochanter and the femoral head are indicated to minimize the risk of avascular necrosis and degenerative joint disease.

The greatest risk factor for sports injury in adolescents is a prior significant sports injury. Several organizational guidelines have addressed sports participation examinations, and a model form is shown in Figure 8-9. The goals of these examinations are to detect potentially life-threatening conditions and previous or incompletely rehabilitated injuries and to direct developing athletes into activities that maximize their opportunity for performance while minimizing their risk of injury. This evaluation should not take the place of regular routine well care, and the

Part C – PHYSICAL EXAMINATION RECORD

NAME ______________ DATE ________ AGE ________ BIRTHDATE ______________

Height ________ Vision: R _____/_____, corrected _____, uncorrected _____

Weight ________ L _____/_____, corrected _____, uncorrected _____

Pulse ________ Blood Pressure ______________ Percent Body Fat (optional) ______________

	Normal	Abnormal Findings					Initials
1. Eyes							
2. Ears, Nose, Throat							
3. Mouth & Teeth							
4. Neck							
5. Cardiovascular							
6. Chest and Lungs							
7. Abdomen							
8. Skin							
9. Genitalia - Hernia (male)							
10. Musculoskeletal: ROM, strength, etc.							
a. neck							
b. spine							
c. shoulders							
d. arms/hands							
e. hips							
f. thighs							
g. knees							
h. ankles							
i. feet							
11. Neuromuscular							
12. Physical Maturity (Tanner Stage)		1.	2.	3.	4.	5.	

Comments re: Abnormal Findings: ______________

____

____

____

PARTICIPATION RECOMMENDATIONS:

1. No participation in: ______________

____

2. Limited participation in: ______________

____

3. Requires: ______________

____

4. Full participation in: ______________

Physician Signature ______________

Telephone Number ______________ Address ______________

A American Academy of Pediatrics

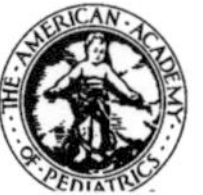

Figure 8-9. Preparticipation sports screening examination form, 1990. Parts A and B show both sides of form. (Courtesy of American Academy of Pediatrics.)

SPORTS PARTICIPATION HEALTH RECORD

This evaluation is only to determine readiness for sports participation. It should not be used as a substitute for regular health maintenance examinations.

NAME ______ AGE ______(YRS) GRADE ______ DATE ______

ADDRESS ______ PHONE ______

SPORTS ______

The Health History (Part A) and Physical Examination (Part C) sections must both be completed, at least every 24 months, before sports participation. The Interim Health History section (Part B) needs to be completed at least annually.

PART A — HEALTH HISTORY:
To be completed by athlete and parent

	YES	NO
1. Have you ever had an illness that:		
a. required you to stay in the hospital?	____	____
b. lasted longer than a week?	____	____
c. caused you to miss 3 days of practice or a competition?	____	____
d. is related to allergies? (ie, hay fever, hives, asthma, insect stings)	____	____
e. required an operation?	____	____
f. is chronic? (ie, asthma, diabetes, etc)	____	____
2. Have you ever had an injury that:		
a. required you to go to an emergency room or see a doctor?	____	____
b. required you to stay in the hospital?	____	____
c. required x-rays?	____	____
d. caused you to miss 3 days of practice or a competition?	____	____
e. required an operation?	____	____
3. Do you take any medication or pills?	____	____
4. Have any members of your family under age 50 had a heart attack, heart problem, or died unexpectedly?	____	____
5. Have you ever:		
a. been dizzy or passed out during or after exercise?	____	____
b. been unconscious or had a concussion?	____	____
6. Are you unable to run 1/2 mile (2 times around the track) without stopping?	____	____
7. Do you:		
a. wear glasses or contacts?	____	____
b. wear dental bridges, plates, or braces?	____	____
8. Have you ever had a heart murmur, high blood pressure, or a heart abnormality?	____	____
9. Do you have any allergies to any medicine?	____	____
10. Are you missing a kidney?	____	____

11. When was your last tetanus booster? ______

12. **For Women**
    a. At what age did you experience your first menstrual period? ______
    b. In the last year, what is the longest time you have gone between periods? ______

EXPLAIN ANY "YES" ANSWERS ______

______

______

______

I hereby state that, to the best of my knowledge, my answers to the above questions are correct.

Date ______

Signature of athlete ______

Signature of parent ______

PART B — INTERIM HEALTH HISTORY:
This form should be used during the interval between preparticipation evaluations. Positive responses should prompt a medical evaluation.

1. Over the next 12 months, I wish to participate in the following sports:
   a. ______
   b. ______
   c. ______
   d. ______

2. Have you missed more than 3 consecutive days of participation in usual activities because of an injury this past year?
   Yes ______ No ______
   If yes, please indicate:
   a. Site of injury ______
   b. Type of injury ______

3. Have you missed more than 5 consecutive days of participation in usual activities because of an illness, or have you had a medical illness diagnosed that has not been resolved in this past year?
   Yes ______ No ______
   If yes, please indicate:
   a. Type of illness ______

4. Have you had a seizure, concussion or been unconscious for any reason in the last year?
   Yes ______ No ______

5. Have you had surgery or been hospitalized in this past year?
   Yes ______ No ______
   If yes, please indicate:
   a. Reason for hospitalization ______
   b. Type of surgery ______

6. List all medications you are presently taking and what condition the medication is for.
   a. ______
   b. ______
   c. ______

7. Are you worried about any problem or condition at this time?
   Yes ______ No ______
   If yes, please explain: ______
   ______
   ______
   ______

I hereby state that, to the best of my knowledge, my answers to the above questions are correct.

Date ______

Signature of athlete ______

Signature of parent ______

B

Figure 8-9. (Continued.)

sports physical can be combined with regular preventive service visits without jeopardizing the importance of the preparticipation safety assessment.

Primary care physicians often are called on to assess sports injuries. Most injuries are sprains, strains, or contusions and can be managed initially with rest, ice, compression, and elevation (RICE). Injuries that should be evaluated by an orthopedist include those with rapid or obvious swelling, a popping or snapping noise at the time of injury, anatomic deformity, limited range of motion, neurovascular compromise, or joint instability.

Rheumatologic Conditions

The most common rheumatologic conditions affecting adolescents are rheumatoid arthritis, systemic lupus erythematosus, and dermatomyositis. Caring for patients with these conditions should usually involve consultation with experts in pediatric rheumatology.

The most common chronic arthritis in adolescent females is pauciarticular rheumatoid arthritis. This condition, affecting fewer than five joints, usually begins between ages 12 and 16. Patients are generally well, with the exception of asymmetric inflammation of the larger lower extremity joints, most commonly the knee. If only one joint is inflamed, septic arthritis, particularly with *N gonorrhoeae*, must be considered in the differential diagnosis. Antinuclear antibody (ANA) is used as a marker for increased risk of uveitis and iridocyclitis, unrelated to the extent of pauciarticular joint involvement. Thus, adolescent females who are ANA positive with pauciarticular arthritis should have eye examinations annually, regardless of the activity of joint inflammation. HLA-B27 antigen is associated with this form of arthritis in less than 10% of girls.

Polyarticular arthritis is characterized by symmetric inflammation of at least five joints, usually the smaller ones of the hands and feet, wrists, and elbows. Positive rheumatoid factor (RF+) is found in only 10% to 15% of cases of juvenile polyarticular arthritis; it is more common in females and, when present, is associated with the onset of progressive joint destruction at a median age of 12 years. RF– disease, on the other hand, is usually marked by exacerbations and remissions, with a good long-term prognosis.

The management of adolescents with juvenile arthritis consists of medications (systemic, intraarticular, or both), physical therapy, and supportive therapy; surgery may be required for destructive forms. Nonsteroidal antiinflammatory drugs are the primary medications used, although low-dose systemic corticosteroids can be a very effective short-term adjunctive. Cytotoxic medications and cyclosporine also have a place in the treatment of juvenile arthritis but should be prescribed only by those familiar with their use.

Systemic lupus erythematosus is a multisystem disease with protean manifestations, sparing no organ. Females are affected five times more commonly than males, with the onset commonly at puberty. There is a familial predisposition to lupus, and HLA loci that are associated with it include A1, B8, and DR3. A positive ANA test, various antinuclear subunit antibodies (particularly *rho* and *la*), and an elevated erythrocyte sedimentation rate are highly sensitive but not specific for the diagnosis. Up to half of adolescents with lupus present with primarily behavioral or psychiatric manifestations. Long-term management can be difficult because of the chronic nature of the illness and the prominence of mental health problems.

Juvenile dermatomyositis is an inflammatory myopathy characterized by vasculitis of the skin and skeletal muscles. Dermatomyositis has a female predominance during adolescence. HLA loci DR3 and B8 are associated with dermatomyositis. A light, violaceous, scaling, mildly edematous "heliotrope" rash usually affects the eyelids. Scaling, erythematous to violaceous papular lesions are usually found over the interphalangeal joints, elbows, knees, and malleoli and may progress to become thickened, smooth, and shiny (Gottron patches). Muscle involvement is primarily proximal and rarely involves the heart. About 25% of affected adolescent females have complications involving the GI tract, joints, or skin (calcinosis cutis). Treatment involves aggressive physical therapy to preserve range of motion and strength, together with systemic corticosteroids and, in resistant cases, immunosuppressive therapy.

Neurologic Conditions

Seizures, nonepileptic paroxysmal disorders, multiple sclerosis (MS), myasthenia gravis, and Wilson disease are among the neurologic conditions that may present in adolescence. All these conditions require close coordination of care between the primary care provider and neurologists and other specialists skilled in managing these conditions.

Epilepsy is a symptom complex defined as recurrent, episodic paroxysms (seizures) due to activation of the cerebral cortex and gray matter. Seizures may be due to tumors, metabolic disturbances, or infection but are often idiopathic. The location and pattern of spread of activity determine the clinical expression. Few forms of epilepsy have their onset in adolescence, but epileptic seizures may worsen during adolescence because of hormonal changes (especially in relation to the menstrual cycle), because of changes in the metabolism of anticonvulsants during puberty, or because of nonadherence to medication regimens due to psychosocial conflicts. These conflicts may include having a chronic illness with few visible manifestations, undesirable side effects of medications, limit-testing with authority, fear of losing control when having a seizure, and being unable to participate in activities.

Syncope and hyperventilation are two common nonictal paroxysmal disorders in adolescent females. There is a prodrome in each, which may be followed by secondary epileptic phenomena. Therefore, the history of events immediately before the attacks must be sought. Syncope is characterized by malaise, vertigo and dizziness, and blurring and fading of vision, followed by the loss of postural tone and passing out; pallor and limpness are often noted by witnesses. Hyperventilation causes a similar lightheadedness and blurring of vision, but patients also characteristically report perioral paresthesias and tingling of the fingertips.

MS, the most common demyelinating disease in adolescent females, is an immune-mediated disorder characterized by demyelination and scarring of white matter in multiple CNS sites over time. The differential diagnosis includes idiopathic optic neuritis, acute disseminated encephalomyelitis, the inherited leukodystrophies, and collagen vascular diseases. Most adolescents with MS have well-delineated exacerbations and remissions, with complete or nearly complete recovery, but a few have a severe, rapidly progressive form of the disease. Although there is no definitive cure, treatment consists of symptomatic management in combination with various immunomodulators.

Myasthenia gravis is an immunologically mediated disorder of the neuromuscular junction that results in episodic or progressive skeletal muscle weakness. Juvenile myasthenia is more common in females than males and is associated with acetylcholine receptor antibodies. The insidious onset of weakness of the ocular, facial, and oropharyngeal muscles is characteristic; often patients complain of ptosis or diplopia, and symptoms tend to worsen late in the day or during stress or fatigue. Generalized muscle weakness, if it occurs, progresses slowly. Intravenous administration of edrophonium chloride (Tensilon) generally results in an abrupt improvement in strength and provides a presumptive diagnosis. Almost all adolescents respond, at least initially, to treatment with cholinesterase inhibitors.

Wilson disease, an autosomal dominant condition resulting from an inborn error of copper metabolism, often presents in adolescents with tremor, chorea, dystonia, and dysarthria. Due to behavioral abnormalities, it may initially be mistaken for a primary psychiatric condition. Copper deposition in the cornea produces the pathognomonic Kayser-Fleischer ring, which is always present when neurologic symptoms are evident. The diagnosis is confirmed by finding excessive copper concentration and a decreased serum ceruloplasmin level in the blood.

Psychological Conditions

Among the many mental health issues important to the care of women, two are particularly relevant to primary care practice: depression and somatoform disorders.

Depression in older adolescents presents much as it does in adults, with sadness, depressed mood, sleep disturbances, anhedonia, and other vegetative (or agitated) symptoms. However, in younger and middle adolescents, depression may present in a masked form and may be hard to differentiate from oppositional behavior or other acting-out or behavioral problems. In young adolescents in particular, depression often does not present as sadness but as irritability, aggression, or acting-out behavior. As adolescents mature, their increasing cognitive ability makes it possible to think about thinking, and thus to express sadness and manifest more adult-like depressive symptoms.

Many adolescents experience transient depression: as many as 25% to 66% of adolescents report feeling sad or depressed. However, younger adolescents with depression may report being bored as their only symptom. Additionally, as many as 15% of 10th graders report having tried to commit suicide (many of these youths never receive medical or mental health services for their attempts). Major depression is defined by either depressed mood or loss of interest or pleasure in nearly all activities for at least 2 weeks. The prevalence of major affective disorders in adolescents has been estimated at 4% to 6%. Although bipolar disease is much rarer that depressive illness, the peak period of onset for bipolar disease is between ages 15 and 25. The differential diagnosis of depression includes depressed mood due to a medical or social condition (eg, bereavement) and also must include consideration of organic etiologies for the mood disturbance (eg, hypothyroidism, substance abuse).

Many adolescents who attempt or complete suicide present to primary care providers in the 2- to 4-week period before their attempt, often presenting with vague or nonspecific complaints. Thus, systematic and careful screening for depressed mood and suicidality is an important part of adolescent primary care practice. Mildly depressed mood or occasional suicidal thoughts without specific intent are normal, and adolescents can be reassured as well as informed of the availability of resources should they need more intensive counseling. Most primary care providers should also be comfortable diagnosing and treating depressive illness and managing first-line pharmacologic therapy with either tricyclic antidepressants (eg, imipramine, desipramine, amitriptyline) or selective serotonin reuptake inhibitors (fluoxetine, sertraline, paroxetine). The use of these medications is reviewed in Chapter 153. Primary care providers should also have crisis services available so that adolescents at high risk for self-destructive behaviors can be assessed by mental health professionals without delay.

Somatoform disorders include a variety of conditions in which physical symptoms are attributed to emotional or psychological factors. These disorders are often considered when an adolescent's symptoms suggest a medical problem but her history, physical examination, and laboratory studies do not support an organic cause, giving rise to a presumed psychological etiology. These disorders are often grouped into conditions in which symptoms are under voluntary control (malingering and factitious disorders) and those with involuntary symptoms (somatization disorder, conversion disorder, hypochondriasis). The professional providing primary care to adolescent females must avoid common pitfalls in approaching the diagnosis and management of these disorders.

In clinical practice, it is usually countertherapeutic to label the cause of symptoms as organic or psychological and the control over symptoms as voluntary or involuntary. The rare patient who has malingering or factitious disorder generally seeks care from other sources after her diagnosis is discovered. The vast majority of adolescent females in primary care with somatoform disorders begin to have symptoms as part of an organic process (such as a viral illness or trauma) but then have persistent or gradually changing symptoms as the organic process subsides. They seek care because their symptoms are not under their control and interfere with their daily activities. Thus, attempts to determine if the symptoms are voluntary are met, understandably, with resistance and frustration. Making the diagnosis by exclusion ("I can't find anything wrong. Your symptoms must be due to psychological problems.") rarely is accepted, as it implies that the symptoms are imaginary or are being feigned. Referral to a mental health provider, although possibly worthwhile, is usually rejected because the symptoms are experienced somatically and are not "all in her head."

Perhaps the best example of the futility of making a diagnosis of somatoform disorder by exclusion is provided by adolescent dysmenorrhea. In the early 1970s, a reputable pediatric publication described the cause of adolescent dysmenorrhea as "psychogenic." A decade later, that same publication reported that dysmenorrhea was due to increased and irregular myometrial pressure related to prostaglandin levels. In the intervening decade, there was an increase in knowledge regarding menstrual physiology; in the absence of knowledge, psychogenic causes had been presumed previously. The absence of proof of organic causation does not rule out organic pathology. Thus, symptoms should be assumed to be involuntary unless proven otherwise. Finally, if a psychological conflict is discovered while evaluating a patient, it should be acknowledged and addressed, whether or not there is an etiologic link with the presenting symptoms.

When approaching the adolescent female with a somatoform disorder, communication during the evaluation is part of the intervention; active listening is essential on the part of the primary care provider. A dichotomous, "rule-out," mechanistic approach is counterproductive. When the patient seems disappointed to learn that "all the tests are normal," this does not necessarily mean she wants to be in the sick role (factitious disorder). More likely, she may interpret negative tests as evidence that her symptoms are either not being taken seriously or cannot be relieved.

A functional pathophysiologic explanation is needed and should be based on data obtained during the evaluation. For example, tension headaches in the temporal region are best attributed to sustained contraction of the temporalis and masseter muscles. To emphasize this, it is often helpful to have the patient bite down hard while placing her fingers on the temporal region. The resultant palpable movement of the painful area as her affected jaw and scalp muscles contract demonstrates the biologic substrate of her pain.

Any concomitant developmental or psychological problems should be identified during the evaluation, rather than attempting to identify psychological "causes" of the symptom. Often there is a family member with a similar problem, so it is frequently essential to include the family in the treatment program.

Finally, primary care providers can institute face-saving therapies for the symptoms to resolve. These can include physical therapy, biofeedback, and attention to adequate sleep, nutrition, and exercise. The use of a symptom journal can be effective in documenting the conflicts that may be related to the symptoms. Additionally, seeing these patients regularly (regardless of symptoms), examining the patient on each visit, and performing only those laboratory tests indicated by physical findings help limit unnecessary testing and often help allow for recovery over time.

BIBLIOGRAPHY

American Medical Association. Guidelines for adolescent preventive services. Chicago, 1992.

Emans SJ, Goldstein DP. Pediatric and adolescent gynecology, 3d ed. Boston: Little, Brown & Co., 1990.

Hoffman AD, Greydanus DE. Adolescent medicine, 2d ed. Norwalk, CT: Appleton & Lange, 1989.

McAnarney ER, Kreipe RE, Orr DP, Comerci GD. Textbook of adolescent medicine. Philadelphia: WB Saunders, 1992.

U.S. Congress, Office of Technology Assessment. Adolescent health. OTA-H-468. Washington DC, April 1991.

APPENDIX GUIDELINES FOR ADOLESCENT PREVENTIVE SERVICES

RECOMMENDATIONS FOR DELIVERY OF HEALTH SERVICES

Recommendation 1: From ages 11 to 21, all adolescents should have an annual preventive services visit.

- These visits should address both the biomedical and psychosocial aspects of health and should focus on preventive services.
- Adolescents should have a complete physical examination during three of these preventive services visits. One should be performed during early adolescence (age 11-14), one during middle adolescence (15-17), and one during late adolescence (18-21), unless more frequent examinations are warranted by clinical signs or symptoms.

Recommendation 2: Preventive services should be age- and developmentally appropriate and should be sensitive to individual and sociocultural differences.

Recommendation 3: Physicians should establish office policies regarding confidential care for adolescents and how parents will be involved in that care. These policies should be made clear to adolescents and their parents.

RECOMMENDATIONS FOR HEALTH GUIDANCE

Recommendation 4: Parents or other adult caregivers should receive health guidance at least once during their child's early adolescence, once during middle adolescence, and preferably once during late adolescence.

This includes providing information about:

- Normative adolescent development, including information about physical, sexual, and emotional development
- Signs and symptoms of disease and emotional distress
- Parenting behaviors that promote healthy adolescent adjustment
- Why parents should discuss health-related behaviors with their adolescents, plan family activities, and act as role models for health-related behaviors
- Methods for helping their adolescent avoid potentially harmful behaviors, such as:
  - Monitoring and managing the adolescent's use of motor vehicles, especially new drivers
  - Avoiding having weapons in the home. Parents who have weapons in the home should be advised to make them inaccessible to adolescents. If adolescents have weapons, parents and other adult caregivers should ensure that adolescents follow weapon safety procedures.
  - Removing weapons and potentially lethal medications from the homes of adolescents who have suicidal intent
  - Monitoring their adolescent's social and recreational activities for the use of tobacco, alcohol and other drugs, and sexual behavior.

Recommendation 5: All adolescents should receive health guidance annually to promote a better understanding of their physical growth, psychosocial and psychosexual development, and the importance of becoming actively involved in decisions regarding their health care.

Recommendation 6: All adolescents should receive health guidance annually to promote the reduction on injuries.

Health guidance for injury prevention includes the following:

- Counseling to avoid the use of alcohol or other substances while using motor or recreational vehicles, or where impaired judgment may lead to injury
- Counseling to use safety devices, including seat belts, motorcycle and bicycle helmets, and appropriate athletic protective devices
- Counseling to resolve interpersonal conflicts without violence

- Counseling to avoid the use of weapons or promote weapon safety
- Counseling to promote appropriate physical conditioning before exercise.

Recommendation 7: All adolescents should receive health guidance annually about dietary habits, including the benefits of a healthy diet and ways to achieve a healthy diet and safe weight management.

Recommendation 8: All adolescents should receive health guidance annually about the benefits of exercise and should be encouraged to engage in safe exercise on a regular basis.

Recommendation 9: All adolescents should receive health guidance annually regarding responsible sexual behavior, including abstinence. Latex condoms to prevent STDs, including HIV infection, and appropriate methods of birth control should be made available, as should instructions on how to use them effectively.

Health guidance for sexual responsibility includes the following:

- Counseling that abstinence from sexual intercourse is the most effective way to prevent pregnancy and STDs, including HIV infection
- Counseling on how HIV infection is transmitted, the dangers of the disease, and the fact that latex condoms are effective in preventing STDs, including HIV infection
- Reinforcement of responsible sexual behavior for adolescents who are not currently sexually active and for those who are using birth control and condoms appropriately
- Counseling on the need to protect themselves and their partners from pregnancy, STDs, including HIV infection, and sexual exploitation.

Recommendation 10: All adolescents should receive health guidance annually to promote avoidance of tobacco, alcohol and other abusable substances, and anabolic steroids.

Recommendation 11: All adolescents should be screened annually for hypertension according to the protocol developed by the National Heart, Lung, and Blood Institute Second Task Force on Blood Pressure Control in Children.

- Adolescents with either systolic or diastolic pressures at or above the 90th percentile for gender and age should have blood pressure (BP) measurements repeated at three different times within one month under similar physical conditions to confirm baseline values.
- Adolescents with baseline BP values greater than the 95th percentile for gender and age should have a complete biomedical evaluation to establish treatment options. Adolescents with BP values between the 90th and 95th percentile should be assessed for obesity and their BP monitored every 6 months.

Recommendation 12: Selected adolescents should be screened to determine their risk of developing hyperlipidemia and adult coronary heart disease, following the protocol developed by the Expert Panel on Blood Cholesterol Levels in Children and Adolescents.

- Adolescents whose parents have a serum cholesterol level greater than 240 mg/dL and adolescents who are over 19 years of age should be screened for total blood cholesterol level (nonfasting) at least once.
- Adolescents with an unknown family history or those who have multiple risk factors for future cardiovascular disease (eg, smoking, hypertension, obesity, diabetes mellitus, excessive consumption of dietary saturated fats and cholesterol) may be screened for total serum cholesterol level (nonfasting) at least once at the discretion of the physician.
- Adolescents with blood cholesterol values less than 170 mg/dL should have the test repeated within 5 years. Those with values between 170 and 199 mg/dL should have a repeated test. If the average of the two tests is below 170 mg/dL, total blood cholesterol level should be reassessed within 5 years. A lipoprotein analysis should be done if the average cholesterol value from the two tests is 170 mg/dL or higher, or if the result of the initial test was 200 mg/dL or greater.
- Adolescents who have a parent or grandparent with coronary artery disease, peripheral vascular disease, cerebrovascular disease, or sudden cardiac death at age 55 or younger should be screened with a fasting lipoprotein analysis.
- Treatment options are based on the average of two assessments of low-density lipoprotein cholesterol. Values below 110 mg/dL are acceptable; values between 110 and 129 mg/dL are borderline, and the lipoprotein status should be reevaluated in 1 year. Adolescents with values of 130 mg/dL or greater should be referred for further medical evaluation and treatment.

Recommendation 13: All adolescents should be screened annually for eating disorders and obesity by determining weight and stature and asking about body image and dieting patterns.

- Adolescents should be assessed for organic disease, anorexia nervosa, or bulimia if any of the following are found: weight loss greater than 10% of previous weight; recurrent dieting when not overweight; use of self-induced emesis, laxatives, starvation, or diuretics to lose weight; distorted body image; or body mass index (weight/height) below the fifth percentile.
- Adolescents with a body mass index (BMI) equal to or greater than the 95th percentile for age and gender are overweight and should have an in-depth dietary and health assessment to determine psychosocial morbidity and risk for future cardiovascular disease.
- Adolescents with a BMI between the 85th and 94th percentile are at risk for becoming overweight. A dietary and health assessment to determine psychosocial morbidity and risk for future cardiovascular disease should be performed if:
  - their BMI has increased by two or more units during the previous 12 months;
  - there is a family history of premature heart disease, obesity, hypertension, or diabetes mellitus;
  - they express concern about their weight;
  - they have elevated serum cholesterol levels or blood pressure.

If this assessment is negative, these adolescents should be provided general dietary and exercise counseling and should be monitored annually.

Recommendation 14: All adolescents should be asked annually about their use of tobacco products, including cigarettes and smokeless tobacco.

- Adolescents who use tobacco products should be assessed further to determine their patterns of use.
- A cessation plan should be provided for adolescents who use tobacco products.

Recommendation 15: All adolescents should be asked annually about their use of alcohol and other abusable substances and about their use of over-the-counter or prescription drugs for nonmedical purposes, including anabolic steroids.

- Adolescents who report any use of alcohol or other drugs or inappropriate use of medicines during the past year should be assessed further regarding family history; circumstances surrounding use; amount and frequency of use; attitudes and motivation about use; use of other drugs; and the adequacy of physical, psychosocial, and school functioning.
- Adolescents whose substance use endangers their health should receive counseling and mental-health treatment, as appropriate.
- Adolescents who use anabolic steroids should be counseled to stop.
- The use of urine toxicology for the routine screening of adolescents is not recommended.
- Adolescents who use alcohol or other drugs should also be asked about their sexual behavior and their use of tobacco products.

Recommendation 16: All adolescents should be asked annually about involvement in sexual behaviors that may result in unintended pregnancy and STDs, including HIV infection.

- Sexually active adolescents should be asked about their use and motivation to use condoms and contraceptive methods, their sexual orientation, the number of sexual partners they have had in the past 6 months, if they have exchanged sex for money or drugs, and their history of prior pregnancy or STDs.
- Adolescents at risk for pregnancy, STDs (including HIV), or sexual exploitation should be counseled on how to reduce this risk.
- Sexually active adolescents should also be asked about their use of tobacco products, alcohol, and other drugs.

Recommendation 17: Sexually active adolescents should be screened for STDs.

- STD screening includes the following:
  - A cervical culture (females) or urine leukocyte esterase analysis (males) to screen for gonorrhea
  - An immunologic test of cervical fluid (female) or urine leukocyte esterase analysis (male) to screen for genital chlamydia
  - A serologic test for syphilis if they have lived in an area endemic for syphilis, have had other STDs, have had more than one sexual partner within the last 6 months, have exchanged sex for drugs or money, or are males who have engaged in sex with other males
  - Evaluation for human papilloma virus by visual inspection (males and females) and by Pap test.
- If a presumptive test for STDs is positive, tests to make a definitive diagnosis should be performed, a treatment plan instituted according to guidelines developed by the CDC, and the use of condoms encouraged.
- The frequency of screening for STDs depends on the sexual practices of the individual and the history of previous STDs.

Recommendation 18: Adolescents at risk for HIV infection should be offered confidential HIV screening with the ELISA and confirmatory test.

- Risk status includes having used intravenous drugs, having had other STD infections, having lived in an area with a high prevalence of STDs and HIV infection, having had more than one sexual partner in the last 6 months, having exchanged sex for drugs or money, being male and having engaged in sex with other males, or having had a sexual partner who is at risk for HIV infection.
- Testing should be performed only after informed consent is obtained from the adolescent.
- Testing should be performed only in conjunction with both pre- and posttest counseling.
- The frequency of screening for HIV infection should be determined by the risk factors of the individual.

Recommendation 19: Female adolescents who are sexually active or any female 18 or older should be screened annually for cervical cancer by use of a Pap test.

Adolescents with a positive Pap test should be referred for further diagnostic assessment and management.

Recommendation 20: All adolescents should be asked annually about behaviors or emotions that indicate recurrent or severe depression or risk of suicide.

- Screening for depression or suicidal risk should be performed on adolescents who exhibit cumulative risk as determined by declining school grades, chronic melancholy, family dysfunction, homosexual orientation, physical or sexual abuse, alcohol or other drug use, previous suicide attempt, and suicidal plans.
- If suicidal risk is suspected, adolescents should be evaluated immediately and referred to a psychiatrist or other mental-health professional, or should be hospitalized.
- Nonsuicidal adolescents with symptoms of severe or recurrent depression should be evaluated and referred to a psychiatrist or other mental-health professional for treatment.

Recommendation 21: All adolescents should be asked annually about a history of emotional, physical, and sexual abuse.

- If abuse is suspected, adolescents should be assessed to determine the circumstances surrounding abuse and the presence of physical, emotional, and psychosocial consequences, including involvement in health risk behaviors.

- Health providers should be aware of local laws about the reporting of abuse to appropriate state officials, in addition to ethical and legal issues regarding how to protect the confidentiality of the adolescent patient.
- Adolescents who report emotional or psychosocial sequelae should be referred to a psychiatrist or other mental-health professional for evaluation and treatment.

Recommendation 22: All adolescents should be asked annually about learning or school problems.

- Adolescents with a history of truancy, repeated absences, or poor or declining performance should be assessed for the presence of conditions that could interfere with school success. These include learning disability, attention deficit hyperactivity disorder, medical problems, abuse, family dysfunction, mental disorder, or alcohol or other drug use.
- This assessment and the subsequent management plan should be coordinated with school personnel and with the adolescent's parents or caregivers.

Recommendation 23: Adolescents should receive a tuberculin skin test if they have been exposed to active tuberculosis, have lived in a homeless shelter, have been incarcerated, have lived in or come from an area with a high prevalence of tuberculosis, or currently work in a health-care setting.

- Adolescents with a positive tuberculin test should be treated to CDC treatment guidelines.
- The frequency of testing depends on risk factors of the individual adolescent.

Recommendation 24: All adolescents should receive prophylactic immunizations according to the guidelines established by the federally convened Advisory Committee on Immunization Practices.

- Adolescents should receive a bivalent dT vaccine 10 years after their previous DPT vaccination.
- All adolescents should receive a second trivalent MMR vaccination, unless there is documentation of two vaccinations earlier during childhood. An MMR should not be given to pregnant adolescents.
- Susceptible adolescents who engage in high-risk behaviors should be vaccinated against hepatitis B virus. This includes adolescents who have had more than one sexual partner during the previous 6 months, have exchanged sex for drugs or money, are males who have engaged in sex with other males, or have used intravenous drugs. Widespread use of the hepatitis B vaccine is encouraged because risk factors are often not easily identifiable among adolescents. Universal hepatitis B vaccination should be implemented in communities where intravenous drug use, adolescent pregnancy, or STD infections are common.

Adapted from American Medical Association. Guidelines for Adolescent Preventive Services. December 1992.

Primary Care for Women, edited by Phyllis C. Leppert and Fred M. Howard. Lippincott-Raven Publishers, Philadelphia © 1997.

9

The Reproductive Age Woman

PHYLLIS C. LEPPERT

For more than half her life, a woman is physiologically capable of bearing children. In North America, this physiologic reproductive age extends, in general, from age 12 to age 55. However, this entire period of time is not optimal for childbearing: the optimal time for reproduction is from 20 to 29, as pregnancy outcomes for women younger than 20 and in their 30s and over are not as successful. A U-shaped curve describes pregnancy outcome by age, with the least desirable and more complicated pregnancies occurring in young teens and in women age 35 and older.

In addition to the physiologic readiness to conceive and bear healthy children, women of reproductive age face the social and psychological aspects of pregnancy, birth, and childrearing as well. Human infants are extremely dependent at birth, and human childhood is long compared to that of other species. At a fundamental level, a woman needs a partner in the process of childrearing. All human societies have understood this and have stressed within their cultures the importance of the family unit. The family unit was not only a nuclear family of biologic parents and children, but also included grandparents, aunts, uncles, and other kin as well. This basic unit reinforced the importance of social and economic support of women in their reproductive role. In modern society, this need for social and economic support continues.

Modern society has presented challenges to women and to families. More than anything else in the lifetime of women living in the last half of the 20th century, modern methods of contraception have contributed to the ability of women to develop roles in the world that do not depend solely on motherhood. This change has come about due to the scientific understanding of reproductive biology. All forms of contraception, including and most especially the concept of natural family planning espoused by several religious groups, are based on the tremendous scientific advances in reproductive biology that have occurred over the past 50 years or so. Without a fundamental scientific understanding of the complexities of the menstrual cycle, modern contraception would not be possible. In this essential way, modern women owe a great deal to the basic sciences. They have advanced reproductive health and, thus, the general health of women. Since 1900, the number of pregnancies each individual woman will have in a lifetime has been reduced. Also, the number of children born to each woman has decreased. Therefore, reproductive-age women have been freed from the stress of endless pregnancies and childbearing without rest between children. This has enhanced women's health overall and has allowed women to pursue education and careers, in addition to motherhood.

Pregnancy and lactation produce numerous physiologic and psychological alterations, but they also protect from certain diseases, such as breast cancer. Lifetime issues, including the more sedentary behavior of our times, contributes to diseases women acquire as well. The environmental pollution in industrial societies is also associated with disease occurrence.

Despite changing societal roles and lifestyle changes, women still link health and well-being with their reproductive health. Given the centrality of reproductive hormones to female physiology, this is inevitable. As long as a woman is actively menstruating, pregnancy is possible, and this physiologic fact creates a sense of psychological vulnerability in many women. Modern women need to assimilate these facts of reproductive physiology into their lives and accept them. Unfortunately, some women have tended to embrace pregnancy and motherhood for its own sake, often at an inappropriate point in their lives. Conversely, some modern women have assumed an unbalanced view toward motherhood and have ignored their reproductive potential. Thus, primary care providers for women must guide each woman toward an integrated and "appropriate for her" approach to reproduction and reproductive health. This integrated approach does not negate the role of a woman's reproductive health in her total health and well-being, and does not mean that all women should be mothers. It means simply that all women ought to be encouraged to discern the right decision for them regarding pregnancy and birth in a responsible manner.

THE MENSTRUAL CYCLE

For a reproductive-age woman, menstruation is a central reality, and the primary care provider, whether obstetrician/gynecologist, internist, pediatrician, family practitioner, physician assistant, midwife, or nurse practitioner, must be knowledgeable regarding menstrual physiology.

Changes in the Endometrium

During the menstrual cycle, the endometrium undergoes distinct changes. The first day of bleeding is customarily considered the first day of the menstrual cycle, a convention important for the prescribing of contraceptive pills.

The endometrial lining of the uterus is divided into two layers. The upper, or functional layer, makes up two thirds of the lining, the lower basalis layer one third. The basalis layer provides for regeneration of the endometrium after menstruation. A sequence of specific histologic and functional changes occurs within the glandular, vascular, and stromal parts of the endometrium. These five phases occur in concert with the changes occurring in the ovary, pituitary gland, and hypothalamus. The menstrual endometrium phase occurs between days 1 and 4 of the cycle; the proliferative phase begins at day 4 or 5; the secretory phase occurs after ovulation, followed by the implantation preparation and endometrial

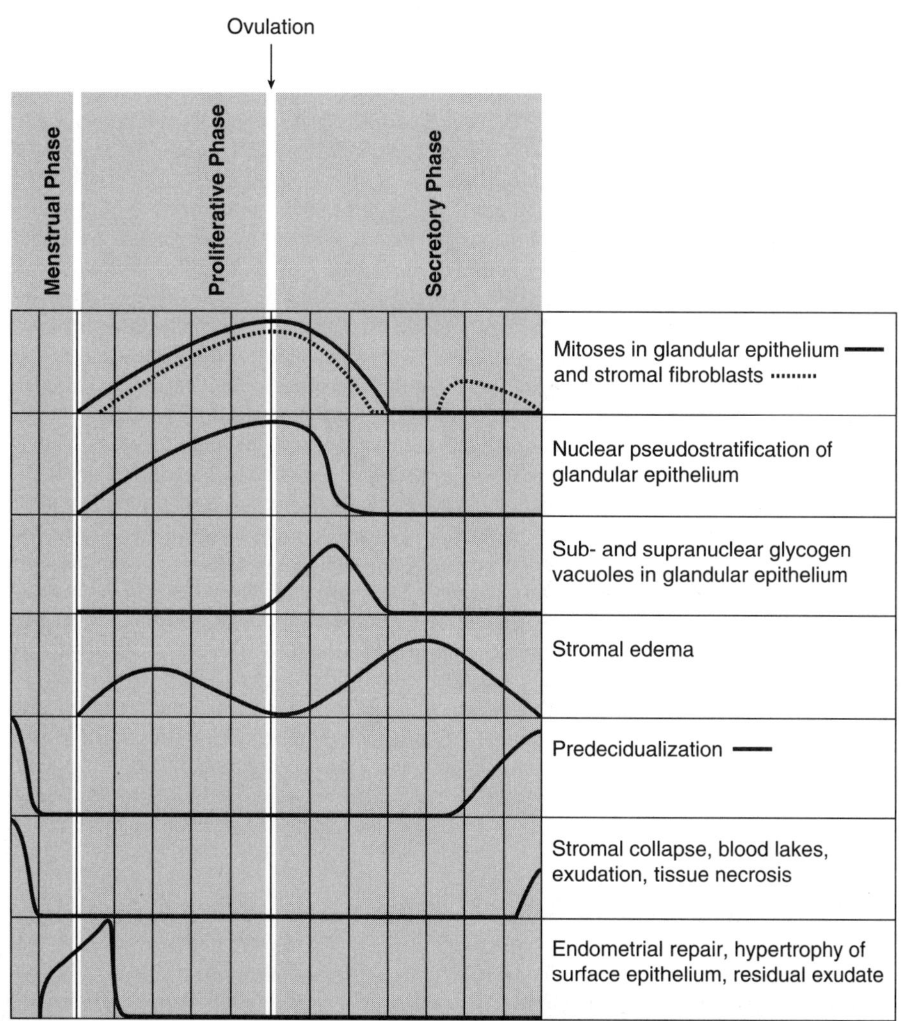

Figure 9-1. Dating the endometrium. (Redrawn from Speroff L, Glass RH, Kase NG. Clinical gynecologic endocrinology and infertility, 5th ed. Baltimore: Williams & Wilkins, 1994:120.)

breakdown phases. Figure 9-1 shows the endometrial changes throughout the 28-day cycle.

Menstrual Phase

The endometrium of the menstrual phase consists of tissue that demonstrates fragmented blood vessels and disarray and breakage of the glands. Throughout the tissue there is evidence of stromal necrosis, white cell infiltration, and interstitial diapedesis of red cells. There is a collapse of the supporting matrix as well. As much as two thirds of the functioning endometrium is lost during menstruation. A short duration of menstrual flow occurs with rapid tissue loss, whereas a heavier flow and greater blood loss is seen when there is delayed or incomplete shedding. During endometrial shedding in normal menstrual cycles, evidence of tissue repair can be seen along with the loss of the functional endometrium. Rapid growth of new epithelium is noted beginning on days 2 to 3 of the cycle. By days 5 to 6, the entire endometrium has acquired new epithelium.

Proliferative Phase

The proliferative phase occurs in conjunction with the growth of the ovarian follicle and increased estrogen secretion. The endometrial glands are lined by low columnar epithelial cells and are narrow and tubular. In these cells, mitosis develops and becomes predominant. A pseudostratification of these cells is seen. The glandular epithelium extends and the glands become linked with the adjacent glands. The endometrial stroma is densely cellular during the menstrual phase. For a brief time, it is edematous and becomes at the end a loose syncytial-like tissue. The blood vessels course through the stroma. The spiral arteries extend in an unbranched manner to just below the epithelial binding membrane, where they form a loosely organized capillary network. The proliferative phase peaks at day 8 to 10. This peak of markedly increased mitotic cytoplasmic RNA synthesis is followed by a peak of intranuclear concentrations of estrogen and progesterone receptors at midcycle, just before ovulation.

Secretory Phase

An early sign of ovulation is the appearance of glycogen vacuoles in the glandular epithelium. These glycogen vacuoles are seen in the subnuclear intracytoplasmic compartment of the glandular cells. There is an unfolding of the nuclear membranes under the influence of progesterone into a nucleolar channel system.

The tissue continues to grow, but because it is confined in a fixed area, progressive tortuosity of the glands and a progressively intense curling of the spiral cells occur. Glycoproteins and peptides are secreted into the endometrial cavity. A plasma transudate also is noted in the secretions. Circulating immunoglobulins are secreted into the endometrial cavity by an epithelial binding protein. Seven days after the midcycle gonadotropin surge, the peak secretory activity is reached. If conception had occurred, this peak secretory activity would coincide with the implantation of the blastocyst.

Implantation Phase

On days 21 to 27 (or days 7 to 13 postovulation), marked changes occur. At the beginning of this phase, tortuous secretory glands are seen with very little stromal tissue between them. At day 13 postovulation, the endometrium develops three separate zones. One fourth of the tissue is basalis, in which there are straight blood vessels and spindle-shaped stroma. The middle part, making up half of the endometrium, is the stratum spongiosum, a lace-like layer composed of loose edematous stroma and tightly coiled, densely packed spiral vessels and ribbons of exhausted glands. Over the spongiosum is the stratum compactum, the remaining fourth of the total tissue. In this layer, the stromal cells have become large and polyhedral, with one cell compressing the other. The glands in this area are compressed; the subepithelial capillaries and spiral vessels are prominent and engorged. Receptors for estrogen and progesterone are located in this phase in the walls of the endometrial blood vessels. The enzymes necessary for prostaglandin synthesis are present in the muscle walls and endothelium of the endometrial arteriolae.

If a pregnancy occurs, the stromal cells are transformed into decidua, producing a multitude of hormones and growth factors. They produce prolactin, relaxin, renin, insulin-like growth factor, and insulin-like growth factor binding proteins. Decidual cells are derived from primitive uterine mesenchymal stem cells. The process of decidualization begins in the late luteal or implantation phase under progesterone influence. On day 23 of the menstrual cycle, predecidual cells can be identified.

Endometrial Breakdown Phase

If conception and implantation and the secretion of human chorionic gonadotropin (HCG) from the trophoblast do not ensue, the corpus luteum dies and estrogen and progesterone levels fall. By day 25, the upper compactum layer is transformed. As the progesterone level falls, endometrial cell lysosomal membranes rupture and acid phosphatase and other lytic enzymes are released into the cytoplasm. Tissue necrosis, vascular thrombosis, and extravasation of red blood cells are seen. Matrix metalloproteinases degrade the extracellular matrix and basement membrane.

As estrogen and progesterone withdrawal begins, three responses occur. First, the tissue height shrinks, blood flow within the spiral vessels decreases, venous drainage is decreased, and vasodilatation occurs. Then the spiral arterioles rhythmically constrict and relax. Each spasm is more prolonged, leading finally to endometrial blanching and to endometrial ischemia and stasis. Red blood cells escape into the interstitial space. This occurs 24 hours before menstruation. White cells migrate into the tissue and the prostaglandin content in the secretory endometrium peaks. Thrombin platelet plugs are seen in the vessels. Finally, breaks in the superficial arteriolae and capillaries occur. New thrombin platelet plugs are formed. Further tissue breakdown is noted. The endometrium shrinks further, and the coiled spiral arteries are compressed and buckled. Thus, ischemic breakdown progresses. A cleavage plane between the basalis and spongiosum is breached, and the spongiosum desquamates and collapses. Menstrual flow stops then because of combined vasoconstriction, tissue collapse, vascular stasis, and estrogen-stimulated repair and clot formation over the stumps of the endometrial spiral arteriolae. The basalis endometrium remains, and repair occurs from this layer.

Menstrual flow consists of red blood cells, inflammatory exudate, proteolytic enzymes, and autolysed functionalis.

Ovarian Changes

The menstrual cycle is divided into the follicular phase and the luteal phase. An average or typical cycle is said to be 28 days, although there is considerable variation, both among women and among cycles in one individual woman. The follicular phase is the more variable; the duration of the luteal phase is more constant in duration, lasting 13 to 15 days.

Follicular Phase

In the follicular phase, a new group of primordial follicles begins to grow and develop. However, these follicles have begun to be "recruited" during the luteal phase of the preceding menstrual cycle. In the preceding luteal phase, a number of antral follicles (2 to 4 mm in diameter) are active. These antral follicles develop an aromatase activity stimulated by follicle-stimulating hormone (FSH). These follicles, usually three to five in number, form the cohort of follicles developed in the next follicular phase. FSH is the hormone that provides the fundamental stimulus to follicular granulosa growth. Stimulated by FSH, androgens in the granulosa cells are converted into estrogen. Thus, 17β-estradiol concentrations increase during the follicular phase.

During the first 5 days of the menstrual cycle, a selection process occurs. Only one of the three to five FSH-stimulated follicles from the previous luteal phase grows and becomes the preovulatory graafian follicle. This one follicle develops increased vascularization and blood flow. The increasing estradiol concentration in the follicle increases the sensitivity of the granulosa cells to FSH because the FSH receptors increase. Over time, this dominant follicle secretes sufficient estradiol to elevate peripheral estradiol concentrations. When this happens, FSH is suppressed and the growth of the nondominant follicles ceases. As the follicular phase continues, the dominant follicle grows in diameter to 10 to 20 mm, its final size. As a result, the secretion of estradiol increases exponentially. This great increase in estrogen (Fig. 9-2) causes the proliferation of the glandular endometrium. The estrogen rise also causes increased secretion of cervical mucus, a decrease in its viscosity, and an increase in its pH. There is also cornification of the vaginal smear. These changes are the basis of a simple, indirect test of normal ovulation.

The peak of estradiol secretion is associated with the maturation of the graafian follicle that communicates the readiness of the reproductive tract for ovulation to the brain and the pituitary gland. Estrogen then stimulates the gonadotropin surge of luteinizing hormone (LH) and FSH. This surge persists for 1 to 2 days and leads to the final stage of maturation of the graafian follicle. The high concentrations of the gonadotropins stop granulosa cell growth and secretory activity. As the granulosa cells arrest, estradiol secretion abruptly ceases. LH induces theca luteinization, leading to a small preovulatory rise in progesterone. Follicle rupture and ovulation occur 24 to 36 hours after the beginning of the LH and FSH surge (see Fig. 9-2). At the time of ovulation, the first meiotic division is completed and a secondary oocyte has formed.

Luteal Phase

The luteal phase is characterized by major changes in the dominant follicle. Shortly after the LH and FSH surge, the secretory activity in the granulosa cell stops. The basal lamina is invaded by the capillaries of the theca interna. A new structure, the corpus luteum, forms. The corpus luteum secretes both progesterone and 17β-estradiol. Progesterone dominates the luteal phase. Changes in

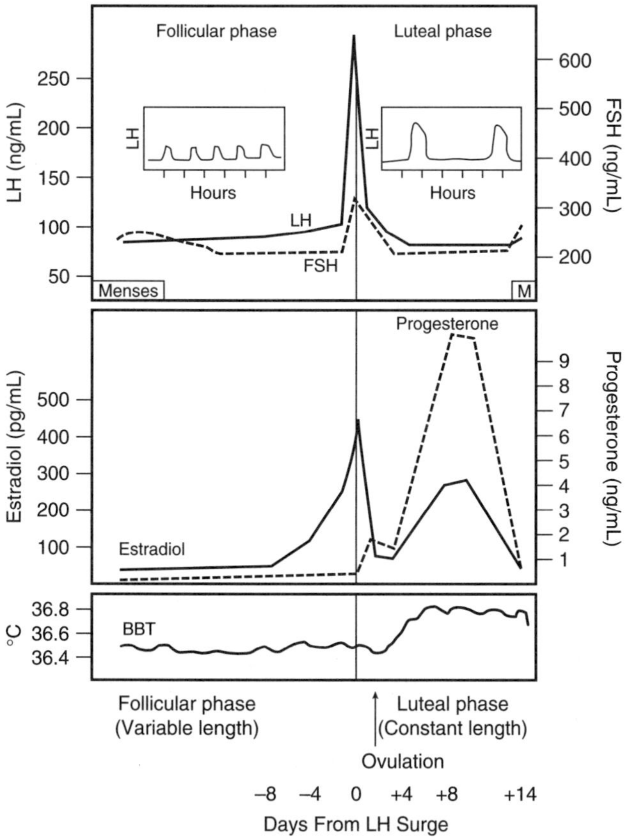

Figure 9-2. The human menstrual cycle. (Redrawn from Speroff L, Glass RH, Kase NG. Clinical gynecologic endocrinology and infertility, 5th ed. Baltimore: Williams & Wilkins, 1994.)

the reproductive tract occur in preparation for the potential implantation of a fertilized ovum. Increased secretory activity of the endometrial glands is seen and the cervical mucus becomes thick and viscous. Progesterone affects the hypothalamic thermoregulatory center, and an increase in basal body temperature occurs (see Fig. 9-2).

The corpus luteum reaches maturity in 8 to 9 days after ovulation. Midway through the luteal phase, the levels of estradiol and progesterone decrease. Thus, menstruation follows ovulation by 13 to 15 days. When and if a pregnancy occurs, HCG extends the life of the corpus luteum and maintains the secretion of estrogen and progesterone (Fig. 9-3). In nonfertile cycles, luteolysis occurs. A decrease in luteal hormonal secretion is followed by an increase in FSH.

Hormonal Changes

The menstrual cycle is under the control of positive and negative reproductive hormone feedback. As in other endocrine systems, the major feedback is inhibitory. Estradiol and progesterone secreted by the target organ, the ovary, inhibit gonadotropin-releasing hormone (GnRH) and gonadotropin secretion from the hypothalamus and the pituitary gland. This is the negative or inhibitory feedback loop. In the positive or stimulatory feedback loop, the increase of ovarian steroids increases gonadotropin secretion. In the first negative feedback system, 17β-estradiol inhibits gonadotropin secretion from the anterior pituitary. Small increases in estradiol cause a decrease in gonadotropins. In the follicular phase of the menstrual cycle, LH and FSH levels are determined by circulating estradiol concentration (see Fig. 9-2). At menopause, or after surgical removal of the ovaries, LH and FSH secretion is increased in a continuous fashion.

The second or positive feedback loop is indicated by the fact that during the late follicular phase, large increases in estradiol initiate the midcycle gonadotropin (LH and FSH) surge. Experimental studies indicate that a preovulatory rise in progesterone plays an important role in the midcycle gonadotropin surge. However, large amounts of circulating progesterone inhibit the estrogen-induced LH surge.

LH and FSH are released from the anterior pituitary in a pulsatile manner (see Fig. 9-2). Estradiol and progesterone affect this pulsatile release of gonadotropin. Estradiol affects the pulse amplitude; progesterone affects its frequency. However, over time the estradiol negative feedback loop selectively suppresses FSH more than LH.

The anterior pituitary secretion of LH and FSH is regulated by the hypothalamus. Neurohormones are secreted and transported via the portal blood vessels to the anterior pituitary sinusoids. GnRH is a small protein of ten amino acids. Its prohormone contains 92 amino acids and is degraded before release as the decapeptide, GnRH. GnRH cells are located in the arcuate nucleus of the hypothalamus. These cells extend to the portion of the hypothalamus known as the median eminence. Although some GnRH cells originate in the preoptic area of the hypothalamus, it appears that in women the GnRH neurons in the arcuate nucleus are the most important cells. During embryogenesis, GnRH cells originate in the olfactory placodes outside the brain and then migrate into the CNS. This is of interest because Kallmann syndrome (hypogonadotropic hypogonadism, delayed puberty, and anosmia) may reflect a defect in the migration of GnRH during embryogenesis.

GnRH secretion occurs in a pulsatile fashion and is related to the pulsatile secretion of LH and FSH. The pulsatile GnRH release mechanism is present at birth but is suppressed. During the prepubertal period, the pulsatile pattern of gonadotropin release begins, stimulated by the GnRH pulse-generator region of the hypothalamus. At first, the phenomenon occurs during sleep at night; in adulthood, LH secretion occurs throughout a 24-hour period. A new hormone, inhibin, a glycoprotein with α and β subunits, is found in follicular fluid and is secreted into the circulation. This hormone inhibits FSH secretion.

Finally, the frequency of the GnRH pulse affects LH and FSH secretion in different ways. High GnRH frequencies contribute to LH release; low GnRH frequencies contribute to FSH release.

Declining inhibin in the peripheral circulation and the type of GnRH pulse frequency seen at the end of the luteal phase stimulate the early rise of FSH in a new follicular phase. Thus, the menstrual cycle begins again.

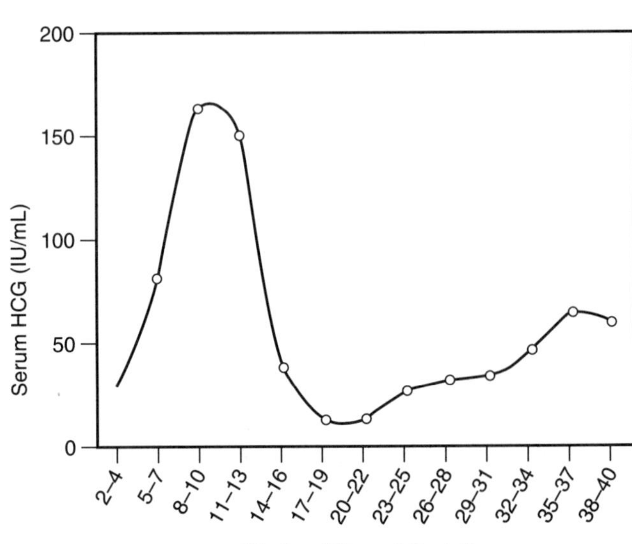

Figure 9-3. Fluctuation of serum human chorionic gonadotropin (HCG) during normal intrauterine gestation. (Redrawn from Speroff L, Glass RH, Kase NG. Clinical gynecologic endocrinology and infertility, 5th ed. Baltimore: Williams & Wilkins, 1994.)

COMMON ABNORMALITIES OF THE MENSTRUAL CYCLE

Small disturbances of the feedback systems regulating the ovary and anterior pituitary affect the menstrual cycle.

If the FSH release at the end of one cycle is less than normal, difficult follicular growth occurs. This produces subnormal estrogen concentration and a short luteal phase. Progesterone levels are low then as well. Sometimes a premature LH surge occurs, halting follicular maturation. In obese women, androstenedione is converted to estrone in adipose and other tissue, such as skin, leading to anovulation. In polycystic ovarian syndrome, the extraovarian production of estrogen increases, thus allowing abnormal feedback regulation to modify the LH pulse; again, anovulation results. Abnormalities of the hypothalamus or pituitary gland may also produce anovulatory cycles.

The menstrual cycle can be suppressed by pituitary tumors, especially prolactin-secreting adenomas and craniopharyngiomas. Severe postpartum hemorrhage and ischemic shock are associated with Sheehan syndrome. Amenorrhea can be caused by hypothalamic tumors and by head trauma.

Hypothalamic amenorrhea is associated with poor nutrition and is seen as a result of anorexia nervosa, stress, and strenuous exercise. Psychological stress can produce chronic amenorrhea. The mechanism is thought to be due to corticotropin-releasing hormone inhibition of the GnRH pulse generator. This inhibitory effect is the result of activation of endogenous opioid peptides, which are endorphins.

Chapter 7 of this book discusses congenital and genetic causes of menstrual cycle abnormalities. Premenstrual syndrome is discussed in Chapter 32.

The complex interaction of the hypothalamic-pituitary unit, the pituitary-ovarian unit, and the positive and negative feedback regulatory systems make the diagnosis of menstrual irregularities a challenge. Therefore, if amenorrhea persists despite treatment for 6 months, or if symptoms of headache, visual disturbances, or galactorrhea occur, a referral to a specialist is necessary.

PREGNANCY

In women of reproductive age, the single most common cause of amenorrhea is pregnancy. Because pregnancy is a time of major physiologic change for women, ideally every woman should plan for pregnancy and for childbearing to occur at the optimal time in her life. The woman should be as physically and psychologically healthy as possible and should be in a stable economic and social environment with supportive family and friends.

Preconceptual Counseling

Because women have fewer pregnancies than in previous generations, it is essential to the future of our race that each child born is wanted, loved, and treasured by parents who love and support each other. This is the ideal, but of course as humans not all ideals are met. The goal, then, of preconceptual counseling is to maximize the chances of a successful pregnancy outcome for each woman.

Preconceptual counseling should include the woman's family and especially her spouse or significant other. By including the others, the primary care provider emphasizes the fact that childbearing is a shared endeavor. To be a parent is a joyful privilege, but it is also a responsibility. When this responsibility is a shared one, the woman, her partner, and the child all benefit.

Preconceptual counseling includes a careful medical history, focusing on familial medical problems and the woman's past medical and reproductive history. While obtaining this information, the provider can observe areas of concern and can begin educating the couple regarding health matters. One short but to-the-point remark made at the appropriate time by a physician can be a powerful agent of change in behavior toward a more healthy lifestyle. Health care providers who take care of childbearing-age women find that pregnancy and birth is one of the most important times in a woman's life to effect change to a healthy lifestyle.

Women contemplating a successful pregnancy must be counseled to obtain appropriate weight, so nutritional education is essential. The food pyramid concept shown in Figure 9-4 is an excellent educational aid and suggests eating three fruits and five vegetables a day, a complex carbohydrate, such as breads, rice, pasta, and a moderate amount of meat and poultry. The diet of the average North American tends to include sizable portions, so it is wise to advise eating smaller servings at each meal. The meat serving should be no larger than a deck of cards. Pregnancy is not a time to lose weight. Conversely, if a woman is underweight before pregnancy or does not gain enough weight during pregnancy, the outcome is usually suboptimal. Women who take 0.4 mg/day of folic acid around the time of conception could reduce the risk of having an infant with spina bifida by about 50%.

Exercise is important and must be carried out routinely and in moderation. Many women now work outside the home, so diet and exercise counseling and education must include strategies for the workplace. Women need to know how to select healthy food at restaurants and workplace cafeterias. Working women should be encouraged to walk and climb stairs during their working hours. Some helpful strategies are to walk upstairs rather than to take elevators, and in fair weather to take a walk outdoors at lunch.

In many health care settings, preconceptual classes are held for women contemplating a pregnancy, and many women benefit from a referral to these for additional information. Table 9-1 lists the content of preconceptual classes held at Rochester General Hospital.

Before a pregnancy, the woman should stop smoking cigarettes. Cigarette smoking is responsible for more low-birthweight infants than any other drug. Chapter 6 discusses helpful smoking cessation techniques. Because binge consumption of alcoholic beverages and the use of illicit drugs are harmful, the complete preconceptual counseling session covers these areas as well. It is easiest to touch on these aspects of education during counseling sessions. By asking questions about smoking, alcohol consumption, and recreational drug use, the health care provider can ascertain which women would benefit from referrals to other resources.

A history of genetic and congenital diseases in the families of the woman and her partner is ascertained. Genetic diseases now include many problems such as colon cancer and some breast and ovarian cancers. The primary care provider must understand basic genetic concepts, but definitive counseling should be done by genetic centers.

As the human genome becomes understood and, thus, genetic disease becomes more complex, large regional referral centers that serve numerous academic medical centers will be the rule. They will house the vast databases from which genetic counseling advice will be available to persons contemplating a pregnancy. Genetic testing must be voluntary. Women over age 35 must fully

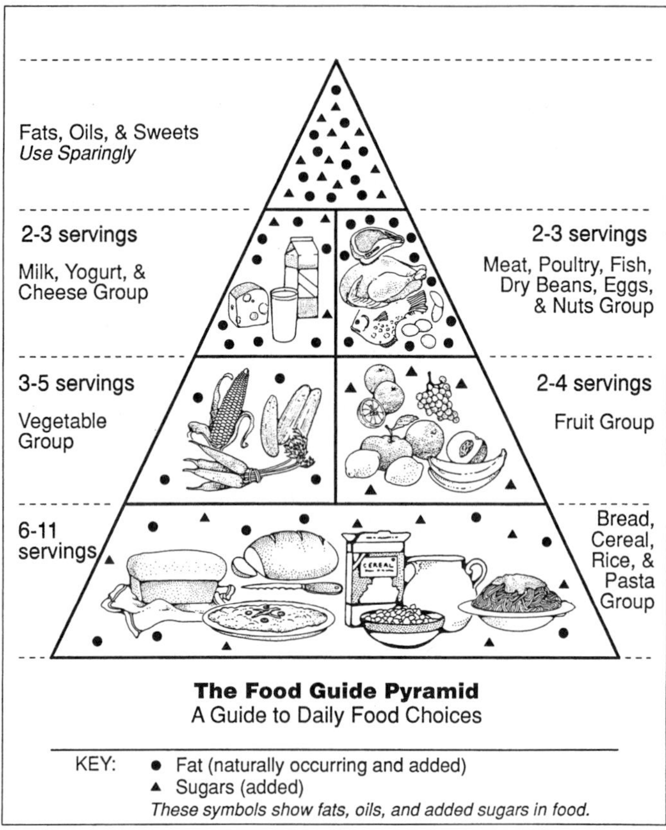

Figure 9-4. Food pyramid.

appreciate the genetic risks of a pregnancy. Amniocentesis and chorionic villus sampling should be explained. People interpret relative risks of disease in ways that are acceptable to them in their individual circumstances, and the right of a woman and her partner to make their own choices is an important ethical consideration. The age of the potential mother should be explored. If she is a teenager, it should be pointed out that it would be advisable to wait several years. On the other hand, a woman nearing her mid-30s should be encouraged to have a child as soon as possible.

A thorough history of infectious diseases that would affect a pregnancy is taken. Rubella vaccine is given to any woman who has not already had the disease. Past exposure to sexually transmitted disease, including HIV and herpes simplex, should be discussed in a matter-of-fact and nonjudgmental manner. Most women are extremely honest with their care provider regarding this history when they appreciate how important this information is to having a healthy childbearing outcome. If a woman is in a profession, such as health care, where she might acquire hepatitis B, she should be immunized rather than run the risk of becoming infected during pregnancy.

The workplace environment should be discussed in some detail. The possibility of exposure to environmental toxic chemicals should be explored. There are still workplaces where cigarette smoking continues, so the need to avoid passive smoke should be indicated. The possibility of acquiring infectious diseases potentially harmful to an embryo or fetus in the first months of pregnancy should be mentioned. For instance, nurses working in a neonatal intensive care nursery have acquired cytomegalovirus infections that have damaged a fetus. Workers in child day-care centers are also exposed to infectious disease. The aim is to help each woman determine her own particular risks, and the actual plan for dealing with these risks must be individualized. Primary care providers must be aware that for many women, work is an economic necessity.

Women in professional careers, such as medicine, law, business, and the clergy, need to understand the demands their careers will place on their roles as mothers. Often these women are extremely goal-oriented and are high achievers. Realistic plans for parenthood need to be part of their lives. At a preconceptual counseling session, a woman needs to look at these issues and find the right solutions. She must be aware of the availability of day-care facilities for infants and toddlers. Professional women do not have the option, as do women in other careers, of dropping out for several years to raise children, because they would lose too much career momentum. Professional musicians and others in the enter-

Table 9-1. Planning for Pregnancy

Reproduction
Fetal growth and development
Nutrition
Exercise
Substance use or abuse (illegal drugs, alcohol, cigarettes)
Medication use (prescription, over-the-counter)
Infectious diseases (eg, STDs, HIV, rubella, toxoplasmosis)
Medical history (eg, diabetes, hypertension)
Genetics
Environmental issues
Specific issues and concerns of males
Parenting issues
Childbirth options
Community resources

tainment field face the same dilemma. Each woman makes her own choice, but these issues must be addressed.

The potential father must be a part of these discussions. His role is to maintain a caring and loving partnership throughout pregnancy, to provide emotional support and company during labor, and to be a caring and dependable member of the extended family. Childbirth is a time when families can be strengthened. At a time when society seems to make it extremely difficult for families, it is a privilege and responsibility of health care providers, especially primary care physicians, to use childbearing as a way to strengthen the family. The patient's family may not be a traditional one, but there is always a family that can be strengthened.

It is helpful to recommend childbirth classes and preparation for parenthood classes as important experiences during pregnancy. Some mention of health care—pediatrician, family physician, pediatric nurse practitioner—for the planned-for infant is helpful in preconceptional counseling as well.

Any special needs of the mother must be addressed. A diabetic should be instructed that she must have good glucose control before conception. Her eyes should be examined for retinopathy and her renal status obtained. Women with chronic hypertension should be in good normotensive control. Women with this disease should not stop their antihypertensive medication when they conceive. Women on thyroid medication should continue their thyroid replacement as well. The goal for women with medical disease is to prevent as many complications as possible. If the primary care physician does not understand the specific risks, a referral should be made to the appropriate specialist, or a computer search can be made. No physician, especially a primary care physician, can know everything and rely on memory, or even textbooks, and large data banks can be of help. Primary providers are excellent persons to do the initial preconceptual counseling, because they know the woman and her partner best and have established some trust in an ongoing relationship.

Preconceptual counseling should offer the woman and her partner the concept of a maternity care team. The woman's primary care provider is one member of the team, and other physicians, midwives, nurses, health educators, and nutritionists on the team are there to provide the best care for an optimal pregnancy outcome. Isolated care by one or two physicians is a thing of the past. The team approach gives an appropriate, caring, and scientifically up-to-date pregnancy experience. Each member of the team has his or her own special expertise to bring to the care of the childbearing woman, and this should be conveyed during the preconceptual counseling session.

Childbearing has been a central part of women's lives in the past. Although most modern women have only two or three children on the average, pregnancy and birth remains a terribly important part of the total health of individual women. First, the physiologic changes of pregnancy affect all organ systems, and some of the effects are long term. Second, for women to maintain their modern roles and careers, the goal should be for every pregnancy to be healthy.

Conception and Diagnosis of Pregnancy

Classically, amenorrhea is the most significant sign of pregnancy in a healthy woman. Slight bleeding at the time of implantation can be mistaken for a menstrual period. Therefore, the woman should be carefully questioned regarding the duration and characteristics of the last vaginal bleeding episode. This is especially important because abnormal vaginal bleeding often is associated with an ectopic pregnancy.

Other subtle signs of pregnancy are a slight tingling in the breasts, noticed especially by primigravid women. Morning sickness occurs at any time in the day, usually from the fourth to 14th week of gestation, but it occurs in only about 50% of pregnant women. Many pregnant women describe a bladder irritability in the first 12 weeks of pregnancy, usually noted as an increased frequency of urination, unaccompanied by pain or burning. Some women note skin changes of chloasma, linea nigra, and a darkening of the primary areola and formation of a secondary areola of the breasts. It is not uncommon for a woman to tell her health care provider, "I just know I am pregnant. I feel pregnant." A careful and thorough physician does not ignore such a comment, but takes it seriously and follows up with the appropriate diagnostic evaluation.

On physical examination, classical probable signs of pregnancy can be noted (Table 9-2). In our era of accurate ultrasound and immunologic tests for pregnancy, it is tempting to ignore these signs, but they are helpful adjunct findings and should not be overlooked.

Physical signs are important clues to the need to obtain further diagnostic tests. Primary care providers for women must appreciate them, especially in a managed care environment; if they are overlooked or not appreciated, a pregnancy will not be diagnosed as early as it could be. Especially in the early weeks, not all pregnancies are normal. Ectopic pregnancies and incomplete spontaneous abortions are life-threatening because of hemorrhage (see Chap. 18). Without immunologic tests and a vaginal probe ultrasound, these two abnormalities of pregnancy cannot be diagnosed until late in their course. When a pregnancy is suspected, an

Table 9-2. Signs of Pregnancy

SIGN	TIME OF OCCURRENCE	DESCRIPTION
Hegar sign	6th to 12th weeks	Because of the softness of the isthmus at this stage, the two fingers of the vaginal hand almost meet the abdominal hand of the examiner. It helps to establish gestational age.
Jacquemier sign*	8th week	A blue to violet discoloration of the vaginal mucous membrane
Osiander sign*	8th week onward	Increased pulsation palpated in the lateral fornices
Uterine signs	8th week onward	Enlarged, soft uterus, globular in shape
Cervical softening	10th week	The cervix has a consistency of the lips. In nonpregnant women, it has the consistency of the tip of the nose.
Uterine souffle*	16th week onward	A blowing sound heard on auscultation and synchronous to the mother's pulse

*Can also be seen in other clinical circumstances.

immunologic test of pregnancy should be performed. If abnormal results are obtained, a vaginal probe ultrasound can then usually confirm the diagnosis.

Immunologic Tests for Pregnancy

Immunologic tests measure HCG. HCG is produced by the syncytiotrophoblast of the placenta, and the amount of placental HCG corresponds to the amount in the urine. HCG has a characteristic pattern in normal pregnancy (see Fig. 9-3). The tests are reliable to determine pregnancy if they are done on urine collected 14 days or more after a missed, expected menstrual period. However, HCG appears in urine about 9 days after conception. A positive test does not mean a viable embryo or fetus, as women with hydatidiform mole, invasive mole, and choriocarcinoma, as well as a blighted ovum, test positive as well.

The definitive diagnosis is made when the fetal heart tones are heard. They may be heard by Doppler auscultation as early as 10 weeks. By 14 weeks, this method detects fetal heart tones in almost all women except the very obese. The most reliable method for the detection of fetal heart pulsation in early gestation is by real-time ultrasound, especially if done by vaginal probe. Unfortunately, ultrasound scanning has been a source of controversy. One reason for this is that in North America physicians have traditionally charged a fee for the procedure. It has been argued that if there were no fee for the procedure, ultrasound examination might be used more appropriately. However, a scan should not be done at every obstetric visit: this does not help pregnancy outcomes and is not cost-effective under our current system of reimbursement. However, obstetric ultrasound has a significant place in prenatal care.

Fetal movement felt by the mother is not a positive sign of pregnancy, as she might be imagining movement. However, if the examiner feels fetal parts and fetal movement, usually at 22 weeks, this is a positive sign of pregnancy. Reliable diagnostic measures of pregnancy are summarized in Table 9-3.

PRENATAL CARE

The concept of antenatal care was initiated in the early decades of the 20th century as a means to prevent severe preeclampsia, eclampsia, and maternal mortality. Before the universal acceptance of prenatal care, pregnant women were urged to stay home. They would go on errands to a butcher, for instance, very early in the morning. To be "in the family way" was not a time to be in society. Women would see a midwife or physician infrequently in pregnancy, if at all. It is a tremendous achievement that prenatal care has achieved its goals. Although other factors, such as availability of blood products, good anesthesia, and improved delivery practices, contributed, maternal mortality fell from 376 deaths per 100,000 births in 1940 to 8.2 deaths per 100,000 births in 1990.

Table 9-3. Reliable Diagnostic Measures of Pregnancy

Positive immunologic test
Auscultation of fetal heart
10–14 weeks by Doppler auscultation
Ultrasound evidence
Fetal heart beat
Gestational sac
Fetal movement and fetal parts
Palpated by examiner at 22 weeks' gestation
X-ray
Fetal skeleton noted at 16 weeks
Not recommended because of the hazards of radiation to the fetus

Prenatal care was not inaugurated specifically to prevent the poor pregnancy outcomes of low-birthweight infants and premature delivery. This has become a modern expectation of prenatal care, with conflicting evidence as to its success. Prenatal care currently encompasses many activities. The traditional activities of weighing women, taking their blood pressure, and checking urine for albumin or protein all are aimed at the early diagnosis and treatment of preeclampsia. Until science understands totally what role molecular, biochemical, and physiologic events play in the initiation of labor and preterm labor, prenatal care cannot be expected to eradicate the problem of low birthweight. About a third of cases of preterm labor are associated with an infectious etiology. Therefore, activities to eradicate and prevent prenatal infections should be included in prenatal care. It is also necessary to continue to fund basic research into the physiology of parturition.

The most important aspect of prenatal care may be the education of childbearing women and their families, as well as the motivation of each woman to become responsible for her own health. This becomes a complex task in a society where the average reading ability is fifth-grade level, and where many women and their families are not completely conversant in English. Physicians have not been taught principles of education, and until recently medical schools have not traditionally taught principles of communication and interviewing techniques well. Primary care providers must learn to be effective teachers and communicators. Nurses, midwives, social workers, dietitians, and genetic counselors often learn teaching principles as part of their basic professional education.

Most hospitals and health care facilities have prenatal education programs established in the 1950s and 1960s. These programs usually started as classes to teach preparation for labor and delivery and emphasized methods and ways to cope with labor. These programs should now include all the necessary information for a healthy pregnancy, with an emphasis on diet, rest, recreation, exercise, and avoidance of cigarette smoke, alcohol, and illicit drugs. Education regarding sexually transmitted diseases is also essential. These important programs complement but do not replace the ongoing prenatal education and emphasis on lifestyle change that should occur at each prenatal visit to the primary care provider.

Managed care plans should provide a way to individualize each woman's risk of untoward pregnancy outcomes and provide special educational and social assistance for the pregnant woman as needed. Figure 9-5 shows the risk-assessment tool used by one HMO; it includes medical, obstetric, and social risk factors, and case managers are provided for the highest-risk families. Managed care plans promote collaborative practice among different medical specialists and among physician and nonphysician providers. For this concept to succeed, there must be respect for each provider's various roles. For instance, modern midwives are trained to act as an educator to expectant mothers, to provide professional companionship, and to encourage preventive medicine in obstetrics. Many physicians practice the art of midwifery as well.

Prenatal care in 1995 has three aspects: education about pregnancy and infant care, along with advice on how to reduce risks; screening and risk assessment; and treatment of medical conditions throughout pregnancy.

Name________________ Provider ________ EDC ___ CONTRACT # _________

DOB:__________ MONROE PLAN— GROUP HEALTH— OTHER ____________

Initial Assessment Form

Age & Parity						
	Age > 40 Primip		Age < 15 Primip		Age < 14 Primip	
	Age > 45 Multip		Age < 17 Multip			
	Age < 19 Multip		< 18 Not in School			

Documented Problems in Maternal Medical History

Cardio-vascular	Mitral Valve Prolapse				Chronic Hypertension	
					Heart Disease	
					Pulmonary Embolus	
					Cong. Heart Defects	
Urinary	> 3 Uncomplicated Urinary Tract Infections in last 12 months		Chronic Pyelonephritis prior to this pregnancy		Renal Disease mod. to severe, including Nephritis or Chronic Renal Disease	
Psycho-Neurological	Severe Recurring Migraines		Psychiatric Evaluation for documented Mental Health Disorder		Epilepsy or Seizure Disorder on anticonvulsent drugs	
			Previous Psychotic Episode		Drug Addiction (heroin, barbiturates, alcohol) current use	
			Hx. of Seizure Disorder with no seizure activity within last year		Suicide Attempt	
			Hx. of depression or Post Partum depression		Chronic Psychiatric Disorder on medications	
Endo-crine	Thyroid Disease > 1 yr. controlled		Thyroid Disease Less than 1 yr. (controlled)		Diabetes Mellitus	
			Hx of DES Exposure		Hx of Autoimmune Disorder	
Respiratory	Asthma or Chronic Pulmonary Disease within last 2 yrs. without inhaler therapy		Asthma or Chronic Pulmonary Disease within last 2 yrs. with inhaler therapy		Tuberculosis active or history of Tuberculosis	
	Past Hx of Cigarette Smoking		Current Use of Cigarettes		Heart Disease	
	Past hx of marijuana use		Current use of marijuana		Pulmonary Embolus	
					Asthma on systemic meds	
					Congenital Heart Disease	
Social Demographic	Living in same residence < 12 months		Residence vhanged >twice in past 12 months		No recent or current stable living arrangement	
	Employed or DSS < 6 months		Unemployed or DSS > 6 months		Unemployed or DSS >12 months	
	Telephone disconnected once in last 12 months		No telephone in residence		No access to telephone	
	Secondary smoke in residence		> 2 Persons smoking in residence		Present or past: Physical and/or Sexual Abuse	
	< 2 Supportive persons over age 18		Living alone – no support		Hx of foster care, past or current	
	> 18 Yrs no HS disploma		< 18 Yrs no diploma or GED not in school		< 16 Yrs. not in school	

Figure 9-5. (A) This assessment form, used by one HMO, helps identify mothers with the potential for a complicated pregnancy. **(B)** This 30- to 34-week reassessment tool is used to check status before mothers give birth. **(C)** The social intake form is used for mothers who may need to be referred to a caseworker.

Education includes advice to eliminate or reduce alcohol intake, to eliminate smoking, and to avoid illegal drugs. Advice should be given about the proper foods to eat, the appropriate weight gain, and the taking of vitamin and mineral supplements. The woman should also be encouraged to prepare for childbirth and breast feeding.

Screening should include blood-pressure monitoring, Pap smear, urinalysis, recording of weight gain, a physical examination, including a pelvic examination, and a health history. Screening should also be undertaken for genetic disease or congenital anomalies by ultrasound, α-fetoprotein, estradiol, and β-HCG. Amniocentesis is appropriate for women with a family history of genetic disorders, as well as for women over age 35. Women who take care of cats should avoid their litter to prevent toxoplasmosis.

The adequacy of prenatal care is defined not only by how many of the above procedures are done, but by when prenatal care is initiated. The Kessner index is a widely used standard to ascertain the adequacy of prenatal care. Under this classification, "adequate" care begins in the first trimester and includes nine or more visits during a pregnancy that lasts 36 or more weeks. "Intermediate" care is care that was started in the second trimester and includes five to eight visits for a pregnancy that lasts at least 36 weeks. "Inadequate" is care that starts in the last trimester or has only four visits or less. However, it is unclear which aspects of prenatal care contribute most to good outcomes. Further research needs to be

Other						
	Sensitivity to local anesthetics		Chronic Medical Illness, identify:		Bleeding Disorder	
					HIV+ with or without associated Syphilis	
					Hemolytic Disease	

Documented Problems in Maternal Obstetrical History						
	<12 Months between births		Prev. Uterine Surgery		Rh Sensitization/other Antibody Sensitization	
	Term Preg. > 5		Prev. Abortions 2nd Trimester		Severe Hypertension During Prev. Preg.	
	PTL < 35 wks no tocolytics		Hx of PTL <35 weeks with tocolytics		> PTL < 32 weeks with tocolytics	
	Hx of Anemia		Prev. Gestational Diabetes		Pica/History of Eating Disorder	
	Pregnancy Induced Hypertension		Placenta Previa		Preclampsia with ITP or HELLEP	
			History of Sexually Transmitted Diseases		Hx of Secondary or Tertiary Syphillis	
	PROM > 24 hours		Abruptio Placenta		> 4 Cesarian Sections	
					Group B Strep with previous pregnancy	

Documented Physical Findings in Previous Infants						
			Stillbirth >28 wks. gestation			
			Birthweight < 2500 gms			
			Birthweight > 4000 gms			
			Genetic Metabolic Disorder			

Maternal Physical Findings						
	Maternal Weight less than or greater than ideal body weight		Physically Challenged		Major Medical Problem identified not specified elsewhere, Identify:	
	Registered for Prenatal Care this preg. 12-15 wks.		Registered for care this pregnancy 16-20 wks.		Registered for care > 28 wks.	
			Uterine, Abdominal, or Adnexal Abnormality		Hypertension > 130/90	
			Mentally Challenged		Current Pica	
			Cardiac Murmur grade II or higher		Current Eating Disorder	

Please add any components of the history or physical examiniation that you as the provider feel place this patient at risk for this pregnancy not detailed in the tables above.

List Here: ____________________

Type of Provider completing form: Please circle.

MD PA NP CNM RN LPN Med. Assist. Other ____________

Please enter weeks gestation by Lmp ________Wks., and by exam ________Wks.

❑ Yes, I would recommend case management/resource assistance from Monroe Plan.

❑ No, this case does not require case management/resource assistance from Monroe Plan.

Figure 9-5A. (Continued)

done to determine if screening for disease and treatment of underlying medical problems, or more education, or better nutrition, is most effective in lowering infant mortality.

The first prenatal visit is an extremely important one, as the establishment of trust and communication is initiated then. The primary care provider must allow enough time so that the visit is not hurried and the pregnant woman's questions may be answered to her satisfaction. Time must be provided to listen to the woman and her partner. Their concerns, fears, and anxieties may be discerned and can then begin to be addressed. It is essential as well to understand and accept her dreams and expectations. The goal of this visit is to establish a mutual partnership that will work toward a healthy outcome of the pregnancy and birth for both the mother and child.

A thorough medical history should be obtained and documented, and a complete medical examination should be conducted. A careful pelvic examination should ensue, including an assessment of the adequacy of the pelvis for childbirth. Individual pregnancy risk should be obtained and documented. Educational material and counseling on healthy lifestyle should be provided at this first visit. It is essential to obtain some idea of family traditions surrounding pregnancy and birth and to begin the process of developing a safe but culturally appropriate plan for the birth experience. Expectations of both the mother and the physician should be clearly stated. The importance of good nutrition for the mother and of breast feeding for the infant should be stressed. Table 9-4 lists the screening tests that should be obtained.

Subsequent visits should be planned to monitor the growth and well-being of the fetus and to monitor the pregnant woman's health. Table 9-5 lists tests to be done at subsequent visits. Blood pressure, weight, and urine protein monitoring are conducted to diagnose and

Name______________________________ DATE ______________

DOB:__________ EDC:__________

PROVIDER: __________ CONTRACT# __________

Monroe Plan ______

GVGHA ______

Other ______

30 Wk – 34 Wk Reassessment Tool

Laboratory Data

Anemia (Hct 27 or 30 more than 3 pt. drop since initial assessment)	Anemia less than Hct 27	+ PPD with abnormal chest xray
Gestational Diabetes confirmed by abnormal GTT	Sickle Cell Disease or hemoglobinopathy causing Hemolytic Disease of newborn	HIV+ with or without associated Syphilis
	Cervical culture + for Group Beta Strep	Hepatitis B Antigen +
Rh Neg		Rh sensitization
Sexually Transmitted Diseases - identify:	Syphilis + current or history of Syphilis	Syphilis with rising titers
Pap smear min to mod dysplasia	Pap smear - severe dysplasia	Idiopathic Thrombocytopenic Purpura
Asymptomatic Bacteruria or single UTI	Recurrent UTI > 1 once this pregnancy	

Antepartum Factors

Weight Gain < 10 lb. at 20 wks	Weight Gain < 10 lb. at 30 wks.	Fetal Chromosomal Disorder confirmed by u/s, AFP analysis
Multiple Gestation – total #:	Weight Gain > 40 lb. at 30 weeks	Mild PIH/developing signs of Pre-eclampsia
Varicose Veins – 1st degree	Cervical Cerclage in place	Severe of superimposed Pre-eclampsia
Polyhydrammnios confirmed by u/s	Superficial Thrombosis	Cervix dilated 2 cm. at < 34 weeks
		PROM less than 34 weeks
Gestational Diabetes confirmed by 3h GTT - diet controlled	LGA confirmed US and clinical findings	Major trauma or surgery during pregnancy
>2 documented ED or Labor Floor visits	PTL controlled with bedrest >32 weeks	PTL > 26 weeks controlled with tocolytics
	Marginal Placenta Previa	PTL < 26 weeks
Missed 1 or 2 Appointments	Missed appointments > 2	Continue to miss appointments despite counseling
Poor diet	Pyelonephritis once	Placenta Previa – complete
Continued cigarette use	Continued use of alcohol	Heavy use of alcohol or Rx drugs
Greater than 2 Labor Deck visits		
	2nd or 3rd trimester bleeding – not Previa	Heroin or Crack Addiction
Irritable Uterus necessitating evaluation		IUGR confirmed by U/S and clinical findings
Oligohydramnios		Unable to locate, out of care
		Deep Vein Thrombosis
		Intrauterine Fetal Demise > 24 weeks

Please add any conditions that have been identified as risks that you as the provider feel place this patient at risk at this point in the pregnancy. List here: ______________________________

____

How many weeks pregnant was patient when form was completed? __________ wks.

❑ Yes, I would recommend case management/resource assistance from Monroe Plan.

❑ No, this case does not require case management/resource assistance from Monroe Plan.

Figure 9-5B.

treat preeclampsia during its earliest stages. Current studies indicate that weight gain in pregnancy should not be limited to 20 or 25 pounds; however, excessive weight gain is inappropriate and is ultimately harmful, because many women first become obese at the time of their pregnancies. Obesity is a serious health problem for women in the United States, and primary care providers for women must educate women about the need for appropriate weight gain to enhance the welfare of both the mother and fetus.

The traditional pattern of prenatal care visits once every month until the 28th week, then every 2 weeks in the 28th to 36th weeks, followed by once a week from 36 weeks until delivery should be modified depending on the circumstances. Women who have increased educational needs, serious social difficulties such as the use of illicit drugs, or medical complications such as diabetes should be seen more frequently.

A postdate pregnancy should be followed carefully, with biweekly antenatal testing for fetal well-being. Accepted management is to induce labor in patients with a softened cervix at 42 weeks gestational age. If the cervix is not favorable, prostaglandin E_2 gel is most commonly used to prepare the cervix for induction.

The aims of prenatal care are to ensure a healthy mother, to prepare her for labor and childbirth, and to ensure a viable, healthy baby born no earlier than 36 weeks.

COMMON PROBLEMS OF PREGNANCY AND DANGER SIGNS

Nausea and vomiting, or "morning sickness," is a common complaint and may occur at any time of the day. Pregnant women should eat frequent light meals. It is useful to have dry foods such as toast or crack-

Date________ **Provider____________________**
Contract #________________ **Plan ________________________**

SOCIAL INTAKE FORM

Many woman face situations that make their lives Difficult. We are here to help you. We can also refer you to others who can help you. Your answers to these questions will help us understand your needs. Your health care providers will then be able to go over your answers and talk with you about them. Please do not worry about sharing your concerns with us. Everything you tell us is confidential.

Please print

NAME: ____
first middle last

DATE OF BIRTH:____________________

1. People in your household:

NAME	AGE	RELATIONSHIP
____________	____	____________
____________	____	____________
____________	____	____________
____________	____	____________
____________	____	____________
____________	____	____________

If more room is needed - please use the back of this page

2. Who can help you if needed ?

Name:________________ Name:________________
Relationship:________________ Relationship:________________
Phone Number:________________ Phone Number:________________

3. Do You have a Job ?:________________Where do you work ?____________

Hours:____________ Type of work:________________________

Figure 9-5C.

ers during the time of nausea. Pregnant women with constant vomiting or diarrhea need urgent evaluation by a primary care physician.

In the first trimester, the growing uterus puts pressure on the bladder, causing the pregnant woman to urinate more frequently. Reassurance should be given.

Backaches may occur during the second and third trimesters. Excellent posture, wearing low-heeled, comfortable shoes, sleeping on a good firm mattress, and instruction in pelvic rocking as an exercise are helpful strategies to reduce the problem.

Leg muscle cramps are usually caused by increased pressure on veins, but they may be due to low levels of calcium and high levels of phosphorus. Pregnant women should drink milk and eat dairy products and should take a vitamin and mineral supplement. Leg cramps may be relieved by lying on the back with the affected leg extended. The knee should be kept straight and the foot flexed up and down.

Heartburn may occur, especially after a large meal. It is relieved by antacids and reduced by eating frequent small meals throughout the day.

When a pregnant woman stands or moves quickly, a pulling pain in the right or lower left abdomen is caused by tension in the round ligament. Pregnant women should rise slowly from a sitting or lying position. Lying on the side of the pain helps lessen this round ligament pain.

Most pregnant women notice some swelling of the ankles and feet, especially in hot weather. It helps to elevate the feet and to walk rather than stand to ensure better circulation. Facial and hand edema should be reported to the physician.

Braxton-Hicks contractions of the uterus typically become more noticeable as pregnancy progresses toward delivery. They are usually irregular and last about 30 seconds. They are self-limited.

Varicosities are common during pregnancy and are treated by support stockings. Pregnant women should be encouraged to take "walk breaks" at least twice a day and should drink plenty of fluids. The legs may be raised against a wall above the heart for 15 to 20 minutes a day.

Constipation and hemorrhoids are common complaints. Fluids and a mild laxative may help. Because progesterone can cause

4. What was the last grade in school you completed? __________

5. Are you going to school or class now ?______ If yes, name of school __________

6. Is it hard for you to keep appointments? Yes ☐ *Why - Please check* No ☐

Medical Provider	☐	No Health Insurance	☐	Inadequate Clothing	☐
Transportation	☐	No Child Care	☐	Other	☐

8. Are you receiving any of these services ? If No would you like a referral ?

	Yes /No	→	Yes / No
Community Health Nurse	___	I would like a referral	___
WIC	___	I would like a referral	___
Public Assistance/Food Stamps	___	I would like a referral	___
Counseling / Social Work	___	I wouldlike a referral	___

9. Have you been denied services or been sanctioned? yes____ no_____
Please list______________________________________

____

10. If you are under 21, who is responsible for your finances:

Name:________________ Relationship:________________

11. Have you ever experienced any of the following?

Sexual Abuse	☐	Physical Abuse	☐
Depression	☐	Stress from a recent loss	☐
Thoughts of hurting self	☐	Slapping or hitting by your boyfriend	☐
or others	☐	Forced sex by a partner or stranger	☐

12. Would you like to know more about ? *Please Check*

Finding a Job	☐	Child care	☐
AIDs/HIV	☐	Domestic violence	☐
Adoption	☐	Parenting classes	☐
Self breast exam	☐	Family Planning	☐
Sexually transmitted diseases	☐	Pregnancy Planning	☐

13. I would help with:
Food ☐ Clothing ☐ Transportation ☐ Housing ☐

14. When do you think your baby is due? ________________
Date

Figure 9-5C. (Continued)

some decreased intestinal motility, walking and exercise are important. Sitz baths and analgesic ointments are helpful for hemorrhoids. The pregnant woman should be able to reduce hemorrhoids easily herself; if they become thrombosed, she must be evaluated.

A "pregnancy mask" of dark blotches around the eyes, mouth, and forehead may occur but disappears after delivery. Many women worry about stretch marks. The skin discoloration of these marks also disappears after delivery. They are due to hormonal changes, not to the size of the fetus.

Pregnant women should call their obstetric provider immediately if vaginal bleeding or spotting occurs. In the first trimester, it can indicate a threatened abortion. Late in pregnancy it can indicate abruptio placentae or placenta previa. Headache and blurred vision can be a sign of preeclampsia. Severe abdominal pain may be a sign of abortion, ectopic pregnancy, or infection. Chills and a fever of 38.3°C (101°F) without symptoms of upper respiratory infection point to pyelonephritis, especially if the woman has a history of urinary tract infections. Fluid escaping from the vagina can indicate rupture of membranes.

NORMAL BIRTH

Physicians must learn the mechanisms and physiology of normal birth as part of their fundamental medical knowledge. Just as a noncardiologist must have a fundamental appreciation of normal cardiac and circulatory physiology, all physicians must understand the process of childbirth, as birth deeply affects women at many levels, physiologically, emotionally, and spiritually.

Every woman has a deep need to share her own childbirth story. One woman will tell another her story, even among strangers. Childbirth is a major life event, and women tell it to each other as a way of coming to terms with the experience. It is not unusual for a health care provider taking a history from a postmenopausal woman to encounter a detailed and complete account of that woman's childbirth history. Such storytelling helps the woman understand exactly what happened to her, and puts the experience, whether it was a normal birth or an operative delivery, into context in her life. Birth to women is not just a medical or physiologic event: it is a social, psychological, and spiritual event.

15. How do you feel about being pregnant? Check all that apply

Happy ☐ Unhappy ☐ Scared ☐
Depressed☐ Angry ☐ Unsure ☐

16. Different drugs may effect you and your baby's health. In the past six months, have you used any of the following?

Prescribed medicine ☐ Marijuana ☐
Caffeine (coffee, soda)☐ Cocaine ☐
Cigarettes ☐ Heroin ☐
Alcohol, list please ☐ Other drugs ☐

17. The father of the baby:

Name:____________________ Are you and the father together?_________

18. How do you think he feels about your being pregnant? (Check all that apply).

Happy ○ Unhappy ○ Scared ○
Depressed ○ Angry ○ Unsure ○

Does he support/helpful to you? Yes___ No___ He doesn't know ____

Will he be helping you care for the baby? Yes ___ No___

19. How do you think your family feels about you being pregnant? (Check all that apply).

Happy ☐ Unhappy ☐ Angry ☐ O.K ☐ I don't know ☐
I haven't told them ☐

Are they supportive/helpful ? Yes ☐ No ☐

Do you think they will help you care for the baby ? Yes ☐ No ☐

Figure 9-5C. (Continued)

Both positive and negative feelings need to be expressed. Expressing through storytelling her disappointment with any aspect of birth allows these feelings to be resolved.

Retelling a birth experience allows the new mother to accept her baby as a separate human, not just the fetus she carried for 9 months. New babies are often different from what the new mother expected. Retelling her story lets each woman acknowledge her strength. Labor and birth is one of the most incredible and physically and emotionally challenging life events. Women, after birth, discover what they are capable of, and it is not unusual for women to use this strength as a basis for renewing their lives. Women see themselves in a new light. Birth is a physical triumph. All physicians need to understand this very fundamental aspect of the birth experience.

Retelling the childbirth story also aids in the woman's transition to the new role of mother and helps the woman relate to her own mother as well. Finally, in telling her birth story every woman shares with others the miracle of life. All physicians need to respect and revere this sense of the miracle of birth as part of life and to encourage it in our patients.

No primary care text can present in great detail all aspects of labor and delivery, so the student is encouraged to read and study further. What follows is a description of the essential events of normal birth.

Stages of Labor

Before onset of parturition, the cervix softens and the presenting part of the fetus descends into the pelvis. In normal pregnancy, the cervix becomes soft, easily admits one finger on examination, and becomes effaced or thin, usually to less than 1.3 cm in length. This process may be evaluated by a Bishop score (Table 9-6); a score of 9 or greater indicates that the cervix is ready for parturition because it is easily dilatable with the onset of contractions. The mucus that has plugged the cervix throughout pregnancy is passed and is usually noted as dark, bloody mucus.

Women often describe irregular contractions of the uterus that increase in intensity and frequency as pregnancy advances toward term (36 to 41 weeks). Other signs of impending labor include a spurt of energy that usually occurs 24 hours before the onset of contractions that dilate the cervix. Because of the decrease in progesterone levels, women tend to lose 1 to 1.5 pounds about 1 to 2 days before the onset of labor.

Table 9-4. Screening Tests

Hematocrit
Type and Rh and antibody screen
VDRL test
Rubella titer
Hepatitis B screening
Urine culture
Cervical cytology
Cervical cultures for gonorrhea (and β-streptococcus and Chlamydia, as indicated)
Sickle-cell screening in women at risk
HIV counseling and testing
Genetic counseling and amniocentesis for women over 35 or with family history of genetic disease
Tuberculin testing

Table 9-5. Prenatal Studies at Subsequent Visits

Screen for neural tube defects and trisomy 21	(14–16 wks)
α-fetoprotein, estradiol, and β-HCG	
Complete obstetric ultrasound encouraged	(18–20 wks)
1-hour 50-g glucose screen	(26 wks)
Herpes culture in symptomatic patients or in patients with history of herpes	

Labor begins as a series of mild but regular uterine contractions that start out usually 20 or 30 minutes apart. They are experienced as pressure, cramps, or sometimes a backache. Over time, these contractions become stronger, more noticeable, and closer together. At some point, they hurt, and the pregnant woman involuntarily stops what she is doing and must rest and breathe deeply to cope with the contraction pain. In early labor, women feel the need to be active and to eat and drink. However, as labor progresses to a more active phase, the digestive process slows and most women are not hungry. The woman begins to focus her energies on her labor and turns inward in her concentration.

Labor is divided into three stages. The *first stage* is further subdivided into the latent phase and the active phase. The latent phase varies in length and starts with the onset of contractions and cervical change. During this phase, contractions become stronger, efficient, and polarized and are accompanied by softening of the cervix. The cervix becomes thinner and is easily stretched. In nulliparas, the average length of the latent phase is 8.6 hours; in multiparas, it is 5.3 hours. The Friedman curve in Figure 9-6 demonstrates this. The normal limit of the latent phase is 20 hours in nulliparas and 14 hours in multiparas. The length of this phase is correlated with the state of cervical softness at the onset of labor.

The active phase starts when the cervix is 3 to 4 cm dilated. The extracellular matrix of the cervix has been altered to allow more rapid dilatation; thus, the active phase of labor is 5.8 hours in nulliparas and 2.5 hours in multiparas (see Fig. 9-6). This phase normally should not exceed 12 hours in nulliparas and 6 hours in multiparas.

A transition phase of varied but short duration occurs between the first and second stages. The transition phase from stage one to stage two corresponds to the time between 8 and 10 cm, or full dilatation. At this time, it is normal for women to have a full gamut of emotions that range from feeling wonderful, happy, powerful, and elated, to angry, sad, overwhelmed, and scared.

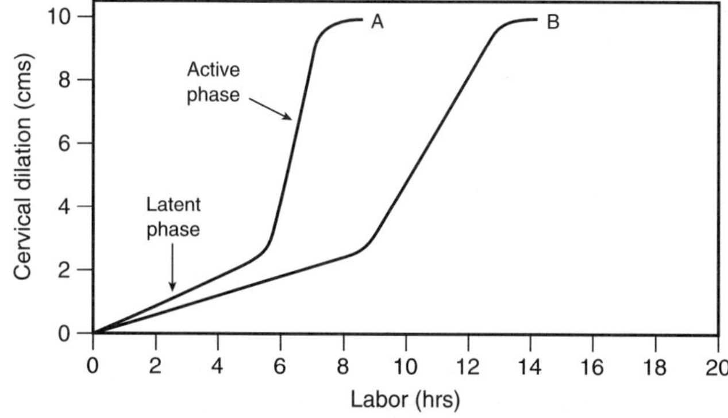

Figure 9-6. First stage of labor: Friedman curves. *A,* multipara; *B,* nullipara.

Table 9-6. Bishop Score

	POINTS			
FACTOR	*0*	*1*	*2*	*3*
Dilatation of cervix (cm)	0	1–2	3–4	5–6
Effacement of cervix (%)	0–30	40–50	60–70	80
Consistency of cervix	Firm	Medium	Soft	
Position of cervix in the vagina	Posterior	Mid	Anterior	
Station	–3	–2	–1.0	+1, +2

Oxorn H. Oxorn-Foote human labor and birth; 5th ed. Norwalk, CT: Appleton & Lange, 1986.

The *second stage* of labor begins with full dilatation of the cervix and ends with the birth of the baby. Once transition is completed and the cervix is fully dilated, the second or expulsive stage commences. The laboring woman feels an instinctive urge to push. Pushing, accomplished by a Valsalva maneuver, extends the force of the contractions by 20% to 30% to allow the fetus to pass through the pelvis. Progress of the second stage of labor is measured by the station of the presenting part (Fig. 9-7). The membranes, if not ruptured artificially, usually rupture spontaneously in the active phase. In some cases, membranes rupture before the onset of labor, and in most of these cases contractions begin spontaneously within 12 hours. The time between spontaneous rupture of the membranes and onset of labor normally does not exceed 24 hours.

The normal mechanisms of labor that allow the fetus to pass through the pelvic bones are descent and flexion, internal rotation, extension, restitution, and external rotation, followed by delivery. These classic mechanisms occur because the force of the mother's expulsive efforts and of the contractions causes the fetal presenting part to meet the resistance of the pelvis. Thus, passively the fetal presenting part turns as it makes its way through the pelvic canal. The mechanisms of labor are illustrated in Figures 9-8 through 9-10.

The *third stage* of labor is the delivery of the placenta. In a normal birth, this stage is accomplished easily, with spontaneous separation and expulsion of the placenta. The upper limit of this stage is 30 minutes; the placenta should be removed manually under anesthesia after 30 minutes. Care must be taken to ensure that the complete placenta is delivered, because even small portions of retained membranes can cause postpartum hemorrhage. Normal blood loss is 200 to 250 mL.

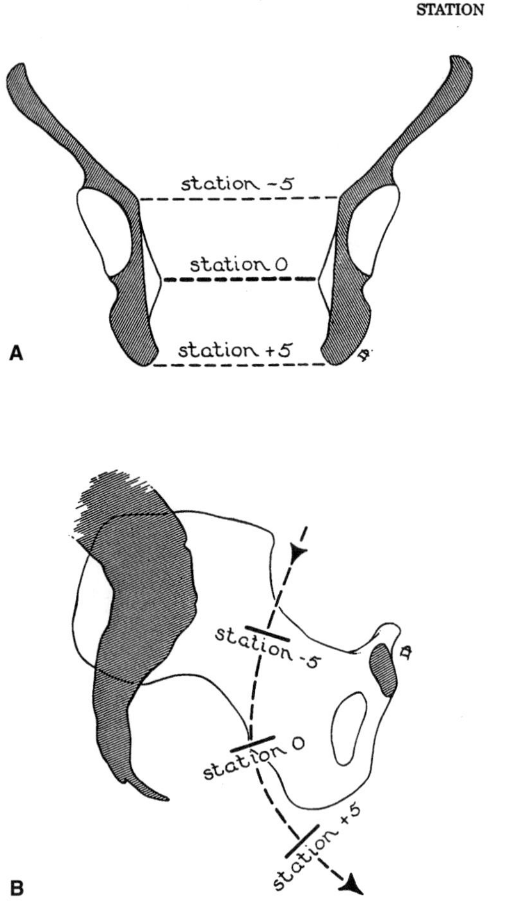

Figure 9-7. Station of presenting part. **(A)** Anteroposterior view. **(B)** Lateral view.

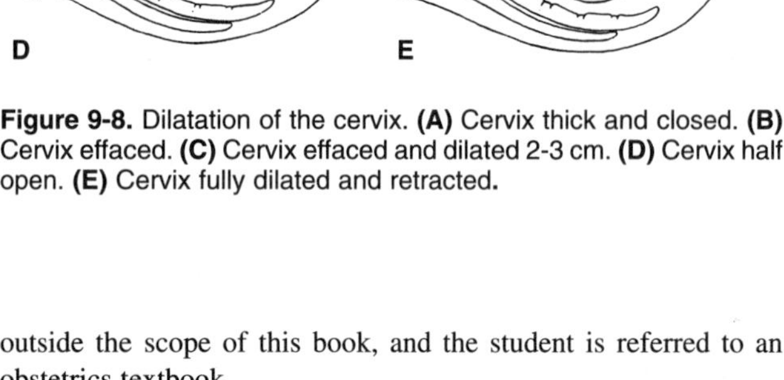

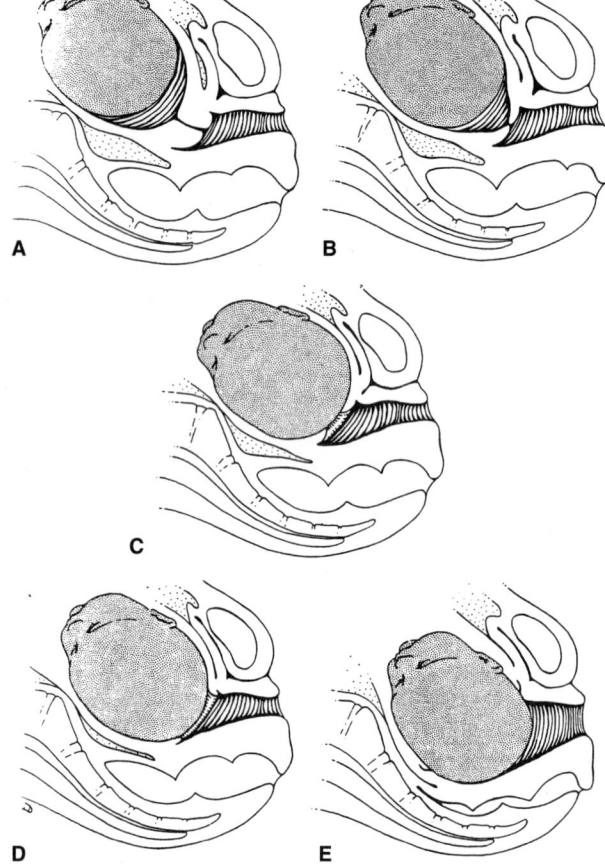

Figure 9-8. Dilatation of the cervix. **(A)** Cervix thick and closed. **(B)** Cervix effaced. **(C)** Cervix effaced and dilated 2-3 cm. **(D)** Cervix half open. **(E)** Cervix fully dilated and retracted.

After the birth of the infant, the physician or midwife must ensure that the mother's uterus is well contracted to prevent hemorrhage. This is accomplished by giving the mother 20 units of oxytocin (Pitocin) intravenously, putting the infant immediately to the breast, or both.

Care of the Fetus/Infant

During labor, the well-being of the fetus is monitored carefully. There is controversy concerning whether electronic fetal monitoring is necessary for normal labor. However, if auscultation is done, it must be done religiously every 15 minutes in the first stage and after every contraction in the second stage. If this is not feasible, electronic monitoring must be initiated. The primary care provider must know what is accepted as a normal fetal heart rate tracing and, when deviations occur, how to manage care appropriately. This may mean a consultation with a specialist. At birth, the physician or midwife suctions the infant's nasopharynx of secretions and mucus and helps the infant adjust to extrauterine life. The infant must be kept warm.

Abnormal labor and delivery, which includes malpresentation, such as breech and occiput posterior, and multifetal pregnancies, is outside the scope of this book, and the student is referred to an obstetrics textbook.

This summary of normal birth is not meant to present obstetric management and the conduct of labor, including methods of pain management and appropriate anesthesia: these belong to the realm of specialists in the field. However, all physicians should have an understanding of the birth process.

OTHER ISSUES OF REPRODUCTIVE HEALTH

Family planning and contraceptive care, essential to women of reproductive age, are discussed in Chapter 16. Abnormalities of pregnancy, such as ectopic pregnancy and spontaneous abortion, are discussed in Chapter 18.

The reproductive health of women must always address the issue of termination of pregnancy. Unfortunately, in our society abortion has become a polarizing topic. Most women take a position somewhere in the middle, acknowledging women's needs and the fact that in some cases a pregnancy is detrimental to a woman physically or psychologically but at the same time understanding that using abortion as a means of birth control undermines a woman's health as well. This position acknowledges the fact that

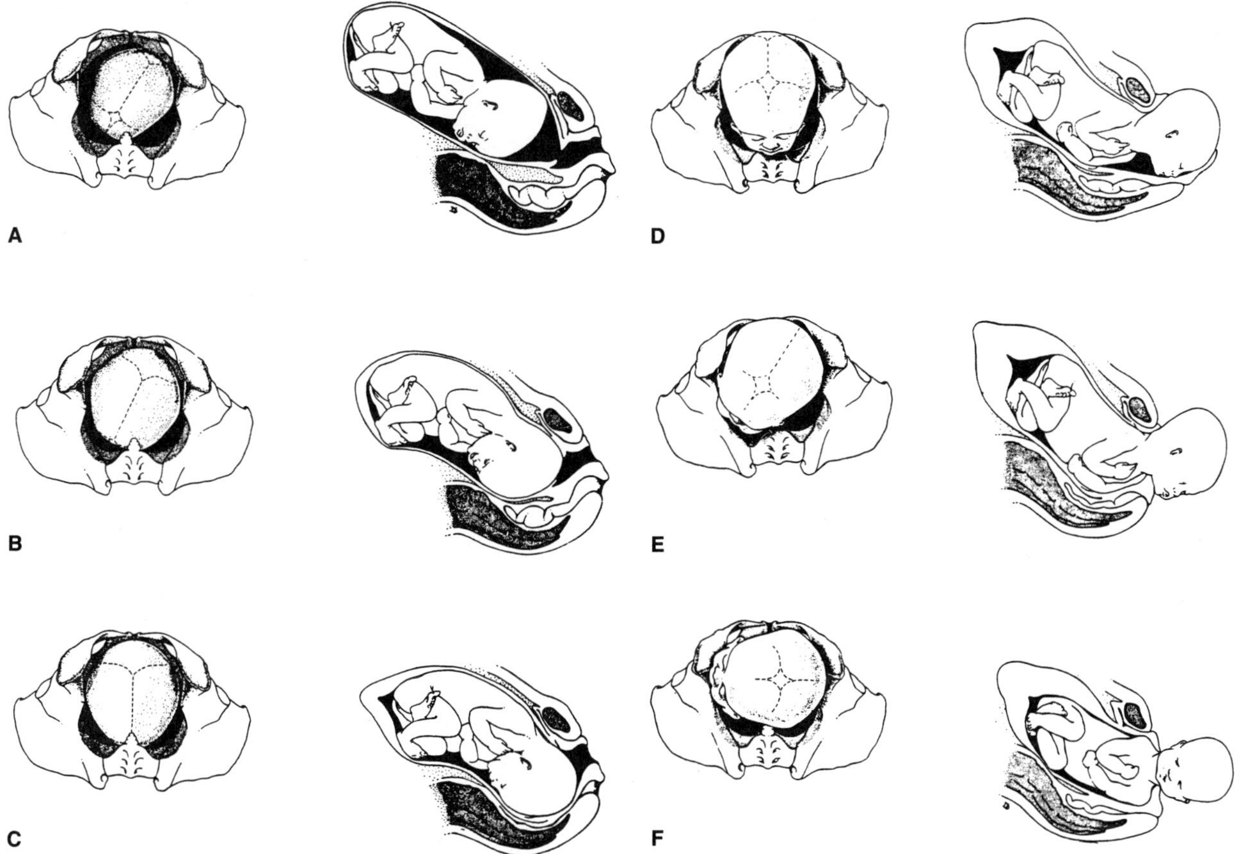

Figure 9-9. Summary of mechanism of labor. (**A through C**) Anterior positions of the occiput. (**A**) Onset of labor. (**B**) Descent and flexion. (**C**) Internal rotation: left occipital anterior (LOA) to occipito-anterior (OA). **(D through F**) Left occiput anterior. (**D**) Extension. (**E**) Restitution; OA to LOA. (**F**) External rotation: LOA to left occipital transverse (LOT).

the decision to terminate a pregnancy is a difficult one and one that a woman does not make lightly. Counseling is an indispensable part of all abortion services. In an open society with diverse opinions, respect for the individual's choice and beliefs must be paramount, and part of this respect is providing access to safe clinical services for abortion. All cultures have practiced termination of pregnancy. Even when abortion was illegal, women sought abortion providers, at great risk to their health. The American College of Obstetricians and Gynecologists has stated that their residents must have exposure to and education in the proper management of termination of pregnancy. Residents with religious or moral objections to the procedure are not obligated to perform abortions but must state their reasons in writing.

CHRONIC MEDICAL CONDITIONS AND REASONS FOR HOSPITALIZATION FOR REPRODUCTIVE-AGE WOMEN

The most common reason for hospitalization for women aged 18 to 44 is complications of pregnancy, followed by other genital tract problems and diseases of the female pelvic organs. The fourth most common reason for hospitalization is for spontaneous abortion and termination of pregnancy. This emphasizes the importance of reproductive health in this age group.

The reasons for hospitalization are completely different from the most common chronic conditions of reproductive age. These conditions are most often treated on an ambulatory basis. The ten most common chronic conditions are: chronic sinusitis; hay fever without asthma; chronic obstructive pulmonary disease, which includes chronic bronchitis, asthma, and emphysema; orthopedic deformities, especially of the back; migraines; arthritis; disease of the female genital tract; hemorrhoids; high blood pressure; and dermatitis. When chronic medical conditions that impair activity are considered, the most common conditions of women aged 18 to 44 are back deformity; lower extremity deformity; chronic obstructive pulmonary disease; arthritis; intervertebral disc disorders; high blood pressure; visual impairment; upper extremity orthopedic deformity; heart disease, including congestive heart disease but not ischemic disease; diabetes; and hearing impairment.

The variation in this list points to the fact that ambulatory care and hospital care facilities treat and manage different problems in this age group. It is tempting to think, therefore, that health care providers for women could easily and rationally be divided into two groups, primary care ambulatory care providers and specialized hospital care providers. The problem with this analysis is that it is incomplete: prenatal care is recorded as complete care including delivery, so prenatal care is not counted in ambulatory care statis-

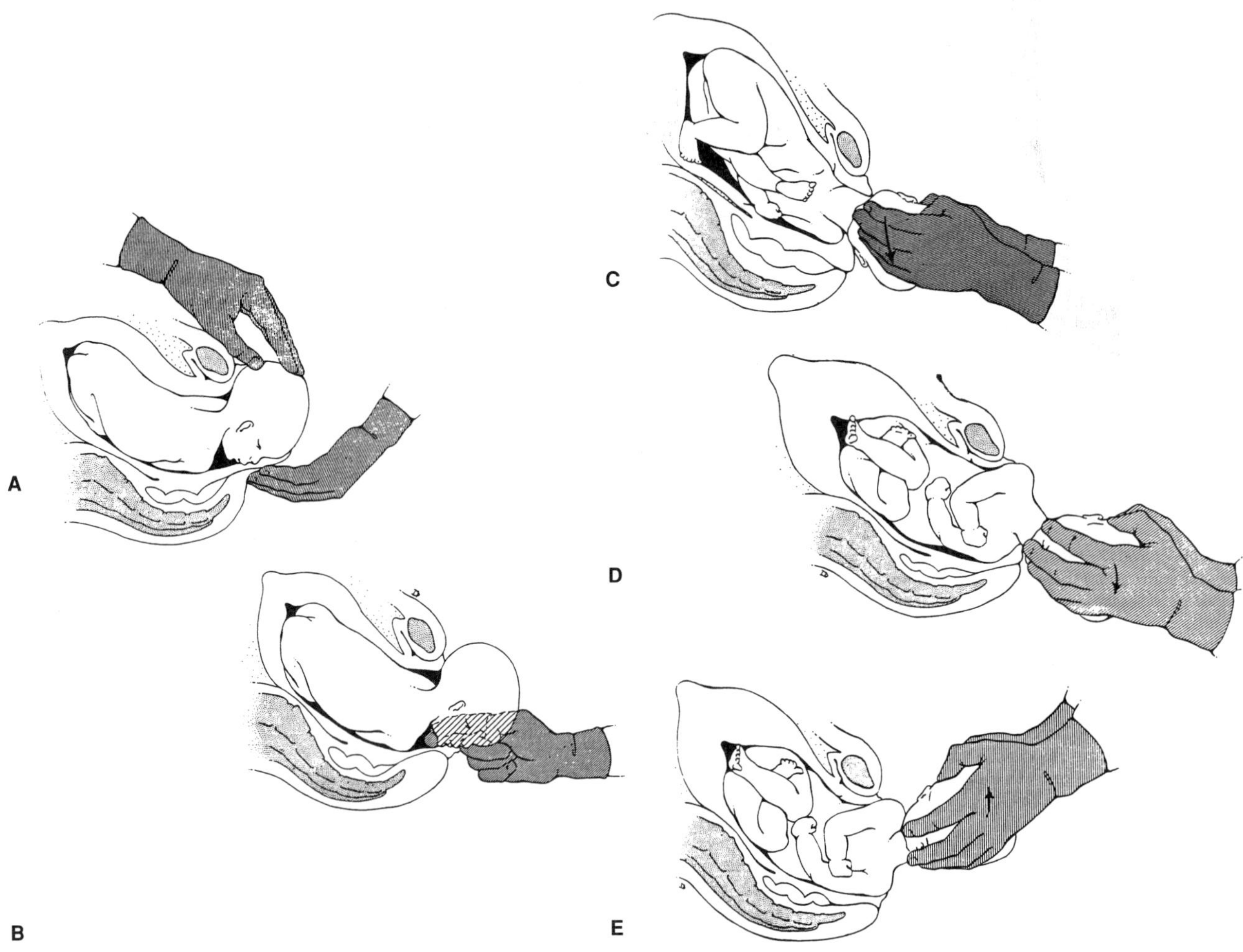

Figure 9-10. Birth of head and delivery of shoulders. (**A**) Rigen maneuver. (**B**) Hooking out of chin. (**C**) Lowering of fetal head. (**D**) Delivery of anterior shoulder. (**E**) Delivery of posterior shoulder.

tics. Because pregnancy-related problems are the most common reasons for hospitalization, it follows that prenatal care is a common reason for women to seek ambulatory care.

BIBLIOGRAPHY

Anderson HF. The prenatal record and the initial prenatal visit. In: Sciarra J, ed. Gynecology and obstetrics, vol. 2. Philadelphia: JB Lippincott, 1994.

Cooper RL, Goldenberg RL, DuBard MB, Davis RO, and the collaborative group on preterm birth prevention. Risk factors for fetal death in white, black, and Hispanic women. Obstet Gynecol 1994;84:490.

Farook AA. Colour atlas of childbirth and obstetric techniques. Aylesbury, England: Wolfe Publishing, 1990.

Herschel M, Hsieh H, Mittendorf R, Khoshnood B, Covert RF, Lee K. Risk factors for fetal death in white, black and Hispanic women [letter]. Obstet Gynecol 1995;85:318.

Luke B. Maternal nutrition. In Reece EA, Hobbis ID, Mahoney MJ, Petrie RH, eds. Medicine of the fetus and mother. Philadelphia: JB Lippincott, 1992:869.

Myles MF. Textbook for midwives with modern concepts of obstetric and neonatal care, 10th ed. Edinburgh: Churchill Livingstone, 1985.

Oxorn H. Oxorn-Foote human labor and birth, 5th ed. Norwalk, CT: Appleton & Lange, 1986:918.

Pridjian G. Diagnosis of pregnancy. In: Sciarra J, ed. Gynecology and obstetrics, vol 2, chap. 2. Philadelphia: JB Lippincott, 1992.

Robert Wood Johnson Foundation. Special report: the Medicaid expansions for pregnant women and children. Princeton, NJ, 1995.

Shyken JM, Petrie RH. Antepartum fetal rate monitoring. In: Reece EA, Hobbins JC, Mahoney MJ, Petrie RH, eds. Medicine of the fetus and mother. Philadelphia: JB Lippincott, 1992:757.

Speroff L, Glass RH, Kase NG. Clinical gynecologic endocrinology and infertility, 5th ed. Baltimore: Williams & Wilkins, 1994:109.

Sullivan LE. The birth experience. Working Mothers, June 1995.

Primary Care for Women, edited by Phyllis C. Leppert and Fred M. Howard. Lippincott-Raven Publishers, Philadelphia © 1997.

10
The Menopausal Woman

CAROL ACHILLES
PHYLLIS C. LEPPERT

The life transition of menopause occurs sometime around age 50. Menopause is the cessation of menstruation secondary to the diminution of ovarian steroids. It heralds the end of the female fertile period of life. The time immediately before and after the cessation of menses is referred to as perimenopause. The climacteric is a term used for the time in life when a woman goes through the physiologic transition from the reproductive age to the postmenopausal age and is also associated with changes due to diminished ovarian function.

The actual age of menopause varies. The median age is about 50 to 52, based for the most part on histories of women obtained in a retrospective fashion. One small prospective study found that the median age of the onset of the perimenopausal period was 47.5 years. Most women in this study reported irregularity of menses during perimenopause, with only 10% having an abrupt cessation of menstruation.

There is no evidence that the age of menopause has changed greatly over the centuries. Likewise, there is no evidence of a correlation between the age of menarche and the age of menopause, nor does race or parity have any relation to the age of onset of menopause. However, some factors can lead to earlier menopause. Undernourished women and women who live at high altitudes have earlier menopause. There is a correlation between early menopause and the number of cigarettes smoked, as well as the duration of smoking.

The perimenopausal signs and symptoms associated with diminished ovarian hormones are of concern to the women experiencing these changes. Public health concerns regarding preventive health care and quality-of-life issues for these "baby boomers" occur as the number of women born during the post-World War II era enter their perimenopausal years (Fig. 10-1). As more and more women age, the primary care provider will be increasingly responsible for the care of perimenopausal women. Thus, such caregivers must be cognizant of the essentials of preventive care, as well as the principles of disease screening and the fundamental management of common problems and diseases for women of this age.

PHYSIOLOGY OF MENOPAUSE

Before the cessation of menses, the length of the menstrual cycle changes compared to that of younger women. In the perimenopausal period, both short cycles, due to short follicular phases, and long cycles, associated with an inadequate luteal phase or anovulation, can be seen. As the cycles become irregular, vaginal bleeding may occur at the end of a short luteal phase, or after a peak of estradiol in the circulation during an anovulatory cycle. In their mid-40s, women start to have anovulatory cycles that begin 2 to 8 years before menopause.

The changes in the menstrual cycle are associated with high follicle-stimulating hormone (FSH) levels, but levels of luteinizing hormone (LH) and estradiol remain normal, unchanged from the younger years. Estradiol levels remain in the normal range until follicular growth and development stop. As the ovary ages, fewer and fewer follicles develop during each cycle until the follicular supply is depleted. In addition, the aging ovary produces less inhibin, which allows the rise in FSH. The decline in inhibin secretion by ovarian follicles begins around age 35, and secretion is greatly diminished after age 40. The decline in inhibin is a more sensitive marker for the aging ovary than the FSH rise. Because the ovary's production of inhibin is diminished at menopause, FSH is not suppressed by hormone replacement therapy. Thus, FSH cannot be used to determine the appropriate postmenopausal hormone replacement dose. Because occasional corpus luteum formation may occur, a perimenopausal woman is not completely safe from unwanted pregnancy. However, shortly after the cessation of menses, no ovarian follicles remain, marking the onset of loss of fertility.

One to 3 years after menopause, there is a ten- to 20-fold increase in FSH and about a threefold increase in LH. After this peak, slight, gradual declines in FSH and LH levels are seen. These elevated levels of FSH and LH in postmenopausal women are definite evidence of ovarian failure.

In postmenopausal women, the circulating levels of androstenedione is half that in the premenopausal period. Most of this androstenedione is secreted by the ovary. Testosterone levels do not fall very much. In some postmenopausal women, more ovarian testosterone is secreted than in the premenopausal period, due to the elevated FSH and LH levels, which stimulate the ovarian stroma tissue to secrete this hormone. However, because peripheral conversion of androstenedione to testosterone is reduced, the total amount of testosterone secreted after menopause is decreased. Ovarian estrogen production ceases at menopause. However, circulating estrogen levels in postmenopausal women are 10 to 20 pg/mL, mostly derived from the peripheral conversion of estrone. Extraglandular conversion of androstenedione and testosterone to estrogen also occurs. There is great individual variation in the degree of extraglandular production of estrogen and, therefore, a variation in clinical effect from woman to woman. Because fat cells can convert androgen to estrogen, there is an association of obesity with endometrial cancer.

As women age further, the steroid production of the ovarian stroma effectively ceases, and because the adrenal gland does not provide an adequate amount of estrogen precursors, estrogen levels are diminished. In this last postmenopausal stage, secondary sex tissues atrophy (Fig. 10-2).

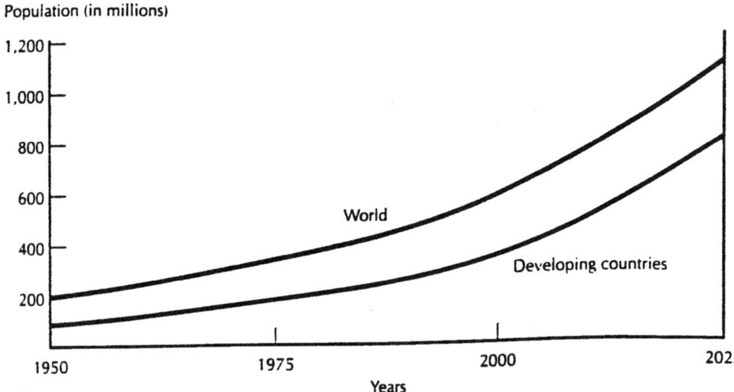

Figure 10-1. Projected size of world population age 60 and older. (Speroff L, Glass RH, Kase NG. Clinical endocrinology and infertility, 5th ed. Baltimore: Williams & Wilkins, 1994:585.)

SIGNS AND SYMPTOMS

There is considerable variation in the signs and symptoms of menopause. Some women experience many symptoms, others few. The symptoms discussed in this chapter should be carefully evaluated and all differential diagnoses suggested by symptoms should be considered. For example, if a primary care provider is not thorough, the sweating and anxiety that can accompany coronary artery disease might easily be attributed to the vasomotor instability and psychological symptoms of menopause. Alternatively, bleeding can be due to endometrial cancer.

One of the primary symptoms of the menopausal period is a change in the pattern of the menses. There may be decreased flow caused by anovulatory cycles, irregularity of menses, or hypermenorrhea. During the perimenopause, estrogen excess may lead to dysfunctional uterine bleeding, endometrial hyperplasia, and perhaps endometrial cancer.

Vasomotor instability caused by estrogen depletion causes hot flushes and night sweats. In many women, these are mild annoyances, but in others they are severe and cause disruption in sleep and inability to concentrate. Some women may be acutely embarrassed if excessive hot flushes and sweating occur in the workplace.

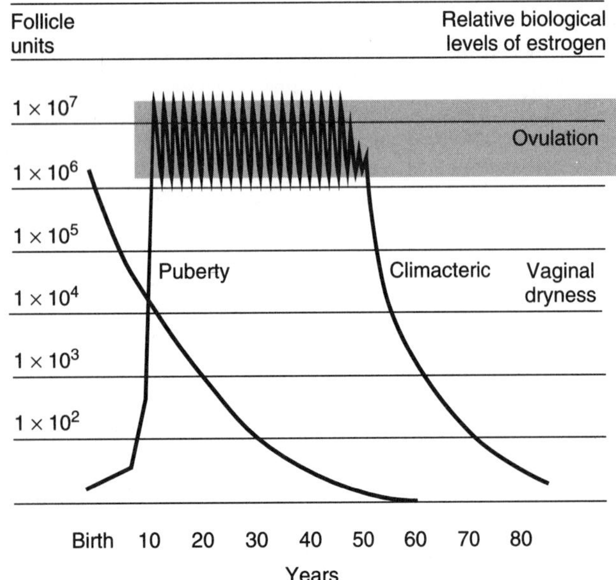

Figure 10-2. Relative biologic levels of estrogen. (Speroff L, Glass RH, Kase NG. Clinical endocrinology and infertility, 5th ed. Baltimore: Williams & Wilkins, 1994:591.)

Estrogen depletion also leads to atrophy of the vaginal epithelium and enhances the formation of urethral caruncles. General skin atrophy occurs. Vulvar, introital, and vaginal atrophy lead to pruritus and dyspareunia. This estrogen depletion may cause urinary problems, such as urgency, urethritis, and cystitis.

There has been no scientific proof that estrogen depletion has a direct cause-and-effect relation on increased psychological symptoms, but anxiety, increased tension, and depressed mood are reported in perimenopausal women. Many of these symptoms are directly associated with life stresses, such as children leaving home.

Finally, estrogen depletion is linked to the other health problems of menopausal and postmenopausal women—specifically, cardiovascular disease and osteoporosis are serious sequelae to estrogen depletion.

In evaluating a woman of menopausal age, the caregiver must perform a careful history and physical examination and obtain the appropriate laboratory tests, including an endometrial biopsy if necessary because of dysfunctional endometrial bleeding. When the uterus is normal on examination, the endometrial biopsy should be performed as an office procedure. A vaginal probe ultrasound examination is an essential component of the pelvic examination in perimenopausal women. As more clinicians use this procedure, the sizing of the uterus will be more accurate. This ultrasound examination should be conducted as an adjunct to the pelvic examination and should not be billed as a distinct procedure separate from the pelvic examination. An endometrial biopsy for vaginal bleeding carried out in the office is accurate and cost-effective. An in-hospital dilatation and curettage (D&C) is not indicated for a woman with a normal-size uterus who needs an endometrial tissue sampling.

The endometrial biopsy is done with the use of a plastic endometrial suction curet or device. Because it is small (3 mm in diameter), no cervical dilatation is needed. The use of a suction curet is usually painless, as the initial attempt to insert the plastic suction cannula is done without the use of a tenaculum on the cervix. In most women, this is successful, and it avoids the often considerable discomfort of the tenaculum grasping the cervix and the sensation of discomfort as traction is placed on the cervix during the insertion of the cannula. After suction is applied, the endometrial cavity is curetted thoroughly in all directions. When one cannula is filled, authorities recommend the use of two or even three suction devices until no further endometrial tissue is obtained. This procedure may cause cramps in a few women, usually limited to 5 to 10 minutes. Prostaglandin synthetase inhibitor is not indicated for routine use, but it may be given about 20 minutes before the procedure in women needing repeat biopsies and those known to have problems with cramping.

Fewer than 10% of women cannot be adequately evaluated by office endometrial biopsy. The usual reason for inadequate evaluation is the inability to enter the uterine cavity. These women must then undergo an in-hospital D&C. The other group of women who must undergo an in-hospital D&C are women found to have an abnormal uterus on pelvic examination.

If the vulva, vagina, and cervix seem normal on inspection and the cervical cytology from a Pap smear is normal, bleeding is assumed to be intrauterine in origin. Because the primary sign of endometrial cancer is abnormal vaginal bleeding, postmenopausal bleeding is considered to be a serious finding and must be evaluated, although only about 2% of endometrial biopsies in postmenopausal women are diagnosed by the pathologist as carcinoma. In addition, the histologic diagnoses in endometrial biopsy samples are 3% polyps, 14% endometrial hyperplasia, and 50% normal endometrium.

If the health care provider is certain of the technique, endometrial biopsies with a histologic report of little or no tissue may be reassuring. If the woman is on estrogen-progestin therapy, then a pathologic evaluation of "tissue insufficient for diagnosis" is due to atrophic, decidualized endometrium. In this situation, however, the clinician must be certain that the technique used was complete.

Other office procedures used to evaluate vaginal bleeding in perimenopausal and postmenopausal women are colposcopy and cervical biopsy, done for abnormal cytology or lesions seen on inspection; endocervical curettage for abnormal cytology; and hysteroscopy for persistent bleeding to observe for the presence of endometrial polyps or submucosal fibroids. These are standard procedures recommended by all authorities.

Treatment of uterine bleeding is determined by the total clinical picture, including the endometrial biopsy findings. If definite organic disease is present, appropriate surgical intervention is warranted. Any adnexal mass in a postmenopausal woman is abnormal and is considered cancer until proven benign. Referral to a specialist for surgical preparation and intervention is essential. Table 10-1 lists treatment modalities for women with dysfunctional bleeding in the absence of marked abnormalities.

It has been stated that clinicians should not be afraid to prescribe low-dose oral contraceptives to anovulatory perimenopausal women. It is not a good idea to give women with irregular menses estrogen-progestin therapy, because this causes the endometrium to be exposed to high doses of estrogen. Expert clinicians who care for perimenopausal women on oral contraceptives follow FSH levels and switch to estrogen-progestin therapy when the FSH level exceeds 30 IU/L. This is done only for women on oral contraceptives, not all women. It is prudent to educate all perimenopausal women taking birth-control pills to cease cigarette smoking.

Hot flushes (the vasomotor flush) are noted by about half of postmenopausal women. They are seen as a sudden reddening of the skin of the head, neck, and chest, along with a sensation of increased body heat. They can be followed by profuse perspiration. They appear to be more severe at night, and usually a woman suffering from such a hot flush is awakened from sleep. Hot flushes are noted in about 10% of women during the perimenopausal period and in about 50% of women just after menopause. Hot flushes last 1 to 2 years in most of these women, but in others they may last longer than 5 years. The physiology of the hot flush is incompletely understood, but it seems to originate in the hypothalamus and is associated with a decrease in circulating estrogen. Estrogen replacement therapy effectively treats hot flushes. However, it is essential for all primary care providers to be aware that there are other causes of hot flushes besides menopause. If the clinical situation is unclear, elevated FSH levels document estrogen deficiency.

Genital and urinary tract mucosal atrophy in the late postmenopausal years can lead to vaginitis, pruritus, dyspareunia, and stenosis. Urgency incontinence and frequency are other symptoms. Recurrent urinary tract infections are effectively prevented by postmenopausal estrogen treatment. Some but not all authorities state that genuine stress incontinence is improved with estrogen therapy, but many older women have a mixed cause of urinary incontinence.

Dyspareunia can be a significant problem for older women. They are often reluctant to discuss this problem, so an open attitude and gentle questions by the primary care provider are helpful. Hormone replacement therapy treats vaginal atrophy and enhances sexual pleasure. Although significant improvement occurs in 1 month, it takes 6 to 12 months for complete restoration of the genitourinary tract. Sexual activity itself increases the circulating response of vaginal tissues. Thus, sexually active older women have less atrophy even if they do not take hormones.

Finally, there is no scientific evidence that emotional health is harmed by menopause. Fatigue, nervousness, headaches, insomnia, depression, irritability, dizziness, palpitations, and joint and muscle pain are not symptoms of menopause and should be evaluated thoroughly for organic and psychosomatic origin.

Table 10-1. Treatment of Dysfunctional Uterine Bleeding in the Absence of Organic Disease

FINDINGS	TREATMENT
Proliferation	Medroxyprogesterone acetate 10 mg qd, first 10 days of the month
Hyperplastic endometrium (without atypia or biopsy, dysplastic elements)	Medroxyprogesterone acetate 10 mg qd, first 10 days of the month, followed by aspiration, endometrial biopsy curettage.
	If hyperplasia is still present, formal D & C is indicated before deciding on a therapeutic surgical procedure.
	Continue monthly progestin therapy until withdrawal bleeding ceases.

Modified from Speroff L, Glass RH, Kase NG. Clinical gynecologic endocrinology and infertility, 5th ed. Baltimore: Williams & Wilkins, 1994.

MENOPAUSE AND CARDIOVASCULAR DISEASE

Menopause is associated with an increased risk of coronary heart disease. In women over age 55, coronary heart disease becomes a major cause of morbidity and mortality. Prevention of cardiovascular disease by reducing risk is extremely important, in view of the fact that 40% of coronary events in women are fatal. In 1991, cardiovascular disease, defined as heart disease, stroke, and atherosclerosis, was responsible for 46% of deaths in women and only 40% of deaths in men. As the proportion of menopausal and postmenopausal women increases in the population, the problem of cardiovascular disease in women will be even more significant.

The Framingham Heart Study, begun in 1948 for the purpose of determining within a community environment the risk factors leading to cardiovascular disease, continues to provide physicians with important information. From this study, it was learned that women develop symptoms of heart disease one decade later than men. At age 75, the incidence of coronary heart disease in the United States is equal in men and women, but before this the incidence is higher in men. For instance, the incidence of coronary heart disease is three times higher in men than in women age 45 to 54. Women age 55 or older had a tenfold higher risk of developing coronary heart disease than women ages 35 to 54. One in nine women age 45 to 64 had some type of cardiovascular disease, and this increased to one in three after age 65.

Cardiovascular disease is also a leading cause of disability and morbidity. One reason for the increased mortality in women is that the signs and symptoms of coronary heart disease appear to be different than in men. In one study, fatigue and symptoms ascribed to indigestion were more often described by women with coronary heart disease than were the classic signs and symptoms. Historically, women's symptoms often have been attributed to problems other than coronary heart disease. Women are less likely than men to have angiography performed. Thus, a delay in diagnosis often occurs. Women and health care providers alike tend to believe that cancer is more of a threat than heart attack and stroke, although the opposite is true. Mortality from heart disease increases with age, although one third of heart disease-related deaths occur in women under age 65. Death from heart disease among black women is highest at all ages; this may be attributable to diminished access to health care as well as to delayed diagnosis.

From the few studies of risk for cardiovascular disease that have included women, we have gained some understanding of factors that contribute to cardiovascular disease in women. These risks include cigarette smoking, hypertension, increased levels of total serum cholesterol and low-density lipoprotein, and decreased levels of high-density lipoprotein (HDL). Obesity and a sedentary lifestyle are also associated with an increased risk of heart disease. The low estrogen levels of surgical or natural menopause seem to increase the risk of heart disease among women. This understanding comes from the Framingham study, which found an increased risk after menopause. The later Nurses' Health Study demonstrated that women who had surgical menopause had an increased risk of coronary heart disease. Diabetes, hypertriglyceridemia, and low HDL levels also seem to increase the risk of coronary heart disease more in women than in men.

Because prevention of disease is paramount in primary care, physicians and other health care providers must use principles of prevention, including knowledge of health education methods, to effect change in women's lifestyles. Smoking is common among women of all ethnic and racial groups, and the trend in the reduction of cigarette smoking seems to be slowing. Most worrisome is a 45% increase in smoking among women 65 and older. Public health authorities have taken the lead in educating the public and in advocating smoke-free environments. This is an important trend, in light of the evidence that passive smoking may also be a factor in disease etiology. Despite the ever-increasing sophistication of health education campaigns, health workers face a challenge, in view of the resources spent in advertising cigarettes to women of all ages. Primary care providers must emphasize repeatedly to their patients the harmful effects of smoking.

Hypertension is a consistent risk factor for heart disease and thus must be identified and treated. Women must be reminded that hypertension may have no symptoms initially and that appropriate blood-pressure examinations are essential as they age.

High serum cholesterol (240 mg/dL or higher) is associated with an increased risk of heart disease. Cholesterol levels increase with age and become markedly elevated in women age 50 or older. Thus, HDL levels predict cardiovascular disease risk in women better than in men. Higher levels of HDL are correlated with a decreased risk of heart disease. Lifestyle changes such as diet, weight control, and exercise are the preventive health measures needed to maintain healthy cholesterol levels and to raise HDL levels, but these changes do not modify lipoprotein levels in women as well as they do in men. Estrogen replacement in postmenopausal women has a protective effect and is thus an essential preventive measure.

Some major studies show that diabetes in women is a risk factor for death from cardiovascular disease. The reason is not completely understood. It may be due to the fact that diabetes in women raises the level of low-density lipoprotein and triglycerides. Another reason may be cofactors such as hypertension and obesity.

BREAST DISEASE

As women age, the incidence of breast cancer, the most common malignancy of women, increases. More than 50%, probably close to 65%, of breast cancers are detected after age 50. The risk of developing breast cancer is one in 15 in women age 60 to 79. These figures vary, depending on a woman's risk factors. Breast cancer is more common in white women over age 45 than in black women in the same age group. It is also more common in women with a family history of breast cancer, in women who have never had a child, and in women who first delivered an infant at age 30 or greater. Breast cancer is more common among women of upper socioeconomic status, and some cite early menarche and late menopause as a risk factor. Women with a confirmed histologic diagnosis of proliferative breast disease, such as moderate hyperplasia and papilloma with fibrovascular core, are at two times the risk for breast cancer. Those with atypical hyperplasia of the breast, or those exposed to high doses of ionizing radiation, are also at risk.

There does not appear to be an increased risk of breast cancer in women who have used oral contraceptives. It appears that estrogen therapy at 0.625 mg/dL or less of conjugated estrogens does not increase the short-term risk for breast cancer. The role of dietary fat as a risk for breast cancer is controversial. A 10-year study of the National Institutes of Health, the Women's Health Initiative, was designed to answer these questions, but it has not been completed. Some completed studies indicate no association of dietary fat and the development of breast cancer.

The most important preventive measure for breast cancer morbidity and mortality is early detection. Women over age 40 must undergo an annual clinical breast examination. This examination should also be carried out any time a woman has a breast complaint. Women of all ages should be taught breast self-examination, because 80% to 85% of breast cancers are found first by the woman. However, breast self-examination alone is not a primary prevention screen: it is an adjunct to the clinical breast examination and the screening mammography.

Screening mammography, usually limited to two views (craniocaudal and lateral oblique), has clearly been shown to decrease breast cancer deaths. Although controversy exists regarding the initial age of screening and the optimal screening interval to maximize detection of breast cancer, current American Cancer Society recommendations include a baseline mammogram from age 35 to 39, but from age 30 for women at high risk; mammography at 1- to 2-year intervals from age 40 to 49; and an annual mammogram for women age 50 and over.

The sensitivity of mammography is about 90%. False-negative results occur in 10% to 15% of cases. It is thought that a lesion detected on mammography would be clinically detected in 2.5 to 3.5 years. Thus, all palpable masses require investigation, no matter what the mammogram image demonstrates. Palpable breast masses should be evaluated and a biopsy or aspirate obtained. A screening mammogram is not helpful in this situation. It is helpful, though, for radiographic localization for a directed needle biopsy performed for suspicious masses or lesions.

Many menopausal and postmenopausal women do not obtain screening mammograms, and this is unfortunate. Some women do not have insurance coverage for screening mammograms, although several states now mandate such coverage. Medicare recipients are covered. However, economic access through insurance coverage will not ensure compliance. Women must be educated that breast cancer increases with age, and they must understand and be reminded of the recommended screening intervals. Many menopausal and postmenopausal women are unaware of these guidelines, and many think screening mammography is unnecessary unless symptoms are present. Many fear radiation exposure or discomfort. Some do not obtain a mammogram because their physician failed to remind them or failed to recommend it. Minority women often are less likely to receive appropriate mammograms.

Breast cancers detected early have a favorable prognosis. When discovered at an early stage before axilla metastasis occurs, cure is possible and more therapeutic options are available.

OSTEOPOROSIS

Osteoporosis (see Chap. 97) is age-related and is a state of deficiency of bone mass. It should be prevented. When it occurs, predominantly in menopausal women but also in amenorrheic young girls, it should be identified and treated. This condition is related to genetic background, nutritional state, exercise, and estrogen levels. Bone loss is inevitable and occurs at midlife onward. It begins about 10 years before menopause, but it can start at age 20. Loss is 0.3% to 0.5% per year for cortical bone and 1.2% per year for trabecular bone. After menopause, bone loss accelerates by an average of 2% to 3% or more per year, and this rate lasts for 6 to 10 years. Bone loss leads to enhanced fragility and, thus, to an increased risk of fractures.

Cortical bone is 80% of the total bone mass. Trabecular bone, the bone in the spinal column, is a honeycomb structure. Bone is living tissue undergoing constant loss and replacement in a bone remodeling cycle of resorption and formation. Trabecular bone remodeling occurs eight times as fast as in cortical bone. Bone remodeling involves resorption of bone by osteoclasts and bone formation by osteoblasts. In this process, osteoclasts secrete an acid-like substance that digests the matrix and minerals of the bone. When a certain resorption cavity depth is reached, the resorption process stops and bone formation then begins. The osteoblasts synthesize collagen and other matrix proteins to which hydroxyapatite and other crystals adhere. Bone mass is maintained when resorption and formation remain equal. Hormones such as estrogen, calcitonin, and parathyroid hormone, as well as mechanical stress, affect the bone remodeling cycle. Bone loss accelerates after menopause because of enhanced osteoclast activity and bone turnover. Estrogen administration increases calcitonin, which directly inhibits osteoclast activity; therefore, bone resorption is reduced. Estrogen may lead to a decreased sensitivity of bone to parathyroid hormone, also reducing bone resorption. Osteoblasts produce certain cytokines that activate osteoclasts. Estrogen directly inhibits osteoblastic secretion of the cytokines, thus inhibiting osteoclast formation. The result is the inhibition of bone loss.

As a function of aging, a woman could lose up to 50% of her bone mass by age 70. Osteoporosis is asymptomatic until fractures occur. The most common sites of fractures are the distal radius, vertebral body, and femoral neck. Hip fractures are the most serious, as approximately 27% of women with hip fractures die within 1 year of the fracture. For those who do not die, long-term care is usually necessary for permanent disabilities. Therefore, osteoporosis is a serious public health problem.

HORMONE REPLACEMENT THERAPY

The relative risk of coronary heart disease is decreased 56% in women who take estrogen. Estrogen replacement alone or in combination with a progestin lowers fibrinogen levels and decreases lipoproteins. Unopposed estrogen is the optimal treatment for reduction of HDL cholesterol, but this regimen causes endometrial hyperplasia and thus can be used only in women without a uterus. In women with a uterus, conjugated equine estrogen with cyclic medroxyprogesterone acetate produces no excess risk of endometrial hyperplasia and has the most favorable effect on HDL cholesterol.

Hormone replacement therapy prevents bone loss when given as 0.625 mg of conjugated estrogens daily, 1 mg/d of 17 β-estradiol, or transdermal estradiol in doses of 0.05 to 0.1 mg.

Estrogen benefits the cardiovascular system, prevents bone loss, and relieves vasomotor symptoms. A progestin given with the estrogen protects the endometrium from hyperplasia. The long-term effect of estrogen-progesterone therapy on the breast is not yet completely understood. The progesterone is given as 10 mg methylmedroxyprogesterone acetate cyclically, 200 mg micronized progesterone cyclically, or 2.5 mg methylmedroxyprogesterone acetate continuously. Progesterone protects women against endometrial cancer.

There continues to be debate as to how long hormonal therapy should be prescribed. Those concerned with the risks of endometrial and breast cancer suggest treatment for a short time; however, when estrogen is withdrawn, there is rapid bone loss. Because estrogen-progesterone therapy protects against osteoporosis and

Table 10-2. Common Hormone Replacement Therapy Regimens

SEQUENTIAL*	CONTINUOUS‡
(daily first through 25th day of each month)	(daily)
0.625 conjugated estrogen	0.625 mg conjugated estrogen
or	or
1.0 mg micronized estradiol	0.625 mg estrone sulfate
Plus	or
	1.0 mg micronized estradiol
10 mg medroxyprogesterone acetate (MPA)†	*Plus*
first 14 days of month	2.5 mg MPA
or	or
last 10 days of estrogen administration	0.35 mg norethindrone
or	
200 mg micronized progesterone	
first 14 days	
Transdermal estradiol 0.05 to 0.1 mg	
q 3 days plus a progestin	

*Progestin withdrawal bleeding occurs in 80% to 90% of women in this regimen.

†May use 5 mg MPA if breast tenderness, fluid retention, and depression become clinically significant.

‡Reportedly no bleeding in 80% of women. However, in first 6 months, 40% to 60% of women have breakthrough bleeding.

cardiovascular disease, menopausal women should continue hormonal replacement therapy as long as there are no contraindications to the treatment.

Table 10-2 lists common hormone replacement regimens. The primary care provider should consult specialists when questions arise about hormone replacement therapy. Examples of patients to refer to a specialist include women with a history of breast cancer, uterine or ovarian cancer, or cardiovascular disease. Patients with significant side effects would also benefit from a consultation with a specialist.

REFERENCES

Healy B. PEPI in perspective: good answers spawn pressing questions. JAMA 1995;273:240.

Horton JA. Osteoporosis. In: Women's health data book: a profile of women's health in the United States, 2d ed. Washington DC: Jacobs Institute of Women's Health, 1995.

Kuhn FE, Rackley CE. Coronary artery disease in women: risk factors, evaluation, treatment, and prevention. Arch Intern Med 1993;153:2626.

Speroff L, Glass RH, Kase NG. Clinical gynecologic endocrinology and infertility, 5th ed. Baltimore: Williams & Wilkins, 1994:583.

Tan G, Ma HK. Menopausal osteoporosis. Int J Gynecol Obstet 1994;46:203.

Walsh BW, Schiff I, Rosner B, Greenberg LM, Ravnikar V, Sacks M. Effects of postmenopausal estrogen replacement on the concentrations and metabolism of plasma lipoproteins. N Engl J Med 1991;325:1196.

Wolf SA. Hormone replacement and osteoporosis. Clin Consult 1992;4:37.

Writing Group for the PEPI Trial. Effects of estrogen or estrogen/progestin regimens on heart disease. Risk factors in postmenopausal women. JAMA 1995;273:199.

Primary Care for Women, edited by Phyllis C. Leppert and Fred M. Howard. Lippincott-Raven Publishers, Philadelphia © 1997.

11
The Elderly Woman

MICHELLE CARPENTER BRADLEY, MARIE AYDELOTTE, BRENDA L. JOHNSON

The field of geriatrics is not limited to the practice of the geriatrician or internist. With the exception of the pediatrician, all medical specialties care for elderly patients. Before the twentieth century, few people lived beyond the age of 75 years, whereas more than 50% of the United States population now reaches age 75. It is estimated that as many as 35 million people in the United States will be older than 65 by the year 2000, and this number may reach 67 million by the year 2050. By virtue of their increased longevity, the majority of these people will be women.

The scope of geriatrics is much too large to include in its entirety here. Virtually every organ system is affected by both the normal and pathologic changes of aging. We have attempted to cover a few specific topics that, because of their incidence of severity, impact greatly on the elderly woman. By no means, however, are these the only important issues concerning the elderly woman.

Screening and Preventive Care

Over the last century, the periodic health exam, cancer screening, and preventive care have been studied, and guidelines have been developed by several organizations based upon the efficacy of the test or intervention. Most of these apply to adults up to age 65, and some go up to age 75, but few recommendations are made beyond this age. As the population ages, this type of data and assessment takes on greater importance. For example, when should a healthy elderly woman be counseled to stop having mammograms?

Healthy, that is, disease-free, old age is not uncommon. The life expectancy at age 65 is 17 more years; at age 75, it is 11 more years; at age 85 it is 6 years; at age 90 it is 4 years; and at age 100 it is 2 years. Only 30% of people over age 85 are impaired in one of the activities of daily living, and only 20% reside in nursing homes. Dysfunction may become more common with age, but age alone is not an explanation for dysfunction.

Assessment of functional status has gained acceptance as an important reflection of an elderly person's overall health. The goal of including this type of assessment in the periodic health exam for patients over age 65 is to diagnose problems early, target appropriate areas of intervention, and reduce morbidity and mortality. The questions and observations deal with areas commonly affecting the elderly population. These areas are vision, hearing, use of arms, use of legs, continence of urine, nutrition, mental status, depression, activities of daily living (ADL-IADL), home environment, and social support (Table 11-1.)

The United States Preventive Services Task Force (USPSTF) has evaluated screening tests for older persons who are asymptomatic and lack clinical evidence of the target condition. The evaluation included consideration of the impact on the elderly population of the disease being screened, noting, for example, that heart disease is much more prevalent than cervical cancer. See Table 11-2 for their findings.

The USPSTF finds that there is insufficient evidence to make a recommendation regarding fecal occult blood testing and sigmoidoscopy for screening for colorectal cancer. Other groups, such as the American Cancer Society, recommend digital rectal exam and fecal occult blood testing yearly starting at age 50, and sigmoidoscopy every 3 to 5 years starting at age 50.

Not recommended as screening tests in asymptomatic person were ECG, carotid evaluation, chest x-ray or sputum analysis, pelvic examination for ovarian cancer, cholesterol, examination or diagnostic tests for pancreatic cancer, hemoglobin and hematocrit.

Advance directives and identification of a *health care proxy* should be addressed in one or several discussions, and documented in the chart, including any legal documents that have been completed. The patient, the physician, and the proxy should discuss specific issues and attempt to have an optimal understanding of the patient's wishes in various circumstances such as cardiac or respiratory arrest, or vegetative state.

In making decisions regarding screening tests for elderly patients, as with all age groups, it is wise to inform them of the significance of a positive test, and the likely recommended follow-up, such as colonoscopy, breast biopsy, or chemotherapy. Some individuals may not agree to these invasive tests in the absence of an established problem, making performance of the initial screening test unnecessary. The elderly population is heterogeneous, and care must be taken to individualize treatment based on multiple factors, such as functional status, comorbid illness, and the patient's goals for successful aging, rather than on age alone.

Osteoporosis and Hip Fracture

Progressive loss of bone mass begins in all women after the third decade of life, and rapidly accelerates in the years after menopause. Clinically significant osteoporosis resulting in fracture occurs in about 1 in 4 women over the age of 65. Morbidity, mortality and costs associated with this disease are tremendous. Chapters 97 (Osteoporosis) and 98 (Hip Fracture) discuss these topics in greater detail.

Multiple factors affect the development of osteoporosis. These include hormonal, nutritional, genetic, and lifestyle influences. In postmenopausal women, estrogen lack causes bone resorption and net calcium loss. With aging, calcium and vitamin D malabsorption commonly occur, both of which may increase the likelihood of osteoporosis. Lifestyle factors such as alcohol and tobacco use are associ-

Table 11-1. Procedure for Functional Assessment Screening in the Elderly

TARGET AREA	ASSESSMENT PROCEDURE	ABNORMAL RESULT	SUGGESTED INTERVENTION
Vision	Test each eye with Jasger card while patient wears corrective lenses (if applicable).	Inability to read greater than 20/40.	Refer to ophthalmologist.
Hearing	Whisper a short, easily answered question such as "What is your name?" in each ear while the examiner's face is out of direct view.	Inability to answer question.	Examine auditory canals for cerumen and clean if necessary. Repeat task; if still abnormal in either ear, refer for audiometry and possible prosthesis.
Arm	Proximal: "Touch the back of your head with both hands." Distal: "Pick up the spoon."	Inability to do task.	Examine the arm fully (muscle, joint, and nerve), paying attention to pain, weakness, limited range of motion. Consider referral for physical therapy.
Leg	Observe the patient after instructing as follows: "Rise from your chair, walk 10 feet, return, and sit down."	Inability to walk or transfer out of chair.	Do full neurologic and musculoskeletal evaluation, paying attention to strength, pain, range of motion, balance, and traditional assessment of gait. Consider referral for physical therapy.
Continence of urine	Ask, "Do you ever lose your urine and get wet?"	"Yes."	Ascertain frequency and amount. Search for remarkable causes, including local irritations, polyuric states, and medications. Consider referral.
Nutrition	Ask "Without trying, have you lost 10 lb or more in the last 8 months?" Weigh the patient. Measure height.	"Yes," or weight is below acceptable range for height.	Do appropriate medical evaluation.
Mental status	Instruct as follows: "I am going to name three objects (pencil, truck, book). I will ask you to repeat their names, now and then again a few minutes from now." (See text discussion.)	Inability to recall all three objects after 1 minute.	Administer Folstein Mini-Mental Status Examination. If score is less than 34, search for causes of cognitive impairment. Ascertain onset, duration, and fluctuation of overt symptoms. Review medications. Assess consciousness and effect. Do appropriate laboratory tasks.
Depression	Ask, "Do you often feel sad or depressed?" or "How are your spirits?"	"Yes" or "Not very good, I guess."	Administer Geriatric Depression Scale. If positive (score above 5), check for antihypersensitive, psychotropic, or other pertinent medications. Consider appopriate pharmacologic or psychiatric treatment.
ADL-IADL	Ask, "Can you get out of bed yourself?" "Can you dress yourself?" "Can you make your own meals?" "Can you do your own shopping?"	"No" to any question.	Corroborate responses with patient's appearance; question family members if accuracy is uncertain. Determine reasons for the inability (motivation compared with physical limitation). Institute appropriate medical, social, or environmental interventions.
Home environment	Ask, "Do you have trouble with stairs inside or outside of your home?" Ask about potential hazards inside the home with bathtubs, rugs, or lighting.	"Yes."	Evaluate home safety and institute appropriate countermeasures.
Social support	Ask, "Who would be able to help you in case of illness or emergency?"	—	List identified persons in the medical record. Become familiar with available resources for the elderly in the community.

ADL-IADL, Activities of daily living-instrumental activities of daily living.
(Modified from Lache MG et al: A simple procedure for general screening for functional disability in elderly patients. Ann Intern Med 1990;112:899.)

ated with an increased incidence of the disease. Weight-bearing exercise may be protective. Causes of secondary osteoporosis include medications (eg, corticosteroids, phenytoin, excess thyroid hormone, heparin) and medical conditions such as hyperparathyroidism, Cushing's disease, hyperthyroidism, athletic amenorrhea, and others (see Chap. 97). Genetic heritage primarily affects the attainment of peak bone mass during the third decade of life. Women with slight stature or positive family history are more likely to develop osteoporosis.

The clinical evaluation and treatment of osteoporosis are discussed in detail in Chapter 97. Given adequate calcium and vitamin D intake, the major treatment option for perimenopausal women is estrogen replacement therapy, although results from large randomized, controlled trials are still awaited. Estrogen therapy decreases the incidence of coronary artery disease and may or may not increase breast cancer risk (see Chap. 97). Other treatment options for osteoporosis include calcitonin, the bisphosphonates, and sodium fluoride.

Hip fracture is the most dreaded complication of osteoporosis for many elderly women. One in seven women who reach the age of 80 suffers a hip fracture. Disability after hip fracture is common. Up to 50% of hip fracture patients require short- or long-term nursing home care, and 35% will be able to ambulate only with a cane or walker. Mortality is also increased in the months after fracture, and may be as high as 15% to 30%. Risk of death is highest in those with advanced age or severe comorbid medical illness.

Hip fracture is multifactorial in etiology. The major contributors to risk of hip fracture are osteoporosis and falls, with lesser factors including fall orientation and body habitus. Falls are discussed in depth later in this chapter. Fall prevention may be of major benefit in the avoidance of hip fracture. Some particularly important ways to decrease fall risk include correction of visual impairment and minimization of medication use (especially of benzodiazepines, narcotics, and medications that cause orthostatic hypotension). Use of

Table 11-2. Recommendations for Screening in the Elderly Woman—the U.S. Preventative Services Task Force

Recommendations for Asymptomatic Persons

Counseling
- Diet and exercise
- Tobacco and alcohol use
- Protection from exposure to sunlight

History
- Functional assessment (see Table 11-1)
- Medication evaluation with attempts to simplify
- Ask regarding history of TIA or other neurologic illness
- Ask regarding history of falls
- Assess risk of osteoporosis, and counsel regarding calcium intake (1500 mg/day) and vitamin D (400–500 IU/day, amount in most multivitamins), and weight-bearing exercises
- Assess for bereavement and abnormal grief
- Assess benefits of low dose aspirin use

Physical Examination
- Blood pressure measurement, yearly, with recommended treatment of both systolic and diastolic hypertension, and isolated systolic hypertension
- Height and weight and dietary counseling
- Visual acuity
- Ophthalmologic exam for glaucoma
- Hearing evaluation, including exam for cerumen
- Dental evaluation and counseling regarding routine care
- Breast exam, every 1 to 2 years

Laboratory and diagnostic testing:
- Mammography, yearly until age 75, with insufficient data to advise beyond this age (subsequent study supports no restriction based on age alone)
- Pap smear if not done in the last decade, stop at age 65 if previous testing has been consistently normal
- TSH and free T_4, especially in women
- Dipstick and microscopic urinalysis for asymptomatic bacteriuria, hematuria, and proteinuria

Immunization
- Influenza yearly
- Pneumococcal once
- Tetanus every 10 y

Recommendations for Persons in High-risk Groups

- Serum cholesterol in persons with established coronary heart disease
- EKG in persons with two or more cardiac risk factors
- Exercise test for sedentary or high-risk persons who are planning to start an exercise program
- Carotid auscultation in persons with established risk factors for cerebrovascular disease or coronary disease (increased age, HTN, smoking, CAD, atrial fibrillation, diabetes mellitus, neurologic symptoms, history of cerebrovascular disease)
- Complete skin exam for persons with a family or personal history of skin cancer, evidence of precursor lesions, and increased exposure to sunlight
- Oral exam for cancerous or precancerous lesions in persons with exposure to tobacco or excesive alcohol
- Testing plasma glucose in persons with obesity, family history of DM, or a history or gestational diabetes
- PPD for persons at increased risk of developing tuberculosis, including those living in nursing homes
- Fecal occult blood testing and sigmoidoscopy in persons at high risk

more than four medications concurrently has also been shown to increase the rate of falling. Correction of environmental hazards, such as poor lighting or throw rugs, may be beneficial.

Types of hip fracture and management techniques are discussed in Chapter 98. Preoperative medical evaluation and the prevention of postoperative complications are helpful in ensuring a good outcome. Delirium, infection, congestive heart failure, and depression are common occurrences following fracture repair and should be recognized and treated. Deep venous thrombosis prophylaxis is routine in the postoperative period. Early weight-bearing is usually permitted. Intensive rehabilitation therapies begun immediately after surgery are crucial in helping patients achieve the best functional outcome.

Falls

Falls are a common and serious problem in the elderly. At least 30% of those elderly living in the community will fall one or more times each year. This percentage goes up to 50% in the nursing home population. The National Safety Council lists accidents as the sixth leading cause of deaths in the elderly. The vast majority of these accidents are the result of falls.

Although falls are not a problem only in elderly women, the chances of a serious injury is higher in elderly women than in men of the same age because of osteoporosis. Elderly women are at some increased risk of falling compared to men, probably secondary to a number of factors to be discussed later.

The economic cost is huge. In a study performed in Washington state by Alexander and coworkers, $53 million in hospital charges in 1989 were attributable to fall-related trauma in patients over 65 years of age. This cost did not take into account the long-term sequelae of falls. Falls may result in nursing home placement. The cost of a fall does not end with the hospital discharge.

FALL INJURIES

Only about 5% of falls result in a fracture. Conversely, the vast majority of hip fractures are the result of falls.

Even if there is no fracture, significant soft tissue injuries can cause serious disability. Other consequences include dehydration or rhabdomyolysis from a prolonged time spent on the floor. This extended contact with a hard surface may also cause serious pressure ulcers.

A fall often triggers a further cascade of disability. Bed rest or limited activity following an injury leads to deconditioning. This, in turn, can worsen a person's gait and increase the risk for further falls. An elderly person's ability to take care of herself deteriorates. The loss of independence can be devastating.

The most serious consequence of falls is death. This can occur as a direct result of the fall—for example, a serious head injury. It may result from the implications of a fall—for example, hip fracture leading to deep vein thrombosis leading to pulmonary embolism and death. Mortality is higher in fallers compared to near-fallers, partly secondary to the falls but also reflecting the overall increased frailty of those who fall.

PSYCHOLOGICAL SEQUELAE

Many of those who have fallen, and even those who have not fallen, develop a fear of falling. Studies have reported that as many as 48% of those who have fallen are fearful of falling again. The fear may be disproportionately large compared to the degree of injury in the preceding fall. Those who express a fear of falling, but have not personally had a fall, probably are influenced by the knowledge of a family member's or acquaintance's fall.

To varying degrees, this fear limits people's lives and affects their quality of life. It affects their ability to perform activities of daily living and their physical functioning, and even limits activities they will engage in. When severe, the fear limits engaging in social activities as well.

TYPES OF FALLS

Commonly, falls are grouped into two categories, based on their etiology. *Extrinsic falls* are those precipitated by factors outside of the person. These include environmental causes, such as tripping over objects on the floor, slipping on loose throw rugs, and getting tangled in phone and electric cords. Outdoor hazards are also included, such as slippery sidewalks, loose stones, and automobiles.

Intrinsic falls are those caused by risk factors present within the person. These are outlined further in the next section. Many falls occur because of a combination of extrinsic and intrinsic factors. For example, an elderly person with decreased vision and slower reflexes is not able to see and avoid quickly enough the obstacle in her path.

RISK FACTORS

A number of risk factors are intrinsic to the elderly patient. Increased disability and frailty contribute greatly to falls. An elderly person may be getting along without falls when another disability, such as an acute illness, is added and precipitates a fall.

Neurologic factors are strong contributors to falling. Poor vision is a powerful risk factor. Lower extremity weakness and gait disturbances also predispose the elderly to falling. A previous stroke acts to increase falls by its effect on lower extremity strength, balance, vision, and judgment. A fall can often be the presenting symptom of an acute stroke. Neurologic changes seen with normal aging, such as increased reaction times and a less organized response to a presented obstacle, can cause falls. Parkinson's disease, with its gait abnormalities, predisposes to falls. Cerebellar atrophy causes falls through gait and balance abnormalities. Any vestibular disturbances, including labyrinthitis, Meniere's disease, drugs, and benign positional vertigo, affect balance and thus increase falls.

Another very strong risk factor for falls is dementia. This acts through a number of mechanisms, including impaired judgment and decreased attention span. The demented patient is unable to devise or carry out an effective movement strategy.

Depression also is a risk factor, probably secondary to the decreased attention span of the depressed person.

Joint disease in the elderly contributes to falls. The joints and muscles have less flexibility and increased stiffness, leading, in turn, to lower extremity disability and falls.

Medications are also implicated in the occurrence of falls. Both the number of medications and the types are factors. More than four prescription drugs and sedatives being taken concurrently have been associated with increased risk. Cardiac drugs as a class may not be a risk, but the orthostatic blood pressure changes seen with many of these medications are a problem. Heavy alcohol use is a problem with falls, too.

Decreased hearing is common in the elderly. This contributes to falls by decreasing sensory input that can warn the potential faller of hazards.

Cardiovascular disease can predispose to falls. Syncope can result from arrhythmias, aortic stenosis, or hypotension and precipitate sudden falls. This can also occur in the setting of an acute myocardial infarction. Carotid atherosclerosis acts as a risk factor through its consequences of cerebral hypoperfusion and strokes.

Some metabolic causes contribute to falls. Hypoglycemia with a decrease in mental status is one of these. Hyponatremia results in unsteadiness. Dehydration, and subsequent hypotension, leads to falling. Malnutrition indirectly influences falls by contributing to muscle weakness and fatigue.

All or this would imply that the greater the burden of disease, or frailty, the greater the risk of falling. This is true, but research has shown that the vigorous elderly are more likely to be seriously injured when they do fall. The more vigorous elderly are more likely to encounter hazardous extrinsic factors, and they are more likely to fall on the stairs and away from the home. Thus, concern and education about falls needs to be extended to all elderly patients.

THE FEMALE FALLER

Elderly women are at some increased relative risk of falling compared to elderly men, from a number of intrinsic and extrinsic factors.

Elderly women differ from men in which risk factors are more important in causing a fall. For women, they are increased age, use of psychotropic medications, inability to rise from a chair without using the arms, polypharmacy, and living alone. Men are more influenced by arthritis of the knees, a past history of stroke, and weak grip strength.

Elderly women living alone probably have an increased risk of falls for several reasons. An elderly woman who lives alone is more likely to undertake more physical tasks that put her in danger of falling, such as taking the garbage out or climbing up on a stool. She may also experience fatigue from these physical efforts and be more likely to fall as a result. Or she may limit her activities outside of the home because of a reluctance to do things on her own and so become deconditioned and fall more. An elderly woman living alone does not have the benefit of an arm to support her or steady her during a walk or catch her if she trips.

ASSESSMENT

It is important to assess the elderly person who has fallen. As with all illnesses, a good history and physical examination is critical. In the majority of cases, this reveals the cause of the fall.

Particular attention should be given to the circumstances of the fall to determine where the fall occurred and what, if any, extrinsic factors played a role. Information as to whether a person's shoes fit, if the apartment is cluttered, or they were outside shovelling, is helpful.

What symptoms were experienced just before the fall? Dizziness, palpitations, and chest pain can all help point to the etiology. The patient's baseline is important—how is her vision and hearing?

A medication history is necessary. One or several medications may be the culprit. The faller should be questioned as to her alcohol use. Light to moderate alcohol intake may be of no significance, but heavy use probably is.

Symptomatology of acute illness should be sought. Respiratory illness and urinary tract infections are common etiologies of falls.

Questions concerning unilateral weakness, slurred speech, or new gait disturbances are helpful in determining if a neurologic event has occurred.

Once a careful history has been obtained, an examination should be performed. Orthostatic vital signs should be done. If there are orthostatic changes, the underlying cause should be sought. Is there evidence of bleeding, dehydration, or diabetes with an autonomic neuropathy, or are medications causing these changes? The patient's temperature must be checked to look for infectious illnesses.

A meticulous cardiopulmonary examination is important. The lung examination provides information as to an acute respiratory illness or congestive heart failure. The cardiac examination helps determine the presence of valvular disease or arrhythmias. Listening for carotid bruits helps in picking up carotid disease.

The abdominal examination may reveal a source of infection. Suprapubic tenderness and costovertebral angle tenderness suggest a urinary tract infection as the culprit leading to a fall. The symptom of urinary incontinence also helps in this diagnosis. Incontinence also could indicate that the person had seized and fallen as a result of the seizure.

The musculoskeletal examination, particularly of the lower extremities, is very important. Muscle strength must be tested. The feet should be checked for deformities and for evidence of ill-fitting shoes, corns, callouses, erythema, and pressure ulcers. The knees must be examined for range of motion, deformities, and inflammation. Hips should be checked for the same things. Upper body strength should also be evaluated—particularly in those who use assistive devices for ambulation, because good arm and shoulder strength are needed for this.

The neurologic examination should start with evaluation of the special senses. It is important to check vision, because decreased vision is such a strong risk factor for falls. Hearing should be evaluated. The presence of otitis media or impacted cerumen may be causing vertigo.

Muscle testing and reflexes may reveal the presence of a recent or past stroke. Cogwheeling, rigidity, and a tremor may help with diagnosing Parkinson's disease. Cerebellar testing may indicate balance problems. When assessing balance, see how the patient stands alone, and nudge her a bit, with and without her eyes closed, to see if she is able to recover her balance. Nystagmus may be the clue to vestibular disease.

Sensation to pain and vibration should be examined to determine the presence of neuropathy. Proprioception is an essential sensory input in preventing falls and should be tested.

A functional examination includes gait and body sway evaluation. The patient should be observed as she gets out of a chair to see whether she can get up out of a chair, with or without using the arms, or if she needs assistance to get up. She should be observed to see if her feet slide out from under her when she tries to stand. Once she is up, it is important to see if she stands firmly over her feet or leans backward or forward. A patient's gait is critical. Simple observation of the patient ambulating, with or without an assistive device, can give the examiner a good idea of whether she has a gait disorder.

Although a number of other maneuvers have been devised by researchers, a good, careful examination reveals the cause or causes of many falls. Sometimes further evaluation with laboratory testing, ECGs, and x-rays is indicated. Anemia may be detected. A chemistry profile may aid with the diagnosis of dehydration, malnutrition, and other metabolic derangements. An ECG is helpful in determining if there is an arrhythmia. Radiologic procedures can delineate orthopedic deformities. CT or MRI scans of the head may be necessary to diagnose central nervous system disorders.

TREATMENT

Any acute illnesses precipitating the fall should be treated first. Because falls are often the result of the cumulative effect of a number of factors, treating the acute event can be of benefit in preventing further falls.

Efforts should be made to decrease the total number of medications the patient is taking. Individual medications should be evaluated for adverse effects. If orthostatic hypotension is a problem, consideration should be given to decreasing or discontinuing diuretics or antihypertensive medications. Antidepressants should be chosen from or changed to those with the least effect on orthostasis. Anticholinergic medications should be avoided, because they cause or increase confusion in the elderly. Sedatives should be discontinued, if possible. Psychotropic medications, with their side effects of increased rigidity and sedation, make falls more likely and should be stopped if possible.

Improving vision is very helpful in preventing further falls. An eye examination should be performed and new glasses prescribed, if necessary. It may also be necessary to improve the lighting in the patient's home.

Education of the faller is important. She should be advised concerning slow postural changes from lying to standing, with pauses of a few minutes in between each change. This allows the vascular system to adjust and prevents falls secondary to orthostasis. The patient should be advised to avoid hazardous activities, such as climbing a ladder.

Attempts should be made to modify the patient's environment if possible. Hazards such as clutter on stairs, in rooms, and in hallways can be removed. Loose throw rugs should be taped down or removed. Bathroom safety can be improved with a raised toilet seat, bedside commode, shower, or tub seat, and grab bars as needed. Enhancing visual contrast with tape on the stairs or patterned flooring may help.

Physical therapy can strengthen lower extremities and improve gait. The physical therapist evaluates whether a mobility aid, such as a cane or walker, will facilitate ambulation.

Plans must be individually tailored to each patient. It should be realized, however, that many causes of falls are not reversible or treatable, and the patient will remain at risk for falls.

Previously, studies have not shown particularly positive results of interventions tried. A study by Tinetti and coworkers in 1994 involving a multifaceted intervention had encouraging results, however. They addressed muscle weakness and balance impairment. The experimental group was assessed by trained nurse practitioners and physical therapists. Recommendations were made to the patient's physician regarding medications, and exercises were taught by the physical therapists. The control group received only social visits by a social worker. The experimental group had a longer time to first fall and a significant decrease in risk factors. They also experienced fewer hospitalizations and had shorter stays when they were hospitalized.

This study reinforces that efforts need to be made to fully evaluate those who are falling and help to prevent further falls. Because evidence suggests all people over 65 years old are at risk, they all should be educated concerning risk factors and means to reduce them.

Dementia

The occurrence of dementia has a huge impact on the elderly woman. She not only is at risk for developing dementia herself, but is also more likely to be the primary caregiver for a spouse with dementia. Although the risk of dementia increases with age, dementia is not a characteristic of normal aging.

Dementia is defined as a clinical syndrome remarkable for acquired decline of cognitive function. This cognitive decline is characterized by a decline in memory and other deficits of higher cortical functioning, including language or visuospatial function. There are approximately 60 diseases associated with dementia, but the two most common are Alzheimer's disease and multi-infarct dementia. Alzheimer's disease accounts for 50% to 60% of all dementias, and multi-infarct dementia accounts for about 10% to 20%.

There is a higher incidence of dementia in elderly women, but this is a function of increasing age rather than a true increased risk associated with the female sex. There are approximately 2½ million people in the United States with dementia. With the aging of the population, this may increase to 9 million people by the year 2040. In economic terms, the direct and indirect costs are on the order of $38 billion per year. The emotional and physical costs to the caregivers is indeterminable.

DIFFERENTIAL DIAGNOSIS AND TYPES OF DEMENTIA

Dementia must be differentiated from other disorders that cause cognitive decline. Delirium is commonly mistaken for dementia, particularly in hospitalized patients, where it may occur in as many as 33% of elderly people admitted. Delirium can present both in those without an underlying dementia and in those with dementia. It is critical to diagnose delirium, because it has an associated mortality of approximately 25%. Delirium is characterized by its acute or subacute presentation of a confusional state in which inattentiveness and a reduced level of consciousness are the hallmarks. Agitation or lethargy may be present, and the patient is likely to be very distractable. Visual hallucinations are common. Tremors and myoclonus can be seen. Delirium is caused by medications, worsening of the underlying medical condition, or both.

Depression also may mimic dementia in the elderly. Depressed elderly patients may demonstrate bradykinesia and amotivation. Agitation often accompanies depression in the elderly. However, a depressed person has minimal or no memory deficits and no abnormalities in other cortical functions on testing.

Structural defects of the central nervous system can both cause and mimic dementia. These include normal pressure hydrocephalus, meningiomas, and subdural hematomas. Although these are considered "reversible" causes of dementia, the cognitive dysfunction often persists after surgical correction of these disorders.

Alzheimer's disease is the most common dementing illness. It is associated with a 95% 5-year mortality. Absolute diagnosis of this disease depends on histoneuropathologic changes of neurofibrillary tangles and plagues seen on biopsy or postmortem examination of brain tissue. The term Alzheimer's disease is something of a misnomer, as the condition likely represents a group of diseases that result in this pathology. Alzheimer's disease is discussed in detail later in this chapter.

Multi-infarct dementia may be increasing in incidence with the increased survival of those who have strokes. Multi-infarct dementia (MID) is characterized by abrupt onset with or without a history of a cerebrovascular accident. It usually has a fluctuating course with a stepwise deterioration. It is associated with hypertension and coronary artery disease. Focal neurologic signs are seen on examination. These include dysarthria, increased tone or spasticity, an abnormal small-stepped gait, positive Babinski reflex, hemiparesis, and, often, a labile affect. Laboratory tests may indicate end-organ damage such as renal disease with an elevated BUN and creatinine. The treatment focus is on the underlying disorders: control of hypertension, smoking cessation, antiplatelet agents, control of arrhythmias, and anticoagulation for atrial fibrillation. It is important to diagnose and treat MID, because most of these people will die of their cardiac disease.

Parkinson's disease is often associated with dementia. Parkinson's dementia demonstrates slow mentation on examination, but with preservation of language function. Speech may be difficult to understand because articulation is affected. Bradykinesia, increased rigidity, pill-rolling tremor, mask-like facies, and cogwheeling are other findings that suggest the diagnosis of Parkinson's disease. Treatment of Parkinson's disease does not cure the dementia.

Other diseases that are generally felt to be causes of reversible dementia are thyroid disease, vitamin B_{12} deficiency, neurosyphilis, thiamine deficiency, and other metabolic causes, such as hypercalcemia. Some diseases, such as B_{12} deficiency, have an increased incidence with age and may just coexist with Alzheimer's disease. Thus, treatment of reversible causes may improve the person's cognitive abilities but not cure them.

Infections such as Jakob-Creutzfeld disease and herpes encephalitis can cause dementia. Jakob-Creutzfeld disease is very rare and is passed by human-to-human transmission. Its onset is sudden, with rapid progression over weeks to months. Bizarre behavior, clumsiness, spasticity, myoclonus, and cortical blindness are seen. Laboratory data, cerebrospinal fluid, and head CT scan may all be normal, but an EEG shows a characteristic burst-suppression pattern. Herpes encephalitis has a subacute presentation of fever, headache, and seizures associated with memory or language deterioration. Cerebrospinal fluid examination demonstrates an elevated red blood cell count and protein level. A head CT may show rarefication of the temporal lobes. If clinical suspicion is high for herpes encephalitis, acyclovir should be started immediately.

RISK FACTORS AND THEORIES REGARDING THE ETIOLOGY OF ALZHEIMER'S DISEASE

Age is the biggest risk factor for the development of Alzheimer's disease. Before the age of 65 years, the incidence of Alzheimer's is very low. This increases after the age of 65 to estimates as high as 45% of those over than 85 years of age.

Head trauma has been implicated as a potential risk factor for the development of Alzheimer's disease. Boxers can develop a similar type of dementia. Surveys of patients with Alzheimer's disease have indicated that many have a history of serious head trauma before the development of the disease.

An infectious agent has been sought, but no causative organism has been found. Efforts to transmit Alzheimer's disease have been unsuccessful.

Toxic causes have been postulated. Aluminum is one potential toxin that has been considered, but evidence implicating this has been variable. It is not clear whether increased aluminum concentration in brain tissue is a cause or a sequela of the disease.

There probably is a genetic predisposition for the development of Alzheimer's disease. Virtually all individuals with trisomy 21 (Down syndrome) develop Alzheimer's disease by their 40s. Chromosome 21 has been implicated in those who present with early Alzheimer's disease; there is a defect located on chromosome 21 that has been identified in these people. The gene for the precursor of Alzheimer's amyloid protein, which may play a part in causing the disease, has also been located on chromosome 21, but is not near the gene that is found in early Alzheimer's disease. A marker on chromosome 19 has been identified in some people with late Alzheimer's disease. An individual's risk for developing Alzheimer's diseases increases from 10% if one first degree relative has Alzheimer's to 10% to 50% if two to three relatives have the disease.

There are a number of neurotransmitter derangements in Alzheimer's disease. The most affected is the cholinergic system. Presynaptic acetylcholine is decreased, with a relative sparing of cholinergic receptors. There is a reduction of neurons in a number of areas of the brain. Noradrenergic, serotoninergic, and GABA systems are also affected. The cause or causes of these changes are unknown. They do provide the basis for ongoing research into treatments for Alzheimer's disease.

CLINICAL PRESENTATION OF ALZHEIMER'S DISEASE

The presentation of Alzheimer's disease is often subtle, with memory deficits causing the patient to have difficulty balancing the checkbook, paying bills, or finding her way home along a familiar route. The family may bring the person in for evaluation for this, but often just attribute it to "getting old." A more radical behavioral change, such as agitation, sleep-wake cycle disturbances, or hallucinations, is more likely to trigger evaluation.

In Alzheimer's dementia, people maintain their primary motor and sensory modalities until late in the disease. The dementia is characterized in the early phase by memory loss and personality and psychiatric changes such as anxiety, depression, apathy, and withdrawal. In this phase, social skills are relatively well preserved.

Memory is affected in virtually all people with Alzheimer's. If there is no memory impairment the diagnosis should be doubted. Patients with early Alzheimer's disease usually have mild anomia, ie, difficulty naming objects.

As the disease progresses to the middle phase, intellectual function deteriorates further. Apraxia, difficulty or inability to perform complex motor tasks, such as manipulating forks or toothbrushes, develops. Agnosia, the inability to recognize or interpret what is seen, felt, or heard, also worsens. Language disorders develop or worsen and can progress to complete aphasia. Visuospatial problems become more severe, impairing the patient's ability to recognize or navigate through familiar environments. The ability to recognize close family members may be lost. Urinary incontinence develops secondary to loss of inhibitory fibers from the cerebral cortex. Hallucinations, delusions, and paranoia may escalate. Disruptive behaviors, including agitation, wandering, and sleep-wake cycle disturbances, are frequent.

In the late stages of Alzheimer's disease, double incontinence (bowel and bladder) develops. Awareness to self and environment is lost. Patients can become bedridden in a fetal position. They may stop eating. Aspiration becomes a problem. Death often results as a consequence of sepsis and malnutrition.

EVALUATION

The first step in evaluation is a complete history and physical examination. The history should include information from the family as to the person's acuity and progression of symptoms. This can give clues as to whether the patient may have more acute and potentially reversible dementia. Attention should be paid to all medications, including over-the-counter medications. The history of caffeine, alcohol, tobacco, and other substance abuse should be elicited. A nutritional history is valuable. A previous history of head trauma may be pertinent.

A functional history is necessary. It is important to know a person's previous cognitive function. An education and employment history and the patients's age at and reason for retirement aid in establishing this. Details as to a person's ability to perform the activities of daily living (ADL) such as bathing and dressing are important. Instrumental activities of daily living (IADLs) include using the phone and operating of a stove. These should also be determined. A driving history must be taken.

Psychosocial history is important. The support system of a patient with Alzheimer's disease is critical and will determine how the person will be cared for.

The physical examination must be thorough, including weighing the patient and evaluating orthostatic blood pressure and pulse changes. Close attention should be paid to the cardiovascular examination.

The neurologic examination is of paramount importance. Focal neurologic signs may give clues as to whether the patient's dementia is multi-infarct dementia rather than Alzheimer's. Alzheimer's disease occasionally presents atypically with focal neurologic deficits, dominant hemispheric signs including aphasia, or non-dominant signs including visual agnosia, dressing apraxia, and constructing apraxia. Although rigidity, cogwheeling, postural instability, and loss of facial expression may indicate Parkinson's disease, approximately 30% of Alzheimer's disease patients have these Parkinsonian features.

Formal mental status testing must be performed. A tool such as the Tolstein mini-mental status (MMSE) exam (Fig. 11-1) is useful because it is standardized and can be duplicated by other examiners. The MMSE gives the most information in the greatest number of domains, although it does not specifically assess goal setting behavior. The domains to be evaluated are attention, recent memory, cortical functioning (includes language and visuospatial skills), and goal setting or executive function. Executive function is responsible for motivation, intention, and organizational skills. The total score on the MMSE is not necessarily of value, but the specific areas of deficits provide clues to the diagnosis. For example, performance of serial 7s may be poor secondary to educational level rather than as a result of dementia.

The MMSE can be supplemented by additional questions. A forward digit span test asking for immediate recall and repetition of at least 5 digits can be helpful in circumventing the educational influence. Inability to repeat 5 numbers implies significant inattention problems. The naming section of the MMSE is insensitive to picking up early language problems. This can be expanded by asking the parts of a watch, eg, face, hands, wrist band. The patient's executive function can be tested by asking her to list for 1 minute items to buy in the supermarket. This test is invalidated if the examiner prompts the patient with "what else?"

Ideally, a functional assessment should be performed in the home. This is most helpful in determining home care needs or need

MINI-MENTAL STATE EXAM ADAPTED FROM FOLSTEIN 1975

SCORE=one point for each correct response unless otherwise specified. — MAXIMUM SCORE — ACTUAL SCORE

ORIENTATION

1. Ask for the date. Then specifically ask for parts omitted.
   "What is the (year) (season) (date) (month) (day) ?" (5) ______
2. "Can you tell me the name of the (state) (country) (town) (hospital) (floor) ?" (5) ______

REGISTRATION

SCORE=number of words correct on first attempt (0–3) Allow up to 6 trials.
Ask the patient if you may test his/her memory. Then say the words clearly and slowly.

3. "Remember these 3 words: cup, pencil, airplane."
   After you have said all 3, ask him/her to repeat them.
   (NUMBER OF REPETITIONS REQUIRED____) (3) ______

ATTENTION and CALCULATION

SCORE both tasks, but count only the best one toward the total score

4. "I want you to count backwards from 100 by 7's." Stop after 5 subtractions.
   (93,86,79,72,65)
   (SCORE=one point for each correct subtraction of 7 from the previous number____)
   "Now spell 'WORLD' backwards."
   (SCORE=number of letters in correct order. ie. DLROW=5, DLORW=3 ____) (5) ______

RECALL

5. "Do you remember the words I gave you earlier? What were they?" (3) ______

LANGUAGE

6. NAMING: Point to a wrist watch and ask him/her what it is. Repeat for pencil. (2) ______
7. REPETITION: Ask the patient to repeat "No ifs, ands, or buts." (1) ______
8. COMPREHENSION: Place a piece of paper in front of the patient and say, "Take the paper in your right hand, fold it in half, and put it on the floor." (3) ______
9. READING: CLOSE YOUR EYES.
   Ask the patient to read it and to do what it says. (1) ______
10. WRITING: Ask the patient to write a sentence on the back of the page. Do not dictate a sentence. It should contain a subject and a verb and make sense. Correct grammar and punctuation are not necessary. (1) ______

VISUO-SPATIAL

11. Ask the patient to copy the design. All 10 angles must be present and they must intersect in order to get credit. Tremor and rotation are ignored.
    Allow 1 minute to start and 1 minute to complete task (1) ______

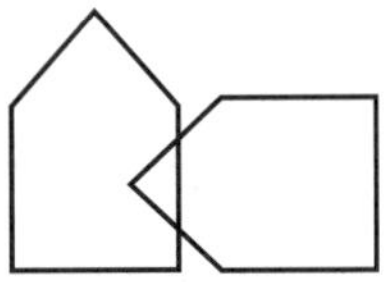

TOTAL SCORE (30) ______

Figure 11-1. Mini-Mental State Exam. (Adapted from Folstein MF, Folstein SE, McHugh PR. "Mini-mental state." A practical method for grading the cognitive states of patients for the clinician. Psychiatr Res 12:189.)

for alternate living arrangements. Assessment of a person's ability to safely use a stove can be lifesaving. Often physicians are unable to perform this assessment, but they can be assisted in this by a home care nurse or an occupational therapist.

The National Institutes of Health (NIH) recommend further testing. Routine laboratory tests recommended are a complete blood count with platelet count, electrolytes, metabolic panel, thyroid function test, B_{12} level, syphilis serology, folate level, and urinalysis. Other tests, including drug levels, toxin screen, HIV testing, and cortisol levels can be done depending on diagnostic suspicion. A lumbar puncture is indicated if neurosyphilis or infectious process is suspected. The NIH also recommends an ECG and a chest x-ray. A head CT is often performed to evaluate for structural lesions and mult-infarct dementia. PET and SPECT scans give functional information about CNS metabolism, which has been shown to be impaired in Alzheimer's disease. These tests are very expensive and experimental.

TREATMENT

There are no restitutive or curative treatments for Alzheimer's disease. Most therapies are aimed toward alleviating symptoms. Therapy should be tailored for specific symptoms or behaviors. Not all behaviors are amenable to pharmacologic therapy.

Wandering, sexual inappropriateness, disrobing, hoarding and hiding objects, and repetitive questioning are examples of behaviors poorly responsive to drug treatment. Behavioral approaches can be successful at managing some of these behaviors. A safe wandering path can be established, or a walking group to provide safe exercise.

Behavioral approaches should be attempted before pharmacologic treatment. Searching for the precipitant of agitation can be productive. Pain, for example, can cause agitation in a person who is not able to tell anyone about it. Environmental factors, such as being too hot or too cold, can also cause agitation. Agitation is the only expression left in a severely demented person's repertoire. Relieving the discomforts can calm the agitation.

To avoid agitation, a person with Alzheimer's disease should be approached with a quiet, friendly, soothing manner. Although she may no longer understand the content of language, she is still responsive to tone.

A structured environment with limited changes in routine and people is often helpful. Catastrophic deterioration often is seen when a person is placed in a new environment, such as the hospital or a nursing home. Meals should be offered in a setting as devoid of distractions as possible—ie, fewer people, no television, and a quiet room.

Agitation and hyperactivity sometimes respond to pharmacologic treatment. Neuroleptics are most often used, although the side effects of these medications are numerous and often severe. Haloperidol, the most potent, has a high incidence of extrapyramidal effects that can lead to gait difficulties and falls. In addition, neuroleptics can cause hypotension and sedation. Neuroleptics are more clearly indicated in delusional and hallucinating subjects. A common mistake is giving doses of these medications that are too large, with disastrous results. As with most medications in the elderly, the "start slow, go slow" approach is best. With haloperidol, it is best to start with a dose of 0.25 to 0.5 mg and slowly increase as needed. If the targeted symptom has not shown improvement after 6 to 8 weeks, the medication should be stopped. The same applies to other symptomatic medications discussed in this chapter.

Benzodiazepines are often used with mixed success for the sleep-wake disorders. These medications often do not work after a few weeks, secondary to habituation. Rebound may also be seen, with resultant increased wakefulness. Withdrawal is also a problem. Benzodiazepines are indicated if anxiety is the target symptom. Shorter- and intermediate-acting benzodiazepines are the preferred drugs to use in the elderly. Over-sedation is the most serious side effect; again, this often leads to falls.

Serotoninergic medications are being used increasingly for agitation. The exact mechanism of action is unclear. Decreased levels of serotonin may be a factor in aggressive behavior, so increasing the level may be the mechanism that controls agitation. The antidepressant effects may also improve behavior. Trazodone, with its mild sedative properties, may be a good choice at bedtime.

Antidepressants are indicated if clear depressive symptomatology is seen. It should be kept in mind that social withdrawal is common in Alzheimer's disease and does not necessarily imply depression. Antidepressant therapy should be chosen keeping the side effect profiles in mind. First-generation tricyclics should be avoided because of their strong anticholinergic properties. Nortriptyline, a second-generation tricyclic, is often a good choice, starting with a low dose at bedtime. Levels of the drug and ECGs should be followed. Trazodine and the newer serotoninergic antidepressants can be very useful.

Anticonvulsants such as carbamazepine may be useful in decreasing impulsiveness and aggression. The mechanism of action is not clear. These drugs must be used with caution because of their potentially fatal side effects of leukopenia, agranulocytosis, Stevens-Johnson syndrome, and hepatotoxicity. Other side effects include thyroid abnormalities, ataxia, dizziness, cardiac problems, and skin rashes. Further studies to evaluate the effectiveness of carbamazepine are ongoing.

Restitutive strategies for treatment of Alzheimer's disease are aimed at restoring imbalances in neurotransmitters. At this time, tacrine, which acts as an anticholinesterase inhibitor, is the only approved drug in this class. Tacrine was tested only on subjects with mild to moderate dementia and without concomitant medical conditions. Over all, these studies showed significant effects on the groups, but individually, only a minority of people showed moderate improvement of mental status and functional activities. Gastrointestinal side effects and transaminase elevations necessitated the discontinuation of tacrine in a large number of study subjects. Its use should be considered in people with mild to moderate dementia. Careful documentation of mental status exams done periodically and review of functional skills with the primary caregiver should be done over a 6-month trial to determine clinical benefit. Liver function tests must be closely monitored. The drug should be discontinued after 6 months if no improvement is seen. There is no evidence to suggest tacrine slows the rate of cognitive decline.

Another restitutive strategy currently being studied is the use of L-doprenyl. This drug is clearly of benefit in slowing the progression of Parkinson's disease and may help in Alzheimer's disease. Through its action as an MAO inhibitor, it has a positive effect on elevating CNS levels of dopamine and other neurotransmitters, which may help preserve surviving neurons.

Other avenues for further studies include nootropics, which are GABA (another neurotransmitter) derivatives. These may have neuroprotective effects against hypoxia and may enhance microcirculation by decreasing platelet activity. Neurotropic factors such as nerve growth factor are being explored. Fibroblasts can be genetically altered in cell culture to produce nerve growth factor, so donor tissue for potential transplant is not a problem.

Treatment of intercurrent illnesses is important. Often an acute medical illness worsens the behavior of a person with Alzheimer's disease. Treatment of more chronic medical illnesses may also improve mentation, for example, by improving oxygenation and thus mental status in a person with emphysema or congestive heart failure. Attention must be paid to the medication regimen, with elimination of medications which can affect mental status. Medications with anticholinergic properties, such as antihistamines, are particular offenders.

PSYCHOSOCIAL ISSUES

The person with Alzheimer's disease should be informed of the diagnosis and involved in as much decision making as possible. Issues such as health care guidelines concerning resuscitation and artificial intubation should be addressed while the person is still able to comprehend. Even with significant mental impairment, a person is often

be dealt with early before the patient is no longer able to make decisions concerning finances or appoint a power of attorney.

Finally, the primary caregivers of these patients should be considered at all times and given as much support as possible. They need to be kept informed of all services and options available to them. They need financial guidance through federal regulations concerning Medicaid if placement issues arise. There are a number of support groups and agencies available to help. Social workers are vital in providing support and assisting with obtaining services. The emotional needs of the caregivers should not be ignored. Alzheimer's disease is as devastating, if not more, to the family as it is to the person herself. The primary care provider should be as helpful as possible in guiding both through this difficult disease process.

Coronary Heart Disease

For many years coronary heart disease has been viewed primarily as a disease of men. Women have been perceived as unlikely to die of a heart attack, even if they have known coronary disease. This perception is wrong.

Coronary heart disease accounts for 250,000 to 500,000 deaths per year in women in the United States. This amounts to one third to one half of all deaths in women.

Until menopause, the incidence of coronary disease in women lags well behind that of men. By the age of 75 years, the incidence is about equal, but because the number of women is higher than men, more women than men are dying of coronary disease. Coronary heart disease in women is mostly a disease of elderly women.

RISK FACTORS

The incidence of coronary disease in women increases with aging due to the changes in their risk factors. Estrogen is the major protective influence in women. That protection changes with menopause. The influence of estrogen lingers, however, pushing the presentation of disease to older ages.

Estrogen favorably affects the lipid profile. In the age group prior to menopause, men have a higher incidence of hypercholesterolemia. After menopause, hypercholesterolemia becomes more prevalent in women than in men. Women do continue to have higher HDL levels than men, but their levels of HDL decline after menopause.

Estrogen may have a direct effect on the vasculature. Estrogen may alter thrombotic mediators, thereby decreasing the risk of thrombosis and infarction. This effect is decreased or lost with the estrogen deficiency state in the postmenopausal woman.

The incidence of hypertension increases with aging in women. The use of antihypertensive medication is a predictor of coronary disease in elderly women, probably reflecting the risk entailed by long-term effects of hypertension, even if current blood pressures are controlled. A number of studies have demonstrated that hypertension is not a benign norm in the elderly and that treatment is important.

Smoking is another risk factor that shows a crossover effect with age. Higher numbers of young men and older women die. Again, this contributes to the increased incidence of coronary disease in elderly women. Even those women who have not smoked but who have lived with smokers are at increased risk.

Hyperglycemia is a very strong risk factor for coronary disease. It, too, is seen in increasing incidence in the older woman. Direct effects on the vasculature, as well as its associated lipid abnormalities, make diabetes a major contributor to coronary disease.

Obesity is another major risk factor, probably through its association with hypertension, hypercholesterolemia, and diabetes. Weight does increase with age in women, at least until extreme old age, when it tends to decrease. Harris and coworkers demonstrated that women 65 to 74 years old who have the highest Quetelet index (weight in kg divided by height in m^2) have the highest incidence of coronary disease. Interestingly, those with the lowest weight who also reported the most previous weight loss had the second highest incidence, suggesting that weight fluctuation is also a risk.

Different factors play roles in mortality from coronary disease in women than in men. Seeman and coworkers found that the strongest predictors of mortality in women were diabetes and current smoking. Other influences, although less strong, were hypertension and known cardiac disease. In men, only the use of hypertensive medications had a significant association with cardiac mortality.

The Seeman study also demonstrated that in women there is a stronger association between risk factors and myocardial infarction and/or coronary artery disease mortality. It may be that the risk factors have stronger biologic effects in postmenopausal women or that all the men susceptible to these risk factors have already died at an earlier age.

CLINICAL PRESENTATION

Silent ischemia presents more frequently in the elderly, particularly in diabetics. Thus, the elderly woman with diabetes as a significant risk factor is somewhat more likely to present atypically without chest pain as a prominent factor.

Dementia in the elderly also plays a role in the atypical presentation. This is less a result of a lack of symptoms than it is an interpretation problem of nonverbal signs and symptoms. Agitation may be the only clue to a problem.

In the elderly woman the only indication of angina often is exertional shortness of breath. For other women, congestive heart failure, resulting from ischemia and subsequent diastolic dysfunction, is the presenting symptom. Other atypical presentations include palpitations, syncope, and sweating with exertion.

Most elderly women do present with typical anginal symptoms as their first indication of coronary disease (ie, chest pain, SCB, radiation to the left arm). Men are more likely to present first with a myocardial infarction or sudden death. Elderly women report more disability from their anginal symptoms than do men. Their symptom complex also tends to be more aggressive.

There is some evidence that women have a poorer prognosis than men after acute myocardial infarction. This increase in mortality is probably related to the increased age of women with coronary disease and to their concurrent illnesses.

DIAGNOSIS

Considering the often less straightforward presentation in elderly women, the diagnosis of coronary disease may be more difficult. It is much easier to diagnose coronary disease in the setting of an acute myocardial infarction than in atypical angina. The history is still important and helpful in women with typical anginal symptoms.

The physical examination may not be particularly helpful. Often, the findings are nonspecific. The resting ECG may also be unhelpful with only nonspecific ST-T wave changes, often in association with left ventricular hypertrophy.

Women do tend to have more noncoronary arterial causes of chest pain. These include mitral valve prolapse and angina sec-

tributes to the unreliability of the initial and most frequently used test for coronary artery disease, the exercise tolerance test (ETT).

The ETT has a lower positive predictive value in women than in men. There is a higher incidence of false positive results in women secondary to the noncoronary causes mentioned previously. Elderly women are less likely to be able to perform to a level adequate to achieve a high enough work load. They are limited not only by their coronary disease but also by other factors such as deconditioning and degenerative joint disease. ECG criteria for a positive ETT may differ for women. Rather than rely only on ST depression to define a positive test, a change in R wave height may be more predictive.

A thallium ETT may to add improved diagnostic ability. However, shadowing of the breast can decrease the accuracy of the test.

In general, noninvasive tests are less accurate in women, particularly elderly women. Clinicians need to consider invasive testing earlier in elderly women with possible coronary disease.

The decision to do angiography is complicated by the increased risk and difficulty performing the procedure in the elderly. Technically, the procedure can be more difficult to perform secondary to generalized arteriosclerosis with plaques in the iliac and aortic arteries. Decreased renal function is seen in the normal aging process and often is worsened by concurrent illnesses and medications. The elderly patient is at higher risk of renal compromise from the administration of contrast dye required for angiography.

Taking these factors into consideration, coronary angiography is the most informative test. Before angiography is performed, it should be determined if the person is a candidate for surgery. If concurrent medical illness contraindicates surgery, or the patient is not willing to undergo surgery, then angiography is probably not indicated.

Many times in the frail elderly, empiric treatment and the person's subsequent response is the only, and best, diagnostic tool available.

SEX BIAS

A number of studies done in recent years suggest a sex bias against women in the diagnosis and treatment of coronary artery disease. Much of the bias stems from the misconception that women do not have as high an incidence or severity of coronary disease as men. Another school of thought questions whether women are actually being diagnosed and treated more appropriately and men are being overtreated. Some earlier studies reported higher mortality of coronary artery bypass grafting in women, and this may have played a role in dissuading physicians from referring women to angiography and subsequent surgery.

The answer probably lies somewhere in the middle. Women are initially referred less for noninvasive testing. Even when they are referred and have a positive ETT, fewer are referred for angiography. This holds true when adjusted for age differences between men and women.

After myocardial infarction, women are less likely to have thrombolytic therapy than men. Elderly women, in particular, are less likely to have thrombolytic therapy because the trials have been in populations younger than age 70 and have included few women. The effect of sex bias on angioplasty in the past MI population is less evident but still present.

Angiography following a myocardial infarction is one area in which the sex bias is less operational. Once age has been controlled for, women are equally likely to be referred for angiography after MI. This does imply that age limits the referral to angiography.

After angiography, women are almost as likely to be referred to surgery as men. Studies have been conflicting as to whether surgery. This may be appropriate, because the sickest patients have the most to gain from surgery.

The referral bias probably has its biggest impact in early diagnosis of coronary artery disease. The question arises: how much morbidity and mortality could be avoided by earlier diagnosis of coronary disease in the elderly woman?

Older women are also less likely to be referred for cardiac rehabilitation following myocardial infarction, despite evidence that older women benefit as much as men in terms of increasing their maximal exercise capacity.

TREATMENT

Risk reduction as primary prevention of coronary disease in elderly women is important. This includes treatment of hypertension, decreasing hyperlipidemia, and avoidance of weight gain, and, thus, avoiding hyperglycemia. Discontinuing smoking is also of paramount importance. It is not clear that aggressive treatment of elevated cholesterol levels in the general elderly population is warranted, but it is indicated in the elderly patient with established coronary disease. Reduction of hyperlipidemia before old age would be most useful in risk reduction.

Exercise also probably continues to be of value in risk reduction in the elderly woman. There is some evidence that exercise slows age-related increases in coronary disease. This benefit is probably derived by the effect of exercise on lowering blood pressure and increasing HDL cholesterol. Exercise is important in the elderly woman who has had a myocardial infarction because it will help her to avoid deconditioning and improve exercise tolerance. This is why a cardiac rehabilitation referral is helpful. The better conditioned an elderly woman is, the more likely she will be able to continue to function independently.

Once a woman has developed coronary disease, medical management is usually the first-line therapy. This is more problematic in the elderly with polypharmacy and subsequent drug interaction and increased side effects in general. There is also decreased clearance of drugs in the elderly secondary to decreased renal function and decreased hepatic perfusion, which leads to increased drug levels and potential toxicity.

Nitrates are often effective in treating ischemia. Hypotension and severe headaches must be watched for. Clear instructions should be given to the patient and to the primary caregiver, if indicated, in order to ensure a nitrate-free interval.

The use of beta blockers is effective in treating angina and decreasing postmyocardial infarction mortality. Their use is more problematic in the elderly woman because of the increased incidence of congestive heart failure. Bradycardia is another potential side effect that can be devastating to the elderly when it results in a fall. Postural hypotension can also result, and this, too, can precipitate falls. Beta blockers also are more likely to cause CNS effects in the elderly with confusion and generalized fatigue.

As a general class, calcium channel blockers exert a less negative inotropic effect and thus less adverse effect on congestive heart failure. However, verapamil and, to a lesser degree, diltiazem can have negative inotropic effects. Calcium channel blockers also can cause postural hypotension. The constipating effect of some calcium channel blockers is a concern in the elderly. The effect on AV node conduction and possible heart block is also a bigger worry in the elderly patient who is already more likely to have underlying conduction abnormalities.

As a consequence of coronary disease, arrhythmias are common

wide array of side effects, including central nervous system effects with confusion, arrhythmias, and anorexia, which are more pronounced in the elderly. Procainamide more easily accumulates to toxic levels in elderly patients with their decreased renal function.

Treatment of an acute myocardial infarction should include more aggressive therapy if indicated. Thrombolysis in acute MI has been shown to decrease mortality in both sexes. There is little information available as to its efficacy in the elderly, as most studies excluded patients over age 70. The risk of thrombolysis does increase in the elderly because of concurrent illnesses such as hypertension, congestive heart failure, and peptic ulcer disease.

Women have greater procedural morbidity than men with angioplasty. They have an increased incidence of internal tears and coronary dissections. This may be secondary to small arterial size and balloons that are oversized for them. Concurrent illnesses also increase risk.

Several studies have been done concerning the question whether women do have an increased mortality following coronary artery bypass grafting (CABG), with conflicting results. Earlier reports indicated that the smaller body size of women influenced mortality, but this has not been supported in more recent studies. This discrepancy may be accounted for by improvements in surgical techniques since the original studies were done.

There may be increased mortality following CABG in women because of the lower frequency of internal mammary grafts. Women also tend to be referred in a worse functional class, and this increases operative mortality. Because women are older when they manifest cardiac disease, their operative mortality is higher. This age effect may be the most important factor.

However, the benefits of surgery are greatest in those with the worst disease, so older women may have the most to gain. Possibly, women with less severe disease, who are not being referred, are missing out on improved quality of life which could have been gained by earlier surgery.

Finally, estrogen therapy causes a risk reduction of coronary artery disease. The studies done have been on women starting in the early postmenopausal stage. There are no data on whether elderly women with coronary disease who are many years past menopause benefit from estrogen.

Coronary artery disease is far from being a benign and rather rare disease in the elderly woman. It is a leading cause of death and of significant morbidity. Treatment options and decisions are made more complex by advancing age.

BIBLIOGRAPHY

Screening

Mandelblatt JS, et al. Breast cancer screening for elderly women with and without comorbid conditions. A decision analysis model. Ann Intern Med 1992;116:722.

Resnick N. Geriatric medicine. In: Tierney LM, McPhee SJ, Papadakis MA, eds. Current Medical Diagnosis and Treatment, 35th edition. 1996:36.

Woolf SH, et al. The periodic health examination of older adults: the recommendations for the US Preventive Services Task Force. Part II: Screening tests. J Am Geriatr Soc 1990;38:933.

Falls

Alexander BH, Rivara FP, Wolf ME. The cost and frequency of hospitalization for fall-related injuries in older adults. Am J Public Health 1992;82:1020.

Arfken CL, Lach HW, Birge SJ, Miller JP. The prevalence and correlates of fear of falling in elderly persons living in the community. Am J Public Health 1994;84:565.

Campell AJ, Spears GF, Borrie MJ. Examination by logistic regression modelling of the variables which increase the relative risk of elderly women falling compared to elderly men. J Clin Epidemiol 1990;43:1415.

Cutson TM. Falls in the elderly. Am Fam Physician 1994;49:149.

O'Loughlin JL, Robitaille Y, Boivin JF, Suissa S. Incidence of and risk factors for falls and injurious falls among the community-dwelling elderly. Am J Epidemiol 1993;137:342.

Rubenstein LZ, Josephson KR, Robbins AS. Falls in the nursing home. Ann Intern Med 1994;121:442.

Speechley M, Tinetti M. Falls and injuries in frail and vigorous community elderly persons. J Am Geriatric Society 1991;39:46.

Tinetti ME, Baker DL, McAvay G, et al. A multifactorial intervention to reduce the risk of falling among elderly people living in the community. N Engl J Med 1994;331:821.

Tinetti ME, Speechley M, Ginter SF. Risk factors for falls among elderly persons living in the community. N Engl J Med 1988;319:1701.

Dementia

Bennett DA, Knopman DS. Alzheimer's disease: a comprehensive approach to patient management. Geriatrics 1994;49:20.

Davis KL, Thal LJ, Gamzu ER, et al. A double-blind, placebo-controlled multicenter study of tacrine for Alzheimer's disease. The Tacrine Collaborative Study Group. N Engl J Med 1992;327:1253.

Eisdorfer C, Olson EJ, eds. Management of patients with Alzheimer's and related dementias. Med Clin North Am 1994;78:4.

Farlow M, Gracon SL, Hershey LA, et al. A controlled trial of tacrine in Alzheimer's disease. JAMA 1992;268:2523.

Gorelick PB, Bozzola FG. Alzheimer's disease: clues to the cause. Postgrad Med 1991;89:231.

Harrell LE. Alzheimer's disease. South Med J 1991;84:S32.

Odenheimer GL. Acquired cognitive disorders of the elderly. Med Clin North Am 1989;73:6:1383.

Coronary Heart Disease

Bickell NA, Pieper S, Lee KL, et al. Referral patterns for coronary artery disease treatment: gender bias or good clinical judgement? Ann Intern Med 1992;116:791.

Eysmann SB, Douglas PS. Reperfusion and revascularization strategies for coronary artery disease in women. JAMA 1992;268:1903.

Harris TB, Ballard-Barbasch R, Madans J, Makuc DM, Feldman JJ. Overweight, weight loss, and risk of coronary heart disease in older women. The NHANESI Epidemiologic Follow-Up Study. Am J Epidemiol 1993;137:1318.

Krumholz HM, Douglas PS, Lauer MS, Pasternak RC. Selection of patients for coronary angiography and coronary revascularization early after myocardial infarction: is there evidence for a gender bias? Ann Intern Med 1992;116:785.

Oettgen P, Douglas PS. Coronary artery disease in women: diagnosis and prevention. Advances in Internal Medicine 1994;39:467.

Nachtigall LE, Nachtigall LB. Protecting older women from their growing risk of cardiac disease. Geriatrics 1990;45:24.

Seeman T, Mendes de Leon C, Berkman L, Ostfeld A. Risk factors for coronary heart disease among older men and women: a prospective study of community-dwelling elderly. Am J Epidemiol 1993;138:1037.

Steingart RM, Packer M, Hamm P, et al. Sex differences in the management of coronary artery disease: survival and ventricular enlargement investigators. N Engl J Med 1991;325:226.

Wei J. Cardiovascular system. In: Rowe JW, Besdine RW, eds. Geriatric Medicine. 2nd edition, Boston: Little, Brown and Company, 1988: 167.

Williams EL, Winkleby MA, Fortman SP. Changes in coronary heart disease risk factors in the 1980s: evidence of a male-female crossover effect with age. Am J Epidemiol 1993;137:1056.

Primary Care for Women, edited by Phyllis C. Leppert and Fred M. Howard. Lippincott-Raven Publishers, Philadelphia © 1997.

III

Reproductive Tract Problems

12

Abnormal Vaginal Bleeding

ROSALIND HAYES

Abnormal vaginal bleeding refers to any bleeding from the vagina that is not part of normal menses (Table 12-1). Variations in bleeding from cycle to cycle may be a part of normal menstruation, but a woman appropriately interprets changes in bleeding patterns, including excess or paucity from her norm, as a potential danger sign and seeks help.

Interval abnormalities outside the ranges given in Table 12-1 include oligomenorrhea (infrequent and usually irregular episodes of bleeding, occurring at intervals of 35 days or more), polymenorrhea (frequent and usually regular episodes of bleeding, occurring at intervals of 21 days or less), metrorrhagia (bleeding at irregular intervals), and intermenstrual bleeding (bleeding between otherwise regular menstrual periods). Abnormal amounts of bleeding include hypomenorrhea (regular bleeding that is decreased in amount), hypermenorrhea or menorrhagia (bleeding at regular intervals that is excessive in amount and duration of flow), and menometrorrhagia (bleeding that is excessive and prolonged at frequent and irregular intervals).

ETIOLOGY AND DIFFERENTIAL DIAGNOSIS

Normal vaginal bleeding results from complex hormonal events requiring communication among the hypothalamus, pituitary, and ovary to produce a sequence of follicular, ovulatory, and luteal phases of a dominant follicle. The signals released by the dominant follicle and subsequent corpus luteum orchestrate the endometrial progression from proliferative to secretory to menstrual endometrium. The endometrium proliferates in response to estrogen secreted by the dominant follicle. The endometrium undergoes secretory changes from progesterone synthesized and secreted by the corpus luteum. Progesterone peaks in the midluteal phase. Regression of the corpus luteum causes a fall in both progesterone and estrogen levels. The withdrawal of estrogen and progesterone causes the breakdown of the endometrium, seen as menses. Menstrual bleeding stops on its own, because resumption of the next menstrual cycle is associated with an increase in estrogen levels to help regenerate the endometrial lining; vasoconstriction and clotting factors aid in hemostasis as well. Any disruption of the controls of the menstrual cycle or of the stability of the endometrium may result in abnormal bleeding.

The differential diagnosis for abnormal vaginal bleeding is broad. It is helpful to categorize abnormal vaginal bleeding by the following characteristics: the patient's age (Table 12-2); ovulatory or anovulatory causes (Table 12-3); and uterine or nonuterine causes. Nonuterine causes of vaginal bleeding include cervical (erosions, polyps, cervicitis, and cancer), vaginal (traumatic vaginal lesions, vaginal infections, and foreign bodies), and other (external genitalia, urinary tract, and gastrointestinal tract).

It is important to rule out pregnancy complications. Important considerations include ectopic pregnancy, spontaneous abortion, complications of elective abortion, retained products of conception, molar pregnancy, other trophoblastic disease, and complications of intrauterine pregnancy, such as placenta previa or placental abruption.

HISTORY

A thorough history is essential in guiding the diagnosis, evaluation, and treatment. Noting the patient's age immediately helps focus the differential diagnosis. The bleeding abnormality can be characterized by asking about the onset of the last menstrual period, as well as the frequency and duration of bleeding. Inquiring about the amount of blood loss is appropriate, but there is a poor correlation between a patient's estimate of blood loss and the measured blood loss. Age of menarche or menopause should be ascertained. Molimina symptoms such as mittelschmerz, breast tenderness, bloating, or mood changes support the presence of ovulatory cycles. Bleeding may be painless or associated with pelvic or abdominal pain.

A history of chronicity, prior similar events, or acuteness with a temporally related event may be helpful. Other obstetric and gynecologic history is useful, such as pregnancy history, abnormalities noted on prior pelvic examinations, sexual activity, and contraceptive method. The rest of the history should include ascertaining current medications, history of bleeding disorders, chronic illness, endocrine disorders, family history, and review of systems, along with weight, exercise, nutrition, and stress.

TABLE 12-1. Characteristics of Normal Menses

	AVERAGE	RANGE
Menarche	12.8 years	8–16 years
Interval	29.5 days	21–35 days
Duration	4 days	2–8 days
Amount	35 mL	20–80 mL
Menopause	51.4 years	35–60 years

PHYSICAL EXAMINATION AND CLINICAL FINDINGS

A routine physical examination is performed, with particular attention paid to the thyroid for goiter, the breasts for galactorrhea, and the abdomen for masses or pain. In cases of acute or substantial bleeding, orthostatic blood pressure, pulse, and pallor are noted, as for any hemorrhage with the potential for shock.

A thorough pelvic examination is performed, noting activity of bleeding, potential extrauterine bleeding sources, palpable uterine or adnexal abnormalities such as masses, tenderness, and deviations in size or position.

The diagnosis of dysfunctional uterine bleeding (DUB) is made in the reproductive-age woman after organic causes have been ruled out. DUB is most common in perimenarcheal and perimenopausal women, as well as in patients with polycystic ovary disease. The stage for bleeding is set by anovulation and the resultant chronic unopposed estrogen stimulation to the endometrium.

LABORATORY AND IMAGING STUDIES

A pregnancy test should be done; a positive test determines further evaluation and treatment. Virtually all pregnancies, normal and abnormal, cause a positive pregnancy test by the time of a missed menses.

Useful hematologic studies are a complete blood count (CBC) and ferritin levels, which reflect current hemoglobin levels and iron storage. Blood losses of more than 80 mL per cycle generally produce anemia. A platelet count and coagulation studies are indicated in adolescents and in other cases suspicious for blood dyscrasia. An elevated erythrocyte sedimentation rate may reflect inflammatory states, neoplasms, or chronic illness.

Several endocrine tests may be informative. A thyroid-stimulating hormone elevation implies hypothyroidism; low levels are consistent with hyperthyroidism. An elevated prolactin level may cause a luteal-phase defect. Gonadotropin levels may reveal findings consistent with polycystic ovaries and chronic anovulation if the ratio of luteinizing hormone to follicle-stimulating hormone (FSH) is greater than 3; ovarian failure if the FSH is elevated into the menopausal range; or hypothalamic or pituitary dysfunction if hypogonadism is detected. Estradiol reflects the level of stimulation to the uterine lining. Cortisol elevation may prompt evaluation for Cushing syndrome.

Infectious disease evaluation may involve vaginal wet preparation or cervical cultures to detect extrauterine causes for vaginal bleeding. Cervical sources of bleeding can be further evaluated by Pap smear or cervical biopsy. An endometrial biopsy is used to diagnose endometritis.

Ovulation may be documented by basal body temperature charts, endometrial biopsy, or luteal-phase progesterone levels.

Imaging studies may be useful for diagnosis. Transvaginal ultrasonography can aid in visualizing endometrial thickness, polyps, and submucous myomas. Myometrial abnormalities, such as intramural myomas or adenomyosis, may be seen. A search for intrauterine and extrauterine pregnancy should occur when a pregnancy test is positive.

Adnexal anatomy is usually well visualized with transvaginal ultrasonography. Most ovarian masses are apparent and can be characterized based on their appearance on a sonogram. Normal fallopian tubes are not seen on ultrasound; therefore, the presence of hydrosalpinx indicates a past or present pelvic inflammatory state. Magnetic resonance imaging may be used to clarify or confirm pelvic or abdominal ultrasound if necessary.

Hysterosalpingography provides an x-ray that demonstrates the contour of the uterine cavity by radiographic contrast. It displays filling defects that may represent polyps, fibroids, or scarring as causes of abnormal bleeding.

An endometrial biopsy is a sampling of uterine lining performed with a small plastic catheter in the office. Its accuracy in diagnosing secretory endometrium, hyperplasia, or neoplasia is comparable to that of a more involved dilation and curettage (D&C) and therefore is the preferred diagnostic approach.

A hysteroscopy, an endoscopic visualization of the uterine cavity, can be performed in the office or the operating room. Hysteroscopy detects about 10% to 25% of diagnoses that the blind procedure of D&C misses. Operative hysteroscopy has the advantage of offering simultaneous treatment and diagnosis.

Laparoscopy, similarly, is an endoscopic visualization of the pelvis. It allows diagnosis of adnexal, uterine, and peritoneal pathology and also permits treatment.

TABLE 12-2. Age-Related Categories of Abnormal Vaginal Bleeding

AGE	ETIOLOGY
Newborn	Maternal estrogen
Childhood	Genital trauma, infection, foreign body, tumor, precocious puberty
Adolescence	Hypothalamic-pituitary dysfunction, blood dyscrasia
Reproductive age	Ovulatory or anovulatory, pregnancy-related
Perimenopausal and postmenopausal	Uterine cancer, endometrial polyps, hormone replacement therapy

TREATMENT

Treatment is tailored to the underlying cause of bleeding. The course of action is influenced by the patient's age, desire for contraception or fertility, severity or chronicity of bleeding, and other conditions.

Profuse bleeding requires hemodynamic stabilization. The immediate course of action should include administering intravenous fluids and inserting a Foley catheter. Essential laboratory studies include a CBC with clotting studies, pregnancy test, typing and cross-matching. A history and physical examination, along with imaging studies if needed, should complete data collection; then a decision for medical or surgical treatment can be made.

Medical treatment involves estrogens (Table 12-4). Estrogens at least temporarily stop most acute uterine bleeding, but they do

TABLE 12-3. Causes of Abnormal Bleeding

OVULATORY	ANOVULATORY
Blood dyscrasia (idiopathic thrombocytopenic purpura, von Willebrand disease)	Endocrine-hypothalamic-pituitary disorders, including chronic anovulation, polycystic ovary disease, hyperprolactinemia, thyroid and adrenal disease
Neoplasm (benign or malignant)	Ovarian failure
Infection (endometritis)	Neoplasms of hypothalamus or pituitary
Trauma	Chronic illness
Iatrogenic (intrauterine devices, drugs)	Stress reactions (exercise, eating disorders)
Endometriosis or adenomyosis	Hormonal treatment (oral contraceptives, hormone replacement therapy)
Luteal phase deficiency	
Persistent corpus luteum (Halban syndrome)	

not correct the underlying cause. Estrogen can be administered orally or intravenously with equal effectiveness. Treatment regimens may be 1.25 mg of estrogen (Premarin) orally every 4 hours for 24 hours, followed by 1.25 mg/day for 7 to 10 days; or 25 mg of Premarin intravenously every 4 hours until bleeding stops, or for 12 hours. Cessation of bleeding is a sign that estrogen has caused proliferation of the uterine lining. Estrogen administration should be followed by a progestin to induce withdrawal bleeding.

Surgical treatment may be needed in acute uterine hemorrhage for profuse bleeding, particularly when the bleeding is unresponsive to medical treatment. A D&C stops bleeding in most cases, except if it is caused by blood dyscrasia, malignancy, or submucous myoma. If medical treatment and initial surgical treatment fail to stop bleeding and conservation of fertility is important, hypogastric or uterine artery ligation or embolization may be tried. Hysterectomy is the treatment of last resort.

For less severe acute or chronic bleeding, estrogen therapy followed by a progestin controls most cases.

In DUB, the uterine lining has been exposed to estrogen and the bleeding is an example of estrogen breakthrough bleeding. The level of estrogen exposure often correlates with the amount of bleeding. The uterine lining has thereby lost the hemostatic control typically present when the sequence of estrogen followed by progestin provides structural stability and shedding occurs as a universal event. Progestins provide effective treatment in most cases of DUB and are the treatment of choice when contraception is not desired. Progestins stabilize the proliferated endometrium that is breaking down in an asynchronous fashion.

Endometrial biopsy should be considered in women at high risk for endometrial hyperplasia and malignancy. The high-risk group consists of women who are obese, nulliparous, and have a history consistent with chronic anovulation. Biopsy should be performed on women over age 40, and consideration should be given to the procedure for women who are younger, because risk is primarily related to duration of exposure to unopposed estrogen.

Examples of treatment with a progestin for DUB are 10 mg of medroxyprogesterone (Provera) orally every day for 10 days; or 5 to 10 mg norethindrone orally every 6 hours for 1 to 2 days, then 5 mg twice each day for 10 days. Treatment is repeated every 1 to 2 months in chronic anovulation. Bleeding due to withdrawal of progestin is expected after completion of the progestin, usually within 7 days.

Progestins are available in oral forms: medroxyprogesterone acetate, norethindrone, and norethindrone acetate. Injectable progestins and intrauterine devices impregnated with progestin are available when sustained action is desired.

Oral contraceptives offer multiple benefits in the treatment of DUB. They contain a combination of an estrogen, such as ethinyl estradiol, and a progestin, such as norethindrone. The predominant action on the endometrium is progestational. Oral contraceptives typically used are low-dose monophasics with less than 50 mg of estrogen. An example of treatment with an oral contraceptive is one pill four times a day for a week, followed by a withdrawal bleed; then one pill a day is resumed in a cyclic fashion.

The benefits of using cyclic oral contraceptives to control DUB in women of reproductive age include reduction in menstrual blood loss by about 60%, predictable bleeding, reduction of androgens, decreased risk of anemia, contraception, and decreased risks of endometrial hyperplasia and endometrial and ovarian cancer. For reproductive-age women with DUB who desire pregnancy, ovulation induction is indicated. The agents available include clomiphene citrate, human menopausal gonadotropins, or pulsatile gonadotropin-releasing hormone.

TABLE 12-4. Estrogen Equivalents

GENERIC NAME	TRADE NAME	CLINICALLY EQUIVALENT DOSE (mg)	AVAILABLE FORMULATIONS
Conjugated estrogen	Premarin	0.625	Oral, IV, vaginal cream
Estradiol	Estrace	1.0	Oral, transdermal, parenteral, vaginal cream
Esterified estrogens	Estratab, Menest	0.625	Oral
Ethinyl estradiol	Estinyl	0.05	Oral
Estropipate Diethyl-stilbestrol	Ogen	0.75	Oral, vaginal cream

In patients with ovulatory menorrhagia, useful agents may include cyclic oral contraceptives, nonsteroidal antiinflammatory drugs (particularly mefenamic acid 500 mg three times each day on days 1 through 3, which can reduce blood loss by 30%), and progestins, administered for the week preceding menses. Ergot derivatives are not effective treatment.

In menorrhagia associated with coagulopathies, two less common treatments may be useful in selected patients. Tranexamic acid, an antifibrinolytic agent, functions as a competitive inhibitor of plasminogen activation, reducing blood loss by about 50%. It is administered as 1 g four to six times a day on days 1 through 4. The second agent, desmopressin acetate (DDAVP), is a synthetic analog of arginine vasopressin. It is considered a last-resort medical treatment and is given 0.3 mg/kg in a 50-mL saline solution over 15 to 30 minutes. Treatment results in a rise of factor VIII that lasts about 6 hours. The drug may be given every 12 to 24 hours, but efficacy decreases with continued use.

SURGICAL TREATMENT

D&C is indicated in bleeding unresponsive to medical treatment, profuse bleeding, or when endometrial biopsy reveals premalignant neoplasia. Hysteroscopy may be a useful adjunct in identifying and treating endometrial polyps or submucous myomas, or in directing a biopsy of a suspicious lesion.

If the D&C is unsuccessful in controlling bleeding, uterine or hypogastric arteries can be surgically ligated or embolized under fluoroscopic guidance. These measures reduce arterial pressure to improve the efficacy of normal hemostatic mechanisms.

Hysterectomy is used as a final option when medical treatment and conservative surgery have been ineffective in controlling bleeding. The decision may be influenced by coexisting conditions where hysterectomy may be indicated, such as uterine fibroids or uterine descensus.

Endometrial ablation is an alternative to hysterectomy when there are no coexisting uterine conditions and major surgery is to be avoided, due to patient preference or to conditions of the patient that make surgery a high-risk procedure. Endometrial ablation is usually performed through the hysteroscope, with either a cautery or a laser. About 90% of women with menorrhagia improve; 50% become amenorrheic.

Additional considerations in the management of abnormal vaginal bleeding involve the treatment of secondary anemia with iron supplementation, as well as correction of any underlying contributory conditions, such as extragenital sources of bleeding (cervical polyp or vaginitis), or medical factors such as thyroid dysfunction or hyperprolactinemia.

Sometimes observation is warranted. One example is the menarcheal patient in whom fertility or contraception is not needed and bleeding has not been excessive. She may be counseled that in most adolescents, normal ovulatory cycles are established within 2 years, but further evaluation and treatment are available if the bleeding becomes heavier or persists.

Any bleeding in pregnancy requires referral for obstetric evaluation and management.

Abnormal vaginal bleeding can be a diagnostic and therapeutic challenge. The need for consultation may arise based on the desires of the physician or patient. Situations that may prompt a consultation involve calling a hematologist when faced with a bleeding diathesis in an adolescent, a gynecologist or reproductive endocrinologist when medical therapy is ineffective, or a gynecologist or gynecologic oncologist in cases of reproductive tract cancer. For the physician untrained in obstetric care, referral to an obstetrician in cases of pregnancy-associated bleeding is always appropriate.

It is also appropriate to honor a patient's request for a second opinion.

BIBLIOGRAPHY

Herbst AL, Mishell Jr. DR, Stenchever MA, Droegmueller W. Comprehensive gynecology, 2d ed. St. Louis: Mosby Year Book, 1992:1079.

Rivlin ME. Handbook of drug therapy in reproductive endocrinology and infertility, 1st ed. Boston: Little, Brown & Co., 1990:15.

Speroff L, Glass RH, Kase NG. Clinical gynecologic endocrinology and infertility, 5th ed. Baltimore: Williams & Wilkins, 1994:531.

Zuspan FP, Quilligan EJ. Current therapy in obstetrics and gynecology, 4th ed. Philadelphia: WB Saunders, 1994:25.

Primary Care for Women, edited by Phyllis C. Leppert and Fred M. Howard. Lippincott-Raven Publishers, Philadelphia © 1997.

13

Amenorrhea

G. WILLIAM BATES

Amenorrhea is the absence of menstruation. If menstrual cycles are not established by age 16 in an adolescent woman with other signs of secondary sexual maturation, this is called primary amenorrhea. If menstrual cycles cease for longer than 6 months in women with established menstruation, this is called secondary amenorrhea. However, these definitions have little bearing on the diagnosis and prognosis—amenorrhea is best understood and evaluated by knowing the pathophysiology of failure to menstruate.

Dysfunction of the hypothalamus, pituitary gland, ovaries, adrenal glands, or thyroid gland can cause amenorrhea, as can atrophy or scarring of the endometrium or obstruction of the genital tract. The cause of amenorrhea can often be ascertained by history and physical examination. Laboratory studies, imaging studies, and dynamic testing should substantiate the cause in most cases and should not be relied on as the primary method for diagnosis.

THE FEMALE REPRODUCTIVE CYCLE

The female reproductive cycle results from the cyclic interaction of hypothalamic, pituitary, and ovarian hormones. Hypothalamic-pituitary secretion of gonadotropin-releasing hormone (GnRH) and the gonadotropins, follicle-stimulating hormone (FSH) and luteinizing hormone (LH), is held in abeyance during childhood. By unknown mechanisms, gonadotropin stimulation begins during puberty and the female reproductive cycle is established. For ovulation to occur, there must be cyclic interaction between pituitary gonadotropins and ovarian sex-hormone secretion. Figure 13-1 shows the cyclic hormone interaction during the course of a female reproductive cycle. Any alteration in this cyclic secretion of pituitary gonadotropins or sex-steroid hormones results in anovulation and amenorrhea. When any gonadotropin or sex-steroid hormone becomes tonically elevated or tonically suppressed, the reproductive cycle is disrupted. For example, in pregnant women, progesterone is tonically elevated and gonadotropin secretion is suppressed; she does not ovulate. In women with polycystic ovarian disease (PCOD), tonic production of estrone causes tonic secretion of LH, leading to chronic anovulation and amenorrhea.

CAUSES OF AMENORRHEA

Hypothalamic Dysfunction

Disruption of GnRH or gonadotropin secretion leads to anovulation and amenorrhea. The common types of hypothalamic-pituitary dysfunction are presented here.

Kallmann syndrome (DeMosier syndrome in females) is the most common genetic cause of hypothalamic-pituitary dysfunction. This disorder is characterized by anosmia, sexual infantilism, and primary amenorrhea. Olfactory tract hypoplasia results in anosmia. During fetal life, the secretory cells of the anterior hypothalamus migrate with the olfactory tracts to the portal plexus, allowing secretory communication between the anterior hypothalamus and pituitary gland. In Kallmann syndrome, this secretory linkage is not established; therefore, there is no hypothalamic oscillator to stimulate gonadotropin secretion.

The diagnosis of Kallmann syndrome is suspected when diminished or absent olfactory function is demonstrated by challenging the patient with known odors such as coffee or rubbing alcohol. If the patient cannot recognize these common odors, the diagnosis is almost certain. FSH and LH levels are in the hypogonadotropic range. Treatment consists of administration of estradiol-17β to simulate estradiol secretion during puberty, followed by administration of a progestin to stimulate progesterone receptors. Because ovarian follicles are present, the woman with Kallmann syndrome can be reassured that ovulation can be induced when pregnancy is desired.

Low body weight is the most common cause of hypothalamic-pituitary dysfunction in women who have established reproductive cycles. Anorexia nervosa is the extreme form of weight loss and amenorrhea. However, marginal loss of body fat can result in amenorrhea or oligomenorrhea with associated infertility, vaginal dryness, and loss of bone mass. Therapy is directed at restoring body fat to appropriate levels (lean : fat = 3 : 1). Women with marginal loss of body fat often resist the recommendation to gain

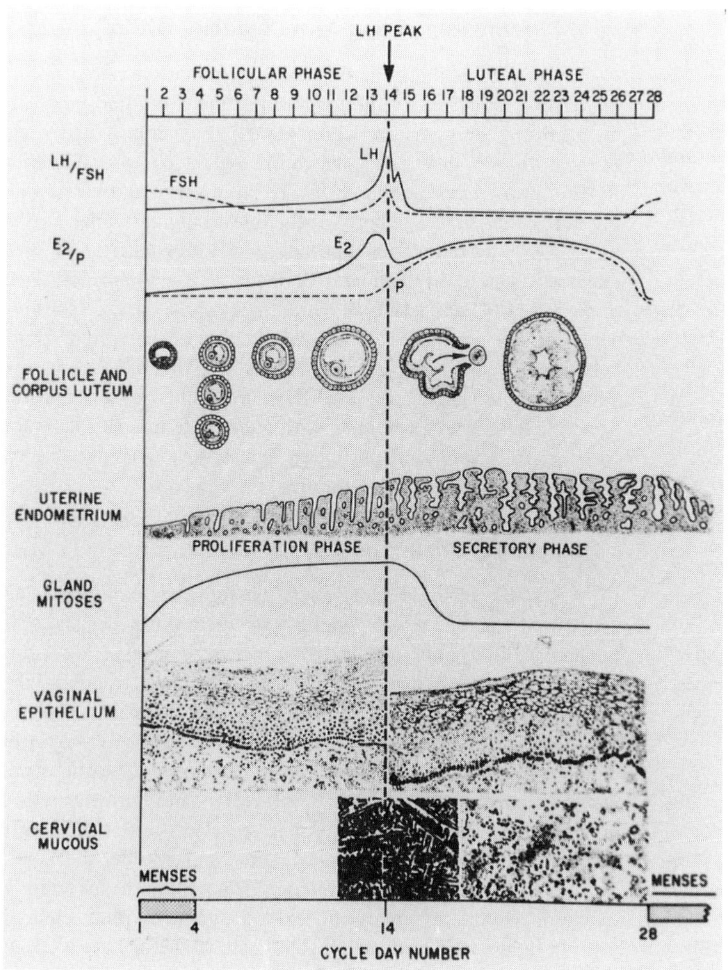

FIGURE 13-1. Cyclic hormone interaction during the reproductive cycle. (DeGroot LJ. Endocrinology 1989;3:1946.).

weight, but no other therapy is successful in restoring ovulation and cyclic menstruation.

Marijuana blocks the secretion of GnRH. Men who smoke marijuana can experience infertility and impotence; women who smoke marijuana can experience anovulation and amenorrhea. Inquiry about marijuana use should be part of the evaluation of amenorrhea, anovulation, and infertility. The only treatment is cessation of marijuana use.

Suprasellar tumors such as craniopharyngioma and hamartoma and inflammatory disorders such as sarcoidosis interrupt pituitary portal plexus blood flow. Thus, there is functional isolation of the hypothalamus from the pituitary gland. Suprasellar tumors usually occur during childhood and lead to sexual infantilism and primary amenorrhea; inflammatory conditions can occur at any time. The diagnosis of suprasellar tumors is made by imaging studies. These studies should not be obtained until hypogonadotropic hypogonadism is demonstrated by laboratory studies and the other causes of hypogonadotropic hypogonadism have been excluded. Surgical removal of suprasellar tumors is not indicated unless there is evidence of increased intracranial pressure or visual disturbance. Treatment can be accomplished by administration of appropriate sex-steroid hormones to bring about secondary sexual maturation, and ovulation induction can be initiated when required for pregnancy.

Pituitary Dysfunction

Prolactin-secreting adenoma with subsequent hyperprolactinemia is the most common pituitary cause of amenorrhea in adolescents and sexually mature women. The diagnosis should be suspected when gonadotropins are suppressed below physiologic levels and should be strongly suspected when there is accompanying galactorrhea and elevated serum prolactin levels. If the serum prolactin concentration exceeds 100 ng/mL, a magnetic resonance imaging scan of the pituitary gland is indicated to exclude a large pituitary microadenoma or a pituitary macroadenoma. Otherwise, bromocriptine, a dopamine agonist, should be administered to restore normal hypothalamic-pituitary function. Ovulation is quickly restored in women with serum prolactin concentrations of less than 50 ng/mL, so these women need contraceptive counseling if they do not plan to conceive.

Isolated gonadotropin deficiency, a rare cause of pituitary dysfunction, may cause primary amenorrhea. The diagnosis is established by intravenous bolus infusion of GnRH with demonstrated failure of the pituitary gland to respond with gonadotropin secretion.

Sheehan syndrome is associated with postpartum hemorrhage and resultant anterior pituitary necrosis. There is generalized pituitary failure, usually beginning with failed lactation, followed by gonadal, thyroid, and adrenal dysfunction. The treatment of Sheehan syndrome necessitates replacement of all deficient hormones.

Ovarian Dysfunction

Genetic information that determines the rate of ovarian follicular atresia is carried on the long arm of the X chromosome. (Somatic information is carried on the short arm of the X chromosome.) Any deletion of the X chromosome, complete or partial, results in premature ovarian failure, somatic abnormalities, or both. Turner syndrome, the most frequent cause of sexual infantilism and premature ovarian failure, evidences these facts.

Turner Syndrome

Turner syndrome is characterized by a 45X chromosomal karyotype. Short stature, webbed neck (pterygium colli), increased carrying angle (cubitus valgus), and shield chest with a thick torso are the common physical features. The disorder can usually be recognized during childhood, but diagnosis may be delayed until secondary sexual characteristics fail to appear at puberty. Ovarian follicular atresia is accelerated; ovarian failure is usually complete at birth.

Treatment with sex-steroid hormones should begin at the expected time of breast development (age 10 or 11 years). Low doses of estradiol should be initiated to simulate ovarian estrogen secretion. Excessive estradiol dosage can produce premature closure of the epiphyses, with a resultant shorter stature than usual. Bone age films of the hands should be obtained before starting therapy and the rate of increase in height monitored. When menarche occurs after estrogen administration, a progestin should be added to the regimen to bring about adult breast development.

Women with mosaic Turner syndrome (46XX/45X) present with varying features, depending on the predominant cell line. Some have few characteristics of Turner syndrome; in others, the features are obvious. If the affected woman presents with sexual infantilism, treatment is the same as that for Turner syndrome. If she presents with the classic signs of ovarian failure (hot flushes, vaginal dryness, sleep disturbance), treatment is the same as for any other woman with ovarian failure.

X-Chromosome Long-Arm Deletion (46XXq-)

Because genetic information that determines the rate of follicular atresia is carried on the long arm of the X chromosome, any loss of the long arm results in premature ovarian failure. The extent of long-arm loss determines the chronologic age at which ovarian failure occurs. For example, if the loss is substantial, ovarian failure may occur before puberty. If the loss is slight, ovarian failure may occur after the woman has had several pregnancies. The first diagnostic step in the evaluation of any woman with amenorrhea is to measure FSH and LH levels. If these are elevated, then chromosomal studies are indicated. Banding studies of the chromosomes help distinguish chromosomal deletions. The treatment of women with X-chromosome long-arm deletion should be based on the same guidelines as for women with pubertal failure (if that is the case) or for women with secondary sexual development who present with premature ovarian failure.

Alkylating Chemotherapy

Alkylating chemotherapy alters the follicular membrane surrounding the oocyte to make the membrane resistant to gonadotropin stimulation. Thus, women who receive alkylating chemotherapy for hematologic neoplastic diseases (Hodgkin lymphoma, leukemia), breast cancer, and other neoplastic diseases may experience symptoms of ovarian failure, and this should be anticipated. If a woman experiences a change in the menstrual cycle or hot flushes, FSH and LH levels should be measured. If gonadotropins are elevated, she must be placed on estradiol-17β therapy. This should be administered continuously, and she should be monitored with basal body temperature charts to ascertain if ovulation occurs. Women who exhibit symptoms and signs of ovarian failure as a result of alkylating chemotherapy are likely to ovulate when given estradiol. If pregnancy is desired, restoration of ovulation is the best possible outcome. If pregnancy is not desired, then contraception must be implemented. Nevertheless, estrogen (preferably estradiol) must be given to alleviate the symptoms of estrogen deficiency.

Polycystic Ovarian Disease

Polycystic ovarian disease (PCOD) can present as primary or secondary amenorrhea. There is an androgen excess (manifested by acne, hirsutism, and increased muscle mass), obesity, and estrogen excess. The excessive estrogen is estrone, not estradiol-17β. Obesity is a characteristic feature of PCOD and may be the initiating cause because of the increased conversion of androstenedione to estrone in obese men and women. In this disorder, the production of estrogen is tonic, not cyclic. Thus, stimulation of the endometrium by estrogen is gradual, which results in irregular shedding of the endometrium. There may be long episodes of amenorrhea followed by episodes of severe menorrhagia.

If PCOD is established at the time of puberty, menarche may be delayed, creating the impression that the young woman has primary amenorrhea. However, menarche does occur eventually, and the first menses may be unusually heavy in the amount and duration of flow.

During the pelvic examination, the physician can observe signs of estrogen excess—a heavily rugated vaginal epithelium and abundant endocervical mucus and vaginal secretions. Administration of a progestin such as medroxyprogesterone acetate (Provera) induces withdrawal bleeding.

ANATOMIC CAUSES OF AMENORRHEA

Vaginal Agenesis (Rokitansky-Küster-Hauser Syndrome)

Vaginal agenesis is a birth defect resulting from failure of fusion and cannulization of the müllerian ducts. Unless the defect is recognized at birth (and it usually is not), the presenting sign is primary amenorrhea. In 95% of cases, the uterus as well as the vagina is absent. Because there is normal ovarian function, sexual hair growth, growth spurt, and breast development occur at the expected times. If the uterus is present, the presenting sign is pelvic pain associated with an abdominal mass, as the menstrual blood cannot escape the uterine cavity except through the fallopian tubes. The uterine cavity becomes distended, producing pelvic pain. In these cases, the diagnosis is usually made by age 12 or 13.

Imperforate Hymen

In cases of imperforate hymen, the menstrual fluid is obstructed at the vaginal introitus. The vaginal vault can accumulate a large amount of menstrual effluent before symptoms begin. A bluish, bulging imperforate hymen is the characteristic feature. This problem can be resolved by incising the hymen, allowing evacuation of the accumulated effluent and providing immediate and long-term resolution of the problem.

Asherman Syndrome

Asherman syndrome usually follows dilatation and curettage of a postpartum uterus for retained products of conception. It presents as secondary amenorrhea. Curettage of a postpartum uterus several days after delivery can denude the endometrium, making it impossible for it to regenerate; without endometrial regeneration, menstruation cannot occur. The diagnosis is made by hysterosalpingography or hysteroscopic visualization of the endometrial cavity. On hysterosalpingogram, the endometrial cavity shows signs of attenuation and scarring. If endometrial scarring is minimal, lysis of adhesions by hysteroscopy restores cyclic menstruation and fertility. However, if scarring is extensive, the prognosis is poor for restoring menstruation and fertility.

In Asherman syndrome, as in other anatomic causes of amenorrhea, ovarian function is preserved, and affected women continue to experience cyclic changes of ovarian function such as breast fullness, fluid retention, mood changes, and changes in libido. In contrast, women with endocrine causes of amenorrhea have no cyclic secretion of estrogens and progesterone.

Androgen Insensitivity Syndrome

Women with androgen insensitivity syndrome have a 46XY chromosomal constitution but lack receptors for testosterone. The sexual assignment at birth is female. Breast development occurs near the expected time of puberty, but menarche does not occur. Because the intraabdominal testicles secreted müllerian duct inhibiting factor during fetal life, there is no uterus, fallopian tubes, or vagina, so menstruation cannot occur. Once the diagnosis is established, the gonads must be removed because of the risk of neoplastic change, and estradiol must be administered to maintain secondary sexual characteristics. Vaginoplasty is required to establish a functional vagina for sexual intercourse.

EVALUATION

The caregiver should begin by obtaining a history of the stages of secondary sexual development. Failure of secondary sexual development to occur by age 13 or 14 suggests that the hypothalamic-pituitary axis has failed to secrete GnRH or gonadotropins, or that the ovaries have failed to respond to the hypothalamic-pituitary signal. If secondary sexual development has occurred partially—for instance, breast development and sexual hair growth have begun but have not been completed—the pubertal process was initiated but was interrupted before completion of secondary sexual maturation. In most such cases, the ovaries have failed prematurely. If full secondary sexual maturation has been completed and there is a history of menstrual molimina (cyclic breast fullness, cyclic mood changes, cyclic acne, cyclic bloating), it is likely that there is obstruction of the genital outflow tract.

Illicit drug use, especially the use of marijuana, can alter hypothalamic-pituitary function to produce cessation of ovarian function. Alterations in body weight, both rapid weight gain and rapid weight loss, can interfere with estrogen metabolism to produce amenorrhea. Body weight alterations can result from altered caloric intake and exercise, and these issues must be covered in the medical history.

Physical Examination

A careful physical examination often uncovers clues that suggest the etiology of amenorrhea. First, the body habitus is noted. A slender or obese habitus is frequently linked to amenorrhea because of the alterations in estrogen production and metabolism associated with these conditions. The skin is examined for acne, hirsutism, hair loss, and acanthosis nigricans. These conditions suggest androgen excess of adrenal or ovarian origin. Hair loss (telogen effluvium) is found in men and women who experience changes in sex-steroid hormone concentrations. This condition is commonly seen at puberty, in pregnancy, when hormone therapy is initiated, and at menopause. Loss of axillary and pubic hair is found in patients with anorexia nervosa, marijuana use, and ovarian failure. Striae on the abdomen are found in conditions of cortisol excess, due either to endogenous secretion or exogenous administration of glucocorticoid therapy.

A woman's breast configuration changes as she undergoes hormonal changes. In pregnancy, the breasts become full and rounded in the lateral quadrants. In conditions of estrogen excess (PCOD, iatrogenic estrogen excess), the breasts become tubular. Conversely, in conditions of estrogen deficiency, the breasts may undergo partial involution. The nipples and areolae become tan and pale compared with the pink color found with normal ovarian function.

The pelvic examination reveals conditions of estrogen production. In women with excess estrogen, the vagina is heavily rugated, with abundant vaginal secretions. The cervical mucus, clear and watery, pours from the cervical os. When estrogen is deficient, the opposite conditions are found. The vaginal epithelium is thin, pale, and dry; the cervix is dry. If the cervical mucus is thick, viscous, and opaque, the woman is in the luteal phase of the cycle, is pregnant, or is using a progestin contraceptive method. There are no signs on the bimanual examination that give clues to the etiology of amenorrhea.

Laboratory Evaluation

Hormonal studies are useful in distinguishing the etiology of amenorrhea. The clinician can begin by measuring gonadotropins—FSH and LH, along with prolactin, androstenedione, testosterone, and dehydroepiandrosterone. The levels of gonadotropins place the etiology in either the hypothalamic-pituitary axis or the ovaries.

Hyperprolactinemia suppresses gonadotropin secretion. Ovarian failure is manifested by elevated gonadotropins. Women with low body weight, those who live under chronic stress, and those who use marijuana have suppressed gonadotropins. Women with PCOD have normal FSH, elevated LH, and elevated androstenedione levels; the testosterone level is in the upper range of normal or is mildly elevated. Many physicians think that testosterone must be elevated to make a diagnosis of PCOD, but this is incorrect. Obese women often meet the laboratory criteria for the diagnosis of PCOD, even in the absence of hirsutism.

In women with late-onset adrenal hyperplasia, the dehydroepiandrosterone level is at the upper limit of normal or is elevated. An elevated dehydroepiandrosterone level is followed by an ACTH stimulation test. The subject with suspected late-onset adrenal hyperplasia is given 1 mg of dexamethasone at 10 p.m. The next morning, blood is drawn at 8 a.m. Immediately after blood is drawn, 250 μg of ACTH (Cortrosyn) is injected by intravenous bolus. One hour later, another blood sample is obtained. The two samples are assayed for 17-hydroxyprogesterone. If the value obtained after ACTH stimulation exceeds the baseline value by more than 2.8 times, this is a positive ACTH stimulation test and meets the criteria for the diagnosis of late-onset adrenal hyperplasia.

Women with anatomic abnormalities such as Asherman syndrome, vaginal agenesis, and imperforate hymen have laboratory studies that are in the normal range for an ovulating woman. A basal body temperature record can be used to verify ovulation in women with these conditions; blood studies are not needed.

Women with intersex problems such as testicular feminization have testosterone concentrations in the range of a normal male. The diagnosis of an intersex problem should be suspected by the clinician before large sums of money are spent on establishing the diagnosis in the laboratory. Laboratory studies should not be used as a "fishing trip" to make a diagnosis. In most cases, the diagnosis should be closely approximated by the history and physical examination before laboratory studies are obtained.

TREATMENT

The patient's desires should be the basis for treatment of amenorrhea. Some women want restoration (or initiation) of cyclic menses; some want pregnancy; some want resolution of hirsutism; some want freedom from hot flushes, vaginal dryness, and sleep disturbances; some want elimination of galactorrhea; and others simply want information. It is important to ascertain the woman's desires when she presents with a complaint of absence of menstruation.

Once the cause of amenorrhea is established, the clinician must try to meet her expectations or explain why they cannot be met. For example, if a woman with PCOD wants both relief from hair growth and pregnancy, these expectations cannot be met simultaneously. If an obese woman with amenorrhea wants pregnancy through clomiphene citrate ovulation induction, this expectation is unrealistic until she can reduce her body fat. Because clomiphene citrate is lipid-soluble, it is stored in body fat, and adequate blood levels cannot be achieved to stimulate an FSH surge. If a slender woman wants ovulation induction for pregnancy, she is best advised to gain weight before expecting ovulation to occur. The administration of ovulation induction agents to obese or slender women creates unrealistic expectations and does not address the fundamental problem—obesity or slimness.

There are several judgments the clinician must make about the long-term consequences of amenorrhea on a woman's health. Prolonged estrogen deficiency can lead to osteoporosis and cardiovascular disease, even in young women. Therefore, the cause of the estrogen deficiency should be established if possible and definitive treatment instituted. Anorexia nervosa has a mortality rate approaching 5%; estrogen administration is warranted to prevent osteoporosis and heart disease and to facilitate weight gain. Estrogen excess, as is found in PCOD, is associated with endometrial hyperplasia, menometrorrhagia, and endometrial carcinoma. Women with estrogen excess should be placed on oral contraceptives to reduce LH secretion and to protect the endometrium from excessive estrogen. Women with androgen excess continue to have new terminal hair growth, along with stimulation of existing terminal hair. They may experience a change in body habitus, taking on a more masculine appearance. By administering oral contraceptives to women with PCOD, weight loss is facilitated by the suppression of ovarian androgens. Androgens are anabolic steroids that promote weight gain.

Women with late-onset adrenal hyperplasia are best managed by the administration of low-dose glucocorticoids (eg, prednisone, 2.5 mg/day given at bedtime). This therapy restores ovarian function to normal, prevents new hair growth, and restores fertility. This dose of prednisone does not suppress ACTH secretion and does not produce signs of glucocorticoid excess.

The treatment of anatomic causes of amenorrhea is surgical and was discussed previously.

SUMMARY

Amenorrhea results from dysfunction of the hypothalamic-pituitary axis, the ovaries, or the genital outflow tract. Evaluation of amenorrhea requires obtaining a thoughtful medical history, performing a thorough physical examination, and selecting the appropriate laboratory studies. From these sources of information, the clinician should be able to establish the etiology of amenorrhea and implement proper treatment. It is important to understand the woman's desires in evaluating and treating amenorrhea, and to help her understand the long-term consequences of amenorrhea.

BIBLIOGRAPHY

Bates GW, Bates SR, Whitworth NS. Reproductive failure in women who practice weight control. Fertil Steril 1982;37:373.

Bates GW, French GM, Humphries BB, Blackhurst DW. Outcome of ACTH stimulation testing in women with androgen excess and ovulatory dysfunction. Am J Obstet Gynecol 1992;167:308.

Bates GW, Whitworth NS. Effects of body weight reduction on plasma androgens in obese, infertile women. Fertil Steril 1982;38:406.

Blackwell RE. Diagnosis and management of prolactinomas. Fertil Steril 1985;43:5.

Damewood MD, Grochow LB. Prospects for fertility after chemotherapy or radiation for neoplastic disease. Fertil Steril 1986;45:443.

Federman DD. Mapping the X chromosome: mining its p's and q's. N Engl J Med 1987;317:161.

Rugarli EI, Ballabio A. Kallmann syndrome. From genetics to neurobiology. JAMA 1993;270:2713.

Saenger P. The current status of diagnosis and therapeutic intervention in Turner's syndrome. J Clin Endocrinol Metab 1993;77:297.

Smith CG, Smith MT. Substance abuse and reproduction. Semin Reproduct Endocrinol 1990;8:55.

Stein IF, Leventhal ML. Amenorrhea associated with bilateral polycystic ovaries. Am J Obstet Gynecol 1935;29:181.

Treloar AE, Boynton RE, Benn BG, Brown BW. Variations of human menstrual cycle through reproductive life. Int J Fertil 1967;12:77.

Wilson JD, Harrod MJ, Goldstein JL, Hemsell DL, MacDonald PC. Familial incomplete male pseudohermaphroditism, type I. N Engl J Med 1974;290:1097.

Wiser WL, Bates GW. Management of vaginal agenesis: a report of 92 cases. Surg Gynecol Obstet 1985;159:108.

Primary Care for Women, edited by Phyllis C. Leppert and Fred M. Howard. Lippincott-Raven Publishers, Philadelphia © 1997.

14

Dysmenorrhea

RAHUL LAROIA
FRED M. HOWARD

Dysmenorrhea is defined as severe, cramping pain in the lower abdomen that occurs just before or during menses. The term is derived from a Greek root meaning difficult monthly flow and first appeared in the English language in 1810. Until recently, painful menstruation was considered a woman's lot by many professionals. However, attitudes toward this problem have changed greatly over the past 30 years due to serious scientific work on its etiology and treatment.

Much of the epidemiologic work on dysmenorrhea has been carried out in Scandinavia, where the prevalence is as high as 75%, with about 15% of affected women having severe symptoms that limit daily activities. In the United States, work absenteeism due to dysmenorrhea is estimated at 600 million work hours, and the economic consequences are estimated to be $2 billion per year.

Primary dysmenorrhea, a diagnosis of exclusion, is made when no pelvic pathology is found that accounts for painful menstruation. It is generally a problem of young women, with onset at less than age 20. Improvement in symptoms of primary dysmenorrhea after age 25 is more common in married women; however, pregnancies and vaginal deliveries do not necessarily cure primary dysmenorrhea. Secondary dysmenorrhea is diagnosed in women with pelvic pathology that causes pain with menstruation. It is more common in women over age 20.

ETIOLOGY

Hippocrates believed that stagnation of menstrual blood caused by cervical obstruction led to painful menstrual periods. Cervical stenosis, leading to increased intrauterine pressure and retrograde flow at menses, can cause lower abdominal discomfort and dysmenorrhea. However, this is not the cause of primary dysmenorrhea, although in rare instances it may be a cause of secondary dysmenorrhea. Hysterosalpingographic studies carried out during menstruation fail to demonstrate any differences in tightness of the cervical canal in women with primary dysmenorrhea compared to those without dysmenorrhea.

In 1940, Smith described an extract of menstrual discharge, "menstrual toxin," that caused severe vasoconstriction, fibrinolysis, and an inflammatory reaction and was a powerful muscle stimulant. Pickles called this substance "menstrual stimulant" in 1954 and subsequently showed that it contained prostaglandins E and F. An association between increased uterine prostaglandin $F_{2\alpha}$ ($PGF_{2\alpha}$), increased myometrial activity, and dysmenorrhea is now well established. $PGF_{2\alpha}$ is present in higher concentrations in the menstrual fluid of dysmenorrheic women. The intravenous injection of $PGF_{2\alpha}$ reproduces uterine cramps and pain. $PGF_{2\alpha}$ can also produce diarrhea, vomiting, headache, and syncope, symptoms common with primary dysmenorrhea. Also, prostaglandin synthetase inhibitors relieve dysmenorrhea and decrease menstrual flow and uterine contractility.

Prostaglandins are specialized unsaturated fatty acids with a cyclopentane ring and two side chains. Of the several compounds in this group, prostaglandin E_2 (PGE_2) and $PGF_{2\alpha}$ have been extensively evaluated. Their synthesis is from arachidonic acid and is controlled by microsomal enzymes called prostaglandin synthetase.

There are two major pathways of synthesis of prostaglandins (Fig. 14-1). In the cyclooxygenase pathway, arachidonic acid is converted into cyclic endoperoxides, then into PGE_2, $PGF_{2\alpha}$, prostacyclin, or thromboxane A_2. The other metabolic pathway

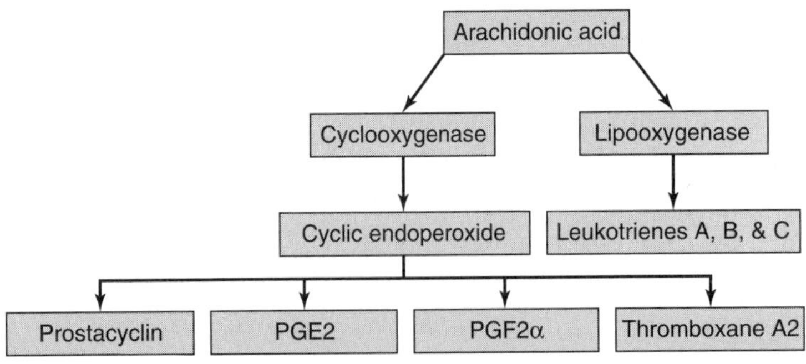

FIGURE 14-1. Biosynthesis of prostaglandins and leukotrienes.

for arachidonic acid metabolism, the lipoxygenase pathway, leads to the formation of leukotrienes. Leukotrienes cause uterine muscle contractions and are potent vasoconstrictors and bronchoconstrictors.

The cyclooxygenase pathway can be blocked by many nonsteroidal antiinflammatory drugs (NSAIDs). NSAIDs, however, do not block the lipoxygenase pathway, explaining why these drugs do not relieve primary dysmenorrhea in some patients.

In addition to prostaglandins, several other factors may play a role in the etiology of dysmenorrhea. One is vasopressin, a powerful stimulant of the uterus, particularly at the onset of menstruation. There is a fourfold increase in circulating vasopressin levels during menstruation in women with dysmenorrhea over the levels in asymptomatic women. The effect of vasopressin is not thought to be mediated by prostaglandins. Vasopressin levels are not decreased when the pain of dysmenorrhea is controlled by prostaglandin synthetase inhibitors.

There may be a familial tendency, as it is common to find that dysmenorrheic mothers have dysmenorrheic daughters. This condition seems to be more prevalent among women who have early menarche, have increased duration of menses, and smoke cigarettes. Pregnancy does not seem to affect its prevalence.

Much has been written about psychological factors in dysmenorrhea. Although purely psychological causes of dysmenorrhea occur rarely if ever, psychological factors may intensify or diminish the severity of pain (see Chap. 22).

The afferent sensory innervation of the uterus runs primarily with the autonomic sympathetic nerves. Transecting the sympathetic autonomic nerves (eg, in presacral neurectomy) promotes vasodilatation, interrupts sensory input from the uterus, and relieves the pain of dysmenorrhea. Also, relief of primary dysmenorrhea in some women after childbirth may be explained by the fact that short adrenergic neurons in the myometrium tend to be destroyed in pregnancy and do not regenerate afterward.

CLINICAL SYMPTOMS AND FINDINGS

Primary Dysmenorrhea

Primary dysmenorrhea usually begins 6 to 12 months after menarche, almost invariably coinciding with the onset of ovulatory cycles. Patients complain of spasmodic or cramping lower abdominal pain that may radiate suprapubically or to the inner aspect of the thighs. They may have backache of varying severity. They may also have other accompanying symptoms, such as headache, nausea, vomiting, diarrhea, or fatigue. Symptoms typically last 48 hours or less, but sometimes may last up to 72 hours.

A careful history and detailed examination are the key to diagnosing primary dysmenorrhea. It is a diagnosis of exclusion. The general physical examination and pelvic examination reveal no abnormality. Sometimes a laparoscopy may have to be performed to rule out pelvic pathology, particularly endometriosis.

Secondary Dysmenorrhea

Secondary dysmenorrhea is caused by identifiable pathologic conditions acting on the internal genital organs or pelvic peritoneum (Table 14-1). It tends to start at a later age than primary dysmenorrhea. However, endometriosis may be present soon after menarche and may be the cause of more cases of "primary" dysmenorrhea than generally recognized. Patients with secondary dysmenorrhea may have a history of menorrhagia, past pelvic inflammatory disease, infertility, dyspareunia, or use of an intrauterine contraceptive device.

The physical examination may reveal findings consistent with anemia secondary to heavy menstruation. A careful pelvic examination should be performed to look for uterine enlargement or irregularity, pelvic masses, or pelvic tenderness. A rectal examination should be done to assess nodularity and tenderness along the uterosacral ligaments and cul-de-sac, findings suggestive of endometriosis. The presence of an intrauterine device may be confirmed by finding its string at the cervix.

TABLE 14-1. Common Causes of Secondary Dysmenorrhea

Uterine
Adenomyosis
Leiomyomata
Endometrial polyps
Congenital malformation (ie, redundant uterine horn)
Cervical stenosis
Extrauterine
Endometriosis
Pelvic inflammatory disease
Pelvic congestion syndrome
Allen-Masters syndrome
Iatrogenic
Intrauterine contraception device
Psychogenic
Uncommon (learned behavior?)

LABORATORY AND IMAGING FINDINGS

No laboratory tests are diagnostic or specific to primary or secondary dysmenorrhea. Ca-125 levels may be elevated with endometriosis or leiomyomata, but there are several other causes of Ca-125 elevation that are not related to dysmenorrhea. Although prostaglandin levels have been measured experimentally in menstrual fluid, this is not a clinically useful test.

Ultrasonography, especially when performed transvaginally, may be useful to look for uterine leiomyomata, uterine enlargement, adnexal masses, endometrial polyps, or an unsuspected intrauterine device. It may also be useful for the nonoperative diagnosis of adenomyosis, but further investigation is needed. Hysterosalpingography often detects uterine anomalies, endometrial polyps, or Asherman syndrome. Cervical cultures for gonorrhea and cervical chlamydial antigen testing may be positive and helpful if pelvic inflammatory disease is suspected. Computed tomography and magnetic resonance imaging may be useful, but further experience with these modalities is needed to determine their role in the evaluation of dysmenorrhea.

Laparoscopy remains the most important diagnostic procedure to assess the pelvis for any pathology. Simultaneous hysteroscopy to evaluate the uterine cavity may also be useful.

TREATMENT

Successful management of dysmenorrhea can be challenging. For appropriate selection of treatment, it is usually helpful to determine if dysmenorrhea is primary or secondary.

Primary Dysmenorrhea

Oral contraceptives provide significant relief of primary dysmenorrhea. They suppress ovulation, resulting in lower levels of prostaglandins, and also markedly reduce spontaneous uterine activity. Oral contraceptives are a good first-line therapy for many young women, especially if contraception is also needed.

The NSAIDs that inhibit prostaglandin synthetase have had a pivotal role in treating primary dysmenorrhea for the last 20 years (Table 14-2). Unlike oral contraceptives, they need to be taken only 2 or 3 days per month and do not suppress the hypothalamic-pituitary-ovarian axis. Their primary therapeutic benefit is inhibition of prostaglandin formation. They provide relief in up to 80% of patients. It is hypothesized that patients whose pain is not relieved by NSAIDs have increased activity of the alternate lipoxygenase pathway of prostaglandin production.

The choice of a particular NSAID depends on the clinical efficacy, side effects, patient acceptance, and individual clinical experience. NSAIDs should be started at or just before the onset of pain and continued regularly during the symptomatic period. They should be taken on an "as needed" basis. If pain is inadequately controlled, the loading dose may be increased by up to 50% during the next cycle, but the maintenance dose should be kept the same. A trial of up to 6 months may be needed to demonstrate effective relief of symptoms.

The side effects of NSAIDs include gastric irritation, heartburn, abdominal pain, nausea, vomiting, headache, occasional visual disturbances, allergic reactions, and blood disorders. However, these are unusual when these drugs are used on an intermittent basis for dysmenorrhea.

TABLE 14-2. Nonsteroidal Antiinflammatory Drugs Commonly Used for Dysmenorrhea

DRUG	TRADE NAME	RECOMMENDED DOSAGE
Ibuprofen	Motrin, Advil, Rufen	400–800 mg q6-8h
Naproxen	Naprosyn	250–500 mg q6-8h
Mefenamic acid	Ponstel	250–500 mg q6h
Diclofenac	Voitarel	50 mg q8h
Naproxen sodium	Anaprox	275–500 q6-8h

Calcium antagonists such as verapamil and nifedipine reduce uterine activity and contractility. They have produced relief in some resistant cases of dysmenorrhea.

Transcutaneous electrical nerve stimulation effectively relieves pain in various conditions, including dysmenorrhea. It seems to act by blocking the transmission of pain impulses through the dorsal nerve horns and by its antiischemic effects. It relieves primary dysmenorrhea without any significant reduction of uterine activity and represents a nonpharmacologic treatment option. Acupuncture also effectively treats primary dysmenorrhea, probably via a similar mechanism.

Surgical interruption of neural pathways from the uterus may be done to decrease the pain of dysmenorrhea. Presacral neurectomy has greater than 80% efficacy in relieving midline dysmenorrhea. Uterine nerve ablation by transecting the uterosacral ligaments may be more easily performed than a presacral neurectomy, but it is less reliable in efficacy. Cervical dilatation has been historically used to relieve dysmenorrhea thought to be secondary to cervical stenosis. Its value is debatable, but it may act by promoting blood flow, by disrupting sensory nerves from the cervix, or by decreasing intrauterine pressure secondary to obstruction.

A healthy lifestyle, including nutritional supplements, and aerobic exercise such as brisk walking, swimming, and bicycling may produce an overall benefit and decrease the impact of dysmenorrhea on the patient's daily activities.

Secondary Dysmenorrhea

Therapy should be directed at the underlying condition. Women using intrauterine devices can be treated with NSAIDs or can have the device removed. NSAIDs may also offer an added benefit of reduced menstrual flow. Naproxen, mefenamic acid, and ibuprofen are used most commonly (see Table 14-2). It is important to rule out pelvic inflammatory disease in women with intrauterine devices.

Endometriosis is treated medically or surgically, depending on the severity of symptoms and the patient's age and parity. This is discussed in more detail in Chapter 22.

Leiomyomata uteri may be treated surgically with myomectomy or hysterectomy, again depending on the patient's age, parity, and symptom severity. Adenomyosis is usually treated by hysterectomy but may respond to conservative treatment with NSAIDs. Endometrial polyps may be removed via hysteroscopy or dilatation and curettage.

BIBLIOGRAPHY

Akerlund M, Stromberg P, Forslin MD. Primary dysmenorrhea and vasopressin. Br J Obstet Gynaecol 1979;86:484.

Aspland J. The uterine cervix and isthmus under normal and pathological conditions. Acta Radiol (Suppl) 1952;91:1.

Cibils LA. Contractibility of the non-pregnant human uterus. Obstet Gynecol 1967;30:441.

Dawood MY. Ibuprofen and dysmenorrhea. Am J Med 1984:87.

Goldstein DP, Cholkony C, Emanus JS. Adolescent endometriosis. J Adolesc Health Care 1980;1:37.

Pickles VR, Hall WJ, Bes FA, Smith CN. Prostaglandins in endometriosis and menstrual fluid from normal and dysmenorrheic subjects. Br J Obstet Gynaecol 1965;72:185.

Smith OW, Mass B. Menstrual toxin. Am J Obstet Gynecol 1947:54:201.

Sundell G, Milson I, Andersch B. Factors influencing the prevalence and severity of dysmenorrhea in young women. Br J Obstet Gynaecol 1990;97:588.

Primary Care for Women, edited by Phyllis C. Leppert and Fred M. Howard. Lippincott-Raven Publishers, Philadelphia © 1997.

15

Infertility

ROSALIND HAYES

Although infertility is not a life-threatening condition, it is a serious medical concern that affects quality of life and plagues about 10% to 15% of reproductive-age couples. The desire for childbearing has compelled millions of couples to seek competent care from physicians.

Infertility implies subfertility, a prolonged time to conceive, as opposed to sterility, which means inability to conceive. Multiple studies have shown that a normally fertile couple has approximately a 25% chance of conception in each ovulatory cycle. Guttmacher's classic 1956 study showed that 85% of couples attain pregnancy in 1 year and 93% by 2 years. Infertility is defined as failure to conceive within 1 year of unprotected intercourse. Primary infertility applies to a woman who has never been pregnant; secondary infertility applies to a woman who has been pregnant in the past.

This chapter will discuss the basic concepts involved in the diagnosis and treatment of the infertile couple.

ETIOLOGY

Infertility is commonly a multifactorial problem. Multiple factors in a female or at least one male and one female factor contributing to infertility may be identified. This highlights the need for a complete and systematic evaluation of the couple.

For women, about 40% of infertility cases involve ovulatory dysfunction, 40% involve tubal and pelvic pathology, 10% remain unexplained, and 10% are attributed to less-common problems. When couples have had a complete evaluation, the causes of infertility involve a male factor in 35%, tubal and pelvic pathology in 35%, and ovulatory dysfunction in 15%; 10% remain unexplained and 5% involve unusual problems. Unexplained infertility is perplexing and frustrating for patients and physicians. This does not imply that there is nothing wrong, rather that the explanation for failure to conceive is beyond the sensitivity of current testing and state of knowledge.

HISTORY

Historical information regarding fertility issues may help formulate a diagnosis and direct the evaluation and treatment. Pertinent avenues of questioning regarding ovulatory function include current age; age of menarche; pattern of menses; evidence suggestive of ovulation, including mittelschmerz, increase in midcycle cervical mucus, or molimina symptoms (premenstrual breast tenderness, abdominal bloating); current or past use of medications; or any breast discharge. Past use of oral contraceptives does not cause changes in ovulatory function. Questioning involving tubal or pelvic pathology is intended to elicit risk factors for pelvic adhesions or endometriosis. Patients should be asked about a history of in utero diethylstilbestrol (DES) exposure, intrauterine device use, pelvic inflammatory disease, genital infection or sexually transmitted disease, prior pelvic surgery, family history of endometriosis, pelvic pain, dysmenorrhea, and dyspareunia. Recording a male factor history involves inquiring about age; prior paternity; impotence or other sexual dysfunction; drug, heat, or toxin exposure; and reproductive organ congenital abnormality, infection, injury, or operation.

A history of adequate coital exposure should confirm that at least two acts of intercourse per cycle in the periovulatory period took place on repeated monthly attempts over the course of a year. Lubricants known to be spermicidal, such as K-Y Jelly, should not have been used.

PHYSICAL EXAMINATION

Important areas to evaluate during the physical examination include the reproductive tract and organs that interact with the reproductive hormones. The thyroid should be evaluated, particularly for goiter. Thyroid dysfunction is associated with ovulatory abnormalities. The breasts should be examined for galactorrhea. Hyperprolactinemia and galactorrhea are also associated with ovulatory dysfunction. Hirsutism, most commonly seen as facial hair and a male escutcheon, reflects the elevated free androgens characteristic of chronic anovulation.

When doing a pelvic examination, the clinician should inspect for genital malformations, vaginal and cervical abnormalities characteristic of in utero DES exposure, vaginal or cervical discharge, and other pathology, such as cervical polyps. A bimanual examination evaluates the size, mobility, positioning, and tenderness of the uterus and adnexa. Pertinent findings include nodularity of the uterosacral ligaments suggestive of endometriosis, fixation of the uterus or adnexa, uterine masses suggestive of fibroids, and adnexal masses requiring evaluation for ovarian pathology.

The physical examination in the male includes evaluation for anatomic abnormalities such as varicocele, hypospadias, and congenital absence of the vas deferens. Evaluation for infection includes checking the genitourinary tract for potential sources, including urethritis, epididymitis, prostatitis, or pyelonephritis.

LABORATORY AND IMAGING STUDIES

The basic infertility evaluation includes the following examinations:

- Assessment of ovulation: prolactin and thyroid-stimulating hormone (TSH), basal body temperature (BBT) charting, ovulation predictor kits, sonographic identification of follicle development, luteal-phase progesterone levels, and endometrial biopsy
- Assessment of uterine and tubal status: hysterosalpingography (HSG), hysteroscopy, and laparoscopy
- Cervical factor: postcoital test
- Male factor: semen analysis
- Peritoneal factor: laparoscopy.

Testing in the female is performed in specific time frames. HSG is scheduled in the midfollicular phase, after menstrual flow has stopped, typically between days 5 and 10 of a cycle. Postcoital testing is performed in the periovulatory period, preferably on the day before or the day of ovulation. An ultrasound performed at this time will confirm follicle development and appropriate timing of this test. Endometrial biopsies are done in the midluteal to late luteal phase, usually between days 21 and 27. Progesterone levels are obtained in the midluteal phase on day 21.

The reference to dates in the cycle is based on an idealized 28-day menstrual cycle. This is adapted to each woman according to her BBT chart. BBT recording is performed by using a BBT thermometer to record temperatures on first waking in the morning. Temperature charting is a useful exercise to track cycle length, estimate the time frame of ovulation, document the presence and length of the temperature rise in the luteal phase, evaluate the timing of intercourse retrospectively, and plan appropriate timing for the infertility evaluation. For those who cannot perform BBT charting, the evaluation is planned based on an estimated date of ovulation.

In women who have irregular, infrequent (> 35 days), or absent menstrual cycles, ovulation induction is required before an assessment of ovulatory adequacy can be made. Lack of adequate ovulation is generally made by history and can be confirmed if necessary by monophasic BBT charts, preovulatory levels of progesterone in the latter part of a cycle, a proliferative-phase reading on an endometrial biopsy, or lack of follicle development on ultrasound. About 5% of women who have apparent menstrual cycles are anovulatory. An elevated day 3 follicle-stimulating hormone level may reflect a perimenopausal state as the underlying cause of the ovulatory dysfunction.

Hysterosalpingography

HSG is performed in a radiology suite with fluoroscopic guidance. One or more x-rays are made for a permanent record. The patient may be instructed to take a dose of a nonsteroidal anti-inflammatory drug 30 to 60 minutes before the examination to act as an antispasmodic, as some cramping is commonly associated with the procedure. Local anesthesia applied to the anterior lip of the cervix with either a 3-mL injection of 1% lidocaine or a topical application of 2% lidocaine jelly will also help alleviate discomfort and decrease the false-positive occurrence of cornual obstruction due to tubal spasm.

With the patient in the lithotomy position, a speculum is placed, followed by cleansing of the cervix, administration of anesthesia, and then grasping the anterior lip of the cervix with a tenaculum. The cervix is cannulated with an acorn or Jarcho cannula or with a similarly designed apparatus for injecting contrast. The speculum is removed from the vagina to prevent obscuring the uterine contour. Oil- or water-based contrast is injected slowly and steadily while observing the uterine and tubal patterns under fluoroscopy. If possible, the x-rays are shown to the patient and the findings explained at the time of examination.

Important uterine findings include congenital abnormalities such as a unicornuate or septate uterus or acquired abnormalities seen as filling defects, which represent polyps, fibroids, or synechiae (intrauterine scarring). Tubal observations include patency or obstruction, the site of obstruction, the degree of tubal dilation, the presence of ampullar rugae, other tubal abnormalities such as cornual polyps, salpingitis isthmica nodosa, atypical tubal positioning, and the pattern of contrast dispersion. Loculated contrast dispersion suggests adnexal adhesions; free dispersion suggests their absence.

Abnormalities detected on a hysterosalpingogram require verification by endoscopic examination. Hysteroscopy allows a visual diagnosis of the etiology of the filling defects. Most uterine polyps, adhesions, septa, and many submucosal fibroids can be relieved by operative hysteroscopy at the time of diagnosis. Laparoscopy with chromotubation can confirm tubal obstruction and give a visual assessment of the fimbriae and the rest of the pelvis.

Postcoital Testing (Sims–Huhner Test)

Postcoital testing (PCT) is the only in vivo test to evaluate the interaction between the sperm and the cervical mucus. The patients should be instructed to have intercourse the day before or the day of expected ovulation. Optimally, the male should abstain from ejaculation 2 to 3 days before PCT. The female should be examined about 2 to 12 hours after intercourse. Showering before the PCT has no effect on the results, but douches and vaginal lubricants should not be used.

Mucus is collected from the cervical canal with either a tuberculin syringe without a needle or a nasal speculum. The mucus is placed on a glass slide, covered with a cover slip, and examined under 200× magnification. If a transvaginal ultrasound is performed to confirm correct timing of the PCT, the mucus sample should be collected before introduction of the probe.

Cervical mucus at midcycle should appear clear, acellular, thin, and stretchable (spinnbarkeit) to 8 to 10 cm and should display a fern pattern on drying, which reflects a high salt content. Sperm should be present and display linear motion. A finding of one or more motile sperm per high-power field (HPF) falls within the range of normal; more than 20 motile sperm/HPF indicates an increased likelihood of conception. A clearly abnormal PCT shows no sperm, no motile sperm, or no sperm with forward progression (shakers). Shakers can be further evaluated with sperm antibody testing. A normal PCT confirms appropriate coital technique, correct timing at midcycle, good-quality cervical mucus, absence of hostile mucus factors, and ability of sperm to survive in cervical mucus. An abnormal PCT may indicate incorrect timing of the test, poor mucus quality or poor semen quality, the presence of sperm antibody, or improper coital exposure, such as nonvaginal ejaculation. The most common reason for an abnormal PCT is incorrect timing of the test.

Evaluation of Ovulation

All infertile patients should have ovulatory function assessed, because a history of monthly menses is inadequate to conclude that ovulation is occurring and is optimal for conception. Prolactin and TSH should be checked when an ovulatory abnormality is suspected. Abnormal findings in the infertile population are common and can be effectively treated medically in most patients. BBT charts are also used to evaluate ovulation. These charts show a biphasic pattern, depicting a temperature rise at ovulation and maintenance of that temperature for 12 or more days. This indicates ovulation with an adequate luteal phase. Ovulation predictor kits or luteinizing hormone (LH) assays that detect the LH surge in a urine sample or in the serum, respectively, also help predict ovulation.

An ultrasound in the late follicular phase should show a mature follicle more than 18 mm in diameter. A postovulatory ultrasound should show disappearance of the follicle. Postovulation ultrasound characteristics may include a shrunken, collapsed, or absent follicle. Echolucency of the follicle may be replaced by echodensity, indicative of organizing hemorrhage or luteinizing tissue. Fluid around the ovary or in the cul-de-sac may be observed. Unchanged ultrasound appearance in the luteal phase may indicate an unruptured follicle.

Luteal phase evaluations include progesterone levels and endometrial biopsies. Progesterone levels peak in the midluteal phase on day 21 of an idealized 28-day cycle. Progesterone levels greater than 10 ng/dL are compatible with establishing a normal pregnancy; a level greater than 3 to 5 ng/dL is consistent with ovulation. Progesterone undergoes pulsatile secretion, which limits the value of a single reading representing only one point in time.

An endometrial biopsy provides histologic evaluation of the endometrium. It is performed with a plastic endometrial suction curet. The biopsy is a brief procedure but may cause cramping. The histology is judged by the criteria of Noyes and associates. The biopsy is performed 2 to 3 days before the expected menses, when the cumulative hormonal effects of that menstrual cycle are evident on the endometrium. Some argue that dating is more sensitive in the midluteal phase, when the state of the endometrium at the time of implantation can be seen.

A pathology report of the biopsy may identify proliferative endometrium, which indicates anovulation or endometritis that precludes dating. Patients with endometritis should be treated with 100 mg doxycycline twice each day for 14 days and undergo biopsy again to confirm resolution. An adequate report indicates a secretory endometrium characteristic of a postovulatory day. The patient is instructed to call to report the day of onset of menses after the biopsy. For purposes of interpreting the endometrial biopsy, the first day of bleeding is called day 28; the clinician must count backwards from the day of menses to the day the biopsy was performed. For example, if the biopsy was performed 3 days before the onset of menses, it should appear as a secretory day 25 endometrium. Alternatively, dating can be counted forward from the time of ovulation if a urine or serum LH surge was detected, counting day 14 as the day of ovulation.

A histologic lag of more than 2 days on two endometrial biopsies leads to a diagnosis of luteal-phase defect. The ambiguity of this diagnosis stems from the large number of isolated cycles fitting this criteria in normally fertile women, as well as from the high rate of interobserver discrepancies in dating the endometrium. The diagnosis is more substantial as the lag in dating increases to 5 days or more, as evidenced by a higher conception rate in response to treatment.

Laparoscopy

Laparoscopy is an endoscopic evaluation of the pelvis. The procedure is invasive and requires anesthesia, usually general. Because this test involves surgical risks and disability from work or other activities for 2 to 4 days, it is usually reserved as the last diagnostic procedure, but history, physical examination, HSG, or ultrasound findings that suggest tubal or peritoneal factors may indicate laparoscopy as an appropriate procedure earlier in the evaluation.

Diagnostic laparoscopies identify pelvic abnormalities in about 50% of cases. The most common findings are pelvic adhesions and endometriosis. Most findings can be treated laparoscopically at the time of diagnosis. A few diagnostic laparoscopies lead to a future laparotomy due to the location or extent of the pathology.

Preparing a patient for laparoscopy includes acquiring informed consent. The patient should understand that the risks of surgery include anesthesia complications, bleeding, infection, or damage to internal organs. Rarely, serious complications are encountered during laparoscopy that transform outpatient surgery into major surgery.

Male Factor

Every couple requesting an infertility evaluation should have the male evaluated by ordering a semen analysis (SA). The man is instructed to collect a masturbated semen specimen in a sterile container. For men who cannot do this, nonspermicidal condoms are available to collect a sample during intercourse.

The World Health Organization criteria are generally accepted guidelines for interpretation of SA:

- Volume: > 2 mL
- Sperm concentration: > 20 million/mL
- Motility: > 50% with forward progression
- Morphology: > 30% normal forms
- White blood cells: < 1 million/mL.

Men with an analysis outside these guidelines are asked to obtain a repeat test, because each ejaculate is different. There may be large fluctuations between samples due to individual variation or other influences, such as a febrile illness or medication exposure. A persistent abnormality in the SA should prompt a recommendation for urologic evaluation. Urologists may be helpful in defining congenital, acquired, hormonal, or infectious abnormalities.

TREATMENT

Cervical Factor

If a cervical factor, as defined by an abnormal PCT, is the sole reason for infertility, it is effectively treated by intrauterine insemination, which has a cumulative pregnancy rate of 35% in three or four cycles. A less reliable treatment alternative involves the addition of estrogen during the follicular phase, such as 0.625 to 1.25 mg conjugated estrogen daily. Guaifenesin is a mucolytic agent used to treat thick cervical mucus, but there are no data to show that such treatment results in increased pregnancy rates.

If cervical cultures are positive for *Chlamydia trachomatis* or *Ureaplasma urealyticum*, the patient and her partner are treated with 100 mg doxycycline orally twice a day for 7 days. If external lubricants are needed to have intercourse at midcycle, vegetable oil can be used without detrimental effects on sperm.

There is no method at this time for removing sperm antibodies. Potentially beneficial therapy involves intrauterine insemination, particularly with superovulation, or assisted reproduction technologies such as in vitro fertilization (IVF), with or without micromanipulation.

Ovulatory Dysfunction

The treatment for anovulation involves ovulation induction using clomiphene citrate, human menopausal gonadotropins, or pulsatile gonadotropin-releasing hormone. Ovulatory abnormalities, such as oligo-ovulation or luteal-phase defect, are treated with ovulation enhancement using the same agents. Hyperprolactinemia is treated with bromocriptine. Thyroid dysfunction is treated to produce a euthyroid state. Empiric treatment with bromocriptine or thyroid replacement in the face of normal thyroid function tests and prolactin levels is not helpful.

Uterine Factor

Corrective surgery for uterine septa, leiomyomata, polyps, or synechiae may be useful to optimize the endometrium for implantation. Surgery may involve hysteroscopy, laparoscopy, or laparotomy. Bicornuate, unicornuate, or hypoplastic uteri due to DES exposure usually do not benefit from surgical intervention.

Peritoneal Factor

Adnexal adhesion lysis by laparoscopy or laparotomy is advocated to optimize pickup of the ovum by the fallopian tube. Removal of endometriosis by laser vaporization, cauterization, or sharp excision is performed to restore functional adnexal anatomy, inhibit disease progression, and minimize toxic peritoneal factors.

Tubal Factor

The prognosis for pregnancy after tubal surgery varies inversely with the degree of tubal damage. Multiple sites of internal obstruction in a fallopian tube preclude surgical repair.

Proximal tubal obstruction may be relieved by tubal cannulization, resection and reanastomosis, or implantation. Isthmic and ampullar obstructions require resection and reanastomosis. Distal tubal surgery may involve fimbrioplasty or neosalpingostomy.

If surgical repair is impossible, if a failed attempt at repair occurs, or if tubal patency is present after repair but conception does not occur, IVF is indicated. IVF involves ovarian hyperstimulation, ovum retrieval, fertilization, and embryo transfer into the uterus. This procedure bypasses the fallopian tubes' function of gamete and embryo transport and location for fertilization.

Male Factor

Reproductive tract infections require antibiotic treatment. Consideration of varicocelectomy should be given to varicoceles associated with infertility and a compromised SA. Hypogonadotropic hypogonadism may respond to hormonal treatment with clomiphene citrate or human chorionic gonadotropin.

The most common semen abnormality is asthenospermia (low motility), followed by oligoasthenospermia (low count and low motility). Identifiable exacerbating factors should be relieved, including excess heat in the environment (from sources such as hot tubs, saunas, spas, and heated waterbeds), medications, recreational drugs, alcohol, and tobacco. Improved pregnancy rates result from a combination of superovulation and intrauterine insemination. If this treatment is unsuccessful, assisted reproductive technologies may be needed. .

Cervical inseminations or intrauterine inseminations in a natural cycle have not proven to be more beneficial than intercourse alone in the treatment of asthenospermia or oligoasthenospermia. Situations involving aspermia, severe compromises in the SA, or failed fertilization in IVF, or IVF with ICSI (intracytoplasmic sperm injection) are indications for the use of donor sperm.

Unexplained Infertility

When factors contributing to infertility cannot be identified, it is reasonable to offer empiric treatment. This treatment may involve measures with multiple effects intended to enhance a couple's chance of conceiving. Ovulation enhancement with clomiphene citrate or human menopausal gonadotropins, with or without intrauterine insemination, or assisted reproductive technologies with IVF or gamete intrafallopian transfer may be tried.

REFERRAL

Any patient who has tried to conceive unsuccessfully for a year or who has a known impediment to conception, such as amenorrhea, and desires a pregnancy requires evaluation. The evaluation and treatment may be undertaken by any physician trained to do so. Referral for evaluation and treatment of infertility should occur when the patient requests a referral or when the physician feels it is appropriate, considering his or her own training, facilities, comfort, and willingness to provide care for infertile patients. The time at which referrals should be made to gynecologists or reproductive endocrinologists varies widely.

It is reasonable to inform patients that 15% of couples have not conceived after 1 year and only 7% have not conceived after 2 years. Therefore, about half of couples conceive without active intervention between their first and second year of conception attempts. But it is inappropriate to inform couples that if they just relaxed and forgot about trying, they would be able to have a baby. Timely evaluation, treatment, and referral must be instituted for all patients requesting care. Advancing age is one of the more pressing issues.

BIBLIOGRAPHY

Herbst AL, Mishell Jr DR, Stenchever MA, Droegmueller W. Comprehensive gynecology, 2d ed. St. Louis: Mosby Year Book, 1992.

Keye Jr WR. Unexplained infertility. Endocrine and Fertility Forum 1993;16:1.

Rowe PJ, Comhaire FH, Hargreave TB, Mellows HJ. WHO manual for standardized investigation and diagnosis of the infertile couple. Cambridge: Cambridge University Press, 1993.

Seibel MM. Infertility: a comprehensive test. East Norwalk: Appleton & Lange, 1990.

Speroff L, Glass RH, Kase NG. Clinical gynecologic endocrinology and infertility, 5th ed. Baltimore: Williams & Wilkins, 1994.

16

Contraception

DEREK TENHOOPEN

Primary Care for Women, edited by Phyllis C. Leppert and Fred M. Howard. Lippincott-Raven Publishers, Philadelphia © 1997.

Primary care physicians must help prevent the 3.5 million unplanned pregnancies that occur in the United States each year. Although the ideal method of contraception will probably never be developed, various effective methods of birth control now exist. When providing information about contraception, the clinician must carefully explain the advantages and disadvantages of each method.

Because male contraceptive choices are so limited, the clinician generally counsels the female partner. Data from the National Survey of Family Growth reveals that about 39 million women are at risk for unintended pregnancy. Of these, 90% use some form of contraception; unfortunately, the 10% of women who do not account for 53% of the unintended pregnancies, half of which end in abortion.

The choice of contraception often depends on whether the couple plans to have additional children. Women who do usually choose oral contraceptives; those who do not usually choose sterilization.

Thus, the percentage choosing one particular method (and the choices currently available) varies widely. The estimated percentage using oral contraceptives is 27.7%; tubal sterilization, 24.8%; vasectomy, 10.5%; barrier methods, 13.1%; long-acting progestins, 8.0%; natural family planning, 2.1%; withdrawal, 2%; the intrauterine device (IUD), 1.8%; and spermicides, 1.7%. Those using no method account for about 9.9%. The contraceptive sponge was recently removed from the market.

Contraceptives vary widely in effectiveness. Failure rates range from as low as 0.1% to as high as 52%. Education and counseling by the primary care physician play a major role in lowering the failure rate and increasing the compliance rate. With proper guidance and accurate information, every couple may make an informed decision and rationally choose the method most appropriate for them.

ORAL CONTRACEPTIVE PILLS

Oral contraceptive pills (OCPs), chosen by about 28% of women, are the most widely chosen form of reversible contraception. This is due in part to their extremely high rate of effectiveness and ease of administration. There are three major types of OCP formulations: fixed-dose combination, multiphasic combination, and daily progestin-only. OCPs are derived from synthetic steroids and contain no natural estrogens or progestins. The only estrogen used (except for two higher-dose brands) is ethinyl estradiol. In contrast, five longstanding progestins (norethindrone, norethindrone acetate, ethynodiol diacetate, norethynodrel, and levonorgestrel) and three recently approved progestins (desogestrel, norgestimate, and gestodene) are present in current formulations. The newer progestins were approved by the FDA in 1993 and reportedly have greater progestational activity but are less androgenic.

The combination formulations are the most widely used and the most effective. They consist of tablets containing both an estrogen and a progestin taken continuously for 3 weeks, followed by a 1-week steroid-free interval that allows withdrawal bleeding to occur. The multiphasic combination OCPs were developed to lower the total dose of steroid, primarily the progestin, without increasing the incidence of breakthrough bleeding. These formulations contain two or three different amounts of the same estrogen and progestin.

The progestin-only formulations consist of tablets containing a progestin without any estrogen. They must be taken daily without a steroid-free interval. They are used in women who cannot tolerate estrogen or if estrogen intake is contraindicated. The incidence of breakthrough bleeding and the pregnancy rate are slightly higher.

Many of the most common symptoms produced by combination OCPs are due to the estrogen component. These include nausea, breast tenderness, and fluid retention. However, the incidence of these side effects is lower because current formulations contain less estrogen than previous ones; in fact, current OCPs have a three- to fourfold lower dose of estrogen and a tenfold lower dose of progestin. Because failure rates remained constant despite these changes, there was no longer a need to manufacture or prescribe higher-dose pills.

The effectiveness of OCPs is primarily based on consistent inhibition of the midcycle gonadotropin surge, thus preventing ovulation. Other effects include alteration of the cervical mucus, which makes it viscid and scanty, retarding sperm penetration. They also alter motility of the uterus and fallopian tubes, impairing transport of both ova and sperm. The endometrium is altered so that its glandular production of glycogen is diminished and less energy is available for the blastocyst to survive in the uterine cavity.

OCPs also have substantial metabolic effects—in fact, the estrogen component and the progestin component have different, and sometimes opposite, effects. The symptoms most commonly caused by the estrogen component include nausea, breast tenderness, and fluid retention (from decreased sodium excretion). Less common are mood changes, sleepiness, and depression. The progestins, because they are structurally related to testosterone, may produce weight gain, acne, and nervousness.

OCPs also offer many noncontraceptive health benefits. Due to the antiestrogenic action of progesterone, the endometrium is thinner than that seen in a normal cycle, resulting in less blood loss and a 50% reduction in the risk of iron-deficiency anemia. Users are less likely to develop menorrhagia or irregular menstruation and about half as likely to develop endometrial cancer. By inhibiting ovulation, OCPs decrease dysmenorrhea and premenstrual tension and protect against functional ovarian cysts. OCP users have a 40% reduced risk of developing ovarian cancer. The incidence of clinical salpingitis among OCP users is 50% less than that of a control group using no method.

OCPs have not been shown to interfere with the action of other drugs, despite their metabolism in the liver. However, some drugs can interfere clinically with the action of OCPs, decreasing their effectiveness. These include barbiturates, cyclophosphamide, sulfonamides, and rifampin. Women should be instructed to use some form of barrier contraception while taking these drugs. It is less clear whether the penicillins or cephalosporins have such an effect; generally, the use of additional barrier methods of contraception is not recommended to women taking these antibiotics.

OCPs may be prescribed to most healthy women of reproductive age. The few absolute contraindications are a present or past history of vascular disease, including thromboembolism, deep thrombophlebitis, atherosclerosis, and cerebrovascular accident; a systemic disease that may affect the vascular system, such as hemoglobin SS disease or systemic lupus erythematosus; tobacco use by women over age 35; hypertension; diabetes mellitus with vascular disease; severe hyperlipidemia; and active liver disease (however, women with a history of liver disease whose liver function test results are normal may use OCPs).

Relative contraindications to OCP use include heavy cigarette smoking (> 15 cigarettes per day), depression, and migraine headaches. Women who develop frequent or severe headaches, fainting, paresthesias, or loss of speech or vision should stop taking OCPs immediately. In addition, many women develop mild hypertension while using OCPs and likewise should be advised to stop them. For this reason, the woman's blood pressure should be rechecked 3 months after starting this form of contraception.

Prescribing guidelines for OCPs are relatively simple. At the initial office visit, a history and physical examination should be performed. The physical examination must include a breast and pelvic examination with a Pap smear. The blood pressure and weight should be recorded as well. If there is no medical contraindication to the use of OCPs, the patient should be informed of the benefits, risks, and alternatives. These should likewise be noted in the patient's chart. At the end of 3 months of OCP use, the patient should be seen again and the blood pressure measured. The patient should be seen at least once a year, at which time a nondirected history should be taken, blood pressure and body weight measured, and a physical examination performed. Again, this must include a breast, abdominal, and pelvic examination with a Pap smear.

In determining which formulation to use, it is best initially to prescribe a formulation with less than 50 μg of ethinyl estradiol, as these agents have fewer estrogenic side effects. (Theoretically, this may also lessen the chance of a thromboembolic event.) The formulation with the lowest dose of a particular progestin should be chosen because this mitigates progestational metabolic and clinical adverse effects. Many women cease using OCPs due to these progestational effects, which often include androgenic side effects. Thus, the OCP formulations that contain the newer progestins (including desogestrel, norgestimate, and gestodene, as noted earlier) may increase compliance rates.

Primary care physicians must improve patient compliance with OCPs. Discontinuation falls into the category of noncompliance and contributes to the alarming number of unintended pregnancies seen each year. About 25% of OCP users in the United States discontinue use of this method during the first year, many without adopting an alternative means of birth control. Reducing the user failure rate by just 1% would prevent nearly 170,000 accidental pregnancies each year in the United States alone. Among women who stop using OCPs, side effects or fears of potential side effects are cited as the most frequent reason. Careful education and anticipatory guidance as to the nuisance side effects are a necessity. Women must be made aware of the fact that breakthrough bleeding, amenorrhea, actual or perceived weight gain, nausea, headaches, and mood changes are often transient.

A woman should take the pill at night (which lessens the possibility of nausea) and should use a given OCP for at least three cycles to evaluate its effects. During the first month of use, up to 30% of women may have breakthrough bleeding; the proportion drops to less than 10% during the third month. Other clinical recommendations for improving oral contraceptive compliance are given in Table 16-1.

Any woman who does not fulfill one of the absolute contraindications to the use of OCPs is a candidate for their use. However, the woman must be compliant and must remember to take a pill each day.

The failure rate for OCPs, if used properly, is among the lowest of all forms of birth control: they are about 99.9% effective.

Table 16-1. Clinical Recommendations for Improving Oral Contraceptive Compliance

1. All oral contraceptive users should know three things before they start taking their pills:
   a. How to take the oral contraceptive prescribed
   b. What to do if they miss a pill or pills
   c. Which side effects are common and usually transient (breakthrough bleeding and nausea), and which are potentially serious and should be brought immediately to their clinician's attention.
2. Simple instructions should be provided to all patients both verbally and in writing; a copy of written instructions should be discussed with the patient point by point during the visit. Another copy of written instructions should be offered at each follow-up visit.
3. Show each patient who is starting a new brand of pill (and especially first-time oral contraceptive users) how to use the specific package being prescribed. Use of the 28-day package enhances compliance.
4. Help women select a specific time of day to take their pills; a brief discussion of their daily schedules may help identify an optimal time of day. Taking the pill after dinner or with a bedtime snack lessens the possibility of nausea. Patients who skip breakfast may find that taking the pill in the morning leads to nausea and sometimes vomiting.
5. The refill prescription should include an additional cycle to accommodate missed pills or lost packets.
6. The use of a back-up method and the availability of emergency contraception should be discussed.
7. Discuss prevention of sexually transmitted diseases (STDs). Provide the OC user with a condom and discuss its proper use.
8. On follow-up visits, ask patients if they have had any problems taking their pills; ask what they did when they missed pills. A nonjudgmental approach encourages honesty and can help uncover and solve potential problems.
9. Oral contraceptive users who have repeated difficulty remembering to take their pills, or other serious compliance problems, should be counseled about other available methods.

(Grimes DA. Oral contraceptive compliance: strategies for ensuring correct and continued use of the pill. Contraception Report 1994;5:3.)

LONG-ACTING CONTRACEPTIVE STEROIDS

Chosen by about 8% of couples, this method of contraception includes the injectable progestational suspensions and the subdermal implant (Norplant). They provide a highly effective, long-acting, estrogen-free, reversible method of contraception.

Of the injectable steroid formulations, three types are available, but only one, depo-medroxyprogesterone acetate (DMPA), has been approved for use in the United States. DMPA (Depo-Provera) is an aqueous suspension of microcrystals that is given by intramuscular injection every 12 weeks (not every 3 months). Contraceptive protection is immediate. It acts by inhibiting the midcycle surge of luteinizing hormone. Mean serum estradiol levels remain higher than menopausal levels so that patients do not develop signs and symptoms of estrogen deficiency (eg, vaginal dryness or atrophy, hot flushes, decreased bone density). The first injection is generally given within the first 5 days after menses. This should exclude pregnancy and lessen menstrual irregularities (the most common reason for discontinuing this method). Other side effects include amenorrhea, mild weight gain, and headache. Less common untoward reactions include abdominal discomfort, nervousness, dizziness, depression, and acne. In addition, the return of fertility may be delayed in some women, depending on the number of months of use.

DMPA may be used in postpartum women; those who are not breastfeeding may be given the injection within 5 days after delivery. These women should receive the injection before being discharged from the hospital. In nursing mothers, the injection should be delayed until lactation is well established.

Candidates for DMPA use include women in whom exogenous estrogen is contraindicated or those who cannot tolerate estrogens, women who dislike taking a pill daily or simply cannot remember to do so (often making this an ideal method for teenage women), or women who want a long-acting, coitus-independent, convenient method of birth control.

The second method of contraception in this category is the subdermal implant system. This form of birth control consists of the subdermal placement of six Silastic capsules containing levonorgestrel. It too is a highly effective, estrogen-free, long-term method of contraception. Insertion is performed on an outpatient basis by implanting six capsules just under the skin in the upper, inner area of the arm. They are effective for 5 years. Its primary mechanism of action is the inhibition of the midcycle surge of luteinizing hormone, thus preventing ovulation. Other actions include effects on cervical mucus and sperm penetration, as well as effects on the endometrial lining and implantation. The major side effect is similar to that of DMPA—menstrual irregularities. Other untoward effects include headache, weight gain, acne, depression, anxiety, abdominal discomfort, and hirsutism.

Controversy surrounds the use of Norplant, especially in the lay press. It has been blamed for a whole host of atypical side effects. Compounding the problem are its cost (about $650, but this should include both insertion and removal) and the difficult decision-making process in early removal. Many clinicians recommend a trial of DMPA for several months. If the patient tolerates the injectable progesterone well, she will probably tolerate the subdermal implants. The manufacturer is also aware of some of the problems and has attempted to improve the current product. Removal is often difficult, given the need to locate six capsules. The second-generation product, Norplant 2, consists of two 40-mm solid silicone rods impregnated with the same progesterone as the original (levonorgestrel). However, it is reportedly more easily inserted and removed than the conventional Norplant, while retaining the earlier product's safety and efficacy.

Candidates for Norplant are women who are seeking long-term birth control, such as those who have completed their families, but who do not want permanent sterilization. In addition, teenage mothers, noncompliant patients, and women who must avoid estrogen are other excellent candidates.

Failure rates for these two long-acting contraceptive steroids are similar, at about 0.1%.

BARRIER CONTRACEPTION

Barrier contraception, chosen by about 13% to 15% of couples, includes the diaphragm, the cervical cap, and the male and female condoms. Two new devices, the Femcap and the Lea's shield, are entering final clinical trials and may be on the market in the near future.

Diaphragm and Cervical Cap

The diaphragm must be carefully fitted by the practitioner. The largest size that does not cause discomfort or undue pressure on the vaginal mucosa should be used. The cervical cap comes in four sizes. It is smaller than the diaphragm, fits closely over the cervix, and relies on suction to stay in place. Its advantages includes comfort and the ability to be left in place for up to 48 hours. A spermicide should be used and placed inside each device. Both devices should be left in place for at least 8 hours after the last coital act, but no longer than 24 hours or 48 hours, respectively. If repeated intercourse takes place or if coitus occurs more than 8 hours after insertion, additional contraceptive cream or jelly should be used. Diaphragm users have a lower risk for developing clinical gonococcal infection but have a higher rate of cystitis than nonusers.

Effectiveness requires motivation, and failure rates decline with increasing age and increasing usage. Failure rates range from 6% to 21%.

Male Condom

The male condom is made of latex rubber. It should not be applied too tightly. The tip should extend beyond the end of the penis by about a half-inch to collect the ejaculate. Latex condoms can reduce the transmission rate of sexually transmitted diseases, including HIV, gonorrhea, chlamydia, and herpes. The incidence of cervical neoplasia is also reduced. For men or women with an allergy to latex or men who desire greater sensitivity, condoms made of lamb's intestine are available, but they do not protect against HIV.

Candidates for the use of the condom as the primary form of birth control include couples with a high level of motivation, as it is coitus-dependent. Any man or woman with multiple sexual partners should be encouraged to use a condom, regardless of whether another form of birth control is also being used.

Effectiveness depends on the user and may be as high as 98% in the motivated couple. However, the overall failure rate approaches about 18%.

Female Condom

The female condom is made of polyurethane that resists tearing during use. It too reduces the transmission rate of sexually transmitted diseases, including HIV. It is disposable and designed for a single coital act. It can be inserted several hours before sexual intercourse. Again, the ideal candidates are highly motivated couples. The failure rate is reportedly as high as 25%, but this is believed to result primarily from improper use.

SPERMICIDES

Chosen by about 2% of couples, vaginal spermicides include foams, creams, suppositories, and jellies. Also included in this category was the contraceptive sponge, recently removed from the market. All spermicides contain a surfactant, usually nonoxynol-9, that immobilizes or kills sperm on contact. Because they also provide a chemical barrier, they must be placed into the vagina before each coital act. They are most effective when used with a device to hold them in place. Spermicides may inhibit certain sexually transmitted diseases as well as the development of cervical cancer. The disadvantage is that this method is messy and sometimes difficult to use.

Vaginal spermicides require a moderate degree of motivation, and thus effectiveness increases with age. The ideal candidates are older women who are unable or unwilling to use other forms of birth control. They should be instructed to use this method in combination with a barrier contraceptive. The failure rate may approach 22% to 26% and is believed to result from incorrect or inconsistent use.

NATURAL FAMILY PLANNING OR PERIODIC ABSTINENCE

Chosen by about 2% of couples, this method involves no drugs, devices, or surgery. To be effective, it requires a highly motivated couple who can accurately predict their most fertile interval. This method requires abstinence by most women with regular menstrual cycles for almost one third of the days of each cycle; thus, it has a high failure rate and a high rate of discontinuation.

There are four techniques for determining the fertile interval: the calendar rhythm method, the basal body temperature method, the cervical mucus method, and the symptothermal method. Only the latter should be used. The symptothermal method uses several indices to determine the fertile period rather than relying on a single physiologic index. It uses both calendar calculations and changes in the cervical mucus to estimate the onset of the fertile period and changes in the mucus and basal temperature to estimate its end. Although more effective, this method is more difficult to learn.

With the need to abstain from sexual intercourse for many days during the menstrual cycle, many women choose to use barrier methods or spermicides during the fertile period. In addition, home ovulation predictor kits may help define the fertile interval more accurately. Because such assays lead to a reduction in the number of days of abstinence, this may improve the effectiveness and acceptance of this method.

Candidates for natural family planning are limited to highly motivated couples intelligent enough to comprehend the subtleties of this method. It may also be the only method available to strict practicing Roman Catholics and other religious couples. The overall failure rate approaches 15% to 20%.

INTRAUTERINE DEVICE

Chosen by about 2% of couples, the IUD is a highly effective method of birth control that has recently gained some resurgence in popularity. The advantages include a lack of systemic metabolic effects, no coitally related responsibility, and the need for only a single act of motivation for long-term use. For these reasons, combined with the need for a second visit to a health care professional for removal, IUDs have one of the highest continuation rates of all reversible methods of birth control. Classic contraindications to its use include nulliparity, a history of pelvic infection, current involvement in a nonmonogamous relationship, and uterine malformation, but more recent studies challenge these long-held concepts. For example, some believe it is no longer contraindicated to place an IUD in a properly selected nulliparous woman.

Two IUDs are approved for use in the United States: the progesterone-releasing IUD known as the Progestasert, which must be replaced annually; and the Copper T-380A, known as the Paragard, which was recently approved for 10 years of use (the presence of copper increases its effectiveness).

The IUD's main mechanism of action is spermicidal, produced by a local sterile inflammatory reaction caused by the presence of a foreign body in the uterus. This inflammatory reaction also impedes the ability of the blastocyst to implant. Adverse effects include uterine bleeding, perforation of the uterus at the time of insertion, infection-related complications, pregnancy-related complications, and expulsion. During the first year of IUD use, the expulsion rate is about 10%, but up to 20% of all expulsions go unnoticed by the user. Thus, clinicians must stress the importance of periodic palpation of the string. The incidence of all major adverse events, including unplanned pregnancy, steadily diminishes in subsequent years and with increasing age.

Several epidemiologic studies have confirmed that if pregnancy occurs with an IUD in place, it is more likely to be an ectopic pregnancy. Thus, if a pregnancy does occur, the patient must be followed diligently with serum quantitative β-hCG levels and early transvaginal ultrasound to confirm viability.

Resumption of fertility after IUD removal is not delayed. It occurs at the same rate as the resumption of fertility after discontinuation of mechanical methods of contraception, such as the condom or diaphragm.

The best candidates for IUD use are parous women with stable, monogamous sexual relationships. For women who have completed their families but do not opt for sterilization, or women who cannot take OCPs, this may be the method of choice. The first-year failure rate ranges from less than 1% to 3.7%, but as noted this declines steadily in subsequent years.

SURGICAL STERILIZATION

Surgical sterilization, chosen by about 35% of couples, is the most widely used form of contraception. In contrast to the other forms of birth control, which are reversible or temporary, sterilization should be considered permanent. Voluntary sterilization is legal in all 50 states, and the decision to be sterilized should be made solely by the patient in consultation with the physician. An informed consent discussing the risks, benefits, permanence, irreversibility, and failure rate and a detailed list of alternative methods of contraception must be obtained.

Female Sterilization

Female sterilization, which is chosen by about 25% of couples, may be performed on an outpatient basis, usually by the laparoscopic two-puncture technique or as an inpatient following a vaginal delivery. It may also be performed at the time of cesarean section. Sterilization of the female, regardless of technique, is more complicated than sterilization of the male. The laparoscopic technique requires general anesthesia, with its inherent risks. In addition, although rare, the risk of bowel or bladder injury exists. The failure rate is about 0.2%.

Male Sterilization

Male sterilization or vasectomy, chosen by about 10% of couples, is an outpatient procedure that takes about 20 minutes and requires only local anesthesia. Complications include hematoma, sperm granulomas, infection, and spontaneous reanastomosis (if this is to occur, it does so within a short time after the procedure). Unlike female sterilization, effective male sterilization is not immediate. The male is not considered sterile until two sperm-free ejaculates have been produced. Semen analyses should be performed 1 and 2 months after the procedure. Usually about 15 to 20 ejaculations are required after the operation before the male is sterile. The failure rate is about 0.1%.

The ideal candidate for sterilization, male or female, has completed childbearing and is certain he or she wants no additional children, regardless of the possibility of remarriage.

POSTCOITAL CONTRACEPTION

Postcoital or "morning after" contraception is used to prevent pregnancy after unprotected intercourse, failure of a barrier method, or rape. Although there is debate about the magnitude of the protective effect, few people question the important role that postcoital contraception can play in preventing unwanted pregnancy and thus maternal mortality and morbidity resulting from unsafe abortion. Every primary care practitioner concerned with improving women's reproductive health should be familiar with and should provide postcoital contraception.

The development of hormonal methods of postcoital contraception dates back to the 1960s, when the first human trials of postcoitally administered high-dose estrogens were undertaken. Given in the postovulatory period, this should prevent implantation. The most popular regimen involves the administration of a combined high-dose estrogen-progesterone pill. Its popularity is based on proven safety with minimal side effects. Although the choice of which hormone should be used varies, treatment should begin as soon as possible after coitus. If initiated within 72 hours after an isolated midcycle act of intercourse, its effectiveness is very good. If more than one episode of coitus occurred or if treatment is initiated 72 hours after intercourse, the method is much less effective.

Other compounds that have been tested more recently include danazol, levonorgestrel, and the antiprogesterone mifepristone (RU-486). Some have even advocated the placement of an IUD. The current recommendation is that the combination oral contraceptive Ovral should be given in doses of two tablets 12 hours apart.

CONCLUSION

Although the ideal method of contraception will probably never be available, current methods are such that with proper education, counseling, and support every patient should have the opportunity to prevent an unwanted or unplanned pregnancy. Because of their unique relationship with patients, primary care physicians can obtain a proper and thorough sexual history and can help prevent the 3.5 million unplanned pregnancies that occur in the United States each year.

BIBLIOGRAPHY

Chi I. What we have learned from recent IUD studies: a researcher's perspective. Contraception 1993;48:81.

Dickey RP. Managing contraceptive pill patients, 7th ed. Durant, OK: CIP Inc, 1993:12.

Fertility Control Precis V: An Update in Obstetrics and Gynecology, 5th ed. Washington DC: American College of Obstetrics and Gynecology, 1994:56.

Grimes DA. Oral contraceptive compliance: strategies for ensuring correct and continued use of the pill. Contraception Report 1994;5:3.

Grimes DA. Thirty years of change: the current perspectives on cardiovascular risks and oral contraceptives. Contraception Report 1995;6:4.

Mishell DR Jr. Contraception, sterilization, and pregnancy termination. In: Herbst AL, Mishell DR Jr, Stenchever MA, Droegemueller W, eds. Comprehensive gynecology, 2d ed. St. Louis: Mosby Year Book, 1992:295.

Mishell DR Jr. Noncontraceptive benefits of oral contraceptives. J Reprod Med 1993;38:1021.

Stampfer MF, Willet WC, Colditz GA, Speizer FE, Hennekens CH. A prospective study of past use of oral contraceptive agents and risk of cardiovascular disease. N Engl J Med 1988;319:1313.

Van Look PF, von Hertzen H. Emergency contraception. Br Med Bull 1993;49:158.

17
Sterilization

REINALDO SANCHEZ

Primary Care for Women, edited by Phyllis C. Leppert and Fred M. Howard. Lippincott-Raven Publishers, Philadelphia © 1997.

Sterilization is one of the most common methods used for contraception. As shown in Table 17-1, combined female and male sterilization accounted for 48.7% of contraceptive use by 1988, with female sterilization being chosen by 31.4% for married couples and 27.5% for all women aged 15 to 44 years.

Female sterilization is an effective method for preventing future pregnancies, with a failure rate of 1 to 3 per 1000. It is also relatively simple and safe, with major complications occurring in less than 1% of cases.

Different surgical techniques have comparable efficacy and safety. Therefore, in the selection process, the surgeon's preference and expertise combined with individual patient's needs determine the technique of choice in each particular case. It is important as primary care givers to be able to explain to patients the different

Table 17-1. Percentage Distribution and Number (in Thousands) of All Contraceptive Users Aged 15 to 44 Years and of All Currently Married Users, by Current Method, 1990

METHOD	ALL USERS		CURRENTLY MARRIED USERS	
	%	*No.*	*%*	*No.*
Sterilization	39.2	13,686	48.7	10,561
Female	27.5	9614	31.4	6806
Male	11.7	4069	17.3	3755
Oral contraceptive	30.7	10,734	20.4	4409
IUD	2.0	703	2.0	427
Diaphragm	5.7	2000	6.2	1335
Condom	14.6	5093	14.3	3103
Foam	1.1	371	1.4	293
Per. abstinence	2.3	806	2.8	603
Withdrawal	2.2	778	2.3	503
Other	2.1	76	1.9	423
Total	100.0	34,912	100.0	21,657

(Modified from: Mosher WD. Contraceptive practice in the United States, 1982–1988. Fam Plann Perspec 1990;22:198.)

options and modalities when permanent surgical contraception is considered.

PREOPERATIVE EVALUATION

A complete history and physical examination are mandatory. Furthermore, significant emphasis needs to be given to identify anesthesia, surgical, and psychosocial risk factors. Gynecologic pathology such as abnormal cervical cytologic findings, menstrual disorders, symptomatic pelvic relaxation, and neoplasia must be excluded or, if identified, treated appropriately.

Risk factors for regret after sterilization should be considered during the preoperative counseling (Table 17-2). It has been well documented that age at the time of the surgery has an inverse relationship to the percentage of patients regretting a surgical sterilization.

Long-term effects of tubal sterilization should be part of the counseling. Data on long-term effects on menstrual patterns are controversial, with some studies showing an increase in menstrual dysfunction and others showing no effect. Some studies show a small increase in the likelihood of future hysterectomy for these patients. Whether this is secondary to differences in the type of patient who decides to have a tubal sterilization or a decreased threshold for hysterectomy from the patient or physician is not clear.

Evaluation of preexisting medical conditions influences the anesthesia of choice. The most commonly used surgical techniques have been successfully done under sedation and local anesthetic, but the preferred anesthesia method is general anesthesia.

Tubal sterilization should be presented as a permanent procedure. Failure rates, whether intrauterine or ectopic pregnancies, and complications related to the surgical technique require adequate discussion and documentation. In the case of mental retardation or psychiatric disorder, consultation is warranted to determine the capability of the patient to understand and give consent for the procedure.

Table 17-2. Regret After Tubal Sterilization, by Selected Baseline Characteristics*

CHARACTERISTIC	RATE	ODDS RATIO	CI
Age (y)			
< 20	6.5	2.9	1.2–7.0
20–24	4.3	1.9	1.4–2.5
25–29	3.1	1.3	1.0–1.7
30–34	2.4	1	Referent
> 34	1.2	0.5	0.4 to 0.7
Timing of sterilization			
Interval	2.1	1	Referent
Postvaginal delivery	3.0	1.4	1.0–2.0
Postcesarean section	4.4	2.1	1.5–2.9
Postabortion	2.6	1.2	0.7–2.1
History of abortion			
Yes	3.0	1.3	1.1–1.7
No	2.3	1	Referent
Method of payment			
Private insurance	2.1	1	Referent
Medicaid	3.7	1.8	1.4–2.3
Time after sterilization (y)			
1	1.8	1	Referent
2	2.8	1.5	1.3–1.8
3	2.5	1.4	1.2–1.7
4	2.2	1.2	0.9–1.6
5	3.1	1.7	1.4–2.1
Marital status			
Married	2.3	1	Referent
Not married	2.7	1.2	0.9–1.5
Education (y)			
< 13	2.4	1	Referent
13–16	2.3	0.9	0.7–1.2
> 16	3.4	1.4	0.9–2.4
Employed			
Yes	2.7	1	Referent
No	2.1	0.8	0.6–1.0
No. of living children			
0	1.9	0.8	0.5–1.4
1	2.7	1.2	0.9–1.6
2	2.2	1	Referent
> 2	2.5	1.1	0.9–1.4
Race			
White	2.4	1.0	Referent
Black	2.4	1.0	0.8–1.3
Other	2.2	0.9	0.5–1.8

*Adjusted rate per 100 women, adjusted odds ratios, and 95% CI rates and odds ratios adjusted for all other characteristics listed in table and for institution.

CI, confidence interval.

(Wilcox LS, Chu SY, Eaker ED, Zeger SL, Peterson HB. Risk factors for regret after tubal sterilization: 5 years of follow up in a prospective study. Fertil Steril 1991;55:930.)

SURGICAL TECHNIQUES

The pelvis can be accessed through the vaginal or the abdominal route. Minilaparotomy and laparoscopy are the choices for interval abdominal surgery, infraumbilical incision for postpartum tubal sterilization, and posterior colpotomy if the procedure is done vaginally.

For the laparoscopic approach, either a closed or an open technique can be used. The closed method is preferred by most gynecologic laparoscopic surgeons. The patient is placed in low dorsolithotomy position, the abdomen and vagina are cleansed, the bladder is emptied, and a uterine manipulator is inserted. For the closed technique, a small periumbilical incision is done, the abdominal wall is elevated, and direct trocar insertion of a 10- or 11-mm trocar follows. Under direct visualization, a pneumoperitoneum is developed by insufflating with carbon dioxide. The pneumoperitoneum can be developed before the insertion of the trocar by using a Veress needle if preferred by the surgeon. The open technique uses a similar periumbilical incision, but the incision is continued in layers until the peritoneal cavity is entered, the fascia is sutured with 0 synthetic absorbable suture in each corner, and a special trocar designed for the open method is inserted and secured. The main advantage of open laparoscopy is that it prevents major vascular injury. Although rare, such injury is a very serious complication, requiring immediate laparotomy. For patients with documented abdominopelvic adhesive disease or with risk factors for it, a left upper quadrant entrance is an excellent option. Once the laparoscope is inserted, the operator decides the number of punctures and the size of the extra trocars required for the type of surgical procedure selected, with single puncture or double puncture being the most popular.

If the selected incision is minilaparotomy, a 3-cm transverse incision is done 2 to 3 cm above the superior aspect of the symphysis pubis in layers. A transverse incision of the fascia of the rectus abdominis exposes the muscles, which then are separated in the midline, followed by opening the peritoneum and entering the abdominopelvic cavity. Using a uterine manipulator greatly facilitates minilaparotomy sterilizations.

For vaginal tubal sterilizations, the cervix is grasped at the posterior lip with a tenaculum or it is sutured temporarily with any 0 suture material (I prefer modern synthetic absorbable). This allows the operator to retrovert the uterus, exposing the fallopian tubes through a posterior colpotomy incision of 3 to 4 cm made transversely between the uterosacral ligaments 1 to 2 cm under the cervicovaginal junction. After securing hemostasis, vaginal retractors are inserted and the tubes are exposed with the further help of ring forceps.

With the significant advances in laparoscopic instrumentation, almost any technique developed for minilaparotomy (eg, Pomeroy) can be done laparoscopically with only minor modifications. Also, a significant number of techniques designed for minilaparotomy or laparoscopic sterilizations are done safely and successfully through the vaginal route.

Regardless of the incision or method selected for the tubal sterilization, appropriate identification of the relevant anatomic structures and the fimbriated end of each fallopian tube is mandatory. Although tubal sterilization is considered permanent, it is inappropriate to select surgical techniques that involve excessive and unnecessary destruction of the fallopian tube, thus impairing the possibility of a tubal reversal. It is important to be sensitive to the fact that when a woman decides on a tubal reversal, that decision might be surrounded by a personal tragedy such as loss of a child or change in marital status.

The remainder of this chapter discusses the most commonly used surgical techniques and their preferred incisions.

Silastic Band (Falope Ring)

The preferred incision for the Silastic band technique is laparoscopy. The Falope-ring applicator is loaded with two Silastic bands and inserted through the operative laparoscope with a single puncture technique, or through a 7- or 8-mm trocar placed 3 cm above the symphysis pubis in the midline with a two-puncture technique. A midportion of the fallopian tube is grasped with the tongs of the applicator, and a Silastic band is applied. The same procedure is done on the contralateral side (Fig. 17-1). The presence of tubal engorgement (eg, in postabortal sterilization) makes this technique difficult because of the limitation of the diameter of the applicator. Also, adequate mobility of the tube is required to prevent transection of the fallopian tube. Severe tubal ischemic pain is one of the most common problems with this method. The preoperative use of nonsteroidal antiinflammatory medications and spraying the tubes or injecting the mesosalpinx with local anesthetics help to reduce immediate postoperative pain.

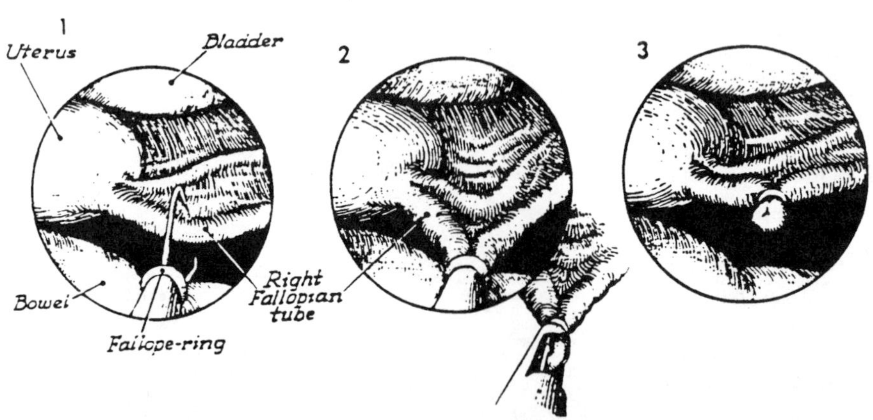

Figure 17-1. Silastic band technique (Falope ring). (From Wheeless CR. Atlas of pelvic surgery, 2nd ed. Philadelphia: Lea & Febiger, 1988: 2581.)

Bipolar Electrocoagulation (Kleppinger Forceps)

Coagulation of a midsegment of the fallopian tube with the bipolar cautery is one of the preferred methods for sterilization laparoscopically (Fig. 17-2). This technique also has been successfully used during vaginal sterilization. The current flows from the active tong to the ground tong of the forceps, eliminating spread to other structures. The advantages of bipolar electrocoagulation are as follows: (1) it is fast and easy to master; (2) size of the tube or its mobility is not an issue; (3) it minimizes the possibility of bowel injury and excessive destruction of the tube found with the use of unipolar current; (4) it is probably the least painful technique; and (5) only 6 to 8 mm of tissue is destroyed, making the probability for reversal as good as that with Falope ring or Hulka clip sterilizations.

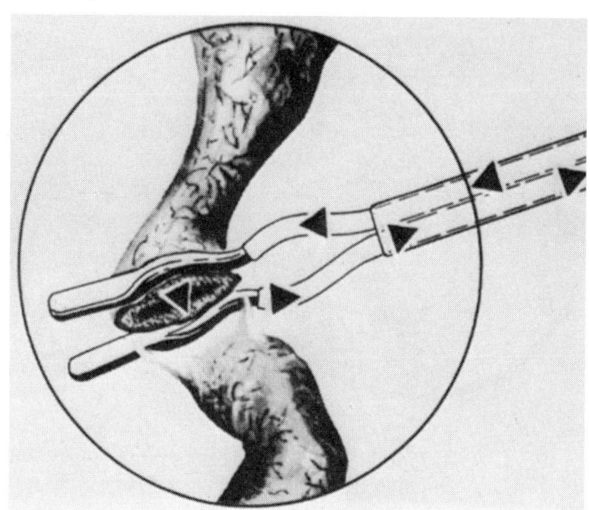

Figure 17-2. Bipolar electrocoagulation (Kleppinger forceps). (From Thompson JD, Rock JA. TeLinde's operative gynecology, 7th ed. Philadelphia: JB Lippincott, 1992:343.)

Unipolar Electrocoagulation

The unipolar technique is very similar to bipolar electrocoagulation (Fig. 17-3). The main difference is that with unipolar technique, the current flows from the tip of the forceps through the body to a grounding pad or return electrode placed on the patient's thigh. The disadvantages compared with bipolar coagulation were already mentioned.

Hulka Clip

The Hulka clip technique was introduced in 1972 as a method for laparoscopic sterilization. The greatest advantage of this procedure is that less than 1 cm of tissue is destroyed in the isthmic area; therefore, the potential for reversal is excellent.

With this technique, a plastic clip with interlocking teeth is loaded into a special applicator. The spring-loaded clip is then applied perpendicular to the fallopian tube in the isthmus (Fig. 17-4).

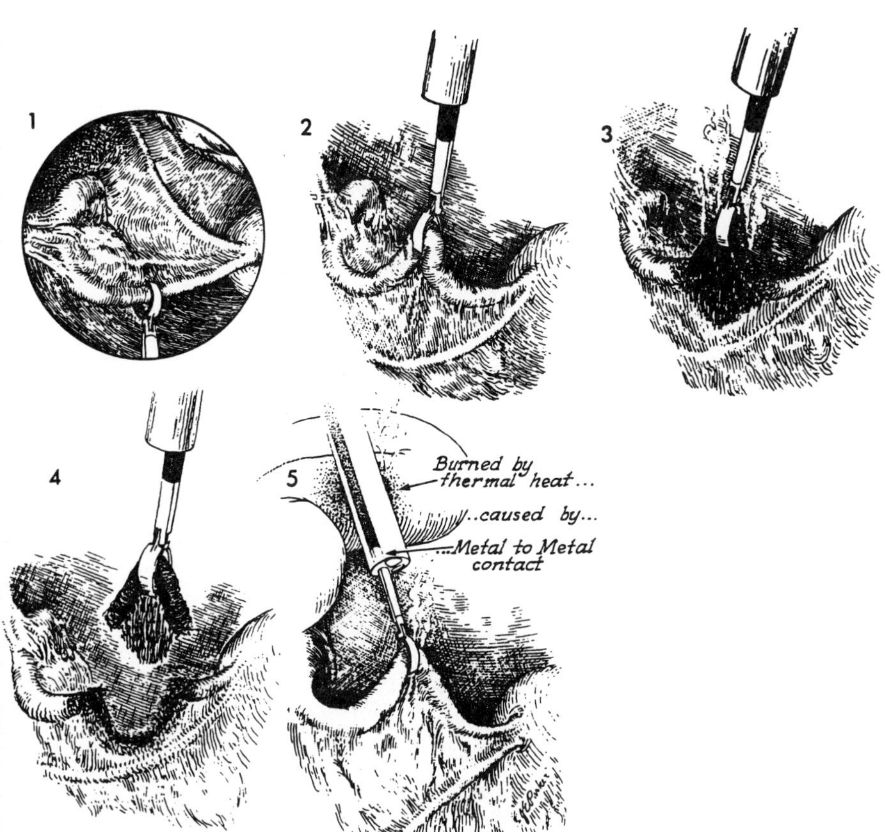

Figure 17-3. Unipolar electrocoagulation. (From Wheeless CR. Atlas of pelvic surgery, 2nd ed. Philadelphia: Lea & Febiger, 1988: 258.)

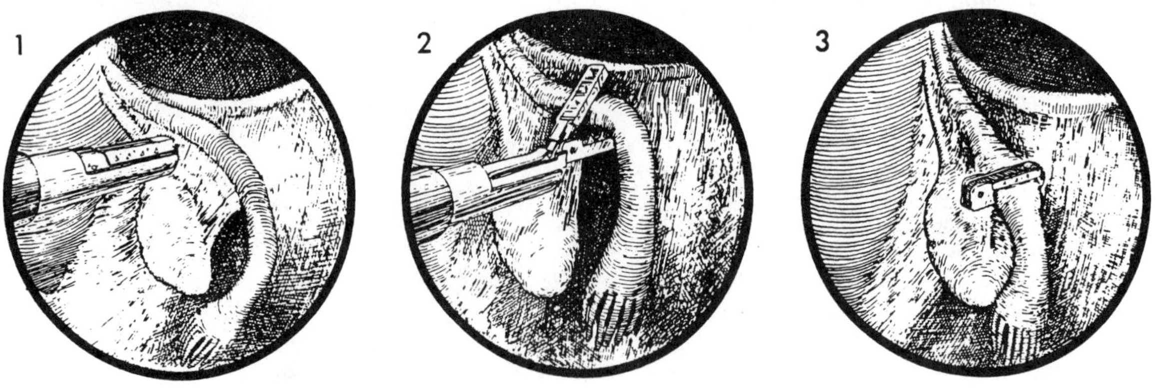

Figure 17-4. Hulka clips technique. (From Wheeless CR. Atlas of pelvic surgery, 2nd ed. Philadelphia: Lea & Febiger, 1988: 258.)

Pomeroy

The Pomeroy method is one of the most popular and simple techniques for tubal sterilization. After adequate identification of the fallopian tubes with their respective fimbriated ends, the midportion of one tube is grasped with a Babcock clamp, the tube is elevated and a loop is formed. A single strand of absorbable suture material is placed around the 1.5-cm knuckle and tied firmly, followed by excision of the loop with the scissors (Fig. 17-5). The same procedure is done on the contralateral side. In the initial description of this method, 0 plain catgut was the suture of choice. Currently, we have the option of using high-quality rapidly absorbable synthetic suture material of smaller diameter, with the advantage of less tissue reaction. This technique can easily be carried out through a minilaparotomy or vaginal incision during interval sterilization, or through a small infraumbilical incision during the early puerperium. The availability of endoloop sutures allows this method to be done laparoscopically as well.

Parkland Procedure

Although most commonly used for postpartum sterilization, the Parkland procedure is an easy and effective choice for interval sterilizations done by minilaparotomy. The fallopian tube is identified, grasped, and elevated as described for the Pomeroy. The mesosalpinx is entered through an avascular space with a small Kelly

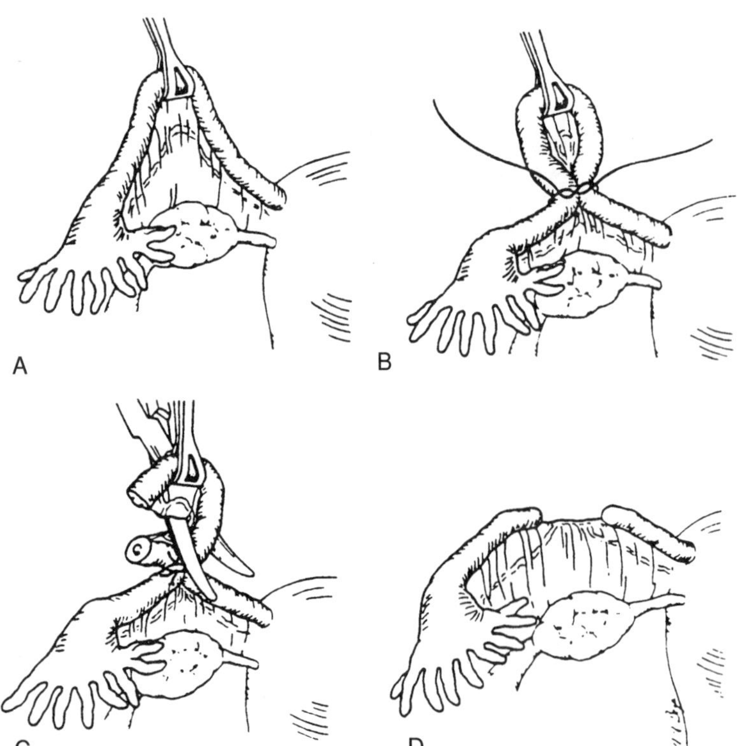

Figure 17-5. Pomeroy technique. (From Sciarra JJ, Surgical procedures for tubal sterilization. In Sciarra JJ, Steege JF, eds. Gynecology and obstetrics, vol 6. Philadelphia: Lippincott-Raven, 1996:3.)

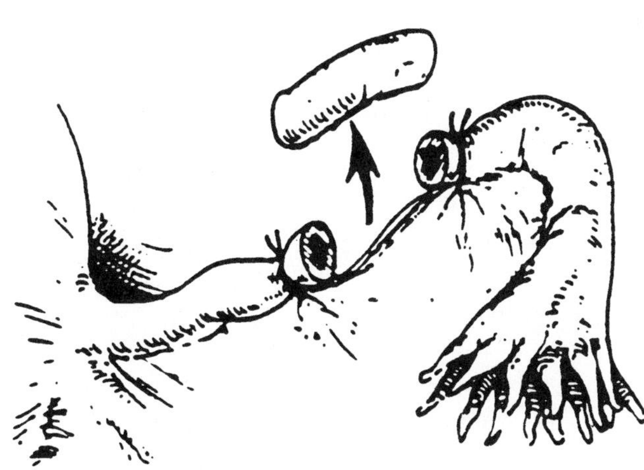

Figure 17-6. Parkland procedure. (From Cunningham FG, MacDonald PC, Gant NF. Williams obstetrics, 19th ed. Norwalk, CT: Appleton & Lange, 1993:1354.)

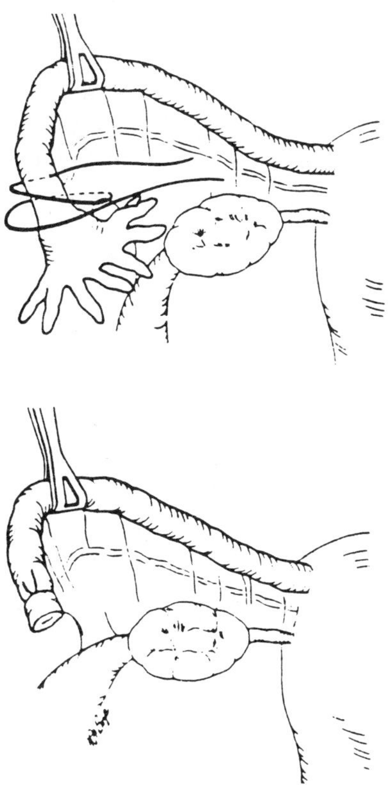

Figure 17-7. Kroener fimbriectomy. (From Sciarra JJ. Surgical procedures for tubal sterilization. In: Sciarra JJ, Steege JF, eds. Gynecology and obstetrics, vol 6. Philadelphia: Lippincott-Raven, 1996:3.)

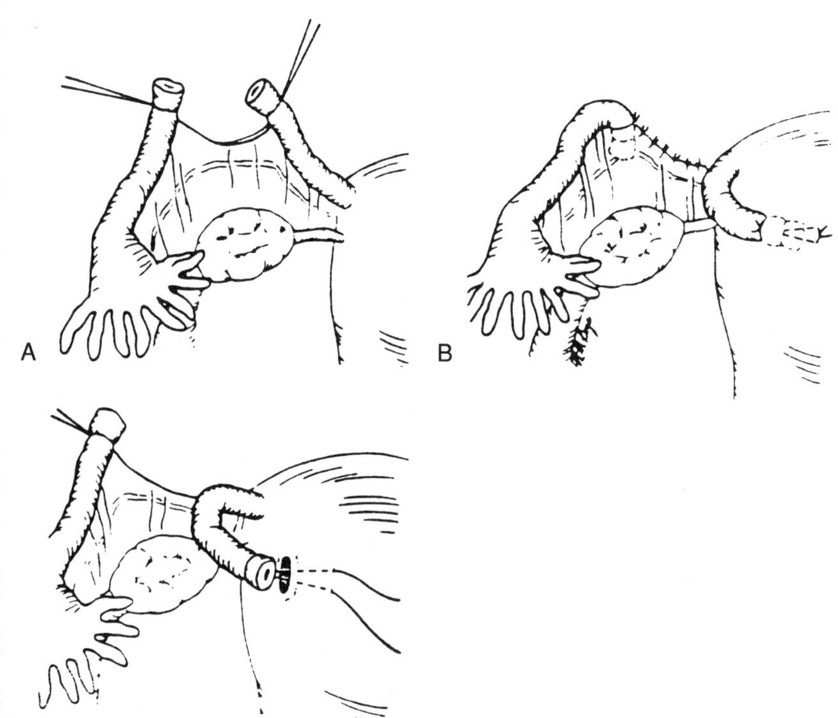

Figure 17-8. Irving procedure. (From Sciarra JJ. Surgical procedures for tubal sterilization. In: Sciarra JJ, Steege JF, eds. Gynecology and obstetrics, vol 6. Philadelphia: Lippincott-Raven, 1996:3.)

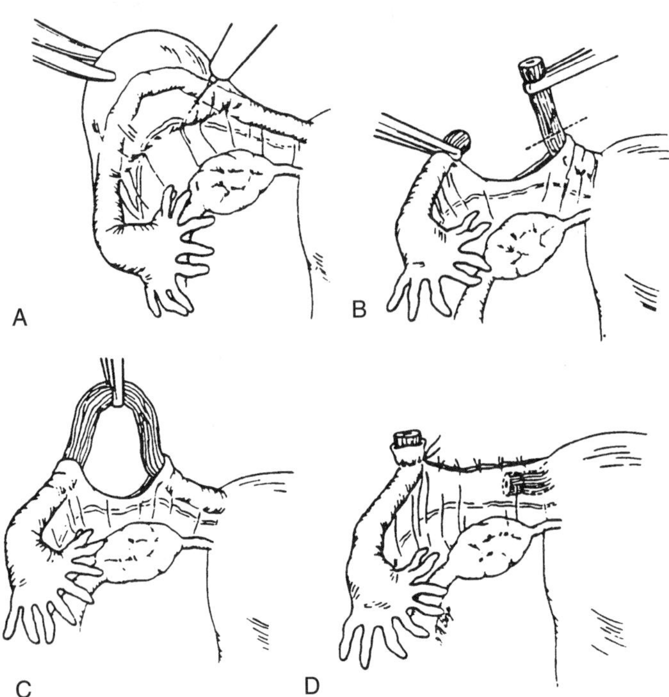

Figure 17-9. Uchida technique. (From Sciarra JJ. Surgical procedures for tubal sterilization. In Sciarra JJ, Steege JF, eds. Gynecology and obstetrics, vol 6. Philadelphia: Lippincott-Raven, 1996:3.)

clamp. The isolated portion of the tube is excised after ligating proximally and distally with absorbable suture material (Fig. 17-6).

Kroener Fimbriectomy

Kroener fimbriectomy involves excision of the distal portion of the ampulla with its fimbriated end. It is a simple procedure that can easily be carried out through a minilaparotomy or through the vaginal route. The distal end of the fallopian tube is grasped with a Babcock clamp; it is then double sutured or clamped and double ligated, followed by excision with scissors (Fig. 17-7). This technique has lost popularity in view of an almost nonexistent potential for reversal.

Other Techniques

The Irving procedure and the Uchida technique are shown in Figures 17-8 and 17-9, respectively. They are highly effective methods for sterilization with low failure rates. Nevertheless, the higher complexity of these procedures makes them less popular.

Hysteroscopic sterilization has been beautifully reviewed by Dr. Cooper, but the different techniques are under research and none of them has become widely accepted. It is exciting, though, to think about the possibility of a future technology that might allow patients to be sterilized without major surgery or anesthesia.

BIBLIOGRAPHY

Blimandimala PP, Mumford SD, Feldblum PJ. A comparison of different laparoscopic sterilization occlusion techniques in 24,439 procedures. Am J Obstet Gynecol 1982;144:319.

Cooper JM. Hysteroscopic sterilization. Clin Obstet Gynecol 1992;35:282.

Cunningham FG, MacDonald PC, Gant NF. Williams Obstetrics, 19th ed. Norwalk, CT: Appleton & Lange, 1993:1354.

Hartfield JV. Female sterilization by the vaginal route: a positive reassessment and comparison of 4 tubal occlusion methods. Aust N Z J Obstet Gynaecol 1993;33:408.

Nisanian A. Outpatient minilaparotomy sterilization with local anesthesia. J Reprod Med 1990;35:380.

Peterson HB, Hulka JF, Spielman FJ, Lee S, Marchbanks PA. Local versus general anesthesia for laparoscopic sterilization: a randomized study. Obstet Gynecol 1987;70:903.

Peterson LS. Contraceptive use in the United States: 1982–1990. In: Advance data from vital and health statistics, no. 260. Hyattsville, MD: National Center for Health Statistics, February 14, 1995.

Platz-Christensen JJ, Transtad SE, Johansson O, Carlsson SA. Evaluation of regret after tubal sterilization. Int J Gynaecol Obstet 1992;38:223.

Sciarra JJ. Surgical procedures for tubal sterilization. In: Sciarra JJ, Steege JF, eds. Gynecology and obstetrics, vol 6. Philadelphia: Lippincott-Raven, 1996:3.

Smith EM, Friedrich E, Pribor EF. Psychosocial consequences of sterilization: a review of the literature and preliminary findings. Compr Psychiatry 1994;35:157.

Smith RP, Maggi CS, Nolan TE. Morbidity and vaginal tubal cautery: a report and review. Obstet Gynecol 1991;78:209.

Stergachis A, Shy KK, Grothaus LC, et al. Tubal sterilization and the long term risk of hysterectomy. JAMA 1990;264:2893.

Thompson JD, Rock JA. TeLinde's operative gynecology, 7th ed. Philadelphia: JB Lippincott, 1992:343.

Wheatley SA, Millar JM, Jadad AR. Reduction of pain after laparoscopic sterilisation with local bupivacaine: a randomised, parallel, double-blind trial. Br J Obstet Gynaecol 1994;101:443.

Wheeless CR. Atlas of pelvic surgery, 2nd ed. Philadelphia: Lea & Febiger, 1988:258.

Wilcox LS, Chu SY, Eaker ED, Zeger SL, Peterson HB. Risk factors for regret after tubal sterilization: 5 years of follow up in a prospective study. Fertil Steril 1991;55:927.

Primary Care for Women, edited by Phyllis C. Leppert and Fred M. Howard. Lippincott-Raven Publishers, Philadelphia © 1997.

18

Abortion and Ectopic Pregnancy

FRED M. HOWARD

Abortion

Abortion is the termination of pregnancy before 20 gestational weeks. Another definition is loss of a fetus weighing less than 500 g. Although the true embryonic or fetal wastage rate is much higher, clinically recognized spontaneous abortion occurs in about 15% to 20% of known human pregnancies. (Elective or therapeutic abortion is discussed in Chapter 19.) Most abortions (80%) are early abortions—that is, they occur in the first trimester. Abortions between 12 and 20 weeks gestation, or late abortions, are less common. The abortion rate is relatively constant from 5 to 12 weeks gestation, but it drops steadily and rapidly after 12 weeks.

Several stages of abortion may be clinically defined. Threatened abortion is uterine bleeding at less than 20 weeks gestation without cervical dilation or effacement. This occurs in about 30% of pregnancies; about half of patients with threatened abortion miscarry. Inevitable abortion is uterine bleeding at less than 20 weeks gestation with cervical dilation but without passage of placental or fetal tissue. Incomplete abortion is uterine bleeding with expulsion through the cervix of some but not all placental and fetal tissue at less than 20 weeks gestation. Complete abortion is the expulsion through the cervix of all placental and fetal tissue at less than 20 weeks gestation. Septic abortion is an abortion in which there is uterine infection.

Ultrasonography, especially performed transvaginally, provides significantly more information than the clinical history and examination. It provides evidence that with first-trimester abortion, most fetuses die before 8 weeks and are retained in the uterus for several weeks before clinical symptoms occur. This situation is termed an intrauterine fetal death and may be sonographically diagnosed when a fetus with a crown–rump length of 15 mm or more does not have fetal cardiac activity. Ultrasound also allows the detection of a blighted ovum (anembryonic gestation), a pregnancy of more than about 7 weeks with a gestational sac but without a fetus. If the fetus is shown by sonography to be viable at less than 12 weeks, the incidence of abortion is only 2% to 3%.

The risk of abortion is increased by both maternal and paternal age. For maternal age, the risk at over 40 years of age is twice that of a woman less than 25 years old (25% to 30% versus 10% to 15%, respectively). For paternal age, risk of abortion at 45 or more years is about double that of a man less than 25 years old (23% versus 12%, respectively).

Reproductive history is the best predictor of miscarriage risk. The risk of abortion is increased by a history of prior abortion, particularly if there is no history of a prior pregnancy past 20 weeks gestation. The risk of abortion is only slightly increased with a history of one prior abortion. However, with a history of two prior abortions, the risk is about 35%; with three, it is about 50% (in women with no parity). Having at least one live birth decreases the statistical risk of recurrent abortion after three prior abortions to 30%. Women with three or more abortions are sometimes diagnosed as having recurrent or habitual abortion. In clinical practice, however, couples with two consecutive abortions warrant an evaluation for treatable causes of abortion (Fig. 18-1).

ETIOLOGY

Numerous diseases and abnormalities, congenital and acquired, can lead to abortion (Table 18-1).

Abortions are most commonly caused by genetic abnormalities. Cytogenetic studies show that chromosomal anomalies account for about 50% of all abortions. Most of these anomalies are aneuploidies—in other words, numeric abnormalities with greater or less than the normal 46 chromosomes. Table 18-2 summarizes the most common chromosomal abnormalities associated with spontaneous abortion. Autosomal trisomies are the most common abnormality; about one third of the trisomies are trisomy 16. Monosomy 45,X is the most common single chromosomal abnormality associated with abortion. About one in 300 conceptuses with a 45,X karyotype survive (Turner syndrome). Only about 5% of chromosomal anomalies are structural, with a euploid 46-chromosome karyotype. This has clinical relevance, as this is the group in which a chromosomal carrier state may be detectable in one of the members of a couple with recurrent spontaneous abortion.

Increasing maternal and paternal age both independently increase the risk of spontaneous abortion. However, paternal age does not correlate with an increase of chromosomal anomalies as a cause of abortion. Maternal age correlates only with an increase in trisomies, particularly of groups D and G chromosomes, as a cause of miscarriage. The relation of age to the incidence of chromosomally abnormal abortion is not intuitive.

Most chromosomally abnormal abortions occur in the first trimester. Generally, chromosomally normal fetuses abort later in gestation than those with abnormal chromosomes; the peak incidence is at 12 to 13 weeks for chromosomally normal fetuses versus 11 weeks for chromosomally abnormal fetuses.

The other general category of causes of abortion may be called environmental or maternal (see Table 18-1). These are less common causes of abortion, although they are often causes of recurrent abortion. Anomalies of uterine development are due to abnormal fusion of the müllerian system and probably occur in one in 200 to 600 women. About 25% of women with müllerian anomalies have reproductive problems. Most of these anomalies may cause reproductive problems, but unicornuate uterus (Fig. 18-2) carries the greatest risk of abortion (about 50%). Bicornuate and septate uteri (Fig. 18-3) are the anomalies most amenable to surgical correction, but carry only about a 25% risk of causing abortion. Resection of uterine septae can usually be done hysteroscopically with subsequently normal rates of abortion. Bicornuate uteri usually require a transabdominal Strassman reunification procedure. Resultant abor-

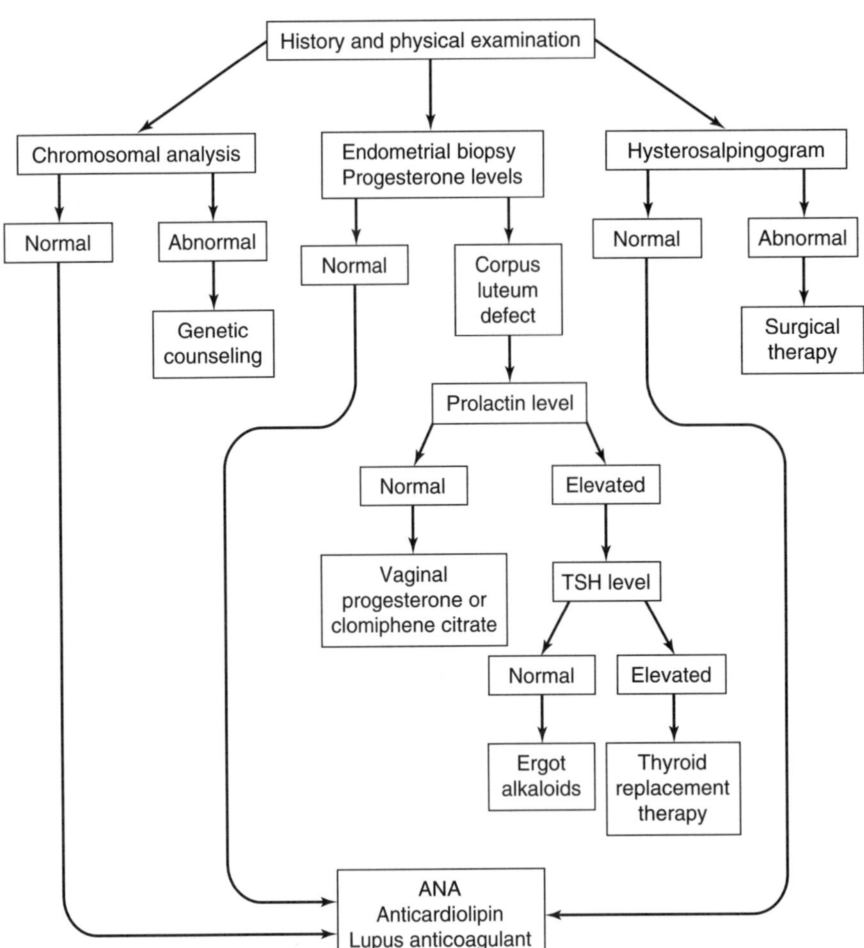

Figure 18-1. One possible evaluation scheme for recurrent abortions.

tion rates are decreased to 12% to 25%. Uterine anomalies usually cause second-trimester abortions.

Leiomyomata are present in about 25% of women of reproductive age and are not a frequent cause of abortion. However, in occasional cases, particularly with submucosal myomata, they may be a cause of miscarriage. Myomectomy may improve pregnancy outcomes.

Incompetent cervix refers to a syndrome of asymptomatic cervical dilation leading to pregnancy loss in the second trimester. It may be congenital, including association with congenital uterine anomalies, or it may be acquired secondary to traumatic cervical dilatation. Placement of a cervical cerclage is often an effective treatment (Fig. 18-4).

Intrauterine adhesions may cause infertility or recurrent abortion. These adhesions most often occur after vigorous postpartum uterine curettage but have also been reported after curettage for incomplete abortion, missed abortion, and diagnostic evaluation. Genital tuberculosis may also be an etiology. To prevent this problem, vigorous sharp endometrial curettage is best avoided.

In utero exposure to diethylstilbestrol (DES) may cause subsequent müllerian abnormalities, but this should now be a rare clinical occurrence. The risks of anomalies and of vaginal adenocarcinoma are well known, and therefore DES should not be used during pregnancy. In utero exposure to DES leads to a small endometrial cavity, possibly with a T-shaped uterus, and to an increased chance of cervical incompetence.

Endocrine dysfunctions may also be an etiology of abortion, especially recurrent abortion. Viability during the first 7 weeks of gestation depends on production of progesterone by the corpus luteum. If this production is insufficient (luteal insufficiency), then abortion may result. Midluteal progesterone levels are normally greater than 9 ng/mL. Consistently lower midluteal levels, or a discrepancy of 3 or more days between expected and actual histologic dating of the endometrium (usually done for at least two menstrual cycles), suggests a diagnosis of luteal insufficiency as a cause of recurrent abortion.

Uncontrolled diabetes mellitus increases the rate of abortion and of fetal anomalies. However, when blood glucose levels are well controlled, women with diabetes have no increase in the risk of abortion. There is a direct correlation of risk of abortion and elevated glycosylated hemoglobin ($HgbA_1$) levels.

Hypothyroidism is another endocrine dysfunction often included as a cause of abortion, although there is little objective evidence for such a relation. Some evidence suggests that women with thyroid dysfunction and thyroid autoantibodies are at increased risk of abortion.

The presence of lupus anticoagulant activity or anticardiolipin antibodies has been associated with an increased risk of abortion, as well as intrauterine fetal death. The mechanism by which these factors cause abortion is unclear, but evidence supports testing women with recurrent abortion for lupus anticoagulant activity and anticardiolipin antibodies.

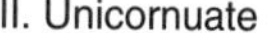

Table 18-1. Classification of Causes of Spontaneous Abortion

Chromosomal
Autosomal trisomy
Monosomy 45,X
Triploidy
Tetraploidy
Structural abnormality
Uterine Abnormalities
Congenital
Unicornuate
Bicornuate
Septate
DES exposure
Acquired
Leiomyomata
Incompetent cervix
Intrauterine adhesions (Asherman syndrome)
Progesterone deficiency (corpus luteum defect)
Thyroid disease
Diabetes mellitus
Immunologic factors
Lupus anticoagulant activity
Anticoagulant antibodies
Infections
Smoking

Endometritis due to certain bacteria, viruses, and parasites may be a cause of spontaneous abortion, although infections are probably not a common cause. *Toxoplasma gondii*, herpes simplex, and *Ureaplasma urealyticum* appear to be proven to cause abortion. *U urealyticum* and possibly *Mycoplasma hominis* may be an occasional cause of recurrent abortion.

Cigarette smoking, alcohol consumption, and possibly radiation or environmental toxin exposure increase the risk of abortion.

DIFFERENTIAL DIAGNOSIS

Ectopic pregnancy is the major diagnosis that the clinician may easily confuse with a possible abortion (Table 18-3). Both may present with a positive pregnancy test, abdominopelvic pain, and irregular bleeding. Often, clinical evaluation by historical and physical findings does not allow differentiation, but current methodologies with ultrasounds and quantitative βHCG (human chorionic gonadotropin) levels usually allow an accurate diagnosis.

Molar pregnancy may also present similarly to abortion. Again, ultrasound and quantitative βHCG levels generally allow an accurate diagnosis preoperatively. Also, routine histologic evaluation of aborted products of conception allows identification of hydatidiform molar pregnancies, including partial and incomplete molar pregnancies, in most cases.

The most common causes of bleeding in the first 20 gestational weeks of pregnancy are summarized in Table 18-3.

Table 18-2. Abnormal Karyotypes Observed in Spontaneous Abortions

KARYOTYPE	FREQUENCY (%)
Autosomal trisomy	50
Monosomy 45,X	20
Triploidy	15
Tetraploidy	10
Structural abnormality	5

II. Unicornuate

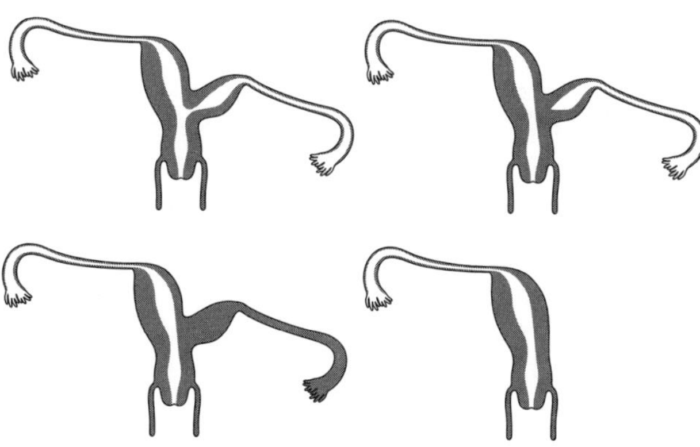

Figure 18-2. Variations of possible types of unicornuate uteri. (Roman numeral indicates the AFS classification of the anomalies.)

HISTORY

Patients with abortion have a history of amenorrhea or irregular bleeding. Their chief complaints at presentation are usually vaginal bleeding and cramping lower abdominopelvic pain. Women with

V. Septate

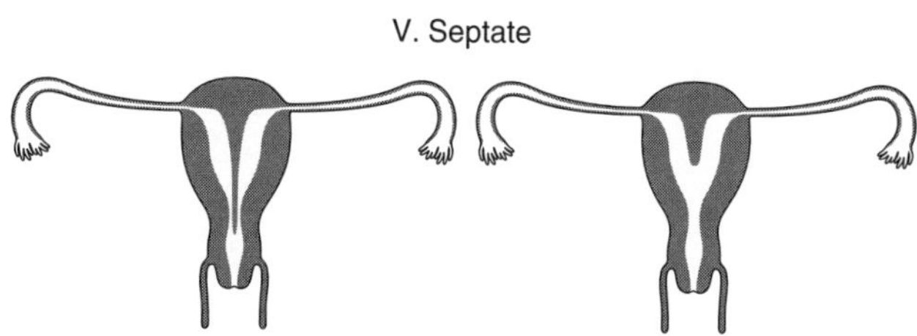

IV. Bicornuate

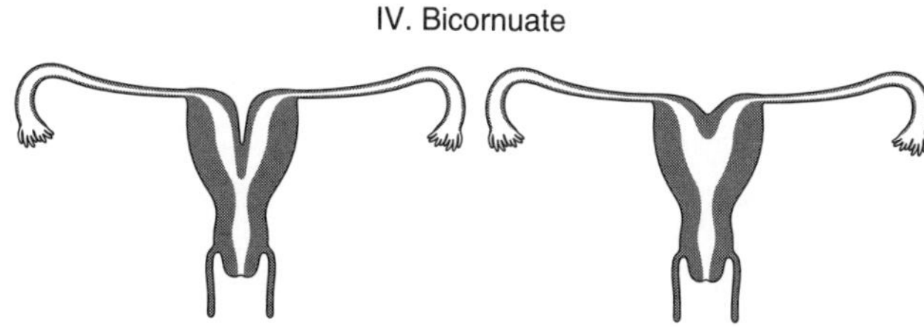

Figure 18-3. Variations of types of septate and bicornuate uteri. (Roman numerals indicate the AFS classification of the anomalies.)

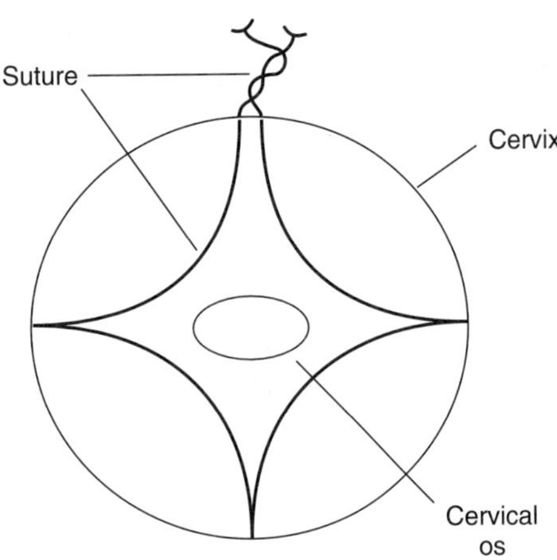

Figure 18-4. McDonald cerclage placement for incompetent cervix.

threatened abortion who do not subsequently miscarry usually do not have cramping pain.

Although 15% to 20% of pregnancies abort, twice this number have bleeding in the first half of pregnancy. Thus, bleeding by itself is a symptom of abortion only half the time—in other words, a pregnant woman with bleeding in the first 20 weeks of pregnancy has about a 50% chance of miscarrying. Bleeding for 3 or more days is associated with a greater risk of abortion than if bleeding lasts only 1 or 2 days.

Associated fever and foul vaginal discharge, especially with a history of uterine instrumentation, should raise a concern of possible septic abortion. Indeed, any symptoms suggestive of infection without a clear origin outside the genital tract should evoke this worry.

PHYSICAL EXAMINATION AND CLINICAL FINDINGS

The status of the cervix at the time of examination may allow a definitive diagnosis. If the cervix is dilated without a history of passage of tissue, the diagnosis is inevitable abortion. If tissue has passed or is in the cervical os and the cervix is dilated, the diagnosis is incomplete abortion. If all fetal and placental tissue has passed and the cervix is closed, usually with a decrease to minimal bleeding and cessation of cramping, the diagnosis is complete abortion.

Abortions after 14 weeks or before 6 weeks of gestation are more likely to be complete. Those between 6 and 14 weeks are often incomplete.

Table 18-3. Causes of Vaginal Bleeding Before the 20th Week of Gestation in 1549 Patients

DIAGNOSIS	NUMBER	%
Threatened abortion	211	13.6
Inevitable and incomplete abortion	951	61.4
Complete abortion	203	13.1
Septic abortion	67	4.3
Missed abortion	27	1.7
Hydatidiform mole	12	0.8
Tubal ectopic pregnancy	78	5.1

(Cavanagh D, Fleisher A, Ferguson JH. Am J Obstet Gynecol 1964;90:216.)

If there is cervical motion tenderness, foul cervical discharge, and marked abdominopelvic tenderness, then septic abortion is likely. Pelvic inflammatory disease can occur during pregnancy but is uncommon. If pelvic inflammatory disease is thought to be the explanation for these findings, treatment should be in the hospital with intensive observation. Patients with septic abortion can develop septic shock rapidly due to gram-negative endotoxins.

LABORATORY AND IMAGING STUDIES

With the use of ultrasonography, particularly transvaginal ultrasound, it is almost always possible to identify a gestational sac by 5 weeks of gestation (34 days) and a fetal pole by 6 weeks (40 to 42 days) in a normal pregnancy. Generally, this correlates with a βHCG level of 1800 to 2000 mIU/mL. Fetal heart activity can usually be seen within another week (at 7 weeks or 47 to 49 days). Thus, ultrasound can diagnose intrauterine death or anembryonic gestation and allow a clear differentiation of threatened abortion from incomplete or missed abortion. Indeed, the use of ultrasound makes the term "missed abortion" irrelevant, as it can diagnose fetal death and allow uterine evacuation rather than the continued observation and delay that lead to missed abortion.

Although the usual abortion rate is about 15%, once fetal viability is sonographically established at 8 or more weeks of gestation, the abortion rate is only 3% to 4%.

Although parental chromosomal abnormalities are an uncommon cause of abortion, if a couple has had two or more consecutive abortions there is a 3% prevalence of major chromosomal anomalies. About half of these are balanced translocations and about a fourth are robertsonian translocations. Thus, with such a history, parental karyotyping is indicated. If a translocation is found, then 80% of pregnancies will abort; of those that do not abort, 3% to 5% have unbalanced fetal chromosomes. Because of this, amniocentesis for fetal karyotyping is indicated in the second trimester in a couple with a parental translocation.

In couples with two or more consecutive abortions, hysterosalpingography and hysteroscopy may be indicated to evaluate for intrauterine adhesions, especially if there is a history of prior curettage. Hysterosalpingography may also demonstrate uterine anomalies as a cause of abortion. Complete blood count, thyroid-stimulating hormone (TSH) levels, lupus anticoagulant activity, anticardiolipin antibody levels, and midluteal progesterone levels or endometrial biopsies may also be indicated in patients with multiple miscarriages (see Fig. 18-1).

TREATMENT

Threatened Abortion

No specific treatment has been shown to alter the course of threatened abortion, but most clinicians recommend bed rest, no coitus, and restricted activities anyway. Increasing pain or bleeding necessitates reevaluation.

Progesterone supplementation is indicated only in cases with a prepregnancy diagnosis of luteal insufficiency. Initiating progesterone after a diagnosis of pregnancy has already been made, whether for bleeding, low progesterone levels, or a history of recurrent abortion, is of no proven benefit. If a prepregnancy diagnosis of luteal insufficiency is made, progesterone vaginal suppositories, 25 mg twice daily, or intramuscular progesterone, 12.5

mg/day, may be effective if started about 3 days after ovulation and continued through the first 8 to 12 weeks of gestation.

Inevitable Abortion

Outpatient suction curettage is probably the best treatment for inevitable abortion, particularly in the first trimester. As the cervix is open, this can be done comfortably and safely with conscious sedation or local anesthesia. Although an intravenous line and intravenous fluids are ideal, they may sometimes be avoided if bleeding is not profuse. Sedation with meperidine, 50 to 75 mg, and diazepam, 5 to 10 mg, can be used, as well as a paracervical block with 20 mL of 1% lidocaine. Care must be taken to avoid intravascular injection of the local anesthetic. Various methods of paracervical block have been shown to be efficacious. The injection of 1 mL into the anterior cervical lip allows painless grasping of the cervix with a Jacobs or single-tooth tenaculum; the remaining anesthetic can then be injected at 3 and 9 o'clock at the cervicovaginal junction. A suction curet is then introduced just through the internal cervical os, suction is initiated to about 60 cm H_2O pressure, and the curet is gently rotated 360° several times. When tissue and blood stop passing through the curet and frothy bubbles start appearing, the procedure is usually finished. A gentle curettage with a sharp curet may be done to ensure that all products of conception have been evacuated, but this must not be vigorous or deep. Ergonovine (0.2 mg intramuscularly) or oxytocin (10 to 20 units intravenously or intramuscularly) is usually given during or at the end of the procedure.

The patient should be observed for bleeding, with vital signs measured for 2 to 8 hours, depending on her preoperative and intraoperative blood loss and her level of consciousness. At discharge, the patient is given ergonovine, 0.2 mg every 4 hours for six doses, and doxycycline, 100 mg twice daily for 2 or 3 days. Prophylactic antibiotic treatment may decrease the risk of postoperative infection after elective abortion. Discharge instructions include rest for 24 to 72 hours and nothing per vagina for 2 weeks.

Incomplete Abortion

Between 6 and 14 weeks gestation, most clinicians recommend curettage for incomplete abortion. However, a recent Swedish study suggests that expectant management without curettage may decrease the risk of infection, with an average of only 1.5 days more bleeding than with traditional curettage treatment. Duration of pain, time of convalescence, and need for transfusion were not different with expectant versus surgical management.

It has been reported that conception within the first 3 months after a live birth results in an increased rate of abortion. Extrapolation from this information has led to a clinical recommendation that women not attempt conception for at least 3 months after a spontaneous abortion, although there is no clear evidence for this recommendation.

Septic Abortion

If the history, physical examination, and laboratory findings suggest septic abortion, the patient and physician must recognize this as a potentially fatal condition. Hospital admission is mandatory. Cultures of the cervix and blood should be obtained. Complete blood count, electrolytes, chemistries, and coagulation studies are advisable. Broad-spectrum antibiotics should be immediately initiated. A preferred regimen is triple antibiotic coverage with ampicillin, gentamicin, and clindamycin. After antibiotics have been started, dilatation and suction curettage or evacuation are done. Rarely, the infection is severe enough to necessitate hysterectomy. If the patient develops septic shock or disseminated intravascular coagulation, intensive care is needed, possibly including Swan-Ganz catheterization, vasopressors, and blood products.

Recurrent Abortion

A couple with two consecutive abortions, especially if they have no live births, should be evaluated and treated for recurrent abortion. Most of the known causes and the evaluation of recurrent abortion were discussed previously. Treatment is based on the results of the diagnostic evaluation (see Fig. 18-1).

A history and physical examination specifically directed toward incompetent cervix, cigarette smoking, alcohol, and environmental toxins should be completed. Then a complete blood count, TSH level, lupus anticoagulant activity, anticardiolipin antibody level, and several midluteal progesterone levels are obtained. A hysterosalpingogram should be performed to look for intrauterine adhesions, leiomyomata, or uterine anomalies. If all these studies are normal, then chromosomal abnormalities in either the man or woman should be sought by karyotyping both.

If a diagnosis of luteal insufficiency is made based on midluteal progesterone levels of less than 9 ng/mL, progesterone vaginal suppositories, 25 mg twice daily, or intramuscular progesterone, 12.5 mg/day, may be effective if started 3 days after ovulation and continued through the first 8 to 12 weeks of gestation.

If TSH levels are high, then thyroid replacement should be initiated and studies to evaluate possible autoimmune thyroid disease obtained.

If intrauterine adhesions are diagnosed, surgical treatment is indicated. Hysteroscopic adhesiolysis, followed by endometrial distention with a Foley catheter, then high-dose estrogen (eg, 2.5 mg of conjugated estrogen) for 30 to 60 days, results in a normal abortion rate postoperatively.

Lupus anticoagulant activity or anticardiolipin antibodies have been associated with recurrent abortion. If either of these is present in a woman with abortion, treatment is probably indicated, although there is no general agreement as to the best therapy. Corticosteroids, aspirin, and heparin have all been used.

Rh Immune Globulin

The patient's blood type should be known with any of the categories of abortion. Patients with Rh-negative blood should be administered prophylaxis against Rh sensitization with Rh immune globulin. There is debate as to the need for Rh immune globulin with threatened abortion, but prophylaxis is clearly indicated in all other cases. In the first trimester, a decreased dose (50 mg) may be adequate rather than the usual 300-mg dose.

Postabortion Counseling

It has been reported that conception within the first 3 months after a live birth results in an increased rate of abortion. Extrapolation from this information has led to a clinical recommendation that women not attempt conception for at least 3 months after a spontaneous abortion, although there is no clear evidence for this recommendation.

If the abortion is the woman's first, she can be counseled that there is no increased risk of abortion with the next pregnancy. However, with two or more abortions the subsequent risk is 30% to 50%.

The clinician must be aware of the loss that the patient suffers with an abortion. Most women have bonded with their baby, even in the first trimester, and grieve for the loss of their child. Physicians and other providers involved in the woman's care should be sensitive to this suffering and offer the woman appropriate psychosocial support and counseling. Many locales have active support groups that are helpful to many women. Well-intentioned comments are often painful to the woman and are best avoided; examples are, "At least this happened before it was a real baby" and "Don't worry, you can always get pregnant again." Every effort should be made to make the woman's medical experience with an abortion as supportive as possible.

Ectopic Pregnancy

Ectopic pregnancy is a pregnancy that develops after implantation of the blastocyst at any site other than the endometrium of the uterine cavity. The most common site of ectopic implantation is the fallopian tube, accounting for 97% to 98% of all ectopic pregnancies. The remaining 2% to 3% are abdominal, ovarian, cornual (interstitial), and cervical implantations (Fig. 18-5).

Ectopic pregnancy is a life-threatening disease. With the availability of early diagnosis, blood transfusions, and effective surgical and medical therapies, the death rate has decreased by more than sevenfold over the past three decades and is now less than five per 10,000 cases. However, there are still 40 to 50 deaths per year in the United States due to ectopic pregnancy, and it is the leading cause of maternal mortality in black women. As this is a disease of young women with 50 to 70 more years of life expectancy, any deaths are particularly tragic. Early diagnosis and treatment are essential if serious or fatal complications are to be avoided. Primary care physicians must always consider the possibility of ectopic pregnancy in any woman of reproductive age with irregular vaginal bleeding or abdominopelvic pain.

Over the past two decades, the rate of ectopic pregnancy appears to have increased by three- to fourfold and is currently 16 to 20 per 1000 pregnancies in the United States. The rate is higher in nonwhite than white women and higher in parous than nulligravid women.

ETIOLOGY

Normally, the fertilized ovum passes through the fallopian tube to implant in the decidual endometrium at about 7 days of age. It appears that any factor that impedes this migration may lead to tubal implantation (Table 18-4). The most common factor seems to be tubal damage due to acute salpingitis. About half of all women with a first episode of ectopic pregnancy have morphologic changes attributed to previous acute salpingitis. Further evidence contributing to the hypothesis that acute salpingitis is a major cause of ectopic pregnancy comes from a 1981 study by Westrom and colleagues, who followed 900 women with laparoscopically confirmed salpingitis and observed a rate of ectopic pregnancy of 68.8 per 1000 conceptions, a sixfold increase over the rate in a control population without prior salpingitis. Scarring and agglutination

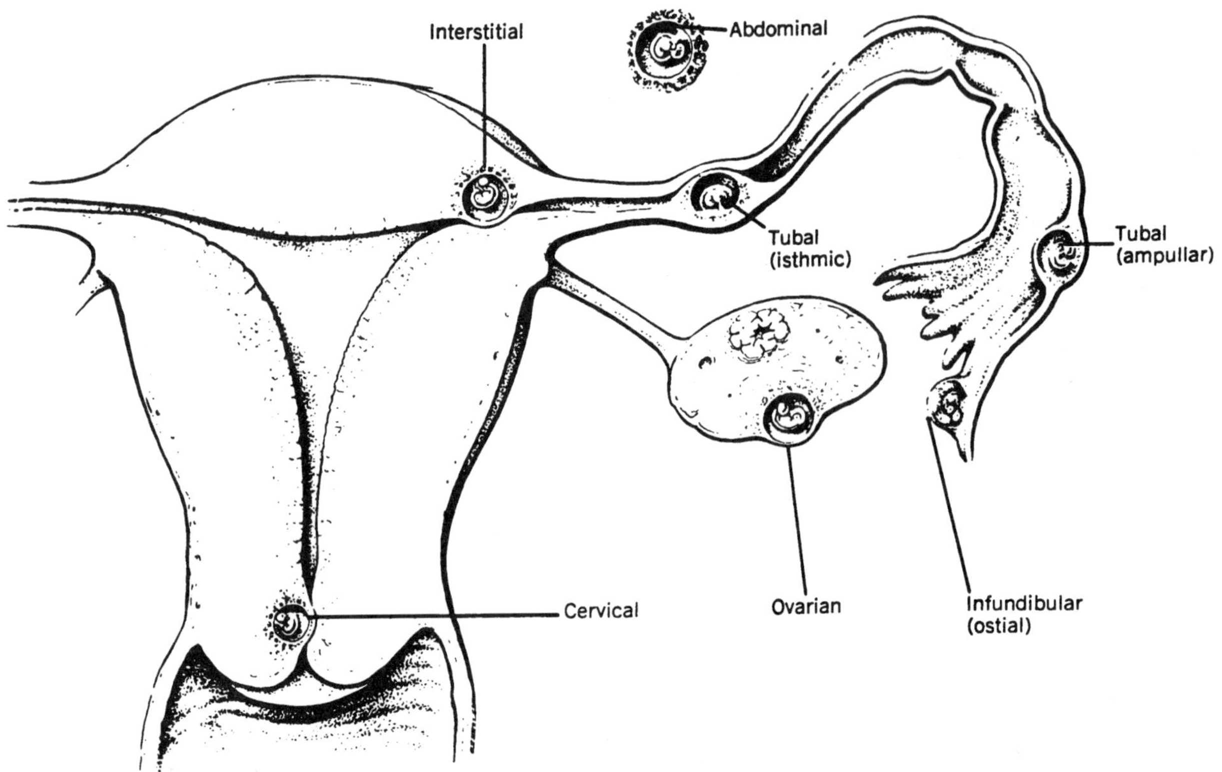

Figure 18-5. Possible locations of ectopic pregnancies.

Table 18-4. Risk Factors for Ectopic Pregnancy

Risk factor
History of salpingitis
Prior ectopic pregnancy
Progesterone-releasing IUD
Progestin-only birth-control pill failure
Pharmacologic ovulation induction
Pelvic adhesions
Prior pelvic surgery
Prior tubal surgery (tubal sterilizations or tuboplasties)
Two or more induced abortions

of the endosalpinx probably are the mechanisms by which salpingitis leads to tubal implantation. Adhesions of the tubal serosa to the bowel or peritoneum often occur after salpingitis and may also impede normal tubal motility and play a role. Such adhesions may also arise in women with prior pelvic surgery, a history that also appears to increase the chance of ectopic pregnancy.

Any surgery on the fallopian tube increases the risk of tubal ectopic pregnancy. Often this is because the surgery is done to treat infertility due to salpingitis; however, the surgery does not correct the endosalpingeal damage secondary to salpingitis, so that if conception occurs, the same factors discussed previously lead to tubal implantation. When the tubal surgery is done on a relatively normal tube (eg, for tubal reanastomosis after sterilization), the risk of ectopic pregnancy is less than when done on an abnormal tube. However, the risk is still higher than in the normal population, as surgery on the tube, even with the most meticulous technique, inevitably causes some damage.

Tubal sterilization is a particularly important risk factor for ectopic pregnancy. Although tubal sterilization is an effective method of permanent contraception, when it fails there is a particular risk of tubal implantation. Tubal coagulation and Falope ring techniques may carry a higher risk of ectopic pregnancy when they fail than do other methods of tubal sterilization. As tubal sterilization has become a more popular family planning method, it has also become a more common etiology for ectopic pregnancy.

Another suspected factor in the etiology of tubal ectopic pregnancy is hormonal imbalance, with excessive levels of estrogen or progesterone or both. These levels are thought to impede normal tubal motility and contractility, slowing the transit of the fertilized ovum through the tube. This mechanism probably accounts for the increase of ectopic pregnancies in women who conceive on progestin-only oral contraceptives, ovulation-inducing drugs such as clomiphene and human menopausal gonadotropin, and progesterone-releasing IUDs. The magnitude of the risk of these factors is less than that of salpingitis, ranging from a 50% to 300% increase in the rate of ectopic pregnancy. These contraceptive methods do not place a woman at risk of ectopic pregnancy: they decrease the chance of pregnancy and thus decrease the chance of an ectopic pregnancy. However, when they fail, the progestin-only pill and the IUD carry a higher risk of tubal implantation. Failures of diaphragms, condoms, and combination oral contraceptives carry no increase in the rate of ectopic pregnancy over that in women who do not use contraception.

Etiologic mechanisms of other types of ectopic pregnancies—cervical, ovarian, interstitial, and abdominal—are less well understood. Abdominal pregnancies are thought to occur often after abortion of a tubal pregnancy, with reimplantation and development (secondary abdominal ectopic). However, both abdominal and ovarian pregnancies appear to occur primarily as well, with direct implantation of the blastocyst on the peritoneum or ovary, respectively.

DIFFERENTIAL DIAGNOSIS

There are numerous other causes of abdominopelvic pain or bleeding in young women. The most common differential diagnoses are listed in Table 18-5. It is worth dividing the differential into diagnoses directly related to pregnancy and those that may occur in nonpregnant women as well. (This assumes that a positive pregnancy test is obtained; modern sensitive pregnancy tests are almost never negative in women with ectopic pregnancy.) These diagnoses are extensively covered in Chapter 21, so only those specific to pregnancy are reviewed here.

Abortion is a common cause of bleeding and pain in the first half of pregnancy. Pain is usually cramping and midline and accompanied by vaginal bleeding, often heavy with clots. An open cervical os with obvious products of conception often allows a clinical diagnosis without further laboratory or imaging tests. However, a decidual cast, passed in about 10% of women with ectopic pregnancy, may lead to an incorrect diagnosis of abortion. Histologic evaluation of any passed or curetted tissue is a safeguard against such a misdiagnosis. Frozen section evaluation can be done in uncertain cases and reveals chorionic villi in most cases of abortion. Floating the tissue on saline is a useful clinical technique to help identify chorionic villi, but a histologic evaluation must still be done. Permanent sections may show an Arias-Stellas reaction (hypersecretory endometrial glands with hyperchromatism, pleomorphism, increased mitotic activity, and hypertrophy), which in the absence of obvious chorionic villi should make the clinician highly suspicious of an ectopic pregnancy rather than an abortion.

Heterotopic pregnancy is the presence of both an intrauterine and ectopic pregnancy. Although rare (one in 4000 to 30,000 pregnancies), this may occur with increased frequency after ovulation induction. Only with a high index of suspicion, leading to further laboratory and imaging studies, can the clinician make the correct diagnosis.

Appendicitis during the first trimester of pregnancy may be confused with ectopic pregnancy. As with ectopic pregnancy, pain is usually unilateral early in the disease (right lower quadrant). Bleeding is not a characteristic symptom of appendicitis. Fever is usually higher with appendicitis than with ectopic pregnancy, as temperature elevations with ectopic pregnancies are usually minimal. White blood cell counts with appendicitis are usually ele-

Table 18-5. Differential Diagnosis of Ectopic Pregnancy

Diagnosis
Abortion
Heterotopic pregnancy
Acute salpingitis
Functional ovarian cyst
Ovarian tumor
Appendicitis
Adnexal torsion
Endometriosis
Pelvic adhesions
Leiomyomata
Cystitis
Polycystic ovarian disease
Urinary calculus
Gastroenteritis

vated above the normal pregnancy range of up to 14,000/mL. Both diseases may present with anorexia, nausea, and vomiting.

HISTORY

The classic symptoms of ectopic pregnancy are abdominopelvic pain, absence of menses, and irregular vaginal bleeding (Table 18-6). Pain is almost always present. Usually it starts as unilateral pain, and as the course progresses it becomes bilateral or generalized. The quality of the pain is not characteristic. At first it may be colicky or vague; at times it is sharp or stabbing. The pain characteristically becomes intense with tubal rupture. There may be associated right shoulder pain due to diaphragmatic irritation by a hemoperitoneum. Occasionally patients complain of rectal pain or the urge to defecate.

Amenorrhea is present in more than 75% of patients but occasionally is hard to elicit due to a history of irregular bleeding, also present in about 75% of patients. With careful inquiry, most women are found at the time of clinical presentation to be 6 weeks or more from their last normal menstrual period. The irregular bleeding is characteristically of a spotting nature but occasionally is heavy enough to resemble menstrual flow. It is not usually as heavy as that associated with miscarriage. As noted earlier, up to 10% of women pass a decidual cast that resembles tissue passage with a spontaneous abortion.

Before diagnosis, about 25% of women complain of dizziness or syncope. Ideally, the diagnosis should be made before this symptom, as most young, healthy women can compensate for significant blood loss before true syncope.

Pregnancy molimina are common: breast tenderness, nausea, and constipation are not unusual complaints.

PHYSICAL EXAMINATION AND CLINICAL FINDINGS

Vital signs reveal tachycardia or low-grade fever (38°C or less) in up to 20% of patients. Orthostatic changes in pulse and blood pressure are also found in up to 20% of patients.

Most patients have abdominal tenderness that may be unilateral, bilateral, or generalized. Rebound tenderness may also be present, but this does not necessarily mean the patient has a hemoperitoneum; conversely, the patient may have a hemoperitoneum and not have rebound tenderness. Pelvic tenderness is usually present and may be unilateral, bilateral, or diffuse. Cervical motion tenderness is not unusual. An adnexal mass is palpable in about half of patients but usually represents a corpus luteum cyst, not the ectopic pregnancy—in fact, in up to 20% of patients, the mass is on the contralateral side. The uterus is usually enlarged, but almost never greater than 8 weeks gestation in size. Uterine bleeding may be noted but is usually not heavy. The cervical os is

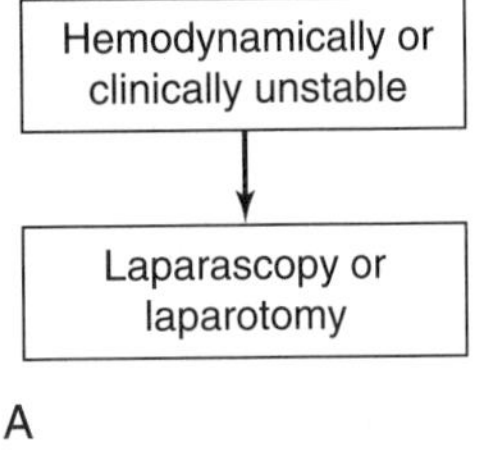

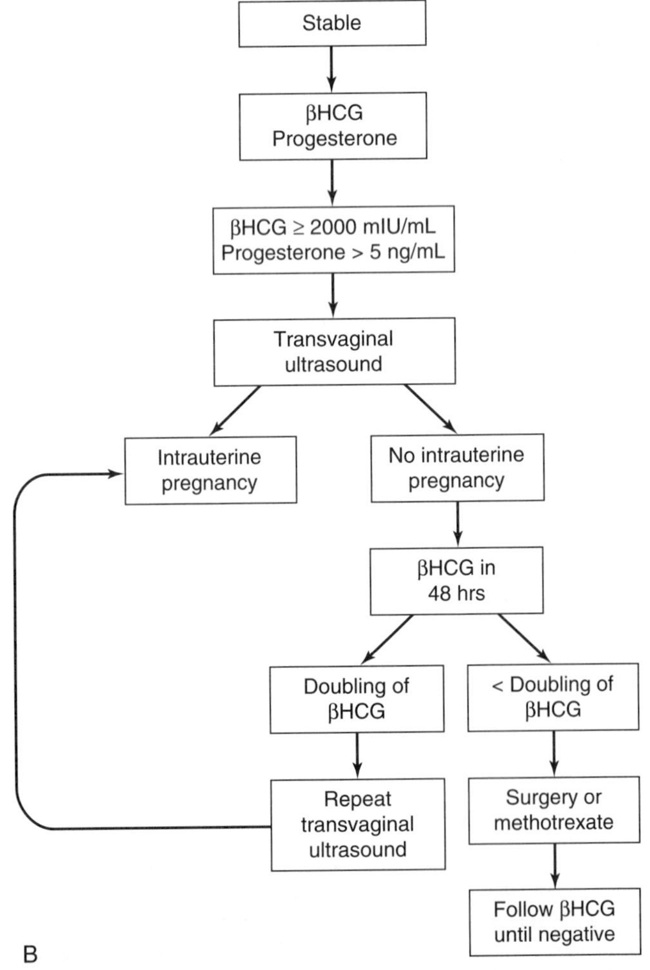

Figure 18-6. Algorithms for evaluation and treatment of patients with suspected ectopic pregnancy, using βHCG levels, progesterone levels, and transvaginal ultrasound. (***A***) Evaluation and treatment of patients with suspected ectopic pregnancy who are unstable—in other words, clinical findings make the diagnosis of ectopic very likely or the patient is hemodynamically unstable. All the other algorithms assume the patient is stable. If the patient becomes unstable during the evaluation adhering to any of the other algorithms, then this algorithm should be followed instead of continuing to adhere to the original algorithm. (***B***) Evaluation and treatment of patients with suspected ectopic pregnancy and βHCG levels of 2000 nIU/mL or more and progesterone levels of 5 ng/mL or more. *(continued)*

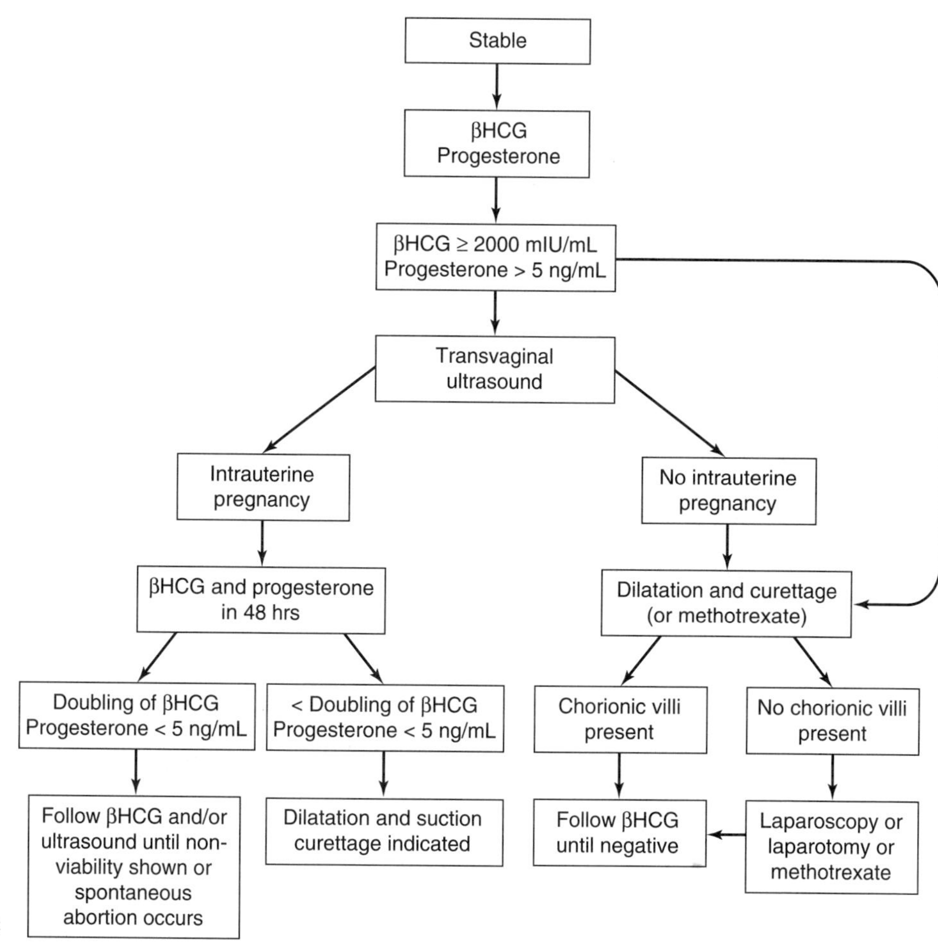

Figure 18-6. *(Continued)* (***C***) Evaluation and treatment of patients with suspected ectopic pregnancy and βHCG levels of 2000 mIU/mL or more and progesterone levels of less than 5 ng/mL. Two options are possible: immediate dilatation and curettage or continued conservative evaluation, depending on the clinician's evaluation. *(continued)*

almost always closed; an exception may be with passage of a decidual cast.

LABORATORY AND IMAGING STUDIES

For all intents and purposes, all women with an ectopic pregnancy have a positive serum pregnancy test if a sensitive radioimmunoassay-type test is performed. A negative serum assay for HCG makes the diagnosis quite unlikely. In addition to a pregnancy test, women suspected of having an ectopic pregnancy should have a complete blood count, blood type, and Rh. About 25% of women have a hematocrit of 30% or less at presentation. Consistent with pregnancy changes, up to a third have a white cell count of 10,000 to 15,000/mm^3. Less than 20% have a significant leukocytosis of greater than 15,000/mm^3.

If the diagnosis is not apparent and the patient is clinically not deemed to be in imminent danger, the diagnosis may be established with a rational, judicious approach using a combination of serial βHCG measurements and transvaginal ultrasound. A baseline βHCG is always obtained if an ectopic pregnancy is suspected and the patient is stable, but this value is rarely diagnostic. Although βHCG levels are usually lower than normal with an ectopic pregnancy, the variation of levels at a given gestational age and the usual uncertainty about the date of conception do not allow a diagnosis with one level. If the turnaround time for the βHCG level is short, then the clinician may wish to wait for the value before ordering an ultrasound. With a βHCG level of 1800 to 2000 mIU/mL, an intrauterine pregnancy can be seen by transvaginal ultrasound in almost 100% of cases of normal intrauterine pregnancy. If no intrauterine pregnancy is seen, then the diagnosis is almost certainly an abortion or an ectopic pregnancy. If transvaginal ultrasound is unavailable, then an abdominal ultrasound may be done, but it does not reliably detect an intrauterine pregnancy until the βHCG level is 6500 mIU/mL or higher. Most patients with ectopic pregnancy do not achieve a βHCG level this high.

If the initial βHCG level is less than 1800 mIU/mL, the fact that βHCG levels double about every 48 hours may be used to aid in diagnosis (Table 18-7). A classic study found that only 15% of normal pregnancies failed to show an increase of 66% or more in 2 days, and only 13% of ectopic pregnancies showed this normal increase of βHCG. Following doubling times allows continued observation as long as the patient is stable until a βHCG of 2000 mIU/mL is reached and an ultrasound can confirm that an intrauterine pregnancy is present. A drop-off of the normal doubling time allows diagnosis of an abnormal pregnancy and intervention with dilatation and curettage or laparoscopy, if clinically indicated, to allow definitive diagnosis and treatment.

Progesterone levels have also been suggested as useful in the evaluation of patients who may have an ectopic pregnancy. A single measurement may be useful if it is pathologically low; in this case, it suggests an inevitable abortion or an ectopic pregnancy. Published pathologically low values are 5 to 9 mg/mL, but each

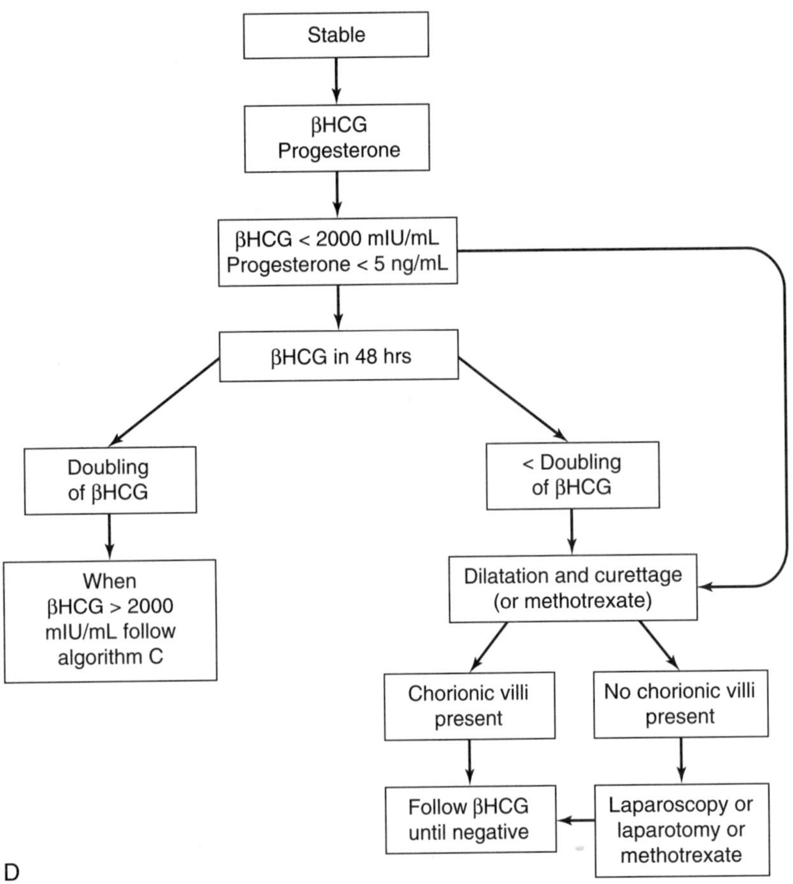

Figure 18-6. (*Continued*) (***D***) Evaluation and treatment of patients with suspected ectopic pregnancy and βHCG levels of less than 2000 mIU/mL and progesterone levels of less than 5 ng/mL. Two options are possible: immediate dilatation and curettage or continued conservative evaluation, depending on the clinician's evaluation. *(continued)*

institution should establish its own levels. A normal progesterone level is not diagnostic, as it may be consistent with normal pregnancy, inevitable abortion, or ectopic pregnancy. Following progesterone levels to observe a pathologic decline does not seem to offer any additional benefit over simply following βHCG levels.

Ultrasonography is probably most useful in combination with βHCG levels. However, in some cases it shows an adnexal gestational sac and leads to a direct diagnosis of ectopic pregnancy. This was reported in up to 65% of cases in one series, but ultrasonography usually leads to a direct diagnosis much less commonly than this. Ultrasonography may also show free blood in the pelvis, suggesting ectopic pregnancy and leading to surgical exploration.

Laparoscopy as a diagnostic technique is accurate but has been reported to miss 2% to 5% of ectopic pregnancies. It has the advantage of allowing treatment via laparoscopy if ectopic pregnancy is diagnosed.

Many algorithms for the diagnosis of ectopic pregnancy have been proposed (Fig. 18-6) and may assist the clinician in organizing the diagnostic evaluation. The clinician caring for a woman with a differential diagnosis that includes ectopic pregnancy should fully understand the utility and pitfalls of the available diagnostic tests, particularly βHCG levels and ultrasonography, and should tailor the evaluation to the clinical situation.

TREATMENT

Surgical removal remains the mainstay of current therapy, but medical management is assuming a promising and increasingly prevalent role. Radical surgical therapy refers to removal of the involved fallopian tube, sometimes with the ipsilateral ovary or with hysterectomy and salpingo-oophorectomy. Radical therapy is not usually indicated, but if the fallopian tube has ruptured or if no further pregnancies are desired, then complete or partial salpingectomy may be appropriate. If the ovary is intimately involved in the adnexal pathology, oophorectomy is occasionally necessary. There is no evidence that removing the ipsilateral ovary decreases the risk of a subsequent ectopic pregnancy, so prophylactic oophorectomy is not indicated. Occasionally, significant uterine pathology coincident with ectopic pregnancy may justify a hysterectomy, but in general the additional morbidity of a hysterectomy is not justified, particularly in an unstable patient with hemorrhage due to an ectopic pregnancy.

Conservative surgical therapy refers to treatment with preservation of the fallopian tube. Either salpingostomy (incision into the tube without subsequent closure of the incision) or salpingotomy (incision into the tube with subsequent closure of the incision) may be done. Because the outcomes and sequelae appear to be the same with either procedure, salpingostomy is usually preferred as it is simpler and faster. Sometimes hemostasis is difficult to obtain with either procedure, requiring a segmental salpingectomy; this may also be necessary in cases of tubal rupture. If preservation of fertility is desired, segmental resection is preferred to complete salpingectomy, as it allows the potential of future reanastomosis.

Laparoscopy is usually preferable to laparotomy, as it decreases blood loss and the hospital stay. Salpingostomy, salpingotomy, segmental salpingectomy, and total salpingectomy may

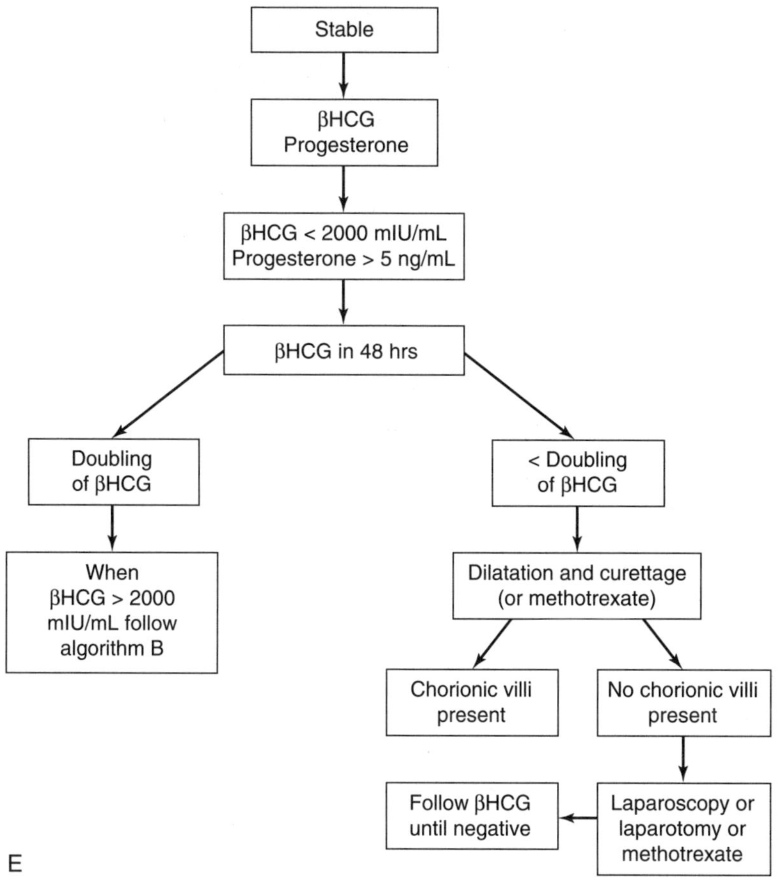

Figure 18-6. *(Continued)* (***E***) Evaluation and treatment of patients with suspected ectopic pregnancy and βHCG levels of less than 2000 mIU/mL and progesterone levels of 5 ng/mL or more.

all be done laparoscopically. If the patient is hemodynamically unstable or if a skilled laparoscopic surgical team is unavailable, laparotomy is still appropriate. Regardless of the incisional approach, if fertility is to be preserved, then microsurgical principles of fine nonreactive suture material, complete hemostasis, and minimal tissue trauma, destruction, and drying should be followed.

Table 18-6. Symptoms and Signs of Ectopic Pregnancy

> 75% of Patients Have:

Abdominopelvic pain
Abnormal uterine bleeding
Normal-sized uterus
Adnexal tenderness

50%–75% of Patients Have:

Generalized abdominopelvic pain
Amenorrhea

25%–50% of Patients Have:

Unilateral abdominopelvic pain
Syncopal symptoms
Unilateral adnexal mass
Cervical motion tenderness

< 25% of Patients Have:

Shoulder pain
Passage of uterine cast
Fever
Tachycardia
Orthostatic changes

In interstitial or cornual implantation, wedge or cornual resection is usually necessary. Bleeding preoperatively and intraoperatively may be massive due to involvement of the myometrium and large uterine vessels. These cases have been done laparoscopically but are more difficult and should be treated via laparotomy except by a very skilled laparoscopic team. Attempts to reimplant the tube at the time of the primary operation are discouraged; this may be done later if indicated.

Medical therapy of unruptured ectopic pregnancy with methotrexate was introduced in 1982 and has been growing in popularity. Its major advantage is the avoidance of surgery and anesthesia. Early studies suggest that it may result in improved subsequent conception rates (up to 90%) and intrauterine pregnancy rates (up to 60%). Numerous protocols have been used, but

Table 18-7. Lower Limits of Percentage Increase of βHCG Levels Early in Pregnancy*

SAMPLING INTERVAL (DAYS)	PERCENT INCREASE IN βHCG
1	29
2	66
3	114
4	175
5	255

*85% of normal pregnancies show an increase greater than these lower limits.

(Adapted from Kadar N, Caldwell BV, Romero R. A method of screening for ectopic pregnancy and its indications. Obstet Gynecol 1981;58:162.)

Table 18-8. Multiple-dose Methotrexate Regimen With Citrovorum Rescue for Treatment of Ectopic Pregnancy

DAY	TIME	THERAPY & LABORATORY TESTS
1	0800	Methotrexate IM, 1.0 mg/kg CBC, SGOT, type & Rh, creatinine, BUN, βHCG
2	0800	Citrovorum IM, 0.1 mg/kg βHCG
3	0800	Methotrexate IM, 1.0 mg/kg βHCG
4	0800	Citrovorum IM, 0.1 mg/kg βHCG
5	0800	Methotrexate IM, 1.0 mg/kg βHCG
6	0800	Citrovorum IM, 0.1 mg/kg βHCG
7	0800	Methotrexate IM, 1.0 mg/kg βHCG
8	0800	Citrovorum IM, 0.1 mg/kg βHCG, CBC, SGOT, type & Rh, creatinine, BUN

Table 18-9. Single-dose Methotrexate Regimen for Treatment of Ectopic Pregnancy

DAY	THERAPY & LABORATORY TESTS
1	Methotrexate IM, 50 mg/m^2 βHCG, CBC, SCOT, BUN, creatinine
2	βHCG
4	βHCG
7	βHCG
8	Repeat protocol if <15% drop in βHCG between days 4 and 7

two seem to be the most clinically practical: high-dose methotrexate with citrovorum rescue and single low-dose methotrexate. Tables 18-8 and 18-9 show two examples of such protocols. Failures of methotrexate occur in up to 10% of cases, sometimes with hemorrhage requiring transfusion and emergency surgery. These complications may be avoided by careful patient selection and follow-up. It is probably wisest not to give methotrexate if there is an adnexal mass over 3 cm, a sonographically visible fetal heartbeat in the adnexa, evidence of hemoperitoneum by ultrasound, or a pretreatment βHCG level over 2000 to 3000 mIU/mL. Daily or alternate-day measurements of βHCG levels are important. Failure of levels to decline by 15% to 20% every 2 to 3 days, or plateauing or rising levels, may indicate the need for retreatment or surgical intervention. Side effects of methotrexate therapy occur in about 20% of patients, but with the regimens used these are minor and transient. Bone marrow suppression does not occur, and the reported side effects have not altered or stopped the treatment.

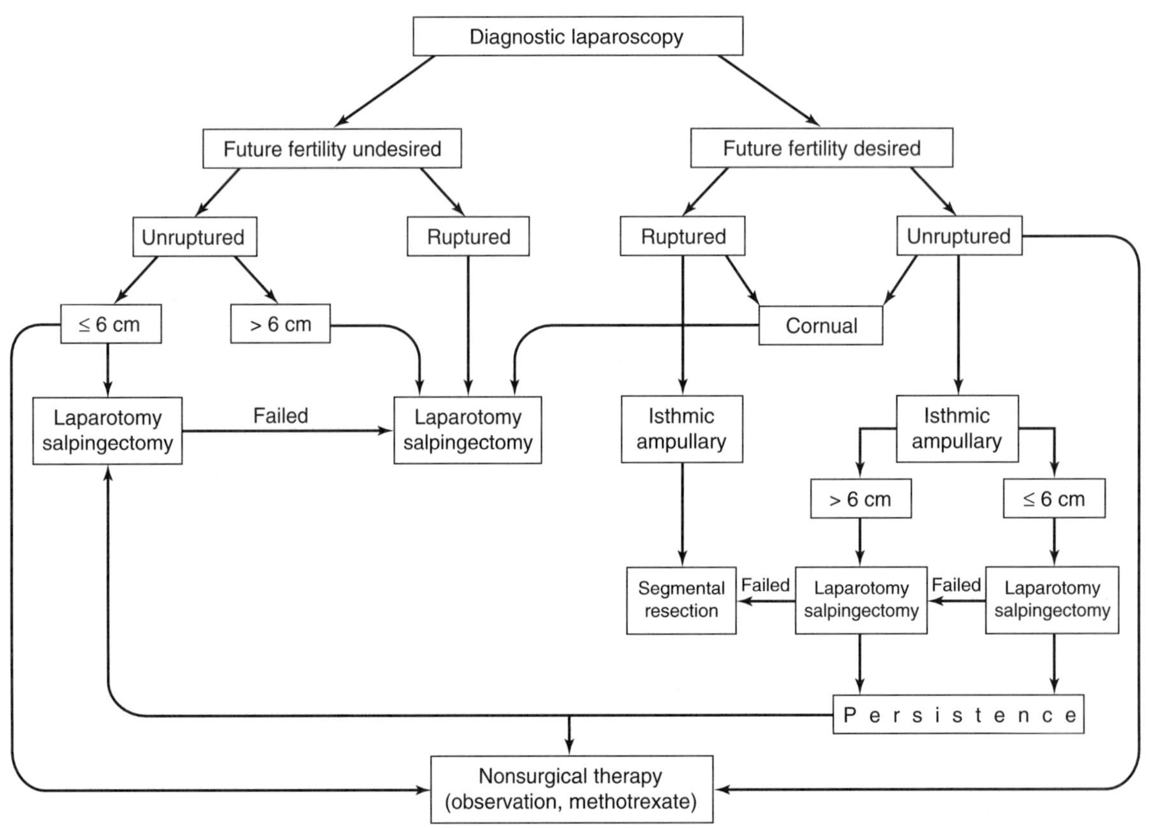

Figure 18-7. Algorithm for the operative management of tubal ectopic pregnancy. (Adapted from Vermesh M. Conservative management of ectopic pregnancy. Fertil Steril 1989;51:559.)

After conservative therapy for ectopic pregnancy, whether surgical or medical, βHCG levels must be followed until they are negative. Due to persistent trophoblastic tissue, subsequent surgical or medical retreatment is necessary in up to 7% of cases managed conservatively. A rising or persistent βHCG level or acute abdominal signs and symptoms may mean that there is persistent trophoblastic tissue. Even in cases of persistent ectopic pregnancy, the βHCG levels may initially decline rapidly. However, if the βHCG level exceeds 10% of the pretreatment level 12 days after conservative therapy, the possibility of persistent ectopic gestation should be considered likely. Similarly, increasing levels after 6 days are very suggestive of persistence. The choice of surgical or medical treatment of persistent trophoblastic tissue depends on the patient's condition and preference.

Observation may be appropriate in selected cases of ectopic pregnancy: up to 60% of cases resolve without surgical or medical therapy. However, the potential for life-threatening hemorrhage is significant, so hospitalization seems wisest if this approach is chosen. A major drawback to this approach is that the average time of hospitalization to document resolution exceeds 1 month.

Many treatment algorithms have been proposed, but again a fundamental understanding of the disease and the treatment options and the physician's experience are most important. The algorithm proposed by Vermesh and Presser (1992) is useful for the clinician who is planning treatment for a woman with an ectopic pregnancy (Fig. 18-7).

Rh screening should be done on all women with ectopic pregnancy. Rh sensitization may occur secondary to ectopic pregnancy, although the magnitude of this risk is unknown. However, as the risk of administration of Rh immune globulin is nil, any patient with an ectopic pregnancy should be given Rh immune globulin if she is Rh negative. At less than 12 weeks gestation, a 50-mg dose may be used, but the full 300-mg dose is advised at more than 12 weeks gestation.

It is difficult to counsel the woman subsequent to an ectopic pregnancy about her fertility prognosis, as many factors (eg, age, prior infertility, tubal disease, adhesions, ruptured or unruptured tube) influence the statistics. Repeat ectopic rates are 8% to 20%, with a mean of about 15%. Subsequent intrauterine pregnancy rates range from 45% to 70%. If the ectopic pregnancy occurred in the presence of an IUD, there appears to be no increased risk of a subsequent ectopic pregnancy. If the woman is parous, the subsequent fertility rate is higher than if she has an ectopic pregnancy with her first pregnancy. Gross evidence of salpingitis also predicts a lowered fertility rate and higher recurrence rate. Diagnosis and treatment before rupture of the fallopian tube improves the prognosis, so every effort should be made to diagnose the situation early and provide immediate treatment.

BIBLIOGRAPHY

Abortion

Ben-Baruch G, Schiff E, Moran O, Mehashe Y, Mashiach S, Menczer J. Curettage vs. nonsurgical management in women with early spontaneous abortions. J Reprod Med 1991;36:644.

Ohno M, Maeda T, Matsunobu A. A cytogenetic study of spontaneous abortion with direct analysis of chorionic villi. Obstet Gynecol 1991;77:394.

Simpson JL. What management for repeated spontaneous abortion? Contemp Ob/Gyn 1985;100.

Quenby SM, Farquharson RG. Predicting recurring miscarriage: what is important? Obstet Gynecol 1993;82:132.

Von Stein GA, Munsick RA, Stiver K, Ryder K. Fetomaternal hemorrhage in threatened abortion. Obstet Gynecol 1992;79:383.

Ectopic Pregnancy

Barnhart K, Mennuti MT, Benjamin I, Jacobson S, Goodman D, Coutifaris C. Prompt diagnosis of ectopic pregnancy in an emergency department setting. Obstet Gynecol 1994;84:1010.

Ory SJ. New options for diagnosis and treatment of ectopic pregnancy. JAMA 1992;267:534.

Shalev E, Romano S, Peleg C, Bustan M, Tsabari A. Spontaneous resolution of ectopic tubal pregnancy: natural history. Fertil Steril 1995;63:15.

Shepherd RW, Patton PE, Novy MJ, Burry KA. Serial βHCG measurements in the early detection of ectopic pregnancy. Obstet Gynecol 1990;75:417.

Stovall TG, Ling FW. Ectopic pregnancy. Diagnostic and therapeutic algorithms minimizing surgical intervention. J Reprod Med 1993;38:807.

Stovall TG, Ling FW, Gray LA. Single-dose methotrexate for treatment of ectopic pregnancy. Obstet Gynecol 1991;77:754.

Vermesh M, Presser SC. Reproductive outcome after linear salpingostomy for ectopic gestation: a prospective 3-year follow-up. Fertil Steril 1992; 57:682.

Washington AE, Katz P. Ectopic pregnancy in the United States: economic consequences and payment source trends. Obstet Gynecol 1993;81:287.

Westrom L, Bengtsson LPH, Mardh P-A. Incidence, trends and risks of ectopic pregnancy in a population of women. Br Med J 1981;282:15.

Primary Care for Women, edited by Phyllis C. Leppert and Fred M. Howard. Lippincott-Raven Publishers, Philadelphia © 1997.

19

Elective Termination of Pregnancy

MORRIS WORTMAN

Elective termination of an unwanted pregnancy is one of the oldest surgical procedures known, but even today the ethical, moral, and religious debates that accompany this issue continue to rage. In recent years, the worldwide trend has been toward liberalization of abortion laws. Well known, for example, are recent changes in Canada, Greece, Hungary, Romania, and Vietnam. According to the Alan Guttmacher Institute, 40% of the world's population lives in countries where induced abortion is permitted on request (the "least restrictive" category) and 25% lives in countries where abortion is allowed only if the woman's life is in danger (the "most restrictive" category). Countries in the least restrictive category include China, Russia, the United States, Turkey, Greece, Singapore, France, Germany, Austria, Denmark, Sweden, and Canada. The countries with the most restrictive abortion laws include Angola, Botswana, Chad, Libya, Mali, Mozambique, Nigeria, Somalia, Sudan, Zaire, Iran, Iraq, Laos, Lebanon, Pakistan, Syria, Guatemala, Haiti, Mexico, Brazil, Colombia, and Venezuela.

In 1973 the U.S. Supreme Court legalized abortion in this country. That year, 744,000 abortions were performed. Since 1980, more than 1.5 million pregnancies per year are reportedly terminated, making abortion the most common surgical procedure in the United States. Despite this fact, and largely because of the stigma associated with this procedure, scant scientific literature is available on the subject of elective pregnancy termination. Fewer still are textbooks, review articles, and organized meetings for those who wish to practice this service in a medically safe manner. Even as this text is written, there is congressional debate concerning whether obstetrics and gynecology residency training programs should be required to teach this procedure.

This chapter focuses on the medical and surgical techniques needed to perform abortions safely in the first and second trimesters.

HISTORICAL ASPECTS

Abortion had been legally practiced since colonial times under the common law of England. The practice of legalized abortion continued after the birth of the United States and well into the 19th century, at which time numerous states began passing restrictive abortion laws. In 1830, the state of New York enacted the nation's first statute making it illegal to perform a pregnancy termination after "quickening." The person performing the abortion was criminally liable, not the woman. Early abortion remained legal. By 1850, 17 states had similar laws, and by the end of the 19th century, every state except Kentucky had passed antiabortion legislation. Abortion had effectively been forced into the medical underground, both in the United States and England.

All this began to unravel in the famous Rex vs. Bourne decision in England, handed down in 1939. The defendant, a prominent London obstetrician, performed an abortion on a 14-year-old girl whose pregnancy resulted from a gang rape by three British soldiers. The trial judge, in an unusual move, had instructed the jury to consider a broader definition of "preserving the life of the woman" than simply the prevention of her imminent death. The jury was asked, for the first time, to consider that the preservation of the woman's life also meant preventing her from becoming a "physical or mental wreck." The defendant was acquitted and a new concept of "preservation of life" emerged.

The effect of Rex vs. Bourne was eventually felt in the United States, but 28 years passed until Colorado became the first state to pass a liberalized abortion statute. For the first time, the need to consider preservation of the mother's mental health was added to the consideration to preserve her life. By 1971, 17 states had followed Colorado's lead. A patchwork quilt of state laws varied widely in their restrictions to abortion. Even among states that allowed abortion, requirements varied with respect to gestational limits, the need for hospitalization, parental consent, and residency. When the U.S. Supreme Court rendered its historic Roe vs. Wade (Texas) and Doe vs. Bolton (Georgia) decision on January 22, 1973, it effectively stripped the states of power to prohibit abortion, except after the onset of fetal viability. The states' powers were limited to ensuring adequate facilities and duly licensed physicians.

PREOPERATIVE COUNSELING

Preoperative counseling must be individualized from one woman to the next. Counseling should be adjusted to reflect the patient's needs, education, and emotional state. Some patients are resolute in their choice to terminate a pregnancy; others are ambivalent and require considerable guidance. The counselor must maintain complete neutrality about the patient's decision. The counselor's role is not to advocate a particular outcome but to facilitate the patient's decision-making process. Counseling should always include some inquiry into the circumstances surrounding the pregnancy—was it the result of contraceptive failure, unwillingness to use contraception, forcible sex, or the sudden departure of a sexual partner? In other cases, counseling requires some assessment of the risk of x-ray, chemical, or alcohol exposure. Counseling may provide information that seriously affects a patient's decision to undergo a pregnancy termination. Perhaps the most important role of the counselor is to help the patient separate the medical realities from the emotional realities surrounding this difficult decision.

The counselor should be sensitive to the fact that for many couples, a pregnancy termination represents a turning point in a relationship. For a single woman, a pregnancy may highlight her wish to enter a more permanent bond or impel her to leave a partner whom she senses would be an inadequate father. For some women, confronting the partner with the fact that she is pregnant often underscores opposing wishes, leaving each little room to maneuver and compromise. For a newly married couple, an unplanned pregnancy confronts them with even greater commitment. I often explain to couples that many newlyweds get married twice, once at the altar and a second time when they choose to start a family. The deepening commitment that attends the birth of a child may catapult one out of the marriage. Still other marriages begin with the premise that children will not be a part of the relationship. These marriages are often tested when the partners are confronted with an unplanned pregnancy. For a stable couple who already have children, an unplanned pregnancy may herald the decision to complete their family.

The counselor must respect a woman's desire to maintain her privacy, even if that means an unwillingness to disclose information regarding the circumstances surrounding her choice.

INFORMED CONSENT

Physicians often misunderstand the meaning of informed consent, generally mistaking it for a signed document. Informed consent is a conversation that occurs between a health care provider and a woman who has elected to terminate a pregnancy. Physicians have the obligation to explain, in terms the patient understands, the substantive risks, benefits, and alternatives associated with elective abortion. The informed consent document, which the patient signs, is merely supportive evidence that such a conversation occurred.

In most states, a minor may give informed consent for an elective pregnancy termination. In New York, the Public Health Law provides that minors are considered emancipated from their parents once they become pregnant. Other states may require some form of notification of a parent or legal guardian. If there is doubt as to whether a minor, or an adult, is competent (based on that individual's mental or emotional ability) to give informed consent for an abortion, the court has indicated that parental or judicial consent may be required.

FACILITIES FOR PREGNANCY TERMINATION

Pregnancy terminations may be performed in various facilities, ranging from a private practice setting to a hospital inpatient unit. With careful patient selection and proper staffing, most elective pregnancy terminations can be safely carried out to the 18th week of gestation in an office or outpatient setting.

Wherever abortions are carried out, certain critical needs must be met:

- Properly trained counselors

- A practice-specific protocol
- Well-trained, compassionate, and experienced staff
- Proximity to a hospital with blood-banking facilities
- Availability of parenteral sedation, narcotic analgesics, uterotonic agents, and crystalloid solution and antibiotics
- Emergency equipment (including oxygen, resuscitation equipment, narcotic antagonists, intravenous catheters, and atropine)
- Pulse oximetry
- Immediate access to ultrasound equipment
- An adequate sterilizer
- Means to transfer the patient to the hospital in an emergency
- Access to contraception and information regarding contraceptive use.

In many communities, there is considerable hesitation to perform elective pregnancy terminations in an office environment beyond the 12th week. Often patients are treated in hospital outpatient or inpatient departments that have the "hardware" but lack the trained and compassionate staff that are critical to the patient's well-being. The patient's physical and emotional needs must be entrusted to professionals with proper credentials. Abortion providers must be dedicated to the patient's physical and emotional safety.

ANALGESIA AND ANESTHESIA

Women require a range of analgesic and anesthetic choices for a pregnancy termination. It makes little sense to offer a service that can be provided only under paracervical block anesthesia; it is equally punitive to insist that all patients undergo general anesthesia. A variety of choices should be offered, ranging from simple paracervical block anesthesia, intravenous conscious sedation (with or without narcotics), to a full general anesthetic provided by a board-certified anesthesiologist. This approach applies to both the first and second trimesters.

Occasionally, patients arrive at a facility in terror brought on by innumerable issues, including fear of surgery, anesthesia, and loss of control. Such fear may be compounded by guilt arising from political, moral, and religious concerns about abortion. Such patients must hear several important reassurances immediately on arrival:

- Every precaution will be taken to minimize the risk of complications.
- The patient can choose from a variety of analgesics and anesthetics.
- The patient will be treated with dignity and respect in a confidential, nonjudgmental manner.
- All possible precautions will be made to safeguard their future reproductive choices.
- All possible precautions will be made to safeguard the patient's privacy and confidentiality surrounding their medical record.

Some women have difficulty deciding, in advance, whether they wish to undergo a pregnancy termination under paracervical block, intravenous sedation, or general anesthesia. I recommend that for patients less than 10 weeks pregnant, the procedure may be initiated under paracervical block, with the understanding that intravenous conscious sedation may be added at any time. Patients are therefore asked to avoid food or liquids for at least 4 hours before the procedure. They must have someone to drive them home.

IMPORTANCE OF ACCURATE DETERMINATION OF FETAL GESTATIONAL AGE

Safe abortion services demand accurate preoperative information regarding the gestational age of the fetus. The need for accurate information must be balanced, however, against the cost of expensive technology. For example, the use of routine ultrasound examinations is not recommended in the first trimester when a simple urine pregnancy test, combined with the hands of an experienced examiner, often suffices. However, the selective use of transvaginal ultrasound in the first trimester is highly recommended when assessing a pregnancy complicated by bleeding, pelvic pain, syncope, hyperemesis gravidarum, or uncertain dates. Additionally, teenagers, poor historians, and obese and difficult-to-examine patients are best served with careful sonographic examinations.

The potential risks that accompany second-trimester abortions demand routine sonographic dating. The importance of routine ultrasound examination for these patients cannot be overstated. A miscalculation or an inaccurate bimanual examination may result in an illegal abortion, beyond the limits established by a state or municipality.

PREGNANCY TERMINATION IN THE FIRST TRIMESTER

First-trimester abortions are those performed before the 13th week of gestational age, as measured from the first day of the last menstrual period (LMP). These can be subdivided into three groups: those performed before 8 weeks, between 8 and 10 weeks, and between 10 and 13 weeks (ending at the onset of the 13th week).

Before 8 Weeks

A growing body of evidence suggests that during the first 8 weeks, many pregnancy terminations may be safely managed with medical, rather than surgical, intervention. At least two drug regimens are under study. Mifepristone (RU-486), an antiprogestin studied in Europe since 1979, is being used in formal multicenter clinical trials in the United States. The second regimen consists of a combination of methotrexate, an antifolate known for its use in gestational trophoblastic disease, and misoprostol, a prostaglandin known for its salutary effect on peptic and gastric ulcers. Both agents have been well studied under different clinical settings and are being used in combination as an abortifacient with encouraging results.

Medical abortifacients are important because they can eliminate most surgical interventions before the 8th week of gestation and may reduce the cost, complications, and fear of an invasive alternative. Another advantage of a medical abortifacient may be its ability to reduce the number of "failed abortions" within the first 42 days of gestation (measured from the patient's LMP). Medical abortions may more effectively protect a woman's privacy while making this critical decision. Further study is needed before these medications become a standard of care in the United States, but early experience suggests that they may be an important solution to the declining availability of abortion services in rural areas.

Abortions before 8 weeks are usually performed by dilatation and suction curettage. The safety of suction curettage during the first 8 weeks has been well established and is often a surprise to health professionals: during this period, it is associated with a mortality rate of 0.5 per 100,000 population—less than the mortality associated with a single oral dose of penicillin.

From 8 to 10 Weeks

From 8 to 10 weeks, the use of medical abortifacients is not recommended because of the increased pain, bleeding, and incidence of retained products of conception. The safest technique is simple dilatation and suction curettage during a 1-day procedure.

Up to 10th week of gestation, I prefer to perform most procedures at a single visit without the insertion of laminaria tents. With some exceptions, most abortions can be performed safely with the careful use of a paracervical block anesthetic, with or without conscious sedation (usually intravenous midazolam). Lidocaine 1% is recommended because of its excellent safety record. The procedure is begun as 1 to 2 mL is injected just under the anterior cervical mucosa to facilitate tenaculum placement. The rest of the lidocaine (9 to 14 mL) is slowly injected in the midline just beneath the posterior cervical mucosa and is allowed to diffuse across the uterosacral ligaments and the accompanying nerve plexus. The patient is allowed to rest for 5 to 10 minutes in the presence of a trained medical assistant or nurse. Dilatation is accomplished with the gentle use of Hank or Denniston dilators (Fig. 19-1). This is normally followed by suctioning with an appropriate disposable plastic suction curet.

Uterine perforation is rare, provided that tissues are handled delicately and the position of the uterus has been correctly assessed. Occasionally, ultrasound is necessary to gain this information in the obese or difficult-to-examine patient.

From 10 to 13 Weeks

Pregnancy terminations performed during the interval from 10 to 13 weeks require two visits to the physician's office: one for laminaria insertion and a second for the suction procedure. These visits can be scheduled 24 hours apart so that cervical dilatation can be safely accomplished beginning the day before the suction procedure. Some physicians prefer to use hygroscopic dilators, which accomplish dilatation within 3 to 4 hours. This allows procedures in this interval to be performed in a single day, which is a consideration if the patient must travel a long distance. Both of these methods promote safe dilatation of the cervix and minimize the risk of tears and subsequent stenosis.

Although laminaria tents are occasionally inconvenient and time-consuming, they obviate many complications that result from aggressive and overzealous dilatation of the cervix. Among these complications are rupture of the cervix, lacerations of the anterior cervical lip, uterine perforation, and incomplete removal of the products of conception. The use of laminaria, therefore, provides an important margin of safety that should not be overlooked. Often, women who have recently delivered vaginally or who have a soft, patulous cervix may undergo a procedure during this interval without undue concern for cervical tears. Patients who have demonstrated poor compliance in keeping appointments may be better served by not using laminaria, as prolonged retention of these devices may result in life-threatening sepsis.

After selecting an appropriate anesthetic or sedative-hypnotic, the laminaria is removed. Occasionally some mechanical dilation is necessary after the cervix has been secured with a tenaculum. After selecting an appropriate suction catheter, a thorough curettage is performed. A good rule for determining the appropriate size of a suction catheter is to select one whose diameter in millimeters equals the gestational age in weeks. For example, at 12 weeks gestation, a suction catheter 12 mm in diameter is used. In most instances, an abortion during this interval does not require the use of intrauterine manipulation with forceps.

PREGNANCY TERMINATION IN THE SECOND TRIMESTER

The safety principles for middle trimester abortions are identical to those for abortions performed in the first trimester. I prefer to perform most abortions up to the 18th week of gestation in an office setting. Experience has shown this to be safe, as long as appropriate facilities are maintained and highly trained personnel are available. However, physicians who are ill equipped would better serve their patients by using an appropriate hospital or clinic facility. Although the maternal risks and consequences associated with midtrimester abortions increase with gestational age, they do not exceed those associated with continued uninterrupted pregnancy to term. Most large studies in the United States and Canada demonstrate an increase in maternal mortality from one per 100,000 in the first trimester to two to five per 100,000 in the middle trimester. The lower range of maternal mortality applies to abortions per-

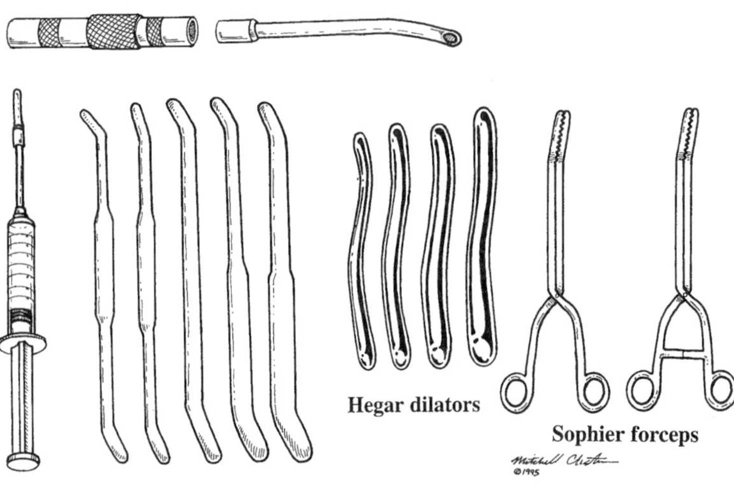

Figure 19-1. Commonly-used instruments for first and second trimester abortions.

formed before 18 weeks. Morbidity, in contrast, does not vary widely between the first and second trimesters.

Abortions performed in the middle trimester are said to confront the provider with the destructive nature of this procedure, which may explain the paucity of providers who perform this service. Most studies support the notion that midtrimester abortions by dilatation and evacuation are safer than other methods of pregnancy termination. During this procedure, the cervix is dilated with one or more laminaria tents, followed by the use of limited suction curettage. The use of destructive instruments such as Sophier forceps (see Fig. 19-1) is necessary to assist in the evacuation of all fetal and placental tissue. The uterus must be completely emptied of all products of conception. This is done by several methods, including examination of all fetal parts, digital examination of the uterine cavity, or sonographic examination of the uterus.

An increasing number of midtrimester abortions have been performed under ultrasound guidance (Fig. 19-2). This generally reduces the length of the procedure and may play an important role in reducing uterine perforations.

Midtrimester abortions demand meticulous attention to the patient's well-being. The use of sedative-hypnotics, narcotic analgesics, and parenteral nonsteroidal antiinflammatory agents must be strongly considered. Many physicians prefer to use a general anesthetic for abortions performed in this interval. Except in the most difficult cases, complicated by massive obesity or vaginismus, I prefer to use sedative-hypnotics, such as midazolam, as this avoids the uterine atony and associated blood loss that occurs with general anesthesia. Although many physicians question the use of midazolam in an office environment, fearing its potential for respiratory depression, such fears are unfounded when this agent is administered without a narcotic analgesic.

PROPHYLACTIC ANTIBIOTICS

The incidence of infections associated with pregnancy termination varies with factors such as socioeconomic class, race, marital status, and geographic location. Several authors advocate the use of routine prophylactic antibiotics as a way to reduce the incidence of subsequent endometritis/salpingitis. This has been my practice since 1990. For pregnancy terminations performed in a single office visit (eg, without laminaria tents), women are asked to begin a regimen of doxycycline 100 mg orally twice a day for 5 days immediately after laminarian insertion. For patients unable to tolerate doxycycline and who are not allergic to penicillin, ampicillin 500 mg orally twice a day for 5 days can be given. Reported side effects are few with either regimen. Patients who have intolerable gastrointestinal side effects are asked to discontinue the medication.

COMPLICATIONS

Because of the political debate that surrounds the abortion issue and also because it is the most commonly performed surgical procedure in the United States, few, if any, surgical procedures have been as extensively studied. Among the organizations that regularly track abortion and abortion complications are the Alan Guttmacher Institute, the National Abortion Federation, and the Centers for Disease Control. Most state health departments collect and analyze data on the demographics of abortion facilities, as well as complications secondary to abortion.

Morbidity and mortality associated with abortion vary with gestational age. The mortality associated with first-trimester abortion is about one per 100,000. This increases to 1.2 per 100,000 at 13 to 15 weeks gestation and 5.8 per 100,000 beyond 16 weeks.

The most common morbidities associated with first-trimester abortions are upper genital tract infections and excessive blood loss. The latter may require resuctioning, blood transfusions, or both. Perforation injuries are uncommon and vary inversely with operator experience. Rarely, perforation injuries lead to subsequent hysterectomy. Other complications of first-trimester abortion include failure to terminate the pregnancy, failure to diagnose an ectopic pregnancy, and severe vasovagal reactions.

Second-trimester abortions carry equivalent complications. However, because of the more advanced gestation, uterine perforation injuries and incomplete abortion take on much greater significance. Some physicians use prostaglandin gels or suppositories to

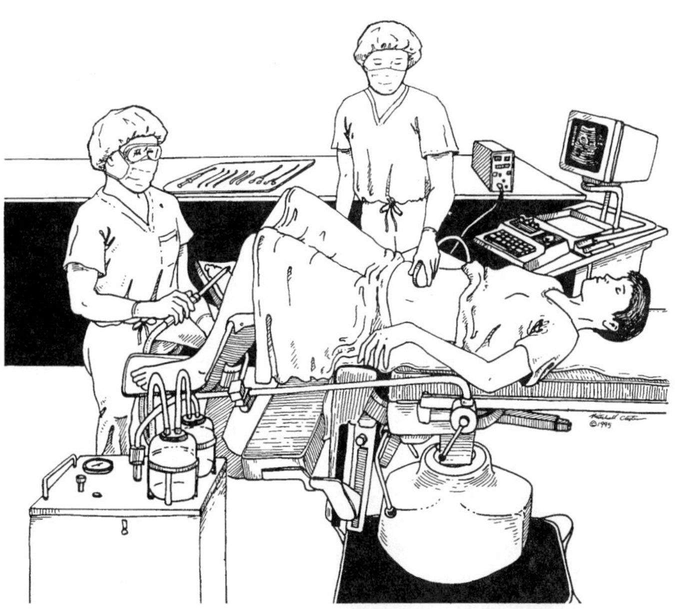

Figure 19-2. Office operating room setup for pregnancy termination under ultrasound guidance.

facilitate midtrimester abortions. These have been associated with hypertonic uterine contractions resulting in lower segment ruptures. On rare occasions, prostaglandins have been associated with the unplanned birth of a live fetus.

Midtrimester abortions are best handled by highly experienced physicians in an optimal clinical environment. For physicians learning to perform this demanding procedure, proper credentialing demands close work with an experienced gynecologist to supervise training.

Many women who present for midtrimester abortion are extremely ambivalent about their choice, making the need for gentle psychological support extremely important. Other patients require greater education about the need to avoid, when possible, abortion in the middle trimester. For some patients, midtrimester abortion is a difficult choice made after learning of a significant congenital malformation or even fetal demise. Care must be individualized, and this often requires the abortion provider to coordinate consultations from genetic counselors and perinatal experts.

CONTRACEPTION

Abortion providers must dispense information about the use of various contraceptive methods. Many women accept contraceptive counseling readily when faced with the difficult decisions regarding a pregnancy termination. For others, the fear that may accompany the process of pregnancy termination does not allow them to absorb and weigh additional medical information at this time. Instead, they might be better served with some written information and a follow-up appointment to discuss various contraceptive choices. For a more complete discussion of contraceptive choices, see Chapter 16.

STERILIZATION AND ABORTION

Although the safety of simultaneous abortion and sterilization procedures has been well established, it is important to recognize the difficulty in making these two decisions simultaneously. Patients who elect to undergo simultaneous pregnancy termination and sterilization must be carefully counseled. The physician must obtain a history regarding the circumstances surrounding the decision to terminate a pregnancy. Often, a pregnancy termination represents a turning point in a relationship. For single women, it often precipitates a separation from their partner. For married women, it may tip the scales from a stable to an unstable marriage. For this reason, it is important that the physician carefully counsel women who seek simultaneous abortion and sterilization procedures. If the patient or her provider has doubts about the wisdom of this procedure, it may be best to involve an outside consultant or agree to provide only the pregnancy termination at the present time, while more thought is given to an elective sterilization procedure. Although a woman may be very strong in her demand that the two procedures be carried out simultaneously, she must occasionally be reminded that the physician also has the right to exercise his or her choice in agreeing to this demand.

BIBLIOGRAPHY

Atrash HK, MacKay HT, Binkin NJ, Hogue CJ. Legal abortion mortality in the United States: 1972–1982. Am J Obstet Gynecol 1987;156:605.

Butler JD, Walbert DF. Abortion, medicine, and the law, 4th ed. New York: Facts on File, 1992.

Cates W. Legal abortion: the public health record. Science 1982;215:1586.

Cheng M. The safety of combined abortion-sterilization procedure. Am J Obstet Gynecol 1977;129:548.

Grimes DA, Cates W. Complications from legally induced abortion: a review. Obstet Gynecol Surv 1979;34:177.

Grimes DA, Schultz KT. The comparative safety of second-trimester abortion methods. Ciba Foundation Symposium 1985;115;83.

Grimes DA, Schulz KF, Cates W, Tyler CW. Midtrimester abortion by intraamniotic prostaglandin F2, safer than saline? Obstet Gynecol 1977;49:612.

Jacobsen J. Promoting population stabilization: incentives for small families. Worldwatch Paper 54, June 1983.

Lanman JT, Kohl SG, Bedell JH. Changes in pregnancy outcome after liberalization of the New York State abortion law. Am J Obstet Gynecol 1974;118:485.

Lauersen NH, Tiberius D, Scher J, Iliescu C, Wilson KH. A new abortion technique: intravaginal and intramuscular prostaglandin. Obstet Gynecol 1981;58:96.

MacKenzie IE, Bibby JG. Critical assessment of dilatation and curettage in 1209 women. Lancet 1978;2:566.

McFarlane DR. On avoiding the abortion issue. Am J Gynecol Health 1992;6:9.

McFarlane DR. U.S. abortion policy since Roe v Wade. Am J Gynecol Health 1993;7:17.

Rovinsky JJ. Impact of a permissive abortion statute on community health care. Obstet Gynecol 1973;41:781.

Spreet H. Obstetrics and gynecology in America: a history. Chicago: American College of Obstetricians and Gynecologists, 1980.

20

Dyspareunia

DAVID BARAM

Primary Care for Women, edited by Phyllis C. Leppert and Fred M. Howard. Lippincott-Raven Publishers, Philadelphia © 1997.

Dyspareunia ("difficult mating" or "badly mated") is pain or discomfort in the labial, vaginal, or pelvic region that occurs before, during, or after intercourse in the absence of vaginismus. The repeated experience of pain during intercourse can cause marked distress, anxiety, and interpersonal difficulties, leading to anticipation of a negative sexual experience and eventually to decreased sexual frequency or sexual avoidance. As with other sexual dysfunctions, dyspareunia can be generalized (not limited to a specific partner or situation) or situational, primary (pain present from initial intercourse) or secondary (acquired after a period of pain-free sexual functioning). Secondary dyspareunia occurs, on average, about 10 years after the onset of sexual activity.

Dyspareunia is one of the most common sexual dysfunctions seen by gynecologists and is estimated to affect about two thirds of women during their lifetime. Women usually discuss the pain with their sexual partner, but fewer than half consult a physician about their dyspareunia. Because dyspareunia is a psychophysiologic condition, both psychological and physical factors must be considered when assessing patients with this condition. In many cases, no exact physical cause can be found. Even when a source of pain is identified and successfully treated, fear of pain and the presence of anxiety before and during intercourse can inhibit arousal, causing lack of vaginal lubrication and further discomfort.

ETIOLOGY

Causes of pain on stimulation of the external genitalia include chronic vulvitis, the vulvar dystrophies, and clitoral irritation and hypersensitivity (Table 20-1). Pain at the introitus caused by penile entry can be caused by a rigid hymenal ring, scar tissue in an episiotomy repair, vaginal stenosis, a müllerian abnormality, or vaginitis caused by one of the many common vaginal pathogens such as *Candida*, *Trichomonas*, or *Gardnerella* or by irritation from over-the-counter vaginal sprays, douches, or contraceptive devices. Other causes include Bartholin gland inflammation, radiation vaginitis, infection with human papillomavirus (HPV), urethritis, urethral syndrome, cystitis, trauma, chronic constipation, or proctitis. Common causes of vaginal dyspareunia are friction due to inadequate sexual arousal and lack of vaginal lubrication and vaginal atrophy after surgical or natural menopause. Vulvar vestibulitis syndrome is a constellation of symptoms consisting of severe pain or burning on vestibular touch and attempted vaginal entry. In addition to dyspareunia, these patients may have pain with tampon insertion or with pressure from a bicycle seat. On examination, diffuse or focal vulvar erythema is noted around the orifices of the Bartholin, Skene, periurethral, or vestibular glands. This syndrome may be caused by an infection (subclinical HPV, bacterial vaginosis, chronic candidiasis), irritants (soaps, detergents, douches, or vaginal sprays), or altered vaginal pH secondary to a decrease of lactobacilli. Vulvar vestibulitis may be secondary to treatment of HPV with podophyllin, trichloroacetic acid, or laser.

Vaginismus, according to the DSM-IV, is the recurrent or persistent involuntary contraction of the perineal muscles surrounding the outer third of the vagina when vaginal penetration with a penis, finger, tampon, or speculum is attempted. Vaginismus is an involuntary reflex precipitated by real or imagined attempts at vaginal penetration. It can be global (the woman cannot place anything inside her vagina) or situational (she can use a tampon and can tolerate a pelvic examination but cannot have intercourse). Many women with vaginismus have normal sexual desire, experience vaginal lubrication, and are orgasmic, but cannot have intercourse. Vaginismus can be primary (the woman has never been able to have intercourse) or secondary (often due to acquired dyspareunia). Some couples may cope with this difficulty for years before they decide to seek help. They usually seek treatment because they desire children or decide they would like to consummate their relationship. Vaginismus is relatively rare, affecting about 1% of women. It can be a conditioned response to an unpleasant experience such as past sexual abuse, a painful first pelvic examination, or a painful first attempt at intercourse, or may be secondary to religious orthodoxy or sexual orientation concerns. Many women with vaginismus have an extreme fear of penetration and misconceptions about their anatomy and about the size of their vagina. They may believe that their vagina is too small to accommodate a tampon or penis, and that great physical harm will result from placing anything inside of them.

Medical conditions are rarely the cause of vaginismus, but conditions such as endometriosis, chronic pelvic inflammatory disease, partially imperforate hymen, and vaginal stenosis must be ruled out by a careful pelvic examination. The pelvic examination, which should be done if possible in the presence of the woman's partner, allows the physician to help educate the couple about normal female anatomy and may help dispel misconceptions about the size of the introitus and vagina. Providing the patient with a mirror so she can observe the examination is helpful. Because the etiology of vaginismus is usually psychophysiologic, patients with this condition should not have surgery to enlarge their introitus unless they have a partially imperforate hymen or another valid indication for surgery.

Causes of midvaginal pain include a congenitally shortened vagina and interstitial cystitis, a chronic idiopathic inflammatory condition of the bladder. Pain with orgasm may be associated with uterine contractions.

Dyspareunia with deep vaginal penetration can be associated with inadequate vaginal lengthening and lubrication secondary to inadequate sexual arousal, pregnancy, menopause, or the use of oral contraceptives. Chronic pelvic inflammatory disease, endometriosis, a fixed retroverted uterus, a pelvic mass, an enlarged uterus secondary to myomata or adenomyosis, inflammatory bowel disease, irritable bowel syndrome, or pelvic relaxation are also possible causes of deep dyspareunia.

Psychological factors contributing to dyspareunia include developmental factors, such as an upbringing that invested sex with guilt and shame; traumatic factors such as rape, childhood sexual abuse, or other sexual assault; and relationship factors, such as anger or resentment toward a sexual partner or fear of pregnancy.

Lazarus uses the mnemonic "Basic ID" to describe his multimodal approach to the assessment of dyspareunia: **B**ehavior (faulty technique), **A**ffect (guilt, anger, fear, and shame), **S**ensation (where is the pain), **I**magery (do intrusive thoughts or negative images disrupt sexual enjoyment), **C**ognition (do dysfunctional beliefs or misinformation play a role in undermining sexual participation), **I**nterpersonal (how do the partners communicate and relate in both sexual and nonsexual settings), and **D**rugs (is the patient on any medication that would diminish vaginal lubrication, such as an antihistamine).

HISTORY

A careful history should be directed toward a complete chronology of the discomfort, an assessment of the impact of the dyspareunia on the patient and her partner, and any prior attempts to treat the condition. What effect has the pain had on the couple's sexual functioning? The patient should be asked about the specific location of the pain (where on the vulva or in the vagina the pain occurs), when in the course of lovemaking the pain occurs (during foreplay, on penile entry, throughout intercourse, after intercourse, or only on deep thrusting), how long the pain lasts, the nature and quality of the pain (burning, stabbing), and the severity of the pain. Is the pain always present, or are there times when intercourse is not painful? What relieves or aggravates the discomfort? It often helps to ask the patient about her theory of how the pain began and to assess her expectations and goals for treatment. The patient's understanding of sexual physiology and sexual behavior should

Table 20-1. Causes of Dyspareunia

Pain on Insertion
Vaginal atrophy secondary to menopause or surgery
Chronic vulvitis (allergy to lubricant or contraceptive)
Vulvar dystrophy
Vulvar vestibulitis
Vulvodynia
Rigid hymenal ring
Episiotomy scar
Mullerian abnormality
Vaginismus
Bartholin's gland infection
Inadequate sexual arousal and lubrication
Mid-vaginal Pain
Urethritis
Shortened vagina
Interstitial cystitis
Following surgery or radiation
Deep Dyspareunia
Pelvic inflammatory disease
Endometriosis
Fixed uterine retroversion
Pelvic adhesions
Ovarian pathology
Bowel disease
Pelvic relaxation
Myomas, adenomyosis

also be assessed and any myths or misinformation addressed. Patients must be carefully asked about a history of childhood sexual or physical abuse or adult sexual assault, as they may be associated with dyspareunia. Patients who are anxious about sexuality because of sexual misconceptions, guilt, fear of pregnancy or sexually transmitted disease, or prior unpleasant sexual experiences may be unable to relax during lovemaking, leading to impaired arousal and lubrication.

Significant relationship or couple communication problems may also contribute to dyspareunia. It is often useful to think of dyspareunia as a couple problem, and it is helpful to interview the couple together. Couples often can provide useful clues about the etiology of the dysfunction. Conflicts about family size, contraception, sexual frequency, and sexual technique may lead to anger, distrust, misunderstanding, depression, and ultimately pain. The patient's partner may pick an inconvenient time or may not spend enough time on foreplay for the patient to become adequately sexually aroused and lubricated.

PHYSICAL EXAMINATION

During the physical examination,attempts should be made to identify any, often subtle, organic factors contributing to the discomfort. A careful, thorough, and systematic abdominal, low back, and pelvic examination should be carried out. Physiologic changes that occur during sexual arousal may account for pain that is present during intercourse but absent at other times, such as during a routine pelvic examination. Examples are Bartholin gland cysts, which swell during intercourse, and adhesive bands that form between portions of the hymenal ring only during arousal.

The physical examination should evaluate and educate the patient. She should be examined while sitting upright and in the presence of her partner if possible, and should be given a hand mirror to observe the pelvic examination and to indicate where her pain is coming from. The physician should watch the patient's face while performing the pelvic examination to see if pain is elicited and if the pain of intercourse is re-created by palpation of specific anatomic sites. Careful inspection of the external genitalia can identify ulcerations, erythema, or pigment changes. Palpation with a moist cotton-tipped swab can identify sites of vulvar vestibulitis, which are exquisitely tender to palpation. Colposcopy with application of 5% acetic acid may help identify abnormal areas on the vulva and introitus.

The vagina should be gently and carefully examined with one finger, checking for any scars from previous surgery or an episiotomy and any involuntary spasm of the muscles of the introitus or the levator sling. Having the patient contract the muscles of her pelvic floor (Kegel exercises) while the examiner places a finger inside her vagina helps assess the tone of the pelvic floor and helps identify these muscles as a possible source of the dyspareunia. Stroking the bladder base and urethra may reproduce pain caused by trigonitis, interstitial cystitis, chronic urethritis, or a urethral diverticulum. A speculum examination should be done to obtain cervical cultures and vaginal secretions for wet-mount examination and to assess the vagina for atrophy.

The bimanual and rectovaginal examination should be carried out in a systematic manner. Pain with manipulation of the cervix may identify it as a source of dyspareunia, possibly due to chronic pelvic inflammatory disease. Uterine pain with palpation may be due to adenomyosis or uterine myomata. A fixed, tender, and retroverted uterus may be caused by endometriosis. Tender adnexa, possibly caused by endometriosis or an ovarian cyst, may be the cause of deep thrust dyspareunia. A rectovaginal examination may help identify endometriosis, retroperitoneal lesions, inflammatory bowel disease, and rectal masses.

In patients who are difficult to examine because of obesity, tenderness, or anxiety, a pelvic ultrasound may provide further evaluation of the pelvic organs and possible clues to the etiology of the pain. Many patients who do not tolerate pelvic examinations well may be survivors of childhood sexual abuse or adult sexual assault or may have had a traumatic and uncomfortable first pelvic examination. These patients must be approached in a gentle, sensitive, and reassuring way, allowing them as much control as possible over the examination.

TREATMENT

Many physicians have anxiety about discussing sexual issues with their patients and believe they lack the basic skills to provide counseling for sexual dysfunction, but most sexual concerns can be treated by the primary care physician. The "PLISSIT" model is a useful sexual counseling and therapy method consisting of four levels of therapeutic intervention. Using the first three levels of this model, about 80% to 90% of sexual concerns can be treated. The first level, **P**ermission, validates the patient's feelings and gives her permission to address her sexual concerns. The second level, **L**imited **I**nformation, provides the patient with information about sexual physiology and behavior. The third level, **S**pecific **S**uggestions, involves specific reeducation regarding the patient's sexual attitudes and practices. For example, a woman with dyspareunia secondary to inadequate vaginal lubrication because of inhibited sexual desire is first given permission to address the situation with her partner and to look at her genitalia and touch her clitoris. She is then given limited information about the genital anatomy and the physiology of the sexual response. Specific suggestions are then offered about using fantasy (specific self-help books may be suggested), prolonging foreplay, improving communication, using water-soluble lubricants during intercourse, and having the patient and her partner stimulate her clitoris before and during intercourse.

The fourth level, referral for **I**ntensive **T**herapy, is reserved for patients who do not respond to the first three levels of intervention and who may require intensive individual or couple therapy. Patients who are sexual abuse survivors and those who have significant anxiety or depression, sexual aversion, or significant marital dysfunction should be referred to a therapist who specializes in these areas.

Vaginal atrophy secondary to natural or surgical menopause rapidly responds to systemic or vaginal estrogen replacement. Kegel exercises help the patient improve control over her vaginal muscles and increase the elasticity of the vaginal canal. Treatment of the vulvar dystrophies is based on diagnosis by biopsy. Lichen sclerosis is treated with topical 2% testosterone ointment, hypertrophic lesions with topical corticosteroids.

In treating vulvovaginitis, attempts should be made to diagnose a specific pathogen with the use of vaginal cultures, wet preps, and vaginal pH. If a specific organism, such as *Trichomonas*, is identified, both the patient and her partner should be treated. In many cases, a specific organism is not found, but the patient may often become less symptomatic by changing some hygiene habits. She should use unperfumed soap, avoid using soap in her vaginal area, dry her vulva after bathing with a hair dryer, and not use douches, vaginal sprays, or scented tampons. Wearing cotton underwear and loose-fitting clothing often helps. Because many detergents contain enzymes, which can be irritating to the skin, she should wash her underwear in Dreft or Woolite.

In treating vulvar vestibulitis syndrome, efforts should be made to identify and treat a specific cause, such as HPV. Other symptomatic treatments include topical steroid ointments, anesthetic creams, injection of a long-acting local anesthetic, antidepressants, or antihistamines. Surgery (vestibulectomy with vaginal advancement) should be reserved for patients with severe dyspareunia who do not respond to conservative management.

Chronic urethritis due to inadequate estrogen support or an unrecognized infection with *Chlamydia trachomatis* responds to estrogen replacement or antibiotic treatment. Patients with urinary urgency, frequency, and dysuria without an identifiable infection may respond to urinary antispasmodics, low-dose antibiotics, or tricyclic antidepressants.

Vaginal strictures or vaginal shortening following surgery or radiation therapy can be treated with estrogen vaginal cream and progressive dilatation of the vagina with vaginal dilators.

Treatment of vaginismus is directed toward extinguishing the conditioned involuntary vaginal spasm. This can be accomplished by helping the woman become more familiar with her anatomy and more comfortable with her sexuality; teaching her techniques to help her relax when she anticipates vaginal penetration; instructing her in the use of Kegel exercises to gain control over the muscles surrounding her introitus; and instructing her how to use graduated rubber dilators (fingers can also be used as dilators).

The protocol for use of the dilators is explained to the patient while she is in the office, but the actual placement of the dilators is done by the patient at home. It is important for the patient to maintain total control over the use of the dilators and to use them in an environment that is comfortable and safe. The dilators should be covered with a warm, water-soluble lubricant such as K-Y Jelly. She should initially try to place the dilators (or her finger) in her vagina when she is alone and relaxed. If she cannot relax enough to place the smallest dilator in her vagina, she may be able to reduce her anxiety by learning relaxation or self-hypnosis techniques. Medications, such as propranolol or alprazolam, may also help reduce anxiety. Once she has been able to place the smallest dilator in her vagina, she can progressively insert the larger dilators, practicing Kegel exercises while they are in place. When she is comfortable inserting the larger dilators, she can instruct her partner how to place the dilators in her vagina while she maintains control over how quickly they are placed. She may then be ready to proceed to intercourse. Again, this must be under her control, with her sitting or kneeling over her partner and inserting his penis herself. The majority (90%) of couples who follow this protocol are successful and able to have intercourse.

Deep thrust dyspareunia can be caused by endometriosis, pelvic adhesions, pelvic relaxation, symptomatic uterine retroversion, or adnexal pathology. The treatment of endometriosis is described elsewhere, but improvement or worsening of dyspareunia can be a guide to the success or failure of treatment. With laparoscopic lysis of pelvic adhesions, many patients note improvement in chronic pelvic pain and dyspareunia. Laparoscopy can also be used to diagnose and treat adnexal masses and to suspend a fixed, retroverted uterus.

In addition to treating specific physical problems, the physician can assign the patient and her partner behavior therapy exercises they can practice at home. These exercises can help desensitize the patient to the discomfort she may anticipate with vaginal penetration and help her extinguish the learned pain response to intercourse. Suggested exercises might include assigned readings, progressive sexual fantasies, instruction in deep muscle relaxation, and couple pleasuring exercises ("sensate focus"). As in the treatment of vaginismus, Kegel exercises and the use of graduated vaginal dilators can help the patient overcome her discomfort. Once the patient has gained voluntary control over her levator muscles, she may want to proceed to intercourse, eventually incorporating sexual responsiveness and a variety of coital positions into lovemaking.

SUMMARY

Inquiries about sexual dysfunction, childhood sexual abuse, and adult sexual assault should be part of every routine gynecologic history. Physicians will feel more comfortable talking to their patients about sex if they understand the normal sexual response and know how to approach the evaluation and treatment of common sexual dysfunctions. Asking about sexual concerns gives physicians an opportunity to educate patients, dispel sexual myths and misconceptions, and gives patients permission to address sexual issues in a professional, confidential, and nonjudgmental setting. When evaluating and treating patients with dyspareunia, physicians should be aware that psychological, physical, and relationship factors all contribute to this condition. After a careful and systematic physical examination, developmental, intrapersonal, and relationship issues should be explored. It is important to help the patient set realistic goals and expectations for treatment and to realize that treatment is an ongoing process that may require more than one treatment approach. Most patients with primary and secondary dyspareunia improve when treated by an interested, empathetic, and knowledgeable physician.

BIBLIOGRAPHY

American Psychiatric Association. Diagnostic and statistical manual of mental disorders, 4th ed. Washington DC: American Psychiatric Association, 1994.

Dewitt DE. Dyspareunia. Postgrad Med 1991;89:67.

Franger AL. Taking a sexual history and managing common sexual problems. J Reprod Med 1988;33:639.

Glatt AE, Zinner SH, McCormack WM. The prevalence of dyspareunia. Obstet Gynecol 1990;75:433.

Kaplan HS. The evaluation of sexual disorders: psychological and medical aspects. New York: Brunner/Mazel, 1983.

Lamont J. Vaginismus. Am J Obstet Gynecol 1978;131:632.

Lamont JA. Dyspareunia and vaginismus. In: Sciarra JJ, Droegemueller W, eds. Gynecology and obstetrics. Philadelphia: JB Lippincott, 1990.

Lazarus AA. Dyspareunia: a multimodal psychotherapeutic perspective. In: Leiblum SR, Rosen RC, eds. Principles and practice of sex therapy, 2d ed. New York: Guilford Press, 1989:89.

Marinoff SC, Turner MLC. Vulvar vestibulitis syndrome: an overview. Am J Obstet Gynecol 1991;165:1228.

Peckham BM, Maki DG, Patterson JJ, Hafez G. Focal vulvitis: a characteristic syndrome and cause of dyspareunia. Am J Obstet Gynecol 1986;154:855.

Pion R, Annon J. The office management of sexual problems: brief therapy approaches. J Reprod Med 1975;15:127.

Sarazin SK, Seymour SF. Causes and treatment options for women with dyspareunia. Nurse Practitioner 1991;16:30.

Spector IP, Carey MP. Incidence and prevalence of the sexual dysfunctions: a critical review of the empirical literature. Arch Sex Behav 1990;19:389.

Steege J. Dyspareunia and vaginismus. Clin Obstet Gynecol 1984;27:750.

Steege JF, Ling FW. Dyspareunia. Obstet Gynecol Clin North Am 1993;20:779.

Stevenson RWD, Szasz G, Maurice WL, Miles JE. How to become comfortable talking about sex to your patients. Can Med Assoc J 1983;128:797.

Walling MK, Reiter RC, O'Hara MW, Milburn AK, Lilly G, Vincent SD. Abuse history and chronic pelvic pain in women: I. Prevalences of sexual abuse and physical abuse. Obstet Gynecol 1994;84:193.

Primary Care for Women, edited by Phyllis C. Leppert and Fred M. Howard. Lippincott-Raven Publishers, Philadelphia © 1997.

21

Acute Abdominopelvic Pain

RAYMOND J. LANZAFAME
CESAR BARADA

The evaluation and diagnosis of abdominal and pelvic pain form one of the greatest clinical challenges in the care of women. For ease of presentation, we shall split our discussion into two sections: abdominopelvic pain in nonpregnant and pregnant patients.

Abdominopelvic Pain in the Nonpregnant Patient

To paraphrase the great clinician William Osler, listen to the patient and she will often give you the diagnosis. In other words, a careful and complete history is an essential component of the assessment of the patient with abdominal pain. The clinician should elicit a history of the onset of symptoms, with reference to their chronologic appearance from the last time the patient felt well. Acute abdominal crises usually present with a combination of symptoms and signs that may include pain, vomiting, muscular rigidity, abdominal distention, or shock. However, pain may be the sole symptom. The severity and sequence in which the signs and symptoms appear are important, as is the presence of fever, diarrhea, constipation, and urinary or vaginal symptoms in conjunction with the patient's primary complaint.

Defining the onset and character of the abdominal pain is key. One should determine whether the pain is cramping, steady, sharp, or burning and whether it radiates to other areas. Does it change with position or motion? Have its location and character changed since the patient first noticed the discomfort? Various nonabdominal conditions may present with abdominal pain, including pneumonia, myocardial infarction, syphilis (tabes dorsalis), herpes zoster, and even acute glaucoma. Therefore, the patient whose sole complaint is severe central or epigastric abdominal pain should be reevaluated and reexamined every 2 to 3 hours. Many of the surgically relevant conditions manifest other clinical signs and findings as their course unfurls.

Severe epigastric or central (periumbilical) abdominal pain may indicate intestinal colic or gastroenteritis, early acute appendicitis, early small bowel obstruction, mesenteric thrombosis or ischemia, or acute pancreatitis. The pain of acute appendicitis may be followed by nausea, then vomiting, then right lower quadrant tenderness and a low-grade fever. Pelvic appendicitis may have a much longer interval before the appearance of right lower quadrant pain. A rectal examination in these patients reveals right iliac tenderness.

Severe central abdominal pain accompanied by collapse, pallor, lowered blood pressure, and below-normal temperature without muscular rigidity of the abdominal wall indicates acute pancreatitis, mesenteric ischemia or thrombosis, ruptured aortic aneurysm, dissecting aortic aneurysm, myocardial infarction, internal hemorrhage, or ectopic pregnancy.

Pain associated with multiple episodes of emesis and increasing distention without rigidity is usually associated with intestinal obstruction. Persistent vomiting associated with distention and abdominal rigidity is found in spreading peritonitis. In suspected obstruction, the patient must be examined carefully for inguinal or femoral hernias or scars from prior operations. The character of the vomitus (eg, bilious, green, or feculent) may help differentiate gastroenteritis from early or late small bowel obstruction. An abdominal free air series (upright chest x-ray and abdominal flat plate with upright or decubitus views) helps make the diagnosis.

Abdominal pain accompanied by constipation with steadily increasing distention but little or no emesis indicates large bowel obstruction. The patient with an incompetent ileocecal valve exhibits feculent emesis in the case of large bowel obstruction. Again, a free air series helps in the diagnosis. Rapid development of large intestine obstructive symptoms, particularly in an elderly patient, should lead the clinician to suspect sigmoid or cecal volvulus.

Uremia may also present with abdominal distention and vomiting. Ureteral obstruction due to tumor encasement (eg, ovarian carcinoma) should be considered.

Severe abdominal pain with collapse and generalized rigidity of the abdominal wall is usually related to a perforated viscus such as the stomach or duodenum due to peptic ulcer disease. However, acute perforations may also occur in the patient taking high-dose steroids or ulcerogenic drugs such as nonsteroidal inflammatories. Other conditions that must be considered include perforated diverticulitis, stercoraceous perforation of the colon, perforation due to carcinoma, and bilateral pneumonia. The characteristic sudden, severe abdominal pain that becomes generalized with board-like rigidity is well known with a perforated ulcer. As peritonitis develops, the patient exhibits tachycardia and vomiting with distention. She often complains of shoulder pain, and liver dullness may diminish or disappear. The free air series demonstrates air beneath the diaphragm.

Pain associated with localized rigidity is considered separately. Right hypochondrial pain and rigidity may occur with cholecystitis or a leaking duodenal ulcer. Chest examination is necessary to rule out lower lobar pneumonia, particularly in the elderly or debilitated patient. Although rare in the United States, amebic abscess or hydatid disease of the liver commonly present in this manner and should be considered in the foreign traveler or immigrant from endemic areas. Left upper quadrant pain and rigidity may occur secondary to localized gastric perforation, rupture of a splenic artery aneurysm, an inflamed jejunal diverticulum, or splenic rupture. However, the most common cause of left upper quadrant peritoneal signs is acute pancreatitis. Right lower quadrant pain and peritoneal signs may be secondary to acute appendicitis. However, pancreatitis, perforated ulcer (duodenum), ruptured or gangrenous cholecystitis, Meckel diverticulitis, diverticulitis, regional enteritis (Crohn disease), salpingitis, ectopic pregnancy, and other conditions of the right fallopian tube and ovary may produce similar symptoms and findings. Left lower quadrant pain with tenderness, with or without peritoneal signs, may occur with diverticulitis, Crohn disease, inflammation or perforation of colonic carcinoma, diseases of the left fallopian tube or ovary, ectopic pregnancy, or perforated pelvic appendix. An ascending urinary tract infection, particularly in a so-called pelvic kidney, may localize to the lower quadrants. Pain in the hypogastrium may be due to early appendicitis or conditions involving the uterus, ovaries, or fallopian tubes. Similarly, suprapubic or lower midline pain may arise from a variety of etiologies, as was discussed for the lower quadrants and hypogastric region. Cystitis must also be considered.

Although an exhaustive discussion of the myriad of conditions that can produce acute abdominal and pelvic pain is beyond the scope of this chapter, the more common conditions are discussed in detail.

ACUTE APPENDICITIS

Acute appendicitis is the most common emergent operation of the nongravid patient and is the most common nonobstetric emergency of pregnancy. The diagnosis of appendicitis remains one of clinical judgment, despite an increasing array of diagnostic studies and algorithms. Classic teachings indicate that the clinician is accurate 80% of the time. However, the correct diagnosis may be made in only 40% of menstruating young females. It has generally been felt that the removal of 15 to 20 normal appendices per 100 is justifiable and prudent when one compares the low morbidity of appendectomy versus that of perforated appendicitis with significant peritonitis.

History and Clinical Findings

The sequence of the signs and symptoms of appendicitis is epigastric pain followed by the development of anorexia, nausea, and emesis (usually emesis occurs only once or twice), right lower quadrant tenderness, right lower quadrant peritoneal signs, and the later development of generalized peritonitis (Table 21-1). The order of development is so consistent that deviation from it should lead one to question the diagnosis.

The patient may describe the occurrence of vague symptoms of indigestion or flatulence for a few hours or a day before the onset of the acute attack. Many patients describe one or more prior episodes of lesser attacks of right lower quadrant abdominal pain in the past. Unusual irregularity of the bowels occurs often. Both constipation and diarrhea may be presenting complaints, as an inflamed pelvic appendix may irritate and stimulate the rectum. Pelvic peritonitis or pelvic abscess may produce frequent episodes of mucoid diarrhea, usually small in volume.

The pain of acute appendicitis is first noted in the epigastric or umbilical region in most cases. Initially, the pain is vague and may resemble that of indigestion or flatulence. The patient may note the sensation that the passage of stool or flatus would relieve the discomfort, but the passage of either or both fails to do so. A retrocecal appendix may present first with right iliac or right lower quadrant pain. Localization of the pain to the right lower quadrant in most cases occurs hours after the onset of the more diffuse periumbilical or epigastric pain. Typically, this is 12 to 18 hours after the onset of periumbilical pain.

If present, vomiting usually occurs a few hours after the onset of abdominal pain. Many patients have nausea, loss of appetite (anorexia), or repulsion for food. These symptoms are so common that a patient with hunger and abdominal pain should cause one to question the diagnosis of appendicitis. Similarly, vomiting that precedes the onset of pain is rare in acute appendicitis.

Physical Examination

Physical examination over the site of the appendix often fails to elicit tenderness at the onset of the attack. Early deep tenderness is most often found at McBurney's point or along a line from the anterior superior iliac spine to the umbilicus. Gentle percussion is helpful in locating the point of maximal tenderness. Retrocecal appendicitis may present with diminished tenderness on abdominal examination due to its insulation by the cecum. Pelvic appendicitis may present with localized tenderness on rectal examination and minimal abdominal tenderness. The physical examination in sus-

Table 21-1. Typical Symptoms of Acute Appendicitis and Their Sequence of Occurrence

1. Epigastric or periumbilical pain
2. Anorexia
3. Nausea or vomiting
4. Tenderness localizing to the right lower quadrant, pelvis, or adjacent areas
5. Fever (usually low-grade)
6. Leukocytosis (usually 10,000–18,000/mL)

pected appendicitis should include pelvic and rectal examinations. Hyperesthesia of the right abdominal wall in the distribution of T10, T11, T12, and L1 may be present.

Local muscular rigidity may be present in the patient with nonperforated appendicitis. However, this finding is variable and must be differentiated from voluntary guarding. Guarding is present when the parietal peritoneum is irritated by the inflammatory process. The psoas sign is elicited by extending the right thigh with the patient positioned on her left side. The obturator sign is elicited by abduction and external rotation of the hip. The Rovsing sign is present when right lower quadrant pain is elicited after releasing the deeply palpating hand from the left lower quadrant; however, the clinician should be careful not to startle the patient, as this may produce a false-positive result.

Fever is not generally present at the onset of the attack. A low-grade fever (elevation of 1° or 2°C) may occur within 24 hours of the onset of symptoms in uncomplicated appendicitis. The rate of temperature elevation is typically gradual as the clinical course progresses. Temperatures of 38.5°C (101.5°F) or greater are uncommon before 24 to 36 hours from the onset of symptoms. However, once perforation has occurred, rigors and temperature elevation are likely. If fever precedes the onset of pain or if vomiting occurs before the development of pain, the patient generally does not have appendicitis.

Gaseous distention of the cecum or localized ileus is most common when the appendix is in a retrocecal position or closely embedded to the wall of the cecum. This is noted as tympany on percussion and is also noted on the abdominal x-ray. Diffuse abdominal distention appears as a late consequence of perforation.

The signs and symptoms of appendicitis with a retrocecal appendix are generally less than those of classic appendicitis. Pain and tenderness are usually noted only in the right lower quadrant. The signs of localized peritonitis, such as muscular guarding or rigidity, are less than would be expected.

Laboratory and Imaging Studies

The laboratory evaluation should include a complete blood count with differential, urinalysis, SMA-7, amylase, and a pregnancy test. The latter is particularly important in the sexually active female of childbearing age, with or without the presence of gynecologic symptoms or irregularities. The kidney-ureter-bladder (KUB) or abdominal flat plate film may be useful if an appendiceal fecalith (appendicolith) is noted or if a renal calculus is present. The presence of an appendicolith with right lower quadrant pain should be considered diagnostic of appendicitis. The KUB film may also demonstrate cecal distention or localized distended loops of bowel in the right lower quadrant.

Leukocytosis is generally modest, with the white cell count ranging from 9000 to 18,000/mL. Many patients have white counts of 12,000 to 16,000/mL, but with early diagnosis leukocytosis may be absent.

The barium enema examination has been suggested by some to be useful in the difficult case. The findings of cecal spasm, edema, extrinsic compression of the cecum by a mass, partial visualization or nonvisualization of the appendix, and irregular filling of the appendiceal lumen have been considered diagnostic. However, nonfilling of the appendix as the sole abnormality on the full-column barium enema examination is a nonspecific finding; 20% of normal adults have an obliterated appendiceal lumen. The barium enema is helpful in differentiating appendicitis from regional enteritis involving the terminal ileum and from colon carcinoma involving the cecum or ascending colon.

Improvements in ultrasound techniques have led to increased use of ultrasonography in female patients. The findings of distention of the appendiceal lumen, thickening of the appendiceal or cecal walls, and localized fluid collections are considered diagnostic. The ultrasound examination can also yield useful information as to the presence or absence of ovarian cysts, pelvic fluid or hemorrhage, tuboovarian abscess or other abnormalities, and ureteral calculi or obstruction, as well as the presence of an ectopic pregnancy.

Nuclear imaging techniques have been used in some centers but are not readily available in most hospitals, especially in off-hours. The indium-labeled white cell scan, the most promising study, is based on the localization of inflammatory cells to the area of the inflamed appendix. The abdominal and pelvic computed tomography (CT) scan may be helpful in the evaluation of right lower quadrant or pelvic masses but is not generally cost-effective or useful in the diagnosis of uncomplicated appendicitis. Diagnostic laparoscopy is extremely useful in the management of abdominopelvic pain, particularly in the female, because various processes of the female genital tract may confuse the clinical picture.

Differential Diagnosis

The differential diagnosis of appendicitis can present challenges in women. Bacterial or viral gastroenteritis can be mistaken for appendicitis, particularly in the early stages. Viral and bacterial enteritis often present with prominent episodes of diarrhea as a major component of the presenting complaints. The patient often experiences crampy periumbilical or lower abdominal pain that may be colicky but is relieved by the passage of stool. Bacterial gastroenteritis often presents with a fever of 38° to 39°C and may be accompanied by several episodes of vomiting. Often the nausea, vomiting, and diarrhea precede the onset of pain; appendicitis presents with pain first. Slight abdominal tenderness may be elicited, but localized or generalized peritoneal signs do not occur. Typically, the white count is normal or slightly elevated, and the patient experiences progressive clinical improvement after intravenous rehydration and being maintained NPO. Similarly, influenza and various flu-like syndromes may manifest with severe abdominal pain and tenderness. They may present with a febrile course and may exhibit a varying degree of myalgia.

Acute gastritis can generally be traced to an inciting event related to food, drug, or alcohol consumption. Gnawing abdominal pain may be experienced. The pain tends to be poorly localized and is associated with significant nausea and emesis.

Hepatitis may present with anorexia, nausea, abdominal pain, and abdominal tenderness, especially when the liver capsule is compressed on abdominal palpation. Jaundice occurs but may not present initially.

Diabetic ketoacidosis and uremia are two metabolic conditions that may present with significant abdominal symptoms. Careful history and laboratory evaluation confirm the diagnosis. However, intraabdominal infection or missed appendicitis may precipitate these conditions in the diabetic or end-stage renal disease patient, respectively. Therefore, the clinician must carefully note the resolution of abdominal complaints with treatment.

Acute intermittent porphyria, although uncommon, can present with attacks of abdominal pain that can be quite severe. Patients may give an antecedent history of consumption of alcohol, barbiturates, or sulfonamides and may not be aware of a familial trait. Typical symptoms include severe colicky abdominal pain, vomiting, and constipation. The pain is often central but may radiate widely. The patient may have noticed prior episodes of rash or intolerance to sun exposure and red-brown urinary discoloration on exposure to sunlight. Fever and leukocytosis may be present. The patient may have experienced similar symptoms previously, and right lower quadrant localization of pain does not occur.

Several conditions specific to women bear consideration (Table 21-2). Dysmenorrhea characteristically presents with a relation to the menstrual cycle and is often recurrent. Pain is often referred to the lumbar, sacral, and hypogastric regions. Mild tenderness to palpation may be noted, but localized peritoneal signs do not occur.

Threatened abortion presents with previous amenorrhea and crampy lower abdominal or perineal pain that may also radiate to the lumbar, sacral, and hypogastric areas. Vaginal bleeding may be minimal at first. A positive pregnancy test or characteristic pelvic ultrasound facilitates the diagnosis.

Similarly, ectopic pregnancy may present with severe right lower quadrant abdominal pain and tenderness. Menstrual irregularities, an episode of syncope, and anemia may be present. Pelvic examination occasionally demonstrates the characteristic clinical cervical softening of pregnancy and may document enlargement of the fallopian tube or a tender, mobile, pelvic adnexal mass or displacement of the uterus. The onset of abdominal pain is sudden, and ongoing bleeding may precipitate tachycardia, low or low-normal blood pressure, faintness or actual syncope, and shoulder strap pain due to subdiaphragmatic irritation by blood. Lower abdominal tenderness is present in what is described as a "flaccid" abdomen. The pregnancy test is positive and a pelvic ultrasound may confirm the diagnosis and the degree of free abdominal fluid present.

Acute salpingitis due to *Neisseria gonorrhoeae* or other organisms presents with signs and symptoms of pelvic peritonitis. Patients experience hypogastric pain, nausea or vomiting, and fever (up to 39°C). A vaginal discharge may be present. Cervical motion tenderness or the so-called "chandelier sign" is unreliable, as it is not specific for salpingitis and may be present in all cases of pelvic peritonitis. Cervical examination may show signs of gonorrheal infection, and a purulent or foul discharge may be observed. Palpation of the lateral fornices may elicit pain. Leftward-oriented or more bilateral abdominal pain may be experienced. Ultrasonography may demonstrate enlargement of the salpinx with or without pelvic fluid. Pyosalpinx and tuboovarian abscess may result and may require surgery.

Table 21-2. Sources of Lower Abdominal Pain That May Mimic Appendicitis in the Female Patient

Ectopic pregnancy
Torsion of ovarian cyst
Torsion of hydrosalpinx
Ruptured pyosalpinx
Tubovarian abscess
Salpingitis
Ruptured follicle cyst (mittelschmerz)
Ruptured corpus luteum cyst
Torsion of uterine fibroid
Ruptured chocolate cyst (endometrioma)

Torsion of an ovarian cyst presents with the acute development of hypogastric pain, vomiting, and the presence of a tender mass in the lower abdomen. Vomiting occurs with the onset of pain but is not always present. A sitting position may reduce the symptoms, but a supine position may accentuate the pain. Ultrasound and laparoscopy are diagnostic. Torsion of a hydrosalpinx has a similar presentation but is usually less severe.

Rupture of an endometrioma of the ovary or pelvis can result in hypogastric pain, vomiting, and low-grade fever. Bimanual pelvic examination may demonstrate unilateral or bilateral swelling of the pouch of Douglas. A history of endometriosis is helpful but may not be noted. Ultrasonic evidence of pelvic fluid may be present, and other smaller lesions may be documented. Laparoscopy is diagnostic.

The pain of a ruptured graafian follicle (mittelschmerz) or corpus luteum cyst is distinguished by the fact that the former occurs at or near midcycle and the latter occurs at or near the onset of menses. A history of cyclic or similar pain in relation to the menstrual cycle is helpful. The pain is gradual in onset but becomes steady. It is aggravated by motion, cough, or the Valsalva maneuver. It is typically felt low in the iliac fossa and may radiate to the groin. Pelvic examination documents ovarian tenderness with or without slight ovarian enlargement. Overt peritoneal signs are rare. Ultrasound may document pelvic fluid, and laparoscopy is diagnostic in severe or confusing cases. Observation and the use of nonsteroidal antiinflammatories can be helpful, as the latter may significantly decrease or eliminate the abdominal symptoms and pain.

Treatment

The appropriate management of acute or suspected appendicitis is prompt surgery. The traditional surgical approach is to perform one of several right lower quadrant muscle-splitting incisions and to remove the vermiform appendix, regardless of the presence or absence of appendicitis. Exceptions to this rule are appendiceal abscess, wherein the appendix cannot be removed safely if a significant inflammatory reaction or phlegmon is present, and Crohn disease involving the caput cecum. The latter condition remains a management controversy in the surgical literature. The surgeon must rule out the presence of other surgically relevant processes by systematic abdominal exploration if appendicitis is not found. Laparoscopic approaches to appendectomy are particularly useful in these cases, as the surgeon has a clear field of view and can evaluate the abdominal and pelvic organs under direct vision. The recent surgical literature supports the utility of laparoscopy as a means of establishing the diagnosis in patients with right lower quadrant abdominal pain in whom appendicitis cannot be ruled out. In addition, patients who undergo laparoscopic appendectomy appear to derive the same benefits of low morbidity and rapid recovery that have been demonstrated dramatically with laparoscopic cholecystectomy.

RENAL COLIC AND ACUTE PYELONEPHRITIS

These entities are considered together, although their etiologies are different. Both may present with severe abdominal pain and associated nausea. Flank pain is present and tenderness is elicited by percussion over the costovertebral angle. The patient with renal colic may have a prior history of ureteral calculi, gout, or other metabolic disorders. Both conditions may present with urinary frequency. Renal colic due to calculus presents with hematuria. In the menstruating patient, a straight catheter specimen allows differentiation between true hematuria and contamination of the urine by menstrual flow. Pyuria and a history of cystitis or dysuria, frequency, and urgency often precede an episode of pyelonephritis. Acute pyelonephritis presents with fever and often with rigors due to bacteremia. Hydronephrosis may be present with either a calculus or pyelonephritis. Ureteral calculi may produce pain that radiates to the ipsilateral groin. Sometimes a calculus at the pelvic brim produces tenderness on examination that simulates acute appendicitis. Ultrasound examination may demonstrate hydroureter or hydronephrosis. Plain abdominal x-rays can demonstrate opacified calculi. Calcium oxalate stones account for over 85% of urinary stones. However, small calculi may be missed unless an intravenous pyelogram is performed.

In both cases, intravenous hydration and parenteral analgesics are needed. Acute pyelonephritis requires prompt treatment with appropriate antibiotics, modified according to the urine culture and sensitivity and the patient's clinical course. Untreated or inadequately treated infection of the ascending urinary tract can lead to sepsis or a perinephric abscess. The latter requires surgical or percutaneous drainage.

In most cases of renal or ureteral calculus, the stone eventually passes, but stone manipulation is required in some cases. Electrohydraulic shock wave lithotripsy is effective in fragmenting larger calculi as well as stones located in a favorable position in the ureter (positions not obscured by bony prominences that would interfere with triangulation of the sonic shock waves). Laser-based and direct contact piezoelectric lithotripsy techniques are also effective in shattering calculi throughout the urinary tract, thereby facilitating their passage.

MESENTERIC ADENITIS

Mesenteric adenitis may present with acute lower abdominal pain and tenderness. A febrile course may be present. The pain may be colicky but should not progress to signs of localized peritonitis. Both viral and bacterial etiologies have been implicated. *Yersinia* infection accounts for many such cases in adults.

MECKEL DIVERTICULUM

A Meckel diverticulum is found in about 2% of the population. The "rule of two's" is enumerated as 2 inches long, 2% of the population, 2 to 5 feet from the ileocecal valve, and a male:female ratio of 2:1. The diverticulum is a remnant of the vitelline duct and may contain aberrant gastric or pancreatic tissue. Although many patients are asymptomatic, Meckel diverticulitis can present with an acute abdomen as a result of infection, bleeding, perforation, or bowel obstruction due to intussusception, torsion, or volvulus about a band-like remnant of the vitelline duct. The patient may present with periumbilical pain or may have signs and symptoms difficult to distinguish from those of acute appendicitis. Bleeding due to a Meckel diverticulum occurs due to ulcer formation in the adjacent distal ileum.

A suspected Meckel diverticulum can be localized by radionuclide scanning with technetium. The test is based on the fact that H_2 blockade of gastric acid production occurs in the normal stomach but not in the aberrant gastric tissue contained in the diverticulum.

Resection is required for Meckel diverticulitis or its complications. The routine removal of an asymptomatic Meckel diverticulum continues to be controversial, but many authors suggest that the morbidity of diverticulectomy is minimal, particularly with the use of stapling devices.

VASCULAR DISORDERS

A complete discussion of cardiovascular disorders is beyond the scope of this chapter, but a few bear mention.

Splenic artery aneurysm may present with a pulsatile or expanding mass in the upper abdomen. The lesion can produce sudden collapse due to massive intraabdominal hemorrhage (abdominal apoplexy). Splenic artery aneurysm rupture has a predilection for pregnant women or women on oral contraceptives. A calcified lesion may be noted on abdominal x-ray or CT scan. Prompt surgical intervention is required for expanding, leaking, or ruptured aneurysms. Arteriography may be helpful in establishing the diagnosis.

Abdominal aneurysm formation is increasing in frequency in women, particularly in hypertensive patients and smokers. The pulsatile abdominal mass of a small aneurysm can be difficult to palpate, particularly in an obese patient. Patients may present with abdominal or back pain and may or may not have other symptoms of peripheral vascular disease. Plain films can demonstrate aortic calcifications; CT scanning, arteriography, and ultrasonography better define the anatomy and size of the aneurysm. Most aneurysms are fusiform rather than saccular and are located in the infrarenal aorta. Most patients have few if any symptoms, unless the aneurysm is rapidly dilating, or in cases of impending or contained rupture. The pain of impending rupture may be throbbing or aching and may be more significant in the back or lumbar region.

Aneurysms 6 cm or more in diameter are in danger of rupture more than half the time. Resection and elective vascular reconstruction are necessary. Smaller aneurysms (4.5 to 5.5 cm) should also be repaired electively, as the natural course is progressive dilation of the aorta over time. However, the urgency of repair is not as great as for larger aneurysms.

Tenderness of the aneurysm or significant pain in a patient with a known aneurysm should lead to immediate referral for surgical evaluation and intervention, as leakage or impending rupture must be presumed unless proved otherwise. Free rupture of an aneurysm into the abdominal cavity can result in sudden shock and death. Patients who are successfully operated on and resuscitated have considerable perioperative morbidity due to renal failure and other sequelae of sudden and profound cardiovascular collapse.

Mesenteric ischemia and embolic disease can result from several conditions. The index of suspicion should be increased in an elderly patient, a patient with a known cardiovascular disease or arrhythmia or coagulopathy, and a patient who has sustained a hypotensive insult due to sepsis or trauma. The pain is often sudden in onset, severe, and unrelenting. The patient may writhe about the bed, and the physical examination is generally much less impressive than the degree of the complaints. Prompt diagnosis and surgery are necessary. The classic symptoms and signs of bloody diarrhea, metabolic acidosis, elevated CPK or amylase values, pneumatosis intestinalis, or "thumb printing" of the bowel on x-ray are variable and are nonspecific or absent in many cases. Many of these signs occur late and may herald an irreversible course. Vigorous fluid resuscitation, prompt arteriography, and surgery are the keys to survival. Irreversible necrosis of the bowel is invariable after 6 hours of warm ischemia. Segmental ischemia can be treated successfully with judicious resection and "second-look" procedures. The survival of patients with short-gut syndrome after massive small bowel resection has been greatly improved with the use of total parenteral nutrition and elemental diets.

OTHER SYNDROMES

Other disorders that may produce acute abdominal symptoms include cholecystitis, diverticulitis, regional enteritis and inflammatory bowel disease, pancreatitis, hepatitis, pneumonitis, myocardial infarction, intussusception, peptic ulcer disease, carcinoma, mesenteric ischemia, and aortic aneurysm.

Trauma can result in profound injury that requires particular vigilance on the part of the clinician. Careful, methodical serial abdominal examinations and the judicious use of radiologic and other studies (eg, peritoneal lavage, laparoscopy) are recommended. CT scans can provide useful information in the stable patient, particularly in the evaluation of retroperitoneal and pelvic structures.

Various hemolytic disorders can result in acute abdominal pain and tenderness. These episodes tend to occur in proportion to the degree of anemia or developing jaundice. Sickle-cell crisis is a classic example. The patient may also have development of pigmented gallstones, which can give rise to symptomatic cholecystitis.

Acute withdrawal from narcotics, opiates, and other drugs can result in severe, cramping abdominal pain. Other signs may be present, such as tachycardia, diaphoresis, pupillary dilation or constriction, and evidence of drug use (eg, pockmarked skin, needle tracks, absence of patent upper extremity vessels). Oral or inhaled drugs may be used, however. The clinician should remember that drug abuse occurs in all social strata.

Tuberculosis can produce tuberculous peritonitis, and this is relevant with the increase in HIV-positive and immunocompromised patients. This disease is called "the great mimicker" because it produces a wide variety of complaints and signs. The patient may present with vague abdominal pain, abdominal distention, and ascites. Evidence of pulmonary tuberculosis can be helpful in establishing the diagnosis. Tuberculosis can also result in intestinal perforation or obstruction that requires surgical intervention in addition to antitubercular drugs. The emergence of resistant strains is of great concern.

SUMMARY

The ability to distinguish an acute process that requires surgical intervention or referral to a specialist is based on the clinical skills of the provider. This requires a complete history, a careful physical examination (including rectal and pelvic examinations), the judicious use of laboratory and radiologic studies, and frequent reevaluation until a firm diagnosis is reached. The clinician should have a low threshold for seeking advice from a surgeon, gynecologist, or other specialist.

Acute Abdominopelvic Pain in the Pregnant Patient

The pregnant patient with acute abdominal pain can present one of the most difficult diagnostic challenges to both the obstetrician and primary care practitioner. The clinical evaluation is generally confounded because the symptoms typical of these illnesses are common to pregnancy itself, and the physical examination of the abdomen is hampered by the pregnant state.

ANATOMIC AND PHYSIOLOGIC CHANGES

The primary care provider must be familiar with the anatomic and physiologic changes of pregnancy. By 12 weeks gestation, the uterine fundus rises from the pelvis and becomes an abdominal organ. The adnexal structures also become abdominal organs. As the uterus enlarges, it displaces superiorly and laterally the intestines and the omentum. By late pregnancy, the appendix is much more likely to be closer to the gallbladder than to McBurney's point. The anterior abdominal wall is also elevated, so that any underlying inflammation is less likely to exert its usual symptoms due to direct parietal peritoneal irritation.

The leukocyte count varies considerably during normal pregnancy. The normal white cell count during pregnancy is elevated to 12,000 to 16,000/mL, a level that overlaps with expected levels for intraabdominal inflammatory conditions.

The etiology of acute abdominal pain in pregnancy can be separated into obstetric and nonobstetric causes. The most common etiologies for nonobstetric causes of acute abdominal pain in the pregnant patient are appendicitis, cholecystitis, pyelonephritis, hepatitis, pancreatitis, and degenerating uterine myomata.

NONOBSTETRIC CAUSES

Acute Appendicitis

Acute appendicitis complicates about one in 1600 pregnancies and is the most common nontraumatic, nonobstetric surgical condition that complicates pregnancy. The diagnosis during pregnancy is often challenging because the typical symptoms (anorexia, nausea, and vomiting) mimic those of normal pregnancy, and because the location of the appendix differs from its location in the nonpregnant state (Fig. 21-1). Appendicitis should always be considered when a pregnant woman presents with abdominal pain, nausea, vomiting, fever, and leukocytosis. Laparotomy should not be delayed when the clinical suspicion is high. The differential diagnosis includes preterm labor, abruptio placentae, degenerating myoma, and adnexal torsion. Postoperative antimicrobial agents are recommended for perforation, peritonitis, or periappendiceal abscess. Tocolysis is indicated in the postoperative period with evidence of preterm labor and absence of clinical infection.

Cholecystitis/Cholelithiasis

Asymptomatic cholelithiasis occurs in 3.5% of pregnant women and is the cause of over 90% of cases of cholecystitis in pregnancy. Acute cholecystitis usually presents with the abrupt onset of right upper quadrant or epigastric pain described as colicky or stabbing. Associated symptoms include nausea, vomiting, fever, and abdominal tenderness. Laboratory findings include leukocytosis and elevated serum amylase and bilirubin levels. Cholelithiasis may be diagnosed by ultrasonography.

The medical management of acute cholecystitis consists of intravenous hydration, nasogastric suction, and analgesics. Surgical therapy is reserved for patients with recurrent attacks of biliary

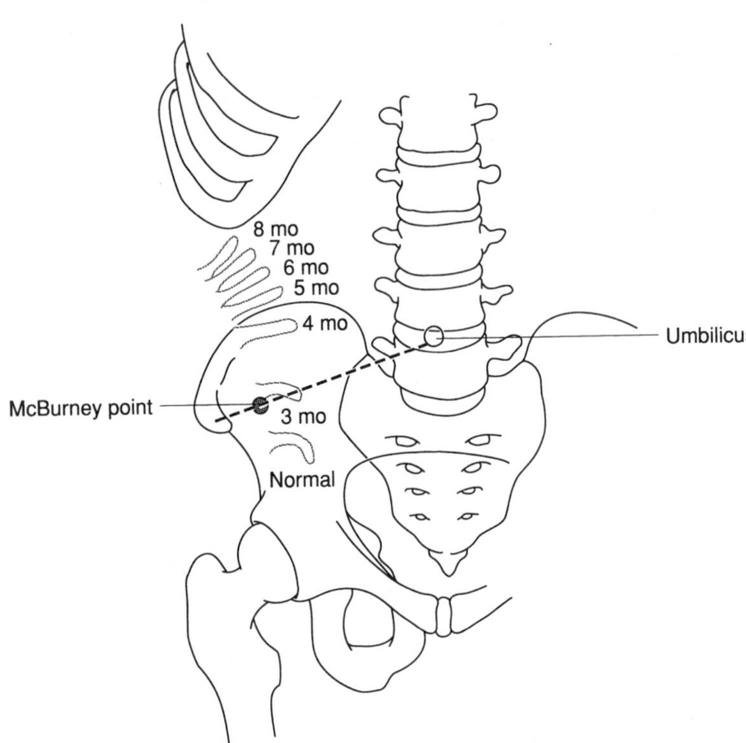

Figure 21-1. Location and orientation of the appendix in pregnancy. (Greenfield LJ, Mulholland MW, Oldham KT, Zelenock GB, eds. Surgery; scientific principles and practice. Philadelphia: JB Lippincott, 1993:1135.

colic, suspected perforation, sepsis, or peritonitis. Prophylactic antibiotics in the preoperative period are recommended.

Hepatitis

Viral hepatitis is the most common serious liver disease in pregnant women. There are five types of viral hepatitis: hepatitis A, hepatitis B, hepatitis B-associated δ agent, and two types of non-A, non-B hepatitis—one blood-borne (hepatitis C) and the other enterically transmitted. With all of these forms, symptoms may precede jaundice by 1 to 2 weeks and include nausea, vomiting, headache, and malaise. When jaundice develops, symptoms usually improve and there may be pain and tenderness over the liver. Serum aminotransferase levels are elevated, but the levels vary. Hepatitis profile is diagnostic, and treatment is supportive.

Pancreatitis

Acute pancreatitis complicates one in 1000 to 10,000 pregnancies. Gallbladder disease is the most common cause; medications, infection, and hyperlipidemia are less frequent causes. Signs and symptoms include epigastric pain that radiates to the back and left flank and is accompanied by nausea, vomiting, and fever. Physical examination includes abdominal distention, hypoactive bowel sounds, guarding, and tenderness. Amylase levels are elevated. Ultrasonography, CT scanning, and magnetic resonance imaging may identify pancreatic edema and enlargement, abscess, phlegmon, or pseudocyst to support the diagnosis. Medical management includes bowel rest with nasogastric suction, pain relief, and correction of fluid and electrolyte imbalances. Patients with pancreatic abscess, ruptured pseudocyst, or hemorrhagic pancreatitis may require surgery.

Pyelonephritis

Pyelonephritis is identified in 1% to 2% of all pregnancies. The diagnosis is made by the presence of symptoms and signs in combination with a positive urine culture. The most common symptoms are fever, chills, nausea, vomiting, and flank pain that may radiate to the upper and lower quadrants. Treatment includes parenteral antibiotics, intravenous hydration, and close monitoring for complications (renal impairment, hematologic abnormalities, septic shock, and pulmonary dysfunction). Ampicillin is no longer recommended as single-agent therapy due to high degrees of bacterial resistance. Extended-spectrum penicillins or cephalosporins are safe and typically result in cure rates of 85% to 90%, with resolution of symptoms within 24 to 48 hours.

Uterine Leiomyomata

The most important complication of myomata is red or carneous degeneration, which is hemorrhagic infarction usually due to acute inadequacy of blood supply to the myoma. The pain and tenderness are usually localized. Low-grade fever and leukocytosis can occur. Preterm labor may be initiated due to irritation of adjacent myometrium. Ultrasound is helpful in making the diagnosis. Management is nonsurgical and includes analgesics and observation of preterm labor.

OBSTETRIC CAUSES

Preterm Labor

The cyclic nature of contraction pain, with a rapid building to an acme and then complete resolution, is characteristic of regular uterine contractions. A history of regular uterine contractions (eg,

Table 21-3. Laboratory Findings in Common Liver Diseases in Late Pregnancy

TEST	AFMP	PREECLAMPSIA	ICP	HEPATITIS
Alkaline phosphatase	S1↑	S1↑	7–10×↑	Variably↑
Total bilirubin	2–5-mg/dL	1–5 mg/dL	1–5 mg/dL	20–30 mg/dL
SGOT	300–500 IU	<500 IU	<250 IU	500–3000 IU
Fibrinogen	↓↓	↓	WNL	↓↓
Prothrombin time	2–5×↑	WNL-2×↑	WNL-2×↑	2–3×↑
Glucose	↓	WNL	WNL	↓
Arterial ammonia	↑	WNL	WNL	↑
Platelets	20–100K	Variable	WNL	20–100K

AFMP, acute fatty metamorphosis of pregnancy; *ICP,* intrahepatic cholestasis of pregnancy; *SGOT,* serum glutamic oxaloacetic transaminase; *WNL,* within normal limits.

(Varner MW. Laboratory findings in common liver diseases in late pregnancy. Contemp Ob/Gyn 1995;12.)

four contractions in 20 minutes, or eight contractions in 1 hour) associated with cervical dilatation (2 cm) or effacement (80%) is diagnostic of labor or preterm labor. Treatment includes tocolysis between 20 and 34 weeks gestation and antenatal steroids (dexamethasone or betamethasone) between 24 and 34 weeks gestation.

Abruptio Placentae

Acute abdominal pain could signal premature separation of the placenta. The frequency of this condition averages about one in 150 deliveries. The etiology is unknown. Associated conditions include age, multiparity, pregnancy-induced or chronic hypertension, preterm prematurely ruptured membranes, external trauma, cigarette smoking, cocaine abuse, and uterine leiomyoma.

The signs and symptoms include vaginal bleeding, uterine tenderness or back pain, high-frequency contractions, hypertonus, and idiopathic preterm labor. Symptomatic abruptio placentae can produce profound blood loss, anemia, coagulopathy, and fetal death; the latter usually occurs when the degree of separation exceeds 50%.

Treatment varies depending on the status of the mother and fetus. In general, with the development of massive external bleeding, intense therapy with blood plus electrolyte solution and prompt delivery to try to control the hemorrhage can be lifesaving for the mother and fetus. With slower blood loss, the management is influenced by the status of the mother and fetus. If the fetus is alive without evidence of fetal compromise and if maternal hemorrhage is not causing serious hypovolemia or anemia, close observation, with facilities for immediate intervention, can be practiced.

The difficulties of diagnosing abdominal pain in pregnancy are well known. Prompt clinical diagnosis and surgical intervention when indicated are necessary to minimize maternal and fetal mortality. When the diagnosis is uncertain, liberal use of surgical and obstetric consultants is warranted.

Preeclampsia

Hepatic involvement is reported to occur in 10% of women with severe preeclampsia. The patient typically presents in the middle to late portion of the third trimester with right upper quadrant and epigastric pain, nausea and vomiting, hypertension, and proteinuria. Tender hepatomegaly is found on physical examination. Alkaline phosphatase and transaminase levels are elevated. Serum bilirubin is elevated in 10% of cases. Thrombocytopenia and disseminated intravascular coagulation with microangiopathic hemolytic anemia may be present. In patients who present in hypovolemic shock, hepatic hematoma and ruptured liver should be considered immediately. Hepatic rupture has an associated maternal mortality rate of 70%.

Delivery is the recommended management of severe preeclampsia and should be done once the patient has been medically stabilized. In a patient with suspected hepatic rupture, surgical intervention is mandatory. Hepatic artery ligation, partial hepatic resection, laceration repair, and packing are the suggested intraoperative treatment.

Acute Fatty Liver of Pregnancy

This complication of one in 10,000 to 15,000 pregnancies usually occurs in the third trimester. Patients typically present with an abrupt onset of nausea, persistent vomiting, abdominal pain, and jaundice. Laboratory findings include hyperbilirubinemia, elevated alkaline phosphatase and serum transaminase levels, thrombocytopenia, hypoglycemia, elevated serum ammonia levels, and prolonged coagulation studies (Table 27-3). The initial management is medical, with correction of fluid, electrolyte, and coagulation abnormalities. Prompt delivery is the only known cure. Recurrences in subsequent pregnancies are unusual.

BIBLIOGRAPHY

Acute Abdominopelvic Pain in the Nonpregnant Patient

Burnett ALS. Gynecologic causes of the acute abdomen. Surg Clin North Am 1988;68:385.

Chappius CW, Cohn I. Acute colonic diverticulitis. Surg Clin North Am 1988;68:301.

DeGown EL, DeGown RL. Bedside diagnostic examination, 2d ed. London: Collier Macmillan, 1969.

Jordon PH, Morrow C. Perforated peptic ulcer. Surg Clin North Am 1988;68:315.

Koch MO, McDougal WS. Urologic causes of the acute abdomen. Surg Clin North Am 1988;68:399.

Maddus MA, Ahrenholz D, Simmons RL. The biology of peritonitis and implications for treatment. Surg Clin North Am 1988;68:431.

Mannick JA, Whittemore AD. Management of ruptured or symptomatic abdominal aortic aneurysms. Surg Clin North Am 1988;68:377.

Meredith JN, Trunkey DD. CT scanning in acute abdominal injuries. Surg Clin North Am 1988;68:255.

Nylander WA. The acute abdomen in the immunocompromised host. Surg Clin North Am 1988;68:457.

Potts JR. Acute pancreatitis. Surg Clin North Am 1988;68:281.

Richards WD, Williams LF. Obstruction of large and small intestine. Surg Clin North Am 1988;68:355.

Schwartz SI, Shires GT, Spencer FC, Husser WC, eds. Principles of surgery, 6th ed. New York: McGraw-Hill, 1994.

Shaff MI, Tarr RW, Partain CL, James AE. Computed tomography and magnetic resonance imaging of the acute abdomen. Surg Clin North Am 1988;68:233.

Silen W. Cope's early diagnosis of the acute abdomen, 18th ed. New York: Oxford University Press, 1991.

Williams LF. Mesenteric ischemia. Surg Clin North Am 1988;68:331.

Acute Abdominopelvic Pain in the Pregnant Patient

Baaknia A, Hussein P, Woodruff JD. Appendicitis during pregnancy. Obstet Gynecol 1977;50:40.

Baer JL, Reis RA, Aren S. Appendicitis in pregnancy with changes in position and axis of the normal appendix in pregnancy. JAMA 1932;98:1359.

Bis K, Waxman B. Rupture of liver associated with pregnancy: a review of the literature and report of 2 cases. Obstet Gynecol Surv 1976;3111:763.

Creasy RK, Resnik R. Maternal-fetal medicine: principles and practice, 3d ed. Philadelphia: WB Saunders, 1994:494.

Cunningham FG, MacDonald PC, Gant NF, et al, eds. Williams' obstetrics, 19th ed. Norwalk: Appleton & Lange, 1993:210.

Gilstrap LC, Cunningham FG, Whalley PJ. Acute pyelonephritis in pregnancy: an anterospective study. Obstet Gynecol 1981;57:409.

Gilstrap LC, Henkins GDV, Snyder RR, et al. Acute pyelonephritis in pregnancy. Comp Ther 1986;12:38.

Gomez A, Wood MD. Acute appendicitis during pregnancy. Am J Surg 1979;137:180.

Mabie WC. Acute fatty liver of pregnancy. Gastroenterol Clin North Am 1992;21:951.

McKay AJ, O'Neill J, Imrie CW. Pancreatitis, pregnancy, and gallstones. Br J Obstet Gynaecol 1980;87:67.

Nathan L, Huddleston JF. Acute abdominal pain in pregnancy. Obstet Gynecol Clin North Am 1995;22:55.

Sharp HT. Gastrointestinal surgical conditions during pregnancy. Clin Obstet Gynecol 1994;37:306.

Simon JA. Biliary tract disease and related surgical disorders during pregnancy. Clin Obstet Gynecol 1983;26:810.

Stauffer RA, Adams A, Wygal J, et al. Gallbladder disease in pregnancy. Am J Obstet Gynecol 1982;6:661.

Varner MW. Laboratory findings in common liver diseases in late pregnancy. Contemp Ob/Gyn 1995;12.

Weinstein L. Syndrome of hemolysis, elevated liver enzymes, and low platelet count: a severe consequence of hypertension in pregnancy. Am J Obstet Gynecol 1982;142:159.

Primary Care for Women, edited by Phyllis C. Leppert and Fred M. Howard. Lippincott-Raven Publishers, Philadelphia © 1997.

22

Chronic Pelvic Pain

FRED M. HOWARD

Pelvic pain that lasts more than 3 months is considered chronic. Sometimes dysmenorrhea and dyspareunia are included in this definition, but here dysmenorrhea and dyspareunia are considered separately and discussed in Chapters 14 and 20, respectively. The duration of 3 months is an arbitrary convention. Acute pelvic pain rarely lasts more than 1 month without crisis, resolution, or cure, so in a sense any pain lasting more than 1 month could be considered chronic. However, the rationale is that after 3 months, pain can become an illness in itself rather than just a symptom of some other disease.

Chronic pelvic pain is a significant problem and is estimated to account for 10% of all referrals to a gynecologist. It may lead to years of disability and suffering, with loss of employment, marital discord and divorce, and numerous untoward and unsuccessful medical misadventures. As many as 40% of all laparoscopies and 12% of hysterectomies are performed for chronic pelvic pain. The mean age of women with chronic pelvic pain is 30 years, making it an affliction of women during the peak of their productive years. It is estimated that direct and indirect costs of chronic pelvic pain in the United States exceed $2 billion per year.

Chronic pelvic pain is frustrating for most physicians, as most think of pain within the context of the classic cartesian model. This model postulates that pain is the direct result of tissue trauma, activating specific neuroreceptors and neural pain fibers. It also postulates that the severity of pain is directly proportional to the severity of the traumatic insult. As a corollary, pain that is not associated with identifiable tissue injury is regarded as spurious or psychogenic. Although this model is useful in acute pain, it is not applicable to chronic pain. Attempts to find enough organic pathology to explain chronic pain have routinely been frustrating, and somatic pathologies, such as endometriosis, adhesions, or leiomyomata, have at best an uncertain relation to chronic pelvic pain. Considering chronic pain solely a psychiatric disorder is also frustrating and is not supported by scientific evidence. The current consensus is that a biopsychosocial model that takes into account the influences of nociceptive stimulation, individual psychological characteristics, and social and cultural determinants of pain is most useful as a model for chronic pain.

Melzack and Wall's gate control theory is the model most frequently used in trying to understand chronic pain. In oversimplified terms, this theory states that afferent neural impulses from the periphery may be modulated by spinal and cortical signals ("gates"). The modulation may be either enhancement or diminution of the afferent impulse. The neurophysiologic events that gate or modulate the pain impulses are influenced by numerous factors, both peripheral and central. The gates may be affected by the level of firing of the visceral afferent nerves, by afferent input from cutaneous and deep somatic structures, by endogenous opioid and nonopioid analgesic systems, and by various central excitatory and inhibitory influences from the brain stem, hypothalamus, and cortex. This pain theory provides a neurologic basis for both somatic and psychogenic factors—in other words, anxiety, depression, physical activity, mental concentration, marital discord, and so forth may increase or decrease the perception of pain. Although neurophysiologic and biochemical research has resulted in significant modifications of this theory since its original proposal, it still serves as a good (but not the only) model for the clinical observations in chronic pain patients and provides a more productive approach to therapy than the classic cartesian model.

For example, the common association of depression and chronic pain may be explained as due to the dysregulation of neurotransmitters associated with depression, which "opens" the CNS gate, increasing sensitivity to nociception. Conversely, this model allows an explanation of chronic pain as a cause of depression. Chronic somatic nociception may deplete the descending CNS of modulators of pain (eg, endogenous opioids), and this depletion may biochemically lead to depression. Thus, mechanisms for depression leading to chronic pelvic pain and for chronic pelvic pain leading to depression can be postulated, and there is neurophysiologic evidence to support both.

Such theoretical concepts may have clinical relevance. For example, Steege has found depression to be a significant indicator of the clinical responsiveness of chronic pelvic pain patients and has included it as one of the major criteria for diagnosing chronic pain syndrome. Patients with chronic pain syndrome have a much poorer response to traditional treatment, such as surgical lysis of abdominopelvic adhesions, than do patients with chronic pain without chronic pain syndrome. Furthermore, it has been noted that major depressive illness is sometimes seen in chronic pain patients, with a cycle of pain, depression, and withdrawal.

Observations of such psychological changes have led to a search for identifiable psychosocial characteristics of chronic pelvic pain patients. Psychological interviews suggest these patients are anxious and depressed and have low self-esteem, high somatization, and high dependency. Psychometric testing (eg, the Minnesota Multiphasic Personality Inventory) shows that chronic pelvic pain patients have a characteristic personality profile, with high scores on the hysteria, hypochondriasis, and depression scales. These personality profiles are noted both in patients in whom organic pathology can be found and in those in whom no such pathology is noted. Such psychological changes tend to maintain or increase the level of pain, regardless of the degree of physical disease. Additionally, when pain treatment is successful, the high scores on hysteria, hypochondriasis, and depression revert to normal. However, such research has been difficult due to the heterogeneity of patients with chronic pelvic pain.

The clinical relevance of biopsychosocial pain theories is that diagnosis and treatment must integrate many influences, including the patient's personality and affect; cultural influences; stress; organic changes that may trigger nociceptive signals, sensory thresholds, or gates; and the patient's cognition about pain. For chronic pain, no clear distinction between psychological and physical causes of pain can be made, nor are attempts to make such a distinction useful. Rather than trying to establish organic versus functional etiologies, it is more useful to ask in each case whether there is any physical disease or abnormality that requires medical or surgical treatment and whether there is emotional or psychological distress that requires treatment.

DIAGNOSES AND ETIOLOGIES

Every disorder has several determinants; the notion of a single cause for any illness has been abandoned.—Doyle, 1963

Patients with chronic pelvic pain often either lack a demonstrable organic injury or disease that may account for their pain or have organic pathologies of uncertain relation to the pain. Because of this, in contrast to the usual search for one etiology, a useful approach is to evaluate the pain itself as a diagnosis, with the potential of several organic contributors, and to assess the person with chronic pain as someone with a unique exposure history, taking into account the many factors that lead to her biopsychosocial situation. For the primary care physician, this is particularly important. Women suffering from chronic pelvic pain are a heterogeneous group, and the possible diagnoses are numerous and varied (Table 22-1). Occasionally, the primary care physician is the first to evaluate the patient and a single diagnosis can be made with curative treatment, but more often the pain is longstanding with numerous prior diagnoses and treatments. In such cases, pain becomes an illness in itself, and several contributing factors need evaluation and treatment. The primary care physician may need to serve as the organizer of a multidisciplinary team. For example, urethral syndrome, irritable bowel syndrome, poor posture, and emotional stresses may all be contributing factors in a single patient, with the need for simultaneous urologic, gastroenterologic, and physical therapy and psychological treatment.

Women with chronic pelvic pain are no less likely than the rest of the population to develop acute and serious illnesses, such as appendicitis or cystitis. Thus, with acute exacerbations of pain, it is important to review the symptoms and reevaluate the patient appropriately to rule out acute medical or surgical conditions.

Adenomyosis

Adenomyosis is the presence in the uterine myometrium of ectopic tissue that has the histologic structure and function of uterine mucosa. It is most commonly a cause of dysmenorrhea and menorrhagia, not chronic pelvic pain, but it occasionally presents with persistent nonmenstrual pain as well. Traditionally, the diagnosis is confirmed only by histologic evaluation after hysterectomy, but recent studies suggest it may be diagnosed by resectoscopic or laparoscopic myometrial biopsies. Also, it has been suggested that relief of pain with bilateral uterosacral (paracervical) block may empirically confirm adenomyosis as a source of chronic pelvic pain. Hysterectomy is suggested if this results in appropriate anesthetic pain relief.

Adhesions

Classically, the causes of adhesions are pelvic inflammatory disease, endometriosis, perforated appendix, prior surgery (particularly with associated hemoperitoneum), and inflammatory bowel disease. There is minimal objective evidence that abdominopelvic adhesions cause chronic pelvic pain or that adhesiolysis is therapeutic. The best current speculation regarding the role of adhesions in chronic pelvic pain is that in susceptible patients, adhesions may be a source of nociceptive signals and thereby contribute to pain.

Chronic Appendicitis

Chronic appendicitis is a controversial diagnosis. If it exists, it presents with recurrent, severe, cramping right lower quadrant pain, with or without pyrexia. It is thought to be caused by incomplete luminal obstruction secondary to inspissated fecal material. It accounts for at most 0.6% of appendectomy cases. Histologic findings in cases diagnosed as chronic appendicitis include fecalith, torsion, fibrosis of the lumen, and inspissated material in the lumen.

Table 22-1. Diseases That May Cause or Contribute to Chronic Pelvic Pain in Women

Gynecologic—Extrauterine

Adhesions
Adnexal cysts
Chronic ectopic pregnancy
Chlamydial endometritis or salpingitis
Endometriosis
Ovarian retention syndrome (residual ovary syndrome)
Ovarian remnant syndrome
Ovarian dystrophy or ovulatory pain
Pelvic congestion syndrome
Postoperative peritoneal cysts
Residual accessory ovary
Subacute salpingo-oophoritis
Tuberculous salpingitis

Gynecologic-Uterine

Adenomyosis
Atypical dysmenorrhea or ovulatory pain
Cervical stenosis
Chronic endometritis
Endometrial or cervical polyps
Intrauterine contraceptive device
Leiomyomata
Symptomatic pelvic relaxation (genital prolapse)

Urologic

Bladder neoplasm
Chronic urinary tract infection
Interstitial cystitis
Radiation cystitis
Recurrent, acute cystitis
Recurent, acute urethritis
Stone/urolithiasis
Uninhibited bladder contractions (detrusor dyssynergia)
Urethral diverticulum
Urethral syndrome
Urethral caruncle

Gastrointestinal

Carcinoma of the colon
Chronic intermittent bowel obstruction
Colitis
Constipation
Diverticular disease
Hernias
Inflammatory bowel disease
Irritable bowel syndrome

Musculoskeletal

Abdominal wall myofascial pain (trigger points)
Chronic coccygeal pain
Compression of lumbar vertebrae
Degenerative joint disease
Disk
Faulty or poor posture
Fibromyositis
Hernias: ventral, inguinal, femoral, spigelian
Low back pain
Muscular strains and sprains
Neoplasia of spinal cord or sacral nerve
Neuralgia of iliohypogastric, ilioinguinal, or genitofemoral nerves
Pelvic floor myalgia (levator ani spasm)
Piriformis syndrome
Rectus tendon strain
Spondylosis

Other

Abdominal cutaneous nerve entrapment in surgical scar
Abdominal epilepsy
Abdominal migraine
Bipolar personality disorder
Depression
Familial Mediterranean fever
Neurologic dysfunction
Porphyria
Shingles
Sleep disturbances
Somatic referral

Endometriosis

Endometriosis is the presence of ectopic tissue that has the histologic structure and function of the uterine mucosa. It can be diagnosed only at the time of laparoscopy or laparotomy. Biopsies with histologic confirmation of endometriosis are advisable due to the potential error of 25% or more with solely visual diagnosis of both typical and atypical lesions at laparoscopy. Additionally, biopsies of atypical peritoneal lesions increase the chance of diagnosing endometriosis by about 25%. Endometriosis does not always cause pelvic pain, but it appears that endometriosis, like a number of other abnormalities associated with pain (eg, adhesions), may be a source of nociceptive signals that result in pain in certain patients. Deep dyspareunia, postcoital pain, and recurrent pain are more common in women with laparoscopically diagnosed endometriosis than in women without endometriosis. Although the literature on endometriosis is extensive, most of it does not specifically address chronic pelvic pain.

The etiology of endometriosis is unknown. Several risk factors have been epidemiologically identified that may be helpful to the primary care physician in counseling patients for prevention of primary or recurrent disease. Women who have intercourse during menses are about twice as likely to have endometriosis. Women with menstrual cycles of less than 28 days are twice as likely to have endometriosis as those with cycles of 28 to 34 days. Aerobic exercise for more than 7 hours per week decreases the odds of endometriosis by fivefold over that of women who do not exercise.

Menstrual Pain (Atypical Dysmenorrhea or Ovulatory Pain)

Luteal phase pain associated with premenstrual syndrome, protracted dysmenorrhea, protracted mittelschmerz, and recurrent functional ovarian cysts may all present as cyclical chronic pelvic pain. This diagnosis is difficult without a detailed pain diary. Such atypical menstrual pain may account for the symptoms of up to 20% of patients with a negative laparoscopy. Treatment via hormonal suppression of the menstrual cycle is usually successful.

Musculoskeletal Dysfunction

Some of the musculoskeletal dysfunctions that have been reported as causes of chronic pelvic pain are listed in Table 22-1, but little objective evidence has been published substantiating that these abnormalities are etiologically linked to chronic pelvic pain. Certainly, the musculoskeletal structures of the pelvis and lower abdomen have coincident innervation with the pelvic viscera (T12, L1-5, and S1-3), so it theoretically makes sense that chronic musculoskeletal pathologies may account for chronic pelvic pain.

The muscles most commonly involved in chronic pelvic pain are the iliopsoas, piriformis, obturator internus, pubococcygeus, abdominals, and quadratus lumborum. Frequent periods of prolonged sitting, unilateral standing patterns, inactive lifestyles, and side and stomach sleeping are physical habits observed to be common to many chronic pelvic pain patients. These may lead to poor posture, particularly a posture termed "typical pelvic pain posture," a persistent lordosis or kyphosis/lordosis with anterior pelvic tilt. This posture leads to several musculoskeletal dysfunctions: stretching and weakening of the abdominal muscles; shortening of the thoracolumbar fascia; shortening of the posterior muscles of the trunk; compression of the posterior articulations of the lumbar spine; and shortening of the iliopsoas, obturator internus, coccygeus, and piriformis muscles. The prolonged shortening of the latter group of muscles causes muscular strain and pain. As previously noted, these muscle groups are innervated by T12 to L3 (as are the pelvic viscera and lower abdominal wall) and may produce pelvic pain both directly and by referral to the pelvic organs and lower abdomen.

Other musculoskeletal abnormalities may be important in some patients. For example, the asymmetric pelvic posture due to an anatomic short leg may cause traction forces on the abdominal, paravertebral, and gluteal muscles, resulting in muscular strain and pain that may present as chronic pelvic pain. Treatment with a heel lift to the short limb is indicated. Most primary care physicians need orthopedic and physical therapy consultation for the diagnosis and treatment of such patients.

Pelvic floor myalgia is a form of tension myalgia that produces pain much as tension headaches cause pain. The tension or spasm involves the musculature of the pelvic floor and causes pain in these muscles or in their areas of attachment to the sacrum, coccyx, ischial tuberosities, and pubic rami. Several names have been used for syndromes that appear to be similar: piriformis syndrome, levator ani spasm syndrome, diaphragma pelvis spastica, and coccydynia. Several factors are believed to cause habitual contraction or chronic spasm of the pelvic floor muscles: inflammatory processes such as urethritis, anal fissures, or hemorrhoids; general muscular deconditioning and poor posture as described above; and prior orthopedic or gynecologic surgery. This syndrome is more common in women than men (5:1 ratio) and occurs most frequently at 40 to 50 years of age. Symptoms are often vague, but most patients complain of aching, throbbing, or heavy discomfort in the pelvis, rectum, or lower back. Leg pain, pain with bowel movements, and constipation are present in less than half of patients. Dyspareunia is an occasional complaint. The pain is most consistently exacerbated by sitting for more than a half-hour. Anxiety and physical exercise occasionally increase the pain. It has also been reported due to overzealous Kegel pelvic exercises. Physical examination reveals tenderness on rectovaginal evaluation of the piriformis muscles, coccygeus muscles, levator ani muscles, sacrococcygeal ligaments, the attachments of these muscles to the sacrum or coccyx, or a combination of these loci. Numerous treatments have been recommended with varying success, including rectal diathermy, Thiele massage (rectal massage of the levators), relaxation exercises, hot-tub immersion twice a day, and biofeedback pelvic floor training.

Myofascial or trigger point pain syndrome is a not uncommon finding in chronic pelvic pain patients. In this syndrome, there are discrete 1- to 2-cm hyperpathic areas deep to the subcutaneous fat. These focal areas of marked tenderness are generally found on the anterior abdomen within the T11, T12, and L1 dermatomes, but sometimes are also noted posteriorly over the same dermatomes on the midback or in the dermatomes of S2, S3, and S4 over the sacrum. Several etiologies are suggested, including focal spasms due to the postural dysfunctions described earlier, an as-yet-unidentified chronic viral infection, and abdominal cutaneous nerve entrapment. Although nerve entrapment and myofascial pain may be due to previous abdominal surgical incisions, this is not always the case. Slocumb has written extensively on trigger points and in a referral population found them in 74% of patients. Others have reported a lower incidence. Physical findings with this syndrome are described later in this chapter. Palliative treatment is reported with local anesthetic injections (with or without steroid injections), transcutaneous electrical nerve stimulation, acupuncture, ultrasound, and physical therapy. These modalities are not universally successful, nor are they curative.

Hernias may cause chronic abdominopelvic pain that is generally intermittent and accompanied by abdominal distention. Incisional hernias may develop after any abdominal surgery but are more common with vertical than transverse incisions. Spigelian hernias are small, spontaneous ventral hernias with protrusion through the transversus abdominis aponeurosis lateral to the edge of the rectus muscle but medial to the spigelian line. The spigelian line is the point of transition of the transverse abdominal muscle to its aponeurotic tendon. This fascia starts at the level of the ninth costal cartilage and has its widest point just below the umbilicus, the site where spigelian hernias occur most commonly. They are often difficult to palpate and diagnose. Ultrasound evaluation may be helpful in diagnosis in some cases. Inguinal hernias, either direct or indirect, are also occasionally a source of abdominopelvic pain. Often the defect is palpable at the time of physical examination if care is taken to perform the examination both standing and with tensing of the abdominal muscles. Such hernias may also be noted on laparoscopy.

The pain of musculoskeletal problems may mimic that of gynecologic disease in many ways. It may be altered by hormonal influences and therefore be cyclic. It may be dull, aching, stabbing, or cramping in character. It may vary with posture, position, and specific activities, particularly decreasing with rest.

Ovarian Remnant Syndrome

After prior hysterectomy and bilateral oophorectomy, recurrent pain may be due to ovarian remnant syndrome. The diagnosis is sometimes confirmed by measuring follicle-stimulating hormone levels when the patient is not on hormonal replacement therapy. This syndrome has also been reported after unilateral oophorectomy, with persistence of ovarian tissue and pelvic pain on the ipsilateral side. Pain may be relieved by gonadotropin-releasing hormone agonist (GnRH-a) therapy, but definitive treatment requires surgical removal of the remnant tissue. Such surgery is often difficult and complicated. Castrating doses of radiation have also been used for treatment.

Ovarian Retention Syndrome (Residual Ovary Syndrome)

Ovarian retention syndrome is the presence of persistent pelvic pain, dyspareunia, or a pelvic mass after conservation of one or both ovaries at the time of hysterectomy. Ovarian retention syndrome is also called residual ovary syndrome, but both of these terms lend themselves to easy confusion with ovarian remnant syndrome. Pain due to ovarian retention syndrome is usually relieved by complete ovarian suppression with GnRH-a treatment. Sometimes suppression with oral contraceptives or high-dose progestins is effective. Definitive treatment is surgical extirpation. In young women in whom preservation of ovarian function is desired, adhesiolysis and ovarian cystectomy may be tried.

Pelvic Congestion Syndrome

Pelvic congestion syndrome is characterized by delayed or slow venous return in the ovarian veins. It is not synonymous with pelvic varicosities. It may be diagnosed by pelvic venography and possibly by Doppler flow studies or applied potential tomography. Symptoms of pelvic congestion syndrome are vague and nonspecific and include dull, aching pelvic pain, congestive dysmenorrhea, postcoital pain, backache, excessive vaginal discharge, pelvic pressure, deep dyspareunia, and urinary symptoms. Almost all patients have either postcoital aching pain in the lateral lower abdomen or ovarian tenderness on palpation. It has been suggested that pain improves with knee-chest positioning, but the diagnostic usefulness of this has not been studied.

Pelvic Inflammatory Disease

Chronic or recurrent pelvic inflammatory disease is not uncommonly diagnosed in women with chronic pelvic pain. Although up to 30% of women who develop pelvic inflammatory disease subsequently experience chronic pelvic pain, this chronic pain is not due to a chronic or recurrent infectious process. Thus, empiric antibiotic therapy has little if any role in the evaluation or treatment of women with chronic pelvic pain. In fact, more than half of women diagnosed with chronic or recurrent pelvic inflammatory disease as the etiology for their chronic pelvic pain have no objective evidence at the time of laparoscopy of prior pelvic inflammatory disease.

Pelvic Relaxation

Relaxation of the pelvic floor with development of cystocele, rectocele, enterocele, or uterine descensus may cause pelvic and perineal pain. However, the pain is usually not severe and is most commonly described as pressure. It is relieved by a pessary or surgical repair.

Postoperative Peritoneal Cysts

Postoperative peritoneal cysts are rare causes of chronic pelvic pain; only 17 such cases have been reported. All but one patient had undergone prior surgery, and the woman without surgery had a history of pelvic inflammatory disease. When such cysts occur, they develop many months to years after surgery. They are generally demonstrated only by ultrasound or computed tomography (CT), as all other laboratory and radiographic studies tend to be normal. Histology shows a cyst lining of cuboidal or flat mesothelial cells.

Tuberculous Salpingitis

Tuberculous salpingitis is an insidious infection that may cause chronic pelvic pain, as well as abnormal uterine bleeding or infertility. Diagnosis is difficult in some cases, but it may be confirmed by a positive tuberculin skin test, an endometrial biopsy showing tuberculous granulomas and acid-fast bacilli, and possibly a positive culture from menstrual blood. Findings at laparoscopy of miliary pelvic visceral and peritoneal disease are characteristic of tuberculous salpingitis. Although a rare disease at present, the incidence of tuberculous pelvic infections may increase with the recent increase in cases of pulmonary tuberculosis.

Urologic Diagnoses

Urinary calculi generally cause acute, not chronic, abdominopelvic pain. Rarely, stones lodge at the ureterovesical junction and present with insidious pain. Urethral diverticula are not usually a source of chronic pelvic pain, although low-grade infection or inflammation could present this way. More commonly, the pain due to diverticula is dyspareunia. Urethral syndrome and interstitial cystitis are not infrequent causes of pelvic pain.

HISTORY AND PHYSICAL EXAMINATION

Often, the diagnostic approach to the woman with chronic pelvic pain is directed as much by the specialty of the evaluating physician as by the woman's clinical characteristics. The diversity of potential etiologic or contributing diagnoses demands a more general approach. The primary care physician may not have the expertise to diagnose or manage all the possible diagnoses, but he or she can do a thorough, explorative history that will direct further evaluation and requisite referrals. Although the history is directed to the patient's pain, a thorough review of systems must not be neglected. Particular attention should be given to a review of symptoms of the gastrointestinal, reproductive, urologic, and musculoskeletal systems.

The location of pain is a crucial part of the history. The patient should also be asked about any radiation of the pain. A useful technique at the initial interview and at intervals during care is to have the patient do a "pain map" on a human anatomy diagram (Fig. 22-1). Other pain locations are often revealed in this manner. For example, up to 60% of women with chronic pelvic pain also have headaches, and up to 90% have backaches. The location of chronic pain is sometimes useful in the differential diagnosis. Visceral pain is not as well localized as dermatomal pain, so patients with chronic pain and visceral pathology may have trouble localizing their pain. Lateral pelvic pain is commonly of adnexal or sigmoid colonic origin. Midline infraumbilical pain is often due to pathology of the uterus and cervix. Pain from the bladder or vagina may localize over the mons pubis, pubic bone, or groin. Lower sacral and midline pain may be from the uterosacral ligaments and posterior cul-de-sac. Complaints of pain both ventrally and dorsally often suggest intrapelvic pathology, whereas only dorsal low back pain suggests an orthopedic or musculoskeletal origin.

The severity, frequency, and timing of pain should be investigated. Determining consistency or cyclicity of pain is useful by asking, for example, if symptoms are the same 24 hours a day, 7 days a week, every week. Stress-related and musculoskeletal-associated pain may differ depending on the day of the week and corresponding work or activity level. Accurate records are useful during the initial history, as well as during follow-up and treatment evaluations. Asking the patient to keep a diary of symptoms, with timing and severity of pain, medication use, and other potentially related factors, is often useful. The patient should use some type of rating system for her pain and other symptoms. A visual or verbal analog scale, with a 0 to 10 rating, is most commonly used for pain, with 0 representing no pain, 4 or 5 moderate pain, and 10 the worst pain imaginable. A simple "no pain, mild pain, moderate pain, severe pain" rating system may also suffice. The American Fertility Society has suggested for endometriosis-associated pain a "mild," "discomforting," "distressing," "horrible," and "excruciating" system, noted as A through E, respectively. Although more

Patient's Name ______________________ Age __________ Date __________

PRE-OPERATIVE ASSESSMENT OF PELVIC PAIN

Complaints ____

Describe the patient's symptoms of pain quality and position, and any limitation caused by these symptoms. Abbreviate quality of pain as **A = mild, B = discomforting, C = distressing, D = horrible, E = excruciating.** On the anatomic drawings below, draw a **SOLID LINE** around the area(s) of pain described by the patient, and mark the most intense area(s) with an **X.**

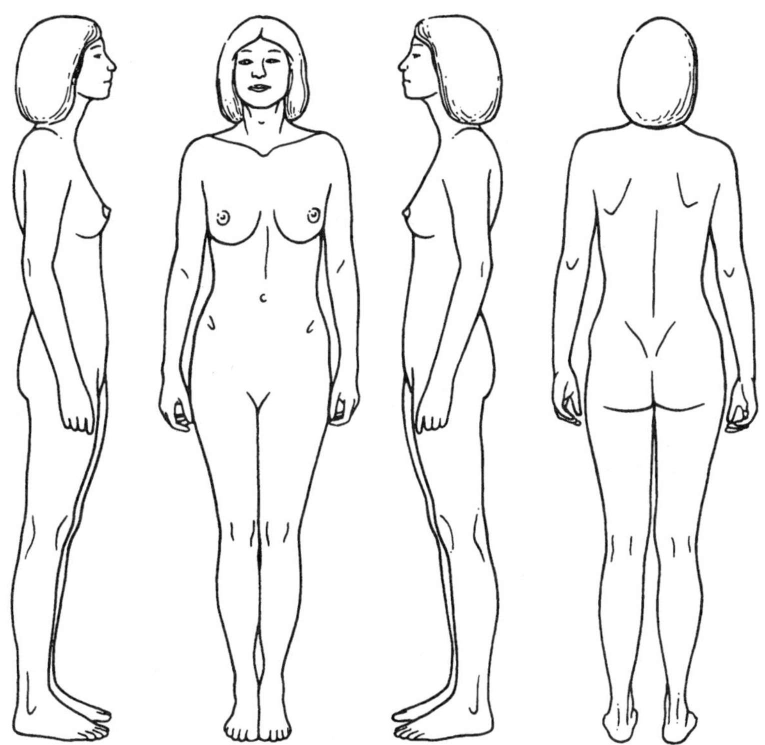

Physical findings ____

Identify the quality and site of tenderness caused by palpation, extent of nodularity, diffuse or focal distribution, and/or fixation of uterus/adnexa. On the anatomic drawings above, draw a **BROKEN LINE** around the area(s) of tenderness found on examination.

Figure 22-1. Example of an instrument to document the location of chronic pelvic pain.

complicated rating systems are used for research and in chronic pain clinics, these relatively simple scales are sufficient for primary care purposes.

The quality or nature of pain should be sought. Patients sometimes have difficulty with this part of the history, and the physician may need to supply possible descriptors. Some of the terms used in the McGill Pain Questionnaire (Table 22-2) may be useful. For example, the pain of cutaneous nerve entrapment is often described as sharp, piercing, or burning. Further suggesting this etiology is pain that radiates along the distribution of the entrapped nerve. With the iliohypogastric or ilioinguinal nerve, pain radiation is medially along the lower abdomen into the labia or upper inner aspect of the thigh.

The patient should be asked about factors that provoke, intensify, and palliate the pain. For example, rest often decreases pain of musculoskeletal or adnexal origin but has no effect on pain of mostly psychological origin. The amount, type, and effectiveness of pain medications should be included in this part of the history.

Aspects of the psychosocial history should be explored by the primary care physician. Sexuality, abuse (physical or sexual), health habits, sleep habits, depression, and anxiety are some of the areas that may be evaluated. It is important to assess the consequences of the patient's pain on her functional ability. The degree of incapacity caused by the pain, especially as it affects work and family roles, appears to be a significant indicator of success of traditional treatment. Symptoms of depression are particularly important to seek. This is important not only because of the association of depression and chronic pain previously noted, but also because many depressed patients consult their primary care physician 1 to 2 months before they commit suicide.

A history of dyspareunia is frequently sought during the history and variously interpreted as pathognomonic of psychological disease, marital problems, endometriosis, vulvodynia, and so forth. In fact, dyspareunia is present in about 50% of women with chronic pelvic pain, but this may not be elicited without direct questioning. It occurs with all the above-noted problems as well as with irritable bowel disease, inflammatory bowel disease, adhesions, and pelvic floor defects. It is not specific for any particular disease.

During the history and discussion, nothing should be dismissed as ridiculous, impossible, or unimportant. Stating such things to the patient is counterproductive and creates distrust. Tolerance is important in listening to the patient's telling and interpretation of her history. A major goal in caring for women with chronic pelvic pain is establishing rapport. Because of this, even though a questionnaire may be very helpful for the busy primary care practitioner, it must not replace allowing the patient to tell her history to the physician directly.

CLINICAL FINDINGS

A major goal of the examination in patients with pain is to detect the exact location or locations of pain and tenderness. This requires a systematic and methodical attempt to duplicate the pain by palpation. The physician may find it useful to record these findings on a human anatomy diagram similar to that used by the patient for recording her pain location (see Fig. 22-1).

Ideally, the examination should start as the patient enters the office or examination room. Her gait and posture are observed, especially noting limp, altered or asymmetric gait, lordosis, kyphosis/lordosis, scoliosis, or one-leg standing. Evaluation of forward bending may be helpful: normally, this causes a reversal of the concave lumbar lordotic curve, but in patients with the typical pelvic pain posture (lordosis or kyphosis/lordosis), this reversal does not occur and the curvature remains convex with forward bending. The physician can also evaluate unequal iliac crest heights by placing the flattened palms on the superior aspects of the iliac crests and noting asymmetry; a difference of more than 0.25" is significant and may occur with short leg or unilateral standing habit. Also in the standing position, evaluation for femoral and inguinal hernias is done by palpation both with and without Valsalva maneuvers. The standing position is also useful for evaluation of pelvic floor relaxation defects, by placing the index finger of one hand in the vagina and the index finger of the other hand in the rectum while the patient bears down. Occult enterocele, rectocele, cystocele, and uterine prolapse may be diagnosed with this procedure more accurately than if the patient is in the lithotomy position.

Posture should also be noted in the sitting position. Palpation for tenderness of the upper and lower back and sacrum should be done, including single-digit palpation for trigger points.

After the patient lies down, inspection and palpation for lordosis or pelvic tilt are done again. Surgical scars should be noted. Leg flexion, knee to chest, can be done to elicit low back dysfunction, low

Table 22-2. McGill Pain Questionnaire Descriptors for Quality of Chronic Pain

1. Flickering Quivering Pulsing Throbbing Beating Pounding	5. Pinching Pressing Gnawing Cramping Crushing	9. Dull Sore Hurting Aching Heavy	14. Punishing Grueling Cruel Vicious Killing	18. Tight Numb Drawing Squeezing Tearing
2. Jumping Flashing Shooting	6. Tugging Pulling Wrenching	10. Tender Taut Rasping Splitting	15. Wretched Blinding	19. Cool Cold Freezing
3. Pricking Boring Drilling Stabbing Lancinating	7. Hot Burning Scalding Searing	11. Tiring Exhausting	16. Annoying Troublesome Miserable Intense Unbearable	20. Nagging Nauseating Agonizing Dreadful Torturing
4. Sharp Cutting Lacerating	8. Tingling Itchy Smarting Stinging	12. Sickening Suffocating	17. Spreading Radiating Penetrating Piercing	
		13. Fearful Frightful Terrifying		

back pain, and abdominal muscle weakness. Head raise and leg raise can be similarly used. Abdominal palpation should initially be superficial, noting hyperesthesias. Next, single-digit palpation for trigger points is carefully and systematically done, including the inguinal areas. This technique is also used for localizing cutaneous nerve entrapment. The point of maximum tenderness is localized with one finger, and the patient confirms that this palpation duplicates her pain. The abdominal wall tenderness test may be useful in distinguishing abdominal wall (myofascial) tenderness from visceral tenderness. In this test, while the area of abdominal tenderness is palpated, the patient tenses the abdominal muscles voluntarily or by raising her head or legs. If the pain is unchanged or increased, it suggests there is no intraabdominal disease and that the pain is of myofascial origin; if the pain is decreased, it suggests intraabdominal disease. Myofascial pain suggested by the abdominal wall tenderness test may be due to muscular strain, nerve entrapment, viral myositis, trauma, epigastric artery rupture, or an abdominal wall hernia, as well as myofascial trigger points.

Palpation for hernial defects should be done, including careful palpation of any surgical scars. This may necessitate having the patient stand, as previously described, for complete evaluation. Spigelian hernias have been reported as potential causes of abdominopelvic pain but are difficult to diagnose. There may be tenderness at the location, but these fascial defects are small and hard to palpate.

The usual components of the abdominal examination should not be neglected. Examination for distention, bowel sounds, shifting dullness, vascular bruits, and palpation for deep tenderness, guarding, or rigidity are essential. A palpable, tender sigmoid colon may suggest irritable bowel syndrome.

Visual inspection of the external genitalia should be performed with particular attention to any redness, discharge, abscess formation, excoriation, atrophic changes (thinning, paleness, loss of vaginal rugae, protruding urethral mucosa), or signs of trauma. A cotton-tipped applicator may be used to evaluate the vestibule for the localized tenderness of vulvar vestibulitis. Fistulas and fissures should be noted and are occasionally the first objective evidence of inflammatory bowel disease.

Pain or tension in the pelvic muscles can be assessed by inserting a single blade of the speculum into the posterior vagina. While the patient is asked to relax, the resistance to downward or posterior pressure can be evaluated to reveal increased muscle tone, tension, or spasm. This maneuver may also reproduce part of the patient's symptom complex. Examination with a single speculum blade or a Sims-type retractor may also reveal evidence of pelvic relaxation. The traditional speculum examination is done to provide full visual inspection and to obtain requisite cytologic and bacteriologic specimens.

The pelvic examination should always be initiated with a single index finger, first noting any introital tenderness or spasm. Next, the levator ani muscles are directly palpated for tone and tenderness. The insertion of the levators should also be palpated if possible, both laterally at the arcus tendineus and anteriorly at the pubic rami. The urethral and trigonal areas should be gently palpated to elicit any areas of tenderness, induration, or thickening. The urethra should also be massaged to elicit any secretions. Then the gutter on either side of the urethra should be evaluated for any fullness, fluctuance, or discomfort that might suggest a urethral diverticulum or vaginal wall cyst. The bladder base is also evaluated for tenderness. With deeper palpation, evaluation for cervical or vaginal forniceal tenderness is done. The piriformis, coccygeus, and obturator internus should also be palpated for tenderness that reproduces pelvic pain.

The traditional bimanual examination is the last portion of the pelvic examination in the pelvic pain patient. A fixed, retroverted uterus may suggest endometriosis or cul-de-sac adhesions. Endometriosis is also suggested by tenderness of the posterior uterus, nodularity of the uterosacral ligaments and cul-de-sac, and narrowing of the posterior vaginal fornix. Pelvic nodularity is, however, not diagnostic of endometriosis and may occur with other conditions, particularly ovarian carcinoma. Asymmetric, enlarged ovaries, particularly if fixed to the broad ligament or pelvic sidewall, may imply the presence of endometriosis. Bilateral or unilateral ovarian tenderness almost always occurs with pelvic congestion syndrome. Marked discomfort with digital rectal examination often accompanies irritable bowel syndrome or chronic constipation, as may hard feces in the rectum. The function of the internal and external anal sphincters should be evaluated by reflex "wink" and voluntary constriction. The rectal examination should also include evaluation for rectal masses, as many colorectal carcinomas are palpable this way.

Basic sensory testing to sharpness, dullness, and light touch may be indicated, as well as muscle strength testing and deep tendon reflexes of the trunk and lower extremities. Further neurologic, musculoskeletal, gastrointestinal, gynecologic, and urologic aspects of the physical examination may be needed, based on the clinical history. Consultation outside the primary care physician's areas of expertise should be liberally obtained.

LABORATORY AND IMAGING STUDIES

Most women with chronic pelvic pain should have cervical cultures or smears for gonorrhea and chlamydia, a complete blood cell count, sedimentation rate, stool guiaic testing, urinalysis, and urine culture. Other tests depend on the history and physical findings.

Imaging studies are mostly useful to rule out specific diagnoses suggested by the clinical findings. For example, intravenous pyelography, cystography, skeletal or pelvic x-rays, ultrasound, and CT scans may be useful in certain patients but should not be done routinely.

TREATMENT

Not uncommonly, the primary care physician is the one to assist the chronic pelvic pain patient in setting clear goals of treatment that are short of a cure. Examples of such goals are to relieve suffering by treatment of identifiable symptoms and concurrent psychological morbidity; to restore normal function, without specific goals regarding pain level; to improve quality of life and minimize disability by managing pain and other symptoms with analgesics, physical therapy, acupuncture, nerve blocks, and so forth; and to prevent recurrence of chronic symptoms and disability via ongoing compliance and treatment.

Also, as previously mentioned, the primary care physician may need to assemble a multidisciplinary team to treat the chronic pelvic pain patient. Special multidisciplinary chronic pain clinics are not available to all patients due to geographic, time, and financial constraints, but the physician may be able to accomplish similar care using appropriate referral and consultation. In such a setting, the primary care physician serves as the consistent care provider and resource person for the patient.

Although the placebo effect may play a role in many of the therapies used for treatment of chronic pelvic pain, the deliberate use of placebo medication has no role in the diagnosis or treatment. It is not true that if a patient responds to placebo, then the pain is of psychological origin.

Surgery

Various surgical procedures, including neurolytic and neuroextirpative operations, organ extirpative procedures, and removal of specifically abnormal tissue, remain a mainstay of treatment of chronic pelvic pain. Although surgery is a part of the management of chronic pelvic pain, its limitations must be recognized by both the surgeon and the patient.

Laparoscopy

As a diagnostic procedure, laparoscopy serves at least three useful functions: diagnostic confirmation, histologic documentation, and patient reassurance. It also may prevent unnecessary laparotomy and allow simultaneous surgical treatment via operative laparoscopy. More than half of women with abnormal findings at the time of laparoscopy have normal physical examinations. However, routine laparoscopy for all women with chronic pelvic pain may be unnecessary. Considering the benefits and risks of laparoscopy, reasonable indications are an abnormal examination; failure of initial management to provide significant resolution of symptoms; fixed attributions on the patient's part regarding the cause of the pain that may interfere with treatment; or strong suspicion of disease (eg, endometriosis) that is best diagnosed or treated surgically.

Hysterectomy

By discharge diagnosis data, about 12% of all hysterectomies in the United States are done for pelvic pain. Hysterectomy has a useful role in the treatment of many women with chronic pelvic pain. In the Maine Women's Health Study, 74 (18%) of 418 women had hysterectomies for a primary indication of chronic pelvic pain. Furthermore, 45% of the women with hysterectomies for leiomyomata had more than 8 days of pain per month, and 66% of those with bleeding as the preoperative indication had similar pain, suggesting that many women have pelvic pain as a primary or secondary diagnosis for hysterectomy. Although not extensively studied, it appears that 75% of women with hysterectomy for chronic pelvic pain are relieved of pain at the time of follow-up 1 year later.

Oophorectomy

Bilateral oophorectomy must be undertaken with great caution in young women because the long-term risks of osteoporosis and cardiovascular disease represent serious diseases that may result from noncompliance with estrogen replacement therapy. However, oophorectomy is sometimes necessary, for example with endometriosis involving the adnexae or pelvic congestion syndrome.

Regrettably, in cases with a gynecologist as the primary care physician and with failure of hysterectomy and bilateral salpingo-oophorectomy to ameliorate pain, the surgery sometimes results in discontinuation of further primary care.

Ovarian Cystectomy

Rarely are benign ovarian cysts other than those due to endometriosis a cause of chronic pelvic pain. Adnexal surgery results in significant adhesive disease, so caution must be exercised in deciding to perform ovarian cystectomies for chronic pelvic pain in young women of reproductive age.

Adhesiolysis

Fifty percent to 70% of patients with chronic pelvic pain and abdominopelvic adhesions have significant relief of pain symptoms for more than 6 months after laparoscopic adhesiolysis. However, when a patient has either vegetative signs of depression (particularly sleep disturbance) or significant alterations of her role in the family, relief of pain after adhesiolysis is less likely. About 25% of patients with initial pain relief after adhesiolysis have recurrence of pain over the first 3 to 5 months after surgery. The only randomized study of adhesiolysis (performed by laparotomy after diagnostic laparoscopy) failed to show any effectiveness of adhesiolysis of pelvic visceral adhesions.

Presacral Neurectomy

Innervation from the superior hypogastric plexus (presacral nerve) supplies the cervix, uterus, and proximal fallopian tubes with afferent nociception, so not surprisingly this operation is particularly useful for central dysmenorrhea unresponsive to other treatment. About 75% of patients with this symptom have a greater than 50% decrease in pain after presacral neurectomy. However, the response of nondysmenorrhea pain is lower: 60% of patients or fewer have decreased central chronic pelvic pain after presacral neurectomy. This response is similar whether or not specific pathology (eg, endometriosis or adhesions) is present. Pain that is localized in the lateral pelvic area, as opposed to central pelvic pain, has a notably lower response to treatment by presacral neurectomy.

Indications for presacral neurectomy are limited and include dysmenorrhea from endometriosis or adenomyosis, dysmenorrhea unresponsive to nonsurgical treatments, deep dyspareunia, sacral backache associated with menses as part of conservative surgery for endometriosis and pelvic pain, and chronic recurrent central pelvic pain from fibrosis or leiomyomata in the region of the uterosacral ligaments.

Excision or Destruction of Endometriosis

Conservative surgical treatment of endometriosis results in complete pain relief for 1 year or more in 45% to 70% of patients. A small study of laparoscopic electrosurgical treatment of endometriosis versus no treatment showed 64% pain relief for 1 year with surgical treatment compared to 20% in the group with laparoscopy only. The recurrence rate of endometriosis after conservative surgical treatment is variously reported as 15% to 100%. The average time to recurrence after initial surgery by laparotomy is 40 to 50 months. However, the time to recurrence may reflect the thoroughness of the original surgery or the effectiveness of subsequent medical treatment. Surgical or medical treatment of endometriosis is recommended even in asymptomatic patients, as placebo-controlled studies have shown that 48% of untreated (placebo-treated) patients have worsening of their disease over 24 weeks of observation. Surgical treatment is mandatory for acute rupture of an endometrioma, ureteral obstruction, large bowel compromise, or adnexal enlargement to 8 cm or more.

Uterosacral Nerve Resection or Ablation

The controversial procedure of uterosacral nerve resection or ablation has mixed results. There are no controlled clinical trials available that evaluate its effectiveness. Specific indications for paracervical uterine denervation are when a nodule of endometriosis or a myoma is present at the base of the uterosacral ligament, necessitating excision of part of the ligament; when exposure for presacral neurectomy is inadequate; when pain recurs after a presacral neurectomy; and when intractable primary dysmenorrhea is unresponsive to medical treatment in a young woman.

It is not useful to combine this procedure with presacral neurectomy, as it does not improve the results over those obtained with presacral neurectomy only.

Uterine Suspension

Uterine suspension is usually done to establish and maintain anteversion of the fixed, retroverted uterus as part of the overall surgery for nonuterine pathology such as endometriosis or adhesions. Rarely, it is indicated for the patient with a retroverted and mobile uterus. If dyspareunia or pelvic pain is thought to be secondary to a mobile retroverted uterus, then repositioning with a pessary (eg, a Smith-Hodge pessary) for 4 to 6 weeks is recommended. If this relieves the pain, then uterine suspension may be helpful. The procedure may be done via laparotomy or laparoscopy.

Appendectomy

Chronic appendicitis or periappendiceal adhesions as causes of chronic pelvic pain are controversial. Endometriosis of the appendix occurs in up to 15% of endometriosis patients but is rarely an isolated finding. In patients with persistent right lower quadrant abdominopelvic pain and appendiceal endometriosis, adhesions, or a suspicious history for chronic appendicitis, laparoscopic appendectomy has been reported to result in pain relief in up to 80%.

Trigger Point Therapies

Trigger point injections should not be considered curative. They are methods of diagnostic evaluation and temporizing or modulating the pain response. Reports of effectiveness vary, but Slocumb has reported that 80% to 90% of patients with trigger points obtain relief or significant improvement with local anesthetic injection. However, if repeat injections are needed, the rate of response declines notably. Most patients have recurrences related to stress or specific activities within a few months after successful treatment. When trigger points are due to nerve entrapment, surgical resection of a neuroma or of the entrapped nerve may result in permanent relief.

Hormonal Therapies

GnRH-a and danazol have been shown to result in complete pain relief in 50% to 60% of endometriosis patients and to decrease pain in up to 90%. Continued decreased pain levels up to 6 months after discontinuation of GnRH-a or danazol therapy have been reported in 70% to 80% of patients. However, more than 40% of patients have full recurrence of pelvic pain symptoms within 3 years of completion of danazol treatment. GnRH-a and danazol are contraindicated with undiagnosed abnormal uterine bleeding, pregnancy, or breastfeeding; danazol is also contraindicated with impaired renal, cardiac, or hepatic function. GnRH-a and high-dose danazol should not be continued beyond 6 months of therapy due to concerns about osteoporosis.

Suppression of the normal hormonal changes of the menstrual cycle may be useful in women with functional menstrual pain, either atypical dysmenorrhea or pain with premenstrual syndrome. This may be accomplished with oral contraceptives, gonadotropin-releasing hormone agonists, danazol, or high-dose medroxyprogesterone acetate.

The short-term use of GnRH-a may be helpful for both therapeutic and diagnostic evaluation of cycle-based pain. If a trial of several months does not result in resolution of pelvic pain, then it is unlikely that hysterectomy and salpingo-oophorectomy will be beneficial.

Dihydroergotamine is effective for acute pain exacerbations in women with pelvic congestion syndrome. This treatment may have diagnostic as well as therapeutic utility in some cases.

Drug Therapy

Antidepressants

Antidepressants, particularly the tricyclics, have been shown in placebo-controlled studies to improve pain levels and pain tolerance in various chronic pain syndromes. The most commonly used are imipramine, amitriptyline, and doxepin. Doses lower than those used for the treatment of depression seem effective for chronic pain. The analgesic effect of antidepressants appears to require 2 to 3 weeks, similar to the antidepressant effect. Fluoxetine, which is not a tricyclic, has also been used empirically for chronic pelvic pain, but less clinical experience has been reported.

Little study of the use of antidepressants specifically for chronic pelvic pain has been done. In one uncontrolled evaluation of nortriptyline for chronic pelvic pain, a decrease of pain intensity and duration and a change of pain character were noted. However, half of the enrolled patients discontinued nortriptyline before completing the study due to drug side effects at doses of 100 mg or less.

Analgesics

Optimization of analgesic therapy is sometimes overlooked with initial treatment of chronic pelvic pain. Particularly with nonsteroidal antiinflammatory medications, a scheduled regimen rather than an as-needed regimen may be more effective. An as-needed regimen may be less successful because the patient may delay self-medication until the pain is severe, resulting in less effective analgesia, and because having the patient focus on pain symptoms may in itself result in increased pain.

Although opiate analgesics are indicated for acute pain, with chronic pain their use leads to tolerance and dependence as well as debilitating side effects such as apathy, lethargy, constipation, and depression. Additionally, their sedating effects limit restoration of normal function and activity. It seems best to avoid their use for chronic pelvic pain.

Anxiolytics

Anxiolytics, particularly the benzodiazepines, should be used only for specific diagnoses of anxiety syndromes or for their muscle relaxation properties in some cases of pain secondary to muscle spasm. Their general use for chronic pelvic pain is not advised due to problems of drug dependency and the likelihood of rebound symptoms of anxiety, sleeplessness, and abdominal pain on withdrawal.

Antibiotics

Antibiotic therapy should be used only with suspected upper genital tract infection, positive cervical cultures, or urinary tract symptoms and bacteriuria. Some effectiveness of prolonged antibiotic treatment for urethral syndrome has been suggested. Empiric antibiotic treatment for "chronic pelvic inflammatory disease" is ill advised, as such therapy is ineffective. Furthermore, the diagnosis is controversial and greatly overused, as there is evidence that no chronic infectious process is present in women with chronic pelvic pain after acute salpingitis. Attribution of chronic pelvic pain to prior pelvic inflammatory disease should be made only with objective laparoscopic evidence.

Psychological Treatments

Psychogenic chronic pelvic pain is uncommon, but psychological factors are always important in patients with chronic pelvic pain. Unfortunately, referral for psychological evaluation is difficult. Many of these women have been told "the pain is in your head," a statement that only angers them, as they tend to have a persistent focus on a physical diagnosis and medical cure. Because of this, when the physician fails to deduce a specific physical diagnosis and suggests the diagnosis is psychiatric, the patient continues to fear an occult disease continuously missed by physicians and seeks a new physician to pay attention anew to her perceived occult physical disease. Even when sufficient rapport is established to suggest psychological evaluation and therapy as an adjunct to pain treatment, ambivalence often makes this difficult to accomplish. The cost of such care may also be an impediment.

Traditional individual psychiatric care for women with chronic pelvic pain who are not psychotic has not been particularly useful. As already mentioned, most women refuse to consent to psychiatric treatment. Those who do consent to such care have the same rate of improvement as those that refuse. Behavior-oriented, psychological pain programs with a rehabilitation approach that includes family dynamics interventions may be more useful. Table 22-3 summarizes some of the goals and techniques that may be applicable to chronic pelvic pain patients. The primary care physician may be comfortable working with the patient on some of these but may find it helpful to involve a psychologist trained in pain treatment and therapy, if the patient is willing.

Use of relaxation techniques at the first signs of a painful episode may be useful to manage chronic pelvic pain and may be accomplished via several modalities, such as biofeedback, self-hypnosis, or meditation. Many women with prior Lamaze technique training for childbirth can benefit by applying the same breathing and relaxation techniques to chronic pain management.

Table 22-3. Goals of Psychological Pain Management

• Control pain	Relaxation techniques Stress management Pain coping strategies Pain attributions Attention diversion Distraction techniques
• Reduce disability	Progressive activities Pain behavior modification Reemployment Treat substance abuse
• Promote wellness	Eating behavior and nutrition Sleep Hygiene Physical exercise
• Treat psychological morbidity	Treat depression and anxiety Treat abuse survivors Marital and family counseling Sex therapy

Multidisciplinary Clinics

In planning the treatment of patients with chronic pelvic pain, it is useful to stress the differentiation between acute pain and chronic pain, both psychologically and physiologically, and to recognize chronic pain as a diagnosis in itself, rather than as a symptom. With the current incomplete understanding of chronic pain, it is necessary to accept that chronic pelvic pain must be managed, rather than cured, in many patients. As previously noted, this management is best accomplished with a multifaceted, biopsychosocial approach that involves a multidisciplinary team of health care providers. To meet this need, pain centers have been developed that use the expertise of psychologists, anesthesiologists, neurologists, and physical therapists. Clinics dedicated to chronic pelvic pain often also involve gynecologists and gastroenterologists.

Such multidisciplinary clinics are not a panacea. For example, in the Mayo Clinic pain center, using a cognitive-behavioral approach, 25% of patients regressed within a few months after completing treatment. Three years after treatment, two thirds of the patients who completed the program either failed initially or could not maintain improvement of attitude, activity, or medication usage. This clinic's approach resulted in no significant improvement in pain levels. (Only 9% were patients with pain of the abdomen or perineum.)

Also, many women do not have access to or cannot afford multidisciplinary clinics or pain centers. Even outpatient clinics require 3 to 5 hours per week, a time demand that many women have trouble meeting. In such cases, the primary care physician may need to try to mimic the multidisciplinary pain clinic approach using a select pool of consultants and a multidisciplinary treatment plan.

BIBLIOGRAPHY

Beard RW, Reginald PW, Wadsworth J. Clinical features of women with chronic lower abdominal pain and pelvic congestion. Br J Obstet Gynaecol 1988;95:153.

Beard RW, Kennedy RG, Gangar KF, et al. Bilateral oophorectomy and hysterectomy in the treatment of intractable pelvic pain associated with pelvic congestion. Br J Obstet Gynaecol 1991;98:988.

Black WT. Use of presacral sympathectomy in the treatment of dysmenorrhea. A second look after 25 years. Am J Obstet Gynecol 1964;89:16.

Candiani GB, Fidele L, Vercellini P, Bianchi S, DiNola G. Repetitive conservative surgery for recurrence of endometriosis. Obstet Gynecol 1991;77:421.

Dmowski WP, Radwanska E, Rana N. Recurrent endometriosis following hysterectomy and oophorectomy: the role of residual ovarian fragments. Int J Gynecol Obstet 1988;26:93.

Henzyl MR, Kwei L. Efficacy and safety of nafarelin in the treatment of endometriosis. Am J Obstet Gynecol 1990;162:570.

Howard FM. The role of laparoscopy in the evaluation of chronic pelvic pain: promise and pitfalls. Obstet Gynecol Survey 1993;48:10.

Longstreth GF, Preskill DB, Youkeles L. Irritable bowel syndrome in women having diagnostic laparoscopy or hysterectomy. Relation to gynecologic features and outcome. Digest Dis Sci 1990;35:1285.

Monafo W, Goldfarb W. Postoperative peritoneal cysts. Surgery 1963;53:470.

Peters AAW, van Dorst E, Jellis B, van Zuuren E, Hermans J, Trimbos JB. A randomized clinical trial to compare two different approaches in women with chronic pelvic pain. Obstet Gynecol 1991;77:740.

Reiter RC. A profile of women with chronic pelvic pain. Clin Obstet Gynecol 1990;33:130.

Renaer M, Vertommen H, Nijs P, Wagemans L, Van Itemelnjck T. Psychological aspects of chronic pelvic pain in women. Am J Obstet Gynecol 1979;134:75.

Rolland R, van der Heijden PFM. Nafarelin versus danazol in the treatment of endometriosis. Am J Obstet Gynecol 1990;162:586.

Slocumb JC. Chronic somatic, myofascial, and neurogenic abdominal pelvic pain. Clin Obstet Gynecol 1990;33:145.

Steege JF. The psychological component of chronic pelvic pain. The Female Patient 1986;11:139.

Steege JF. Ovarian remnant syndrome. Obstet Gynecol 19

Stovall TG, Ling FW, Crawford DA. Hysterectomy for c pain of presumed uterine etiology. Obstet Gynecol 19

Stripling MC, Martin DC, Chatman DL, VanderZwaag R. Subtle appearance of pelvic endometriosis. Fertil 49:427.

Tjaden B, Schlaff WD, Kimball A, Rock JA. The efficacy of presacral neurectomy for the relief of midline dysmenorrhea. Obstet Gynecol 1990;76:89.

Primary Care for Women, edited by Phyllis C. Leppert and Fred M. Howard. Lippincott-Raven Publishers, Philadelphia © 1997.

23

Vaginitis

PAUL NYIRJESY

For any clinician involved in women's health care, vaginitis remains an unavoidable problem. It is estimated that vaginitis accounts for more than 10 million office visits each year, and it is the most common reason why a patient visits her obstetrician-gynecologist. OTC antifungal therapies rank among the top ten best-selling OTC products, with about $160 million dollars yearly in sales. Despite these numbers, vaginitis is trivialized by many within the medical community. This lack of interest results in misdiagnosis and mistreatment, which in turn complicates efforts at further evaluation and treatment of vaginal symptomatology.

Most studies confirm that the three most common vaginal infections are bacterial vaginosis (30% to 35%), vulvovaginal candidiasis (20% to 25%), and trichomoniasis (15% to 20%). The remaining causes of vaginitis include a host of miscellaneous conditions; the most common of these are a heavy but physiologic discharge, atrophic vaginitis, and vulvar disorders.

Estrogen plays a crucial role in determining the vagina's microbial flora (Table 23-1). As the dominant microorganisms in healthy women, vaginal lactobacilli and their role in regulating the vaginal environment have been extensively scrutinized. Colonization of the vagina by lactobacilli has been thought to be due to the increased glycogen in vaginal epithelial cells, in turn a result of estrogen. Although previous theories had focused on the production of lactic acid by lactobacilli and its effects, recent evidence shows that the presence of lactobacilli that produce hydrogen peroxide can inhibit the growth of other organisms in vitro and in vivo.

However, even in the reproductive years, a woman's flora contains a wide variety of organisms. For example, the skin and fecal organisms present during the prepubertal years, such as *Staphylococcus epidermidis* or *Escherichia coli*, remain as part of the normal flora and can be isolated from vaginal cultures with relative ease. Indeed, pathogenic organisms such as *Streptococcus agalactiae* (group B streptococci), *Mycoplasma hominis*, *Ureaplasma urealyticum*, *Gardnerella vaginalis*, and *Candida albicans* are each present in about 20% of healthy asymptomatic women, with wide variations depending on the patient population.

EVALUATION

All too often when seeing women with vaginal symptoms, physicians avoid obtaining a complete history, perhaps out of fear of embarrassing the patient or physician. However, just as with any disorder, such a history is essential to obtaining an accurate diagnosis. Symptoms related to vaginitis include a broad spectrum of manifestations, not just vaginal discharge, irritation, itching, or burning. A thorough historian asks about the nature, quantity, and color of discharge, but then focuses on symptoms other than discharge, as those are often the cause of the patient's distress. Pertinent areas include the location of the symptoms (vulvar, introital, or vaginal), their duration, variations with the menstrual cycle, their association with sexual relations, and their response to past therapy. With the widespread use of OTC antifungal agents, a particularly important question is when the patient last used any treatment, to determine if she is partially treated. These nuances within the history often allow a better evaluation.

The physical examination should begin with a careful evaluation of the vulva and vestibule, particularly if they are the focus of symptoms. Palpation with a cotton-tipped applicator helps discern areas of tenderness. After insertion of the speculum, the vagina and cervix are inspected thoroughly. If secretions are present, an effort is made to determine if they are cervical or vaginal in origin.

The laboratory evaluation of vaginal symptoms is summarized in Table 23-2. Each part of this work-up is an essential component of the office visit. The experienced clinician can perform all these tests in at most 5 minutes, and they yield an accurate diagnosis the vast majority of the time.

When sampling the vagina, it is important to swab the middle third of the vagina, not the pooled vaginal secretions in the posterior fornix. Because the latter are composed of cervical and vaginal secretions, they may hinder the ability to assess vaginal pH and to examine the saline smear. By touching the swab to pH paper with a range of 3.5 to 5.5, not nitrazine paper, the characteristic color change of a high pH is unmistakable. A whiff test for the presence of amines is most easily performed by obtaining an additional swab and placing a drop of 10% KOH on the swab itself, then checking for the characteristic fishy odor. Just as with the vaginal pH, this simple test is easy, unequivocal, and underused.

In a few complicated patients, adjunctive studies may be indicated. These include a culture for herpes simplex in the case of ulceration or in the presence of mucopurulent cervicitis, as well as cultures for *Trichomonas vaginalis* and yeast. Given the wide range of organisms that can be part of the normal flora and the potential for being misled, vaginal bacterial cultures play little role in the evaluation of vaginal symptoms.

Table 23-1. Effect of Estrogen on the Vaginal Environment

AGE	ESTROGEN SOURCE	DOMINANT FLORA	VAGINAL pH
Newborn	Maternal	Lactobacilli	<4.5
Prepubertal	Peripheral fat	Skin organisms	>4.5
		Fecal flora	
Reproductive	Ovaries	Lactobacilli	<4.5
Menopausal	Peripheral fat	Variable	Variable
	Hormone therapy	Lactobacilli	<4.5

A physiologic discharge, the result of secretions from the uterus, including the cervix and fallopian tubes, the glands that line the vagina, and the vestibular glands, can sometimes be quite heavy. Any alteration in these organs can result in a change in the physiologic discharge; the classic example is the heavy discharge associated with fallopian tube carcinoma. More common factors affecting normal vaginal discharges are the patient's age, her menstrual cycle, use of oral contraceptives, and pregnancy. In general, a physiologic discharge is described as odorless; clear or white; viscous, flocculent, or homogeneous; and with little vaginal pooling. However, wide variations in the normal discharge occur, even in the same patient over time. Because American society is often unwilling to acknowledge the existence of normal discharges, women may present for evaluation who do not have any infection. Only with a thorough evaluation can potential infections be excluded and the patient reassured that her discharge is normal. Although it sounds as if it would be easier to take a quick look and write a prescription, the lack of response to inappropriate and unnecessary therapy will frustrate the patient and physician alike in the longer term.

TRICHOMONIASIS

Trichomonas vaginalis is the one of the most common protozoan infections in the United States, with an estimated 3 million annual cases. Although nonsexual transmission (eg, fomites) has been suggested as an occasional source of infection, the primary mode of transmission is sexual. Therefore, the prevalence of the disease depends in large part on the overall level of sexual activity of the group of women being studied, with a range of 5% in family planning clinics to 75% in studies of prostitutes. Asymptomatic men represent a large reservoir for reinfection.

Even in women, trichomoniasis is an infection that is often harbored asymptomatically. When symptomatic, it can cause an abnormal purulent, frothy, or bloody discharge. Vaginal malodor, pruritus, and dyspareunia are relatively frequent complaints as well. *T vaginalis* can invade the bladder and urethra, so some women have dysuria or urinary frequency as well.

Findings on examination include varying degrees of erythema and excoriations of the vulva, erythema and edema of the vagina, an abnormal discharge, and punctate hemorrhages of the cervix ("strawberry cervix"). In most offices, the diagnosis ultimately rests on microscopic examination of the wet smear showing live motile trichomonads. Additional microscopic findings include an increase in white blood cells and a shift away from the normal bacillary flora. However, recent data show that the wet smear has a relatively poor sensitivity (22% to 76%). Although a positive whiff test and an elevated pH are helpful clues if the smear is negative, they do not allow the clinician to distinguish between trichomoniasis and bacterial vaginosis. A Pap smear has a higher sensitivity, but its false-positive rate is about 20%. The gap between these two methods of detection can be bridged by culture systems, a sensitive method of detection. They are affordable and easy to use, but unfortunately are not always readily available.

The only medication in the United States that is effective against *T vaginalis* is metronidazole. The most commonly prescribed regimen is a single oral 2-g dose, which achieves cure rates in over 90% of cases if sexual partners are treated simultaneously. In treatment failures, the standard therapy consists of 250 mg three times a day for 7 days, after excluding reinfection from the partner as the source of infection. In metronidazole-resistant infections, increasing doses may be required. Common side effects of metronidazole, especially at higher doses, include nausea, a disulfiram-like effect if alcohol is ingested, and a metallic taste.

Although case-control studies have failed to reveal an association between birth defects and metronidazole, this drug is generally avoided in the first trimester of pregnancy because it has mutagenic activity in in vitro assay systems. In the severely symptomatic patient in early pregnancy, topical clotrimazole or pH-lowering solutions such as vinegar douches may inhibit growth sufficiently to alleviate symptoms.

BACTERIAL VAGINOSIS

Bacterial vaginosis (BV), formerly known as nonspecific vaginitis or *Gardnerella* vaginitis, is a polymicrobial infection of the vagina. As its

Table 23-2. Evaluation of Acute Vaginal Symptoms

TEST	POTENTIAL DIAGNOSTIC USE
History	Extent, nature, location, and duration of symptoms
Physical examination	Localization of symptoms, abnormal physical findings
Cervical samples for chlamydia test, *Neisseria gonorrhoeae* culture	Cervicitis
Vaginal pH	Hormonal status, bacterial vaginosis, trichomoniasis
Whiff test	Bacterial vaginosis, trichomiasis
Saline smear	WBC: Epi ratio Vaginal cytology Bacterial floral pattern Trichomonads Clue cells
10% KOH smear	Hyphae, blastospores

name suggests, this is an abnormal condition of the vagina marked by a paucity or absence of hydrogen peroxide-producing lactobacilli and an overgrowth of facultative anaerobic organisms. Gardner and Dukes initially implicated *Gardnerella vaginalis* (then known as *Haemophilus vaginalis*) as the causative organism, but subsequent studies and the realization that they did not actually fulfill Koch's postulates demonstrated that *G vaginalis* is not the cause of this syndrome. Rather, a multitude of organisms seem to be acting synergistically to produce this syndrome, including *G vaginalis*, genital mycoplasmas, *Mobiluncus* spp, *Bacteroides* spp, and other anaerobes.

The prevalence of this infection is highly variable. As with trichomoniasis, the prevalence seems to be related to the general level of sexual activity, with 5% in college populations and up to 60% in STD clinics. However, whether BV is sexually transmitted remains controversial. It is rare in women who have never been sexually active and it is associated with multiple sexual partners. However, it has been found in virginal women, and treatment of the male partner has not prevented recurrences.

Up to 50% of women with BV are asymptomatic. Symptomatic women complain of a profuse, malodorous discharge. The fishy odor may be more noticeable during menses or after intercourse, when the high pH of blood or semen volatilizes the amines that are its cause. Although it is not part of the classic description, itching is present in up to 67% of cases.

The diagnosis of BV is made on clinical grounds, not on the basis of a positive culture for *Mycoplasma* or *Gardnerella*. Three out of the four following conditions should be met: a homogeneous gray or white discharge, a vaginal pH above 4.5, a positive whiff test, and more than 20% clue cells on a wet prep. In addition, a shift from the normal bacillary flora to a coccobacillary pattern is noted, along with an increase in the flora noted on the smear.

Acceptable treatment regimens include metronidazole, 500 mg twice a day for 7 days; clindamycin, 300 mg twice a day for 7 days; clindamycin cream 2%, one 5-g applicator at bedtime for 7 days; or metronidazole gel 0.75%, one 5-g applicator twice daily for 5 days. Vulvovaginal candidiasis as a sequela to therapy occurs in up to 10% of treated patients. *Clostridium difficile* colitis has occurred rarely after therapy with clindamycin cream.

In the past decade, there has been an increasing awareness of BV because of its consistent association with many of the infectious morbidities of the female genitourinary system. In nonpregnant women, it is associated with a higher risk for recurrent urinary tract infections, posthysterectomy cuff cellulitis, and pelvic inflammatory disease. In pregnant women, it is a risk factor for some of the most common causes of perinatal morbidity and mortality: premature labor, premature rupture of membranes, preterm delivery, and postpartum endometritis. Antepartum treatment with metronidazole results in a significant decrease in these morbidities in patients with a history of previous preterm birth. Less clear is whether to treat the asymptomatic gynecologic patient. Because of a fairly high risk of recurrence within a year after treatment and because the goal of therapy is to alleviate symptoms, the CDC does not recommend treatment for these patients. Most clinicians do not treat partners of women with BV.

VULVOVAGINAL CANDIDIASIS

Vulvovaginal candidiasis (VVC) is one of the most common infections of the female genital tract. About 75% of women at some time in their lives experience the discomfort of a vaginal yeast infection. For most, these infections are rare and respond to a multitude of therapies. However, an estimated 5% suffer chronic or recurrent episodes of VVC, despite the absence of underlying medical illnesses or predisposing factors. Theories to explain these repeated infections have focused on vaginal reinfection, either from a gastrointestinal source or from sexual transmission, or on vaginal relapse, which hypothesizes that recurrent infections are due to the same infecting organism, suppressed only temporarily by antifungal therapy. Although a precipitating factor such as pregnancy, the use of oral contraceptives, diabetes mellitus, systemic diseases requiring the use of antibiotics or corticosteroids, or HIV infection is sometimes found, most of these women have no underlying medical disorders.

C albicans is the cause of about 95% of cases of VVC, but other yeast species have been implicated in selected cases. In centers that treat chronic vaginitis, non-*C albicans* species such as *Candida (Torulopsis) glabrata*, *C parapsilosis*, *C tropicalis*, and *Saccharomyces cerevisiae* (baker's or brewer's yeast) account for up to a third of infections. Although competing claims of clinical efficacy against these non-*C albicans* organisms are being made, no adequate clinical studies have been done to show that any of the drugs on the market are effective against anything other than *C albicans*. Anecdotal evidence suggests that non-*C albicans* cases are more resistant to imidazole and triazole therapy.

Patients with candidiasis complain primarily of vulvar or vaginal pruritus, irritation, or burning. In chronic cases, dyspareunia may become a more prominent symptom. Although a white discharge resembling oral thrush is sometimes found, many patients with VVC notice no change in their discharge.

Vulvar or vaginal erythema should prompt a search for candidiasis, as should the presence of vaginal thrush. The vaginal pH is normal with VVC. Diagnosis is made on the basis of hyphae or blastospores, visualized either on wet mount or KOH prep. Although *C albicans* can produce either blastospores (budding yeast) or hyphae on clinical samples, smears positive for *C glabrata* and *S cerevisiae* contain only blastospores. In these cases, as well those in which the history is strongly suggestive for VVC but the smears are unrevealing, fungal cultures may help confirm the diagnosis as well as identify the species of the pathogen. However, because yeast can be present as part of the normal vaginal flora, asymptomatic patients with yeast on either a vaginal culture or a Pap smear should not be treated.

Various therapies are effective in the treatment of VVC (Table 23-3). The imidazoles and triazoles are the mainstay of therapy, usually applied as a topical regimen of 1 to 7 days. They are generally well tolerated, but 5% of patients note itching and burning from the therapy. A single oral dose of fluconazole, in initial studies, was shown to be as effective as a week of miconazole, clotrimazole, and terconazole in uncomplicated cases of VVC. Side effects such as headaches, nausea, and diarrhea tend to be self-limited. There are insufficient data to support its use in pregnancy. There are also interactions with other drugs, particularly rifampin, theophylline, phenytoin, warfarin, cyclosporine, and oral hypoglycemic agents.

For patients with recurrent VVC, a 6-month course of ketoconazole decreases the risk of recurrent infection. Early studies of fluconazole suggest that it is also effective as a maintenance regimen, and there is a lower risk of hepatotoxicity with this medication. Treating the partners of such women does not seem to decrease the risk of recurrent disease. In non-*C albicans* infection, therapy with boric acid suppositories seems to be of use.

Table 23-3. Therapy for Vulvovaginal Candidiasis

DRUG	FORMULATION	DOSE
Nystatin	100,000-U vaginal tablet	100,000 U × 14d
Butoconazole	2% cream	5 g × 3d
Clotrimazole	1% cream	5 g × 7d
	100-mg vaginal inserts	100 mg × 7d
	500-mg vaginal tablet	500 mg × 1d
Miconazole	2% cream	5 g × 7d
	100-mg vaginal suppository	100 mg × 7d
	200-mg vaginal suppository	200 mg × 3d
Terconazole	0.4% cream	5 g × 7d
	0.8% cream	5 g × 3d
	80-mg vaginal suppository	80 mg × 3d
Tioconazole	6.5% cream	5 g × 1d
Fluconazole	150-mg oral tablet	150 mg × 1d PO

Table 23-4. Pitfalls in the Treatment of Vaginitis

Patient self-diagnosis and treatment
Failure to see the patient (telephone diagnosis)
Patient seen but not examined
Failure to examine vulva and vestibule
Failure to perform laboratory tests
Treating *Escherichia coli,* enterococcus, *Gardnerella vaginalis,* and other normal flora as pathogens
Use of shotgun therapy
Guessing at therapy
Overuse of topical steroids
Relying on Pap smear to make diagnosis
Failure to recognize that topical therapy may exacerbate symptoms

(Adapted from Sobel JD. Vaginal infection in adult women. Med Clin North Am 1990;74:1573.)

ATROPHIC VAGINITIS

As noted earlier, estrogen plays a central role in maintaining the homeostasis of the vaginal environment. Therefore, any woman who no longer produces estrogen is theoretically at risk for developing atrophic vaginitis.

Atrophic vaginitis should be suspected in any postmenopausal woman who complains of abnormal vaginal discharge, dryness, itching, or burning. Examination may reveal atrophy of the labia minora or majora, vaginal pallor, or loss of rugal folds. However, the genitalia often appear normal. The diagnosis is relatively easy to make by routinely checking the vaginal pH and looking at vaginal cytology when examining saline smears. With estrogen deficiency, the pH rises above 4.5. On the microscopic wet mount, many of the vaginal epithelial cells are parabasal or intermediate cells. The vaginal flora is scant and often is composed of bacilli and cocci, as opposed to the normal predominantly bacillary flora. A whiff test is negative.

The only therapy that truly reverses atrophic changes is estrogen therapy, either topical or oral. It may take several weeks before the patient begins to notice an improvement in symptoms, and once she stops therapy, her symptoms are likely to recur.

CHRONIC VAGINITIS

With the treatment approaches discussed here, most women should achieve a satisfactory resolution of their symptoms. However, when the patient fails to respond to seemingly appropriate therapy, the clinician must reassess the initial evaluation and diagnosis (Table 23-4) before proceeding with further therapy. It is sometimes helpful to discontinue all therapy to see whether the remaining symptoms are due to the treatment itself. In the first year of our vaginitis center at Temple University, the most commonly overdiagnosed condition was VVC. Although over 90% of patients had been given a prior diagnosis of VVC, by the time they came to the clinic, only 22% actually had yeast infections. The most common causes of "chronic vaginitis" other than VVC were physiologic discharge (16%) and vulvar vestibulitis (15%). This experience is similar to that of others who treat women with chronic vaginal symptoms, and it underlines the need to question the active diagnosis and to pursue a thorough evaluation at every visit.

BIBLIOGRAPHY

CDC. 1993 sexually transmitted diseases treatment guidelines. MMWR 1993;42(RR-14):1.

Gardner HL, Dukes CD. *Haemophilus vaginalis* vaginitis: a newly defined specific infection previously classified "nonspecific" vaginitis. Am J Obstet Gynecol 1955;69:962.

Grossman JH III, Galask RP. Persistent vaginitis caused by metronidazole-resistant trichomonas. Obstet Gynecol 1990;76:521.

Hillier SL, Krohn MA, Klebanoff SJ, Eschenbach DA. The relationship of hydrogen peroxide-producing lactobacilli to bacterial vaginosis and genital microflora in pregnant women. Obstet Gynecol 1992;79:369.

Kent HL. Epidemiology of vaginitis. Am J Obstet Gynecol 1991;165:1168.

Klebanoff SJ, Hillier SL, Eschenbach DA, Waltersdorph AM. Control of the microbial flora of the vagina by H_2O_2-generating lactobacilli. J Infect Dis 1991;164:94.

Morales WJ, Schorr S, Albritton J. Effect of metronidazole in patients with preterm birth in preceding pregnancy and bacterial vaginosis: A placebo-controlled, double-blind study. Am J Obstet Gynecol 1994;171:345.

Nyirjesy P, Seeney SM, Grody MHT, Jordan CA, Buckley HR. Chronic fungal vaginitis: the value of cultures. Am J Obstet Gynecol 1995;173:820.

Piper JM, Mitchel EF, Ray WA. Prenatal use of metronidazole and birth defects: no association. Obstet Gynecol 1993;82:348.

Schaaaf VM, Perez-Stable EJ, Borchardt K. The limited value of symptoms and signs in the diagnosis of vaginal infections. Arch Intern Med 1990;150:1929.

Sobel JD. Vaginal infections in adult women. Med Clin North Am 1990;74:1573.

Sobel JD. Candidal vulvovaginitis. Clin Obstet Gynecol 1993;36:153.

Primary Care for Women, edited by Phyllis C. Leppert and Fred M. Howard. Lippincott-Raven Publishers, Philadelphia © 1997.

24

Benign Breast Disease

JAMES V. FIORICA

State-of-the-art health care for women must include screening for breast diseases. Primary care physicians should be able to diagnose common benign breast conditions and to screen and diagnose breast malignancies. This chapter presents a clinically oriented evaluation of the most common breast diseases.

HISTORY AND PHYSICAL EXAMINATION

A thorough initial history is oriented toward risk factors for breast cancer (Table 24-1). The most recognized epidemiologic risk factors include previous breast cancer in the opposite breast or breast cancer in a first-degree relative. The incidence of breast cancer in a contralateral breast is about 1% per year. A family history of breast cancer increases the risk by two to three times to as high as nine times in cases of bilateral premenopausal breast cancer. Nulliparous women, women whose menopause began after age 55, and women who had their first pregnancy after age 35 have a two to three times higher risk of developing breast cancer. Age is probably the most significant risk factor, because the breast cancer risk increases with age throughout the woman's life.

However, only 12% of breast cancer patients have any known risk factor; in other words, 88% have no antecedent risk. Therefore, all women should be considered at risk for the disease, and the physician should conduct the physical examination keeping this in mind.

Most lumps are discovered by the patient. If a patient notices a breast lump, pertinent historical factors include the duration, the relation to menses, the presence or absence of pain, and the presence of dimpling of the skin. Pain is most common in cystic disease and is less common in carcinoma. Persistent unilateral pain in a postmenopausal patient who is not taking estrogen should be viewed with more suspicion. A premenstrual tender thickening is more likely to be benign engorgement, fibrocystic disease, rather than malignant disease. Skin dimpling is nearly always pathognomonic of carcinoma and results from shortening of Cooper ligaments.

Nipple discharge must be evaluated. Malignant discharges are unilateral, spontaneous, or bloody. Postmenopausal nipple discharges deserve special attention as well. Previous injury, surgery, infection, or inappropriate lactation are all pertinent breast-related questions.

The clinical breast examination should be performed in the upright and supine positions. Lack of proper training is widespread among physicians. One third of the 80 physicians surveyed in all major specialties stated that their training in medical school or residency was not adequate. Eighty-four percent said they needed to improve their abilities in detecting breast lumps.

The best time to perform the breast examination is immediately after menstruation and before ovulation to avoid evaluating an engorged, tender breast. The breasts are inspected in the upright position, looking for precancerous abnormalities such as retraction, deviations, or inverted nipples, as well as dermatologic disorders that might indicate more serious conditions such as nevi, edema, erythema, ulcers, or eczematoid reactions. A scaly red eruption around the areola suggests Paget disease. The breasts should be inspected with the patient's hands down at her side, then with her arms elevated, and finally with her arms tensing at her hips, contracting the pectoralis muscles. These maneuvers best reveal subtle contour and skin abnormalities and retractions.

In the sitting position, attention is directed toward the supraclavicular area and axilla. Digital palpation is performed beneath the lateral pectoralis muscles into the axillary contents. This is best performed in the upright position. In breast cancer patients, a clinically negative axilla contains metastatic lymph nodes about 40% of the time, emphasizing the need for a careful examination of this region.

The breast examination is then repeated with the patient in the supine position, covering the entire breast, chest wall, and axilla. This is the ideal time to instruct the patient about breast self-examination. Compliance is significantly improved when the patient is instructed by a physician rather than obtaining a pamphlet in the waiting area, although both forms of teaching are important. During this patient education, the physician has the opportunity to individualize the examination and reinforce "normal versus abnormal" to the patient. Digital palpation is then carried out using the index and middle fingers, applying varying amounts of pressure with the flats or pads of the finger. A thorough examination covers the entire breast and chest wall, first superficially at the skin, then intermediately within the breast stroma and subcutaneous tissue, and finally deep against the chest wall (triple-touch technique). The entire breast must be examined systematically. This examination can be done in a circular, clockwise, or stripwise manner. Particular attention must be focused beneath the nipple/areola complex and within the axilla. Breast cancer occurs most often in the upper outer quadrant (50%), beneath the nipple/areola (18%), and in the upper inner quadrants (15%).

If no lesions are noted on examination, it is critical to document those negative findings, discuss cancer screening, and plan follow-up. Pertinent negative findings can be summarized as, "No dominant masses, no retractions, no nipple discharge, or lymphadenopathy was noted in the sitting and supine positions." It is also useful to write the date of last mammogram, whether hormones were administered, and any pertinent risk factors. Hormones should not be renewed unless a breast examination and mammogram are performed. Also, oral contraceptives should not be renewed without a documented annual breast examination. These practices are good for the patient and protect the physician, as most litigation results from failure to diagnose breast cancer. The Physician Insurers Association of America's breast cancer claims study, conducted in 1988, found that 75% of successful malpractice lawsuits involved primary care

Table 24-1. Risk Factors for Breast Cancer

FACTOR	RISK*
Family History	
Primary relative with breast cancer	1.2–3.0
Premenopausal	3.1
Premenopausal and bilateral	8.5–9.0
Postmenopausal	1.5
Postmenopausal and bilateral	4.0–5.4
Menstrual History	
Age at menarche < 12	1.3
Age at menopause > 55 with > 40 menstrual years	1.48–2.0
Pregnancy	
First child after age 35	2.0–3.0
Nulliparous	3.0
Other Neoplasms	
Contralateral breast cancer	5.0
Cancer of the major salivary gland	4.0
Cancer of the uterus	2.0
Benign Breast Disease	
Atypical lobular hyperplasia	4.0
Lobular carcinoma in situ	7.2
Previous Biopsy	1.86–2.13

*General population risk, +1.0.

(Data from Love SM, Gelman RS, Silen W. Sounding board: fibrocystic "disease" of the breast: a nondisease? N Engl J Med 1982;307:1013.)

physicians with practices in family medicine, internal medicine, or obstetrics and gynecology. One third of the cases involved inadequate chart documentation.

THE DOMINANT MASS

Once a lesion is discovered, it must be pursued and the analysis documented. If a mass is palpated, the physician must determine whether the lesion is a discrete three-dimensional mass versus the thickening commonly noted in breasts with fibrocystic changes. Discrete masses are commonly referred to as dominant masses. Once a mass is identified, a diagnosis must be assigned and cancer ruled out.

The first step is to measure the size of the lesion. This can sometimes be done by compressing the lesion against the adjacent rib to stabilize and help quantitate the lesion. The next step is to determine whether the lesion is solid or cystic. A simple cyst aspiration can be performed in the office. The breast is prepped with an alcohol pad. A 23-gauge needle connected to a 10-cc syringe is placed directly into the mass while the opposite hand stabilizes the lesion. Once the needle has passed through the skin, negative pressure is applied. If the mass is cystic, the fluid is completely evacuated and the lesion should disappear completely. The suction is then taken off the syringe and the needle removed from the patient. The fluid is discarded if it is serous and nonbloody. The patient is instructed to return in 4 to 6 weeks for reexamination.

If the lesion is noncystic, it is presumed to be solid and a fine-needle aspiration (FNA) is performed. Using the same technique, the needle, once placed in the mass, is moved back and forth eight to ten times while applying full suction. The plunger of the syringe is then released and the negative pressure normalized. The needle is withdrawn and a smear is prepared for cytologic evaluation. Usually, two or three separate specimens are obtained on solid lesions to sample the mass adequately and increase the cell collection. Cytologic preparation can be a monolayer smear, similar to a Pap test. However, the yield can be improved by lavaging the syringe in a specimen jar containing cytofixative, where a cell block is created for cytologic analysis.

The differential diagnosis of solid breast lesions is shown in Table 24-2. The sensitivity, specificity, positive predictive value, and negative predictive value of FNA are 82%, 97%, 95%, and 96%, respectively. A false-positive rate of 1.2% and a false-negative rate of 7.7% are generally seen. The number of satisfactory collections varies from 50% to 87%. Thus, the physician must not rely on a negative FNA. The accepted standard of care is to remove all solid three-dimensional masses unless a definitely benign diagnosis can be made by FNA. An open biopsy is also required if the cystic lesion does not disappear completely on fluid aspiration, if bloody cyst fluid is obtained on aspiration, if the cyst recurs after one or two aspirations, if a solid dominant mass is not diagnosed as a fibroadenoma, or if the patient has a bloody nipple discharge, nipple ulceration, or skin edema suspicious of carcinoma. The purpose of FNA is to determine if a malignancy is present so that the patient may be counseled and triaged for immediate cancer treatment. If the lesion is cystic, the aspiration is therapeutic and diagnostic and the patient's anxiety is relieved.

Table 24-2. FNA Diagnosis of Breast Masses

Inflammatory
Acute mastitis
Plasma cell mastitis
Subareolar abscess
Fat necrosis
Benign Tumors
Fibrocystic change
Cyst contents
Apocrine metaplasia
Epithelial hyperplasia
Lactating adenomas
Intraductal papilloma
Fibroadenoma
Cystosarcoma phylloides
Adenoma of nipple
Rare tumors
Granular cell tumor
Malignant Tumors
Ductal carcinoma
Lobular carcinoma
Sarcomas
Metastatic tumors

(Data from Walloch J. Technique and interpretation of breast aspiration cytology. Clin Obstet Gynecol 1989;32(4):795.)

Mammography should be performed before any open biopsy. The mammogram may better delineate the palpable lesion and can identify other lesions in the same or opposite breast that may need treatment.

If the palpable mass is not a discrete dominant mass, but rather thickening within the breast, the physician must determine whether the findings are consistent with fibrocystic changes versus asymmetric breast parenchyma that must be biopsied. If the patient is premenstrual, sometimes a reexamination after the next menstrual cycle can make the diagnosis.

MAMMOGRAPHY

Film screen mammography is the uniformly accepted radiologic screening test for breast cancer. In diagnostic mammography, breast x-ray images are obtained in patients with symptoms or palpable or mammographic abnormalities. The radiologist is present at the examination and is available to order additional films as necessary. Screening mammography is performed only on asymptomatic women. The x-rays are taken by a technician, and the radiologist, who is not always present, reads them later, thus reducing the cost. Specific screening guidelines for breast cancer are discussed in Chapter 26.

Mammographic abnormalities are grouped into three categories: densities, microcalcifications, and parenchymal asymmetry. Nonpalpable mammographic densities are handled in the same manner as their palpable counterparts. The densities are either solid or cystic, and new or old. An ultrasound can determine simple cysts, which are generally left alone unless a complex pattern is seen. Previous films can help distinguish old from new findings and can determine if a solid lesion is enlarging. The radiologist can assist in further recommendations about whether to biopsy. All new, enlarging, or irregular lesions should have histologic analysis.

Microcalcifications can be scattered or clustered. They can be coarse or fine, and old or new. Again, previous films and additional magnification views may be helpful. Clustered, fine, increasing, or new calcifications are generally removed.

Parenchymal asymmetry can be the most difficult radiologic abnormality encountered. Previous films and additional compression films of the breast are often helpful. A skilled breast radiologist should make the final recommendation about the need to biopsy. Subtle abnormalities, including lobular cancers, can be concealed within the asymmetric parenchymal breast.

Newer mammography equipment offers better-quality images with less than 0.1 cGy of radiation exposure. The false-negative rate for mammography is 10% to 15%, but this figure varies with the density of the breast parenchyma, the patient's age, and the amount of compression that can be applied.

If nonpalpable mammographic abnormalities require a biopsy, a needle localized breast biopsy, a two-step outpatient procedure, is performed. In the radiology unit, a localizing wire is placed under mammography. Then, in the surgical suite, the wire, together with the suspicious breast tissue, is surgically removed under local anesthesia. A specimen radiograph is taken to confirm that the area of concern has been removed.

A newer technique, stereotactic needle localized biopsy, is becoming available at specialized hospitals. Rather than performing a surgical biopsy, a specialized mammogram machine, often connected to a computer monitor, identifies the abnormal coordinates within the breast and a core biopsy is performed within the radiology unit, thus saving the patient surgical costs. The technique and indications are still being defined. The patient may experience moderate discomfort during the procedure. Once the details have been ironed out, stereotactic breast biopsies may prove useful.

FIBROADENOMAS

Fibroadenomas are common benign tumors generally seen in women under age 25. They may be present for years. These well-circumscribed dominant masses are noted on examination or mammography and should be treated like all solid dominant masses: excision is required unless the lesion can be histologically proven to be fibroadenoma and stable in size by examination or mammography.

FIBROCYSTIC CHANGES/MASTALGIA

The most common benign condition of the breast is fibrocystic change (FCC), an enhanced or exaggerated reaction by breast tissue in response to the fluctuating levels of ovarian hormones. The phrase "fibrocystic breast disease" is a catch-all term; the term "fibrocystic change" replaces this nebulous phrase because fibrocystic breast disease is noncancerous. The incidence of FCC is greatest in women aged 20 to 50 years who are in their reproductive, premenopausal years.

The most common symptom of FCC is pain (mastodynia). The pain is often bilateral and particularly noticeable during the premenstrual phase. The lumpiness (nodularity) may be localized or generalized, unilateral or bilateral. Occasionally, a spontaneous nipple discharge is present.

The pathogenesis is not precisely known, but it seems to be due to an imbalance in estrogen and progesterone levels. The cyclic changes of the breast tissue under the influence of hormones may induce epithelial and stromal changes. Age, parity, genetic makeup, and lactational history may all have a bearing on FCC. Risk factors include nulliparity, late age of natural menopause, and high socioeconomic class.

There are several histologic variants of FCC, but all involve hyperplasia. Fibrocystic changes are histologic and can be divided into three prognostic categories: nonproliferative, proliferative changes with no atypia, and proliferative changes with atypia. Seventy percent of breast biopsies showing FCC are nonproliferative lesions (no increased risk for cancer), and 30% are proliferative lesions. Twenty-six percent are proliferative lesions with no cellular atypia and no apparent increased risk for breast cancer; 4% show both atypia and proliferative changes on biopsy, which appears to have a fivefold increased risk for breast cancer. Women at the highest risk of developing cancer were those that had both cellular atypia and a positive family history for breast cancer; this carries an 11-fold increased risk. Unless proliferative changes with atypia are present, FCC is not a risk factor for cancer, and fortunately this is the case in the vast majority of women.

Women who present with complaints of FCC should have a thorough breast examination. Most symptoms are treated by medical management, but a tissue biopsy is mandatory for a three-dimensional lump. Medical therapy for FCC includes the use of a support bra, worn all day and night, to mitigate pain and heaviness. The use of diuretics, especially premenstrually, may transiently alleviate discomfort.

Studies by Minton and colleagues showed a correlation between the consumption of methylxanthines (eg, caffeine) and tobacco and FCC. There was a 24% improvement in clinical symptoms by decreasing intake of methylxanthines and tobacco. Although this therapy has been refuted by others, discontinuing caffeine does no harm and may benefit symptomatic patients.

The use of oral contraceptives and supplemental progestogens during the secretory phase of the menstrual cycle has had some effect on pain control. The preferred drug for the treatment of severe FCC is danazol (Danocrine). A 3- to 6-month trial of 100 to 400 mg/day eliminates pain and nodularity in about 69% of women and reduces signs and symptoms in another 30%. A course of danazol may focus attention on a dominant lump to be biopsied, reducing the need for additional biopsies as the other nodules respond to therapy. At the low doses recommended, side effects are minimal. Danazol's effects can last several months after discontinuation.

NIPPLE DISCHARGE

A nipple discharge is not a common complaint. It is a true drainage expelled directly from the mammary duct or ducts and appears on the surface of the nipple. To be significant, the nipple discharge should be true, spontaneous, persistent, and nonlactational. Nonspontaneous discharge from multiple ducts of both breasts is generally due to pharmacologic or endocrinologic causes. The drainage is milky, sticky, and consistent with galactorrhea.

Mammary duct ectasia produces a multicolored (green, yellow, white, brown, gray, or reddish-brown) nipple discharge. It is thought to be due to an increase in glandular secretions with the production of an irritating lipid fluid that can produce a nipple discharge. The median age for this type of discharge is 43 years. The reddish-brown discharge is often mistaken for a bloody discharge.

Nonpuerperal mastitis is the next most common cause of a multicolored, sticky nipple discharge. The transient types are associated with periareolar inflammation; the persistent type involves inflammation in deeper portions of the breast. If the inflammation develops into an inflammatory mass, surgical excision and drainage are necessary. When infection is suspected, however, medical management with local care, avoidance of all nipple manipulation, and the use of nonsteroidal antiinflammatory agents, bromocriptine, and antistaphylococcal antibiotics is often successful.

Bloody and persistent discharges warrant further investigation. Intraductal papillomas are the most common cause of bloody nipple discharge. The cancer risk is increased if the discharge is unilateral from a single duct, if it occurs in a postmenopausal patient, or if a mass is present.

Although a mass is usually present when the discharge is due to cancer, there is no palpable mass in 13% of cancers with nipple secretions. The physician should not rely solely on the cytology of the discharge, because there is an 18% false-negative rate and a 2.6% false-positive rate with standard cytology alone. Mammography has a 9.5% false-negative rate and a 1.6% false-positive rate for detecting cancer in patients with a nipple discharge. Galactography (injecting radiopaque contrast into the discharging duct and then performing mammography) offers better visualization of small intraductal papillomas but cannot differentiate benign from malignant lesions, and a surgical procedure is still necessary.

The initial history and physical examination should determine whether the discharge is spontaneous, unilateral, or recurrent. If the drainage first appeared in the patient's bra or nightgown on awakening, this finding is more significant than discharge during an aerobic workout at the gym. Postmenopausal discharges are always significant.

During the breast examination, the physician should look for an associated periareolar mass. It is important to reproduce the discharge and demonstrate the quadrant of breast from which it emanates. The examination consists of gently and carefully palpating the subareolar region to identify the pressure point that produces the discharge. All significant nipple discharges warrant referral for tissue biopsy.

MASTITIS

Mastitis is common in postpartum lactating women but is occasionally seen in nongravid, nonlactating women. *Staphylococcus aureus* (penicillin-resistant) and *Streptococcus* spp are the most common organisms that are colonized in the nasopharynx and oropharynx of the nursing infant. Pain, fever, erythema, and a palpable mass are the most common signs and symptoms. Treatment consists of the prompt use of antibiotics (dicloxacillin or equivalent). Lactating mothers should nurse from the unaffected breast and express and discard the milk from the affected breast. If symptoms do not resolve rapidly, a breast ultrasound should be performed to rule out a breast abscess and intravenous antibiotics should be instituted.

BIBLIOGRAPHY

American College of Obstetricians and Gynecologists. Nonmalignant conditions of the breast. ACOG Technical Bulletin #156. Washington DC: American College of Obstetricians and Gynecologists, 1991.

Berkowitz GS, Kelsey JL, Livols VA, et al. Exogenous hormone use and fibrocystic breast disease by histopathologic component. Int J Cancer 1984;34:443.

Ciatto S, Cariaggi P, Bulgaresi P. The value of routine cytologic examination of breast cyst fluids. Acta Cytol 1987;31(3):301.

Cross MJ, Evans WP, Peters GN, Cheek JH, Jones RC, Krakos P. Stereotactic breast biopsy as an alternative to open excisional biopsy. Ann Surg Oncol 1995;2:195.

Fiorica JV. Breast disease. Curr Opin Obstet Gynecol 1992;4:893.

Fiorica JV. Nipple discharge. Obstet Gynecol Clin North Am 1994;21:453.

Fiorica JV. Fibrocystic changes. Obstet Gynecol Clin North Am 1994;21:445.

Fletcher SW, O'Malley MS, Bunce LA. Physicians' abilities to detect lumps in silicone breast models. JAMA 1985;253:2224.

Greenblatt RB, Samaras C, Vasquez JM, et al. Fibrocystic disease of the breast. Clin Obstet Gynecol 1982;25:370.

Henderson IC, Danner D. Legal pitfalls in the diagnosis and management of breast cancer. Hemat Oncol Clin North Am 1989;3:823.

Leis HP Jr. Management of nipple discharge. World J Surg 1989;13:736.

Lubin F, Ron E, Wax Y, et al. A case-control study of caffeine and methylxanthines in benign breast disease. JAMA 1985;253:2388.

Marchant DJ. Breast disease and the gynecologist. Curr Probl Obstet Gynecol Fertil 1992;15:5.

Minton JP, Foecking MC, Webster DJT, et al. Caffeine, cyclic nucleotides and breast disease. Surgery 1979;86:105.

Zarbo RJ, Howanitz PJ, Bachner P. Interinstitutional comparison of performance in breast fine-needle aspiration cytology. A Q-probe quality indicator study. Arch Pathol Lab Med 1991;115(8):743.

25
Breastfeeding

CYNTHIA HOWARD
RUTH A. LAWRENCE

Primary Care for Women, edited by Phyllis C. Leppert and Fred M. Howard. Lippincott-Raven Publishers, Philadelphia © 1997.

Nourishing a child to provide for its proper growth and development is an essential task of parenthood. Parents judge their competency by how well or poorly their infant grows, and physicians use growth as an overall indicator of an infant's health. Issues surrounding the choice of an infant feeding method are thus of great concern to expectant and new parents. Although many mothers make their decision regarding infant feeding before pregnancy, a substantial proportion seek the advice of their physician. Women in the United States are increasingly choosing to breastfeed, making lactation management a common part of clinical practice for primary care physicians. This chapter discusses the management of breastfeeding mothers and infants and the treatment of common lactation problems.

Breast milk is the ideal food for infants. Breastfeeding is acknowledged by the American College of Obstetricians and Gynecologists, the American Academy of Pediatrics, and the World Health Organization as the optimal way to nourish an infant. The Institute of Medicine of the National Academy of Sciences recommends breastfeeding for all infants in the United States under ordinary circumstances and believes that exclusive breastfeeding is the preferred method for feeding most infants from birth to age 6 months.

Breastfeeding is considered to be so important to the health of mothers and infants that national health goals for the year 2000 include the objective that 75% of women initially breastfeed their infants, and 50% breastfeed until age 5 to 6 months. Currently, only about 57% of women in the United States initially breastfeed, and as few as 20% are still breastfeeding at 6 months.

Infant feeding methods in the United States, however, have changed dramatically during this century. During the early 1900s, industrialization, urbanization, and the emancipation of women led to an increased demand for artificial infant feeding methods. Technologic and public health advances resulted in the development of proprietary infant formulas that made artificial feedings safe and convenient. Breastfeeding rates subsequently declined from nearly 100%, reaching a low point in the 1970s, when only 30% of infants were breastfed at age 1 week. A range of actions, including changes in physician practices, hospital routines, educational programs, and government initiatives, subsequently produced a resurgence of breastfeeding that peaked in 1982, when over 60% of mothers initially breastfed.

Rates of breastfeeding are increasing with the recognition of breastfeeding as preventive health care for mothers and infants. However, many of the most vulnerable women and children are the least likely to experience its benefits. Disproportionately large declines in breastfeeding occurred between 1984 and 1989 among women with low education and low income, and breastfeeding rates among participants in the Women, Infants and Children (WIC) Supplemental Food Program are about half those of nonparticipants. Clearly, we are far from reaching our national health goals, especially in at-risk mothers and infants. The promotion of breastfeeding as optimal infant nutrition must be a priority for physicians, public health officials, and organizations with an interest in maternal and child health.

BENEFITS TO MOTHER AND INFANT

Human milk is species-specific and thus is the ideal source of nourishment for human infants. Various components of breast milk, such as the concentrations of cholesterol and taurine and the specific amino acid profile, are believed to be essential for optimal CNS development, nerve myelinization, and retinal development. The stable presence of cholesterol, which is quite high in human milk, is thought to be a factor in the ability to metabolize cholesterol in later life. Also, active enzymes in human milk facilitate digestion and absorption of nutrients for breastfed infants while enhancing gut maturation and repair.

Women who breastfeed experience health benefits, including concurrent fertility reduction, lower risks of breast cancer, and probable protection against osteoporosis and adult-onset obesity. In the United States, postpartum women tend to be heavier than their ideal body weights, and breastfeeding may help with postpartum weight loss. It is normal for lactating women to lose an average of 0.5 to 1.0 kg (1 to 2 lb) per month during the first 6 months of breastfeeding. Breastfeeding may also help women who stop smoking during pregnancy maintain their resolve to abstain.

Breastfeeding also provides benefits to the infant. Among the most important is enhanced protection against many common infectious diseases. Human milk reduces exposure to contaminated food sources, enhances the nutritional status of at-risk infants, and prevents infection via several antiinflammatory, immunologic-stimulating, and antimicrobial factors.

The preventive effects of breastfeeding are especially evident in the Third World, where infant mortality rates are many times higher in artificially fed than in breastfed infants. Several studies have documented the value of breast milk in preventing and ameliorating diarrhea. Infants are protected against gastrointestinal infections caused by diarrheal agents, including *Vibrio cholerae* and rotavirus. Protection against respiratory infections has also been reported, including those caused by respiratory syncytial virus.

Although the protective effects of breastfeeding are more difficult to document in industrialized nations, several studies have demonstrated a decreased risk of gastrointestinal and lower respiratory tract disease, otitis media, and bacteremia and sepsis in breastfed infants living in developed nations.

Infants also experience long-term health benefits from breastfeeding. It appears to protect against the development of food allergies, and recent studies suggest that breastfeeding provides long-term protection against some chronic diseases, including childhood-onset diabetes mellitus, lymphoma, and Crohn disease.

The evidence remains inconclusive regarding other possible benefits, such as increased intelligence and protection against atherosclerosis and sudden infant death syndrome. Future research may confirm these, as well as other currently unrecognized benefits.

ANATOMY AND PHYSIOLOGY OF THE LACTATING BREAST

Breast development, under the influence of estrogen, progesterone, and lactogenic hormones, begins in early fetal life and extends into puberty and adult life. Only during pregnancy does the breast become fully mature, with rapid growth of ducts and alveoli in response to prolactin and placental lactogen. Small amounts of milk synthesis and secretion begin during the second trimester of pregnancy. Lactogenesis, the onset of copious milk secretion around parturition, is triggered by the decrease in progesterone after delivery (Fig. 25-1).

Once milk production begins, prolactin and oxytocin provide the hormonal environment for its maintenance. Prolactin is produced in response to the amount and frequency of suckling and controls milk synthesis and secretion. Suckling also promotes the release of pituitary oxytocin. Oxytocin causes the myoepithelial cells in the breast to contract and causes milk ejection or "letdown" to occur. During milk ejection, milk moves from the alveoli into the lacteal sinuses of the breast, where it is easily removed by the infant (Fig. 25-2).

Milk production also responds to local negative feedback in the breast. Local distention and increases in pressure in the breast, such as those experienced with engorgement, may lead to decreased milk production. The major effect of engorgement is to decrease vascular flow in the breast and thus to slow the transport of prolactin and oxytocin to target cells in the breast. In animals, a constituent of milk, whey protein, inhibits milk secretion in a dose-dependent manner. As milk accumulates in the breast between feedings, inhibitor concentration rises, retarding production. Milk removal decreases the concentration of inhibitor and results in increased production.

Most women can successfully breastfeed, but a few experience primary lactation failure due to inadequate glandular tissue, neurohormonal disruption, or prolactin deficiency. Normal breast changes during pregnancy include an increase in breast size, increased pigmentation of the nipple and areola, and hypertrophy of the Montgomery tubercles. A lack of normal changes during pregnancy should alert the clinician to possible lactation problems. These women and their infants benefit from close postpartum follow-up to ensure adequate milk production.

Women who have had surgical procedures that interrupt ducts and sever or damage nipple nerves may also produce inadequate supplies of milk. Conversely, women who have undergone augmentation procedures usually have few problems breastfeeding. Although studies are inconclusive, esophageal motility problems have been reported in breastfed infants of mothers with silicone implants. Silicone, however, is present in many substances, including some antacid preparations. Unless the implant has ruptured and the mother's serum levels are elevated, breastfeeding is not contraindicated.

MANAGEMENT

Maternal Nutritional Needs and Milk Production and Composition

Milk production on the first postpartum day ranges from about 50 to 150 mL. Production rapidly increases starting about 36 hours postpartum. The volume of milk produced does not appear to be affected by maternal nutrition, body composition (adiposity), and energy or nutrient intake. Average milk production is about 750 to 800 mL/day by women of widely varying dietary intakes and nutritional status. If a lactating woman is overweight, a weight loss of up to 2 kg (4.5 lb) per month is unlikely to affect milk volume; however, women should be alert to signs that the infant's appetite is not being satisfied. In general, women can produce much more breast milk than an infant is likely to require.

Infant characteristics, such as ineffective or infrequent suckling by low-birthweight or preterm infants, can affect the amount of milk produced. In the early postpartum period, frequent suckling (10 ± 3 sessions/day) is important to the establishment of an adequate milk supply. Mothers whose infants are hospitalized can develop an adequate supply by pumping their breasts (using an electric breast pump) about five times a day (90 minutes total pumping time) in the first postpartum month.

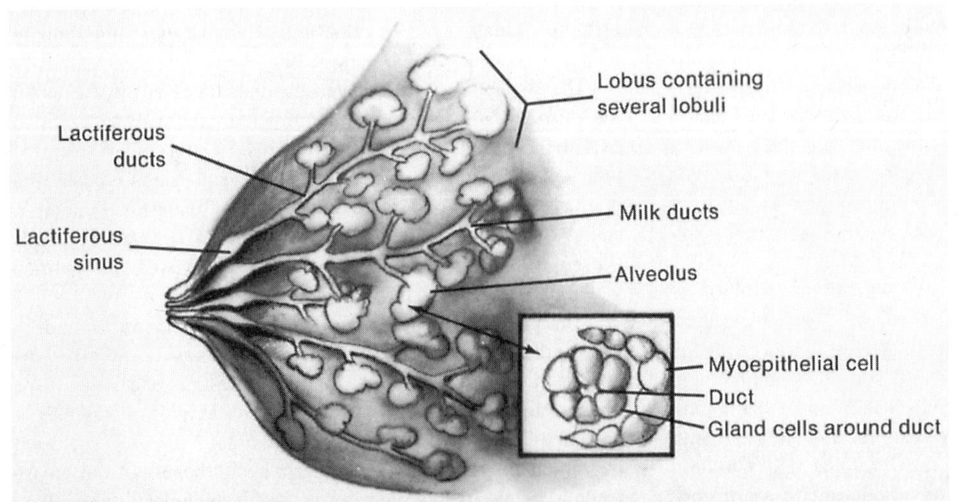

Figure 25-1. Anatomy of the breast. (Lawrence RA. Breastfeeding: A guide for the medical profession, 4th ed. St. Louis: Mosby,1994.)

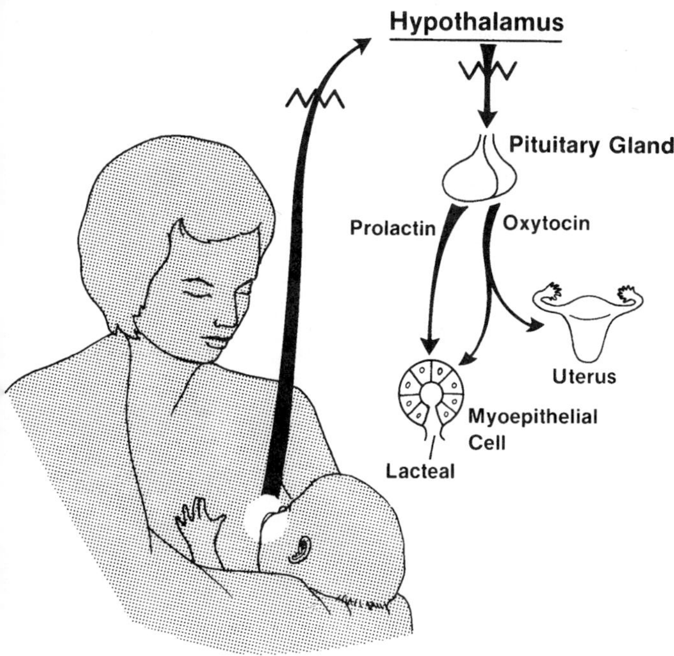

Figure 25-2. Ejection reflex arc. (Lawrence RA. Breastfeeding: A guide for the medical profession, 4th ed. St. Louis: Mosby, 1994.)

Maternal factors that may contribute to inadequate milk production include pain, stress, fatigue, and the use of alcohol, cigarettes, or some oral contraceptives. Pain, stress, and fatigue inhibit oxytocin release and thus milk ejection. The use of progestin-only contraceptives is compatible with breastfeeding, but combination pills with more than 50 micrograms of ethinylestradiol or 100 micrograms of mestranol have been associated with declines in milk production. Smoking may also decrease milk volume by decreasing the prolactin and oxytocin response. Although sipping small amounts of alcohol has traditionally been recommended to enhance letdown, ethanol in sufficient amounts inhibits oxytocin release. For the average 60-kg woman (132 lb), an alcohol dose of 0.5 g/kg or about 2 to 2.5 oz of liquor, 8 oz of wine, or two cans of beer inhibits oxytocin release. (However, breast milk production was enhanced in a study of Mexican women consuming small amounts of a traditional alcohol-containing drink.) Although nursing mothers should maintain adequate fluid intake, fluids consumed in excess of thirst do not appear to increase milk volume, and forcing fluids may decrease production.

Milk composition varies between women and with stages of lactation, although individual differences in well-nourished women are insignificant. Over 200 different constituents make up human milk, providing both nutritive and nonnutritive benefits for the infant. The constituents of milk are synthesized in the mammary secretory cells from precursors in the plasma, produced by other cells in the mammary gland, or transferred directly from the plasma to milk. Milk composition is thus influenced by physiologic and biochemical processes that affect the plasma and by hormonal and biosynthetic processes in the mammary gland. Table 25-1 lists the components of human milk.

Milk composition changes most rapidly in the first few weeks of lactation. Colostrum is the fluid secreted by the mammary gland immediately after delivery. It is produced in smaller quantities than mature milk and is higher in protein, minerals, and immunoglobulin. Beginning on about day 7, milk composition begins a slow transition over about 2 weeks to mature milk.

By using their body stores, women can produce milk with adequate amounts of protein, fat, carbohydrate, and most minerals even if their own supply of nutrients is limited. Maternal diet strongly affects the fatty acid content of human milk, but the total fat and cholesterol content is independent of diet. Human milk content is most likely to be affected by low maternal intakes of vitamins, especially vitamins B_6, B_{12}, A, and D. Breastfeeding women should consume good sources of all essential nutrients for their own health and to replenish their body stores.

The total amounts of nutrients that a lactating mother secretes are directly related to the amount and duration of breastfeeding. If nutrient intake is inadequate, maternal body stores of macronutrients, many minerals, and folate may be sacrificed to maintain milk composition. Due to the substantial safety margin included in the Recommended Daily Allowances (RDAs) for lactating women, women's needs are easily met by an average American diet containing 2700 kcal/day. At energy intakes of less than 2700 kcal/day, the nutrients most likely to be deficient are calcium, magnesium, zinc, vitamin B_6, and folate. Table 25-2 list food sources rich in these nutrients, and women should be encouraged to consume these foods. Iron-rich foods are important once the mother's menstrual cycle returns. Adolescents, women who are complete vegetarians (vegans), and those who avoid dairy products, diet to lose weight during lactation, or are impoverished may be at risk for nutritional deficiencies during lactation. Table 25-3 contains suggestions for increasing nutrient intake in women at risk for nutritional deficiencies during lactation. Current evidence does not warrant recommending routine vitamin-mineral supplementation for lactating women.

Prenatal Preparation

A knowledgeable, supportive physician is an essential part of any effort to promote breastfeeding. Because most women make decisions about infant feeding before the third trimester, physicians caring for women are in an ideal situation to influence the choice

Table 25-1. Constituents of Human Milk

Nitrogen Compounds	Water-Soluble Vitamins	Lipids
Proteins	Thiamine	Triglycerides
Caseins	Riboflavin	Fatty acids
α-Lactalbumin	Niacin	Phospholipids
Lactoferrin	Pantothenic acid	Sterols and Hydrocarbons
S IgA, Immunoglobulins	Biotin	Fat-soluble vitamins A, D, E, K
β-Lactoglobulin	Folate	**Minerals**
Lysozyme	Vitamin B_6	Calcium
Enzymes	Vitamin B_{12}	Phosphorus
Hormones	Vitamin C	Magnesium
Growth factors	Inositol	Potassium
Nonprotein Nitrogen	Choline	Sodium
Urea	*Cells*	Chlorine
Creatine	Leukocytes	Sulfur
Creatinine	Epithelial cells	Iodine
Uric acid	**Carbohydrates**	Iron
Glucosamine	Lactose	Copper
α-Amino nitrogen	Oligosaccharides	Zinc
Nucleic acids	Bifidus factors	Manganese
Nucleotides	Glycopeptides	Selenium
Polyamines		Chromium
		Cobalt

(Reprinted with permission from Nutrition during lactation. © 1991 by the National Academy of Sciences. Courtesy of the National Academy Press, Washington D.C.)

to breastfeed. Although the physician must support the mother's decision either way, he or she also must educate her so that her decisions are based on facts. Except for some sophisticated families, most infant feeding discussions are initiated by the physician. Given the overwhelming evidence in support of breastfeeding, physicians should sensitively but openly encourage women to choose breastfeeding.

The physical examination early in pregnancy provides a good opportunity to discuss breastfeeding and any breast abnormalities. Any questions about lactation or the mother's ability to produce sufficient milk should be addressed at this time. The size of the mammary gland does not predict a mother's ability to nourish her infant, although failure of the gland to enlarge with pregnancy may be associated with inadequate production. If there are anatomic abnormalities or previous breast surgery, however, potential problems should be discussed. Particular attention should be paid to the nipple and areola. Nipples should be tested for their ability to protrude. Inverted nipples are caused by persistent fibers from the invagination of the mammary dimple in the embryo and become evident when the areola is squeezed or compressed (Fig. 25-3).

A prenatal visit with a pediatric care provider may provide expectant patients with useful information about infant feeding. Many hospitals also conduct prenatal education classes that are excellent sources of information about breastfeeding. Additionally, Lamaze classes and La Leche League representatives may serve as educational resources. The American Academy of Pediatrics, the American College of Obstetricians and Gynecologists, and La Leche League publish patient education materials about breastfeeding. Patient education materials published by formula companies may not be appropriate sources of breastfeeding information.

The Lactation Study Center at the University of Rochester School of Medicine and Dentistry (716-275-0088) provides information on medications and lactation and lactation management issues and maintains a computer data bank on lactation literature. Wellstart International (619-295-5192) provides educational programs and handouts and information regarding lactation management issues.

Preparation of the Breasts

In general, no special preparation of the breasts is necessary in anticipation of breastfeeding. Women should avoid the use of soap, alcohol, or other drying agents on the nipples. Secretions from the Montgomery glands cleanse and lubricate the areola and nipple. Studies have not shown ointments or creams to be effective in preventing sore nipples; in fact, they may cause the nipples to macerate and become more susceptible to irritation. In extremely dry climates where lubricating ointments are necessary for skin integrity, however, such an ointment might be indicated. Nipple rolling and other manipulations are also ineffective in preventing sore nipples and should be avoided due to the risk of inducing uterine contractions and premature labor.

As many as 10% of pregnant women have inverted (nonprotractile) nipples that may make it difficult for an infant to get a proper

Table 25-2. Food Sources for Nutrients Most Likely to be Deficient in the Diet of the Lactating Woman

Calcium	Zinc	Magnesium	Vitamin B_6*	Thiamine*	Folate
Milk	Meat	Nuts	Bananas	Pork	Leafy vegetables
Cheese	Poultry	Seeds	Poultry	Fish	Fruit
Yogurt	Seafood	Legumes	Meat	Whole grains	Liver
Fish with edible bones	Eggs	Whole grains	Fish	Organ meats	Green beans
Tofu made with calcium sulfate	Seeds	Green vegetables	Potatoes	Legumes	Fortified cereals
Bok choy	Legumes	Scallops	Sweet potatoes	Corn	Legumes
Broccoli	Yogurt	Oysters	Spinach	Peas	Whole-grain cereals
Kale	Whole grains		Prunes	Seeds	
Collard greens			Watermelon	Nuts	
Mustard greens			Some legumes	Fortified cereal grain	
Turnip greens			Fortified cereals		
Breads made with milk			Nuts		
Seeds and nuts					

*In general, this nutrient is widely distributed in food rather than concentrated in a small number of foods.
(Reprinted with permission from Nutrition during lactation. © 1991 by the National Academy of Sciences. Courtesy of the National Academy Press, Washington D.C.)

grasp on the breast. Hoffman exercises (stretching and pulling of the nipple and areola) are not very effective and are contraindicated due to the potential of inducing uterine contractions. Women with flat or inverted nipples may, however, benefit from treatment with breast shells (plastic discs with holes in the center and a domed cover). The inner ring of the shell fits over the areola, causing the nipple to protrude through the hole in the center. The gentle pressure produced causes stretching of the fibrous tissue and causes the nipple to evert slowly. Small air vents in the dome allow air circulation around the nipple. Daytime use during the last trimester may alleviate attachment problems when breastfeeding begins.

After delivery, flat or inverted nipples may be treated by use of an electric breast pump. The breast is pumped before breastfeeding, using low settings, until the nipple is drawn out and with the areola the teat is formed. Pumping is usually required only temporarily. Mothers can be taught to use a hand-held manual pump for the same purpose if continued pumping is needed at home. Nipple shields, made of thin latex, usually interfere with proper attachment.

Ideally, prenatal preparation for breastfeeding includes an early breast examination and discussion encouraging breastfeeding as the optimal infant feeding method, early discussion about and treatment of any breast problems, a prenatal visit later in pregnancy with a pediatric care provider, and referrals to helpful community resources (eg, breastfeeding classes, La Leche League).

Care in the Hospital

Hospital policies and routines greatly influence breastfeeding success. An experienced nursing staff is critical to the management of the nursing mother and infant in the first few days after birth. All

Table 25-3. Suggested Measures for Improving Nutrient Intake of Women With Restrictive Eating Patterns

EATING PATTERN	CORRECTIVE MEASURES
Excessive restriction of food intake (ie, ingestion of < 1800 kcal of energy per day, which ordinarily leads to unsatisfactory intake of nutrients compared with the amounts needed by lactating women)	Encourage increased intake of nutrient-rich foods to achieve an energy intake of at least 1800 kcal/day; if the mother insists on curbing food intake sharply, promote substitution of foods rich in vitamins, minerals, and protein for those lower in nutritive value. In individual cases, it may be advisable to recommend a balanced multivitamin-mineral supplement. Discourage the use of liquid weight-loss diets and appetite suppressants.
Complete vegetarianism (avoidance of all animal food, including meat, fish, dairy products, and eggs)	Advise intake of a regular source of vitamin B_{12}, such as special vitamin B_{12}-containing plant food products or a 2.6-µg vitamin B_{12} supplement daily.
Avoidance of milk, cheese, or other calcium-rich dairy products	Encourage increased intake of other culturally appropriate dietary calcium sources, such as collard greens for blacks from the southeastern U.S. Provide information on the appropriate use of low-lactose dairy products if milk is being avoided because of lactose intolerance; if correction by diet cannot be achieved, it may be advisable to recommend 600 mg of elemental calcium per day taken with meals.
Avoidance of vitamin D-fortified food, such as fortified milk or cereal, combined with limited exposure to ultraviolet light	Recommend 10 µg of supplemental vitamin D per day.

(Reprinted with permission from Nutrition during lactation. ©1991 by the National Academy of Sciences. Courtesy of the National Academy Press, Washington D.C.)

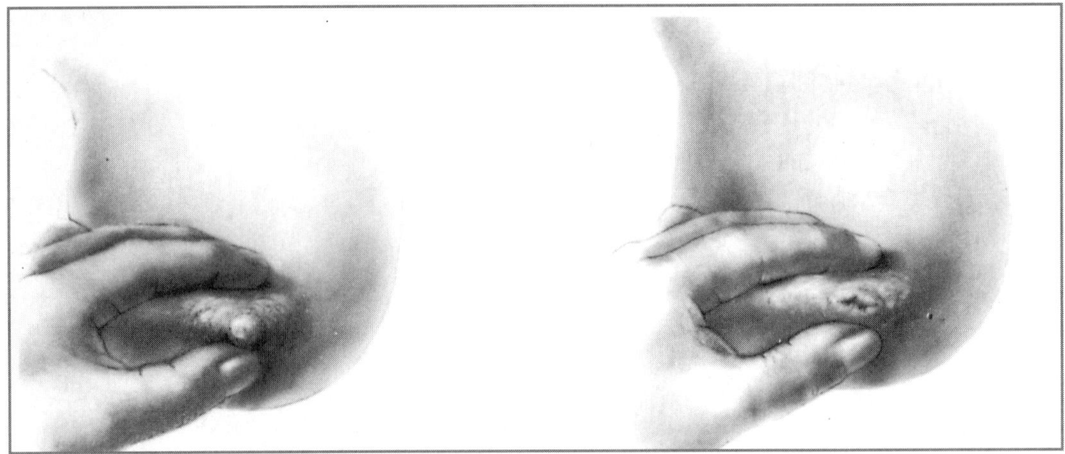

Figure 25-3. **(*A*)** Normal nipple everts with gentle pressure. **(*B*)** Inverted or tied nipple inverts with gentle pressure. (Lawrence RA. Breastfeeding: a guide for the medical profession, 4th ed. St. Louis: Mosby,1994.)

labor and delivery, newborn nursery, neonatal intensive care, and postpartum nurses should be adequately trained to assist the nursing mother. Care should be taken to ensure that advice given in the hospital is consistent between providers. A written breastfeeding policy with input from physicians and nurses ensures that advice given to mothers is consistent and accurate. Policies that encourage breastfeeding success include early (as soon as possible, preferably within a half-hour of delivery), frequent opportunities to breastfeed, rooming-in, "demand" feeding schedules, and the avoidance of routine water or formula supplements.

Some mothers, such as those who become ill postpartum, have a difficult delivery, or deliver multiple infants, may be at risk for breastfeeding problems such as sleepy infants, late initiation of breastfeeding, increased needs for supplementation, less frequent night feedings, and delayed increases in milk supply. Excellent supportive care is essential for these at-risk mothers. Key factors in early management include:

- *Proper positioning at the breast*: Mothers must be taught to position the infant properly at the breast. The infant's abdomen should be against the mother's abdomen, and the infant's head should be well supported and kept in line with his or her body. After eliciting a rooting response by stimulating the infant's lower lip with the nipple, the mother should bring the infant's head toward her breast by moving her arm or hand. The head should not be pushed toward the breast, as it may cause the infant to arch back. If the infant's arms are not swaddled, they should be around the mother's thorax.
- *Supporting the breast*: The mother should be taught to support her breast using a palmar or scissors grasp (whichever works best for her). The mother's grasp must not interfere with the infant's position on the breast. The infant's lips should be positioned on the areola about 1" or 1.5" from the base of the nipple. The infant's lower lip should not be folded in so that he or she sucks on the lip.
- *Detaching the infant from the breast*: The mother should be taught to break the suction at the breast by inserting her finger in the infant's mouth when removing the infant from the breast.
- *Waking a sleepy baby*: Mothers should be taught ways to awaken a sleepy infant for feedings such as unwrapping, diapering, or gentle stimulation.
- *Frequency of feedings*: Feedings should be frequent, every 2 to 2.5 hours from the start of a feeding to the start of the next. To equalize stimulation of the breasts, mothers should alternate the breast that is offered first at each feeding.
- *Length of feedings*: Some mothers benefit from general guidelines to nurse about 10 to 15 minutes per side in the first few days. Generally, infants need to suckle about 2 or 3 minutes before the mother experiences milk letdown, especially in the first week or two. Frequent small feedings provide good breast stimulation and avoid undue tiredness in the mother. If rooming-in is impossible, infants should be taken to their mothers to nurse at night.

Breastfed infants should not be given supplementation that is not medically indicated, as early supplementation is consistently associated with shortened duration and increased rates of early cessation of breastfeeding. Supplementation interferes with the supply-and-demand nature of breastfeeding by lessening demand and reducing milk production. Also, mechanical differences between breastfeeding and bottle feeding may cause an infant to refuse the breast or to learn to suckle ineffectively. Commercial formula discharge packs should not be given to breastfeeding mothers. The distribution of advertising and formula samples to breastfeeding women in the hospital lessens the duration of exclusive and overall breastfeeding and hastens the introduction of solid foods to the infant.

Many women discontinue breastfeeding within the first postpartum month; thus, early (5 to 7 days) follow-up with a pediatric care provider is essential. Additionally, La Leche League representatives, hospital hotlines, and lactation consultants may all be useful to mothers in the early postpartum period. Issues related to breastfeeding should also be a regular part of obstetric postpartum care. Table 25-4 lists factors that promote successful breastfeeding.

Supplements in the Breastfeeding Infant

Vitamin K prophylaxis should be administered to all infants regardless of feeding method to prevent hemorrhagic disease of the newborn. Vitamin D levels in the breast milk of a well-nourished mother are adequate for the healthy term infant. However, if the mother's vitamin D nutrition or exposure to sunlight is inadequate,

Table 25-4. Factors that Promote Breastfeeding

PRENATAL	IMMEDIATE POSTPARTUM	INFANCY
General health information	Early maternal-infant contact	Counseling and support
Breastfeeding education	Rooming-in	Avoidance of exposure to formula samples and advertising
Encouragement by health professional	"Demand" feeding schedules	Information about breast pumping; counseling regarding return to work
	Avoidance of supplementation	
	Supportive atmosphere for breastfeeding women	

(Adapted from Kramer MS. Poverty, WIC, and promotion of breastfeeding. Pediatrics 1991;87:399.)

or if the infant does not benefit from adequate ultraviolet light exposure, the mother's diet should be improved or supplements of vitamin D provided. If this is impossible, the breastfed infant should receive a vitamin D supplement.

Neonatal iron stores meet the needs of a term infant for the first 6 months of life. Iron in human milk is very bioavailable, delaying the depletion of these stores until after 6 months of life. After that time, other sources of iron, such as iron-fortified infant cereal, should be added to the diet.

Fluoride supplements are no longer recommended for infants less than 6 months of age. Infants and children 6 months to 3 years old living in areas where the fluoride content of the water is less than 0.3 parts per million should receive a supplement of 0.25 mg/day.

Postpartum Follow-Up

The nursing mother and infant should be assessed frequently throughout their hospital stay for the successful establishment of lactation. With the increasing frequency of early hospital discharge, however, many mothers and infants go home before the mother's milk supply increases. These women and infants require close outpatient monitoring. Ideally, breastfed infants discharged 48 to 72 hours after delivery should be seen in follow-up between 5 to 7 days of age. Infants discharged from the hospital earlier require follow-up within 48 hours and again at 1 week of age.

Some useful clinical criteria that signal the successful establishment of breastfeeding at 5 to 7 days include:

- The mother's milk has increased in quantity. Mothers generally experience their milk "coming in" between postpartum day 2 to 4 and note that their breasts become firm and full.
- The mother and infant have established an appropriate feeding schedule of every 2 to 3 hours, with one longer sleep interval of about 5 hours. The infant should not be receiving any supplemental feedings (water or formula).
- Any nipple tenderness the mother experienced in the first postpartum days should be mild and resolving.
- The infant should be having at least three or four breast milk stools (mustard-colored seedy stools) and six to eight clear voids per day (at least one diaper per day should be soaked). Urate crystals (the color of brick dust) in the urine are a clue to inadequate hydration.
- The infant's weight loss since birth should be no more than 7%. After the mother's milk increases in quantity, the infant should gain about 30 g/day. Birth weight should be regained by 2 weeks of age.

CONTRAINDICATIONS TO BREASTFEEDING

Contraindications to breastfeeding are rare. However, some medications, infectious agents, and toxic substances may appear in breast milk and pose a risk to the nursing infant. The assessment of any exposure must weigh potential risks against the many benefits of breastfeeding. Mothers with life-threatening illnesses, however, must give their own medical treatment priority.

Most medications are safe for use during breastfeeding. The risk a medication poses to the infant depends on the pharmacokinetics of the substance; the route by which the mother is exposed, as well as her absorption, metabolism, and excretion of the substance; and the infant's physiologic maturity (his or her ability to absorb, metabolize, and excrete the substance).

Drugs contraindicated during breastfeeding include therapeutic radiopharmaceuticals, lithium, lactation-suppressing drugs, some antithyroid drugs, illicit or street drugs, and synthetic anticoagulants. Short courses of medications such as radiopharmaceuticals, antiprotozoal compounds, and a few antibiotics (eg, chloramphenicol) may require mothers to pump their breasts temporarily and discard the milk. Other drugs may be contraindicated depending on the infant's age (eg, sulfa-containing medications should be avoided in an infant less than 1 month of age).

If the mother has been exposed to high levels of insecticides, heavy metals, or other contaminants that appear in breast milk, breastfeeding is not recommended without evaluation of levels. Pesticides such as DDT, PCBs, hexachlorobenzene, dieldrin, and heptachlor epoxide have been identified in the milk of women with heavy exposures. Heavy metals such as lead, mercury, arsenic, and cadmium, although a matter for concern, are generally found in lower levels in breast milk than in water. If a mother has undergone a heavy metal exposure, levels in breast milk and infant serum should be measured.

Infectious diseases are rarely a contraindication to breastfeeding. Neither cytomegalovirus nor hepatitis B is a contraindication. Although infants of mothers infected with hepatitis C should not breastfeed, infants whose mothers are hepatitis B antigen positive are unlikely to acquire the infection via breast milk. These infants should be vaccinated and protected against infection with immune globulin (0.5 mL HBIG) as soon as possible after birth. If a mother requires rubella immunization after delivery, she may still breastfeed.

Of more concern is the possible transmission of HIV infection through breast milk. Transplacental transmission of HIV from infected mothers to their infants during pregnancy occurs in about 10% to 15% of cases (with AZT). Several cases of transmission of HIV-1 to infants via breast milk have been reported. Therefore, the Public Health Service and the Centers for Disease Control and Prevention recommend that women who test seropositive for HIV antibody in the United States should not breastfeed to avoid postnatal transmission to an infant who may not be infected. In developing countries, because of the protective effects of breastfeeding and the greater risk of infant mortality from diarrheal and other diseases if not breastfed, mothers are encouraged to breastfeed regardless of HIV status.

Mothers who develop mastitis may with rare exceptions continue to breastfeed. Women should be counseled to seek early medical care at the first signs of infection (mastitis is discussed later in this chapter). Mothers of infants diagnosed with galactosemia should not breastfeed; a milk substitute with a nonlactose sugar source should be chosen.

COMMON PROBLEMS

Sore Nipples

Mothers commonly experience some discomfort in the early days of breastfeeding with the initial grasp and suckling of the breast. The discomfort is caused by the negative pressure on empty ductules and typically resolves as the milk supply increases. Any nipple pain that persists throughout a breastfeeding or fails to resolve within the first week may indicate more serious problems and needs evaluation.

Early in breastfeeding, the most common cause for nipple trauma and subsequent pain is poor positioning of the infant at the breast. Common causes of nipple pain associated with poor positioning include the infant who attaches only to the nipple with suckling, the infant who sucks in his or her lower lip and irritates the underside of the nipple, and the mother who does not break the suction before removing the infant from the breast.

Sometimes the infant's nursing style causes pain. A very vigorous infant suckling at the breast may result in temporary discomfort for the mother. Especially delicate tissues may benefit from air drying after nursing or from brief dry heat, especially in climates with high humidity. A hair dryer set on warm and fanned across the breast for 2 or 3 minutes at 6" to 8" provides relief for many mothers. Because human milk has many antiinfective and healing properties, expressing a few drops of milk and allowing them to dry on the areola may also help.

Candidal infection is associated with stabbing pain, radiating throughout the breast. This type of infection often presents after antibiotic treatment (mother or infant) or in the mother of an infant with a candidal infection (eg, thrush, diaper rash).

Addressing an underlying cause such as poor positioning is the first step in treatment of soreness, but careful assessment of any other contributing factors is also important. Soaps or self-prescribed treatments may lead to drying of the area and subsequent contact dermatitis. If the skin is particularly dry, the area may benefit from lubrication, but routine use of ointments is not recommended, as the sebaceous glands and Montgomery glands are easily plugged. A and D Ointment is not harmful to the infant, but vitamin E and local anesthetic creams should not be used. Lanolin may cause a severe contact dermatitis in women allergic to wool. Purified lanolin ointments that are free from alcohol and allergens are safe if an ointment is indicated. Some dermatologists recommend moist healing of sore and cracked nipples, citing insufficient moisture coupled with poor positioning of the infant as the cause. Certainly, surface moisture due to milk or occlusive plastic in nursing pads aggravates the problem and should be avoided. After gentle drying, however, the area may benefit from the application of a nonirritating ointment to restore moisture in the tissues.

Nipple shields are devices made of rubber or synthetic material designed to be worn over the areola while the infant is nursing. They reduce the amount of milk the infant receives and may cause the infant to learn to suckle improperly. Subsequent weaning back to the bare breast may be difficult. In general, the use of these devices should be avoided.

Flat or inverted nipples may make it difficult for an infant to grasp the breast properly. Compressing the areola between two fingers to allow the nipple to protrude as much as possible helps the infant grasp the breast. Expressing a small amount of milk before a feeding to soften the areola and entice the infant is also helpful. Additionally, breast shells may be worn between feedings to encourage the nipple to protrude. If the above techniques fail to produce results, the nipple can be drawn out before breastfeeding with an electric pump. Inverted nipples often respond to these measures within the first 1 or 2 postpartum days.

If the mother has cracked, bleeding, or blistered nipples, she may also benefit from shorter, more frequent feedings and the use of a short-acting analgesic before nursing. She should begin the feeding with the breast that is less sore, limiting the amount of nonnutritive sucking (that not associated with swallowing) by the infant. If the nipple is in the precracked stage, dry heat followed by lubrication with cream or ointment between feedings is most effective. Cracks are often caused by poor positioning combined with excessive dryness. Pain is eased by proper positioning and by application of a therapeutic ointment such as A and D Ointment, purified lanolin, or a synthetic corticoid (by prescription). If nursing is stopped on the involved side, the breast is prone to engorgement, reduced flow, and plugged ducts.

When the nipple is severely affected and fungal and bacterial infections have been ruled out, the physician may wish to prescribe 1% cortisone ointment or a synthetic corticoid (halobetasol propionate 0.05% or mometasone furoate 0.1%) to be rubbed into the nipple and areola after each feeding. The underlying cause of the problem, such as poor positioning, should always be addressed. Usually only a short course of treatment (2 days) is needed. The infant receives an insignificant amount of medication from such treatment.

Engorgement

Engorgement involves congestion, increased vascularity, and accumulation of milk in the breast. It may involve primarily the areola or the entire breast. Some amount of fullness and swelling, however, is normal as milk quantity increases in the early postpartum period. A woman who does not experience such changes in her breasts may be at risk for lactation failure. The best treatment for engorgement is prevention, with early frequent nursing to enhance milk quantity and to empty the breast adequately. Engorgement often becomes evident when the infant has been left in the nursery overnight so that the mother can rest.

In areolar engorgement, swelling flattens the nipple, making attachment difficult for the infant. If the infant attaches improperly, sucking only on the nipple, breastfeeding is painful and the nipple may be traumatized. Improper attachment to the nipple also makes milk withdrawal inefficient, and the infant receives little nourishment.

The treatment of engorgement is directed at emptying the breast. Often, manual expression of a small amount of milk allows the infant to grasp the breast properly and nurse efficiently. Warm compresses applied to the breast before expression facilitate blood flow and letdown. Mothers may also find a warm shower a helpful place to express milk manually. During manual expression, the mother compresses the breast just behind the areola back into the chest and then brings her fingers gently together to express milk. When presenting an engorged breast to the infant, the areola should be softened by expression and compressed between two fingers to help the nipple protrude.

Engorgement involving the entire breast usually occurs on the second postpartum day and is largely due to increased vascularity. The mother complains of throbbing pain in breasts that are full, hard, and tender. Breast swelling may extend from the clavicle to the lower ribcage and into the axilla. Treatment, as before, involves adequate emptying of the breast. In addition to milk expression, a well-fitting bra is important to support the breast and provide comfort. Analgesics, including acetaminophen, aspirin, or codeine, may provide further relief; if taken a half-hour before nursing, the infant will receive little medication in the milk. It is important to empty the breast adequately to prevent milk stasis and back-pressure, with subsequent decreased milk production. Frequent feeding around the clock to empty the breast is essential in the treatment of engorgement. Milk production and vascularity stabilize over a few days of treatment. Between feedings, cool compresses may provide additional relief.

Plugged Ducts

The lactating breast is lumpy, but the lumps appear in different places and are not tender. Mildly tender lumps in the breasts of a lactating women who shows no other systemic signs of illness are probably due to a plugged collecting duct. She should continue to nurse to ensure adequate emptying of the breast. Warm compresses and massage of the affected area before nursing may further aid in emptying the breast. Women may also be counseled to alternate nursing positions, as different areas of the breast empty better depending on the infant's position at the breast (Madonna, cross cradle, or football hold). A good nursing bra is helpful, as regular bras with wire stays or constricting straps may contribute to milk stasis in a compressed area.

Mastitis

Mastitis is an inflammation of the lactating breast, with cellulitis, commonly caused by *Staphylococcus aureus* or *Escherichia coli* and less commonly by *Streptococcus* and coagulase-negative *Staphylococcus*. Bacteria infect a secreting lobule in the breast by way of the lactiferous ducts, through a traumatized nipple to the periductal lymphatics, or by hematogenous spread. The clinical signs and symptoms include a fever of 38.5°C or greater, systemic flu-like illness (chills, aching, headache, nausea, malaise), and a pink, tender, hot, swollen wedge-shaped area of the breast. Certain conditions may predispose to mastitis, including milk stasis (engorgement or plugged ducts) and lowered maternal defenses secondary to fatigue and stress. Cracked or sore nipples may lead to milk stasis when a woman avoids nursing on a painful breast. Engorgement, plugged ducts, and sore nipples should be treated vigorously to prevent the development of mastitis. The onset of mastitis varies widely, from several days to several months postpartum.

Early diagnosis and treatment are essential to prevent progression of the disease to abscess formation or chronic mastitis. Midstream cultures of milk and cell counts (bacteria $> 10^3$ and leukocytes $> 10^6$) may be helpful in diagnosis, but antibiotic therapy should not await culture results. Uninfected human milk normally contains 1000 to 4000 cells/mm^3. Adverse outcomes such as recurrent mastitis and abscess formation are clearly associated with delays between the onset of symptoms and treatment.

The affected breast should be regularly emptied by nursing or pumping. The woman may continue to nurse, beginning with the unaffected breast, to enhance letdown on the affected side and lessen the discomfort when the infant latches on. The breastfed infant generally remains well during episodes of acute mastitis, and the choice of antibiotics should be compatible with continued breastfeeding. Sulfa drugs should be avoided if the infant is less than 1 month of age. The antibiotic therapy chosen should account for likely organisms, local sensitivities, and exposure to resistant organisms. Staphylococcal disease responds readily to dicloxacillin or nafcillin, streptococcal disease to penicillin. Acute uncomplicated mastitis presenting after 1 month postpartum responds readily to dicloxacillin or erythromycin therapy. Antibiotics should be given for at least 10 to 14 days. Adequate rest and stress reduction are essential. Warm compresses often hasten drainage of the involved area and provide additional pain relief. Analgesics such as aspirin or acetaminophen and a supportive bra are also helpful.

Chronic Mastitis

Chronic mastitis can result from inadequate or delayed treatment of acute mastitis. The clinician must stress the importance of a full 10 to 14 days of treatment for acute mastitis. A breast milk culture, best obtained as a midstream sample, should guide antibiotic therapy. The woman should manually express her milk after carefully washing her hands and cleansing the breast with water. The first 3 mL of expressed milk is discarded and a midstream sample obtained for culture.

Recurrent mastitis should be aggressively treated with antibiotics for at least 2 weeks. Treatment should also include the measures discussed under acute mastitis. If treatment fails, chronic bacterial infection, fungal infection, or underlying breast disease such as a tumor or cyst must be considered. Cysts or tumors present as unchanging masses in the lactating breast. Rarely, fungal infections cause mastitis and require treatment with oral and local antifungal agents.

Monilial Infection

Monilial infection of the breast typically presents as stinging, burning pain radiating throughout the breast during and after nursing. The infection is a common secondary complication of recent antibiotic treatment, maternal candidal vaginitis, or fungal infection in the infant (thrush or candidal diaper rash). The nipple may be normal or appear pink and shiny with typical satellite lesions. A 2-week course of treatment with a topical antifungal agent rubbed into the nipple and areola after breastfeeding is usually effective. Other sources of infection in the mother such as vaginitis should also be treated. The infant should always be treated simultaneously with oral nystatin to prevent recurrences. Such therapy is indicated even if there is no evidence of concurrent thrush or candidal diaper rash in the infant.

Colic and Breast Rejection

Some breastfed infants exhibit colicky symptoms believed to be associated with specific foods in the mother's diet, such as garlic, onions, cabbage, turnips, broccoli, or beans. Other often-cited foods are apricots, rhubarb, prunes, melons, peaches, and other fresh fruits. Strong spices in foods or teas may also produce symptoms. If a mother has questions regarding foods in her diet, she should carefully document any effects in the 24 hours after ingestion of the suspected irritant. Caffeine, which appears in breast milk, may cause irritability, but most infants tolerate maternal intake of one or two cups of a caffeinated beverage without problems. Smoking decreases milk production and may also cause irritability, as cotinine (a metabolite of nicotine) appears in breast milk.

Colic in breastfed infants has also been attributed to cow milk in the mother's diet. Numerous components of cow milk appear in breast milk. A positive family history of allergies, especially to cow milk, suggests this diagnosis, and the infant may benefit from the mother's eliminating cow milk from her diet; a week-long trial of elimination is usually diagnostic. Often just eliminating drinking milk is effective, although if the infant fails to respond to such measures, the mother may need to eliminate all dairy products, especially yogurt, from her diet. Alternative sources of calcium and vitamin D may be necessary for the mother who eliminates all dairy products.

Infants 3 to 4 months old sometimes temporarily refuse to breastfeed for several days. The rejection is often associated with strong foods in the mother's diet, illness in the infant, or the return of menstruation in the mother. Breast rejection is usually temporary. Addressing dietary causes and underlying disease and increasing cuddling and soothing during breastfeeding usually remedies the situation. Breast rejection secondary to menses usually lasts only the first 1 or 2 days of the cycle. Rarely, one breast is permanently rejected; the milk supply in that breast declines and the supply in the opposite breast increases to meet the infant's demands.

BIBLIOGRAPHY

American Academy of Pediatrics, Committee on Drugs. Transfer of drugs and other chemicals into human milk. Pediatrics 1994;93:137.

Flores-Huerta S, Hernandez-Montes H, Argote RM, et al. Effects of ethanol consumption during pregnancy and lactation on the outcome and postnatal growth of the offspring. Ann Nutr Metab 1992;36:121.

Human Milk Banking Association of North America, Inc. Recommendations for collection, storage and handling of a mother's milk for her own infant in a hospital setting. West Hartford, CT: HMBANA, 1993.

Institute of Medicine. Nutrition during lactation. Washington DC: National Academy Press, 1991.

Lawrence RA. Breastfeeding: a guide for the medical profession, 4th ed. St. Louis: Mosby, 1994.

Marshall BR, Hepper JK, Zirbel CC. Sporadic puerperal mastitis: an infection that need not interrupt lactation. JAMA 1975;233:1377.

Neville MC, Neifert MA. Lactation: physiology, nutrition, and breastfeeding. New York: Plenum Press, 1983.

Walker M. How to evaluate breast pumps. Am J Matern Child Nurs 1987;12:270.

Walker M, Driscoll JW. Sore nipples: the new mother's nemesis. Am J Matern Child Nurs 1989;14:260.

Zinaman MJ. Breast pumps: ensuring mothers' success. Contemp OB-GYN 1998 (special issue):55.

26

Breast Cancer

JAMES V. FIORICA

Primary Care for Women, edited by Phyllis C. Leppert and Fred M. Howard. Lippincott-Raven Publishers, Philadelphia © 1997.

Breast carcinoma is the most common cancer in women, with 182,000 new cases and 46,000 deaths reported in 1995 in the United States. Early diagnosis is the key to survival. The American College of Obstetricians and Gynecologists requires all obstetrics and gynecology residency training programs in the United States to have formal training in the diagnosis and treatment of early breast cancer; other primary care residency programs are also mandating these standards. Breast cancer is so prevalent that the diagnosis of a small percentage of early breast cancers could save several hundred lives every year.

Primary care providers must know the risk factors for breast cancer, must be able to perform a satisfactory breast examination, and must understand the diagnostic studies, including screening of asymptomatic patients. Physicians should also know how to evaluate a breast lump, when to refer the patient, and how to counsel the patient regarding the treatment of early breast cancer.

SCREENING FOR BREAST CANCER

Next to cervical cancer, screening for breast cancer is the most extensively studied cancer screening program. The goals of screening are to detect clinically unrecognized cancer in asymptomatic women, to interrupt the natural course of the disease with early detection, and to reduce the mortality rate of the disease. Screening includes patient education with breast self-examination, a clinical breast examination (CBE), and mammographic surveillance. There is debate over the guidelines for screening, based not so much on the merits of the procedure as it is on the cost.

Breast self-examination may be advantageous if performed on a monthly basis, as it can detect cancers that arise between the annual CBE and mammography. Detection by CBE or self-examination depends on the tactile appreciation of differences between a tumor and surrounding tissue, so a thorough understanding of this examination is essential. The proper method of examining the breast is described in Chapter 24.

The American Cancer Society's screening guidelines for asymptomatic women are shown in Table 26-1. Annual mammography at earlier intervals is generally recommended for high-risk groups such as breast cancer patients (the contralateral breast after radical therapy, both breasts after conservative therapy), women with a strong family history of breast cancer, and women with a history of severe proliferative breast disease. Mammography is also indicated in women with known breast abnormalities.

Nearly all medical organizations agree to mammographic screening of women over age 50. Breast cancer survival depends

Table 26-1. American Cancer Society Guidelines for Breast Cancer Screening

TEST	AGE (YR)	FREQUENCY
BSE	≥20	Every month
CBE	20–39	Every 3 years
	≥49	Every year
Mammography	40–49	Every 1–2 years
	≥50	Every year

BSE, breast self-examination; *CBE,* clinical breast examination.

strongly on tumor size, lymph node status, and stage. Screening detects cancer at an earlier stage and decreases the incidence of nodal disease among the screened groups. In randomized trials, mortality was reduced by 30% after 10 to 12 years in screened women age 50 to 69. Screening mammography has a sensitivity rate of greater than 80%, a specificity rate of over 95%, and a positive predictive value of over 20% and is safe, with a negligible risk of radiation-induced carcinogenesis.

Mammography is technically easier to interpret in elderly women, and the incidence of breast cancer increases with age. Because women over age 70 still have a significant life expectancy, some experts argue that although there are no data to demonstrate the benefits of screening in this age group, benefits probably exist.

The real debate about screening focuses on women under age 50. Eight major randomized controlled trials have been conducted worldwide. Six of the eight trials with follow-up of 7 to 12 years and five of the six trials with follow-up of 10 years have shown mortality reductions of 22% to 49% (Table 26-2). Deficiencies in these trials include excessively long screening intervals, single mediolateral oblique x-ray views rather than two-view mammograms, poor-quality mammography, lack of CBE, and short follow-up. Nevertheless, all randomized trials except the Canadian National Breast Screening Study showed an 18% mortality reduction for women age 40 to 49. Major criticisms of the Canadian trial include technically poor mammography, inappropriate randomization bias, too few patients in the 40-to-49 age group, and insufficient follow-up for the effects to become apparent.

There is no biologic or scientific rationale indicating that age 50 is a critical point. The number of breast cancers diagnosed in women age 40 to 49 is significant, and because the information available from clinical trials is insufficient, many organizations remain firm in recommending screening mammography for women age 40 to 49. The full answers will not be known until the completion of new clinical trials designed to answer these questions.

GENETIC SCREENING

Advances in genetic technology have been encouraging. A tumor suppressor gene, BRCA1, has been demonstrated from chromosome 17q21. The absence of both wild-type copies of this tumor suppressor gene could allow for malignant growth. Information about the BRCA1 mutation status might be used to inform some women from high-risk families about an inherited predisposition to breast cancer. In one study of 214 families, the penetrance or cumulative risk associated with BRCA1 was 59% by age 50 and 82% by age 70. The ethical, social, and legal implications of genetic susceptibility testing are being defined. Familial cancer risk counseling may become available in the near future, but there may be several phases until nationwide implementation occurs. A well-thought-out treatment plan must be agreed on before implementation, and this plan is in its experimental stage and not widely available.

MANAGEMENT OF EARLY BREAST CARCINOMA

Breast cancer is divided histologically into two noninvasive categories (ductal carcinoma in situ and lobular carcinoma in situ) and two invasive categories (infiltrating ductal and invasive lobular). Infiltrating ductal carcinoma accounts for 72% of breast cancers, followed by infiltrating lobular (10% to 15%); ductal in situ, including Paget disease (5%); lobular in situ (3%); inflammatory carcinoma (2% to 4%); and sarcomas (0.5% to 1%). The most common locations within the breast are the upper outer quadrant (50%), beneath the nipple (18%), and the upper inner quadrant (15%).

Once the diagnosis of breast cancer is established and confirmed by a pathologist, the cancer is staged and treatment decisions begin. The most widely accepted clinical staging system, approved by the American Joint Commission on Cancer, uses the TNM classification.

TABLE 26-2. Metanalysis of Randomized Clinical Trials That Included Women Aged 40–49 Years*

STUDY (DATES)	NO. OF MAMMOGRAPHY VIEWS	SCREENING FREQUENCY (MO)	FOLLOW-UP (YR)	RELATIVE RISK	95% CONFIDENCE INTERVAL	MORTALITY (%)
HIP, NY (1963–69)	2	12	18	0.77	0.53–1.11	–23
Malmo, Sweden (1976–86)	1 or 2	18–24	12	0.51	0.22–1.17	–49
Kopparberg, Sweden (1977–85)	1	24	13	0.73	0.37–1.41	–27
Ostergotland, Sweden (1977–85)	1	24	13	1.02	0.52–1.99	+2
Edinburgh, Scotland (1979–88)	1 or 2	24	11	0.78	0.46–1.51	–22
Stockholm, Sweden (1981–85)	1	28	8	1.04	0.53–2.05	+4
Gothenburg, Sweden (1982–88)	2	18	10	0.60	0.34–1.08	–40
All Trials				0.76	0.62–0.95	–24

*National Breast Screening Study of Canada excluded.

(Feig SA. Estimation of currently attainable benefit from mammographic screening of women aged 40–49 years. Cancer 1995; 75: 2412.)

The most common treatment options for invasive breast cancer include modified radical mastectomy or conservative breast-preservation surgeries, including quadrantectomy or wide local excision with axillary node dissection. A modified radical mastectomy is complete removal of the breast, pectoralis major fascia, and level I and II axillary lymph nodes, with preservation of the pectoralis muscles. A breast-conserving operation is a wide local excision and resection of the tumor with 1 or 2 cm of adjacent breast tissue. A quadrantectomy is the resection of the tumor with the overlying skin and the involved quadrant of the breast. These procedures are coupled with an axillary lymphatic dissection of level I and II lymph nodes (removal of the axillary content from the tail of the breast to the latissimus dorsi, the axillary vein superiorly, and the lateral border of the pectoralis to beneath the pectoralis minor medially) (Fig. 26-1).

When breast cancer is detected early, breast preservation is an option for most patients. Breast-preservation surgery is generally coupled with adjuvant whole breast radiation therapy when the patient has healed.

Several factors influence the choice of surgical treatment, including the size and location of the tumor and the size of the breast. Poor candidates for breast preservation are women with large tumors, multifocal diffuse tumors, or small breasts. Age is not a contraindication to breast preservation.

Breast reconstruction should be discussed with all patients who are considering mastectomy. The reconstruction may be performed in conjunction with the primary surgery or delayed, waiting until completion of adjuvant chemotherapy or radiation therapy. Cancer is a potential killer, but the threat of death is abstract and vague. Thoughts of disfigurement are ever-present, and the physical and mental adjustment to the diagnosis of breast cancer and the removal of the breast is an important part of the recovery process. Breast reconstruction is a vital aspect of that recovery process. The options for reconstruction include prosthetic augmentation with saline-filled implants and reconstruction with a myocutaneous flap, such as the rectus abdominis muscles. These decisions are made by the patient and her surgical team and vary according to her body habitus, medical problems, and prior surgery.

Breast-preservation procedures result in survival rates equal to those of modified radical mastectomies. In a randomized trial comparing breast-conserving surgery without and without radiation therapy to mastectomy for tumors up to 4 cm, there was no difference in distant relapses or mortality among the three study groups, with a 10-year survival of 38% in stage I and II patients. There was a substantial rate of local breast relapse in the breast-conservation patients who did not receive radiation therapy (36% versus 5% for node-positive patients and 30% versus 10% for node-negative patients). The study concluded that breast-conserving surgery is comparable to mastectomy and that 50-cGy whole breast radiation therapy is recommended in breast-conservation patients. The radiation therapy is well tolerated and has a proven benefit and minimal side effects. The 1990 National Cancer Institute of Health Consensus Conference on Early Breast Cancer concluded that breast-conserving surgery was the preferred treatment option for most patients.

In the era of managed care, cost may become an important issue, as breast conservation with radiation therapy is more expensive than mastectomy. However, the patient's cosmetic results and psychological well-being should be the highest considerations when discussing the treatment course in curable cancer patients.

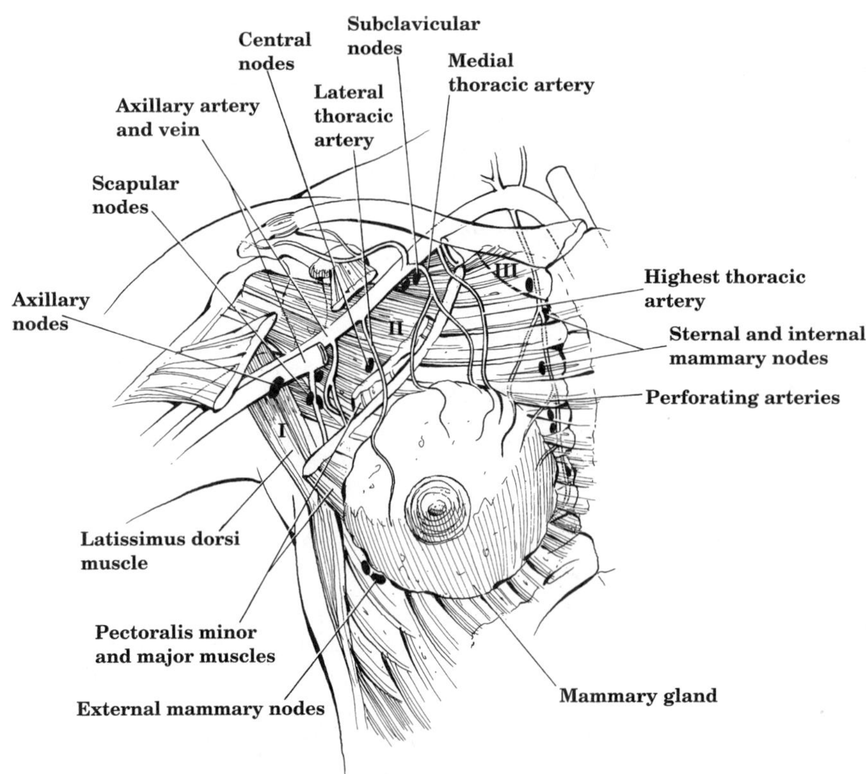

Figure 26-1. Lymphatics and blood supply of the breast. (Rock JA, Thompson JD, eds. Te Linde's operative gynecology, 8th ed. Philadelphia: Lippincott-Raven, 1996; with permission.)

ADJUVANT THERAPY

Tumor size and axillary nodal status are the most important prognostic factors affecting breast cancer survival. Patients with negative axillary nodes have 78% 5-year and 65% 10-year crude survival rates and an 82% 5-year disease-free survival rate. When axillary nodal disease is present, the crude survival rates drop to 46% at 5 years and 25% at 10 years, with a 35% 5-year disease-free survival. The number of nodes involved is important as well.

Therefore, all node-positive patients should receive adjuvant treatment. For premenopausal patients, chemotherapy is recommended, regardless of hormone-receptor status. Ovarian suppression may be considered for patients who do not become ovulatory after chemotherapy. In postmenopausal node-positive patients who are positive for estrogen receptor (ER), tamoxifen citrate therapy is indicated. ER-negative postmenopausal patients should be offered chemotherapy, assuming they are in good health. These women might also benefit from the addition of tamoxifen.

Adjuvant therapy—such as chemotherapy, ovarian ablation, tamoxifen, or immunotherapy—can also be of benefit in several groups of node-negative patients. These node-negative patients are generally stratified into menopausal status and then are divided into risk categories according to prognostic factors; the 5-year recurrence rate for node-negative patients varies according to these factors:

- Low risk (5-year recurrence risk < 10%): Noninvasive tumor, tumor size less than 1 cm, nuclear grade I, low S-phase fraction
- Intermediate risk (5-year recurrence risk 10% to 27%): tumor size less than 2 cm, nuclear grade II, ER-positive tumor
- High risk (5-year recurrence risk 25% to 35%): nuclear grade II, high S-phase fraction, ER-negative tumor
- Extremely high risk (5-year recurrence risk 55%): combination of high HER-2, ER-positivity, tumor size less than 3 cm.

Node-negative patients at minimal or low risk need no additional treatment. The moderate-risk group should receive tamoxifen. Patients at high risk are divided into premenopausal and postmenopausal subgroups. All high-risk premenopausal patients should receive chemotherapy, regardless of ER status. Tamoxifen might be added with ER-positive tumors. For postmenopausal node-negative patients, ER receptor status becomes more important. Chemotherapy has been the treatment of choice for ER-negative tumors, possibly with the addition of tamoxifen, although further investigation is needed. Tamoxifen is recommended for ER-negative, node-negative, high-risk menopausal patients. Chemotherapy may be beneficial with tamoxifen, but further evaluation is needed. The final category is the elderly node-negative patient. These patients are divided into low, good, and high risk, and their therapy is individualized according to their medical health.

Tamoxifen reduces recurrence by 25% and mortality by 17%. Longer-duration tamoxifen therapy is more effective than its short-term use, although the exact duration is still being defined, as are the side effects, including the risk of endometrial cancer. Polychemotherapy reduces recurrence by 28% and death by 16%, with a greater effect seen in premenopausal patients. Combined chemoendocrine therapy may be more effective than either one used alone. Immunotherapy does not seem to show benefits in the adjuvant treatment of breast cancer.

Ovarian castration can be performed surgically with oophorectomy or medically with gonadotropin-releasing hormone agonists. No benefit is seen in postmenopausal patients, but premenopausal patients undergoing surgical ovarian ablation have a 30% improvement in disease-free survival and overall survival, similar to the results with polychemotherapy. Randomized trials are underway comparing ovarian ablation to tamoxifen therapy in ER-positive, node-negative patients. The long-term side effects of castration need further investigation, especially osteoporosis and heart disease.

HORMONE REPLACEMENT THERAPY

The debate regarding the risk of hormone replacement therapy (HRT) and breast cancer continues. Numerous studies concerning the risk of breast cancer have failed to provide clear answers. The Nurses' Health Prospective Cohort Study, which involved a questionnaire sent to 121,700 female registered nurses, found that the relative risk of breast cancer was 1.32 for the estrogen-alone groups when compared with postmenopausal women who had never used hormones. The addition of progesterone to estrogen therapy did not reduce the risk. Another study compared white women age 50 to 64 with histologically confirmed breast cancer to a matched control group; it failed to show an increased risk of breast cancer associated with current or long-term (20 years or more) use of estrogen alone or combined estrogen-progestin therapy. An elevated risk was observed in the users of combined HRT who had undergone hysterectomy with bilateral oophorectomy. However, the number of these patients is small and the duration of HRT was short in this group, so the significance remains uncertain.

Pregnancy is a highly estrogenic state. Breast cancers diagnosed during pregnancy do not appear to have a worse prognosis than those in nonpregnant patients when matched by stage.

One study showed that HRT may even have a protective effect against breast cancer. The mortality rate for cardiovascular disease among U.S. women is ten times that of breast cancer. It is estimated that cardiac mortality can be reduced by 50% with the use of postmenopausal estrogen replacement therapy. Osteoporosis mortality can also be reduced with the addition of exogenous estrogens.

The risks and benefits of HRT must be thoroughly discussed with the patient. No woman can be guaranteed protection from a recurrent breast cancer, nor can she be guaranteed not to suffer a myocardial infarction while on HRT. Primary care providers must keep current with the literature, research the individual patient's risk of recurrent cancer and of subsequent heart disease, and factor in quality-of-life issues before deciding to prescribe or withhold hormones for postmenopausal women.

BIBLIOGRAPHY

American College of Obstetricians and Gynecologists. The role of the obstetrician-gynecologist in the diagnosis and treatment of breast disease. ACOG Committee Opinion #140, June 1994.

Barrett-Connor E, Bush TL. Estrogen and coronary breast disease in women. JAMA 1991;265:1861.

Beahrs OH, Henson DE, Hutter MD, Kennedy BJ (eds). Manual for staging of cancer, ed 4. Philadelphia: JB Lippincott, 1992.

Cambrell RD Jr, Maier RC, Sanders BI. Decreased incidence of breast cancer in postmenopausal estrogen-progestogen users. Obstet Gynecol 1983;62:435.

Colditz GA, Hankinson SE, Hunter DJ, et al. The use of estrogens and progestins and the risk of breast cancer in postmenopausal women. N Engl J Med 1995;332:1589.

Consensus Development Conference on the Treatment of Early-Stage Breast Cancer. J Natl Cancer Inst Monogr 1992;11:1.

Easton DF, Bishop DT, Ford D, et al. Genetic linkage analysis in familial breast and ovarian cancer: result from 214 families: The Breast Cancer Linkage Consortium. Am J Hum Genet 1993;52:678.

Feig SA. Mammographic screening of women aged 40–49 years: is it justified? Obstet Gynecol Clin North Am 1994;21:587.

Fisher B, Redmond C, Fisher ER, et al. Ten-year results of a randomized clinical trial comparing radical mastectomy and total mastectomy with or without radiation. N Engl J Med 1985;312:674.

Henderson IC, Canellos GP. Cancer of the breast. The past decade. N Engl J Med 1980;302(1):17.

Hortobagyi GN, Buzdak AU. Current status of adjuvant systemic therapy for primary breast cancer: progress and controversy. CA Cancer J Clin 1995;45:199.

Kopans DB, Feig SA. The Canadian National Breast Screening Study: A critical review. AJR 1993;161:755.

Lee JM. Screening and informed consent. N Engl J Med 1993;328:438.

McGuire LW, Clarke MG. Prognostic factors and treatment decisions in axillary node-negative breast cancer. N Engl J Med 1992;326:1756.

Murphy WA Jr, Destrovet JM, Monsees BS. Professional quality assurance for mammography screening programs. Radiology 1990;175:319.

Stanford JL, Weiss NS, Voigt LF, Daling JR, Habel LA, Rossing MA. Combined estrogen and progestin hormone replacement therapy in relation to risk of breast cancer in middle-age women. JAMA 1995;274:137.

Wingo PA, Tong T, Bolden S. Cancer statistics 1995. CA Cancer J Clin 1995;45:8.

27

Premalignant Lesions of the Cervix

REINALDO SANCHEZ

Primary Care for Women, edited by Phyllis C. Leppert and Fred M. Howard. Lippincott-Raven Publishers, Philadelphia © 1997.

Over the past 30 years, there has been a significant reduction in the incidence of cervical cancer, but the prevalence of premalignant lesions of the cervix has increased, particularly among young women in their childbearing years. Therefore, accurate diagnoses and treatments that preserve fertility potential are important. The Pap smear and colposcopy have been responsible for the decrease in the incidence of cervical cancer, because they allow lesions to be detected in the premalignant stages.

Several epidemiologic studies have shown the following risk factors: early onset of first coitus, multiple sex partners, high parity, low socioeconomic group, use of oral contraceptive pills, history of sexually transmitted disease, and history of previous vulvar intraepithelial neoplasia and cervical intraepithelial neoplasia (CIN). Factors that affect the patient's immunologic competency also put her at risk for CIN (eg, HIV infection, smoking, vitamin deficiencies, treatment with immunosuppressive drugs).

The most significant finding in the last decade is the correlation between human papilloma virus (HPV) infection and CIN. Figure 27-1 shows a proposed model for HPV infection followed by progression to CIN into invasive disease. Some strains of HPV are more often associated with cervical neoplasia (eg, HPV 16, 18, 31). Whether DNA typing will affect how aggressive or conservative the treatment should be for a particular patient remains under investigation.

DIAGNOSIS

Pap Smear

Cervical cytology is an excellent screening test. It is cost-effective, simple to do, and well accepted by patients and providers; it offers adequate specificity and sensitivity; and, most importantly, it is very effective in detecting premalignant disease. The frequency for screening remains controversial. The American Cancer Society suggests that low-risk groups be screened every 3 years. The American College of Obstetricians and Gynecologists recommends that patients who are or have been sexually active, or are 18 years or older should have cervical cytology annually and a complete pelvic examination. After three normal Pap smears and pelvic examinations, the test may be performed at the discretion of the physician. This group also recommends annual examinations for those who are at high risk.

Physicians must become familiar with the terminology used by their cytopathology laboratory (Table 27-1) and should know the laboratory's false-negative and false-positive rates.

Figure 27-2 shows the most common method used for collecting cervical cells. Immediate fixation of the material is important to prevent air-drying artifacts. Once a squamous intraepithelial lesion (SIL) is reported, arrangement for colposcopic evaluation should immediately follow. In the case of a gross cervical lesion identified with the naked eye, biopsy rather than a Pap smear should be performed immediately.

Abnormal Pap Smear in Pregnancy

In an abnormal Pap smear in pregnancy, immediate evaluation by colposcopy should be done. The goal is to exclude microinvasive or invasive disease of the cervix as early as possible during the pregnancy. In view of the vascular changes that occur during pregnancy, the colposcopic evaluation must be performed by a colposcopist with vast experience in doing colposcopies in pregnant patients. The physiologic changes in the cervix and the hormonally induced eversion permit good visualization of the transformation zone and the squamocolumnar junction. Evidence supports the safety and reliability of colposcopically directed biopsies during pregnancy. Some experienced colposcopists perform biopsies only when invasive or microinvasive disease is suspected. Once microinvasive or invasive carcinoma is excluded, treatment is deferred to the postpartum period, and management during the rest of the pregnancy consists of interval Pap smears or colposcopy.

Colposcopy

The colposcope is a microscope designed to visualize the cervix under six- to 40-fold magnification. High-intensity illumination and a green filter allow the visualization of vascular changes characteristic of squamous cervical intraepithelial lesions. Its use

Table 27-1. Terminology in Cervical Cytology

Clinical Diagnosis	Histologic and Cytologic Diagnosis	Bethesda System
Normal	Normal	Normal
Atypical metaplasia	Atypical cells	ASCUS†
CIN I*	Mild dysplasia	Low-grade squamous intraepithelial lesion (HPV included)
CIN II	Moderate dysplasia	High-grade squamous intraepithlial lesion
CIN III	Severe dysplasia Carcinoma in situ	

*Cervical intraepithelial neoplasia
†Atypical squamous cells of undetermined significance

has been expanded to the evaluation of the entire lower genital tract, including the vagina and vulva.

The basic equipment, besides the colposcope, consists of Graves speculums of different sizes, cotton swabs, sponges, ring forceps, an endocervical speculum, endobrushes, an endocervical curet, punch biopsy forceps (eg, Burke, Tischler, Kevorkian), 3% acetic acid solution, Lugol's iodine solution, and Monsel's solution or silver nitrate sticks for hemostasis.

The patient is placed in the dorsolithotomy position and the speculum is inserted. The acetic acid is applied by spraying the cervix with a 5-mL syringe or with the cotton swab. The acetic acid solution makes it easy to remove the cervical mucus and accentuates the difference between squamous epithelium and columnar epithelium, making the latter turn white, so the squamocolumnar junction can be easily identified. Also, abnormal tissue in the transformation zone appears as aceto white epithelium, contrasting with the pink color of normal squamous epithelium. Vascular patterns contrast with the white background, making it easy to identify areas of punctation, mosaicism, or atypical vessels (Fig. 27-3). Any of these lesions must be biopsied. An endocervical specimen is obtained either by endobrush or endocervical curettage. The iodine test is helpful when no apparent lesion is seen on the initial part of the procedure. It stains dark cells with a high content of glycogen, such as normal squamous epithelium, leaving the abnormal cells and the columnar cells basically unstained. If a lesion extends inside the endocervical canal, an effort should be made to visualize

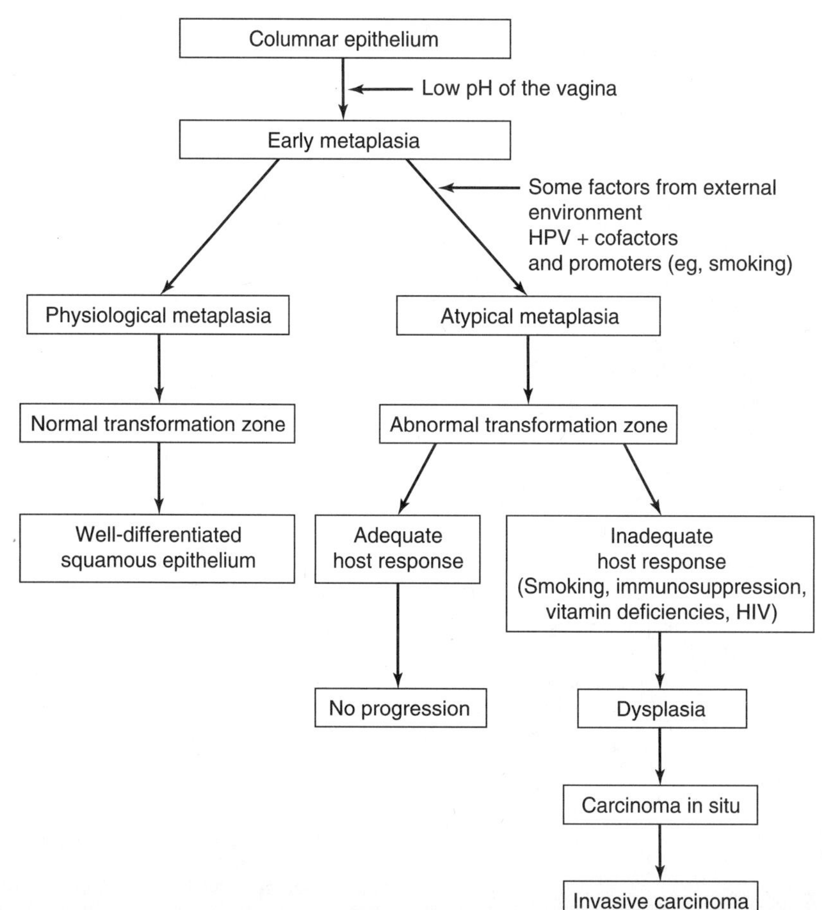

Figure 27-1. Pathogenesis of cervical neoplasia. (Modified from Stafl A, Mattingly RF. Vaginal adenosis. Am J Obstet Gynecol 1974;120:666.)

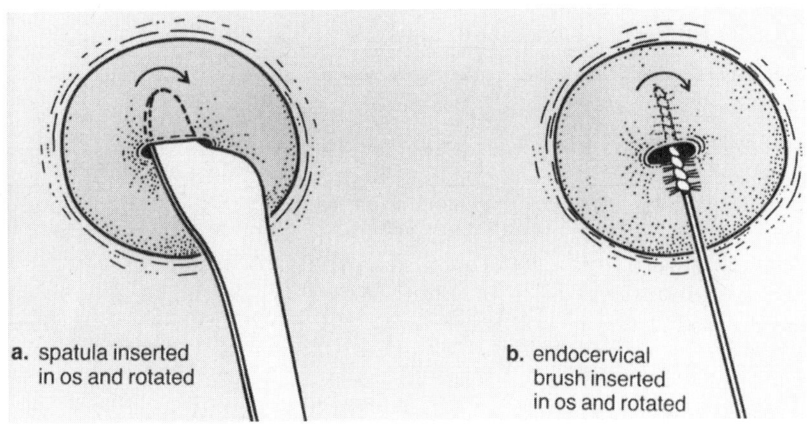

Figure 27-2. Obtaining a cervical smear, using (***a***) a spatula and (***b***) an endocervical brush. (Anderson M, Jordan J, Moore A, Sharp F. A text and atlas of integrated colposcopy. St. Louis: Mosby-Year Book, 1991.)

the lesion in toto; this can be achieved by using the endocervical speculum.

A colposcopy is considered satisfactory if the squamocolumnar junction and the entire transformation zone are identified, as well as any lesion. If the colposcopy was unsatisfactory because of inability to recognize the new squamocolumnar junction, or because the lesion was not completely delineated, then punch biopsies might be deferred, as that patient requires a more advanced diagnostic procedure such as a top-hat large loop excision of the transformation zone (LLETZ) or a cone biopsy (laser or cold knife cone). If invasive disease is suspected, a punch biopsy should be done even if the lesion was not completely visualized. Other indications for any of these

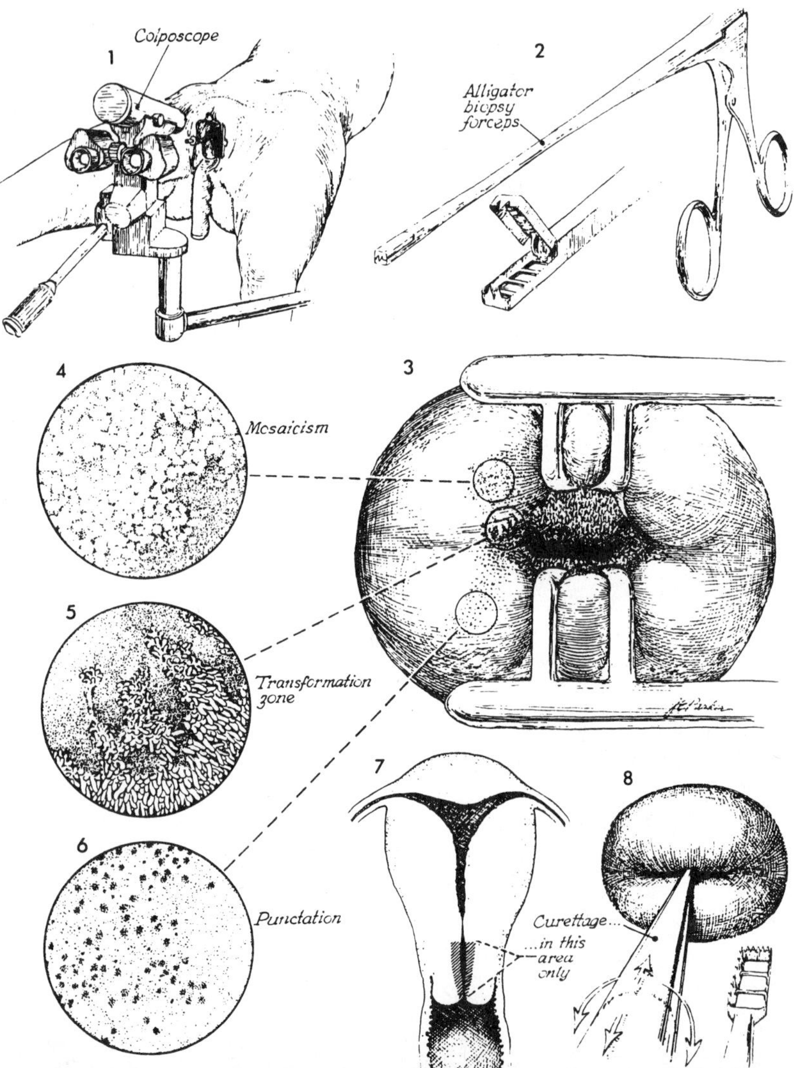

Figure 27-3. Colposcopy. (Modified from Wheeless CR. Atlas of pelvic surgery, 2nd ed. Philadelphia: Lea & Febiger, 1988:183.)

three types of conization include a positive endocervical specimen, colposcopy suspicious for occult invasive disease regardless of the results of the punch biopsy, discrepancy of two grades between cytology and histology, and microinvasive disease on punch biopsy. In microinvasive disease, cold knife cone biopsy is the diagnostic procedure of choice to avoid any thermal damage that could impair an accurate histologic diagnosis by the pathologist.

After the colposcopy, the patient is instructed to avoid vaginal intercourse or the use of tampons for 2 weeks, and a follow-up appointment is scheduled for 2 to 4 weeks later to discuss the results and follow up.

If the Pap smear reports glandular atypia or dysplasia, the diagnosis is more challenging. Colposcopy, endocervical curettage, and endometrial sampling should be performed, because the disease can be coming from either the endocervix or endometrium. If all of the above are negative, with an endocervical curettage showing normal endocervical glands, an argument can be made for close surveillance with repeated Pap smears and perhaps endocervical curettage or aggressive endocervical brush. Nevertheless, if the endocervical curettage is nondiagnostic or if the glandular atypia persists, a diagnostic conization is warranted (top-hat LLETZ, laser or cold knife cone).

TREATMENT

A complete colposcopic evaluation of the cervix must be done by an experienced colposcopist before the use of any of the therapeutic modalities available for premalignant conditions of the cervix. The Pap smear is a screening test, not a diagnostic test.

Cryotherapy

Cryosurgery is one of the most popular methods for the treatment of CIN. It is an office procedure that usually does not require anesthesia. It offers cure rates above 90% for CIN I and CIN II; for CIN III, other therapeutic modalities are preferred. The equipment consists of a gas tank containing nitrous oxide connected to a pistol that delivers the gas to the cryotip, producing temperatures below −70°C (Fig. 27-4)

The patient is placed in a dorsolithotomy position. The cervix is inspected and the extension of the lesion is defined. A cryotip that will cover the entire lesion is selected and applied to the affected area. Freezing is continued until the iceball extends 5 mm away from the edges of the cryotip, which correlates with a 4- to 5-mm depth of tissue destruction. The other option is the 3-minute freeze, 5-minute thaw, and 3-minute freeze described by Creasman and coworkers in 1973.

During and immediately after the procedure, the patient might experience mild uterine cramps that usually respond to nonsteroidal antiinflammatory agents. It is important to explain to the patient that a profuse watery vaginal discharge with an odor is to be expected for 4 weeks. Tampons and intercourse should be avoided for 3 to 4 weeks. If fever or pelvic pain beyond mild cramps develops, immediate evaluation is warranted, because infection is the most common complication of this procedure. Three to 4 months after the procedure, a repeat Pap smear is performed, followed by Pap smears at 6-month intervals. After two or three negative cytology results, the patient can go back to routine screening.

Although the procedure is highly successful, one of the disadvantages is that after the healing process is finished, stenosis and

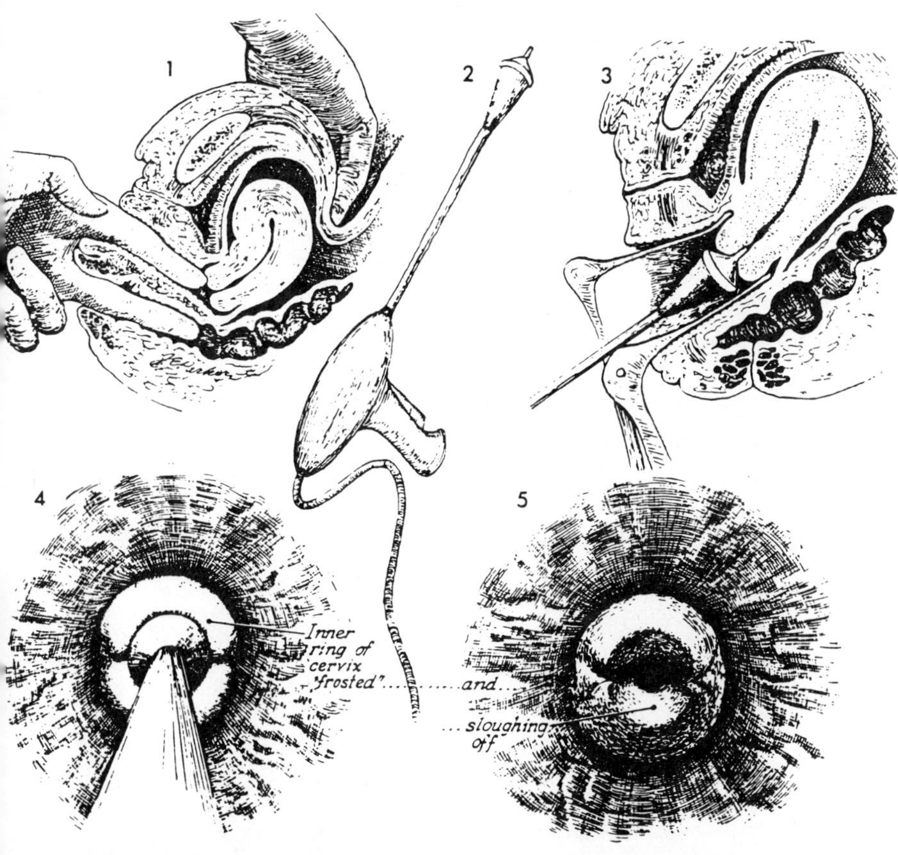

Figure 27-4. Cryosurgery of cervix. (Modified from Wheeless CR. Atlas of pelvic surgery, 2nd ed. Philadelphia: Lea & Febiger, 1988:185.)

scarring preclude the visualization of the new squamocolumnar junction.

CO_2 Laser Ablation

The CO_2 laser machine has an output of up to 100 watts and can be adjusted to a continuous or pulsatile flow of energy, depending on the procedure. The amount of wattage to use depends on whether the laser is being used as an ablative instrument or a cutting device—low wattage (10 to 30) is preferred for ablation. The laser is used for the treatment of genital warts or extensive cervical lesions that are difficult to excise by the LLETZ technique.

All personnel in the room, including the patient, must wear glasses designed for CO_2 laser protection. The patient is prepared for a vaginal procedure and a nonreflective speculum is placed. The cervix is reevaluated either by another colposcopy or by staining the cervix with Lugol's iodine solution. A cervical block is given by using 10 mL of 1% lidocaine with epinephrine, or any other equivalent solution of local anesthetic with vasoconstrictive medication. This is not a paracervical block: the goal is to infiltrate the cervical stroma, and a waiting period until complete blanching is seen is recommended. The laser joystick can be attached to the colposcope or it can be used freely. The transformation zone is identified and marked with 3 mm of clearance of normal tissue. It is divided into quadrants, and each quadrant is worked on independently until a complete vaporization is achieved, all the way down to 7 mm of depth (Fig. 27-5). If bleeding occurs, hemostasis can be obtained by defocusing the laser beam or by using electrocautery.

Large Loop Excision of the Transformation Zone

Large loop excision of the transformation zone is used commonly for the treatment of CIN II and III. It is both curative and diagnostic, therefore decreasing the chance of missing a more advanced lesion. It is an office procedure done under local anesthesia, and it can be done in the same visit as the colposcopy, an important strategy for clinics with a significant number of noncompliant patients. The success rate is 90% to 98% for the treatment of SIL. It is well accepted by patients; mild discomfort is reported by a minority of patients.

A diathermy ground plate is attached to the patient. A nonconductive speculum is applied and a suction tube is attached to it to aspirate fumes and to allow adequate visualization. The cervix is inspected with the colposcope or with Lugol's solution and the extension of the lesion is assessed. An appropriate size of loop is selected. Whether the lesion is taken in toto or in parts depends on its extension. For lesions extending into the canal, a follow-up excision of the canal with a smaller square loop (1 × 1 cm) in a top-hat fashion is recommended after the initial excision. The power setting is selected depending on the size of the loop (Fig. 27-6). A stromal infiltration with 1% lidocaine with epinephrine is used, and after complete blanching of the cervix is seen, the procedure is performed (Fig. 27-7). Hemostasis is secured by using the ball cautery.

The patient is instructed to avoid tampons, vaginal douches, or intercourse for 4 weeks. A discharge similar to the one seen after cryosurgery might occur. The patient is instructed regarding fever or excessive pain and is told to report any bleeding to the provider immediately. A follow-up Pap smear is recommended as for cryosurgery.

Laser Cone

Conization of the cervix can be done with the laser. The power is increased to high wattage, decreasing the spot diameter and making the laser beam work as a knife. This procedure can be done under local anesthesia, using the same approach described above. The patient is positioned and a nonreflective speculum is inserted with the suction tube attached to it. The lesion and the transformation zone are identified and then marked, with 3-mm margins left around the lesion. With a small hook device, the specimen is mobi-

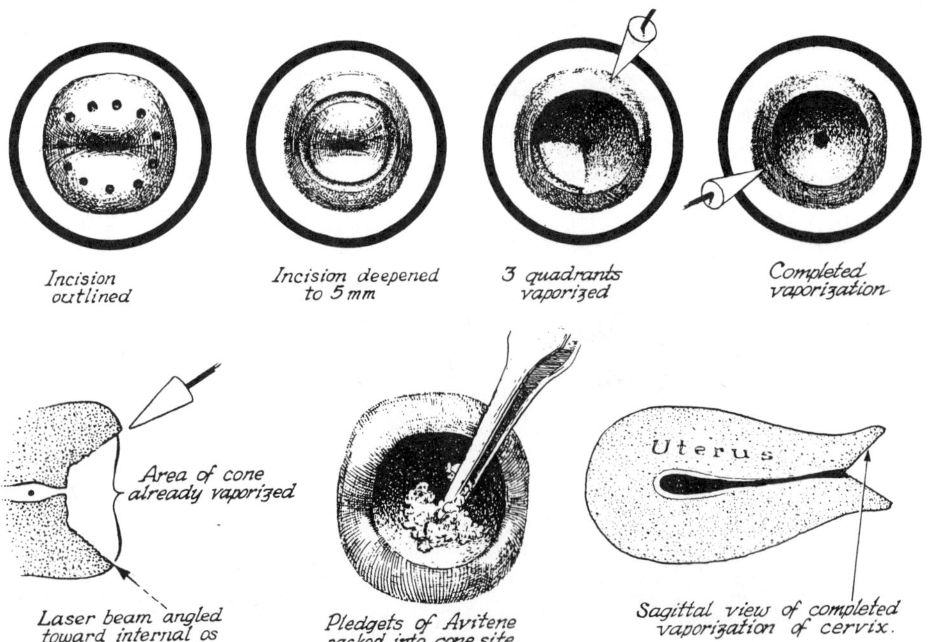

Figure 27-5. CO_2 laser ablation technique. (Modified from Wheeless CR. Atlas of pelvic surgery, 2nd ed. Philadelphia: Lea & Febiger, 1988:191.)

Loop	Width & depth (mm)	Wire length (mm)	Finesse power setting (W)	Force 2 power setting (W)
	10×10	26	50	25
	15×12	33	60	30
	20×12	35	60	40
	20×15	41	60	40
	20×20	51	70	45

Figure 27-6. Suggested power settings for full-depth cuts. Blend 1, for Utah Medical's Finesse ESU and Valleylab's Force 2 ESU. The power output needed depends on the length of wire contact with the tissue at any point in time. Some newer units have a feedback system that continuously recognizes the resistance in the tissue and adjusts the output accordingly. (Prendiville W. Bailliere's Clin Obstet Gynecol 1995;9:194.)

lized to facilitate the progression of the procedure until the specimen is completely excised. Although it is a good technique, it has lost popularity due to the simplicity of the LLETZ technique.

Cold Knife Cone

Conization has been considered the standard of care and definitive treatment for carcinoma in situ and high-grade lesions. Nevertheless, it has been replaced by some of the techniques described above, such as laser cone and LLETZ, particularly in young patients in whom postsurgical stenosis of the cervix might impair future fertility. Although usually performed under general anesthesia, it can be done with a combination of conscious sedation and a similar block as described above. It remains a useful technique for patients with a nonvisible lesion inside the endocervical canal that cannot be visualized with an endocervical speculum.

The cervical branches of the uterine artery are bilaterally ligated with a hemostatic figure-of-eight suture with 1-0 absorbable synthetic material. This initial ligation helps minimize bleeding and aids in traction and exposure of the cervix. The stroma of the cervix is infiltrated with a local anesthetic with a vasopressive solution of epinephrine. With a scalpel, a cone is done and the specimen, whether a strict cone shape or a narrow but cylindrical one, is obtained (Fig. 27-8). Hemostasis is secured by using a suction cautery device or by placing individual figure-of-eight sutures of synthetic absorbable material. In contrast to laser cone and the LLETZ technique, the cervical margins must be free of disease.

Hysterectomy

Although widely used in the past as treatment for premalignant conditions of the cervix, hysterectomy is not as popular today in view of the highly successful, less invasive therapeutic options. It is still indicated in microinvasive carcinoma. It can also be considered in patients with CIN III, carcinoma in situ, or glandular dysplasia

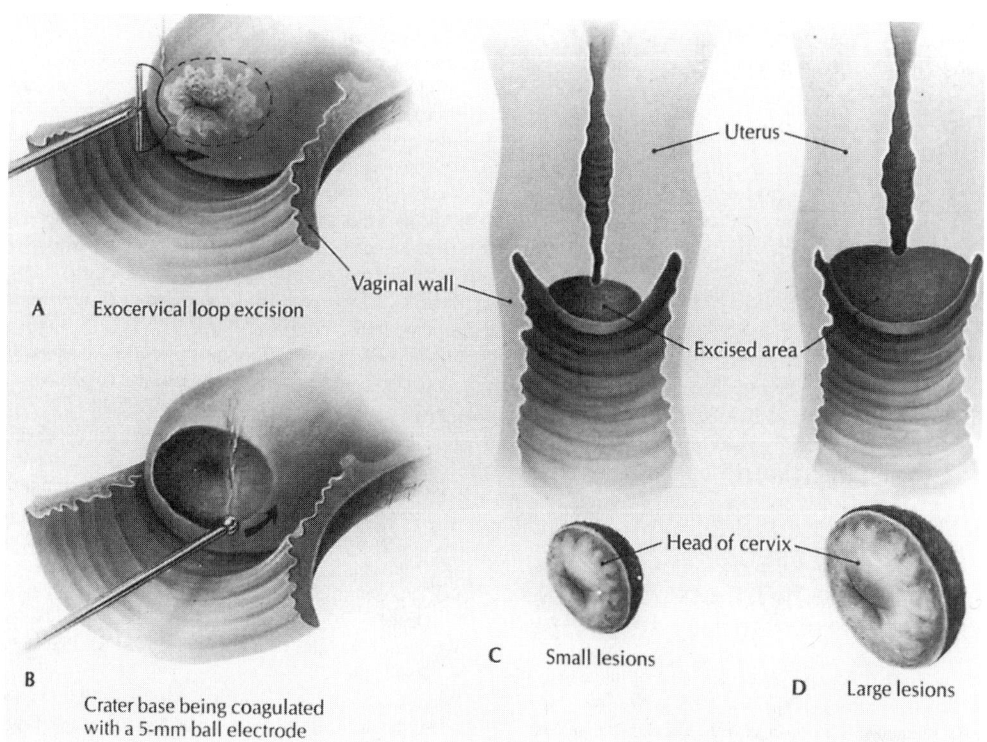

Figure 27-7. Large loop excision of the transformation zone (LLETZ technique). (Apgar B, Wright T, Pfenninger J. Loop electrosurgical excision procedure for CIN. Am Fam Physician 1992;46:514.)

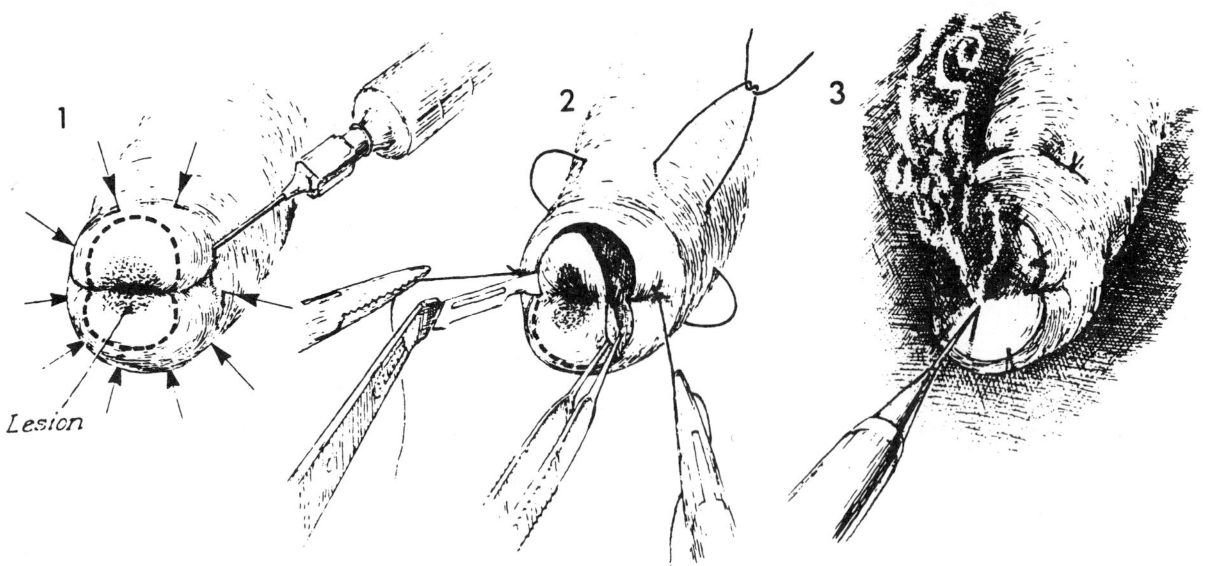

Figure 27-8. Cold knife cone technique. ((Modified from Wheeless CR. Atlas of pelvic surgery, 2nd ed. Philadelphia: Lea & Febiger, 1988:187.)

when further fertility is not an issue, particularly if other gynecologic pathology coexists. It can also be considered if the margins of the cone (cold knife) are involved with disease, and when several more conservative therapies have failed. The type or route of the hysterectomy (abdominal, vaginal, laparoscopically assisted vaginal) depends more on the surgeon's preferences and skills. After the hysterectomy, it is important to continue Pap smear surveillance in these patients, as vaginal dysplasia, although rare, has been reported. Furthermore, the same etiologic factors that induced the cervical changes are still present in the lower genital tract.

SUMMARY

Premalignant conditions of the cervix can be successfully treated by the techniques described above, thus preventing cervical cancer. Adequate colposcopic evaluation of the cervix and endocervix with appropriate biopsies to rule out microinvasive or invasive disease of the cervix should always precede any therapeutic modality. Cryosurgery is the most commonly used technique for low-grade SIL, and LLETZ is becoming the preferred technique for high-grade SIL. The LLETZ technique is replacing cone biopsy (laser or cold knife cone) as a diagnostic tool for unsatisfactory colposcopy in young patients.

BIBLIOGRAPHY

ACOG Committee Opinion. Recommendation on frequency of Pap test screening. Internat J Gynecol Obstet 1995;49:210.

Andersen W, Frieson H, Barber S, Tabbarah S, Taylor P, Underwood P. Sensitivity and specificity of endocervical curettage and the endocervical brush for the evaluation of the endocervical canal. Am J Obstet Gynecol 1988;159:702.

Anderson M, Jordan J, Morse A, Sharp F. A text and atlas of integrated colposcopy, 1st ed. St. Louis: Mosby-Year Book, 1991.

Apgar BS, Wright TC, Pfenninger J. Loop electrosurgical excision procedure for CIN. Am Fam Physician 1992;46:505.

Berek JS, Hacker NF. Practical gynecologic oncology. Baltimore: Williams & Wilkins, 1989:195.

Brisson J, Morin C, Fortier M, et al. Risk factors for cervical intraepithelial neoplasia: differences between low- and high-grade lesions. Am J Epidemiol 1994;140:700.

Brotzman GL, Apgar BS. Cervical intraepithelial neoplasia: current management options. J Fam Prac 1994;39:271.

Economos K, Perez Veridiano N, Delke I, Loh Collado M, Tancer ML. Abnormal cervical cytology in pregnancy: a 17-year experience. Obstet Gynecol 1993;81:915.

Herbst AL. The Bethesda System for cervical/vaginal cytologic diagnosis. Clin Obstet Gynecol 1992;35:22.

Hoffman MS, Sterghos S, Gordy LW, Gunasekaran S, Cavanagh D. Evaluation of the cervical canal with the endocervical brush. Obstet Gynecol 1993;82:573.

Jones HW. Cervical intraepithelial neoplasia. Bailliere's Clin Obstet Gynecol 1995;9:1.

Lonky NM, Navarre GL, Saunders S, Sadeghi M, Walde-Tsadik G. Low-grade Papanicolaou smears and the Bethesda System: a prospective cytohistopathologic analysis. Obstet Gynecol 1995;86:716.

Mayeaux EJ, Harper MB. Loop electrosurgical excisional procedure. J Fam Prac 1993;36:214.

Mayeaux EJ, Harper MB, Abreo F, Pope JB, Phillips GS. A comparison of the reliability of repeat cervical smears and colposcopy in patients with abnormal cervical cytology. J Fam Prac 1995;40:57.

Thompson JD, Rock JA. TeLinde's operative gynecology, 7th ed. Philadelphia: JB Lippincott, 1992:1141.

Raju KS, Henderson E, Trehan A. A study comparing LETZ and CO_2 laser treatment for cervical intraepithelial neoplasia with and without associated human papilloma virus. Am J Gynec Oncol 1995;16:92.

Stafl A, Mattingly RT. Vaginal adenosis: a precancerous lesion. Am J Obstet Gynecol 1974;120:666.

Wheeless CR. Atlas of pelvic surgery, 2d ed. Philadelphia: Lea & Febiger, 1988:180.

Widra EA, Dookhan D, Jordan A, McCue P, Bibbo M, Dunton CJ. Evaluation of the atypical cytologic smear. Validity of the 1991 Bethesda System. J Repro Med 1994;39:682.

Wilkinson EJ. Pap smears and screening for cervical neoplasia. Clinical Obstet Gynecol 1990;33:817.

Primary Care for Women, edited by Phyllis C. Leppert and Fred M. Howard. Lippincott-Raven Publishers, Philadelphia © 1997.

28

Cervical Carcinoma

BRENT DUBESHTER

Invasive cervical carcinoma is arguably the most preventable malignancy in women. Although more widespread screening has led to a reduced incidence in the United States, cervical cancer remains the fourth most common female malignancy. Despite a long and treatable preinvasive phase (cervical intraepithelial neoplasia [CIN]), 15,000 new cases and 4600 deaths were expected in 1994. Early detection of CIN is critical, and fortunately Pap smear screening is widely available.

Risk factors strongly associated with the development of cervical carcinoma, such as early age of first coitus and multiple partners, have supported the view that a sexually transmitted agent is an important causative factor. Although an association between herpesvirus type II and cervical cancer has been found, an etiologic role has not been confirmed. Human papillomavirus (HPV) is considered an important cofactor in the development of cervical cancer. HPV types 16, 18, 31, 33, 35, and 39 have been associated with high-grade dysplasia and carcinoma, but the role of HPV subtyping in the management of dysplasia and carcinoma is uncertain.

ETIOLOGY

The cause of cervical cancer is unknown. However, it would appear that women are particularly susceptible to some inciting event associated with coitus for several years after menarche, a time during which the transformation zone of the cervix is undergoing active squamous metaplasia. Epidemiologic studies strongly support a sexually transmitted agent, probably HPV, as an important cofactor. The risk of cervical cancer in women beginning intercourse before age 15 is double that of those whose first coitus was after age 20. Squamous cell carcinoma of the cervix is virtually unknown among nuns. A "male factor" also may be important: the risk is three times higher for the current wife of a man whose previous wife had cervical cancer. These facts are all consistent with the theory that a sexually transmittable agent, probably HPV, has a role in cervical carcinogenesis.

SCREENING

No consensus has been reached regarding the optimal, most cost-effective program of cervical cytologic screening. The American College of Obstetricians and Gynecologists recommends that Pap smears be performed in women at age 18 or when sexually active, and annually thereafter. In patients who have had three or more annual normal smears, the interval of testing may be increased at the discretion of the physician. However, the false-negative rate of cervical cytology is 20% to 30% for squamous lesions and up to 40% for adenocarcinomas. In most patients, therefore, an annual pelvic examination and Pap smear is the most prudent recommendation.

In the past, cervical cytology results were reported as class I to V (Table 28-1). The 1988 Bethesda system of reporting cervical/vaginal cytology was introduced in an attempt to standardize cervical cytologic results. In this system, smears with HPV atypia and mild dysplasia are reported as LSIL (low-grade squamous intraepithelial lesions). High-grade squamous intraepithelial lesions (HSIL) include moderate and severe dysplasia and carcinoma in situ. LSIL and HSIL results require further evaluation by colposcopy and biopsy.

PRECURSORS OF CERVICAL CANCER

The site where the columnar epithelium of the endocervix meets the squamous epithelium of the portio of the cervix is known as the squamocolumnar junction. During a female's life, this junction progressively migrates from the cervical portio in newborns to well within the endocervical canal in postmenopausal women. The transformation zone where this occurs, through a process called squamous metaplasia, is the part of the cervix most prone to the development of malignancy. The metaplastic squamous epithelium in this zone is abundant early in the postmenarchal period and is undoubtedly susceptible to oncogenic triggers such as HPV exposure.

Cervical intraepithelial neoplasia (CIN), or cervical dysplasia, is a precursor of cervical cancer that may antedate invasive cervical cancer by 10 or more years. Although at one time it was thought that there was a progression of malignant change from mild dysplasia (CINI) to severe dysplasia and carcinoma in situ (CINIII), it is impossible to correlate the degree of dysplasia with the eventual risk of malignancy or the time to progress into a cancer. Therefore, in most patients, appropriate management is to treat any dysplasia confirmed by biopsy. However, up to two thirds of cases with mild dysplasia regress spontaneously. Consequently, selected patients with mild dysplasia may be monitored by periodic Pap smears and colposcopy if reliable follow-up is ensured.

The initial evaluation of all patients with LSIL or HSIL should include colposcopic evaluation of the cervix and vagina (after the application of 3% acetic acid), with directed biopsies, including an endocervical curettage (ECC). Therapy should be undertaken for biopsy-proven dysplasia only; it depends on the results of biopsies and the colposcopic findings.

In cases with an adequate colposcopy (the entire transformation zone and lesion are fully visualized) and a negative ECC, various ablative methods can be used with success. Cryocautery of the cervix is acceptable but usually results in the transformation zone being located well in the endocervical canal after healing; this may make recurrent dysplasia more difficult to evaluate. Laser ablation of the cervix is particularly well suited to patients whose lesions extend onto the vaginal fornices. The most widely used treatment of CIN is the loop electrosurgical excision procedure (LEEP), in which a loop cautery is used to excise the entire lesion and transformation zone. This method has become popular because it is simple, can be performed in an office setting, and is applicable to cases with both adequate and inadequate colposcopy.

Table 28-1. Bethesda Classification of Pap Smears

CLASS	DYSPLASIA	BETHESDA
I	Normal	Normal
II	Atypical	Reactive or reparative changes
III	Mild dysplasia	Low-grade SIL
	Moderate dysplasia	High-grade SIL
	Severe dysplasia	High-grade SIL
IV	Carcinoma in situ	High-grade SIL
V	Invasive cancer	Invasive cancer

SIL, squamous intraepithelial lesion.

An invasive cancer must be excluded in cases with a positive ECC, inadequate colposcopy, or cytologic evidence of an invasive process. A cone biopsy is mandatory in these instances. In the past, this was performed in the operating room using a scalpel, but currently LEEP is used in most instances.

HISTORY

CIN and early cases of cervical cancer are usually asymptomatic, so early detection of these patients depends on routine cytologic screening.

Abnormal vaginal bleeding is the most common symptom associated with cervical cancer. All patients who complain of abnormal bleeding should undergo a pelvic examination, and often a Pap smear, cervical biopsy, and endometrial biopsy are indicated. Vaginal discharge and odor frequently accompany bleeding but may be the primary complaint. The classic complaint of postcoital spotting is seldom the only symptom, although an occasional patient with an early cervical carcinoma presents in this fashion.

Weight loss, pelvic pain, fatigue, and weakness are not uncommon in patients with more advanced cancers. Flank pain may accompany obstructive uropathy.

PHYSICAL EXAMINATION/CLINICAL FINDINGS

Many early cervical cancers and most cases of CIN do not have any abnormalities detectable on a routine physical examination. Occasionally, an area of cervical leukoplakia may be seen on speculum examination, but usually these early cases are detectable only by colposcopy, with application of acetic acid to the cervix.

More advanced cervical cancers are virtually always accompanied by an abnormality in the appearance or consistency of the cervix. Although exophytic lesions are usually easily detected, endophytic growth patterns may have normal overlying mucosa, making diagnosis more difficult. In most of these cases, the cervix is abnormally enlarged and firm. Biopsy is mandatory whenever a cervical lesion is detected, and the clinician should not be reassured by a normal Pap smear. Even in the presence of invasive cervical cancer, only inflammatory changes may be noted on the Pap smear, particularly with an endophytic growth pattern.

The size of the tumor and the presence of vaginal or parametrial involvement should be noted. Parametrial involvement, manifest by thickening of tissue adjacent to the cervix, is accompanied by fixation of the cervix and is best detected on rectovaginal examination.

Systemic disease may be manifest by an enlarged supraclavicular lymph node. When this is detected, aspiration or biopsy is warranted.

LABORATORY AND IMAGING STUDIES

Patients with preinvasive disease (CIN) or very early cancers that do not have metastatic potential require no special laboratory or radiologic assessment. In the presence of an invasive cancer, a complete blood count and SMA-12 are routine.

Although various radiologic procedures have been used in patients with invasive cervical carcinoma, most are of limited usefulness and should be used only in specific circumstances (Table 28-2). A chest x-ray and urography (intravenous pyelography [IVP] or computed tomography [CT] scan) are routine. Other tests, such as magnetic resonance imaging, ultrasound, and radionuclide bone scans should be performed only for specific indications.

A tumor marker, squamous cell carcinoma antigen, has been found to correlate with tumor status in patients with invasive cervical carcinoma. However, it is unclear whether this test is useful in the management of patients with cervical cancer, and its routine use is discouraged.

STAGING

The staging of cervical carcinoma is clinical and depends primarily on the results of the pelvic examination and the routine radiologic tests (eg, chest x-ray, IVP) allowed by the International Federation of Gynecology and Obstetrics (FIGO) staging system (Table 28-3). In most cases, an examination under anesthesia with cystoscopy and proctoscopy is performed to assess the extent of local disease. A chest x-ray and a CT scan are the only tests routinely used to detect metastatic disease. Although CT scanning has supplanted IVP in most centers, abnormal findings are uncommon in patients with early-stage cancers.

TREATMENT

The treatment of cervical cancer depends on stage, with surgical excision the predominant mode in patients with early cancers and radiation therapy in those with more advanced cancer. Various other factors, such as age, histology, the patient's desire for childbearing, and her medical condition, are used in forming an individualized treatment plan.

Cervical Intraepithelial Neoplasia

Local methods including cryotherapy, laser ablation, sharp knife conization, and more recently LEEP have been the predominant methods used to treat CINI to CINIII. The type of local method used depends on the results of colposcopy with biopsy and ECC. Ablative methods such as cryotherapy and laser ablation, which do not permit comprehensive pathologic assessment, are appropriate only if an invasive cancer has been excluded. Routine hysterectomy is not indicated for CIN but may be appropriate in postmenopausal patients with persistent disease or in cases of recurrent disease where prior treatment has compromised the ability to use a local method.

Stage IA

Stage IA is meant to encompass so-called "microinvasive" cervical carcinoma, which has a limited potential for metastatic spread. However, the subgrouping IA_1 and IA_2 does not adequately distinguish between cases with a negligible risk of lymph node

Table 28-2. Radiologic Assessment in Cervical Carcinoma

METHOD	USE	RECOMMENDED
Chest x-ray	Exclude metastases	Routine
IVP	Exclude hydronephrosis	Routine
CT scan	Detect lymphadenopathy, hydronephrosis, liver metastases	Routine for advanced-stage or large tumors
MRI	Define tumor extent	Optional
Ultrasound	Define tumor extent	Optional
Skeletal x-rays	Confirm suspicious bone scan	With equivocal bone scan
Bone scan	Detect bony metastases	Increased alkaline phosphatase or bone pain

spread. In 1974, the Society of Gynecologic Oncologists adopted a more useful definition of microinvasive carcinoma: "A microinvasive lesion is one in which the neoplastic epithelium invades the stroma in one or more places to a depth of 3 mm or less below the base of the epithelium, and in which lymphatic or blood vessel involvement is not demonstrated."

Substage IA_1 is in accordance with this definition of microinvasive carcinoma, and this type of early cervical cancer has a very limited (< 1%) risk of lymph node spread. In patients who desire childbearing, cervical conization is adequate treatment if the margins of resection are uninvolved. In older patients or those who do not want more children, hysterectomy may be considered.

In substage IA_2, up to 5 mm of stromal invasion is allowed. With 1 to 3 mm of stromal invasion, treatment is similar to that for stage IA_1. However, with 4 to 5 mm of stromal invasion, the risk of lymph node spread is about 5%, so more radical treatment methods are usually employed: radical hysterectomy with pelvic lymphadenectomy or pelvic radiation may be appropriate.

Stage IB or IIA

Tumors clinically confined to the cervix make up stage IB. Treatment depends on the patient's age and medical condition and tumor size. In general, young patients who are good surgical candidates are treated with radical hysterectomy. Selected stage IIA patients, with minimal vaginal involvement, are also candidates for radical surgical treatment. In other cases, pelvic radiation is used. In cases with a bulky cervical lesion, combined radiation and surgery may be appropriate.

Table 28-3. FIGO Staging of Cervical Carcinoma

FIGO STAGE	DESCRIPTION
IA_1	Microinvasive with minimal stromal invasion
IA_2	Invasion < 5 mm
IB	Tumor confined to cervix
IIA	Vaginal involvement confined to upper two thirds
IIB	Parametrial involvement
IIIA	Lower third vaginal involvement
IIIB	Hydronephrosis or parametrial involvement to sidewall
IV	Bladder or rectal mucosal involvement, metastatic beyond pelvis

Stage IIB-IV

With tumor extension beyond the cervix, pelvic radiation in conjunction with radiosensitizing chemotherapy is usually employed. Cisplatinum, alone or in combination with infusional 5-FU, is administered during external beam treatment. One or two brachytherapy implants are routinely performed after external beam treatment.

CONSIDERATIONS IN PREGNANCY

The diagnosis of CIN during pregnancy is uncommon, and invasive cancer complicating pregnancy occurs in only one in 2200 pregnancies. The treatment of cervical cancer in pregnant patients depends entirely on the extent of tumor and the length of gestation. Although normal delivery can be anticipated for preinvasive lesions, cesarean section may be appropriate in more advanced cases.

The pregnant patient with a Pap smear showing either a low- or high-grade intraepithelial lesion should be referred to an experienced colposcopist for evaluation. If an invasive lesion is excluded, periodic reevaluation during pregnancy with anticipation of a normal delivery is appropriate. When a suspicious lesion is found colposcopically, biopsy is necessary and management depends on whether invasion is identified.

Microinvasive carcinoma of the cervix can be managed expectantly during pregnancy. This diagnosis can be made only by cervical conization. Conization should be performed during pregnancy only when a biopsy has shown an early invasive lesion or when there is a strong suspicion of invasive cancer.

The treatment of more advanced invasive cancers during pregnancy depends on the length of gestation. If the cancer is discovered in the third or late in the second trimester, treatment may be delayed until fetal viability. In these cases, cesarean section is usually employed to avoid hemorrhage from the tumor. If cancer is discovered during the first trimester, treatment is initiated without regard to the fetus.

BIBLIOGRAPHY

Berek JS, Hacker NF, eds. Practical gynecologic oncology, 2d ed. Baltimore: Williams & Wilkins, 1994.

DeVita VT, Hellman S, Rosenberg SA, eds. Cancer, principles & practice of oncology. Philadelphia: JB Lippincott, 1993.

DuBeshter B, Lin JY, Angel C. Tumors of female reproductive organs. In: Rubin P, ed. Clinical oncology: a multidisciplinary approach for physicians and students, 7th ed. Philadelphia: WB Saunders, 1993.

Hoskins WJ, Perez CA, Young RC, eds. Principles and practice of gynecologic oncology. Philadelphia: JB Lippincott, 1992.

Morrow CP, Curtin JP, Townsend DE. Synopsis of gynecologic oncology, 4th ed. New York: Churchill Livingstone, 1987.

Primary Care for Women, edited by Phyllis C. Leppert and Fred M. Howard. Lippincott-Raven Publishers, Philadelphia © 1997.

29

Uterine Carcinoma

GIUSEPPE DEL PRIORE

Uterine cancer is the most common female genital tract malignancy in the United States, with one in 100 women developing it over their lifetime. Each year nearly 32,000 women are diagnosed with this neoplasm. Although generally found in early (curable) stages, nearly 5000 women die from this disease each year in the United States. The peak incidence occurs around age 65, when it approaches 200 cases per 100,000 women per year. Although uterine cancer is a disease of older women, up to 15% of cases occur in women less than age 40. Prevalence and incidence data vary at least fourfold between different nationalities and ethnic groups and are highly dependent on socioeconomic factors and race. For instance, Caucasians may have a rate of endometrial cancer twice that of minorities in the United States.

The uterus consists of a smooth muscle outer layer, the myometrium, and an inner lining of glandular tissue, the endometrium. Malignant neoplasms are much more common in the endometrium than in the myometrium. About 95% of uterine neoplasms are adenocarcinomas of the endometrium; sarcomas make up only about 3% of uterine cancers.

ETIOLOGY

Risk factors for adenocarcinoma of the endometrium include early menarche, late menopause, ovarian granulosa cell tumors, polycystic ovarian syndrome, and nulliparity. Each of these conditions is probably related to endometrial cancer through unopposed estrogen stimulation of the endometrium or an imbalance of normal estrogen/progesterone production. This imbalance may be due to either excess estrogen or decreased progesterone, as in polycystic ovary syndrome.

Unopposed estrogen, whether exogenous or endogenous, has been unequivocably linked to the development of endometrial cancer. Estrogen replacement therapy in postmenopausal women has multiple benefits but should always be administered in conjunction with progestin treatment in women with an intact uterus. Progestin treatment is probably unnecessary in a woman whose uterus has been removed. In obese women, endogenous estrogen production can occur via peripheral conversion of androstenedione into estrone in adipose cells. Other endogenous sources of estrogen production are hormonally active ovarian tumors and polycystic ovary syndrome.

Tamoxifen is a synthetic steroid with weak estrogenic activity on the endometrium. It is also associated with endometrial hyperplasia and adenocarcinoma, although the causal relation is controversial. The epidemiologic association between tamoxifen use and uterine neoplasms may be genetic, in that women with breast cancer receiving tamoxifen may have a genetic predisposition to uterine cancer. Until more information is available, women receiving tamoxifen who have uterine bleeding should undergo periodic surveillance by ultrasound or endometrial biopsy.

The most significant risk factor for development of adenocarcinoma of the uterus is the presence of complex endometrial hyperplasia with atypia. Hyperplasia results from excessive estrogen stimulation, as found in many of the above conditions. Hyperplasia can be simple or complex, with or without atypia. If left untreated, up to 30% of patients with atypical hyperplasia progress to cancer; consequently, hysterectomy is usually recommended for these patients. The risk of simple hyperplasia without atypia progressing to a malignancy is less than 2%.

Numerous genetic abnormalities have been described in all histologic types of uterine cancer. These include abnormal expression of p53 and the retinoblastoma genes. Multiple cytogenetic abnormalities have also been found using routine chromosome banding techniques. A syndrome associated with an inherited predisposition to certain cancers, the Lynch type II syndrome, has been described and includes endometrial cancer as well as mammary, colonic, and ovarian neoplasms. There are no guidelines for recommending prophylactic hysterectomy for women at increased risk of endometrial cancer by virtue of their family history.

Supplemental progestins are extremely effective in eliminating the excess cancer risk associated with high estrogen states. Hormonal contraceptives (eg, birth-control pills and parenteral progestins) are associated with up to a 50% reduction in endometrial cancer risk through the inhibitory effect of progesterone on endometrial proliferation. This risk reduction persists for many years after stopping the oral contraceptive.

Smoking may modestly decrease the risk of an estrogen-dependent endometrial cancer by lowering circulating estrogen levels.

HISTORY

The initial history should focus on the patient's age, the age of menarche and menopause, the number of pregnancies, and the use of steroid contraceptives or hormone replacement therapy. The most common presenting symptom of uterine cancer is postmenopausal bleeding, but in some patients the only complaint is discharge or odor.

Most postmenopausal women with vaginal bleeding do not have endometrial cancer. The risk is age-related and ranges from 10% in women age 50 to 59 to greater than 50% in women older than age 80. Overall, about 30% of women with postmenopausal bleeding have a malignancy. Postmenopausal bleeding is always an indication for endometrial biopsy or dilatation and curettage (D&C).

PHYSICAL EXAMINATION

Most patients with endometrial cancer have no abnormalities on physical examination. An enlarged uterus is the most common abnormality but is not specific. Adnexal masses are unusual but may occur in cases of simultaneous ovarian endometrioid adenocarcinoma or ovarian granulosa cell tumor. Cervical or vaginal involvement may be

Table 29-1. Surgical Staging of Uterine Cancer

STAGE	CHARACTERISTICS
IA	Confined to the endometrium. No uterine invasion.
IB	Myometrial invasion < 50% of uterine wall.
IC	Myometrial invasion > 50% of uterine wall.
IIA	Tumor involves endocervical glands.
IIB	Tumor involves endocervical stroma.
IIIA	Tumor involves uterine serosa or adnexa.
	Cytology positive for malignant cells.
IIIB	Tumor metastases to the vagina.
IIIC	Positive retroperitoneal lymph nodes.
IVA	Tumor metastases to the bowel or bladder.
IVB	Other distant metastases or positive inguinal nodes.

noted and is associated with a more advanced stage. Manifestations of distant metastases, such as dyspnea from pulmonary involvement, seizures from brain metastases, or pain from bone metastases, are rare. Other physical findings are nonspecific and are usually related to coexistent obesity, hypertension, or diabetes.

LABORATORY AND IMAGING STUDIES

A speculum examination with a biopsy of any suspicious lesion, a Pap smear, and a pelvic examination are mandatory in any patient with postmenopausal bleeding. In addition, an in-office endometrial biopsy should be obtained using small flexible catheters. If in-office endometrial sampling is unsatisfactory, further evaluation is warranted. Transvaginal ultrasonography is usually performed; if a thickened endometrium is found, hysteroscopy with D&C is warranted. Due to a change in staging, according to the International Federation of Gynecologists and Obstetricians (FIGO), a fractional D&C is no longer required for staging. An endometrial stripe less than 3 mm usually excludes a significant cancer.

Although a Pap smear is not a screening test for endometrial carcinoma, abnormal findings occasionally lead to the diagnosis of endometrial cancer in the asymptomatic patient. The presence of endometrial cells on the Pap smear of a postmenopausal patient is abnormal and requires endometrial evaluation. In addition, the presence of malignant endometrial cells on cervical cytology in patients with endometrial cancer indicates a more advanced lesion that warrants referral to a gynecologic oncologist.

The only metastatic survey routinely indicated for patients with uterine cancer is a chest x-ray. If the pelvic examination is difficult or a mass is suspected, pelvic ultrasound may be helpful. Screening for other malignancies with mammography, stool guaiac, and flexible sigmoidoscopy may be warranted. CA-125 is elevated in a minority of patients, and although not routinely performed, is a marker in advanced stage.

TREATMENT

For patients with simple hyperplasia and no atypia, first-line treatment should consist of periodic progestins such as medroxyprogesterone acetate (Provera) 10 to 20 mg/day for 14 days each month. A repeat biopsy should be performed in about 4 months to exclude persistent hyperplasia. Because simple hyperplasia without atypia is sometimes seen in younger women with infertility due to anovulation, induction of ovulation may be the therapy of choice in these patients. In older patients in whom ovulation induction is not an objective, continuous progestin therapy with megestrol acetate (Megace) 40 to 160 mg/day for 12 weeks, followed by repeat endometrial sampling, may be appropriate.

Endometrial hyperplasia with atypia requires a more thorough evaluation and treatment. If this diagnosis is made by in-office endometrial biopsy, coexistent cancer should be excluded by D&C or hysteroscopy. In a premenopausal woman who desires fertility, management by ovulation induction or long-term administration of megestrol acetate may still be appropriate. If progestin treatment is chosen, it must be continued indefinitely, as up to 50% of patients who discontinue treatment develop recurrent hyperplasia or carcinoma. Postmenopausal patients or those not desirous of childbearing are often better treated by hysterectomy.

The mainstay of treatment of endometrial cancer is total abdominal hysterectomy and bilateral salpingo-oophorectomy, with lymph node sampling in most cases. Selected patients who are not operative candidates may be treated solely with pelvic radiation, but the chance of cure may be compromised. During hysterectomy, lymph node biopsies should be obtained from the pelvis and periaortic areas especially in patients with myometrial invasion or high-grade disease to identify patients who may benefit from postoperative adjuvant therapy. Omental biopsy or removal may be indicated if an advanced stage is suspected (Table 29-1).

After surgery, patients at high risk for recurrence and those with extrauterine disease should receive radiation treatment to the pelvis and vaginal apex. Patients with evidence of cancer in the upper abdomen may be offered systemic chemotherapy or whole abdomen radiation treatment. Chemotherapy is preferred for large unresectable lesions.

Most patients with uterine cancer are cured, but recurrence in the pelvis is associated with a 50% mortality. As most recurrences occur in the first 2 years after treatment, close surveillance in this interval may be warranted. Physical examination with a pelvic examination and Pap smear three or four times a year for 2 years and every 6 months thereafter is appropriate. Routine metastatic surveillance is not indicated, as systemic disease is usually not curable. For disseminated disease, either chemotherapy or progestins may be useful. Patients with an isolated recurrence of disease, usually at the vaginal apex, may be treated with radiation if no prior radiation was used, or exenteration if the recurrence is isolated and occurs in a previously irradiated field.

CONSIDERATIONS IN PREGNANCY

Pregnancy is associated with a lifetime risk reduction in developing endometrial adenocarcinoma. Vaginal bleeding is common during pregnancy but is rarely due to a neoplastic process. When it is, it is almost always a result of cervical neoplasms. Therefore, uterine cancer is not usually included in the differential diagnosis of bleeding during pregnancy.

BIBLIOGRAPHY

Gal D. Endometrial hyperplasia. In: Sciarra JJ, ed. Gynecology and obstetrics. Philadelphia: JB Lippincott, 1994.

Endometrial cancer. In: Morrow CP, Curtin JP, Townsend DE, eds. Synopsis of gynecologic oncology, 4th ed. New York: Churchill Livingstone, 1993.

Hacker NF. Endometrial cancer. In Berek J, Hacker NF, eds. Practical gynecologic oncology, 2d ed. Baltimore: Williams & Wilkins, 1994.

30
Ovarian Carcinoma

DAVID P. WARSHAL

Primary Care for Women, edited by Phyllis C. Leppert and Fred M. Howard. Lippincott-Raven Publishers, Philadelphia © 1997.

In the United States, ovarian carcinoma is the sixth most common malignancy among women and the second most frequent gynecologic cancer, with an estimated 26,700 new cases diagnosed in 1996. Ovarian cancer–related mortality for 1996 was predicted to be 14,900 women, making it the leading cause of death from gynecologic malignancies. A woman is estimated to have a 5% to 7% chance of developing an ovarian neoplasm and a 1 in 70 risk of ovarian carcinoma over the course of her lifetime.

The neoplastic potential of the ovary is among the most diverse for any organ system. The classification system adopted by the World Health Organization has been a useful framework for clinicians and pathologists (Table 30-1). Neoplasms intrinsic to the ovary have been divided into three broad categories based on their cellular origin.

Epithelial tumors primarily arise from the coelomic epithelium of the ovary, which undergoes metaplastic transformation to müllerian- and nonmüllerian-derived histologic subtypes. On occasion, epithelial malignancies, primarily endometrioid and clear cell histologic types, arise from endometriosis. Epithelial tumors comprise 60% to 70% of ovarian neoplasms and approximately 90% of ovarian malignancies.

Sex cord–stromal tumors develop from the sex cords and specialized stroma, or mesenchyme, of the ovary. They often are functional, producing estrogen, progesterone, or various androgens. They make up 5% to 10% of ovarian tumors and approximately 2% of malignancies. Most of these malignancies are indolent.

Germ cell tumors derived from the primitive germ cells of the ovary can replicate embryonic, extraembryonic, or adult-type tissue. Approximately 20% of ovarian neoplasms are germ cell derived. The dermoid cyst is the most common ovarian neoplasm of childhood and constitutes up to half of all benign ovarian tumors in women of reproductive age. Primitive germ cell malignancies occur predominantly in young women, with half occurring in women younger than 20 years of age. Recent advances in the use of chemotherapy have significantly reduced the mortality associated with these tumors.

ETIOLOGY

The biology of ovarian carcinoma is an area of intense research. Although not well understood, the process of malignant transformation seems to be multifactorial with reproductive, behavioral, and genetic elements involved.

The major reproductive risk factor for epithelial ovarian carcinoma is nulliparity. Multiple studies have reported an approximately 40% reduction of risk from a single full-term pregnancy. Subsequent pregnancies seem to reduce the risk by an additional 14% each. The benefit of incomplete pregnancies and breast-feeding have not been uniformly demonstrated. The effects of early age at menarche and of late menopause also are unclear. Oral contraceptive use has been shown to reduce the risk of ovarian carcinoma by 20% to 75%. Increasing duration of use confers greater risk reduction. Infertility has been associated with increased risk. However, many of these studies have failed to document the basis of the infertility.

An attempt to explain the relationship between reproductive history and ovarian carcinoma has led to the theory of incessant ovulation. Disruption of the ovarian epithelium occurs with each ovulation. It is hypothesized that the risk of aberrant epithelial repair leading to malignant transformation increases as the number of ovulations rises. A second theory proposes that persistent ovarian stimulation by pituitary gonadotropins increases the risk of ovarian cancer. Consistent with these theories is the increased risk of ovarian carcinoma with the use of clomiphene, as suggested by two recent studies.

Behavioral risk factors for epithelial ovarian carcinoma have been extensively studied. A high fat diet, obesity, and high galactose consumption in patients with low levels of galactose transferase activity have been associated with an increased risk of ovarian carcinoma. Exposure of the perineum to talc may double the risk. Smoking, alcohol use, and coffee consumption have shown no clear relationship to ovarian carcinoma.

Three hereditary epithelial ovarian carcinoma syndromes have been identified based on pedigree: (1) site-specific ovarian carcinoma involving only the ovary; (2) breast–ovarian carcinoma; and (3) the Lynch II syndrome, which includes familial nonpolyposis colorectal carcinoma (Lynch I syndrome), ovarian, breast, and endometrial carcinomas. These syndromes account for less than 5% of all cases of ovarian epithelial carcinomas. All three syndromes manifest an autosomal dominant pattern with variable penetrance. They can be inherited through the male, who may himself have an increased risk of prostate carcinoma.

One first-degree relative with ovarian carcinoma increases a woman's lifetime risk from 1.7% to 5%. Lifetime risk increases to 50% with two or more affected first-degree relatives. In estimating risk, it must be recognized that only 3% of women with two or more family members with ovarian carcinoma have a familial ovarian cancer syndrome.

Developments in the field of molecular genetics have made possible the identification of genetic aberrations that seem to be associated with the development of ovarian carcinoma and the transmission of its familial forms. Most of this research involves proto-oncogenes and tumor suppressor genes.

Proto-oncogene–derived proteins promote and regulate cell growth. Specific genetic alterations of proto-oncogenes produce oncogenes that promote aberrant growth and malignant transformation. Over 50 oncogenes have been identified. Those most strongly associated with ovarian carcinoma include c-*myc*, K-*ras*, and HER-

2/NEU. Overexpression of the HER-2/NEU gene product in ovarian carcinoma has been associated with a poor prognosis.

Tumor suppressor genes inhibit cellular proliferation. Mutation of these genes eliminates their regulatory function, which may result in malignant transformation. A limited number of tumor suppressor genes have been described. Overexpression of p53 has been detected in almost 50% of ovarian epithelial carcinomas. The prognostic implications of p53 overexpression is unclear.

Multiple tumor suppressor genes associated with familial ovarian cancer syndromes have been characterized. BRCA1 mutations have been implicated in the site-specific ovarian syndrome, in the breast–ovarian cancer syndrome, and in approximately half of all inherited cases of breast carcinoma. Four genes have been associated with the Lynch II syndrome. Still in the research phase, clinical testing for these genes will allow more precise identification of patients at high risk for these syndromes.

HISTORY

The development of ovarian carcinoma is insidious, with only 25% of patients presenting with disease confined to the ovaries. Presenting symptoms are nonspecific and most often related to advanced disease. Abdominal discomfort and distention caused by a large pelvic mass or ascites are the most common symptoms. Constipation, urinary frequency, and dyspareunia can develop as the mass enlarges. Rapidly enlarging masses occasionally present as surgical emergencies due to torsion, intracystic hemorrhage, or rupture. Gastrointestinal complaints of early satiety, dyspepsia, and nausea are common. Shortness of breath and fatigue are occasionally noticed and may be related to massive ascites or pleural effusions. The clinician may rarely encounter manifestations of paraneoplastic syndromes.

Sex cord–stromal tumors, often hormonally active, can present with precocious puberty in the premenarchal patient. Menstrual cycle irregularity is the most common presentation in women of reproductive age. Postmenopausal women often develop symptoms and signs of estrogenization, including vaginal bleeding. Occasionally, virilization is present.

Germ cell tumors occur primarily in young women. They present on occasion with symptoms and signs of abnormal endocrine activity, including precocious puberty, hyperthyroidism, and carcinoid syndrome.

PHYSICAL EXAMINATION

An annual pelvic examination is recommended for all women as part of their routine health care. Ovarian carcinoma sometimes is first detected during these examinations. Less than 5% of adnexal masses in reproductive-age women are malignant. In women older than 50 years of age, about half are malignant.

Rectovaginal examination is an essential component of the pelvic examination, allowing palpation of small adnexal masses and evaluation of the cul-de-sac, uterosacral ligaments, rectovaginal septum, and distal sigmoid colon. An increased risk of malignancy is associated with adnexal masses found to be bilateral, solid, fixed, or nodular. Ascites also is suggestive of malignancy and can be distinguished from an adnexal mass by the fluid wave test or by the distribution of dullness and tympany with percussion of the abdomen. Relevant aspects of the general physical examination include palpation of the inguinal and supraclavicular lymph nodes, evaluation for pleural effusions, and attention to signs of abnormal hormonal activity. Breast examination is necessary as this is a common primary site for metastatic disease to the ovary.

Table 30-1. Modified WHO Classification of Ovarian Tumors

Epithelial tumors
Serous
Mucinous
Endometrioid
Clear cell
Brenner
Mixed
Undifferentiated
Sex cord–stromal tumors
Granulosa stromal cell
Granulosa cell
Thecomoma-fibroma
Sertoli-Leydig cell tumors
Lipid cell tumors
Gynandroblastoma
Germ cell tumors
Dysgerminoma
Endodermal sinus tumor
Embryonal carcinoma
Polyembryoma
Choriocarcinoma
Teratomas
Immature
Mature
Monodermal (struma ovarii, carcinoid)

LABORATORY AND IMAGING STUDIES

The primary modalities used to evaluate adnexal masses are ultrasound and CA 125. Basic ultrasonographic features and mass size initially were used to predict the likelihood of malignancy. Recent studies employing high-resolution transvaginal ultrasonography have developed detailed morphologic scoring systems. Positive and negative predictive values of 37% and 100% have been reported, but it remains unclear whether these scoring systems will alter standard management of an adnexal mass.

A promising development in ultrasonography involves transvaginal color-flow Doppler measurement of blood flow in vessels within the adnexal mass. Results are reported in terms of resistance to flow with low resistance associated with a higher risk of malignancy. Tumors growing to greater than 2 to 3 mm require neovascularization to maintain continued growth. Vessels developed as a result of neovascularization have a relative deficiency of smooth muscle in their walls. The reduced resistance in these vessels allows greater blood flow, which is measured by color-flow Doppler. Initial studies have reported positive predictive values ranging from 50% to 98%. Negative predictive values generally have been in the middle to high 90s. Measurement of resistance to flow of vessels within the center or septum of the adnexal mass and a diffuse arrangement of vessels have been shown to improve diagnostic accuracy. Color-flow Doppler remains an investigational tool in evaluating adnexal masses.

CA 125 is the most commonly used tumor-associated antigen in the evaluation of adnexal masses. Values are elevated in over 80% of advanced ovarian epithelial carcinomas but are normal in 50% of cases of early stage disease. In addition to its generally poor sensitivity, specificity also is lacking, particularly in premenopausal patients for whom a wide variety of benign conditions can result in elevated levels. The benefit of combining CA 125 with ultrasound in the evaluation of postmenopausal masses has been demonstrated. However, the most valuable use of CA 125 is in monitoring patients with ovarian carcinoma for response to therapy and for recurrent disease. A frequent exception is mucinous tumors, which are not associated with elevations of CA 125 but do have a much higher incidence of carcinoembryonic antigen (CEA) elevation.

Several studies evaluating the feasibility of mass screening for ovarian carcinoma using ultrasound and CA 125 are ongoing. As noted by the recent National Institutes of Health Consensus Development Conference Statement, a representative screening study performed 65 laparotomies for each case of ovarian carcinoma discovered. They recommend at least annual screening, including a rectovaginal examination, transvaginal ultrasound, and CA 125 level for women presumed to have a familial syndrome. Screening of all other women should be performed within the framework of a clinical trial.

Nonepithelial ovarian tumors have been associated with several other tumor markers. Germ cell tumors are known to produce β-human chorionic gonadotropin (β-HCG), α-fetoprotein (AFP), human placental lactogen (HPL), placental alkaline phosphatase, and fast fraction lactic dehydrogenase (LDH). Sex cord–stromal tumors can be hormonally active with granulosa cell tumors notable for production of estrogen and associated with serum elevations of inhibin.

Routine preoperative studies should include a chest x-ray to rule out pleural effusions and metastatic disease. Liver function tests are used in the evaluation of metastatic disease and ascites. Elevated levels necessitate imaging of the liver. Computed tomography (CT) of the abdomen and pelvis allows evaluation of the retroperitoneal lymph nodes, liver, urinary tract, and omentum. However, most authors conclude that CT is of limited benefit relative to ultrasound. Cervical cytologic examination should be performed if not done recently. Some authors recommend a barium enema in patients older than 45 years of age due to the risk of colon carcinoma. Results are also helpful for planning surgery. A recent mammogram is indicated to rule out metastatic carcinoma of the breast.

TREATMENT

The initial management of a medically fit patient with an adnexal mass suspicious for ovarian carcinoma is surgical exploration. The aims of operative management are confirmation of the diagnosis, accurate staging, and maximal tumor resection if advanced disease is discovered. Consultation with a gynecologic oncologist often is beneficial. Mechanical bowel preparation with preoperative antibiotics and deep venous thrombosis prophylaxis are indicated.

A surgical–pathologic staging system for ovarian carcinoma has been adopted by the International Federation of Gynecology and Obstetrics (Table 30-2). Accurate staging, especially in cases of apparently early stage disease, requires a systematic approach based on an understanding of patterns of dissemination.

Direct spread of disease along peritoneal surfaces is the most common mechanism of tumor dissemination. Upper abdominal involvement is facilitated by the circulation of peritoneal fluid through the abdomen in a clockwise pattern. Lymphatic metastasis occurs primarily via the infundibulopelvic ligaments to the periaortic nodes and along the broad ligament and parametria to the pelvic nodes. Obstruction of peritoneal lymphatics may play a role in the development of ascites. Hematogenous spread, most frequently to the liver or lung, is less common. Surgical exploration should be performed through a midline vertical incision, allowing maximum exposure of the pelvis and upper abdomen. If gross upper abdominal disease is not apparent, ascites or peritoneal washings from the

Table 30-2. FIGO Staging of Ovarian Cancer (1988)

Stage I	Growth limited to the ovaries
Stage IA	Limited to one ovary; no malignant ascites, no tumor on external capsule, capsule intact
Stage IB	Limited to both ovaries; no malignant ascites, no tumor on external capsule, capsule intact
Stage IC	Limited to ovaries; malignant ascites or washing, tumor on external capsule, or capsule ruptured
Stage II	Growth involving one or both ovaries with pelvic extension
Stage IIA	Extension to uterus, tubes, or both
Stage IIB	Extension to other pelvic tissues
Stage IIC	Stage IIA or IIB with malignant ascites or washings; or tumor on capsule; or capsule ruptured
Stage III	Extrapelvic peritoneal implants or positive retroperitoneal or inguinal nodes; extension to small bowel or omentum
Stage IIIA	Tumor grossly limited to true pelvis with negative nodes but microscopic seeding of abdominal peritoneal surfaces
Stage IIIB	Nodes negative; implants on abdominal peritoneal surfaces or omentum ≤ 2 cm in diameter
Stage IIIC	Nodes positive or implants on abdominal peritoneal surfaces or omentum > 2 cm in diameter
Stage IV	Growth involving one or both ovaries with distant metastases; malignant pleural effusion or parenchymal liver metastases

pelvis and upper abdomen should be collected for cytologic evaluation. After verification of malignancy, total abdominal hysterectomy and bilateral salpingo-oophorectomy are routinely performed. Meticulous examination of all peritoneal surfaces, the bowel and its mesentery, the liver, and the omentum is necessary. Adhesions and roughened surfaces often are indicative of metastatic disease and should be sampled. Staging of early stage disease is completed with pelvic and periaortic lymph node sampling, infracolic omentectomy, and random biopsies from the pelvis, pericolic gutters, and the diaphragm.

Operative efforts in advanced-stage epithelial disease are directed toward removal of as much tumor as possible. Optimal cytoreduction has been demonstrated in multiple studies to improve prognosis. Cytoreduction to residual tumor nodules no greater than 1 cm in maximum diameter generally is considered optimal. Approximately 50% of patients with advanced disease can be optimally cytoreducted. Resection of tumor in patients unable to be optimally cytoreducted may provide palliative benefit, such as reduced ascites production and relief from impending bowel obstruction. Prognosis has not been shown to improve with cytoreduction when tumor nodules greater than 2 cm remain.

Conservative surgical management of early stage ovarian carcinoma is acceptable in younger women who desire preservation of their reproductive potential. Unilateral oophorectomy with complete surgical staging, including ipsilateral pelvic and bilateral periaortic lymph node sampling, is adequate for well-differentiated stage IA disease. Cystectomy has been demonstrated to be effective therapy for similar patients with borderline malignancies. Biopsy of the normal-appearing contralateral ovary is controversial. Close follow-up with removal of the retained ovary is recommended once childbearing is completed. Bilateral oophorectomy with uterine preservation is possible for stage IB disease.

Ovarian germ cell malignancies involve young women and are usually stage I. They are usually unilateral with the exception of dysgerminomas, which are grossly bilateral in 10% of cases and covertly bilateral in an additional 10% of cases. After unilateral oophorectomy and staging, preservation of the contralateral ovary and the uterus is indicated, except when disease involving these sites is discovered.

In a well-selected patient population, laparoscopic evaluation of an adnexal mass is appropriate. When cancer is suspected, effort is made to remove the ovary intact, avoiding tumor spill. However, recent studies have failed to confirm intraoperative tumor rupture to be a poor prognostic factor in early stage disease. Patients must be prepared for a laparotomy if cancer is discovered.

Patients with well-differentiated stage IA or IB epithelial carcinoma with no poor prognostic factors are at low risk for recurrence, and adjuvant therapy is not recommended. Factors increasing the risk for recurrence include high-grade disease, capsular excrescences or adhesions, clear cell histologic type, and malignant peritoneal cytologic findings. Therapy for patients with early stage disease who are at high risk may be individualized. Options include using platinum-based combination chemotherapy, intraperitoneal ^{32}P, or observation in selected cases.

The mainstay of postoperative therapy for advanced-stage disease has been platinum-based combination chemotherapy. The effects of dose intensification and extended duration of therapy remain points of controversy. Whole-abdominal radiation therapy has a limited role in advanced-stage disease. A recent randomized trial involving patients with suboptimal cytoreduction has established cisplatin and paclitaxel (Taxol) as standard therapy for patients with advanced epithelial ovarian carcinoma. Improved clinical response (73%), progression-free survival (median, 18 months), and overall survival (median, 38 months) were demonstrated for the cisplatin-paclitaxel arm. Intraperitoneal chemotherapy for optimally cytoreduced disease and high-dose chemotherapy with autologous bone marrow support are potentially beneficial therapies currently under study.

Monitoring for response to chemotherapy is generally by means of physical examination and serial serum CA 125 levels. An elevated CA 125 more than 3 months beyond the start of chemotherapy is a strong predictor of persistent disease at the completion of chemotherapy. CT scanning and other radiographic examinations are not used routinely but occasionally may be useful in evaluating symptoms in patients with a normal physical examination and CA 125 level.

The role of second-look surgery in patients treated for advanced disease with no clinical evidence of persistence is unclear. Under study circumstances, it allows evaluation for a complete pathologic response because up to 65% of patients clinically free of disease after standard chemotherapy have persistence documented at the time of second-look surgery. In addition, approximately half of all patients with negative findings on second-look will have a recurrence. Efforts to reduce this relapse rate have included the use of consolidation chemotherapy and intraperitoneal ^{32}P. Despite these measures and the earlier initiation of salvage therapy for patients with persistent disease, second-look surgery has not yet been shown to improve patient survival.

Patients with a complete response to therapy should be examined every 3 months for 2 years. Examinations every 6 months for the subsequent 3 years are recommended with yearly follow-up thereafter. CA 125 levels should be obtained at each visit. A rising CA 125 level is a strong indicator of recurrent disease and often occurs 3 or more months before disease is detected by other clinical means. Some authors recommend biannual CT scans for the first 2 years because 80% of recurrences develop during this period.

Salvage chemotherapy for recurrent disease is individualized according to the agents used previously and the length of the disease-free interval. Extended survival for patients with recurrent disease is rare.

Postoperative therapy usually is not recommended for most patients with ovarian epithelial tumors of low malignant potential and sex cord–stromal tumors. Malignant germ cell tumors, with the exception of early stage dysgerminomas and immature teratomas, require aggressive multiagent chemotherapy.

CONSIDERATIONS IN PREGNANCY

Most ovarian masses discovered during pregnancy are benign. CA 125 levels are unreliable in pregnancy. Surgical exploration at 16 to 18 weeks gestation is recommended for adnexal masses greater than 6 cm in diameter. Masses discovered during the third trimester may be managed by exploration at the time of delivery or postpartum. Of patients undergoing exploration, less than 5% have malignancies.

The most common malignancies during pregnancy are germ cell tumors and epithelial tumors of low malignant potential. Conservation of the pregnancy usually is possible. Postoperative therapy is similar to that for the nonpregnant patient. Chemotherapy may be administered in the last two trimesters as no well-documented teratogenic or long-term effects have been found.

BIBLIOGRAPHY

Berek JS, Hacker NF (eds). Practical gynecologic oncology, 2nd ed. Baltimore: Williams & Wilkins, 1994.

DeVita VT, Hellman S, Rosenberg SA (eds). Cancer: principles & practice of oncology, 4th ed. Philadelphia: JB Lippincott, 1993.

DuBeshter B, Lin JY, Angel C. Tumors of female reproductive organs. In: Rubin P, ed. Clinical oncology: a multidisciplinary approach for physicians and students, 7th ed. Philadelphia: WB Saunders, 1993.

Hoskins WJ, Perez CA, Young RC (eds). Principles and practice of gynecologic oncology. Philadelphia: JB Lippincott, 1992.

Morrow CP, Curtin JP, Townsend DE. Synopsis of gynecologic oncology, 4th ed. New York: Churchill Livingstone, 1987.

31
Vulvar Diseases

PAUL NYIRJESY

Primary Care for Women, edited by Phyllis C. Leppert and Fred M. Howard. Lippincott-Raven Publishers, Philadelphia © 1997.

Vulvar disorders are a disparate group of entities with a wide variation in manifestations. Certain disorders, such as squamous cell carcinoma of the vulva, may present as a large asymptomatic ulceration or lump in the vulvar area; others, such as vulvar vestibulitis, may cause tremendous burning and pain but present with findings on examination that are quite subtle. In evaluating a woman with a vulvar disease, it is helpful to keep in mind a differential diagnosis (Table 31-1) to determine the cause of symptoms and the most appropriate treatment. Table 31-1 is by no means an exhaustive list, but represents the more common entities that the primary care practitioner is likely to encounter.

HISTORY AND PHYSICAL EXAMINATION

A careful history is essential to a correct diagnosis. Not realizing that there is a difference between vaginal and vulvar diseases, many women who present with a vulvar disease think that the term that best describes the location of their symptoms is the vagina; closer questioning reveals that their symptoms are actually on the outside of the vagina (the vulva) or around the opening to the vagina (the vulvar vestibule). If this potential for misunderstanding is not appreciated, selecting appropriate therapy becomes a hit-or-miss affair instead of a process based on an accurate examination and workup.

A patient with vulvar symptoms should also be questioned about any abnormal lumps or sores she may have noticed; whether she has mainly itching, which connotes a need to scratch or touch the area, or burning or irritation, where she wishes to avoid contact with the area; the type of soap she uses and how often she washes the vulvar area; and the type and number of treatments she has had for her condition, and whether each one makes her feel better or worse.

A sexual history is particularly important, not only to evaluate the potential for sexually transmitted diseases, but also because intercourse can be viewed as a stress in the vulvar area that may make subtle symptoms more obvious to the patient. Any patient with dyspareunia should be asked whether her pain is mainly with penetration, which suggests a vulvar or vestibular problem, or with deep thrusting, which may be a symptom of an intraabdominal process such as endometriosis.

During the pelvic examination, the vulva and vestibule should be examined routinely in both the symptomatic and asymptomatic patient. Inspection should focus on areas of hyperpigmentation, erythema, ulceration, or excrescence. Palpation with a cotton-tipped applicator helps localize areas of tenderness. Any abnormal lesions can be grasped between the thumb and index finger to determine the size, texture, and depth of the abnormality. If the patient complains of a lump that cannot initially be seen, it sometimes is useful to have her point it out during the examination. The use of a simple magnifying glass or, if available, a colposcope allows a more detailed look at the vulva in the patient with vulvar symptoms but no obvious findings.

Because a vaginal disease such as candidiasis or trichomoniasis can have vulvar manifestations, the evaluation described in Table 23-2 in Chapter 23 should be undertaken in the symptomatic patient. In the presence of ulcerations or excoriations, adjunctive studies such as cultures for herpes simplex virus, yeast, or *Trichomonas vaginalis* should be considered. If a syphilitic chancre is suspected, a serologic test for syphilis should be obtained, but these tests are negative in many cases of primary syphilis. The diagnosis of chancroid is usually made on clinical grounds, as culture media for *Haemophilus ducreyi* are not widely available and have a sensitivity no higher than 80%.

If the diagnosis is still unclear, the clinician should strongly consider performing a biopsy on any lesion that is raised, ulcerated, erythematous, or hyper- or hypopigmented. This is particularly true if the lesion fails to respond to one or perhaps two attempts at medical therapy. Biopsies of the vulva require 1% lidocaine, a punch biopsy instrument, fine-toothed forceps, fine scissors, and either silver nitrate sticks or Monsel solution to coagulate the biopsy site. The biopsy technique is straightforward. After injecting the area with lidocaine, the biopsy instrument, which resembles a coring device, is pressed against the lesion and twirled back and forth until the desired biopsy depth has been reached. The forceps and scissors are used to grasp and excise the core of tissue. If needed, pressure in combination with the application of silver nitrate or Monsel solution stops whatever bleeding occurs. The biopsy site heals on its own without the need for primary closure. Usually, a 4- or 6-mm punch biopsy yields a sufficient sample for diagnosis; if necessary, multiple sites can be biopsied. Whenever feasible, efforts should be made to review the biopsy specimen in person with the pathologist to get the most information possible from the sample.

Using such an approach, it is possible to establish the proper diagnosis. Some conditions, such as vulvar intraepithelial neoplasia or vulvar carcinoma, require immediate referral to a specialist. However, most conditions fall well within the primary care practitioner's ability to diagnose, treat, and follow.

Table 31-1. Common Types of Vulvar Diseases

Contact Dermatitis	**Infectious**
Vulvodynia	Vulvovaginal candidiasis
Vulvar vestibulitis	Trichomoniasis
Dysesthetic vulvodynia	Herpes simplex virus
Nonneoplastic Epithelial Disorders	Syphilis
Squamous cell hyperplasia	Chancroid
Lichen sclerosus	Venereal warts
Other dermatoses	
Neoplastic Disorders	
Vulvar intraepithelial neoplasia	
Vulvar carcinoma	
Melanoma	

DIAGNOSIS AND TREATMENT

Chapter 23 provides a detailed discussion of vulvovaginal candidiasis and trichomoniasis.

Contact Dermatitis

When the patient complains primarily of vulvar itching or burning, the clinician should exclude an irritant dermatitis or an allergic dermatitis. The distinction is based on whether the offending agent is likely to be irritating to anyone with prolonged contact or whether the particular patient is allergic to the substance. The former condition, marked primarily by burning, can be the result of many potential causes, including any type of topical antifungal or corticosteroid therapy, various soaps, shampoos and perfumes, laundry detergents, toilet papers, and spermicidal agents. Allergic reactions tend to take longer to develop and are often more severe. Possible culprits include chemicals in sanitary napkins (the "minipad syndrome") and latex. Practically any substance applied to the vulvar area may cause an irritant or an allergic reaction, so the history should include a search for possible causes.

On examination, the patient with contact dermatitis has varying amounts of vulvar erythema and edema. Women with severe cases may even have areas of skin breakdown or blistering. The rest of the examination is unrevealing.

The first course of treatment is to try to identify and remove the offending agent. In some cases, the patient can be counseled to discontinue all self-medication and to avoid the use of all soaps in the vulvar area for 1 month to see if her symptoms resolve. Various soothing measures can be suggested to alleviate the symptoms, such as sitz baths with 4 to 5 tablespoons of baking soda, cool compresses with Domeboro solution, and emollients such as ointments used for diaper rash (if the perfume from these proves to be irritating, vegetable shortening can be applied as an ointment as often as needed). If the symptoms are more severe or fail to respond to initial measures, topical corticosteroid ointments may be prescribed, but the patient should be warned to beware of symptom exacerbation.

Herpes Simplex Virus Infection

Herpes simplex virus (HSV), a double-stranded DNA virus that belongs to the herpesvirus group, is one of the most common sexually transmitted diseases. Although the initial distinction between HSV-1 and HSV-2 was based on the site of infection (oral versus genital), it has been established that both types can infect either site. Based on serologic studies, the Centers for Disease Control and Prevention estimate that about 30 million people in the United States may have HSV infection; most of those infected are never diagnosed because they never become symptomatic or have only a single mild episode that they never bring to the attention of a health care worker.

In evaluating a patient with herpes, it is important to distinguish between a first episode and a recurrent one. When the first episode of genital herpes occurs in someone who has had a prior HSV infection and has HSV antibodies present (usually as a result of a nongenital herpes infection), it is described as nonprimary. Primary episodes tend to be more severe and long-lasting, and they are often associated with systemic complaints such as fever, malaise, headaches, or myalgias.

Classically, the patient with an active HSV infection exhibits clusters of small vesicles on an erythematous base. Left untreated, they rupture and leave an ulcer that heals without scarring. However, in many patients, the presentation is milder, with a small isolated ulcer associated with mild burning or irritation. In recurrent disease, the entire process may last only 3 to 5 days, but it may take several weeks in a primary first episode. Thereafter, the virus remains latent and reactivates symptomatically and asymptomatically.

Because of the tremendous psychological distress associated with the diagnosis of herpes, it is essential to identify this infection accurately. Although commonly used in clinical practice, serologic tests can be used only to confirm a past infection with HSV. Furthermore, because HSV-1 and HSV-2 share many antigens and may cross-react in the laboratory, serologic diagnosis may not distinguish between viral types, nor can it determine whether a positive test is a result of a past oral or genital infection. Viral culture of the herpes virus remains the gold standard, with a false-negative rate of 5% to 30%. Factors that enhance the likelihood of obtaining a positive culture include seeing the patient early in the course of an episode and ensuring that the specimen is inoculated into viral medium as quickly as possible.

Acyclovir, a viral thymidine kinase inhibitor, remains the mainstay of treatment for HSV infections. Treatment with oral acyclovir, 200 mg five times a day for 7 to 10 days, in a first episode of herpes decreases the duration of viral shedding and shortens the duration of the symptomatic episode. However, it does not eradicate latent virus nor affect the risk of subsequent reactivation. Symptomatic recurrences occur in up to 90% of patients in the first year; asymptomatic shedding occurs in up to 23% of women with a recent first episode of herpes. In patients with frequent (six or more per year) recurrences, suppressive treatment with oral acyclovir, 400 mg twice a day, decreases episodes of viral reactivation. After the first year of continuous suppressive therapy, it may be discontinued to assess the need for further therapy. If such a need is still present, daily therapy can be reinstituted. Although such an approach has raised concerns about the development of acyclovir-resistant strains of HSV, such strains have not yet been found in immunocompetent persons.

Although it is beyond the scope of this chapter to examine the numerous issues surrounding perinatal herpes, the traditional approach of performing a cesarean section on any woman who did not have a recent negative viral culture has been abandoned.

Human Papillomavirus Infection

Infection with the human papillomavirus (HPV) is even more common than HSV infection. Depending on the population studied and the techniques used for virus identification, HPV is present in 10% to 50% of patients. Infection with this virus is of concern because of its consistent association with abnormal Pap smears and cervical cancer, as well as its role in the development of vulvar warts. In general, different types of HPV are associated with different manifestations. For example, HPV 6 and 11 are seen more often with exophytic warts, whereas HPV 16 and 18 are associated with a high risk of cervical cancer.

As noted by Stone (1995), "perhaps the greatest morbidity associated with genital warts, aside from that caused by treatment, is not physical but psychosocial." Certainly, the patient will seek treatment for warts, but the symptoms she may have may simply be an asymptomatic lump, itching, burning, pain, or bleeding. Frequently of greater concern to her will be the potential impact on her risk of cervical cancer, the effect on a future pregnancy, and the possibility of transmission to and need for evaluation of a sexual partner. In terms of cervical cancer, women diagnosed with genital warts can be reassured that in general warts are linked with different types of HPV than those associated with cervical cancer. These women, therefore, have the same risk of developing cervical cancer as women without warts, and they can be reassured that the general guidelines for cervical cancer screening apply to them.

During pregnancy, genital warts may become larger as a result of estrogen stimulation. Apart from podophyllin preparations, which are contraindicated, the treatment options for genital warts in pregnancy are the same as for the nonpregnant patient. However, as they often regress postpartum, some clinicians treat exophytic warts only if they have the potential to impede a vaginal birth. A woman with HPV infection theoretically may transmit the virus to a newborn, resulting in either genital warts or laryngeal papillomatosis. These risks, however, are difficult to quantify, and despite the ubiquity of HPV infection, reported cases of newborn infection remain rare. Cesarean delivery to prevent transmission to the newborn remains untested, and it is not recommended in current CDC guidelines.

There are insufficient data to address the risk of sexual transmission and the role of the partner. Although up to 68% of male sexual partners of women with warts may have HPV-associated lesions, it is less clear whether treating the partner has an effect on subsequent recurrence in the female patient, or even if the partner was the source of the original infection. Although condoms may decrease the risk of transmission of HPV, many partners may be subclinically infected even before entering their present relationship; the extent to which condoms are used to prevent HPV transmission depends on the couple's tolerance for the risks, which remain difficult to estimate. The need for controlled studies to answer these important and common questions is clear.

On examination, genital warts appear as exophytic lesions of varying dimensions. Their texture is rough or cauliflower-like. Common locations include the periclitoral area, the posterior fourchette, and the perianal area. The finding of genital warts mandates a careful inspection of all these areas. Biopsy confirmation is not usually necessary if the lesion appears typical, but should be considered for an uncertain diagnosis, a lesion that fails to respond to therapy, or in older patients, where the risk of warts is lower and the risk of vulvar cancer is greater.

Various treatment modalities (Table 31-2) have been proposed to treat vulvar warts. Response rates of 40% to 80% have been reported with all these modalities, and deciding on the appropriate therapy should focus on patient motivation, the extent of lesions, side effects, and cost. In general, topical therapies are associated with irritation and mild to moderate discomfort, but they represent the least expensive and most convenient therapy. Podofilox 0.5% solution is applied by the patient; in a patient who is motivated and can examine and treat herself, it obviates the need for weekly office visits and allows the patient to treat lesions early on. However, its use is contraindicated in pregnancy and, because of fears of systemic absorption and neurotoxicity, in the treatment of vaginal warts. For patients who fail topical therapy, the other modalities listed in Table 31-2 can be considered; these patients should be referred to someone who treats these problems frequently.

Table 31-2. Therapies for Genital Warts

Chemotherapy	Podophyllin in tincture of benzoin
	Podofilox 0.5% solution
	Trichloroacetic acid, 80%–90%
	Topical 5-fluorouracil
Immunotherapy	Intralesional interferon
Destructive therapy	Cryotherapy
	Electrodesiccation/electrocautery
	CO_2 laser vaporization
Excisional therapy	Cold knife excision
	Loop electrosurgical excision

Vulvodynia and Vulvar Vestibulitis

With headlines such as "The Bizarre Disease That Almost Ruined My Life" (*Good Housekeeping*, February 1993) and a write-up in the science section of *The New York Times*, vulvar vestibulitis and vulvodynia have achieved a certain notoriety. As defined by the International Society for the Study of Vulvovaginal Diseases, vulvodynia is characterized by the patient's complaint of burning, stinging, irritation, or rawness of the vulva. Vulvodynia is a descriptive term, and various conditions can cause these symptoms; the most common are vulvar dermatoses, recurrent candidiasis, squamous papillomatosis, vulvar vestibulitis, and essential vulvodynia. Although the last two terms are often used interchangeably, there is a difference in terms of management and treatment.

Essential or dysesthetic vulvodynia is considered a neurologic problem, marked by a chronic burning vulvar pain in the presence of a normal physical and laboratory examination. Although the condition waxes and wanes, most women who have it are rarely symptom-free, and contact with the vulvar area does not increase their pain. As with other neurologically mediated pain syndromes, many patients with essential vulvodynia respond to low-dose amitriptyline.

Vulvar vestibulitis, however, is often or minimally asymptomatic unless the patient is touched in the vestibular area. As a result, the most common complaints of women with vulvar vestibulitis are of entry dyspareunia and of pain with tampon insertion or when wearing tight clothes. Some of these women also have dysuria, either because of contact of urine with the vestibule or because of coexisting interstitial cystitis. Examination reveals areas of erythema in the vestibule, and touching these areas with a cotton-tipped applicator reproduces the pain they have at other times.

The etiology of vulvar vestibulitis remains undetermined. HPV infection, initially proposed as the cause, does not seem to be more common in patients with vulvar vestibulitis in controlled studies. Because the cause of this disorder is unknown, selecting appropriate medical therapy is difficult and often involves the issues listed in Table 31-3. The primary care practitioner may consider a trial of a regimen similar to the one used for irritant dermatitis before referring her to a specialist in vulvar diseases. For patients who fail medical therapy, vestibulectomy with advancement of the vaginal mucosa offers a 90% chance of significant improvement or cure. Anecdotal reports of laser surgery have also been encouraging.

Nonneoplastic Epithelial Disorders

Nonneoplastic epithelial disorders of the vulvar skin and mucosa, formerly known as vulvar dystrophies, are relatively chronic conditions of the vulva. They are divided into three distinct categories: squamous cell hyperplasia, lichen sclerosus, and other dermatoses.

Squamous cell hyperplasia is marked by thickening and hyperkeratosis of the skin. Although the cause is unknown, it is thought to be the result of a "scratch-itch-scratch" cycle: an initial insult leads to pruritus, which in turn leads to scratching and resulting hyperkeratosis, which then causes increased itching. As this cycle progresses, the patient develops thickened skin with varying amounts of erythema, edema, and excoriations. By the time she presents for evaluation, an underlying etiology is rarely determined. Although the disorder can be suspected on the basis of the history and examination, biopsy is generally recommended to confirm the diagnosis.

Treatment of squamous cell hyperplasia consists initially of removing any aggravating factors, such as trichomoniasis, candidiasis, allergy, and improper hygiene. Soothing preparations such as emollient creams or dressings with Burow's solution may alleviate the symptoms. In refractory or severe cases, topical corticosteroid therapy is indicated. Weaker steroids include triamcinolone ointment 0.025%, but some patients require more potent agents such as clobetasol cream 0.05%. With potent agents such as this one, the potential for skin atrophy, adrenal suppression, candidiasis, and rebound burning after stopping therapy are concerns. Cautious use and tapering of therapy to weaker corticosteroids are important. Many patients who successfully respond to therapy may require a maintenance regimen with hydrocortisone 1% or 2.5% to remain comfortable.

At the other extreme of the spectrum from squamous cell hyperplasia is lichen sclerosus, whose hallmark is a thinning of the skin. Although the primary complaint may again be pruritus, these patients have skin with a white, parchment-like appearance. If the process is extensive, adhesions may form in such a way as to cover the clitoris completely. Scarring around the labia minora may lead to their resorption, and many women complain of dyspareunia because of the scarring and loss of flexibility of the tissues around the introitus. On biopsy, the epithelium is thinned and atrophic, with a band of inflammatory cells below the basement membrane. These findings are thought to result from an immunomediated disorder, although the association with systemic autoimmune diseases is inconsistent.

In the past, testosterone cream in a petrolatum base was the mainstay of treatment. More recently, it has been suggested that testosterone cream has few if any effects apart from the soothing nature of the cream, and a 3-month course of clobetasol propionate 0.05% has been recommended. Thereafter, moderately potent steroids or emollient creams may be used to maintain remission.

SUMMARY

The amount of time a primary care practitioner wishes to invest in vulvar disorders depends on his or her level of interest and expertise. Each patient deserves appropriate initial evaluation and diagnosis. In women whose diagnosis is unclear, who may require therapies with potentially serious side effects, or who fail to respond to treatment, referral to a gynecologist or dermatologist experienced in treating these conditions is essential. Although most of these conditions are not life-threatening, their impact on the patient's quality of life and sense of well-being can be tremendous and should never be underestimated.

Table 31-3. Suggested Causes and Possible Medical Therapies for Vulvar Vestibulitis

	CAUSE	TREATMENT
Infectious	*Candida albicans*	Suppressive antifungal therapy
	Human papillomavirus	5-FU, intralesional interferon
Environmental	Topical antifungal therapy	Avoidance of self-medication
	Urinary oxalate excretion	Diet, calcium citrate pills
	Chronic irritant dermatitis	Topical corticosteroids
	Early sexual intercourse	
	Early contraceptive use	
	Atrophic vestibular skin	Topical estrogen cream
Autoimmune	"Urogenital sinus syndrome"	Topical corticosteroids
Neurologic	"Sympathetically maintained pain"	Tricyclic antidepressants

BIBLIOGRAPHY

American College of Obstetricians and Gynecologists Technical Bulletin #139. Vulvar dystrophies, 1990.

Bazin S, Bouchard C, Brisson J, Morin C, Meisels A, Fortier M. Vulvar vestibulitis syndrome: an exploratory case-control study. Obstet Gynecol 1994;83:47.

Carli P, Bracco G, Taddei G, Sonni L, DeMarco A, Maestrini G, Cattaneo A. Vulvar lichen sclerosus: immunohistologic evaluation before and after therapy. J Reprod Med 1994;39:110.

CDC. 1993 Sexually transmitted diseases treatment guidelines. MMWR 1993;42(RR-14):1.

Gibbs RS, Amstey MS, Sweet RL, Mead PB, Sever JL. Management of genital herpes infection in pregnancy. Obstet Gynecol 1988;71:779.

Koelle DM, Benedetti J, Langenberg A, Corey L. Asymptomatic reactivation of herpes simplex virus in women after the first episode of genital herpes. Ann Intern Med 1992;116:433.

Krebs HB, Helmkamp BF. Treatment failure of genital condylomata in women: role of the male sexual partner. Am J Obstet Gynecol 1991;165:337.

Mann M, Kaufman RH, Brown D, Adam E. Vulvar vestibulitis: significant clinical variables and treatment outcomes. Obstet Gynecol 1992;79:122.

McKay M. Subsets of vulvodynia. J Reprod Med 1988;33:695.

Reeves WC, Rawls WE, Brinton LA. Epidemiology of genital papillomaviruses and cervical cancer. Rev Infect Dis 11;1989:426.

Stone KM. Human papillomavirus infection and genital warts: update on epidemiology and treatment. Clin Infect Dis 1995; 20(Suppl. 1):S91.

32
Premenstrual Syndrome

G. WILLIAM BATES

Primary Care for Women, edited by Phyllis C. Leppert and Fred M. Howard. Lippincott-Raven Publishers, Philadelphia © 1997.

Premenstrual syndrome (PMS) is a complex of psychosomatic changes that occur during the late luteal phase of a woman's reproductive cycle—usually in the week before the onset of menses with continuation of symptoms during the first 1 or 2 days of menstruation. Because PMS is not observed in girls who have not initiated puberty and established ovulatory cycles, and because PMS is not observed in menopausal women, PMS is linked to ovulation. PMS symptoms begin after the luteinizing hormone (LH) surge when the corpus luteum has formed and begun secreting progesterone. Thus, the PMS symptom complex is linked to the corpus luteum.

CLINICAL FINDINGS

Most ovulating women notice symptoms of PMS during the last week of the reproductive cycle. The most common symptoms are breast fullness, abdominal bloating, fluid retention, lethargy, and mood swings with mild irritability and depression. Although 30% to 40% of reproductive-age women complain of some symptoms of PMS, approximately 3% to 8% of women have accentuation of one or more of these symptoms that interferes with interpersonal relationships, job performance, mood, and affect. These women seek medical consultation for relief from these symptoms.

ETIOLOGY

Many theories have been advanced to explain the complex of PMS symptoms. Most of these theories provide an explanation for individual symptoms, but none provides a unified explanation of all of the PMS symptoms. Because of the relationship of PMS symptoms to corpus luteum function, the most likely explanation for PMS is the effects of progesterone on brain, breast, gut, and kidney.

Progesterone relaxes smooth muscle. During pregnancy, progesterone relaxes the myometrium to maintain uterine quiescence. Progesterone relaxes other smooth muscle as well. For example, progesterone produces vasodilatation, relaxation of gut smooth muscle, and relaxation of the ureteral smooth muscle. Moreover, progesterone acts on the acinar glands of the breasts to produce fullness of the breasts and rounding of the lateral quadrants of the breasts. Progesterone also induces depression and mood changes. Finally, progesterone is a substrate for deoxycorticosterone (DOC)—a potent mineralocorticoid. Renal 21-hydroxylase converts progesterone to DOC in the kidney. This extraglandular DOC (produced in tissue other than the adrenal glands) promotes sodium retention, potassium excretion, and obligatory water retention.

When these actions of progesterone are interpreted in light of the symptoms and signs of PMS, many of the symptoms and signs of PMS can be attributed to corpus luteum secretion of progesterone. Women who complain of PMS describe breast fullness, abdominal bloating, constipation, mood changes and depression, and fluid retention. All of these changes correlate with the metabolic actions of progesterone or the conversion of progesterone to DOC. Moreover, PMS symptoms occur *only* in ovulating women and occur *only* during the luteal phase of a reproductive cycle. Thus, corpus luteum secretion of progesterone may be the unifying explanation for PMS.

There may be a relationship between declining estradiol-17β and the degree of PMS symptoms. Although PMS is seen in women of all reproductive ages—from puberty through menopause—many women report beginning or worsening of symptoms in the late reproductive years. Moreover, Reid and others report that 90% of symptomatic women with PMS reported hot flushes during the luteal phase of the cycle compared with 17% of asymptomatic women without PMS symptoms, indicating that PMS symptoms may be related to ratio of estradiol to progesterone.

Most investigators and clinicians acknowledge that changes in sex steroid hormone secretion bring about the symptoms of PMS. However, investigators continue to seek mediators to explain the symptoms.

Endorphins, prostaglandins, and serotonin have been the substances most widely investigated to explain these symptoms. There is some correlation between each of these substances and PMS symptoms.

Endorphin levels are affected by sex steroid hormone secretion. Naloxone, an opiate antagonist, has been administered to women with PMS and found to exacerbate the symptoms. Thus, there may be a correlation between declining endorphins and PMS.

Progesterone withdrawal initiates prostaglandin synthesis with subsequent release of prostaglandin $F_{2\alpha}$. Several clinical studies have been reported in which women with PMS symptoms were given the precursor for prostaglandin synthesis, linolenic acid, to reduce PMS symptoms. No clear therapeutic efficacy was established.

Serotonin is related to mood changes and irritability. Some clinical data suggest a role for decreased central nervous system serotonin in women with PMS. On this basis, buspirone (BuSpar)—a serotoninergic agent—has been used to treat PMS.

DIAGNOSIS

To establish a diagnosis of PMS, symptoms must occur in *ovulating* women during the luteal phase of the menstrual cycle. If symptoms are continuous, or if symptoms are acyclic (and not occurring during the luteal phase of the cycle), the diagnosis of PMS cannot be made.

Many women present with a self-diagnosis of PMS. Some may be correct; others may not be correct. The woman who has made a self-diagnosis or a woman suspected to have PMS should be asked to maintain a calendar of symptoms that can be correlated with the reproductive cycle. In addition, there are questionnaires and calendars that have been developed specifically to establish a diagnosis of PMS. These include the Moos' Menstrual Distress Questionnaire and the University of California–San Diego Calendar of Premenstrual Experiences. These tools have been used in research protocols and in clinical evaluation of women suspected to have PMS. Daily records confirming the severity, impact, and timing of symptoms are essential to confirm the diagnosis and rule out more chronic disorders of mood or behavior that may worsen during the premenstrual period. Since many women experience premenstrual molimina, the diagnosis of PMS requires that symptoms have a substantial impact on psychologic function, interpersonal relationships, or both during the premenstrual period.

TREATMENT

A variety of treatments have been proposed for PMS. Progesterone supplementation during the luteal phase of reproductive cycle has been the most widely used and promoted treatment for PMS. This treatment was developed by Katherina Dalton, who coined the term *premenstrual syndrome* in 1953. For years, women were given massive doses of progesterone in the form of vaginal suppositories. Maddocks and coworkers performed a double-blind placebo-controlled trial of progesterone vaginal suppositories in the treatment of PMS and reported in 1986 that they found no significant difference in the effects of progesterone suppositories compared with placebo.

No single therapy has emerged as best for PMS. Women have been advised to avoid alcohol, animal fats, caffeine, refined sugar, salt and high-sodium foods, and dairy products. Complex carbohydrates as well as vitamins A, E, and B_6 have been promoted as providing partial relief from symptoms.

Agents to give individual symptomatic relief abound. Bromocriptine has been tried to alleviate breast fullness. Diuretics have been used for edema. Tranquilizers have been used to alleviate mood changes, depression, and anxiety. No uniformly successful psychotropic agent has been identified.

Oral contraceptive tablets to suppress ovulation have been used with some success, although some oral contraceptive formulations may cause symptoms of PMS. One is best advised to use low progestin activity oral contraceptives.

The author has found that administering continuous, low-dose estradiol-17β (50-μg patches [Estraderm]) is an effective treatment for most women who complain of PMS symptoms. The patch is applied on day 16 of a 28-day cycle and continued through the first 2 days of menstruation. The patch is changed every 3 days.

The best treatment for refractory PMS is administration of gonadotropin-releasing hormone (GnRH) agonists. These agents ablate pituitary gland secretion of follicle-stimulating hormone (FSH) and LH, thereby suppressing ovulation. However, GnRH agonists produce symptoms of ovarian failure such as hot flushes, sleep disturbance, and vaginal dryness, and may not be welcomed by a woman who is trying to eliminate symptoms of PMS. Moreover, GnRH agonists cannot be used for more than 6 months because bone demineralization has been associated with GnRH administration for extended periods of time.

Mortola and associates report the successful use of GnRH agonists combined with estrogen and progestin replacement. This therapy was successful in more than 75% of the subjects studied and can be used for extended periods of time.

Hysterectomy is an aggressive therapy for PMS and should not be entertained until *all* other treatments have failed. Hysterectomy alone does not alleviate PMS symptoms. However, when a hysterectomy is combined with bilateral oophorectomy, symptoms are relieved.

The physician caring for women with PMS symptoms must be cognizant of the relationship of corpus luteum function to PMS symptoms. Moreover, the physician must provide emotional support for women whose lives are altered for 7 to 10 days each month.

BIBLIOGRAPHY

Backstrom CT, Boyle H, Baird DT. Persistence of symptoms of premenstrual tension in hysterectomized women. Br J Obstet Gynaecol 1981;88:530.

Casson P, Hahn PM, Van Vugt DA, Reid RL. Lasting response to ovariectomy in severe intractable premenstrual syndrome. Am J Obstet Gynecol 1990;162:99.

Dalton K. The premenstrual syndrome and progesterone therapy. London: William Heinemann Medical Books, 1984.

DeVane GW. Premenstrual syndrome. J Clin Endocrinol Metab 1991;72:250.

Facchinetti F, Genazzani AD, Martignoni E, Fioroni L, Nappi G, Genazzani AR. Neuroendocrine changes in luteal function in patients with premenstrual syndrome. J Clin Endocrinol Metab 1993;76:1123.

Freeman EW, Sondheimer S, Weinbaum PJ, Rickels K. Evaluating premenstrual syndrome symptoms in medical practice. Obstet Gynecol 1985;65:500.

Ginsburg KA. Some practical approaches to treating PMS. Contemp Obstet Gynecol 1995;40:24.

Hammarback S, Backstrom T. Induced anovulation as a treatment of premenstrual tension syndrome: a double blind crossover study with LRH-agonist versus placebo. Acta Obstet Gynecol Scand 1988;67:159.

Maddocks S, Hahn P, Moller F, Reid RL. A double-blind placebo-controlled trial of progesterone vaginal suppositories in the treatment of premenstrual syndrome. Am J Obstet Gynecol 1986;154:573.

Moos RH. The development of a menstrual distress questionnaire. Psychosom Med 1968;30:853.

Mortola JF, Girton L, Fischer U. Successful treatment of severe premenstrual syndrome by combined use of gonadotropin-releasing hormone agonist and estrogen/progestin. J Clin Endocrinol Metab 1991;71:252A.

Rapkin AJ. The role of serotonin in premenstrual syndrome. Clin Obstet Gynecol 1992;35:629.

Reid RL. Premenstrual syndrome. N Engl J Med 1991;324:1208.

Reid RL, Greenway-Coats A, Hahn PM, et al. Menopausal-like hot flushes in women of reproductive age: a possible clue to the etiology of PMS. Presented at the Annual Meeting of the American Fertility Society/Canadian Fertility Society. Toronto, September 27–October 1, 1986.

Seifer DB, Collins RL. Current concepts of β-endorphin physiology in female reproductive dysfunction. Fertil Steril 1990;54:757.

Smith S, Schiff I. The premenstrual syndrome: diagnosis and management. Fertil Steril 1989;52:527.

Woods NF, Most A, Dery GK. Prevalence of premenstrual symptoms. Am J Public Health 1982;72:1257.

33
Genital Prolapse

KATHLEEN MARTIN

Primary Care for Women, edited by Phyllis C. Leppert and Fred M. Howard. Lippincott-Raven Publishers, Philadelphia © 1997.

Understanding the pathophysiology of genital prolapse and being able to evaluate the female pelvic floor are essential parts of providing care for women. Fifty percent of parous women have some degree of genital prolapse, of which 10% to 20% is symptomatic. Genital prolapse is most prevalent among white women and least prevalent in black women, with Asian women being at intermediate risk. Genital prolapse becomes more prevalent as women age. In 1980 12% of the population was older than 65 years of age, but by the year 2000 20% of the population will be older than 65. Moreover, it is estimated that 50% of women who are currently 50 years old will live to be at least 90 years old.

For clinicians who participate in the care of the female patient, a thorough pelvic examination that includes evaluation of genital prolapse is crucial. Some contend that a thorough primary evaluation is superfluous; they therefore refer the patient to a urologist if she experiences urinary incontinence, a gynecologist if she has a "bulge down there," and to a colorectal surgeon if she has fecal incontinence. Woe to the woman who has all three. This is not to say that specialists are not important, but a global view of the female pelvic floor is critical to proper management and referral. Also, there are nonsurgical preventative and therapeutic measures that the primary care physician can initiate before referral. The goal of this chapter is to help the primary care physician do just that.

ANATOMY

Pelvic floor anatomy is fundamental to understanding genital prolapse. The pelvic floor is supported by a muscular plate called the levator ani. The name is derived from one of the functions of this muscle, namely to elevate the anus. Indeed, when a patient is being coached on proper Kegel technique, it is this muscle that she is contracting. The clinician uses descriptors such as "lifting the anus internally" in describing the sensation to the patient. This muscular plate lies between the pubic bone and extends to the pelvic sidewalls and posteriorly to the ischial spine and coccyx. It is subdivided into three muscle groups according to where they attach to the pelvis (Fig. 33-1). The pubococcygeus muscle extends from the pubic bone to the coccyx. The puborectalis is a U-shaped muscle that extends from the pubic bone posteriorly behind the rectum and inserts back into the pubic bone. This portion of the levator ani is important in maintaining fecal continence. It maintains a rectal angle that straightens only during defecation, at which time the levator ani relax. Finally, the iliococcygeus extends laterally to the pelvic sidewall, inserting into a fascial condensation called the "white line" or arcus tendineus. These muscles as a group are in a constant tonic state except during urination and defecation. The levator ani act as a hammock that supports the bladder, vagina, and rectum. In the standing woman, this plate is nearly horizontal. The tonic contraction of the levator ani pulls the rectum and vagina forward, creating a nearly horizontal axis of both the vagina and rectum. This effectively closes the levator hiatus. The levator hiatus is the opening through which the urethra, vagina, and rectum pass. The levator ani interdigitate with the urethra, vagina, and anus, giving another level of support. In addition, condensations of endopelvic fascia enmesh the pelvis. These condensations contain collagen and smooth muscle and have erroneously been called fascia and ligaments. Examples of these structures include the uterosacral ligaments, pubourethral ligaments, and bladder and rectal fascia. This meshwork adds a level of stability to the pelvic floor structures. Dr. Delancey's "boat at the dock" analogy best explains this interplay: the boat represents the pelvic organs, the water represents the levator ani, and the ropes holding the boat to the dock represent the ligaments. What would happen to the tension on the ropes should the water level fall? The ropes would stretch and perhaps break. Analogously, should the pelvic floor muscles become lax, for reasons discussed later, the ligaments stretch and break because the major support of the pelvic floor has been lost.

RISK FACTORS

Many factors lead to genital prolapse. The underlying principle, however, is that it is usually not one event that leads to the development of genital prolapse, but a lifetime of incidents and accidents that lead to this culmination. In the most basic sense, this condition represents a hernia. However, this hernia does not have a simple fascial defect that can be easily oversewn. To complicate matters, it is located in the worst possible place in terms of gravitational and force vectors. Remembering the dictum that to be forewarned is to be forearmed, let us examine the risk factors for the development of genital prolapse.

Thirty percent of the American population is morbidly obese. Recalling the boat analogy, the more cargo put on the boat the deeper it sets in the water, and the more stress and strain is placed on the ropes. Clearly, obesity is a major public health concern, and its presence complicates and compromises health. The presence of

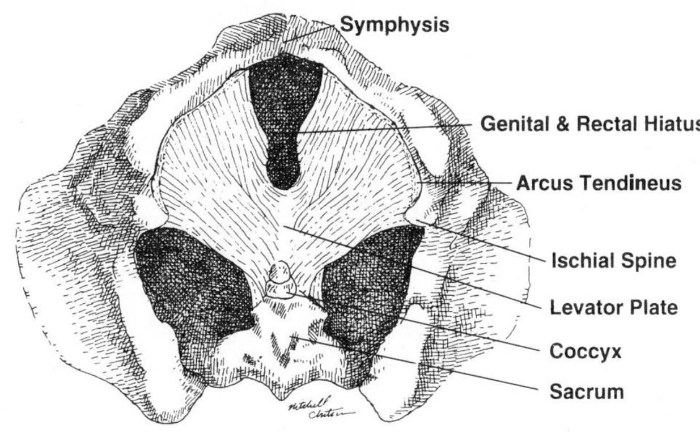

Figure 33-1. Diagrammatic respresentation of the levator ani muscles in a nulliparous woman showing the levator plate, the levator crura, and the prerectal fibers, which course between the rectum and the posterior vaginal wall. (Adapted from Nichols DH, Milley PS. Clinical anatomy of the vulva, vagina, lower pelvis, and perineum. In: Sciarra JJ, ed, Gynecology & obstetrics, vol. 2. Philadelphia: JB Lippincott, 1993:1.)

obesity decreases the likelihood of success of any therapeutic intervention that may be employed for genital prolapse.

Vaginal delivery is the biggest risk factor for the development of genital prolapse. Only 2% of prolapse cases in North America occur in nulliparas. Many aspects of parturition have been implicated, including prolonged second stage of labor, difficult forceps delivery, the macrosomic infant, and large laceration or episiotomy with suboptimal repair. Experts in the field are investigating the role of pudendal nerve injury during parturition. The pudendal nerve is the major innervation of the levator ani. Branches of the pudendal nerve innervate the external anal sphincter and the periurethral striated muscles. The pudendal nerve arises from sacral nerves 2, 3, and 4. It then courses to the back of the pelvis between the coccygeus and piriformis muscles. It exits the pelvis through the greater sciatic foramen, crosses behind the ischial spine, and then reenters the pelvis through the lesser sciatic foramen. The pudendal nerve then passes through the Alcock canal, created by a split in the obturator fascia. It is here that the nerve is relatively fixed. Finally, the nerve divides into the inferior rectal nerve, the perineal nerve, and the dorsal nerve of the clitoris. The perineal nerve further divides into a superficial branch to the labia and a deep branch to the periurethral sphincter. During parturition, as the fetus descends into the pelvis it produces traction and pressure on this nerve, which may cause injury. Depending on the size and configuration of the pelvis and the size and position of the fetus, this process can have variable and unpredictable results. Most women notice that their pelvic floors are never the same after vaginal delivery. It is a goal of researchers in this area to analyze the many variables involved with parturition and to minimize the damage incurred by vaginal delivery.

Injury to the nerves supplying the pelvic floor, whether from childbirth, trauma, or organic disease, can result in levator ani laxity. In its most severe form, this condition is called perineal descent syndrome, whereby the entire pelvic floor descends, obscuring the normal anal recess and making the anus the most caudal structure extending below the ischial tuberosities.

Chronic pressure on the pelvic floor incurred by the chronic cougher is another risk factor for prolapse. Here is another reason to encourage the smoker to quit. Controlling chronic coughing in any patient with chronic lung disease is also important. It is the chronicity of the condition that leads to the development of genital prolapse. Parenthetically, iatrogenic causes of chronic cough, such as the use of angiotensin converting enzyme inhibitors, should be avoided if possible.

Anything that causes an increase in abdominal pressure over time can lead to genital prolapse. This includes occupations that require heavy lifting and chronic straining with defecation and urination. Many women strain with defecation and urination not because they are having difficulty with elimination, but because they are in a hurry and do not want to waste time in the bathroom. To illustrate this behavioral phenomenon, it is uncommon to see a woman go to the bathroom with a magazine in her hand, a common custom among her male counterparts. This is a socialized behavior that requires behavioral modification to overcome.

Many women experience genital prolapse after menopause. There are estrogen receptors throughout the tissues of the pelvic floor, and with estrogen deprivation these tissues become atrophic and their blood supply diminishes, thus compromising tissue strength.

Previous hysterectomy can place a patient at risk for prolapse, especially if the surgeon is not diligent in supporting the vagina carefully. This is estimated to occur in 1% of patients with hysterectomies; however, it is most likely an underestimate. Repairing any coexistent defects of the pelvic floor at the time of hysterectomy is also important. There is no difference in the risk of posthysterectomy prolapse after abdominal or vaginal hysterectomy.

Finally, it is common for a patient to state that many women in her family have had similar problems with genital prolapse. There is likely to be a genetic component to the strength and elasticity of collagen. This is demonstrated in the obstetric clinics daily in that some women develop extensive striae with pregnancy and others develop none.

PATHOPHYSIOLOGY

When evaluating a patient with genital prolapse, the goal is to precisely define where the defects in support are located. Before discussing how to examine the patient, the possible defects and their possible locations should be analyzed. The vagina is a fibromuscular tube that is held in place by its attachments laterally to the pelvic sidewall, by its attachments apically to the uterosacral "ligaments" and bladder, by its attachment posteriorly to the rectovaginal septum, and by its attachment distally to the perineal body. These "attachments" are the condensations of endopelvic "fascia" previously described. Remember that although these support structures are referred to as ligaments and fascia, they are really made up of smooth muscle, collagen, and neurovascular pedicles and are not the classic fascia that overlies muscle. Defects in the support of the vagina can occur in any one of these areas and are usually multiple. These defects are called cystocele, rectocele, uterovaginal prolapse, enterocele, and rectal prolapse, depending on which pelvic organ has prolapsed (Fig. 33-2). As Figure 33-3 demonstrates, midline and sidewall breaks may occur in the tissues supporting the bladder and rectum. First, directing attention to the anterior vaginal wall, the anterior vagina may be seen ballooning down without the normal rugal vaginal folds. This finding is consistent with a midline break in the vesicovaginal fascia overlying the bladder. The anterior vaginal

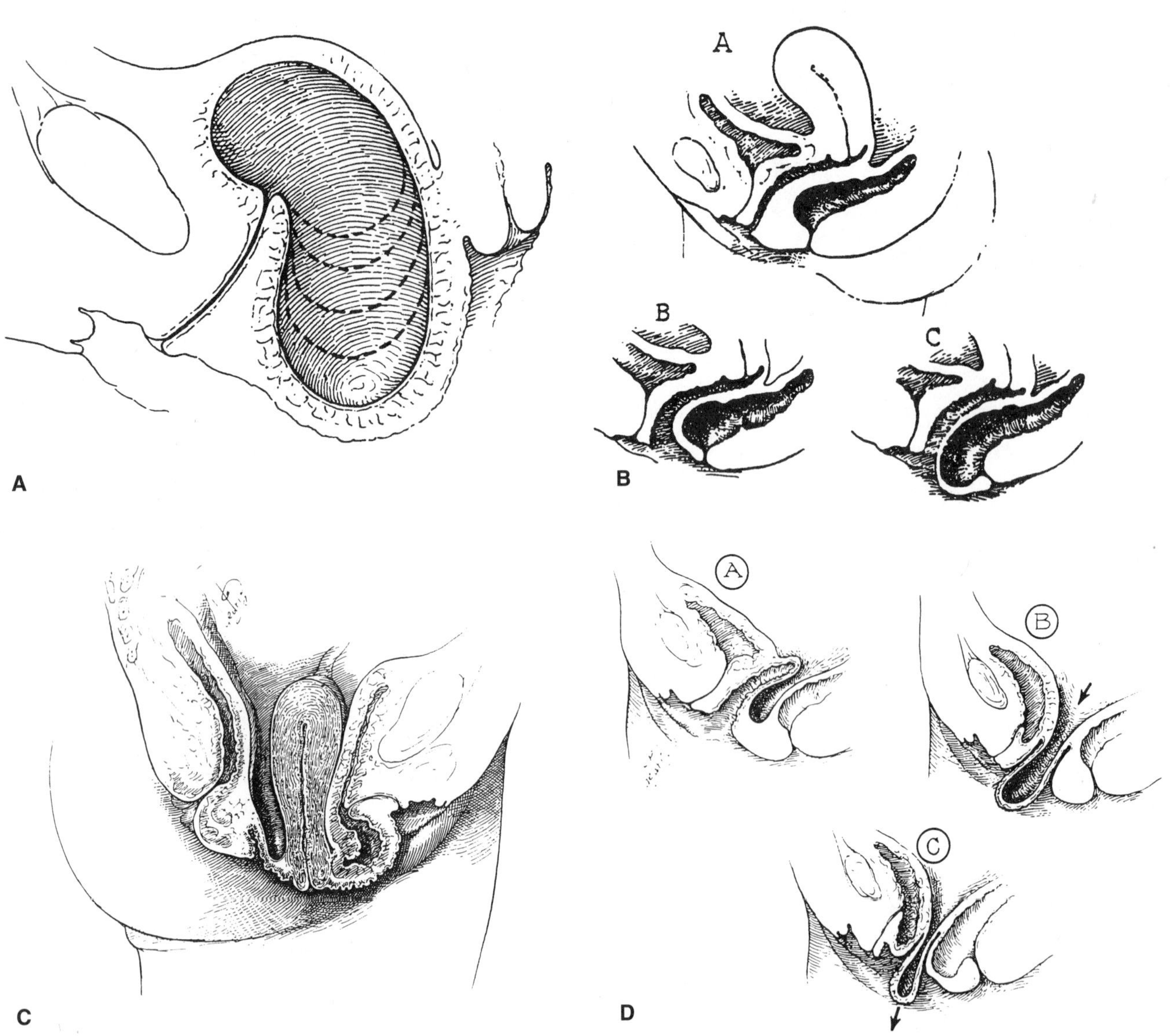

A

B

C

D

Figure 33-2. (***A***) Varying degrees of posterior distention–type cystocele are shown by the broken lines. (***B***) A normal relationship between vagina, perineum, and rectum is depicted in *A*. A major perineal defect is seen in *B*, there is no rectocele, but restoration of the nerineal body is indicated. A major perineal defect with rectocele is shown in *C* and, in this cirumstance, perineorrhaphy should be accompanied by an appropriate posterior colporrhaphy. (***C***) Uterovaginal or sliding prolapse is depicted. There is enterocele but no rectocele present. The uterosacal ligaments are long and strong. Note the position of the uninvolved anterior rectal wall. (Adapted from Nichols DH, Randall CL, eds. Vaginal surgery, 3rd ed. Baltimore: Williams & Wilkins, 1989.) (***D***) *A*, posterior enterocele without eversion of the vagina. *B*, with pulsion enterocele, the upper vagina is everted and the enterocele sac follows the everted vault. Cystocele and rectocele are minimal. *C*, with traction enterocele, there is eversion of the vagina with enterocele, cystocele, and rectocele. (From Nichols DH. Obstectics and gynecology. New York: Elsevier Science Publishing, 1972:257.)

wall also may descend with the rugal folds intact. This finding is suggestive of a sidewall (ie, paravaginal) or apical tear in the supporting structures. The former defect, without normal rugal folds, is referred to as a distention cystocele, and the latter, with intact rugal folds, a displacement cystocele. Analogous defects may occur on the posterior vaginal wall; however, they are not classified as displacement or distention rectoceles, but rather are described in terms of location (ie, low, mid-, high, or full length). One of the most common causes of low rectocele is detachment of the rectovaginal septum from the perineal body. This usually occurs during vaginal delivery.

The apical supports of the vagina and cervix may be compromised, allowing the uterus and cervix to descend. In its most extreme form, the entire uterus and cervix prolapse out of the vagina. This is called procidentia. Remember that the uterus is the innocent passenger and not the cause of the prolapse. Additionally, small bowel may interpose between the vagina and rectum in the rectovaginal space, causing an enterocele. The two types of enteroceles are classified according to the forces that generate the defects. In a pulsion enterocele, intraabdominal pressure forces small bowel into the rectovaginal space. In a traction enterocele,

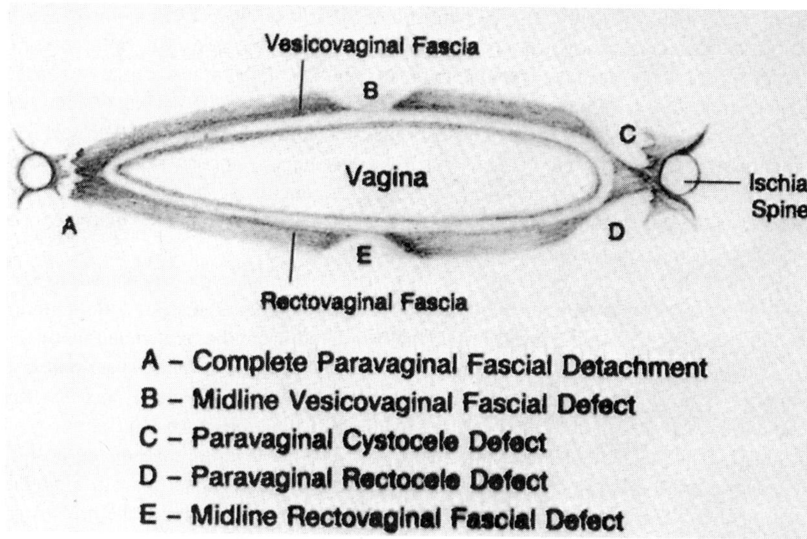

Figure 33-3. Vagina support loss. Sites of midline and paravaginal defects: The following locations are shown: (***A***), paravaginal, (***B***), anterior, (***C***), lateral vesicovaginal, (***D***), rectovaginal, and (***E***), posterior midline fascial defects. (From Baden WF, Walker T. Surgical repair of vaginal defects. Philadelphia: JB Lippincott, 1992:47.)

the cul-de-sac and rectovaginal space are pulled down by other pelvic floor defects that allow development of the enterocele.

Rectal prolapse also may be present, wherein the rectal mucosa intususscepts through the anus. This can be differentiated from prolapsed hemorrhoids by the circumferential folds present in the rectal mucosa. Hemorrhoidal prolapse exhibits vertical folds.

THE PATIENT INTERVIEW

The classic complaint of a patient with genital prolapse is that of a bulge. The bulge at first is present only intermittently, but as time and gravity take their toll the bulge becomes progressively worse. The patient also may complain of a backache that is not present in the morning but becomes progressively worse throughout the day. Another common symptom is that of progressive pelvic pressure throughout the day. The patient may have urinary incontinence. Often the patient states that she had problems with incontinence until the bulge became worse and then no further incontinence was noted. This occurs because as the bladder descends the urethra kinks. Concomitant with progressive prolapse, the patient may notice a slow stream of urine or difficulty with defecation. As the prolapse progresses even further, the patient may require manual reduction of the prolapse to urinate, defecate, or both. With long-standing prolapse, the exposed vaginal mucosa develops ulcerations that may be painful and infected. Remember that many women with less severe degrees of prolapse are entirely asymptomatic and are unaware of the impending descent. In this group of patients, clinicians have the chance of preventing further prolapse if pelvic floor evaluations are performed to identify the women at risk.

THE PHYSICAL EXAMINATION

The complete pelvic floor examination is done in both the dorsolithotomy and standing positions, with the patient performing a Valsalva maneuver in both positions. This is a difficult examination for the patient, especially if she also has urinary or fecal incontinence, because she will be afraid of having an "accident" during the examination. To do an adequate examination, the clinician has to be sensitive to this and reassure the patient. The pelvic floor examination can easily be incorporated into the normal pelvic examination. To be able to measure the various components of the pelvic floor, it is helpful to use the distance between the interphalangeal joints of the clinician's dominant index finger. The following system has been endorsed by the International Continence Society (ICS) to standardize the way clinicians describe the pelvic floor, improve communication between physicians, and objectify findings to facilitate research in this area.

The components of the pelvic floor examination include the genital hiatus, perineal body, anterior vaginal wall, posterior vaginal wall, cervix, cul-de-sac, total vaginal length, levator ani tone, and external anal sphincter tone (Fig. 33-4). First, careful inspection of the vulva is performed to look for atrophy and to assess the size of the genital hiatus and perineal body. The genital hiatus is measured from the urethral meatus to the 6 o'clock position on the

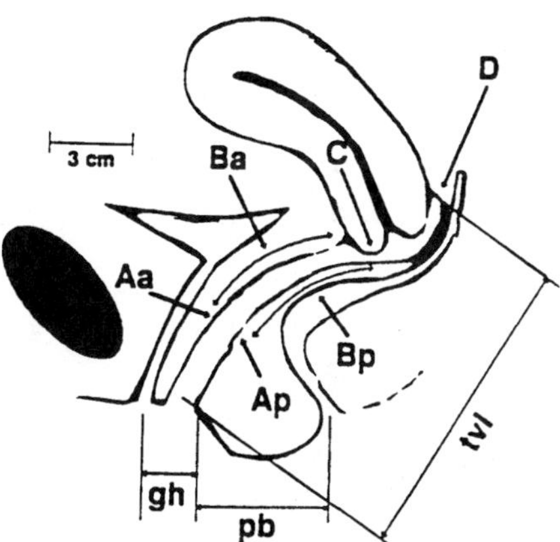

Figure 33-4. Six points, genital hiatus (gh), perineal body (pb), and total vaginal length (tvl) used for prolapse quantitation. (Adapted from The International Continence Society. The standardization of terminology of female pelvic organ prolapse and pelvic floor dysfunction. Bristol UK: The International Continence Society, 1994.)

hymenal margin. The perineal body is measured from 6 o'clock position on the hymenal margin to the anus. Nulliparous values are about 1.5 and 4 cm, respectively. Next, a speculum is placed to assess the vaginal walls and cervix. A pap smear is taken at this time if appropriate. Vaginal walls that are collapsing around the edges of the speculum indicate a lack of paravaginal support.

The speculum is then taken apart, with only the bottom half of the speculum used for traction. Alternatively, a Sims retractor can be used. The posterior vaginal wall is gently depressed, allowing full visualization of the anterior vaginal wall. The patient is then asked to perform a Valsalva maneuver. Usually her first Valsalva attempt is weak, and, therefore, several Valsalva maneuvers should be done to note the maximum degree that the anterior vaginal wall descends. The ICS has described two points on the anterior vaginal wall. One is located 3 cm from the urethral meatus and corresponds to the approximate location of the urethral vesical junction. It is designated point Aa and has a value of −3 in the nonprolapsed state. The hymen is the reference point, and anything distal to it is measured in positive centimeters and anything proximal is measured in negative centimeters. The capitalized letter *A* refers to that point on the anterior vaginal wall that lies 3 cm from the urethral meatus, and the subscript *a* refers to the anterior vaginal wall. Point B on the anterior vaginal wall (ie, Ba) refers to the lowest point on the anterior vaginal wall proximal to point Aa. For instance, if there is no prolapse of the anterior vaginal wall, then both point Aa and point Ba are −3. Distinguishing between point Aa and Ba is difficult. Theoretically, it is important to observe where the urethrovesical junction is relative to the remainder of the anterior vaginal wall. However, the entire wall often descends in such a fashion as to make this distinction difficult. It may be easier to measure the lowest point of prolapse of the anterior vaginal wall relative to the hymen and call this point A. The examiner uses the known interphalangeal distance of the index finger to assess the distance relative to the hymen. Recall that it is necessary to observe whether there is loss of the rugal folds of the vagina, which is consistent with a distention cystocele, versus no loss of the rugal folds, which characterizes a displacement cystocele. Determining where the defects lie with a displacement cystocele is out of the scope of this chapter. The interested reader is referred to the many texts and journals on this subject.

Next, attention is turned to the posterior vaginal wall. Again, two points have been defined. Point Ap is measured in the midline of the posterior vaginal wall 3 cm from the hymen and has a value of −3 in the nonprolapsed state. Point Bp is the lowest point of the posterior vaginal wall proximal to point Ap and is also −3 in the nonprolapsed state. Again, the distinction of Ap and Bp may be difficult. A solution is to measure the leading edge of the posterior vaginal wall prolapse during maximum Valsalva, with the hymen as the reference point. Remember, too, that it is helpful to note whether it is a low, mid-, high, or full-length rectocele. Figure 33-5 demonstrates the ICS grading system for normal support and for complete vaginal vault eversion.

A bimanual examination then is performed in the routine fashion to assess the uterus and adnexa and to note any pelvic masses. During this portion of the examination, the clinician may assess levator tone by asking the patient to squeeze the examining fingers with her vagina. The clinician may be surprised to learn how many patients perform a Valsalva maneuver instead of the classic Kegel squeeze. The patient is reminded not to flex her abdomen, adductors, or gluteus muscles during this Kegel maneuver. Many patients think that they are doing a proper Kegel when really they are flexing every muscle but the levator ani. With proper instruction at this

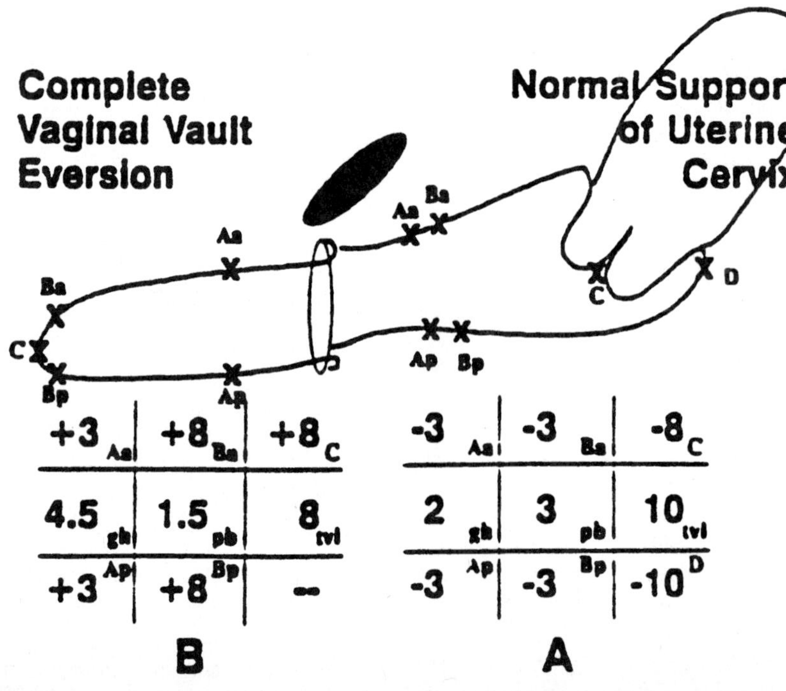

Figure 33-5. (*A*) Normal support. (*B*) Complete eversion. (Adapted from The International Continence Society. The standardization of terminology of female pelvic organ prolapse and pelvic floor dysfunction. Bristol, UK: The International Continence Society, 1994.)

point in the examination, many women can be reeducated as to the proper technique, which they can then practice at home. With the examining finger touching the cervix, the patient is then asked to perform a Valsalva maneuver. The examiner "follows" the cervix down with the "measured" index finger and notes where, relative to the index finger, the cervix descends, remembering that ground zero is the hymen (see Fig. 33-5, point *C*). A similar procedure is then performed, placing the finger on the cul-de-sac behind the cervix and following its descent with Valsalva (see Fig. 33-5, point D). If the patient has no cervix, then just the vaginal cuff is assessed (see Fig. 33-5, point C). Finally, the total vaginal length is assessed at rest without a Valsalva maneuver. This measurement is important because if a patient has a foreshortened vagina, a pessary is less likely to be successful.

The final part of the examination is a rectovaginal examination in the standing position. This allows the clinician to assess for the presence of an enterocele and also to note whether the degree of prolapse was underestimated in the dorsolithotomy position. The clinician places a finger in the vagina and in the rectum and again asks the patient to perform a Valsalva maneuver. If a bulge descending between the vagina and rectum is detected, then this is evidence for an enterocele. External anal sphincter tone is also assessed, and stool for guaiac is obtained. The presence of stool in the rectum is a sign of abnormal bowel emptying, whether it be secondary to the presence of a rectocele, constipation, or other bowel motility disorder. The most common cause stems from improper diet, which leads to constipation.

In truth, the physical examination is not a reliable way to assess for the presence of an enterocele. To absolutely define whether an enterocele is present, a modified defecogram can be obtained as popularized by Drs. Linda Brubaker and J. Thomas Benson. Contrast is placed in the small bowel, bladder, vagina, and rectum, and then the patient is instructed to defecate and radiographs are taken. Documenting the presence of an enterocele is important only if surgery is being planned and the findings on examination are not straightforward. All defects of the pelvic floor are demonstrated with this type of defecography. Parenthetically, this test reveals the presence of a sigmoidocele wherein the sigmoid—not the rectum or small bowel—has prolapsed into the rectovaginal space. Some estimate that this occurs in about 1% of cases thought to be rectocele or enterocele. Again, the importance of knowing that this defect exists is when surgical repair is planned.

MEDICAL MANAGEMENT

As observed earlier, the finding of genital prolapse may indeed be asymptomatic. At this point the primary care provider has a chance to impact its further development. Counseling on weight reduction, smoking cessation, lifting precautions, and regular Kegel exercise may prevent further progression. If the patient is unable to perform Kegel exercise, she may benefit from pelvic floor rehabilitation via biofeedback and electrical stimulation. Perhaps the patient is able to flex her levator ani, but only weakly. This is a patient who may benefit from vaginal cone therapy. These vaginal cones are of graduated weights, and the patient is instructed to place this weight in her vagina 15 minutes twice a day. The heaviest cone she is able to retain is where she starts. As her Kegel ability improves, the weight is gradually increased. See Chapter 80 for more details on urinary incontinence.

The patient should understand that she does not have to have surgery for her condition. The exception would be failed pessary management of severe genital prolapse that causes ureteral obstruction or chronic vaginal ulcerations. These cases are fortunately rare. It is the patient's symptoms and quality of life issues that determine what, if any, treatment is required for her prolapse. Reassuring the patient that she does not have a serious rare disease is important. Should the patient be symptomatic, a pessary trial can be offered. If the condition is severe enough or symptomatic enough that referral is necessary, the clinician should seek a specialist who has expertise in the entire pelvic floor and not just one part of it. Usually the bladder, vagina, and rectum are all involved to varying degrees, and all are impacted by treatment.

The pessary device has been around for eons and certainly has a role, should the patient opt for nonsurgical intervention. Figure 33-6 shows a Gellhorn, donut, ring, and cube pessary. Many others are on the market. The right pessary for a particular patient is the one that works. A pessary should cause no pain and be totally asymptomatic after placement. Patients with foreshortened vaginas or large rectoceles typically have a difficult time retaining a pessary. If the levator hiatus is abnormally widened or the perineal defect is exceptionally large, the patient will also have a difficult time retaining a pessary. These patients are most likely to require surgery, should their symptoms warrant such intervention. The most successful pessary for genital prolapse is the Gellhorn. The downside is that it is difficult to remove and to place. It is difficult to teach a patient to do this on her own, although not impossible in the motivated patient. This is not an issue for the patient who is not sexually active, however. In that subset of patients, the pessary may be placed and left in for 3 months at a time. The patient is instructed to use estrogen vaginal cream once a week at bedtime (2 g) and return for pessary checks every 3 months. She is carefully advised that pain with a pessary is never acceptable and must be evaluated at once. The patient is also advised to call if she experiences a vaginal discharge. The risks of the pessary include ulceration, failure to support the prolapse, and urinary incontinence. The patient who has a contraindication to estrogen use may be treated with Trimo-san (oxyquinoline sulfate, sodium lauryl sulfate, boric

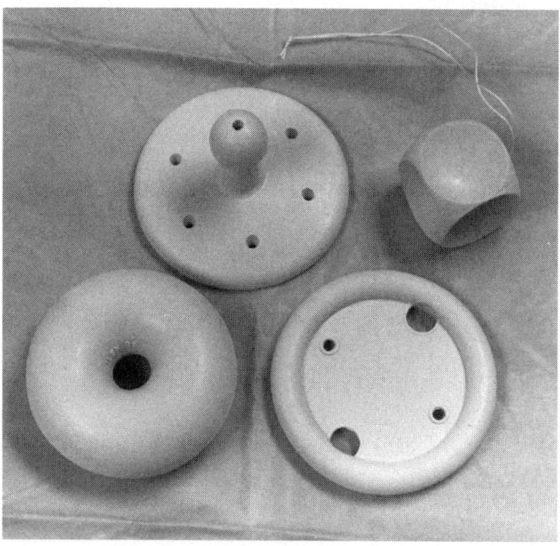

Figure 33-6. Examples of commonly used pessaries.

acid, and borax) or Sultrin (sulfathiazole, sulfacetamide, and, sulfabenzamide) vaginal cream one night per week. If a Gellhorn is used for genital prolapse in which the cervix is still present, a polyp on the posterior lip of the cervix will almost certainly develop. This is of no clinical relevance but may cause some nuisance bleeding. Of course, a biopsy must be performed on a lesion of questionable pathology; however, development of this "pressure polyp" should not be unexpected. The key to placing and removing a pessary is to instruct the patient that it will be slightly uncomfortable, and to place and remove the device slowly and gently. I have had the best success with Gellhorn pessaries. A patient who is sexually active most likely will be unable to remove and replace the Gellhorn pessary on her own, and therefore the ring or cube pessary may be effective. A precautionary note on the cube pessary is in order. This pessary maintains its position by suction and therefore must be removed nightly or every other night to prevent the development of ulcerations.

The Gellhorn pessary is placed so that the knob lies in the axis of the vagina. The round circle lies above the levator ani behind the pubic bone at a 45° angle to the floor while the patient is in the dorsolithotomy position. The ring and donut pessaries are placed similarly, except there is no knob. The orientation of the cube pessary is unimportant. After placement of the pessary, the patient is asked to sit on the toilet and bear down. If the pessary is too small it will fall out with this maneuver. The patient is advised that if the pessary falls out at home she should retrieve the pessary before flushing the toilet. She is told not to panic but to call the office for placement of a larger size. Usually if the pessary is going to fall out it will do so with Valsalva maneuvers in the office. The patient should be warned about incipient urinary incontinence with pessary placement. This occurs because the kinking of the urethra that occurs with a large cystocele is removed with reduction of the prolapse. If the patient was relying on that kink for continence, incontinence will follow. This also indicates what would result from surgical intervention should no attention be paid to the bladder during repair of the prolapse. This highlights the importance of a thorough urodynamic evaluation before pelvic reconstructive surgery. Certainly, if the patient has problems with chronic constipation efforts to alleviate this should be undertaken concurrently with pessary management.

Pelvic floor rehabilitation is discussed in Chapter 80. This involves both biofeedback and electrical stimulation to retrain the patient on how to flex her levator ani so that she may strengthen this muscle complex. Clearly, in the patient with severe pudendal neuropathy, this therapy has no benefit. No prospective studies have been undertaken to evaluate the effect of pelvic floor rehabilitation in patients with asymptomatic prolapse. However, this is an important area for future research. It is reasonable to presume that since the levator ani are the primary support of the pelvic floor, strengthening this muscle should be beneficial to maintain this support.

SUMMARY

This chapter has highlighted the importance of genital prolapse as a public health issue and has clarified its evaluation. Certainly, there is much that the primary health care provider can do to help in the prevention of its development. Further, patients should be referred to specialists in the field who, when considering surgical intervention, consider the entire pelvic floor and not just a portion of it.

BIBLIOGRAPHY

Delancey JO. Anatomy and biomechanics of genital prolapse. Clin Obstet Gynecol 1993;36:897.

Harris TA, Bent AE. Genital prolapse with and without urinary incontinence. J Reprod Med 1990;35:792.

Kelvin FM, Maglinte DT, Benson JT. Evacuation proctography (defecography): an aid to the investigation of pelvic floor disorders. Obstet Gynecol 1994;83:307.

Nichols DH, Genadry R. Pelvic relaxation of the posterior compartment. Curr Opin Obstet Gynecol 1993;5:458.

Nichols DH, Randall CL. Vaginal surgery, 3rd ed. Baltimore: Williames & Wilkins, 1989.

Stanton S. Prolapse. Baillieres Clin Obstet Gynaecol 1988;2:385.

The Standardisation of Terminology of Female Pelvic Organ Prolapse and Pelvic Floor Dysfunction. ICS Final Draft 1994.

Timmons MC, Addison WA. Pelvic relaxation involving the middle compartment. Curr Opin Obstet Gynecol 1993;5:452.

Wall L. Medical management of pelvic relaxation. Curr Opin Obstet Gynecol 1993;5:440.

34
Environmental Hazards to Reproduction

MAGGIE D. VILL

Primary Care for Women, edited by Phyllis C. Leppert and Fred M. Howard. Lippincott-Raven Publishers, Philadelphia © 1997.

Infertility is by no means a simple problem. It has multiple etiologies, which, in many cases, are never elucidated. Oligospermia, azoospermia, or anovulation can be diagnosed, but what factors contribute to these states? Many physicians do not think of environmental exposure as a possible etiology of the inability to reproduce. Heat, chemicals, metals, and radiation have been shown to adversely affect reproductive capabilities. Is the possibility of environmental exposure entertained during the investigation for repetitive spontaneous abortions or continued inability to conceive?

Every physician cannot be an expert in occupational medicine. However, every physician should be capable of eliciting a good occupational history.

Environmental exposure may be involved in the development of disease. To determine if an environmental hazard or exposure is a contributing factor, a good occupational history is required. Suspicion leads to further investigation.

As a screening tool, questions addressing current or past exposure to any chemicals, fumes, radiation, loud noises, excessive heat, or biohazards may be asked. These questions elicit information on possible exposure at home and work, and the answers may indicate the need for a more thorough occupational history.

When inquiring about the details of the chief complaint, any relationship between activities at work or home (eg, hobbies) and the time of onset of symptoms should be noted. If symptoms are ameliorated during vacations or on weekends, job-related exposure may be a factor. Does the patient have any other complicating factors, for example, cigarette smoking or medications taken at work or home? Occasionally a patient's reason for consultation may involve questions of occupational exposure and its impact on her health. For example, a patient at her first prenatal visit may inquire if chemicals handled at work will affect her baby.

A thorough occupational history includes current and past employment with a detailed description of the job performed by the patient, the nature of the manufactured product, and whether other workers experience similar symptoms or illnesses. Find out if special equipment is used in carrying out tasks and if special ventilation is used within the occupational environment. Does the patient need special personal protective equipment? If so, must personal protective equipment be used continuously or only when performing certain tasks? Has the employee been compliant with equipment use? Is the personal protective equipment comfortable? (Discomfort may be a key to noncompliance.) Is the equipment inspected or tested periodically? Are filters used that must be changed after a certain period of time? If so, what indicates the need for filter change? Is the indication time elapsed or is an odor perceived (and is the allowable limit of exposure exceeded when the odor is perceptible)? Although hazardous materials are handled on the job, hazardous exposure has not necessarily occurred. What has to be determined is if the employer has complied with Occupational Safety and Health Administration regulations for occupational exposure. This is where consultation with an industrial hygienist is valuable. The worker and care provider have the right to obtain results of industrial hygiene measurements and biologic monitoring that has been performed at the workplace. The physician has the right to request a worksite tour to better understand the work performed by the patient as well as the conditions under which there may be toxic exposure. The employer may also be asked to perform measurements of exposure. If this request is denied, federal and state regulatory agencies in occupational health can perform workplace inspections and environmental monitoring at the request of a concerned employee.

If the patient does not have knowledge of the specific chemicals used on the job, the physician or patient may obtain material safety data sheets (MSDS) from the employer that explain chemical components and possible health effects of the substances handled by the patient. MSDS, however, often do not contain information about reproductive effects. Additional data may be obtained from hotlines, databases, published references, and occupational medicine specialists. An experienced occupational health physician in the local area can be consulted to help obtain and analyze data and suggest strategies. Such strategies may be a temporary job transfer or compensated leave. Information services such as TERIS (Seattle), Perinatal Environmental & Drug Consultation Service (Rochester, NY), Centers for Disease Control (Atlanta), and REPROTOX (Washington, DC) are valuable sources of information.

Lead, mercury, and pesticides are discussed in greater detail as examples of substances that may be sources of reproductive hazard in the occupational or home setting.

LEAD

All practitioners should be aware of the adverse effects of lead exposure on reproduction. Lead was believed to be an abortifacient during the late 19th and early 20th centuries in women in the pottery and white lead industries. That lead crosses the placenta was illustrated by Timpo and associates, who reported a case of congenital lead intoxication when a pregnant patient ate paint chips during the last few months of her pregnancy. The patient underwent chelation therapy during pregnancy and delivered 8 days after the therapy was completed. The cord blood level was found to be 60 μg/dL, and neonatal x-rays revealed metaphysitis, submetaphyseal lucencies, and sclerosis of the shafts. Bellinger and associates, in a prospective cohort study, looked at the early cognitive development of children with low (< 3 μg/dL), medium (6 to 7 μg/dL), or high (≥ 10 μg/dL) prenatal exposure based on umbilical cord blood levels. At all ages, infants in the high–prenatal exposure group scored lower than infants in the other two groups on developmental tests. The current Occupational Safety and Health Administration Lead Standard states that the maximum allowable blood lead levels for newborns is < 30μg/dL, which is much higher than the levels observed by Bellinger and coworkers found to affect cognitive development in children up 2 years of age.

Lead is found in paint, water, food, air, and soil. Although the level of lead in paint was decreased in 1971, it continues to be a significant source of exposure because it is found in older homes in the United States. Those engaged in renovation of older homes must be advised to take the proper precautions to limit exposure to lead. This is illustrated by the report by Marino and coworkers of lead poisoning in a family who had levels of lead requiring chelation therapy although they were not actively participating in the renovation. The family was exposed to the dust and fumes generated by sanding and torching to remove the old layers of paint. Drinking water also can be a significant source of lead, because it leaches out of lead pipe service connections or lead solder used to join copper pipes.

Lancranjan and others studied the effects of lead on spermatogenesis. One hundred fifty men working in a storage battery plant were investigated. Semen analyses showed an increased frequency of asthenospermia, hypospermia, and teratospermia in the men who had lead poisoning and in the men with moderately increased absorption of lead. Urinary excretion of gonadotropins were within the limits of normal, indicating that the hypothalamic–pituitary axis was not affected and that lead had a direct effect on the gonads.

MERCURY

Mercury is another metal to which patients may be exposed. Mercury can be found in three states: elemental mercury (Hg^0) which is a silver gray liquid at room temperature, inorganic mercury salts (mercurous Hg^{+1} and mercuric Hg^{+2}), and organic mercury (most important of which is methyl mercury).

Elemental Mercury

Elemental mercury is used in thermometers, thermostats, sphygmomanometers, and batteries. Elemental mercury is a liquid at room temperature and is easily vaporized when heated. It is about 80% absorbed when inhaled and has a biologic half-life of about 60 days. Elemental mercury is more neurotoxic than mercury salts because it has a greater ability to cross cell membranes. Occupational exposures are usually through inhalation of mercury vapor. Folk medicines used by Mexican-Americans and Asian populations also may be a source of mercury exposure. A case of early prenatal exposure to elemental mercury was reported by Thorp and colleagues. The patient was exposed during the first trimester and presented for evaluation at 17 weeks' gestation, at which time a 24-hour urine specimen yielded levels of 230 μg/L (normal < 25). At the time of term delivery, maternal urine levels were undetectable. The cord blood yielded a level of 1.4 ng Hg/mL (normal < 1.6), and neonatal hair levels were 3 ng/g (normal < 0.008). Thorp and associates concluded that whereas inorganic and organic forms of mercury may cross the placenta, the organic form passes more easily. The form of mercury exposure is important when advising mothers. Several factors contribute to the development of symptoms with exposure to elemental mercury and include the concentration of vaporized mercury, length of exposure, and individual susceptibility. With acute exposure, symptoms include metallic taste, burning, irritation, salivation, vomiting, diarrhea, upper gastrointestinal tract edema, abdominal pain, and hemorrhage.

Inorganic Mercury

Mercuric salts (Hg^{+2}) are used to inhibit bacterial or fungal growth. They are used as preservatives in eye drops, eye ointments, nasal sprays, and vaccines. Mercuric salts were once used as cathartic, antisyphilitic, antipruritic, and antiinflammatory medications. Interior latex paint manufactured before 1990 and outdoor paint before 1991 may contain mercury compounds used to prevent bacterial and fungal growth.

Organic Mercury

Most human exposure to organic mercury is through food (eg, fish or contaminated grain). Microorganisms found in soil and water can potentially methylate any mercury compound released into the environment to methylmercury. Methylmercury found in water accumulates in fish by their eating contaminated food and through their gills. Biomagnification occurs as small fish are eaten by larger fish. This is a concern in the face of the now-popular dietary consumption of fish to reduce cholesterol. Ingestion of fish from contaminated waters can lead to significant exposures. Limiting the ingestion of fish from these areas to one meal per month is recommended. The department of health in the patient's area can provide information on the water conditions found locally. Several examples of mercury poisoning through ingestion of contaminated food have been reported.

In late 1953 in and around Minamata, a town in southern Japan, a nervous disorder began afflicting villagers. The manifestations included mental confusion, convulsions, and coma with death in about 38% of individuals. Between 1955 and 1959, about 6% of the children born in the area developed cerebral palsy. Chorea, ataxia, tremors, seizures, and mental retardation were additional symptoms seen in these children. The fish from Minamata Bay was found to contain 9 to 24 μg/g of methylmercury.

In 1972, an epidemic of methylmercury poisoning occurred in Iraq due to ingestion of bread prepared from wheat treated with a methylmercury fungicide. Among those evaluated were 15 infant–mother pairs exposed to methylmercury during pregnancy. Blood and milk samples obtained from these patients as well as clinical examinations were the basis of the report. Amin-Zaki and coworkers report that infants born during and shortly after maternal consumption of contaminated bread received maximum exposure late in gestation and had a relatively large postnatal intake from milk. Infants born 6 to 9 months after maternal consumption of methylmercury were maximally exposed in early pregnancy. As reported by the Amin-Zaki group, the most frequent symptoms in the adults included malaise, vague muscle and joint pains, and loss of sensation in the perioral regions and extremities. Motor weakness and exaggerated reflexes also were observed. Of the infants, the oldest was 6.5 months of age whereas the youngest was 6 days of age. No congenital anomalies were noted, and weight and length measurements were within normal ranges. Five severely affected infants had evidence of gross impairment of motor and mental development, with cerebral palsy, deafness, and blindness in four. The results obtained by Amin-Zaki and colleagues indicate that methylmercury passes the placenta readily since 14 of 15 blood samples obtained from the mother–infant pairs showed infant levels of mercury at birth and up to 4 months after birth that were equal to or higher than the concentrations in maternal blood.

PESTICIDES

Pesticide exposure can occur anywhere since they are sold over the counter and are used in the home, at work, and in the agricultural setting. Various occupational settings may incur exposure. A worker who handles pesticides or is in contact with crops that are sprayed has the greatest exposure. Examples are those employed in greenhouses, as chemical lawn sprayers, as workers on golf courses or parks, and as farm workers.

At home, potential exposures may occur in those living in rural communities comprised of orchards, vineyards, citrus groves, or vegetable fields that are regularly sprayed with a variety of pesticides.

When used in the home, proper precautions must be taken since pesticides can be absorbed through the skin and respiratory or gastrointestinal tract.

1,2-Dibromo-3-chloropropane (DBCP) is an example of a pesticide that has been shown to cause male infertility. Whorton and associates studied a number of workers in a California pesticide factory. Length of time worked at the plant was used as a measure of exposure. Semen samples were examined for sperm count, motility, and morphology. Other laboratory tests included blood chemistries, urinalysis, complete and differential blood counts, thyroxine, testosterone, follicle stimulating hormone (FSH), and luteinizing hormone (LH) assays. Men with indisputably low sperm counts (≤ 1 million) were compared with men with normal sperm counts (≥ 40 million) by age; time worked in the plant; and serum LH, FSH, and testosterone levels. Additionally, bilateral open testicular biopsies were performed on nine volunteers who represented a spectrum of chemical exposure times and sperm counts. Workers with sperm counts ≤ 1 million had been exposed at least 3 years, whereas none with sperm counts above 40 million had been exposed for more than 3 months. The men with low sperm counts were found to have significantly higher levels of FSH and LH. Measurements of airborne DBCP were conducted and found to be less than 1 ppm.

Potashnik and coworkers evaluated six men at a DBCP factory and found results similar to the Whorton group. All six men had azoospermia, elevated FSH levels, normal testosterone levels, but also normal LH levels. Bilateral testicular biopsy was performed in four of the six men and revealed that the seminiferous epithelium had undergone complete atrophy and most of the tubules were lined by Sertoli cells only. There was no evidence of active spermatogenesis. Effects in women have not been evaluated. This insecticide has been banned in the United States.

HEAT

Maternal hyperthermia early in gestation has been thought to be associated with an increased incidence of neural tube defects. Retrospective studies suggest that significant maternal hyperthermia (defined as temperature of 38.9°C or above) during the first trimester is associated with central nervous system and facial defects. Prospective studies, however, do not show a significantly increased incidence of congenital anomalies or neurologic abnormalities in women who experienced hyperthermia in the first trimester. Comparing women who experienced first-trimester febrile illnesses with temperature elevations to 38.9°C or higher with women who did not report febrile illnesses during pregnancy, Clarren and associates found no differences in the incidence of congenital malformations, preterm birth, growth retardation, stillbirth, or postnatal neurologic deficits.

Harvey and others studied nonpregnant women to assess the possibility of maternal hyperthermia due to bathing in a hot tub or sauna during the first trimester. They used two hot tubs: an indoor tub set at 39°C, and an outdoor tub at 41.1°C. The sauna that they used had an average temperature of 81.4°C with a relative humidity of 15%. The subject's temperature was recorded before entering the tub or sauna, every 5 minutes during her stay, immediately before she left the heated environment, and 10 minutes thereafter. Harvey and colleagues conclude that healthy women of childbearing age are able to remain in a hot tub at 39°C for at least 15 minutes and at 41.1°C for at least 10 minutes without risk of their core temperature reaching 38.9°C. All of the subjects left the sauna and most left the hot tubs because of discomfort before their vaginal temperatures reached 38.9°C.

The generation of heat during exercise was studied by Lotgering and associates. Under normal resting conditions, the temperature of the fetus is about 0.5°C higher than that of the mother in humans and sheep. By exercising sheep, Lotgering and coworkers found that fetal temperature lagged behind maternal temperature, such that at the beginning the fetal–maternal temperature difference was reduced or even reversed, whereas a larger temperature difference existed after exercise. With higher levels of exercise, the maternal temperature increased more rapidly and these changes were more prominent. Prolonged (40 minutes) exhaustive exercise led to a slow return of the fetal temperature to control values, requiring more than 1 hour. No large, well-controlled prospective studies have addressed the issue of physical activity and its effect on fetal outcome. The American College of Obstetricians and Gynecologists recommends that women can continue to exercise on a regular basis and derive health benefits from mild-to-moderate exercise routines. Exercise in the supine position should be avoided after the first trimester, as should exercising to exhaustion. Women who have any risk factors for adverse maternal or perinatal outcomes (ie, premature rupture of membranes, preterm labor during the prior or current pregnancy or both, incompetent cervix or history of cerclage, persistent second- or third-trimester bleeding, intrauterine growth retardation, or pregnancy induced hypertension) should not exercise during pregnancy.

In men, elevated testicular temperature has been shown to affect spermatogenesis. Levine and others suggest that summer heat has a deleterious effect on spermatogenic cells or on epididymal spermatozoa, which may reduce male fertility. A total of 1235 samples were collected after a 2- to 4-day period of abstinence. Of these, 1159 samples were analyzed after exclusion of 52 specimens because they were incomplete, partially liquefied, obtained by methods other than masturbation, or azospermic (24 specimens). A highly significant depression of semen quality was found in summer relative to all other seasons combined with respect to the following parameters: sperm concentration, total sperm per ejaculate, percent motile sperm, motile sperm concentration, and percentage of sperm with normal morphologic features.

Zorgniotti and associates demonstrated that scrotal hypothermia improves poor semen so that pregnancy can occur in "hard core" infertile couples, but found no differences in temperature rise between wearers of "jockey" versus "boxer" undershorts.

Many questions need to be answered about the etiology of infertility or reproductive failure that go beyond adequacy of sperm, absence or presence of ovulation, or the patency of the fallopian tubes. Environmental hazards to reproduction are many and varied, and sometimes may be a factor in the inability to produce viable offspring. Clinicians owe it to their patients to keep in mind that environmental exposures may be involved in a couples' reproductive failure and ask appropriate questions to uncover this remote possibility. If appropriate, an investigation of an environmental exposure may yield a factor that can be modified to yield a desired outcome.

BIBLIOGRAPHY

Agency for Toxic Substances & Disease Registry. US Department of Health and Human Services, Public Health Service. Mercury toxicity. Am Fam Physician 1992;46:1731.

American College of Obstetricians and Gynecologists. Exercise during pregnancy and the postpartum period. In: ACOG technical bulletin 189. Washington, DC: ACOG, 1994.

Amin-Zaki L, Elhassanni S, Majeed M, Clarkson TW, Doherty RA, Greenwood M. Intrauterine methylmercury poisoning in Iraq. Pediatrics 1974;54:587.

Bellinger D, Leviton A, Waternaux C, Needleman H, Rabinowitz M. Longitudinal analysis of prenatal and postnatal lead exposure and early cognitive development. N Engl J Med 1987;316:1037.

CDC. Mercury exposure in a residential community: Florida 1994. MMWR 1995;44:436.

Clarren SK, Smith DW, Harvey M, Ward RH, Myrianthopoulos NC. Hyperthermia: a prospective evaluation of a possible teratogenic agent in man. J Pediatr 1979;95:81.

Dixon RL, ed. Reproductive toxicology. New York: Raven Press, 1985.

Fisher NL, Smith DW. Occipital encephalocele and early gestational hyperthermia. Pediatrics 1981;68:480.

Harvey MAS, McRorie MM, Smith DW. Suggested limits to the use of the hot tub and sauna by pregnant women. Can Med Assoc J 1981;125:50.

Koos BJ, Longo LD. Mercury toxicity in the pregnant woman, fetus, and newborn infant. Am J Obstet Gynecol 1976;126:390.

Koren GM, ed. Maternal–fetal toxicology: a clinicians' guide. New York: Marcel Dekker, 1990.

Lancranjan I, Popescu H, Gavanescu O, Klepsh I, Servanescu M. Reproductive ability of workmen occupationally exposed to lead. Arch Environ Health 1975;30:396.

Levine RJ, Bordson BL, Mathew RM, Brown MH, Stanley JM, Starr, TB. Deterioration of semen quality during summer in New Orleans. Fertil Steril 1988;49:900.

Lotgering FK, Gilbert RD, Longo LD. The interactions of exercise and pregnancy: a review. Am J Obstet Gynecol 1984;149:560.

Marino P, Landrigan P, Graef J, et al. A case report of lead paint poisoning during renovation of a Victorian farmhouse. Am J Public Health 1990;80:1183.

NIOSH. Occupational safety and health guidelines for chemical hazards. DHHS (NIOSH) pub. nos. 81–123, 88–118, suppl 1-OHG; 89–104, suppl 11-OHG. Washington, DC: US Superintendent of Documents, Government Printing Office.

Paul M. Occupational and environmental reproductive hazards: a guide for clinicians. Baltimore: William & Wilkins, 1992.

Paul M, Himmelstein J. Reproductive hazards in the workplace: what the practitioner needs to know about chemical exposures. Obstet Gynecol 1988;71:921.

Paul M, Kurtz S. Analysis of reproductive health hazard information on material safety data sheets for lead and the ethylene glycol ethers. Am J Ind Med 1994;25:403.

Pleet H, Graham JM, Smith DW. Central nervous system and facial defects associated with maternal hyperthermia at 4 to 14 weeks' gestation. Pediatrics 1981;67:785.

Potashnik G, Ben-Aderet N, Israeli R, Yanai-Inbar I, Sober I. Suppressive effect of 1,2-dibromo-3-chloropropane on human spermatogenesis. Fertil Steril 1978;30:444.

Rom W. Effects of lead on the female and reproduction: a review. Mt Sinai J Med 1976;43:542.

Scialli A, ed. Pregnancy and the workplace. Semin Perinatol 1993;19:18.

Scialli AR. A clinical guide to reproductive and developmental toxicology. Boca Raton, FL: CRC Press, 1992.

Thorp JM, Boyette DD, Watson WJ, Cefalo RC. Elemental mercury exposure in early pregnancy. Obstet Gynecol 1992;79:874.

Timpo A, Amin J, Casalino M, Yuceoglu A. Congenital lead intoxication. J Pediat 1979;94:765.

Whorton D, Krauss RM, Marshall S, Milby TH. Infertility in male pesticide workers. Lancet 1977;ii:1259.

Zorgniotti AW, Reiss H, Toth A, Sealfon A. Chronic scrotal hypothermia as a treatment for poor semen quality. Lancet 1980:i:904.

Zorgniotti AW, Sealfon AI, Toth A. Effect of clothing on scrotal temperature in normal men and patients with poor semen. Urology 1982;19:176.

Primary Care for Women, edited by Phyllis C. Leppert and Fred M. Howard. Lippincott-Raven Publishers, Philadelphia © 1997.

IV

Endocrine Problems

35

Thyroid Disease

PHYLLIS C. LEPPERT

Women are affected more commonly by thyroid disorders than are men. Estrogens enhance the physiologic response to thyroid-releasing hormone (TRH) by increasing TRH receptor number. In general, women—especially those older than 40 years of age—seem to have a greater response to TRH administration with increased thyroid-stimulating hormone (TSH) secretion. Thyroid goiters are more common in the female life cycle when there are physiologic hormonal changes such as pubescence, pregnancy, and menopause.

Age also affects the presentation of thyroid symptomatology. In older women, for instance, hyperthyroidism may be difficult to diagnose because the classic symptoms may be blunted. Thyroid cancers are usually slow growing, and therefore decades may separate the inciting event, such as irradiation, from the clinical diagnosis of the carcinoma.

The thyroid is probably the largest endocrine gland. The thyroid is comprised of two lobes joined by an isthmus. It is 2.0 to 2.5 cm thick at its widest and 4 cm in length. The right lobe is more vascular than the left. In the normal adult, it usually weighs 20 g. However, in some pathologic states, weights of 45 kg (100 lb) have been reported. The thyroid metabolizes iodine. Its function is controlled by positive and negative feedback from the pituitary. TSH stimulates secretion of thyroxine (T_4). The pituitary is in turn stimulated by TRH, which is secreted by the hypothalamus. The thyroid's metabolism of iodine results in the biosynthesis of thyroid hormones. First, there is active transport of iodine into the gland. This is followed by the oxidation of iodine and iodination of tyrosine within thyroglobulin. This step leads to the formation of iodotyrosines, which are hormonally inactive. Finally, the iodotyrosines are linked or coupled to form iodothyronines (T_3 and T_4), the active thyroid hormones. The actual metabolic turnover rate for T_4 is low; however, the thyroid gland stores T_4 before secretion. Some T_3 is produced by peripheral conversion from T_4. The thyroid hormone T_4 changes the activity and concentration of numerous enzyme systems; it influences the metabolism of vitamins and minerals as well as affects the production, secretion, and degradation of most other hormones and changes the responses of their target organs to them. If that were not enough metabolic activity, T_4 also increases protein synthesis, carbohydrate metabolism, lipid synthesis, and degradation in addition to increasing the body's demand for vitamins and numerous coenzymes. Therefore, the clinical symptoms of thyroid disorders are numerous and affect all organ systems.

ETIOLOGY AND DIAGNOSIS

Disorders of the thyroid gland, such as thyroid cancers or benign nodules, may or may not affect thyroid metabolism and therefore may be asymptomatic. Aberrations of thyroid metabolism lead to hyperthyroid and hypothyroid states. These metabolic alterations produce multiple systemic symptoms because of the effect of T_4 on so many physiologic functions.

Thyroid disorders include hyperthyroid states, hypothyroid states, cancer of the thyroid, and benign growth of the gland. Each category includes numerous well-defined diseases with specific pathophysiologic characteristics (Table 35-1).

Hyperthyroid conditions include toxic multinodular goiter, or Plummer disease. This is a disorder where the overproduction of the thyroid hormones occurs over a fairly long period of time in a previously enlarged thyroid. The symptoms of hyperthyroidism may appear abruptly. The thyroid gland in this disorder develops areas of hyperfunction accompanied by areas of nonfunction. The nonfunctioning areas of the gland result from suppression of TSH, which occurs by the hyperfunction in other areas of the gland.

Graves disease is responsible for approximately 90% of hyperthyroidism in persons younger than 40 years of age. This disease is caused by an autoimmune phenomenon. Basically, there is a deficiency of thyroid-specific suppressor T-cell lymphocytes. Because of this deficiency, a thyroid-stimulating antibody (TS ab) is produced. The TS ab then is bound to thyrotropin receptors, and excess thyroid hormone synthesis occurs.

Hyperthyroidism may be caused by one or more adenomas of the thyroid. These adenomas occur in an otherwise normal gland. Most often this condition is caused by a single solitary adenoma. Thus, this disorder also is referred to as hyperfunctioning solitary nodule. These toxic adenomas are follicular adenomas, which can

Table 35-1. Disorders Associated With Thyrotoxicosis

TYPE OF THYROTOXICOSIS	PATHOGENIC MECHANISM
Thyrotoxicosis Associated With Hyperthyroidism	
States of TSH excess	
Tumor	Thyroidtrophic adenoma
Nontumor	Resistance to T_4 by thyrotrophs
Abnormal thyroid stimulation	
Graves disease	TSH receptor antibody
Choriocarcinoma	Chorionic gonadotropin release
Intrinsic thyroid autonomy	
Toxic adenoma	Benign tumor
Toxic multinodular goiter	Foci of functional autonomy
Thyroid cancer	Foci of functional autonomy
Inflammatory disease	
Silent thyroiditis	Release of preformed hormones
Subacute thyroiditis	Release of preformed hormones
Extrathyroidal source of hormone	
Exogenous hormone use	Hormone in medication or food
Ectopic thyroid tissue	Dermoid tumor (struma ovarii)

Table 35-2. Common Causes of Hypothyroidism

Primary Hypothyroidism
Destruction of thyroid tissue
Chronic autoimmune thyroiditis (atrophic and goitrous forms)
Radiation–radioiodine therapy, neck irradiation for lymphoma, head and neck cancer, environmental exposure
Subtotal and total thyroidectomy
Infiltrative diseases of the thyroid (amyloidosis, scleroderma)
Thyroid hormone biosynthetic defects
Iodine deficiency and excess
Use of antithyroid drugs
Inherited enzymatic defects
Central Hypothyroidism
Pituitary disease, Sheenhan syndrome
Hypothalamic disease
Generalized Thyroid Hormone Resistance
Transient Hypothyroidism
Silent thyroiditis
Subacute thyroiditis

function without TSH stimulation. The basic underlying etiology or pathogenesis is unclear.

Hyperthyroidism also occurs in women with hydatidiform mole and choriocarcinoma. This neoplasm produces a thyroid stimulator, which produces a hyperthyroid state. Hyperthyroidism also may be produced by the hypersecretion of TSH by a pituitary adenoma or by increased secretion of TRH, but this is rare.

In women with an endemic iodine deficiency goiter, iodine administration can result in overproduction of thyroid hormone. This iodine-induced hyperthyroidism is a common disorder in the parts of the world where there is a deficiency of dietary iodine.

Finally, thyroid tissue may occur in teratomas. Struma ovarii is a disorder in which ectopic thyroid tissue occurs in the ovary and may produce a hyperthyroid state. Ingestion of amounts of thyroid hormones by persons with a history of underlying psychiatric disease has led to a hyperthyroid state and thyrotoxicosis.

Severe thyrotoxicosis (thyroid storm) is uncommon, but it is extremely serious and is life-threatening. It is abrupt in onset and is caused by a precipitating event: trauma, infection, surgical emergencies, diabetic ketoacidosis, preeclampsia, or childbirth. The clinical picture is one of *severe* hyperthyroidism.

Hypothyroid disorders or thyroid hormone deficiencies have multiple causes, which include primary idiopathic hypothyroidism, thyroid aplasia and dysplasia, and hypothyroidism after thyroid surgery (Table 35-2). Other conditions are caused by pituitary disorders such as Sheehan syndrome and hypothalamic disorders that decrease TSH, TRH, or both. In some cases, hypothyroidism follows a hyperthyroid state, as may be seen with Graves disease.

In addition, hypothyroid conditions are caused by thyroiditis, iodine deficiency, iodine goiter, genetic defects in thyroid synthesis and action, and peripheral resistance to thyroid hormone. Paraaminosalicylic acid, phenylbutazone, resorcinol, and lithium are antithyroid agents, and their administration may produce hypothyroidism as a side effect. The overingestion of cruciferous plants and cascara has been associated with hypothyroidism.

The etiologies of thyroid nodules are multiple and varied. They range from carcinoma, to adenomas, to lymphomas, to multinodular goiter, to thyroiditis.

Thyroid cancer frequently is noticed first as a asymptomatic thyroid nodule. This fact causes difficulty in diagnosis because nontoxic nodular goiter is common in adult women in the United States. Thyroid malignancies are epithelial in origin and are therefore carcinomas. Thyroid cancer is rare and is mostly slow growing. The most malignant tumors, however, occur in older women. These aggressive cancers are rare since most subjects with thyroid cancer develop their disease between 25 and 65 years of age.

Fifty percent to 70% of thyroid carcinomas are papillary. Women are more often affected. Irradiation of the head and neck plays a role in its pathogenesis. This carcinoma is the slowest growing of the thyroid malignant tumors.

Ten percent to 15% of carcinomas are follicular. These tumors occur at an older age than papillary carcinomas and also affect more women than men. A highly malignant lesion is anaplastic carcinoma, which is usually discovered in persons 50 years of age and older. Women are just slightly more apt to develop this carcinoma than men. Ten percent of all thyroid carcinomas are anaplastic.

Medullary carcinoma usually occurs in persons older than 40 years of age and again is slightly more common in women. This malignancy represents only 1% to 2% of all thyroid carcinomas and is more malignant than follicular carcinomas.

Thyroid lymphoma is rare and is a curable malignancy as compared with anaplastic carcinoma, with which it may be confused.

Table 35-3. Forms of Primary Hypothyroidism

Transient Thyroiditis
Subacute thyroiditis
Silent (painless) thyroiditis
Postpartum thyroiditis
Infiltrative Diseases of the Thyroid
Riedel thyroiditis (invasive fibrous thyroiditis)
Cystinosis (cystine storage disease)
Hemochromatosis
Progressive systemic sclerosis (scleroderma)
Sarcoidosis
Amyloidosis
Thyroidal Infections
Thyroidal Irradiation
External radiation therapy
Radioiodine therapy
Postoperative Hypothyroidism
Drug-Induced Hypothyroidism
Iodide
Lithium
Carbamazepine and phenytoin
Amiodarone
Other drugs
Industrial and Environmental Chemicals
Struma Ovarii

HISTORY

Patients with hyperthyroidism present invariably with nervousness, tremor, heat intolerance, weight loss and increased appetite, muscle weakness, excessive sweating, and lid lag and stare (Table 35-5). This classic picture may not be seen in the elderly. Instead, the elderly person with hyperthyroidism is apathetic and has weight loss, and consequently may be misdiagnosed as depressed. The elderly patient with hyperthyroidism may present to her primary care physician with atrial fibrillation. The clinical history given by the patient with hyperthyroidism may suggest exacerbations and remissions. Toxic multinodular goiter, common in the middle aged and elderly, may have predominately cardiovascular symptoms. An elderly woman with a large nodular goiter is likely to develop thyrotoxicosis with ingestion of iodides. Subacute thyroiditis usually follows a viral illness and has an abrupt onset. In this disease, the symptoms of hyperthyroidism are mild and self-limiting. The hyperthyroidism is usually followed by hypothyroidism in this disease.

The history of a patient with hypothyroidism is usually one of gradual onset. The patient complains of fatigue, heavy menstrual periods, slight weight gain despite minimal appetite, and cold intolerance. There are complaints of moderately dry skin, impaired mental activity, coarse hair, and hoarseness. Depression also may occur (Table 35-6).

Thyroid nodules—both malignant and benign—are most often asymptomatic and painless. They may become painful because of rapid growth or hemorrhage or because of inflammation.

Table 35-4. Classification of Causes of Hypothyroidism

Thyroprivic
Postablative hypothyroidism
Primary idiopathic hypothyroidism
Sporadic athyreotic cretinism (thyroid aplasia or dysplasia)
Trophoprivic
Sheehan syndrome
Infiltrative disorders of pituitary or hypothalamus
Goitrous
Hashimoto thyroiditis
Endemic iodine deficiency
Antithyroid agents (para-aminosalicylic acid, phenylbutazone, resorcinol, lithium; cruciferous plants; cassava)
Iodide goiter and hypothyroidism
Heritable defects in hormone biosynthesis and action
Peripheral resistance to thyroid hormone (may be nongoitrous)

PHYSICAL FINDINGS

Careful observation of the patient is the first and an important step in the physical examination. Not only is observation of the thyroid gland conducted, but thorough inspection of other organ systems that are affected by thyroid abnormalities is performed. These include, but are not limited, to skin, body habitus, and eyes. Marked exophthalmos is usually obvious, but subtle forms exist. The eyes are observed for lid lag. A goiter may be obvious to visual observation; however, in most situations inspection may give the examiner no real information. Performing a careful visual observation of the patient is crucial despite the rarity of findings, because when subtle abnormalities are noted they are helpful clues to diagnosis and further testing.

Palpation of the thyroid gland is performed with both hands placed on either side of the gland. It may be palpated with the examiner standing immediately in front of the patient or behind her. The patient is asked to swallow during the examination to determine the mobility of the gland. Often the thyroid is not easily palpable. The exception to this is when a goiter is present (caused by thyroiditis, congenital T_4 synthesis defects, or use of certain medications such as lithium or iodides). The consistency of the thyroid gland has no significance, but the presence of one or more nodules is highly meaningful. Usually, a solitary nodule is palpated in cases of benign and malignant neoplasms. Thyroid cancer is most often palpable as an irregular mass, greater than 2 cm, that is fixed and does not move with swallowing. The cervical lymph nodes are palpated carefully because enlargement of these nodes may point to thyroid cancer. In cases of Hashimoto thyroiditis, multinodular goiter, subacute lymphocytic thyroiditis, and occasionally thyroid carcinoma or lymphoma, multiple nodules are palpable. It must be cautioned that it is possible to palpate only one nodule in multinodular disease.

Notable physical findings of hyperthyroid states are warm skin, warm moist feet, rosy complexion, palmar erythema, patchy vitiligo, thin hair, early gray hair, soft and friable nails, stare (caused by a rim of sclera between lid and limbus), jerky lid movements, and lid lag (upper lid lags behind eye globe on slow down-

Table 35-5. Common Clinical Manifestations of Hyperthyroidism

Symptoms
Nervousness
Fatigue
Weakness
Increased perspiration
Heat intolerance
Tremor
Hyperactivity
Palpitation
Appetite change (usually increase)
Weight change (usually loss)
Menstrual disturbances
General Signs
Hyperactivity
Tachycardia or cardiac arrhythmia
Systolic hypertension
Warm, moist, smooth skin
Stare
Eyelid retraction
Tremor
Hyperreflexia
Muscle weakness
Signs Associated With Specific Causes of Thyrotoxicosis
Diffuse, uninodular, or nodular goiter
Thyroid pain and tenderness
Ophthalmopathy (Graves disease)
Localized myxedema (Graves disease)

Table 35-6. Clinical Features of Hypothyroidism

Symptoms
Fatigue
Lethargy
Sleepiness
Mental impairment
Depression
Cold intolerance
Hoarseness
Dry skin
Decreased perspiration
Weight gain
Decreased appetite
Constipation
Menstrual disturbances
Arthralgia
Paresthesia
Signs
Slow body movements
Slow speech
Hoarseness
Bradycardia
Dry skin
Nonpitting edema (myxedema)
Hyporeflexia
Delayed relaxation of reflexes
Signs Associated With Specific Causes of Hypothyroidism
Diffuse or nodular goiter
Signs of pituitary tumor

ward gaze). Further findings are tachycardia, even at rest or sleep (pulse ≥ 90 beats per minute); widened pulse pressure; and loud heart sounds, usually accompanied by a systolic or late diastolic murmur. These findings are the result of hypermetabolism and the direct cardiac stimulatory effect of thyroid hormones. Cardiac arrhythmias are common whereas congestive heart failure is rarely seen, except in persons with preexisting heart disease. Toxic multinodular goiter typically occurs after 50 years of age and has mainly cardiovascular symptoms and findings. Toxic adenoma, on the other hand, occurs in those 30 to 40 years of age and has milder cardiovascular and ophthalmopathic manifestations.

Muscle weakness and wasting are seen in persons with severe thyrotoxicosis but may not be universally present.

Symptoms of typical and often severe thyrotoxicosis are noted in thyrotoxicosis factitia, which is seen more frequently in women than men. There is a history of underlying psychiatric disease. Access to thyroid medication is available, but the patient typically denies it.

In thyrotoxic crisis, extreme fever occurs along with marked tachycardia. Frank psychosis and delirium may be noted. If this disorder is not recognized and treated, stupor and coma followed by hypotension and death occurs.

The hypothyroid state also affects all organ systems. The skin becomes puffy, and features become thickened (myxedema, which is an accumulation of hyaluronic acid, which binds water). The myxedema causes thickening of the tongue. The skin is dry, cool, and pale (because of anemia), and is yellow tinged (because of hypercarotenemia). Hair is dry and brittle, as are the nails, which grow slowly. When the hypothyroid state is caused by a deficiency of TSH, the skin changes are less noticeable.

Blood volume is reduced so that pulse pressure is narrowed. Bradycardia is noted. Weight gain is not marked but results from fluid retention, which occurs in myxedema. Reduced bowel peristalsis occurs, and gaseous distention of the abdomen may be noted. This may mimic a mechanical ileus.

A characteristic physical finding in hypothyroid states is slow speech and intellect. Lethargy and somnolence are noteworthy, and dementia may occur. Agitation, paranoia, and depression may be present. Movements are slow and clumsy. "Hung up" tendon reflexes are observed, caused by a slow rate of contraction and relaxation.

Severe hypothyroidism in infancy is called cretinism, with mental and growth retardation as classic findings. Findings include feeding problems, failure to thrive, constipation, a hoarse cry, somnolence, and

Table 35-7. Circumstances Associated With Alterations in Binding of T_4 by TBG

Increased Binding
Pregnancy
Neonatal state
Estrogens and hyperestrogenemic states
Tamoxifen treatment
Oral contraceptives usage
Acute intermittent porphyria
Infectious and chronic active hepatitis
Biliary cirrhosis
Genetic conditions
Perphenazine usage
HIV infection
Decreased Binding
Androgenic or anabolic steroid use
Large doses of glucocorticoids
Active acromegaly
Nephrotic syndrome
Major systemic illness
Genetic conditions
Asparaginase

HIV, human immunodeficiency virus; T_4, thyroxine; *TBG*, thyroid-binding globulin.
(Modified from Larsen PR, Ingbar SH. In: Wilson JD, Foster DW, eds. Williams textbook of endocrinology, 8th ed. Philadelphia: WB Saunders, 1992:357.)

delayed developmental milestones. These are irreversible; thus, early recognition by the routine measurement of neonatal T_4 or TSH concentrations is essential to make the diagnosis.

LABORATORY AND IMAGING STUDIES

Diagnosing hyperthyroidism may be difficult on clinical grounds because of subtle or mild symptomatology; thus, serum tests are necessary for diagnosis.

The serum free T_4 is elevated, and the TSH suppressed or absent. A normal TSH in a few circumstances may suggest thyrotoxicosis factitia, in which the person tested has ingested exogenous thyroid hormone. This serum value is sometimes noted in euthyroid patients with an autonomously functioning thyroid nodule. TSH is measured in most laboratories with an immunoradiometric technique able to detect small amounts of TSH. Thus, TSH testing is an excellent screening test for hyperthyroidism. When a patient is clinically thyrotoxic but the T_4 is normal or only slightly elevated, a serum total T_3 is helpful. This should not be ordered routinely, however. Total T_4 is not of value to the clinician because it measures both the free T_4 available to tissues and the T_4 bound to thyroid-binding globulin (TBG). Many clinical states are associated with changes in the binding of T_4 by TBG (Table 35-7)

About one third of T_4 is converted to T_3 during metabolism. In fetal and early neonatal life, the conversion of T_4 to T_3 is slower than in the adult. This peripheral conversion of T_4 to T_3 may be physiologically reduced in old age as well. Fasting, malnutrition, systemic illness, trauma, the postoperative state, and hepatic and renal dysfunction all are associated with impaired conversion of T_4 to T_3. Thus, free T_4 concentrations in these conditions are elevated.

A thyrotoxic patient with a nodular goiter or any patient with a thyroid nodule benefits from a thyroid scan (Table 35-8). Benign and malignant thyroid nodules cannot be diagnosed based on clinical grounds, and a biopsy is necessary. Based on the clinical picture, a fairly accurate judgment can be made to determine if a specific nodule is malignant. When a cytopathologist with experience in the evaluation of fine-needle aspiration is available, this approach to diagnosis is employed. In the absence of specialists, a different approach may be taken where ultrasonography plays a role. Because thyroid cancer is slow growing and rarely causes death, surgery for all patients with a solitary nodule cannot be justified. Suspicion of malignancy is increased in patients with irradiation to the face and neck in childhood, a family history of tumors, a recent change in size of the gland, hypothyroidism, Hashimoto thyroiditis, thyrotoxicosis, tracheal deviation or hoarseness, thyroid fixation and tenderness, and lymphadenopathy. All patients with these symptoms should undergo needle biopsy or surgical exploration. Be aware that a solitary nodule in a woman has a greater chance of being benign than a solitary nodule in a man, however.

TREATMENT

Treatment of nontoxic goiter depends on its etiology. However, as this is often unclear, authorities advise thyroid administration as the first and most helpful approach. This empiric approach is

Table 35-8. Causes of Thyroid Nodules

CAUSES	APPEARANCE OF NODULE ON ^{123}I THYROID SCAN
Solitary Nodule	
Adenoma	
Nonfunctioning	Absent or low uptake
Functioning	Moderate uptake, remainder of gland normal
Toxic	"Hot" nodule with remainder of gland without uptake
Cyst	No uptake
Follicular carcinoma	No uptake
Papillary carcinoma	No uptake
Anaplastic carcinoma	No uptake
Medullary carcinoma	No uptake; may be multicentric; upper part of the gland
Lymphoma	No uptake
Congenital anomaly	No uptake
Multiple Nodules	
Hashimoto thyroiditis	Heterogenous uptake
Multinodular goiter	Heterogenous uptake, including areas without uptake
Subacute lymphocytic thyroiditis	Low or absent uptake diffusely
Cancer in a multinodular goiter	

(From Goroll AH. Evaluation of thyroid nodules. In: Goroll AH, May LA, Mulley AG Jr, eds. Primary care medicine, 2nd ed. Philadelphia: JB Lippincott, 1987:457.)

Table 35-9. Hyperthyroidism: Therapeutic Recommendations

Initial symptoms and preparation for surgery
Beta-blocking agent—propranolol 80 mg/d; increase dose until control attained
Add
SSKI 60 mg tid in preoperative patients if resting heart rate >90 bpm and exercise tachycardia persists. Do not use for prolonged periods
For Grave disease:
Add antithyroid therapy (methimazole or PTU)
Use lowest dose to maintain control
Continue for 4–8 wk then taper
Monitor carefully elderly and pregnant patient
Monitor with clinical status (tremor, appetite, weight, resting heart rate, heat intolerance, and free T_4. TSH monitors overtreatment and avoids hypothyroidism)
Taper antithyroid therapy after 3 to 5 mo; if relapse occurs in 12–24 mo after stopping therapy, switch to another modality
Check WBCs every 2–4 wk initially; after 4 mo check every 4–6 mo and stop if neutrophils fall below 1500/mL
Consider ^{131}I for patients with solid toxic nodules
Pregnant patients are treated with antithyroid medication
Refer patients with obstructive symptoms, or a failure of or contraindication of antithyroid medication
Monitor for postoperative hyperthyroidism

SSKI, saturated solution of potassium iodide; *PTU,* propylthiouracil.

essentially a therapeutic trial. Before thyroid medication is initiated, however, the basal secretion of TSH is obtained. The amount of thyroid hormone prescribed is that amount that does not reduce the TSH concentration lower than 0.2 to 0.5 mU/L. In patients in whom the concentration is not greater than 1 mU/L, a therapeutic trial of thyroid hormone is too risky and is not attempted. The exogenous thyroid hormone is given to decrease the size of the goiter. The dose is usually 0.2 to 0.3 mg/day of L-thyroxine. Initially, 0.05 mg/day is given, and the amount is increased gradually. This therapeutic approach is not usually given to the elderly or to those with coronary disease. Surgery is not indicated unless obstructive symptoms occur or unless carcinoma is suspected.

Toxic goiter is treated with either radioiodine or surgery. Because radioiodine is potentially carcinogenic in young persons, it is mainly prescribed to the elderly, since thyroid cancer does not become clinically apparent for decades.

Newly diagnosed hyperthyroid patients obtain prompt relief of symptoms from treatment with beta-blocking agents. Propranolol is the most widely used of the agents, but atenolol, metoprolol, and nodal are also successful. Beta-blockade controls the adrenergic effects of thyroid hormones but has little direct effect on the thyroid gland itself. At high doses, however, beta-blockade does slow peripheral conversion of T_4 to T_3.

If surgery is necessary, it may be conducted in 1 to 2 weeks after the initiation of beta-blocking agents.

The antithyroid medications, methimazole and propylthiouracil (PTU), interfere with T_4 synthesis. Of the two drugs, methimazole is more potent than PTU. The initial PTU dosage in adults is 300 mg/day in divided doses every 8 hours. Methimazole is given in a 15-mg/day dose once a day. Biochemical control occurs in 1 to 2 weeks, whereas a clinical response usually takes 4 to 8 weeks. Treatment is given for 12 to 24 months and then is stopped. If a relapse occurs, further treatment is indicated: either radioiodine or surgery.

Because agranulocytosis is a serious side effect of PTU therapy, patients taking this medication need to be monitored closely. Methimazole does not cause agranulocytosis. Potassium iodide (SSKI) has been prescribed to prepare patients for surgery because this medication interferes with the synthesis and release of T_4. It can be used as an adjunct to beta-blocking agents or antithyroid medication. SSKI should not be given long term because it can cause a paradoxical rise in thyroid hormone secretion with subsequent thyrotoxicosis.

Radioactive iodine (^{131}I) is widely used for therapy in Graves disease, especially for elderly persons or persons who have not adhered to the prescribed medication regimen. A common complication is hypothyroidism. This treatment has a 70% success rate in the first year. In the eastern United States, it appears to be highly effective for both toxic multinodular goiter and diffuse toxic goiter. However, in the Great Lakes region, where goiter was endemic in the past, toxic multinodular goiter has been considered to be resistant to radioiodine, but little scientific evidence supports this supposition (Table 35-9).

Ophthalmopathy, if symptomatic, is treated with steroids, often prednisone 120 to 140 g/day, which is tapered to a lower dose. If the patient's lids do not close completely during sleep, 1% methylcellulose can be instilled. Sunglasses are in order for persons with photophobia.

Hypothyroidism, if mild, is treated gradually (Table 35-10). L-thyroxine is potent, and full replacement doses are 100 to 150 g/day. Younger patients are begun on 50 g/day, which is increased in 25- to 50-g increments every 2 weeks until the person is euthyroid. Caution is necessary in patients older than 50 years of age because thyroid medication may produce angina, tachycardia, or atrial fibrillation.

L-thyroxine is the drug of choice. It is cost-effective and safe. Furthermore, the serum T_4 value reflects directly the dosage used.

Table 35-10. Hypothyroidism: Therapeutic Recommendation

Confirm diagnosis with TSH and free T_4 (stop any exogenous or antithyroid medication if unclear why patient is taking drug)
Test for pituitary insufficiency if TSH is not appropriately elevated
Primary Hypothyroidism
Replacement therapy initiated with L-thyroxine 50 μg/d give 25–50 μg/d in persons with coronary artery disease
Increase dose by 25–50 μg every 2–3 wk according to clinical response and TSH-free T_4 levels; increase by less in elderly
Monitor with TSH and free T_4 levels (during first 6 mo of therapy these may be high)
Switch to another brand of L-thyroxine if inadequate response
Secondary Hypothyroidism
Perform ACTH stimulation test to access adrenal response; if low, give cortisol acetate *before* thyroid replacement
Replace thyroid hormone and monitor therapy as in primary hypothyroidism

TSH, thyroid stimulating hormone; *T_4,* thyroxine; *ACTH,* adrenocorticotrophic hormone.

Some of L-thyroxine is converted peripherally to T_3. Variations in biological activity may be present in some commercial preparations. Thus, often a therapeutic benefit is obtained by switching brands. Monitoring of the therapy necessitates following TSH, T_4, and free T_4 levels. TSH monitors the adequacy of the preparation; after 6 months, free T_4 measures excess hormone replacement. Women with solitary thyroid nodules who are euthyroid should have a prompt fine-needle biopsy by a skilled practitioner. Many primary care physicians are able to do fine-needle biopsies; however, the biopsy specimen needs to be evaluated by an experienced cytopathologist. Biopsy should be performed on multinodular thyroid glands when the patient gives a history of neck irradiation, cervical adenopathy, rapid growth of the nodule, or the presence of obstructive signs such as recurrent laryngeal nerve palsy. Referral to a specialist for ablative surgery or ablative radioactive iodine treatment is essential for persons with a toxic or greater than 3 cm autonomously functioning thyroid.

CONSIDERATIONS IN PREGNANCY

The pregnant state is similar to hyperthyroidism in that in both cases thyroid enlargement, hyperdynamic circulation, and hypermetabolism occur. In both situations, the total serum T_4 and T_3 values are elevated. There are differences, however. An office screening abdominal ultrasound or a urine human chorionic gonadotropin (hCG) diagnoses pregnancy in an amenorrheic woman of childbearing age. The primary care provider must be cognizant that whereas hyperthyroidism may be associated with amenorrhea, pregnancy is the most common reason for absence of menses in a young woman. In pregnancy, secretion of TBG is increased; therefore, an increase of total T_4 and T_3 occurs. The increase results from the increase of these thyroid hormones that are bound to TBG, but the free T_4 and T_3 levels are not significantly increased over the nonpregnant state. Furthermore, in pregnancy the glomerular filtration rate increases, causing an increase in the excretion of iodide. Plasma iodide levels fall. However, the thyroid gland increases its uptake of iodine. If a pregnant woman's iodine intake is insufficient, a goiter develops. In most regions of the world where the iodine intake is high—either because of an adequate intake of dietary iodine or the routine marketing and consumption of iodized salt—goiter is uncommon in pregnancy.

TSH produced by the thyroid gland does not cross the placenta and is not elevated in pregnancy; however, chorionic thyrotropin is synthesized by the placenta. In pregnancies complicated by hydatidiform mole, hCG may stimulate the thyroid gland sufficiently to produce a clinically apparent hyperthyroid state.

Primary care providers need to be cognizant that TRH released by the hypothalamus does cross the placenta and stimulates the production of TSH by the fetal pituitary. Iodine also readily crosses the placenta and is necessary for fetal thyroid activity. If a pregnant woman increases dietary intake of iodine or takes iodine for any reason, the fetus is at risk for the development of fetal goiter and hypothyroidism.

A primary care physician should consult with and refer a pregnant patient having hyperthyroidism to a specialist with expertise in maternal–fetal medicine for management. The treatment of choice is medical rather than surgical. Usually, the dose of antithyroid drug needed to control hyperthyroidism in late pregnancy is less than that required by the same woman when she is not pregnant. Propylthiouracil and methimazole cross the placenta and concentrate in the fetal thyroid and also can produce fetal goiter and hypothyroidism. Therefore, a pregnant woman is given the smallest does of antithyroid medication necessary to control her disease. Pregnant patients with Graves disease need careful monitoring of the fetus for fetal thyroid disturbance. Fetal heart rate monitoring, ultrasound for assessment of fetal growth, and examination of fetal thyroid for goiter are performed. Fetal disease can be treated in utero by large doses of methimazole, but this must be done by a specialist at a referral center.

A fetus of a mother with Graves disease who has received ablative treatment is still at risk for developing neonatal thyrotoxicosis because there may still be high maternal titers of antithyroid antibodies. Mothers who are taking antithyroid medication in general should not nurse their infants, considering that significant amounts of methimazole appear in breast milk. PTU is not secreted as readily in breast milk, however.

Postpartum thyroiditis syndrome is found to occur in approximately 10% of women with positive antimicrosomal antibodies. A transient thyrotoxicosis occurs within several months of delivery, and is followed by a hypothyroid state of several months' duration and then a return to a euthyroid state. Many women experience only the hypothyroid phase. Recurrences are common after subsequent pregnancies and may occur between gestations as well. This syndrome is associated with Graves disease and Hashimoto disease. Radioactive iodine is not given during pregnancy because the isotope concentrates in the fetal thyroid after the 12th week of pregnancy. Thyroid surgery, if necessary, is ideally performed in the second trimester.

It is rare to find pregnancy associated with hypothyroidism, primarily because of the infertility associated with the amenorrhea and anovulation, both of which usually occur with hypothyroidism. Primary hypothyroidism in pregnancy is commonly caused by Hashimoto thyroiditis, although idiopathic myxedema related to Hashimoto disease also may occur. Hashimoto disease may be seen in patients with diabetes mellitus and other endocrine disorders such as Addison disease.

Treatment is initiated with L-thyroxine. Usual doses are 120 to 150 g/day. TSH levels are obtained every 3 weeks. The TSH is maintained below 6 U/mL. T_4 concentrations should be maintained at the normal pregnancy range. The euthyroid state should be maintained throughout gestation.

NEONATAL HYPOTHYROIDISM

Although infants with neonatal hypothyroidism appear to be normal at birth, fetal and neonatal thyroid deficiency is associated with developmental retardation. When diagnosed and treated before 3 months of age, most of the children develop normally. Referral to a specialist is indicated. Replacement therapy is 10 g/kg of L-thyroxine a day in single dose. T_4 concentrations should be kept at 8 to 12 g/100 mL. Neonates are monitored carefully, and the thyroid replacement is decreased gradually over the first year of life.

BIBLIOGRAPHY

Braverman LE, Utiger RD. Werner and Ingbar's the thyroid, 6th ed. Philadelphia: JB Lippincott, 1991:1365.

Cavalieri R, Pitt-Revees R. The effect of drugs on the distribution and metabolism of thyroid hormones. Pharmacol Rev 1981;33:55.

Cohen JH, Ingbar SH, Braverman LE. Thyrotoxicosis due to ingestion of excess thyroid hormone. Endocrinol Rev 1989;10:113.

Dowling JT, Appleton WG, Nicholoff JT. Thyroxine turnover during human pregnancy. J Clin Endocrinol Metab 1964;27:1749.

Falk S, ed. Thyroid disease: endocrinology, surgery, nuclear medicine, and radiotherapy. New York: Raven Press, 1990;644.

Favus MJ, Schneider AB, Stachura ME, et al. Thyroid cancer occurring as a late consequence of head and neck irradiation. N Engl J Med 1976;294:1019.

Fisher DA, Burrow GN, Dussault, JH, et al. Recommendations for screening programs for congenital hypothyroidism. J Pediatr 1976;89:692.

Fisher DA, Klein AH. Thyroid development and disorders of thyroid function in the newborn. N Engl J Med 1981;304:702.

Galway AB, Burrow GN. Endocrine disorders in pregnancy. In: Reece EA, Hobbins JC, Mahoney MJ, Petrie RH, eds. Medicine of the fetus and mother. Philadelphia: JB Lippincott, 1992:1021.

Goroll AH. Evaluation of thyroid nodules. In: Goroll AH, May LA, Mulley AG Jr, eds. Primary care medicine, 2nd ed. Philadelphia: JB Lippincott, 1987:455.

Goroll AH. Management of hyperthyroidism. In: Goroll AH, May LA, Mulley AG Jr, eds. Primary care medicine, 2nd ed. Philadelphia: JB Lippincott, 1987:484.

Goroll AH. Management of hyperthyroidism. In: Goroll AH, May LA, Mulley AG Jr, eds. Primary care medicine, 2nd ed. Philadelphia: JB Lippincott, 1987:491.

Hamburger JI. The autonomously functioning thyroid nodule: Goetsch's disease. Endocrinol Rev 1987;8:439.

Larsen PR. Feedback regulation of thyrotropin secretion by thyroid hormones: thyroid pituitary interaction. N Engl J Med 1982;306:23.

Larsen PR, Ingbar SH. Thyroid. In: Wilson JD, Foster DW, eds. William's textbook of endocrinology, 8th ed. Philadelphia: WB Saunders, 1992:357.

Leeper RD. Thyroid cancer. Med Clin North Am 1985;69:1079.

Marchant B, Brownlie BEW, Hart DM, et al. The placental transfer of propylthiouracil, methimazole, and carbimazole. J Clin Endocrinol Metab 1977;45:1187.

Miller JM, Hamburger JI, Kine S. Diagnosis of thyroid nodules: use of fine-needle aspiration and needle biopsy. JAMA 1979;241:481.

Mulley AG Jr. Screening for thyroid cancer. In: Goroll AH, May LA, Mulley AG Jr, eds. Primary care medicine, 2nd ed. Philadelphia: JB Lippincott, 1987:452.

Oppenheimer JA. Thyroid hormone action at the cellular level. Science 1979;203:971.

Salvi M, Fukazawa H, Bernard N, et al. Role of autoantibodies in the pathogenesis and association of endocrine autoimmune disorders. Endocrinol Rev 1988;9:450.

Wang C, Vickery AA Jr, Maloof F. Needle biopsy of the thyroid. Surg Gynecol Obstet 1976;143:365.

Wood LC, Ingbar SH. Hypothyroidism as a late sequelae in patients with Graves' disease treated with antithyroid agents. J Clin Invest 1979;64:1429.

Yoshikawa N, Nichikawa M, Horimoto M, et al. Thyroid-stimulating activity in sera of normal pregnant women. J Clin Endocrinol Metab 1989;69:891.

36

Adrenal Disorders

GEOFFREY P. REDMOND

Primary Care for Women, edited by Phyllis C. Leppert and Fred M. Howard. Lippincott-Raven Publishers, Philadelphia © 1997.

There is a mystery and obscurity about adrenal disorders that, combined with their infrequency, makes their diagnosis and treatment seem more esoteric than it really is. The location of the adrenals—deep in the trunk—enhances this mystery, as they are not easily imaged and are not palpable.

The most straightforward approach to the adrenal is physiologic rather than anatomic; indeed, this is true for most aspects of endocrine diagnosis. Knowing the actions of each hormone makes apparent the effects of hypo- and hypersecretion. From the disorder of function, one can reason back to the causative hormonal secretory abnormality and then to the anatomic lesion that might be responsible.

The classically described adrenal disorders—Cushing syndrome, adrenal hyperplasia, Addison disease, pheochromocytoma—are uncommon. In the primary health care of women, their main importance is as conditions to be ruled out in women presenting with obesity, acne, hirsutism, fatigue, or anxiety attacks. Although these symptoms, with the exception of androgenic skin and hair changes, are rarely due to adrenal disease, one cannot honestly reassure the patient until these endocrine causes have been ruled out. In most cases this can be done with clinical evaluation, supplemented when necessary by simple and relatively inexpensive laboratory tests. The complete evaluation of patients with adrenal conditions often requires extensive testing, but this is unnecessary simply to rule the condition in or out.

The emphasis in this chapter is not on detailed descriptions of adrenal diseases, but rather on useful clinical and laboratory procedures for initial evaluation.

The adrenal is best thought of as not one organ, but four. It regulates the metabolism of fat, carbohydrate, and protein, the microcirculation, and response to stress via secretion of cortisol by the zona fasciculata. The regulation of electrolyte balance by secretion of mineralocorticoids, principally aldosterone, is accomplished by the zona glomerulosa, and androgen production by the zona reticularis. The zona fasciculata also contributes to androgen and mineralocorticoid production. Hence, function does not correspond exactly to these histologic zones but is relatively close. The adrenal medulla, essentially a separate organ enclosed in the adrenal cortex, is involved in metabolic regulation and the response to stress via secretion of the catecholamine hormone epinephrine and, to a lesser extent, norepinephrine. Many adrenal disorders involve changes in the secretion of only one steroid hormone, but others, especially neoplastic or destructive processes and inborn errors, may affect several aspects of adrenal function.

It is physiologically efficient to house these functions together, but the effects exerted are quite different. Because the cortical functions all involve steroid hormones, it is biochemically understandable for them to be placed together, despite the diversity of their physiologic actions. It is important for the medulla to be bathed in high levels of cortisol to make proper proportions of epinephrine and norepinephrine. However, the medulla is histologically quite different and subject to different disease processes than the cortex.

Cortisol is concerned with making fuel available for stress situations (eg, fasting or starvation) or situations of increased need (eg, fever). Its actions result in the net conversion of protein to glucose for use as substrate (gluconeogenesis) or for storage as fat. This is seen clinically as muscle weakness due to the protein depletion, higher blood glucose levels due to increased production, and accumulation of fat, particularly in the centripetal distribution, with truncal obesity and facial rounding. The skin is also affected. Thinning of the skin results in increased visibility of capillaries and in striae. These are the result of stretching due to the combined effects of weight gain and decreased structural strength of the skin. Striae in glucocorticoid excess look different than those found with pregnancy or exogenous obesity. They are redder due to capillary visibility, and the amount of injury appears greater, making the striae look as if the skin might actually pull apart. In very mild or temporary glucocorticoid excess, the changes may be less dramatic.

Androgens are essential for male sexual development at puberty and for testicular spermatogenesis. Their effects in women are familiar—the appearance of hair on the axillary and pubic skin and increased facial sebum production—but the biologic value of androgen action in women is poorly understood. There is a weak relation between testosterone levels and libido in women, but testosterone's role in the sex drive is far less central than it is for men. Some women with low testosterone levels have a high libido; others with high values have none. In women, testosterone and other androgens may be involved in bone and muscle development, as they are in men. The effects, if any, of testosterone deficiency in women remain unclear; in fact, it is unclear whether such a condition can be said to exist at all. It has become popular to treat perimenopausal women with depression or low libido with testosterone "replacement," but the efficacy and safety of this are not established. There is particular concern about the action of androgens to induce unfavorable changes in lipoproteins (an increase in low-density lipoprotein cholesterol and a decrease in high-density lipoprotein cholesterol). In women, adrenal androgens mainly show themselves when they are exerting excessive action. Indeed, mild androgen hypersecretion is the most common endocrine disorder of women, although it is not the most written about.

DHEA and DHEA-S are secreted by the adrenal in large quantities. When levels are very excessive, androgenization can result. There has been considerable interest as to whether DHEA is an antiaging hormone. In animals, carcinogenesis is inhibited and there may be antiaging effects on the circulation as well. Human studies of DHEA administration have not shown clear benefits. As with testosterone, it is unclear whether DHEA deficiency in women has any clinical significance.

Mineralocorticoids, of which aldosterone is the principal one in humans, are involved in the regulation of plasma volume and blood pressure. Aldosterone stimulates sodium retention and potassium excretion. Its deficiency results, as one might expect, in low sodium and high potassium levels.

Epinephrine and norepinephrine are involved in preparing the body for stress. Increased cardiac output, mobilization of glucose, and a subjective sensation of foreboding are the effects of adrenal catecholamines. A slight excess may be involved in anxiety states; the symptoms are attributable less to the hormones than to the patient's psyche. Tumors such as pheochromocytomas produce marked catecholamine excess. Deficiency states have been demonstrated only in rare metabolic errors, but some think that idiopathic orthostatic hypotension is due to an inadequate adrenaline response to postural change. This is not universally accepted; in any case, the fraction of cases of dizziness or anxiety due to demonstrable organic lesions of the adrenal medulla is infinitesimal.

Because of the multiple functions of the adrenal, this chapter considers each separately, with respect to physical signs, testing, and treatment.

ANDROGEN EXCESS

Androgenic disorders are the most common endocrine disorder of women, although their presence goes undiagnosed more often than not. They are due to the increased androgen effect, resulting in skin and hair changes such as persistent or severe acne, hirsutism, and androgenic alopecia. There may also be associated metabolic changes (insulin-resistent diabetes and dyslipidemia). In many women with androgenic disorders, the level of circulating androgens is normal, at least on a single determination, but androgenic skin and hair changes are present. In such cases, the abnormality is end-organ sensitivity rather than hypersecretion of androgens. Some androgenized women with apparently normal blood levels of testosterone and DHEA-S probably have subtle hypersecretion with increased integrated androgen levels. When androgen levels are elevated, an actual endocrine disorder is present.

There has been much debate about the relative roles of the adrenal and the ovary in androgenic disorders. Studies have given conflicting results for various reasons, the chief of which is the use of dissimilar patient populations and inadequate suppressive testing. Our work indicates that an adrenal source is slightly more prevalent than an ovarian source. However, symptoms are in general milder when the adrenal is the source, making detection less likely.

Clinical Presentation

There are two basic patterns of androgenic disorder. Women with polycystic ovary syndrome (PCO) tend to be obese, have oligoamenorrhea due to anovulation, and have higher elevations of androgens. Onset is usually in the teens. Those with adrenal hyperandrogenism tend to have a later onset and presentation, menstruate regularly. They are less likely to have associated infertility or the abnormalities of carbohydrate and lipid metabolism. These generalizations are useful, but there are exceptions. In some hyperandrogenic women, both the ovary and adrenal contribute. The distinction is made by means of adrenal suppression testing, in which dexamethasone is given in a dose of 0.375 mg four times daily for at least 6 days. The androgen level is measured before and after dexamethasone administration, and cortisol is measured again at the end to verify compliance.

Women with androgenic disorders usually seek medical advice for the visible changes in skin or hair and for menstrual irregularity and infertility. Many affected women find these changes extremely disruptive to their quality of life, but all too often physicians do not take the appearance changes seriously and do not attempt diagnosis or offer treatment. Androgenic disorders are extremely distressing to many affected women, not because of vanity but because of a threatened loss of feminine characteristics.

Acne is easily recognized. The presence of a few comedones does not suggest an androgenic disorder, but a more significant degree does. When an adolescent or adult woman has frequent inflammatory lesions, scarring gradually accumulates, eventually producing skin injury, which is difficult to conceal. Hirsutism is increased hair in androgen-sensitive areas (the face, especially the chin, neck, and upper lip, the chest, the abdomen, and the back). Androgenic alopecia is the mild, female form of male pattern baldness. In women with this condition, the anterior hair line is preserved but thinning occurs on the crown, vertex, and temples. Hair on the sides of the head tends to be spared. There are many nonhormonal causes of alopecia, but they are uncommon; the exception is alopecia areata, an autoimmune condition. With androgenic alopecia, there is diffuse but incomplete thinning in affected regions. In alopecia areata, hair is lost completely from affected areas, which may be small or may represent most of the body's hair covering.

Obesity is a common cause of visits by women to physicians. It is important to be aware of two distinct patterns of female obesity. The more common form, gynecoid or lower segment obesity, manifests as exaggeration of the normal female fat distribution, with thickening of the hips, thighs, and buttocks. The hips are wider than the waist. In contrast, android or upper segment obesity affects mainly the upper body, with the waist being wider than the hips and the hips, thighs, and buttocks being relatively thin. This latter form is associated with a greatly increased incidence of adult-onset diabetes, unfavorable lipid profiles, coronary heart disease, and breast and endometrial cancer. It is often noted in women who have other indications of PCO. Women with android obesity need more intense scrutiny for the diseases just enumerated. Obesity in Cushing syndrome resembles the android type, with the legs being relatively spared; however, facial rounding is more striking.

Although the presence of menstrual dysfunction (usually oligo-amenorrhea) in a woman with androgenic changes usually suggests PCO, it can be present with adrenal androgen excess, especially when severe, as well as with Cushing syndrome. Menstrual abnormalities in women with androgenic disorders must be taken seriously because they usually are due to anovulation, which can lead to endometrial cancer. Appropriate intermittent progestin therapy is essential. Oral contraceptives are an alternative, especially for younger affected women, if no contraindications are present.

Laboratory Testing

Laboratory testing for androgenic disorders can be elaborate in complex cases but need not be at the initial stages. Measurement of free testosterone and DHEA-S levels is sufficient for most patients and detects nearly all cases with significant hyperandrogenism. When menstrual abnormalities are present, prolactin and FSH levels should be measured. It is not unusual to find hyperprolactinemia, sometimes due to a pituitary adenoma, coexisting with an androgenic disorder. Testosterone can be of either adrenal or ovarian origin; only a dexamethasone suppression test can make the distinction. DHEA-S is essentially of adrenal origin. A high DHEA-S level does not necessarily mean that an elevated testosterone level is of adrenal origin. DHEA-S levels are much higher in younger patients. Levels over 400 μg/dL probably contribute to androgenic skin and hair changes, and tumor must be ruled out with a level over 500 μg/dL. The level that should trigger suspicion is somewhat lower in patients in their mid-30s or older. Testosterone probably begins to produce unwanted androgenic effects at levels just below the usual upper normal limit. Often when this is the case, the free testosterone level is elevated. Levels over 150 ng/dL should prompt a more complete laboratory evaluation to rule out tumor or late-onset adrenal hyperplasia. The latter has been frequently reported but in our experience accounts for only a few cases of androgen excess. A single determination of 17-hydroxyprogesterone detects most cases, but in borderline ones, ACTH stimulation is necessary because the baseline 17-hydroxyprogesterone may be normal. The upper normal limit is about 500 ng/dL. Laboratory results must be read carefully, as the test is reported in various units. Other forms of late-onset adrenal hyperplasia are less common. In 3β-hydroxysteroid dehydrogenase deficiency, the criteria for diagnosis are unclear. Most cases of mild to moderate adrenal androgen excess are due to hyperfunctional states, not to tumors.

Treatment

When elevated androgens are of definite adrenal origin, suppression can be achieved with daily use of a glucocorticoid. Dexamethasone in a single bedtime dose of 0.125 to 0.375 mg is preferred. Higher doses are unnecessary and often produce cushingoid side effects. The dose should be titrated up at 1-month intervals until the originally elevated androgen is in the normal range (about 35 ng/dL for total testosterone and 300 μg/dL for DHEA-S). Suppression to lower levels is unnecessary and greatly increases the chance of adverse effects.

Even when androgens are normalized with suppression, hirsutism and alopecia usually improve only slightly unless a concomitant antiandrogen is given. No drugs are officially labeled for this indication in the United States, but spironolactone has long been used with good results. There is theoretical concern regarding teratogenicity, because androgen blockade might interfere with masculinization of an XY fetus. This has not been reported to our knowledge, however. Nonetheless, antiandrogens should be given only to women who understand the need for effective contraception. Doses of spironolactone range from 75 to 200 mg daily. Side effects include polymenorrhea, which can be prevented by simultaneous use of an oral contraceptive, and dizziness and fatigue, which are due to inadequate water intake in the face of the mild diuresis induced by the drug. Oral contraceptives have some effectiveness in mild adrenal androgen excess because they reduce total testosterone levels by decreasing the ovarian contribution. Additionally, they reduce the free fraction by increasing sex hormone binding globulin (SHBG). They are often the best treatment for anovulation. The patient and physician must understand that treatment results usually take several months to appear.

GLUCOCORTICOID EXCESS

Obesity is the most important clinical sign of Cushing syndrome, but because obesity is so common, the clinician's task is to distinguish cortisol excess from exogenous obesity or other disorders associated with obesity, such as PCO. Some patients with Cushing syndrome do not develop marked obesity. In children, glucocorticoid excess halts growth, but exogenous obesity may slightly accelerate it. The combination of weight gain and growth failure should arouse strong suspicion of Cushing syndrome.

Clinical Presentation and Differential Diagnosis

A cushingoid appearance is common, but Cushing disease and syndrome are not. The most common cause of true cushingoid changes is exogenous glucocorticoid use, but this presents no problem in diagnosis. Most women thought to have Cushing syndrome actually have an androgenic disorder such as PCO. Both are associated with obesity that may be truncal, especially in the common android pattern seen in many women with androgenic disorders. The seborrhea due to increased androgen action causes redness and sometimes visible capillaries on the same general facial area as the thinning of the skin that results from glucocorticoid excess. Both may be associated with hirsutism and oligoamenorrhea.

It is important to be able to distinguish the common androgenic disorders from the uncommon Cushing syndrome. An important differentiating factor is the proximal muscle weakness found in Cushing syndrome but not in androgen excess. Testing consists of asking the patient to get up from a squatting position.

Cushing disease usually has a discrete onset, but androgenic disorders begin in adolescence with gradually increasing manifestations. The pitfall here is that obesity is common and may predate the onset of Cushing syndrome.

When Cushing syndrome is of adrenal origin, there may be increased secretion of androgens and mineralocorticoids as well as cortisol. This can result in signs of androgenization and hypertension, respectively. Libido is usually diminished in Cushing syndrome, which is not the case in androgenic disorders. However, many female patients complain of lack of libido and some may have exogenous obesity with or without an androgenic disorder. Oligomenorrhea can occur in Cushing syndrome but is usual with PCO.

The major cause of death with Cushing syndrome is cardiovascular complications. The disorder is often associated with hypertension and sometimes with edema or congestive heart failure. Of course, these may be found with exogenous obesity as well.

These remarks are not meant to instill pessimism about the possibility of diagnosing Cushing syndrome but to point out overlap in signs and symptoms with far more common clinical entities. Perhaps the most important feature of Cushing syndrome is that patients with it are, once the condition is established, quite ill. The proximal weakness contributes significantly to loss of function. Often there are mental changes that are hard to characterize. Cortisol promotes protein anabolism; this is apparent in the muscle weakness and skin changes. The skin becomes very thin, sometimes to the point of looking as if it will pull apart. Striae are bright purple due to the exposure of capillaries, and there may be easy bruisability. Striae in obesity are much less severe, and in androgenic disorders the skin structure and muscle strength are unaffected.

Another change that differentiates Cushing syndrome from exogenous obesity and androgenic disorders is osteopenia. The former two conditions are protective, but bone loss may be dramatic in the latter, resulting in vertebral compression fractures or aseptic necrosis of the femoral head. In children and adolescents, glucocorticoid excess artifactually delays bone age by interfering with mineralization.

Factitious Cushing syndrome due to concealed glucocorticoid intake occurs rarely. Cortisol excretion is characteristically low due to suppression by the exogenous glucocorticoid. Ethanol is a cortisol secretagogue, and pseudo-Cushing syndrome can occur in alcoholics.

Laboratory Testing and Imaging Studies

Testing for Cushing syndrome has two phases. The first aims to rule in or out the diagnosis; the second aims to determine its anatomic source and pathophysiology. The second stage is complex and need not be described here. Complicating all testing is the fact that cortisol is secreted in pulsatile fashion and normal blood levels vary considerably. In most laboratories, cortisol levels range from 0 to 25 or 30 ng/dL. In most patients with Cushing syndrome, random cortisol levels are not above the upper limit of normal; rather, the integrated concentration, something not readily measured in the clinical setting, is increased. Cortisol is at the upper normal limit more often than it should be. The popular a.m.-p.m. cortisol test is intended to look for a lack of diurnal variation but includes only two samplings; this is inadequate to characterize the complex secretory pattern of the hormone. Random blood levels of cortisol may be low at times in people with Cushing syndrome and high in normals, due to apparently random secretory episodes or to known secretagogues such as fasting, fever, or stress. The most common cause of mildly increased cortisol levels is depression.

The simplest and most useful screening test for Cushing syndrome is the 24-hour urinary free cortisol: it sums up the cortisol secretion for a 24-hour period. When suspicion is high, at least two separate 24-hour urine values should be determined. The principal confounding factor is obesity, which is associated with an elevation of free cortisol excretion due to complex changes in the metabolism of this steroid. This can present difficulties because the test is usually done on obese patients. With Cushing syndrome, the elevation is usually substantial; in simple exogenous obesity, it is minimal.

Cushing disease, which is a cortisol excess due to a pituitary tumor secreting ACTH, can be associated with only mild or intermittent cortisol excess. If suspicion is high, more elaborate testing may be needed, or urinary cortisol tests can be repeated a few months later. In the common overnight dexamethasone suppression test, a 1-mg dose of dexamethasone is given at bedtime and a single cortisol level obtained in the morning. A value above 2.5 to 5.0 suggests Cushing syndrome. This test is abnormal in about 75% of people with depression, and there are also false-negative results in patients with mild pituitary Cushing disease. However, positive results on the 24-hour free cortisol and overnight suppression suggest a high likelihood of Cushing syndrome, sufficient to make definitive testing mandatory.

Imaging studies are useful when the diagnosis of excess glucocorticoid secretion has been made and it is necessary to identify the anatomic location of the abnormal production. Because "incidentalomas" (apparent masses on magnetic resonance imaging or computed tomography [CT] that do not represent clinically significant tumors) are notoriously common in both locations, the presence of a small mass in either location does not by itself establish the diagnosis of Cushing syndrome. A large tumor in either location is far more likely to be significant.

Definitive laboratory diagnosis of Cushing syndrome is complex and involves stepwise low- and high-dose dexamethasone suppression and the use of corticotrophin releasing hormone, metyrapone, and sometimes petrosal sinus sampling. These must be performed by an endocrinologist at a center experienced with the diagnosis and treatment of pituitary Cushing disease.

Adrenal carcinoma can present as Cushing syndrome, although often the androgenic changes are striking and rapidly advancing. Dissemination is usually present by the time of diagnosis, and cure is infrequent. The diagnosis can be made with an adrenal CT scan. ACTH-dependent Cushing syndrome can be caused by ACTH-secreting tumors, most commonly carcinoid of the bronchus or thymus.

Treatment

The treatment of Cushing syndrome and its variants is vital but not always satisfactory. Mortality is high, most often from cardiovascular complications. When it is caused by a tumor, tumor removal is the obvious approach. Most ACTH-secreting pituitary tumors can be removed, but not always totally. A single adrenal adenoma can be removed, but with carcinoma surgery is rarely curative. Peri- and postoperative care of these patients is complex and should be managed by a physician experienced in this area. Various drugs are available that destroy adrenal tissue or inhibit ACTH secretion or cortisol-synthesizing enzymes. These are used when a surgical cure cannot be attained and include mitotane (which is adrenolytic), cyproheptadine, and aminoglutethimide. Their use is complex; they are not simple cures for Cushing syndrome and should be used only by physicians experienced with this condition.

MINERALOCORTICOID EXCESS

Excess secretion of aldosterone presents as hypertension with spontaneous hypokalemia. The hypokalemia may be mild (3.5 to 4.0 mEq/L), but the hypertension is sometimes severe. Laboratory testing shows an elevated level of aldosterone with suppression of plasma renin activity. The underlying adrenal abnormality is an isolated adenoma (Conn syndrome) or bilateral adrenal hyperplasia. Treatment consists of unilateral adrenalectomy for Conn syndrome and medical management with spironolactone and additional antihypertensive agents as required for bilateral hyperplasia.

GLUCOCORTICOID DEFICIENCY

Deficiency of cortisol can result from destruction of the adrenal glands (primary adrenal insufficiency or Addison disease) or lack of pituitary ACTH secretion (secondary adrenal insufficiency). The principal clinical signs are weakness and lack of energy, which are unfortunately entirely nonspecific. Nausea and vomiting are common. With primary adrenal insufficiency, there is excessive secretion of POMC, the precursor of ACTH, due to lack of feedback inhibition. POMC causes hyperpigmentation, which is present in most patients with primary adrenal failure. The pigmentation is most conspicuous at minor trauma areas, principally skin folds. The belt line is most characteristic because in normal patients pigmentation there is slight. Sun exposure increases the hyperpigmentation, which is sometimes confused with normal tanning.

Etiology

The characteristic electrolyte disturbances are depression of sodium and elevation of potassium. These findings occur only in patients with primary adrenal insufficiency; the zona glomerulosa is not dependent on ACTH for stimulation of aldosterone release, so mineralocorticoid deficiency does not occur. However, circulatory compromise occurs because in the absence of cortisol, endothelial cells lose their cohesion and capillaries become leaky, resulting in hypotension. This is a primary mechanism of adrenal crisis. In patients with primary adrenal insufficiency, the characteristic electrolyte disturbances may not be present, except in crisis.

With adrenal crisis, circulatory compromise occurs because of salt loss and capillary leakiness. Hypoglycemia may occur, particularly if vomiting prevents retention of nutrients. Patients with adrenal insufficiency tolerate vomiting poorly because adaptive mechanisms depend on normal adrenal and pituitary function; the same is true for fever. What might seem to be minor illnesses accompanied by vomiting or fever can be life-threatening in patients with primary or secondary adrenal insufficiency. The hyponatremia and hyperkalemia are often incorrectly attributed to vomiting and dehydration, dangerously delaying diagnosis. Often the diagnosis is made by a specialist only after several admissions for vomiting and dehydration in which hyperkalemia was present but ignored. Misdiagnosis as a functional disorder is common because the vague complaints of weakness mimic neurosis.

The diagnosis of primary adrenal insufficiency is suggested by the characteristic electrolyte disturbances. However, this sign is often absent in patients who are not in crisis. Random serum cortisol levels are not useful because they are often very low in normals. The 24-hour urinary free cortisol level is most useful as a screening test. In primary adrenal failure, levels are quite low. Diagnosing mild adrenal insufficiency and adrenal insufficiency due to pituitary hypofunction is more difficult. ACTH stimulation using a single intravenous dose may not separate partially deficient patients from normals. More elaborate stimulation tests require administration of ACTH over 48 hours and usually are done in the hospital because of the supposed possibility of precipitating adrenal crisis. Insulin hypoglycemia is the definitive test for secondary adrenal insufficiency but must be performed with great care.

An important clue to the presence of primary adrenal failure is the presence of another autoimmune endocrine disease. Hashimoto thyroiditis, gastric parietal cell dysfunction with or without pernicious anemia, autoimmune ovarian failure (which presents as premature menopause), and, occasionally, insulin-dependent diabetes may suggest the presence of endocrine autoimmunity. Signs and symptoms of Addison disease in patients with these conditions should prompt a thorough work-up. Most patients with autoimmune combined endocrine failure presenting in adulthood do not have associated mucocutaneous candidiasis. Nonautoimmune causes of primary adrenal failure include tuberculosis (now rare but the cause of Addison's original case), AIDS, and replacement by metastatic cancer. Adrenoleukodystrophy and adrenomyeloneuropathy are inborn errors of metabolism, but because they are sex-linked recessives are rare in females. Presentation is in childhood, adolescence, or occasionally young adulthood.

In pituitary disease, ACTH secretion is most resistant to injury. Accordingly, secondary adrenal insufficiency is rarely the presenting manifestation; rather, it is usually found in patients with known pituitary disease. Pituitary insufficiency in women may be caused by Sheehan syndrome (postpartum pituitary necrosis), associated with postpartum hemorrhage. The most obvious sign is failure of return of menses after childbirth. Unfortunately, amenorrhea is often ignored and the diagnosis may be considerably delayed. In these and other patients with pituitary disease, the defect in ACTH secretion may be partial and can become clinically apparent only with physical stress such as fever, vomiting, or general anesthesia or with a long duration of disease. Amenorrhea, weakness, and fatigue may be mistakenly dismissed as functional.

Other pituitary disorders that may include adrenal insufficiency include idiopathic hypopituitarism (usually present from early childhood), pituitary tumors, or rare disorders such as histiocytosis X. Pituitary microadenomas and most macroadenomas, such as those that often cause hyperprolactinemia, do not cause secondary adrenal insufficiency.

Treatment

Treatment of adrenal insufficiency is straightforward and depends on certain basic principles. Physiologic replacement doses are just a fraction of the doses used more commonly for pharmacologic effect. For an adult, typical replacement doses of glucocorticoid are hydrocortisone 10 to 37.5 mg/day, prednisone 2.5 to 5.0 mg/day, and dexamethasone 0.125 to 0.375 mg/day. The lower doses are appropriate for patients with partial or secondary adrenal insufficiency. Individual dose titration is essential. Patients are fatigued on inadequate doses but may develop subtle cushingoid features (eg, facial rounding, weight gain) if the dose is excessive. With replacement therapy, in contrast to pharmacologic use, an adequate replacement dose does not produce these changes; when they occur, the dose must be reduced. Generally the glucocorticoid is divided into morning and evening doses, but with dexamethasone a single evening dose is sufficient. The higher dose should be given in the evening because normally cortisol levels peak in the early morning. Symptoms of adrenal insufficiency, especially when they are of pituitary origin, tend to peak in the morning and are best controlled by an adequate bedtime dose. Giving the larger dose in the morning to mimic the diurnal rhythm of cortisol is fallacious: by the time the morning dose is absorbed, it is far past the time when the cortisol peak normally occurs.

Patients with Addison disease usually require mineralocorticoid replacement as well. Fludrocortisone 0.05 to 0.3 mg/day is given. Without this, weakness and orthostatic symptoms may persist and hyperpigmentation may not be well controlled. In Addisonian patients, this drug is unlikely to cause hypertension and edema. In the rare situation in which these occur, resolution is rapid after dose reduction. Addisonian patients often also require a substantial salt intake. They should be encouraged to salt their food as heavily as they like, something most fear doing because of widespread public health advice to limit salt intake.

Certain physical stresses increase the cortisol requirement, principally a fever over 100°F, vomiting more than once or twice, and general anesthesia. Fasting is tolerated poorly by patients with adrenal or pituitary disease. In these situations, glucocorticoid doses should be at least doubled and a reliable route of entry used. Adrenal crisis is often exacerbated by the patient's inability to retain oral glucocorticoid due to vomiting. Vomiting of any persistence requires intravenous fluids with glucose and adequate amounts of sodium. The sodium maintenance requirement in an addisonian patient may be twice what is calculated by usual clinical formulas. Intravenous hydrocortisone can be given with a bolus of 50 to 100 mg and 100 to 200 mg/24 hours as a continuous drip.

ADRENAL MEDULLA

Disorders of the adrenal medulla are uncommon. The most important is pheochromocytoma. This is found rarely in primary care, but similar symptoms are common because the effects of epinephrine secretion are universal and can be quite disturbing to some patients. Such effects include an increase in cardiac rate and output (usually noticeable by the patient); vasodilatation or constriction (depending on the tissue or specific catecholamines released), resulting in flushing or pallor; elevation of blood pressure, which may be sustained or episodic and can be severe; sweating; elevation of blood glucose; and headache, which has a sudden onset and may be severe. Headache is the most common symptom, followed by diaphoresis, palpitations, pallor, and nausea. There may be a sense of overwhelming anxiety or doom, although not all patients report these subjective symptoms. Orthostatic hypotension can occur, presumably as a result of the decreased plasma volume resulting from chronic catecholamine excess.

The difficulty with the diagnosis of pheochromocytoma is that the symptoms mimic those of anxiety attacks, presumably because both involve a sudden release of catecholamines (although more severe in pheochromocytoma). The diagnosis of pheochromocytoma is often considerably delayed. Paroxysmal episodes with pheochromocytoma are not usually precipitated by stress but may be by body movement. However, ordinary panic or anxiety attacks may also occur without an apparent provocative event, or at least the patient is unaware of one. Women with panic attacks often have a low baseline blood pressure; in pheochromocytoma, the blood pressure is elevated, at least during episodes. Women with panic attacks usually have a long history of anxiety-related symptoms. Small doses of tricyclic antidepressants or selective serotonin reuptake inhibitors often prevent panic attacks. The former probably should not be used because of occasional cardiac arrhythmias and are contraindicated in possible pheochromocytoma because they may increase catecholamine action by preventing reuptake. Some women with severe anxiety-related symptoms are reluctant to accept nonorganic diagnosis. In such cases, testing for pheochromocytoma may be necessary for reassurance.

Laboratory testing for possible pheochromocytoma is simple now that it is possible to measure plasma catecholamines, but it is important to use a laboratory skilled in this assay. The patient should lie quietly in the supine position without elevating the body for 20 to 30 minutes before the venipuncture. Measurement of urinary catecholamines is also useful. If borderline levels occur, more elaborate tests are available.

Treatment of pheochromocytoma should be done by a team experienced with the condition. It consists of adrenergic blockade followed by surgery when the patient is stable.

BIBLIOGRAPHY

Dluhy RG. The growing spectrum of HIV-related endocrine abnormalities. J Clin Endocrinol Metab 1990;70:563.

Opocher G, Rocco S, Carpene G, Matero F. Differential diagnosis in primary aldosteronism. J Steroid Biochem Mol Biol 1993;45:49.

Orth DN. Cushing's syndrome. N Engl J Med 1995;332:791.

Redmond GP. The good news about women's hormones. New York: Warner Books, 1995.

Redmond GP. Androgenic disorders. New York: Lippincott-Raven, 1995.

Thomas JE, Rooke ED, Kvale WF. The neurologists' experience with pheochromocytoma: a review of 46 cases. J Urol 1974;111:715.

Tsigos C, Papanicolaou DA, Chrousos GP. Advances in the diagnosis and treatment of Cushing's syndrome. Clin Endocrinol Metab 1995;9:315.

Tyrrell JB, Wilson CB. Cushing's disease: therapy of pituitary adenomas. Endocrinol Metab Clin North Am 1994;23:925.

Weigel RJ, Wells SA, Gunnells JC, Leight GS. Surgical treatment of primary hyperaldosteronism. Ann Surg 1994;219:347.

37

Ovarian Endocrine Disorders

THOMAS M. PRICE
G. WILLIAM BATES

Primary Care for Women, edited by Phyllis C. Leppert and Fred M. Howard. Lippincott-Raven Publishers, Philadelphia © 1997.

The functions of the ovary include the production of sex steroids, including androgens, estrogens and progesterone, and the cyclic production of a mature oocyte for reproduction. During childhood, the ovary remains quiescent due to the lack of gonadotropin stimulation from the brain. During the reproductive years, the ovary secretes androgens, estrogens, and progesterone in an orchestrated cyclic fashion, resulting in ovulation. In the postmenopausal years, ovulation and estrogen production from the ovary cease but androgen production persists. This chapter discusses disorders that result in disruption of the ovulatory process through excessive ovarian androgen production and those that result in premature cessation of ovarian estrogen production.

DISORDERS OF ANDROGEN EXCESS

Etiology

The adrenal glands and the ovaries contribute to the circulating androgens, androstenedione and testosterone, in the reproductive-age woman. Dihydrotestosterone (DHT) is produced from testosterone by the enzyme 5α-reductase in target tissues; it is primarily responsible for the androgenic action on skin structures that results in body hair growth and acne formation.

Table 37-1 outlines several conditions that result in androgen excess. Of these conditions, polycystic ovarian syndrome (PCOS) is the most common, affecting about 5% to 10% of reproductive-age women. Classically, PCOS is characterized by hirsutism, ovulatory dysfunction with infertility, obesity, and insulin resistance (Fig. 37-1, Table 37-2). Hyperthecosis, a variant of PCOS, involves more severe androgen excess and ovarian thecal cell hyperplasia but is still a functional disorder driven by gonadotropins from the brain. Congenital adrenal hyperplasia (CAH), resulting from 21-hydroxylase or 11β-hydroxylase deficiency, is a rarer cause of androgen excess. Patients with severe CAH are recognized at birth due to sexual ambiguity, but patients with milder forms of enzyme insufficiency may have a peripubertal onset of androgen excess. Hypothyroidism and hyperprolactinemia may be associated with mild hirsutism. Cushing syndrome may also cause hirsutism, but other signs and symptoms such as diabetes, hypertension, muscle wasting, and cutaneous striae tend to be more impressive. Neoplasms of the ovary or adrenal gland may cause androgen excess, but such neoplasms are rare compared to the functional disorders.

History and Physical Examination

Signs of androgen excess due to functional disorders begin at puberty and progress slowly. In contrast, androgen excess caused by neoplasms may occur at any age and usually has a more rapid progression. Mild androgen expression in women is characterized by body hair growth, acne, and seborrhea. Hirsutism consists of hair growth in locations such as the face, breasts, chest, and abdomen and more than average growth on the extremities. About one third of reproductive-age women have pigmented hair growth of the upper lip; 6% to 10% have other facial hair growth. The degree of hirsutism depends on the levels of circulating androgens such as free testosterone and on the activity of 5α-reductase that leads to production of DHT at the hair follicle. Ethnic differences in body hair growth may be due to differences in 5α-reductase activity. For example, Asian women have significantly less body hair than North American Caucasian and black women.

In women, peripubertal acne should not be considered part of normal puberty. Even though many factors—such as infection, abnormal keratinization, and immune reaction—influence acne problems, teenagers with significant acne should be evaluated for androgen excess. Peripubertal acne and sebum production correlate best with levels of dehydroepiandrostenedione sulfate (DHEAS) produced by the adrenal gland, but other androgens such as androstenedione and testosterone also contribute to the condition.

More severe androgen expression is manifested by alopecia, an increase in muscle mass, clitoral hypertrophy (Fig. 37-2), deepening of the voice, and an increase in aggression. Androgen expression of this severity tends to be caused by androgen-secreting tumors or is associated with hyperthecosis.

Most patients with androgen excess have ovulatory dysfunction leading to menstrual abnormalities. Ovarian production of progesterone after ovulation synchronizes endometrial development in preparation for a pregnancy. When pregnancy does not occur, progesterone levels fall, initiating menses. Because women with androgen excess infrequently ovulate, they may have prolonged periods of time without menses. Continuous stimulation of the endometrium by estrogen leads to a thickened endometrium that may break down, causing unpredictable and prolonged uterine bleeding. This chronic estrogen exposure without progesterone exposure increases the risk of endometrial hyperplasia and endometrial carcinoma. Endometrial carcinoma is usually a disease of the fourth through sixth decades, but women with PCOS may have an earlier onset, in the third decade.

Obesity and abnormal adipose distribution are associated with androgen excess in at least 50% of cases. Normally, women have a lower body (gynoid, low waist-to-hip ratio) fat distribution with adipose tissue deposition primarily in the gluteofemoral area. Women with androgen excess tend to have an upper body (android, high waist-to-hip ratio) adipose distribution characterized by fat deposition in the upper abdomen, similar to that in males. Upper body adiposity is associated with an increased risk of diabetes, hypertension, arteriosclerosis, gallbladder disease, endometrial cancer, and possibly breast cancer.

Table 37-1. Possible Etiologies of Androgen Excess in Women

Polycystic ovarian syndrome
Hyperthecosis
Hypothyroidism
Hyperprolactinemia
Ovarian tumors Sertoli-Leydig cell Lipoid cell Hilar cell Thecoma Granulosa-theca cell
Cushing syndrome
Congenital adrenal hyperplasia 21-hydroxylase deficiency 11β-hydroxylase deficiency
Adrenal tumors Adenomas Adenocarcinomas
Exogenous androgens or progestins

Table 37-2. Symptoms of Polycystic Ovarian Syndrome

SYMPTOMS	MEAN INCIDENCE (%)
Infertility	74
Hirsutism	69
Amenorrhea	51
Obesity	41
Functional bleeding	29
Dysmenorrhea	23
Corpus luteum at surgery	22
Virilization	21
Biphasic body temperature	15
Cyclic menses	12

(Adapted from Carr BR. Disorders of the ovary and female reproductive tract. In: Wilson JD, Foster DW, eds. Williams textbook of endocrinology. Philadelphia; WB Saunders, 1992:769, and Goldzieher JW, Axelrod LR. Clinical and biochemical features of polycystic ovarian disease. Fertil Steril 1963;14:631.)

Obesity with upper body adiposity is strongly associated with insulin resistance. Even nonobese women with PCOS have greater insulin resistance than nonobese women without PCOS, but obesity with upper body adiposity greatly increases insulin resistance. Insulin resistance appears to be due to receptor abnormalities that lead to an inappropriately low number of receptors per cell and a corresponding circulating hyperinsulinemia. Women with PCOS account for about 10% of premenopausal women with glucose intolerance. The fat distribution associated with androgen excess appears to be the important determinant of insulin resistance, as correction of hyperandrogenism with drug therapy does not improve insulin resistance. In contrast, drug therapy that lowers insulin levels improves hyperandrogenism. This difference may be due to the fact that insulin increases ovarian androgen production by cross-reactivity with insulin-like growth factor receptors.

Acanthosis nigricans is another marker of insulin resistance. This condition of hyperpigmented-appearing skin is due to hypertrophy and exaggerated folding of normal skin, most commonly in areas of skin creases such as the posterior neck, axillae, and antecubital regions.

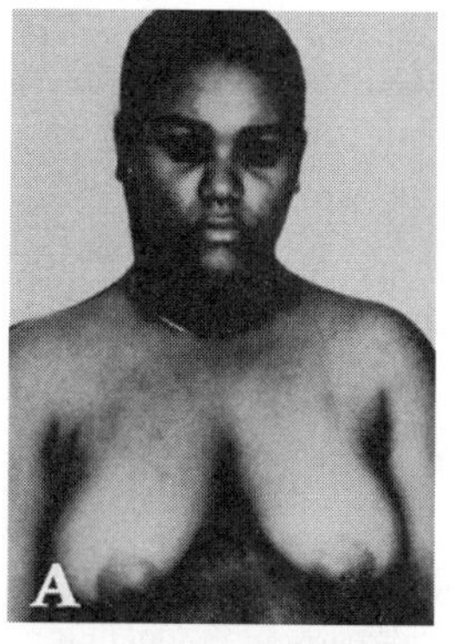

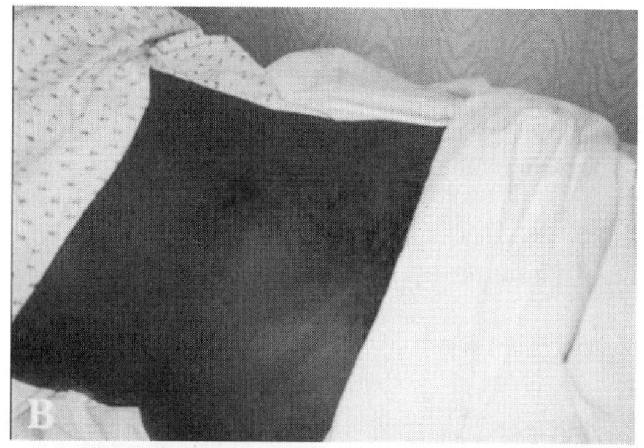

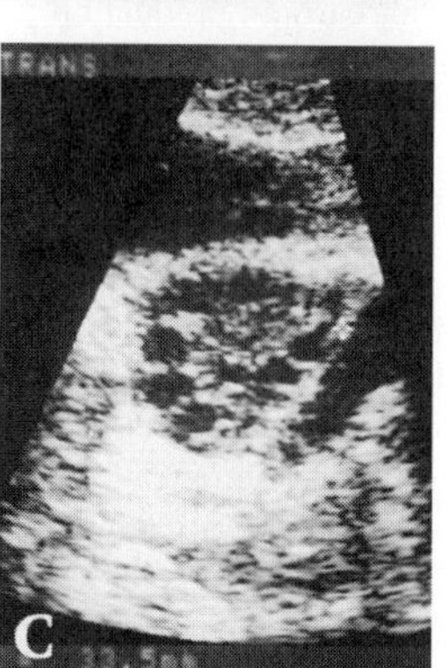

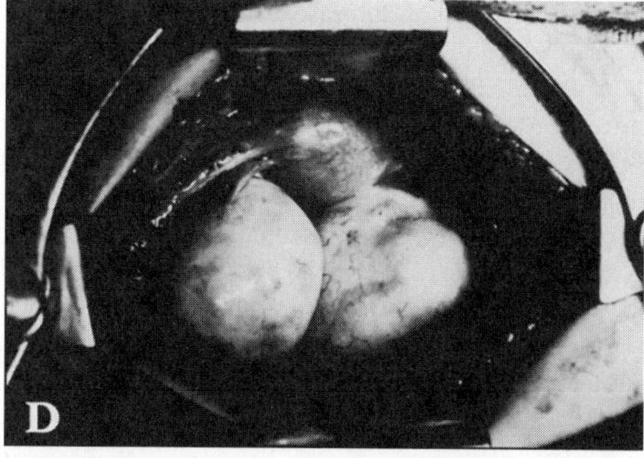

FIGURE 37-1. Typical signs of androgen excess, such as those seen in polycystic ovarian syndrome. ***(A)*** Facial acne and acanthosis nigricans. ***(B)*** Abdominal hirsutism. The ovaries on ultrasound evaluation show characteristic multiple peripheral follicles ***(C)*** and are often significantly enlarged with a thickened, glistening capsule ***(D)***.

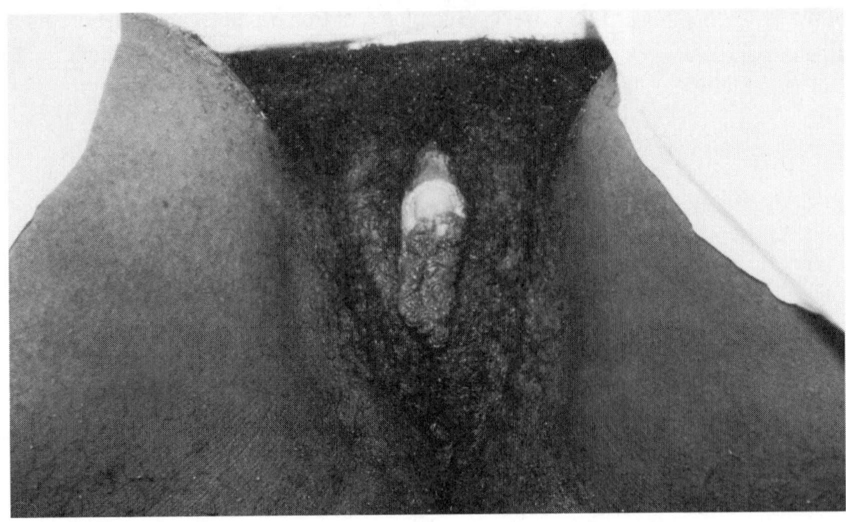

FIGURE 37-2. Clitoral hypertrophy is often seen with more severe androgen excess, as in hyperthecosis, androgen-producing tumors, and congenital adrenal hyperplasia.

Diagnostic Studies

The purposes of diagnostic testing are to establish the source of the androgen excess and to evaluate for glucose intolerance, hypertension, endometrial abnormalities, and lipid abnormalities. Hormonal testing may include tests for thyroid-stimulating hormone, prolactin, DHEAS, androstenedione, testosterone, luteinizing hormone (LH), and follicle-stimulating hormone (FSH). In women who appear to be ovulatory, laboratory testing should be done in the follicular phase of the cycle.

In patients with androgen excess, the LH:FSH ratio is often increased to above 3:1; this is a hallmark of PCOS. This increased ratio is not, however, specific for PCOS and may be seen with other conditions, such as CAH. In a patient with PCOS, the androstenedione level commonly ranges from 270 to 450 ng/dL; the testosterone level may range from 50 to 150 ng/dL. The polycystic ovary has a characteristic ultrasound appearance with multiple small peripheral follicles; however, this appearance is not specific for one cause of androgen excess and may be seen with PCOS, hyperprolactinemia, and CAH. DHEAS levels may be elevated in patients with PCOS but usually remain less than 500 μg/dL. Levels above 500 μg/dL suggest the need to evaluate for CAH or an adrenal tumor.

Screening for 21-hydroxylase CAH should include a morning 17-hydroxyprogesterone (17-OHP) during the follicular phase if the subject is ovulatory. A 17-OHP level below 200 ng/dL generally rules out CAH, but a higher level warrants more sensitive ACTH stimulation testing. The presence of hypertension suggests the possibility of an 11β-hydroxylase deficiency, and ACTH stimulation testing of deoxycorticosterone levels should be performed. Cushing disease is suggested by other symptoms; the patient should be screened with a 24-hour urine study for free cortisol. Testosterone-producing tumors are suggested by signs of virilization, testosterone levels above 200 ng/dL, and low androstenedione-to-testosterone ratios. Pelvic ultrasound may be useful for ovarian evaluation, but androgen-producing tumors may be very small, leading to difficult diagnostic dilemmas. DHEAS levels above 700 μg/dL warrant adrenal imaging to rule out the rare neoplasm. Women in the third decade or older who experience infrequent uterine bleeding (fewer than six or eight a year) should be evaluated with an endometrial biopsy to exclude endometrial hyperplasia and carcinoma.

Evaluation for glucose intolerance may include a 2-hour blood glucose after a 75-g glucose load. Levels above 140 but below 200 mg/dL suggest impaired glucose tolerance; levels above 200 mg/dL are consistent with diabetes mellitus. A fasting lipid profile—including total cholesterol, triglycerides, high-density lipoprotein (HDL), low-density lipoprotein (LDL), and very-low-density lipoprotein—is necessary to evaluate for hyperlipidemia.

Treatment

The multiple symptoms associated with androgen excess often lead the patient to see multiple physicians. The dermatologist focuses on acne and directs therapy at skin structures rather than androgen excess, the underlying cause. The gynecologist focuses on irregular menses, hirsutism, and risk of endometrial cancer. The internist thinks mainly of obesity, diabetes, hypertension, and lipid abnormalities. Therapy should be geared toward correcting the androgen excess and insulin resistance and normalizing body weight.

Androgen excess is treated by decreasing androgen production, by inhibiting binding to the receptor, and by decreasing 5α-reductase activity. Androgen excess of ovarian origin, such as PCOS and hyperthecosis, is treated by inhibiting gonadotropin production to decrease ovarian stimulation. Classically, a low-dose oral contraceptive (OCP) has been used. Newer OCPs containing the progestins desogestrel or norgestimate appear to be the least androgenic pills available, and they create the most favorable lipid changes, especially an increased HDL:LDL ratio. The most effective therapy for treating ovarian androgen excess appears to be the use of a gonadotropin-releasing hormone (GnRH) analog (to ablate pituitary FSH and LH production) in combination with "add-back" therapy of estrogen and a progestin to prevent complications of estrogen deficiency. However, because the FDA has not approved the use of GnRH for this indication and because GnRH analogs are expensive, this therapy cannot be used for most patients.

In contrast to the treatment of patients whose androgen excess originates in the ovary, patients with CAH are treated with a low-dose glucocorticoid to suppress ACTH and thus decrease adrenal androgen production. A dose of 0.5 mg dexamethasone or 2 to 5 mg prednisone nightly may be used. Levels of 17-OHP and DHEAS should be monitored during therapy.

Because they compete with DHT for binding of the androgen receptor, the antiandrogens—spironolactone, cimetidine, flutamide, and cyproterone acetate—may decrease hirsutism. Cyproterone acetate is unavailable in the United States. Flutamide appears to have more liver toxicity than spironolactone and has not had widespread use. Spironolactone 100 to 200 mg/day is the most common therapy. Because these drugs are potential teratogens, they should not be used without adequate birth control.

The most common treatment for PCOS in women not desiring to remain fertile is a low-dose OCP with or without spironolactone. Patients on this regimen need to be advised that improvement of hirsutism is slow and that visible changes should not be expected for 4 to 8 months.

To decrease the risk of endometrial cancer in women with chronic anovulation, treatment with either OCPs or cyclic progestins should be initiated. Medroxyprogesterone acetate 10 mg/day or norethindrone 2.5 to 5 mg/day for 10 to 12 days of the month may be used.

Specific 5α-reductase inhibitors, such as finasteride, have been introduced for the treatment of prostate cancer. Due to possible teratogenicity, the use of this drug in women has not been recommended.

Demonstrable glucose intolerance should be treated by encouraging weight loss and prescribing oral antidiabetic agents such as glipizide and glyburide. Patients with significant hyperlipidemia should consider lipid-lowering drugs. The most difficult problem to treat in these patients is obesity with upper body adiposity. Weight loss improves the situation but does not reverse body fat distribution. Weight is the most important and the most difficult symptom to control.

Pregnancy Considerations

Women with PCOS are often infertile because of ovulatory dysfunction. Restoration of normal ovulation through therapy such as clomiphene citrate significantly increases pregnancy rates. In general, maternal excessive androgens are not a risk to the fetus because the placenta converts androgens to estrogens. Pregnancy does not change the underlying condition, and after delivery the original symptoms reappear.

Because CAH is an autosomal recessive disease, prenatal diagnosis must be considered if both partners are affected. Because males with CAH are often asymptomatic, the partner of a patient with CAH should be screened for the disease. If both partners have biochemical evidence of CAH, prenatal counseling is recommended.

PREMATURE OVARIAN FAILURE

Etiology

The natural lifespan of the ovary is genetically programmed and is about 52 years. However, the ovary may lose the ability to produce oocytes and estrogen during childhood or during the reproductive years. Cessation of ovarian function before age 40 is considered premature. Prepubertal ovarian failure is almost always due to a chromosomal abnormality, most commonly Turner syndrome. Rarer causes include childhood chemotherapy treatment, abdominopelvic radiation therapy, 17α-hydroxylase deficiency, galactosemia, and lack of gonadotropin production. Postpubertal ovarian failure may also be due to these causes but more commonly is associated with autoimmune phenomena. Women may develop antibodies to gonadotropins or to gonadotropin receptors. Other associated autoimmune diseases include hypothyroidism, hypoadrenalism, myasthenia gravis, and hypoparathyroidism. Cigarette smoking may lead to menopause at an earlier than average age but, without other factors, does not cause ovarian failure before age 40.

History and Physical Examination

The time of premature ovarian failure (POF) determines the presentation. Prepubertal ovarian failure is noted at puberty, when secondary sexual characteristics fail to develop and primary amenorrhea becomes evident. Women with peripubertal ovarian failure may present with incomplete sexual development and either primary or secondary amenorrhea. Adult women present with secondary amenorrhea and other signs of loss of estrogen (vasomotor symptoms of hot flushes, vaginal dryness with dyspareunia, mood changes, and sleep dysfunction). Vasomotor symptoms are observed only in women who have previously been exposed to endogenous or exogenous estrogen. Secondary amenorrhea is usually not abrupt and is preceded by irregular menstrual cycles.

Physical examination of patients with prepubertal ovarian failure reveals lack of breast development and often a less than average amount of pubic hair. The stigmata of Turner syndrome—short stature, webbed neck, low-set ears, low posterior hair line, high-arched palate, cubitus valgus, and widely spaced nipples—should be sought (Fig. 37-3). Some patients with Turner syndrome have a later onset of POF and present with secondary sexual development and a history of previous menstrual bleeding. With peripubertal ovarian failure, breast examination may show halted development at Tanner stage III or IV, as well as poor development of the labia minora compared to the labia majora. In adults, evidence of estrogen loss includes lack of cervical mucus, atrophy of the vaginal mucosa with loss of rugae and luster, and urethral caruncle. Breast atrophy is a late sign of estrogen deprivation.

Diagnostic Studies

The most efficient test for POF is the measurement of FSH levels. FSH levels in excess of 30 IU/L indicate POF. The only time a woman still capable of normal reproduction would have a similar FSH level is at ovulation. To rule out this unlikely coincidence, an LH level may be measured, or FSH levels from different times may be assayed. Determination of the FSH level is much more efficient than measuring the estrogen level.

In general, the younger the patient's age when presenting with POF, the higher the chance of a chromosomal abnormality. There is no universally accepted age below which a karyotype should be obtained. In patients without physical abnormalities, a karyotype is usually performed in women less than age 30. Patients with Turner syndrome need additional diagnostic testing to evaluate for cardiac abnormalities such as coarctation of the aorta, renal abnormalities, thyroid disease, and diabetes mellitus.

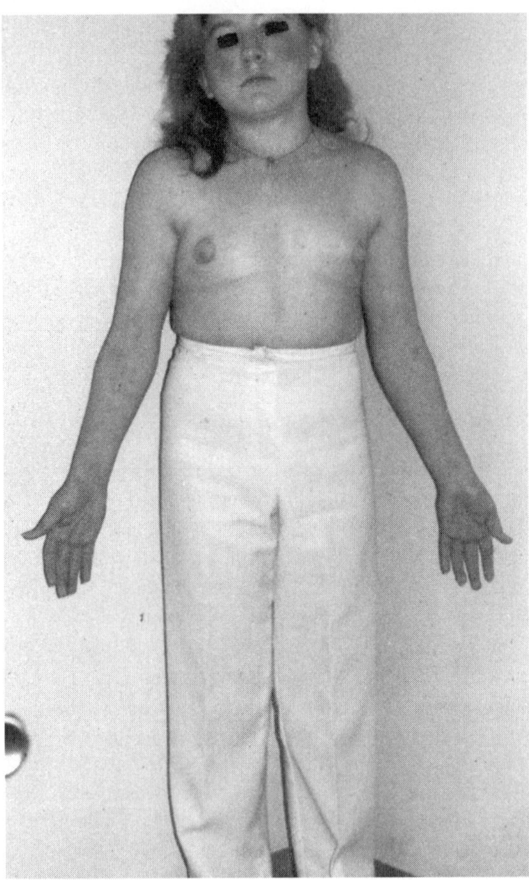

FIGURE 37-3. Typical female with Turner syndrome, exhibiting short stature, cubitus valgus, sexual infantilism and wide-spaced nipples.

In women thought to have autoimmune-related POF, additional testing of other endocrine pathways is warranted. Thyroid function tests should be obtained, and evaluation for hypoparathyroidism should be carried out through serum calcium and serum phosphate tests. Some have recommended testing for adrenal reserve with corticotropin-releasing factor or ACTH stimulation testing, but the cost-effectiveness of this testing in the absence of signs or symptoms of hypoadrenalism is not established. Evaluation for antithyroid antibodies is prudent. Although the presence of thyroid antibodies with normal thyroid function tests does not require therapy, it does suggest the need for periodic retesting of thyroid function. Widespread clinical testing for antibodies directed against the ovary or adrenal is unavailable.

Some women with POF have unstimulated ovarian follicles and elevated gonadotropins, a condition termed "resistant ovary syndrome." To evaluate for this condition, some have suggested ovarian biopsy through diagnostic laparoscopy. However, therapy for resistant ovarian syndrome is no different from that for other causes of POF, and ovarian biopsy should not be performed. Nor is there a role for ovarian imaging in women with POF, at least not in women who have a normal pelvic examination and no chromosomal abnormalities.

Treatment

The main goal of treatment is correction of estrogen deficiency and treatment of associated diseases. Sexually infantile women need stimulation of breast growth with low-dose estrogen therapy. Theoretically, OCP therapy is not optimal for breast development because of the presence of the progestin. In general, hormonal replacement therapy is preferable to the use of OCPs for POF. Although low-dose OCPs carry a low risk, the risk is still higher than standard hormone replacement regimens. Women with an intact uterus need combination therapy with continuous estrogen and monthly progestin therapy to ensure orderly sloughing of the endometrium. Various doses and combination strategies using conjugated estrogens or micronized 17β-estradiol with medroxyprogesterone acetate are available.

Occasionally, initiation of therapy may result in ovulation due to initial changes in gonadotropin levels. Although uncommon, patients should be counseled to use barrier contraceptives for the first few months if pregnancy is not desired.

POF is not always irreversible. Transient POF is not uncommon and may be due to fluctuating autoimmune antibodies. Patients with this condition tend to be in their second or third decade and have mildly elevated gonadotropins. Transient secondary amenorrhea and vasomotor symptoms may be followed by resumption of normal menses. Hormonal therapy does not influence the ultimate course of POF.

Pregnancy Considerations

In patients with POF, conception is obviously difficult. Treatment with low-dose estrogen may occasionally lead to ovulation but does not do so predictably. However, due to both the low cost and low risk of low-dose estrogen, treatment for 3 to 4 months in an attempt to induce ovulation is not unreasonable, as long as the patient does not have unrealistic expectations. In vitro fertilization using donor oocytes has offered a new opportunity to women with POF; it has a per-cycle pregnancy rate of 30% to 40%. Women with POF who do conceive do not face any additional obstetric risks.

BIBLIOGRAPHY

Buyalos RP, Watanabe RM, Geffner ME, et al. Insulin and insulin-like growth factor-1 responsiveness in polycystic ovarian syndrome. Fertil Steril 1992;57:796.

Carr BR. Disorders of the ovary and female reproductive tract. In: Wilson JD, Foster DW, eds. Williams textbook of endocrinology. Philadelphia: WB Saunders, 1992:760.

Dunaif A, Green G, Futterweit W, Dobrjansky A. Suppression of hyperandrogenism does not improve peripheral or hepatic insulin resistance in the polycystic ovary syndrome. J Clin Endocrinol Metab 1990;70:699.

Haseltine F, Wentz AC, Redmond GP, Wild RA. Androgens and women's health. Clinician: National Institutes of Health Continuing Medical Education 1994;12:1.

Jaffe RB. The menopause and perimenopausal period. In: Yen SSC, Jaffe RB, eds. Reproductive endocrinology. Philadelphia: WB Saunders, 1991:401.

Levine LS, Dupont B, Lorenzen F, et al. Genetic and hormonal characterization of cryptic 21-hydroxylase deficiency. J Clin Endocrinol Metab 1981;53:1193.

Nestler JE, Barlascini CO, Matt DW, et al. Suppression of serum insulin by diazoxide reduces serum testosterone levels in obese women with polycystic ovarian syndrome. J Clin Endocrinol Metab 1989;68:1027.

New MI, Lorenzen F, Lerner AJ, et al. Genotyping steroid 21-hydroxylase deficiency: hormonal reference data. J Clin Endocrinol Metab 1983;57:320.

Palmer CG, Reichman A. Chromosomal and clinical findings in 110 females with Turner syndrome. Hum Genet 1976;35:35.

Rosenwaks Z, Navot D. Oocyte donation in ovarian failure. In: Rosenfield RG, Grumbach MM, eds. Turner syndrome. New York: Marcel Dekker, 1990:109.

38

Diabetes Mellitus

PHYLLIS C. LEPPERT

Primary Care for Women, edited by Phyllis C. Leppert and Fred M. Howard. Lippincott-Raven Publishers, Philadelphia © 1997.

Diabetes comprises several distinct disease states (Table 38-1). Type I diabetes, or insulin-dependent diabetes mellitus (IDDM), occurs early in life; it was previously called juvenile-onset diabetes. The lack of or ineffectiveness of insulin produces severe disturbances in carbohydrate, protein, and lipid metabolism. Therefore, exogenous insulin therapy is necessary to maintain normal glucose levels in the peripheral circulatory system. Type II diabetes, or non–insulin-dependent diabetes mellitus (NIDDM), may be controlled by diet and oral sulfonylurea to maintain glucose level. This mature-onset diabetes usually occurs after age 40, with a peak age of onset at age 65. In a few persons, the age of onset is in adolescence or early adulthood; this type is called maturity-onset diabetes of youth (MODY). The National Diabetes Data Group further classifies diabetes mellitus into type III, or malnutrition-related diabetes, and type IV, or other forms of diabetes, including gestational diabetes.

ETIOLOGY

Type I (IDDM) and type II (NIDDM) are distinct diseases genetically. IDDM is diagnosed in 6% to 10% of all persons with diabetes. It is fairly common in Caucasians but rare in Japanese, Chinese, and Inuit. Autoimmunity plays a significant role in its etiology. Insulin autoantibodies and islet cell antibodies are produced, and over time these cause a complete destruction of pancreatic beta cells. Studies of twins demonstrate that there is a genetic susceptibility for IDDM. This susceptibility is polygenic in both human leukocyte antigen (HLA) and non-HLA gene regions. HLA-DR_3/DR_4 genotype persons have the highest risk of developing IDDM, but other genetic factors are also involved. IDDM is not inherited; the susceptibility to develop the disease is inherited, but the onset of the disease depends on environmental factors as well. This genetic susceptibility to IDDM is transmitted to offspring of diabetic fathers more than to the offspring of diabetic mothers.

NIDDM is not linked with HLA. In this form of diabetes, impaired insulin secretion and insulin antagonism are present. There is a much stronger genetic component in NIDDM than in IDDM. Studies of monozygotic twins show an almost 100% concordance for type II diabetes; the concordance for IDDM varies from 20% to 50%. The protein PC-1, which is thought to interfere with the body's response to insulin, is overproduced in NIDDM. The subgroup of NIDDM, MODY, is transmitted in an autosomal dominant fashion. The etiologies of type III and type IV diabetes are multifactorial.

Gestational diabetes is genetically heterogeneous. In most cases, gestational diabetes represents a preclinical form of NIDDM, but in some cases it is early-stage or preclinical IDDM. Up to 3% of women with gestational diabetes have circulatory antiislet cell antibodies. More women with these antibodies are positive for HLA-DR_3/DR_4. Over half of persons with islet cell antibodies developed type I diabetes 1 to 11 years after the diagnosis of gestational diabetes mellitus.

Among Pima Indians, a group of people with a high incidence of NIDDM, there is a greater prevalence of this form of diabetes in the offspring of women who had NIDDM in pregnancy compared to the offspring of women who were not diabetic at the time of pregnancy but who developed NIDDM later. Thus, factors surrounding the in utero environment of the offspring of diabetic mothers plays a part in the etiology of this form of the disease.

Human placental lactogen (HPL) is a polypeptide hormone secreted by the syncytiotrophoblast of the placenta. Maternal blood levels of this protein steadily increase during pregnancy until the last 4 weeks of gestation. They peak around 24 to 28 weeks of gestation. HPL mobilizes lipids to provide free fatty acids as a source of energy for maternal metabolism. It is thought that this increase in maternal free fatty acids interferes with insulin action and the uptake of glucose by maternal cells. HPL has an amino acid structure similar to that of human growth hormone and reduces insulin binding to specific insulin receptors. Thus, HPL has a diabetogenic effect on pregnancy.

NATURAL HISTORY

The natural history of diabetes mellitus in susceptible persons is one of insidious onset that slowly progresses to complete destruction of the pancreatic beta cells of the islets due to an autoimmune process. Circulatory cytoplasmal islet cell antibodies and insulin autoantibodies are seen early in the disease. Viral infections and possibly chemical agents and other environmental factors trigger the disease onset. Clinical symptoms appear abruptly when the insulin insufficiency becomes severe. Within a few weeks, fatigue, sudden weight loss, polyuria, polydipsia, and polyphagia appear. Diabetes mellitus can be diagnosed earlier by testing siblings of diabetics for elevated fasting blood sugar or, in an even better approach, by a postprandial blood sugar or glucose tolerance test. In IDDM, exogenous insulin is essential to prevent spontaneous ketosis, coma, and death.

Within 10 to 15 years of onset, peripheral arterial disease develops. Atherosclerotic disease occurs earlier than usual in dia-

Table 38-1. Classification of Diabetes

	TYPE	ETIOLOGY
Diabetes Mellitus		
Type I	Insulin-dependent (juvenile-onset): IDDM	Islet cell antibody
		Insulin autoantibody; over time, complete destruction of pancreatic beta cells
Type II	Non–insulin-dependent (maturity-onset): NIDDM: MODY (maturity-onset diabetes of youth)	Strong genetic component.
		May be caused by increased PC-1 protein, which interferes with body's response to insulin.
		Autosomal dominant
Type III	Malnutrition-related diabetes	Protein deficiency fibrocalculus diabetes
Type IV	Pancreatic disease	
	Hormone-induced	
	Drug- or chemical-induced	
	Some genetic syndromes	
	Insulin receptor abnormalities	
Impaired Glucose Tolerance		
Gestational Diabetes	Diagnosed in pregnancy	Human placental lactogen promotes a diabetogenic state.

(Modified from Rifkin H, Porte D, eds. Ellenberg and Rifkin's diabetes mellitus, 4th ed. New York: Elsevier, 1990.)

betics and it involves the smaller, more distal and peripheral vessels. Intimal thickening of the basement membranes of vessels occurs in both diabetics and nondiabetics. However, the microcapillary angiopathy varies from one diabetic to another. As diabetes progresses, retinopathy and nephropathy occur.

In poorly controlled diabetics, a form of metabolic imbalance occurs. During acute episodes of hyperglycemia, decreased tissue oxygen use is seen as glucose is shunted through the sorbitol pathway instead of the glycolytic pathway. Thus, there is decreased energy production and decreased pyruvate use in the mitochondria. In episodes of acute hyperglycemia lasting longer than 4 hours, intracellular levels of fructose, sorbitol, and lactate are elevated. These high levels are associated with impairment of neural, skeletal, and smooth muscle cells, along with increased capillary permeability. This phenomenon is hyperglycemia-induced pseudohypoxia, and it can help explain why diabetics are prone to foot ulcers and other problems involving skin integrity breakdown in the peripheral extremities. Over a long time, the increased capillary permeability resulting from pseudohypoxia probably accelerates atherogenesis by allowing atherogenic proteins and fatty acids access to the subendothelial space.

Peripheral neuropathies occur in about 55% of persons with IDDM. As the disease progresses, the incidence of neuropathies increases. The initial clinical symptoms of diabetic peripheral neuropathies vary but are usually paresthesia and hypersensitivity to touch (unpleasant dysesthesia). In some diabetics, this progresses to complete loss of sensation. The mechanisms causing these neuropathies are unclear. It has been postulated that a prostaglandin precursor, linolenic acid, plays a role, as large population studies have shown that either prostaglandin E_1 or δ-linolenic acid prevents progression of diabetic neuropathy. In some situations, treatment with one of these substances improves diabetic retinopathy. Some postulate that an element of compressive neuropathy is also involved in the pathogenesis of diabetic neuropathy. This peripheral neuropathy predisposes diabetics to unrecognized injury, especially to the foot.

Diabetic Ketoacidosis

One of the most serious complications of diabetes mellitus is diabetic ketoacidosis (DKA). It is most often seen in patients with IDDM, but in certain circumstances may occur in NIDDM. DKA was described in 1886 and had a 100% mortality rate until insulin was discovered in 1922. Today the mortality rate is less than 5%. DKA is characterized by three metabolic abnormalities: high blood glucose, high ketone bodies, and metabolic acidosis. Situations that precipitate DKA, in order of frequency of occurrence, are infection, omission or inadequate use of insulin, new-onset diabetes, and other events. Modern management of diabetes, including patient education and a multidisciplinary health care team, has reduced the incidence of DKA to a very low level.

Other forms of ketosis that should be in the differential diagnosis are ketotic hypoglycemia, alcoholic ketosis, and starvation ketosis. Metabolic acidosis may be due to lactic acidosis, salicylism and other drug-induced acidoses, uremia, and hyperchloremic acidosis. Hyperglycemia may occur in nonketotic hyperosmolar coma, stress hyperglycemia, and impaired glucose tolerance. Diabetics may have a relatively high blood glucose level without ketosis. In a severe hyperosmolar state, the pathogenesis of DKA is due to severe perturbations in intermediate metabolic pathways and in fluids, electrolytes, and acid-base status. The lack of or ineffectiveness of insulin results in hyperglycemia. In addition, the counterregulatory hormones, glucagon, catecholamines, and cortisol are elevated. Catecholamines, without effective insulin, cause triglyceride breakdown (lipolysis) to free fatty acids and glycerol. These two substances are used to produce glucose in gluconeogenesis (glucose production from noncarbohydrates). Thus, increased hyperglycemia occurs. Peripheral tissues do not use glucose in DKA because of inadequate insulin. The accumulated free fatty acids lead to ketone body formation. Ketogenesis is increased further by decreased malonyl coenzyme A. Low levels of the enzyme allow carnitine palmitoyl transferase to become more active, and thus more ketones are produced. Protein is also broken down into amino acids. The effect of these metabolic abnormalities is to switch the insulin-dependent cells of the body from carbohydrate metabolism to fat metabolism.

Hyperglycemia causes glycosuria and an osmotic diuresis (polyuria). This causes a loss of glucose in urine and a progressive loss of fluids and electrolytes, leading to polyphagia. As the metabolic disturbances accelerate, weight loss and dehydration occur. Increased free fatty acids stimulate the increased formation of ketone bodies by beta oxidation. The ketones are buffered by extracellular and intracellular buffer systems, resulting in metabolic acidosis. Normally, the cells of liver, muscle, and fat are capable of gluconeogenesis and free fatty acid and ketone body formation to provide glucose to the brain in starvation states. These cells produce glucose in DKA because without insulin, glucose does not get into cells. Thus, in DKA, liver, muscle, and fat cells are functioning in a "starved" state.

Because of the osmotic diuresis, sodium chloride and potassium are also excreted in the urine, along with severe water loss. As DKA develops, glucose accumulation in the extracellular space draws water into that compartment from the intracellular space. At this point, the plasma sodium concentration falls. However, as hyperglycemia increases, the water losses due to osmotic diuresis exceed the NaCl losses. Finally, the fluid losses from the intracellular and extracellular spaces equalize. Thus, plasma sodium concentrations are often low or normal in DKA despite the profound water losses. Furthermore, the severe hyperlipidemia seen in DKA displaces plasma water, with the effect of spuriously lowering the plasma sodium concentration. Total body potassium loss is severe, but plasma potassium concentrations are normal or elevated in DKA. Potassium is shifted from the intracellular to the extracellular space. This potassium shift is aggravated by the breakdown of protein and the presence of acidosis. A secondary hyperaldosteronism that develops in DKA further increases potassium loss.

Ketones produce ketoacids at physiologic pH. The H^+ ions cause metabolic acidosis. They are buffered, however, by extracellular and intracellular buffers. Ketones are excreted in the urine. Patients with a better dietary intake of NaCl and fluid during the development of DKA have less volume depletion and, therefore, lower plasma ketoanions. There is a greater degree of hyperchloremic metabolic acidosis. As DKA is treated with insulin, ketoanion is metabolized, resulting in the regeneration of plasma bicarbonate and the correction of the metabolic acidosis.

Nonketotic Hypertonicity

In poorly controlled diabetes, there are two causes of hypertonicity. In the first, glucose is added to the extracellular space and hypotonic osmotic diuresis then decreases total body water. This may lead to hypertonicity without ketosis. Extracellular glucose cannot enter the cell, and therefore intracellular water flows into the extracellular space. Eventually, both extracellular fluid and the intracellular space lose water, creating hypertonic fluid on both sides of the cell membrane.

Normally, the glucose filtered in the kidney is reabsorbed until the tubular fluid glucose reaches about 180 mg/dL. As glucose becomes elevated above this level, it is not reabsorbed but remains in the tubal fluids, where it induces a hypotonic osmotic diuresis. Urine in this circumstance contains 50 to 70 mEq/L sodium and increased calcium, phosphate, magnesium, urea, and uric acid. Volume contraction occurs, resulting in decreased glomerular filtration of glucose and greater hyperglycemia. This leads to nonketotic hypertonicity (NKH).

In young diabetics who can drink water freely, the blood volume, glomerular filtration rate, and glycosuria are maintained; thus, the blood glucose level may reach 300 mg/dL before a new steady state develops. The glomerular filtration rate decreases with age, so the renal threshold for glucose increases. Thus, in the elderly diabetic, a higher blood glucose level is found before osmotic diuresis begins.

In NKH, the hyperosmolarity suppresses lipolysis and thus ketosis. Patients with NKH also have lower levels of counterregulatory hormones (growth hormone, glucagon, epinephrine, and cortisol) and higher intraportal insulin than patients with DKA. These factors account for the lack of ketosis.

NKH usually is seen in elderly patients (age 57 to 69) with NIDDM, but it also is found in IDDM patients, especially those who have received intermediate-acting insulin 15 hours or less before the diagnosis of NKH. In 33% to 60% of patients, the diabetes is newly diagnosed. NKH is associated with female sex, new-onset diabetes, and infection. Infection is the most common precipitating event (pneumonia, usually with a gram-negative organism, in 40% to 60% of cases, a urinary tract infection in 5% to 10% of cases). Other illnesses that trigger NKH are cerebrovascular accident, myocardial infarction, pancreatitis, uremia, burns, heatstroke, ectopic ACTH syndrome, and subdural hematoma.

PHYSICAL EXAMINATION

The primary care provider must be alert for persons at risk for IDDM and NIDDM. Young persons with a family history of IDDM should be examined with the thought in mind that they could have diabetes. For example, a young woman with a diabetic brother who has recurrent and persistent vaginal and vulvar candidiasis should be evaluated for glucose intolerance. Patients at risk for diabetes should have a postprandial blood sugar or a glucose tolerance test, as early mild diabetes is asymptomatic and the progression of the disease is slow.

Two of every five Americans over age 65 have abnormal glucose homeostasis. Furthermore, one of every five older persons has diabetes; of that number, half are undiagnosed. In such older persons, the presentation of diabetes is subtle: the classic symptoms of polyuria, polydipsia, and polyphagia are less common, but weight loss and fatigue are prominent. In older women, cataracts, paresthesia, heart disease, autonomic dysfunction, and peripheral vascular disease should trigger a search for undiagnosed glucose intolerance.

Women with a history of gestational diabetes are at risk for the development of diabetes in their later years. Most women with gestational diabetes have a preclinical form of NIDDM. However, some women with gestational diabetes seem to have circulating islet cell antibodies. About half of these women eventually develop IDDM. Women with overt IDDM are thin; those with NIDDM tend to be obese.

In patients initially presenting with DKA, signs of dehydration, such as decreased skin turgor, tachycardia, and low-grade temperature elevation, are apparent; on the other hand, a patient with DKA and an infection may be hypothermic. Lethargy and coma may occur. Thus, diabetes should be considered in anyone presenting in coma, especially a young girl or woman. Except for tachycardia, the examination of the cardiac system may be normal. A funduscopic examination determines the degree of involvement of the peripheral vascular system and must be done on all diabetics regardless of age. This examination is critical in patients with longstanding IDDM. Examination of the respiratory tract in patients with uncontrolled diabetes may at first be normal, but after adequate hydration, the clinical signs of pneumonia or pleural effusion may be noted. In 40% of patients presenting with NKH, there is no prior history of diabetes mellitus. Respiratory and urinary tract or other infections often coexist. Often the history is incomplete or unavailable and the physician must be alert to the possibility of NKH in any elderly obtunded patient. CNS disturbances occur in this condition, and patients may present with hallucinations and other psychic disturbances. One quarter of patients present with focal or generalized seizures, such as gaze-induced visual seizures or occipital seizures. Any seizure resistant to anticonvulsant therapy should raise the suspicion of diabetes. Phenytoin given for seizure disorders may exacerbate the disease by inhibiting insulin release. Finally, the hypertonicity of NKH causes gastric dilatation with accompanying nausea, distention, and pain from gastroparesis.

A well-controlled diabetic is at no greater risk of infection than is a nondiabetic. Hyperglycemia, however, appears to lead to diminished humoral defense, and high plasma glucose levels may actually promote the virulence of some microbes. Other factors that contribute to increased infection in poorly controlled diabetics are dehydration secondary to osmotic diuresis, poor nutritional status, and long-term complications of vascular insufficiency and neuropathy.

Phagocytosis and bacterial killing by polymorphonuclear cells is severely diminished in DKA and can be impaired in NKH. Peripheral vascular disease associated with microangiopathy and neuropathy is common in patients with advanced diabetes. This leads to impaired circulation, which delays host response, retards wound healing, and slows the delivery of antibiotics or antifungal drugs to the infected tissue. Diabetic patients have increased numbers of potential pathogens, such as *Staphylococcus aureus*, in normal skin and mucous membrane flora. Any foot infection in a diabetic patient is a serious complication.

Every primary care provider must be aware of the rare but life-threatening infections that can occur in diabetics (Table 38-2).

LABORATORY EVALUATION

The diagnosis and management of diabetes depend to a large extent on the proper use and interpretation of laboratory tests, especially plasma glucose evaluations. Table 38-3 lists the persons who should receive a screening test for diabetes. A random plasma glu-

Table 38-2. Life-Threatening Infections in Diabetics

INFECTION	SIGNS, SYMPTOMS, AND COURSE	CAUSATIVE ORGANISM
***Malignant External Otitis:* Occurs almost exclusively in diabetics**	Severe otalgia, otorrhea, and periauricular swelling and tenderness Infection begins in the external auditory canal and then rapidly invades surrounding tissue, mastoid cells, and cranial nerves (facial, glossopharyngeal, vagal, spinal accessory, and hypoglossal).	Usually *Pseudomonas aeruginosa.* Can be *Aspergillus* spp, *Enterobacter, Klebsiella,* and *Staphylococcus aureus.*
***Rhinocerebral Mucormycosis:* Occurs in poorly controlled type I diabetics**	Associated with marked hyperglycemia and dehydration. Disease begins on nasal mucosa or palate and extends to paranasal sinuses and retroorbital space and into the brain. Characterized by black necrotic eschars on infected tissue.	Fungal organisms: *Rhizopus, Rhizomucor, Mucor,* and *Absidia* (funguses that cause gray-black mold on bread)
***Emphysematous Cholecystitis:* One third of patients are diabetics**	Highly virulent form of acute cholecystitis with gas production around the gallbladder. Diabetic vascular disease plays a role. More common in males. Mortality rate is 15%.	Predominantly *Clostridium* species; occasionally caused by *Escherichia coli,* staphylococci, streptococci, and *Pseudomonas aeruginosa.*
Emphysematous Pyelonephritis	Rare gas-forming infection of renal collecting system, parenchyma, and perinephric tissue. Occurs more often in women. Involves left kidney more frequently. 21% develop renal papillary necrosis.	*E coli* most frequent organism
Necrotizing Soft-Tissue Infection Includes nonclostridial gas gangrene necrotizing fasciitis, and necrotizing cellulitis	Patients are severely ill with high fevers. Frequently associated with DKA. Skin anesthesia, draining ulcers, and skin necrosis are seen. In some cases of necrotizing cellulitis, the skin may be deceptively normal in appearance.	Polymicrobial infections caused by a mixture of anaerobic and aerobic organisms that may include *Bacteroides* spp, anaerobic streptococci, *Clostridium* spp, and *Pseudomonas aeruginosa* and other gram-negative rods: *Streptococcus, Enterococcus,* and *Staphylococcus.*

Table 38-3. Persons Who Should Be Screened For Diabetes

Persons with a strong family history of diabetes
Markedly obese persons
Women with a history of stillbirth, neonatal death, large-for-gestational-age infant (over 10 lb), toxemia of pregnancy, and glycosuria (if known)
All pregnant women between 24 and 28 wk
Patients with recurrent genital, urinary tract, and skin infections.

cose level of 200 mg/dL or greater in the presence of polydipsia, polyuria, polyphagia, weight loss, fatigue, or blurred vision is diagnostic of diabetes at any age. An elevated fasting blood sugar of 140 mg/dL or greater in a nonpregnant woman is specific for the diagnosis of diabetes but lacks sensitivity. In the "mild" diabetic, the fasting plasma glucose level is normal; therefore, a 2-hour postprandial or a glucose tolerance test is a more sensitive indicator.

The oral glucose tolerance test (OGTT) remains the most sensitive and practical test for the early recognition of asymptomatic diabetes. Venous blood should be used, as a capillary blood glucose reading used to monitor the therapy of diabetes can be 20 to 70 mg/dL higher than in nonvenous blood. Table 38-4 summarizes laboratory evaluation.

Impregnated paper test strips with glucose reflectance meters cannot be used for diagnostic purposes. Plasma is used, as it reflects the extracellular glucose concentration more accurately and is independent of hematocrit. If the hematocrit is normal, whole blood glucose can be converted to plasma by multiplying by 1.15. The blood sample must be chilled to prevent glycolysis of glucose by the blood cells. Fluoride in collection tubes inhibits glycolysis but should not be used because it interferes with enzymatic methods of glucose determination. The glucose-specific enzyme methods produce values 10 mg/dL lower than does the copper reduction method used in the past.

The OGTT is performed on ambulatory patients. Moderate walking during the test is permitted, but excessive exercise is prohibited. The glucose load in nonpregnant women is 75 g given in a chilled solution of 300 mL water to prevent nausea. In pregnant women, the loading dose is 100 g, again given as a chilled solution. Lemon juice may be added to enhance the palatability of these loading doses. In children, the loading dose of glucose is 1.75 g/kg of ideal body weight, up to a total dose of 75 mg. The test is timed from the first swallow, but the glucose solution is ingested over a 5-minute period. Venous blood samples are obtained at 0.5, 1, 1.5, and 2 hours. The 1.5-hour value may be the most useful in the interpretation of borderline tests. In pregnant women, a 3-hour glucose tolerance test is performed. Women with histories of reactive hypoglycemia 2 or more hours after a meal should undergo a 5-hour test with half-hour intervals and an interval timed to coincide with the time of hypoglycemic symptoms.

The test is always performed in the morning after a 10- to 14-hour fast, as glucose tolerance deteriorates in the afternoon. No coffee ingestion or smoking should be done before the test. The test is not accurate in and should not be done on anyone with an acute or chronic disease such as infection, acute cardiovascular or cerebrovascular disease, renal disease, or an active endocrine disease. Patients should not be taking birth-control pills. Hyperlipoproteinemia may give an inappropriately abnormal test. Table 38-4 outlines the diagnostic criteria for abnormal OGTTs.

Table 38-4. Laboratory Evaluation for Diabetes

Diabetes Mellitus	
FPG < 140 mg/dL and 2 OGTTs with 2 hr P ≥ 200 mg/dL and one other interval value ≥ 200 mg/dL	
Impaired Glucose Tolerance	
FPG < 140 mg/dL and	
PG ≥ 140 mg/dL and < 200 mg/dL and one other interval value ≥ 200 mg/dL after standard 75-g glucose load OGTT	
Gestational Diabetes Glucose Screen	
50-g oral glucose load at 24–28 wks or at first visit for patients at risk. Repeat negative test in these patients at 24–28 wks	
1-hour PG ≥ 150 and < 185 requires OGTT	
1-hour PG ≥ 185 diagnostic	
Consider retesting women with ≥ 120 and < 139 at 34 weeks gestation	
OGTT 100-g load	
FPG 105	
1 hr 190	2 or more values greater than upper limits of normal
2 hr 165	
3 hr 145	

FPG, fasting plasma glucose; *OGTT*, oral glucose tolerance test; *PG*, plasma glucose.

In the past, carbohydrate loading of patients undergoing OGTT was done 3 days before the test, based on the theory that this would prevent a plateau of plasma glucose and false diabetic results in normal patients. This is no longer necessary for most patients. However, patients with anorexia nervosa or those on a reducing diet should be given a diet of 200 g of carbohydrates 1 week before the OGTT. Pregnant patients should have at least 3 days of a diet with more than 150 g of carbohydrates before the OGTT.

In diabetics, a hexose can attach as a ketamine to the N-terminal valine of the normal beta chain of hemoglobin A_1 (HbA_1). Thus, the HbA_1C, or glycosylated hemoglobin, detects marked hyperglycemia. The rate of formation of HbA_1C is directly proportional to the average concentration of glucose within the erythrocyte. The time to return to normal after hyperglycemia in a controlled diabetic is 5 to 6 weeks. HbA_1C is not useful in the diagnosis of diabetes, nor are plasma insulin levels.

Once the diagnosis of diabetes is made, the woman and her physician monitor glucose values on a daily basis using impregnated paper test strips with a glucose reflectance meter. Diabetic patients need periodic urinalysis for albuminuria, urine cultures, and laboratory tests of renal function as their disease progresses. Creatinine clearance should be monitored, as diabetic nephropathy occurs in stages. Similarly, careful examination of the retina to diagnose and monitor diabetic retinopathy is essential.

Any diabetic who presents with evidence of DKA or NKH must have, at a minimum, immediate urinalysis, blood chemistries (electrolytes, glucose, and bicarbonate levels), glucose by a finger-stick method, blood and urine ketones by nitroprusside reaction, appropriate bacterial cultures, an electrocardiogram, and an arterial blood gas analysis (Table 38-5)

Table 38-5. Criteria for Diagnosis of Diabetic Ketoacidosis

Plasma glucose > 250 mg/dL
Low bicarbonate < 15 mEq/L
pH < 7.3
Ketonemia (positive at 1:2 dilution)
Moderate ketonuria
Usually WBC = 25,000/mL without left shift in absence of infection; WBC > 25,000/mL with shift in presence of infection

TREATMENT

The treatment of diabetes includes diet and exercise. In type I and some other diabetics, it includes insulin. Oral hyperglycemia agents are used in NIDDM but never in a pregnant woman. Successful treatment necessitates the establishment of routines. Ideally, the insulin dose, the level of activity, and the number of calories used are the same each day. Some flexibility is necessary, but it demands a significant understanding of the multiple facets of diabetes on the part of the patient, her family, and her physician. For the physician caring for a diabetic, taking the time to pay attention to small details is extremely important. Often the dietary prescriptions are overwhelming to a new diabetic. The American Diabetes Association, in their 1986 *Nutritional Recommendations and Principles for Individuals with Diabetes Mellitus*, called for limited fat, restriction of protein to the recommended daily intake for the patient, and carbohydrates to fill the rest of the needed calories. A good, understanding physician-patient relationship, a dietitian skillful in diabetic diets, and expert nurses are essential to help the diabetic woman accomplish the goals of her diet.

The caloric needs of the diabetic are no different from those of a normal person. Patients should maintain the appropriate weight for their height, bone structure, and age. Children need an adequate caloric intake to grow. Many diabetics, especially children, pregnant women, and some adults, require snacks between meals to prevent plasma glucose fluctuations. It is then necessary to subtract the calories in snacks from the main meals to keep weight at appropriate levels. Overweight women should be encouraged to restrict calories, as this improves glycemic control.

There appears to be no reason to restrict carbohydrates in a diabetic diet. Complex carbohydrates should make up 50% to 60% of total calories. Diabetics must control their fat intake because of their predisposition to vascular disease and lipid disorders. Ideally, the diet should have only 30% of calories as fat. The ratio of polyunsaturated to saturated fat should be 0.8 to 1.2. The diet needs to contain enough fiber to prevent an increase in synthesis of plasma triglycerides and serum cholesterol. Some antilipemic drugs, such as nicotinic acid, may impair glucose tolerance. For diabetics, the recommended daily protein intake is 0.8 g/kg; most Americans eat 1.4 g/kg of protein each day. The lower intake of protein in diabetic patients may prolong the slow but steady decrease in creatinine clearance once renal disease or stage III "incipient" nephropathy exists. At this stage, decreased protein intake may have a beneficial effect, although control of hypertension is the single most important factor in the treatment of renal disease.

Fiber in the diet helps to improve constipation, delay gastric emptying, and alter intestinal transit time. It also binds water, drugs, cation, and bile salts. Soluble fibers slow the rate of food absorption from the small intestine and significantly reduce the postprandial glucose level. Insoluble fibers, such as cellulose, increase stool bulk, thereby shortening the transit time and reducing constipation. Large amounts of fiber must be avoided in children, the elderly, and women with gastrointestinal disease. Foods rich in fiber are legumes, fruits, vegetables, oats, wheat, and bran.

Diet and sufficient exercise for the maintenance of weight are keys to the successful treatment of diabetics. Patients who meet with the dietitian regularly have a better understanding of their disease than those taught only by a physician. A diabetic diet is really an eating plan. The classic "exchange lists" help diabetics avoid boredom with their diet. Because such an eating plan is actually healthy for everyone, the entire family of the diabetic should benefit from following it. Compliance is best when ethnic and social customs and the patient's eating habits are taken into account. Children and adolescents need special help with their diet. Teenagers with diabetes may do better if the parents allow them to manage the disease. Finally, the person in the household who does the cooking must understand the disease.

Insulin is a requirement for patients with IDDM. It may be required for patients with NIDDM who cannot maintain euglycemia on oral hypoglycemic drugs. Insulin is also given to gestational diabetics who have consistently elevated fasting plasma glucose levels or an elevated postprandial glucose level despite diet therapy. Every insulin-treated woman and a family member should be taught to monitor the blood glucose level, generally two to four times a day. These values should be recorded by the patient and discussed with the provider at each visit. All patients need instruction and monitoring in the technique of insulin administration. It is important for the nurse instructing the patient to note that she can accurately draw up the insulin. Errors in insulin administration occur 10% to 20% of the time.

Table 38-6 lists the insulin regimens in common use. Oral hypoglycemic agents include tolbutamide, tolazamide, chlorpropamide, glipizide, and glyburide (Table 38-7).

Table 38-6. Common Insulin Regimens for Nonpregnant Diabetics

REGIMEN	INSULIN ADMINISTRATION	COMMENT
Morning insulin	Intermediate/regular combination given at breakfast	If this does not adequately control p.m. glucose, split/mixed regimen is required.
Split/mixed insulin	Intermediate/regular combination given before breakfast and supper	Usually 70/30 split
Evening insulin	NPH or Lente at bedtime	Dose is increased every 3 to 5 days until optimal fasting glucose is reached
Insulin/sulfonylurea	NPH or Lente at bedtime added to a sulfonylurea	

Table 38-7. Oral Hypoglycemic Agents in Common Use

AGENT	DURATION OF ACTION (H)	SUGGESTED STARTING DOSE (mg)§	MAXIMAL DOSAGE (mg/d)	USUAL DOSING (PER DAY)
First Generation				
Tolbutamide* (Orinase)	6 to 12	250 up to 2000	3000	2 to 3
Tolazamide (Tolinase)	12 to 24	100–250	1000	1
Chlorpropamide† (Diabinese)	24 to 60	100–250	500	1
Second Generation				
Glipizide‡ (Glucotrol)	10 to 16	2.5–5	40	1 to 2
Glyburide (Diabeta, Micronase)				
Nonmicronized	24	1.25–5.0	20	1 to 2
Micronized	24	0.75–2.5	12	1 to 2

*Lowest cost, best in renal failure.
†Not recommended in elderly due to long half-life.
‡Short half-life may minimize silent hypoglycemia.
§Individualize according to patient's age and clinical status.
(Modified from Brown DF, Jackson TW. Diabetes "tight control" in a comprehensive treatment plan. Geriatrics 1994;49:24.)

When a diabetic is ill, the stress of the sickness increases her insulin needs, even if she cannot maintain oral intake. Insulin should never be omitted during an illness. All diabetics should carry diabetic identification.

Diabetics may travel without problems. They should carry snacks in case they miss a meal. Insulin should be stored in a cool place, never in a car trunk. Diabetics can give themselves insulin injections in a restaurant restroom before the serving of an appetizer. When traveling abroad, it is a good idea to carry a letter from the physician and a prescription when passing through customs with syringes, needles, and other supplies.

Finally, diabetics should be encouraged to exercise, preferably in the morning, with warm-up and cool-down periods. A social, noncompetitive attitude toward exercise is helpful. Injecting insulin away from the exercising muscle and eating 15 to 20 g of carbohydrates before exercise prevents hypoglycemia.

The aim of therapy in diabetic patients is to control blood glucose. Tight control of both type I and type II nonpregnant diabetics targets a fasting glucose level of less than 140 mg/dL. This tight control has been demonstrated to prevent acute and long-term complications. Because patients age 65 to 69 live another 15 years on the average, women of this age should also be encouraged to control their blood glucose tightly. Some persons, such as women with cognitive impairment, those in isolated social situations, those at increased risk for silent asymptomatic hypoglycemia, or those who for any reason cannot comply with treatment, are not good candidates for tight glucose control, and a target glucose level for them might be 150 to 200 mg/dL.

CONSIDERATIONS IN PREGNANCY

During normal gestation, the fasting glucose level decreases the first few weeks of pregnancy and reaches its lowest level by the 12th week of gestation. Thereafter, the levels remain unchanged until delivery. This decrease is about 15 mg/dL in the pregnant woman who has fasted overnight, compared to a nonpregnant woman. In contrast to nonpregnant women, pregnant women respond to a meal with an increased postprandial glucose level. This is thought to facilitate glucose transport to the fetus across the placenta. Insulin levels in a basal state are no different from those in nonpregnancy during the first and second trimesters, but they increase by 50% in the third trimester. There is an insulin resistance in pregnancy. These changes are related to the effect of increased estrogen and estrogen in pregnancy, in addition to the effect of HPL. The free cortisol level is increased in pregnancy, and this increase reduces the effectiveness of insulin.

During late gestation, there is a greater postprandial increment and preprandial decrease in the plasma glucose level than in nonpregnant women. Women with diabetes (usually type I) need special preconceptual and prenatal care to maintain glucose control well within that seen in normal pregnant patients. Before pregnancy, the diabetic woman should be evaluated for general medical status and for signs of retinopathy, nephropathy, hypertension, and ischemic heart disease. An ophthalmologic examination, an electrocardiogram, and renal function tests should be performed. Patients should be told to stop oral hypoglycemia medication and begin insulin. The goal is to have optimal diabetic control before conception.

The frequency of major congenital anomalies among infants of diabetic mothers is thought to be 6% to 10%, or a twofold to fivefold increase over those born to nondiabetic mothers. These congenital malformations account for about 40% of all perinatal deaths in the United States and involve many organ systems. Cardiac anomalies are the most common. In women who have achieved excellent and tight glucose control before conception, the incidence of these fetal anomalies may be reduced to nearly zero (0.8%).

Pregnant diabetic patients should be followed closely during pregnancy by experts in the management of complicated high-risk pregnancies and diabetic control. By maintaining euglycemia with mean blood glucose levels below 100 mg/dL, perinatal mortality is reduced. The target maternal glucose to maintain in pregnancy is the blood glucose seen in normal pregnancy: this means that fasting plasma glucose levels should be 60 to 80 mg/dL. The mean diurnal glucose level should be 85 mg/dL, and postprandial levels should rarely exceed 120 mg/dL.

Table 38-8. Complications in Newborn of Diabetic Mother

Significant macrosomia
Birth trauma
Hypoglycemia
Hypocalcemia and hypomagnesemia
Polycythemia
Hyperbilirubinemia
Respiratory distress syndrome
Intrauterine chronic hypoxia leading to neonatal asphyxia
Cardiomyopathy

Insulin in pregnancy is given usually as a split dose of neutral protein Hagedorn (NPH) insulin and regular insulin, on a regimen of two, three, or four injections daily. The three-injection regimen may be most effective. NPH and regular insulin is given before breakfast, regular is given before dinner, and NPH or Lente is given at bedtime to prevent nocturnal hypoglycemia and for early-morning glucose control. Human insulin is used in pregnant diabetics. The diabetic pregnant woman should be taught self-monitoring of blood glucose and maintained on a recommended diet of 35 kcal/kg of ideal body weight, 20% protein, 30% fat, and 50% carbohydrates. This diet usually consists of three meals and one to three snacks. The bedtime snack is made up of complex carbohydrates that prevent nocturnal hypoglycemia. In pregnant diabetics requiring insulin, a fiber-enriched diet may decrease the frequency of hypoglycemic reactions.

A birthweight in excess of 4000 g, or a birthweight above the 90th percentile of gestational age, occurs in 30% of all diabetic pregnancies. These infants have a higher morbidity and mortality. Among these infants, the incidence of diabetes in later life is markedly increased. Macrosomia can be prevented by tight glucose control during pregnancy. The fetus of a diabetic mother requires careful surveillance, including ultrasound and antenatal fetal heart rate testing and biophysical scores. An insulin-requiring diabetic woman must give birth in a hospital with expert professional staff capable of caring for her and her newborn.

The newborn is at risk for complications during early life (Table 38-8). Maternal complications of diabetic pregnancy include DKA, hypoglycemia, pyelonephritis, and polyhydramnios. The pregnant woman is at increased risk for spontaneous abortion and preterm labor. Diabetic retinopathy may develop and progress during pregnancy, but these changes may regress. Careful, well-designed epidemiologic studies need to be conducted to determine the influence of pregnancy on diabetic retinopathy.

Gestational diabetics have carbohydrate intolerance of variable severity first recognized during pregnancy. The diagnosis is based on the results of the 100-g OGTT, and screening is conducted with the 50-g oral glucose load. Gestational diabetes is also associated with increased perinatal mortality. Most women with gestational diabetes achieve good control with diet alone, although prophylactic insulin may be of some benefit in reducing neonatal morbidity.

SUMMARY

The primary care aspects of diabetes involve making the diagnosis and understanding its natural history. Because diabetes in its early stages is asymptomatic, the primary care provider must be alert for persons at risk. All pregnant women over age 25—according to some, all pregnant women—should be screened for diabetes at 24 to 28 weeks of gestation. Women at risk for diabetes benefit from screening at the initial prenatal visit.

The treatment of diabetes is highly complex and involves an expert multidisciplinary team. The education of the patient and her family is paramount for optimal outcome.

BIBLIOGRAPHY

Bridges RM Jr, Deitch EA. Diabetic foot infections: pathophysiology and treatment. Surg Clin North Am 1994;74:537.

Brown DF, Jackson TW. Diabetes "tight control" in a comprehensive treatment plan. Geriatrics 1994;49:24.

Hagay ZJ, Reece EA. Diabetes mellitus in pregnancy. In: Reece EA, Hobbins JC, Mahoney MJ, Petrie RH, eds. Medicine of the fetus and mother. Philadelphia: JB Lippincott, 1992:982.

Kitabchi AE, Wall BM. Diabetic ketoacidosis. Med Clin North Am 1995;79:9.

Lorber D. Nonketotic hypertonicity in diabetes mellitus. Med Clin North Am 1995;79:39.

Quinn S. Diabetes and diet: we are still learning. Med Clin North Am 1993;77:773.

Rifkin H, Porte D, eds. Ellenberg and Rifkin's diabetes mellitus: theory and practice, 4th ed. New York: Elsevier, 1990:972.

Smitherman KO, Peacock JE Jr. Infectious emergencies in patients with diabetes mellitus. Med Clin North Am 1995;79:53.

39

Hypoglycemia

PHYLLIS C. LEPPERT

Primary Care for Women, edited by Phyllis C. Leppert and Fred M. Howard. Lippincott-Raven Publishers, Philadelphia © 1997.

Hypoglycemia is a clinical situation in which various symptoms occur in association with a plasma glucose level of 40 mg/dL or less. There are two major groups of these symptoms: one group is due to the activation of the autonomic nervous system; the other is caused by the effects of neuroglycopenia. Not all persons with a low plasma glucose level develop symptoms of hypoglycemia. Many persons with low glucose levels of 35 to 45 mg/dL are asymptomatic. Glucose levels below 50 mg/dL have been reported in normal persons without the occurrence of symptoms during glucose tolerance testing.

ETIOLOGY

Hypoglycemia is the most common medical emergency, primarily because of the number of diabetics in the general population who are at risk for hypoglycemia as a result of their treatment. The very young and the very elderly are particularly susceptible. The seriousness of this complication is related to the fact that when the brain is deprived of its essential nutrient—glucose—cognitive dysfunction and neurologic deficits occur. The high brain glucose requirements of the very young make them vulnerable when plasma glucose falls to low levels. The elderly may have underlying health problems, such as liver disease or renal disease, that increase the hypoglycemic action of many therapeutic drugs. Their increased susceptibility to hypoglycemia is due in part to the fact that they also may have a reduced cognitive function exacerbated by even slight degrees of hypoglycemia.

Other clinical entities also associated with hypoglycemia are listed in Table 39-1.

Hypoglycemia may result from increased insulin secretion (or use of exogenous insulin), enhanced glucose use, or inadequate functioning of one or more of the glucoregulatory mechanisms. In addition, autoantibodies to insulin may occur. Glucose is the essential fuel for normal brain function. Only in very exceptional circumstances, such as prolonged severe starvation, does the brain switch to the use of ketone bodies. The liver constantly produces glucose through gluconeogenesis and glycogenolysis. These metabolic processes are stimulated by glucagon and epinephrine. Growth hormone secreted by the pituitary inhibits muscle use of glucose. Growth hormone also enhances lipolysis, in which fats are broken down into glucose. The pituitary also secretes ACTH, the hormone that stimulates glucocorticoid production. The increase in cortisol diminishes muscle use of glucose and also stimulates gluconeogenesis.

Table 39-1. Causes of Hypoglycemia

Exogenous insulin and oral sulfonylureas in persons with diabetes mellitus.
Ethanol ingestion (especially in a fasting state)
Abnormal beta cell function
Islet cell tumors (insulinoma)
Non–islet cell tumors (especially in the older person)
Hepatic insufficiency
Renal insufficiency
Ingestion of hypoglycemic agent (accidental, malicious, surreptitious)
Hypopituitarism
Congestive heart failure
Inborn errors of metabolism
Strenuous exercise
Gastroparesis
Postpartum state (in a known type I diabetic)
ACTH or growth hormone deficiency
Total parenteral nutrition
Extensive burns
Neoplasia
Sepsis
Severe malaria
Postprandial hypoglycemia in a postgastrectomy patient
Treatment of hyperkalemia with insulin
Severe HELLP syndrome (hemolysis, elevated liver enzymes, and low platelet count)
Severe hypothyroidism
Idiopathic

Glucose metabolism in the brain is tightly linked to that organ's oxygen consumption. Falls in plasma glucose are associated with similar reductions in oxygen consumption in the brain. Glucose is transferred across the blood–brain barrier by a carrier-facilitated mechanism. Glucose-transport proteins carry glucose across the blood–brain barrier down a concentration gradient. There are regional differences in the brain's glucose metabolism; therefore, different brain areas have different potentials for adverse outcomes with hypoglycemia. Hypoglycemia causes nonspecific electroencephalographic abnormalities, and experimentally induced hypoglycemia impairs cognitive function, especially decision making and reaction time. If prolonged and severe enough, hypoglycemia causes neurologic deficits that may continue for days or weeks after euglycemia. Pathologic alterations in the brain in hypoglycemia are cortical and are seen predominantly in the temporal lobes and middle layers of the cerebral cortex and hippocampus. Chronic or recurrent hypoglycemia results in a sensorimotor peripheral neuropathy. Hypoglycemia also leads to elevated tissue pH, in contrast to hypoxia, which leads to tissue acidosis. Coma and death occur if hypoglycemia is not treated. Neurologic deficits are more common among diabetics who develop hypoglycemia than among nondiabetics with hypoglycemia.

Postprandial hypoglycemia usually is caused by postgastrectomy syndrome and adult-onset diabetes (type II diabetes). Addison disease, hypopituitarism, and alcoholism and end-stage renal disease complicated by poor nutrition cause hypoglycemia by means of impaired glycogenolysis or gluconeogenesis. The rapidity and magnitude of the decrease in plasma glucose contributes to the onset of symptoms.

Some divide hypoglycemia into postprandial and fasting types. In fasting hypoglycemia, symptoms occur after prolonged exercise or in the fasting state. In the postprandial form, an abnormal response to the intake of food causes the low glucose level. There is also a form of hypoglycemia called "idiopathic postprandial hypoglycemia" or "functional reactive hypoglycemia."

HISTORY AND CLINICAL PRESENTATION

The symptoms of hypoglycemia are grouped into two categories. Symptoms attributed to autonomic nervous system activation include sweating, trembling, nausea, anxiety, restlessness, palpitations, and a sensation of hunger. Neuroglycopenia symptoms include headache, weakness, vertigo, fatigue, difficulty speaking, and inability to concentrate. The symptoms of drowsiness, weakness, and blurred vision cannot be placed easily into these categories. Diabetics have autonomic symptoms more often; patients with insulinomas have more neuroglycopenia symptoms. The neurologic deficits associated with hypoglycemia are hemiparesis, convulsions, severe confusion, coma, decortication, decerebration, choreoathetosis, ataxia, and locked-in syndrome.

In mild hypoglycemia, many persons develop warning symptoms and can institute immediate treatment. In severe hypoglycemia, the situation is extremely urgent: as cognition becomes progressively impaired, hypoglycemic persons cannot help themselves and often they cannot recognize the seriousness of the situation. When assistance is offered, patients may be belligerent and combative due to their impaired neurologic functioning.

There are usually few physical findings, and often the physician may not be able to obtain a cogent history initially. The physician should carefully evaluate the patient for goiter, jaundice, hyperpigmentation, signs of hyperthyroid and liver disease, and alcoholic breath or a breath odor characteristic of some inborn errors of metabolism. The extremities and other possible injection sites should be observed for needle marks. Convulsions are more common in diabetics, especially children, as a result of hypoglycemia. Because neurologic sequelae may occur and may persist before resolution, a thorough neurologic examination must be done.

The patient's perception of hypoglycemic symptoms may be blunted or blocked by ethanol, sedatives, or β-adrenergic blockers, and sometimes by a supine position. Persons with longstanding diabetes and those with insulinoma have defective counterregulation (ie, decreased secretion of glucagon and epinephrine); this produces hypoglycemic unawareness.

LABORATORY EVALUATION

The diagnosis is made when the symptoms are consistent with neuroglycopenia, autonomic adrenergic stimulation, and a low glucose concentration. Symptoms are relieved when the glucose level returns to normal.

The diagnosis of hyperinsulinism due to abnormal beta cell function can be confirmed by demonstrating raised plasma insulin, C-peptide, and proinsulin levels in peripheral blood in the presence of hypoglycemia. Patients given exogenous insulin have raised plasma insulin but low C-peptide levels. Hypoglycemia associated with non–islet cell tumors tends to occur in older patients. The laboratory work-up shows depressed plasma insulin, C-peptide, and proinsulin levels, but the ratio of plasma IGF-II to IGF-I is high. Furthermore, the E- domain of pro-IGF-II is raised. Autoimmune hypoglycemia does occur and is usually due to autoantibodies to insulin. Autoantibodies to the insulin receptor and autoantibodies that stimulate pancreatic beta cells have also been reported.

Idiopathic hypoglycemia is rare and is characterized by a low glucose level in plasma collected during a symptomatic episode but not at any other time.

TREATMENT

Preventive treatment includes educating diabetics to be aware of their symptoms of hypoglycemia and to take corrective action by eating. In diabetics, 20 g of oral glucose or 40 g of carbohydrates, as found in orange juice, corrects hypoglycemia. Fifteen grams of carbohydrates as glucose solution or in tablets is also effective. Patients with exercise-induced hypoglycemia should eat 15 to 30 g of carbohydrates before exercise. Persons with postgastrectomy hypoglycemia may benefit from anticholinergic medications.

Emergency treatment of hypoglycemia requires the delivery of glucose. If oral glucose is not accepted, parenteral therapy is necessary. One mg of intravenous glucagon or 25 g of intravenous glucose should be given to diabetics experiencing severe hypoglycemia. Intravenous glucose is more rapid (about 2.5 minutes) than intravenous glucagon in restoring consciousness during coma.

When hypoglycemia is due to any underlying disease, as listed in Table 39-1, specific treatment for that disease is necessary.

CONSIDERATIONS IN PREGNANCY

The very tight control of diabetes necessary to prevent complications of pregnancy places pregnant diabetic women at risk for hypoglycemic episodes. There is good evidence that the glucose counterregulatory mechanisms in pregnant patients with insulin-dependent diabetes mellitus are suppressed. In the first trimester of pregnancy, there tends to be an increased incidence of hypoglycemic episodes. In the first trimester, insulin action is enhanced by estrogen and progesterone, leading to lower fasting plasma glucose levels. Short episodes of hypoglycemia at 26 to 34 weeks' gestation were not found to change the fetal heart rate significantly, nor were fetal movements affected. At glucose levels below 70 mg/dL, fetal breathing was temporarily increased. Thus, it seems that the fetus tolerates short-lived hypoglycemia. However, hypoglycemia during organogenesis may be teratogenic. Further studies on this issue are needed.

BIBLIOGRAPHY

American Diabetes Association. Statement on hypoglycemia. Diabetes Care 1982;5:72.

Campbell IW. Hypoglycemia and type 2 diabetes sulfonylurea. In: Frier BM, Fisher BM, eds. Hypoglycaemia and diabetes: clinical and physiological aspects. London: Edward Arnold, 1993:387.

Hagay ZJ, Reece AE. Diabetes mellitus. In: Reece EA, Hobbins JC, Mahoney MJ, Petrie RH, eds. Medicine of the fetus and mother. Philadelphia: JB Lippincott, 1992:986.

Kaminer Y, Robbins DR. Insulin misuse: a review of an overlooked psychiatric problem. Psychosomatics 1989;30:19.

Marks V, Teale JD. Hypoglycaemia in the adult. Baillieres Clin Endocrinol Metab 1993;7:705.

Persson B, Hansson U. Hypoglycaemia in pregnancy. Baillieres Clin Endocrinol Metab 1993;7:731.

Service FJ. Hypoglycemia: endocrine emergencies. Med Clin North Am 1995;79:1.

Stellon A, Townell NH. C-peptide assay for factitious hyperinsulinism. Lancet 1979;2:148.

Primary Care for Women, edited by Phyllis C. Leppert and Fred M. Howard. Lippincott-Raven Publishers, Philadelphia © 1997.

40

Hirsutism

EBERHARD KARL MUECHLER

Hirsutism is the excessive growth of coarse, terminal, and pigmented hair on the face, trunk, or extremities. The hair follicle in androgen-responsive zones of the skin produces coarse, terminal hair, and there is increased secretion of sebaceous and sweat glands as a result of overproduction of androgens. Common sites of excessive hair growth in women include the sideburn area, upper lip, chin, neck, chest, lower abdomen, lumbosacral area, thighs, and forearms.

The incidence of hirsutism is estimated to be 5% to 10%. Observations by McKnight (1964) showed that 84% of normal women have terminal hair on the arms and legs, 26% have terminal hair on the facial skin, 17% have periareolar hair, and 35% have hair on the linea alba. To classify the intensity of hirsutism, Ferriman and Galloway (1961) defined 11 zones of surface areas of skin and graded hair density from one to four in each area. The numbers are multiplied to arrive at a score for the severity of hirsutism.

ETIOLOGY AND DIFFERENTIAL DIAGNOSIS

The most important androgen, testosterone, is produced in normal women by ovarian secretion (25%), adrenal secretion (25%), and extragonadal conversion from precursors (50%), primarily androstenedione. The daily production rate of testosterone in normal women is 230 ± 30 μg. Testosterone is reduced in the liver to androsterone and etiocholanolone, which are excreted in the urine and measured as 17-ketosteroids. Liver metabolism of testosterone in normal women occurs at saturation of the enzyme system. Extrahepatic sites such as the hair follicle and the sebaceous glands accommodate increases in androgen production by metabolizing testosterone to dihydrotestosterone. This local conversion stimulates the dormant hair follicle to produce terminal hair.

Hirsutism is classified by identifying the source of overproduction of androgens as ovarian, adrenal, or combined and by identifying the disease process as the result of hyperplasia or tumor. The most common cause of hirsutism is polycystic ovary syndrome (PCOD). An estimated 5% to 10% of all premenopausal women have PCOD. This syndrome is characterized by hirsutism, obesity, chronic anovulation, oligomenorrhea, and insulin resistance. Follicle development is arrested at an early antral stage and shows ultrasound changes of multiple small follicles in the ovarian periphery.

Indirect evidence for the causal relation of insulin resistance in the development of hyperandrogenism in PCOD is derived from selective suppression studies. When androgen production is suppressed, there is no change in abnormal insulin resistance in women with PCOD. However, when insulin resistance is suppressed by treatment with metformin, androgen production is reduced.

Laboratory confirmation of the clinical symptomatology in PCOD includes increased serum or urine androgens, a ratio of luteinizing hormone (LH) to follicle-stimulating hormone (FSH) of 2 or higher, and the absence of increased androgenic hormones of adrenal origin, such as dehydroepiandrosterone sulfate (DHEAS). Variations of PCOD have been described historically using terms such as Stein-Leventhal syndrome, ovarian hyperthecosis, and idiopathic hirsutism.

Hyperplastic disorders of the adrenal cortex are the second most common cause of hirsutism due to overproduction of androgens. There are two forms of adrenal hyperplasia, according to age of onset. Congenital adrenal hyperplasia occurs in one of 14,000 newborns and is the most common cause of ambiguous external genitalia in newborns. Signs and symptoms of overproduction of androgens are present at birth, continue in childhood and puberty, and persist throughout adult life. Several enzyme defects have been identified as causes of congenital adrenal hyperplasia associated with ambiguous external genitalia and hirsutism later in life. 21-Hydroxylase deficiency accounts for 95% of all cases. Less common enzyme defects associated with ambiguous external genitalia and hirsutism are 11β-hydroxylase deficiency and 3β-ol-dehydrogenase deficiency. All these enzyme defects have in common a block in the synthesis of cortisol from cholesterol, with accumulation of androgenic byproducts in the chain of steroid hormone biosynthesis. Hyperplasia of the adrenal cortex results from overproduction of ACTH in the pituitary gland due to inadequate feedback from enzymatically blocked cortisol levels.

Prenatally, the diagnosis is made by amniocentesis or chorionic villus biopsy when the family history suggests a fetus at risk. Treatment of the mother with dexamethasone before sex differentiation in the ninth week of gestation may prevent sexual ambiguity. There has not been much experience with this treatment, and referral to subspecialists, with geneticists, pediatric endocrinologists, and perinatologists working in collaboration, is required.

Adult-onset adrenal hyperplasia occurs when enzyme deficiencies in the biosynthesis of cortisol from cholesterol become symptomatic in late puberty or early adult life. Compensatory feedback of cortisol to pituitary ACTH suppression becomes inadequate in early adulthood and adrenocortical hyperplasia develops, with its signs and symptoms of overproduction of androgens. Hirsutism, oligomenorrhea, anovulation, and obesity are similar to those seen in PCOD. Only laboratory evaluation allows a distinction between the disease entities.

Ovarian or adrenal tumors are uncommon but more serious causes of hirsutism. They are associated with additional manifestations of excessive overproduction of androgens such as clitoromegaly, profound facial beard growth, temporal hair line recession, and balding. The diagnosis requires a combination of biophysical procedures such as ultrasound, computed tomography (CT) scanning, magnetic resonance imaging (MRI), and biochemical measurements of androgens in blood, serum, or urine.

Cushing syndrome is associated with hirsutism, but clinical signs such as moon facies, buffalo hump, striae, and petechiae should direct the clinician to the appropriate diagnostic tests (cortisol and ACTH measurements). Finally, abnormalities of thyroid function, prolactin regulation, and growth hormone secretion must be considered in the differential diagnosis. Symptoms of hirsutism, oligomenorrhea, amenorrhea, anovulation, and obesity overlap to some extent with PCOD and adrenal hyperplasia. Specific diagnostic studies to rule out endocrine disorders other than ovarian or adrenal disease may include serum T_4, thyroid-stimulating hormone, prolactin, or growth hormone.

HISTORY

The initial interview should include a detailed personal and family history. The presentation of symptoms overlaps frequently between changes in appearance, menstrual irregularities, infertility, and metabolic disorders. Because treatment by hormonal suppression of increased androgen production is incompatible with stimulation of ovulation to treat infertility, it is important to address the priority in treatment.

Three specific events associated with puberty must be identified: thelarche, adrenarche, and menarche. When hirsutism begins slowly at puberty and progresses gradually, it is usually due to LH- or ACTH-dependent overproduction of androgens in the ovaries or adrenal glands, not to androgen-producing tumors. The family history is important, as in most cases of hirsutism there is evidence of familial variants of the condition in several female family members. The precise genetic pattern of transmission has not been identified.

A careful history of medication intake is required. Pharmacologic agents with stimulatory effects on hirsutism include androgens, anabolic agents such as danazol, phenytoin, minoxidil, diazoxide, and cyclosporine A.

PHYSICAL EXAMINATION AND CLINICAL FINDINGS

Several categories of clinical findings are associated with hirsutism and androgen overproduction: changes in appearance, irregular menstruation and anovulation with infertility, and changes in metabolism.

Obesity in women with hirsutism is typically android or wedge-shaped. The preponderance of fat accumulation in the upper body leads to an increased waist-to-hip ratio. The distribution of coarse, terminal hair on the entire integument must be carefully inspected and classified. If the woman shaves or bleaches her facial hair, hirsutism may elude detection if it is not suspected. Seborrhea and acne are usually induced by androgen's action on the pilosebaceous unit. Excessive keratin formation and increased sebum secretion lead to bacterial colonization and the formation of pustules. Androgen-dependent alopecia is inherited in autosomal dominant fashion. The most common locations are the vertex and the crown. Usually there is a pattern of diffuse hair thinning in women. Acanthosis nigricans may be linked to insulin resistance and the overproduction of androgens. The typical skin change of acanthosis nigricans is hyperpigmentation and skin hypertrophy with thickening in the nuchal area, axillae, and inner thighs.

Menstrual irregularities are associated with anovulation and infertility. The pattern of abnormal menstruation varies between patients and sometimes within the same patient. Oligomenorrhea and amenorrhea are commonly observed in patients with PCOD or adult-onset adrenal hyperplasia. Menometrorrhagia occurs more often in obese women with PCOD. Weight reduction may result in changes in androgen metabolism, with improvement of hirsutism and correction of menstrual disorders. Even ovulation and fertility are improved after weight loss in obese women with PCOD. More often, treatment of anovulation and infertility requires pharmacologic agents to overcome follicular arrest in the antral stage in PCOD patients.

Glucose intolerance is observed in 20% of obese women with PCOD but only 5% of all premenopausal women. The impact of hyperandrogenism on cardiovascular disease is unclear. There is a weak correlation between androgen and lipoprotein levels. Testosterone stimulates lipoprotein lipase activity, which results in increased HDL_3 levels.

LABORATORY AND IMAGING STUDIES

The goal of biochemical and biophysical diagnostic studies is to identify the source of the overproduction of androgens. Because ovarian or adrenal tumors are the most serious concern, the hyperandrogenic state must be evaluated using criteria that separate androgen-producing tumors from hyperplastic abnormalities of the ovaries and adrenal cortex. Androgen-producing tumors should be suspected when virilizing symptoms such as clitoromegaly, balding, and facial beard growth are observed.

Palpatory findings during the pelvic examination require biophysical confirmation by ultrasound examination of the pelvic organs and kidneys with the adjacent adrenal glands. The presence of a solid mass in one ovary or one adrenal gland in a virilized woman is preliminary evidence for an androgen-producing tumor. Further information about the location and tissue characteristics may be obtained by a CT scan or MRI examination. Biochemical baseline studies to screen for the presence of androgen-producing tumors include, at a minimum, serum total testosterone, free testosterone, and DHEAS. When the blood level of total testosterone exceeds 200 ng/dL or the level of free testosterone exceeds 2 ng/dL, there is a high probability of an androgen-producing ovarian tumor such as arrhenoblastoma, lipoid cell tumor, or hilus cell tumor. When serum DHEAS values exceed 700 micrograms/dL, there is a strong suspicion for an androgen-producing adrenal tumor. In PCOD or adult-onset adrenal hyperplasia, baseline androgen levels in blood serum are slightly elevated in about two thirds of hirsute women; they are normal in the rest. This difference is explained by variations in the metabolic clearance rates in women with variable degrees of hirsutism and obesity.

Much has been written about provocative stimulation and suppression tests using human chorionic gonadotropin, ACTH, oral contraceptives, and dexamethasone for distinguishing ovarian from adrenal tumors or androgen-producing tumors from hyperplasia of the ovaries and adrenal cortex. Paradoxic results have been obtained for all lesions with provocative tests. Therefore, selective ovarian and adrenal vein catheterization should be performed with analysis of ovarian and adrenal vein blood for androgens. When a ten- to 20-fold difference or greater is found between androgen levels in ovarian or adrenal vein effluent compared to peripheral blood, the diagnosis of a tumor is very likely.

Baseline studies of modest value in evaluating hirsutism include, in order of importance, serum 17-hydroxyprogesterone, androstenedione, LH:FSH ratio, cortisol, urinary testosterone glucuronide, urinary 17-ketosteroids, and urinary free cortisol. In suspected 21-hydroxylase deficiency, 17-hydroxyprogesterone should be measured in blood serum as a baseline test and 60 minutes after giving 0.25 mg ACTH.

Figure 40-1 shows a decision tree in the diagnostic work-up of hirsutism.

TREATMENT

Except for androgen-producing tumors, treatment for hirsutism consists of medication and depilatories. Surgical treatment of androgen-producing ovarian tumors involves laparotomy with tumor resection or extirpation of the ovary. The contralateral ovary requires careful inspection and in some cases bisection because bilateral tumors are infrequently found. Androgen-producing tumors of the adrenal cortex are referred to the general surgeon for removal. Many years ago, it was common practice to treat hirsutism associated with PCOD with bilateral ovarian wedge resection. This treatment has been abandoned because of the transient nature of improvement and a 25% to 35% rate of ovarian adhesions. If infertility is the primary concern in a hirsute patient with PCOD, it may be useful to perform laparoscopic cauterization of multiple follicles in selected cases. Medical therapy of hirsutism must be oriented toward specific goals and toward specific androgen-producing glands. The patient must be prepared for a slow and delayed onset of treatment effects: it usually takes 3 to 6 months before clearly visible results become noticeable.

There are three treatment categories: suppression of the ovaries, suppression of the adrenal cortex, and competitive inhibition of androgens on the pilosebaceous unit. Suppression of ovarian androgen production is achieved with the use of pharmacologic agents that inhibit the hypothalamic-pituitary-ovarian axis. Some drugs also enhance the metabolic clearance of androgens. The most widely used drugs in the United States are oral contraceptives and gonadotropin-releasing hormone agonists and antagonists. In other countries, there have been favorable reports with antiandrogens such as cyproterone acetate in combination with synthetic estrogen.

Among oral contraceptives, a drug whose progestational component has a low androgenic potential is preferred. The newer progestins, desogestrel and norgestimate, are well tolerated and do not have undesirable side effects on lipid metabolism. Adrenal overpro-

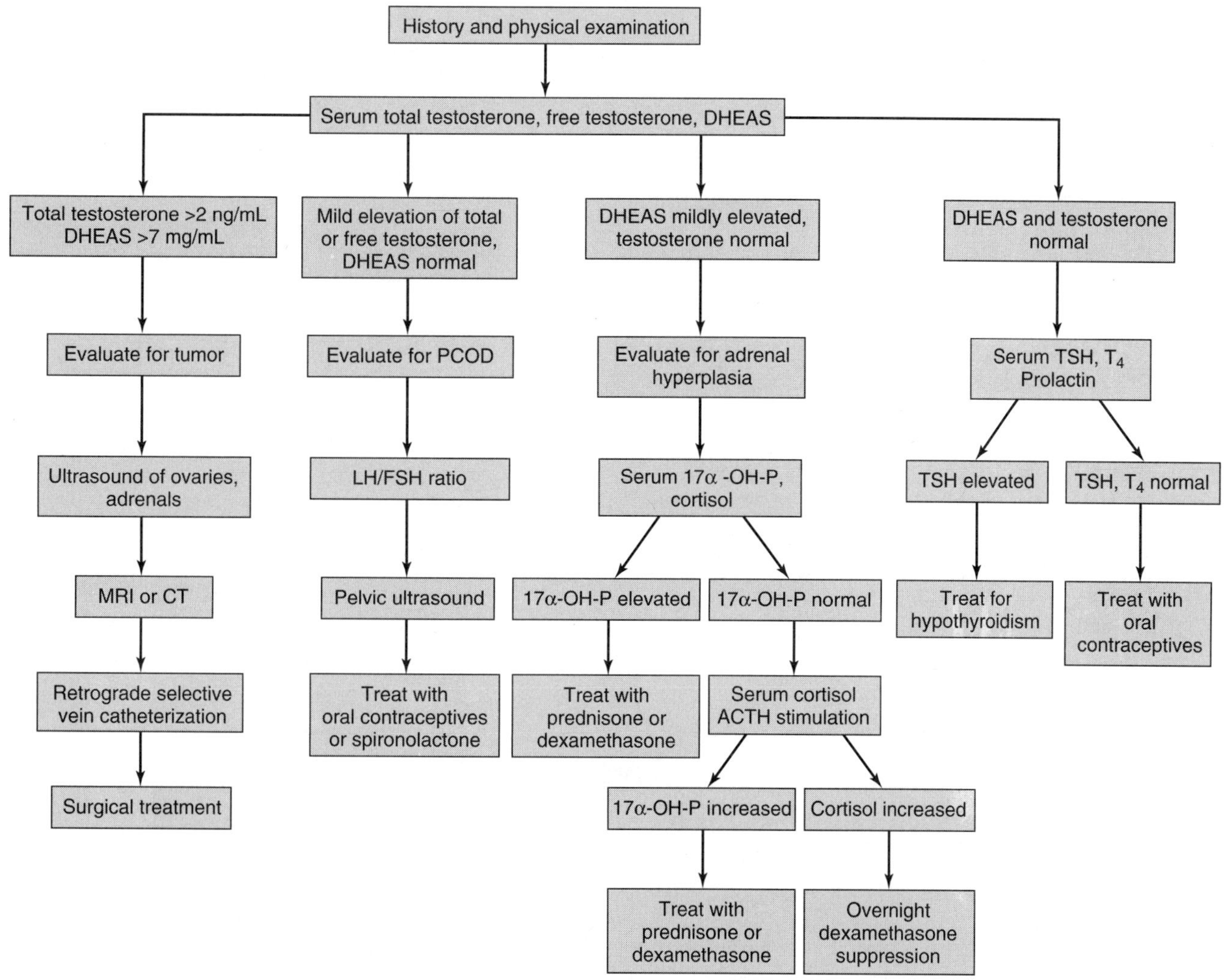

Figure 40-1. Algorithm for hirsutism.

duction of androgens is suppressed with the use of prednisone, 5 to 7.5 mg daily or on alternate days. Dexamethasone suppression is used at a dose of 0.25 to 0.5 mg daily or on alternate days.

When there is no specific identification of a glandular source of androgens, or if side effects to the aforementioned drugs become apparent, the choice of drug treatment is the antiandrogen spironolactone, 100 mg twice daily for 25 days each month. This medication competes with testosterone for the androgen receptor in the pilosebaceous unit.

Additional treatment methods include shaving, waxing, the use of hair-removal creams, and electrolysis. These methods remove existing hair and must be combined with hormone suppression to prevent new hair growth. Psychological support may help the patient maintain a normal body image of femininity.

CONSIDERATIONS IN PREGNANCY

Hirsutism is unlikely to progress during pregnancy. Large amounts of circulating estrogen stimulate testosterone-binding globulin and prevent increases in metabolically active free testosterone. If hirsutism progresses in pregnancy, the index of suspicion for an androgen-producing tumor is high. If the pregnant woman with an androgen-producing tumor carries a female fetus, there is concern about masculinization of the baby's external genitalia. Surgical treatment of an androgen-producing tumor during pregnancy is justified to prevent virilization of the female fetus.

BIBLIOGRAPHY

Aziz R, Gay F. The treatment of hyperandrogenism with oral contraceptives. Semin Reprod Endocrinol 1989;7:246.

Dunaif A. Insulin resistance and ovarian hyperandrogenism. Endocrinologist 1992;2:258.

Ferriman D, Galloway JD. Clinical assessment of body hair growth in women. J Clin Endocrinol Metab 1961;21:1440.

McKnight E. The prevalence of hirsutism in young women. Lancet 1964;1:410.

Moltz I, Schwartz U, Sorensen R, Pickartz H, Hammerstein J. Ovarian and adrenal vein steroids in patients with nonneoplastic hyperandrogenism: selective catheterization findings. Fertil Steril 1984;42:69.

Muechler EK. Testosterone-producing ovarian tumor associated with erythrocytosis, hyperuricemia and recurrent deep vein thrombosis. Am J Obstet Gynecol 1977;129:467.

Muechler EK, Fichter J, Zongrone J. Human chorionic gonadotropin, estriol and testosterone changes in two pregnancies with hyperreactio luteinalis. Am J Obstet Gynecol 1987;157:1126.

Muechler EK, Gillette MB, Cary D, et al. Ovarian lipoid cell tumor: steroid hormones and ultrastructure. Diag Obstet Gynecol 1982;4:209.

Muechler EK, Kohler D, Grove S. Steroid hormones in ovarian vein and cyst fluid of a virilizing gonadal stromal tumor. Obstet Gynecol 1978;62:609.

Rittmaster RS, Thompson DL. Effect of leuprolide and dexamethasone on hair growth and hormone levels in hirsute women. J Clin Endocrinol Metab 1990;70:1096.

Siegel SF, Finegold DN, Lanes R. ACTH stimulation tests and plasma dehydroepiandrosterone sulfate levels in women with hirsutism. N Engl J Med 1990;323:849.

Speiser PW, Laforgia N, Kato K, et al. First-trimester prenatal treatment and molecular genetic diagnosis of congenital adrenal hyperplasia (21-hydroxylase deficiency). J Clin Endocrinol Metab 1990;70:838.

Tagatz GE, Kopher RA, Nagel TC, Okagaki T. The clitoral index: a bioassay of androgenic stimulation. Obstet Gynecol 1979;54:562.

Velazquez EM, Mendoza S, Hamer T, Sosa F, Glueck CJ. Metformin therapy in polycystic ovary syndrome reduces hyperinsulinemia, insulin resistance, hyperandrogenemia, and systolic blood pressure, while facilitating normal menses and pregnancy. Metabolism 1994;43:647.

Wild RA, Demers LM, Applebaum-Bowden D, Lender R. Hirsutism: metabolic effects of two commonly used oral contraceptives and spironolactone. Contraception 1991;44:113.

Primary Care for Women, edited by Phyllis C. Leppert and Fred M. Howard. Lippincott-Raven Publishers, Philadelphia © 1997.

V

Cardiovascular Disease

41

Hypertension

RICHARD S. CONSTANTINO

Hypertension is a common disease among women in the United States. According to various studies, more than 20% of adults have blood-pressure levels of 160/95 mm Hg or higher. For women, the prevalence varies from less than 2% for white women under age 25 to more than 70% for elderly black women. The prevalence of high blood pressure increases with age and is greater for black women than for white women. In young adulthood and early middle age, the prevalence of high blood pressure is greater for men than for women; thereafter, the reverse is true. Nonfatal and fatal cardiovascular diseases, as well as renal disease and all causes of mortality, increase progressively with higher levels of both systolic and diastolic blood pressure. It is important to screen for and treat even mildly elevated blood pressure, as the risk for end-organ damage with stroke, myocardial infarction, and renal dysfunction rises with increased blood pressure.

FACTORS ASSOCIATED WITH HYPERTENSION

Excess weight is associated with hypertension in women, as is the distribution of body fat. Hypertension is more frequently associated with intraabdominal upper body obesity, as compared with obesity of the hips and buttocks.

Insulin resistance is also associated with hypertension, independent of weight and age. Type II diabetes occurs twice as frequently in hypertensive patients, compared with matched normotensive patients. Insulin resistance occurs commonly in whites, but not as commonly in Native Americans or blacks.

Race is associated with different patterns of hypertension in Americans. Blacks have a higher prevalence of hypertension and a higher proportion of uncontrolled hypertension, as well as a higher incidence of stroke, renal failure, and heart involvement. The risk of end-stage renal disease is much greater for hypertensive blacks than for hypertensive whites. Response to medications may also vary by race.

It has long been believed that sodium intake accounted for a significant percentage of hypertension. Although dietary sodium may be important in some hypertensive patients, particularly those with renal failure, the role of salt in raising blood pressure may be less than previously thought. Studies have shown an inverse relation between dietary potassium and blood-pressure levels, with small increases in potassium intake resulting in small decreases in systolic blood pressure. Sodium and potassium intake may be a significant factor in some salt-sensitive patients, including blacks, the elderly, and first-degree relatives of hypertensive patients. Several studies have indicated a relation between low calcium intake and elevated blood pressure. Calcium supplementation may lower blood pressure in some patients, particularly those who consume less than the recommended daily doses for calcium.

DIFFERENTIAL DIAGNOSIS

Many patients are falsely labeled hypertensive as a result of transient anxiety, recent intake of stimulants, or use of inappropriate blood-pressure measuring equipment. As many as 20% of patients classified as hypertensive have "white coat hypertension" and manifest increases in blood pressure only in the physician's office. Many of these patients display normal blood pressures when tested outside the physician's office or in less stressful situations.

Home monitoring of blood pressure is an important adjunct to physician values in determining the true state of hypertension. In addition, ambulatory monitoring is an important means of measuring 24-hour blood pressures and assessing the presence of true hypertension. In ambulatory monitoring, the patient wears a blood-pressure cuff and a recording monitor for 24 hours. Activities and emotions are also recorded during this time. Studies indicate that ambulatory blood-pressure readings may correlate better with certain complications of high blood pressure, specifically left ventricular hypertrophy, than do office or home values. Ambulatory pressure monitoring is an important adjunct in identifying patients with true white coat hypertension and certain patients with borderline hypertension. It can also help assess response to therapy in patients with labile hypertension.

Many patients who present with apparent hypertension have only transiently elevated values as a result of recent ingestion of medications or other drugs. Theophylline preparations, corticosteroids, over-the-counter asthma preparations (eg, ephedrine), and over-the-counter common cold preparations containing phenylpropanolamine or pseudoephedrine can also raise blood pressure. Nonsteroidal antiinflammatory drugs reportedly raise blood pressure an average of 5 to 8 mm Hg and are commonly used by ambulatory patients who may have borderline blood-pressure elevations. Cyclosporine- and estrogen-containing compounds, including birth-control pills, may raise blood pressure, as may nasal decongestants, appetite suppressants, erythropoietin, tricyclic antidepressants, and monoamine oxidase inhibitors.

Blood pressure should be determined precisely and should be measured in such a way that the values obtained represent the patient's usual levels. Patients should be seated with their arm bared and supported at heart level. They should not have smoked or ingested caffeine within 30 minutes before the measurement. Patients should be allowed to rest quietly for 5 minutes before blood-pressure determinations are made.

A blood-pressure cuff of appropriate size must be used for women. Normal-size cuffs and, particularly, larger cuffs can underestimate blood pressure; small or pediatric cuffs may overestimate it. An appropriate-size cuff should almost completely encircle the arm, or at least 80% of it. Measurements should be taken with the mercury sphygmomanometer, a recently calibrated aneroid manometer, or an electronic device. Systolic and diastolic pressures should be recorded, with the diastolic value being the disappearance of sound. At least two readings separated by 2 minutes should be averaged. If the first two readings differ by more than 5 mm Hg, additional readings should be obtained and averaged to yield a more representative value.

The diagnosis of hypertension should not be based on a single measurement. Ideally, the patient is seen on at least two subsequent visits 1 to 4 weeks after the additional readings are made, unless the blood pressure is stage 3 or 4. The time of the patient's visits should vary to ensure a spectrum of times during the day. The patient's three initial visits should be divided between morning, midday, and afternoon.

LEVELS OF HYPERTENSION

Attempts have been made to grade levels of hypertension to ensure appropriate therapy and follow-up. The following classifications have been established by the Joint National Committee on Detection, Evaluation, and Treatment of High Blood Pressure:

- Less than 130/85 mm Hg: normal
- 130 to 139/85 to 89 mm Hg: high normal
- 140 to 159/90 to 99 mm Hg: hypertension stage 1 (previously termed "mild")
- 160 to 179/100 to 109 mm Hg: hypertension stage 2 (previously termed "moderate")
- 180 to 209/110 to 119 mm Hg: hypertension stage 3 (previously termed "severe")
- Greater than 210/120 mm Hg: hypertension stage 4 (previously termed "very severe")

EVALUATION

Once the patient has been identified as hypertensive, it is important to consider whether she has primary or secondary hypertension. The latter is potentially reversible, so diagnosis of this category is critical. Secondary hypertension should be considered in a relatively young patient whose history and physical examination or severity of hypertension suggests secondary causes. Patients whose blood pressures respond poorly to drug therapy should be considered to have secondary hypertension. Patients who were previously well controlled and whose blood pressure begins to rise precipitously despite therapy should also be evaluated for a secondary cause. Secondary hypertension should be considered when blood pressure is accelerated or malignant and when someone has a sudden onset of hypertension.

Most hypertensive patients have primary, essential hypertension. Fewer than 10% have secondary causes, and most of these patients have kidney disease. The history should include questions regarding types of medications, including over-the-counter preparations and illegal drugs such as cocaine. The physical examination should attempt to identify patients who have abdominal or flank masses suggestive of polycystic kidneys. It should also identify abdominal bruits that may indicate renovascular disease. Delayed or absent femoral pulses and decreased blood pressure in the lower extremities may be compatible with aortic coarctation. Truncal obesity with purple striae may denote Cushing syndrome. Tachycardia, tremor, orthostatic hypotension, sweating, and pallor may indicate a pheochromocytoma.

Once it is determined if hypertension is primary or secondary, it is important to identify the target organ disease or dysfunction. This requires assessment of the fundi, kidneys, and heart in all hypertensive patients.

After identifying the presence or absence of target organ dysfunction, it is important to identify cardiovascular risk factors. Coronary artery disease and stroke are more likely to occur where hypertension exists with other risk factors, including hypercholesterolemia, family history, cigarette smoking, diabetes, and obesity or sedentary lifestyle. The presence of cardiovascular risk factors, in addition to the degree of blood-pressure elevation, determines the absolute risk level and, therefore, how aggressively blood pressure may need to be reduced.

Medical History

The evaluation begins with a complete medical history. Historical data should include information regarding family history of hypertension, premature coronary heart disease, stroke, diabetes mellitus, dyslipidemia, and cigarette smoking. Symptoms of cardiovascular disease, pending stroke or transient ischemic attack, renal disease, diabetes, dyslipidemia, or gout should be sought. It is also important to identify how long and to what degree the patient's blood pressure has been elevated. Information regarding the level of physical activity, recreational drug use, sodium intake, consumption of alcohol, and level of fat in the diet is also important, as are questions regarding the patient's psychosocial status. The information gained may affect the subsequent level of control with treatment and may identify issues preventing adequate control. The history should also include questions about the patient's use of medications that could raise the blood pressure, as listed earlier.

Physical Examination

The physical examination for hypertensive patients should include multiple blood-pressure determinations separated by 2 minutes with the patient either supine or seated and after the patient has been standing for at least 2 minutes. Blood pressure should be taken in both arms, with the higher value used as a baseline. The examination should include estimates of height, weight, and variation from ideal body weight. A critical part of the examination is the funduscopic examination. This attempts to identify arteriolar narrowing, arteriovenous nicking, hemorrhages, exudates, or even papilledema. It includes examination of the neck for carotid bruits, distended veins, and enlarged thyroid indicative of metabolic disease. The examination of the heart should include an estimate of the point of maximal impulse and should identify clicks, murmurs, arrhythmias, and additional heart sounds, including S_3 and S_4. Examination of the abdomen should identify bruits, enlarged organs (particularly the kidneys), and the presence or absence of an abnormal aortic pulsation. The examination of the extremities is intended to identify diminished or absent peripheral pulses, bruits, or edema.

The baseline examination should also include a neurologic examination appropriate to the patient's condition. If evidence of hypertensive encephalopathy exists, then a full neurologic examination with mental status determination is appropriate.

Laboratory Evaluation

Routine laboratory studies in patients presenting with hypertension should include urinalysis, complete blood cell count, fasting blood glucose, creatinine clearance, calcium, potassium, uric acid, fasting lipid profile with total cholesterol, high-density lipoprotein, and triglyceride levels. An electrocardiogram should be done on all patients to provide a baseline.

More extensive evaluations for secondary causes of hypertension may be appropriate in the following settings:

- Females less than age 25 with marked hypertension should be evaluated for renovascular etiology.
- Patients with evidence of advanced atherosclerosis with new-onset hypertension should be evaluated for renovascular hypertension.
- Patients with spontaneous or low-dose diuretic-induced persistent hypokalemia should be evaluated for aldosteronism.
- Patients with headache, flushing, diaphoresis, and marked blood-pressure lability should be evaluated for pheochromocytoma.
- Patients with malignant hypertension should be evaluated for renovascular hypertension.
- Patients who have resistant hypertension (hypertension not amenable to conventional therapy) should be evaluated for renovascular hypertension or other secondary causes.

A cardiac echo may be appropriate for patients believed to have had long-term hypertension or those who have evidence of left ventricular hypertrophy on the electrocardiogram. Cardiac echo may also be a useful monitor of response to therapy and may identify left ventricular hypertrophy, which is associated with a greatly increased risk of cardiovascular morbidity. However, it is unclear if regression of left ventricular hypertrophy reverses the risk. Plasma renin and urinary sodium determination may also be appropriate in cases where it is important to assess the vascular status, as in renovascular hypertension.

Evaluation of Renovascular Hypertension

Renovascular disease is a rare cause of hypertension, occurring in fewer than 5% of hypertensive patients. Because it is potentially curable, however, the diagnosis should be considered in young white women with hypertension who may have fibromuscular hyperplasia; older hypertensive patients with hypertension of recent onset or those refractory to therapy; and patients who have evidence of advanced atherosclerotic disease, or abdominal bruits.

Evaluation of renovascular causes of hypertension should be considered only in patients who are candidates for surgical or angioplastic correction of renoartery stenosis. Opinions vary regarding the preferred evaluation, but random plasma renin activity, intravenous pyelography, and renography without converting enzyme assay are not considered useful. Venous digital subtraction angiography cannot be interpreted in up to 25% of cases. Both hippuran renography, after administration of converting enzyme inhibitor and furosemide (Lasix), and diethylenetriamine pentaacetic acid (DPTA) renography, after administration of converting enzyme inhibitors, have about 90% sensitivity and specificity for renovascular causes. Positive converting enzyme inhibitor renography should be confirmed by arteriography.

Not all stenotic lesions are functionally significant; therefore, split renal vein renin determinations after administration of converting enzyme inhibitor are useful in predicting responses to surgery or angioplasty.

TREATMENT

Complications, including stroke, heart failure, and myocardial infarction, are common in hypertensive patients. Several studies, including the Veterans Administration Cooperative Study, have shown a decrease in mortality and morbidity when patients whose diastolic blood pressures exceeded 104 mm Hg had their pressures lowered with drugs, lifestyle changes, or both. The most striking benefits from treatment of mild hypertension come from prevention of stroke, rather than from reductions in myocardial infarction. However, metanalyses of randomized trials indicate that the rates of fatal and nonfatal myocardial infarction are decreased by about 20% when mild to moderate hypertension is treated.

The goal of treatment is to prevent the morbidity and mortality associated with high blood pressure, using measures that have the least impact on quality of life. Ideally, blood pressure should be maintained below 140/90 mm Hg, and lower levels may be pursued in selected instances. The goal of therapy should be to reduce and modify cardiovascular risk factors.

Diet and Lifestyle Changes

Lifestyle modifications (weight reduction, moderation of dietary sodium and alcohol intake, increased physical activity, enhanced intake of potassium and calcium where safe and appropriate) may be adequate to control hypertension. These initiatives are consistent with good general health and also, in some instances, with reduction in cardiovascular risk. In many instances, they are adequate to control mild to moderate hypertension (stage 1 or 2). Even if lifestyle modifications are not adequate to control elevated blood pressure, they are still important adjuncts to therapy for all levels of hypertension.

Weight reduction should be recommended for all patients who are more than 10% above ideal weight. A blood-pressure reduction usually occurs early, with a weight loss of as small as 10 pounds. In patients with stage 1 hypertension, an attempt to control blood pressure with weight loss and other lifestyle modifications is a reasonable approach and should be tried for at least 3 to 6 months before initiating pharmacologic therapy.

Moderation of alcohol intake is recommended for all patients with hypertension. Alcohol can raise blood pressure and can also cause resistance to antihypertensive therapy. Patients should be counseled to drink no more than 1 oz of ethanol, 8 oz of wine, or 24 oz of beer in a 24-hour period.

Regular aerobic exercise is important in achieving fitness, helping to lower blood pressure, and reducing the risk of cardiovascular disease and all causes of mortality. Unfit normotensive patients have a 20% to 50% increased risk of developing hypertension, when compared with their more active and fit counterparts. Moderately intense physical exercise at 40% to 60% of maximal oxygen consumption can lower hypertensive patients' systolic blood pressure by 10 mm Hg. For most sedentary patients, brisk walking 30 to 45 minutes three to five times per week will achieve these goals. It may also help promote weight loss and minimize other cardiovascular risks. However, patients with known cardiac disease or other more serious health problems should undergo a thorough examination before proceeding with even moderate exercise.

Dietary changes, with limitation of saturated fat and total calories, should be recommended for patients who have elevated lipids and for those above ideal body weight. In addition, sodium restriction seems prudent. Patients who reduce their daily sodium intake to less than 2.3 g of sodium, or about 6 g of sodium chloride, may be able to reduce their systolic blood pressure by up to 5 to 10 mm Hg. Black women and elderly women seem to benefit most from reductions in dietary sodium chloride. Dietary counseling to achieve this level of sodium reduction is usually required. Sodium avoidance may be adequate in and of itself to control stage 1 hypertension, but also benefits patients treated with antihypertensive medications.

Although there is an association between dietary potassium and calcium intake in the prevention and control of blood pressure, formal supplementation is not recommended. Patients should ingest the usual daily allowance of these substances, preferably from food sources. Diuretics that enhance hypokalemia may complicate hypertensive therapy. In addition, patients with renal impairment should avoid high-potassium regimens.

Although much has been written about magnesium supplementation in hypertensive patients, there are no convincing data to justify recommending an increased magnesium intake in an effort to lower blood pressure. Similarly, claims of near-magical effects of garlic and onion supplements in lowering blood pressure have not been confirmed in controlled trials.

Many patients with hypertension suffer from variable levels of anxiety. In some cases, stress plays a role in inducing and maintaining hypertension. Stress reduction and management is an appropriate goal to maximize the quality of life, but there is little evidence that behavior modification and stress management are effective in controlling hypertension. For certain patients, however, antianxiety therapy may be an appropriate adjunct to hypertension treatment.

Several studies suggest that nonpharmacologic therapy is not as effective as pharmacologic therapy in controlling blood pressure. In the Trial of Antihypertensive Interventions and Management (TAIM) Study, short-term blood-pressure control was used as an end point. Use of a diuretic and β-blocker was more successful in controlling blood pressure than were weight loss, decreased sodium intake, and increased potassium supplementation. These agents also did not seem to compromise the quality of life.

Smoking cessation is critical for patients with essential hypertension. Although blood pressure may not be significantly lowered by smoking cessation, it reduces the cardiovascular risks in hypertensive patients, as smoking has a multiplicative effect when combined with hypertension in increasing coronary and vascular risks.

Drug Therapy

The goal of therapy is to lower blood pressure to 140/90 mm Hg or below. Lowering of blood pressure protects against stroke, coronary events, congestive heart failure, and progression to more severe heart failure, and reduces mortality from all causes. A metanalysis of randomized trials indicated a 42% reduction in stroke from a diastolic reduction of just 5 to 6 mm Hg. A similar reduction in diastolic blood pressure effected a 14% decrease in coronary heart disease during 6 years of follow-up.

Various agents in multiple drug classes effectively lower blood pressure. Tables 41-1 and 41-2 describe medications, dosages, and dosing intervals. Several factors should be taken into consideration when selecting an initial antihypertensive drug, including efficacy, cost, compliance, adverse effects, organ involvement, and atherosclerotic risk factor modification. About half of all patients can be expected to respond to monotherapy. When a second drug from a different class is added, 70% to 90% of patients achieve blood-pressure control.

Confusion may exist as to when to add a second agent rather than substituting a different drug for the initial one. In patients who respond to the initial medication with a reduction in blood pressure of 15 mm Hg systolic or 10 mm Hg diastolic, but who do not achieve their goal blood pressure, additive therapy is recommended. If, however, the initial drug used in monotherapy did not result in significant reduction in blood pressure, then substituting a different class of drug is often effective. Two drugs from a similar class are generally not recommended for routine control of blood pressure. The addition of a third medication, frequently a diuretic, is not uncommon to control stage 3 or 4 hypertension. Frequently, adding a third medication not only facilitates the desired further decrease in blood pressure, but also deals with the side effects of the two others. Diuretics may be used as a second or third class of drug when hypertension is not yet under adequate control and significant edema has occurred as a result of certain classes of medications, such as calcium channel blockers. Diuretics also may be used to control the mild potassium elevations that may occur with the use of angiotensin-converting enzyme (ACE) inhibitors in certain patients.

In many patients, it is undesirable to reduce the diastolic blood pressure below 80 mm Hg because of the J-curve phenomenon. In this hypothesis, it is believed that lowering diastolic blood pressure too much may increase the risk of coronary heart disease, possibly by lowering diastolic perfusion pressure in the coronary circulation. However, an increase in mortality in this setting is probably not caused by reduced diastolic blood pressure specifically, but by underlying coronary artery disease and subsequent hypoperfusion.

If blood pressure remains at or above 140/90 mm Hg despite vigorous efforts at lifestyle modification, pharmacologic agents should be started. This is especially true in patients who have target organ dysfunction, cardiovascular disease, or other cardiovascular disease risk factors. If patients do not have target organ dysfunction or other risk factors and pressures are 149/94 mm Hg or below, they may be observed for another 3 to 6 months with

Table 41-1. Initial Antihypertensive Drugs, Dosage, and Frequency

TYPE OF DRUG	USUAL DOSAGE RANGE (TOTAL mg/d)*	FREQUENCY (TIMES/d)
Diuretics		
Thiazides and related agents		
Bendroflumethiazide	2.5–5	1
Benzthiazide	12.5–50	1
Chlorothiazide	125–500	2
Chlorthalidone	12.5–50	1
Cyclothiazide	1.0–2	1
Hydrochlorothiazide	12.5–50	1
Hydroflumethiazide	12.5–50	1
Indapamide	2.5–5	1
Methyclothiazide	2.5–5	1
Metolazone	0.5–5	1
Polythiazide	1.0–4	1
Quinethazone	25.0–100	1
Trichlormethiazide	1.0–4	1
Loop diuretics		
Bumetanide	0.5–5	2
Ethacrynic acid	25.0–100	2
Furosemide	20.0–320	2
Potassium-sparing		
Amiloride	5–10	1 or 2
Spironolactone	25–100	2 or 3
Triamterene	50–150	1 or 2
Adrenergic inhibitors		
β-Blockers		
Atenolol	25–100†	1
Betaxolol	5–40	1
Bisoprolol	5–20	1
Metoprolol	50–200	1 or 2
Metoprolol (extended release)	50–200	1
Nadolol	20–240†	1
Propranolol	40–240	2
Propranolol (long-acting)	60–240	1
Timolol	20–40	2
β-Blockers with ISA		
Acebutolol	200–1200†	2
Carteolol	2.5–10†	1
β-Blockers with ISA (Continued)		
Penbutolol	20–80†	1
Pindolol	10–60†	2
α-β Blocker		
Labetalol	200–1200	2
α_1-Receptor blockers		
Doxazosin	1.0–16	1
Prazosin	1.0–20	2 or 3
Terazosin	1.0–20	1
ACE inhibitors		
Benazepril	10.0–40†	1 or 2
Captopril	12.5–150†	2
Cilazapril	2.5–5.0	1 or 2
Enalapril	2.5–4.0†	1 or 2
Fosinopril	10.0–40	1 or 2
Lisinopril	5.0–40†	1 or 2
Perindopril	1.0–16†	1 or 2
Quinapril	5.0–80†	1 or 2
Ramipril	1.25–20†	1 or 2
Spirapril	12.5–50	1 or 2
Calcium antagonists		
Diltiazem	90–360	3
Diltiazem (sustained release)	120–360	2
Diltiazem (extended release)	180–360	1
Verapamil	80–480	2
Verapamil (long-acting)	120–480	1 or 2
Dihydropyridines		
Amlodipine	2.5–10	1
Felodipine	5–20	1
Isradipine	2.5–10	2
Nicardipine	60–120	3
Nifedipine	30–120	3
Nifedipine (GITS)	30–90	1

In all patients, lifestyle modifications should also be advised. *ACE*, angiotensin-converting enzyme; *ISA*, intrinsic sympathomimetic activity; *GITS*, gastrointestinal therapeutic system.

*The lower dose indicated is the preferred initial dose, and the higher dose is the maximum daily dose. Most agents require 2 to 4 weeks for complete efficacy, and more frequent dosage requirements are not advised except for severe hypertension. The dosage range may differ slightly from the recommended dosage in the *Physicians' Desk Reference* or package insert.

†Indicates drugs that are excreted by the kidney and require dosage reduction in the presence of renal impairment (serum creatinine $\geq$221 µmol/L $\geq$2.5 mg/dL).

(Adapted from The fifth report of the Joint National Committee on Detection, Evaluation, and Treatment of High Blood Pressure (JNC V). Arch Intern Med 1993;153:154.)

nonpharmacologic therapy. These patients should be observed closely and not lost to follow-up, as blood pressure in these patients often rises and may lead to target organ dysfunction before appropriate therapy is initiated.

When therapy in stage 1 and 2 hypertension has been deemed necessary, monotherapy is recommended. Diuretics and β-blockers have been studied extensively and shown to reduce cardiovascular morbidity and mortality. Therefore, these drugs are preferred for initial drug therapy. Other agents, including ACE inhibitors, calcium antagonists, α_1-receptor blockers, and α-β-blockers are equally effective in reducing blood pressure, but have not yet been used in long-term controlled trials. They have, therefore, not

Table 41-2. Supplemental Antihypertensive Drugs

TYPE OF DRUG	USUAL DOSAGE RANGE (TOTAL mg/d)*	FREQUENCY TIMES/d)
Centrally acting α_2-agonists		
Clonidine	0.1–1.2	2
Clonidine patch	0.1–0.3	1 weekly
Guanabenz	4–64	2
Guanfacine	1–3	1
Methyldopa	250–2000	2
Peripheral-acting adrenergic antagonists		
Guanadrel	10–75	2
Guanethidine	10–100	1
Rauwolfia alkaloids		
Rauwolfia serpentina	50–200	1
Reserpine	0.05†–0.25	1
Direct vasodilators		
Hydralazine	50–300	2 to 4
Minoxidil	2.5–80	1 or 2

*The lower dose indicated is the preferred initial dose, and the higher dose is the maximum daily dose. Most agents require 2 to 4 weeks for complete efficacy, and more frequent dosage adjustments are not advised except for severe hypertension. The dosage range may differ slightly from the recommended dosage in the Physicians' Desk Reference or package insert.

†A 0.1-mg dose may be given every other day to achieve this dosage.

(Adapted from The Fifth report of the Joint National Committee on Detection, Evaluation, and Treatment of High Blood Pressure [JNC V]. Arch Intern Med 1993;153:154.)

demonstrated their efficacy in reducing morbidity and mortality, as have diuretics and β-blockers. For this reason, these alternative agents should be used when diuretics and β-blockers have proved unacceptable or ineffective.

Thiazide diuretics effectively reduce stroke, myocardial infarction, and cardiovascular mortality in patients with mild to moderate hypertension. They tend to be inexpensive. However, they may worsen insulin resistance, cause hypokalemia, and affect lipid status.

β-Blockers are particularly useful in young white females who are hyperadrenergic. They may be less effective in older black women.

ACE inhibitors are effective in controlling hypertension. Their cost is significant, however, and they may cause intractable cough and electrolyte abnormalities. None is more effective than others in controlling hypertension. Generally, these agents have not been documented to reduce left ventricular hypertrophy, as other drugs have. The effectiveness of ACE inhibitors is enhanced by sodium avoidance and use of diuretics.

Calcium channel blockers are also effective as first- or second-line antihypertensives. They have not been demonstrated to have an adverse effect on lipid or carbohydrate metabolism. Agents in this class reduce left ventricular hypertrophy and increase renal blood flow. A study involving a relatively small number of patients indicated that calcium channel blockers may be associated with a higher rate of myocardial infarction than β-blockers. It is unclear how this applies to patients being treated with these agents for hypertension. Further studies are underway that could affect the use of calcium channel blockers.

Various coexisting medical conditions may influence the choice of initial antihypertensive agents; these are listed in Table 41-3.

Therapeutic regimens for stage 3 and 4 hypertension consist of starting with medications as for stage 1 and 2 hypertension, but the addition of a second or third agent is often necessary. The intervals between redocumentation of blood pressure and changes in the regimen should be decreased. In some cases, it may be necessary to use more than one agent for initial therapy. In patients whose diastolic pressure exceeds 120 mm Hg, more aggressive therapy may be required. If significant target organ dysfunction is present, these patients may benefit from hospitalization and consultation.

Follow-Up of Hypertensive Patients

After patients have been diagnosed with hypertension, follow-up at appropriate intervals is required. Recommendations for follow-up based on the initial set of blood-pressure measurements are outlined in Table 41-4. Although patients should be started on the lowest dosages listed in Table 41-1 to minimize side effects, increases in dosage may be required to effect adequate control. The clinician should not be discouraged if the patient does not initially respond to pharmacologic therapy. One may increase the medication to the next dosage level and subsequently to maximal dosages over several weeks to months. This presumes that the patient has tolerated the medication well in terms of not having significant adverse effects: if the patient does not tolerate a low dose of an initial therapeutic agent, she certainly will not tolerate a higher dose. Under these circumstances, it may be appropriate to switch to an alternative drug. If the agent is well tolerated but blood-pressure control is inadequate, the dosage should be increased over several weeks to months to achieve a maximally recommended and tolerated dose.

If the patient experiences no reduction in blood pressure or a reduction of less than 15/10 mm Hg, despite maximal dosages of the medication, then it is appropriate to discontinue the medication. If the initial drug causes no significant adverse effects and maximal doses lower the blood pressure but not to effective or optimal levels, then it is appropriate to add a second drug. Again, if the initial drug does not result in a significant drop in blood pressure, it is not reasonable to add a second drug; instead, the first should be discontinued.

Combining antihypertensive drugs with different modes of action often allows smaller doses of drugs to be used, thereby minimizing potential adverse effects. If the addition of a second agent produces satisfactory blood-pressure control, an attempt should be made to withdraw the first agent, as monotherapy controls blood pressure in at least half of all patients.

When therapy is inadequate to control blood pressure, the clinician should consider the causes of a lack of response to therapy, listed in Table 41-5.

When prescribing antihypertensives, the clinician should be acutely aware of drug interactions and adverse drug effects, listed in Table 41-6.

When patients have been well controlled on antihypertensive medications, attempts should be made to decrease the dosage of these medications or their number, or both. When blood pressure has been effectively controlled during at least four visits over a 1-year period, a deliberate, slow withdrawal of medication is prudent. The patient must continue lifestyle modifications. Many

Table 41-3. Medical Conditions and Preferred Initial Therapy

CLINICAL SITUATION	PREFERRED	SPECIAL MONITORING	CONTRAINDICATED
Cardiovascular			
Angina pectoris	β-Blockers, calcium antagonists	—	Direct vasodilators
Bradycardia/heart block, sick sinus syndrome	—	—	β-Blockers, labetalol, verapamil, diltiazem
Cardiac failure	Diuretics, ACE inhibitors	—	β-Blockers, calcium antagonists, labetalol
Hypertrophic cardiomyopathy with severe diastolic dysfunction	β-Blockers, diltiazem, verapamil	—	Diuretics, ACE inhibitors, α_1-blockers, hydralazine, minoxidil
Hyperdynamic circulation	β-Blockers	—	Direct vasodilators
Peripheral vascular occlusive disease	—	β-Blockers	—
After myocardial infarction	Non-ISA β-blockers	—	Direct vasodilators
Renal			
Bilateral renal arterial disease or severe stenosis in artery to solitary kidney	—	—	ACE inhibitors
Renal insufficiency			
Early (serum creatinine, 130–221 μmol/L [1.5–2.5 mg/dL])	—	—	Potassium-sparing agents, potassium supplements
Advanced (serum creatinine ≥ 221 μmol/L [≥ 2.5 mg/dL])	Loop diuretics	ACE inhibitors	Potassium-sparing agents, potassium supplements
Other			
Asthma/COPD	—	—	β-Blockers, labetalol
Cyclosporine-associated hypertension	Nifedipine, labetalol	Verapamil,* nicardipine,* diltiazem*	—
Depression	—	α_2-Agonists	Reserpine
Diabetes mellitus			
Type I (insulin dependent)	—	β-Blockers	—
Type II	—	β-Blockers, diuretics	—
Dyslipidemia	—	Diuretics, β-blockers	—
Liver disease	—	Labetalol	Methyldopa
Vascular headache	β-Blockers	—	—
Pregnancy			
Preeclampsia	Methyldopa, hydralazine	—	Diuretics, ACE inhibitors
Chronic hypertension	Methyldopa	—	ACE inhibitors

ACE, angiotensin-converting enzyme; *ISA,* intrinsic sympathomimetic activity; *COPD,* chronic obstructive pulmonary disease.

*Can increase serum levels of cyclosporine.

(Adapted from The fifth report of the Joint National Committee on Detection, Evaluation, and Treatment of High Blood Pressure (JNC V). Arch Intern Med 1993;153:154.)

patients can be maintained under adequate control with a small dosage of a single medication; if multiple drugs had been used, many patients can be maintained with monotherapy.

The clinician must carefully weigh the risks of myocardial ischemia and cerebral hypoperfusion that can occur with overly aggressive intervention. In the absence of target organ dysfunction or system failure symptoms, a less aggressive approach may be appropriate. The goal of therapy should be to reduce blood-pressure levels *toward* normal but not necessarily *to* normal. In general, it is safe to reduce blood pressure under these circumstances to about 160/90 mm Hg.

HYPERTENSION IN SELECTED SITUATIONS

Isolated *systolic hypertension* is frequently seen in elderly women. When systolic hypertension without diastolic hypertension occurs in younger females, it indicates a hyperdynamic circulation and may predict future diastolic elevations. When the systolic blood pressure consistently exceeds 160 mm Hg but the diastolic blood pressure is less than 90 mm Hg, therapy should be considered. If lifestyle modification does not lower values to acceptable levels, then antihypertensive drug therapy is indicated for older women. Younger patients without evidence of target organ dysfunction should be continued on lifestyle modification and close observation.

Pseudohypertension is occasionally encountered in elderly patients with rigid brachial arteries. Because the sphygmomanometer cuff cannot compress the brachial artery, artificially high readings are obtained. This condition should be suspected in elderly women who have not previously been hypertensive and who manifest no evidence of target organ dysfunction despite very high blood pressures. This condition can be confirmed by observing the pulseless radial artery to be palpable, even though the sphygmomanometer cuff is inflated to pressures high enough to occlude the brachial artery.

Table 41-4. Recommendations for Follow-up Based on Initial Set of Blood-Pressure Measurements for Adults

INITIAL SCREENING BLOOD PRESSURE (MM HG)*		
Systolic	*Diastolic*	FOLLOW-UP RECOMMENDED†
<130	<85	Recheck in 2 y
130–139	85–89	Recheck in 1 y
140–159	90–99	Confirm within 2 mo
160–179	100–109	Evaluate or refer to source of care within 1 mo
180–209	110–119	Evaluate or refer to source of care within 1 wk
≥210	≥120	Evaluate or refer to source of care immediately

*If the systolic and diastolic categories are different, follow recommendation for the shorter-time follow-up (eg, 160/85 mm Hg should be evaluated or referred to source of care within 1 mo).

†The scheduling of follow-up should be modified by reliable information about past pressure measurements, other cardiovascular risk factors, or target organ disease.

Note: Consider providing advice about lifestyle modifications.

(Adapted from The fifth report of the Joint National Committee on Detection, Evaluation, and Treatment of High Blood Pressure [JNC V]. Arch Intern Med 1993;153:154.)

Hypertension emergencies are an important category to consider but are beyond the scope of this chapter. The primary care physician should seek appropriate consultation and referral for these patients.

Hypertensive encephalopathy results from excessive perfusion of the brain when its autoregulatory mechanism is exceeded. Sodium nitroprusside administration may be used to reduce blood pressure over 3 to 4 hours to 160/100 mm Hg; however, blood pressure should not be reduced by more than 25% of initial levels. The tables in this chapter list alternative medications and regimens.

Use of several *illicit drugs*, including cocaine, crack, amphetamines, phencyclidine hydrochloride (PCP), or diet pills, may acutely raise blood pressure. Frequently, the patient presents with stroke, seizures, myocardial infarction, or encephalopathy. Sodium nitroprusside is the treatment of choice, as noted in Table 41-7. Phentolamine is alternative therapy. β-Blockers should be avoided because of the potential for coronary spasm as a result of unopposed α-adrenergic receptor activation.

Most women experience a slight rise in blood pressure with use of *oral contraceptives*. However, their blood pressure usually does not rise out of the normal range. Hypertension may be as much as three times more common in women taking oral contraceptives for more than 5 years than in those never exposed to oral contraceptives. Risks of hypertension appear to increase with duration of use, age, and increased body mass. Many practitioners discourage women above age 35 from taking oral contraceptives if they cannot stop smoking. Most of the cardiovascular deaths attributable to oral contraceptives have occurred in women over age 35 who have continued to smoke. However, much of this data resulted from studies done using birth-control pills with higher doses of estrogen and progesterone than currently used. Hypertension among women taking oral contraceptives should result in discontinuation of these drugs and close monitoring of subsequent blood pressure. Prophylactic hormonal therapy with estrogen compounds in postmenopausal women has generally not been associated with the development of hypertension. These patients, however, should have blood-pressure levels determined 1 month and 6 months after starting therapy.

Table 41-5. Common Causes of Therapy Failure

Nonadherence to therapy
Cost of medication
Instructions not clear or not given to patient in writing
Inadequate or no patient education
Lack of involvement of patient in treatment plan
Side effects of medication
Organic brain syndrome (eg, memory deficit)
Inconvenient dosing

Drug-related causes
Doses too low
Inappropriate combinations (eg, two centrally acting adrenergic inhibitors)
Rapid inactivation (eg, hydralazine)

Drug interactions
Nonsteroidal antiinflammatory drugs
Oral contraceptives
Sympathomimetics
Antidepressants
Adrenal steroids
Nasal decongestants
Licorice-containing substances (eg, chewing tobacco)
Cocaine
Cyclosporine
Erythropoietin

Associated conditions
Increasing obesity
Alcohol intake (>1 oz/day of ethanol)

Secondary hypertension
Renal insufficiency
Renovascular hypertension
Pheochromocytoma
Primary aldosteronism

Volume overload
Inadequate diuretic therapy
Excess sodium intake
Fluid retention from reduction of blood pressure
Progressive renal damage

Pseudohypertension

(Adapted from The fifth report of the Joint National Committee on Detection, Evaluation, and Treatment of High Blood Pressure [JNC V]. Arch Intern Med 1993;153:154.)

Table 41-6. Selected Drug Interactions with Antihypertensive Therapy*

Diuretics

Possible situations for decreased antihypertensive effects
Cholestyramine and colestipol decrease absorption; NSAIDs (including aspirin and over-the-counter ibuprofen) may antagonize diuretic effectiveness.

Possible situations for increased antihypertensive effects
Combinations of thiazides (especially metolazone) with furosemide can produce profound diuresis, natriuresis, and kaliuresis in renal impairment.

Effects of diuretics on other drugs
Diuretics can raise serum lithium levels and increase toxic effects by enhancing proximal tubular resorption of lithium. Diuretics may make it more difficult to control dyslipidemia and diabetes.

β-Blockers

Possible situations for decreased antihypertensive effects
NSAIDs may decrease effects of β-blockers. Rifampin, smoking, and phenobarbital decrease serum levels of agents primarily metabolized by the liver due to enzyme induction.

Possible situations for increased antihypertensive effects
Cimetidine may increase serum levels of β-blockers that are primarily metabolized by the liver due to enzyme inhibition. Quinidine may increase risk of hypotension.

Effects of β-blockers on other drugs
Combinations of diltiazem or verapamil with β-blockers may have additive sinoatrial and atrioventricular node depressant effects and may also promote negative inotropic effects on failing myocardium. Combination of β-blockers and reserpine may cause marked bradycardia and syncope.

β-blockers may increase serum levels of theophylline, lidocaine, and chlorpromazine due to reduced hepatic clearance. Nonselective β-blockers prolong insulin-induced hypoglycemia and promote rebound hypertension due to unopposed α-stimulation; all β-blockers mask adrenergically mediated symptoms of hypoglycemia and have the potential to aggravate diabetes.

β-Blockers may make it more difficult to control dyslipidemia.

Phenylpropanolamine (which can be obtained over the counter in cold and diet preparations), pseudoephedrine, ephedrine, and epinephrine can cause elevations in blood pressure due to unopposed α-receptor-induced vasoconstriction.

ACE inhibitors

Possible situations for decreased antihypertensive effects
NSAIDs (including aspirin and over-the-counter ibuprofen) may decrease blood pressure control. Antacids may decrease the bioavailability of ACE inhibitors.

Possible situations for increased antihypertensive effects
Diuretics may lead to excessive hypotensive effects (hypovolemia).

Effect of ACE inhibitors on other drugs
Hyperkalemia may occur with potassium supplements, potassium-sparing agents, and NSAIDs. ACE inhibitors may increase serum lithium levels.

Calcium Antagonists

Possible situations for decreased antihypertensive effects
Serum levels and antihypertensive effects of calcium antagonists may be diminished by these interactions: rifampin–verapamil; carbamazepine–diltiazem and verapamil; phenobarbital and phenytoin–verapamil

Possible situations for increased antihypertensive effects
Cimetidine may increase pharmacologic effects of all calcium antagonists due to inhibition of hepatic metabolizing enzymes, resulting in increased serum levels.

Effects of calcium antagonists on other drugs
Digoxin and carbamazepine serum levels and toxic effects may be increased by verapamil and possibly by diltiazem. Serum levels of prazosin, quinidine, and theophylline may be increased by verapamil.

Serum levels of cyclosporine may be increased by diltiazem, nicardipine, and verapamil; cyclosporine dose may need to be decreased.

α-Blockers

Possible situations for increased antihypertensive effects
Concomitant antihypertensive drug therapy (especially diuretics) may increase chance of postural hypotension.

Sympatholytics

Possible situations for decreased antihypertensive effects
Tricyclic antidepressants may decrease effects of centrally acting and peripheral norepinephrine depleters. Sympathomimetics, including over-the-counter cold and diet preparations, amphetamines, phenothiazines, and cocaine, may interfere with antihypertensive effects of guanethidine and guanadrel. The severity of clonidine withdrawal reaction can be increased by β-blockers.

Monoamine oxidase inhibitors may prevent degradation and metabolism of norepinephrine released by tyramine-containing foods and may cause hypertension; they may also cause hypertensive reactions when combined with reserpine or guanethidine.

Effects of sympatholytics on other drugs
Methyldopa may increase serum lithium levels.

*This table does not include all potential drug interactions with antihypertensive drugs.

ACE, angiotensin-converting enzyme; *NSAID*, nonsteroidal antiinflammatory drug.

(Adapted from The fifth report of the Joint National Committee on Detection, Evaluation, and Treatment of High Blood Pressure [JNC V]. Arch Intern Med 1993;153:154.)

CONSIDERATIONS IN PREGNANCY

According to a classification recommended by the National High Blood Pressure Education Program's Working Group Report on High Blood Pressure in Pregnancy, hypertension in pregnancy may be placed in one of four categories: chronic hypertension, preeclampsia-eclampsia, chronic hypertension with superimposed preeclampsia, and transient hypertension.

It is important to diagnose and treat hypertension during pregnancy effectively, as it may result in life-threatening consequences for mother and fetus. The criteria for diagnosing hypertension in pregnancy are blood-pressure measurements of 140/90 mm Hg.

Chronic hypertension is the state observed before pregnancy or diagnosed before the 20th week of gestation. The patient's prepregnancy medication may be continued, except for ACE inhibitors, which may cause serious neonatal problems, including renal failure and death. For patients who were not previously on a medication and who do not respond to rest and moderate sodium restriction, antihypertensive drug therapy should be instituted when the diastolic blood pressure is 100 mm Hg or higher. Aggressive pressure-lowering regimens are discouraged to avoid compromising the uteroplacental blood flow. Methyldopa has been used extensively in pregnancy and is considered safe. β-Blockers are as effective as methyldopa in

Table 41-7. Adverse Side Effects of Antihypertensive Agents

DRUGS	SIDE EFFECTS*	PRECAUTIONS AND SPECIAL CONSIDERATIONS
Diuretics		
Thiazides and related diuretics	Hypokalemia, hypomagnesemia, hyponatremia, hyperuricemia, hypercalcemia, hyperglycemia, hypercholesterolemia, hypertriglyceridemia, sexual dysfunction, weakness	Except for metolazone and indapamide, ineffective in renal failure (serum creatinine ≥221 μmol/L [2.5 mg/dL]); hypokalemia increases digitalis toxic effect; may precipitate acute gout
Loop diuretics	Same as for thiazides except loop diuretics do not cause hypercalcemia	Effective in chronic renal failure
Potassium-sparing agents	Hyperkalemia	Danger of hyperkalemia in patients with renal failure, in patients treated with ACE inhibitor or with NSAIDs
Amiloride	—	—
Spironolactone	Gynecomastia, mastodynia, menstrual irregularities, diminished libido in males	—
Triamterene	—	Danger of renal calculi
Adrenergic inhibitors		
β-Blockers†	Bronchospasm, may aggravate peripheral arterial insufficiency, fatigue, insomnia, exacerbation of CHF, masking of symptoms of hypoglycemia; also hypertriglyceridemia, decreased high-density lipoprotein cholesterol (except for drugs with ISA); reduces exercise tolerance	Should not be used in patients with asthma, COPD, CHF with systolic dysfunction, heart block (greater than 1st degree), and sick sinus syndrome; use with caution in insulin-treated diabetics and patients with peripheral vascular disease; should not be discontinued abruptly in patients with ischemic heart disease
α-β-Blocker (labetalol)	Bronchospasm, may aggravate peripheral vascular insufficiency, orthostatic hypotension	Should not be used in patients with asthma, COPD, CHF, heart block (greater than 1st degree), and sick sinus syndrome; use with caution in insulin-treated diabetics and patients with peripheral vascular disease.
α_1-Receptor blockers	Orthostatic hypotension, syncope, weakness, palpitations, headache	Use cautiously in older patients because of orthostatic hypertension.
ACE inhibitors	Cough, rash, angioneurotic edema, hyperkalemia, dysgeusia	Hyperkalemia can develop, particularly in patients with renal insufficiency; hypotension has been observed with initiation of ACE inhibitors, especially in patients with high plasma renin activity or receiving diuretic therapy; can cause reversible, acute renal failure in patients with bilateral renal arterial stenosis or unilateral stenosis in solitary kidney and in patients with cardiac failure and with volume depletion; rarely can induce neutropenia or proteinuria; absolutely contraindicated in 2nd and 3rd trimesters of pregnancy
Calcium antagonists		
Dihydropyridines (Amlodipine, felodipine, isradipine, nicardipine, nifedipine)	Headache, dizziness, peripheral edema, tachycardia, gingival hyperplasia	Use with caution in patients with CHF; may aggravate angina and myocardial ischemia
Diltiazem, verapamil	Headache, dizziness, peripheral edema, (less common than with dihydropyridines), gingival hyperplasia, constipation (especially verapamil), atrioventricular block, bradycardia	Use with caution in patients with cardiac failure; contraindicated in patients with 2nd- or 3rd-degree heart block or sick sinus syndrome
Centrally acting α_2-agonists (clonidine, guanabenz, guanfacine hydrochloride)	Drowsiness, sedation, dry mouth, fatigue, orthostatic dizziness	Rebound hypertension may occur with abrupt discontinuance, particularly with previous administration of high doses or with continuation of concomitant β-blocker therapy.
Clonidine patch	Same as for clonidine; localized skin reaction to patch	—
Methyldopa	—	May cause liver damage, fever, and Coombs-positive hemolytic anemia
Peripheral-acting adrenergic antagonists		
Guanadrel sulfate, guanethidine monosulfate	Diarrhea, orthostatic and exercise hypotension	Use cautiously because of orthostatic hypotension.
Rauwolfia alkaloids, reserpine	Lethargy, nasal congestion, depression	Contraindicated in patients with history of mental depression or with active peptic ulcer
Direct vasolidators	Headache, tachycardia, fluid retention	May precipitate angina pectoris in patients with coronary artery disease; generally, use with diuretic and β-blocker
Hydralazine	Positive antinuclear antibody test	Lupus syndrome may occur (rare at recommended doses).
Minoxidil	Hypertrichosis	May cause or aggravate pleural and pericardial effusions

See Table 41-1 for a list of drugs. *ACE,* angiotensin-converting enzyme; *NSAID,* nonsteroidal antiinflammatory drug; *COPD,* chronic obstructive pulmonary disease; *ISA,* intrinsic sympathomimetic activity; *CHF,* congestive heart failure .

*The listing of side effects is not all inclusive, and clinicians are urged to refer to the package insert for a more detailed listing. Sexual dysfunction, particularly impotence in men, has been reported with the use of all antihypertensive agents. Few data are available on the effect of antihypertensive agents on sexual function in women.

†Some of the metabolic side effects of diuretics and β-blockers can be minimized by appropriate dietary counseling.

(Adapted from The fifth report of the Joint National Committee on Detection, Evaluation, and Treatment of High Blood Pressure [JNC V]. Arch Intern Med 1993;153:154.)

lowering blood pressure, but their safety in early pregnancy has been questioned.

Preeclampsia is a state of hypertension associated with proteinuria and edema and frequently with abnormalities of coagulation and liver function. Preeclampsia must be recognized, as it may evolve to eclampsia. Further details regarding preeclampsia and eclampsia can be found in appropriate obstetric texts.

Gestational or transient hypertension involves blood-pressure elevations that usually occur late in pregnancy and disappear after delivery. Often these patients are overweight and have a family history of hypertension, and they often become hypertensive in later years. They must be observed closely during pregnancy, with frequent determinations of blood pressure, as well as detection of urinary protein, serum uric acid, creatinine clearance, and blood urea nitrogen, to identify progression to preeclampsia. Methyldopa or β-blockers are usually effective in lowering blood pressure if nonpharmacologic efforts are unsuccessful and the diastolic blood pressure remains above 100 mm Hg.

REFERRAL OF HYPERTENSIVE PATIENTS

Primary care physicians should feel comfortable in managing most patients with hypertension, but referral of patients to a hypertension specialist, either a cardiologist or a nephrologist with an interest in hypertension, is appropriate in the following situations:

- Refractory blood-pressure elevations despite multiple trials with maximal-dose agents in a combination of two or more of these medications in different classes
- Strong suspicion of renovascular hypertension
- Evidence of ongoing target organ dysfunction or organ system deterioration (eg, evidence of myocardial ischemia or infarction, progressive left ventricular dysfunction with or without acute pulmonary edema, hypertensive encephalopathy, transient ischemic attack, cerebrovascular accident, progressive proteinuria, deterioration of blood urea nitrogen and creatinine clearance, and other end-organ dysfunctional agents)
- Any patient whose blood pressure has been reasonably well controlled but who has intolerable side effects despite attempts at multiple alternative agents.

Patients suspected of having aldosteronism, pheochromocytoma, or other endocrine states resulting in hypertension should be referred to an endocrine specialist for definitive diagnosis and treatment. Hypertension in pregnancy is a serious complication and mandates referral to or consultation with a perinatologist or obstetrician experienced in the management of hypertensive diseases of pregnancy.

BIBLIOGRAPHY

Aviv A. The roles of cell Ca^{2+}, protein kinase C, and the $Na^{(+)}$-H^{+} antiport in the development of hypertension and insulin resistance. J Am Soc Nephrol 1992;3:1049.

Burker EJ, Fredrikson M, Rifai N, Siegel W, Blumenthal JA. Serum lipids, neuroendocrine, and cardiovascular responses to stress in men and women with mild hypertension. Behav Med 1994;19:155.

Choo MH. Problems and solutions in diagnosing systemic hypertension. Ann Acad Med Singapore 1990;19:113.

Collins R, Peto R, MacMahon S, et al. Blood pressure, stroke, and coronary heart disease. Part 2: Short-term reductions in blood pressure: overview of randomized drug trials in their epidemiological context. Lancet 1990;335:765.

Conde-Agudelo A, Lede R, Belizan J. Evaluation of methods used in the prediction of hypertensive disorders of pregnancy. Obstet Gynecol Surv 1994:49:210.

Croog SH, Elias MF, Colton T, et al. Effects of antihypertensive medications on quality of life in elderly hypertensive women. Am J Hypertens 1994;7:329.

Drory Y, Pines A, Fisman EZ, Kellermann JJ. Exercise response in young women with borderline hypertension. Chest 1990;97:298.

Eison H, Phillips RA, Ardeljan M, Krakoff LR. Differences in ambulatory blood pressure between men and women with mild hypertension. J Hum Hypertens 1990;4:400.

Enstrom I, Lindholm LH. Blood pressure in middle-aged women: a comparison between office-, self-, and ambulatory recordings. Blood Press 1992;1:240.

Epstein FH. The hypertensive patient beyond blood pressure. J Hum Hypertens 1992;6:459.

Fifth report of the Joint National Committee on Detection, Evaluation, and Treatment of High Blood Pressure (JNC V). Arch Intern Med 1993;153:154.

Falkner B. Differences in blacks and whites with essential hypertension: biochemistry and endocrine. Hypertension 1990;15:681.

Greene J. NSAIDS and blood pressure: five not-so-silly millimeters. Internal Medicine Alert 16:169.

Hall PM. Hypertension in women. Cardiology 1990;77:25.

Jamerson K, Julius S. Predictors of blood pressure and hypertension. General principles. Am J Hypertens 1991;4:598S.

Karpanou EA, Vyssoulis GP, Georgoudi DG, Toutouza MG, Toutouzas PK. Ambulatory blood pressure changes in the menstrual cycle of hypertensive women. Significance of plasma renin activity values. Am J Hypertens 1993;6:654.

Knott C. The treatment of hypertension in pregnancy. Clinical pharmacokinetic considerations. Clin Pharmacokinet 1991;21:233.

Langford HG, Davis BR, Blaufox D, et al. Effect of drug and diet treatment of mild hypertension on diastolic blood pressure. The TAIM Research Group. Hypertension 1991;17:210.

Manhem K, Jern C, Pilhall M, Hansson L, Jern S. Cardiovascular responses to stress in young hypertensive women. J Hypertens 1992;10:861.

Mann SJ. Systolic hypertension in the elderly. Pathophysiology and management. Arch Intern Med 1992;152:1977.

Mann SJ, Pickering TG. Detection of renovascular hypertension. Ann Intern Med 1992;117:845.

Mundal HH, Nordby G, Lande K, Gjesdal K, Kjeldsen SE. Effect of cold pressor test and awareness of hypertension on platelet function in normotensive and hypertensive women. Scand J Clin Lab Invest 1993; 53:585.

National High Blood Pressure Education Program Working Group on High Blood Pressure in Pregnancy. Working group report on high blood pressure in pregnancy. Am J Obstet Gynecol 1990;163:1689.

O'Brien E, O'Malley K, Mee F, Atkins N, Cox J. Ambulatory blood pressure measurement in the diagnosis and management of hypertension. J Hum Hypertens 1991;5:23.

Os I, Nordby G. Hypertension and the metabolic cardiovascular syndrome: special reference to premenopausal women. J Cardiovasc Pharmacol 1992;20:S15.

Parodi O, Neglia D, Sambuceti G, Marabotti C, Palombo C, Donato L. Regional myocardial blood flow and coronary reserve in hypertensive patients. The effect of therapy. Drugs 1992;44:48.

Phillips RA. Etiology, pathophysiology, and treatment of left ventricular hypertrophy: focus on severe hypertension. J Cardiovasc Pharmacol 1993;21:S55.

Verdecchia P, Porcellati C. Defining normal ambulatory blood pressure in relation to target organ damage and prognosis. Am J Hypertens 1993;6:207S.

42
Chest Pain

PATRICIA G. FITZPATRICK

Primary Care for Women, edited by Phyllis C. Leppert and Fred M. Howard. Lippincott-Raven Publishers, Philadelphia © 1997.

The evaluation of chest pain is a common and diagnostically challenging problem facing primary care physicians. The potential etiologies are numerous, and the diagnosis relies on a careful history and physical examination to direct further investigation. Serious disorders such as acute myocardial infarction and unstable angina must be recognized and treated expediently. In the remainder of patients, the process of determining the presence or absence of coronary artery disease and the associated prognosis requires assessment of a variety of factors, including the patient's presentation, risk factor evaluation, pretest probability of disease, physical examination, and response to a therapeutic trial of medication or preliminary diagnostic testing. The difficulty in arriving at a diagnosis is compounded by the marked variation in presentation that is seen among patients who are later documented to have coronary artery disease.

Cardiac disease is the leading cause of death in men and women, with about 550,000 deaths annually in the United States. At least half of these deaths occur in women, and most of these are related to coronary artery disease. In addition, although mortality associated with cardiac disease has declined in recent years, the rate of decline has been less rapid in women and black men. Until recently, chest pain, the usual manifestation of coronary disease, has been perceived as a relatively benign process in women, since, when studied angiographically, up to 50% of women presenting with "angina" have been shown to have no or minimal coronary artery disease. However, in women of advanced years, classic angina pectoris carries the same prognosis as in their male counterparts, with similar or greater associated morbidity and mortality.

DIFFERENTIAL DIAGNOSIS

Angina pectoris is a term first used by Heberden in the 18th century to describe a strangulation or choking sensation, triggered by exertional effort and relieved with rest. The differential diagnosis of chest pain is extensive, and some of the more common etiologies are listed in Table 42-1. Obtaining a detailed, accurate history is the most important way to assess the significance and likely causes of chest pain. Chest pain is the most common manifestation of coronary artery disease; however, more vague symptoms such as fatigue, dyspnea on exertion, or no discomfort, such as in silent ischemia, may predominate. The chest discomfort of angina pectoris is typically not "painful," but rather, a pressure, squeezing, or tightness in the chest, occurring with or without associated symptoms such as shortness of breath, diaphoresis, nausea, and lightheadedness. Characterization of factors, such as location and quality of the discomfort, its intensity and duration, associated symptoms, and factors that precipitate or relieve symptoms aid in the categorization of chest pain as typical angina, atypical angina, or nonanginal pain (Table 42-2).

Esophageal Disorders

Gastroesophageal reflux is relatively common and can cause inflammation of the esophageal mucosa. Patients also may develop esophagitis in other ways (Barrett esophagitis, lower esophageal sphincter disorders). Symptomatically, patients may experience retrosternal burning that may be confused with angina. Typically, however, this discomfort is nonradiating and continuous, is often precipitated by eating or swallowing certain foods and aggravated by lying down, is not related to exertion, and is relieved with food or antacids. Note that, whereas esophageal spasm may be relieved by sublingual nitroglycerin, other features more typical for esophageal pain usually help differentiate this from a cardiac source. The two disorders occur concomitantly in approximately 10% of patients, however, so a diagnosis of hiatal hernia or gastroesophageal reflux does not exclude the diagnosis of coronary artery disease. Adding to the diagnostic difficulty, when angina does develop in patients with gastrointestinal symptoms, the location of discomfort is the typically the same.

Other Gastrointestinal Causes of Chest Pain

Biliary colic, caused by a rapid increase in biliary pressure due to obstruction of the bile or cystic duct, causes symptoms that may be confused with angina pectoris. The discomfort is usually constant, with a longer duration than typical angina (hours), and is more prominent in the right upper quadrant, although it may radiate to the substernal area as well as the epigastrium, left abdomen, and scapula. It typically occurs spontaneously, although there may be a history of dyspepsia or fatty food intolerance, and usually resolves spontaneously as well. *Peptic ulcer* discomfort usually is an epigastric or substernal burning that persists for hours; it is typically aggravated by lack of food or by foods with high acidity and is relieved with antacids or food.

Musculoskeletal Disorders and Chest Wall Syndromes

Costochondritis is a common musculoskeletal disorder that can mimic angina pectoris. It is characterized by localized, superficial discomfort, which is aggravated by movement and palpation of the costochondral junctions, and typically is relieved by antiinflammatory medication and rest. *Tietze syndrome*, where there is actual swelling of the costochondral junction, is uncommon. Other uncommon musculoskeletal disorders also may produce symptoms similar to angina but are usually easily differentiated by a careful history and physical examination. *Cystic mastitis* is a common cause of chest wall pain, reproduced by pressure over tender areas of breast tissue.

Table 42-1. Differential Diagnosis of Chest Pain

Cardiac Causes

Myocardial infarction/acute ischemic syndromes (including coronary artery spasm or Prinzmetal angina)
Mitral valve prolapse
Aortic valvular stenosis
Pericarditis
Hypertrophic cardiomyopathy
Microvascular angina (or syndrome X)

Pulmonary Causes

Pulmonary embolism ± infarction
Pneumothorax
Bronchitis, pneumonia, carcinoma
Pleuritis

Esophageal Causes

Esophagitis, reflux, or other causes
Esophageal spasm
Esophageal motility disorders
Esophageal rupture
Tumor, foreign body
Zenker diverticulum

Other Gastrointestinal Causes

Cholecystitis, cholelithiasis
Pancreatitis
Peptic ulcer disease

Musculoskeletal/Chest Wall Causes

Costochondritis (including Tietze syndrome)
Fracture, neoplasm, osteomyelitis
Manubriosternal or xiphisternal arthralgia
Cervicothoracic spinal disorders
Thoracic outlet obstruction
Cystic mastitis

Miscellaneous Causes

Aortic dissection/aneurysm
Hyperventilation syndrome
Anxiety states

Pulmonary Disorders

Pulmonary embolism typically causes a substernal chest discomfort that may be confused with angina, but usually the predominant symptom is dyspnea. It often occurs spontaneously, without association with exertion. With *pulmonary infarction* there may be a pleuritic component to the pain, so that deep inspiration aggravates symptoms, and a pleural rub may be heard on auscultation. Duration of symptoms is often prolonged and usually relieved with rest over time. Patients with severe *pulmonary hypertension* may describe chest pain similar to angina, but typically have findings on physical examination (parasternal lift, palpable or loud pulmonary component of the second heart sound) and electrocardiography (right ventricular hypertrophy) that distinguish this from true angina.

Functional or Psychogenic Chest Pain

Often referred to as Da Costa syndrome or neurocirculatory asthenia, the functional or psychogenic chest pain accompanying this anxiety state is typically localized to the left chest and is characterized as a prolonged, dull, persistent ache with intermittent sharp, stabbing pain of brief duration accompanied by fatigue, emotional strain, light-headedness and breathlessness, and has little relationship to exertion. Its response to intervention is variable, but sometimes is helped by rest, exercise, analgesics, or anxiolytic medications.

Cardiovascular Disorders Unrelated to Coronary Artery Disease

Mitral valve prolapse is one of the most common cardiac valvular abnormalities, affecting 5% to 10% of the population, resulting from a variety of abnormalities of the mitral valve apparatus. It is more common in women. Chest discomfort is a common symptom in mitral valve prolapse and is typically prolonged, not associated with exertion, may be associated with intermittent sharp, stabbing pain, and typically resolves spontaneously. At times, the pain may be difficult to distinguish from angina, however, and the two disorders may coexist. Chest pain also may accompany other valvular disorders, with or without associated coronary artery disease, such as *severe aortic stenosis*, where coronary blood flow is reduced or unable to provide adequate supply to the hypertrophied muscle. Typically, dyspnea is a more prominent feature in aortic stenosis compared with coronary artery disease. The pain of *acute pericarditis* also may resemble angina; however, it is usually sudden in onset, prolonged and severe, with pleuritic components, such that it is aggravated by inspiration, cough, reclining, and is relieved by sitting forward. A pericardial friction rub, when auscultated, aids in the diagnosis. *Aortic dissection* is typically characterized by severe, persistent retrosternal discomfort radiating to the back. A history of hypertension is usually present. *Microvascular angina* (also called *syndrome X*) has been identified in a subset of patients with typical—and sometimes atypical—angina who have normal epicardial

Table 42-2. Features of Typical Angina and Noncardiac Chest Pain*

FEATURE	ANGINA	NONCARDIAC PAIN
Location of pain	Substernal, diffuse, often radiates	Localized
Quality of pain	Dull, constricting, deep weight on chest; burning band across chest	Sharp, shooting, knife-life, jabbing
Intensity and duration	Steady, with gradual changes in intensity, typically lasts 5–15 min	Fluctuates in intensity, with rapid changes, lasts seconds to hours
Provoking factors	Physical or emotional stress	Single movement or action, related to meal
Relief	After several minutes of rest and/or nitroglycerin	Often spontaneously, within seconds or after prolonged rest, usually not by nitroglycerin

*Atypical angina may have features of both noncardiac chest pain and typical angina, with the noncardiac features usually more prominently weighed in consideration of the differential diagnosis.

vessels at angiography and an abnormally increased coronary vascular resistance when atrially paced after the administration of intravenous ergonovine. This affects both men and women, although typically the ratio of women to men is higher than would be expected from coronary artery disease data. Symptoms often are characteristic of angina, although there may be more rest pain, prolonged pain, and a variable response to nitrates. Electrocardiographic changes may be present at rest, and are frequent after exercise or pharmacologic stress testing. Effective treatment usually involves a standard antianginal regimen, and the long-term prognosis is excellent for most patients. *Cocaine abuse* also must be considered in the differential diagnosis of chest pain. Cocaine can trigger intense coronary artery spasm, with or without superimposed thrombus formation, resulting in unstable angina pectoris or myocardial infarction.

HISTORY

In determining the probability of coronary artery disease, it is important to risk-stratify the patient using a variety of clinical factors, including description of symptoms as discussed earlier, age, gender, risk factors associated with heart disease, and physical findings. Evaluation of chest pain, however, can be particularly challenging in women (Fig. 42-1). Even when women present with symptoms of typical angina, defined as chest pressure or tightness, substernal in nature with or without radiation to the jaw, neck, or left arm, with a duration of 2 to 15 minutes, studies of the natural history of disease, such as the Framingham Heart Study, have demonstrated a low frequency of evolution to myocardial infarction when compared with men (14% in women with angina versus 25% of men with angina). Part of this discrepancy may be related to the policy of equating symptoms of angina with the presence of coronary artery disease in women. In the Coronary Artery Surgery Study Registry, only 50% of women believed to have angina had evidence of coronary disease compared with 83% of men. Women have a higher prevalence of conditions that can mimic atherosclerotic heart disease, such as coronary artery spasm, mitral valve prolapse, and microvascular angina, which adds to the complexity of diagnostic evaluation. However, when symptomatic women are stratified by age, the probability of disease increases. For example, the subset of women in the Framingham Heart Study 60 to 69 years of age with typical angina symptoms had a prognosis similar to that of men. Thus, the occurrence of coronary disease is much more age dependent in women compared with men, with a low prevalence of coronary disease in the 35- to 44-year-olds, whereas by 75 years of age, morbidity related to coronary disease is similar in men and women (Table 42-3).

Major risk factors for the development of cardiac disease have undergone extensive study. However, most of these studies have focused on men. Whereas women tend to have a lower prevalence of classic cardiac risk factors for coronary artery disease, differences in risk profile, changes with age, and the influences of potential risk factors unique to women have not been well examined (Table 42-4). Major risk factors affect men and women in similar ways, with some interesting differences. Diabetes mellitus, for example, is more prevalent in women, and the risk of developing coronary artery disease is higher in female diabetics compared with male diabetics. As a consequence, the prevalence of coronary artery disease is similar in male and female diabetics, even when younger, premenopausal women are compared with men of similar age. Contributions of certain potential risk factors unique to women, such as oral contraceptive use, pregnancy, hysterectomy with or without oophorectomy, menopause, postmenopausal hormone replacement therapy, and the mechanisms by which they may confer risk or benefit, have not been well studied.

PHYSICAL EXAMINATION

In patients with coronary artery disease and angina pectoris, the physical examination may be entirely normal. The focus of the examination is directed toward differentiating the probable causes of chest pain, and searching for evidence that may help to corroborate a suspicion of coronary artery disease. The presence of a corneal arcus on inspection of the eyes is known to correlate with increased levels of cholesterol and low-density lipoprotein. Xanthelasmas, which are deposits of lipid intracellularly in the skin, correlate with increased triglyceride levels and a deficiency of high-density lipoprotein. The blood pressure may be elevated, chronically or acutely, in patients with angina. Peripheral arterial

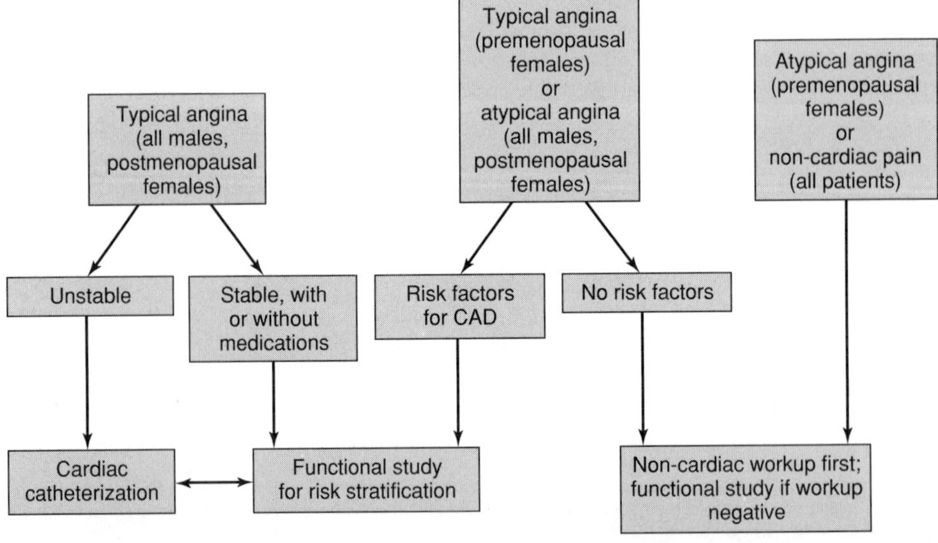

Figure 42-1. Strategy for evaluation of chest pain. *CAD*, coronary artery disease.

Table 42-3. Use of Probability Analysis in the Diagnosis of Coronary Artery Disease

AGE	NONANGINAL CHEST PAIN* Male	NONANGINAL CHEST PAIN* Female	ATYPICAL ANGINA* Male	ATYPICAL ANGINA* Female	TYPICAL ANGINA* Male	TYPICAL ANGINA* Female
Pretest likelihood of disease (%)						
30–39	5	1	22	4	70	26
60–69	28	19	67	54	94	91
Posttest likelihood of disease (%)						
With ST depression 0–0.5 mm						
30–39	1	0	6	1	24	7
60–69	8	5	32	21	79	69
With ST depression 1.0–1.5 mm						
30–39	10	2	38	8	83	42
60–69	45	33	81	72	97	95
With ST depression 2.0–2.5 mm						
30–39	38	8	76	33	96	79
60–69	81	72	96	93	99	99

**Typical angina:* (1) pressure or squeezing discomfort, substernal with or without radiation to jaw, neck or left arm, lasting 2–15 min and (2) precipitated by exertion or stress and relieved by rest. *Atypical angina* (1) or (2) but not both. *Nonanginal chest pain:* neither (1) or (2).

(Modified from Diamond GA, Forrester JS. Analysis of probability as an aid in the clinical diagnosis of coronary artery disease. N Engl J Med 1979;300:1350.)

disease often is a clue to more extensive atherosclerosis and is frequently present in coronary artery disease. The cardiac examination can provide useful information in the differential diagnosis of chest pain. A sustained cardiac impulse on palpation often is seen in patients with left ventricular dysfunction. The presence of a heart murmur can help distinguish the pain associated with aortic stenosis or hypertrophic cardiomyopathy. Transient apical systolic murmurs may indicate papillary muscle dysfunction in the presence of ischemia. A third or fourth heart sound can be heard in patients with angina pectoris, even when other obvious causes are not present. A midsystolic click with or without a late systolic murmur is characteristic of mitral valve prolapse. A continuous murmur over the precordium is uncommon, but may be attributed to turbulent flow across a stenotic proximal coronary artery.

LABORATORY STUDIES

Appropriate laboratory testing is directed by the results of the history and physical examination. Several studies are available to determine the presence or absence of coronary artery disease.

Table 42-4. Risk Factors for Coronary Artery Disease

	MEN	WOMEN
Major risk factors		
Age	45 y or older	55 y or older; premature menopause, without estrogen replacement
Family history	MI or sudden death in 1st-degree relative before age 55 y (male) or 65 y (female)	
Current cigarette smoking		Combination of smoking and oral contraceptive use increases risk of MI
Hypertension	BP 140/90 mm Hg or greater, or taking antihypertensive medications	
	More common in men < 45 y	More common in women > 45 y
Diabetes mellitus		More prevalent in women; confers risk of CAD equal to men across all age groups
Lipid disorders	Total cholesterol > 200, HDL < 35, LDL > 130	
	Total cholesterol and LDL tend to stabilize at age 45	Total cholesterol and LDL tend to rise at age 45 y and exceed levels of men beyond age 55 y; HDL levels run higher than men, but drop slightly after menopause
Other factors		
High triglycerides	May be independent risk factor	Independent risk factor in postmenopausal women
Obesity		
Stress		
Sedentary lifestyle		

BP, blood pressure; *CAD,* coronary artery disease; *HDL,* high-density lipoprotein; *LDL,* low-density lipoprotein; *MI,* myocardial infarction.

Electrocardiogram

A resting electrocardiogram (ECG) is normal in at least one third of patients with angina pectoris. Evidence of prior myocardial infarction or nonspecific ST-T wave changes, particularly if these changes were not present on a previous ECG, may aid in the diagnosis. Ambulatory ECG recordings may be useful in detecting ST segment depression associated with ischemia, which frequently occurs in the absence of symptoms, as in silent ischemia.

Exercise Electrocardiography

The exercise tolerance test (ETT) is most useful when there is at least an intermediate pretest probability of coronary artery disease. However, in general, up to 30% to 40% of results may be falsely positive, depending on the population being tested. Several factors reduce the diagnostic accuracy of exercise testing in women, including the following: factors that reduce the specificity of the test, such as the lower incidence of coronary artery disease in premenopausal women and the higher prevalence of mitral valve prolapse with its nonspecific ECG changes, ECG changes with hyperventilation, and vasospasm; and factors that reduce the sensitivity of the test, such as a higher incidence of single-vessel disease in women and the tendency for women to attain a lower cardiac workload with exercise testing compared with men. A normal finding on exercise study in women is useful and highly specific for the absence of coronary artery disease, comparable with the specificity rate described in men (93%). In addition, the ETT is valuable in assessing the severity and prognosis of the disease, as judged by duration of exercise, symptom provocation, blood pressure response to exercise, and extent and duration of ECG changes with exercise.

Radionuclide Angiography

Radionuclide imaging performed during exercise and/or with pharmacologic intervention improves the sensitivity and specificity of routine stress testing for the detection of coronary artery disease, and provides additional prognostic value. In women with perfusion abnormalities and atypical chest pain, the sensitivity is increased to 85%, whereas with typical angina, the sensitivity is 93%. Recognition of breast attenuation artifact and use of newer agents, such as technetium-99 sestamibi, has improved the specificity rate to 91%. Women have been shown to have a greater incidence of side effects during pharmacologic testing with agents such as dipyridamole or adenosine. This is believed to be related to the greater proportion of adipose tissue and smaller intravascular volume of distribution in women compared with men, even though doses are weight-adjusted. Further study is necessary.

Radionuclide Ventriculography

Use of radionuclide ventriculography for the detection of coronary artery disease is based on the principle that in patients with normal coronary arteries, left ventricular ejection fraction is augmented by at least 5% at peak exercise. When ejection fraction fails to augment or falls, coronary artery disease has been shown to be present in men, with a sensitivity of 82% and a specificity of 73%. Although the sensitivity in women is 78%, the specificity is only 46%, because the physiologic response of healthy women to exercise varies from men and there is frequently no augmentation of ejection fraction. The high rate of false-positive study results therefore limits the usefulness of this screening tool in women.

Stress Echocardiography

Echocardiography can be used to detect regional changes in contractility during stress (exercise or pharmacologic) compared with rest. This is a relatively new diagnostic tool, and information regarding gender differences is limited. Early studies are encouraging, however, with sensitivity and specificity rates of 79% to 88% and 84% to 93%, respectively, in groups of women with moderate pretest probability of disease. The predictive accuracy of the technique also appears to be preserved for single-vessel versus multivessel disease.

Coronary Angiography

Coronary angiography generally is restricted to patients who have symptoms refractory to medical therapy, patients who are believed to be at high risk for a coronary event based on noninvasive testing, or patients who are unable to undergo risk stratification in any other way. Several studies show that women tend to be referred for diagnostic angiography less often that men, even when they have classic symptoms of angina and equivalent ECG changes on stress testing, perfusion defects on nuclear imaging, or both, with higher subsequent morbid event rates. On the other hand, women, even when they have classic angina, have a higher frequency of normal angiograms when studied.

TREATMENT

Once the cause of chest pain has been elucidated through a careful history, physical examination, and supplemental laboratory studies, the treatment can be more specifically directed. Treatment of nonanginal chest pain is not covered here. Treatment of coronary artery disease generally is divided into medical therapy versus revascularization with either coronary artery bypass surgery or angioplasty.

Medical Therapy

Standard treatment of angina pectoris involves the use of nitrates, beta-blockers, calcium channel blockers, and aspirin. Aspirin, in a dose of 160 mg/day or 325 mg every other day, has been shown to decrease the incidence of death and nonfatal MI. Benefit also has been recently demonstrated in women. Nitrates have a dual action of increasing oxygen supply and reducing oxygen demand, resulting in relief of anginal symptoms. These are useful in patients with fixed-threshold angina, where symptoms are predictably reproduced with certain types of activity, as well as with variable-threshold angina, where vasospasm may play a more important role in producing angina. Sublingual nitroglycerin or inhaled spray is used to treat individual episodes. When angina occurs more than two to three times per week, or when silent ischemia is documented, longer acting nitrates often are employed, either in a transdermal preparation or orally. A 10- to 12-hour nitrate-free interval (usually overnight) is important to limit nitrate tolerance and improve effectiveness. Intravenous preparations are available for use in unstable angina.

Beta-blockers are particularly useful in effort-related angina. These work by inhibiting the effects of circulating catecholamines on beta-adrenergic receptors, thereby reducing heart rate and contractility, resulting in reduced myocardial oxygen demand, particularly during periods of activity or excitement. Use of beta-blockers in the setting of congestive heart failure, bradyarrhythmias, significant depressive illness, asthma, severe diabetes mellitus, severe peripheral vascular disease, or when a strong vasospastic component to the angina is suspected may be limited by side effects. Calcium channel blockers work by causing relaxation of vascular smooth muscle in both the systemic and coronary arteries. Entry of calcium into myocardial cells is opposed, resulting in a negative inotropic effect. Generally, if vasospasm is suggested and the heart rate is normal, calcium channel blockers are preferred over beta-blockers, whereas if resting tachycardia or arrhythmias are present, beta-blockers may be more effective. Simultaneous use of beta-blockers and calcium channel blockers, in addition to nitrates, often are needed to control anginal symptoms but should be done cautiously due to the risk of severe bradycardia, atrioventricular block, hypotension, and congestive heart failure.

Other agents, such as the histamine antagonist cyproheptadine, may be useful in Prinzmetal angina, and angiotensin converting enzyme inhibitors have been successfully employed in unstable angina. Aggressive cholesterol lowering has been shown to alter vascular tone favorably and may have a direct effect on control of symptoms. There are relatively little data on the usefulness of medical therapy in women versus men with angina pectoris, nor has relative effectiveness of combination therapy been examined by gender. Hormone replacement therapy in postmenopausal women has been shown to confer benefit in prolonging life in women with coronary disease compared with women who have never used estrogen. Further studies are ongoing.

Table 42-5. Markers of High Risk for Cardiac Event

Electrocardiographic criteria
Failure to complete 6.5 METS or attain HR > 120 bpm
ST depression > 2 mm
Flat or decreasing blood pressure response to exercise
ST depressions that persist > 6 min postexercise
ST depressions that occur in multiple leads
Exercise-induced ventricular tachycardia
ST elevation in leads without Q waves
Radionuclide criteria
New redistribution defects at low workload (≤ 6.5 METS or HR ≤ 120 bpm)
Multiple redistribution defects
Increased lung uptake of isotope
Redistribution defects remote from an infarct zone
Redistribution defect in a zone of non-Q wave MI
Increase in cardiac pool of isotope
Echocardiographic criteria
Ejection fraction ≤ 35%
Multiple new wall motion defects
New wall motion defects at low workload (≤ 6.5 METS or HR ≤ 120 bpm)
Exercise increase in ejection fraction < 5%

Revascularization

Revascularization generally should be considered for any patient who has acceptable coronary anatomy for revascularization and either fails a trial of medical management or has markers for high risk of a major cardiac event on noninvasive testing (Table 42-5). The choice of angioplasty versus coronary artery bypass surgery (CABG) depends on the extent, distribution, and severity of disease; left ventricular function; other comorbid disease; and physician and patient preference.

Percutaneous transluminal coronary angioplasty (PTCA) has been available for over a decade as an alternative treatment to CABG in selected patients with refractory angina who have suitable coronary anatomy. Newer devices, such as atherectomy and stents, have broadened the indications for the procedure, although typically PTCA is recommended in patients with normal or mildly depressed left ventricular function, with focal stenoses involving one or more vessels. Women presenting for PTCA tend to be older, with a higher prevalence of congestive heart failure, more severe symptoms of angina, and more cardiac risk factors compared with their male counterparts. In the early registry of patients undergoing PTCA, women tended to have lower procedural success rates, with higher rates of complications, including mortality. It was believed that much of this difference could be explained by the higher risk profile of women presenting for PTCA. Over subsequent years, this gender gap has narrowed. Whether the apparent increased risk of PTCA in women is related primarily to vessel size remains to be determined. Long-term follow-up of PTCA patients reports no differences in survival, rates of myocardial infarction, or occurrence of severe angina, although women seem to be more likely to have ongoing anginal symptoms and be treated with antianginal medications.

CABG has been shown to improve survival in patients with left main, three-vessel coronary artery disease, or with significant left ventricular dysfunction. As with PTCA, women who present for CABG tend to be older, with more severe and more unstable anginal symptoms, although left ventricular function in more often preserved with fewer diseased vessels compared with men. Women have more comorbid disease preoperatively, and a higher operative mortality compared with men, with a relative risk of 1.5 to 2.5 in most studies. These differences may be related to differences in age, comorbid disease, body surface area, and coronary artery size. Symptomatically, women seem to have similar long-term results after CABG, with no apparent differences in 5- or 10-year survival based on gender. Clearly, ongoing study of treatment options in women, with an emphasis on earlier recognition of disease, management of comorbid conditions, and use of techniques to improve acute revascularization outcomes is needed.

CONSIDERATIONS IN PREGNANCY

Whereas shortness of breath and fatigue are common manifestations of the major hemodynamic alterations that occur during pregnancy, chest pain and ischemic heart disease are unusual in women of childbearing potential, and when seen typically occur in women older than 35 years of age. Aortic dissection is a rare cause of chest pain that can occur in pregnancy. When necessary, diagnostic evaluation using exercise tolerance testing at a submaximal level usually can be performed safely. The effects of radionuclide isotopes, such as thallium or sestamibi, on the unborn fetus have not been well studied and should be avoided when the diagnosis can be made another way. When the baseline ECG finding is not normal, stress echocardiography may provide additional information safely. Cardiac catheterization and angiography should be avoided if the patient is medically stable, because of the radiation exposure to the fetus.

For treatment of angina pectoris during pregnancy, calcium channel blockers are generally recommended. Beta-blockers can depress uterine contraction, cause bradycardia, hypotension, and hypoglycemia in the newborn and should be avoided. When required for stabilization of symptoms, beta-1–selective blockers are preferred. Nitrates are relatively ineffective in the presence of the marked vasodilation and decreased peripheral vascular resistance already present during pregnancy.

BIBLIOGRAPHY

Ayanian JZ, Epstein AM. Differences in the use of procedures between women and men hospitalized for coronary artery disease. N Engl J Med 1991;325:221.

Bell MR. Coronary artery disease in women: the safety and efficacy of coronary angioplasty. Cardiovascular Reviews and Reports 1995; January:15.

Cannon RO III, Camici PG, Epstein SE. Pathophysiological dilemma of syndrome X. Circulation 1992;85:883.

DeSanctis RW. Clinical manifestations of coronary artery disease: chest pain in women. Cardiovascular Reviews and Reports 1994;May:10.

Diamond GA, Forrester JS. Analysis of probability as an aid in the clinical diagnosis of coronary artery disease. N Engl J Med 1979; 300:1350.

Eysmann SB, Douglas PS. Coronary heart disease: therapeutic principles. In: Douglas PS, ed. Cardiovascular health and disease in women. Philadelphia: WB Saunders, 1993:43.

Eysmann SB, Douglas PS. Reperfusion and revascularization strategies for coronary artery disease in women. JAMA 1992;268:1903.

Kannel WB, Wilson PWF. Risk factors that attenuate the female coronary disease advantage. Arch Intern Med 1995;155:57.

Lerner DJ, Kannel WB. Patterns of coronary heart disease morbidity and mortality in the sexes: a 26-year follow-up of the Framingham population. Am Heart J 1986;111:383.

Matthews KA, Wing RR, Kuller LH, Meilahn EN, Plantinga P. Influence of the perimenopause on cardiovascular risk factors and symptoms of middle-aged healthy women. Arch Intern Med 1994;154:2349.

Pepine CJ. Angina pectoris. In: Freed M, Grines C, eds. Essentials of cardiovascular medicine. Birmingham, MI: Physicians' Press, 1994:54.

Rutherford JD, Braunwald E. Chronic ischemic heart disease. In: Braunwald E, ed. Heart disease: a textbook of cardiovascular medicine, 4th ed. Philadelphia: WB Saunders, 1992:1292.

Wenger NK. Coronary heart disease: diagnostic decision-making. In: Douglas PS, ed. Cardiovascular health and disease in women. Philadelphia: WB Saunders, 1993:25.

Williams MJ, Marwick TH, O'Gorman D, Foale RA. Comparison of exercise echocardiography with an exercise score to diagnose coronary artery disease in women. Am J Cardiol 1994;74:435.

Primary Care for Women, edited by Phyllis C. Leppert and Fred M. Howard. Lippincott-Raven Publishers, Philadelphia © 1997.

43
Angina and Myocardial Infarction

CYNTHIA REDDECK

After decades of misperceptions and misinformation, it has become clear that heart disease is as common and serious in women as in men. In the United States, cardiovascular disease is the leading cause of death in women, with coronary disease accounting for about one third of all female deaths. This amounts to over 250,000 deaths annually. Coronary artery disease (CAD) may manifest as angina, congestive heart failure, or myocardial infarction (MI). Women's primary care physicians must be alert to the symptoms and signs of heart disease so that timely recognition and treatment can be initiated. The recognition of heart disease is more difficult in women, who often exhibit less typical and less dramatic symptoms of coronary disease compared with men. Also, noninvasive diagnostic testing is less reliable in women. The disease, however, is more debilitating and more often fatal in women, whether treated medically or surgically. This is partly due to women's older age at the time of onset, with a known higher associated likelihood of comorbid illnesses.

ATHEROSCLEROSIS

Coronary artery disease usually results from atherosclerosis, a slowly progressive disease that may begin as early as childhood and worsen over decades before becoming symptomatic. The primary basis for atherogenesis is endothelial injury, and it is by this stimulus that risk factors such as diabetes, hypertension, smoking, and elevated low-density lipoprotein (LDL) cholesterol contribute to atherosclerosis. Endothelial disruption triggers a variety of cellular and hormonal mediators (platelets, thromboxane A_2, prostacyclin, platelet-derived growth factor, and other substances) that initiate cellular proliferation. Simultaneously, macrophages play a role by engulfing oxidized plasma lipids to form "foam cells," which coalesce into fatty yellow streaks. Cellular proliferation, along with lipid accumulation, ultimately results in fixed atherosclerotic plaques.

Many hormonally regulated factors also affect coronary flow, with platelet "stickiness" and coronary artery vasomotor tone influencing instantaneous flow dynamics.

The inciting event in acute MI is rupture of the atherosclerotic plaque or hemorrhage within the plaque, with resultant acute occlusive thrombus formation. Complete occlusion of a coronary artery due to clot results in the classic Q wave or transmural MI, with necrosis of the full thickness of a myocardial segment. However, intracoronary clot is not always static, but may from minute to minute expand or shrink as the body's intrinsic lytic mechanisms attempt to dissolve the clot. Incomplete or nonsustained occlusion can thereby result in the syndrome of unstable angina or a non–Q wave (subendocardial) infarct.

Angina and MI are unusual in premenopausal women, suggesting a protective effect of estrogen against atherosclerosis. Beyond a favorable effect on the lipid profile, estrogen mediates coronary vasodilation, acts as an antioxidant, and alters LDL uptake. Estrogen affects insulin levels, coagulation factors, and prostaglandins. These effects of estrogen and its role in delaying atherogenesis are under active investigation with the hope of learning more about the pathophysiologic mechanism of heart disease and the role of hormonal therapy in preventing coronary disease in postmenopausal women.

RISK FACTORS FOR CORONARY HEART DISEASE

Several factors increase statistical risk for atherosclerotic heart disease. However, in any individual patient, the presence of risk factors does not mandate that coronary disease exists, nor does their absence absolutely preclude heart disease.

Because of estrogen's strong protective effects, coronary disease is rare until natural or surgical menopause, lacking other overwhelming risk factors. Therefore, coronary disease is much more a function of age in women than in men, and occurs 10 to 15 years later than in men. In epidemiologic and observational trials, lack of postmenopausal hormonal supplement confers an increased risk of coronary disease. Other risk factors for atherosclerosis are shared by both men and women.

A family history of premature coronary disease in first-degree relatives is strongly predictive. A male relative with disease before 50 years of age or a female relative diagnosed before 60 years of age is a serious risk factor for coronary disease.

Although familial hyperlipidemia or hypertension in some cases mediates the genetic tendency to atherosclerosis, a positive family history is an independent risk factor for CAD. Diabetes is a powerful risk factor for coronary disease and virtually negates the protective effect of gender. Diabetes often coexists with other risk factors, particularly elevated cholesterol and hypertension. Hyperinsulinemia per se may play an important role in atherosclerosis development in diabetes, and diabetes may impair estrogen binding. A diabetic woman with chest pain requires prompt cardiac evaluation.

Hypercholesterolemia is a risk factor for coronary disease in women as it is in men. Estrogen confers a beneficial effect on the lipid profile, so that "good" cholesterol (high-density lipoprotein [HDL]) levels are higher in women that in men, with generally lower LDL levels. After menopause, however, LDL levels rise and are implicated in the increased risk for CAD development in older women. Interestingly, HDL cholesterol is a more potent protector against CAD in women than in men. On the other hand, high triglyceride levels confer a higher CAD risk for women. Recent cholesterol-lowering trials have included larger numbers of women and show significant benefits to lowering cholesterol in women as well as in men, particularly in secondary prevention. In postmenopausal women, hormonal replacement along with diet should be considered as first-line therapy for hypercholesterolemia. Estrogen clearly lowers LDL cholesterol and raises HDL levels. The addition of progestin to estrogen, necessary for prevention of uterine cancer, unfortunately abolishes much of the beneficial rise in HDL, but the favorable effect on LDL lowering persists.

Hypertension, either systolic or diastolic, is a risk factor for CAD in women as in men. If hypertension is mild, weight reduction and exercise may be adequate therapy, otherwise antihypertensive medications are indicated along with evaluation to exclude underlying causes.

Cigarette smoking is clearly atherogenic and a serious risk for coronary disease. Smoking also is thrombogenic and can cause coronary artery spasm, which may explain the cases of MI in women smokers who have no evidence of coronary stenoses on angiography. The risk of developing atherosclerotic coronary disease is proportional to the amount smoked and is not lessened by low-nicotine brands. It is disturbing that young women comprise the only group in the United States in whom smoking is on the rise. Primary care providers must educate women as to the substantial risk of cigarette smoking. Three to 4 years after cigarette cessation, the risk of a first heart attack equals that of a nonsmoker. Quitting should be vigorously encouraged, therefore, regardless of how long the patient has smoked.

Obesity and a sedentary lifestyle appear, in observational studies, to be important risk factors in women. Obesity as an independent risk factor seems in particular to be a stronger predictor of coronary disease for women than for men. The mechanisms of association of these factors with CAD may be largely through other commonly affiliated risks, such as hypertension, hyperlipidemia, or insulin resistance. Obesity is incompletely understood as far as atherosclerosis risk, but there are many reasons to encourage patients to maintain ideal weight and an active lifestyle.

Although there was once concern that oral contraceptives enhanced coronary risk, oral contraceptive dose and potency have changed significantly over the last few years. Older, stronger preparations may have conferred some increased risk in smokers older than 35 years of age, and it seems prudent to use oral contraceptives with caution, if at all, in this subgroup, pending further study. Otherwise, birth control preparations present no significant cardiac risk.

Cardiovascular disease is the leading cause of death in women, but many risk factors for atherosclerosis are modifiable. The primary care physician's role in addressing these factors in women cannot be overemphasized. Whereas the need for risk factor modification is obvious in women already diagnosed with cardiovascular disease, *primary* prevention must be a compelling goal for women's health care providers.

ANGINA

Typical angina has been classically described as a sensation of pressure or heaviness or dull discomfort precipitated by physical exertion and relieved with rest or nitroglycerin. Emotional upsets, cold, or a heavy meal also may trigger angina. Usually, the sensation is substernal but may radiate to or manifest solely as arm, neck, or jaw discomfort. An accompanying sensation of breathlessness is common. Angina generally lasts 2 to 5 minutes. Symptoms lasting only a few seconds or for hours are unlikely to be angina. A patient who is questioned only about "pain" may not report angina symptoms, since angina is often perceived as more of an uncomfortable sensation, rather than severely painful.

When angina conforms to the above definition, diagnosis may be obvious. However, angina symptoms may be less typical, a phenomenon reported more frequently in women than in men.

In some women, angina may manifest as a sharper pain or only as dyspnea, without discomfort, or it may be nonexertional. Diagnosis may be more difficult in these patients. The primary care provider must be alert to atypical symptoms that may be an angina equivalent, particularly in the woman with coronary risk factors.

Variant or Prinzmetal angina refers to angina that occurs because of coronary vasospasm, that is, spasm due to contraction of the muscular wall of the artery. A resultant decrease in intraluminal size can then occur, even in the total absence of atherosclerosis. Prinzmetal angina seems to be more common in women than in men, with symptoms occurring primarily at rest, often at night, and defined by ST elevation on the electrocardiogram (ECG) during pain. Vasospastic angina can be precipitated by such stimuli as cold, emotional stress, smoking, or certain drugs such as cocaine. Vasospasm probably plays a significant role in the MIs that occur with illicit drug use.

The term *unstable angina* refers to angina that is increasing in frequency or duration, or is of recent onset, or has started to occur at rest. When following patients with coronary disease, be attuned to descriptions of worsening angina. Unstable angina may presage MI and therefore generally mandates hospitalization and aggressive evaluation and therapy in consultation with a cardiologist.

Remember that despite the symptomatic description of angina, the occurrence of "silent" angina is common in patients with coronary atherosclerosis. Cardiac ischemia (inadequate cardiac perfusion) may be present at times without symptoms. In fact, in most patients with significant coronary disease, angina probably represents only the "tip of the ischemic iceberg." Most ischemic episodes, documentable by continuous monitoring, are asymptomatic. Also remember that little correlation exists between the perceived frequency and severity of angina and the severity of angiographically documented coronary disease. For these reasons, even infrequent episodes of angina imply potentially serious disease, demanding a thorough evaluation.

Diagnostic Testing in Coronary Disease

The physical examination in a patient with chest pain may reveal evidence of atherosclerosis elsewhere in the vascular system or may identify cardiac abnormalities such as signs of cardiac enlargement, gallops, or accompanying valvular disease. The examination results in a patient with coronary disease, however, may be entirely normal. The resting ECG findings also may be normal, but should be obtained at baseline to identify the heart rhythm and assess for left ventricular hypertrophy or Q waves from prior MI. During angina, most patients have identifiable ischemic ST or T wave abnormalities that often normalize once the ischemia has resolved; the transient appearance of ST or T wave abnormalities during chest pain means that the pain is likely due to coronary ischemia.

The New York State Heart Association classification is a useful shorthand for describing the clinical status of a patient with chronic angina (Table 43-1).

Diagnostic testing is required in patients believed to have coronary disease to confirm or exclude the diagnosis and to better define the severity of the disease. In some contexts, the immediate referral of the patient to a cardiologist for angiography is appropriate. This is the case when the patient's symptoms appear to represent unstable angina. When it is unclear whether the patient has angina or if a patient's symptoms are chronic, stable, and mild, noninvasive diagnostic studies should be considered.

The most commonly used form of stress testing in the ambulatory patient is the exercise tolerance test. A standardized treadmill protocol is used, usually the Bruce protocol, which increases cardiac workload by adjusting the treadmill speed and incline (Table 43-2). Ischemic ST depression occurring with exercise, particularly when associated with typical symptoms, is strongly correlated with the presence of CAD. Patients with severe disease tend to have marked ST depression at fairly low levels of exercise. A drop in blood pressure or serious ventricular arrhythmias with exercise usually implies severe, often multivessel disease. Unfortunately, the treadmill test is not 100% accurate: the overall sensitivity rate for exercise testing in detecting CAD is about 60% to 70%, with a test specificity rate of about 75% to 90%. The accuracy of the test is much lower if the patient is unable to exercise to an age-defined target heart rate. The test also is less accurate if the resting ECG is abnormal such as in left ventricular hypertrophy or bundle branch blocks, or with a variety of medications such as digoxin, antidepressants, antiarrhythmics, or diuretics. Also, false-positive test results occur in patients with mitral valve prolapse and some healthy individuals have confounding ST abnormalities with hyperventilation. The statistical accuracy of stress testing also depends on the prevalence of the disease in the population being tested. This means that in young or middle-aged women, a negative stress test finding is reliable. However, a positive result on stress testing is likely to be false positive, since the prevalence of CAD is low in premenopausal women. Conversely, in postmenopausal cigarette smokers, a positive stress test finding is reliable, but the likelihood of a false-negative test result increases. These statistical realities mean that the stress test is only one tool in the total evaluation of a woman with possible heart disease. The stress test result must be interpreted in the total context of the patient's symptoms and risk factors. In women with significant risk factors and typical symptoms, the clinical information should not be totally abandoned in the face of a negative test result, nor should a positive test result in a premenopausal woman with atypical symptoms lead to a diagnosis of heart disease.

Stress testing is significantly less reliable in women than men due to the problem of false-positive test results in young women, and the difficulties older women may have in exercising to their target heart rate. Other imaging techniques known to improve the accuracy of stress testing can therefore be helpful. These include exercise radionuclide scans or stress echocardiography.

Exercise radionuclide testing is performed by intravenous (IV) injection of a radioisotope (generally thallium or sestamibi) during exercise. The radioisotope is taken up only by viable heart muscle

Table 43-1. New York State Heart Association Functional Classification of Angina

FUNCTIONAL CLASS	CLINICAL STATUS	APPROXIMATE EXERCISE TOLERANCE (METS)*
Class I	Symptoms with unusual activity, little impairment	7 METs or more
Class II	Symptoms with moderate activity, capable of light work	5–6 METs
Class III	Symptoms with daily activities, capable of sedentary work	3–4 METs
Class IV	Symptoms at rest, severely disabled	1–2 METs

*Physical work is often expressed in METs. 1 MET = 3.5 mL of oxygen uptake/kg body weight/min, and is the metabolic cost of standing quietly at rest.

Table 43-2. Bruce Treadmill Protocol: Three-Minute Stages

STAGE	SPEED (MPH)	GRADE (%)	WORKLOAD (METs)
1/2*	1.0	5	3
I	1.7	10	5
II	2.5	12	7
III	3.4	14	9
IV	4.2	16	13
V	5.0	18	16

*The standard Bruce protocol begins at stage I. However, the protocol is sometimes modified to start at a lower level of exercise for elderly patients or patients who have had a recent MI.

that is normally perfused. Gamma camera scans of the heart are made from several angles and then compared with resting images. Nonviable or scarred myocardium appear as a "cold" spot on the scan on both resting and exercise images. Ischemic myocardium is normal at rest but cold after exercise. The sensitivity rate of exercise radionuclide testing is about 80% to 90% with a specificity rate of about 80% to 90%. Radionuclide stress testing is equally accurate in men and women, as long as the interpreting radiologist is familiar with the sometimes confounding breast tissue artifacts on scan.

A more recent alternative to stress radioisotope testing is stress echocardiography. This test uses the occurrence of ischemic-induced left ventricular wall motion abnormalities by echo to detect coronary disease. Stress echocardiography is probably equivalent in sensitivity and specificity to radioisotope testing. Stress echo has some advantages in that no IV injections are required, and the test provides additional structural information about the heart, including chamber sizes and assessment of valve function. The echocardiogram may help to identify other potential sources of chest pain such as mitral valve prolapse, pericarditis, aortic stenosis, or hypertrophic cardiomyopathy.

For patients who cannot exercise on a treadmill, other forms of noninvasive testing can be used, including dipyridamole (Persantine) radionuclide scanning or dobutamine echocardiography. Dipyridamole given intravenously dilates normal coronary arteries but not stenotic vessels, so that disparities between normal and ischemic segments become apparent after radioisotope injection. Dipyridamole is contraindicated, however, in patients with a history of bronchospasm. During dobutamine echocardiography, insufficient left ventricular wall motion response to IV dobutamine allows identification of underperfused myocardium.

Remember that unstable angina is a contraindication to any form of stress testing because of the potential for precipitating an MI. Such patients generally require stabilization and evaluation in the hospital. Significant aortic stenosis and severe hypertension also are contraindications to exercise testing.

When coronary disease is likely, based on clinical presentation or stress testing, it is usually appropriate to refer the patient to a cardiologist for an initial evaluation. The cardiologist can help decide the need for coronary angiography and assist with formulation of a management strategy appropriate to the patient's age and general medical condition. Angiography is done to confirm the diagnosis, define the prognosis, and assess the need for interventions such as angioplasty or coronary bypass surgery. The decision to perform angiography is influenced by many factors, including the following: (1) the individual patient's lifestyle and activity level; (2) the patient's age and other medical problems; (3) the severity and stability of the angina; and (4) the likelihood of severe disease, specifically triple-vessel disease or disease of the left main coronary artery where bypass surgery is likely to improve longevity as well as symptoms. Since coronary angiography does carry some small risk (MI, stroke, arterial damage, allergic reactions, nephrotoxic dye effect, and, rarely, death) the benefit-to-risk ratio must be assessed for each patient. The primary care provider must communicate to the cardiologist information that may affect the aggressiveness of therapy. This includes the patient's other medical problems, the patient's activity level and lifestyle, and the patient's own wishes regarding therapy.

An accumulating and convincing body of evidence shows that there has in the past been a "gender gap" in the treatment of women with heart disease. This gap can be pinpointed to occur primarily as a bias in referral of women to coronary angiography after the confirmation of an abnormal noninvasive diagnostic test. Multiple studies show that fewer women are sent for cardiac catheterization after an abnormal stress test results compared with men. The reasons for this are uncertain, but some explanation lies in the fact that women develop coronary disease 7 to 10 years later than men and have other comorbid illnesses on presentation. However, there is concern that delays in referral for angiography, and, therefore, for balloon angioplasty or bypass surgery, may explain the known increased morbidity and mortality for these procedures in women compared with men. Statistics show that women often undergo cardiac surgery for an unstable or emergency condition, rather than more electively. This accounts, at least in part, for the 9% mortality rate in women for bypass surgery compared with the rate of about 4.5% for men. These observations should encourage primary caregivers to refer their female patients earlier to the consultant. Delaying to a time when the woman's disease may be more severe or unstable may put the patient at greater risk for complications during interventions.

Treatment of Angina

Treatment of chronic stable angina includes correction of risk factors, counseling and education of the patient, and antiangina medications.

Coronary risk factors should be identified and vigorously treated in the woman with angina. Cigarette cessation is imperative. Hypertension and diabetes should be well controlled, and a dietary regimen established to reach ideal weight. Cholesterol lowering probably decreases the risk of cardiovascular events in women with CAD, although clinical studies have disproportionately enrolled men. If the patient's HDL level is low, or if the LDL is higher than 100 to 130 mg/dL, a low-fat, low-cholesterol diet should be prescribed, with consideration of drug therapy if necessary to lower the LDL to less than 100 mg/dL. Estrogen improves the lipid profile and appears to decrease the risk of cardiovascular events in the postmenopausal woman with CAD. This beneficial effect is probably blunted but not eliminated by the addition of progesterone to the regimen.

Modification of work responsibilities and physical activities may be necessary. Patients need to recognize their ischemic symptoms and know to stop activities when angina occurs. Patients should avoid angina precipitants such as temperature extremes, large meals, emotional stresses, or heavy isometric exercise. Regular aerobic exercise should, however, be encouraged since physical conditioning may allow patients to be more active within the bounds of their anginal threshold. Exercise enhances collateral circulation development and is an adjunct to risk factor modification. Long-term commitment to an exercise program can be accomplished through a formal cardiac rehabilitation or by the patient at home with a physician's guidance. Limitations can be established based on symptoms and stress test results. The stress test provides a good objective measurement of the workload that a given patient can safely tolerate (see Table 43-2). The patient can monitor her own pulse during exercise and aim for a target heart rate. This target rate is equal to the resting heart rate added to 40% to 50% of the difference between the resting and peak heart rate achieved on formal exercise stress testing. Angina has a circadian pattern, so that the pace and nature of activities should be modified during early morning hours when angina is more likely to occur.

Women and their spouses are frequently concerned about the safety of maintaining an active sexual life. Sexual intercourse is generally not a problem if the patient can tolerate a flight of stairs or exercise to a heart rate of about 120. Nitroglycerin may be used prophylactically when the patient is concerned about an angina attack during sexual activity or before other activities that may cause angina.

If angina occurs, the patient should cease activity and take nitroglycerin for any symptoms persisting more than a minute. Women using nitroglycerin should know about the potential orthostatic blood pressure effects of nitroglycerin and about the benign but aggravating headaches that may accompany nitroglycerin use. Often patients are reluctant to take nitroglycerin if their symptoms are mild or if they are uncertain whether their discomfort is angina. It is important to stress that nitroglycerin is not just a pain reliever but actually improves coronary flow and cardiac hemodynamics. It is not "addictive," and there is no harm in using the pills, even if the symptoms are indeed noncardiac.

Nitroglycerin should be replaced with a fresh supply every 6 months to ensure potency. The tablets may be used sublingually every 5 minutes for chest discomfort, up to a total of three tablets. Patients should seek emergency room care for symptoms that persist after three nitroglycerin tablets. It is important to stress the benefit of early medical care in the event of a heart attack. Studies have suggested that, compared with men, women often delay seeking emergency care during an MI. This may explain why women are less likely to receive thrombolytic therapy, which requires early administration to be effective.

The psychosocial issues faced by the patient with heart disease are significant and must be addressed in the context of the patient's age, career, lifestyle, other medical problems, and family situation. A patient's reaction to her disease may include fear, depression, or anger. It is important to maintain effective ongoing communication to establish a realistic perspective for the patient and family.

Several classes of antiangina medications are used in long-term management, including aspirin, beta-blockers, calcium blockers, and nitrates (Table 43-3).

All patients with coronary disease, without a significant contraindication such as a true allergy, are treated with daily aspirin, 81 to 324 mg per day, as an antiplatelet agent. Enteric coated preparations may allow for fewer gastrointestinal side effects during long-term use. Beta-blockers are considered by most cardiologists to be first-line therapy for angina, except where their use is contraindicated because of severe asthma, significant bradycardia, or severe left ventricular dysfunction. In general, calcium blockers may be added to beta-blockers or substituted in patients in whom beta-blockers cannot be used. Calcium blockers should not be used if left ventricular function is abnormal, although some of the newer calcium blockers, specifically amlodipine, may not have the same negative inotropic effect as the other drugs in that class. Long-acting nitrate preparations come in several forms (oral, ointment, and patches); tachyphylaxis can occur unless an adequate nitrate-free interval is prescribed. Use of chronic nitrate preparations does not obviate the need for sublingual nitroglycerin during acute angina attacks.

The choice of antiangina medications is largely determined by the existence of other medical indications for a specific type of drug, as well as the side effect profiles and contraindications for a given patient (Table 43-3).

Table 43-3. Antianginal Medications for Chronic Angina

MEDICATION CLASS	MODE OF ACTION	OTHER BENEFITS	SIDE EFFECTS
Aspirin	Antiplatelet agent to reduce risk of intracoronary clot and MI	Decrease in neurologic events with carotid disease. Reduces risk of recurrent MI.	GI side effects and bleeding
Beta-blockers, e.g., metoprolol, atenolol, propranolol, nadolol	Decrease cardiac workload by decreasing HR, BP, and contractility during exercise	Post-MI decreases risk of recurrent MI and death; antiarrhythmic and antihypertensive	Negative inotropic effect may worsen CHF if LV function is poor; may cause bronchospasm with lung disease; can cause fatigue, bradycardia, depression, and can worsen claudication; can mask hypoglycemia in diabetics
Calcium blockers, e.g., diltiazem, verapamil, amlodipine, nifedipine	Decrease myocardial oxygen demand; increase coronary flow by vasodilatation	Antihypertensives; some (verapamil and diltiazem) are used for supraventricular arrhythmias	Hypotension; worsening CHF (should not be used if serious LV dysfunction); bradycardia with verapamil and diltiazem; constipation, flushing and peripheral edema
Long-acting nitrates, e.g., isosorbide dinitrate or isosorbide mononitrate po, or transdermal nitroglycerin patches	Vasodilators; prevent coronary spasm; increase collateral and subendocardial flow; decrease venous return to lower intracardiac pressures	May help CHF symptoms by lowering intracardiac pressures	Headache, postural hypotension; tachyphylaxis can occur, therefore must have a nitrate-free interval

Unstable angina, as defined previously, is treated as a potentially impending MI and usually requires hospitalization for urgent evaluation and aggressive therapy. Underlying precipitating or aggravating factors such as anemia, tachyarrhythmias, infection, heart failure, hypoxia, or hyperthyroidism require correction. Bed rest with telemetry rhythm monitoring is appropriate, and IV nitroglycerin helps with pain relief. Only IV heparin and aspirin have been proven to decrease both mortality and morbidity in unstable angina. This is consistent with the known pathogenetic role of partial or intermittent intracoronary clot in unstable angina. Lacking contraindications, heparin and aspirin often are prescribed concurrently with appropriate monitoring for bleeding complications. Consideration should be given to coronary angiography in patients with unstable angina, with the timing dictated by the patient's clinical course.

MYOCARDIAL INFARCTION

A MI usually occurs due to clot formation at the site of intracoronary atherosclerotic plaque; vasospasm and coronary emboli are rare causes. Thrombus formation occurs due to plaque rupture (resulting in exposed collagen and platelet adhesion), or due to subintimal plaque hemorrhage with eventual stasis. When intracoronary clot occludes an artery, the myocardium supplied by that artery receives little or no blood flow and is damaged. The amount of permanent myocardial injury depends on many factors but can be limited if coronary flow can be reestablished quickly to that region.

The care of the woman with an MI is often complicated and intensive. Decisions regarding initial therapy, management of complications, and decisions regarding post-MI risk stratification usually require the input of a cardiologist.

Diagnosis of Acute MI

The history and physical in a patient presenting with possible MI should be abbreviated, since the earlier the therapy, as measured in minutes, the better the survival rate. The classic MI is described as chest pressure or pain, sometimes radiating to the left arm or neck, and often accompanied by diaphoresis, nausea, and a sensation of impending doom. Unfortunately, some patients present with less typical pain, and silent unrecognized MIs are not rare. In the emergency room, the patient's risk factors for coronary disease are an important part of the history; chest pain in a postmenopausal cigarette smoker would be more likely to be cardiac than in a premenopausal woman without other risks. Besides musculoskeletal and gastrointestinal causes of chest pain, the history taking also should address the possibility of other causes for chest pain, including pulmonary embolus, pericarditis, and aortic dissection.

The physical examination findings in acute MI may be normal, especially if the infarct is small. In other cases, signs of hemodynamic instability may be present such as hypotension, bradycardia, tachycardia, ventricular gallops, rales, or murmurs (due to papillary muscle dysfunction causing mitral regurgitation or due to an infarct-related ventricular septal defect). The physical also should be focused to assess the possibility of the other causes of chest pain noted earlier. Does the patient have a rub suggesting pericarditis? Is there a differential in arm blood pressures suggesting the possibility of aortic dissection?

Simultaneous to beginning a short history and physical examination on the patient, an ECG should be recorded. The presence of significant convex ST elevation in two or more contiguous leads is consistent with an acute MI. ST elevation in leads II, III, and aVF, often with reciprocal ST depression in the precordial leads, indicates an inferior infarct, usually due to occlusion of the right coronary artery. ST elevation in the precordial leads generally is seen with occlusion of the left anterior descending artery, resulting in an anterior MI. Occlusion of the circumflex artery may be more subtle electrocardiographically; ST elevation may occur in leads I and aVL, or in leads II, III, and aVF. ST depression may represent ischemia or a subendocardial infarction, or if localized to the pre-

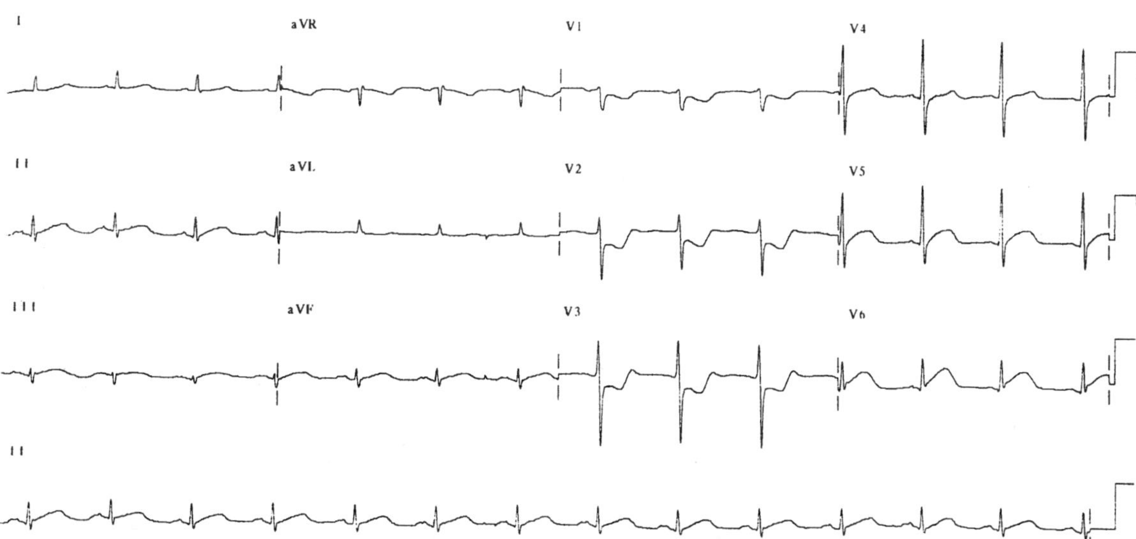

Figure 43-1. Electrocardiogram in a 63-year-old postmenopausal cigarette smoker with a history of hypertension and high cholesterol. Patient presented with ventricular fibrillation from which she was successfully cardioverted. There is ST elevation in leads V4–V6, with slight elevation in leads II, III, and aVF, and ST depression in leads V1–V3, consistent with an acute inferolateral MI. Catherization showed disease in the circumflex artery.

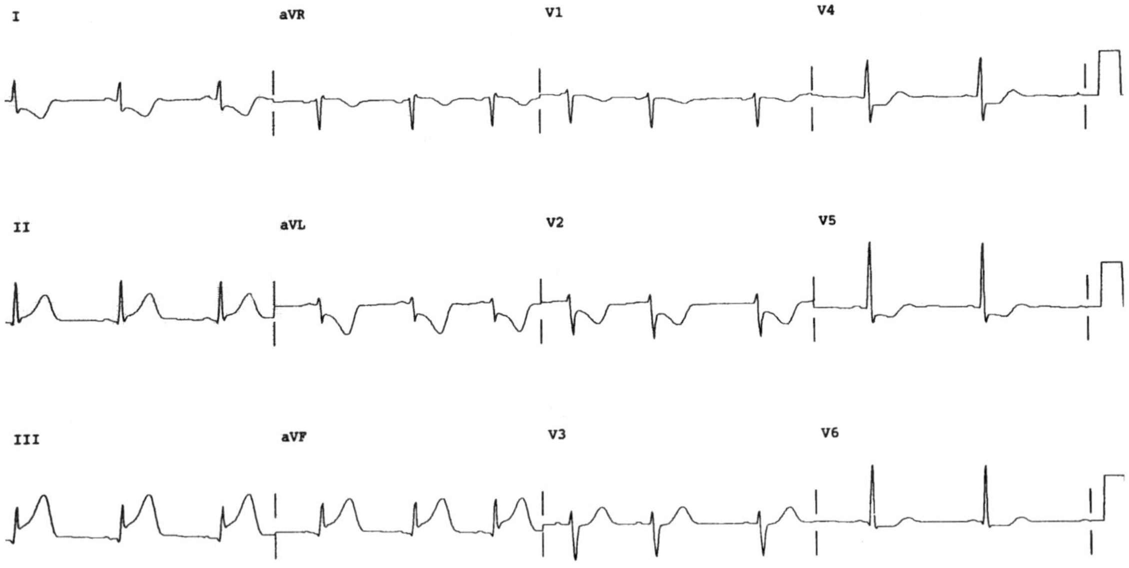

Figure 43-2. Electrocardiogram in a 35-year-old woman who was a long-standing heavy cigarette smoker on birth control pills, with high cholesterol and a family history of premature coronary disease. Electrocardiogram shows ST elevation in leads II, III, and aVF with reciprocal depression in leads I, aVL, and V2, diagnostic of an acute inferior wall MI. At cardiac catherization, patient had a right coronary artery stenosis.

cordial leads, could represent a true posterior MI. ST depression is less specific than ST elevation and can, in fact, occur with other conditions such as left ventricular hypertrophy, electrolyte abnormalities, or certain drugs (Figs. 43-1 through 43-3).

If the ECG in a patient with suspected MI is nondiagnostic, repeat tracings should be obtained every 10 or 15 minutes, since diagnostic changes may become apparent with time.

An acute MI is confirmed on blood sampling by demonstration of the classic pattern of cardiac enzyme evolution. However, therapy usually precedes laboratory confirmation because of the time delay inherent in awaiting results and the necessity for expedient treatment. A cardiac subtype of creatine kinase isoenzyme, CK-MB, is present in myocardium and can be detected by blood test, with blood levels usually peaking at 10 to 18 hours after coronary occlusion. Early in the course of an MI, CK-MB levels still may be normal; blood levels are usually obtained every 6 to 8 hours for the first 24 to 48 hours after presentation with chest pain. The absolute CK-MB levels do not always correlate with the ultimate size of the MI for various reasons. Reestablishment of coronary artery patency can result in early peaking high CK-MB values due to a washout phenomenon, without necessarily implying a large amount of permanent myocardial damage.

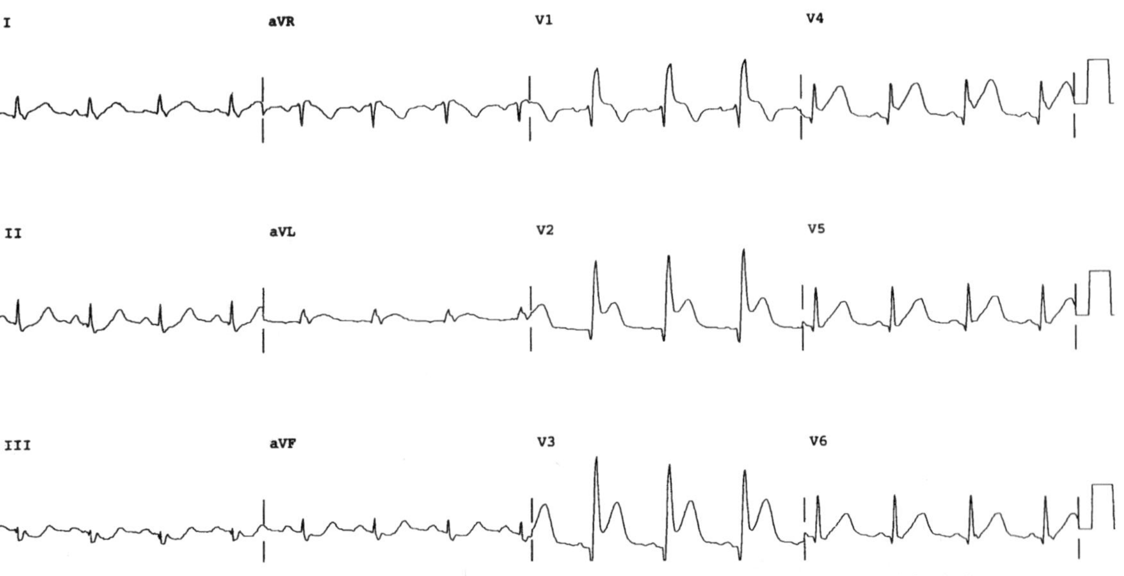

Figure 43-3. Electrocardiogram in a 53-year-old postmenopausal smoker who had a high cholesterol level. Note ST elevation in leads V1 through V5 with mild reciprocal ST depression in leads II, III, and aVF, diagnostic of an acute anterior wall MI. A right bundle branch block is also noted. At coronary angiography, patient had a stenosis in the left anterior descending artery.

Treatment of Acute MI

Because occlusive intracoronary thrombus is usually the cause of an acute MI, it follows that the key to effective treatment is thrombolytic therapy. All patients having a MI should be considered for "clot-busting" enzyme therapy, usually with tissue plasminogen activator or sometimes with streptokinase. Thrombolytic therapy has been shown to limit the size of the MI and reduce MI mortality by about 30%. The faster that the clot can be lysed, the sooner arterial patency is reestablished and the less is the potential for irreversible myocardial damage. This means that the earlier the drug is given, the greater the benefit on left ventricular function and mortality. The likelihood of myocardial salvage during an MI declines during every minute that arterial occlusion persists, so that ideally thrombolytic therapy should be given immediately. Practically speaking, due to delays in patient presentation and time needed to diagnosis, the goal is to begin thrombolytic therapy within 4 to 6 hours after the onset of an MI. Some degree of survival benefit can be demonstrated, however, even up to 12 hours after the onset of the MI.

Because of the risk of serious bleeding, there are several contraindications to thrombolytic therapy, including the following:

- Active bleeding
- Suspected aortic dissection
- Significant trauma or surgery within the preceding 2 weeks
- Pregnancy
- Recent head trauma or known intracranial tumor
- Prolonged or traumatic cardiopulmonary resuscitation
- Hemorrhagic retinopathy
- History of stroke or transient ischemic attack
- Persistent hypertension with systolic blood pressure greater than 180 mm Hg.
- Menstrual bleeding does not appear to be a contraindication to thrombolytic therapy.

Intracranial bleeding, the most dreaded complication of lytic therapy, is somewhat more likely to occur in women. This may be due to lower body weight, and dosing of thrombolytic medication should be modified by weight following the manufacturer's package insert. The incidence rate of intracranial bleeding in women is about 0.1% and is still statistically outweighed by the dramatic reduction in MI mortality with lytic therapy. Patients who have contraindications to thrombolytic therapy should be considered for emergency balloon angioplasty to open the occluded artery where these facilities are available. Emergency angiography has become a more commonly used alternative to thrombolytic therapy for acute MI. "Primary angioplasty" has been advocated not only in situations where thrombolytic therapy may be contraindicated, but preferentially in some patients with large infarcts.

Adjunctive Therapy in Acute MI

Several other medications are adjuncts to thrombolytic therapy in the patient with acute MI. Some are used fairly routinely whereas others must be individualized, depending on the patient's hemodynamic status. These drugs also are crucial in patients with an MI who are not candidates for thrombolytic therapy or where diagnosis has been confirmed too late for reperfusion therapy with lytic drugs or angioplasty. Table 43-4 describes these classes of drugs, their benefit in acute MI, and potential side effects.

Table 43-4. Adjunctive Therapies in Acute Myocardial Infarction

THERAPY	COMMONLY USED DOSES	BENEFITS	CAUTIONS AND COMMENTS
Aspirin	160–324 mg po given with lytic therapy, then qd	Improved mortality (alone or with lytic therapy); prevention of rethrombosis and recurrent MI	Contraindicated if true aspirin allergy; can cause bleeding and GI side effects
Oxygen	2–4 L/min; need to monitor oxygen sats and increase if needed in CHF	Improved oxygenation, esp in CHF	Caution in patients with COPD, who can develop carbon dioxide retention
Nitroglycerin	Initially given in sublingual form, then in IV form starting at 5 μg/min	Increases venous capacitance to lower intracardiac pressures; coronary vasodilatation; may be esp useful for CHF or hypertension	IV dosage rate is adjusted according to BP and pain relief
Morphine	2–5 mg IV q 5–30 min	Anxiolytic and analgesic; decreases preload and afterload and thereby decreases myocardial oxygen consumption; good in CHF	Caution to avoid respiratory depression and hypotension
Beta-blockers (metoprolol)	5 mg IV q 5 min for 3 doses, then 50 mg po q 6 h for 48 h, then 100 mg po bid	Reduce long-term mortality after MI and may reduce acute mortality when used with lytic drugs; reduce reinfarction incidence; reduce HR and cardiac oxygen consumption; may have antiarrhythmic effect	Contraindicated if hypotension, bradycardia, heart block, or severe LV dysfunction
IV heparin	In conjunction with lytic drug, bolus with 5000–10,000 U then start IV drip at 800–1000 U/h; titrate to APTT of 60–80 s; continue for about 48 h	Helps prevent coronary reocclusion; in cases of large, usually anterior MIs, helps prevent LV clot	Usual bleeding precautions; must monitor for thrombocytopenia; in case of large anterior MIs, coumadin is indicated for 4–6 mo after heparin is stopped to prevent LV clot
ACE inhibitors (eg, captopril, enalapril, lisinopril)	Depends on patients BP and EF; if BP is low in patient with poor EF, start at low doses.	Started within 24 h after MI, appears to reduce mortality. After MI, prevents LV expansion and dilatation, especially with anterior infarcts and severe LV dysfunction. Reduces afterload to treat CHF.	Must avoid hypotension, monitor renal function and potassium. Cough is a common but non-serious side effect.

APTT, activated partial thromboplastin time; *ACE,* angiotensin converting enzyme; *EF,* ejection traction; *sats,* saturation levels.

Complications of Acute MI

Potential complications in the patient with an MI include persistence of coronary occlusion after lytic therapy, cardiogenic shock, congestive heart failure, aneurysm formation, pericarditis, arrhythmias, and shock.

Inability to Establish Coronary Patency

It is not always possible clinically to be sure whether thrombolytic therapy has effected coronary artery patency. However, the presence of ongoing chest pain, persistence of ST elevation, or hemodynamic instability at 90 minutes or more after administration of a thrombolytic agent suggests that arterial occlusion persists. This scenario should prompt consideration for "rescue" angioplasty. If the culprit artery causing the MI is demonstrated in the catheterization laboratory to be occluded, emergency angioplasty can be performed to limit infarct size by opening the artery.

Cardiogenic Shock

Cardiogenic shock, defined as persistent hypotension and poor cardiac output despite adequate intravascular volume, confers a poor prognosis. Even with thrombolytic therapy, the mortality rate may be 80% to 90%. This patient subgroup seems to have a better survival if treated with immediate "first-line" angioplasty instead of lytic therapy. These patients require placement of an intraaortic balloon pump in the thoracic aorta, which inflates in diastole to augment coronary perfusion and deflates in systole to decrease afterload and augment forward cardiac output. Right heart catheterization with a Swan-Ganz catheter allows for optimization of intracardiac filling pressures to maximize cardiac output and improve pulmonary edema. An infarct of the right ventricle, which can occur in conjunction with an inferior MI, may be diagnosed when right-sided pressures are high with a low cardiac output. A patient in shock with a heart murmur may have an acute ventricular septal defect, or rupture of a papillary muscle causing acute mitral regurgitation. The Swan-Ganz catheter or echocardiography can confirm these diagnoses, which require surgical repair.

Hospitals without facilities to perform invasive procedures in the patient with shock must consider emergency air transport of their patients to tertiary centers.

Congestive Heart Failure

Congestive heart failure of varying severity is a common complication in the patient with acute MI. Congestive heart failure can occur due to poor systolic pumping function of the heart or can be due to myocardial "stiffness" as a result of ischemia. Diuretics and oxygen are the mainstays of therapy, with morphine intravenously if pulmonary edema is severe. Prescription of longer term therapy for congestive heart failure after an MI is determined by the predischarge evaluation of systolic function by catheterization or echocardiography. If pumping (systolic) function is poor, as defined by a low ejection fraction, then angiotensin converting enzyme inhibitors and diuretics are appropriate. Digoxin is sometimes used as an inotrope.

Aneurysms

Aneurysm formation is another potential complication of MI. Left ventricular aneurysms occur most commonly after anterior MI; a large area of scarred myocardium becomes permanently dyskinetic. Left ventricular clot is common with aneurysm formation, and anticoagulants are therefore indicated. Ventricular arrhythmias and congestive heart failure are common accompaniments of left ventricular aneurysms, but rupture does not occur. This is in contrast to the so-called "false" aneurysm in which spontaneous rupture is a high likelihood. False aneurysms, in fact, represent a subacute tear in the myocardium and temporary walling-off of the hemorrhage by the pericardial sac. These false aneurysms must be treated as surgical emergencies.

Pericarditis

Pericarditis can occur 12 hours to 10 days after an MI and often manifests as chest pain that is worsened by deep inspiration or the supine position, associated with a pericardial rub on examination. Frequently, a pericardial effusion is seen by echocardiography. Heparin or lytic therapy may increase the risk of bleeding into the pericardium and resultant tamponade, and should therefore be used with caution, if at all, when pericarditis is present. The chest pain accompanying pericarditis usually responds dramatically to nonsteroidal antiinflammatory drugs.

Arrhythmias

A variety of rhythm disturbances including bradycardias, tachycardias, and heart block complicate acute MI. The decline in MI mortality over the last several decades is largely due to recognition and treatment of potentially fatal arrhythmias. In general, MI patients must have continual heart rhythm monitoring for at least 48 hours, with longer requirements when the MI has been large or associated with hemodynamic instability. Ventricular fibrillation, which is fatal without immediate DC cardioversion, is most likely to occur within the first few hours of an MI, with declining likelihood thereafter. Ventricular fibrillation in the setting of an MI can occur with a small MI, and therefore does not carry implications for long-term prognosis. IV lidocaine is commonly prescribed for patients who have had ventricular fibrillation or serious ventricular arrhythmias. Because lidocaine does have potential serious side effects and because a survival advantage has not been shown, lidocaine generally is not given prophylactically or for isolated premature ventricular contractions.

Sinus bradycardias are particularly common with inferior infarctions because of increased vagal tone. These require treatment only if associated with hypotension, and IV atropine usually is effective.

Some form of atrioventricular block occurs in about 20% of patients with acute MI. Prolongation of the PR interval or first-degree heart block requires no therapy. There are two types of second-degree heart block: type I (Wenckebach) and type II. Wenckbach is manifest on ECG as progressive PR prolongation followed by a nonconducted P wave and is common with inferior infarcts. This is usually transient and resolves spontaneously. Mobitz type II heart block is more ominous, often a manifestation of a large amount of myocardial damage in the setting of an anterior infarct. Placement of a temporary pacemaker usually is indicated. Third-degree or complete heart block is manifest on ECG as dissociation between P waves and the QRS complex. The QRS complex generally is wide with a slow rate, representing a ventricular escape rhythm. When occurring during an inferior MI, complete heart block usually is well tolerated and generally resolves spontaneously. Recovery may take up to 2 weeks, however. Third-degree heart block, which occurs in the setting of an anterior MI, however, is more serious. Third-degree heart block with an anterior MI usually implies a large amount of myocardial damage and often does not resolve, necessitating a permanent pacemaker.

Bundle branch blocks occurring with an MI may require temporary pacing; this is especially true for left bundle branch blocks and bifascicular blocks (right bundle branch block with left anterior hemiblock), where progression to complete heart block is more likely to occur.

Supraventricular arrhythmias (paroxysmal supraventricular tachycardia, atrial fibrillation, or atrial flutter) that occur with an acute MI may be related to hemodynamic instability with severe left ventricular dysfunction and congestive heart failure, or may be a consequence of electrolyte imbalance, pericarditis, or atrial ischemia. Since tachycardias may lead to extension of infarct size due to increased cardiac work, timely treatment is imperative. Adenosine can be used to treat paroxysmal supraventricular tachycardia. For atrial fibrillation or flutter, short-acting IV beta-blockers such as esmolol or IV calcium blockers such as diltiazem can be used for rate control, but consideration should be given to electrical cardioversion (or overdrive pacing in the case of atrial flutter) for more prompt restoration of normal rhythm. This is especially true if the patient is hemodynamically unstable.

Hospital Convalescence and Post-MI Evaluation

The greatest mortality and morbidity risk in the hospital is immediately after the MI; therefore, the patient is monitored in a coronary care unit for 48 to 72 hours, with marked curtailment of physical activity for the first day or two. Thereafter, the patient can begin gradual ambulation if she has no evidence of congestive heart failure or recurrent ischemia.

Statistically, patients who appear to be at highest risk for recurrent MI or death in the year after an MI are those who either have evidence for severe left ventricular dysfunction with a low ejection fraction, or those who have evidence of ongoing ischemia, that is, residual viable myocardium that is in jeopardy. Recurrent angina, congestive heart failure, or hemodynamic instability therefore should prompt consideration for early angiography to assess the appropriateness of revascularization by angioplasty or bypass surgery. In the patient with an uneventful recovery, noninvasive evaluation is performed to identify patients at highest risk who should then go on to angiography. This evaluation generally includes an echocardiogram to assess systolic function and noninvasive stress testing in the stable patient at 7 to 10 days after the MI to identify provokable ischemia. This is usually accomplished with a "low-level" treadmill test. Radionuclide scans with dipyridamole or dobutamine echocardiography are techniques used to identify ischemia in the patient who is unable to exercise. Most patients who reperfuse with thrombolytic therapy during their MI

Table 43-5. Estimates of Energy Requirements of Avocational and Occupational Tasks

CATEGORY	SELE-CARE OR HOME	OCCUPATIONAL	RECREATIONAL	PHYSICAL CONDITIONING
Very light				
< 3 METs < 10 mL/kg/min < 4 kcal	Washing, shaving, dressing, desk work, writing, washing dishes, driving auto	Sitting (clerical, assembly), standing (store clerk, bartender), driving truck, operating crane	Shuffleboard, horseshoes, bait casting, billiards, archery, golf (cart)	Walking (2 mph), stationary bicycle (very low resistance), very light calisthenics
Light				
3–5 METs 11–18 mL/kg/min 4–6 kcal	Cleaning windows, raking leaves, weeding, power lawn mowing, waxing floors (slowly), painting, carrying objects (6.8–13.5 kg [15–30 lb])	Stocking shelves (light objects), light welding, light carpentry, machine assembly, auto repair, paper hanging	Dancing (social and square), golf (walking), sailing, horseback riding, volleyball (6 man), tennis (doubles)	Walking (3–4 mph), level bicycling (6–8 mph), light calisthenics
Moderate				
5–7 METs 18–25 mL/kg/min 6–8 kcal	Easy digging in garden, level lawn mowing, climbing stairs (slowly), carrying objects (13.5–27 kg [30–60 lb])	Carpentry (exterior home building), shovelling dirt, using pneumatic tools	Badminton (competitive), tennis (singles), snow skiing (downhill), light backpacking, basketball, skating (ice and roller), horseback riding (gallop)	Walking (4.5–5 mph), bicycling (9–10 mph), swimming (breast stroke)
Heavy				
7–9 METs 25–32 mL/kg/min 8–10 kcal	Sawing wood, heavy shoveling, climbing stairs (moderate speed), carrying objects (27–40.5 kg [60–90 lb])	Tending furnace, digging ditches, pick and shovel	Canoeing, mountain climbing, fencing, paddleball, touch football	Jog (5 mph), swim (crawl stroke), rowing machine, heavy calisthenics, bicycling (12 mph)
Very heavy				
> 9 METs > 32 mL/kg/min > 10 kca	Carrying loads upstairs, carrying objects (> 40.5 kg [90 lb]), climbing stairs (quickly), shoveling heavy snow, shoveling 10 min (7.2 kg [16 lb])	Lumberjack, heavy laborer	Handball, squash, ski touring over hills, vigorous basketball	Running (≥ 6 mph), bicycle (≥ 13 mph or up steep hills), rope jumping

(From Haskell WL. Design and implementation of cardiac conditioning programs. In: Wenger NK, Hellerstein HF, eds. Rehabilitation of the coronary patient. New York: John Wiley & Sons, 1978:214.)

have an underlying critical coronary artery stenosis. If this artery is supplying viable but jeopardized heart muscle, then consideration must be given to revascularization.

Patients with small infarcts and no evidence for ongoing ischemia often have sustained an infarct due to thrombotic occlusion at the site of a mild coronary stenosis. These patients should be treated with aspirin and perhaps beta-blockers; repeat stress testing with a standard protocol is recommended at 4 to 8 weeks after the MI to reevaluate for evidence of any ongoing ischemia at higher work levels.

The rehabilitation of post-MI women must address psychosocial adjustment, risk factor modification for secondary prevention, and physical reconditioning. These issues should start to be discussed before discharge from the hospital, with ongoing assessment and education of the patient during the ensuing 3 to 4 months. Smoking, physical inactivity, hyperlipidemia, and lack of estrogen increase the risk of accelerated atherosclerosis. Patients should be strongly advised to discontinue smoking, which is known to increase mortality after MI. Women with low HDL cholesterol levels or LDL levels higher than 130 mg/dL should be counselled on a low fat, low cholesterol diet, and plans should be made for long-term cholesterol follow-up to ascertain need for lipid-lowering drugs. Unless contraindicated, estrogen replacement should be considered in the postmenopausal patient with a history of coronary disease, based on the mortality data from population studies and known beneficial effect on the lipid profile. Patients should be encouraged to enroll in cardiac rehabilitation programs where available. These programs are designed to individualize exercise regimens for the post-MI patient to facilitate attainment of maximal functional capacity, as guided by the patients's baseline exercise test results, known medical history, and monitored progress in the program. Cardiac rehabilitation programs also provide patient education on risk factors and psychosocial support. Where formal programs are not available, MET equivalent charts (Table 43-5 can assist the physician in advising activity parameters based on the work level attained on the post-MI stress test.

The emotional stress of an MI on the patient and her family can be great. Disbelief, denial, fear, depression, anxiety, and sometimes anger are common responses to a life-threatening medical event. Education, reassurance, and early enrollment in a cardiac exercise program can help the patient return to as full a lifestyle as possible, but patients need support in dealing with restrictions, changing their lifestyles, and gaining confidence. Women often have nurturing roles within their immediate and extended family structures, and the changes within the family dynamics during a woman's convalescence may add to the stresses. Family members may be fearful and therefore overprotective, or, on the other hand, may use denial to handle their fears. Most cardiac rehabilitation programs actively involve the patient's family to reassure and educate them as well as the patient. Also remember that women, because they tend to present with MIs at an older age, may live alone and have less family support locally available. Return-to-work questions also must be addressed. These issues must be individualized, based on the woman's occupation and medical condition.

Reassurance, education, and encouragement of physical reconditioning over time can restore the patient's sense of well- being, confidence, and self-worth after an emotionally cataclysmic event such as a heart attack, and deserve the health care team's ongoing efforts.

BIBLIOGRAPHY

ACC/AHA Task Force. ACC/AHA guidelines for the early management of patients with acute myocardial infarction. Circulation 1990;82:664.

Braunwald E. Heart disease: a textbook of cardiovascular medicine. Philadelphia: WB Saunders, 1992:1106.

Braunwald E, Mark DB, Jones RH, et al. Diagnosing and managing unstable angina: quick reference guide for clinicians, no. 10, AHCPR publication no. 94-0603. Rockville, MD: U.S. Department of Health and Human Services, Public Health Service, Agency for Health Care Policy and Research and National Heart, Lung, and Blood Institute, 1994.

Schlant R, Alexander RW, O'Rourke RA, Roberts R, Sonnenblick EH. Hurst's the heart. New York: McGraw Hill, 1994:973.

Thompson M, Ross A. Acute myocardial infarction. In: Conn HF, ed. Conn's Current Therapy. Philadelphia: WB Saunders, 1994:295.

Wenger N, Speroff L, Packard B. Cardiovascular health and disease in women (proceedings of a NHLBI conference). Greenwich, CT: LeJacq Communications, 1993:61.

Primary Care for Women, edited by Phyllis C. Leppert and Fred M. Howard. Lippincott-Raven Publishers, Philadelphia © 1997.

44
Peripheral Vascular Disease

CYNTHIA K. SHORTELL

Peripheral vascular disease encompasses disorders of the arterial, venous, and lymphatic systems. The incidence and manifestations of these disorders frequently differ according to gender. Some vascular diseases, such as atherosclerosis obliterans, have affected predominantly males in the past, but with the increase of smoking and stressful lifestyles these disease have become more prevalent in women. Other diseases, such as aneurysm formation, are more common in men than women for unknown reasons. Finally, some disorders, such as thromboangiitis obliterans and Takayasu disease, are seen virtually exclusively in one sex or the other. This chapter provides an overview of peripheral vascular diseases, as well as elucidating those aspects of disorders that are unique to women.

BASIC CONSIDERATIONS

Clinical Evaluation of the Patient with Vascular Disease

The object of the vascular history is to determine if the patient has a disorder of the arterial, venous, or lymphatic system. A history of intermittent claudication of the upper or lower extremity is suggested by the presence of crampy pain with a fixed degree of exertion, such as walking two blocks. The discomfort is located just distal to the level of the arterial occlusion; thus, calf cramps suggest disease in the superficial femoral artery. Cramps in the absence of exertion are not likely to be vascular in etiology. More severe degrees of ischemia result in rest pain, characteristically affecting the toes or instep and relieved by dependency. The sudden onset of pain is suggestive of acute arterial occlusion. True ischemic rest pain must be distinguished from other pain syndromes, such as diabetic neuropathy, in which the patient typically experiences burning on the plantar surface of the foot. Finally, the patient should be questioned regarding the presence of nonhealing sores or ulcers, and the location of these lesions determined; lesions of the toes and feet suggest arterial disease, whereas perimalleolar lesions suggest a venous etiology. If aneurysmal disease is suspected, the patient should be questioned for a history of abdominal, back, and flank pain, as well as the presence of "blue toes," suggestive of embolic events.

Symptoms of atherosclerotic cerebrovascular disease include the classic hemispheric complaints of transient monocular blindness (amaurosis fugax), hemiparesis or hemiparesthesia, dysphasia, and dysarthria, as well as nonhemispheric symptoms such as blurred vision, ataxia, and syncope.

Patients with venous disorders may present with acute or chronic complaints. The sudden onset of pain, swelling, and cyanosis of an extremity is highly suggestive of deep venous thrombosis. Patients with varicose veins should be questioned regarding the presence of pain, rupture, and superficial phlebitis. Chronic venous insufficiency is characterized by skin pigmentation, edema, and chronic ulceration.

Physical examination of the patient with vascular disease begins with observation of the skin, noting the presence of pallor, dependent rubor, and digital ulceration suggestive of arterial disease, as well as cyanosis, pigmentation, swelling, and malleolar ulceration suggestive of venous disorders. Isolated, painful blue toes indicate an embolic process. Auscultation for bruits over the aorta and its major branches may suggest areas of disease, but are not diagnostic of the presence of stenosis. The patient should next be examined for the presence of all pulses, which should be graded from 1+ to 4+, indicating a diminished-to-aneurysmal quality. Aneurysms of the aorta and popliteal arteries are detected by palpation of the epigastrium and popliteal fossa, respectively.

Noninvasive and Invasive Evaluation of the Vascular System

If vascular disease is suspected on the basis of the history and the physical, noninvasive vascular screening is indicated. Segmental measurement of the blood pressure in the lower extremity provides information regarding the location and severity of arterial disease; a drop in pressure is indicative of occlusive disease proximal to the level of measurement. Duplex evaluation of the carotid arteries and venous systems can determine the presence of a stenosis or valvular incompetency, respectively, with a very high degree of accuracy. Ultrasound is used to identify and quantify aneurysmal changes, usually involving the abdominal aorta. Arteriography is usually reserved for patients in whom operative intervention is planned, as it confers the added risk of arterial puncture and contrast administration.

ARTERIAL DISEASES

Associated Conditions

Patients with significant peripheral vascular disease are rarely without associated medical conditions. Some of these disorders, such as hypertension, tobacco abuse, and diabetes, are etiologic factors associated with atherosclerosis obliterans, while other disorders have a shared etiology with atherosclerosis (eg, coronary artery disease and chronic obstructive pulmonary disease). These concomitant disease processes are significant because they influence the management of patients with peripheral vascular disease. Individuals with severe underlying medical conditions such as coronary artery disease may pose an unacceptable operative risk, precluding consideration for elective procedures such as revascularization for claudication. Alternatively, underlying disease may require additional medical or surgical therapy (eg, coronary artery bypass grafting) before proceeding with nonelective surgery such as repair of a large abdominal aortic aneurysm. Finally, in elderly or terminally ill patients, it may be determined that the patient is likely to die of other underlying medical conditions before succumbing to her vascular problem, rendering intervention by the vascular surgeon futile.

All patients in whom major operative intervention is being considered should be screened for coronary artery disease, even those who are asymptomatic. The most appropriate screening test has not yet been established, but dipyridamole thallium and dobutamine stress echocardiogram have both been successfully employed. Pulmonary function tests should be obtained in all smokers.

Aortoiliac and Lower Extremity Occlusive Disease

The incidence of lower extremity peripheral vascular disease is estimated at 1.5% of all women under the age of 59 years and 5% of all women over the age of 60 years. Of these individuals, 25% will require revascularization and 5% will eventually undergo amputation. Small artery syndrome is a variant of atherosclerotic occlusive disease seen exclusively in slightly built women with a heavy smoking history. These patients experience premature disease onset and an accelerated course, and should be treated aggressively with operative intervention and smoking cessation.

The most common presenting symptom of lower extremity occlusive disease is intermittent claudication. Patients experience cramping pain involving the muscle groups immediately distal to the obstructed arterial segment; thus, thigh and calf claudication are typically experienced by patients with iliac and superficial femoral artery occlusions, respectively. Symptoms are highly reproducible and consistent with respect to walking distance in a given individual. Night cramping is typically seen in elderly and pregnant women and may be due to a variety of factors, but is not vascular in origin. Other conditions involving the lower extremity that are frequently confused with arterial occlusive disease include lumbar disc disease and spinal stenosis. The differential diagnosis is primarily based on a careful history, as older patients may have objective evidence of both disease processes. The major differences between true claudication and pseudoclaudication are outlined in Table 44-1.

Rest pain is the next clinical step in the progression of lower extremity occlusive disease. The pain is characteristically located in the toes, forefoot, and instep, and may awaken the patient at night. Relief is obtained by dangling the feet or walking briefly. Symptoms of this severity usually require occlusive lesions involving two or more arterial segments. The differential diagnosis includes diabetic neuropathy, in which patients experience burning pain in the soles of the feet which is unrelieved by dependency and is often in the presence of normal pedal pulses. Ischemic ulceration

Table 44-1. Claudication Versus Pseudoclaudication

	INTERMITTENT CLAUDICATION	PSEUDOCLAUDICATION
Symptoms	Cramping pain	Paresthesias, weakness, radicular pain
Location	Buttock, thigh, calf	Buttock, thigh, calf
Symptomatic occurrence	With walking only (exercise)	Walking, sitting, standing
Symptomatic relief	Stop walking	Change position

and gangrene represent the ultimate progression of peripheral vascular disease. Lesions are typically found at the tips of toes or over pressure points (such as the metatarsal heads) in contrast to venous ulcerations, which are pretibial or perimalleolar.

If lower extremity occlusive disease is suspected on the basis of the history and the physical, the patient is referred for arterial noninvasive evaluation, with segmental blood pressure recordings at the high thigh, low thigh, calf, and ankle levels. The ratio between the highest brachial pressure and the ankle pressure is referred to as the ankle-brachial index (ABI), and is 1.0 or slightly higher in normal individuals. Claudicants and patients with single level disease usually have an ABI between 0.5 and 0.75, while patients with rest pain and ulceration will usually have an ABI between 0 and 0.3.

The treatment of intermittent claudication due to superficial femoral occlusion involves smoking cessation, exercise, and possibly pentoxifyline. In patients with aortoiliac lesions (Fig. 44-1), surgical intervention is recommended, as these individuals are at risk for retrograde aortic and renal artery thrombosis if progression to complete occlusion occurs. Patients with rest pain and gangrene should always undergo revascularization; this may be performed in conjunction with toe amputation. Amputation of the affected digit without appropriate bypass surgery is unlikely to heal and may lead to progressively higher levels of amputation. Arteriography is reserved for patients undergoing surgery and is always performed prior to operation to provide the surgeon with information regarding the origin and termination of the bypass graft. Aortoiliac occlusive disease requires replacement of the diseased arterial segments using a prosthetic graft originating from the infrarenal aorta and terminating at the common femoral arteries bilaterally (aortobifemoral bypass). Patency of these grafts is 80% to 90% at 5 years. An alternative for short, isolated, incomplete iliac artery occlusions is percutaneous balloon dilatation (angioplasty) and arterial stenting. Infrainguinal disease is treated with a bypass graft beginning at the common femoral artery and extending beyond the occlusive process to the popliteal, tibial, or pedal arteries. Saphenous vein is the preferred conduit, but prosthetic material is acceptable when the distal anastomosis is above the knee joint. Patency of infrainguinal grafts depends on location and conduit, but is between 45% and 75% at 5 years. Angioplasty has not been as successful for arteries below the femoral level. Primary amputation is reserved for patients with irreversible, extensive gangrene, for nonambulatory patients, and for patients in whom major surgery poses an unacceptable risk.

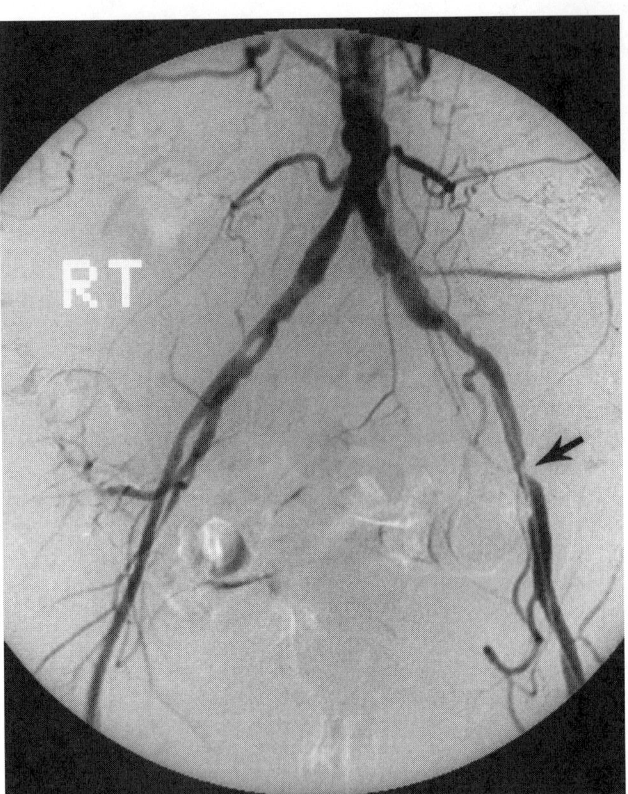

FIG. 44-1. Intraarterial aortogram of a patient with left leg ischemia, demonstrates diffuse disease of both iliac systems, with a severe stenosis of the left iliac artery (*arrow*).

Cerebrovascular Disease

Symptoms of cerebrovascular insufficiency are classified as either hemispheric or nonhemispheric, based on whether they correspond to carotid territory or vertebrobasilar territory disease, respectively. Hemispheric, or carotid distribution symptoms, include contralateral weakness and numbness of the upper and lower extremities and face, dysphasia, and ipsilateral monocular blindness (amaurosis fugax). Nonhemispheric, or vertebrobasilar symptoms, typically involve disorders of gait and vision, including blurred vision, double vision, ataxia, dysarthria, and symptoms of brainstem ischemia such as drop attacks, vertigo, and dizziness. The severity of the event is further classified based on the clinical duration: transient ischemic attacks are defined as symptoms lasting less than 24 hours, reversible ischemic neurologic deficits as symptoms lasting between 24 hours and 2 weeks, and a completed stroke as any deficit persisting for longer than 2 weeks.

There are two possible etiologies for symptoms due to cerebrovascular disease: embolization and flow reduction. Embolic phenomena occur in a hemispheric distribution and are a result of detachment of debris from atherosclerotic plaque located in the proximal internal carotid artery (Fig. 44-2). Flow related symptoms are nonhemispheric in nature, are much less common, and are due to a global reduction in blood flow to the brain. Flow related symptoms are usually due to disorders other than cerebrovascular disease that result in intracerebral hypoxia, such as cardiac arrhythmias and obstructive lung disease, since the collateral flow to the brain is usually adequate to compensate hemodynamically for even severe vascular lesions.

A special case of flow-related symptoms occurs with the subclavian steal syndrome. In this situation, lesions of the subclavian

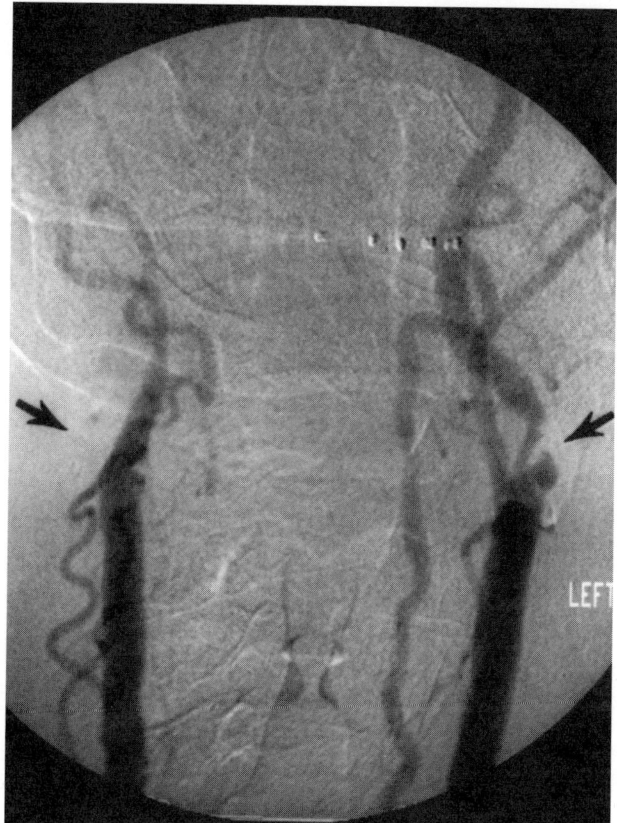

FIG. 44-2. Arteriogram of a patient with left eye amaurosis fugax demonstrates stenosis and complex plaque in the left internal carotid artery and complete occlusion of the right internal carotid artery (*arrows*).

artery proximal to the origin of the vertebral artery result in a pressure gradient which causes reversal of flow in the vertebral artery and diversion of blood away from the brain, especially under circumstances where blood flow to the arm is increased, such as with exercise. Treatment is only indicated in symptomatic patients.

In patients with hemispheric or nonhemispheric symptoms, as well as in those with asymptomatic bruits, the first screening test for determining the presence or absence of cerebrovascular disease is the duplex study, combining B-mode ultrasound and Doppler analysis. This is an extremely sensitive means of identifying stenosis of the carotid arteries and determining the direction of flow in the vertebral arteries. Following duplex evaluation, the decision regarding further work-up and treatment is determined by the presence or absence of symptoms. If no lesion is detected, other etiologies should be considered, including cardiac emboli, lesions of the aortic arch and great vessels (rare), hypertensive strokes, and migraine equivalents. If the patient is asymptomatic, operative intervention is appropriate only if the stenosis is severe (80% to 99%). If the patient is symptomatic, surgery should be considered if the stenosis is greater than 50%, although this remains controversial. Patients with crescendo transient ischemic attacks or thrombus in the internal carotid artery constitute a surgical emergency. Surgery is not indicated for patients with complete occlusions of the carotid artery and should be delayed for 6 weeks following a completed stroke with a positive head computed tomography (CT) scan. Operative intervention consists of internal carotid artery endarterectomy, a procedure that carries a 2% risk of perioperative stroke in asymptomatic patients and an up to 5% risk of stroke in patients presenting with symptoms preoperatively.

Visceral Ischemic Syndromes

The intestinal tract receives its blood supply from three major arterial systems; the celiac axis, the superior mesenteric artery, and the inferior mesenteric artery. A rich plexus of collaterals connects these vascular beds; therefore, occlusion of only one of these vessels rarely results in visceral ischemia, with the exception of acute occlusion of the superior mesenteric artery.

Chronic mesenteric ischemia is typically seen in patients with advanced atherosclerosis of the coronary and peripheral vascular systems. Clinical features include weight loss, severe postprandial abdominal pain, and diarrhea. The diagnosis is confirmed by arteriographic evaluation and treatment consists of bypass grafting from the aorta to the involved arteries, usually superior mesenteric, celiac, or both.

Acute mesenteric ischemia may be due to one of four causes. Treatment is based on diagnosis of the underlying pathology using clinical and arteriographic findings. Regardless of the etiology, the clinical picture is similar—sudden onset of severe abdominal pain, with pain out of proportion to physical findings. With progression of bowel ischemia, leukocytosis, fever, and eventually peritonitis are found. Superior mesenteric artery thrombosis occurs in patients with underlying chronic superior mesenteric artery stenoses. Treatment consists of bypass grafting following arteriographic evaluation. Embolic occlusion of the superior mesenteric artery, usually from a cardiac source, is treated with embolectomy. In patients with both thrombotic and embolic occlusions, the decision regarding bowel resection is made after blood flow is reestablished. Mesenteric venous thrombosis is seen in patients with hypercoagulable states and can be treated with either anticoagulation or venous bypass, with bowel resection as needed. Nonocclusive mesenteric ischemia is due to vasospasm and occurs in patients with severely compromised cardiac output and splanchnic vasoconstriction. It may be associated with the use of digitalis preparations or vasopressor agents. Treatment involves discontinuation of responsible medications and improvement in the underlying condition, and may also include intraarterial papaverine administration in selected cases.

The existence of celiac artery and superior mesenteric artery compression syndromes is controversial, but they almost exclusively involve women and so deserve mention. The celiac axis compression syndrome is characterized by abdominal pain and is due to compression of the celiac artery by the median arcuate ligament, as determined arteriographically. The superior mesenteric artery syndrome, or cast syndrome, is characterized by duodenal obstruction and is caused by compression of the duodenum by the superior mesenteric artery. This syndrome is seen in patients with rapid, severe weight loss or in patients immobilized in body casts, and is diagnosed by upper gastrointestinal series. Operative intervention may be appropriate in very selected cases.

Renovascular Hypertension

Although hypertension is a commonly encountered medical disorder, renovascular disease is rarely the cause, especially in women (< 0.5%). Conversely, the presence of benign (ie, not causing hypertension or renal insufficiency) renal artery stenosis is relatively high, particularly in patients with underlying vascular disease. Renovascular hypertension should be suspected in patients in whom the onset of hypertension is sudden, occurs at an unusually early (younger than 30 years) or late (over 55 years) age, or is difficult to control using standard medications. Causes include atherosclerosis obliterans, and, in women between the ages of 25 and 50, fibromuscular dysplasia. The diagnosis is confirmed with renal artery duplex evaluation. If a lesion is detected, its severity and significance with regard to hypertension and renal function must be evaluated with arteriography, followed by renal vein renin determination and split renal function tests, respectively. If the lesion is found to be responsible for either hypertension or diminished renal function, treatment is appropriate. The treatment of choice for atherosclerotic nonorificeal lesions and for most fibromuscular dysplastic lesions is angioplasty. Lesions not amenable to angioplasty are treated with renal artery bypass grafting in acceptable risk patients. Surgical options include renal endarterectomy, aortorenal bypass, splenorenal bypass, and hepatorenal bypass, and treatment is individualized to reflect the patient's health and anatomy.

Arterial Aneurysms and Dissections

An aneurysm is defined as a localized dilatation of an artery to at least twice its normal size in a given patient. Aneurysms are more common in men than women, and rare in individuals under the age of 50 years. The natural history of arterial aneurysms is expansion over time, and they are rarely benign. Complications include rupture, embolization, and compression of adjacent structures; the relative frequency depends on the type and location of the aneurysm. Aneurysms are classified as true or false. True aneurysms are dilatations that involve all three layers of the arterial wall, develop spontaneously, and are usually fusiform in shape. False aneurysms occur when the full thickness of the arterial wall is disrupted and extravasation of blood is contained by the adventitia and surrounding soft tissue structures. They are usually saccular in shape. The treatment of true aneurysms depends on their size, location, and the patient's health, whereas repair is almost always indicated for false aneurysms because of their unstable structure. The etiology of most aneurysms is atherosclerotic degeneration, although the exact mechanism by which atherosclerosis leads to aneurysm formation is uncertain. A genetic susceptibility to aneurysm formation is believed to play an important role in most patients. This is particularly true in women. When aneurysmal disease occurs in women, all first-degree relatives should be screened for the disorder after 50 years of age. Congenital defects in the arterial wall, such as Ehlers-Danlos and Marfan syndromes, may be a cause of aneurysm formation, as may acquired defects such as vasculitis due to Takayasu disease and polyarteritis nodosa. Infection, once a common factor in aortic aneurysm formation in the form of syphilitic aortitis, is now a rare cause of aneurysmal degeneration, with the most common agent being salmonella in primary infections. Trauma remains an important cause of aneurysm formation and may result in the development of either true aneurysms, in the case of repetitive blunt trauma, or false aneurysms, in the case of penetrating trauma due to violent or iatrogenic causes (eg, catheterization). A special case of traumatic aneurysm formation is postoperative separation of a vascular graft from the native artery, resulting in false aneurysm formation.

Thoracic aortic aneurysms have decreased in incidence with the advent of treatment for syphilis. The most common type of thoracic aneurysm involves the descending thoracic aorta. Most patients with this disorder are asymptomatic and the diagnosis is made unexpectedly as an incidental finding on a chest x-ray. When they occur, the most frequently noted symptoms are upper back pain, chest pain, and hoarseness. The prognosis of untreated thoracic aortic aneurysms is surprisingly poor (25% survival at 3 years); therefore, operative intervention is indicated for patients with aneurysms larger than 6 cm whose life expectancy exceeds 2 years. Urgent intervention is indicated for rapid expansion, larger size, symptomatic aneurysms, and severely hypertensive patients.

Abdominal aortic aneurysms are the most commonly encountered form of aneurysmal disease. They are usually asymptomatic, especially if small in size, and may be discovered by the patient or by the primary care practitioner on physical examination. When present, symptoms usually consist of pain in the abdomen, back, flanks, or groin, or may be related to embolization of debris from the inside of the aneurysm to distal structures (blue toe syndrome). Physical examination may fail to reveal the aneurysm if it is small or if the patient is obese. Conversely, intraabdominal masses overlying a normal aorta, such as a pancreatic carcinoma, may transmit an exaggerated aortic pulse and be confused with an aneurysm. If the diagnosis of abdominal aortic aneurysm is suspected based on clinical or physical findings, the screening test of choice is abdominal ultrasound. This test provides accurate information regarding the presence and size of the aneurysm, and is also an excellent modality with which to follow aneurysm size in patients in whom observation is elected. If rupture is suspected, however, ultrasound is inadequate and abdominal CT scan should be obtained. Similarly, abdominal CT scan is required in preparation for operative intervention as it provides important additional anatomic details to the surgical team (Fig. 44-3). The goal of operative intervention is the prevention of complications and preservation of life; the mortality for elective abdominal aortic aneurysm repair is 5%, as compared with 50% to 75% for ruptured aneurysms. The indications for operative repair include symptoms of pain or embolization, rapid expansion (greater than 1 cm in a year), and size greater than 5 cm in an otherwise healthy patient. In poor-risk patients, the risk of rupture (Table 44-2) must be weighed against the individual patient's estimated operative risk. Elective repair should always be preceded by a thorough evaluation for cardiac, pulmonary, and carotid artery disease, because these disorders are often encountered in patients with abdominal aortic aneurysms and may be asymptomatic. Operative repair consists of graft replacement of the aneurysmal portion of the aorta, usually from the infrarenal abdominal aorta to its bifurcation. Placement of either the aortic cross clamp or the graft itself above the level of the renal arteries significantly increases the operative morbidity and mortality of the procedure.

Thoracoabdominal aneurysms consist of a number of anatomic patterns of aneurysms involving all or part of the thoracic and abdominal aorta. They confer a much higher mortality, both with and without surgery, than either thoracic or abdominal aneurysms alone because of the involvement of great vessels and visceral vessels in many cases and their high rate of rupture. Repair should be undertaken only in those centers that specialize in care of these patients; even in the most experienced hands the incidence of perioperative complications such as stroke, paraplegia, renal failure, myocardial infarction, and gut ischemia is high.

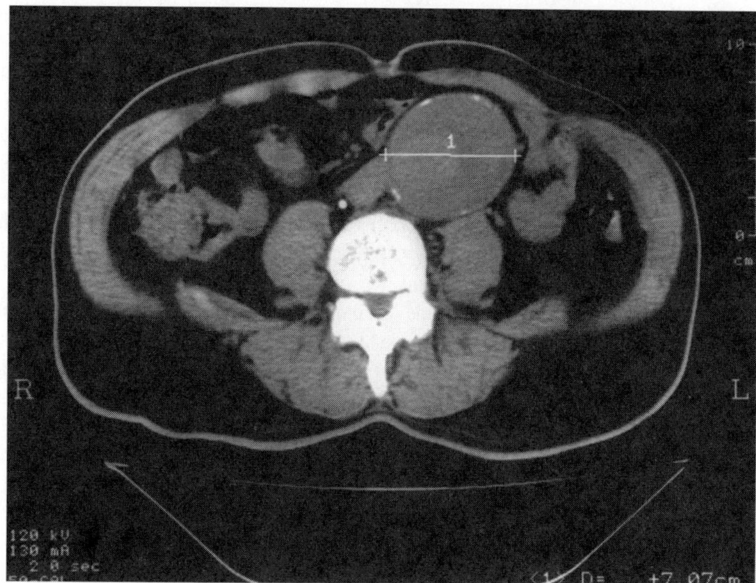

FIG. 44-3. Abdominal CT scan demonstrates a large infrarenal abdominal aortic aneurysm with intraluminal thrombus.

Aneurysms of the iliac arteries are rarely seen in isolation but are frequently associated with abdominal aortic aneurysms. They rarely cause symptoms until rupture occurs or is imminent. When present they should always be repaired, either alone or in conjunction with aortic aneurysm repair.

Aneurysmal degeneration may also occur in virtually any of the visceral arteries, including hepatic, celiac, gastroduodenal, and superior mesenteric. The most common visceral artery to become aneurysmal is the splenic artery, of interest because this is the only site in which aneurysmal degeneration is much more common in women than in men. Splenic artery aneurysms rarely cause symptoms before rupture, with the highest rate of rupture seen during the third trimester of pregnancy. Under these circumstances, maternal and fetal mortality is very high; hence any splenic artery aneurysm larger than 2 cm detected in a woman of child-bearing age should be repaired electively.

The popliteal and femoral arteries are also relatively common sites for aneurysm formation, particularly in individuals with abdominal aortic aneurysms, and repair is almost always indicated to avoid complications. Both of these lesions are extremely rare in women, however.

Arterial dissection may occur in any location but is most common in the thoracic aorta and is rare in other segments of the aorta and its branches. The lesion is initiated by an intimal tear in the vessel, followed by separation of the layers of the media and creation of a false arterial channel. This process should not be confused with aneurysm rupture, as the vessel is not initially aneurysmal but only becomes aneurysmal over time due to the weakness of the arterial wall caused by dissection. The clinical signs and symptoms of aortic dissection reflect two simultaneous events—the expansion of the artery and surrounding structures results in severe chest and upper back pain, while occlusion of arterial branches to the heart, brain, intestines, kidneys, and extremities by the false channel results in ischemia to these organs. Most patients are severely hypertensive as well. The diagnosis is made on the basis of chest x-ray, electrocardiogram, chest CT, and arteriogram. Dissections are classified based on the relationship to the great vessels: type I begins at the level of the aortic root and extends throughout the descending thoracic aorta; type II begins at the aortic root and extends to the origin of the innominate artery; and type III begins distal to the left subclavian artery and involves the descending thoracic aorta. Patients with types I and II dissections should undergo immediate operative repair because of the danger to the coronary and cerebral circulation. Type III dissections may be managed medically, at least in the acute phase, with aggressive antihypertensive therapy and monitoring in the intensive care unit.

Table 44-2. Risk of Rupture of Abdominal Aortic Aneurysm With Increasing Size

ANEURYSM SIZE	5-YEAR RISK OF RUPTURE*
4 cm	10%
5 cm	20%
6 cm	30%
7 cm	50%
8 cm	80%

*Percentages based on estimates from a variety of sources.

Acute Peripheral Arterial Occlusion

The classic signs and symptoms of acute arterial occlusion are described by the "six P's": pain, pulselessness, paresthesias, pallor, paralysis, and poikilothermy (cold temperature). In reality, however, symptoms may vary greatly from patient to patient depending on the arterial anatomy and collateral blood supply to the extremity. The patient with acute thrombosis of a previously stenotic artery often has extensive collateral circulation to the extremity and may experience minimal or no symptoms. By contrast, the patient with sudden occlusion of a previously normal artery is unlikely to have developed significant collaterals and will probably experience severe, limb-threatening ischemia as described by the six P's. As noted, acute arterial occlusion is either thrombotic or embolic in nature, with 90% of emboli to the lower extremity and virtually all emboli to the arm originating from a cardiac source.

Thrombotic occlusion usually occurs in the setting of preexisting atherosclerosis, but may also be a result of traumatic or iatrogenic injury. The diagnosis is made initially based on the history and physical examination, and an attempt is made to assess the etiology. Normal pulses in the contralateral extremity, absence of a history of claudication, and the presence of atrial fibrillation or valvular heart disease suggest an embolic etiology, while abnormal contralateral pulse exam, a history of preexisting vascular disease, and the absence of cardiac pathology suggest a thrombotic cause. Regardless of the etiology, the patient is immediately heparinized to prevent antegrade and retrograde propagation of the thromboembolic process. Embolic occlusions are treated with simple embolectomy, whereas thrombotic occlusions require bypass grafting, as thrombectomy alone is doomed to reocclusion. If the degree of ischemia is severe, or if the etiology is clearly embolic, the patient is taken directly to the operating room. If doubt exists as to the nature and location of the occlusion, however, and the patient's condition permits, arteriography is performed to aid in planning the operation. In patients with embolic occlusions, heparin should be continued postoperatively and a thorough search made for the source of the embolus.

An alternative treatment option in patients without severe ischemia is the use of intraarterial thrombolytic agents to dissolve the offending thrombus. Proponents argue that reduction in the clot volume may reduce the frequency and magnitude of operative interventions required in these patients, but this has yet to be proved.

Vasculitides

The systemic vasculitides encompass a wide variety of inflammatory disorders involving large, medium, and small arteries throughout the body. The inflammatory process may be mediated by immune complex deposition, complement activation, or cellular mechanisms, and the classification of these disorders (Table 44-3) is based in part on these distinctions.

Polyarteritis nodosa is a necrotizing vasculitis involving medium-sized arteries and affecting women slightly less often than men. The disease may be devastating, with multisystem involvement, although survival is now 80% at 5 years with the use of steroids and cyclophosphamide. In the hypersensitivity vasculitides, the inciting agent may be a pharmacologic agent, an immunization, or a chemical agent. The most important entity in this group is the vasculitis associated with underlying medical (usually connective tissue) disorders, such as systemic lupus erythematosus, rheumatoid arthritis, and scleroderma, which affect primarily women. In these patients, the most frequently involved sites are the distal digital arteries, and digital ulceration and even gangrene may result. The vasculitis of the patient with Wegener granulomatosis consists of an inflammation of the small- and medium-sized arteries, with major involvement of the respiratory and renal circulations. Women are affected less often than men (2 : 3). Treatment with steroids and cyclophosphamide has improved the prognosis considerably.

Giant cell arteritis consists of two distinct clinical syndromes characterized by identical vascular histopathology (giant cell infiltration of the vessel wall). Both are much more common in women than men. Temporal arteritis is seen in patients over 50 years of age and is characterized by symptoms of temporal headache and tenderness (unilateral or bilateral), visual disturbances, and jaw claudication. Diagnosis is made by the laboratory finding of an elevated erythrocyte sedimentation rate and by temporal artery biopsy; treatment consists of steroid administration. Takayasu disease affects young women (adolescent to 35 years) and usually begins as a systemic illness with fever, sweats, and malaise. The disorder affects large arteries, including the pulmonary circulation and the ascending and descending aorta and branches, especially the great vessels. The inflammatory process may lead to either stenosis or aneurysm formation. The diagnosis is made based on an elevated erythrocyte sedimentation rate, as well as the clinical and arteriographic findings of vascular disease. Biopsy is rarely possible because of the inaccessible nature of the involved vessels. Treatment is medical, with steroids and cyclophosphamide, unless the arterial pathology mandates surgical intervention.

Table 44-3. Classification of Vasculitides

Necrotizing Vasculitis
Classic polyarteritis nodosa
Allergic granulomatosis
Hypersensitivity Vasculitis Group
True hypersensitivity vasculitis
Henoch-Schönlein purpura
Vasculitis with mixed cryoglobulinemia
Vasculitis with connective tissue disorder
Wegener Granulomatosis Group
Classic and limited Wegener granulomatosis
Lymphomatoid granulomatosis
Benign lymphocytic angiitis
Giant Cell Arteritis
Temporal arteritis
Takayasu arteritis

Raynaud Disease

This vasospastic disorder affecting the digits of the upper and lower extremities is seen almost exclusively in women. It may be classified as either primary, when it occurs in the absence of an underlying systemic disease, or secondary, when it occurs in the setting of an underlying systemic disease, usually a connective tissue disorder.

In patients with Raynaud disease, the digits are extremely sensitive to cold exposure and undergo an excessive vasoconstrictor response under conditions of cold. The classic three phases consist of pallor with cold exposure, followed by cyanosis with initial rewarming, and concluding with a hyperemic rubor. Not all patients exhibit all of these phases, however. The diagnosis is suspected based on clinical findings and is confirmed in the vascular laboratory with measurement of digital pressures and waveforms before, during, and after cold immersion. In patients with Raynaud disease, digital pressures and waveforms are markedly dampened with cold exposure. Reduced digital artery pressures prior to cold immersion are suggestive of fixed occlusion and an underlying connective tissue disorder with associated vasculitis. This finding, or a history of systemic symptoms, should prompt a search for underlying pathology. In addition to the overall implications of an underlying disorder, the prognosis with regard to the digital lesions differs between the primary and secondary forms of the disease.

Patients with primary Raynaud disease virtually never develop ischemic ulceration or tissue loss, while patients with secondary Raynaud disease may develop painful digital lesions, including permanent cyanosis, ulceration, and even gangrene resulting in tissue loss. Treatment of the primary form of Raynaud disease consists of cold avoidance and, in severe cases, the use of calcium channel blockers or sympatholytic agents. In patients with secondary Raynaud disease, treatment of the underlying cause is paramount. Other medical and surgical modalities, including cervical sympathectomy, are of limited benefit.

Thoracic Outlet Syndrome

Thoracic outlet syndrome refers to a group of disorders producing symptoms in the neck, shoulder, and upper extremity due to compression of neurologic, venous, and arterial structures as they exit the thoracic cavity. The disorder is more common in women than men because of the less well-developed shoulder girdle muscles.

The neurologic syndrome is the most common (95%) and results from compression of the brachial plexus by a variety of muscular, fibrous, and skeletal anomalies. The clinical features of neurologic thoracic outlet syndrome include pain and paresthesias of the neck, occiput, and upper extremities, which is exacerbated by activity, particularly elevation of the arm above shoulder level. Symptoms may be precipitated by a seemingly minor injury or may develop spontaneously and occur in the distribution of either the radial or ulnar nerves, depending on whether the upper or lower portion of the brachial plexus is impinged upon by the responsible structures. Physical examination reveals tenderness over the supraclavicular area, the back of the neck, and the shoulder. Of the many "maneuvers" reported, only the elevated arm stress test is actually helpful in diagnosing the syndrome; pulse obliteration with elevation and abduction occurs in 50% of normal patients and is not diagnostic. To perform the elevated arm stress test, the patient stands with the arms held at 90° of abduction and external rotation and is asked to open and close both hands for three minutes. Normal individuals do not experience discomfort with this maneuver; reproduction of symptoms on the affected side is considered diagnostic of thoracic outlet syndrome. The mainstay of diagnosis is a careful history and physical examination, although a chest x-ray is indicated to rule out a cervical rib. Other diagnostic modalities, such as nerve conduction studies, are not helpful. The differential diagnosis includes carpal tunnel syndrome, which is characterized by median nerve involvement, and cervical disc disease, in which pain is radicular in nature, is not exacerbated by activity, and is not associated with tenderness on physical examination. Treatment of neurologic thoracic outlet syndrome is initially conservative, with exercises to strengthen the shoulder girdle muscles and thus relieve pressure on structures exiting the chest. If this is unsuccessful, surgical intervention is employed, removing a cervical rib when present, or, more commonly, removing the first rib to decompress the thoracic outlet.

When structures within the thoracic outlet compromise venous outflow, thrombosis of the subclavian vein may occur (Paget-von Schröetter syndrome, effort thrombosis). This often occurs in the setting of repetitive physical activities, such as weight-lifting or pitching, and is most common in muscular young men. The clinical findings include swelling, cyanosis, and pain of the affected arm, with prominent cutaneous venous collaterals visible around the shoulder. Treatment consists of heparinization and elevation; if more aggressive therapy is desired based on the severity of symptoms or the patient's occupation, surgical or medical (thrombolytic) clot removal in conjunction with first rib resection should be employed.

Arterial thoracic outlet syndrome is the least common (1%) and most serious of the various forms of thoracic outlet syndrome. The etiology is chronic compression of the subclavian artery by one of the bony structures of the thoracic outlet, either a cervical rib or clavicular fracture. If diagnosed early, simple removal of the offending structure is adequate therapy. If, however, the process becomes chronic, the artery is injured and aneurysm formation and embolization occur. Under these circumstances, repair of the aneurysm and removal of the offending bony structure are required.

VENOUS DISORDERS

Venous Thromboembolism

Virchow's triad of stasis, vessel wall injury, and hypercoagulability remains the basis of our understanding of the pathophysiology of venous thrombosis. The clinical significance of venous thromboembolism is reflected in the fact that 500,000 patients in the United States are diagnosed with deep venous thrombosis annually, resulting in 50,000 deaths from pulmonary embolism. Furthermore, the disabling long-term sequela of chronic venous insufficiency occurs in more than 50% of patients with deep venous thrombosis.

The clinical picture varies substantially and is determined by the proximal and distal extent of the thrombotic process. Swelling occurs just distal to the level of obstruction, and the severity of pain and cyanosis is determined by the degree to which the thrombus involves the entire venous system, including collaterals. Initially the limb is firm and tender to touch; the Homan sign is distinctly unreliable, however. Phlegmasia cerulea dolens is a special case of deep venous thrombosis, in which there is massive iliofemoral thrombosis with obstruction of arterial inflow and impending venous gangrene, and constitutes a true emergency.

A variety of diagnostic modalities can be used to detect deep venous thrombosis. The "gold standard" has traditionally been ascending phlebography, but this is painful and tedious and may even cause venous thrombosis. Radiolabeled fibrinogen is associated with a high false-positive rate and is time consuming. Impedance plethysmography is accurate but is not always readily available and may be difficult to interpret by the inexperienced observer. Duplex ultrasound evaluation of the venous system allows for direct visualization of the venous system as well as evaluation of venous flow characteristics. The method is more than 95% accurate for detecting proximal thrombi (including popliteal) and is 90% accurate for calf vein thrombi.

Treatment of venous thrombosis is aimed at preventing pulmonary embolism and decreasing the long-term sequelae of a postphlebitic syndrome. Anticoagulation with heparin acutely followed by 3 months of warfarin therapy, during which the international normalized ration (INR) is maintained at 2 to 3 times normal, is the mainstay of therapy and prevents pulmonary embolism in 95% of patients. In patients with malignancy, long-term anticoagulation with subcutaneous heparin is appropriate, because warfarin is not effective. Initial anticoagulation is instituted in conjunction with 5 to 7 days of bed rest and elevation with elastic compression therapy. Other therapeutic modalities may be employed under certain circumstances; in the patient with phlegmasia cerulea dolens, venous thrombectomy is required to prevent limb loss. Alternatively, thrombolytic therapy may be used within the first 48 hours in selected patients (eg, athletes) to reduce the incidence of a postphlebitic syndrome. Isolated calf vein (infrapopliteal) thrombus in healthy, ambulatory patients may by managed with aspirin, elastic compression stockings, and frequent duplex evaluation.

Mechanical interruption of the inferior vena cava to prevent pulmonary embolism using a percutaneously placed filtration device is absolutely indicated if: (1) the patient experiences pulmonary embolism while on adequate anticoagulation therapy; or (2) a patient with a contraindication to anticoagulation experiences a pulmonary embolism. Relative indications for filter placement include free-floating thrombus within the iliac or femoral system and chronic recurrent pulmonary emboli with pulmonary hypertension.

Appropriate prophylaxis for deep venous thrombosis is determined by the patient's risk level. Patients undergoing low-risk surgical procedures (duration less than 1 hour, no prolonged postoperative immobilization) should receive early ambulation only. Patients at moderate risk (those undergoing major gynecologic or general surgical procedures) should receive subcutaneous heparin pre- and postoperatively, and should wear pneumatic compression stockings intraoperatively. Patients at high risk for perioperative venous thrombosis (those undergoing total joint replacement or with prior history of deep venous thrombosis) should receive warfarin or low-dose intravenous heparin perioperatively.

Chronic Venous Insufficiency and Varicose Veins

The venous circulation is comprised of a deep system, including the femoral, popliteal, and tibial veins; a superficial system comprised of the greater and lesser saphenous veins draining into the deep system; and a set of perforating veins directing blood from the superficial to the deep system within the calf. All of these veins contain valves at regular intervals designed to facilitate forward flow and prevent retrograde flow and venous hypertension. Malfunction of the valves at any level may result in venous insufficiency and varicose veins; patients with varicose veins often have intrinsic degeneration of the venous wall in addition to the above mentioned factors.

Varicose veins may range in severity from mild, cosmetic defects to large, tortuous, bulging lesions. Symptoms vary from none to throbbing, aching, and itching, particularly after long periods of standing, during menses, and during pregnancy, when venous pressure is increased by compression of the iliac veins. As noted earlier, the etiology of varicose veins includes hereditary factors within the vessel wall, greater saphenous valvular insufficiency, and pregnancy. The diagnosis of greater saphenous incompetence can be made using venous duplex scanning. Initial treatment consists of elastic compression stockings. If these fail to control the patient's symptoms, high ligation and stripping of the greater saphenous system and excision of individual varicosities is highly effective. Sclerotherapy (injection) using hypertonic saline is effective only for spider veins and very small varicosities.

With long-standing valvular incompetence in the deep and superficial systems and perforators, changes of chronic venous stasis occur. These begin as thickening of the skin with pigmentation secondary to hemosiderin deposits, and progress to ulceration, edema, and cellulitis which may be difficult to eradicate. If ulcers occur and greater saphenous incompetence is prominent, high ligation and stripping may be helpful. If perforator incompetence is predominant, ligation of perforators is beneficial. Otherwise, as in most patients, the mainstay of therapy is the heavyweight elastic compression stocking, used in conjunction with meticulous wound care and strict bed rest with leg elevation in the acute period.

LYMPHEDEMA

Lymphedema is defined as a swelling of the extremities due to inadequate lymphatic drainage, and can be classified as either primary or secondary.

The primary lymphedemas are further classified based on the patient's age at onset, with earlier age at onset correlating with a more severe clinical picture. Milroy disease (familial lymphedema) usually presents in the first decade of life; lymphedema praecox presents in early adolescence; and lymphedema tarda presents after puberty. In all primary lymphedemas, intrinsic anatomic abnormalities of the lymphatics are causative, including lymphatic aplasia, hypoplasia, or hyperplasia with valvular reflux. Secondary lymphedemas are due to obstruction of previously normal lymphatics by tumor, infection, radiation, or surgical interruption.

Clinically, lymphedema can be differentiated from venous stasis disease by physical examination. In patients with venous disorders, pigmentation and ulceration are prominent; by contrast patients with lymphedema have no pigmentation or ulceration. Swelling of the dorsum of the foot and scaling and redundant skin involving the entire extremity are characteristic of lymphedema and absent in patients with venous disease. Recurrent cellulitis is more common in patients with lymphedema and may become quite troublesome. If the diagnosis still remains in doubt, lymphangiography or lymphoscintigraphy may be employed, but they add little to the management of these patients.

Treatment of lymphedema involves elevation and elastic compression stockings. In more severe cases, the Lymphapress, a graded compression device, may be helpful. Medical therapies have not been proven to be effective and diuretics may actually be harmful. In the most incapacitating cases, operative therapy, consisting of resection of large quantities of subcutaneous tissue and skin grafting, has been of benefit.

BIBLIOGRAPHY

DeWeese JA. Vascular surgery. In: Dudley H, Carter DC, eds. Rob and Smith's operative surgery, 4th ed. London: Butterworths, 1985.

Fields WS, Lemak NA. Joint study of extracranial arterial occlusion. JAMA 1976;235:2734.

Goldman L, Calder DL, Nussbaum SR, et al. N Engl J Med 1977;297:846.

Moore W, ed. Vascular surgery: a comprehensive review. Philadelphia: WB Saunders. 1993.

North American Symptomatic Carotid Endarterectomy Trial Collaborators. Beneficial effect of carotid endarterectomy in symptomatic patients with high-grade carotid stenosis. N Engl J Med 1991;325:445.

Rutherford RB, ed. Vascular surgery. Philadelphia: WB Saunders, 1989.

Sanders RJ, Haug C. Subclavian vein obstruction and thoracic outlet syndrome: a review of etiology and management. Ann Vasc Surg 1990;4:397.

Szilagyi DE, Smith RF, DeRusso FJ, et al. Contribution of abdominal aortic aneurysmectomy to prolongation of life. Ann Surg 1966;164:678.

Wolf PA, Kannel WB, Dawber TR: Prospective investigation: the Framingham Study and the epidemiology of stroke. Adv Neurol 1978;19:107.

Young JR, Graor RA, Olin JW, Bartholomew JR, eds. Peripheral vascular diseases. St. Louis: Mosby-Year Book, 1991.

Primary Care for Women, edited by Phyllis C. Leppert and Fred M. Howard. Lippincott-Raven Publishers, Philadelphia © 1997.

45

Cardiac Arrhythmias

ROY S. WIENER

At rest, the healthy cardiac cell membrane maintains the cell interior electrically negative relative to the extracellular space. During the action potential, the transmembrane voltage becomes depolarized (ie, the cell interior becomes electrically positive). A phase of gradual repolarization occurs next, followed by a return of the cell to its resting state. Heart cells exhibit refractoriness—in other words, time must elapse for recovery before the next activation can occur. The action potential has two primary functions: it triggers contraction and mediates intracardiac conduction.

Normally, the sinus node paces the heart. Next, the atria contract, inscribing the P wave on the electrocardiogram (ECG). During the PR interval, conduction to the ventricles occurs slowly through the atrioventricular (AV) node and then rapidly through the His-Purkinje system. The ventricles contract synchronously, inscribing a narrow QRS complex. The T wave represents the return of the ventricle to its resting electrical state.

One mechanism that produces premature beats and tachycardias is increased automaticity in cells that normally exhibit pacemaker activity. A second cause is triggering; during or after repolarization, repetitive reactivation occurs. The most common etiology is reentry—a cardiac substrate supports circular conduction of activation, with transmission out of the circuit to the atria or ventricles or both. If the myocytes are no longer refractory when excitation returns to its starting point, the tachyarrhythmia may become sustained. Bradycardias occur when there is a decrease in the automaticity of pacemaker cells or block in the conduction system.

ETIOLOGY

Arrhythmia may arise in the setting of underlying disease or with no known cause. It may be the most clinically important part of a patient's illness or of secondary importance. Many conditions contribute to the onset or exacerbation of arrhythmias. When evaluating and managing patients, these factors should be systematically explored.

First, one should establish whether there is structural heart disease, such as coronary artery disease, myocardial infarction, cardiomyopathy, valvular dysfunction, or pericarditis. Underlying disease may trigger arrhythmia or amplify its consequences. For example, supraventricular tachycardia is generally well tolerated in a normal heart but frequently causes serious hemodynamic decompensation in the presence of left ventricular dysfunction or coronary artery disease.

Noncardiac precipitants include hypertension, thyroid disease, anemia, infection, fever, hypoxia, pulmonary disease or embolism, sleep apnea, the postoperative state, and changes in autonomic tone. In some women, arrhythmias can occur or worsen with pregnancy or the phases of the menstrual cycle. Vagal discharge may lead to sinus bradycardia, sinus pauses, and AV block; increased sympathetic tone, anxiety, or emotional stress can precipitate tachycardias. Acid-base derangement and abnormal levels of potassium, magnesium, and calcium should be excluded.

β-Adrenergic agonists, theophylline, and anticholinergic agents cause premature beats and tachycardia. Calcium antagonists and β-adrenergic blockers are associated with bradycardias and conduction block. Paradoxically, antiarrhythmic agents may worsen existing arrhythmias or trigger new ones. Diuretics act indirectly by inducing electrolyte abnormalities. Digoxin, at both therapeutic and toxic levels, may cause premature beats, tachycardias, and AV block. One should specifically inquire about nonprescription and illicit drugs, especially cocaine. Drug discontinuation can also be arrhythmogenic, either by removing a therapeutic effect or inducing a withdrawal syndrome. This is frequently noted when β-adrenergic blockers are abruptly discontinued. Alcohol, tobacco, and caffeine commonly precipitate ectopy and tachycardias.

HISTORY

Asymptomatic arrhythmias may be found when taking the pulse, examining the heart, or recording an ECG on a patient who is being routinely evaluated. Palpitations, syncope, and lightheadedness suggest arrhythmia, but these symptoms also have other causes. Chest pain, dyspnea, and fatigue may also occur during rhythm disturbance, but these symptoms are even less specific. Symptom severity may correlate loosely with some arrhythmias; one patient may be distressed by rare premature beats, but another may be oblivious to frequent ectopy.

Palpitations are not precisely defined, although the term is often used to refer to a sensation that the heartbeat is abnormally strong, fast, slow, or irregular. The patient should be urged to describe her sensations in detail. Premature ventricular contractions may be felt as a flip-flop sensation, as a skipped beat, or as a hyperdynamic postectopic beat. Regular tachycardias are often felt as a steady pounding in the chest; atrial fibrillation may be sensed as an irregular heartbeat. Hyperdynamic states characterized as palpitations include normal pregnancy, anxiety, panic disorder, thyrotoxicosis, anemia, and increased sympathetic tone.

Syncope or lightheadedness may occur when either tachycardia or bradycardia induces hypotension that compromises cerebral perfusion. Common etiologies not directly related to arrhythmia include vasodepression, orthostatic hypotension (especially drug-related), and aortic stenosis (see Chap. 48). Vertigo may be characterized as a sensation of lightheadedness (see Chap. 107). Seizure is usually of primary neurologic origin, but cortical ischemia secondary to arrhythmia and hypotension may also trigger convulsive activity (see Chap. 108).

Ischemic chest pain may result if the hemodynamic consequences of arrhythmia are severe enough to compromise the balance of myocardial oxygen supply and demand. This is most commonly seen when there is coexisting coronary artery disease, aortic stenosis, or left ventricular hypertrophy. At rapid heart rates, even patients with otherwise normal hearts may experience anginal-type discomfort; other patients note chest pain of uncertain mechanism. Dyspnea may result when arrhythmia induces heart failure and pulmonary congestion. A patient with cardiomyopathy who is well compensated in sinus rhythm may develop fatigue and exercise intolerance when atrial fibrillation supervenes.

Symptoms may be ongoing if the patient presents with a chronic arrhythmia or during a paroxysm. Prompt, definitive treatment is needed if abnormal mentation, severe dyspnea, or angina is due to arrhythmia. If the symptoms have remitted, one should document the frequency, duration, and precipitants of the episode, as well as the presence of the triggering factors noted above.

PHYSICAL EXAMINATION

If arrhythmia is present during evaluation, the first priority is to confirm that the vital signs are stable. Once it is established that the patient is not in imminent danger, the examination may provide evidence for associated disease or may suggest the ECG diagnosis. The general appearance may suggest pulmonary disease, a thyroid disorder, or cardiac failure. Hypotension is seen with hypovolemia, pump failure, or medication effects. Resting sinus tachycardia commonly occurs with hyperthyroidism; bradycardia suggests sinus node dysfunction, conduction block, or medication effects. Ectopic beats usually cause skips or weak beats against a background of regularity; a randomly irregular pulse suggests atrial fibrillation. Elevated jugular venous pressure, rales, and peripheral edema raise the issue of heart failure. Irregular cannon *a* waves in the jugular venous waveform suggest AV block or ventricular tachycardia. The cardiac examination may reveal abnormal heart sounds, murmurs, gallops, or rubs indicative of valvular disease, left ventricular failure, or pericarditis. The neurologic examination may reveal abnormal reflexes or muscle weakness suggestive of thyroid disease.

LABORATORY AND IMAGING STUDIES

A 12-lead ECG with a long rhythm strip should be obtained, ideally during arrhythmia. Single-lead monitor strips are often inadequate for determining true QRS duration and defining P waves. During ECG analysis, one must identify and focus on the relation between atrial and ventricular activity, irregularity, prematurity, and pauses. Esophageal or intracardiac recording is occasionally necessary for diagnosis. Carotid sinus massage or other vagal stimuli may uncover atrial activity by transiently slowing tachycardias or decreasing AV conduction. Carotid sinus massage is performed with ECG monitoring; it is contraindicated in the presence of a carotid bruit, and caution is advised in the elderly. Drugs may be used for diagnostic purposes; for example, adenosine can transiently decrease AV conduction and uncover flutter waves obscured by QRS complexes and T waves. Electrolytes, thyroid function, and drug levels should generally be checked.

Symptoms of syncope or hemodynamic instability generally require inpatient monitoring and referral. Frequent, benign symptoms may be evaluated with ambulatory ECG recording; a carefully recorded diary is essential for meaningful correlation of symptoms with arrhythmia. Occasional episodes may be captured with ECG event recorders. One type is placed on the chest when symptoms start; a continuously acquiring loop monitor is useful for episodes that are very brief or lead rapidly to syncope.

Echocardiography and exercise testing may be performed to investigate whether structural heart disease is present. Cardiac catheterization may be needed for diagnosis or when percutaneous or surgical intervention is contemplated. Electrophysiologic testing uses electrode catheters to measure and stimulate intracardiac activity. It is useful when arrhythmia has not been documented despite significant symptoms, or to evaluate drug efficacy or map arrhythmogenic foci in preparation for ablation.

TREATMENT

When the patient is unstable due to tachycardia, immediate cardioversion is usually required. Severe bradycardia requires pacing if there is not an immediate response to intravenous atropine. If possible, however, it is best to document and diagnose the arrhythmia before treatment.

When possible, the best treatment is to remove precipitating factors. Occasional, benign, and mildly symptomatic arrhythmias are often best managed with reassurance and observation. For more frequent and bothersome problems, the therapeutic goals include prevention of recurrence and control of symptoms while improving, or at least not worsening, survival. Caution is necessary, as several recent studies have found that some drugs may decrease an arrhythmia at the cost of increased long-term mortality.

Antiarrhythmic drugs are usually grouped according to the Vaughn Williams classification on the basis of their predominant electrophysiologic effects. Class I drugs (sodium channel blockers) are potent agents best used with cardiology referral. They are subgrouped depending on their effects on action potential duration. Class IA drugs (quinidine, procainamide, and disopyramide) treat both supraventricular and ventricular arrhythmias. Class IB drugs (lidocaine, mexiletine, tocainide, and phenytoin) are effective for ventricular arrhythmias; only intravenous lidocaine is used commonly. Class IC drugs (flecainide, propafenone, and moricizine) are active against supraventricular and ventricular arrhythmias and are especially useful in patients with accessory pathways.

Class II drugs (β-adrenergic receptor blockers) are effective in decreasing the ventricular response in atrial fibrillation, and for arrhythmias triggered by increased sympathetic tone or exercise. They can also be used to suppress supraventricular tachycardias and ectopic beats. Long-acting cardioselective agents such as atenolol and metoprolol are often preferred.

Class III drugs (complex mechanisms of action) may have significant adverse effects and are used with cardiology referral. Amiodarone and sotalol are active against ventricular arrhythmias and atrial fibrillation. Bretylium is used intravenously in the intensive care setting for ventricular tachycardia and fibrillation.

Class IV agents (calcium channel blockers) are used for atrial arrhythmias. Verapamil converts and prevents reentrant supraventricular tachycardia. Diltiazem and verapamil are used to slow AV conduction in atrial fibrillation.

Digoxin is commonly used to control the ventricular response in atrial fibrillation. Atropine is a vagolytic used emergently to treat bradycardias and AV block. Intravenous adenosine slows AV node conduction and is the treatment of choice for conversion of reentrant supraventricular tachycardias. When administered during atrial fibrillation, flutter, or tachycardia, it causes a transient increase in AV node block but does not convert the rhythm to sinus.

Electrical cardioversion depolarizes the heart and allows the sinus rhythm to reemerge. It is used emergently for ventricular tachycardia and fibrillation and hemodynamically unstable supraventricular arrhythmias. It is also frequently used for elective conversion of atrial fibrillation and flutter. Transvenous automatic implantable cardioverter defibrillators are now commonly implanted to prevent sudden death from malignant ventricular arrhythmias.

Pacemakers are commonly used for bradyarrhythmias and occasionally for conversion of tachycardias. Transcutaneous and temporary transvenous pacemakers are used emergently; permanent lead/generator systems are implanted for chronic protection against bradycardia. Most patients with sinus rhythm receive dual-chamber pacemakers that preserve normal AV synchrony.

Radiofrequency current delivered via electrode catheters is routinely used for ablation of accessory pathways, AV node-dependent arrhythmias, and some forms of ventricular tachycardia. Surgical methods for control of atrial fibrillation and resection of ventricular arrhythmogenic foci are used occasionally in specialized centers.

SPECIFIC ARRHYTHMIAS

Atrial Arrhythmias

Normal sinus rhythm is defined as a rate between 60 and 100 beats per minute (bpm) with a P wave morphology consistent with sinus origin. Sinus bradycardia (< 60 bpm) is usually physiologic in otherwise healthy people, unless the rate is low enough to cause hypotension or lightheadedness. Sinus tachycardia (> 100 bpm) is generally a response to a physiologic drive such as exercise, hypovolemia, anxiety, pain, hyperthyroidism, impaired left ventricular function, or shock. Identification and treatment of the underlying cause is indicated.

Sinus arrhythmia denotes periodic variations in sinus rate, often related to the respiratory cycle; it is frequently seen in normal persons. Atrial rhythm occurs when an ectopic atrial focus, characterized by abnormal P waves, paces the heart. Wandering atrial pacemaker is similar, with several atrial foci and P-wave morphologies appearing. These three arrhythmias are generally benign and do not require further investigation or treatment.

Premature atrial contractions (PACs) occur when an atrial focus discharges, usually leading to an early beat with an abnormal P wave morphology and a normal QRS. However, if the His-Purkinje system is partially refractory when the premature depolarization reaches it, a wide QRS complex resembling a premature ventricular contraction (PVC) is inscribed (Fig. 45-1). If the conduction system is completely refractory, conduction to the ventricles does not occur and no QRS is inscribed. This is a common and benign cause of pauses; thus, an early P wave should be carefully sought when a pause is evaluated. PACs arise in both normal and diseased hearts; occasionally, they are the presenting manifestation of significant cardiac dysfunction. Reassurance is appropriate in symptomatic patients and referral is rarely necessary. The patient with frequent PACs is at increased risk for supraventricular tachycardias.

Supraventricular Tachycardias

AV node reentrant tachycardia (AVNRT) is common in both structurally normal and diseased hearts. It is regular, with rates usually between 120 and 220 bpm. Atrial activation is retrograde; inverted P waves with a short RP interval may be noted, but they are often not seen due to superimposition on the QRS complex (Fig. 45-2). Paroxysmal episodes may convert spontaneously or with vagal maneuvers; if not, adenosine is the drug of choice. Recurring episodes can be treated with β-adrenergic blockers, verapamil, diltiazem, or digoxin; occasionally a class IA or IC antiarrhythmic is required. Radiofrequency catheter ablation is also indicated in selected cases.

Atrioventricular reentrant tachycardia (AVRT) is common and requires the presence of a congenital accessory pathway connecting atrium to ventricle. It usually occurs when a reentrant circuit combines antegrade AV node and retrograde bypass tract transmission; preexcitation on the baseline ECG is variably seen. AVRT is regular at 140 to 250 bpm, and the abnormal P wave is usually seen following the QRS with a relatively long RP interval. Management is as for AVNRT, except that the use of digoxin is avoided in the presence of an accessory pathway.

Atrial tachycardia is caused by abnormal automaticity or triggering in an atrial focus with subsequent AV conduction; as the AV node is not part of the arrhythmia mechanism, AV block may occur. It is uncommon and is usually seen in the presence of structural heart disease or digoxin toxicity. A P wave of morphology different than for the sinus mechanism precedes the QRS complex. It is managed with AV blocking agents and primary antiarrhythmics if the underlying causes cannot be controlled. Multifocal atrial tachycardia is a chaotic rhythm with multiple P wave morphologies that often vary from beat to beat; it is usually associated with poorly controlled pulmonary disease and generally resolves as the underlying illness improves.

Atrial flutter occurs when reentry within the atrium cycles at about 250 to 350 bpm, usually accompanied by 2:1 AV conduction in the absence of medications or conduction abnormalities (Fig. 45-3). It is usually seen in association with structural heart disease and should be suspected when evaluating a regular narrow QRS rhythm at 150 bpm. Atrial activity classically has a sawtooth pat-

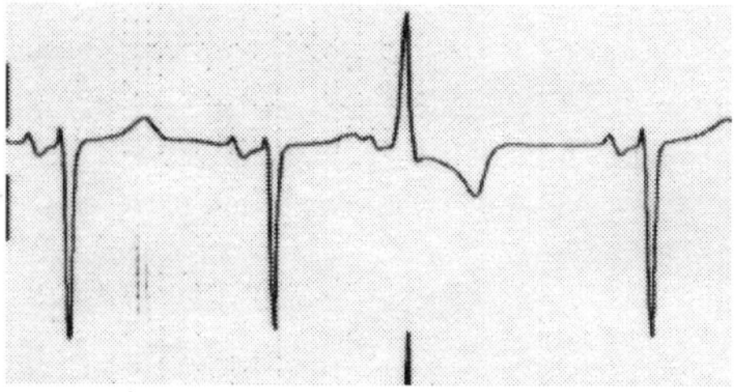

Figure 45-1. Premature atrial contraction (with aberrant conduction).

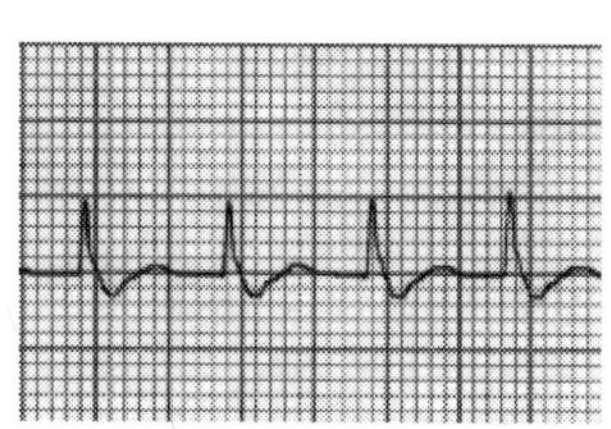

Figure 45-2. AV node reentrant tachycardia.

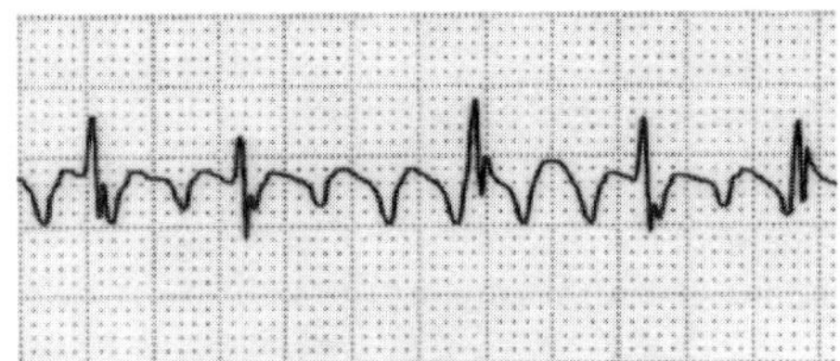

Figure 45-3. Atrial flutter.

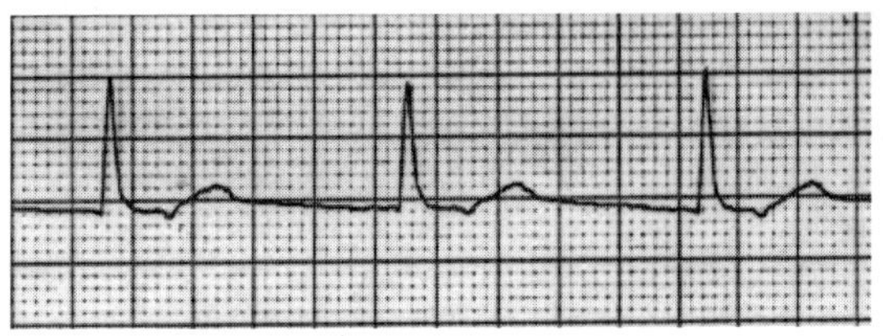

Figure 45-5. Junctional rhythm.

tern in the inferior leads but may resemble a normal P wave in lead V1. Flutter waves blending into the QRS complex and ST-T wave are easily missed by the unwary physician, leading to misdiagnosis as sinus tachycardia, AVNRT, or AVRT. Atrial flutter may be difficult to treat. Initially, the ventricular rate is controlled with AV node blockers, followed by class IA/IC/III antiarrhythmics, electrical cardioversion, or rapid atrial pacing. Although data are scarce, anticoagulation before elective conversion of atrial flutter of more than 48 hours' duration probably decreases the incidence of embolic events.

In atrial fibrillation (AF), atrial electrical activity becomes disorganized, and fine or coarse irregularity of the ECG baseline is seen instead of P waves. The AV node is bombarded by an incoming 400 to 600 impulses per minute and transmits randomly to create a ventricular rate of 140 to 180 bpm (Fig. 45-4). Slower ventricular rates suggest drug effect or intrinsic conduction system disease. The loss of atrial systole may lead to hemodynamic deterioration of marginally compensated patients, and stasis of blood in the atrium predisposes to thrombus formation and embolic events. AF frequently occurs in association with underlying disease, but lone (idiopathic) AF is not uncommon. Common noncardiac causes that are amenable to treatment include hyperthyroidism and alcohol use.

In both chronic and paroxysmal AF, the ventricular rate is controlled as needed with AV node blockers. If the AF is not already known to be chronic, pharmacologic or electrical cardioversion is considered. Factors that favor maintenance of sinus rhythm include short duration of AF, absence of marked left atrial dilation, and control of an identified underlying cause. Many drugs have been used to prevent recurrence, but 1-year success rates are about 50%, and drug toxicity is a significant concern. For example, studies have suggested that quinidine increases the chance of maintaining sinus rhythm at the cost of increased mortality. If the AF is of greater than 48 hours' duration, anticoagulation with warfarin to INR 2.0 to 3.0 for 3 weeks before and 4 weeks after the conversion appears to decrease the risk of embolic events.

Several studies have documented that there is a 5% annual incidence of stroke in AF and that anticoagulation with warfarin to INR 2.0 to 3.0 decreases this risk to 1.5%. Aspirin appears to decrease stroke as well, but not as effectively as warfarin. Therefore, warfarin should be administered to most patients with AF who can safely tolerate anticoagulation. An exception can be made for patients who are at very low risk of stroke without treatment (age <65, with no history of hypertension, diabetes mellitus, stroke, transient ischemic attack, congestive heart failure, angina, valvular disease, or myocardial infarction).

Junctional Rhythms

Premature junctional contractions arise from the AV node and present as early beats with normal QRS morphology but without a preceding P wave. Treatment and evaluation are as for PACs. AV node cells normally pace at about 45 bpm, emerging as an escape rhythm during sinus arrest or AV block (Fig. 45-5). Accelerated junctional rhythms (60 to 120 bpm) appear when this focus becomes faster than the sinus rate, usually secondary to structural heart disease or digoxin toxicity; they are usually well tolerated and treatment is directed at the underlying cause.

Ventricular Arrhythmias

PVCs arise from a ventricular focus and are characterized by wide QRS beats without a preceding P wave and usually with a subsequent pause (Fig. 45-6). They are commonly seen with and without underlying heart disease. In otherwise normal patients, they do not have prognostic significance and do not require treatment. In the occasional patient with severely symptomatic palpitations who cannot be reassured, a trial of β-adrenergic blockers is reasonable. In patients with structural heart disease, an association between the frequency and complexity of ventricular ectopy and mortality has been noted. It was hypothesized that pharmacologic PVC suppression would improve survival, presumably by preventing the triggering of malignant ventricular arrhythmias. Unfortunately, the Cardiac Arrhythmia Suppression Trial demonstrated that class IC agents increased mortality after myocardial infarction, even though PVCs were suppressed. Thus, it seems prudent to avoid antiarrhythmic drugs for PVCs in most patients with an underlying cardiac disorder.

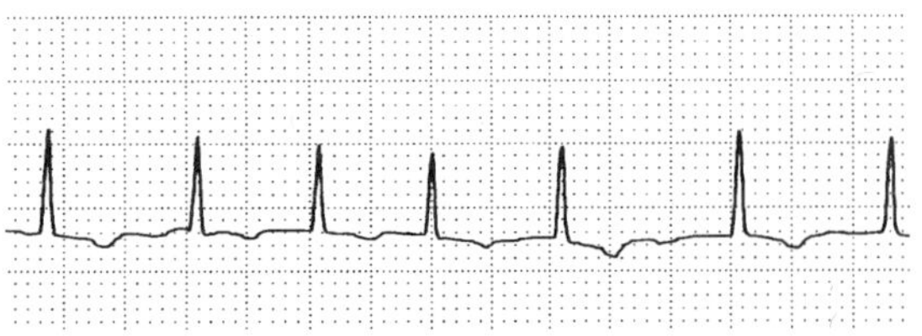

Figure 45-4. Atrial fibrillation.

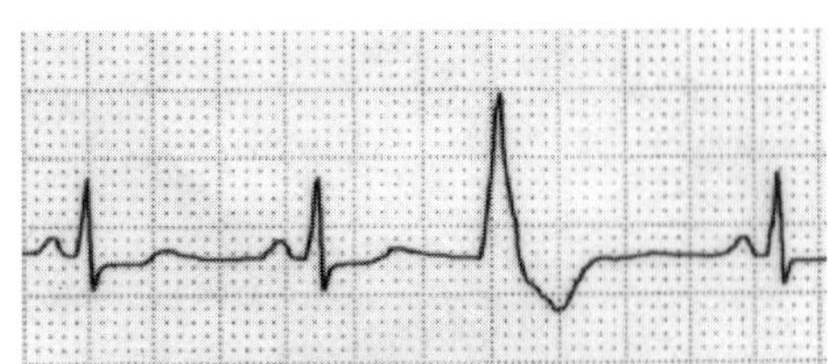

Figure 45-6. Premature ventricular contraction.

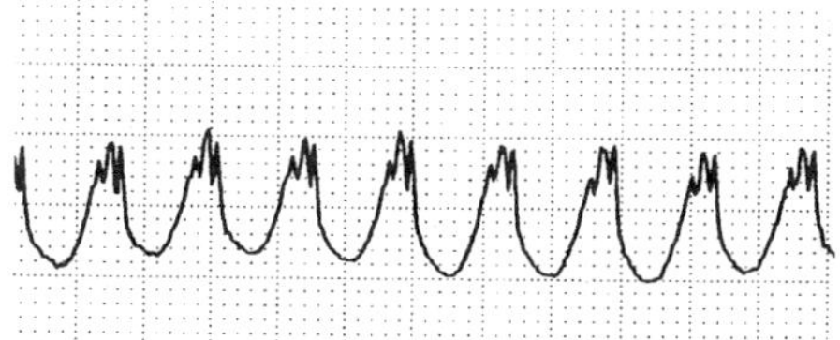

Figure 45-7. Ventricular tachycardia.

Ventricular tachycardia (VT) is defined as three or more ventricular beats in a row at a rate from 100 to 250 bpm; 30 seconds' duration is commonly considered the division between nonsustained and sustained VT (Fig. 45-7). VT is usually reentrant and associated with structural heart disease. Symptoms are sometimes absent but may range from palpitation and brief lightheadedness to syncope and death. When evaluating a wide QRS tachycardia, hemodynamic stability does not exclude the diagnosis of sustained VT. In ventricular fibrillation (VF), ventricular activity is severely disorganized, with the ECG demonstrating fine or coarse irregularity without QRS complexes. Death is immediate without prompt electrical defibrillation. Treatment options for prevention of VF or recurrent runs of symptomatic or sustained VT include class I/II/III drugs and automatic implantable cardioverter defibrillators. Cardiology referral is indicated for the evaluation of VT and VF.

Idioventricular rhythm (20 to 40 bpm) arises from spontaneous pacemaker activity in ventricular cells. A wide QRS bradycardia emerges as an escape rhythm in association with failure of sinus and junctional escape rhythms or His-Purkinje system block. The patient is usually unstable; artificial pacing is indicated. Accelerated idioventricular rhythm (40 to 100 bpm) is a similar rhythm at a faster rate. It is commonly seen during acute myocardial infarction and generally does not require treatment (Fig. 45-8).

Bradycardias

Sinus pauses are noted when the expected P wave fails to appear on time; they may be terminated by return of sinus function or junctional/ventricular escape beats. Severity ranges from short pauses without clinical significance to long periods of asystole associated with syncope or presyncope. Artificial pacemaker placement is indicated for symptoms or long pauses not due to reversible causes.

AV block is first characterized by severity. In 1° AV block, all P waves conduct to the ventricle, but the PR interval is greater than 0.2 seconds. In 2° AV block, some P waves conduct and some are blocked. In 3° AV block, no P waves conduct, and junctional or ventricular escape rhythms emerge. (When diagnosing AV block, it is important to confirm that the P waves are not premature and fail to conduct because of physiologic refractoriness.)

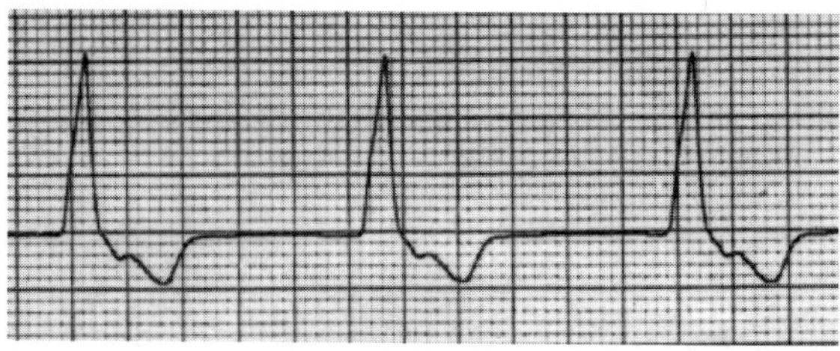

Figure 45-8. Accelerated idioventricular rhythm.

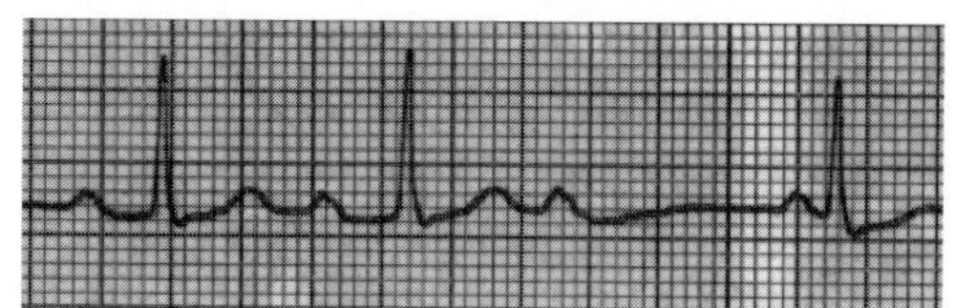

Figure 45-9. Mobitz I second-degree AV block.

Second-degree AV block has several subtypes. Mobitz I (Wenckebach) is characterized by PR interval lengthening before and shortening after the blocked P wave (Fig. 45-9).Usually, block is at the AV nodal level and is responsive to atropine, the QRS width is normal, and a stable junctional escape focus emerges if 3° AV block develops. Mobitz II usually demonstrates PR interval constancy before and after the blocked P wave. Block is typically in the His-Purkinje system; the QRS width is usually prolonged; and unreliable, slow, idioventricular rhythms emerge if progression to 3° AV block occurs. AV conduction ratios of 2:1 may occur in either AV node or His-Purkinje system block; the clinical situation and QRS width suggest the site of the lesion. Third-degree AV block occurs in either the AV node or the His-Purkinje system (Fig. 45-10). As with 2° block, AV nodal block is generally better tolerated due to the presence of junctional escape rhythms.

Etiologies of AV block include myocardial infarction (inferior, Mobitz I; anterior, Mobitz II), cardiomyopathy, calcification or fibrosis of the conduction system, and medications. Treatment is generally artificial pacing if symptomatic or if His-Purkinje system pathology is likely. Cardiology referral is advised.

ARRHYTHMIA SYNDROMES

Sick sinus syndrome, usually seen in the elderly, is characterized by sinus bradycardia and sinus pauses, often severe enough to induce syncope (Fig. 45-11). AV nodal and ventricular escape mechanisms are also frequently abnormally slow or absent. In a variant, bradycardia-tachycardia syndrome, patients also have frequent episodes of atrial tachyarrhythmia. Extremely long pauses may be seen after cessation of tachycardia, as the impaired sinus node function is transiently worsened by the preceding tachycardia. The tachycardias are treated with AV blocking agents and antiarrhythmic drugs; the bradycardias may require pacing if severe or symptomatic. In carotid sinus hypersensitivity, a marked vagal response follows carotid baroreceptor stimulation with bradycardia or vasodepression. The diagnosis is suggested by a long pause following carotid sinus massage. Dual-chamber pacing is frequently effective in preventing recurrent symptoms.

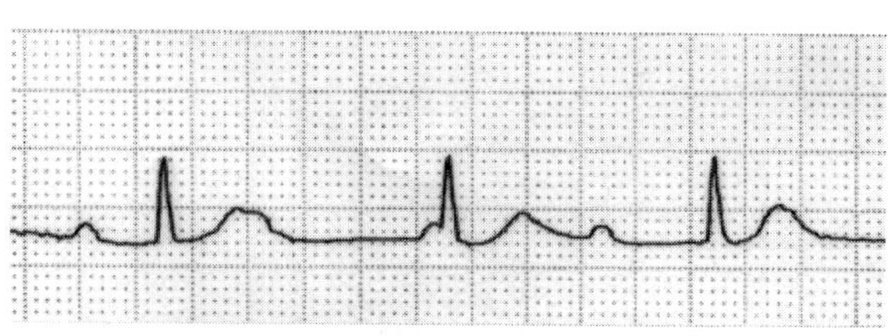

Figure 45-10. Third-degree AV block.

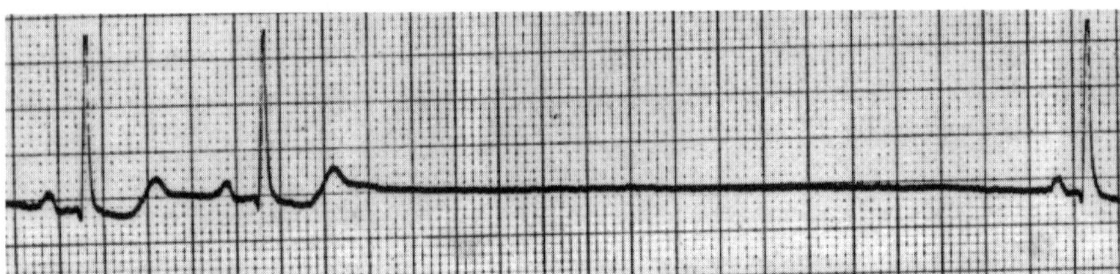

Figure 45-11. Sinus pause characteristic of sick sinus syndrome.

In Wolff-Parkinson-White syndrome, several arrhythmias may arise due to the presence of a congenital accessory bypass tract that connects the atrium and the ventricle. Antegrade conduction through the bypass tract inscribes a delta wave on the ECG, indicating preexcitation of the ventricle and creating a short PR interval/lengthened QRS duration. Orthodromic reciprocating tachycardia (AVRT; see above) occurs when a circuit is formed antegrade through the AV node and retrograde through the bypass tract. Occasionally, the reentry goes antegrade through the bypass tract and retrograde up the AV node (antidromic reciprocating tachycardia), inscribing a wide, preexcited QRS complex. Atrial fibrillation in association with an accessory pathway that conducts antegrade with a short refractory period can lead to rapid ventricular rates that degenerate into ventricular fibrillation and death. Tachycardias with Wolff-Parkinson-White can be treated with drugs, but radiofrequency ablation is being used increasingly as it avoids the side effects of long-term antiarrhythmic use.

Wide QRS tachycardia may be either ventricular tachycardia or a supraventricular tachycardia with bundle branch block/aberrant conduction. Evidence of AV dissociation or a previous history of myocardial infarction favors the diagnosis of ventricular tachycardia. Previously known bundle branch block in sinus rhythm with a similar morphology to the presenting arrhythmia suggests supraventricular tachycardia with aberrancy. Specific ECG morphology criteria have been published that help the physician reach a specific diagnosis. Cardiology referral is usually indicated.

Long QT-interval syndromes may be congenital or induced by drugs, electrolyte abnormalities, severe bradycardia, or abnormal nutritional states. When the QT interval is prolonged, the patient is at significant risk of developing torsade de pointes, a polymorphous ventricular tachycardia with QRS complexes that fluctuate in size and direction in an oscillating pattern (Fig. 45-12). This arrhythmia often causes syncope or death. Causal antiarrhythmic drugs include quinidine, procainamide, disopyramide, sotalol, and amiodarone. Psychotropic drugs that have been implicated include chlorpromazine, thioridazine, and probably tricyclic antidepressants. Terfenadine, macrolides (eg erythromycin), pentamidine, trimethoprim–sulfamethoxazole, ketoconazole, and itraconazole have been associated with torsade de pointes. The combination of terfenadine with macrolide antibiotics, ketoconazole, itraconazole, or hepatic dysfunction is especially likely in this arrhythmia and is absolutely contraindicated. Hypomagnesemia, hypocalcemia, and hypokalemia can trigger torsade de pointes; these electrolyte disturbances may be the cause in cases associated with liquid protein diets and anorexia nervosa. Third-degree AV block and sinus bradycardia/arrest can trigger torsade de pointes due to rate-related QT prolongation. Treatments include discontinuation of the inciting drug, correction of electrolyte abnormalities, artificial pacing to 100 to 110 bpm, and intravenous magnesium sulfate.

Mitral valve prolapse is often associated with palpitations; documented arrhythmias are usually benign and do not require specific treatment. Rarely, clinically malignant tachycardias, generally ventricular in origin, are observed; these patients require cardiology referral.

Left or right bundle branch block occurs when conduction through these components of the His-Purkinje system fails. The ventricle whose bundle branch is blocked activates slowly via intramyocardial conduction from the opposite ventricle, and a prolonged QRS complex is inscribed on the ECG. Left bundle branch block is usually associated with and may be the presenting manifestation of significant underlying structural heart disease. Right bundle branch block may occur with or without associated cardiac disease, and extensive investigation is usually not required if the clinical evaluation is benign.

Permanent artificial pacemakers are now commonly implanted for treatment of bradycardia and occasionally tachycardia; however, these devices may precipitate symptoms or arrhythmias. Ventricular pacemakers often cause loss of AV synchrony; this may lead to lightheadedness, hypotension, and fatigue. Impaired heart rate response to exercise is a problem, although modern pacemakers are usually designed with the ability to respond to increased physiologic demand. Dual-chamber devices are better for duplicating normal cardiac physiology but can produce pacemaker-mediated tachycardias. Cardiology referral is required when symptoms arise in these patients.

CONSIDERATIONS IN PREGNANCY

Pregnancy induces significant maternal changes that may induce arrhythmia in both previously normal persons and in those with preexisting cardiac disease. Cardiac output and blood volume increase, heart rate rises, diastolic and to a lesser extent systolic

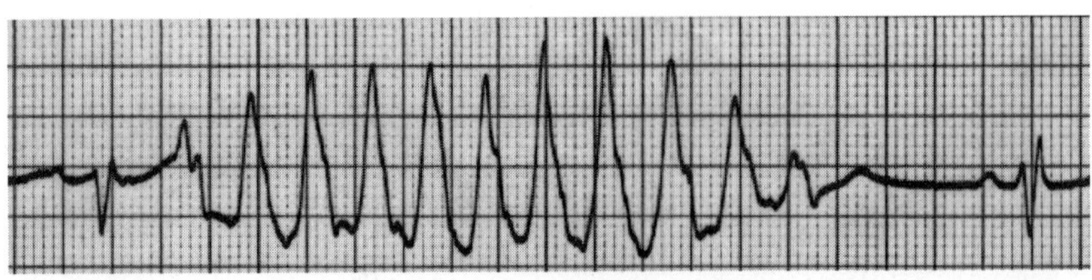

Figure 45-12. Torsade de pointes.

blood pressure falls, and the hormonal milieu changes. Positional compression of the inferior vena cava and abdominal aorta can induce sudden changes in central blood volume. Cardiology referral is advised when sustained or hemodynamically significant arrhythmia requires treatment during gestation.

In general, drug treatment is avoided whenever possible, especially in the first trimester. Drug levels and effects may vary due to changes in intravascular volume, plasma protein binding, renal and hepatic clearance, and gastrointestinal absorption. When predicted efficacy is similar, it is wisest to use older drugs that have been found to be safe over longer periods of experience. Most antiarrhythmic drugs, with the notable exception of amiodarone, appear to be safe for breastfeeding of infants.

Cardioversion and pacing have been used during pregnancy without untoward effects to mother or fetus. Cardiopulmonary resuscitation is initially performed as usual; if it appears that resuscitation will be unsuccessful and the fetus is of viable age, cesarean section should be initiated within 15 minutes of arrest.

Mild sinus tachycardia is normally seen during pregnancy. Premature atrial and ventricular contractions are frequently detected and do not require further evaluation or treatment. Some women have first onset of supraventricular tachycardia in pregnancy; those with a prior history, especially in the setting of Wolff-Parkinson-White syndrome, commonly experience increased frequency and severity of episodes. Rare patients develop continuous automatic atrial tachycardias that resolve after delivery. Acute, sustained episodes of AVNRT or AVRT are approached with vagal maneuvers. First-line drug therapy is adenosine, which is safe, effective, and rapidly metabolized; the next drug used in this setting should be intravenous verapamil. If recurrent episodes are sufficiently frequent or severe, chronic therapy with digoxin (AVNRT only), cardioselective β-adrenergic blockers, verapamil, quinidine, and procainamide have been used safely and effectively. Digoxin is the first choice for ventricular rate control in atrial fibrillation; other options are cardioselective β-adrenergic blockers, verapamil, or diltiazem. Heparin is the preferred method of anticoagulation due to the teratogenicity of warfarin.

Ventricular tachycardia during pregnancy is rare. Initially, the presence or absence of associated cardiac disease should be established. Sustained episodes may be treated with intravenous lidocaine or procainamide. Patients with structurally normal hearts and episodic ventricular tachycardia usually respond to β-adrenergic blockers. When identifiable cardiac pathology is present, treatment proceeds as in the nongravid state. Type IA agents are usually tried first; second-line agents are sotalol and propafenone. Amiodarone is avoided in pregnancy unless necessary.

Bradycardias are uncommon during pregnancy. Occasionally, congenital 3° AV block is encountered; these patients often require temporary or permanent pacing.

BIBLIOGRAPHY

Blackshear JL, Kopecky SL, Litin SC, Safford RE, Hammill SC. Management of atrial fibrillation in adults: prevention of thromboembolism and symptomatic treatment. Mayo Clin Proc 1996;71:150.

Commins RO, ed. Advanced cardiac life support. Dallas: American Heart Association, 1994.

Cox JL, Gardner MJ. Treatment of cardiac arrhythmias during pregnancy. Progr Cardiovascular Dis 1993;36:137.

Elkayam U, Gleicher N, eds. Cardiac problems in pregnancy: diagnosis and management of maternal and fetal disease, 2d ed. New York: Alan R. Liss, 1990.

Page RL. Treatment of arrhythmias during pregnancy. Am Heart J 1995;130:871.

Prystowsky EN, Klein GJ. Cardiac arrhythmias: an integrated approach for the clinician. New York: McGraw-Hill, 1994.

Primary Care for Women, edited by Phyllis C. Leppert and Fred M. Howard. Lippincott-Raven Publishers, Philadelphia © 1997.

46

Cardiac Murmurs

LAURA J. VON DOENHOFF

The finding of a heart murmur on physical examination in a patient not known to have cardiac disease may generate anxiety in the patient and prompt consternation in the physician. Today's informed patient may press for detailed information about the implications of the heart murmur. Her dentist, knowing that a murmur exists, may insist on guidance regarding periprocedural antibiotic prophylaxis. Furthermore, the recent availability of high-quality echocardiography has resulted in additional pressure on the physician to characterize the murmur definitively, to order the test, or both. Most contemporary physicians practice in a litigious climate.

There is no single approach to this clinical problem. The strategy for workup is governed by the characteristics of the murmur as well as other individual factors including the patient's age, overall health, symptomatology, and level of anxiety.

This chapter gives a practical approach to the evaluation and management of heart murmurs. This is intended to be a guide for primary care clinicians in the outpatient setting and not a detailed discussion of valvular or congenital heart disease. The technique of auscultation is briefly described; various murmurs are then discussed in approximate order of prevalence.

PHYSICAL EXAMINATION: A BRIEF GUIDE TO THE TECHNIQUE OF AUSCULTATION

Nonauscultatory aspects of the cardiac physical examination (eg, examination of peripheral arteries, estimation of jugular venous pressure) are not discussed here.

The patient should be placed comfortably in the supine position with the head of the bed elevated to about 30° or 45°. The precordium should be palpated with the entire palm to locate the left ventricular impulse (LVI) and to feel for any thrills (vibrations accompanying a murmur). The patient should then assume the left decubitus position; the LVI again should be located and palpated. In this position, the bell of the stethoscope should be lightly placed over the LVI and the deep-pitched, apical sounds appreciated. These include the first heart sound (S_1), any third heart sound (S_3), the fourth heart sound (S_4), and any mitral diastolic rumble. Auscultation should proceed with the diaphragm of the stethoscope held to the LVI, listening for higher pitched sounds at the apex, such as systolic murmurs. With the patient supine again, auscultation with the diaphragm should proceed from the apex, inching upward toward the base of the heart. One should listen not only in the traditional tricuspid, pulmonic, and aortic areas, but also over the sternum and clavicles, because bony structures transmit high-pitched sounds well. At the base of the heart, attention should be paid to the second heart sound and to higher pitched murmurs (eg, aortic stenosis [AS] or aortic sclerosis, mitral regurgitation, pericardial rubs). Ultimately, the patient should sit up, leaning forward, as the examiner listens with the diaphragm for the high-pitched sounds of rubs and aortic regurgitant murmurs. It may be necessary for the patient to hold expiration. Finally, the patient should stand to allow for characterization of the murmurs of mitral valve prolapse (MVP) and hypertrophic obstructive cardiomyopathy, and (in some patients) to obtain full closure of the second heart sound.

Murmurs have been historically classified as grade 1 (barely audible), grade 2 (faint), grade 3 (moderately loud), grade 4 (accompanied by a thrill), grade 5 (audible with the stethoscope held partly off the chest), and grade 6 (audible with the stethoscope held entirely off the chest).

The patient's body habitus greatly affects the transmission of heart sounds to the chest wall surface. Obesity, increased anteroposterior chest dimension, and hyperinflated lungs, as well as pulmonary adventitious sounds, impede cardiac auscultation.

CLINICAL FINDINGS

Systolic Murmurs

Flow Murmurs (Ejection Murmurs, Innocent Murmurs)

This broad category comprises systolic murmurs heard in the absence of any identifiable disease and connotes benignity. There is no meaningful distinction between flow, ejection, and innocent murmurs. It is not always possible to pinpoint the valvular etiology of these murmurs, even by echocardiography; rarely, if ever, is it necessary to do so. These murmurs often are described as either aortic flow murmurs or pulmonic flow murmurs, depending on the location. They relate to the volume of blood flow, or turbulence, or both.

No symptoms are referable to flow murmurs. Benign systolic murmurs can occur in the setting of hyperdynamic or high-output physiology such as anemia, fever, anxiety, hypertension, and exertion. They also are associated with the increased stroke volume that occurs with pregnancy, obesity, athletic conditioning, and bradycardia.

On auscultation they are systolic; characteristically "crescendo–decrescendo" or "diamond shaped" in their volume profile; relatively low pitched; sometimes musical; often faint (grade 1, 2, or 3, depending on the hemodynamic conditions); and sometimes evanescent. It is typical for the murmur to come and go on serial examinations, depending on the patient's hemodynamic state, and this evanescence may be a tip-off to the diagnosis. (On the other hand, the mitral regurgitant murmur associated with MVP also may vary, but usually more clearly with position.) The murmur may be most prominent at the upper or lower left sternal border, or at the apex. Flow murmurs are common in the young (35 years of age or younger) patient.

Cardiorespiratory (cardiopulmonary) murmurs are soft systolic murmurs that are evident only during inspiration and disappear in expiration or when the breath is held. These murmurs may be of somewhat higher pitch and thus may resemble regurgitant murmurs, except for their phasic nature. They are benign.

If the examiner is confident that the murmur fits these descriptions, then no further workup and no treatment is necessary. Serial auscultation is helpful in confirming the murmur's characteristics and sometimes in establishing its evanescent nature. If an echocardiogram were ordered, results would be benign; it might show an increased stroke volume and (in obese, pregnant, or athletic patients) increased chamber sizes. No valvular disease would be manifest. This point of view concurs with recent work done on outpatients, predominantly women, which suggests that healthy young women (up to 35 years of age) with soft systolic murmurs (up to grade 2) rarely have significant valvular abnormalities on echocardiogram.

Aortic Sclerosis

Aortic sclerosis means the deposition of calcium, visible on echocardiogram, on an otherwise normal, mobile, tricuspid aortic valve. Calcification typically begins in the seventh or eighth decade; it occurs earlier in patients with hypertension, abnormal calcium metabolism, and other conditions. It is a benign entity; no symptoms are referable to it. It could be considered the "flow murmur" of the elderly. It reflects an insignificant degree of AS.

The murmur is systolic and crescendo–decrescendo, but often somewhat harsher and louder (grade 2 or 3) than the previously described flow murmur. It may have a musical quality but, unlike hemodynamically significant AS, high-frequency components are not predominant. The murmur peaks in early to midsystole. The second heart sound is not obscured. It may be best heard at the base of the heart (over the sternum or at the left sternal border). Typically, it is a constant rather than an evanescent finding.

Aortic sclerosis is a benign condition, requiring no workup or treatment. The auscultatory findings in some patients, however, may be hard to differentiate from greater degrees of AS and from mitral regurgitation. In such patients, echocardiography can be helpful. Management depends on the results of the echocardiogram.

Aortic Stenosis

By the eighth and ninth decades of life, age-related calcification of a relatively normal aortic valve in a woman may have progressed to a hemodynamically significant lesion. One could speculate that hypertension and other factors accelerate the rate of stenosis. Younger patients with significant aortic calcification typically have bicuspid or otherwise dysplastic aortic valves; these patients are predominantly male, but bicuspid aortic valve does occur in women. Recent work suggests that these abnormal valves calcify and undergo stenosis at a faster rate than do tricuspid valves.

Moderate AS may cause few, if any, symptoms. Even patients with severe AS may have no cardiac symptoms, especially if they are physically limited for other reasons. Symptoms may include dyspnea or light-headedness on exertion; the classic triad of angina, syncope, and congestive heart failure occurs late in the disease process. The electrocardiogram and the chest roentgenogram may show cardiac enlargement.

On auscultation, the systolic murmur is best heard at the base, that is, over the sternum, over the right clavicle, at the upper right sternal border (the aortic area), or along the left sternal border. It is typically harsh and wheezy or grinding but can be musical. Both high- and low-frequency audio components are present. The timing of the peak of the murmur may help to differentiate mild to moderate AS (early to midsystolic peak) from severe AS (late systolic peak, occasionally obscuring the second heart sound). The milder the stenosis, the more the situation resembles the previously discussed aortic sclerosis.

The murmur of AS commonly radiates to the carotid arteries, especially to the right, but it should not be confused with an arterial (carotid or subclavian) bruit. A bruit should be loudest over the affected artery, and almost inaudible at the base of the heart.

A diastolic murmur (that of aortic regurgitation [AR]) also may be heard; this finding may help localize the systolic murmur to the aortic valve.

The finding of a murmur suggestive of AS warrants echocardiography. In most cases, the aortic valve area, gradient, and other indicators of severity are available from the echocardiogram. Patient management depends on the results of the echocardiogram and may involve cardiology referral.

Rarely, the stenosis is subaortic rather than valvular, and is due to a congenital fibrous subaortic "collar" or membrane. This is known as discrete subaortic stenosis. In childhood, this can be a serious, progressive lesion requiring surgical resection; when it presents in adulthood, it is typically milder. The systolic murmur may be indistinguishable from that of valvular AS. AR, related to deformity of the aortic leaflets by the subaortic jet, can be present. Echocardiography can fully characterize this lesion, which warrants periprocedural antibiotic prophylaxis for the indicated procedures.

Mitral Valve Prolapse

Mitral valve prolapse, also known as Barlow syndrome and the click-murmur syndrome, most often is suspected in young female patients. Estimates of its incidence in the general population range from 5% to 15%. It is an autosomal dominant, congenital trait. Most likely, it is equally common in men and women, but many believe that women are more often symptomatic from it. A history of palpitations, atypical chest pain, cold hands and feet, migraine headaches and other neurologic phenomena, or panic attacks may prompt a search for MVP. On the other hand, many patients are asymptomatic and are found to have a click or characteristic murmur on physical examination.

The pathologic mechanism in classic cases involves elongation, redundancy, and thickening of the mitral leaflets related to myxomatous degeneration. In systole, the leaflets billow, resulting in the characteristic click. Overclosure or faulty closure of the leaflets in systole results in regurgitation into the left atrium.

Much has been made of the tall, thin, asthenic habitus associated with this lesion, but in everyday practice, MVP can be found in a variety of body types. It is, however, notably prevalent in patients with a marked pectus excavatum.

Typically, the electrocardiogram and chest roentgenogram results are normal when the lesion is not hemodynamically significant.

The classic auscultatory findings are a systolic click (literally a high-pitched clicking, "clucking," or snapping sound) followed by an apical regurgitant murmur crescendoing toward the second heart sound. Classically, the click moves earlier in systole and the murmur becomes longer when the patient stands up, because with that maneuver the left ventricular chamber becomes smaller and the disproportion between the small LV chamber and redundant mitral valve increases. In everyday practice, things are less classic. Patients shown by echocardiography to have MVP with significant (ie, mild or worse) mitral regurgitation may have no murmur, even when the body habitus is slender. The murmur may be present, but for some reason is more outflow (diamond shaped and deep pitched) than regurgitant (higher pitched, narrow in frequency range, "whooshy," crescendo or holosystolic, occasionally musical) in character. A coexisting aortic systolic murmur may mask the regurgitant murmur. When the mitral regurgitation is marked, the murmur may be harsh enough to mimic aortic sclerosis or stenosis. The click may be absent.

The presence of a click or multiple clicks, with or without a murmur, indicates a high likelihood of MVP. Other possibilities include that the click is tricuspid in origin (indicating tricuspid valve prolapse) or aortic in origin (the click may be an aortic ejection sound accompanying a bicuspid aortic valve). The latter sound classically occurs earlier in systole than a mitral click and may be associated with the diastolic blow of AR. It is also important not to mistake the sequence of S_4–S_1 for the sequence of S_1–click. This commonly happens in hypertensive patients whose S_4 can be loud. The fourth and first heart sounds are deep pitched; the click is high pitched. A split S_1 also can mimic the S_1–click sequence. Again, both the mitral and tricuspid components of the split S_1 are deep-pitched.

As the regurgitation associated with MVP progresses, the murmur becomes more prominent and assumes an increasingly classic regurgitant character (either crescendo or holosystolic in nature). The click may become relatively less prominent.

Three questions typically arise when MVP is suspected:

1. *Is MVP present*? The finding of a distinctly mitral click is the most powerful clinical indicator of MVP. When the findings are less clear-cut, echocardiography is helpful in establishing or refuting the diagnosis. The finding of MVP may establish an etiology for the patient's chest pain, palpitations, and other symptoms.
2. *Does it require periprocedural antibiotic prophylaxis against infective endocarditis*? The finding of a click and regurgitant murmur establishes that MVP is present and that there is associated regurgitation warranting antibiotic prophylaxis for the indicated procedures. Assuming that a decision to treat prophylactically has been made and that the patient has no exertional dyspnea to suggest hemodynamically significant mitral regurgitation, then echocardiography is not necessary. In most other situations, the echocardiogram provides helpful information. That is, echocardiography can show the degree of mitral regurgitation (which, as mentioned, can exist in the absence of a murmur), can show redundancy (thickening) of the mitral leaflets, and can also *exclude* both the presence of significant (mild or worse) mitral regurgitation and the pres-

ence of MVP itself. By excluding significant regurgitation, echocardiography sometimes allows discontinuation of periprocedural antibiotics currently taken by the patient.

An individual patient's risk of acquiring infective endocarditis after a procedure such as dental cleaning has been shown to depend on several factors. Those at greatest risk (1) are men, (2) are 45 years of age or older, (3) have significant mitral regurgitation, and (4) have redundancy of the mitral leaflets. This information helps the clinician to judge which patients require echocardiograms and which patients require prophylaxis.

3. *Is the mitral regurgitation hemodynamically significant*? Echocardiography to quantitate the degree of regurgitation is warranted in patients who report exertional dyspnea or show signs of congestive heart failure. Patient management depends on the results of the echocardiogram and may involve cardiology referral.

MVP receives attention as a syndrome affecting the young, but as a congenital condition, it is lifelong and equally prevalent in the elderly. As noted, the click may become less prominent with age, possibly because of progressive calcification of the mitral apparatus restricting leaflet motion. The regurgitant murmur may coexist with or be masked by the murmur of aortic sclerosis, but the need to offer antibiotic prophylaxis only increases with age. As the patient ages, the auscultatory findings may be harder to sort out and the echocardiogram may have increasing usefulness.

Hypertrophic Obstructive Cardiomyopathy

Hypertrophic obstructive cardiomyopathy (HOCM), also known as idiopathic hypertrophic subaortic stenosis, originally was described in young patients with rare, severe familial disease. Currently, we have come to understand its greater prevalence in an acquired form. The latter characteristically afflicts hypertensive patients, often elderly women with small, hyperdynamic left ventricles. Exertional dyspnea may be present, especially if there is tachycardia. The electrocardiogram and chest roentgenogram may show left ventricular hypertrophy.

The murmur of either form of this disease is that of dynamic subaortic obstruction. This obstruction, which can be shown on echocardiogram as a subvalvular pressure gradient, is variable with hemodynamic factors such as heart rate, hydration, and blood pressure. If there is a high degree of obstruction at rest (common when there is tachycardia or dehydration), then the systolic murmur may be harsh and on occasion indistinguishable from the murmur of valvular AS. If the patient is elderly, then calcification of the aortic valve and cardiac skeleton is likely, and the murmur of aortic sclerosis (or even significant AS) will be superimposed, confounding the picture.

When lesser degrees of this dynamic subaortic obstruction are present and when significant aortic valvular calcification is absent, diagnosis is facilitated by taking advantage of the change in hemodynamics that occurs with position. That is, the left ventricle becomes smaller when the patient stands. The murmur, which may be soft and "whooshy" with the patient seated (and either holosystolic or late systolic or, perhaps, diamond shaped), becomes more prominent when the patient stands. If late systolic at rest, it may become holosystolic. This is in contrast to the behavior of valvular AS but similar to the behavior of the classic murmur of MVP. The latter condition may be indistinguishable from HOCM on physical examination.

Echocardiography is warranted when HOCM is suspected. Patient management depends on the results of the echocardiogram and may involve cardiology referral. HOCM requires antibiotic prophylaxis.

Papillary Muscle Dysfunction

Women who sustain a myocardial infarction, particularly one involving the inferior wall and inferoseptal papillary muscle, may develop ischemic mitral regurgitation. Failure of the myocardial wall to contract in and around the papillary muscle can result in incomplete leaflet coaptation and leakage. Acute ischemia without infarction can give the same result.

This lesion would not be found in the generally healthy, nonischemic outpatient, but it is mentioned for completeness. The clinical history, electrocardiogram, and echocardiogram as a whole would paint the picture of ischemia or infarction. The murmur is systolic and regurgitant in character. Most believe that it does not warrant periprocedural antibiotic prophylaxis.

Pulmonic Stenosis

Hemodynamically significant congenital valvular pulmonic stenosis (PS) is a congenital lesion that is usually corrected or ameliorated in childhood. Mild degrees of it often persist after surgical or balloon procedures into adulthood. In other cases, the congenital lesion is mild from birth and unsuspected.

In mild PS, the patient is typically asymptomatic. The electrocardiogram and chest roentgenogram may be normal. More severe degrees of PS may give rise to exertional dyspnea, and the electrocardiogram and chest roentgenogram may show right ventricular hypertrophy or enlargement.

The systolic murmur is likely to be most prominent at the upper left sternal border (the pulmonic area). It is outflow in character, sometimes coarse, often grade 3 or 4. As with most right-sided cardiac sounds, it increases on inspiration. It may be associated with a pulmonic ejection sound, which is an early systolic click caused by the doming of a pliable valve. (Paradoxically, the pulmonic ejection sound decreases on inspiration.) There may be an associated diastolic murmur, that of pulmonic regurgitation, particularly in patients who have undergone procedures to lessen the PS; this is also most prominent at the upper left sternal border. There may be a left parasternal lift when significant right heart enlargement is present.

PS and regurgitation do not require periprocedural antibiotic prophylaxis. Lesions confined to the right side of the heart, which functions at pressures much lower than the left side of the heart, typically do not require prophylaxis.

Ventricular Septal Defect

Most congenital hemodynamically significant defects in the interventricular septum are corrected in childhood. Many smaller defects close spontaneously in infancy. Those that persist into adulthood typically are hemodynamically insignificant but require vigilant periprocedural antibiotic prophylaxis. A ventricular septal defect (VSD) is among the lesions at highest risk of infection during bacteremic procedures.

It is rarely a cause of a systolic murmur in an adult. Typically, the patient is asymptomatic. The electrocardiogram and chest roentgenogram may be completely normal. The murmur is prominent (often grade 3 or 4) and typically has been the focus of much attention throughout the patient's life. It is holosystolic, regurgitant, and loud. The smaller the actual defect, the higher the velocities (seen by Doppler echocardiography) across it, and the harsher the murmur.

Echocardiography is warranted if VSD is suspected. When ordering the test, it is crucial to specify what is being sought, as the routine echocardiographic examination may not include a search for a VSD.

Diastolic Murmurs

Aortic Regurgitation

The most common cause of a diastolic murmur is AR. This may be the result of anatomic abnormality of the aortic valve itself, as when the valve is bicuspid or otherwise dysplastic, redundant, or calcified, or is affected by rheumatic processes. It can also result from enlargement of the aortic root; this occurs in hypertension, myxomatous degeneration, and rarely in syphilis.

Mild degrees of AR typically cause no symptoms. Patients with more marked regurgitation, or with uncontrolled hypertension, may report exertional dyspnea. The electrocardiogram and chest roentgenogram results are normal in mild degrees and may show left ventricular enlargement when the AR is substantial. Marked aortic root enlargement can be seen on the chest roentgenogram.

The diastolic murmur of AR is easy to overlook on physical examination. As mentioned earlier, it is best heard over or alongside the sternum as the patient sits up, leaning forward, during expiration. Its intensity and length generally vary with the severity of the regurgitation. What shows on echocardiogram as trace or mild AR often is inaudible, even on careful listening. More severe degrees of AR are likely to be audible, depending on the body habitus; severity generally correlates with pulse pressure (the difference between systolic and diastolic blood pressure).

The murmur is a blow that begins immediately after the second heart sound and that usually has a tambour quality. On occasion, a tambour quality of the second heart sound itself may be the only tip-off to the presence of AR. The blow is decrescendo and high pitched, and may occupy any length of diastole. When the aortic root is substantially enlarged, the blow may be loudest to the right of the sternum.

Significant degrees of AR usually are accompanied by a forward systolic aortic flow murmur, even in the absence of significant AS. On the other hand, hemodynamically significant AS commonly coexists with AR. The presence of an aortic ejection sound, which typically is an early systolic click, signals the presence of a nonstenotic bicuspid aortic valve, as it results from the doming of a pliable valve. As the bicuspid valve calcifies and stiffens, the click typically disappears.

The murmur of AR can be confused with an unusually loud murmur of pulmonic regurgitation, with the murmur of patent ductus arteriosus (PDA), and occasionally with a multicomponent pericardial rub.

Echocardiography is warranted when AR is suspected or when any clearly diastolic murmur is heard. It can delineate the severity of the AR and has been shown to be more accurate than either the chest roentgenogram or the electrocardiogram in measuring the aortic root and the left ventricle. Patient management depends on the results of the echocardiogram and may involve cardiology referral.

Periprocedural antibiotic prophylaxis may not be necessary when the AR is largely due to valve sclerosis or hypertension or aortic root enlargement, and when the valve itself is minimally abnormal. Bicuspid aortic valves, on the other hand, are at high risk of infection during bacteremic procedures, and warrant prophylaxis.

Mitral Stenosis

Now much less common than in the preantibiotic era, but still prevalent in some geographic areas, rheumatic mitral stenosis (MS) is suspected clinically much more often than it is found on echocardiogram. In many patients labeled as having it on the basis of a history of a febrile childhood illness, the diagnosis can be refuted by echocardiography. The typical patient with true MS is an older woman with few symptoms or, in more severe disease, exertional dyspnea and general fatigue.

The auscultatory findings are easy to misinterpret, in part because they are infrequently encountered by the clinician. Making the diagnosis requires careful listening at the cardiac apex and at the left sternal border, with the patient lying on her left side. The most striking finding is usually the accentuated first heart sound. This can be considered the focal point for the entire cadence of MS, which consists of presystolic accentuation, loud S_1, S_2, prominent opening snap, and deep-pitched diastolic rumble. Familiarity with the entire cadence and listening for it as a whole help to establish the diagnosis. The systolic murmur of mitral regurgitation, occurring between S_1 and S_2, often accompanies the findings. As the mitral valve calcifies with age and the stenosis progresses, the auscultatory findings may become more difficult to appreciate.

Echocardiography is warranted whenever MS is suspected and whenever a past diagnosis of it was made on clinical grounds alone. Patient management depends on the results of the echocardiogram and may involve cardiology referral.

Rarely, MS is congenital rather than rheumatic. In the postantibiotic era, the incidence of congenital MS relative to rheumatic MS has increased, especially in young patients. The implication, however, is the same. Echocardiography, which can differentiate the congenital from the rheumatic etiology, is warranted. MS requires periprocedural antibiotic prophylaxis. Rheumatic MS in young patients also requires antibiotic prophylaxis to prevent disease recurrence.

Abnormal Second Heart Sound

Atrial Septal Defect

Failure of the interatrial septum to close during embryonic development can result in a variety of anatomic malformations. Ostium primum defects are often associated with other intracardiac problems and are typically identified and corrected in childhood. Ostium secundum defects may be large and identified early, or relatively small, and undetected until adulthood.

Symptoms of ostium secundum defects may be minimal. The patient may notice exertional dyspnea or palpitations. The chest roentgenogram typically shows right heart enlargement and increased pulmonary vascularity. The electrocardiogram usually shows right bundle branch block and right axis deviation. Atrial arrhythmias may be present. In fact, any patient with right bundle branch block and atrial arrhythmias should be suspected of having atrial septal defect (ASD).

On physical examination, there may be a right ventricular lift at the lower left sternal border. A systolic murmur is usually present; echocardiography has shown that tricuspid regurgitation, increased pulmonic flow, and MVP all are common in ASD. But the striking auscultatory finding is persistent splitting of the second heart sound rather than any murmur.

In the normal patient, the pulmonic component of the second heart sound (P_2) is delayed on inspiration, but superimposed on its aortic component (A_2) in expiration, allowing full closure of

S_2. It may be necessary for the patient to hold expiration and stand for S_2 to close completely. In ASD, wide, fixed splitting of S_2, equal in inspiration and expiration, has classically been described. In everyday practice, what holds true more often is that P_2 is louder and more delayed than normal. The delay of P_2 may be greater on inspiration than expiration, yielding persistent rather than fixed splitting of S_2. In either case, S_2 cannot be made to close fully.

Confounding factors include the fact that right bundle branch block itself—as well as idiopathic, benign right heart enlargement—delays P_2. The suspicion of ASD warrants echocardiography, which clarifies the anatomy. Patient management depends on the results of the echocardiogram. Cardiology referral and transesophageal echocardiography may be necessary.

Murmurs That Are Both Systolic and Diastolic

Pericardial Rub

The visceral and parietal layers of the pericardial sac can become inflamed after viral infection, after transmural myocardial infarction, as a result of a systemic connective tissue disease, or for other reasons. When the two inflamed pericardial surfaces move against each other, a rubbing sound is created. Pericardial effusion often accompanies the inflammation. Large effusions eliminate the rub by preventing contact between the two pericardial layers.

The classic rub is a three-component, high-pitched scratching sound, with one component in systole and two in diastole. The rub often changes or disappears over a matter of hours. One or both diastolic components may disappear, allowing the rub to mimic a systolic murmur.

Pericardial rubs may be best heard over the sternum with the patient leaning forward, in expiration. It may also be useful to have her lie on her left side while the examiner listens at the cardiac apex. Pleural rubs may accompany or mimic pericardial rubs; the former relate clearly to respiratory motion, and the latter, to cardiac motion.

The chest roentgenogram most often is normal. The electrocardiogram may show characteristic repolarization changes. Echocardiography generally is not warranted in the absence of hemodynamic compromise. When performed, the echocardiogram may or may not show pericardial fluid. Management, in the absence of hemodynamic compromise, is directed at the inflammation causing the patient's symptoms and any underlying condition; management is not generally affected by echocardiographic findings.

Patent Ductus Arteriosus

Patent ductus arteriosus is a congenital lesion that is not common, but the consequences of overlooking it are substantial. When the normal fetal connection between the pulmonary artery and the descending thoracic aorta fails to close after birth, a left-to-right shunt develops. Systolic and diastolic shunting and turbulence are detectable by Doppler study of the pulmonary artery.

These patients can be asymptomatic or can report low-grade exertional dyspnea and palpitations. The chest roentgenogram and electrocardiogram results most often are normal, as the amount of the shunt is typically small.

The murmur is continuous, that is, both systolic and diastolic. Classically, this harsh "machinery" murmur is heard at the upper left sternal border or inferior to the left clavicle. It is loudest in late systole and early diastole, with a late diastolic silent interval. The murmur can be subtle. The diastolic component of it can be mistakenly attributed to aortic or pulmonic regurgitation. The diastolic component can be absent, leaving only a systolic murmur. If the body habitus is large, the murmur can be inaudible.

The finding of any diastolic murmur warrants echocardiography, as does any suspicion of PDA. When ordering the test, it is critical to specify what is being sought, because the routine echocardiographic examination may not include a search of the pulmonary artery for disturbed flow signaling the presence of PDA.

A continuous murmur also can be the result of a fistula between a coronary artery and coronary vein, as well as aberrant origin of a coronary artery from the pulmonary artery. These rarer conditions usually are distinguished from PDA by means of transesophageal echocardiography or arteriography.

Cardiology referral is warranted in all three of these conditions. PDA, in particular, is highly correctable in the young. Uncorrected PDA leaves the patient at high risk of bacterial endarteritis after bacteremic procedures. Antibiotic prophylaxis is crucial.

Venous Hum

Venous hum, a benign murmur, is included here for differentiation from PDA. It is heard most often in children and young adults, especially those with hyperdynamic circulation. Typically, the venous hum, although both systolic and diastolic, is deeper pitched, softer, and more nearly continuous than the machinery murmur of PDA. It may be louder in diastole. The venous hum is best heard in the medial aspect of the supraclavicular fossa, especially on the right; it can radiate inferiorly. It is typically obliterated with pressure on the ipsilateral internal jugular vein.

CONSIDERATIONS IN PREGNANCY

The primary hemodynamic alteration in pregnancy is the increase in circulating blood volume, usually to about 50% above the prepregnant state. Accordingly, echocardiography can demonstrate a slight increase in the size of all four cardiac chambers. Cardiac stroke volume increases. Thus, systolic flow murmurs are exceedingly common. It is not clear how soon after delivery the changes return to normal. Cardiac chamber enlargement may persist for 6 months or more and may partly reflect the unreversed maternal weight gain.

Cardiac valvular lesions that restrict cardiac output can become a management problem in the pregnant patient; thus, AS and MS require vigilance by the primary care provider and the cardiologist. Most other cardiac valvular lesions do not present a problem, apart from excessive volume overload produced by the combination of pregnancy and significant valvular regurgitation.

A mammary souffle can be heard late in pregnancy and early in the postpartum period of lactating women. It is high pitched, late systolic or continuous, and heard anywhere on either breast. It reflects arterial blood flow to the breast.

SUMMARY

The stethoscope is not obsolete. The careful clinician develops good judgment in selecting patients for echocardiography referral and cardiology consultation. At times, however, even the seasoned practitioner is confounded by a particular heart murmur. Echocardiography is a powerful diagnostic tool that should be employed whenever the murmur cannot be adequately characterized. The appropriate and cost-effective use of echocardiography and of cardiology consultation is a goal for all clinicians involved in the primary care of women.

BIBLIOGRAPHY

Bates B. A guide to physical examination and history taking, 6th ed. Philadelphia: JB Lippincott, 1994.

Feigenbaum H. Echocardiography, 5th ed. Philadelphia, Lea & Febiger, 1994.

Fink BW. Congenital heart disease: a deductive approach to its diagnosis. Chicago: Year Book Medical Publishers, 1975.

Fink JC, Schmid CH, Selker HP: A decision aid for referring patients with systolic murmurs for echocardiography. J Gen Intern Med 1994;9:479.

Perloff JK. The clinical recognition of congenital heart disease, 4th ed. Philadelphia: WB Saunders, 1994.

Primary Care for Women, edited by Phyllis C. Leppert and Fred M. Howard. Lippincott-Raven Publishers, Philadelphia © 1997.

47

Cardiovascular Antibiotic Prophylaxis

ANN R. FALSEY

Despite the development of antimicrobial agents and modern surgical interventions, infective endocarditis continues to cause significant morbidity and mortality. Approximately 4000 to 8000 new cases of endocarditis are reported per year in the United States. Prevention of endocarditis is highly desirable, because morbidity may be substantial even with treatment. Currently, it is standard practice to administer antimicrobial prophylaxis before dental or other bacteremia-associated procedures to individuals believed to be at risk for developing endocarditis. Because no controlled clinical studies documenting the efficacy of antibiotic prophylaxis in humans have been done or are likely to be done, recommendations by the American Heart Association (AHA) are based on in vitro studies, clinical experience, data from animal models, the bacteriology of endocarditis, and estimates of bacteremia following various medical procedures.

RATIONALE

The rationale for giving antibiotic prophylaxis to prevent bacterial endocarditis is based on several observations. First, patients with certain cardiac abnormalities are at markedly increased risk for endocarditis. Valvulitis or turbulent flow leads to sterile platelet-fibrin thrombi that may be a nidus for infection during bacteremia. Second, 15% to 25% of endocarditis cases occur in temporal association with invasive medical procedures. And last, bacteremias resulting from medical procedures generally are caused by organisms with predictable sensitivity patterns. Thus, it is reasonable to attempt to prevent some cases of endocarditis by using antibiotics before procedures that are associated with bacteremia in individuals at risk. Although "reasonable," one must consider the risk of allergic reactions and cost versus potential benefit to the individual patient. Which specific procedures and cardiac conditions are of sufficient risk to warrant prophylaxis is a source of considerable controversy. Current recommendations are provided in the following sections as guidelines, yet they must be tailored to the individual patient.

CARDIAC DEFECTS

Certain cardiac conditions are more strongly associated with endocarditis than others and, thus, prophylaxis recommendations depend on the cardiac abnormality (Table 47-1). Estimates of risk of endocarditis for specific cardiac defects are based on the frequency with which these conditions are found in patients with documented endocarditis. High-risk conditions include prosthetic cardiac valves, previous bacterial endocarditis, and most congenital cardiac malformations. At the other end of the spectrum are conditions such as atrial septal defects, cardiac pacemakers and implantable defibrillators, and previous coronary artery bypass surgery, all of which are not believed to increase the risk of endocarditis. Antibiotic prophylaxis usually is not recommended for individuals with low-risk conditions, whereas prophylaxis is recommended for those with high or intermediate risk.

Mitral valve prolapse (MVP) deserves special attention because it is clearly associated with bacterial endocarditis and, in many series, is the most common underlying disorder. However, MVP also occurs very commonly in the general population. Depending on the population surveyed and the definition used, the prevalence has been estimated between 2% and 21%. A reasonable approximation of MVP in the general population is between 5% and 8%. Although the risk of endocarditis is increased, the magnitude of the risk is small, roughly 100-fold less than that of rheumatic disease. Not all patients with MVP are at equal risk. Endocarditis seems to occur more frequently in men than in women, and in older patients more frequently than in younger patients. In addition, patients with MVP and an audible regurgitant murmur or echocardiographic findings of thickened, redundant valvular tissue seem to be at highest risk. Risk among patients with a MVP without a murmur is not significantly increased compared with risk of endocarditis among persons with normal valves.

PROCEDURES

Spontaneous transient bacteremias of low intensity and short duration are relatively common. Prophylaxis is feasible only when significant bacteremia can be predicted and, thus, only a few cases of endocarditis are potentially preventable. Not all procedures cause the same frequency or intensity of bacteremia. Additionally, some procedures are associated with bacteremia caused by organisms unlikely to adhere to endothelium, such as gram-negative bacilli.

Table 47-1. Cardiac Conditions*

Endocarditis Prophylaxis Recommended
Prosthetic cardiac valves, including bioprosthetic and homograft valves
Previous bacterial endocarditis, even in the absence of heart disease
Most congenital cardiac malformations
Rheumatic and other acquired valvular dysfunction, even after valvular surgery
Hypertrophic cardiomyopathy
Mitral valve prolapse with valvular regurgitation
Endocarditis Prophylaxis Not Recommended
Isolated secundum atrial septal defect
Surgical repair without residua beyond 6 mo of secundum atrial septal defect, ventricular septal defect, or patent ductus arteriosus
Previous coronary artery bypass graft surgery
Mitral valve prolapse without valvular regurgitation†
Physiologic, functional, or innocent heart murmurs
Previous Kawasaki disease without valvular dysfunction
Previous rheumatic fever without valvular dysfunction
Cardiac pacemakers and implanted defibrillators

*This table lists selected conditions but is not meant to be all inclusive.

†Individuals who have a mitral valve prolapse associated with thickening or redundancy of the valve leaflets may be at increased risk for bacterial endocarditis.

(Dajani AS, Bisno AL, Chung KJ, et al. Prevention of bacterial endocarditis: recommendations of the American Heart Association. JAMA 1990;264:2919.)

When considering the need for prophylaxis based on the planned procedure, three questions should be analyzed: Is the procedure associated with significant rates of bacteremia? Are the organisms likely to cause endocarditis? Is there reasonable clinical evidence that the procedure has been associated with endocarditis? Rates of bacteremia associated with specific procedures are given in Table 47-2.

Dental and Upper Respiratory Tract Procedures

Current recommendations by the AHA for prophylaxis related to dental and surgical procedures are listed in Table 47-3. Because poor dental hygiene can lead to bacteremia even in the absence of a procedure, all high-risk patients should maintain good oral health. Antibiotic prophylaxis is recommended for all dental procedures likely to cause gingival bleeding, including routine cleaning. If a series of procedures is required, a 7-day interval between procedures should be observed to avoid the emergence of resistant organisms. Ill-fitting dentures may result in oral ulcers, which can also lead to bacteremia. Therefore, patients with new dentures should be reexamined periodically. Other upper respiratory tract procedures associated with organisms that commonly cause endocarditis include tonsillectomy/adenoidectomy, bronchoscopy with rigid bronchoscope, and esophageal sclerotherapy and dilation.

α-Hemolytic (viridans) streptococci are the most common cause of bacterial endocarditis following dental and respiratory tract procedures, and therapy should be specifically directed at

Table 47-2. Representative Rates of Bacteremia after Various Dental, Diagnostic and Therapeutic Procedures*

PROCEDURE AND SITE	INCIDENCE RATE (RANGE)
None (spontaneous bacteremia)	< 1 (0–3)
Oral cavity	
Tooth extraction	60 (18–85)
Periodontal surgery	88 (60–90)
Brushing teeth or irrigation	40 (7–50)
Tonsillectomy	35 (33–38)
Respiratory tract	
Tracheal intubation	< 10 (0–16)
Nasotracheal suctioning	16
Bronchoscopy	
Rigid bronchoscope	15
Flexible bronchoscope	0
Genitourinary tract	
Catheter insertion or removal	13 (0–26)
Dilation of strictures	28 (19–86)
Normal delivery	3 (1–5)
Gastrointestinal tract	
Upper gastrointestinal endoscopy	4 (0–8)
Transesophageal echocardiography	1 (0–17)
Endoscopic retrograde cholangiopancreatography	5 (0–6)
Barium enema	10 (5–11)
Colonoscopy	5 (0–5)
Sigmoidoscopy	
Rigid sigmoidoscopy	5
Flexible sigmoidoscopy	0
Proctoscopy	2
Hemorrhoidectomy	8
Esophageal dilation	45
Vascular system	
Cardiac catheterization	2 (0–5)

*Ranges are given, if available. Insufficient data were available to calculate the incidence rate of bacteremia after the removal of tympanotomy tubes or cesarean section.

(Durack DT. Prevention of infective endocarditis. N Engl J Med 1995;332:38.)

these organisms. Standard oral regimes are outlined in Table 47-4. Amoxicillin has been selected over penicillin V because it achieves higher and more sustained levels. Erythromycin–ethyl succinate, erythromycin stearate, or clindamycin are well absorbed and are recommended as alternatives to penicillins. An alternative drug should be given to individuals on chronic penicillin for rheumatic fever prevention because the oral cavity may be colonized with penicillin-resistant streptococci. Tetracycline and sulfonamides are not acceptable prophylaxis. Erythromycin should be given *2 hours* before the procedure.

Alternative prophylactic regimens for dental, oral, and upper respiratory tract procedures for individuals unable to take oral medications are given in Table 47-5. Individuals with cardiac con-

Table 47-3. Dental or Surgical Procedure*†

Endocarditis Prophylaxis Recommended

Dental procedures known to induce gingival or mucosal bleeding, including professional cleaning

Tonsillectomy, adenoidectomy

Surgical operations that involve intestinal or respiratory mucosa

Bronchoscopy with a rigid bronchoscope

Sclerotherapy for esophageal varices

Esophageal dilation

Gallbladder surgery

Cystoscopy

Urethral dilation

Urethral catheterization if urinary tract infection is present‡

Urinary tract surgery if urinary tract infection is present‡

Incision and drainage of infected tissue‡

Vaginal hysterectomy

Vaginal delivery in the presence of infection‡

Endocarditis Prophylaxis Not Recommended†

Dental procedures not likely to induce gingival bleeding, such as simple adjustment of orthodontic appliances or filling above the gum line

Injection of local intraoral anesthetic (except intraligamentary injections)

Shedding of primary teeth

Tympanostomy tube insertion

Endotracheal incubation

Bronchoscopy with a flexible bronchoscope, with or without biopsy

Cardiac catheterization

Endoscopy with or without gastrointestinal biopsy

Cesarean section

In the absence of infection: urethral catheterization, dilation and curettage, uncomplicated vaginal delivery, therapeutic abortion, sterilization procedures, or insertion or removal of intrauterine devices

*This table lists selected procedures but is not meant to be all inclusive.

†In patients who have prosthetic heart valves, a previous history of endocarditis, or surgically constructed systemic-pulmonary shunts or conduits, physicians may choose to administer prophylactic antibiotics even for low-risk procedures that involve the lower respiratory, genitourinary, or gastrointestinal tracts.

‡In addition to prophylactic regimen for genitourinary procedures, antibiotic therapy should be directed against the most likely bacterial pathogen.

(Dajani AS, Bisno AL, Chung KJ, et al. Prevention of bacterial endocarditis: recommendations by the American Heart Association. JAMA 1990;264:2919.)

ditions at highest risk for endocarditis, such as prosthetic valves, previous endocarditis, and surgically corrected systemic–pulmonary shunts, previously were recommended to receive parenteral prophylaxis. In clinical practice, these recommendations are difficult to follow. In addition, data from Great Britain, where oral amoxicillin has been used for patients with high-risk conditions without problem, have prompted the AHA to deemphasize the need for parenteral prophylaxis. However, this option is available for physicians who wish to use it in high-risk patients undergoing high-risk procedures.

Table 47-4. Recommended Standard Prophylactic Regimen for Dental, Oral, or Upper Respiratory Tract Procedures in Patients Who Are at Risk*

DRUG	DOSING REGIMEN
	Standard Regimen
Amoxicillin	3.0 g orally 1 h before procedure; then 1.5 g 6 h after initial dose
	Amoxicillin/Penicillin-Allergic Patients
Erythromycin or	Erythromycin ethylsuccinate, 800 mg, or erythromycin stearate, 1.0 g orally 2 h before procedure; then half the dose 6 h after the initial dose
Clindamycin	300 mg orally 1 h before procedure and 150 mg 6 h after initial dose

*Includes those with prosthetic heart valves and other high-risk patients.

(Dajani AS, Bisno AL, Chung KJ, et al. Prevention of bacterial endocarditis: recommendations of the American Heart Association. JAMA 1990;264:2919.)

Table 47-5. Alternate Prophylactic Regimens for Dental, Oral, or Upper Respiratory Tract Procedures in Patients Who Are at Risk

DRUG	DOSING REGIMEN
Patients Unable to Take Oral Medications	
Ampicillin	IV or IM ampicillin, 2.0 g 30 min before procedure; then IV or IM ampicillin, 1.0 g, or amoxicillin orally, 1.5 g 6 h after initial dose
Ampicillin/Amoxicillin/Penicillin-Allergic Patients Unable to Take Oral Medications	
Clindamycin	IV 300 mg 30 min before procedure and IV or orally, 150 mg 6 h after initial dose
Patients Considered High Risk and Not Candidates for Standard Regimen	
Ampicillin, gentamicin, and amoxicillin	IV or IM ampicillin, 2.0 g, plus gentamicin, 1.5 mg/kg (not to exceed 80 mg), 30 min before procedure; followed by amoxicillin, 1.5 g orally 6 h after initial dose; alternatively, the parenteral regimen may be repeated 8 h after initial dose
Ampicillin/Amoxicillin/Penicillin-Allergic Patients Considered High Risk	
Vancomycin	IV 1.0 g over 1 h, starting 1 h before procedures; no repeated dose necessary

(Dajani AS, Bisno AL, Chung KJ, et al. Prevention of bacterial endocarditis: recommendations by the American Heart Association. JAMA 1990;264:2919.)

Table 47-6. Regimens for Genitourinary and Gastrointestinal Procedures

DRUG	DOSAGE REGIMEN
Standard Regimen	
Ampicillin, gentamicin, and amoxicillin	IV or IM ampicillin, 2.0 g, plus gentamicin, 1.5 mg/kg (not to exceed 80 mg), 30 min before procedure; followed by amoxicillin, 1.5 PO 6 h after initial dose; alternatively, the parenteral regimen may be repeated once 8 h after initial dose
Ampicillin/Amoxicillin/ Penicillin-Allergic Patient Regimen	
Vancomycin and gentamicin	IV vancomycin, 1.0 g over 1 h, plus IV or IM gentamicin, 1.5 mg/kg (not to exceed gentamicin 80 mg) 1 h before procedure; may be repeated once 8 h after initial dose
Alternate Low-Risk Patient Regimen	
Amoxicillin	3.0 g PO 1 h before procedure; then 1.5 g PO 6 h after initial dose

(Dajani AS, Bisno AL, Chung KJ, et al. Prevention of bacterial endocarditis: recommendations by the American Heart Association. JAMA 1990;264:2919.)

Genitourinary and Gastrointestinal Tract Procedures

Surgery or instrumentation of the genitourinary tract may cause bacteremia, but primarily when infection is present. Therefore, prophylaxis is recommended for fairly simple procedures such as urinary catheterization only if an infection is present. Similarly, most obstetric and gynecologic procedures, such as dilation and curettage, therapeutic abortion, cervical brushings or biopsy, sterilization procedures, and insertion or removal of intrauterine devices, do not require prophylaxis unless infection is present (see Table 47-3). One exception is vaginal hysterectomy, for which prophylaxis should be given. Because the incidence of bacteremia following uncomplicated spontaneous vaginal delivery in the absence of pelvic infection is low (1% to 5%), the AHA does not recommend antibiotic prophylaxis in these cases (see Table 47-2). Despite this, the American College of Obstetricians and Gynecologists in the June 1992 *Technical Bulletin* offered a more conservative approach. The committee recommends the standard parenteral regimen for highest risk patients and the alternative oral regimen for patients with all other cardiac abnormalities, with the comment that physicians may wish to use the standard regimen in all pregnant cardiac patients. Certain predisposing factors associated with the development of postpartum endocarditis include premature labor, prolonged rupture of membranes before delivery, prolonged third stage of labor, and manual removal of the placenta. In these situations, the standard parenteral prophylaxis should be administered.

The instrumented gastrointestinal tract seems to be a less common portal of entry for endocarditis-causing organisms than the oral cavity or urinary tract. Endoscopy with or without gastrointestinal biopsy is not sufficient to warrant antibiotic prophylaxis. In addition, barium studies of the gastrointestinal tract and liver biopsy also are believed to be procedures at low risk for bacteremia. However, prophylaxis is indicated for cholecystectomy.

Bacterial endocarditis after genitourinary or gastrointestinal procedures most often is caused by *Streptococcus faecalis* (enterococcus). Although gram-negative bacilli or anaerobic bacteremia may occur after such procedures, these organisms rarely cause endocarditis. Therefore, antibiotic regimens for genitourinary or gastrointestinal procedures should be directed against enterococci (Table 47-6). The AHA continues to recommend parenteral antibiotics in patients at highest risk (prosthetic valves, previous endocarditis, corrected shunts), with an alternative oral regimen for lower risk patients.

The preceding recommendations may be confusing when considering an individual patient's risk. For example: Is prophylaxis indicated in a patient with a high-risk cardiac lesion but undergoing a low-risk procedure? One helpful approach is that of the Durack "two-dimensional" assessment. First, the risk posed by the cardiac lesion is assessed, then the risk posed by the procedure is evaluated. If both risks are high, then prophylaxis should be given. If only one risk is high, then prophylaxis is frequently given but is optional. If neither risk is significant, then prophylaxis should be omitted.

Prevention of all cases of bacterial endocarditis is not possible. Infections do occur, even with optimal prophylaxis. The current AHA recommendations are meant be reasonable guidelines for practicing physicians. However, the individual physician should exercise clinical judgment when tailoring prophylaxis to a specific patient.

BIBLIOGRAPHY

American College of Obstetricians and Gynecologists. Cardiac disease in pregnancy: ACOG technical bulletin 168. Washington, DC: American College of Obstetricians and Gynecologists, 1992

Baker TH, Hubbell R. Reappraisal of asymptomatic puerperal bacteremia. Am J Obstet Gynecol 1967;97:575.

Dajani AS, Bisno AL, Chung KJ, et al. Prevention of bacterial endocarditis: recommendations by the American Heart Association. JAMA 1990;264:2919.

Durack DT. Prevention of infective endocarditis. N Engl J Med 1995;332:38.

Greenman RL, Bisno AL. Prevention of bacterial endocarditis. In: Kaye D, ed. Infective endocarditis. New York: Raven Press, 1992:465.

Marks AR, Choong CY, Sanfilippo AJ, et al. Identification of high risk and low risk subgroups of patients with mitral valve prolapse. N Engl J Med 1989;320:1031.

Seaworth BJ, Durack DT. Infective endocarditis in obstetric and gynecologic practice. Am J Obstet Gynecol 1986;154:180.

Sugrue D, Blake S, Troy P, MacDonald D. Antibiotic prophylaxis against infective endocarditis after normal delivery: is it necessary? Br Heart J 1980;44:499.

Primary Care for Women, edited by Phyllis C. Leppert and Fred M. Howard. Lippincott-Raven Publishers, Philadelphia © 1997.

48

Syncope

AASHA S. GOPAL

Syncope is a common clinical problem, accounting for 3% of emergency department visits and 6% of medical admissions. It is a temporary loss of consciousness due to impaired cerebral perfusion. Because the brain is critically dependent on blood glucose for metabolic fuel, interruption of cerebral blood flow leads to syncope in as little as 8 to 10 seconds. Syncope is more common in elderly patients, as cerebral blood flow declines with aging. Two thirds of patients presenting with syncope are over age 60. In this population, syncope occurs at an annual rate of about 6% to 7%, with a recurrence rate of 30%. Typically, a fall in systolic blood pressure below 70 mm Hg or a mean pressure of 30 to 40 mm Hg results in syncope. Other accompanying factors are pallor, sweating, loss of consciousness, and shallow breathing. The patient is usually motionless and without loss of continence. The syncopal episode may or may not vary with posture, depending on the etiology. Consciousness is regained once cerebral perfusion is restored. Depending on its etiology, symptoms such as impaired vision, weakness, wobbly legs, and a fainting sensation may precede frank syncope. Considerable morbidity can occur, particularly in elderly patients, when trauma is sustained due to an abrupt loss of consciousness.

DIFFERENTIAL DIAGNOSIS

Many acute clinical entities may resemble syncope and must be differentiated from it. It is important to distinguish an episode of syncope from an epileptic seizure. If the syncope is due to vasomotor failure or inadequate cardiac output, the patient's upright posture may be important. Also, syncopal episodes are usually brief, begin gradually, and are not associated with aura, convulsive movements, lip-biting injury, injury from falling, bladder incontinence, or postictal confusion. In contrast, epileptic seizures often last longer, begin suddenly in any position with or without aura, and are associated with injury to the lips and to the body from falling, urinary incontinence, and postictal confusion and somnolence.

Transient ischemic attacks and strokes may also mimic syncopal episodes. The former are usually due to atherosclerosis of the cerebral vessels that produces ischemia, the clinical consequence of which is a neurologic deficit. Neurologic deficits usually affect motor, sensory, visual, or speech faculties. They impair consciousness only when the stroke is large or when it involves the brain stem.

Anxiety disorders, hysterical fainting, and hypoglycemia are other conditions that resemble syncope. Anxiety disorders may produce attacks in which a patient may have dizziness due to reduced cerebral perfusion produced by prolonged hyperventilation. These episodes are not posture-dependent and consequently cannot be remedied by assuming a supine position. Fainting on a hysterical basis is not accompanied by hemodynamic abnormalities attributable to changes in heart rate or blood pressure. Hypoglycemia is often accompanied by signs of sympathetic nervous system overstimulation such as restlessness, tachycardia, and confusion. It may ultimately lead to loss of consciousness that begins gradually but may be prolonged and even progress to coma. The onset of the episode may be 3 to 5 hours after a meal, when there is a reactive surge of insulin, or after a prolonged fast when caused by an islets of Langerhans tumor.

ETIOLOGY

Although autoregulation occurs in the cerebral vasculature, cerebral perfusion is critically dependent on systemic arterial blood pressure, which in turn is related to the product of the cardiac output and systemic vascular resistance. The cardiac output is governed by the product of the heart rate and stroke volume, which in turn is regulated by preload, afterload, and cardiac contractility. Thus, a reduction in systemic blood pressure may be produced by an abnormality in any part of the chain of neural mechanisms for peripheral vascular control: the carotid, aortic, ventricular, and atrial baroreceptors, which carry afferent impulses to the medulla; the central vasomotor centers in the medulla, which receive afferent impulses and transmit efferent impulses; cortical and spinal efferent tracts; peripheral sympathetic or parasympathetic nerves; mechanical factors that normally limit pooling of blood in the peripheral veins; intravascular blood volume; and the heart's ability to maintain cardiac output. These etiologic factors divide the important causes of syncope into five broad categories.

Cardiac Syncope

Disturbances of rate and rhythm, obstruction to flow, and impaired ventricular function are three mechanisms by which cardiac syncope may occur. Disturbances of rate and rhythm may result from asystole due to conduction abnormalities, severe bradycardia, or tachyarrhythmias of atrial and ventricular origin. Arrhythmic disorders are common causes of cardiac syncope. Even among patients with complete heart block, often a superimposed arrhythmia such as transient asystole or ventricular fibrillation eventually culminates in syncope. More than 50,000 new cases of complete heart block occur annually in the United States, and it is estimated that about 50% of these patients experience syncope. Complete heart block in the elderly is most often degenerative in etiology (sick sinus syndrome). Among the causes are Lev and Lenegre diseases; other degenerative etiologies are Friedreich ataxia, progressive muscular dystrophy, myotonic dystrophy, and Duchenne dystrophy. Alternatively, structural abnormalities of the conduction system may result from congenital etiologies, infectious diseases (diphtheria, syphilis, toxoplasmosis, mumps, rheumatic fever), collagen vascular disease, valvular heart disease (endocarditis or postoperative), coronary artery disease with or without infarction, tumors, endocrine and metabolic disorders such as gout with urate deposition in the conduction system, hypo- and hyperthyroidism, hemochromatosis, Addison disease, trauma, and diseases of unknown etiology such as Reiter syndrome, sarcoidosis, amyloidosis, and Paget disease. Electrolyte disturbances such as hyperkalemia, acidosis, and hypomagnesemia may also cause complete heart block. In addition, toxicity from drugs such as digitalis, quinidine, lidocaine, aprindine, phenytoin, and amitriptyline may result in complete heart block.

When syncope occurs in pacemaker-dependent patients, pacemaker malfunction should be considered as an etiology. The lack of atrioventricular synchrony may produce the pacemaker syndrome in patients with single-chamber pacemakers. The pacemaker syndrome may produce syncope due to compromised ventricular filling and reduced cardiac output. Also, a vasodepressor response may occur due to reflex vasodilation produced by atrial contraction and distention occurring against closed atrioventricular valves.

Tachyarrhythmias may occur due to atrial fibrillation, atrial flutter, atrioventricular nodal reentry, Wolff-Parkinson-White syndrome, or coronary artery disease with or without infarction, or due to the presence of electrolyte abnormalities or QT-interval prolongation from drugs or liquid protein diets. In patients with a reduced left ventricular ejection fraction from any cause, self-terminating ventricular tachycardia is a life-threatening cause of cardiac syncope. Less often, ventricular tachycardia occurs in patients with apparently normal hearts. In some patients, ventricular tachycardia is provoked by stress or exercise due to a release of catecholamines. Ventricular tachyarrhythmias may also be caused by metabolic abnormalities such as hypokalemia or hypomagnesemia, drugs such as phenothiazines, antidepressants, or antiarrhythmic agents, and illicit drugs such as cocaine. In young patients, right ventricular dysplasia may produce an isolated right ventricular cardiomyopathy and cause syncope by a tachyarrhythmic mechanism. Polymorphic ventricular tachycardia or torsades de pointes may occur in patients with the long QT syndrome and may cause sudden death. Congenital causes of the long QT syndrome include Romano-Ward syndrome and Jervell and Lange-Nielsen syndrome associated with congenital deafness. Acquired long QT syndrome may be induced by type IA or type III antiarrhythmic agents (quinidine, procainamide, disopyramide, amitriptyline), pentamidine, phenothiazines, antidepressants, trimethoprim-—sulfamethoxazole, or intravenous erythromycin. Repolarization may also be prolonged by hypokalemia, ischemia, myocarditis, severe bradycardia, and CNS disease (subarachnoid hemorrhage). These are other factors that lengthen the QT interval and predispose to torsades. The mitral valve prolapse syndrome may produce tachyarrhythmias in young women.

An obstruction to flow is another mechanism by which cardiac syncope is produced. Depending on the severity of obstruction to flow, symptoms may occur with exercise only or at rest as well. Peripheral arteriolar vasodilation of the muscle beds occurs during exercise and results in a drop in systemic vascular resistance. This normally produces a compensatory increase in cardiac output and arterial blood pressure. However, if there is significant obstruction to outflow, the cardiac output cannot increase sufficiently to compensate for the decline in systemic vascular resistance. Consequently, arterial blood pressure may fall and result in cerebral hypoperfusion and syncope. Common causes of obstruction to flow are aortic stenosis and idiopathic hypertrophic subaortic stenosis. Patients with the former have a fixed valvular orifice area and therefore cannot increase the cardiac output based on demands posed by exercise. Patients with the latter may have fixed or dynamic outflow tract obstruction precipitated by conditions that increase contractility, decrease chamber dimensions, or decrease afterload. Thus, such patients may experience hypotension and syncope when treated with positive inotropes such as digitalis or with arterial and venous vasodilators such as nitroglycerin. Other conditions that lead to obstruction to outflow are pulmonic stenosis (valvular, subvalvular, and supravalvular) and supravalvular aortic stenosis. Obstruction to inflow may occur in a patient with an atrial myxoma or thrombus. The latter is an ominous complication of a prosthetic valve. Primary pulmonary hypertension, pulmonary peripheral branch stenosis, pulmonary emboli, cardiac tamponade, mitral or tricuspid stenosis, a malfunctioning prosthetic aortic or mitral valve, cor triatriatum, tetralogy of Fallot, and Eisenmenger syndrome are other conditions associated with syncope due to obstruction to flow.

Sustained hypotension from impaired ventricular function, most commonly associated with ischemic heart disease, is another mechanism of cardiac syncope. In these patients, intermittent hypotension may arise from conduction disturbances and arrhythmias that are related to a scar from a previous myocardial infarction or from active ischemia. In particular, inferior wall ischemia has been associated with marked bradyarrhythmias due to a surge in parasympathetic activity. Syncope has been reported to be the presenting symptom of myocardial infarction in 7% of patients over age 65.

Decreased Effective Circulating Blood Volume

Syncope may result from reduced effective circulating blood volume produced by conditions such as hemorrhage, dehydration, diabetes insipidus, severe burns, hemodialysis, third trimester of pregnancy, arteriovenous shunt, or venous insufficiency.

Vascular or Neurologic Dysfunction

Reflex syncope results primarily from right heart underfilling produced by peripheral blood pooling, usually occurring in the standing or (less commonly) sitting position. Vasovagal hypotension and vasodepressor syncope, or the common faint, is the most common (55%) cause of syncope in otherwise healthy young persons. It is often precipitated by the sight of blood or loss of blood through trauma, surgery, or phlebotomy or by pain or stress, such as with an arterial puncture or venipuncture. The common faint is more likely to occur in the upright position, associated with hunger and fatigue, particularly in a crowded, hot room. Warning signs suggestive of autonomic nervous system overactivity usually occur before syncope: yawning, pallor, sighing, hyperventilation, epigastric discomfort, nausea, diaphoresis, blurred vision, impaired hearing, mydriasis, unawareness, and rapid heart rate. This type of syncope is characterized by a fall in total peripheral vascular resistance that is not adequately compensated for by a rise in cardiac output. Assuming the sitting or recumbent position usually alleviates the symptoms, and syncope can often be aborted.

Postural hypotension is a common cause of presyncope. When a person stands, the decrease in cardiac output and blood pressure produced by peripheral venous pooling are usually compensated by reflex tachycardia and vasoconstriction mediated by sympathetic stimulation. Usually these intact compensatory mechanisms produce only a transient systolic blood pressure drop of 5 to 15 mm Hg; the diastolic pressure tends to rise. In patients with orthostatic hypotension, however, there is a more profound and persistent decline of systolic pressure (> 20 to 30 mm Hg), with or without a concomitant drop (> 10 mm Hg) in diastolic pressure. Orthostatic hypotension is more prevalent (30% to 50% incidence) in elderly (> 75 years) patients, particularly in those receiving cardiovascular or psychotropic drugs.

Orthostatic hypotension may be an idiopathic disorder. The Bradbury-Eggleston syndrome is characterized by postural hypotension without a compensatory tachycardia, hypohidrosis, impotence, and disturbed sphincter control. It is due to primary degeneration of the autonomic nervous system (primary autonomic insufficiency). Patients often develop postprandial hypotension and presyncope as well as visual impairment while standing or walking. These symptoms become progressive, occurring more frequently in the morning while suddenly assuming an upright posture. Another idiopathic disorder that causes postural hypotension is the Shy-Drager syndrome, in which there is CNS atrophy with involvement of the extrapyramidal tracts and basal ganglia.

Secondary postural hypotension may occur in association with disorders of the peripheral, autonomic, or central nervous system. Such disorders include diabetes mellitus, alcoholism, uremia, pyridoxine deficiency, multiple sclerosis, tabes dorsalis, pernicious anemia, Parkinson disease, vascular lesions in the brain stem, neoplasms and cysts in the parasellar region and posterior fossa, Wernicke encephalopathy, syringomyelia, and other demyelinating disorders.

Familial dysautonomia may also produce postural hypotension. Cardiovascular deconditioning after prolonged recumbency, space flight, or illness, particularly in the elderly, may produce orthostatic hypotension. Diseased or varicose veins cause syncope by producing pooling of blood in the lower extremities. The supine hypotensive syndrome of pregnancy may produce syncope resulting from obstruction of the inferior vena cava, with a reduction in venous return and a decline in cardiac output. Heatstroke, fever, and anorexia nervosa may produce postural hypotension.

Carotid sinus hypersensitivity may produce syncope through inappropriate or excessive activation of vasomotor reflexes. Afferent impulses from the carotid sinuses travel via the glossopharyngeal nerve to the vasomotor and cardioinhibitory centers in the medulla. The efferent limb of the carotid sinus reflex is formed by vagal and cervical sympathetic fibers. Increased pressure on the walls of the carotid vessel leads to an increased frequency of afferent stimulation of the vasomotor center, thereby increasing parasympathetic outflow, reducing sympathetic outflow, and causing systemic vasodilation and bradycardia. The vagal or cardioinhibitory type is the most common form of hypersensitive carotid sinus syndrome, occurring in about 70% of patients. Here, bradycardia, sinus arrest, atrioventricular block, or even asystole may occur to produce dizziness, presyncope, and syncope. The second or vasodepressor type is characterized by marked hypotension without significant bradycardia or atrioventricular block. Pure vasodepressor syncope is uncommon (5% to 10%) except when a tumor involves the carotid sinus. The mixed type includes both cardioinhibitory and vasodepressor responses (20% to 25%). Carotid sinus hypersensitivity usually occurs in the elderly and is more common in men than in women. However, the mere presence of carotid sinus hypersensitivity does not prove that it is the cause of syncope. Atherosclerosis, hypertension, diabetes mellitus, and local pathologic changes such as scars, lymph nodes, and tumors involving the carotid body predispose to carotid sinus hypersensitivity. Turning of the head or pressure on the carotid sinus area may precipitate an episode. Impaired cerebral perfusion due to cerebrovascular disease may also produce syncope from extrinsic compression of neck vessels and must be distinguished from carotid sinus hypersensitivity.

Situational syncope is mediated via the autonomic nervous system reflex mechanisms that lead to a vasodepressor response and syncope. Examples include syncope during micturition, cough, deglutition, defecation, and acute pain states. Micturition syncope is usually caused by rapid emptying of the bladder, which causes reflex vasodilation and decreased cerebral blood flow; this may be further accentuated by the effects of a Valsalva maneuver during voiding. Deglutition syncope can occur in patients with or without esophageal disease. Defecation syncope has been attributed to a reflex mechanism such as a prolonged Valsalva maneuver, leading to decreased cardiac output or reduced cerebral perfusion from a rapid increase in CSF pressure. Glossopharyngeal neuralgia with paroxysmal pain in the posterior pharynx or external auditory canal is occasionally accompanied by syncope secondary to vasodilation and bradycardia. Postprandial hypotension may occur in elderly patients with impaired baroreflex function due to the inability to compensate for pooling of blood in the splanchnic circulation after meals. Cough or tussive syncope may trigger syncope by vagally mediated hypotension and bradycardia produced by prolonged, excessive, violent coughing in patients with chronic obstructive pulmonary disease. In these patients, the propensity for syncope is exacerbated by the decreased venous return produced by the marked increase in intrathoracic pressure from coughing. Rarely, cough syncope may be caused by intracranial or foramen magnum obstructive tumors.

Valsalva syncope related to prolonged increases in intrathoracic pressure during the sustained Valsalva maneuver, oculovagal syncope after ocular compression, sneeze syncope after sneezing, instrumentation syncope occurring during endoscopy, bronchoscopy, or insertion of intrauterine devices, diver's or submersion syncope during underwater diving, Jacuzzi syncope, weightlifter's syncope, and trumpet-player's syncope are other examples of situational syncope.

Hyperventilation, syncope migraine, acute or chronic autonomic neuropathy, and Guillain-Barré syndrome are other causes of syncope mediated by vascular or neurologic dysfunction. Surgical sympathectomy abolishes vasopressor reflex responses and can lead to postural syncope. Idiopathic hypovolemia without an apparent cause but responsive to acute treatment with volume expanders or long-term therapy with mineralocorticoids has also been reported.

Metabolic and Endocrine Disturbances

A reduction of plasma volume, altered adrenergic function, or vasodilation may occur with certain metabolic and endocrine disturbances and may produce hypotension and syncope. Disorders of this type include diabetes mellitus, primary systemic amyloidosis, and acute porphyria. Hypotension due to hypovolemia is seen in adrenal insufficiency, hypoaldosteronism, and salt-wasting nephritis. Altered vascular responses to catecholamines may occur in Addison disease, and angiotensin levels may be diminished in conditions in which plasma renin activity is low. Postural hypotension is common in pheochromocytoma due to depletion of plasma volume. In addition, epinephrine release may mediate vasodilation. Hyperbradykininemia is a familial disorder characterized by severe tachycardia and a narrowed pulse pressure due to an enzyme deficiency resulting in impaired destruction of the circulating peptides. Kinins may also produce hypotension and syncope, seen in the carcinoid syndrome. Serotonin-secreting tumors and electrolyte disturbances such as hypokalemia are other disorders that may produce syncope.

Drug Toxicity

Hypotension may be produced by the administration of vasodilators. All antihypertensive agents may cause postural hypotension, particularly in the setting of dehydration and hypovolemia exacerbated by diuretic administration. The agents that provoke the greatest postural hypotension are ganglionic blockers, depletors of catecholamines such as reserpine, and drugs that block the release of catecholamines such as guanethidine. These agents have largely been replaced by others in clinical practice.

Tranquilizers, sedatives, hypnotics, or antidepressants may cause hypotension by depressing the vasomotor center. Calcium channel blockers and nitrates, often used in the treatment of angina, may produce hypotension. Postural hypotension may also occur in association with the administration of agents such as bromocriptine. Drug toxicity due to barbiturates, vincristine, quinidine, digitalis, marijuana, alcohol, cocaine, and insulin have also been associated with syncope.

HISTORY

The history is a critical part of the initial evaluation of a patient with syncope. The examiner must determine the onset, frequency, and duration of premonitory symptoms; the circumstances surrounding the attacks (eg, relation to meals, alcohol ingestion, cough, micturition, defecation, or movements of the head and neck); associated symptoms such as nausea, vomiting, chest pain, or dyspnea; medications used; and the presence of potentially predisposing disorders such as diabetes mellitus, chronic illness with weight loss, prolonged bed rest, blood loss, or plasma volume depletion.

A cardiac arrhythmia is suggested by an abrupt onset, without premonitory symptoms or signs, that leads to a precipitous fall and major injury. Exertional syncope is associated with cardiac obstructive causes, global myocardial ischemia, or tachyarrhythmias. Relation to meals, alcohol or drug ingestion, cough, swallowing, micturition, defecation, posture, abdominal pain, procedure, or movement of the head and neck suggests situational syncope. Premonitory symptoms (eg, yawning, nausea, epigastric discomfort, pallor, diaphoresis) usually precede the common faint. It occurs commonly in the setting of stress, pain, sight of blood, warmth, hunger, fatigue, crowding, long standing, procedure, or instrumentation.

Recovery from syncope is usually prompt; a seizure is followed by prolonged postictal somnolence and confusion. Atypical tonic or clonic motor activity may accompany syncope due to ventricular tachycardia or fibrillation and complicates the clinical distinction of syncope from seizures.

A detailed medication history is important. First-dose syncope is associated with prazosin, captopril, or nitroglycerin. Postural hypotension is associated with some vasodilators. Some drugs may be proarrhythmic, such as the antiarrhythmic agents themselves, phenothiazines, and tricyclic antidepressants. Drugs that affect the sinus node or atrioventricular node such as methyldopa, β-blockers, and digoxin may aggravate carotid sinus hypersensitivity.

PHYSICAL EXAMINATION AND CLINICAL FINDINGS

A complete physical examination is necessary. Orthostatic vital signs should be obtained in every patient with syncope. Blood pressure and heart rate should be obtained in the supine, sitting, and standing positions. Recordings should be obtained immediately on standing and after several minutes. Evaluation of blood pressure in both arms and legs, as well as recognition of bruits in the carotid, subclavian, supraorbital, and temporal vessels, may identify patients with vascular disorders such as Takayasu disease, aortic dissection, or the subclavian steal syndrome. A careful cardiac examination may detect signs of aortic stenosis, idiopathic hypertrophic subaortic stenosis, mitral valve prolapse, or pulmonary hypertension. Cyanosis, clubbing, and other signs of congenital heart disease should be sought.

The heart rate and blood-pressure response to carotid sinus pressure and simulated movements precipitating syncope should be assessed. Carotid sinus pressure should be done as part of the work-up of any patient with syncope. The presence of carotid bruits or cerebrovascular disease is considered a relative contraindication to carotid sinus pressure, however, as it can cause contralateral hemiparesis. This test may be done in an office setting, provided intravenous access is established and atropine is available before doing the test. Carotid sinus pressure is applied separately on each side for 5 seconds, with electrocardiogram (ECG) and blood-pressure monitoring in the sitting position. A pause of 3 seconds or longer or a systolic blood-pressure drop of more than 50 mm Hg without symptoms (or 30 mm Hg with symptoms) is abnormal. A positive test is confirmatory only if other causes of syncope can be excluded.

Stool testing for occult blood is needed to evaluate gastrointestinal bleeding. This test is particularly important in patients who are orthostatic. A thorough neurologic examination should be performed to exclude focal deficits.

LABORATORY AND IMAGING STUDIES

In up to 50% of patients with syncope, no specific cause is found despite an extensive initial noninvasive evaluation. New diagnostic tests that have been able to uncover a cause in some patients include cardiac electrophysiologic studies (yield 15% to 40%), tilt-table evaluation (yield 25% to 40%), and prolonged ambulatory cardiac rhythm evaluation with loop ECG recorders (yield 25% to 35%).

Hospitalization is advisable when the syncopal episode has resulted in serious injury or when the initial evaluation suggests a serious underlying disorder (eg, a cardiac arrhythmia or myocardial ischemia). Routine blood chemistries should include a complete blood count to evaluate for anemia and infection; electrolyte, blood urea nitrogen, and creatinine levels to evaluate volume and metabolic status; drug and alcohol levels, when appropriate, to detect toxicity; and cardiac enzyme levels to rule out a myocardial infarction, when appropriate. Electroencephalography (EEG) and computed tomography or radionuclide brain scanning have a low diagnostic yield in patients with syncope who have a nonfocal neurologic examination, a negative neurologic history, and no carotid bruits. When a diagnosis of partial complex seizures is suspected in patients with recurrent syncope, a sleep-deprived EEG with nasopharyngeal leads may be helpful. A chest x-ray is not very helpful unless congestive heart failure, pericardial effusion, or mitral stenosis is suspected. Arterial blood gas analysis and lung scanning are not routine but may be helpful if a diagnosis of pulmonary embolism is suggested by the history and physical examination.

An ECG should be obtained routinely to evaluate for the presence of ischemia or infarction, arrhythmia, ventricular hypertrophy, conduction abnormalities, preexcitation, or the long QT syndrome. Echocardiography should also be performed to help confirm or exclude the diagnosis of structural heart disease and left ventricular function, thus directing further testing. Monitoring in a telemetry unit is helpful if a serious arrhythmia is suspected. If the suspicion of a serious arrhythmia is lower, 24-hour ambulatory Holter monitoring is cost-effective and advisable. Two 24-hour Holters performed during the course of the evaluation or a single 48-hour Holter increases the sensitivity of detection of significant arrhythmias. If syncope occurs rarely but is nevertheless recurrent, capturing the cardiac rhythm during a syncopal spell may be possible by prolonged ambulatory transtelephonic monitoring with patient-activated event recorders that may be worn for months at a time. This may help differentiate arrhythmic from nonarrhythmic syncope and has been shown to be very useful in patients with unexplained syncope. The advantage of loop recorders is that their digital or solid-state memory loops can be activated after the syncopal event and can retrieve information about the cardiac rhythm during the preceding 4 minutes.

Exercise testing may be performed to provoke arrhythmias or hypotension in patients with exertional syncope or suspected coronary artery disease. However, this test is relatively nondiagnostic. Exertional syncope in young patients should be evaluated by echocardiography to exclude aortic stenosis, hypertrophic cardiomyopathy, or mitral stenosis. Cardiac catheterization may be warranted if the echocardiogram is abnormal or if an anomalous origin of the left coronary artery is suspected. If a patient presents with syncope and a cardiac abnormality is detected during the initial work-up, referral to a cardiology subspecialist is appropriate due to the relatively high 1-year mortality (20% to 30%) associated with syncope from a cardiac cause.

Another important noninvasive provocative test in reproducing syncope and diagnosing vasovagal or neurally mediated syncope is the head-up tilt test. An upright tilt of 60° to 80° is done for 10 to 60 minutes using a tilt table with a foot board for weight bearing. An intravenous infusion of isoproterenol may be given to enhance the test's sensitivity. A positive result (bradycardia, hypotension, or both) involves the reproduction of symptoms on the tilt table and is thought to invoke a vagally or neurally mediated mechanism for the faint.

The use of signal-averaged ECG is helpful in compiling a risk profile for the patient with syncope. This noninvasive method records, amplifies, and filters the surface ECG to detect low-amplitude, high-frequency signals, called late potentials, at the terminal portion of the QRS complex. These late potentials represent delayed myocardial activation in areas of scar tissue and serve as the electrophysiologic substrate for ventricular arrhythmias. The predictive accuracy for identifying persons at risk for ventricular tachycardia is best in patients with coronary artery disease. The sensitivity of this method for predicting inducible, sustained monomorphic ventricular tachycardia at invasive electrophysiologic testing in patients with unexplained syncope is high (73% to 89%), as is the specificity (89% to 100%). A positive signal-averaged ECG, particularly in patients with known heart disease, warrants invasive electrophysiologic testing. A negative signal-averaged ECG suggests that ventricular tachycardia is unlikely.

Invasive electrophysiologic studies are warranted when the suspicion for cardiac syncope remains high in the face of a nondiagnostic noninvasive evaluation. Electrophysiologic tests are useful in diagnosing conduction abnormalities of the sinus node, atrioventricular node, and the His-Purkinje system. In addition, an attempt is made to provoke supraventricular and ventricular arrhythmias through electrical stimulation. Nevertheless, the diagnosis arrived at by the test is usually presumptive, as the patients's symptoms are seldom exactly duplicated in the electrophysiologic laboratory. Patients with underlying structural heart disease and recurrent unexplained syncope are the best candidates for electrophysiologic studies, as they have a relatively high 1-year mortality (18% to 30%). The diagnostic yield in this population ranges from 18% to 75%. In patients without structural heart disease, clinically significant arrhythmias are induced in only 12% to 20%.

TREATMENT

The prognosis and treatment of syncope largely depend on its etiology. The 1-year mortality is 20% to 30% for cardiac syncope, 5% for noncardiac causes, and up to 10% for unexplained syncope. Simple measures involving the removal of offending agents may be effective for situational or reflex syncope. Postprandial syncope may be treated by eliminating hypotensive drugs before meals and resting in a supine position after meals.

Pharmacologic therapy with anticholinergic agents such as transdermal scopolamine may be helpful in some patients with vasovagal syncope. In some extreme cases in which significant bradycardia or asystole is encountered, implantation of a permanent ventricular pacemaker may be necessary.

Simple measures that may be taken to treat postural syncope include wearing support stockings or pantyhose, eliminating offending vasodilators, minimizing volume depletion, and using high-salt diets or mineralocorticoids (fludrocortisone). β-Blockers (propranolol or pindolol) reduce sympathetic nervous system discharge and have been advocated for some patients with idiopathic orthostatic hypotension. Clonidine is reportedly beneficial in postganglionic idiopathic orthostatic hypotension. Vasopressor agents such as ephedrine, phenylephrine, ergotamine, or hydroxyamphetamine seldom help. Prostaglandin inhibitors such as indomethacin reportedly help prevent the vasodilatory effect of endogenous prostaglandins.

The treatment of cardioinhibitory carotid sinus syncope generally includes permanent pacemaker implantation, preferably the dual-chamber model. Treatment for vasodepressor syncope, on the other hand, has been unsatisfactory, with limited success being reported with dihydroergotamine, ephedrine, irradiation, or surgical denervation of the carotid sinus.

Syncope due to aortic stenosis is an ominous prognostic indicator and is considered an indication for surgical valve replacement or valvuloplasty. Patients with idiopathic hypertrophic subaortic stenosis may be treated with β-blockers, calcium channel blockers, or both. If medical treatment is ineffective, appropriate selection of an atrioventricular interval and timing of ventricular contraction with a pacemaker may be considered. Alternatively, surgical myomectomy of part of the septum may be considered. Because syncope and sudden death frequently occur with strenuous exertion in these patients, strenuous exercise should be avoided. Atrial fibrillation in these patients is usually highly symptomatic due to the loss of the atrial contribution to ventricular filling. Hence, aggressive rate control should be instituted promptly, followed by pharmacologic or electrical cardioversion.

Bradyarrhythmic causes of syncope such as atrioventricular block, His-Purkinje disease, sick sinus syndrome, or the cardioinhibitory carotid sinus syndrome are generally treated with a pacemaker. However, this should be done only after removing agents that may cause bradycardia. Treatment of malignant tachyarrhythmias is usually guided by invasive electrophysiologic testing. Only limited antiarrhythmic agents are available for this purpose. Various nonpharmacologic approaches are being considered for drug-refractory cases, including arrhythmia surgery (aneurysmectomy plus electrophysiologic-guided subendocardial resection), automatic implantable defibrillators, and catheter ablation techniques. The defibrillator can abort sudden death by recognizing ventricular tachycardia or ventricular fibrillation and delivering rescue shocks of 25 to 32 joules directly to the myocardium.

In the acquired long QT syndrome, withdrawal of the offending drug or correction of the metabolic or electrolyte abnormalities is usually successful. Alternatively, patients may be treated with β-blockers for idiopathic or congenital long QT syndrome. Those who fail drug therapy may be considered for left cervicothoracic sympathectomy (stellectomy), permanent pacing, or implantation of an automatic implantable defibrillator.

CONSIDERATIONS IN PREGNANCY

To manage heart disease during pregnancy, the clinician must understand the circulatory and respiratory adaptations to the normal gravid state. The increase in maternal blood volume starts early in pregnancy, peaks at 32 weeks, and plateaus until term. An increase of about 40% to 50% over pregestational levels occurs. The increase in intravascular volume in pregnancy sets the stage for a rise in cardiac output, which increases 30% to 50% over pregravid values. Most of this increase occurs in the first trimester due to an increase in stroke volume, with the peak at 20 to 24 weeks. As pregnancy advances, heart rate continues to rise, and stroke volume declines. Cardiac lesions that cause right or left ventricular outflow tract obstruction (eg, aortic stenosis, mitral stenosis, pulmonic stenosis, and pulmonary hypertension) are poorly tolerated during pregnancy due to the inability to raise cardiac output adequately to meet the increased hemodynamic demands. Hence, the patient may come to medical attention for the first time during pregnancy. Such patients require careful management of fluid status during pregnancy and should be managed jointly with a cardiac subspecialist.

Infrequently, bradycardic hypotensive syncope occurs in the supine position in a pregnant woman (supine hypotensive syncope) during the latter part of pregnancy, when the gravid uterus compresses the inferior vena cava and the abdominal aorta. This dramatic event is promptly reversed by turning the patient on her side. The bradycardia may be attributed to selective vasovagal baroreceptor response to inferior caval expression. Supraventricular and ventricular arrhythmias and orthostatic hypotension also are important causes of syncope during pregnancy.

Arrhythmias during pregnancy fall into two categories: benign rhythm disturbances that occur during an otherwise normal uncomplicated gestation and disturbances in rhythm associated with certain cardiac diseases that prevail in women of childbearing age. Sinus arrhythmia, occasionally sinus bradycardia or tachycardia, and atrial or ventricular premature beats are relatively common benign occurrences. The sensation of "skipped beats" during pregnancy is more likely to be caused by atrial than by ventricular premature beats. Regardless of their site of origin, sporadic premature beats are of no clinical importance if they are not subjectively disturbing and if the patient is appropriately reassured. Even bigeminy or trigeminy is generally unimportant in the pregnant woman without organic heart disease. However, multiform ventricular beats or episodes of ventricular tachycardia, especially near term, should arouse suspicion of peripartum cardiomyopathy.

The most common sustained tachyarrhythmia during pregnancy is paroxysmal reentrant supraventricular tachycardia. This is a relatively common rhythm disturbance, with a peak incidence in women of childbearing age. A history of paroxysmal reentrant supraventricular tachycardia signals the potential for recurrence, to which pregnancy predisposes, especially during the third trimester. Atrial flutter or fibrillation usually denotes the presence of coexisting heart disease, either acquired or congenital. Wolff-Parkinson-White bypass tracts can produce tachycardias during pregnancy. With such tracts, atrial flutter with 1:1 conduction or atrial fibrillation with rapid ventricular rates is of special concern.

Arrhythmias during pregnancy may or may not produce syncope, depending on the patient's ventricular rate and volume status. They may uncover underlying organic heart disease and should be managed in consultation with a cardiac subspecialist.

BIBLIOGRAPHY

Day SC, Cook F, Funkenstein H, Goldman L. Evaluation and outcome of emergency room patients with transient loss of consciousness. Am J Med 1982;73:15.

Eagle KA, Black HR, Cook EF, Goldman L. Evaluation of prognostic classifications for patients with syncope. Am J Med 1985;79:455.

Kapoor W, Karpf M, Levey GS. Issues in evaluating patients with syncope. Ann Intern Med 1984;100:755.

Kapoor WN, Karpf M, Wieand S, Peterson JR, Levey GS. A prospective evaluation and follow-up of patients with syncope. N Engl J Med 1983;309:197.

Manolis AS, Linzer M, Salem D, Estes NA. Syncope: current diagnostic evaluation and management. Ann Intern Med 1990;112:850.

Perloff JK. Pregnancy and cardiovascular disease. In: Braunwald E, ed. Heart disease, 3d ed. Philadelphia: WB Saunders, 1988:1848.

Sobel RE, Roberts R. Hypotension and syncope. In: Braunwald E, ed. Heart disease, 3d ed. Philadelphia: WB Saunders, 1988:884.

Primary Care for Women, edited by Phyllis C. Leppert and Fred M. Howard. Lippincott-Raven Publishers, Philadelphia © 1997.

49

Hyperlipidemia

RICHARD S. CONSTANTINO

Hyperlipidemia, an elevation of total serum cholesterol, triglycerides, or both, is relatively common in American women. Nearly half of the 600,000 deaths occurring annually due to coronary heart disease are associated with hyperlipidemia. Coronary artery disease is the leading cause of death in the United States and the leading cause of death in women over age 65. The diagnosis and treatment of coronary heart disease costs an estimated \$50 to \$100 billion annually, the largest expenditure for any disease entity in the country.

In 1988, 26% of adult women had blood cholesterol levels above 240 mg/dL. Although this percentage fell to 20% in 1991, only 50% of adult females had desirable cholesterol levels of less than 200 mg/dL. Of particular concern is the fact that only a third of the persons with cholesterol levels above 240 mg/dL are receiving any active intervention to lower their cholesterol levels or to alter their lipid profiles.

Serum lipids are composed of various fractions consisting of cholesterol and triglycerides bound in lipoprotein transport molecules. These subfractions include low-density lipoprotein (LDL), also called atherogenic or "bad" cholesterol; high-density lipoprotein (HDL), also known as "good" cholesterol; and very low-density lipoprotein (VLDL), predominantly triglycerides. Chylomicrons and intermediate-density lipoprotein are subfractions beyond the scope of this discussion.

Hypercholesterolemia, particularly an elevated LDL cholesterol level and a diminished HDL cholesterol level, is strongly correlated with the genesis of coronary artery disease. Some risk factors for coronary artery disease cannot be modified, such as age and male gender; however, other risk factors, such as hyperlipidemia, hypertension, smoking, and diabetes can easily be diagnosed and modified. The incidence of coronary artery disease is much lower in premenopausal women than in postmenopausal women and men of the same age. The incidence in women is approximately equivalent to that in men who are 10 to 15 years younger. The risk of coronary artery disease rises in postmenopausal women and approaches the incidence in men by age 70. Although coronary artery disease afflicts both men and women, it is frequently underdiagnosed in women. Similarly, hypercholesterolemia is underdiagnosed in women and is generally treated less aggressively than it is in men.

Risk factors for coronary artery disease are similar in African-American, Hispanic, and white women. Over the past several decades, age-adjusted mortality from coronary artery disease has not declined as dramatically in African-American women as it has in white women. It is believed that less access to medical care, lower rates of smoking cessation, and less tightly controlled lipid-lowering diets are the cause of this disparity. The most cost-effective way to reduce the incidence of coronary artery disease in the entire population is to reduce the prevalence of modifiable risk factors (Table 49-1). Modifying hypercholesterolemia is of great importance in reducing the risk of coronary heart disease. The incidence of coronary artery disease is directly related to levels of LDL and inversely related to levels of HDL. Studies of middle-aged men with mildly to moderately elevated total cholesterol levels have documented that for each 1% reduction in LDL levels and 1% increase in HDL levels, there is an associated 2% to 3% reduction in coronary artery disease. It is thought that a similar relation exists in women, although data are less certain.

In addition to the risk of coronary artery disease, the overall risk of vascular disease in general rises with hypercholesterolemia or low HDL levels. Retinopathy, renal disease, and CNS disease, such as stroke, are also directly or indirectly influenced by serum cholesterol levels. In addition, hypertriglyceridemia with values above 200 mg/dL, predominantly in the VLDL fraction, is commonly associated with reduced levels of HDL cholesterol and attendant vascular risk. There is still debate about whether an elevated serum triglyceride level by itself is an independent risk factor for coronary artery disease. However, current recommendations are to treat specifically if triglycerides are 500 mg/dL or higher. Triglyceride values at this level are frequently associated with xanthelasma and pancreatitis.

DIAGNOSIS

In general, it is desirable to maintain a total serum cholesterol level of 200 mg/dL or less. It is important to perform a fasting lipid profile to determine HDL and LDL levels. Lipoprotein analysis should be done after a 9- to 12-hour fast. Results of two tests taken 1 to 8 weeks apart should be averaged. HDL is considered protective at values of 60 mg/dL or greater. LDL values are considered acceptable if a patient with fewer than two coronary heart risk factors has a value of 160 mg/dL or less. If the patient has no coronary heart disease but has two or more risk factors for coronary artery disease, then optimal LDL levels are less than 130 mg/dL. If the patient has known coronary artery disease, desirable LDL levels are less than 100 mg/dL.

Diet and risk factor modification are in order if HDL levels are less than 35 mg/dL and the patient has no other associated lipid abnormalities, if HDL levels are low and LDL levels are high, or if there are triglyceride abnormalities. For patients failing nonpharmacologic therapy, drug therapy should follow. Treatment recommendations are summarized in Table 49-2.

There is an emphasis on coronary heart disease risk status as a guide to the type and intensity of cholesterol-lowering therapy.

Table 49-1. Risk Factors for Cardiac Heart Disease

Modifiable
Cigarette smoking
Hypertension (≥ 140/90 mm Hg or on antihypertensive medication)
Obesity
Physical inactivity
Diabetes mellitus
Premature menopause without estrogen replacement therapy
Nonmodifiable
Age and gender
Men ≥ 45 years
Women ≥ 55 years
Family history of premature CHD
Father < 55 years
Mother < 65 years

A negative risk factor is the presence of high HDL cholesterol (≥60 mg/dL). In the presence of high HDL cholesterol, one risk factor is subtracted.

(Mattson C, Koentopp C, Jackson K. Treatment of high blood cholesterol. Clinical Pharmacy Review. PCS Health Systems, summer 1995:1.)

Patients with coronary heart disease or other atherosclerotic disease are at highest risk, and lower target levels for LDL should be established. In addition, age 55 or older is a major coronary heart disease risk factor in women. Drug therapy should be delayed in premenopausal women with high LDL levels who are otherwise at low risk for coronary heart disease. Postmenopausal women have a high risk for coronary heart disease as a result of hyperlipidemia, so in general treating older patients, particularly women, pharmacologically is acceptable. Previously, advanced age was a relative contraindication to therapy.

More attention must be paid to HDL levels as a coronary heart disease risk factor. HDL and LDL levels should be included in all cholesterol determinations. A high HDL level should be viewed as a negative risk factor for coronary artery disease and should be considered when selecting drug therapy.

Figures 49-1 and 49-2 outline the initial classification of patients based on total cholesterol and HDL characteristics.

THERAPY

Diet and Exercise

Once the decision has been made to begin therapy for hypercholesterolemia, attempts should be made to ensure that the patient's diet is appropriate. If the patient is overweight, a weight-reduction program is imperative. Weight loss and exercise promote a reduction of cholesterol levels and have other beneficial effects as well, including reduced triglycerides, increased HDL levels, lowered blood pressure, and a decreased risk of diabetes.

Patients without coronary artery risk factors or active coronary artery disease should begin with a stage 1 diet. This approach limits saturated fats to 10% of total calories and total fat to 30% or less. Less than 300 mg of cholesterol should be consumed per day.

Patients who do not achieve desirable cholesterol levels with the stage 1 diet should progress to a stage 2 diet, in which saturated fat is limited to less than 7% of total calories. Total cholesterol intake should be restricted to less than 200 mg/day. The services of a registered dietitian or other qualified nutritional expert are usually necessary to achieve compliance with this intensive diet.

Exercise is effective adjunctive therapy for lowering cholesterol or minimizing cardiac risk factors. Aerobic exercise, achieving a maximal heart rate of 60% to 80% of the age-adjusted pulse rate, for 30 to 45 minutes every other day is adequate. Exercise also promotes weight loss, in addition to its other beneficial effects. Patients at risk for coronary artery disease should be screened before starting a regular exercise regimen.

Pharmacologic Treatment

If diet and exercise do not result in adequate control of cholesterol or triglyceride levels, drug therapy may be appropriate. Primary prevention—prevention of coronary heart disease regardless of risk factors—should be considered for patients with an LDL level of 190 mg/dL or greater. If a patient with more than two other cardiac risk factors has an LDL value above 160 mg/dL, drug therapy should be instituted. Drug therapy should be delayed

Table 49-2. Recommendations for Treating LDL Cholesterol and Low HDL Cholesterol

Recommendations for Treating High LDL Cholesterol	DIETARY THERAPY	
	Initiation Level	*Goal*
Without CHD and <2 risk factors	≥ 160 mg/dL (4.1 mmol/L) ≥ 190 mg/dL (4.9 mmol/L)	< 160 mg/dL (4.1 mmol/L) < 160 mg/dL (4.1 mmol/L)
Without CHD and ≥2 risk factors	≥ 130 mg/dL (3.4 mmol/L) ≥ 160 mg/dL (4.1 mmol/L)	< 130 mg/dL (3.4 mmol/L) < 130 mg/dL (3.4 mmol/L)
With CHD	≥ 100 mg/dL (2.6 mmol/L) ≥ 130 mg/dL (3.4 mmol/L)	< 100 mg/dL (2.6 mmol/L) < 100 mg/dL (2.6 mmol/L)
Recommendations for Treating Low HDL Cholesterol*		
Without other associated lipid abnormalities		Diet and risk factor modification
With associated LDL or triglyceride abnormalities		Diet, risk factor modification; consider drug therapy

*<35 mg/dL.

CAD, coronary artery disease; *LDL,* low-density lipoprotein cholesterol; *HDL,* high-density lipoprotein cholesterol.

(Summary of the second report of the National Cholesterol Education Program (NCEP) Expert Panel on Detection, Evaluation, and Treatment of High Blood Cholesterol in Adults (Adult Treatment Panel II). JAMA 1993;269:3018.)

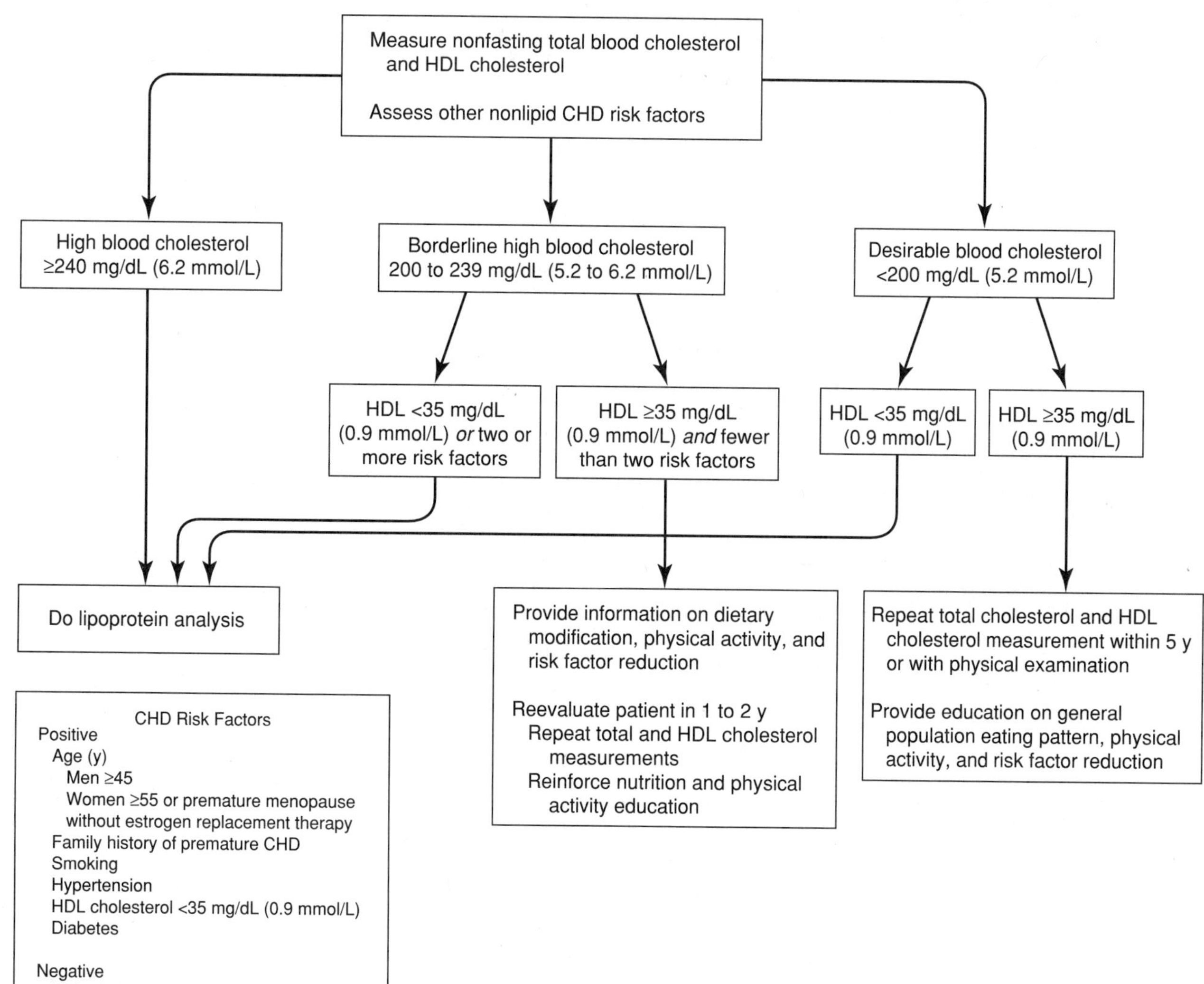

Figure 49-1. Primary prevention in adults without evidence of coronary heart disease (CHD). Initial classification is based on total cholesterol and high-density lipoprotein (HDL) cholesterol levels. (Redrawn from National Cholesterol Education Program. Summary of the second report of the National Cholesterol Education Program Expert Panel on Detection, Evaluation, and Treatment of High Blood Cholesterol in Adults. JAMA 1993;269:3015.)

in premenopausal women without other risk factors whose LDL levels are up to 190 to 220 mg/dL. HDL levels above 60 mg/dL may be considered protective, and a delay in drug therapy may be appropriate.

Secondary prevention—attempts to lower cholesterol in patients who have already developed coronary heart disease—is very important. In general, the goal for LDL should be 100 mg/dL or less in these patients. If the patient has an LDL level of 130 mg/dL or greater and two other cardiac risk factors despite diet and exercise therapy, then aggressive drug therapy to lower the LDL level to 100 mg/dL or below is appropriate.

There are four major categories of drugs used to lower cholesterol, triglycerides, or both, and to raise HDL cholesterol: bile acid sequestrants, niacin, HMG-CoA reductase inhibitors (statins), and other drugs (fibric acid derivatives, probucol, estrogens). Table 49-3 lists certain drug effects on lipoproteins.

Bile Acid Sequestrants

Bile acid sequestrants, such as colestipol and cholestyramine, are effective and safe in lowering total cholesterol and LDL levels by up to 15% to 30% while raising HDL levels by 3% to 5%. These medications are particularly effective in primary prevention when therapy is required in premenopausal women with moderately elevated LDL levels. They may also be used in more severe forms of hypercholesterolemia in combination with other drugs. These medications are generally safe: they are not absorbed from the gastrointestinal tract and therefore lack systemic effects. Constipation and bloating are common but can be minimized by the use of fiber-based stool softeners. Psyllium may minimize these symptoms, and even when used alone it may reduce cholesterol by up to 5% to 10%. Sequestrants may decrease the absorption of certain oral medications, such as HMG-CoA reductase inhibitors,

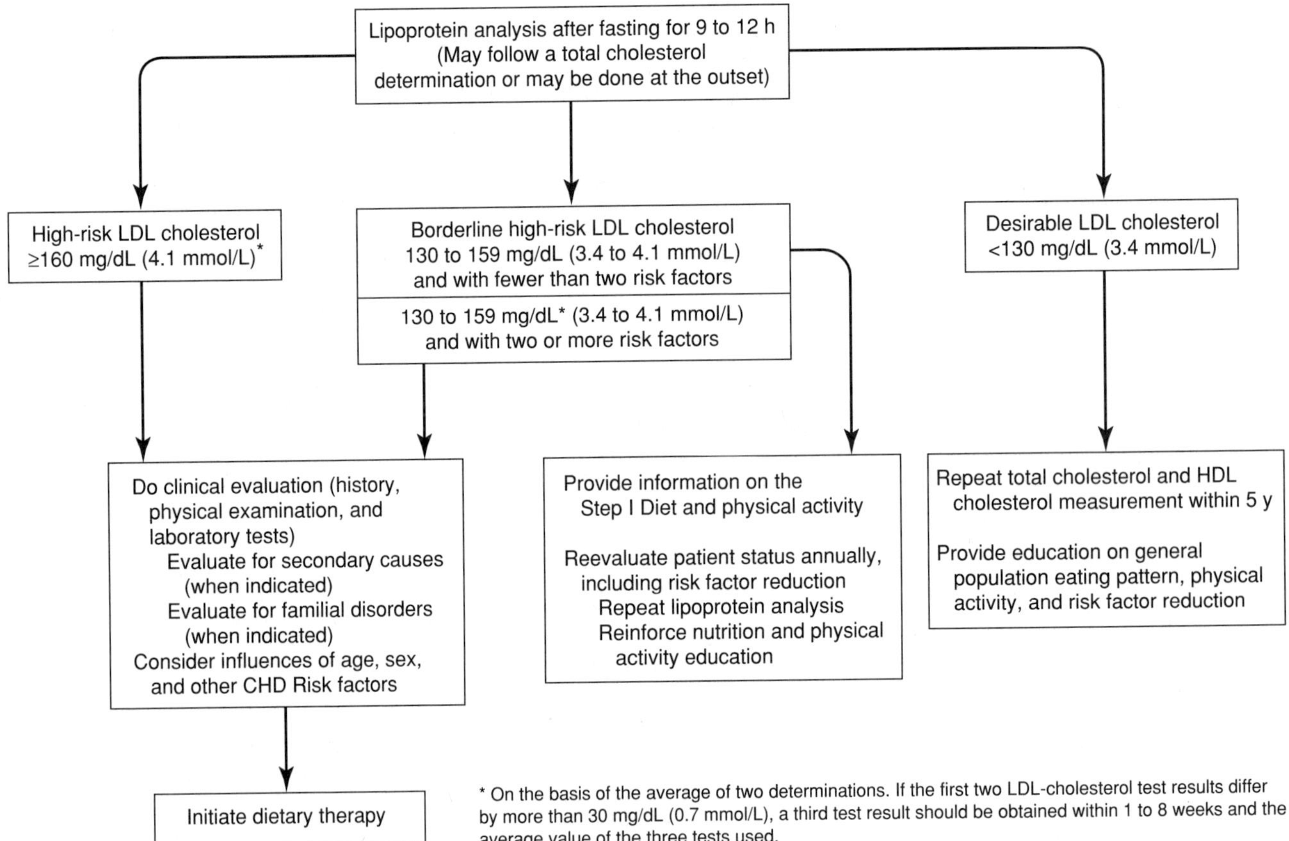

Figure 49-2. Primary prevention in adults without evidence of coronary heart disease (CHD). Subsequent classification is based on low-density lipoprotein (LDL) cholesterol level. (Redrawn from National Cholesterol Education Program. Summary of the second report of the National Cholesterol Education Program Expert Panel on Detection, Evaluation, and Treatment of High Blood Cholesterol in Adults. JAMA 1993;269:3015.)

thiazide diuretics, digoxin, fat-soluble vitamins, and anticoagulants. All other medications taken coincidentally should be taken 1 hour before or 4 hours after the sequestrant dose. Sequestrants are generally most effective and best tolerated when taken before or with meals.

HMG-CoA Reductase Inhibitors

All HMG-CoA reductase inhibitors are relatively similar in efficacy at lower doses. These agents cause a decrease in the total cholesterol level of 20% to 40% and an increase in HDL of 5% to 15%. They may also decrease triglycerides by 10% to 20%. When used as monotherapy, this class of drug is most effective when taken in the evening. These medications are well tolerated by most patients. Gastrointestinal intolerance, with gas, bloating, and constipation, is usually mild and subsides over time. Myopathy is rare, occurring in less than 0.1% of patients. Myopathy becomes much more common when this class of drug is used in combination with cyclosporine, niacin, and gemfibrozil. Abnormal liver function studies occur infrequently and generally resolve completely when the dose is reduced or the drug is discontinued.

Table 49-3. Drug Effects on Lipoproteins

DRUG	TOTAL CHOLESTEROL AND LDL	HDL	TRIGLYCERIDES
Niacin	↓ 15–25%	↑ 15–35%	↓ 20–50%
Sequestrants	↓ 15–30%	↑ 3–5%	0% or slight↑
HMG-CoAs	↓ 20–40%	↑ 5–15%	↓ 10–20%
Gemfibrozil	↓ 10–15%	↑ 10–15%	↓ 20–50%
Probucol	↓ 5–15%	↓ 20–30%	0%

(Mattson C, Koentopp C, Jackson K. Treatment of high blood cholesterol. Clinical Pharmacy Review. PCS Health Systems, Summer 1995:1.)

Prolonged prothrombin times have been reported when HMG-CoA therapy is initiated. Long-term safety data on the use of these drugs are limited, so they should probably be avoided in primary prevention in young females. In severe hypercholesterolemia, or if secondary prevention is required, the use of an HMG-CoA reductase inhibitor with a sequestrant drug or niacin has been shown angiographically to reduce progression and increase regression of coronary artery lesions.

Because abnormal liver function studies may develop, HMG-CoA reductase inhibitors are contraindicated during pregnancy and nursing and in patients with liver disease.

Nicotinic Acid

Nicotinic acid is effective in lowering total cholesterol and triglyceride levels and raising levels of HDL. Niacin may lower cholesterol 15% to 25% and lower triglycerides 20% to 50%. HDL levels may rise as much as 15% to 35% in patients treated with niacin. Nicotinic acid has several side effects, including flushing, pruritus, gastrointestinal disturbances, liver toxicity, hyperuricemia, and hyperglycemia. Patients should be started on low-dose short-acting or immediate-release preparations. Dosage of niacin should start at 250 mg/day and should gradually be increased over several-week intervals to a daily maximal dosage of 1500 to 3000 mg. Low-dose aspirin or a nonsteroidal drug given 60 minutes before the morning dose may mitigate flushing and pruritus when therapy is begun or when the dosage is increased. Niacin given with meals reduces gastrointestinal disturbances.

Niacin should be avoided or used with great caution in patients with a history of gout, peptic ulcer disease, liver disease, and non–insulin-dependent diabetes, and in elderly patients. Postural hypotension may occur in patients, particularly elderly women, who are taking antihypertensive drugs, due to an additive vasodilatory effect. Sustained-release preparations of niacin should be avoided, as they have been associated with an increased incidence of hepatic dysfunction. Because of its significant effect on LDL, HDL, and triglycerides, nicotinic acid is particularly valuable in treating high blood cholesterol levels in patients with low HDL levels or in the treatment of combined hyperlipidemia.

Other Medications

Fibric acid drugs, such as gemfibrozil, lower cholesterol 10% to 15% and raise HDL 10% to 15% as well. They also lower triglyceride levels by 20% to 50%. This class of medication is most effective in lowering triglyceride levels, particularly in patients with familial dysbetalipoproteinemia (type III hyperlipoproteinemia). These drugs also may be effective when used in combined therapy and particularly when used in diabetic patients with elevated triglycerides.

Gemfibrozil is generally well tolerated but occasionally causes gas or mild indigestion. The risk of developing cholesterol gallstones is increased. It can also potentiate the effect of warfarin. Because gemfibrozil has a relatively low impact on total cholesterol and LDL levels, it is generally reserved for use in diabetics and combination drug therapy. Unfortunately, when it is used in conjunction with other medications, particularly HMG-CoA reductase inhibitors, the risk of myositis increases.

Estrogen replacement therapy in postmenopausal women may decrease LDL levels by up to 15% to 20% and raise HDL by a similar amount. In addition, estrogen replacement therapy has been shown to reduce coronary heart disease by up to 25% to 50%. When estrogen therapy is used for hypercholesterolemia and for primary or secondary prevention of coronary heart disease, there is a potential increase in the serum triglyceride level and an increase, presumed small, in the risk of breast and uterine cancer. In postmenopausal women who have not had hysterectomies, combination therapy with progestin is appropriate.

Combination Therapy

When pharmacologic monotherapy, in conjunction with diet and exercise, has failed to yield the desired result, combination drug therapy may be used. It may also be considered if the desired results are achieved but the patient is poorly tolerant of the medication used or the lifestyle imposed by therapy. Combining medications from several lipid-lowering drug classes at lower doses is generally better tolerated and more efficacious and generally increases compliance with the regimen. In addition, it may be more cost-effective to use lower doses of two medications than to use a high dose of a single medication, although this depends on the medications involved. When combination therapy is required, hepatic and renal functions must be monitored.

Common combinations include a bile acid sequestrant with either niacin or an HMG-CoA reductase inhibitor. HMG-CoA reductase inhibitors have also been successfully combined with gemfibrozil, but this combination increases the risk of severe myopathy.

Cost of Therapy

The cost of medication is an important factor in drug selection and may vary greatly. Table 49-4 lists the relative cost of drugs.

Alcohol

Alcohol in moderation may favorably influence lipid levels. "Moderation" is defined as a daily amount not exceeding 2 oz of hard liquor, two 6-oz glasses of wine, or two 12-oz glasses of beer. Several studies have documented a lowering of total cholesterol and an increase in HDL. Some studies have indicated that this benefit occurs only if the calories from alcohol are substituted for other calories, particularly those that contain fat. If alcohol is ingested in addition to a regular caloric load, benefits may also accrue, in terms of diminished coronary artery disease despite persistently elevated cholesterol levels. This phenomenon has been found in certain populations that ingest large quantities of red wine. Some researchers believe the phenol dye created in the production of red wine may be a scavenger for free radicals that ultimately dimin-

Table 49-4. Cost of Pharmacologic Therapy

DRUG	RELATIVE COST
Niacin	+
Gemfibrozil (Lopid)	+
Fluvastatin sodium (Lescol)	++
Pravastatin sodium (Pravachol)	+++
Lovastatin (Mevacor)	+++
Simvastatin (Zocor)	++++
Colestipol (Colestid)	++++
Cholestyramine (Questran Light)	++++

Lowest, +; highest, ++++.

ishes arterial endothelial damage. In any event, some populations ingesting red wine, despite a high fat intake, are relatively protected from coronary artery disease. It is not known if this principle is applicable in all populations.

Alcohol increases triglyceride levels and may increase the risk of coronary artery disease in patients prone to hypertriglyceridemia, particularly when triglyceride levels alone are viewed as a cardiac risk factor.

It seems prudent to recommend the ingestion of low-dose alcohol if patients desire alcohol as part of their daily consumption and if the alcohol is substituted for other calories in a still nutritionally sound diet.

HYPERTRIGLYCERIDEMIA

Elevated serum triglyceride levels are positively correlated with coronary heart disease in univariate analysis, but are not as strongly predictive when other cardiac risk factors are added. There is an association between hypertriglyceridemia, low HDL levels, and very atherogenic forms of LDL. This seems to be the case in women with diabetes and in certain familial combined hyperlipidemias. Patients with triglyceride levels above 500 to 1000 mg/dL have an increased risk of acute pancreatitis.

Nonpharmacologic therapy, with weight reduction in overweight patients and alcohol avoidance and enhanced physical activity for all patients, is generally required. Drug therapy should be considered when triglyceride levels are elevated in association with familial combined hyperlipidemia, or in diabetic patients with high triglyceride levels. Fibric and nicotinic acid medications are generally used in this situation and are also used to prevent acute pancreatitis in patients with triglyceride levels above 1000 mg/dL.

SECONDARY DYSLIPIDEMIA

Diabetes mellitus, chronic renal failure, nephrotic syndrome, and hypothyroidism commonly cause secondary dyslipidemia. Diabetes mellitus is frequently accompanied by an elevated triglyceride level and a low HDL level. It is important to treat diabetic women in this category aggressively, because diabetes seems to negate any benefit of the premenopausal state. Tight control of diabetes and correction of the hypothyroid state generally improve the lipid abnormality. Nephrotic syndrome is usually associated with hypertriglyceridemia and generally can be controlled with nonpharmacologic therapy.

SEVERE FORMS OF HYPERCHOLESTEROLEMIA

Severe elevations of cholesterol occur in the following conditions:

- Familial hypercholesterolemia, which occurs in one in 500 people and is characterized by marked elevations of LDL
- Severe polygenic hypercholesterolemia, which manifests as LDL levels exceeding 220 mg/dL. It occurs in about 1% of the adult population and is commonly associated with premature coronary heart disease.
- Familial combined hyperlipidemia, characterized by elevations of total cholesterol, triglycerides, or both in different members of the same family. It occurs in about 1% of the population and causes premature coronary heart disease.

In any female presenting with these severe forms of hypercholesterolemia, family screening is mandatory to detect other members at risk who may benefit from therapy.

REFERRAL

Most patients can be safely managed by the primary care provider. However, referral to a lipid specialist, commonly an endocrinologist or a cardiologist with an interest in lipids, should be considered if the goals of therapy are not achieved. Referral should also be considered if control is adequate but the patient does not tolerate the medication and lifestyle changes well. In addition, certain patients with complex lipid disorders or responses to medication therapy benefit from referral to a subspecialist.

SUMMARY

The goal of treatment of hyperlipidemia is to reduce the incidence of coronary heart disease and vascular disease. The primary care provider must identify patients at risk for hyperlipidemia-induced coronary heart disease and must reduce the prevalence of other modifiable risk factors that can lead to enhanced coronary disease. Patients must be advised of the need for lipid control, but the clinician must weigh the potential adverse effects of medications against the potential gains.

Hypercholesterolemia is a chronic disease that frequently requires lifelong dietary and drug therapy. Because patients often do not feel any symptoms from hyperlipidemia, it is sometimes difficult to ensure compliance with medications that may cause adverse effects. The clinician must educate the patient in this regard and provide motivation and credibility relative to the importance and benefits of ongoing therapy.

BIBLIOGRAPHY

Denke MA. Individual responsiveness to a cholesterol-lowering diet in postmenopausal women with moderate hypercholesterolemia. Arch Intern Med 1994;154:1977.

Johnson CL, Rifkind BM, Sempos CT, et al. Declining serum total cholesterol levels among U.S. adults. The National Health and Nutrition Examination Surveys. JAMA 1993;269:3002.

Larsen ML, Illingworth DR. Drug treatment of dyslipoproteinemia. Med Clin North Am 1994;78:225.

Medical Knowledge Self-Assessment Program. Cardiovascular medicine. Book 1, Part B. Philadelphia: American College of Physicians, 1994:417.

National Cholesterol Education Program. Summary of the second report of the National Cholesterol Education Program (NCEP) Expert Panel on Detection, Evaluation, and Treatment of High Blood Cholesterol in Adults (Adult Treatment Panel II). JAMA 1993;269:3015.

Sempos CT, Cleeman JI, Carroll MD, et al. Prevalence of high blood cholesterol among U.S. adults. An update based on guidelines from the second report of the National Cholesterol Education Program Adult Treatment Panel. JAMA 1993;269:3009.

Stampfer MJ, Sacks FM, Salvini S, Willett WC, Hennekens CH. A prospective study of cholesterol, apolipoproteins, and the risk of myocardial infarction. N Engl J Med 1991;325:373.

Primary Care for Women, edited by Phyllis C. Leppert and Fred M. Howard. Lippincott-Raven Publishers, Philadelphia © 1997.

50

Venous Thromboembolic Disease

CHARLES W. FRANCIS

Venous thromboembolic disease is a major problem in the United States because of its high incidence and serious health consequences. Symptomatic deep vein thrombosis and pulmonary embolism result in over 250,000 acute hospital admissions per year, and the total incidence is much higher if asymptomatic or undiagnosed cases are included. Pulmonary embolism is the principal or a major contributing cause of death in 15% to 30% of all hospitalized patients and results in 50,000 to 100,000 deaths per year. It contributes significantly to the mortality and morbidity of chronically ill or bedridden patients and also affects otherwise healthy individuals, especially at times of increased risk, such as after surgery or trauma. It also occurs frequently during pregnancy and at parturition, and is the most common cause of maternal mortality associated with live births. Anticoagulant treatment of venous thrombosis requires frequent laboratory monitoring and results in bleeding complications in 5% to 10% of patients, contributing to the high cost of care. Acute venous thrombosis can also lead to permanent vein damage and the postphlebitic syndrome, resulting in the chronic pain, swelling, and leg ulceration that affect approximately 500,000 individuals nationally. The annual cost of treating deep vein thrombosis in the United States has recently been estimated at $6 billion.

The clinical approach to venous thromboembolic disease has undergone rapid evolution as a result of major advances in understanding its pathophysiologic mechanisms and improved clinical management. Increased understanding of hemostatic control mechanisms has led to definition of inherited abnormalities that contribute to a large proportion of cases of idiopathic venous thrombosis. The importance of an accurate objective diagnosis has been documented and new, noninvasive diagnostic approaches introduced. Clinical studies have refined the therapeutic approach, improved anticoagulant therapy, and further defined the roles for thrombolytic and surgical management.

ETIOLOGY

Venous thromboembolism in nearly all patients begins in the deep veins of the calf as small thrombi that are often located in areas of stagnant flow behind vein valve cusps or in relation to sites of vessel wall damage. Such thrombi may extend into larger and more proximal veins, eventually causing leg symptoms, and they may also break free and migrate to the pulmonary artery as emboli. Whereas some pulmonary emboli originate from veins proximal to the legs or from the right heart, these are uncommon, and pulmonary embolism should be viewed as a complication of leg vein thrombosis. The reasons for the remarkable predisposition of leg veins to thrombosis is not well understood, but thrombosis results from an imbalance in the mechanisms that maintain normal blood fluidity. These include the inhibitors of the coagulation system, the nonthrombogenic endothelial cell vessel lining, and the normal flow of blood. Abnormalities in any of these three elements of the "Virchow triad" can contribute to thrombosis, including increased coagulability of the blood, damage to the vessel wall, and abnormalities in flow. Patients who develop venous thromboembolic disease often have abnormalities in more than one of these control mechanisms.

The normal flow of blood in the legs is from superficial to deep veins and from distal to proximal. Flow depends on contraction of the calf muscles to compress veins and cause unidirectional blood flow, because valves in deep and perforating veins prevent retrograde flow. Normal flow inhibits thrombosis by diluting procoagulants that are formed locally and by supplying the vascular lining with necessary nutrients and oxygen. Stasis allows local accumulation of procoagulants that may become sufficient to generate fibrin and activate platelets, and it also contributes to endothelial cell hypoxia, which can stimulate secretion of activators of coagulation. Venous stasis is frequent in hospitalized or injured patients who are often immobilized with little effective calf muscle contraction, resulting in venodilation and blood pooling. Other factors contributing to venous stasis include neurologic disease with paralysis, anesthesia, leg injuries, orthopaedic procedures on the legs, casting, and splints. Slow venous flow also results from proximal obstruction occurring with tumors, pregnancy, congestive heart failure, and venous scarring from prior episodes of leg vein thrombosis.

Vessel wall injury is another contributor to thrombosis, and trauma or surgery that damages the vascular lining can initiate deep venous thrombosis. Whereas the normal venous endothelial lining is thromboresistant, deeper components are prothrombotic. After endothelial cell removal, platelets adhere rapidly to exposed subendothelial proteins, become activated, and promote thrombus formation. Fibroblasts and smooth muscle cells in the vessel wall also express tissue factor, a potent activator of the coagulation system. Endothelial thromboresistance also can be reduced by inflammatory cytokines, hypoxia, or exposure to endotoxin during sepsis.

BLOOD HYPERCOAGULABILITY

The two anticoagulant systems that prevent excessive hemostatic activation and limit clot extension include the antithrombin III–heparin and protein C systems. Inherited deficiencies in either can result in a congenital thrombotic predisposition. Antithrombin III inhibits serine proteases generated during coagulation, and its activity is greatly accelerated by heparin administered either therapeutically or by natural heparin-like molecules present on vascular surfaces. The protein C pathway is activated by thrombin, includes protein S as a cofactor, and results in proteolytic inactivation of factors V and VIII. Inherited deficiencies of antithrombin III, protein C, and protein S occur with a frequency of one in several thousand individuals. More recently described is "activated protein C resistance," which is caused by a mutation in the factor V protein, preventing its inactivation and leading to a hypercoagulable state in approximately 5% of the total population.

These inherited abnormalities may occur in up to 50% of patients with otherwise unexplained venous thromboembolic disease. The likelihood of an inherited hypercoagulable state is increased in individuals with a positive family history of deep vein thrombosis or pulmonary embolism; in those with an early age of onset, with venous thrombosis in unusual locations such as intraabdominal, renal or intracranial thrombosis; and in patients with no other clinical risk factors. The lupus anticoagulant–antiphospholipid antibody syndrome is an acquired hypercoagulable condition caused by the presence of an autoantibody with phospholipid specificity, which often prolongs in vitro coagulation tests but results in an increased risk of both arterial and venous thrombosis and recurrent abortion. Such antibodies may occur in otherwise healthy individuals but are increased in frequency in patients with systemic lupus erythematosus and in the elderly.

These well-defined hematologic abnormalities are found in only a few patients presenting with venous thromboembolic disease. More frequently, these patients have one or more clinical conditions associated with increased thrombotic risk (Table 50-1). These include surgery, trauma, malignancy, immobility, acute myocardial infarction, stroke, congestive heart failure, obesity, inflammatory diseases, and the postpartum state. These risk factors seem to act in an additive way, and multiple factors are often present in patients with venous thromboembolic disease. Identification of these thrombotic risk factors is important both in evaluating the likelihood of venous thromboembolic disease in an individual patient and in judging the need for anticoagulant prophylaxis.

NATURAL HISTORY

Most venous thrombi originate in calf veins, and studies of postoperative patients indicate that they are often asymptomatic. Many resolve without causing symptoms. Symptomatic deep vein thrombosis can be caused by extensive thrombosis limited to calf veins or, more commonly, by proximal extension of thrombus into the popliteal or superficial femoral veins, resulting in interference with venous outflow from the leg. Anticoagulant therapy modifies this natural history by preventing extension of calf vein thrombi, thereby permitting natural resolution through the processes of fibrinolysis and cellular organization. In contrast, thrombolytic therapy actively lyses clot to reduce the amount of thrombus.

Table 50-1. Risk Factors for Venous Thromboembolic Disease

Inherited Hypercoagulable States	Acquired Conditions
Antithrombin III deficiency	Surgery
Protein C deficiency	Trauma
Protein S deficiency	Immobility
Activated protein C resistance (factor V Leiden)	Malignancy
	Pregnancy
	Advanced age
	Lupus anticoagulant
	Obesity
	Prior DVT or PE
	Myocardial infarction
	Congestive heart failure
	Stroke

DVT, deep vein thrombosis; *PE*, pulmonary embolism.

Pulmonary embolism is a complication of deep vein thrombosis, and clinically evident emboli usually originate from proximal leg vein thrombi. Prospective studies indicate that embolism occurs in approximately 50% of patients with proximal leg vein thrombosis, including many in whom embolization is asymptomatic. Another frequent complication of deep vein thrombosis is chronic venous insufficiency, which results from vein scarring, chronic obstruction, and venous valve damage. With valve damage, the venous system is exposed to higher hydrostatic pressures and muscle contraction forces flow into superficial veins, resulting in dilatation, edema, collateral flow, and skin ulceration. Chronic venous insufficiency is most clearly associated with incompetence of valves in the perforating veins connecting the deep and superficial systems and occurs most frequently after extensive iliofemoral thrombosis. It may occur soon after the acute episode, but symptoms often do not appear for up to 5 years or more. Symptoms commonly include chronic leg edema, skin hyperpigmentation, aching pain in the leg relieved by elevation, venous varicosities, and ulceration (most often involving skin near the medial malleolus).

Pulmonary emboli typically resolve rapidly and often cannot be detected within 1 to 2 weeks after an acute event. There is often no clinically apparent functional pulmonary deficit after clinical resolution, although sensitive studies have found minor abnormalities of gas exchange. Because of the dual blood flow to the lungs from both the pulmonary artery and bronchial circulation, infarction is uncommon. In a small number of patients, emboli apparently do not resolve normally and repeated embolization leads to chronic changes in the vasculature and pulmonary hypertension.

CLINICAL SYMPTOMS

The clinical hallmarks of deep vein thrombosis are leg pain and swelling that usually have an acute onset but are sometimes progressive over several days. Patients often complain of tightness or aching in calf muscles and the development of distal edema. Extensive proximal thrombosis can cause symptoms in the thigh, and dramatic swelling may result in bluish discoloration with compromise of arterial flow due to tense edema, resulting in phlegmasia cerulea dolens. Thrombosis confined only to a superficial vein usually presents with localized pain and redness, and a thrombosed vein can often be palpated as a superficial cord. These symptoms should arouse suspicion in the appropriate clinical setting and serve to establish the clinical likelihood of deep vein thrombosis. They are, however, not specific, and prospective studies have established that over 50% of patients with clinically suspected deep vein thrombosis will not have the diagnosis confirmed by objective testing. The differential diagnosis is broad and includes cellulitis, muscle strain, arthritis, ligamentous injury to the ankle or knee, ruptured Baker cyst, muscle hematoma, and congestive heart failure.

Symptoms of pulmonary embolism result from the respiratory and hemodynamic effects of pulmonary artery obstruction, and the severity is proportional to the degree of vascular obstruction. Large emboli cause acute pulmonary hypertension with right heart strain and decreased cardiac output, resulting in chest discomfort, weakness, collapse, or sudden death. Respiratory symptoms often include shortness of breath, wheezing, and cough. Pleuritic chest pain and hemoptysis result from pulmonary infarction and are less common. The most frequent physical findings are tachypnea and tachycardia. Major pulmonary embolism may present with hypotension, shock, and cyanosis. There may be evidence of right heart strain, including a right ventricular lift, gallop, and increased intensity of the pulmonary component of the second heart sound. Pulmonary findings include evidence of atelectasis, and infarction may result in findings of consolidation and a pleural friction rub.

The clinical findings of pulmonary embolism are neither sensitive nor specific, as small emboli may be asymptomatic and at least half of the patients in whom embolus is suspected on the basis of clinical findings do not have the diagnosis confirmed with objective tests. Therefore, a high index of suspicion is required. The chief value of clinical findings is to suggest the diagnosis and thereby lead to objective testing. The differential diagnosis often includes acute myocardial infarction, pneumonia, pleurisy, bronchitis, asthma, congestive heart failure, pulmonary edema, pneumothorax, atelectasis, pericarditis, and musculoskeletal problems.

LABORATORY TESTS AND IMAGING

Patients with suspected deep vein thrombosis should have the diagnosis confirmed by objective tests because of the nonspecificity of the clinical findings (Table 50-2). Ultrasound can be used both to assess flow and image leg veins and is suitable for confirmation of diagnosis in most symptomatic patients. B-mode ultrasound is used to identify proximal leg veins, and gentle compression is applied with the transducer to determine if the vein is fully compressible. Inability to collapse the vein is a sensitive and specific indication of the presence of thrombus. The presence of intraluminal echoes from thrombus and abnormalities in venous flow patterns also provides confirmatory information. In patients with clinical symptoms suggestive of acute deep vein thrombosis, a positive compression ultrasound finding is sufficiently diagnostic to institute treatment. Although compression ultrasound can accurately identify thrombi in the popliteal, superficial, and common femoral veins, its diagnostic value is lessened in patients with thrombi confined to the calf and it is not applicable to pelvic veins. Also, its use is limited in patients with recurrent deep vein thrombosis who may have extensive collaterals and intravascular obstruction due to old clot or scarring that cannot be distinguished from acute thrombosis.

Impedance plethysmography (IPG) is another noninvasive approach to deep vein thrombosis diagnosis based on changes in electrical resistance across the leg in response to compression with a venous tourniquet. The test has reasonable diagnostic accuracy in acute symptomatic proximal leg vein obstruction, but it is insensitive to calf deep vein thrombosis, often fails to detect partially obstructed clots, and can be difficult to interpret in patients with congestive heart failure or other conditions limiting venous outflow. Ultrasound has largely replaced IPG as the noninvasive diagnostic test of choice.

Venography represents the gold standard for deep vein thrombosis diagnosis and routinely provides diagnostic information regarding calf and thigh vein thrombosis. The pelvic veins are not seen well with standard technique, but they can be imaged with special approaches. The presence of an intraluminal filling defect is highly specific for thrombosis. Other abnormalities such as failure to fill veins and the presence of collaterals are suggestive of thrombosis but also can result from technical problems or the effects of previous thrombosis. Limitations of venography include difficulty in cannulating foot veins, pain and inflammation with extravascular extravasation of contrast, allergy to radiographic contrast agents, and the occasional occurrence of postvenography thrombosis. Other useful imaging approaches include computed tomography and magnetic resonance imaging, and venous thrombosis is occasionally identified unexpectedly when imaging is performed for other indications.

In symptomatic patients, compression ultrasound is a reasonable first choice of a diagnostic test, and a positive finding is usually sufficient to initiate therapy. Proximal vein thrombosis is unlikely with a negative test result, but this does not rule out isolated calf vein thrombosis, which may occur in 20% or more of symptomatic patients. The most direct approach to diagnosis of calf vein thrombosis is venography, which immediately confirms or excludes the diagnosis. An alternative approach is to withhold therapy and perform serial compression ultrasounds to detect possible extension into the popliteal or more proximal veins. The importance of treating isolated calf vein thrombosis remains controversial, and the prognosis is good without therapy if the thrombus does not extend proximally. Therefore, withholding therapy is reasonable if repeated compression ultrasound results remain negative.

The diagnosis of pulmonary embolism also requires objective confirmation because clinical findings alone are nonspecific. A chest x-ray is needed in nearly all cases to identify possible alternative diagnoses and as a basis for interpreting lung scan findings, but the findings with pulmonary embolism are highly variable. The chest x-ray findings may be normal or may show atelectasis, infarction, or effusion. Vascular abnormalities are seen occasionally, including an abrupt cutoff of large vessels and areas of

Table 50-2. Tests for Deep Vein Thrombosis

	ADVANTAGES	DISADVANTAGES
Venography	"Gold standard"	Invasive and painful
	Accurate in calf, thigh, and pelvis	Side effects Occasional technical failure
Ultrasound	Noninvasive	Insensitive to calf or pelvic vein thrombi
	Accurate for popliteal and femoral veins in symptomatic patients	
Impedance plethysmography	Noninvasive Accurate for proximal vein obstruction in symptomatic patients	Insensitive to calf DVT Cannot detect partial obstruction False-positive results with other causes of outflow obstruction

DVT, deep vein thrombosis.

increased lucency due to hypoperfusion. Arterial blood gases are of limited diagnostic value as patients frequently are hypoxic, but normal blood gas values do not rule out the diagnosis. The electrocardiographic findings also are nonspecific, but evidence of right heart strain may be seen with large emboli. Cardiac echocardiography can be useful if thrombi are identified in right-sided chambers or in the pulmonary artery, and evidence of right ventricular overload also may be present.

Perfusion lung scanning should be considered as the initial screening test, and the findings often are sufficient to provide a basis for treatment decisions. The most useful finding is normal perfusion, which virtually excludes the diagnosis of pulmonary embolism. A high-probability lung scan showing segmental or larger areas of absent perfusion with normal ventilation is highly predictive of pulmonary embolism in the absence of a likely alternative diagnoses and is sufficient for instituting therapy. Unfortunately, the diagnostic value of intermediate or low probability scans is not sufficiently high to either establish or exclude the diagnosis of embolism, and additional diagnostic tests are then required. Pulmonary angiography can provide a definitive diagnosis of embolism by demonstrating both the presence and extent of pulmonary vascular obstruction. It requires a properly equipped and experienced laboratory and is associated with a small risk of allergic reaction and induction of cardiac arrhythmias. Because of the high association between pulmonary embolism and deep vein thrombosis, an alternative approach is compression ultrasound or venography. Identification of leg vein thrombosis provides a basis for anticoagulant or fibrinolytic therapy and makes the diagnosis of pulmonary embolism highly likely.

The overall diagnostic approach to pulmonary embolism requires an appreciation of the limitations of available imaging modalities and is strongly dependent on the clinical presentation and physician's judgment regarding the likelihood of pulmonary embolism. A chest x-ray and electrocardiogram are required to rule out alternative diagnoses, and characteristic abnormalities may support the diagnosis of pulmonary embolism. The next step is usually lung scanning, which rules out pulmonary embolism if the finding is normal, or provides sufficient evidence for treatment if it is high probability with a high index of clinical suspicion. Patients with other lung scan findings require additional investigation, and proceeding directly to pulmonary angiography is appropriate for acutely ill patients who require prompt and unequivocal diagnosis and aggressive therapy. Definitive angiographic diagnosis also should be considered in patients with strong contraindications to anticoagulation in whom placement of an inferior vena caval filter is considered. An alternative diagnostic approach is to investigate possible deep vein thrombosis, present in approximately 75% of patients. This establishes a need for therapy and greatly increases the likelihood that the respiratory symptoms are due to embolization.

PREVENTION

Prophylaxis is the best approach to decreasing the incidence of venous thromboembolic disease in moderate- and high-risk hospitalized patients. Epidemiologic studies have determined the incidence and clinical outcomes of venous thrombosis in various populations, and advances in understanding the pathogenesis have guided the development of both pharmacologic and nonpharmacologic preventive modalities that are effective and safe. Characterization of risk is the starting point for deciding on prophylaxis for an individual patient. Among surgical patients, those with low risk are younger than 40 years of age with surgery lasting less than 30 minutes and having no additional risk factors (Table 50-3). Patients at moderate risk have an overall incidence rate of calf deep vein thrombosis of 10% to 40%, proximal deep vein thrombosis of 2% to 10%, and pulmonary embolism of 0.1% to 0.7%. These include surgical patients older than 40 years of age undergoing abdominal or thoracic surgery lasting over 30 minutes. Particularly high-risk patients include orthopedic patients with hip fracture or those who are undergoing hip or knee replacement, in whom the total incidence rate of venous thrombosis is 40% to 80%. Surgery for gynecologic malignancies also represents a high-risk procedure. Medical patients are a diverse, moderate-risk group in whom a large number and variety of risk factors for venous thrombosis need to be considered before choosing prophylaxis. For nearly all moderate- and high-risk patients, safe and effective prophylaxis is available, including both pharmacologic and nonpharmacologic approaches.

Venous stasis is common in hospitalized patients, particularly after surgery when the effects of anesthesia, operative pain, and bed rest combine to decrease calf muscle activity. Simple measures to counteract venous stasis can be used in nearly all patients and include leg exercises for bed-bound patients and early ambulation for surgical and postpartum patients. Graded compression stockings exert maximal pressure at the ankle and gradually less pressure toward the thigh, decreasing venous capacitance and preventing blood pooling in leg veins. They are of value in low- to moderate-risk patients. External pneumatic compression employs boots or cuffs that rhythmically inflate to compress the leg; this action results in increased venous blood flow and also activates blood fibrinolytic activity. The absence of side effects makes this approach an attractive prophylactic modality, particularly in patients at high risk of bleeding in whom anticoagulant use is unacceptable. Used in combination with an anticoagulant, the prophylactic effect may be increased without additional risk.

The greatest experience with prophylaxis has been with low doses of heparin, and this is based on the rationale that lower concentrations of anticoagulant are needed to prevent than to treat venous thrombosis. Heparin is administered subcutaneously in a fixed dose of 5000 U every 8 or 12 hours, beginning 2 hours before surgery and continuing until the patient is fully ambulatory. This regimen results in only slight prolongation of the partial thromboplastin time (PTT), and routine monitoring is not required. Its effectiveness in general surgery patients has been documented in many studies, and it results in an overall risk reduction of 67% for deep vein thrombosis and 47% for pulmonary embolism. The main side effect of heparin use is occasional bruising at the injection site and a 2% increase in wound hematomas, most of which are minor. Low molecular weight heparin recently has been introduced and approved for use in prevention of deep vein thrombosis after orthopaedic and high risk surgery. It has a lower mean molecular weight than unfractionated heparin and improved pharmacologic properties. Data are conflicting regarding the relative effectiveness of low molecular weight heparin in comparison with unfractionated heparin in preventing venous thrombosis in general surgical patients. Warfarin is highly effective in preventing venous thrombosis, but its use is restricted primarily to high-risk patients because low dose subcutaneous heparin is effective and simpler to use in patients at moderate risk. Other pharmacologic agents used for prophylaxis include dextran, which is effective but has limited use, and aspirin, for which efficacy data are conflicting.

Table 50-3. Recommendations for Prophylaxis of Deep Vein Thrombosis

CATEGORY	EXAMPLES	APPROXIMATE RISK			RECOMMENDATION
		Calf DVT	*Proximal DVT*	*PE*	
Low	Surgical patients younger than 40 y, surgery lasting < 30 min, no additional risk factors	1–2%	0.5–1%	0–0.1%	Ambulation, leg exercises
	Hospitalized medical patients without risk factors				
Moderate	Surgical patients older than 40 y, having abdominal or thoracic surgery lasting > 30 min	10–40%	2–10%	0.1–0.7%	Low-dose heparin
	Hospitalized medical patients with one or more risk factors				
	Neurosurgery or other patients with high bleeding risk				External pneumatic compression
High	Hip fracture, joint replacement	40–80%	20–40%	5–10%	Warfarin,* low molecular weight heparin or adjusted-dose heparin
	Open prostatectomy and gynecologic malignancy				External pneumatic compression

DVT, deep vein thrombosis; *PE,* pulmonary embolism.
*Given in low-dose regimen.

In deciding on prophylaxis for an individual patient, characterization of risk is the starting point. Recommendations for prophylaxis are given in Table 50-3, which classifies patients into low-, moderate-, and high-risk groups. Among patients at low risk, early ambulation and leg exercises during bed rest may reduce deep vein thrombosis risk further. Most hospitalized medical and surgical patients are in the moderate-risk category and require serious consideration for prophylaxis. Low-dose subcutaneous heparin is appropriate for most patients, whereas external pneumatic compression is an alternative for those with increased bleeding risk. The high-risk category includes those in whom frequent and serious venous thromboembolic complications occur in the absence of effective prophylaxis. Low-dose subcutaneous heparin is generally insufficient in these patient groups, and either warfarin, adjusted-dose heparin, external pneumatic compression, or low molecular weight heparin are appropriate choices.

TREATMENT

The goals of treatment of venous thromboembolic disease are to provide symptomatic relief, to prevent disease extension or recurrence, and to minimize structural damage to deep leg veins and thereby prevent the long-term development of chronic venous insufficiency. Management requires a choice between several effective forms of anticoagulant, fibrinolytic, and surgical therapy to maximize patient benefit. The benefit-to-risk ratio is of central importance in making therapeutic choices, and this always involves difficult issues of clinical judgment focused on individual considerations of disease extent, risk of bleeding, patient ability to comply with long-term therapy, and coexisting medical illnesses that contribute to thrombotic risks or influence drug response. Careful assessment of bleeding risk is particularly important because both anticoagulant and fibrinolytic therapies are associated with bleeding complications that compromise therapy and result in significant morbidity and occasional mortality.

Pulmonary embolism and deep vein thrombosis most often are treated with heparin followed by a period of outpatient oral anticoagulation. For initial therapy, heparin should be administered intravenously in a dose of 5000 U followed immediately by a constant infusion in a dose of approximately 1200 U/hour (Table 50-4). Substantial evidence indicates that an important determinant of the efficacy of initial anticoagulation is the administration of sufficient heparin to prolong the PTT to within the therapeutic range of 1.5 to 2.5 times control. Thus, the PTT should be checked after 4 to 6 hours and the heparin infusion adjusted. Repeated checks and dose adjustments should be made every 4 to 6 hours until the PTT is adequately prolonged. After initial adjustment, the PTT can be checked once daily. Nomograms are available that are useful in heparin dose adjustment. The platelet count should be monitored every other day with heparin use because of the risk of thrombo-

Table 50-4. Anticoagulant Therapy of Deep Vein Thrombosis and Pulmonary Embolism

Initial Therapy With Heparin

1. Administer heparin, 5000 U intravenously, and start an infusion of 1200 U/h
2. Check aPTT after 4–6 h and adjust infusion to prolong aPTT to 1.5–2.5 times control
   Alternative. Administer heparin subcutaneously every 12 h beginning with an initial dose of 18,000 U; check aPTT after 4 h and adjust subsequent doses to prolong aPTT to 1.5–2.5 times control

Maintenance Anticoagulation

Oral anticoagulants

1. Give warfarin, 5–10 mg, during first hospital day
2. Check PT daily
3. Adjust dose to prolong PT to INR of 2–3
4. Discontinue heparin after minimum of 5 d when INR reaches desired range
5. Continue warfarin as outpatient for 3–6 mo

Heparin

1. Heparin subcutaneously every 12 h in a dose to prolonged the mid-interval aPTT to 1.5 times control

aPTT, activated partial thromboplastin time; *INR,* international normalized ratio; PT, prothrombin time.

cytopenia. Warfarin can be started during the first hospital day in a dose of 5 to 10 mg, depending on body weight. The prothrombin time should be checked daily and the dose adjusted to prolong the prothrombin time to an international normalized ratio (INR) of 2 to 3. Heparin can be discontinued after a minimum of 5 days, after the INR has reached the desired range. Warfarin should be continued for a period of 3 to 6 months, depending on the extent of thrombosis and patient predisposition to recurrence. The INR should be checked as an outpatient twice weekly until stable, and then weekly or biweekly as needed. Adjustment of warfarin dose often is needed after hospital discharge, because outpatient diet and medications differ compared with those used in the hospital. Patients should be advised to avoid aspirin-containing medications and to report any medication change to their physician because it may impact on warfarin dosage.

Subcutaneous heparin is an alternative for both the initial and long-term treatment of venous thrombosis. During initial treatment, higher doses of subcutaneous heparin are required in comparison with intravenous administration to achieve comparable prolongation of the PTT. The subcutaneous route has advantages of not requiring an intravenous line and a constant infusion device. A disadvantage is that the PTT must be timed in relation to subcutaneous injections, whereas they can be made at any convenient time during intravenous administration. Also, dose adjustment can be made more rapidly with intravenous therapy. For outpatient anticoagulant management, subcutaneous heparin every 12 hours also can be used. The dose should be initially adjusted to prolong the midinterval PTT to a target of 1.5 times control; this dose then can be given every 12 hours for 3 to 6 months. Thrombocytopenia and osteoporosis are potential risks of long-term heparin therapy. Subcutaneous low-molecular-weight heparin can also be used to manage acute deep vein thrombosis.

Surgical approaches to management of venous thrombosis are limited, but interruption of the venous system proximal to thrombus can prevent an embolus from reaching the lungs and is useful in some patients. Various methods of compartmentalization of the inferior vena cava have been replaced by the development of inferior vena cava filters that can be inserted under local anesthesia through the jugular or femoral veins. In experienced hands, filters are effective in preventing embolization and have a high long-term patency rate. Complications include development of venous stasis and occasional proximal migration of the device. The principal indication for placement of an inferior vena cava filter is deep vein thrombosis or pulmonary embolism in patients with severe bleeding in whom anticoagulation is contraindicated. A filter also should be considered in patients who have recurrent emboli while on optimal anticoagulation.

Bed rest and anticoagulation meet two goals of treatment of deep vein thrombosis by providing symptomatic relief and prevention of recurrence. However, whereas anticoagulation inhibits progression of thrombosis, it does not accelerate physiologic clot dissolution. Also, anticoagulant therapy does little to prevent the valve damage and vein scaring that leads to symptoms of the postphlebitic syndrome. Fibrinolytic therapy offers the potential for rapid clot dissolution, providing rapid relief of vascular obstruction, improving the hemodynamics, and preventing permanent vein damage.

However, despite dramatic advances in fibrinolytic therapy for arterial thrombosis, its application has been limited in venous disease. The primary reasons are an increased risk of bleeding and lack of definitive evidence that mortality is improved in pulmonary embolism or that postphlebitic syndrome can routinely be prevented after venous thrombosis. Despite these appropriate concerns, evidence indicates that there is a clear role for fibrinolytic treatment in both acute pulmonary embolism and deep vein thrombosis. The results of thrombolytic therapy are best if treatment is given to patients most likely to respond and benefit. Because the risk of developing postphlebitic syndrome is highest in patients with extensive proximal deep vein thrombosis, thrombolytic therapy should be considered primarily in this group. The clearest predictor of therapeutic outcome is clot age, as fresh recent thrombi respond best; patients with symptoms lasting more 7 to 10 days are likely to respond poorly. The greatest benefit of thrombolytic therapy for pulmonary embolism is expected in patients with large emboli and hemodynamic compromise, in whom the accelerated early clot lysis results in significant, rapid clinical improvement.

The risk of bleeding is minimized by careful patient selection. Intracranial bleeding is the most serious complication, and patients with recent head trauma, CNS surgery, or history of stroke, subarachnoid bleed, or intracranial metastatic disease should not be treated. Thrombolytic therapy also should be avoided in patients with a major risk of bleeding, such as those with active or recent gastrointestinal or genitourinary bleeding, or major surgery or trauma within 7 days. Minimizing invasive vascular procedure also lowers the bleeding risk. For deep vein thrombosis, urokinase or streptokinase can be administered systemically for durations of up to several days. Recent evidence indicates that catheter-directed thrombosis may be effective for large proximal vein thrombi. Urokinase, streptokinase, and tissue plasminogen activator are effective in treating pulmonary embolism and may be given as a 2-hour regimen. Anticoagulation should be instituted when fibrinolytic therapy is discontinued to prevent recurrence.

CONSIDERATIONS IN PREGNANCY

The risk of venous thromboembolic disease is increased at the time of parturition, and pulmonary embolism is a leading cause of maternal death. Management of venous thrombosis and pulmonary embolism during pregnancy raises unique problems in both diagnosis and treatment. These include risks to the fetus of diagnostic tests and of anticoagulant therapy, as well as danger to the mother of hemorrhage, particularly at the time of delivery. These additional risks of anticoagulant therapy during pregnancy, coupled with the uncertainty of the clinical diagnosis, make accurate objective diagnosis especially important. However, the use of imaging modalities is limited by concerns over potential adverse fetal effects of exposure to ionizing radiation. Also, results from noninvasive tests for venous thrombosis that rely on assessment of flow, such as IPG and Doppler ultrasound, may be abnormal in the third trimester due to extrinsic venous compression from the gravid uterus. Therefore, abnormal noninvasive test results during the third trimester are difficult to interpret, although normal test findings are useful in excluding diagnosis of venous thrombosis. Patients with positive noninvasive tests results can be either treated presumptively, accepting the risk of a false-positive test result or, alternatively, the diagnosis can be confirmed by venography. Venography that is confined to the calf exposes the fetus to a very low dose of radiation, whereas the exposure with a complete venogram of both proximal and distal leg is greater but still low with adequate shielding. Fetal radiation exposure is low from ventilation/perfusion lung scanning.

Anticoagulation during pregnancy is associated with significant risk to the mother and also to the fetus, because oral anticoagulants cross the placenta and enter the fetal circulation. Administration of warfarin during the first trimester of pregnancy, particularly during the sixth to ninth weeks of gestation, can result in warfarin embryopathy, a syndrome characterized by nasal hypoplasia and stippling of the epiphyses that is seen radiographically, primarily in the axial skeleton. CNS abnormalities also may occur with exposure to warfarin at any time during pregnancy, resulting in developmental delay and brain malformations. The fetal coagulation system is sensitive to the anticoagulant effect of warfarin, so that an appropriate level of anticoagulation in the mother can result in fetal hemorrhage and loss. Because of these complications, warfarin should be avoided during pregnancy if possible.

Unlike warfarin, heparin does not cross the placenta to affect the fetus. Most studies of the use of heparin during pregnancy have identified a rate of maternal bleeding complications similar to that in nonpregnant patients and a similar rate of prematurity, abortion, and still births to that in the general population. However, administration of heparin during the 24-hour period before delivery may be associated with increased risk of maternal bleeding. An additional maternal risk of long-term heparin administration is osteoporosis, which may be accelerated by the high calcium requirements during pregnancy.

Because of its effectiveness and safety, heparin is the anticoagulant of choice during pregnancy, and warfarin should be avoided. Anticoagulation for acute venous thrombosis or pulmonary embolism can be provided using the guidelines for nonpregnant patients, with the exception that subcutaneous heparin should be used for long-term therapy rather than warfarin. Heparin should be discontinued at the beginning of labor or 24 hours before elective delivery and should be reinstituted 24 to 48 hours postpartum. Warfarin can be used after delivery and is safe in nursing mothers because it not secreted in breast milk and results in no infant anticoagulation. There is little experience with fibrinolytic therapy during pregnancy and, because of potential for bleeding, its use should be restricted to life-threatening situations.

The risks of venous thrombosis are increased during pregnancy, and women with a prior documented episode of venous thrombosis have a significant risk of developing recurrence. Therefore, consideration should be given to providing prophylaxis with low-dose subcutaneous heparin throughout pregnancy in women at high risk. A careful consideration of the risk factors present in an individual patient is important in minimizing the side effects of bleeding, thrombocytopenia, and osteoporosis with long-term heparin therapy. In a patient with a single prior episode of venous thrombosis and no other risk factors, a reasonable approach is to start prophylaxis at the onset of labor and continue until 6 weeks after delivery. In patients at high risk because of multiple prior episodes of thromboembolism or other risk factors, prophylaxis should be considered soon after diagnosis of pregnancy.

Acknowledgment

Supported in part by grant no. HL-30616 from the National Heart, Lung and Blood Institute, National Institutes of Health, Bethesda, Maryland.

BIBLIOGRAPHY

Anderson FA Jr, Wheeler HB, Goldberg RJ, et al. A population-based perspective of the hospital incidence and case-fatality rates of deep vein thrombosis and pulmonary embolism: the Worcester DVT study. Arch Intern Med 1991;151:933.

Collins R, Scrimgeour A, Yusuf S, Peto R. Reduction in fatal pulmonary embolism and venous thrombosis by perioperative administration of subcutaneous heparin: overview of results of randomized trials in general, orthopedic and urologic surgery. N Engl J Med 1988;318:1162.

Ginsberg JS, Hirsh J. Anticoagulants during pregnancy. Ann Revu Med 1989;40:79.

Ginsberg JS, Hirsh J, Rainbow AJ, Coates G. Risks to the fetus of radiologic procedures used in the diagnosis of maternal venous thromboembolic disease. Thromb Haemost 1989;61:189.

Goldhaber SZ, Morpurgo M for the WHO/SFC Task Force on Pulmonary Embolism. Diagnosis, treatment, and prevention of pulmonary embolism: report of the WHO/International Society of Federation of Cardiology Task Force. JAMA 1992;268:1727.

Hirsh J. Heparin. N Engl J Med 1991;324:1565.

Hirsh J. Oral anticoagulant drugs. N Engl J Med 1991;324:1865.

Lensing AWA, Prandoni P, Brandjes D, et al. Detection of deep-vein thrombosis by real-time B-mode ultrasonography. N Engl J Med 1989;320:342.

The PIOPED Investigators. Value of the ventilation/perfusion scan in acute pulmonary embolism: results of the prospective investigation of pulmonary embolism diagnosis (PIOPED). JAMA 1990;263:2753.

Primary Care for Women, edited by Phyllis C. Leppert and Fred M. Howard. Lippincott-Raven Publishers, Philadelphia © 1997.

51

Secondary Prevention of Coronary Artery Disease

ROBERT A. WILD

Coronary atherosclerotic heart disease is the leading cause of cardiovascular disability and death in the United States. Although men are more often affected than women before age 40, beyond age 70 the ratio is 1:1. In men, the peak incidence of clinical manifestations is at age 50 to 60; in women, it occurs at age 60 to 70.

The classic risk factors for the development of ischemic heart disease include a positive family history (particularly coronary disease occurring before age 50), age, genetic predisposition, blood lipid abnormalities, arterial hypertension, cigarette smoking, diabetes mellitus, and male gender. Other factors of less certain importance include obesity, physical inactivity, and personality type. Patients with clinical manifestations of coronary disease before age 50 tend to have predisposing risk factors, but this is often not the case in older persons. In patients with known disease, management and control of risk factors is termed *secondary prevention*. An algorithm for secondary prevention of coronary heart disease is shown in Figure 51-1.

PATHOPHYSIOLOGY

Knowledge concerning the pathophysiology of atherosclerosis and the clinical presentations of coronary artery disease is accumulating rapidly. Abnormal lipid metabolism or excessive intake of cholesterol and saturated fats, especially when superimposed on a genetic predisposition, initiates the atherosclerotic process. The initial step is the fatty streak, or subendothelial accumulation of lipids and lipid-laden monocytes (macrophages). Low-density lipoproteins (LDLs) are the major atherogenic lipid. High-density lipoproteins (HDLs), in contrast, are protective and probably assist in the mobilization of LDLs. The pathogenetic role of other lipids, including triglycerides, is less clear. LDLs undergo in situ oxidation, which makes them more difficult to mobilize as well as locally cytotoxic. Subsequent steps include altered endothelial function (inhibition of endothelium-derived relaxing factor production), disruption of the endothelium, adherence of platelets and release of platelet-derived growth factor and other growth factors, cell proliferation, and formation of the mature fibrous plaque. These processes are usually slowly progressive over decades. However, the behavior of atherosclerotic plaques may be unpredictable.

The natural history of the mature plaque is less predictable. Plaque ulceration, fracture, or hemorrhage can initiate a cascade of further injury, platelet adherence, and thrombus formation that can either heal, often with more severe luminal obstruction, or cause the various ischemic syndromes described below. "Soft" lipid-laden but nonocclusive plaques are particularly susceptible to rupture, initiating a series of events leading to thrombotic occlusion. These are often the culprit lesions in young persons with acute myocardial infarction or sudden death as their first manifestation of coronary disease, and this abrupt progression explains why most infarctions do not occur at the site of a preexisting critical stenosis. Conversely, the relatively greater reduction in clinical events than lesion severity in lipid-lowering treatment trials is probably explained by the regression or prevention of these early nonfibrotic lesions.

PREVENTION OF ISCHEMIC HEART DISEASE

Reducing certain risk factors, such as smoking and hyperlipidemia, can both prevent coronary disease and delay its progression and complications after it has become manifest. Treatment of lipid abnormalities has been shown to delay the progression of atherosclerosis and in some cases to provide regression.

Another preventive measure is aspirin prophylaxis. Aspirin (80 mg daily) in males over age 50 reduces the incidence of myocardial infarction. Whether this approach should be used for women in the general population or only in those at higher risk is unclear, and the optimal dosage is unknown. A prudent approach would be to administer 80 mg daily or 325 mg every other day in women with known disease (secondary prevention). The value of other platelet-inhibiting agents and dietary supplements, such as fish oil or omega-3 fats, is uncertain. Because LDL oxidation may be a necessary step in trapping these particles in the vessel wall, antioxidant therapy has been advocated as a preventive measure. Suggestive data are available for vitamin E, but more information is required before this approach can be recommended to the general public.

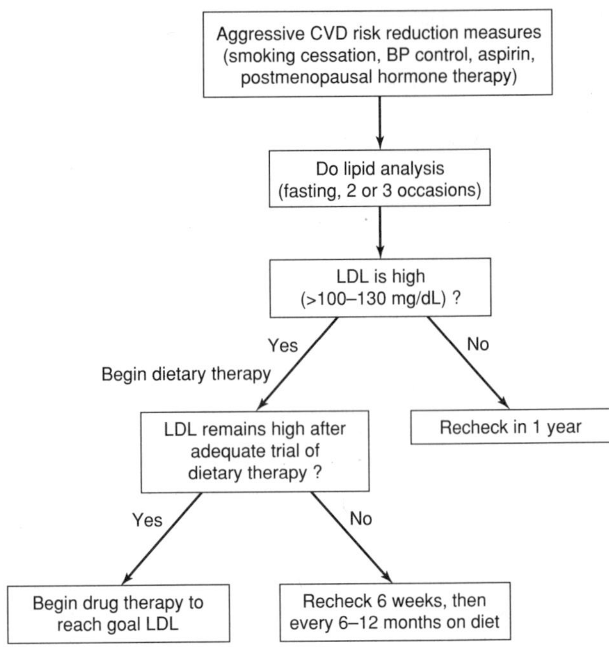

Figure 51-1. Suggested algorithm for screening and management of patients with known cardiovascular disease.

Control of blood pressure has been shown to prevent infarctions. The beneficial role of exercise is understood. The decrease in the number of coronary deaths over the last two decades may be due to a decrease in the prevalence of risk factors but probably also reflects improvements in medical therapy; quick response to the hospital; the role of coronary care units; better treatment of angina, arrhythmias, and heart failure; and improved survival after coronary revascularization in some patients.

PATHOPHYSIOLOGY OF SYMPTOMATIC AND SILENT ISCHEMIA AND CORONARY SYNDROMES

Advanced coronary atherosclerosis and even complete occlusion may remain clinically silent. There is only a modest correlation between the clinical symptoms and the anatomic extent of disease. The only means of determining the location and extent of narrowing is coronary arteriography, although ischemia can be recognized by other less invasive studies. Myocardial ischemia may be provoked by either increased myocardial oxygen requirements (exercise, mental stress, or spontaneous fluctuations in heart rate and blood pressure) or decreased oxygen supply (caused by coronary vasospasm, platelet plugging, or partial thrombosis). Abnormal endothelial function appears to play a role in the fluctuating threshold for ischemia; impaired release of endothelium-derived relaxing factor may permit unopposed vasoconstriction and facilitate platelet adhesion.

Most studies indicate that in angina pectoris, increased oxygen demand is the most frequent mechanism. In contrast, the acute coronary syndromes of unstable angina and myocardial infarction are caused by plaque disruption, platelet plugging, and coronary thrombosis. Of interest is the predilection for these episodes to occur in the early morning or shortly after arising. Whether the vessel becomes occluded or whether thrombolysis occurs and the plaque is stabilized determines the outcome. Thus, therapy is primarily directed toward inhibition of platelet activity (aspirin) and thrombolysis in acute syndromes and toward minimizing myocardial oxygen requirements—as well as preventive measures—in chronic angina.

Some episodes of myocardial ischemia are painful, causing angina pectoris; others are completely silent. Many silent episodes are brought on by emotional and mental stress. In patients with diagnosed coronary disease, as evidenced by prior myocardial infarction or angina, silent ischemic episodes have the same prognostic import as painful ones. The prognosis for patients with only silent ischemia is not well established, nor is the potential benefit of preventing silent ischemia.

ANGINA PECTORIS

Angina pectoris is usually due to atherosclerotic heart disease (see Chap. 43).

Circumstances That Precipitate and Relieve Angina

Angina occurs most commonly during activity and is relieved by resting. Exertion that involves straining the thoracic or upper extremity muscles (eg, lifting) or walking rapidly uphill precipitates attacks most consistently. Patients prefer to remain upright rather than lie down. The amount of activity required to produce angina may be relatively consistent under comparable physical and emotional circumstances or may vary from day to day. It usually occurs after meals, during excitement, or on exposure to cold. The threshold for angina is often lower in the morning or after strong emotion; the latter can provoke attacks in the absence of exertion. In addition, discomfort may occur during sexual activity, at rest, or at night as a result of coronary spasm.

Effect of Nitroglycerin

The diagnosis of angina pectoris is strongly supported if sublingual nitroglycerin invariably shortens an attack and if prophylactic nitrates permit greater exertion or prevent angina entirely. Most patients do not have a risk profile markedly different from that of the general population.

Coronary Vasospasm and Angina With Normal Coronary Arteriograms

Although most symptoms of myocardial ischemia result from fixed stenosis of the coronary arteries or thrombosis or hemorrhage at the site of lesions, some ischemic events may be precipitated by coronary vasoconstriction.

Spasm of the large coronary arteries with resulting decreased coronary blood flow may occur spontaneously or may be induced by exposure to cold, emotional stress, or vasoconstricting medications (eg, ergot derivative drugs). Spasm may occur both in normal and stenosed coronary arteries and may be silent or result in angina pectoris. Even myocardial infarction may occur as a result of spasm in the absence of visible obstructive coronary heart disease, although most instances of coronary spasm occur in the presence of coronary stenosis.

It is important to evaluate risk factors associated with the development of atherosclerosis, particularly serum lipids. Contributing factors such as diabetes, anemia, renal disease, thyrotoxicosis, or myxedema should be sought if suggested by the history and physical examination.

Electrocardiogram Interpretation

The resting electrocardiogram (ECG) is normal in about a quarter of patients with angina. Exercise testing is the most useful noninvasive procedure for evaluating the patient with angina.

The usual ECG criterion for a positive test is 1 mm (0.1 mV) horizontal or downsloping ST-segment depression (beyond baseline) measured 80 ms after the J point. By this criterion, 60% to 80% of patients with anatomically significant coronary disease have a positive test, but 10% to 20% of those without significant disease are also positive. False-positive results are uncommon when a 2-mm depression is present. Additional information is inferred from the time of onset and duration of the ECG changes, their magnitude and configuration, blood-pressure and heart-rate changes, the duration of exercise, and the presence of associated symptoms. In general, patients exhibiting more severe ST-segment depression (2 mm) at low workloads (6 minutes on the Bruce protocol) or heart rates (70% of age-predicted maximum), especially when the duration of exercise and rise in blood pressure are limited or when hypotension occurs during the test, have more severe disease and a poorer prognosis. Depending on symptom status, age, and other factors, such patients should be referred for coronary arteriography and possible revascularization. On the other hand, less impressive positive tests in asymptomatic patients are often false-positive results. Therefore, exercise testing results that do not conform to the clinical picture should be confirmed by stress scintigraphy or echocardiography.

Scintigraphic Assessment of Ischemia

Two nuclear medicine studies provide additional information about the presence, location, and extent of coronary disease. Myocardial perfusion scintigraphy provides images in which radionuclide uptake is proportional to blood flow at the time of injection. Radionuclide angiography images the left ventricle and measures its ejection fraction and wall motion.

Echocardiography

Echocardiography can image the left ventricle and reveal segmental wall motion abnormalities, which may indicate ischemia or prior infarction. It is a convenient technique for assessing left ventricular function, which is an important indicator of prognosis and determinant of therapy. An increasing number of laboratories are performing echocardiograms during supine exercise or immediately after upright exercise; exercise-induced segmental wall motion abnormalities are used as an additional indicator of ischemia. This technique requires considerable expertise, but in experienced laboratories, the increment in test accuracy is comparable to that obtained with scintigraphy, although a higher proportion of tests are technically inadequate. Pharmacologic stress with high-dose (2 to 4 mg/kg/min; start at 10 μg/kg/min) dobutamine can be used as an alternative to exercise.

Ambulatory ECG Monitoring

With current ambulatory ECG recorders and trained technicians, episodes of ischemic ST-segment depression can be monitored.

Coronary Angiography

Selective coronary arteriography is the definitive diagnostic procedure for coronary artery disease. It can be performed with low mortality (about 0.1%) and morbidity (1% to 5%), but the cost is high, and with currently available noninvasive techniques it is usually not indicated solely for diagnosis.

Coronary arteriography should be performed in:

- Patients being considered for coronary artery revascularization because of limiting stable angina who have failed to improve on an adequate medical regimen
- Patients in whom coronary revascularization is being considered because the clinical presentation (eg, unstable angina, postinfarction angina) or noninvasive testing suggests high-risk disease
- Patients with aortic valve disease who also have angina pectoris, to determine whether the angina is due to accompanying coronary disease. Coronary angiography is also performed in asymptomatic older patients undergoing valve surgery so that concomitant bypass may be done if the anatomy is propitious.
- Patients who have had coronary revascularization with subsequent recurrence of symptoms, to determine whether bypass grafts or native vessels are occluded
- Patients with cardiac failure in whom a surgically correctable lesion, such as left ventricular aneurysm, mitral regurgitation, or reversible ischemic dysfunction, is suspected
- Patients surviving sudden death or with symptomatic or life-threatening arrhythmias in whom coronary artery disease may be a correctable cause
- Patients with chest pain of uncertain cause or cardiomyopathy of unknown cause.

Coronary arteriography visualizes the location and severity of stenoses. Narrowing greater than 50% of the luminal diameter is considered clinically significant, although most lesions producing ischemia are associated with narrowing in excess of 70%. This information has important prognostic value, as mortality rates are progressively higher in patients with one-, two-, and three-vessel disease and those with left main coronary artery obstruction (ranging from 1% per year to 25% per year). Among stable patients, 20%, 30%, and 50% have one-, two-, and three-vessel involvement, respectively; left main disease is present in 10%. In those with strongly positive exercise ECGs or scintigraphic studies, three-vessel or left main disease may be present in 75% to 95%, depending on the criteria used. Coronary arteriography also shows whether the obstructions are amenable to bypass surgery or percutaneous transluminal coronary angioplasty (PTCA).

Left Ventricular Angiography

Left ventricular angiography is usually performed at the same time as coronary arteriography. Global and regional left ventricular functions are visualized, as well as mitral regurgitation if present. Left ventricular function is the major determinant of prognosis in stable coronary disease and of the risk of bypass surgery.

Prevention of Further Attacks

Aggravating Factors

Angina may be aggravated by hypertension, left ventricular failure, arrhythmia (usually tachycardias), strenuous activity, cold temperatures, and emotional states. These factors should be identified and treated or avoided where possible.

Nitroglycerin

Nitroglycerin, 0.15 to 0.6 mg sublingually, or nitroglycerin aerosol, 0.4 to 0.8 mg, should be taken 5 minutes before any activity likely to precipitate angina. Sublingual isosorbide dinitrate (2.5 to 5 mg) acts only slightly longer than sublingual nitroglycerin.

Long-Acting Nitrates

Longer-acting nitrate preparations include isosorbide dinitrate (10 to 40 mg every 6 hours or controlled-release 40 to 80 mg every 8 to 12 hours), isosorbide mononitrate (10 to 20 mg orally twice daily or 60 to 120 mg once daily in a sustained-release preparation), oral sustained-release nitroglycerin preparations (6.25 to 12.5 mg two to four times daily), nitroglycerin ointment (7.5 to 30 mg applied two times daily), and transdermal nitroglycerin patches that deliver nitroglycerin at a predetermined rate (usually 0.4 to 0.8 mg/24 hr). The main limitation to chronic nitrate therapy is tolerance, which occurs to some degree in most patients. The degree of tolerance can be limited by using a regimen that includes at least an 8- to 10-hour period without nitrates. Isosorbide dinitrate given three times daily, with the last dose after dinner, is the most commonly used approach in the United States. Isosorbide mononitrate is popular in Europe; because it is the active metabolite of the dinitrate, it has more consistent bioavailability. Transdermal preparations should be removed overnight in most patients. Nitrate therapy is often limited by headache. Other side effects include nausea, dizziness, and hypotension.

β-Blockers

The β-blockers prevent angina by reducing myocardial oxygen requirements during exertion and stress. This is accomplished by reducing the heart rate, myocardial contractility, and, to a lesser extent, blood pressure. The β-blockers are the only antianginal agents that have been demonstrated to prolong life in patients with coronary disease (postmyocardial infarction). They are at least as effective as alternative agents in studies using exercise testing, ambulatory monitoring, and symptom assessment. As a result, they should be considered for first-line therapy in most patients with chronic angina.

In the United States, only propranolol, metoprolol, nadolol, and atenolol are approved for angina. Nonetheless, all available β-blockers appear to be effective for angina, although those with intrinsic sympathomimetic activity, such as pindolol, are less desirable because they may exacerbate angina in some patients and have not been effective in secondary prevention trials. The dosages of all these drugs when given for angina are similar. The major contraindications are bronchospastic disease, bradyarrhythmias, and overt heart failure.

Calcium Entry-Blocking Agents

Verapamil, diltiazem, nifedipine, nicardipine, and amlodipine are chemically and pharmacologically heterogeneous agents that prevent angina by reducing myocardial oxygen requirements and by inducing coronary artery vasodilation. Isradipine and felodipine are not approved in the United States for angina but probably are about as effective as nifedipine and other dihydropyridine agents. Myocardial oxygen demand is lessened by reducing blood pressure, left ventricular wall stress, and, in the case of verapamil and diltiazem, resting or exercise heart rate. Although these agents are all potent coronary vasodilators, it is unclear whether they improve myocardial blood flow in most patients with stable exertional angina. In those with coronary vasospasm, the calcium entry blockers may be the agent of choice.

Most calcium channel blockers have negative inotropic, chronotropic, and dromotropic properties in vitro, but the reflex sympathetic response may obscure these effects in vivo (except in the presence of β-blockade or severely depressed left ventricular function). Several newer calcium channel blockers of the dihydropyridine class, including felodipine and amlodipine, have less negative inotropic action, but their safety in patients with heart failure remains to be demonstrated. Unlike the β-blockers, calcium channel blockers have not reduced mortality postinfarction and in some cases have increased ischemia and mortality rates. This appears to be the case with some dihydropyridines and with diltiazem and verapamil in patients with clinical heart failure or moderate to severe left ventricular dysfunction. Thus, calcium blockers should not be the initial antianginal medication in most patients. Although all have been shown to be efficacious for angina, not all preparations and agents are approved for this indication. Diltiazem and verapamil are preferable as first-line agents because they produce less reflex tachycardia and because the former, at least, may cause fewer side effects. Nifedipine, nicardipine, and amlodipine are also approved agents for angina.

Bepridil is a unique calcium channel blocker similar to verapamil in its effects on automatic tissues but with additional properties similar to those of quinidine (prolonging ventricular refractoriness and the QT interval). It is not approved for hypertension and should be used only for refractory angina because of its potential to induce ventricular arrhythmias.

Combination Therapy

Patients remaining symptomatic when given one class of preventive agent should be treated with combinations. A combination of a β-blocker and a long-acting nitrate or a β-blocker and a calcium channel blocker (other than verapamil, where the risk of atrioventricular block or heart failure is higher) is the most appropriate combination. A few patients have a further response to a regimen including all three agents.

Platelet-Inhibiting Agents

Coronary thrombosis is responsible for most episodes of myocardial infarction and many unstable ischemic syndromes. Several studies have demonstrated the benefit of antiplatelet drugs after unstable angina and infarction. Therefore, unless contraindicated, small doses of aspirin (162 to 325 mg daily or 325 mg every other day) should be prescribed for patients with angina. For patients with ASA sensitivity, use ticlopadine 250 mg by mouth twice a day.

Prognosis

The prognosis of angina pectoris has improved with advances in the understanding of its pathophysiology and in pharmacologic therapy. Mortality rates range from 1% to 25% per year depending on the number of vessels diseased, the severity of obstruction, the status of left ventricular function, and the presence of complex arrhythmias. In patients with stable symptoms and normal ejection fractions (55%, depending on the laboratory), the mortality rate is less than 4% per year. However, the outlook in individual patients is unpredictable, and nearly half of the deaths are sudden. Therefore, risk stratification is often attempted. Patients with accelerating symptoms have a poorer outlook. Among stable patients, those whose exercise tolerance is severely limited by ischemia (< 6 minutes on the Bruce treadmill protocol) and those with extensive ischemia by exercise ECG or scintigraphy have more severe anatomic disease and a poorer prognosis.

Over 90% of patients can be rendered pain-free with revascularization measures. Patients who do not become ischemia-free on medical therapy should have early coronary arteriography and revascularization. Controlled trials have not shown any advantage in increased survival or lower infarction rates with coronary artery bypass grafting (CABG) compared to medical therapy, although many patients treated medically need revascularization later for recurrent symptoms. Depending on the stringency of the definition of unstable angina, 10% to 30% of patients have an early infarction, and the 1-year mortality rate is 10% to 20%. Even in the absence of chest pain, many patients have silent episodes of ST-segment depression or, less commonly, elevation on ambulatory monitoring. These patients have a poorer prognosis.

Because recurrent episodes, infarction, and sudden death may occur after relief of unstable angina, additional evaluations should be performed in patients who have been stabilized, consisting of early exercise or pharmacologic stress testing to identify high-risk subsets for further invasive evaluation, or coronary arteriography. The choice should be individualized based on the patient's age and general health, as well as the severity of symptoms and signs of ischemia. The artery responsible for the ischemia can usually be determined from ECG or scintigraphic changes during pain, and the lesion is often amenable to PTCA. If revascularization is not performed, long-term management is the same as for stable angina pectoris.

Indications for Revascularization

The indications for coronary artery revascularization in patients with stable angina pectoris are often debated. There is general agreement that otherwise healthy patients in the following groups should undergo revascularization:

- Those with unacceptable symptoms despite medical therapy to its tolerable limits
- Those with left main coronary artery stenosis greater than 50% with or without symptoms
- Those with three-vessel disease with left ventricular dysfunction (ejection fraction 50% or previous transmural infarction)
- Those with unstable angina who after symptom control by medical therapy continue to exhibit ischemia on exercise testing or monitoring
- Postmyocardial infarction patients with continuing angina or ischemia on noninvasive testing, particularly if they have received thrombolytic treatment.

In addition, many cardiologists argue that patients with less severe symptoms should be revascularized if they have anatomically critical lesions (90% proximal stenoses, especially of the proximal left anterior descending artery) or physiologic evidence of severe ischemia (early positive exercise tests, large exercise-induced thallium scintigraphic defects, or frequent episodes of ischemia on ambulatory monitoring). This trend toward aggressive intervention has accelerated as a result of the growing availability of coronary angioplasty. Although such patients are at increased risk, it has not been proven that their prognosis is better after coronary revascularization by either surgery or angioplasty. In most, a trial of medical therapy is warranted to determine whether symptoms and other evidence of ischemia improve.

TREATMENT

Type of Procedure

Coronary Artery Bypass Grafting

CABG can be accomplished with a very low mortality rate (1% to 3%) in otherwise healthy patients with preserved cardiac function. However, the mortality rate of this procedure has increased to 4% to 8% or higher in recent years because the proportion of high-risk and older patients is growing. Increasingly, younger patients with focal lesions of one or several vessels are undergoing coronary angioplasty as the initial revascularization procedure.

Grafts using one or both internal mammary arteries (usually to the left anterior descending artery or its branches) provide the best long-term results in terms of patency and flow. Segments of the saphenous vein (or, less optimally, other veins) interposed between the aorta and the coronary arteries distal to the obstructions are also used. One to five distal anastomoses are commonly performed. After successful surgery, symptoms generally abate. The need for antianginal medications diminishes, and left ventricular function may improve.

The operative mortality rate is increased in patients with poor left ventricular function (left ventricular ejection fraction <35%) or those requiring additional procedures (valve replacement or ventricular aneurysmectomy). Patients over age 70, patients undergoing repeat procedures, or those with important noncardiac disease (especially renal insufficiency, diabetes, or poor general health) also have higher operative mortality and morbidity rates, and full recovery is slow. Thus, CABG should be reserved for more severely symptomatic patients in this group. Early (1 to 6 months) graft patency rates average 85% to 90% (higher for internal mammary grafts), and subsequent graft closure rates are about 4% annually. Early graft failure is common in vessels with poor distal flow; late closure is more common in patients who continue smoking and those with treated hyperlipidemia. Antiplatelet therapy with aspirin improves graft patency rates. Long-term dipyridamole therapy is expensive, inconvenient, and of limited value. Vigorous treatment of blood lipid abnormalities is necessary, with a goal for LDL cholesterol of <100 mg/dL and for HDL cholesterol >45 mg/dL.

Repeat CABG or angioplasty is often necessitated by progressive native vessel disease and graft occlusions. Reoperation is technically demanding and less often fully successful than the initial operation.

Percutaneous Transluminal Coronary Angioplasty

Coronary artery stenoses can be effectively dilated by inflation of a balloon under high pressure. This procedure is performed in the cardiac catheterization laboratory under local anesthesia either at the same time as diagnostic coronary arteriography or at a later time. The mechanism of dilation is rupture of the atheromatous plaque, with subsequent resorption of intraluminal debris.

This procedure was at one time reserved for proximal single-vessel disease, but now it is widely used in multivessel disease with multiple lesions, although only rarely in left main disease. PTCA is also effective in CABG stenoses. Optimal lesions for PTCA are relatively proximal, noneccentric, free of plaque dissection, and removed from the origin of large branches. With improved catheter systems, experienced operators can manipulate the balloon catheter across about 90% of approachable lesions and successfully dilate 90% of those. The major early complication is intimal dissection with vessel occlusion. This can sometimes be treated by repeat PTCA, but urgent CABG is required in 3% to 5% of the cases, and morbidity and mortality rates are high. Therefore, these procedures must be done in a laboratory where surgery is available on short notice.

In the United States, the number of PTCA procedures now exceeds that of CABG operations, but the justification for many of these is weak. One controlled study showed PTCA to be superior to medical therapy for symptom relief but not for preventing infarction or death. Controlled studies of PTCA versus either medical treatment or CABG in multivessel disease are not yet available.

The major limitation with PTCA has been restenosis, which occurs in the first 6 months in 30% to 50% of vessels dilated. The mechanism of restenosis is unclear, and it can often be treated successfully by repeat PTCA.

Investigational Revascularization Procedures

There is considerable interest in the use of catheter devices to remove atheromatous material (atherectomy), stents, and laser catheters. These approaches are available on an investigational basis. Current data do not indicate a significant improvement in either initial success or restenosis rates with these experimental techniques, but the technologies are evolving. Intracoronary stents have been used to maintain vessel patency in patients with acute closure during PTCA or with restenosis. Recent studies have suggested that the rate of restenosis can be reduced with primary stenting, but with the added risk of rigorous anticoagulation and the attendant need for longer hospitalization.

Results

The mortality and infarction rates with PTCA and CABG are generally comparable in stable angina. Recovery after PTCA is obviously faster, but the intermediate-term success rate of CABG is higher, because of the high restenosis rate with PTCA. The increasing popularity of PTCA primarily reflects its lower cost, shorter hospitalization, the perception that CABG is best done only once and can be reserved for later, and the preference of patients for less invasive treatment. These arguments make PTCA the procedure of choice for revascularization of single-vessel disease, although this is not usually indicated except when symptoms are refractory. The situation is less clear with multivessel disease. Several randomized studies comparing PTCA and CABG in patients with two- or three-vessel disease have been reported. In general, mortality and nonfatal infarction rates have not differed between treatments. However, the PTCA patients have required substantially more subsequent revascularizations. The early cost savings with PTCA usually disappear over 1 to 3 years because of this higher reintervention rate. Also, the excellent outcome of patients treated medically has made it difficult to show an advantage with either revascularization approach except in patients who remain symptom-limited or have left main lesions or three-vessel disease and left ventricular dysfunction.

UNSTABLE ANGINA

Most clinicians use the term *unstable angina* to denote an accelerating or crescendo pattern of pain in cases where previously stable angina occurs with less exertion or at rest, lasts longer, and is less responsive to medication (see Chap. 43).

Treatment

Treatment of unstable angina should be multifaceted and vigorous. Patients should be hospitalized, maintained at bed rest or at very limited activity, monitored, and given supplemental oxygen. Sedation with a benzodiazepine is usually indicated. The systolic blood pressure is usually maintained at 100 to 120 mm Hg, except in previously severe hypertensives. Patients with heart rates above 70 to 80 beats per minute should be given β-blockers unless heart failure or other medical contraindications are present.

Antithrombotic therapy is an important part of treatment for unstable angina. Heparin may be more effective than aspirin, but the two are probably additive.

Nitroglycerin

The nitrates are first-line antiischemic therapy for unstable angina. Nonparenteral therapy with sublingual or oral agents or nitroglycerin ointment is usually sufficient.

β-Blockers

β-Blockers are effective in unstable angina, particularly when tachycardia is present or precipitated by other medications. If the patient has no history or physical findings of heart failure, these agents can usually be started without measurements of left ventricular function.

Calcium Entry Blockers

Although the data on efficacy of calcium channel blockers are less extensive and less favorable than with β-blockers, these agents are commonly used because alterations in coronary vasomotor tone may play a role in unstable ischemic syndromes. In the presence of nitrates and without accompanying β-blockers, diltiazem or verapamil is preferred, as nifedipine and the other dihydropyridines are more likely to cause reflex tachycardia or hypotension. The initial dosage should be low, but upward titration should proceed rapidly.

Intraaortic Balloon Counterpulsation

Intraaortic balloon counterpulsation can both reduce myocardial energy requirements (systolic unloading) and improve diastolic coronary blood flow. This approach is usually employed to stabilize patients before angiography or revascularization, but the former can generally be accomplished without this intervention. Aortic insufficiency is a contraindication, and this technique must be used cautiously in patients with peripheral vascular disease.

DISTURBANCES OF RATE AND RHYTHM

Abnormalities of cardiac rhythm and conduction can be lethal (sudden cardiac death), symptomatic (syncope, near-syncope, dizziness, or palpitations), or asymptomatic (see Chap. 45). They are dangerous to the extent that they reduce cardiac output, so that perfusion of the brain or myocardium is impaired, or tend to deteriorate into more serious arrhythmias with the same consequences.

Prophylactic Therapy

Postinfarction management should begin with identification and modification of risk factors. Treatment of hyperlipidemia and smoking cessation both prevent recurrent infarctions. Recent guidelines suggest a target LDL cholesterol level below 100 mg/dL for patients with manifest coronary artery disease. Blood-pressure control, weight loss, and exercise are recommended.

Many drugs have been studied, and some have been shown to be beneficial in preventing death or reinfarction. However, their usefulness in the era of thrombolysis and revascularization is unclear. β-Blockers improve survival rates, primarily by reducing the incidence of sudden death in high-risk patients. β-Blockers should be given to such patients, except those with overt heart failure, but are of limited value in uncomplicated patients with small infarctions and normal exercise tests. No advantage of one preparation over another has been demonstrated, except that those with intrinsic sympathomimetic activity have not proved beneficial in postinfarction patients.

Calcium channel blockers have not been shown to improve prognosis overall, but both diltiazem and verapamil appear to reduce mortality rates in patients with preserved left ventricular function. Diltiazem may help to prevent reinfarction after non-Q-wave infarction.

Antiplatelet agents are beneficial; low-dose aspirin is recommended. Warfarin anticoagulation for 3 months reduces the incidence of arterial emboli after large anterior infarctions, and according to the results of at least one study it improves long-term prognosis, but an additive benefit to aspirin after 6 months has not been confirmed.

Antiarrhythmic therapy other than with β-blockers has not been shown to be effective, except in patients with symptomatic arrhythmias; in fact, class IC agents increase the mortality rate in postinfarction patients. However, several small studies and a metanalysis have indicated that low-dose amiodarone may be beneficial.

Cardiac rehabilitation programs and exercise training can be of considerable psychological benefit, but it is unknown whether they alter prognosis.

ACE Inhibitors in Patients With Left Ventricular Dysfunction

Patients who sustain substantial myocardial damage often experience subsequent progressive left ventricular dilation and dysfunction, leading to clinical heart failure and reduced long-term survival. A recent trial demonstrated that in patients with ejection fractions less than 40%, captopril (25 to 50 mg three times daily commencing 3 to 16 days postinfarction) prevents left ventricular dilation and the onset of heart failure and also reduces the mortality rate. Similar data have been collected with ramipril. Although two large trials found a benefit from treating unselected patients beginning on admission, it is unclear how much of this occurs in patients without left ventricular dysfunction and whether there is any advantage to starting treatment while the patient may be hemodynamically unstable.

Revascularization

Because of the increasing use of thrombolytic therapy and accumulating experience with PTCA, the indications for revascularization are rapidly evolving. Postinfarction patients who appear likely to benefit from early revascularization if the anatomy is appropriate are:

- Those who have undergone thrombolytic therapy and have residual symptoms or laboratory evidence of ischemia
- Those with left ventricular dysfunction (ejection fraction 30% to 40%) and evidence of ischemia
- Those with non-Q-wave infarction and evidence of more than mild ischemia
- Those with markedly positive exercise tests and multivessel disease.

The value of revascularization in the following groups is less clear:

- Those treated with thrombolytic agents, with little evidence of reperfusion or residual ischemia
- Those with left ventricular dysfunction but no detectable ischemia
- Those with preserved left ventricular function who have mild ischemia and are not symptom-limited.

Patients who survive infarctions without complications, have preserved left ventricular function (ejection fraction 50%), and have no exercise-induced ischemia have an excellent prognosis and do not require invasive evaluation.

MEDICAL TREATMENT

Lipid Disorders

Serum lipoproteins are important mainly because of their relation to atherosclerotic vascular disease, especially coronary heart disease. Several clinical trials showing that lowering high blood cholesterol reduces the incidence of coronary heart disease have given impetus to nationwide campaigns to reduce serum cholesterol levels. It is important to target LDL concentrations to <100 mg/dL for secondary prevention. There is convincing evidence that this is effective in women. Current therapies have been associated with reduction in total mortality as well (see Chap. 49).

Lipoproteins and Atherogenesis

The plaques found in the arterial walls of patients with atherosclerosis contain large amounts of cholesterol, providing an early clue that serum cholesterol might be an important factor in their development. Epidemiologic studies have established that the higher the level of LDL cholesterol, the greater the risk of atherosclerotic heart disease; conversely, the higher the level of HDL cholesterol, the lower the risk of coronary heart disease. This is true in men and women, in different racial and ethnic groups, and at all adult ages. Because most cholesterol in serum is LDL cholesterol, high total cholesterol levels are also associated with an increased risk of coronary heart disease. As a general approximation in men, each 10-mg/dL increase in cholesterol (or LDL cholesterol) increases the risk of coronary heart disease by about 10%; each 5-mg/dL increase in HDL reduces the risk by about 10%. The effect of HDL cholesterol is greater in women, but the effects of total and LDL cholesterol are smaller. All of these relations diminish with age.

Therapeutic Effects of Lowering Cholesterol

Beneficial effects on the risk of coronary heart disease have been seen with the bile acid-binding resins, with gemfibrozil, and from dietary reduction of cholesterol.

In patients who already have coronary heart disease, the net benefits of cholesterol lowering are clearer, with reductions in the progression of coronary atherosclerosis, fewer subsequent coronary events, less mortality from coronary heart disease, and perhaps a reduction in mortality from all causes. The important exceptions among current therapies are the fibric acid derivatives (clofibrate and gemfibrozil), which have not shown benefits in the secondary prevention of coronary heart disease, and probucol, which has not been studied with clinical end points. Several studies have also shown that cholesterol lowering actually causes regression of atherosclerotic plaques in some women. This effect appears to occur throughout the range of LDL cholesterol levels; the lower the LDL, the greater the regression.

The net benefits from cholesterol lowering depend on the underlying risk of coronary heart disease and of other disease. In patients with manifest atherosclerosis, morbidity and mortality rates associated with coronary heart disease are high.

Low Cholesterol and Other Diseases

Although high cholesterol levels are associated with an increased risk of coronary heart disease, low cholesterol levels (especially <160 mg/dL) are associated with an increased risk of mortality from other causes, including cancer, respiratory disease, injuries and accidents, and liver disease. The biologic explanation for this excess mortality is unknown. Some studies have suggested that low cholesterol represents a preclinical manifestation of the underlying disease (eg, an undiagnosed malignancy). Other analyses have found that the increase in risk persists for at least several years. Thus, the net effect is that the overall relation between cholesterol and mortality is somewhat bow-shaped, with mortality rates highest in those with either low or high cholesterol levels.

Secondary Conditions That Affect Lipid Metabolism

Several factors, including drugs, can influence serum lipid levels (Table 51-1). These are important for two reasons: abnormal lipid levels (or changes in lipid levels) may be the presenting sign of some of these conditions, and correction of the underlying condition may obviate the need to treat an apparent lipid disorder. Diabetes and alcohol use, in particular, are commonly associated with high triglyceride levels that decline with improvements in glycemic control or reduction in alcohol use, respectively. It is unnecessary to rule out each of these secondary causes, but the clinician should consider each possibility.

Table 51-1. Secondary Causes of Lipid Abnormalities

Cause	Associated Lipid Abnormality
Obesity	Increased triglyceride, decreased HDL cholesterol
Sedentary lifestyle	Decreased HDL cholesterol
Diabetes	Increased triglyceride, increased total cholesterol
Alcohol use	Increased triglyceride, increased HDL cholesterol
Hypothyroidism	Increased total cholesterol
Hyperthyroidism	Decreased total cholesterol
Nephrotic syndrome	Increased total cholesterol
Chronic renal insufficiency	Increased total cholesterol, increased triglyceride
Hepatic disease (cirrhosis)	Decreased total cholesterol
Obstructive liver disease	Increased total cholesterol
Malignancy	Decreased total cholesterol
Cushing's disease (for steroid use)	Increased total cholesterol
Oral contraceptives	Increased triglyceride, increased total cholesterol
Diuretics	Increased total cholesterol, increased triglyceride
Beta-blockers*	Increased total cholesterol, decreased HDL

*Beta-blockers with intrinsic sympathomimetic activity, such as pindolol and acebutolol, do not affect lipid levels.

Treatment of High LDL Cholesterol

Reduction of LDL cholesterol is just one part of a program to reduce the risk of cardiovascular disease. Other measures, including smoking cessation and hypertension control, are also of central importance. Less well studied but potentially of great value is raising the HDL cholesterol level. Several healthy habits have more than one benefit. Quitting smoking, for example, reduces the effect of other cardiovascular risk factors (eg, a high cholesterol level); it may also increase the HDL cholesterol level. Exercise (and weight loss) may reduce the LDL cholesterol level and increase the HDL cholesterol level. Modest alcohol use (1 to 2 oz/day) also raises the HDL level and appears to have a salutary effect on coronary heart disease rates. The clinician may not wish to recommend alcohol use to patients, but its safe use in moderation need not be discouraged.

Diet

Dietary modifications play the central role in most algorithms for treatment of elevated lipid levels. The primary recommendation is to reduce the consumption of total dietary fat to less than 30% of total calories, which should be set at the level required to achieve and then maintain ideal body weight. Most Americans currently eat 35% to 40% of calories as fat. In someone eating 2000 kcal/day, 30% of calories as fat would correspond to about 67 g of fat (one pat of butter or margarine contains 15 g). Many clinicians without special expertise and interest in dietary therapy find it advantageous to refer patients to a dietitian. This may be especially helpful if stringent diets (20% calories as fat, with 7% as saturated fat) are prescribed.

In particular, saturated fats (mainly found in animal products, including meats and dairy products) should be reduced to at most 10% of calories. Dietary cholesterol should be reduced to less than 300 mg/day (slightly more than the amount in a single egg yolk). Previous advice to substitute polyunsaturated fats (such as those found in many vegetable oils) or *trans*-monounsaturated fats (as found in margarine) has been changed; instead, foods rich in *cis*-monounsaturated fats, such as olive oil, are now recommended. The average effect of cholesterol-lowering diets varies considerably, suggesting that genetic or other factors influence diet responsiveness. Overall, most studies of free-living patients have shown that low-fat diets result in only modest changes in serum cholesterol levels, with reductions in both the LDL and HDL fractions of a few mg/dL. One recent study comparing a low-fat diet (26% of calories) with a high-fat diet (41% of calories) found a reduction of about 10 mg/dL in LDL cholesterol and a reduction of HDL of about 4 mg/dL in patients eating the low-fat diet.

Soluble fiber, as found in oat bran or psyllium, may reduce LDL cholesterol levels by about 5%. Insoluble fiber (eg, that found in wheat bran) does not affect lipid levels.

Diets should also be rich in antioxidant vitamins, which are found primarily in fruits and vegetables.

Pharmacologic Agents

All patients whose risk from coronary heart disease is considered high enough to warrant pharmacologic therapy of an elevated LDL cholesterol should be given aspirin prophylaxis at a dose of about 325 g every other day, unless there are contraindications such as aspirin sensitivity, bleeding diatheses, or active peptic ulcer disease. Current data suggest that the effect of aspirin in reducing the risk of coronary heart disease is equal to or even greater than that of cholesterol lowering.

Treatment of postmenopausal women with oral estrogen replacement therapy is associated with a reduction in LDL levels and an increase in HDL levels. These lipid effects appear to be responsible for about a third to a quarter of the possible benefit of postmenopausal estrogens on reducing coronary heart disease. The addition of a progestin to the hormone regimen may diminish the beneficial effect on lipids.

If the decision to treat a patient with an LDL-lowering drug is made, the clinician must select an appropriate agent based on the safety, efficacy, cost, and effect on other lipid levels (Table 51-2) and set a goal for treatment (see Chap. 49). Current recommendations do not include drug use to treat low HDL levels in patients who do not also have high LDL levels. As with all therapies for chronic conditions, the therapeutic goal is best approached slowly and steadily, watching carefully for side effects and encouraging continued compliance with nonpharmacologic measures. Combinations of drugs may be necessary. Once the goal is reached, the lipid profile should be monitored every 6 to 12 months, with consideration given to periodic reductions in drug dose or even drug holidays. With the exception of niacin (available generically for a few dollars per month), all of these drugs are expensive and may cost more than $100 per month. Moreover, they may need to be given for decades.

Niacin (Nicotinic Acid)

Niacin has been associated with a reduction in total mortality. Long-term follow-up of a secondary prevention trial of middle-aged men with previous myocardial infarction disclosed that about 52% of those previously treated with niacin had died, compared with 58% in the placebo group. This favorable effect on mortality was not seen during the trial itself, although there was a reduction in the incidence of coronary heart disease in patients with previous myocardial infarction or stable angina.

Niacin reduces the production of very-low-density lipoprotein (VLDL) particles, with secondary reduction in LDL and increase in HDL cholesterol levels. The average effect of niacin is to reduce LDL levels by about 10% to 15% and triglyceride levels by up to half and to increase HDL levels by 10%. It is best to begin at a low dose (at 50 mg/day, using the vitamin preparations of niacin), slowly increasing to the therapeutic range (1000 mg two to three times a day with meals). Niacin causes a prostaglandin-mediated flushing; some patients complain of hot flashes or pruritus. This problem can usually be ameliorated by pretreatment with aspirin (325 mg 30 minutes before each dose) or other nonsteroidal anti-inflammatory agents. Niacin may exacerbate gout and peptic ulcer disease and may provoke hyperglycemia in patients with diabetes. Hepatitis is an important side effect, perhaps especially among patients treated with a sustained-release preparation, which is also more expensive. Whether routine monitoring of liver function tests helps to avoid this side effect is unknown.

Bile Acid-Binding Resins (Cholestyramine, Colestipol)

Treatment with these agents reduces the incidence of coronary events (such as myocardial infarction) in middle-aged men by about 20%, with no significant effect on total mortality (artifact of study power?). The resins work by binding bile acids in the intestine. The resultant reduction in the enterohepatic circulation causes the liver to increase its production of bile acids, using hepatic cholesterol to do so. Thus, hepatic LDL receptor activity increases with a decline in plasma LDL levels. The triglyceride level tends to increase slightly in some patients treated with bile acid-binding resins; they should be used with caution in those with elevated triglycerides and probably not at all in patients who have triglyceride levels above about 500 mg/dL. The clinician can anticipate a reduction of 20% to 30% in LDL cholesterol, with minor changes in the HDL level.

The usual dose of cholestyramine is 8 to 16 g of resin per day in divided doses with meals, mixed in water or, more palatably, juice. The prepackaged 4-g doses are more expensive than the bulk form. Doses of colestipol are 20% higher (the packets each contain 5 g of resin).

These agents often cause gastrointestinal symptoms such as constipation and gas. They may interfere with the absorption of fat-soluble vitamins (thereby complicating the management of patients receiving warfarin) and may bind other drugs in the intestine. Concurrent use of psyllium may ameliorate the gastrointestinal side effects.

HMG-CO Reductase Inhibitors (Lovastatin, Pravastatin, Simvastatin)

The effects of these agents in preventing coronary heart disease have been reassuring: simvastatin has reduced death by 30%. They work by inhibiting the rate-limiting enzyme in the formation of cholesterol. Cholesterol synthesis in the liver is reduced, with a compensatory increase in hepatic LDL receptors (presumably so that the liver can take more of the cholesterol that it needs from the blood) and a reduction in the circulating LDL cholesterol level of

Table 51-2. Effects of Selected Cholesterol-Lowering Drugs

DRUG	EFFECT ON CHD	LONG-TERM SAFETY	EFFECTS ON LDL	EFFECTS ON HDL	EFFECTS ON TRIGLYCERIDE	MONTHLY COST (DOSE)*
Niacin	Reduce	Yes	↓	↑	↓	$5.25 (3 g)
Cholestyramine	Reduce	?	↓	+/–	↑	$67.00 (16 g)†
Colestipol	Reduce	?	↓	+/–	↑	$74.00 (20 g)†
Lovastatin	?	?	↓↓	↑	↓	$60.00 (20 mg)
Simvastatin	?	?	↓↓	↑	↓	$54.00 (10 mg)
Pravastatin	?	?	↓↓	↑	↓	$52.00 (20 mg)
Gemfibrozil	Reduce	Probably not‡	Slight ↓	↑	↓↓	$63.00 (1200 mg)

*Wholesale price of average daily dose, 1993. Costs to patients, or for higher doses, will be higher.

†Cost for individual packets or bars is higher.

‡See text for discussion of fibric acid derivatives and cancer.

up to 35%. There are also modest increases in HDL levels and decreases in triglyceride levels.

Doses of lovastatin are 20 to 80 mg/day; pravastatin and simvastatin doses are 10 to 40 mg/day. These agents are usually given once a day in the evening (most cholesterol synthesis occurs overnight); at the high end of the dose ranges, twice-a-day dosing may be used. Side effects include myositis; the incidence may be higher in patients concurrently taking fibrates or niacin. Manufacturers recommend monitoring liver and muscle enzymes. Several agents (notably erythromycin and cyclosporine) reduce the metabolism of these agents.

Fibric Acid Derivatives (Gemfibrozil, Clofibrate)

In the largest clinical trial that used clofibrate, there were significantly more deaths, especially due to cancer, in the treatment group than in the control. Although still available, clofibrate is rarely used given the availability of its equally effective (but only possibly safer) relative, gemfibrozil. Gemfibrozil reduced coronary heart disease rates in hypercholesterolemic middle-aged men free of coronary disease in the Helsinki Heart Study, perhaps only among those who also had high triglyceride levels. Among men with previous myocardial infarction, however, gemfibrozil increased overall mortality as well as that due to coronary heart disease. Clinicians should also be aware of the trend toward increased numbers of cancer deaths among subjects treated with gemfibrozil in the Helsinki Heart Study.

The fibrates reduce the synthesis and increase the breakdown of VLDL particles, with secondary effects on LDL and HDL levels. They reduce LDL levels by about 10% and triglyceride levels by about 40% and raise HDL levels by about 20%. The usual dose of gemfibrozil is 600 mg twice a day. Side effects include cholelithiasis, hepatitis, and myositis. The incidence of the latter two conditions may be higher among patients also taking other lipid-lowering agents. Given that clofibrate caused a statistically significant increase in cancer mortality, it should not be used.

Probucol

The effects of probucol on coronary heart disease—as well as its long-term safety—are unknown. It reduces the deposition of LDL into xanthomas in humans (and into atherosclerotic plaques in rabbits). The mechanism of action is unclear. It apparently reduces the amount of oxidized LDL (it was originally used as an industrial antioxidant). Probucol reduces LDL levels by 10% to 15% but has the potentially important adverse effect of lowering HDL levels by up to 10%. It also may be cardiotoxic. Probucol, if used at all, should be reserved for patients with a clear genetic disorder who have failed other therapies.

High Blood Triglycerides

Patients with very high levels of serum triglycerides are at risk for pancreatitis. The pathophysiology is uncertain, as some patients with very high triglyceride levels never develop pancreatitis. Most patients with congenital abnormalities in triglyceride metabolism present in childhood; hypertriglyceridemia-induced pancreatitis that first presents in adults is more commonly due to an acquired problem in lipid metabolism.

Although there are no clear triglyceride levels that always result in pancreatitis, most clinicians are uncomfortable with levels above 1000 mg/dL. The risk of pancreatitis may be more related to the triglyceride level after consumption of a fatty meal. Because postprandial increases in triglycerides are inevitable if fat-containing foods are eaten, fasting triglyceride levels in persons prone to pancreatitis should be kept well below that level.

The primary therapy for high triglyceride levels is dietary, avoiding alcohol and fatty foods. Control of secondary causes of high triglyceride levels may also be helpful. In patients with persistent elevations in the pancreatitis range despite adequate dietary compliance—and certainly in those with a previous episode of pancreatitis—therapy with a triglyceride-lowering drug (eg, niacin, in doses as described above) is indicated.

Whether patients with elevated triglycerides (> 250 mg/dL) and no other lipoprotein abnormalities are at increased risk of atherosclerotic disease is unknown. Some of these patients may belong to families with a genetic disorder known as familial combined hyperlipidemia. This disorder is characterized by various lipid abnormalities in different family members: some have high cholesterol levels, some high triglyceride levels, and some both. It appears that the common link is an abnormality in one of the LDL-associated apoproteins (B-100), and that this may be a coronary risk factor. However, the effect on coronary heart disease risk of treating an isolated high triglyceride level in these patients is unknown. Some authorities recommend treating an isolated high triglyceride level in patients with known coronary heart disease, reasoning that such patients are likely to have some abnormality in lipid metabolism. Treatment is primarily nonpharmacologic, with an emphasis on weight loss, a low-fat diet, avoidance of excess alcohol, and exercise.

CONSIDERATIONS IN PREGNANCY

Coronary artery disease is uncommon during pregnancy, but chest pain is not. Usually it is mild and transient and disappears with reassurance. Often its cause is unclear, but thoracic distortion resulting from elevation of the diaphragm and flaring of the ribs is a common explanation. In addition, esophageal reflux occurs more commonly during pregnancy. Similar chest pain, although not otherwise typical, may be associated with prolapse of the mitral valve.

Occurrence

Mortality from coronary artery disease in women in the United States below age 30 is negligible: it is 10 per 100,000 and doubles by age 45. The total incidence of symptomatic coronary disease exceeds 50 per 100,000 at age 40 and increases rapidly thereafter. Predisposing factors are diabetes, hypertension, hypercholesterolemia, or a positive family history.

Cigarette smoking contributes significantly to the incidence of coronary disease in young women. Counseling young women against cigarette smoking is a major responsibility of all health professionals. Sudden death from coronary heart disease is strongly related to cigarette smoking in women.

Oral contraceptives act synergistically with other atherogenic risk factors, particularly cigarette smoking, that predispose to coronary thrombosis. Low-dose combination contraceptive pills apparently do not increase the risk of atherosclerosis.

In recent years, the occurrence of angina pectoris and myocardial infarction in persons with angiographically normal coronary arteries has been recognized. Coronary artery spasm and embolism are two possible mechanisms. The syndrome is more likely to occur in young women than in men.

Effects of Pregnancy

Some of the changes in the circulation that occur during pregnancy may affect the adequacy of oxygen supply to the myocardium. For example, an increased myocardial oxygen consumption would be expected as a result of the changes in heart rate, left ventricular size, and cardiac output. In patients who begin pregnancy with anemia, the hemodilution that usually accompanies pregnancy may require further increases in cardiac work and myocardial oxygen consumption. Additionally, the fall in systemic vascular resistance that accompanies normal pregnancy may divert blood flow from a coronary artery that has been narrowed by atherosclerotic changes. Finally, exercise during pregnancy leads to a greater increase in oxygen consumption than does similar exercise in a nonpregnant patient, and the oxygen requirements of the myocardium for the same workload are probably increased.

On the other hand, vasodilation occurs in some parts of the body during pregnancy, and the total peripheral resistance is lower than in the nonpregnant state. The decline in peripheral resistance reduces the magnitude of the increase in work required of the heart, and the vasodilation of pregnancy may involve the coronary vasculature. The hypothesis is that the balance between myocardial oxygen need and coronary blood flow is unfavorably altered by pregnancy in patients with coronary artery disease.

Some evidence suggests that coronary artery spasm is particularly common in pregnancy, and this cause of myocardial hypoxia deserves attention when the anginal syndrome occurs in a young pregnant woman in the absence of factors that predispose to premature coronary atherosclerosis.

The incidence of symptomatic coronary atherosclerosis in pregnant women appears to be increasing, perhaps because of increased cigarette smoking by women and the advent of oral contraceptives. Additionally, the use of β-adrenergic drugs for the treatment of premature labor is associated with a significant incidence in angina pectoris. The actions of these compounds (terbutaline and ritodrine are the most commonly used), when administered intravenously in the recommended doses, include increases in heart rate and myocardial contractility. Despite an increase in cardiac output, diastolic blood pressure often falls, jeopardizing coronary perfusion. As a result, myocardial hypoxia may occur, especially in women with coronary artery disease.

Chest pain that resembles angina pectoris in location and radiation, when induced by a β-adrenergic agonist, usually disappears promptly when the drug is stopped. These drugs should not be used unless a carefully directed history and physical examination raise no suspicion of heart disease. A pretreatment ECG should be normal, and the occurrence of chest pain during administration of the drug dictates prompt cessation.

The prognosis of a myocardial infarction that occurs during pregnancy depends in part on the time in gestation when it occurs. When myocardial infarction occurred in the first 7 months of pregnancy, death in association with pregnancy was unusual. Eleven of the reported 13 deaths associated with pregnancy occurred among women who suffered a myocardial infarction in the last trimester of pregnancy or during labor. Pregnancy imposes an increased risk to patients with well-documented myocardial ischemia.

If a firm diagnosis of myocardial ischemia is made, pregnancy is contraindicated, because evidence indicates that the risk of maternal death is approximately doubled during pregnancy and the postpartum period.

In planning and implementing medical management, angina pectoris should be seen as a syndrome that is usually precipitated by the superimposition of several burdens. Removal or mitigation of one or more of these burdens may restore the balance between myocardial oxygen supply and demand. In general, obesity, anxiety, and physical activity can be controlled or altered. Smoking and exposure to hot, humid environments are prohibited. In addition, such complicating conditions as hypertension, anemia, hyperthyroidism, and infection must be corrected. Medical management may include sublingual nitroglycerin, calcium channel blockers, or β-adrenergic blocking drugs.

If episodes of angina pectoris continue, and especially if they increase in frequency or severity despite medical management, mechanical intervention should be considered.

If possible, from the fetal standpoint, surgery is best delayed until at least the 12th to 16th week of pregnancy, when organogenesis is nearly complete. Other precautions that are helpful from the fetal standpoint include:

- Performing surgery under normothermic or modestly hypothermic states when possible
- Maintaining extracorporeal circulation at a high flow level
- Instituting fetal monitoring with an obstetric team on standby (if fetal maturity is appropriate)
- Ensuring that the efflux from the coronary sinus does not circulate so as to affect the fetus
- Having a highly experienced cardiac surgeon perform the operation.

Modest rotation of the mother into the left lateral decubitus position should also be done to prevent impedance of flow through caval and aortic compression.

Thrombolytic therapy, the mainstay for treatment of early myocardial infarction in the nonpregnant patient, may potentiate significant bleeding in the mother and fetus. Angioplasty may be more hazardous because of the possible predisposition of the pregnant patient to coronary artery dissection. Even cardiac resuscitation may become more complex, necessitating emptying the uterus, if no response occurs to initial attempts within minutes. Finally, multiple medications used in treatment may affect uterine tone and adversely affect the fetus.

Many recommend that interruption of pregnancy be considered with the hope of prompt symptomatic improvement. Both angioplasty and bypass surgery require coronary angiography and thus pose an added risk for the fetus. When pregnancy has been completed (or interrupted), careful evaluation for long-term management is essential.

When a myocardial infarction occurs during pregnancy, its management should be the same as in nonpregnant patients. If bed rest is necessary, anticoagulation with heparin is probably desirable to minimize the risk of thromboembolism, but anticoagulation should be discontinued as soon as mobilization is possible.

If congestive failure, shock, arrhythmias, or ischemic pain persists after a myocardial infarction despite treatment with β-blockers, long-acting nitrates, and calcium channel blockers, termination of pregnancy before the fourth month is recommended. After the fourth month, the hazards of interruption are probably similar to those of continuing pregnancy. If none of these complications persists, interruption of pregnancy is not justified.

Myocardial infarction in pregnancy is rare. It is frequently overlooked as a diagnostic possibility in the young pregnant patient with chest pain (often ascribed to gastrointestinal causes). The chest pain history should be closely taken. If the pain is not classic for reflux esophagitis, or if it is atypical or crescendo in nature, the potential of a cardiac origin should be entertained. At the very least, an ECG should be obtained and a cardiology consultation considered. In the patient who has had an ischemic event, consultation among the cardiologist, anesthesiologist, and obstetrician should be obtained as early as possible. Labor presents multiple physiologic changes that must be addressed in the patient with left ventricular dysfunction. Pharmacologic manipulations are central to the management of these patients, and the use of the pulmonary artery catheter to adjust several parameters may yield the best outcome. It is hoped that the mortality associated with myocardial infarction can be lowered using these new technologies.

BIBLIOGRAPHY

Amsterdam EA, Hyson D, Kappagoda CT. Nonpharmacologic therapy for coronary artery atherosclerosis: Results of primary and secondary prevention trials. Am Heart J 1994;128:1344.

Despres JP, Lamarche B. Low-intensity endurance exercise training, plasma lipoproteins and the risk of coronary heart disease. J Intern Med 1994;236:7.

Gaziano JM. Antioxidant vitamins and coronary artery disease risk. Am J Med 1994;97(suppl 3A):18S.

Hess DB, Hess LW. Management of cardiovascular disease in pregnancy. Obstet Gynecol Clin North Am 1992;19:679.

Heyden S. Polyunsaturated and monounsaturated fatty acids in the diet to prevent coronary heart disease via cholesterol reduction. Ann Nutrition Metab 1994;38:117.

Hoffman RM, Garewal HS. Antioxidants and the prevention of coronary heart disease. Arch Intern Med 1995;155:241.

Just H, Frey M. Role of calcium antagonists in progression of arteriosclerosis. Evidence from animal experiments and clinical experience. Basic Research in Cardiology 1994;1(suppl 89):177.

LaRosa JC. Dyslipoproteinemia in women and the elderly. Med Clin North Am 1994;78(1):163.

Lavie CJ, Milani RV, Littman AB. Benefits of cardiac rehabilitation and exercise training in secondary coronary prevention in the elderly. J Am Coll Cardiol 1993;22:678.

Metcalfe J, McAnulty JH, Ueland K. Burwell and Metcalfe's heart disease and pregnancy: physiology and management. Boston: Little, Brown, 1986:295.

Nolan TE, Hankins GD. Myocardial infarction in pregnancy. Clin Obstet Gynecol 1989;32(1):71.

Robinson JG, Leon AS. The prevention of cardiovascular disease. Emphasis on secondary prevention. Med Clin North Am 1994;78(1):69.

Rosenson RS, Frauenheim WA, Tangney CC. Dyslipidemia and the secondary prevention of coronary heart disease. Disease-a-Month 1994;40(8):369.

Sacks FM, Rouleau JL, Moye LA, et al. Baseline characteristics in the cholesterol and recurrent events (CARE) trial of secondary prevention in patients with average serum cholesterol levels. Am J Cardiol 1995;75:621.

Seed M. Postmenopausal hormone replacement therapy, coronary heart disease and plasma in lipoproteins. Drugs 1994;47(suppl 2):25.

Truswell SA. Review of dietary intervention studies: effect on coronary events and on total morality. Aust NZ J Med 1994;24:98.

Wood DA. Cholesterol lowering does have a role in secondary prevention. Br Heart J 1995;73(1):4.

Primary Care for Women, edited by Phyllis C. Leppert and Fred M. Howard. Lippincott-Raven Publishers, Philadelphia © 1997.

VI

Respiratory Problems

52

Pneumonia and Acute Bronchitis

CATHERINE F. GRACEY

Pneumonia and bronchitis are both infections of the lower respiratory tract, differing in the areas which are affected. Bronchitis affects the tracheobronchial tree, whereas pneumonia affects the lung parenchyma. Pneumonia and acute bronchitis are addressed separately in this chapter. Although there may be a continuum between pneumonia and bronchitis, differences exist in the frequency of the etiologic agents causing these two conditions. Indications for therapy differ. Both pneumonia and bronchitis are common entities, with bronchitis leading to 12 million office visits to physicians each year in the United States. Costs associated with treating bronchitis are estimated to be about $300 million each year.

Pneumonia is also common, affecting more than three million people per year in the United States and leading to about 500,000 hospital admissions annually. The cost associated with treating pneumonia is over one billion dollars each year. Although it is usually easily treated on an outpatient basis, it still causes significant morbidity and mortality. The mortality in outpatients is approximately 1% to 5%; this goes up to almost 25% in hospitalized patients. About 50,000 people die from pneumonia each year.

It is often necessary to treat pneumonia empirically, because good culture data are usually lacking. In studies, about 50% of pneumonias had no definite etiologic organism identified. Bronchitis also usually does not have a definitively identified etiology. It is therefore crucial to use information from the history, physical examination, laboratory tests, and epidemiology to decide about possible etiology and treatment.

Pneumonia

Pneumonia develops when the normally sterile lower respiratory tract becomes inoculated with organisms, through either inhalation or aspiration. All people aspirate small amounts of oral secretions intermittently, especially during sleep, but if the inoculum of bacteria is high, infection is more likely to develop. Those with poor dentition and a high concentration of oral bacteria are at increased risk. Patients who are debilitated or alcoholic tend to be colonized with more virulent gram-negative bacteria. Aspiration of a small volume may lead to infection, especially if host defenses are not working adequately. Host defenses consist of mucociliary clearance, leukocyte phagocytosis, and antibody and complement production and are affected by viral upper respiratory infections, smoking, and alcohol. Viral infections can affect respiratory epithelium, mucociliary clearance, and neutrophil function. Smoking destroys ciliary clearance and affects macrophage activity, thus preventing the body from responding optimally. Alcohol can cause decreased mobility of neutrophils and abnormal neutrophil function. Age-related changes, malnutrition, acidosis, and uremia also have been shown to affect host defenses.

ETIOLOGY AND DIFFERENTIAL DIAGNOSIS

Cough is present in about 80% of patients presenting with pneumonia. The differential diagnosis of a patient presenting with cough is broad and includes bronchitis, pulmonary embolism, vasculitis or inflammatory disorders, congestive heart failure, chronic obstructive pulmonary disease, asthma, gastroesophageal reflux, pneumothorax, obstructing bronchogenic carcinoma, and sinusitis—postnasal drip. Several of these entities can cause cough, dyspnea, fever, and an abnormal roentgenogram. It is helpful to decide first whether the etiology is infectious or noninfectious, and then to determine the possible cause.

Pneumonia can be caused by bacteria, viruses, atypical bacteria, and mycobacteria. Although pneumonias have often been described as either "typical" (classic) or "atypical," there is much overlap and this distinction does not always help determine etiology. The typical presentation is that of a lobar bacterial pneumonia and consists of the sudden onset of fever, shaking chills, pleuritic pain, dyspnea, and cough productive of purulent "rusty" sputum, as is often seen with *Streptococcus pneumoniae*. The presentation of atypical pneumonia is associated with a longer prodrome, frequently following an upper respiratory infection, and associated with a nonproductive cough (Table 52-1). The patient may look less ill than with the typical pneumonia. Some agents can present in either manner or along a spectrum (Table 52-2). Decision-making based on presentation alone is unreliable in individual cases. It can be helpful, however, to use this classification when thinking about pneumonias as a group.

S pneumoniae is the most common etiology of pneumonias found to have an identified cause. Frequency ranges from 15% to

Table 52–1. Typical Versus Atypical Pneumonia

SIGN/SYMPTOM	TYPICAL	ATYPICAL
Prodrome	No	Yes
Cough	Productive	Dry
Sputum	Purulent	Mucoid
Rigors	Yes	No
Appearance	Ill	Mildly ill
Pain	Pleuritic	Occasionally substernal
Fever	Yes	Yes, or chills
Associated symptoms	No	Yes
Radiographic appearance	Lobar	Diffuse, patchy
Leukocytosis, bandemia	Yes, yes	No, no
Bacteria on Gram stain	Usually	No

60%, depending on the study, and varies depending on whether inpatients as well as outpatients were studied. This number has decreased from the 50% to 90% of cases described in the past. Pneumococcal pneumonia is the usual etiology of the typical pneumonia described earlier. There is usually no history of an antecedent upper respiratory syndrome. The patient may complain of dyspnea and pleuritic pain, and there may be evidence for consolidation (dullness to percussion, increased tactile fremitus, bronchial breath sounds, egophony, whispered pectoriloquy, bronchophony or rales) on physical examination. Leukocytosis is common. Gram stain evaluation of the sputum often shows many leukocytes and gram-positive lancet-shaped diplococci. The roentgenogram usually shows lobar involvement. Bacteremia can occur in 20% of patients and portends a poorer prognosis. Other risks for increased mortality include the involvement of multiple lobes, increased age, and the presence of suppurative complications. Pneumococcus can cause metastatic infections, especially meningitis, endocarditis, and septic arthritis; these were more common before antibiotics were widely used. Mortality ranges from 15% to 20%.

Table 52–2. Usual Etiologic Agents in Typical and Atypical Pneumonia

Typical
S pneumoniae
H influenzae
Aerobic gram-negative bacilli
S aureus
Atypical
M pneumoniae
C pneumoniae
Legionella sp.
Respiratory viruses
M tuberculosis
Either
Legionella sp.
M tuberculosis

Patients older than 65 years of age or those with anatomic or functional asplenia, human immunodeficiency virus (HIV) infection, sickle cell disease, and chronic illnesses including cardiopulmonary disease, cirrhosis, renal disease, and diabetes mellitus are at an increased risk for pneumococcal infection, and it is recommended that they receive the pneumococcal vaccine. This consists of polysaccharide capsule antigen from the 23 serotypes known to cause 90% of the clinical disease. Its efficacy is variable, depending on the antibody-forming ability of the recipient. It is a one-time vaccine except for those patients at higher risk of fatal pneumococcal infection (asplenia), for whom it is recommended that it be given every 6 years. Because the safety of the vaccine has not been established in pregnancy, it should be avoided in pregnant women.

Mycoplasma pneumoniae is another common cause of pneumonia, accounting for 10% to 40% of the cases in which an etiology has been determined. Mycoplasmas are the smallest freeliving microorganisms and are without a cell wall. (This absence is the reason *Mycoplasma* are not demonstrated on Gram stain evaluation.) *Mycoplasma* is the prototype of atypical pneumonia and was originally known as "primary atypical pneumonia." It occurs throughout the year with increased frequency in late summer and fall. There can be great variation in attack rates from year to year. Although typically an illness of children and young adults, it does affect the elderly. It is thought that the body's immune response to infection may cause some of the disease manifestations. The presentation is usually a gradual onset of upper respiratory symptoms, most notably pharyngitis. Headache, fever, and cough ensue, the cough starting out dry or productive of only scant amounts of mucoid sputum. The patient typically looks fairly well, although as the disease progresses she can develop dyspnea. Examination rarely shows evidence for lung consolidation. Bullous myringitis is quite suggestive of *Mycoplasma*; however, it is seen in only 5% to 15% of cases. Gram stain of sputum may show polymorphonuclear leukocytes without any organisms. Chest radiographs usually show patchy disease in an alveolar or reticular pattern in the lower lobes, and perhaps hilar adenopathy or small pleural effusions. Disease visible on chest radiographs may be more extensive than suspected based on physical examination.

Extrapulmonary manifestations include the presence of cold agglutinins in up to 60% of patients. Very high titers of cold agglutinins can lead to hemolysis, which, although usually minimal, has led to death in rare cases. Other rare complications include aseptic meningitis, encephalitis, neuropathy, transverse myelitis, Guillain-Barré syndrome, cardiac abnormalities including EKG changes, dysrhythmias, cardiac dilatation or pericardial effusion, hepatomegaly, splenomegaly, glomerulonephritis, arthritis, and skin rashes. Most patients recover uneventfully, however. *Mycoplasma* is often transmitted within a family, making its way until all have been affected.

Chlamydia pneumoniae is also known as TWAR, the name derived from the laboratory designations of the first two patients from whom the organism was isolated. Epidemiologic studies have shown that *C pneumoniae* is the pathogen responsible for 6% to 12% of community-acquired pneumonia. Infection is usually asymptomatic or mild in younger adults and causes more significant disease in the elderly. Although *C pneumoniae* can spread among a family, usually only one member is affected. Symptoms are of gradual onset, starting with pharyngitis; sinusitis is associated with *Chlamydia* infection in about 5% of patients. Hoarseness is common. Cough is a major manifestation; it is often dry and may persist for weeks despite appropriate antibiotic treatment. As with the other types of pneumonia, disease can be more serious in patients with underlying illnesses. Laboratory data are often unremarkable; the erythrocyte sedimentation rate may be elevated, though not markedly so. Sputum Gram stain demonstrates leukocytes without other organisms. Serologic examination by microimmunofluoresence can demonstrate antibody response and delineate current from past infection, but this test is not widely available. Complement fixation is neither sensitive nor specific, because it will be positive with infection with other *Chlamydia* species.

Legionella pneumophila was first identified in 1977 but was isolated as far back as 1947. More than 30 species have now been identified. *L pneumophila* is a fastidious gram-negative bacillus that tends to be found in aquatic environments such as air conditioners, humidifiers, and water tanks. It can occur either in epidemics or in sporadic cases, and accounts for 1% to 15% of community-acquired pneumonias. People most likely to be affected by *Legionella* are smokers, the elderly, and the immunosuppressed, including those on chronic steroids. The presentation varies, ranging from Pontiac fever, a mild flu-like syndrome without pulmonary involvement, to Legionnaire's disease, a serious illness manifested by pneumonia, high fever, and extrapulmonic disease. Cough is initially nonproductive, although 50% to 75% of patients go on to develop sputum. Diarrhea is a very common occurrence. Other manifestations of disease include headache, lethargy, encephalopathy, and mental status changes in 20% to 30% of patients. Other involvement is secondary to metastatic spread and may include endocarditis, pericarditis, renal disease, abscesses, or sinusitis. Patients are acutely ill-appearing. A relative bradycardia for the degree of fever seen is typically described. Although *Legionella* are gram-negative organisms, they do not stain well with Gram stain; thus, the Gram stain usually shows white blood cells without organisms. Confirmation of disease can be difficult because tests are not entirely sensitive. Culture must be done on special media, and sensitivity of sputum culture is only about 50% to 70%. Tests that rely on sputum are difficult if the cough is nonproductive. Direct fluorescent antibody determination depends on the concentration of organisms in the sputum. Serology is more sensitive, ranging from 70% to 96%, but requires waiting for convalescent samples to see if titers have increased. A titer of greater than 1 : 256 on a single sample, given a background of low community prevalence, may be enough to indicate acute disease. An additional problem with serology is that 20% to 30% of patients will not develop an antibody response.

Viruses also cause lower respiratory tract infections, most notably influenza (types A and B), and much less likely, respiratory syncytial virus, adenovirus, parainfluenza, and rhinovirus. Varicella and measles also can cause pneumonia. Influenza occurs in temperate climates in epidemics lasting for 1 to 2 months each year. Seventy percent of nonimmunized people exposed to influenza will develop the disease. The virus spreads by inhalation of aerosols; it then attaches to the respiratory epithelium, enters the cell, and multiplies, making enough new virus to produce symptoms in several days. Symptoms begin with high fever, exhaustion, myalgias, headache, and sore throat. Cough follows 1 to 2 days later and is usually nonproductive.

Complications of influenza include primary viral pneumonia and secondary bacterial pneumonia. These entities are responsible for most of the deaths associated with influenza epidemics. Primary viral pneumonia can occur in 1% of patients with influenza, and mortality can be up to 30% in this group. Influenza tends to affect those with underlying chronic illnesses; however, healthy pregnant women also are at increased risk. Influenza pneumonia causes a diffuse pneumonitis and clinically one sees significant hypoxia from diffuse alveolar edema.

Secondary bacterial pneumonia also can occur after influenza, usually caused by *S pneumoniae*, *Staphylococcus aureus*, or *Haemophilus influenza*. Clinically one usually sees recurrence of fever and cough productive of purulent sputum after the patient had started to improve, although this biphasic course does not always occur. Patients at increased risk are, again, those with underlying illnesses, especially chronic lung disease, and the elderly. The mortality associated with a secondary bacterial pneumonia can be very high, especially in those cases caused by *S aureus*, so admission to the hospital for intravenous therapy and close monitoring is recommended.

The influenza vaccine is changed yearly to reflect the viral strains which are most likely to cause disease. It is efficacious in preventing or lessening the severity of disease and is recommended for the elderly; those with chronic cardiopulmonary diseases, diabetes, renal disease, malignancy, connective tissue diseases, or HIV infection; and health care workers. It should be obtained in the midfall so that protective antibody has time to develop before the flu season strikes. The only contraindication to influenza vaccine is chicken egg allergy.

Although less common than influenza, other viruses can also cause a diffuse pneumonitis. Varicella can cause a severe diffuse pneumonia, especially in adults and in pregnant women. Mortality and the risk of premature birth and fetal loss is quite high (see Considerations in Pregnancy).

Live attenuated varicella vaccine was licensed for use in 1995. It is felt to be 70% efficacious in preventing disease in adults, and the remaining 30% usually have much milder disease. The vaccine is contraindicated during pregnancy and in immunocompromised individuals. It is recommended that pregnancy be avoided for 3 months after vaccination. As Reye syndrome has been associated with the use of salicylates during varicella infection, it is recommended that salicylates not be used for 6 weeks following vaccination.

H influenza accounts for approximately 10% to 20% of outpatient pneumonias. This number is variable depending on the population studied, however, and is higher in those who are elderly, have chronic bronchitis, or have HIV disease. *H influenza* is a gram-negative coccobacillus on Gram stain examination. There is increasing prevalence of beta-lactamase production, although this varies depending on the community. It is important, therefore, to know the local epidemiology when making a decision regarding therapy.

Gram-negative pneumonias occur with increased frequency in patients who are colonized with gram-negative bacteria, that is, the debilitated, hospitalized, and alcoholic. The elderly are thought to be at increased risk, but that may simply reflect underlying illnesses. Agents most commonly implicated in gram-negative infections include *Klebsiella pneumoniae*, *Pseudomonas aeruginosa*, *Escherichia coli*, *Acinetobacter species*, and *Proteus mirabilis*. The presentation is that of a classic pneumonia; Gram stain evaluation often shows gram-negatives although they are sometimes difficult to see.

Aspiration pneumonias can lead to lung abscess. Sputum is foul-smelling and Gram stain may demonstrate multiple organisms along with leukocytes. These infections are usually caused by mixed aerobes and anaerobes. Organisms often involved include streptococci and anaerobes such as *Bacteroides* spp, *Fusobacterium* spp, and peptostreptococci. Aspiration should be suspected when a chest radiograph demonstrates cavitation (single or multiple) or when an infiltrate is found in the superior or basal segments of the lower lobes or the posterior segments of the upper lobes. Patients at risk for aspiration include those with conditions known to affect the gag reflex (eg, stroke), swallowing mechanism (eg, neuromuscular disorders), or alterations in consciousness (eg, seizures, alcohol or other drug use, anesthesia). Because all people aspirate small amounts of oral secretions intermittently, patients with poor dentition are also at increased risk of introducing pathogenic bacteria into the lower respiratory tract. The presentation may be that of an insidious illness and tends to be associated with weight loss and night sweats.

Mycobacterium tuberculosis should also be considered in those with cough and abnormal chest x-ray, especially as more immunosuppressed patients are in the population and the incidence of tuberculosis is increased. Its presentation can be similar to either typical or atypical pneumonias. Often the time course of symptoms before presentation is prolonged and is associated with more systemic symptoms such as weight loss or night sweats. Hemoptysis may be present. Tuberculosis typically affects the upper lobes preferentially to the lower; a chest x-ray may show an infiltrate rather than cavitation, especially in immunosuppressed patients (HIV infection).

Pneumocystis carinii pneumonia should also be considered in the differential diagnosis of pneumonia, especially as it can be an initial presentation of acquired immunodeficiency disease. As HIV infection increases in prevalence throughout the population, not remaining in defined risk groups, clinicians must keep this in mind. An early complaint may be dyspnea on exertion, or mild dry cough. The physical examination may be nonspecific and may not even demonstrate rales despite the presence of pneumonia. Induced sputum often will show the parasite upon silver staining.

HISTORY

A detailed history is crucial because it gives information about the extent of disease and possible etiologic agents. The tempo of the illness and involvement of other organ systems are important, as are predisposing factors such as comorbid illnesses, HIV status or risk, recent illnesses, travel, exposures, tobacco use, vaccination status (influenza, pneumococcal), and alcohol or other drug use. The history can range from the sudden development of classic symptoms to nonspecific symptoms of malaise or headache. In the elderly, the presentation may be only a change in mental status or an increase in respiratory rate.

In various studies attempting to determine etiologies for community-acquired pneumonias, a definite source is found in only about 50% to 70%, despite extensive testing. As some of these testing methods are not practical in clinical practice, it is necessary to use what is available to narrow down an etiology.

PHYSICAL EXAMINATION

The physical examination is important in diagnosis of the pneumonia and also in looking for signs of compromise that would indicate a need for hospitalization. Evaluation should include vital signs (blood pressure, pulse, respiratory rate, and temperature), mental status examination, and evaluation for presence of cyanosis, skin rash, and use of accessory musculature. The pulmonary examination should search for rales or evidence of consolidation or pleural fluid. It is also necessary to look for evidence of other organ involvement and underlying illnesses.

LABORATORY AND IMAGING

Sputum Gram stain is helpful, rapid, noninvasive, and inexpensive. Although its sensitivity is low, its specificity is high (about 90% for pneumococcus, the most common etiology of community-acquired pneumonia). A proper sputum sample should have > 25 white blood cells and < 10 epithelial cells per low-power field. This decreases the risk of contamination by normal mouth flora and increases accuracy. Sensitivity and specificity of sputum culture are low; however, culture can be helpful, especially if the culture isolates an organism not normally found in oral flora. It is important to interpret the culture data in light of what is seen on the Gram stain. The culture is also helpful for noting what does not grow; gram-negative organisms grow easily in culture so their absence is good evidence that they are not the source of infection.

Sputum can be cultured for *Legionella*; however, this requires special culture techniques and takes several days for a result. *Legionella* cultures have a sensitivity of only about 50% to 70%. Sputum can be examined using direct immunofluorescence to obtain rapid information; however, low sensitivity limits its usefulness. For bacteria, countercurrent immunoelectrophoresis can be done on serum, urine, or sputum samples. However, results on sputum samples do not differentiate between infection and colonization, and tests on urine and serum are less sensitive in patients with pneumonia than in meningitis.

Other laboratory investigations that can be helpful include serology directed at *Mycoplasma*, *Chlamydia*, and *Legionella* species. These examine antibody response and look for a rise in titers. Problems with this method are that it takes time to get results, and serial titers are often necessary, making it impractical for use in making therapeutic decisions. Diagnosis of disease is possible with a fourfold rise in titers to 1 : 128 or more. For *Legionella*, a single titer of 1 : 256 associated with a clinical scenario of Legionnaire disease is also acceptable for the diagnosis. Serologic testing for *C pneumoniae* is not offered by many laboratories.

Blood cultures should be obtained in patients for whom hospitalization is necessary, for help in determining both etiology and prognosis, because those with bacteremia are at increased risk of death.

Other laboratory data that can be helpful in determining the prognosis of patients include measurement of leukocyte count, electrolytes, blood urea nitrogen, and arterial blood gases.

Cold agglutinins at a titer of 1 : 32 are found in about half of patients with *Mycoplasma*, but are nonspecific because these can also be present in patients without *Mycoplasma* infection. Titers of 1 : 256 or greater are more suggestive of *Mycoplasma* infection. The erythrocyte sedimentation rate is usually elevated in *Mycoplasma* and *Chlamydia* infections, but is not specific to these infections.

Chest radiography is not routinely indicated in all patients presenting with cough because the sensitivity is only about 3%. If a patient has an abnormal lung exam, temperature over 37.8°C, heart rate greater than 100 beats per minute, or does not have asthma, the likelihood of a pneumonia is increased. It is also necessary to decide if a chest radiograph will make a difference in treatment (ie, inpatient versus outpatient) or help in determining etiology. It is necessary to remember, however, that there is great overlap in radiologic presentation and radiographic findings alone cannot determine etiology. Radiography is indicated in a patient who does require admission or is at high risk for pneumonia or complications.

There is no need for serial roentgenograms if the patient is clinically improving as the time course for radiographic resolution lags behind clinical findings. For example, it may take 4 weeks for a pneumococcal pneumonia to resolve in a young patient (longer in an elderly patient) and up to 4 months for an infiltrate secondary to *Legionella* to resolve.

TREATMENT

One of the first decisions to be made regarding therapy is whether the patient can be treated as an outpatient or requires inpatient admission. Fine and colleagues published a prospective study in 1990 that attempted to identify subsets of patients who could be safely treated as outpatients. Table 52-3 lists factors that were found to increase morbidity and mortality and that may indicate hospitalization. A study published by the British Thoracic Society in 1987 identified risks for death, including respiratory rate > 30 breaths per minute, diastolic blood pressure < 60 mm Hg, age > 60 years, confusion, previous history of congestive heart failure, leukopenia or leukocytosis, hypoxemia, or blood urea nitrogen > 70 mg/dL. The risk of death was increased 10 to 21 times if two out of three of the following risk factors were present: respiratory rate > 30 at admission; diastolic blood pressure < 60 mm Hg at admission; and presence of confusion or blood urea nitrogen > 70 mg/dL. Table 52-4 lists factors that define a severe pneumonia; any one of these would be an indication for admission to an intensive care unit.

Other factors to consider are the patient's ability to take medication reliably and the patient's social supports. If the decision is made to treat as an outpatient, close follow-up is important to ensure that the patient is improving and not developing any complications. The patient should have instructions to call if she is not improved in 2 to 3 days, her sputum remains purulent (or becomes so), her temperature remains higher than 38.3°C, or if rigors, dyspnea, hemoptysis, or mental status changes develop.

Table 52–3. Reasons to Consider Hospitalization

Severe vital sign abnormality (respiratory rate > 30 breaths per minute, diastolic blood pressure < 60 mm Hg, systolic blood pressure < 90 mm Hg, temperature > 38.3°C)
Altered mental status
Suppurative complication
Hypoxemia (paO_2 < 60 mm Hg on room air)
Acute coexistent medical problem which alone would lead to hospitalization
Severe laboratory abnormality (WBC < 4000/mm^3 or > 30,000/mm^3, creatinine > 1.2 mg/dL, BUN > 20 mg/dL, hematocrit < 30%, or hemoglobin < 9 g/dL
High-risk etiology (staphylococcal, gram-negative rod, aspiration, postobstructive pneumonia)
Immunosuppression
Comorbid illness (diabetes mellitus, chronic pulmonary disease, congestive heart failure, renal insufficiency, chronic liver disease, hospitalization within one year)
Age > 65 years
Chest radiograph demonstrating multilobar involvement, cavity, rapid spreading, pleural effusion.

Table 52–4. Indications for Admission to Intensive Care Unit

Respiratory rate > 30 breaths per minute
Severe respiratory failure (paO_2 < 60 mm Hg on room air or pCO_2 > 50 mm Hg)
Requirement for mechanical ventilation
Chest radiograph showing bilateral involvement or involvement of multiple lobes; increase in size of opacity by 50% or greater in first 48 hours
Shock (systolic blood pressure < 90 mm Hg or diastolic blood pressure < 60 mm Hg)
Requirement for vasopressors
Urine output < 20 cc/h (unless other explanation) or acute renal failure requiring dialysis

Choice of antimicrobial agents depends on the presumed etiology of the pneumonia, based on history, physical examination, laboratory data, and imaging. There are multiple algorithms available to help determine the best antibiotic choice. A key point to remember is that narrow-spectrum antibiotics are usually preferable to broad-spectrum in a patient who is mildly to moderately ill. The patient who is quite ill usually requires broad-spectrum empiric antibiotics while awaiting results of laboratory investigations. Although every effort should be made to obtain culture data before treatment to increase the yield of investigations, therapy should not be unduly delayed. Once a specific etiology is determined, the antimicrobial regimen should be narrowed to the best choice for that organism. Cost is also a factor. Given regimens of equivalent efficacy, a less expensive one should be chosen. Table 52-5 lists initial options for therapy if the etiologic organism is known. Tetracycline should not be used as therapy for pneumococcus, because some isolates have developed resistance to this antibiotic. Of increasing concern is the emergence of penicillin-resistant *S pneumoniae*. This has increased in the United States from 3.6% to 14.5% since 1987, based on culture data from 12 sentinel hospitals. The prevalence of *H influenzae* resistant to beta-lactam antibiotics has also increased markedly over recent years, approaching 30% in some communities. It is important to know community-specific prevalence of drug resistance when empiric therapy is considered.

Table 52–5. Antibiotic Selection Based on Etiologic Organism

ORGANISM	INITIAL	SECOND
S pneumococcus	Penicillin	Erythromycin
M pneumoniae	Erythromycin	Tetracycline
H influenzae	TMP-SMX	2nd generation cephalosporin
C pneumoniae	Tetracycline	Erythromycin
Legionella sp.	Erythromycin	Tetracycline (with addition of rifampin if very ill)

In 1993 the American Thoracic Society published guidelines for the initial treatment of community-acquired pneumonia based on the most likely pathogens for various groups. Patients were stratified into four groups depending on age, comorbid illnesses, and severity of disease. Table 52-6 summarizes these recommendations. Again, as the risk of morbidity and mortality from pneumonia increases, empiric therapy becomes broader.

Other therapeutic goals include maintenance of adequate hydration, control of fever, and suppression of a nonproductive cough by cough suppressants, such as dextromethorphan or codeine, to improve patient comfort. If fever is secondary to influenza or varicella, acetaminophen rather than aspirin should be used to prevent the development of Reye syndrome in young patients.

High-risk individuals who have not received influenza vaccine are often treated with amantidine as prophylaxis against infection. Influenza infections, including viral pneumonia, can be treated with amantidine, and treatment should be started within 48 hours of onset of symptoms. Rimantidine is a newer agent that may be preferred, as it has fewer side effects. Those patients who do contract influenza pneumonia should be considered for hospitalization for therapy and observation.

Varicella pneumonia has a risk of death of 11% to 17% in the nonpregnant patient; thus, hospitalization is recommended for aggressive therapy and observation. Acyclovir is the treatment of choice and, as bioavailability is variable after oral administration, should be given intravenously.

Table 52–6. Usual Organisms and Initial Therapy in Patients Based on Age and Severity of Illness*

USUAL ORGANISMS	INITIAL THERAPY
Outpatient Pneumonia Without Comorbidity and 60 Years Old or Younger	
S pneumoniae	Macrolide† (erythromycin)
M pneumoniae	*or* Tetracycline‡
Respiratory viruses	
C pneumoniae	
H influenzae	
Miscellaneous (*Legionella* sp., *S aureus, M tuberculosis,* endemic fungi, aerobic gram-negative bacilli)	
Outpatient Pneumonia With Comorbidity and/or 60 Years Old or Older	
S pneumoniae	2nd-generation cephalosporin
Respiratory viruses	*or* TMP-SMX
H influenzae	*or* β-lactam/β-lactamase inhibitor with or without macrolide§
Aerobic gram-negative bacilli	
S aureus	
Miscellaneous (*M catarrhalis, Legionella* sp., *M tuberculosis,* endemic fungi)	
Hospitalized Patients With Community-Acquired Pneumonia	
S pneumoniae	2nd- or 3rd-generation cephalosporin‖
H influenzae	*or* β-lactam/β-lactamase inhibitor‡
Polymicrobial (including anaerobic bacteria)	with or without macrolide§,‡
Aerobic gram-negative bacilli	
Legionella sp	
S aureus	
C pneumoniae	
Respiratory viruses	
Miscellaneous (*M pneumoniae, M catarrhalis, M tuberculosis,* endemic fungi)	
Severe Hospitalized Community Acquired Pneumonia	
S pneumoniae	Macrolide#
Legionella sp.	*plus* 3rd-generation cephalosporin with antipseudomonal activity‖,**
Aerobic gram-negative bacilli	*or* other antipseudomonal agents
M pneumoniae	
Respiratory viruses	
Miscellaneous (*H influenzae, M tuberculosis,* endemic fungi)	

*Excludes patients at risk for HIV.

†Consider azithromycin or clarithromycin in those intolerant of erythromycin, or in smokers to treat *H influenzae.*

‡Many isolates of *S pneumoniae* are resistant to TCN; use only if patient cannot take macrolide antibiotic or infection not secondary to *S pneumoniae.*

§ If *Legionella* sp. a concern.

‖3rd generation cephalosporin not as active against *S pneumoniae* or anaerobes as 2nd-generation. Only 3rd-generation cephalosporins with antipseudomonal activity are ceftazidime and cefoperazone.

#May add rifampin if *Legionella* sp. documented.

**Given high mortality of pseudomonal pneumonia would add an aminoglycoside to initial therapy.

Acute Bronchitis

Acute bronchitis is a self-limited inflammatory disorder of the tracheobronchial tree. It should be differentiated from chronic bronchitis, which is defined as the production of sputum on most days for at least 3 months out of the year for more than 2 years. Chronic bronchitis is usually associated with exposure to tobacco smoke or other inhaled toxins, whereas acute bronchitis is usually associated with a viral upper respiratory infection. The peak incidence of acute bronchitis is in the winter, correlating with the highest incidence of viral upper respiratory infections. There appears to be an association between acute bronchitis and asthma. Patients with the diagnosis of bronchitis are more likely to have a history of asthma. They are also more likely to subsequently have findings consistent with asthma.

Pathogenesis is that of hyperemia and edema of the bronchial lining. This leads to increased secretion of mucus and possibly to decreased mucociliary clearance. Exposure to irritants such as tobacco smoke, air pollution, or other inhaled toxins may exacerbate this situation. The role bacterial infection plays in acute bronchitis is unclear. Bacterial growth may be found in sputum samples; this may be secondary to contamination by oral flora, however, or may represent bacterial colonization. Atypical bacteria such as *M pneumoniae* and *C pneumoniae* attach to respiratory epithelium and cause irritation of mucosa. *Mycoplasma* infection can lead to sloughing of epithelium.

ETIOLOGY

The etiology is viral in the majority of cases of acute bronchitis. Viruses usually involved include rhinovirus or coronavirus; less likely pathogens are influenza or adenovirus. In a smaller number of cases the cause is atypical bacteria such as *M pneumoniae* or *C pneumonia*. Bacterial etiologies are much less frequent but can include *S pneumoniae*, *H influenzae*, or *Moraxella catarrhalis*. The actual contribution by bacteria is unknown, because sputum samples are often contaminated by oral flora. Those patients colonized by bacteria (eg, smokers, the chronically ill), may be more likely to have bacterial infection as an etiology of their bronchitis.

HISTORY

History is usually of cough that follows an upper respiratory infection. Fifty percent of people with a viral upper respiratory infection will develop cough, and 50% of those people will have sputum production. The cough may develop as other upper respiratory symptoms abate and can persist 2 to 4 weeks. The cough usually starts out nonproductive but then progresses to be productive of mucoid phlegm. This can be followed by the production of purulent sputum. Infection of the bronchioles can lead to airway hyperreactivity and bronchospasm, leading to wheezing and cough. Some patients may not wheeze but may complain of cough that is made worse by activities such as exercise, taking a deep breath, laughing, or exposure to cold weather. Other symptoms can include fever, burning substernal chest pain, fatigue, and night sweats. The fever is usually low grade but varies depending on the etiologic agent involved. As lung parenchyma is not involved in bronchitis, dyspnea is not seen unless the patient has underlying pulmonary disease. A history of tobacco use or exposure to other inhaled toxins should be sought, as should history of exposure to people with possible respiratory illnesses.

PHYSICAL EXAMINATION

Physical examination should be complete, with a careful search for signs of pneumonia or other cardiopulmonary disease. Parenchymal involvement does not occur with bronchitis; therefore, signs of consolidation or alveolar involvement should be not be present. Rhonchi or wheezes may be present on pulmonary examination. signs of other organ involvement should also be sought.

LABORATORY AND IMAGING STUDIES

Laboratory evaluation is usually deferred given the self-limited nature of this illness. This may be modified, however, depending on the individual patient involved, her degree of illness, and the presence of any comorbid conditions. Evaluation may include viral culture, or possibly serologic studies if *Mycoplasma* or *Chlamydia* is being considered as etiologic agent. Sputum cultures are often difficult to interpret given contamination from nasopharyngeal flora. Chest x-rays and other evaluations are usually deferred unless the symptoms are persistent.

TREATMENT

Treatment is primarily aimed at relief of symptoms. Maintenance of adequate hydration and control of cough are the major goals. Cough can be controlled with dextromethorphan or, if especially bothersome, with codeine. Because cough can be due to the bronchospasm associated with bronchitis, it is necessary to attempt to distinguish this from cough secondary to irritation before trying to suppress it. If the cough is secondary to bronchial hyperreactivity, the use of a beta-agonist inhaler may prove helpful. Although the inhalers are more expensive than oral beta-agonist medications, they have fewer systemic side effects and are better tolerated. The patient must be taught to use the inhaler properly to get its benefit.

The use of antibiotics to treat acute bronchitis in healthy patients is controversial. Because acute bronchitis is a self-limited condition in which the etiology is usually viral, antibiotics are generally not recommended for otherwise healthy patients. In patients with other conditions (ie, pulmonary disease, cardiac disease, diabetes, tobacco use) or more systemic symptoms, a course of antibiotics is often given. There may be a continuum between bronchitis and pneumonia; thus, more systemic symptoms may be a clue to early parenchymal involvement. Choices often include erythromycin (active against *M pneumoniae*, *C pneumonia*, *S pneumoniae*); trimethoprim-sulfamethoxazole, a second generation cephalosporin; or amoxacillin-clavulinic acid (active against *S pneumoniae*, *H influenzae*, *M catarrhalis*), depending on the presumed etiologic agent.

Encouragement of smoking cessation is also important. When a patient is ill with bronchitis she may have less desire to smoke and may be more amenable to attempting smoking cessation. Smokers tend to have more episodes of bronchitis, and their cough is usually more severe and lasts longer than in nonsmokers. This may be in part secondary to increased bronchial irritation and hyperreactivity from the exposure to tobacco smoke.

CONSIDERATIONS IN PREGNANCY

Pneumonia occurs infrequently in pregnancy, although when it occurs it can be serious, for both the pregnant woman and the fetus. Those women at higher risk of developing pneumonia are similar to the nonpregnant population in that smokers, those with prior res-

Table 52–7. Selected Medications and Their Use in Pregnancy (FDA Pregnancy Risk Classification)

Safe to Use in Pregnancy	
Penicillin (B)	
Cephalosporins (B)	
Amoxacillin/clavulinic acid (B)	
Erythromycin base (B) (NOT estolate)	
Clindamycin (B)	
Amantidine (C)*	
Acyclovir (C)*	
Contraindicated for Use in Pregnancy	
Tetracycline (D)	Maternal hepatitis, fetal staining of teeth, bony abnormalities, maternal blood dyscrasias
Chloramphenicol (C)	Fetal gray baby syndrome
Erythromycin estolate	Maternal hepatitis
Quinolones (C)	Fetal arthropathy
Possibly Safe to Use in Pregnancy	
Sulfonamides	(B) During 1st and 2nd trimester, (D) during 3rd trimester-neonatal kernicteris contraindicated during first trimester—folic acid inhibitor
Trimethoprim	(C) in 2nd, 3rd trimesters
Aminoglycosides (C)	Ototoxicity
Nitrofurantoin (B)	Can precipitate hemolysis in G6PD deficiency
Metronidazole (B)	Contraindicated in 1st trimester or in high doses

*To treat life-threatening or systemic infection.

piratory disease, and those with underlying illnesses are most likely to be affected. Etiologies of pneumonia appear to be similar in pregnant and nonpregnant patients, although rigorous epidemiologic studies are lacking. Only a small percentage of pneumonias in pregnant women have an etiologic agent identified. Of those that do, *S pneumoniae*, *H influenzae*, *M pneumoniae*, *C pneumoniae*, *L pneumophila*, influenza, and varicella are most common. There is an increased risk for aspiration around the time of delivery secondary to changes in gastrointestinal physiology and also associated with the use of anesthesia. This should be considered in a woman presenting with pneumonia in the postpartum period.

With pneumonia, the risk of preterm delivery increases, as does the risk of delivering a low-birth-weight infant. Pregnant women who develop pneumonia are also more likely to require mechanical ventilation because they have less pulmonary reserve due to changes in pulmonary physiology in the gravid state. In pregnancy there is decreased functional residual capacity along with increased oxygen consumption; therefore even mild hypoxia is not well-tolerated. Fever, tachycardia, and hypoxemia associated with a pulmonary infection can be hazardous to the fetus.

Not only is a pregnant patient less able to tolerate the infection, but she appears to be more likely to become infected due to changes in her immune status. Lymphocytes show a decreased proliferative response, T4 cells are decreased, there is decreased cell cytotoxicity, and there is a decrease in cell-mediated immunity. This leads to increased virulence of those agents which are controlled by cell-mediated immunity.

Primary varicella infection is complicated by pneumonia in 0.3% to 1.8% of cases in nonpregnant individuals; this increases to up to 9% in pregnant women. It has also been shown that influenza has increased mortality in pregnant women and the risk of developing influenza pneumonia is higher.

Varicella infection affects 0.07% of pregnancies. Pulmonary symptoms may develop 2 to 5 days after the rash occurs, with smokers more likely to develop pulmonary symptoms. Whereas the mortality of varicella pneumonia in nonpregnant patients is 11% to 17%, it is 35% to 40% in pregnant women. Complications tend to be greatest in the third trimester when cell-mediated immunity is at its lowest. Chest x-rays show diffuse miliary or nodular infiltrates. Aggressive therapy is necessary, including intravenous acyclovir in an effort to decrease morbidity and mortality. From 10% to 26% of patients develop intrauterine infection; fetal effects include congenital varicella syndrome, congenital zoster of infancy, or perinatal varicella infection depending on when in gestation infection occurred.

Influenza may also cause increased complications in pregnancy, both from primary viral and secondary bacterial pneumonias. If respiratory symptoms persist longer than usual, the possibility of pneumonia should be considered. The antiviral agents amantidine or rimantidine should be used as prophylaxis in high-risk women who have not received influenza vaccine and to treat influenza. Influenza vaccination is not contraindicated in pregnancy.

It is recommended that the total maternal radiation exposure throughout pregnancy be limited to less than 5 rads. A chest x-ray exposes the patient to 0.2 rads, well under what is deemed safe. Although unnecessary exposure should be avoided, one should not forgo obtaining a chest film if it is important in diagnosis or therapy.

Treatment of pneumonia in a pregnant woman is similar to that in nonpregnant individuals, although special attention is paid to treating hypoxia and in choice of medications. The paO_2 should be kept greater than 70 mm Hg in a pregnant patient to avoid any fetal hypoxemia. Medications must be chosen keeping the effects on both recipients in mind. Pharmacokinetics are different in pregnancy;

Table 52–8. Selected Antibiotics and Use in Breast Feeding

Safe to use
Penicillin
Cephalosporins
Erythromycin
Acyclovir
Trimethoprim
Sulfonamides*
Contraindicated for use
Tetracycline
Quinolones
Chloramphenicol
Amantadine†

*Avoid in premature or stressed infants or those with hyperbilirubinemia or G6PD deficiency.

†Use with caution.

there is an increase in the volume of distribution, decrease in plasma protein concentration, increased renal clearance of medications, increased hepatic metabolism of certain medications, and possibly erratic absorption of medications. This may require that medication dosages and dosing intervals be adjusted in the pregnant patient. This is especially important in the seriously ill patient in whom adequate therapy is crucial; checking drug levels may be advisable.

No medication is without risk, and it must be remembered that the risk of a medication to the pregnancy and fetus must be balanced with the risks to the mother and fetus associated with not treating an illness effectively. Tables 52-7 and 52-8 list selected antibiotics and their recommendations for use in pregnancy and nursing, respectively.

BIBLIOGRAPHY

American Thoracic Society. Guidelines for the initial management of adults with community acquired pneumonia: diagnosis, assessment of severity, and initial antimicrobial therapy. Am Rev Respir Dis 1993;148:1418.

British Thoracic Society. Community-acquired pneumonia in adults in British hospitals in 1982–1983: a survey of aetiology, mortality, prognastic factors and outcome. Q J Med 1987;62:195.

Donowitz GR, Mandell GL. Acute pneumonia. In: Mandell GL, Bennett JE, Dolin R, eds. Principles and practices of infectious diseases. New York: Churchill Livingstone, 1995:619.

Fang GD, Fine M, Orloff J, et al. New and emerging etiologies for community acquired pneumonia with implications for therapy: a prospective multicenter study of 359 cases. Medicine 1990;69:307.

Fine MJ, Smith DN, Singer DE. Hospitalization decision in patients with community acquired pneumonia: a prospective cohort study. Am J Med 1990;89:713.

Gwaltney JM. Acute Bronchitis. In: Mandell GL, Bennett JE, Dolin R, eds. Principles and practices of infectious diseases. New York: Churchill Livingstone, 1995:606.

Luby JP. Pneumonia caused by mycoplasma pneumoniae infection. Clin Chest Med 1991;12:237.

Montella KR. Pulmonary pharmacology in pregnancy. Clin Chest Med 1992;13:587.

Nguyen ML, Yu VL. Legionella infection. Clin Chest Med 1991;12:257.

Pomilla PV, Brown RB. Outpatient treatment of community acquired pneumonia in adults. Arch Intern Med 1994;154:1793.

Rodnick JE, Gude JK. The use of antibiotics in acute bronchitis and acute exacerbations of chronic bronchitis. West J Med 1988;149:347.

Rodrigues J, Niederman MS. Pneumonia complicating pregnancy. Clin Chest Med 1992;13:679.

Simpson ML, Gaziano EP, et al. Bacterial infections during pregnancy. In: Burrow GN, Ferris TF, eds. Medical complications during pregnancy. Philadelphia: WB Saunders, 1988:345.

Sue DY. Community acquired pneumonia in adults. West J Med 1994;161:383.

Thom DH, Grayston JT. Infections with Chlamydia pneumoniae strain TWAR. Clin Chest Med 1991;12:245.

53
The Common Cold

ANN T. RIGGS

Primary Care for Women, edited by Phyllis C. Leppert and Fred M. Howard. Lippincott-Raven Publishers, Philadelphia © 1997.

The "common cold" is the historically designated term for acute viral infection of the upper respiratory system and is characterized by rhinorrhea, congestion, sneezing, cough, and sore throat. The common cold is one of several upper respiratory infections, the other syndromes being sinusitis, otitis media, pharyngitis, tracheobronchitis, laryngitis, and flu syndrome. Unlike the other infections, this benign illness has no age predilection, is self-limited, and usually is self-diagnosed, even by the youngest of children. This seemingly trivial common occurring illness does not carry undo morbidity on an individual level but on a population scale the sheer magnitude of incidence carries a formidable financial and social burden. Upper respiratory illnesses account for approximately one half of all acute illnesses, approximately 20% attributable to the common cold. It is one of the leading complaints in office visits to the physician and is the major cause of school and work absenteeism, accounting for approximately 18 million sick days in 1993, or 15.6 lost work days per 100 employed persons. The cough and cold formula industry is a multibillion dollar industry; approximately $2 billion are spent annually on more than 800 over-the-counter (OTC) medications.

EPIDEMIOLOGY

Over 200 viruses from viral families have been identified as causing the common cold. These include rhinovirus, coronavirus, adenovirus, and the myxoviruses—RSV, parainfluenza, and influenza. Approximately 35% of common colds are caused by one of the 110 identified stereotypes of rhinovirus. Coronavirus is the second leading cause, accounting for 15% to 20%. This is a fastidious organism, and only three serotypes have been identified. Although the myxoviruses and adenoviruses usually produce more of a flu syndrome, they can produce typical cold symptoms and account for approximately 10% of all colds. In addition, milder forms of bacterial infections such as β-hemolytic streptococcus (BHS), *Chlamydia* pneumonia, *Mycoplasma*, and *Haemophilus* influenzae may present with typical cold symptoms. Approximately 35% of colds have no identified source.

The epidemiology of the cold syndrome is one of seasonal variation: prevalence is increased in cold and damp climates. The "cold season" begins in late August, peaks around December, and starts to decline in the early spring. Interestingly, an interseasonal variation exists within this seasonal paradigm. Rhinovirus is seen most commonly in the fall and middle to late spring, and coronavirus and the myxovirus in midwinter. Ambient and core body temperature are not the reason for increased prevalence; rather, transmission is facilitated by indoor crowding during bad weather and the school year. Viral survival during periods of low humidity or changes in host susceptibility secondary to mucous membrane drying also may contribute to seasonal variation. Adults contract an average of *two to four* colds and children *six to eight* per year. Families with young children typically have increased frequency of colds because children seem to be the reservoirs for these agents. Transmission can occur via aerosolization of large or small particles or via direct physical contact with hand-to-nose self-inoculation. Rhinovirus seems to be transmitted predominantly by the latter. It has been shown to last on hands and surfaces for hours, and vigorous handwashing has been shown to markedly reduce the appearance of cold symptoms. Transmission rate is related closely to donor hours of exposure, no matter what route of transmission. The maximum viral excretion coincides with the peak of symptoms.

Clinical Course

The clinical course is fairly predictable. After an incubation period of approximately 72 hours, symptoms of sneezing, malaise, and burning and watery eyes begin. This is followed by nasal stuffiness, congestion, rhinorrhea, and scratchy throat, with symptoms peaking around the second to fourth day. The initial watery discharge eventually becomes purulent, spurring a common misconception that this implies secondary bacterial infection. Within days, the secretions thin again, become watery, and then gradually subside. The course is usually limited to 1 week but may last as long as 2 weeks. Temperatures rarely exceed 0.5°C (1°F) above normal. Higher fever suggests bacterial superinfection or influenza. Smokers and asthmatics may have a protracted course with a prolonged duration of cough, although most studies suggest that they do not have an increased susceptibility to initial infection. Secondary complications of otitis media and sinusitis occur infrequently, 2% and 0.5% respectively. Such complications are heralded by a rise in temperature as well as local symptomatology. Risk factors for complications include duration of cold symptoms greater than 7 days, smoking, and history of asthma. The diagnosis of a cold is usually self-evident, even to young children. Those who seek medical attention do so usually because of protracted symptoms, suspicion of a sinus infection, or simply to fulfill school or work policies that require a doctor's note to excuse an absence.

Pathophysiology

The pathophysiologic course of the common cold has been extensively studied. The rhinovirus has a predilection for the ciliated epithelium of the respiratory passages. It integrates into these cells via the intercellular adhesion molecule (ICAM) receptors, which are predominantly found in epithelium of the nasopharyngeal, posterior pharynx, and sinuses. The initial sequence of events involves viral replication without frank destruction of the cells, leading to cell death, as is seen with influenza or adenovirus. Bradykinin causes increased vascular permeability, leading to hyperemia, edema, and subsequent narrowing of the nasal passages and a feeling of congestion. Stimulation of cholinergic nerves causes increased mucinous and serous nasal discharge that contain the type-specific immunoglobulins IgG and secretory IgA. These are present within 1 to 2 days and provide an immediate immunologic response. Numerous viral immunologic serotypes, however, prevent protection against future colds. Inflammatory mediators cause a brisk infiltration of neutrophils, plasma cells, and lymphocytes into the lamina propria, and the discharge becomes purulent. Sore throat is usually caused by postnasal drip and the inflammatory mediators. Replication of the virus slows ciliary function and transport, which can persist after the infection is gone. The secondary complications of otitis media and sinusitis result from the loss of ciliary function as well as pressure differences, predisposing to bacterial invasion of organisms into normally sterile places.

EVALUATION

Care of the patient who presents to the physician's office with cold symptoms should include the following: differentiating cold symptoms from other causes, determining whether complications have occurred, providing palliative treatment for symptoms, education about prevention, and appropriate use of medical care. Self-care brochures can dramatically reduce office visits due to colds. Careful history and physical examination are usually sufficient to differentiate cold symptoms from other causes. Ancillary tests are rarely needed in initial management decisions. In general, the practitioner must differentiate viral infections from primary or secondary bacterial infections, as antibiotic therapy would be indicated in the latter to avoid further complications. In addition, exclusion of noninfectious causes of rhinorrhea should be sought in the initial interview and physical examination.

The differential diagnosis of congestion, cough, and sore throat includes infectious and noninfectious causes, which can usually be excluded by careful history-taking and physical examination. The viral and bacterial organisms known to cause cold symptoms have been discussed earlier. The noninfectious causes of rhinorrhea to be differentiated from the common cold are commonly categorized into allergic or vasomotor rhinitis, or the inflammatory, mechanical, or hormonal etiologies. Vasomotor rhinitis is further classified by cause and include the following divisions: idiopathic, rhinitis medicamentosa, or chronic cocaine use. Common mechanical causes of rhinitis include polyps, deviated septum, foreign body, and, less commonly, cerebral spinal fluid leak. Rhinitis and congestion may commonly be seen in high-estrogen states, such as pregnancy or oral contraceptive use, and rarely in the hypothyroid state. Chronic inflammatory conditions are infrequent but include Wegner disease, sarcoidosis, or midline granuloma. Finally, commonly implicated drugs include adrenergic blockers, cholinesterase inhibitors, and estrogen preparations.

The physical examination should focus on the upper respiratory system to exclude primary bacterial infections such as bacterial pharyngitis and to evaluate for presence of secondary complications such as bacterial or serous otitis media, sinusitis, or bronchitis. It also can exclude mechanical etiologies such as polyps or foreign bodies. The presence or absence of fever also should be noted. The physical examination is not specific for colds but characteristically shows swollen, red nasal turbinates, mild tonsillar injection without prominent follicles or exudate, an absence of cervical adenopathy, and clear lung fields. Purulent nasal discharge is common in the uncomplicated cold and does not signify sinusitis or bacterial superinfection in the absence of fever or significant facial pain. Prominent tonsillar follicles with exudate and anterior adenopathy suggest BHS, and throat culture should be obtained. A bulging, red tympanic membrane makes the diagnosis of otitis media. Prostration and high fever in the presence of reported myalgia and headache suggest influenza in concordance with a flu epidemic. Clear nasal discharge and conjunctival injection in conjunction with a history of perennial atopy suggests allergic rhinitis. There is no role for laboratory investigation unless an infection with BHS is suspected, in which case a throat culture or rapid strep antigen assay should be obtained. Viral culture or sero-

Table 53-1. Guidelines for Cold Medicines

	DOSES	STRENGTHS	MAXIMUM DAILY DOSE
Decongestants			
Oral			
Phenylpropanolamine	25 mg q 4h	25 mg	150 mg
Short acting	50 mg q 8h	50 mg	
Long acting	75 mg q 12h	75 mg	
Pseudoephedrine			240 mg
Short acting	60 mg q 4–6 h	30 mg, 60 mg	
Long acting	120 mg q 12h	15 mg/5mL, 30 mg/5 mL	
Phenylephrine	10 mg q 4–6h 20 mg q 8–12 h		60 mg
Topical			
Short acting			
Naphazoline HCl	2 Drops q 3 h 2 Sprays q 4–6 h	0.05% sol/20 mL 0.05% spray/15 mL	
Phenylephrine HCl	2–3 drops or sprays of q 4h	0.25%, 0.5%, 1% sol in 15–30 mL	
Long acting			
Oxymetazoline HCl	2 drops q 12h	0.025%, 0.05 drops 0.05%/15–30 mL spray	
Xylometazoline HCl	2–3 drops q 8–10 h	0.05%–0.1%/15 mL spray 0.05–0.1%/15 mL sol	
Antihistamines			
Chlorpheniramine maleate	2–4 mg q 6–8 h 8 mg q 12 h	2, 4, 8 mg	
Brompheniramine maleate	2–4 mg q 6–8h 12 mg q 12 h	2, 4, 12 mg	
Diphenhydramine HCl	25–50 mg q 6–8 h	12.5, 25, 50 mg	
Clemastine fumarate			
Pyrilamine maleate	12.5–50 mg q 6 h	12.5, 25, 50 mg	
Triprolidine HCl	1.25–2.5 mg q 4–6 h	1.25, 2.5 mg	
Antitussives			
Dextromethorphan HBR			120 mg
Codeine sulfate	30 mg q 6–8 h	10, 15.30 mg	120 mg
Hydrocodone bitartrate	30 mg q 6–8 h		
Benzonatate (Tessalon)	100 mg q 6–8 h		600 mg
Expectorants			
Guaifenesin	100–600 mg		2400 mg

BPH, benign prostatic hypertrophy; *CAD,* coronary artery disease; *COPD,* chronic obstructive pulmonary disease; *MOAIs,* monoamine oxidase inhibitors; *STCA,* tricyclic antidepressants.

logic confirmation of the potential viral pathogen is not necessary for treatment, nor is it cost effective. Influenza can be diagnosed clinically in the presence of an influenza epidemic, and there is no need for viral identification. Nasal swabs for eosinophils sometimes can be helpful in differentiating allergic from vasomotor rhinitis or the common cold. Sinus x-rays are not needed to confirm sinusitis before a trial of antibiotic therapy in a young healthy individual. Education should include instructions on preventing secondary spread, such as careful handwashing and avoidance of prolonged exposure to someone with a cold. The patient should be instructed to return if symptoms persist, or if fever or wheezing develops.

TREATMENT

The medical goals of this self-limited illness are to prevent spread, relieve symptoms, and diagnose and treat superinfections. Prevention or treatment of the common cold by medical intervention has not proved successful or financially feasible. Trials of prophylactic doses of vitamin C failed to show efficacy in cold prevention or treatment. Interferon alpha-2, a substance produced by human cells that blocks invasion of the virus into respiratory epithelium, was initially met with great enthusiasm as an agent that could prevent spread and potentially cure the common cold. Clinical trials with this

PRECAUTIONS	PREGNANCY AND LACTATION	CONTAINED IN COMBINATION FORMULA BRAND NAMES
Medical Conditions CAD Hyperthyroidism Hypertension-poorly controlled BPH **Medications** MAOIs TCA Beta-blockers	Avoid 1st trimester Poor fetal reserve	Contac, Coricidin Deconamine, Dimetapp Entex, Ornade, Naldecon Tavist, Triaminic Actifed, Benadryl Cold, Chlor-Trimeton, Novafed, Seldane D, Sudafed Comhist, Dimetane, Dristan, Histaforte, Naldecon, Ru-Tuss
Use of these agents for longer than 3–4 d can cause rebound nasal congestion		Privine Neo-Synephrine, Nostril, Vicks, Sinex Afrin, Dristan, Neo-Synephrine, Vicks Neo-Synephrine, Otrivin
Medical Conditions BPH Angle Closure Glaucoma **Medications** TCA, MAOIs	Avoid 1st trimester and during lactation	
Medical Conditions Avoid with continued high-dose use in asthmatics COPD	Avoid 1st trimester	Benylin, Cerose-DM, Conar, Delsym, Naldecon-DM, Pertussin, Robitussin DM, Tussar, Vicks Actifed-WC, Calcidrine, Dimetane-DC, Naldecon-CY, Novahistane-DH, Nucofed, Pediacof, Robitussin-AC/DAC, Triaminic, Tussar-2 Hydrocodone, Hycomine, Hycuss, P-V-Tussin, Ru-Tuss, Tussionex Breosin, Deconsal, Entex, Glycotuss, Glytuss, Humibid, Hytuss, Naldecon, Robitussin

agent successfully reduced household transmission with modest side effects. However, when used at higher doses, side effects as severe as the cold itself were encountered. For this reason and because of cost concerns, interferon is thought to be untenable for treatment for such a self-limited disease. Likewise, prophylactic vaccines have not been successful because the major cold viruses have too large an antigenic variation to make them effective or worthwhile. Successful vaccination against the common cold awaits the development of a vaccine against the most common rhinovirus types or against shared viral immunogens. Enviroxime, an antiviral spray, shows no protective benefit. Investigational agents that block the ICAM receptor and cellular penetration by the agent into the cell have yet to be proven successful and cost-effective.

Consequently, the current preventive measures are the common sense hygienic practices that have stood the test of time: reducing contact time with infected individuals, frequent handwashing with soap or topical disinfectants, covering the mouth when sneezing, and using disposable tissues. Bed rest is not necessary to facilitate recovery, and avoidance of work and school are necessary only if flu symptoms are present.

Treatment is aimed at palliation of the most unpleasant symptoms of colds: rhinorrhea, congestion, and cough. The five different classes of agents to treat these symptoms include the following:

- Sympathomimetics
- Antihistamines
- Analgesics
- Expectorants
- Cough suppressants.

Table 53-1 shows a breakdown of cold medicines and dosage guidelines.

The consumer is provided with numerous choices. Cough and cold formulas are available in single or combination forms delivered in one of several different vehicles: tablets, capsules, liquids, sprays, or powder. In addition to the classes listed earlier, anticholinergics, caffeine, and vitamins also may be found in combination drugs. Although most combination forms contain only two to three ingredients, some contain as many as eight! In general, it is recommended to treat a particular symptom with a single agent, limiting use of combination medications. This allows individualization of doses and avoidance of polypharmacy, which can produce adverse drug interactions and side effects. Prescription forms contain similar agents but have not applied for or obtained OTC status, although some may be stronger and consequently cannot be sold over the counter. Liquid cold formulas often contain alcohol as a preservative but can be obtained with alternative stabilizing agents. Agents that contain sugar, sucrose, or alcohol can potentially interfere with control of the brittle diabetic; however, metabolic studies suggest that short-term use at the recommended doses does not interfere with control in most diabetics. Indeed, an average of only 70 kcal per day are added. Table 53-2 shows a list of sugar- and alcohol-free forms available for the diabetic. Antibiotics play no role in treating the common cold unless bacterial superinfection is identified.

Sympathomimetics have been shown in controlled studies to decrease nasal congestion, increase nasal patency, and decrease rhinorrhea. Most forms are alpha-adrenergic agonists and act by stimulating release of norepinephrine or directly stimulating adrenergic receptors to produce vasoconstriction of the nasal mucosa. These are available in topical and systemic forms. In general, topical forms are faster acting and of stronger potency but can only be used for a limited time as they can cause rebound congestion after 4 to 5 days of use (rhinitis medicamentosa). Systemic forms provide a sustained duration of action but may be associated with annoying side effects such as elevated pulse rate, palpitations, anxiety, nervousness, dizziness, and anorexia. Susceptible individuals may develop marked tachycardia or arrhythmias and thus use should be limited in individuals with coronary artery disease or hyperthyroidism. Controlled studies have demonstrated that these agents are safe and do not significantly increase blood pressure in normal individuals or those with well-controlled hypertension, but may interfere the antihypertensive effect of certain medications, most notably, beta-blockers. Despite this, labeling precautions continue to advise against the use of these agents in hypertensive individuals. If systemic forms of these agents are chosen, they should be used for short periods and at low doses. Concomitant use of sympathomimetics with monoamine oxidase inhibitors can cause a lethal hypertensive crises. Likewise, use with guanethidine or guanadrel causes marked elevations in blood pressure. Finally, persons with benign prostatic hypertrophy also should avoid these agents because the can increase bladder outlet obstruction and lead to acute urinary retention.

Antihistamines are included in most combination cold formulas, despite their having little therapeutic effect. Viral-induced inflammation is not mediated through the histamine receptor, and therefore antihistamines have little direct benefit. Indirect benefits include modest drying of nasal secretions via atropine-like (anticholinergic) properties and sleepiness via the histamine receptors. Common antihistamines include the following: diphenhydramine (Benadryl), chlorpheniramine, brompheniramine, clemastine fumarate, pyrilamine maleate, and triprolidine HCl. The previously held notion that these agents should be used with caution in persons with asthma or chronic obstructive pulmonary diseases because of potential excessive drying of secretions has not been confirmed. The local anesthetic effect of Benadryl elixir gargles (2 teaspoons every 4 to 6 hours) with a liquid antacid such as magnesium hydroxide (Maalox; 2 teaspoons) is sometimes helpful in relieving pain from sore throat.

Analgesics are another common agent in combination preparations and usually include acetaminophen, a nonsteroidal antiinflammatory agent (NSAID), or aspirin. It is of theoretical concern that aspirin or NSAIDs may increase infection rate and viral shedding by interfering with the cyclooxygenase system and decreasing mucociliary clearance of retained material. However, placebo-controlled double-blind studies do not show this to be true. Instead, use of an analgesic provides significant benefit with decreased symptoms of headache, malaise, and myalgia.

Expectorants have been shown to decrease mucous viscosity in vitro but not in vivo. Doses ten times the recommended dose act as an emetic as well as increase the volume of respiratory secretions and mucociliary action, but at the recommended low doses do not appear to positively affect mucociliary clearance, sputum volume, or clinical course in controlled studies. For example, the most commonly used agent, guaifenesin, was found to be no more effective than placebo in reducing cough frequency or perceived sputum viscosity in controlled studies. These studies, however, were performed at much lower doses than the current recommended doses. Other expectorants work on the emetic principle and include terpin hydrate, the iodides (which have recently been taken off the market because of serious toxicity), and the historical use of ipecac syrup. Of these agents, guaifenesin has no reported serious side effects.

Cough suppressants act centrally to suppress the medullary cough center, or peripherally to anesthetize stretch or cough receptors in the respiratory tract. The centrally acting agents include the narcotics hydrocodone and codeine, and the chemically related but nonnarcotic dextromethorphan. In addition, diphenhydramine is believed to have modest cough-suppressant effects at the central level. Hydrocodone and codeine are controlled narcotic substances, dextromethorphan is available over the counter. Controlled studies show that on a milligram-to-milligram basis, dextromethorphan is equal to codeine in controlling cough. Hydrocodone is three times more potent on a milligram-to-milligram basis than codeine but also has increased addictive properties. These agents are indicated for controlling the bothersome nonproductive cough, nocturnal cough, or forceful cough associated with subconjunctival bleeds. The side effect profile is comparable; however, the psychiatric side effects are not as pronounced with dextromethorphan. Increasing the dose of dextromethorphan to 30 mg increases duration of action but not potency. The peripherally acting agents include benzonatate (Tessalon), which is structurally related to tetracaine and anesthetizes peripheral cough receptors; camphor and menthol, which have

Table 53-2. Sugar- and Alcohol-Free Cough and Cold Formulas

BRAND NAMES	SCHEDULE	AGENTS
Cerose-DM	OTC	Chlorpheniramine maleate 4 mg, phenylephrine HCl 10 mg, dextromethorphan HBr 15 mg
Codegest Expectorant	V	Phenylpropanolamine HCl 12.5 mg, codeine PO_4 10 mg, guaifenesin 100 mg
Conar Oral	OTC	Phenylephrine HCl 10 mg, dextromethorphan HBr 15 mg
Diabetic Tussin Ex		
Dimetapp Elixir	OTC	Brompheniramine maleate 4 mg, phenylephrine HCl 5 mg, phenylpropanolamine HCl 5 mg, Dextromethorphan HBr 15 mg
Entuss-D	III	Pseudoephedrine HCl 30 mg, hydrocodone bitartrate 5 mg
Entuss Ex	III	Hydrocodone bitartrate 5 mg, potassium guaiacolsulfonate 300 mg
Kwelcof	III	Hydrocodone bitartrate 5 mg, guaifenesin 100 mg
Lanatuss	III	Chlorpheniramine maleate 2 mg, phenylpropanolamine HCl 5 mg, guaifenesin 100 mg, sodium citrate 197 mg, citric acid 60 mg
Medatussin	RX	Chlorpheniramine maleate 2 mg, phenyltoloxamine citrate 25 mg, phenylpropanolamine HCl 25 mg, dextromethorphan HBr 20 mg, guaifenesin 100 mg
Naldecon-CX	V	Phenylpropanolamine HCl 12.5 mg, codeine PO_4 10 mg, guaifenesin 200 mg
Naldecon-DX	OTC	Phenylpropanolamine HCl 12.5 mg, dextromethorphan HBr 10 mg, guaifenesin 200 mg
Codiclear DH	V	Hydrocodone bitartate 5 mg, guafenesin 100 mg
Hycomine Syrup	III	Phenylpropanalamine HCl 25 mg, hydrocodone 5 mg
Noratuss II liquid	OTC	Pseudoephedrine HCl 15 mg, dextromethorphan HBr 3.75 mg, guaifenesin 50 mg
Ornade-DM 30	OTC	Chlorpheniramine maleate 2 mg, phenylpropanalamine HCl 15 mg, dextromethorphan 30 mg
Ryna-C Liquid	V	Chlorpheniramine 2 mg, pseudoephedrine HCl 30 mg, codeine PO_4 10 mg
Tussionex Oral Suspension	III	Phenyltoloxamine polistirex 10 mg, hydrocodone polistirex 5 mg

anesthetizing aromatic properties; and throat lozenges, which merely lubricate inflamed mucosa and decrease irritative cough.

Nonmedical remedies are age old but only recently have been studied in a scientific fashion. Humidified air offers an attractive homeopathic, natural remedy with no major side effects. This treatment was hoped to be palliative as well as curative. Rhinovirus replicates best at the lower temperatures found in the nasal passages (33° to 34°C); increasing the temperature above 33°C was intended to reduce viral replication and subsequent shedding. Many people do experience transient amelioration of nasal obstruction with humidity. In fact, initial studies showed promising results of greater than 80% reduction in symptoms. Moreover, viral shedding was reported to be decreased at temperatures of 43°C, but local discomfort became excessive at this temperature. Placebo-controlled trials have been unable to confirm the initial results. Other home remedies include petroleum jelly for sore fissured nostrils and gargling with salt water for sore throats.

CONSIDERATIONS IN PREGNANCY

During pregnancy or lactation cough or cold suppressants should be used with caution, at low doses, and for short periods of time. Single agents targeted to a particular problem should be used if possible. In general, all cough and cold formulas should be avoided during the first trimester, during organogenesis. Bed rest, fluids, and other supportive measures should be tried to alleviate self-limited but aggravating symptoms. The reader is urged to review the references that clearly detail medication use during pregnancy. Most studies regarding use of several cough and cold medications are retrospective; therefore, they can only suggest associations but not causal relationships of minor birth anomalies. Agents implicated with potential birth anomalies if used during the first trimester include codeine, brompheniramine, diphenhydramine, and pseudoephedrine. Acetaminophen is believed to be safe at the recommended doses during the first trimester. Dextromethorphan has not been shown to be associated with birth anomalies, but current recommendations are to avoid use during the first trimester unless cough is severe. Use during the second and third trimester is less worrisome. Pseudoephedrine and dextromethorphan are believed to be safe to use during this time. NSAIDs should not be used to treat cold symptoms during pregnancy because of potential bleeding concerns; they also pose a risk for premature closure of the ductus arteriosus, which can cause fetal pulmonary hypertension if used during the third trimester. Codeine, pseudoephedrine, and other sympathomimetics are safe at low doses during the second and third trimester. No sympathomimetic should be used if there is preexisting hypertension or poor fetal reserve. All agents appear in breast milk in low amounts. Antihistamines with high anticholinergic properties may inhibit milk production in lactating women and may cause newborn agitation.

BIBLIOGRAPHY

Berkowitz RL, Coustan DR, Mochizuki TK. Handbook for prescribing medications during pregnancy, 2nd ed. Boston: Little, Brown, 1986:1, 27, 101, 107, 207, 253, 276

Drugs used to treat upper respiratory tract disorders. In: Drug evaluations annual: 1995. Chicago: American Medical Association, 1995:493.

Gwaltney JM Jr. The common cold: upper respiratory tract infections. In: Mandell GL, Bennett JC, Dolin R, eds. Mandell, Douglas and Bennett's principles and practice of infectious diseases, 4th ed. New York: Churchill Livingstone, 1995:489.

Lowenstein S, Parrino T. Management of the common cold. Adv Intern Med 1987;32:207.

Monto AS. The common cold: cold water on hot news. JAMA 1994;271:1122.

Younbluth M. Infectious mononucleosis and viral infections of the upper respiratory tract. In: Schulman ST, Phair JP, and Sommers HM, eds. The biologic and clinical basis of infectious disease, 4th ed. Philadelphia: WB Saunders, 1991:120.

Primary Care for Women, edited by Phyllis C. Leppert and Fred M. Howard. Lippincott-Raven Publishers, Philadelphia © 1997.

54

Asthma

ANTHONY J. FEDULLO

Asthma is a common chronic respiratory disease, affecting about 5% of adults. It is characterized by reversible airway obstruction, traditionally thought to be due to bronchial muscle hyperreactivity. More recently, inflammation within the airway has been recognized as an important component of obstruction. Asthma can be severe: in 15% to 20% of patients with asthma, the disease limits their activity, and more than 50% of patients with asthma seek help from a health care provider each year. The prevalence and severity of the disease have reportedly increased in the United States recently, particularly in urban areas. This may reflect changes in the urban environment or inadequacies in health care delivery, prevention, and treatment in these areas. An increase in asthma deaths has also been observed, attributed in part to the overuse or abuse of β-agonist medication, but very likely also having a basis in poor care and control of asthma.

The prevalence of asthma does not differ greatly among adult men and women. In childhood and early adolescence, boys are more often affected; women predominate among the elderly. The prevalence of asthma is highest in childhood, but it can appear at any age. Adult-onset asthma or recurrence of asthma in adults after teenage remission is not unusual. The prevalence varies among racial and ethnic groups; African-Americans have a higher prevalence of asthma than do whites.

ETIOLOGY

The precise etiology of asthma is unknown, but it may have a basis in atopy or allergy. Asthmatics have higher rates of reaction to the antigens used in skin testing than do nonasthmatics. Asthmatics also more commonly have a history of other atopic disorders (eg, hay fever, allergic rhinitis, eczema). Fifty percent or more of asthmatics have nasal allergic symptoms as well, and about one third of patients with allergic rhinitis have had episodes of asthma. Asthmatics often have a family history of atopy. The history need not include asthma itself, but many asthmatics have relatives with other allergic disorders, such as hay fever.

Although asthma has a link to allergic conditions, it is not a purely allergic disorder. Allergy is not the major precipitating factor in many asthmatics. Asthma is often exacerbated by cold air, emotional states, and airborne irritants such as cigarette smoke that do not act by allergic mechanisms.

The exact nature of the relation between asthma and allergy remains uncertain, but more is known about the basic mechanisms causing symptoms once asthma is present. Asthma has long been considered a disease of airway hyperreactivity, whereby bronchial smooth muscle contraction would constrict airways, causing the airflow limitation and wheezing associated with the disease. Evidence of bronchial smooth muscle hyperreactivity in asthmatics is found in the increased bronchial constriction occurring with cholinergic agents such as methacholine and with β-sympathomimetic antagonists or blockers such as propranolol. These agents are contraindicated in asthma. Similarly, anticholinergic agents such as atropine and ipratropium and sympathomimetic agents such as epinephrine and albuterol are used therapeutically.

Emphasis has been placed recently on a mechanism of airway obstruction in asthma that is not primarily related to smooth muscle hyperreactivity. Inflammation is increasingly being seen as a predominant factor in asthma, causing excessive mucus hypersecretion, mucus cell and mucus gland hyperplasia, and edema and inflammatory infiltration of the airway wall. This mechanism explains the mucus secretion and productive cough that often accompany asthma in the absence of infection. Evidence of inflammation is seen in the mucus-packed airways of patients who die with severe asthma, as well as the finding of active inflammatory cells in bronchoalveolar lavage specimens from asthmatics. The degree of inflammation does not seem to be related to whether asthma is triggered by allergic or nonallergic factors.

Many mediators can cause the inflammatory changes in the airways as well as bronchoconstriction, although the prime role of any particular one has not been identified. Mast cells and histamine release, prostaglandins and leukotrienes, macrophages, eosinophils, and lymphocyte products all play a role. Specific agents against these or other mediators may someday be available for therapy. At present, nonspecific antiinflammatory agents such as corticosteroids, cromolyn, and nedocromil play an important role in asthma therapy.

The basic mechanisms of inflammation and bronchoconstriction remain uncertain, but asthma attacks or exacerbations are triggered by fairly well-defined clinical variables. *Allergens* remain a prominent factor in inducing an asthma attack. Seasonal allergens such as trees, grass, or weeds are a factor in many asthma attacks, as are the more subtle influences of allergens such as the ubiquitous dust mite or molds containing *Aspergillus* species. Removal or avoidance of these environmental factors or desensitization to specific allergens is a prominent part of asthma therapy. *Air pollution* has been associated with asthma exacerbation. Ozone and sulfur dioxide cause an increase in airway resistance and obstruction; this may play a role in the increased prevalence of asthma in cities. The relation between *occupational triggers* and asthma is often made by obtaining a history of exacerbation with exposure to the offending agent (eg, certain wood dusts in hobbyists or carpenters; chemicals such as toluene diisocyanate used in the plastics industry; flour or animal excreta in flour ["baker's asthma"]). *Viral respiratory infections*, but not bacterial ones, are common precipitants of asthma attacks. *Cold air* and *exercise* are common asthma triggers. The mechanism is thought to be due to cooling and dehydration of the airway mucosa, causing the release of inflammatory mediators. Outdoor jogging in cold, dry, winter air is more likely to cause an asthma exacerbation than is swimming in a heated indoor pool. *Emotional factors* can trigger episodes of acute asthma. The mechanism is uncertain, but anger, anxiety, and unresolved conflicts have been recognized as triggers for asthma exacerbation.

Nocturnal exacerbation of asthma is common. Nocturnal awakening with asthma usually occurs between 2 and 5 a.m. and is thought to be due to circadian differences in ventilation and mediator release. In many asthmatics, nocturnal awakening is a prominent part of their symptomatology. Nocturnal awakening may also represent inadequate daytime asthma control. Many asthmatics can tolerate considerable declines in pulmonary function and not complain of daytime symptoms. The physiologic increase in airway resistance at night may then more easily trigger symptoms as the airways become further narrowed.

There is an interesting relation between asthma and the *menstrual cycle*. Premenstrual worsening of asthma occurs in about a third of women. Studies of airway function do not show large declines in pulmonary function, and the mechanism of the symptomatic exacerbation is uncertain. Fluid retention and changes in circulating progesterone have been suggested, but no convincing physiologic correlates to this clinical observation have been found. *Pregnancy* can affect the severity or frequency of asthma. The complex hormonal and psychological effects of pregnancy must be related to this phenomenon, but the specifics are uncertain. About one third of pregnant asthmatics have worse asthma during pregnancy, one third have improved disease, and one third are unaffected. Good control of asthma is important in pregnancy to ensure adequate fetal oxygenation.

Some asthmatic patients are sensitive to *ingested* material. In adults, this is an uncommon trigger of asthma but should be recognized. Shellfish can produce severe bronchoconstriction. Sulfites, contained in some alcoholic beverages or used in the preservation of foods such as salads, may exacerbate asthma. The mechanism is uncertain, but it is less likely to be allergenic than due to the release of endogenous sulfur dioxide through the airway mucosa. Tartrazine yellow, a food coloring, has been associated with asthma induction. This is thought to be due to effects on prostaglandin metabolism and production.

Drugs can exacerbate or trigger asthma. Any agent that produces anaphylaxis can cause airway edema and wheezing. β-Sympathomimetic blockers, often used in the therapy of hypertension and angina, can affect bronchomotor tone, resulting in enhanced bronchoconstriction. Asthmatics should not take these drugs systemically. Some asthmatics are sensitive even to eye drops that contain them. A few asthmatics are sensitive to aspirin and other antiinflammatory agents. In these asthmatics, the disease is usually of adult onset, with nasal polyposis and rhinitis. The mechanism is thought to be the changes in prostaglandin metabolism and production induced by these drugs. Acetaminophen does not share these effects and can be used safely by asthmatics.

Animal proteins from *pets and dust mites* can be prominent asthma triggers. They can permeate a home and cause asthma in the absence of a pet, indeed even long after a pet has been removed.

These and other possible asthma triggers must be considered when interviewing the asthmatic. Important parts of asthma therapy are recognizing asthma triggers and avoiding them (or instituting prophylactic treatment if avoidance is impossible). This is as important as providing medical therapy for the symptoms.

DIFFERENTIAL DIAGNOSIS

The differential diagnosis of asthma involves the symptoms of cough, shortness of breath, and wheezing. Upper airway obstruction can cause these symptoms; this should be considered in patients who do not have a prior history of asthma. Epiglottitis, for example, should be considered in a patient who has dysphagia and painful swallowing; it is not a disease confined to children. Involvement of the cricoarytenoid joint in rheumatoid arthritis can also present with upper airway narrowing and wheezing, as can laryngeal carcinoma. Stridorous wheezing from an upper airway abnormality should be considered an emergency. The residual airway may be very small (millimeters) by the time wheezing and shortness of breath from an upper airway cause become apparent. These upper airway causes are much less common than asthma but should be considered in adults who have wheezing and shortness of breath without a prior history of asthma. Clues to an upper airway cause for wheezing include a wheeze heard prominently over the central airways in the neck, a predominantly inspiratory component to the wheezing (stridor) rather than the predominantly expiratory wheezing in asthma, and arterial blood gas measurements that show a normal or near-normal oxygen level (taking into account the inspired oxygen concentration) relative to the degree of respiratory distress exhibited.

Congestive heart failure can present with wheezing due to compression of the small airways by interstitial edema. This diagnosis is usually apparent from other physical findings and from the chest x-ray. Pulmonary embolism can sometimes have associated wheezing due to the release of bronchoconstricting mediators.

HISTORY

Patients with asthma complain of intermittent cough, shortness of breath, and wheezing. All these symptoms need not be present in each patient; some patients with asthma have cough as their only complaint. The symptoms are episodic and intermittent, vary in intensity, and are often related to particular events such as exercise, cold air, or exposure to allergens. Patients may describe their asthma as a tightness or heaviness in the chest. This complaint in older asthmatics suggests angina as a differential diagnosis. Nocturnal awakening with shortness of breath and wheezing is common and may suggest congestive heart failure. Symptoms may be chronic in patients who are not adequately treated or who have underlying chronic bronchitis or emphysema, but even in these patients the symptoms vary in intensity when an asthmatic component is present, depending on exposure to exacerbating factors.

The relation of symptoms to asthma severity as measured by pulmonary function tests is imprecise: some patients have symptoms with only slight airway obstruction, and others have few symptoms with severe obstruction. Many patients have no symptoms until airway function, as measured by the forced expiratory volume in 1 second (FEV_1), falls by 30% to 40%. The absence of symptoms, therefore, does not necessarily indicate adequate treatment. Pulmonary function may still be quite abnormal, leaving the patient susceptible to recurrent symptoms.

PHYSICAL EXAMINATION AND CLINICAL FINDINGS

Patients with asthma may have a normal examination, in keeping with the intermittent and episodic nature of the disease. During an asthma attack, findings of airway obstruction such as a prolonged expiratory time or expiratory wheezing are found. These findings can be made more obvious by asking the patient to take a deep breath and perform a forced expiration. The intensity of wheezing is not a good marker for the severity of asthma: slight obstruction may cause easily audible wheezing because of the large volume and velocity of air moving through obstructed airways. A cough may be present, and it may sound congested or "moist." As asthma increases in severity, evidence of tachypnea and respiratory distress becomes evident. Wheezing may not be as prominent because severe obstruction may allow little airflow. An increased pulsus paradoxus (> 20 mm Hg) also reflects more severe asthma. Predominantly inspiratory wheezing suggests upper airway obstruction, and rales and a gallop rhythm suggest congestive heart failure.

LABORATORY AND IMAGING STUDIES

During asthma attacks, pulmonary function tests show a decreased peak expiratory flow (PEF) and a decreased FEV_1, particularly when compared to the forced vital capacity (FVC). Inexpensive PEF measuring devices are available. Measuring the PEF helps patients with asthma monitor their own disease and allows recognition of the early phases of an exacerbation. Reduced PEF and a reduced FEV_1/FVC ratio are nonspecific for asthma and are also found in bronchitis and emphysema. The clinical findings should allow the physician to distinguish emphysema and chronic bronchitis from asthma. Bronchitis and emphysema have chronic symptomatology and evidence of chronic airway obstruction, in contrast to the intermittent and episodic nature of asthma. However, it is sometimes difficult to separate these entities, and they often coexist, particularly in the older patient who has smoked heavily.

One useful characteristic of asthma on pulmonary function tests is improvement after the use of bronchodilator medication. A 15% to 20% improvement in the FEV_1 suggests the presence of reversible airway obstruction, characteristic of asthma. Sometimes the improvement is seen predominantly in the FVC; this is also considered evidence of bronchodilator responsiveness. Absence of bronchodilator response on pulmonary function testing does not exclude asthma, because when patients are severely obstructed, a single treatment with bronchodilator medication may not produce benefit.

If the patient has intermittent symptoms but at the time of the examination or pulmonary function testing has no wheezing or normal airway function, asthma challenge tests can be used. The challenge test most frequently done in pulmonary function laboratories is the inhalation of serial concentrations of methacholine. A positive test is a 20% fall in FEV_1 from baseline. Some laboratories use cold air inhalation or exercise as a challenge. Occasionally, specific challenges are done with agents involved in occupational exposures. However, there is often little need for this in the presence of a history suggesting occupational asthma, and the tests are poorly standardized as to the dose of the agent.

The chest x-ray in asthma is usually normal or shows hyperinflation if the obstruction is severe. Allergic bronchopulmonary aspergillosis, which may affect a few asthmatics, may show infiltrates on chest x-rays, representing mucus impaction.

An increased number of eosinophils on the complete blood count may be seen, but the absence of this finding does not exclude asthma. Immunoglobulin E levels are elevated in many asthmatics. Very high levels (> 1500 ng/mL) suggest allergic bronchopulmonary aspergillosis. Asthmatic patients may have skin test hyperreactivity to antigens, but the antigens causing skin reactions do not correlate well with those that cause symptomatic asthma exacerbation.

TREATMENT

There are two goals of asthma therapy. One goal is to control symptoms so that the patient is asymptomatic at rest and can perform normal daily activities. The second goal is to keep the PEF normal. This is particularly important in the difficult-to-control patient. Treating to symptom relief only can leave a considerable deficit in pulmonary function and can predispose to symptomatic asthma episodes when the patient is exposed to triggering factors.

Treatment of asthma must be tailored to the patient. Avoidance of inciting factors, when possible, is the first step in treatment. Smoking, for example, should be avoided. Some asthmatics are bothered by pets, and removing the animals may be helpful. It often takes a considerable amount of time for the house to be cleaned of all animal products, as animal proteins may be in the carpets and upholstered furniture. Removing mold in the environment and careful cleaning with regard to dust mites are useful. Some asthmatics are sensitive to sulfites in alcoholic beverages, others to aspirin and nonsteroidal antiinflammatory agents, and still others to exposures at work. To avoid or minimize these and other agents triggering asthma, they must first be identified by obtaining a careful history regarding exacerbating factors.

Mild asthmatics with infrequent exacerbations may be treated with inhaled β_2-agonists, two puffs by a metered-dose inhaler. Of the many agents in this class, a commonly used one is albuterol. These agents may be used at the onset of a mild asthma attack or preferably are used prophylactically against factors that consistently result in symptoms.

In patients with more than mild asthma (exacerbations more than a few times a week or exacerbations that last more than an hour or two each), the next step in therapy is to add an inhaled antiinflammatory agent administered by a metered-dose inhaler two to four times daily, not used just when symptoms occur. In children, cromolyn is often chosen; in adults, inhaled corticosteroids are usually the first choice. If on this regimen the patient still has a few attacks of asthma a week, each episode lasting more than a few hours, or has nocturnal asthma, inhaled β-agonists can be taken on a regular basis, not only as needed. Additional use (two or three times daily as needed) may be allowed, but beyond that additional agents are probably necessary, or the patient should seek more definitive care for a refractory attack. The frequent use of inhaled β-agonist medication has been associated with increased mortality in asthma, although this phenomenon may reflect mortality due to uncontrolled asthma in which the patient overused the β-agonist rather than seeking more definitive care. Rather than regular use of a β-agonist, a sustained-release theophylline preparation may be given. Achieving blood levels of 5 to 15 ng/mL is satisfactory. The likelihood of toxicity increases above this point, and additional clinical benefit is not great.

Whether theophylline or regular use of β-agonists is chosen as the next step in therapy after inhaled antiinflammatory medication, the other agent can be added to the regimen if attacks persist more than a few times weekly, if they last more than an hour or two, or if there is nocturnal awakening,

Ipratropium is an anticholinergic bronchodilator available in a metered-dose inhaler. Its use is often advocated in the patient with chronic obstructive pulmonary disease who has a bronchospastic component, but it is efficacious in asthma and has no side effects. Some prefer to add this to regular use of β-agonists rather than theophylline, particularly in patients sensitive to theophylline's side effects.

Antibiotics are not routinely administered to younger patients with asthmatic exacerbations. In older patients with underlying chronic obstructive pulmonary disease, acute bacterial bronchitis is more common and may be associated with exacerbations of dyspnea and wheezing; antibiotics are frequently given in this case.

It is important to treat aggressively asthma that does not respond well to a maintenance therapeutic regimen. Episodes of asthma that do not respond to full-dose inhaler medication and theophylline, or respond only transiently and increasingly poorly, should be recognized within a few days so that a course of oral corticosteroids can be offered. Patients must be instructed to alert their physician to this change and not to use increasingly frequent doses of β-agonist inhalers. The course of steroids can be relatively short if exacerbations that become refractory to routine medication are treated early (within a few days of determining their refractoriness). For example, 40 to 50 mg prednisone given once daily for 3 or 4 days and stopped without tapering can result in amelioration of asthma sufficient to allow control to be again achieved with inhaled medication. If, in a refractory exacerbation, the use of oral corticosteroids is avoided for weeks, the inflammatory component, with mucus hypersecretion and mucosal cell hypertrophy, becomes so prominent that a much longer course of corticosteroids, even hospitalization, may become necessary. The increasing mortality in asthma may reflect avoidance in definitive therapy of refractory exacerbations, hesitancy to use corticosteroids promptly, and overuse of inhaled β-agonists.

Many patients with asthma visit the emergency department or require hospitalization. These patients have acute severe attacks or attacks that have not responded well to outpatient therapy, including a trial of corticosteroids. Unless the patient responds very well in the emergency department, consultation with physicians trained in general internal medicine, pulmonary medicine, or allergy and immunology (depending on the practice patterns in the area) is useful. These specialists can help determine the need for hospitalization, can help manage these often very ill patients, and can give advice on the postdischarge outpatient regimen.

For the very ill patient in the emergency department or one who requires admission, a patient under age 40 may receive subcutaneous epinephrine or terbutaline; this can be repeated every 20 minutes for three doses. Intravenous corticosteroids are started at a dosage of 40 to 60 mg methylprednisolone every 6 to 8 hours. Inhaled β-agonists are given via nebulization four to six times daily. As the patient improves, intravenous corticosteroids are stopped and the patient is switched to oral prednisone 40 to 60 mg/day, to be tapered over 2 to 3 weeks, and the nebulized β-agonist is changed to a metered-dose inhaler.

The use of chronic corticosteroids is sometimes necessary in severe asthma. Because of the side effects associated with long-term use of corticosteroids, it is useful to embark on this therapy in conjunction with help from consulting physicians. Patients who need long-term corticosteroid therapy for control of asthma should be on a maximal regimen of less toxic drugs and should take the lowest dose of corticosteroid to provide asthma control, preferably on an every-other-day basis.

Skin testing and desensitization are controversial in the management of patients with asthma. This therapy should not be offered routinely. Many asthmatics do not have trigger factors that are allergic in nature, and even among asthmatics who have allergic asthma, the results of desensitization are often marginal. Most asthmatics can be treated successfully with inhaled agents, and desensitization adds little to their need for medications or asthma control. Desensitization should be considered only in asthmatics who are difficult to control and have strong seasonal or allergic components to their asthma, as evaluated by history and observation. Before initiating this, the patient should be on a maximal inhaled bronchodilator regimen, perhaps with the use of theophylline as well, and should have the environment investigated thoroughly to avoid exacerbating agents whenever possible.

CONSIDERATIONS IN PREGNANCY

Asthma is the most common chronic disease affecting pregnant women. About 5% to 7% of women of childbearing age have asthma. About equal proportions of women have their asthma improve, worsen, or remain unchanged during pregnancy. Asthma in subsequent pregnancies behaves similarly.

The major risk to the fetus results from maternal hypoxemia. Hypoxemia, which can be significant even in mild asthma, can threaten fetal oxygenation. Respiratory alkalosis from asthma-induced hyperventilation can produce fetal vasoconstriction, further compromising oxygen delivery to the fetus. Poorly controlled asthma in pregnancy has measurable adverse effects on fetal outcome. Epidemiologic studies have shown an increase in preterm births and increased neonatal mortality. Some studies suggest an increased incidence of preeclampsia in women with asthma.

Asthma, although it may not limit the woman's activity, carries a serious risk to the fetus because of the low blood oxygen values. Treatment of asthma in pregnancy is not significantly different than that previously outlined. Epinephrine is avoided because of its constrictive effects on the vasculature, but inhaled β_2-agonists, inhaled corticosteroids and other inflammatory agents, theophylline, and even courses of oral corticosteroids should be used as the clinical circumstances warrant. The goal is asthma control and normalization of pulmonary function tests, just as it is in the non-pregnant woman.

To reiterate, very mild asthmatics may be treated as needed with inhaled β-agonists. Asthmatics with more than a few episodes of asthma weekly, or episodes lasting more than an hour, should begin regular therapy with inhaled corticosteroids. If control is not achieved, regular β_2-agonist use or therapy with a sustained-release theophylline preparation should be instituted. A short course of oral corticosteroids can be used for refractory exacerbations. More severe asthma requiring emergency department visits or hospitalization can be treated with intravenous corticosteroids and bronchodilators given by nebulization.

Consultative help in the care of the pregnant asthmatic is often useful. In addition to assistance in medical management, it offers the opportunity to reinforce patient education regarding the need for good control of asthma and medication compliance, and it can help ease the concern patients feel about taking medication during pregnancy.

BIBLIOGRAPHY

Bailey WC. Symposium on asthma. Clin Chest Med 1984;5:557.

Chan-Yeung M, Lam S. Occupational asthma. Am Rev Respir Dis 1986;133:686.

Corticosteroids: their biologic mechanisms and application to the treatment of asthma. Am Rev Respir Dis 1990;141(suppl):S1.

Executive summary: guidelines for the diagnosis and management of asthma. U.S. Dept. of Health and Human Services, Public Health Service, National Institutes of Health, June 1991. Publication #91-3042A.

Frazier CA, ed. Occupational asthma. New York: Van Nostrand Reinhold Co., 1980.

Holgate S. Mediator and cytokine mechanisms in asthma. Thorax 1993;48:103.

Lang DM, Polansky M. Patterns of asthma mortality in Philadelphia from 1969 to 1991. N Engl J Med 1994;331:1542.

Management of asthma during pregnancy. U.S. Dept. of Health and Human Services, Public Health Service, National Institutes of Health, September 1993. NIH Publication #93-3279.

Martin RJ. Asthma. Semin Respir Critical Care Med 1994;15:97.

Pauli BD, Reid RL, Munt PW, Wigle RD, Forkert L. Influence of the menstrual cycle on airway function in asthmatic and normal subjects. Am Rev Respir Dis 1989;140:358.

Rakel RE, Cockcroft DW, Lieberman P, et al. Improved management of asthma: putting today's knowledge to use. J Respir Dis 1994;15:S1.

Scanlon PD, Beck KC. Methacholine inhalation challenge. Mayo Clin Proc 1994;69:1118.

55

Tuberculosis

ANTHONY J. FEDULLO

Primary Care for Women, edited by Phyllis C. Leppert and Fred M. Howard. Lippincott-Raven Publishers, Philadelphia © 1997.

Disease due to *Mycobacterium tuberculosis* has been known to humankind for thousands of years. Archeologic evidence of bony disease and descriptions of the clinical syndrome from literate societies indicate its long-standing problem as a human pathogen. Tuberculosis as a disease is impacted by the social and economic environment. Urbanization of civilization has resulted in increasing acquisition and death rates from the disease. In the late 1800s, the rates from tuberculosis in urban areas approached 300 to 400 per 100,000, far above levels in the country. Decline in tuberculosis acquisition and mortality began before the antibiotic era, due to improvements in urban crowding, public hygiene, and increased public health awareness with identification of cases and isolation. In the 1940s, streptomycin was shown to be an effective agent in the treatment of tuberculosis. Shortly after its introduction, however, organisms resistant to its use as a single agent appeared, a lesson that remains pertinent to tuberculous therapy today. In the early 1950s, isoniazid was introduced, and by 1985 the number of annually reported patients had fallen from 84,000 in 1953 to 22,000, most of whom had reactivation of previously acquired disease. This decline hid some disturbing statistics, however. Tuberculosis still was distressingly common in some urban communities and among minorities and immigrant groups. Adverse socioeconomic conditions, drug dependency and abuse, and rising rates of HIV infection led to an increase in tuberculosis in certain segments of the urban population. There are 4000 to 5000 more cases of tuberculosis in 1991 than the cases reported in 1984, many due to recent acquisition of disease rather than reactivation of remotely acquired disease, and the increase is predicted to continue. In addition to the increase in the prevalence of disease, strains of mycobacteria resistent to multiple antibiotics have emerged, due to poor compliance with medications as well as importation of resistant strains from areas where single drug therapy has fostered resistance.

ETIOLOGY

There are more than 50 species in the genus Mycobacterium. The pathogenic Mycobacterium tuberculosis complex includes four of these, *Mycobacterium tuberculosis, Mycobacterium bovis, Mycobacterium africanum,* and *Mycobacterium microti.* Most clinical disease in this group is caused by *Mycobacterium tuberculosis,* and the term tuberculosis bacillus henceforth refers to this organism unless noted otherwise.

Mycobacterium species other than *M. tuberculosis* can cause disease. *Mycobacterium avium* complex (which includes *M. avium* and *M. intracellulare*), *M. kansasii, M. scrofulaceium, M. fortuitum,* and *M. chelonae* can cause human disease. These organisms are not usually transmitted from individual to individual, but are likely acquired from soil or water. These and other Mycobacteria can colonize individuals without causing infection or disease, so their presence alone does not necessarily indicate the need for treatment.

Mycobacterium tuberculosis is acquired by inhalation of infected aerosol particles containing the organism. Although deposition of a few organisms in the alveolus can produce infection, tuberculous infection is not acquired by all patients who come into contact with patients who are excreting bacillae in their sputum. It is estimated that even with close contact, only one out of three persons become infected, and with casual contact the likelihood of acquiring tuberculosis is much lower. Proximity, circulation of air, and crowding are important factors in increasing the likelihood of acquiring tuberculosis. The amount of bacilli shed in the sputum is a risk factor for acquiring tuberculosis. Individuals who have negative sputum stains for AFB but are positive on culture are much less infectious than those with positive stains. Patients become noninfectious, even if their sputum is still stain-positive, within 2 weeks of initiation of therapy. Transmission of organisms can be decreased by avoiding open coughing. The major risk of acquiring tuberculosis is in instances in which the disease is not suspected and the patient is coughing into a poorly ventilated environment or is in close contact with other individuals. This may occur in the community before the patient is recognized as requiring medical attention, or in the hospital if tuberculosis is not considered in the differential diagnosis.

After inhalation of tuberculous bacilli, local defense mechanisms in the lung such as macrophages and lymphocytes attack the organism in a fairly nonspecific fashion. If the organism survives, it multiplies locally. Under ideal circumstances, the organism can replicate every 24 hours, but the usual rate of growth is much slower than this due to continuing local defense mechanism. During the first month of infection, local reaction in the lung may cause tuberculous pneumonia with adjacent lymph node involvement. This can often be asymptomatic, or only minimally symptomatic. During this same interval of time, tuberculosis is spread hematogenously throughout the body to areas such as the lung apices, kidney, and meninges, becoming foci for later reactivation. After a month or two of this process, specific cell-mediated immunity develops and attacks the mycobacteria within the lung and wherever hematogenously dispersed. This usually results in containment of the infection and is manifest on the x-ray occasionally by small calcified focus. During this interval, the tuberculin skin test becomes positive as a marker of infection. If the disease cannot be contained by the specific immune response, disseminated disease occurs with multiple areas of tuberculosis throughout the lung (miliary tuberculosis) as well as involvement of other organs such as the meninges, kidneys, and bone. Dissemination occurs more frequently in infants and very young children, those who have specific immunocompromise, such as patients with immunologic malignancies or HIV infection, and in individuals who are non-specifically immunocompromised, such as by old age or malnutrition.

Ordinarily, tuberculous infection is contained rather than disseminated. This sets the stage for reactivation tuberculosis, which is the commonest presentation of clinical disease. Risk of reactivation disease is at its highest in the first few years after acquisition of infection, and may be 3% to 5% in that interval. After that time, the risk is lower, perhaps 0.1% to 0.2% yearly. The specific mechanisms favoring reactivation are unknown, but change in the local and systemic immune status relative to the organisms present in the lung tilt in favor of the organism, and tuberculous bacilli begin to multiply in these areas. In the lung, these areas are usually in the posterior part of the upper lobes of the lung, although it can occur in other areas as well. When the organism begins to grow, the body's immune response often leads to an inflammatory lesion with local necrosis, leading to the cavitary disease that on chest x-ray is characteristic in about half of patients with reactivation pulmonary disease. Reactivation may take place in other areas where the tuberculous bacilli has been disseminated. Approximately 10% to 20% of reactivation tuberculosis may occur in areas outside of the lung parenchyma, although many of these are accompanied by parenchymal reactivation as well. The genitourinary tract, bones and joints, meninges, and gastrointestinal tract are among the areas in which reactivation disease may be seen.

DIFFERENTIAL DIAGNOSIS

The differential diagnosis of tuberculosis can be broad, depending on the phase of the disease. For example, it is in the differential diagnosis of pneumonia, particularly if symptoms are chronic and nonresolving with routine antibiotic therapy. If pulmonary tuberculosis is associated with cavitary disease on chest x-ray, anaerobic lung abscess, fungal infections of the lung, and noninfectious causes such as malignancy, and Wegener's granulomatosis need to be considered. If tuberculosis presents with a pleural effusion, the effusion is often large and unilateral. This differential diagnosis would include malignancy and a parapneumonia effusion or empyema associated with another bacterial infection. When tuberculosis occurs in nonpulmonary sites, fever without apparent cause can be a predominant manifestation, and other causes of persistent fever such as malignancy, bacterial endocarditis, and other occult infections need to be considered.

HISTORY

The history relevant to the acquisition of tuberculosis and can be divided into that which occurs during primary infection and that which can occur with reactivation. Primary infection was usually seen in children when the disease was more endemic in the population. Now, it is often a disease of adults. The primary infection is often asymptomatic. About 25% of patients will have symptoms such as fever, cough, and fatigue. If an x-ray is taken during this time, a mid–lung zone infiltrate may be seen that is noncavitary and is not specific for tuberculosis. This presentation is similar to that of any bacterial pneumonia, and since a natural history is most often toward containment of the infection and resolution of symptoms, the possibility of tuberculosis may not be considered further.

Pleural involvement is usually a manifestation of primary tuberculosis, although it can occur in reactivation disease. Disease may occur from rupture of a subpleural focus of tuberculosis into the pleural space, and usually occurs within weeks to months of acquisition of the infection. Symptoms are nonspecific and include fever, pleuritic chest pain, and shortness of breath if the pleural effusion is large.

Lymph node enlargement may be a symptom of primary disease. The lymph node enlargement is usually not painful, and fever and systemic symptoms may be slight.

Occasionally, the primary infection is not locally contained, and progressive primary tuberculosis ensues. The immunocompromised population, particularly patients with HIV infection with low CD4 counts, are susceptible to progressive disease. Persistent fever, cough and fatigue, and a nonresolving or worsening clinical course and x-ray despite routine antibiotic therapy should raise the question of tuberculosis.

Primary infection, although usually locally contained by the immune system, may present as widely disseminated or miliary disease. Immunosuppresion predisposes to this form of tuberculosis, and young children, the elderly, and those weakened by malnutrition are also at increased risk, Fever may be the predominant symptom, and disseminated tuberculosis is still a prominent cause of "fever of unknown origin." Evidence of dissemination may not be visible on the chest x-ray in the early part of the illness. Because the infection is widely spread, symptoms such as headache or lethargy may indicate meningeal involvement, abdominal pain may indicate intestinal or peritoneal involvement, and pyuria or hematuria may indicate genitourinary tract involvement.

Reactivation pulmonary disease may present with symptoms of cough, hemoptysis, and fever, or more subtle symptoms such as fatigue, anorexia, weight loss, and night sweats. Symptoms may be very slight in reactivation pulmonary disease; an occasional cough may be all that is present. Pleural involvement, again usually a manifestation of primary acquisition of infection, may be seen in reactivation disease, so that shortness of breath or pleuritic chest pain may be presenting manifestations.

Reactivation of tuberculosis in bone is seen in about 10% of individuals with reactivation disease. Pain is the most common complaint, and will be localized at the area of involvement. Any bone can be affected, but the vertebrae are involved in about half the cases. If not diagnosed, vertebral destruction can occur, and symptoms of weakness and paralysis may then occur.

Genitourinary reactivation tuberculosis may be associated with dysuria, hematuria, or flank pain. A minority of patients will have fever or weight loss.

Reactivation in the nervous system often takes the form of meningeal involvement from rupture of a casseous focus into the subarachnoid space. Symptoms may include headache, lethargy, or other changes in mental status. Fever is often, but not invariably, present.

Reactivation tuberculosis in the gastrointestinal tract occurs in about 5% of cases of extrapulmonary tuberculosis. The peritoneum is most often affected; symptoms are abdominal pain or swelling. The ileocecal bowel may be involved, with symptoms of crampy abdominal pain related to intestinal obstruction.

Cardiovascular reactivation tuberculosis is relatively uncommon. It may manifest itself as symptoms of pericarditis, related to rupture of a tuberculous focus from the lung into the adjacent pericardium. Shortness of breath and orthopnea may relate to a pericardial effusion related to tuberculosis.

Rare manifestations of extrapulmonary involvement from reactivation may include hoarseness related to laryngeal involvement, skin ulcerations, and involvement of the adrenal glands with symptoms of Addison's disease.

Disseminated tuberculosis, although usually a manifestation of primary infection that is not controlled by the immune system, can occasionally occur as part of the reactivation process, particularly in patients who are immunocompromised. These patients, in addition to the systemic complaints of fatigue and weight loss, may have symptoms pointing to extrapulmonary sites of dissemination such as headache and cranial neuropathies suggestive of meningitis, or symptoms related to anemia or to bone marrow involvement.

PHYSICAL EXAMINATION AND CLINICAL FINDINGS

Physical findings are often nonspecific for the diagnosis of tuberculosis. Evidence of consolidation on chest x-ray, lymphadenopathy, or tenderness to percussion over the area of bone pain, pericardial rub, and abdominal tenderness are not diagnostic of tuberculous involvement of these organs. These findings may be useful to help pinpoint the site of involvement in a patient in whom tuberculosis is suspected, but rarely will the findings on physical examination be diagnostic.

LABORATORY AND IMAGING STUDIES

The tuberculin test is used to diagnose infection with *M. tuberculosis.* It is not useful in determining whether a patient who is clinically ill has active disease, because patients who are tuberculin positive may have other causes of their acute symptomatology. Similarly, a negative PPD does not exclude active tuberculosis, because of possible malnutrition, immunosuppression, or other factors leading to cutaneous anergy.

The tuberculin test is used to define tuberculous infection so that prophylaxis may be given to avoid later reactivation. The Mantoux intradermal injection of 5 TU of PPD (0.1 mL) is used and is given to patients who are increased risk of acquiring tuberculous infection or who will be at increased risk of reactivation. Such individuals include close contacts of infectious cases; patients with HIV infection; patients with fibrotic disease on chest x-ray consistent with untreated tuberculosis; persons with medical conditions that may increase the risk of tuberculosis, such as prolonged therapy with greater than 20 mg of prednisone daily or other chronic immunosuppressive therapy; residents of long-term care nursing homes; health care workers, individuals born in areas with a high prevalence of TB (eg, Latin American, Asia, and Africa), patients with diseases known to increase the risk of reactivation tuberculosis such as silicosis, malnutrition, and chronic renal failure; and medically underserved, low income populations. It is not recommended that patients who do not have a high likelihood of having been infected or acquiring infection be routinely skin tested. Therefore, not all patients coming to a practice for the first time should have tuberculin skin tests as a routine part of initial laboratory assessment, because tuberculin skin tests may be falsely positive from exposure to nontuberculous mycobacteria. In a population at low risk for acquiring tuberculosis, the chance of false positivity of a skin test becomes close to that of true positivity, with the risk that unnecessary isoniazid prophylaxis will be given.

Skin test positivity is measured by the degree of induration at the injection site measured at 48 to 72 hours. Reactions greater than or equal to 5 mm are positive in individuals with HIV infection, individuals who are close contacts of infectious cases, and individuals with stable fibrotic lesions on chest x-ray, consistent with contained, although advanced, primary infection. A PPD whose induration is greater or equal to 10 mm is positive for adults in the other risk situations listed earlier such as prolonged therapy with steroids, immigrants from areas endemic for tuberculosis, the medically underserved, and residents of long-term care facilities. For other individuals, a PPD greater than or equal to 15 mm is considered positive.

For individuals who are tested at regular intervals with PPD because of risk of exposure (for example, health care workers), a 10 mm or greater increase in induration within a 2-year period in those under age 35 years, and a greater than 15 mm increase for those over 35 years of age is considered positive.

In cases of suspected active tuberculosis, laboratory examination may reveal an elevated blood cell count, low serum albumin reflecting malnutrition, an elevated sedimentation rate, and, occasionally, hyponatremia from inappropriate secretion of ADH, although the latter is nonspecific and is found in many pulmonary inflammatory disorders.

The chest x-ray shows infiltrates in the apical or posterior segment of an upper lobe in most instances, although the superior segment of the lower lobe may be involved as well. Lower lobe disease, although rare, can occur, and its presence on an x-ray should not exclude consideration of tuberculosis in the differential diagnosis. Cavitation occurs in about half of the patients with reactivation disease. Cavitation is less likely to be seen in patients with HIV infection, because cavitation is due in part to the inflammatory reaction against the organism. Occasionally, tuberculosis can appear as a solitary pulmonary nodule (a tuberculoma), mimicking the chest x-ray appearance of a primary lung cancer.

In bone disease, the x-ray may show bony destruction or erosion. Gastrointestinal tuberculosis of the ileocecal area can occur, and contrast studies showing narrowing and irregularity of the lumen can be mistaken for regional enteritis.

The major laboratory test in tuberculosis is identification of the organism on culture or smear. Routine examination of material for bacterial pathogens does not reveal tuberculous organisms unless the appropriate stain is requested for "acid-fast organism." If these stains are performed, the mycobacteria are stained red against a blue background. In most instances of tuberculosis, except in immunocompromised individuals, the acid-fast organisms are not plentiful, and the slide must be examined carefully. In as much as 20% to 30% of pulmonary tuberculosis, the AFB smear is negative. Many of these smears will ultimately grow out acid-fast organisms on culture, but this may take weeks. Bronchoscopy with brushings, washings, and lavage can be useful in patients if routine sputum is smear-negative, because specimens from bronchoscopy have a higher yield for the organism.

The ultimate diagnostic test for tuberculosis is growth of the organism in culture. If tuberculosis is suspect, special culturing must be requested, because tuberculosis will not grow in routine media. It will take tuberculosis 3 to 6 weeks to grow. Biochemical tests are performed to confirm that the organism is *Mycobacterium tuberculosis* and not other Mycobacteria. After growth of the organism, tests for drug susceptibility should be performed in all isolates.

The Bactec System is a relatively new method for identifying *Mycobacterium tuberculosis* that has shortened the time required to identify the organism. The organism is detected by measuring metabolic radioactive carbon dioxide production when colonies are still too small to be visible; by this technique organisms can be identified in 4 to 8 days. Once a Mycobacterium is identified, the Bactec System may selectively provide nutrients to identify which Mycobacterium is present. Drug susceptibility testing can also be done.

TREATMENT

There are two aspects to treatment of tuberculosis. One involves prophylactic treatment of tuberculous infected individuals, and the other involves treatment of active disease.

Prophylactic treatment with isoniazid is offered to patients who have been infected with tuberculosis but do not have active disease. The goal of therapy is to reduce risk of reactivation disease. Drug resistance is not considered a significant problem with this single-drug therapy because the infective load of organisms is small. Standard therapy is 12 months of isoniazid 300 mg a day, although 6-month therapy may be adequate. Patients are offered therapy based on their risk factor and size of the tuberculin test induration, as discussed in the previous section. For example, persons with HIV infection, close contacts of persons with newly diagnosed infectious tuberculosis, and patients with stable fibrotic upper lobe disease consistent with previous tubeculosis who have a PPD greater than or equal to 5 mm should be treated. An individual without known contact who has increased the size of PPD by 10 mm from a previous test and is under the age of 35 is a candidate for treatment. A PPD greater than 10 mm in residents of long-term care facilities, health care workers, immigrants from endemic areas, the medically underserved, and patients with diseases increasing the risk of tuberculosis should also be considered for therapy. In a patient without risk factors, a PPD of 15 mm or more is positive. In these individuals under age 35, therapy should be considered because of their lifelong risk of reactivation tuberculosis. In older individuals with a lower risk of lifetime development of tuberculosis and considering that the risk of isoniazid hepatitis increases with age, therapy is usually not given.

Treatment with isoniazid is expected to reduce the risk of developing reactivation tuberculosis by between 60% and 80%. It is administered as a single daily dose, and has some mild GI upset associated with it. However, the major risk is isoniazid hepatitis, which can be severe, and has caused death. The rate of isoniazid hepatitis seems to increase with age. It is rare under the age of 35, and occurs at a rate of 1% to 2% for patients in their 60s. Because of the isoniazid, patients receiving this medication should be questioned at monthly intervals for symptoms and signs of hepatitis, and if signs are present, should have liver function tests obtained. About 20% of patients receiving isoniazid develop asymptomatic abnormalities of liver function, with SGOT rising two- to threefold. Although asymptomatic rises in liver function are not strictly a cause for discontinuing therapy, many physicians will discontinue isoniazid if the SGOT rises four- to fivefold.

Another form of prevention, which is not used in the United States, is vaccination with BCG, an attenuated strain of *M. bovis*. Protection from vaccination has been variably reported from 10% to 50% and does not seem to provide immunity beyond 15 to 20 years. Because the goal of BCG is to prevent infection, it has not been offered in the United States, since most active cases of tuberculosis have risen as reactivation disease in individuals who were infected in the past. However, with tuberculosis spreading more rapidly in some populations, more interest may appear in the future in preventing primary infection. At present, however, BCG vaccine is recommended only for infants and children who are at high risk of being exposed for long periods to others with untreated tuberculosis, or are being exposed to individuals who have resistant organisms. Such situations could arise, for example, among socially economically deprived childre living in areas where TB is epidemic.

Treatment of active tuberculosis is an area in which expert help should always be sought. The appearance of multiple-drug-resistant tuberculosis has made it imperative that treatment be started with at least two effective drugs so that resistance will not develop to single drug therapy. Drugs that are considered for first-line use in tuberculosis include isoniazid, rifampin, pyridoxine, ethambutol, and streptomycin. The major side effect of isoniazid is hepatitis, the incidence of which increases with age, being 1.2% for patients aged 35 to 50 years, and about 2.3% for patients aged 50 to 64 years. Incidence does not increase much above age 65 years. Peripheral neuropathy is another complication of isoniazid, and the drug should be given with pyridoxine 50 mg daily

Rifampin, like isoniazid, is bactericidal for *M. tuberculosis*. The drug has few side effects, the most common being gastrointestinal upset. Usual dosing for adults is 600 mg daily. In doses greater than 10mg/kg/day some patients may experience a flulike illness and thrombocytopenia. Rifampin is excreted in bodily fluids and colors them orange. This is not harmful, but is alarming to patients if they are not forewarned.

Pyrizinamide is another bactericidal antibiotic. Liver toxicity associated with its use as well, but it does not seem to cause increased liver injury when used in combination with other potentially hepatotoxic drugs such as isoniazid and rifampin. Hepauricemia may occur, although acute gout is uncommon.

Ethambutol is a bactericidal agent. The most serious side effect is retrobulbar neuritis with changes in vision, including changes in color vision acuity. This complication is unusual, however, occurring in less than 1% of individuals given a dose of 15 mg/kg/day.

The 25 mg/kg/day dose of ethambutol is associated with a higher frequency of neuritis, but there is rarely a reason to use ethambutol at this dose.

Streptomycin is another bactericidal agent. It requires parenteral therapy and can be used in twice-weekly dosing regimens when given at a dose of 25 to 30 mg/kg/dose. Dosage must be adjusted if there is any renal impairment. Ototoxicity and vestibular toxicity are side effects of the drug.

Second-line antibiotics effective against tuberculosis include paraminosalicylic acid, ethionamide, capriomycin, cycloserine, and ciprofloxacin.

To treat tuberculosis successfully, the drug should be taken for the appropriate period of time, which is usually many months, and on a regular basis, so that intermittent use does not promote drug resistance. The American Thoracic Society has advocated initial therapy with isoniazid, rifampin, and pyrazinamide for 8 weeks, followed by 16 weeks of isoniazid and rifampin. The New York State Department of Health, because of the incidence of multiple-drug-resistant tuberculosis in New York City, has recommended that all patients who have tuberculosis be started on isoniazid, rifampin, pyrizinamide, and ethambutol. Pyrizinamide and ethambutol are stopped at 2 months; the rifampin and isoniazid are continued for 6 months(9 months in immunocompromised individuals). If drug susceptibility testing shows resistance to isoniazid or other agents, then the ethambutol and pyrizinamide can be continued for the 6- to 9-month total duration of therapy. Medication can be given 2 to 3 times weekly rather than every day, a regimen useful in populations in whom compliance with medication is a problem, as it makes administration under direct observation easier.

When tuberculosis is susceptible to the agents used, patients usually become noninfectious within 2 weeks. The sputum cultures are usually negative by 2 months. Acid-fast organisms may occasionally be found in a sputum specimen for some time after that. Patients do not necessarily need to be hospitalized for 2 weeks of therapy, but if compliant with medication and cough hygiene may be discharged to their home. They have often spent sufficient time at home before diagnosis, in which case infection of family members may already have occurred. If it has not, avoiding close contact and using cough precautions may not result in much further infection risk for the week or two of treatment it takes to become noninfectious. However, in individuals who will have close contact with others, or who will be in situations in which they will be exposed to many people and be unable to avoid this, such as homeless shelters or chronic care facilities, at least the initial 2 weeks of therapy until they are not infectious should be administered in an environment that allows isolation from others.

Extrapulmonary tuberculosis is treated similar to the pulmonary disease, except that the therapeutic course tends to be a bit longer, perhaps 9 to 12 months, since there is not much experience with the shorter courses of chemotherapy that have evolved for the treatment of pulmonary disease.

SPECIAL CONSIDERATIONS IN PREGNANCY

Prophylactic treatment with isoniazid in a pregnant patient with a positive skin test usually is delayed until after delivery. Isoniazid has not been shown to be teratogenic, but for prophylactic use it is not unreasonable to wait until after delivery to begin therapy.

In active tuberculosis, therapy must be initiated during pregnancy. It is not thought that the risk to the fetus from either the disease or therapy warrants therapeutic abortion. Drugs that are used include isoniazid, ethambutol, and rifampin, all of which have been used safely in pregnancy, although rifampin has been associated with isolated reports of fetal malformation. Streptomycin and other aminoglycocides are avoided because of associated fetal hearing and vestibular impairment. There are limited data regarding teratogenicity of pyrizinamide, and it is not used in pregnancy in the United States, although it has been recommended in other countries.

Antituberculous drugs may appear in breast milk, but this is not a contraindication to nursing.

If the mother is on therapy, and thought not to be contagious at delivery, the family members should be carefully checked to make sure there is no reservoir of tuberculosis to affect the newborn. The infant is begun on isoniazid prophylaxis and tuberculin testing is done at 4 to 6 weeks of age. If negative, the test is repeated at 3 to 4 months and again at 6 months, and if negative at 6 months, isoniazid can be discontinued.

If the mother at the time of delivery has active pulmonary disease that has not yet been treated, then the infant should not have contact with the mother until sufficient therapy has been given to reduce the chance of infection, usually about 2 weeks. The child is also begun on isoniazid prophylaxis and skin-tested at the intervals described above.

If the mother has widely disseminated disease with hematogenous spread and multiple organ involvement ("miliary" tuberculosis) the infant may not only be at risk for infection after birth as when the mother has only pulmonary tuberculosis but may have acquired congenital, active, tuberculosis. Clinical evidence of disease in the infant warrants treatment for active tuberculosis with a multiple drug regimen.

In all situations involving treatment of tuberculosis, including during pregnancy, it is wise to seek expert consultative help.

NON-TUBERCULOUS MYCOBACTERIA

Organisms other than *Mycobacterium tuberculosis* can cause human disease. As mentioned earlier, these mycobacteria include the *Mycobacterium avium* complex, *(M. avium* and *M. intracellulare), M. kansasii, M. cheloniae,* and *M. scrofulaceum.* Other Mycobacteria can cause human disease as well. These Mycobacteria have been isolated from soil, water, and animals, but they are not thought to be transmitted human to human. They may be colonizers of the human respiratory tract, and their presence identified on culture does not always mean clinical disease. Most individuals who have disease from these organisms have preexisting pulmonary disease such as preexisting cavitary lesions, chronic obstructive pulmonary disease, and interstitial fibrosis. When these organisms cause disease, it is similar in clinical presentation to that caused by *M. tuberculosis.* In the immunocompromised patient, however, particularly those with HIV infection and low CD4 counts, *M. avium* and *M. intracellulare* can cause rapidly progressive pulmonary disease as well as disease that is widely disseminated hematogenously.

These organisms appear similar to *M. tuberculosis* on acid-fast smears, and they are distinguished from tuberculosis only by culture. These organisms, particularly the *M. avium* complex, may be resistant to multiple drugs, and multiple drug regimens are often necessary for effective treatment.

It is useful to have advice from a specialist when nontuberculous Mycobacteria are isolated from the sputum, or when they are suspected of causing disease in immunocompromised individuals. In immunocompetent individuals consultants can be helpful in deciding whether the organisms represent colonization or true infection, and in cases of disseminated or extensive pulmonary disease in the patient with AIDS or HIV infection, the consultant may provide diagnostic help (eg, bronchoscopy) and help in choice of antimicrobial agents.

BIBLIOGRAPHY

American Thoracic Society. Diagnosis and treatment of disease caused by non-tuberculous Mycobacteria. Am Rev Respir Dis 1990;142:940.

American Thoracic Society/Centers for Disease Control. Diagnostic standards and classification of tuberculosis. Am Rev Respir Dis 1990;142:725.

Barnes PF, Barrows SA. Tuberculosis in the 1990s. Ann Int Med 1993;119:400.

Bass JB (ed.) Mycobacterial disease. Semin in Resp Med 1988;9:1.

Bass JB, Farer LS, Hopewell PC, et al. Treatment of tuberculosis and tuberculosis infection in adults and children. Am J Respir Crit Care Med 1994;149:1359.

Snider DE, Guest ed. Mycobacterial diseases. Clin Chest Med 1989;10:297.

Snider DE Jr, Caras GJ. Isoniazid-associated hepatitis deaths: a review of available information. Am Rev Respir Dis 1992;145:494.

Snider DE, Layde PM, Johnson MW, Lyle MA. Treatment of tuberculosis during pregnancy. Am Rev Respir Dis 1980;122:65.

Primary Care for Women, edited by Phyllis C. Leppert and Fred M. Howard. Lippincott-Raven Publishers, Philadelphia © 1997.

56

Chronic Obstructive Pulmonary Disease

ANTHONY J. FEDULLO

Chronic obstructive pulmonary disease (COPD) is a category of disorders characterized by airflow obstruction. Asthma, bronchitis, and emphysema are the major diseases in this category. Asthma has been included in this category, but there is a tendency to separate it from the more chronic and irreversible causes of obstructive pulmonary disease. Bronchospasm, however, can coexist with bronchitis and emphysema; recognizing a coexisting bronchospastic component in these disorders is important, as it provides an avenue for therapy. The emphasis in this chapter is on emphysema and bronchitis; asthma was discussed in Chapter 54.

COPD is the fifth leading cause of death in the United States and the highest cause of mortality with an avoidable cause, cigarette smoking. In addition to mortality, COPD also causes significant morbidity. Patients are often limited and disabled by dyspnea. The roughly 6 million Americans with COPD make up 5% of office visits and about 10% to 15% of hospitalizations.

Because emphysema occurs after many years of cigarette smoking, most patients present with this disease between ages 55 and 70. COPD has traditionally been considered a disease of older men, but women are equally susceptible and by the late 1980s had a prevalence similar to that of men. More disturbing is the fact that the prevalence of COPD has been stable or declining in men but continues to rise in women, probably reflecting their later development of cigarette smoking.

ETIOLOGY

The main cause of chronic bronchitis and emphysema is cigarette smoking. This evidence is based on epidemiologic studies that attribute 80% to 90% of cases of emphysema and chronic bronchitis to cigarette smoking. There is a strong epidemiologic relation between cigarette smoking and COPD, but only about 15% of smokers develop clinically significant COPD, although a larger number have airway obstruction on pulmonary function tests.

The precise mechanism by which cigarette smoking causes COPD is uncertain. Destruction of lung tissue by products of inflammation plays a role in emphysema by reducing the connective tissue framework that helps to maintain airway integrity and patency. When the supporting framework is not present, airway collapse and limitation of airflow occur. Inhaled irritants are thought to play a role in producing the mucosal hypertrophy and mucous hypersecretion characteristic of chronic bronchitis. These changes result in airway narrowing and airflow limitation.

There are other risk factors in addition to cigarette smoking. The best-defined one is α_1-antitrypsin deficiency, a genetic disorder. Antitrypsin and other serum antiproteases prevent digestion of lung connective tissue by the proteolytic enzymes that are released by inflammatory cells. Patients heterozygous for the gene responsible for α_1-antitrypsin production have levels of α_1-antitrypsin sufficient to protect the lung and do not have an increased rate of emphysema. Homozygous deficient persons, however, are at risk for developing early emphysema. Nonsmokers with homozygous α_1-antitrypsin deficiency may not develop significant or symptomatic COPD until well into later life, but smokers with the deficiency may develop severe emphysema by age 30 or 40. α_1-Antitrypsin deficiency is responsible for only 1% to 3% of cases of emphysema in the United States, but because of the genetic implications and the availability of replacement enzyme, this must be considered, particularly in younger patients with advanced emphysema.

Other risk factors include a poorly understood familial clustering of the disease, not related to a known genetic defect.

Air pollution in urban areas or dust exposure in the workplace increases the incidence of chronic bronchitis but is usually not a factor in clinically significant COPD.

Childhood respiratory infections may increase the risk of developing COPD. Maternal smoking can adversely affect the respiratory status of children living in the home, can increase childhood respiratory infections and bronchial hyperresponsiveness, and perhaps can predispose to the COPD.

The effects of airway obstruction include increased work of breathing, which is partly responsible for the dyspnea patients feel. The airway obstruction also decreases the high peak flow rates that allow cough to clear secretions, predisposing to atelectasis and recurrent chest infection. Destruction of the alveolar/capillary interface in emphysema results in a greater proportion of each breath occurring without gas exchange (increased dead space) and leads to the need for increased ventilatory effort to excrete carbon dioxide. When increased ventilation and the work of breathing it requires can no longer be easily accomplished, carbon dioxide retention develops. Alveolar ventilation to lung capillary perfusion mismatching leads to hypoxemia. Hypoxemia, particularly with a PO_2 below 55 to 60 mm Hg, leads to pulmonary hypertension and the development of cor pulmonale (right-sided heart failure due to pulmonary disease), with peripheral edema.

Patients with advanced COPD often cannot fulfill their ventilatory needs in acute infections such as bronchitis or pneumonia; PCO_2 elevation and respiratory acidosis ensue and the patient may require mechanical ventilation.

DIFFERENTIAL DIAGNOSIS

Because COPD may cause dyspnea and right-sided heart failure, the differential diagnosis includes disorders that cause these findings in smokers or former smokers of middle age or older. Left ventricular heart failure with secondary right-sided heart failure in this age group is often a consideration. Moreover, COPD and left ventricular dysfunction often coexist, both contributing to dyspnea. Pulmonary vascular disease (eg, primary pulmonary hypertension or chronic thromboembolic disease) can cause dyspnea with evidence of right-sided heart failure. Anemia may cause dyspnea but usually does not do so with mild to moderate exertion until the hematocrit level is quite low (often in the upper teens or low 20s) and, unless severe enough to cause heart failure, usually is not accompanied by edema. Large pleural effusions (eg, those associated with malignancy) can cause dyspnea. Obesity is a common cause of complaints of shortness of breath with exertion and may be associated with peripheral edema due to stasis. Other parenchymal lung diseases, such as interstitial lung disease, can cause dyspnea and cor pulmonale. Rarer causes of dyspnea include neuromuscular diseases that inhibit adequate ventilation, such as amyotrophic lateral sclerosis.

Dyspnea in a smoker does not necessarily implicate COPD as a cause, as only about 15% of smokers develop significant COPD. An evaluation still must be done to prove the presence of COPD and to evaluate other potential causes of dyspnea.

HISTORY

Patients with COPD have dyspnea or reduced exercise ability as their prominent complaint. COPD progresses slowly in smokers who are susceptible, but lung function must be reduced considerably before symptoms become noticeable. Early in the disease, many patients decrease their activity level so that they do not perceive any disability or discomfort with exercise. Dyspnea is a subjective complaint, and patients may begin to perceive it only when activities at work or around the home become associated with an uncomfortable shortness of breath. Sometimes the onset of shortness of breath is related to an acute respiratory infection or occurs after a surgical procedure, at which time the decreased respiratory function, muscle weakness, and deconditioning make the symptoms more noticeable.

Nocturnal awakening with dyspnea or orthopnea can occur in COPD but more often reflects asthma or congestive heart failure. In exacerbations of COPD, when the patient is more breathless, many patients want to sit fairly upright: in that position, the chest wall configuration, the positioning of the diaphragm, and respiratory muscle use minimize airflow limitation.

Sputum production is characteristic of chronic bronchitis and defines the disease (3 months of cough for 2 consecutive years). COPD is often associated with wheezing because of the decreased expiratory flow rates. Wheezing does not necessarily mean that a reversible bronchospastic component is present, but asthma can coexist with bronchitis and emphysema. Symptoms that suggest an asthmatic component are intermittent or episodic increases in shortness of breath with wheezing, unrelated to other causes such as acute chest infection or congestive heart failure. Symptomatic relief with bronchodilators also points to a bronchospastic component. It is useful to recognize a reversible bronchospastic component because even mild degrees of bronchospasm may significantly affect a person with an already severe fixed obstructive disease such as emphysema.

PHYSICAL EXAMINATION AND CLINICAL FINDINGS

Early in the disease, when dyspnea is experienced only during moderate exertion, the physical examination reveals little. Auscultation over the trachea during a forced expiration following a full breath often reveals airflow to last more than 4 or 5 seconds, suggesting airway obstruction. Wheezing, either at rest or with forced expiration, may also be heard, although this may be due to asthma, not emphysema or bronchitis. With more advanced disease, dyspnea may be observed with ambulation and an increased resting respiratory rate may be noticed. As the disease progresses and airflow continues to decline, the cough sounds weak and cannot easily raise mucus adequately. Dyspnea at rest and the use of accessory muscles of respiration may be obvious. Pursed-lip breathing may be seen; it may be a mechanism to enhance airway patency and minimize obstruction to airflow.

Elevated jugular venous pressure and peripheral edema suggest cor pulmonale secondary to hypoxemia. The degree of hypoxemia does not correlate well with the severity of airflow obstruction, so cor pulmonale is not necessarily a marker of severe disease. Cyanosis may be seen but many observers find it difficult to detect. A certain amount of desaturated hemoglobin is required for cyanosis to be visible; hence, it is not as obvious in anemic patients and may be due to circulatory causes rather than hypoxemia. The absence of cyanosis does not rule out significant COPD or even significant hypoxemia.

In advanced COPD, weight loss occurs because the work of breathing accounts for a higher proportion of basal metabolism and because the patient experiences shortness of breath with minimal activities such as eating or with gastric distention after a meal. Depression and anxiety due to disabling disease further contribute to poor appetite and weight loss.

Many patients with advanced COPD become depressed, anxious, and dependent. This is understandable in a slowly progressive disease with the symptom of shortness of breath that eventually progresses to the sense of near-suffocation. These patients are often elderly and often lack strong coping mechanisms or outlets.

The terms "pink puffer" and "blue bloater" have been used to describe the stereotypical characteristics of patients with emphysema and bronchitis respectively. These terms describe extremes of presentation and have a demeaning, depersonalized connotation. It is true, however, that some patients with COPD, particularly those with emphysema, resist carbon dioxide retention. To keep their PCO_2 low or normal, these emphysematous patients must ventilate, so they appear to "puff." Oxygenation tends to be better, partly because of their lower PCO_2 and partly because they are usually not obese and have no airway secretions to cause atelectasis; hence, they are "pink." On the other hand, the obese patient with chronic bronchitis and atelectasis has more hypoxemia and is "bluer." Because of the obesity and peripheral edema from cor pulmonale due to the hypoxemia, she appears "bloated." These characteristics cannot be used to quantify the severity of COPD. It is better to characterize each patient by her clinical examination, pulmonary function studies, and arterial blood gas analysis.

LABORATORY AND IMAGING STUDIES

The major characteristic of COPD is airflow obstruction as determined by pulmonary function tests, which should be a routine part of the evaluation of a patient with dyspnea. The fundamental abnormality seen on these tests in COPD is a decrease in the forced expiratory volume in 1 second (FEV_1), particularly as a percentage of the forced vital capacity (FVC). Normal values on pulmonary function tests are derived from population surveys and depend on age, sex, and height. In general, however, most patients in the middle years of life or older exhale 75% of their vital capacity in the first second; hence, the FEV_1 : FVC ratio is 75%. In COPD, the FEV_1 declines at a faster rate than the roughly 40 mL/year that occurs due to aging alone. Therefore, an abnormal FEV_1 : FVC ratio in a smoker in early middle age suggests that significant problems will occur in the ensuing years, as she continues to lose airway function. An abnormal FEV_1 : FVC ratio defines the presence of obstructive lung disease. An abnormal FEV_1 : FVC ratio is also seen in asthma, but in pure asthma this is reversible with therapy.

Correlation of pulmonary function test results with symptoms is not strict, but generally the FEV_1 : FVC ratio may fall to 50% without causing much dyspnea, particularly in older persons who do not exert themselves. As the ratio falls below 50%, most patients note dyspnea with exertion such as climbing stairs, rapid walking, or walking up hills. As the ratio falls to 35%, patients become symptomatic with slight exertion, the cough becomes less effective, and it is difficult to clear mucus well. When the ratio falls under 35%, patients are often symptomatic at rest or with minimal exertion and begin to have frequent emergency department visits or hospitalizations. Respiratory failure may complicate pneumonia or acute bronchitis as the ratio falls below 25%. Symptoms, however, are often a poor guide to the extent of pulmonary dysfunction, and pulmonary function tests are far more accurate in quantifying disease.

Pulmonary function tests need not be done frequently. Smokers and patients with dyspnea should have tests performed as part of the initial evaluation. Tests should be done when the patient is at a stable baseline, and they may be rechecked in 1 or 2 years to give some estimate as to the rate of progression. Some smokers can be motivated to stop smoking when they are shown their declining pulmonary function and are told that disability from emphysema may ensue.

The chest x-ray in emphysema may show hyperinflation, bullae, and a flattened diaphragm, but often it is normal. The chest x-ray cannot be relied on to detect COPD or to quantify its severity.

Oxygen levels on arterial blood gas analysis also do not correlate well with the severity of disease; they may be normal even in severe lung disease. On the other hand, PCO_2 elevation occurs late in the disease and often signifies an FEV_1 under 35% of predicted.

Polycythemia may be present when the PO_2 falls below 50 to 55 mm Hg, but the hematocrit level rarely exceeds 55% to 60%.

α_1-Antitrypsin levels can be obtained when significant airway obstruction occurs in a nonsmoker or a smoker under age 45 or when a chest x-ray shows bullae in a young person, particularly when the bullae are in the lung bases and when there is a familial history of early emphysema.

TREATMENT

The most important therapeutic intervention in COPD is to stop smoking. This is often difficult but very worthwhile. With smoking cessation, bronchitis usually disappears within 2 months and the accelerated decline in pulmonary function stops. Nicotine replacement therapy can be useful in smoking cessation but is not the sole answer. The successful smoking cessation program involves a committed patient and a physician who continuously counsels and encourages her. Some feel that a useful tactic before stopping smoking entirely is to withdraw to five cigarettes daily. The patient often reduces her nicotine addiction by this step, feels some pride in decreasing to this level from her usual 20 or more cigarettes a day, and perhaps can more easily discontinue from that point completely. Self-help groups, hypnosis, and acupuncture have had some success.

The next most important therapy is a trial of bronchodilator medication. A 15% to 20% improvement in the FEV_1 10 to 15 minutes after administration of an inhaled bronchodilator suggests that these medications will be useful. However, a lack of improvement in the FEV_1 does not rule out the use of bronchodilators, because in some patients improvement will occur after days of therapy, rather than at once. Most patients with COPD should be given an inhaled β_2-agonist such as albuterol (two puffs four times/day) or an anticholinergic medication such as ipratropium (two puffs four times/day). Some believe that ipratropium is more beneficial in COPD than β_2-agonists, but most patients who have reversible airway obstruction respond to either in a fairly similar manner. Depending on the severity of the associated bronchospastic component, some patients benefit from routine use of inhaled corticosteroids.

Theophylline is falling out of favor in the treatment of COPD. Older patients commonly have adverse side effects when theophylline levels rise above 15 μg/mL, and many medications and superimposed acute medical processes (eg, a viral infection) can alter theophylline's kinetics.

Short courses of systemic corticosteroids can be given for bronchospastic exacerbations refractory to other medication. Systemic corticosteroids should be used with great caution in patients with COPD and only if there is proof, based on pulmonary function testing, that benefit occurs. Patients on higher doses of steroids often feel euphoric and improved, even though there is no change in pulmonary function. Unfortunately, this effect is not long-lasting, but the initial subjective benefit often commits the patient to long-term use.

Before committing the patient to long-term steroid use, she should just receive maximal therapy for COPD without corticosteroids and then undergo pulmonary function testing. A dose of 30 to 40 mg/day of prednisone is then given for a few weeks, and the pulmonary function tests are repeated. An improvement of 25% or more suggests that the patient will benefit from chronic corticosteroid use. In that case, the steroid dose is reduced gradually as long as the benefit is maintained; ideally, an alternate-day regimen can be achieved. Because of the long-term side effects of corticosteroids, including respiratory and peripheral muscle weakness (which increase dyspnea and decrease exercise tolerance), the advice of a pulmonary medicine consultant is often helpful before committing to their use.

Antibiotics are used when acute bronchitis occurs. They are usually prescribed at the onset of symptoms. Although half of these infections are nonbacterial, treating patients promptly decreases the duration of symptoms and the frequency of hospitalization. The antibiotics could include trimethoprim–sulfamethoxazole, amoxicillin, or amoxicillin with clavulanate if there is a high community incidence of β lactamase producing *Haemophilus influenzae*. Broader-spectrum and more expensive antibiotics are usually unnecessary. If there is no response within a week, a sputum culture is taken to check for resistant organisms. Patients who had recently been in the hospital, perhaps within a month or two, may become colonized with resistant organisms; these patients in particular should be cultured if they fail to respond to an initial course of antibiotics.

Patients with COPD should receive a yearly influenza vaccination; pneumococcal vaccination is also recommended.

Mucolytic agents are generally not useful in COPD patients. The cough is ineffective in patients with severe COPD not because the mucus is thick but because the reduction in airflow reduces the adequacy of cough.

Emphysema due to α_1-antitrypsin deficiency can be treated with a weekly or monthly intravenous infusion of human α-proteinase inhibitor. Therapy with this enzyme costs about $20,000 a year. It is not given to patients who have emphysema and who are heterozygous for α_1-antitrypsin deficiency, as these patients have adequate levels of the enzyme. Homozygous persons with α_1-antitrypsin levels below 70 mg/dL are candidates for therapy if they are nonsmokers and have airflow obstruction on pulmonary function tests.

Oxygen therapy should be given to patients who have a room air resting PO_2 of below 55 mm Hg (saturation 85%) or a PO_2 between 55 and 59 mm Hg (saturation 85% to 89%) when accompanied by polycythemia and cor pulmonale. Oxygen should be given for about 18 hours/day. Patients generally use oxygen all night while sleeping and whatever part of the day they can while at home sitting or resting. Patients do not need portable oxygen 24 hours a day unless their PO_2 is very low (perhaps 40 to 45 mm Hg). Patients with COPD have decreased exercise ability, and a portable oxygen system that they wheel or carry may limit their ability to get out of the home and do routine activities. The goal of oxygen therapy is to reduce the effects of hypoxemia (eg, cor pulmonale, polycythemia); this goal is achieved when using oxygen 16 to 18 hours daily. Dyspnea is not an indication for oxygen unless it is accompanied by a low PO_2.

Oxygen may also need to be considered when a patient with marginal oxygenation changes altitude from a site near sea level to one above 5000 to 8000 feet. At these levels, the oxygen level in the air is reduced by 10% to 20%, which may result in hypoxemia severe enough to cause cor pulmonale. Oxygenation during airline flights—cabins are pressurized to the equivalent of 5000 to 8000 feet above sea level—can be arranged if prior notice is given to the airline.

Patients with chronic and severe dyspnea who have had no relief with other medication and whose lifespan is limited can obtain symptomatic relief with opiates. Because of their potential to depress respiration, opiates and sedatives should be used with great caution in acute exacerbations of COPD or in COPD patients with agitation and confusion (which may occur because of changes in oxygen or carbon dioxide levels). In acute instances of mental status change, opiates and steroids should not be given without checking arterial blood gas measurements and determining that the deterioration in COPD is not the primary cause.

Patients with severe COPD are prone to respiratory failure with acute exacerbations. They often need intensive care unit admission and perhaps mechanical ventilation. Patients with COPD with their first episode of respiratory failure have a fairly high chance of leaving the ventilator in a relatively short time and being discharged home. As COPD becomes severe, exacerbations become more frequent, and the quality of life deteriorates, the likelihood of successful weaning from a ventilator drops. In severe disabling COPD, the difficult issues of whether to continue aggressive care or perform recurrent resuscitation should be openly discussed with the patient.

CONSIDERATIONS IN PREGNANCY

Because COPD is a disease of older persons, smoking women of childbearing age rarely have significant disease unless they are deficient in α_1-antitrypsin.

Smoking in pregnancy has adverse effects. Smoking a pack a day or more may double the risk of delivering a infant weighing less than 2500 g. The growth-retarding effects of smoking are seen at all gestational ages and are probably due to fetal hypoxemia, related to the carbon monoxide in cigarette smoke and to placental vasoconstriction from nicotine exposure. Smoking increases the risk of preterm delivery, spontaneous abortion, placental abruption, and placenta previa. Smoking has not been associated with an increased risk of congenital defects.

Exposure of the child to cigarette smoke after delivery has been associated with an increased frequency of respiratory illnesses, bronchoreactivity, and bronchitis. There is conflicting evidence on whether childhood exposure to smoking in the home predisposes to respiratory disease in adult life.

BIBLIOGRAPHY

Chronic obstructive pulmonary disease. Clin Chest Med 1990 1990;11:363.

Guyatt GH, Townsend M, Pugsley SO, et al. Bronchodilators in chronic airflow limitation. Effects on airway function, exercise capacity, and quality of life. Am Rev Respir Dis 1987;135:1069.

Kellner R, Samet J, Pathak D. Dyspnea, anxiety, and depression in chronic respiratory impairment. Gen Hosp Psychiatry 1992;14:20.

Mahler DA. Evaluation of chronic dyspnea. Clin Pulmon Med 1994;1:208.

Rise in chronic obstructive pulmonary disease mortality. Am Rev Respir Dis 1989;140(suppl):S1.

Rovner MS, Stoller JK. Therapy for alpha 1-antitrypsin deficiency: rationale and strategic approach. Clin Pulmon Med 1994;1:135.

Standards for the diagnosis and care of patients with chronic obstructive pulmonary disease (COPD) and asthma. Official statement of the American Thoracic Society. Am Rev Respir Dis 1987;136:225.

Primary Care for Women, edited by Phyllis C. Leppert and Fred M. Howard. Lippincott-Raven Publishers, Philadelphia © 1997.

57

Lung Cancer

ANTHONY J. FEDULLO

Each year, 160,000 cases of lung cancer are diagnosed and 140,000 lung cancer patients die. Lung cancer is the most common cause of cancer death in men and has replaced breast cancer as the leading cause of cancer death among women. Whereas the incidence of lung cancer among men has reached a plateau, the rate in women has continued to rise, probably due to their increased cigarette smoking. Survival in lung cancer is poor. Five-year survival rates are 10% to 15%. At time of presentation, approximately 70% of patients with non–small cell lung cancer (NSCLC) are not candidates for curative surgical resection; and small cell lung cancer, although responding initially to chemotherapy, is rarely cured. Lung cancer, however, is a preventable disease: 85% to 90% of cases result from cigarette smoking.

ETIOLOGY

Cigarette smoking is a predominant cause of lung cancer. In the 1950s, a study of British doctors showed an increased risk of lung cancer associated with tobacco use, particularly cigarettes. In the United States, *The Report of the Surgeon-General on Smoking and Health* in 1964 demonstrated a correlation to smoking and lung cancer sufficiently strong to argue convincingly for a causal relationship. Historically, a rise in lung cancer was seen following the increase in smoking in the male population during World War I. Women began to increase their smoking later, during World War II and after, and their increase in lung cancer soon followed.

A relationship exists between the number of cigarettes smoked and the risk of developing lung cancer. For the 25% to 35% of the adult population who smoke cigarettes, one-pack-a-day smokers have a death rate of 120 per 100,000 individuals, whereas in those who smoke over one pack a day the rate rises to about 250 deaths per 100,000. Using filtered cigarettes decreases the risk relative to unfiltered cigarettes, but the risk reduction is not as great as expected, because smokers of filtered cigarettes tend to inhale more deeply and frequently, or smoke more cigarettes. This behavior may be related to a need to achieve certain nicotine levels.

Many carcinogenic substances have been found in cigarette smoke. Although it is uncertain which of these is the predominant cause of cancer, this question has little relevance in view that cessation of cigarette smoking would avoid all of them. Nicotine is not the carcinogenic substance, but is the substance that has addictive or habituating potential for cigarette smokers, leading them to continue the habit and leading to some of the withdrawal symptoms associated with smoking cessation.

Concern has arisen recently about risk associated with passive or "second-hand" cigarette smoking. There is evidence that spouses of smokers have a slightly higher risk of lung cancer compared with persons who live in a totally smoke-free environment. The risk is small compared with active cigarette smoking but probably is real. Casual or infrequent contact with cigarette smoke should not cause great concern among nonsmokers, but it is appropriate to segregate smokers from nonsmokers because any added risk, however small, should not be inflicted on nonsmoking individuals.

Whereas cigarette smoking is a predominant cause of lung cancer, it is not the sole cause. It has been well recognized that exposure to certain carcinogens in the occupational setting is associated with lung cancer. Asbestos is a substance with a fairly strong association, although it is particularly dangerous when combined with cigarette smoking. To be a carcinogen, the asbestos fibers must be in inhalable form. Encapsulated or contained asbestos, such as found in intact insulation products, provides no great risk. Great concern by the general public regarding asbestos in the environment is probably unwarranted. Exposure to chromium, certain nickel compounds, and organic compounds such as coal tars, soots, and diesel exhaust also has been associated with an increase in cancer. Women had generally been spared from many of these due to the prominent role of men in occupations where these substances are found. However, as women enter the workplace more broadly, they may be exposed as well. For example, concern has been raised about diesel engine school buses as a new health hazard for women in that many women are drivers.

Radon decay products are one possible cause of lung cancer that has received much attention and that is ubiquitous in the environment. The Environmental Protection Agency (EPA) has released standards for indoor exposure to radon, and most sales of homes require radon measurement as a contingency clause for the sale. Given the widespread possible exposure to radon and patients' concern about it, some discussion is warranted.

Radon is a gas that is a decay product from naturally occurring uranium and radium found in rock. Radon has a half-life of about 4 days, and the radioactive decay sequence generates carcinogenic alpha particles, such as isotopes of polonium and lead. These attach to dust particles, are respirable, and can be mutagenic to airway mucosal cells. It is these intermediate decay products, not radon itself, that are carcinogenic. The increased risk of lung cancer related to radon exposure was first identified in uranium miners. It was not appreciated until recently, however, that radon may be found in home environments. Radon gas enters homes through the ground. Certain areas of the United States have rock structures more predisposed to emit radon, but radon entry can occur in any location. Radon levels are negligible where there is adequate ventilation, so levels on the first floor are much lower than in basements

Radon can be measured by charcoal-containing canisters that trap radon gas and that are placed in a closed basement for a few days. Since radon levels can vary widely in any individual home based on soil moisture, wind speed and direction, atmospheric pressure, and basement ventilation, a more precise measurement can be taken using a tracking device that records the radon decay products. This allows measurements to be made for 1 to 12 months, providing an average reading that is a better estimate of risk.

The EPA has made recommendations for action based on levels. If the short-term screening shows a level of 4 to 8 pCi/L, no action need be taken. Between 8 and 20 pCi/L, it is recommended that longer term measurements be taken by the tracking device, for about 6 to 12 months. If short-term levels are above 20 but below 200, measurements should be taken for 3 months.

If levels on long-term measurement are above 8 pCi/L or if initial screening levels are above 200, prompt remediation should be considered. Remediation involves venting the area below the foundation to the outside atmosphere, and may cost $2000 to $6000.

The risk of lung cancer in the general public from radon exposure is uncertain. Estimates of the risk are extrapolated from information on uranium miners, and do not control other variables well. No literature convincingly demonstrates that the average individual has significant risk from exposure to radon. Radon levels are highest in basements, the source of entry, and most individuals spend only a portion of the day there. Radon levels are reduced considerably above that, as ventilation disperses the gas. It is also thought that the risk of lung cancer from radon is primarily in cigarette smokers. The EPA has estimated that radon causes 13,000 cases of lung cancer a year, but most of these are in cigarette smokers with the radon acting as a cocarcinogen. Although persistently high radon levels are reason for concern, the levels set by the EPA are considered by many to be too stringent. The nonsmoking general population should not worry excessively about lung cancer due to exposure to radon.

CLASSIFICATION

Lung cancer can be divided into two types: (1) small cell ("oat cell") carcinoma, and (2) Non–small cell lung cancer (NSCLC). NSCLC includes squamous cell carcinoma, adenocarcinoma, large cell undifferentiated carcinoma, bronchoalveolar cell carcinoma (a variant of adenocarcinoma), and mixed types. These can be recognized microscopically, but the major clinical importance is that in NSCLC, surgery is the primary curative therapy. Small cell carcinoma, on the other hand, is considered at time of diagnosis not to be surgically curable except in the rare instances where it presents as a peripheral nodule. At the time of diagnosis, 50% of small cell carcinomas have metastasized to the bone marrow, and almost all have metastasized to lymph nodes within the mediastinum. Therapy for small cell lung cancer is chemotherapy in which there is often a good remission rate, although not many long-term survivors.

DIFFERENTIAL DIAGNOSIS

The symptoms associated with lung cancer are often nonspecific. Differential diagnostic possibilities are usually raised by findings on chest x-ray.

A solitary pulmonary nodule may be due to infectious processes such as tuberculoma, histoplasmoma and nocardiosis, vascular malformations, benign tumors such as hamartomas, and bronchial carcinoids. Rheumatoid nodules, Wegener granulomatosis, and metastatic malignancy may present with solitary nodules, although the usual pattern is multiple.

Mediastinal enlargement may be due to lymphoma, and lymphoma also presents as a parenchymal mass. Irregular infiltrative or mass-like lesions also can be seen in tuberculosis, actinomycosis, and histoplasmosis. Lipoid pneumonia, pulmonary sequestration, "rounded atelectasis," and aneurysmal dilatation of central vessels also can have patterns on x-ray that resemble broncho genic cancer.

HISTORY

Lung cancer may be asymptomatic until it is far advanced and uncurable. Hemoptysis in a cigarette smoker, even when associated with an acute bronchitis warrants a chest x-ray. If the chest x-ray finding is negative, studies suggest that 3% to 8% of these individuals have an occult intrabronchial lesion that will be found at bronchoscopy. Cough can be a symptom of lung cancer, but most studies investigating causes of chronic cough have found carcinoma to be low on the list. Recurrent pneumonia in the same anatomic area of the lung may suggest a partially obstructing endobronchial lesion predisposing to infection. Whereas there are other causes of recurrent chest infection, recurrent infections in the same part of the lung in a cigarette smoker warrants referral to a specialist for evaluation. Shortness of breath may be a complaint caused by an obstructed airway or a malignant pleural effusion. Systemic symptoms of weight loss, anorexia, and malaise can be presenting manifestations and often indicate advanced disease. Pain is not a manifestation of lung cancer in its early stage. The lung parenchyma does not contain pain receptors, and only when the tumor involves the pleura or adjacent structures does pain become a symptom.

Unfortunately, many of the presenting complaints in lung cancer represent disseminated or advanced intrathoracic disease that prohibits resection.

For example, hoarseness from compression of the recurrent laryngeal nerve implies mediastinal involvement that precludes surgery. Similarly, bone pain and focal neurologic complaints referable to metastases make the disease inoperable. Central nervous system involvement is common in lung cancer. It has been suggested that 10% of patients with squamous cell carcinoma have asymptomatic central nervous system metastases, and symptomatic metastases to the central nervous system may be the presenting manifestation in 15% of patients. Given the late presentation of lung cancer in an often uncurable state, it is natural to ask whether *screening* for lung cancer is useful. Studies show that chest x-rays performed yearly or every other year, as well as regular sputum cytologic study, do not affect the overall mortality from lung cancer. Therefore, screening for lung cancer by these methods is not recommended as a public health measure. Nonetheless, many physicians obtain chest x-rays yearly or every other year in their patients who are heavy cigarette smokers, hoping to find early evidence of carcinoma, which does not become symptomatic until it is far advanced.

PHYSICAL EXAMINATION

Evidence of a focal wheeze on auscultation of the chest may point to a focal endobronchial lesion. The presence of digital clubbing, although not specific for lung cancer, is consistent with it. Evidence of disseminated disease should be sought so that diagnosis and staging can be made with the least invasive procedure. Enlarged lymph nodes in the supraclavicular area may be found. They can be aspirated for diagnosis and cell type, and if no small cell malignancy is found, this will also stage the disease, excluding curative surgery. Neurologic examination may show signs of focal deficits, consistent with metastatic disease to the brain. Patient complaints of bone tenderness should be evaluated by palpation and percussion to detect focal tenderness and guide imaging studies to detect metastases. Tumors growing in the apex of the lung may involve the cervical sympathetic ganglia and lead to Horner syndrome. Compression of the mediastinal vessels may produce the superior vena cava syndrome, which is characterized by elevated venous pressure with facial plethora, edema of the arm and upper body, and collaterals on the chest wall. The superior vena cava syndrome is a serious complication of lung cancer, usually requiring emergent treatment because brain edema can occur, causing mental status change and coma. Elevated jugular venous pressure also may be caused by a malignant pericardial effusion, which requires urgent intervention if cardiac output is affected.

Blood work may show hypercalcemia. This may not be due to a bony metastases but can be hormonally produced and does not necessarily indicate inoperability.

IMAGING STUDIES

Chest x-ray findings for lung carcinoma may be normal. In cigarette smokers with hemoptysis, a small percentage of patients with a normal finding on chest x-ray have an endobronchial lesion observed on bronchoscopy. Usually, the chest x-ray shows a mass lesion. In a minority of cases, a peripheral nodule is found. These are usually adenocarcinomas, are almost always asymptomatic, and often are found incidentally. If the lesion has not changed in size for a 2-year interval of time, it is unlikely to be lung cancer and can be followed by x-rays over the next 1 to 2 years. If the nodule is new, or at least not known to be old, the risk of carcinoma in a cigarette smoker is sufficiently high to warrant aggressive investigation, usually by exploratory thoracotomy. Patterns of calcification in a pulmonary nodule are rarely diagnostic of benignity. Needle aspiration of these lesions rarely convincingly yield a benign origin, and if results are negative, do not exclude malignancy.

The more common x-ray presentation of lung cancer is evidence of a central mass lesion or irregular infiltrate, hilar enlargement, lobar atelectasis, or mediastinal adenopathy, because cancer arises at the site of carcinogen deposition in these central airways and spreads to adjacent lymph nodes. Approximately 20% to 25% of these central lesions are small cell carcinoma, another quarter is adenocarcinoma, and a third is squamous cell. The remainder is large cell undifferentiated or mixed type.

Pleural effusions can be seen in lung cancer as well. This may be due to pleural involvement with a tumor but also can be due to local lymphatic obstruction without pleural involvement. In non–small cell lung cancer, pleural effusions with malignant cells exclude operability, whereas pleural effusions that are cytologically negative for malignancy still allow the possibility of curative resection.

A third pattern of lung cancer on x-ray is seen in the relatively rare form of lung cancer called bronchoalveolar cell carcinoma. This is a variant of adenocarcinoma in which the malignant cells palisade along alveolar structure, assuming an infiltrative appearance on chest x-ray and resembling a pneumonia or other primary alveolar process.

A computed tomographic (CT) scan of the chest often is obtained as part of an evaluation of a patient with suspected lung cancer. The CT scan is useful in defining the presence and extent of mediastinal adenopathy. Lymph nodes under 2 cm, especially if they occur in a few discreet areas, have about a 50% chance of being benign. Lymph nodes greater than 2 to 3 cm, particularly diffusely involving the mediastinum, have a much higher chance of being malignant. Whereas the CT scan cannot be definitive regarding malignancy in these nodes, the CT scan definition of the mediastinal anatomy allows this area to be approached by fine-needle aspiration or mediastinoscopy to both diagnose and stage the disease, perhaps sparing the need for a thoracotomy.

It is not recommended that patients routinely have bone scans and CT scans of the brain. Bone pain, bone discomfort, and neurologic symptoms or findings on examination, however, should lead to investigation of these areas. The older and more infirm the patient, the more likely one is to search for evidence of inoperability by bone scan or brain CT before thoracotomy.

An important laboratory examination in a patient with suspected lung cancer is pulmonary function testing. Chronic obstructive pulmonary disease increases the risk of postoperative complications and, if severe, may prohibit thoracic surgery and resection of lung. Pulmonary medicine and thoracic surgery consultants usually are involved in deciding fitness for operability. However, as a rule of thumb, if after resection the residual forced expiratory volume in 1 second is less than 700 mL, surgery usually is not considered to be an option.

TREATMENT

At presentation, perhaps only a quarter or third of lung cancer patients have potential for curative treatment because of metastatic disease, mediastinal involvement, or poor pulmonary function. The specific diagnostic and therapeutic approach to the patient with lung cancer usually is multidisciplinary. A physician must be able to help guide the patient through the evaluative process and then through the options for treatment, thoracic surgery, medical oncology, or radiation oncology, depending on the typing and staging of the disease. A pulmonologist often plays this role, although the primary care physician can do so if there is an understanding of the concepts that determine the available options.

The peripheral nodule smaller than 4 to 5 cm in diameter occurs in a minority of patients with lung cancer but is a favorable finding. At presentation, depending on size, the cure rate can be as high as 60% to 80% for these lesions. Therefore, in a cigarette-smoking patient older than 40 years of age for whom the diagnostic workup is usually fairly slight, old chest x-rays should be sought; a lesion unchanged for 2 years is unlikely to be cancer and can be followed by serial chest x-rays. Bronchoscopy has a low yield in diagnosing these peripheral nodules. Moreover, they rarely are small cell cancers, and a positive diagnosis of non–small cell cancer does not change the need for eventual surgery if the patient is otherwise a candidate for curative resection. It has been suggested that bronchoscopy may detect an occult synchronous primary lesion in a more central airway, but that likelihood is so small that routine bronchoscopy is not warranted. Fine-needle transthoracic aspiration of the nodule often can make the diagnosis of lung cancer. However, in a patient who is otherwise a candidate for curative resection, this does not affect the need to undergo surgery. Because a negative result on fine-needle aspiration does not give sufficient confidence to rule out malignancy, the fine-needle aspirate is rarely useful in specifically diagnosing other conditions. The preoperative diagnosis of malignancy in a solitary nodule by needle or bronchoscopy is useful in patients who refuse surgery, cannot tolerate surgery, or have convincing clinical evidence of metastatic disease. A CT scan of the chest is useful to detect mediastinal adenopathy not visible on chest x-ray. Obtaining a biopsy on these nodes by needle aspiration or mediastinoscopy is useful before surgery since mediastinal involvement with tumor would make resection of the nodule unnecessary. The evaluation should include pulmonary function testing to determine operative risk or ability to undergo resection, and good clinical history and physical examination should be performed to determine bone or central nervous system metastases. In the absence of such symptoms, bone scans and brain CTs usually are not routinely obtained. If there is no evidence for metastatic or mediastinal disease from these relatively simple studies and the patient can tolerate surgery based on pulmonary function tests and other medical conditions, then referral to thoracic surgery for thoracotomy follows. Some of these lesions, if sufficiently peripheral, can be removed by thoracoscopy; this is an option left to the individual thoracic surgeon.

In individuals who are extremely elderly, refuse surgery, or have pulmonary function abnormalities prohibiting surgery, a nonsurgical diagnosis should be made. Needle aspiration is usually preferred, although, depending on the location of the nodule in the chest, fluoroscopic-guided bronchoscopy may be useful as well. If there is no evidence of mediastinal or metastatic spread, then the patient can be referred to radiation oncology for curative radiation therapy. The cure rate with full-dose radiation therapy for a solitary pulmonary nodule under 3.0 to 4.0 cm in diameter may be as high as 25%.

The more common presentation of lung cancer is a central mass, for which the prognosis, 15% survival at 5 years, is much poorer than is the case with a peripheral nodule. The focus of the evaluation is to define reasons that will avoid unnecessary thoracotomy. Flexible fiberoptic bronchoscopy is performed because it has a high yield in diagnosing the lesions that arise in the central airways; of equal importance, it can diagnose the 20% to 25% of lesions that are small cell lung cancer, and hence, require chemotherapy rather than surgery. Bronchoscopy also is be useful in showing the extent of the tumor in the airway, defining what degree of resection is necessary, and excluding operability when it involves the carina or subcarinal lymph nodes, which can be aspirated transbronchially. Patients should be interviewed and examined carefully. A supraclavicular node often can be aspirated by needle, and this provides a diagnosis as well as staging, saving an unnecessary thoracotomy. Complaints of bone pain may lead to a bone scan that would reveal foci of metastatic disease. Similarly, eliciting neurologic symptoms leading to a brain CT showing lesions consistent with metastatic disease would stage the disease clinically, even if the brain rarely undergoes biopsy for confirmation. The CT scan of the chest may show mediastinal adenopathy not visible on chest x-ray, which could be approached by possible needle aspiration or mediastinoscopy. If the evaluation reveals no demonstrable metastatic disease and no evident spread to the mediastinum, the patient is referred for thoracotomy. Unfortunately, in large central lesions, many patients who undergo exploration with curative intent are found to be inoperable because of mediastinal extension or invasion diagnosed only at the time of good visualization at thoracotomy.

For patients with NSCLC who are inoperable for cure, alternative therapy does not provide great benefit. Chemotherapy offers some survival advantage to patients with advanced NSCLC, but in studies comparing the best routine supportive care to multidrug chemotherapeutic drug regimens median survival is increased from 4 to 8 months at best, and the toxicity is significant.

Radiation therapy for otherwise unresectable NSCLC does not have a curative role. It is used in palliation to shrink lesions that encroach on the airway and to palliate bony metastases or intracranial lesions.

Endoscopically delivered laser resection also is used for palliation when the tumor mass encroaches on a central airway such as the trachea and causes severe dyspnea with imminent suffocation.

In small cell lung cancer, chemotherapy is the preferred treatment. It results in remission of disease in most patients, lasting as long as 12 to 24 months. The cure rate remains low despite remission, and 5-year cures are rare.

OTHER LUNG CANCERS

In addition to bronchogenic carcinoma, other cancers can arise primarily in the thorax. Carcinoid tumors rise in the airway, can occur at any age, and are unrelated to cigarette smoking. Because of their location in the airway, the presenting manifestations may be recurrent pneumonia in distal lung, cysts, or evidence of persistent atelectasis on chest x-ray. These lesions have some malignant potential and are not truly "benign" adenomas, as they are often labeled. The malignant potential is low, but they can metastasize to regional lymph nodes and even distantly.

Mesothelioma is a primary malignancy of the pleura. It has been strongly related to asbestos exposure and has been predominantly a disease of men working in asbestos-related industries. Mesothelioma presents with recurrent pleural effusion that is often hemorrhagic, thickened pleura on x-ray, and persistent chest wall pain from intercostal nerve involvement. Although they often grow slowly, these lesions are uncurable by either chemotherapy or surgery.

CONSIDERATIONS IN PREGNANCY

Primary bronchogenic carcinoma is unusual in patients younger than 35 years of age. Occasionally, a chest x-ray in a pregnant woman shows a small peripheral nodule that is not known to be old or unchanged because there are no previous x-rays for comparison. In people younger than 35 years of age, even cigarette smokers, these have a low likelihood of being malignant, approximately 5%. Even if the lesion was malignant, there is little evidence that waiting some months will result in a marked deterioration in the probability of cure. It has been estimated, although the data are poor, that every month of waiting may reduce the likelihood of survival by 1%. Patient preference and attitudes relative to the pregnancy play a significant role in how these situations are handled.

Because of the less aggressive malignant behavior of carcinoid tumors, definitive treatment can be deferred until after delivery, unless there are mitigating circumstances such as persistent hemoptysis or uncontrollable pneumonia due to airway obstruction.

BIBLIOGRAPHY

Bains MS. Surgical treatment of lung cancer. Chest 1991;100:826.

Eddy DM. Screening for lung cancer. Ann Intern Med 1989;111:232.

Figlin RA, Holmes EC, Petrovich A, Sarna GP. Lung cancer. In: Haskell CM, ed. Cancer treatment, 3rd ed. Philadelphia: WB Saunders, 1990.

Harley NH, Harley JH. Potential lung cancer risk from indoor radon exposure. Ca 1990;40:265.

Marino P, Pampallona S, Preatoni A, Cantoni A, Invernizzi F. Chemotherapy vs supportive care in advanced non-small-cell lung cancer: results of a meta-analysis of the literature. Chest 1994;106:861.

Matthay RA, Guest ed. Lung cancer. Clin Chest Med 1993;14:1.

Samet JM, Nero AV. Sounding board: indoor radon and lung cancer. N Engl J Med 1989;320:591.

Primary Care for Women, edited by Phyllis C. Leppert and Fred M. Howard. Lippincott-Raven Publishers, Philadelphia © 1997.

58

Cough

ANTHONY J. FEDULLO

Studies examining the etiology of chronic cough have variously defined it as a cough that has been present for longer than 3 to 8 weeks. This time period generally excludes coughs that are due to acute processes such as pneumonia or bronchitis. Chronic cough is a common problem, estimated to be responsible for 30,000,000 physician visits yearly. Whereas a wide variety of disorders can cause cough, the etiology often is determined by history, physical examination, or therapeutic trials directed to its common causes. Radiographic procedures, endoscopic examination, or blood tests play only a minor role in the diagnostic evaluation.

ETIOLOGY AND DIFFERENTIAL DIAGNOSIS

Cough is a protective mechanism, clearing mucus and irritative substances from the lung and guarding against inhalation and retention of foreign material. Submucosal cough receptors richly innervate the pharynx, posterior pharynx, and the airways. Irritation of these, as well as cough receptors on the pleural, pericardial, and diaphragmatic surfaces, can trigger cough.

Cough can be triggered by mechanical stimulation or by irritating fumes. The stimulus is transferred to a cough center in the medulla, and efferent pathways then initiate cough. Coughing involves taking a breath to fill the lungs completely. The glottis is closed while the chest, abdominal muscles, and diaphragm begin to contract, generating intrathoracic pressure. The glottis then opens, letting out an explosive rush of air, clearing the offending material. An effective cough depends on an alert central nervous system, ability to draw a deep breath, ability to close the glottis, and sufficient muscle strength to exert forceful contraction. When irritating stimuli continually trigger the cough receptors or when the receptors become overly sensitive, chronic cough results.

Chronic cough may be productive of purulent sputum ("moist"), indicative of active inflammation and mucous production. Coughs may be nonproductive ("dry"), or productive only of small amounts of thin mucous, suggesting persistent noninflammatory irritation of cough receptors. Whereas causes of cough may overlap in these areas, they provide a useful clinical distinction in investigating cough.

Chronic bronchitis from cigarette smoking is a common cause of productive cough. Most studies evaluating chronic cough have excluded cigarette smokers from analysis, but these patients do not exclude themselves from physicians' offices. It is surprising how frequently cigarette smokers present to the physician complaining of long-standing cough without considering smoking as an etiology. Some of these patients may have their coughs exacerbated by viral or bacterial infections, and may need intermittent antibiotic treatment for the latter. However, the irritating effect of cigarette smoke produces chronic inflammatory change and mucus production, and the cough will not resolve unless cigarette smoking is stopped.

Among nonsmokers, the duration of productive cough following an *acute respiratory infection* such as bronchitis or pneumonia may exceed the 3 to 8 weeks that many studies use to define chronic cough. Patients with cough after an acute respiratory infection usually have the cough slowly improve over 2 to 8 weeks, and as long as the cough is improving, no further diagnostic evaluation or treatment is needed. However, on occasion, postinfectious cough can continue for many months, becoming nonproductive of mucous. It is not clear why some patients develop a *persistent postinfectious cough.* Triggering of latent asthma is a possibility, as well as upper respiratory infection causing postnasal drip, both of which may cause the chronic cough. Severe or persistent coughing during the acute phase of the infection may traumatize the trachea and larynx, making the cough receptors hypersensitive and irritable to any stimulation. Some evidence of hyperirritability is found if the patient communicates that voice use causes the cough and that the cough is triggered by mildly irritating odors or smells that had not caused cough previously.

Bronchiectasis may cause chronic productive cough, often accompanied by large quantities of purulent sputum. Bronchiectasis is a dilatation of bronchioles, usually resulting from previous chest infection that has destroyed surrounding and supporting lung parenchyma. Tuberculosis was a prominent cause in the past, but childhood respiratory illnesses and adult bacterial pneumonias are more frequent causes. The cough in bronchiectasis is characterized by chronic or recurrent sputum production; is often related to body position because the bronchiectatic segment drains into more normal airways, triggering cough; and is often most productive in the morning, when the secretions that accumulate overnight are cleared. Bronchiectasis can be marked by intermittent febrile illnesses with infiltrates on chest x-ray, since the chronic presence of purulent secretions predispose to pneumonia.

Chronic respiratory infections, in addition to bronchiectasis, also cause a chronic productive cough. Tuberculosis can cause chronic cough with sputum production. Often, systemic symptoms such as weight loss, fatigue, fever, and night sweats are present, but in the earlier stages these may be absent. *Cystic fibrosis* can first appear in early adulthood and can present with productive cough.

Chronic coughs that are nonproductive, or only produce small amounts of mucus, are more common than coughs that are productive of purulent mucous. *Postnasal drip* is probably the most common cause of chronic cough. Mucus production may be present but is relatively slight compared with the amount produced in the coughs previously discussed, and the patient and physician can recognize that the mucus is being cleared from the posterior pharynx rather than arising from a source deep within the chest. The etiology of a cough associated with postnasal drip is probably irritation of cough receptors in upper airway structures from postnasal drainage. Because postnasal drip is a common problem, it is not clear why it causes cough in some patients, but it may be that preceding respiratory infection has sensitized the upper airway to be more sensitive to an irritant phenomenon.

In studies examining chronic cough, *asthma* is the second most common etiology. Cough can be the sole manifestation of asthma; wheezing may not be heard on examination, and the patient may not complain of shortness of breath. The cough of asthma may be triggered by factors such as exercise or cold air, may occur nocturnally, and although it usually does not produce mucous, may do so if a significant inflammatory component is present.

Gastroesophageal reflux may cause a chronic cough. This may occur due to reflex bronchoconstriction from acid reflux into the esophagus, or from reflux to the level of the pharynx with laryngeal irritation and aspiration. Esophageal pH monitoring demonstrates the temporal relationship of cough to reflux, although not all studies show this association. Only one half of patients with cough from gastroesophageal reflux, identified by pH monitoring or response to specific therapy, do not have reflux symptoms. Reflux may occur in the upright position, so that although gastroesophageal reflux may cause or exacerbate cough during sleep, it can also be a cause of cough during waking hours.

Postnasal drip, asthma, and gastroesophageal reflux can coexist to play a role in chronic cough. In studies evaluating the etiology of chronic cough, many patients have two or more of these disorders, which need to be treated before cough is improved.

Cough sometimes persists for many months after otherwise uncomplicated respiratory infections. This has been referred to as *postinfectious persistent cough*. Whereas viral respiratory infection may trigger asthma or cause postnasal sinus drainage, these are not the cause of postinfectious cough, as demonstrated by negative results on bronchoprovocation testing and lack of response to treatment trials. The etiology of postinfectious cough may be persistent trauma or irritation of the upper airway from the mechanical effects of coughing itself. Patients often notice that the cough is triggered by using the voice, and that slight hoarseness or loss of voice strength occurs. The vocal cords may appear edematous and inflamed on examination.

Drugs can cause cough. Cough may occur in 5% of patients taking *angiotensin converting enzyme inhibitor* medication. The cough may begin long after the medication is initiated or arise after a change in dose. The mechanism that causes these coughs is unknown, but it does not seem related to bronchial hyperreactivity caused by the agent.

In addition to these common causes of nonproductive cough, *bronchogenic carcinoma* can present with a nonproductive cough. A normal finding on chest x-ray does not exclude cancer; in smokers with hemoptysis, a small percentage of patients have an endobronchial lesion on bronchoscopy with a normal chest x-ray result. Irritation of the *diaphragm*, such as by subphrenic masses or infections, can cause cough; processes involving the *pericardium* also can cause cough, such as pericarditis, although other manifestations of pericarditis are rarely absent. *Pleural effusions*, which are apparent on examination or on the chest x-ray, may have cough as a symptom. *Interstitial lung disease* can have cough as a prominent symptom, but x-ray abnormalities are usually present. *Recurrent aspiration* can be a cause of cough, particularly in patients who have had cerebrovascular accidents and disruption of normal swallowing mechanism. This cough is likely triggered by recurrent aspiration of saliva, and may be more prominent during meals when food also is aspirated. *Congestive heart failure* can cause cough, particularly with exercise or nocturnally. This can be confused with cough associated with asthma, which can occur under similar circumstances. A rare cause of chronic cough is due to a reflex from irritation of the *external ear canal*, such as from ingrown hairs, foreign material, or external otitis.

Finally, a cough may have a *psychogenic* or *habitual* cause. Some patients persistently have a throat-clearing slight cough that does not respond to therapy for postnasal drip. Other patients have dry cough triggered under circumstances of stress or anxiety. Before ascribing cough to this cause, organic etiologies should first be excluded.

HISTORY

The history relating to a patient complaining of cough often is far more helpful in elucidating the cause than are laboratory tests or other interventions beyond a simple chest x-ray. It should first be determined whether the cough is predominantly productive of mucopurulent material or is nonproductive. In a cigarette smoker, a chronic productive cough often is due to irritative bronchitis; in a nonsmoker, bronchiectasis should be considered. Sputum production in bronchiectasis often is greatest on awakening in the morning, when retained secretions are cleared, and the cough of bronchiectasis may be exacerbated by the change in secretions as they empty from the bronchiectatic areas into areas of normal lung having intact cough reflexes. Relationship to a recent respiratory infection should be noted. A productive cough may last for several weeks after an acute respiratory infection. Persistent systemic symptoms of malaise, fever, night sweats, or fatigue raise the question of an indolent infection such as tuberculosis. Productive cough may be a manifestation of occupational-related respiratory irritants, and the relationship of cough to these exposures should be identified.

The presence of hemoptysis in a cigarette smoker suggests the possibility of a bronchogenic carcinoma. Cigarette smokers with hemoptysis and normal chest x-ray findings have an approximately 5% chance of having an endobronchial lesion accounting for an abnormality that is not visible on x-ray. Hemoptysis also may suggest the possibility of indolent infection, particularly tuberculosis. These patients often have systemic symptoms, such as fever and malaise, to suggest infection, but may not, and evidence of parenchymal infiltrates or cavities of tuberculosis are found only when a chest x-ray is obtained.

In patients with a nonproductive cough and who are well except for their complaint of cough, the most common diagnoses are postnasal drip, asthma, gastroesophageal reflux, persistent postinfection cough, or, frequently, a combination of two or more of these. Approximately one half of patients with postnasal drip are asymptomatic. They have no nasal discharge or pharyngeal sense of drainage and, therefore, the exclusion of these findings on history does not exclude the diagnosis. Similarly, asthmatics with a primary complaint of cough may not notice wheezing or shortness of breath. Gastroesophageal reflux causing cough is silent in at least half of the patients who are believed to to have cough on that basis, and conversely, the presence of reflux symptoms are common and do not necessarily implicate reflux as the cause of the cough. Persistent postinfectious cough is identified by its relationship to a previous respiratory infection. Once mucous production associated with the acute infection has stopped, usually within a few weeks, these coughs become dry and are associated with a tickling or "raw" sensation in the upper airway, exacerbation of cough by using the voice, and often a change in voice quality.

Historical information also helps in determining the etiology of less common causes of dry, nonproductive cough. Cough with exertion or occurring nocturnally with orthopnea, or paroxysmal nocturnal dyspnea may point to congestive heart failure as the etiology, although nocturnal asthma can have similar characteristics.

Hypersensitivity pneumonitis is a symptom complex of fever, cough, and shortness of breath that occurs on exposure to organic antigens such as thermophilic *Actinomyces*, *Aspergillus* species, or other antigens. This disease has several names that are associated with the specific exposures, such as farmer lung, bird fancier disease, and humidifier lung. Patients usually have symptoms of shortness of breath, fever, and cough, but occasionally cough may be the predominant complaint. If a history of exposure is not obtained, these patients can go on to develop chronic interstitial fibrosis with permanent loss of lung function.

A complete drug history should be obtained. Drugs such as nitrofurantoin, thiazide diuretics, amiodarone, bleomycin, and methotrexate cause pulmonary infiltrates. These are generally associated with dyspnea, but cough may be the initial symptom. Angiotensin converting enzyme inhibitors, which are commonly used in adults for treating hypertension or congestive heart failure, are frequently associated with causing a cough. These drugs do not cause pulmonary infiltrates or other manifestations such as cough, wheezing, or shortness of breath. The cough may begin some months or even longer after initiation of the drug, and patients may notice the onset after switching from one drug in the family to another. Cough is usually described as an irritating dry cough accompanied by a tickling or raw sensation in the upper airway. The exact mechanism for the cough is uncertain, but the cough is not due to asthma induction by the medication. The cough resolves on cessation of the drug; it takes days to see some effect but may take weeks for the cough to resolve fully.

PHYSICAL EXAMINATION AND CLINICAL FINDINGS

Auscultation of the chest may be helpful. In patients with asthma, a prolonged expiratory time or wheezing may be heard. In patients with interstitial fibrosis, dry rales may be heard, and moister rales may be heard in patients with congestive heart failure. A focal wheeze with expiration suggests the possibility of an obstructing endobronchial lesion. Localized evidence of consolidation suggests a pulmonary infiltrative process such as pneumonia, and dullness and decreased breath sounds suggest a pleural effusion. Focal rales or rhonchi suggest the presence of bronchiectasis.

Examination of the pharynx and upper airway may show evidence of postnasal drainage. However, this is a common and nonspecific finding, so its presence does not implicate postnasal drip as the cause of cough.

An S_3 gallop on examination of the heart and pedal edema may suggest congestive heart failure as a cause of the cough. With some patients, examination of the ear canal elicits brisk cough, and in these sensitive individuals, pathologic elements in the ear canal such as external otitis or irritating hairs may be an etiology of the cough.

LABORATORY AND IMAGING STUDIES

A chest x-ray is a useful part of the evaluation of a patient with chronic cough. A chest x-ray shows most carcinomas that are associated with a chronic cough. Abnormalities suggesting chronic infection, such as tuberculosis, interstitial lung disease, hypersensitivity pneumonitis, or congestive heart failure, may be found. Bronchiectasis sometimes produces findings on chest x-ray such as thickened bronchial walls or cystic spaces, which can suggest that diagnosis. Mediastinal masses, pericardial disease, and pleural effusions also can be seen when either the history or physical examination does not reveal them.

Most of the time, however, the chest x-ray does not give positive results in patients who have a chronic cough, particularly if the cough is not productive and the patient is otherwise feeling well. If the history suggests that asthma may be present, then pulmonary function tests should be performed to demonstrate airway obstruction. If airway obstruction is absent and asthma is still suspected, then a methacholine challenge to induce asthma can be performed. If cough is productive and purulent, then a sputum culture is useful to demonstrate bacterial infection in bronchiectasis, which may require specific antibiotic treatment as therapy.

Bronchoscopy has only a limited role in evaluating patients with cough, with the exception of smokers with hemoptysis. It is usually considered only after interventions directed toward the common etiologies of chronic cough have not benefited the patient.

TREATMENT

Even after careful and complete history, physical examination, chest x-ray, and sputum culture, the etiology of cough often is not precisely determined. In these patients, a program of staged treatment directed toward the commonest causes of cough serves both a treatment and diagnostic purpose. Since postnasal drip is the commonest cause of chronic cough, the initial step is treatment with an antihistamine–decongestant preparation. With this therapy, cough may improve within weeks, but occasionally months may be needed for the cough to completely resolve. As long as the patient shows some improvement, this therapy can be continued. If there is no improvement after weeks of therapy or if some improvement has occurred but the cough persists, further evaluation is warranted. Because asthma in most studies has been shown to be the next most common cause of chronic cough, a trial of inhaled albuterol, 2 puffs four times daily for 1 to 2 weeks, is given. If the cough responds promptly, this confirms asthma as an etiology, and asthma treatment can be continued. If the cough is not better or is only partially better, pulmonary function tests with bronchoprovocation challenge should be performed. If results are positive, a short trial of prednisone, 20 to 30 mg/day for 1 week, can be used to treat asthma that has been refractory to bronchodilators. If the pulmonary function tests and bronchoprovocation tests give negative results and there is a history of onset of cough after respiratory infection, then the same dose of steroids can be given to treat "postinfectious, persistent cough." The antiinflammatory action of steroids works fairly effectively in coughs of this nature, often stopping the cough completely or ameliorating it significantly.

If cough is not improved, then patients are treated for gastroesophageal reflux with an H_2 blocker, along with routine antireflux measures, such as avoidance of caffeine, alcohol, and chocolate, avoidance of eating before sleep, and raising the head of the bed by 15 to 20 cm (6 to 8 inches). If the cough is not improved after a few weeks of this therapy, some authorities suggest 24 hour esophageal pH monitoring, and if reflux is present, treatment with H_2 blockers should be continued, with the addition of omeprazole.

After this staged approach, most patients who meet the entry criteria, that is, having a nonproductive cough lasting for more than 1 to 2 months and no other symptoms, have the cough relieved. Cough recurs in a few of these, but responds again to therapeutic trials.

In patients who continue to have a nonproductive cough after this sequence of treatment, bronchoscopy is indicated to evaluate the possibility of an endobronchial lesion and to obtain secretions. If no abnormality is found and the cough still persists, another trial of corticosteroids and an inhaled bronchodilator could be performed, with reconsideration of the more uncommon causes of cough. It is best to consider causes such as bronchiectasis, tuberculosis, congestive heart failure, interstitial lung disease, and drug-related cough before empirically embarking on what may be a many-week course of a graded treatment trial, so that if no benefit is achieved, the former have already been carefully considered.

While specific therapy is being attempted, nonspecific treatment for cough can be helpful when the cough is severe, annoying, and disturbs sleep. Soothing treatment for upper airway irritation from coughing itself can be useful. Over-the-counter preparations, cough drops and lozenges, and home remedies can provide relief. More potent cough suppression in the form of medications containing opiates or opiate analogues can be useful. They often allow sleep when the cough is nonproductive and irritating. During the daytime, however, cough suppression by these medications may cause drowsiness. Cough-suppressant medications usually do not affect cough to such a degree that the ability to assess the response to progressive trials of various medications is lost.

CONSIDERATIONS IN PREGNANCY

The etiology of the cough may produce effects that pertain to pregnancy. Cough due to asthma, for example, can result in hypoxemia even when there is minimal shortness of breath, and in pregnant patients with cough, it is useful to ensure that arterial blood oxygen tension or oxygen saturation by oximetry is normal. The greatest consideration in pregnancy and cough is to make sure that a systemic disease is not causing the cough, and to ensure that the cough is not associated with hypoxemia. Coughing itself is associated with increased intraabdominal pressure because of the contraction of the abdominal and the thoracic musculature. The pressure increase is usually not so large as to cause any mechanical problems to the fetus or placenta. Urinary incontinence with coughing can occur and may be exacerbated in pregnancy. In late pregnancy, whether the sudden loud sound of cough disturbs the fetus in any psychologic or developmental way is unknown, but seems unlikely.

Medications used in the sequential approach to cough, as described earlier, may need to be modified in pregnancy. It may be prudent to avoid vasoconstrictive decongestants, such as pseudoephedrine, that are used to treat postnasal drip. Among antihistamines, diphenhydramine, brompheniramine, loratadine, and cyproheptadine are category B agents. Bronchoprovocation challenge with methacholine is not advised in the pregnant asthma suspect. Antacids and H_2 blockers for gastroesophageal reflux are not contraindicated in pregnancy and are rated as category B drugs, except for nizatidine, which is category C. There is insufficient experience with omeprazole in pregnancy, and it is a category C drug. Treating asthma in pregnancy is advisable to avoid hypoxemia, and most agents, including systemic corticosteroids, can be used safely. Fiberoptic bronchoscopy, if necessary, can be performed safely. Short-term use of opiates for cough suppression is safe in pregnancy.

BIBLIOGRAPHY

Corrao WM. Chronic cough: when to take the less traveled path. J Respir Dis 1993;14:273.

Corrao WM, Braman SS, Irwin RS. Chronic cough as the sole presenting manifestation of bronchial asthma. N Engl J Med 1975;292:555.

Doan T, Patterson R, Greenberger PA. Cough variant asthma: usefulness of a diagnostic-therapeutic trial with prednisone. Ann Allergy 1992;69:505.

Ing AJ, Ngu MC, Breslin AB. Chronic persistent cough and gastro-oesophageal reflux. Thorax 1991;46:479.

Irwin RS, Curley FJ. The treatment of cough: a comprehensive review. Chest 1991;99:1477.

Irwin RS, Curley FJ, French CL. Chronic cough: the spectrum and frequency of causes, key components of the diagnostic evaluation, and outcome of specific therapy. Am Rev Respir Dis 1990;141:640.

Poe RH, Harder RV, Israel RH, Kallay MC. Chronic persistent cough: experience in diagnosis and outcome using an anatomic diagnostic protocol. Chest 1989;95:723.

Poe RH, Israel RH, Utell MJ, Hall WJ. Chronic cough: bronchoscopy or pulmonary function testing? Am Rev Respir Dis 1982;126:160.

Pratter MR, Bartter T, Akers S, DuBois J. An algorithmic approach to chronic cough. Ann Intern Med 1993;119:977.

Primary Care for Women, edited by Phyllis C. Leppert and Fred M. Howard. Lippincott-Raven Publishers, Philadelphia © 1997.

VII

Gastrointestinal Problems

59

Gastrointestinal Bleeding

DONALD R. BORDLEY

Gastrointestinal (GI) bleeding is a common and serious medical problem, leading to more than 300,000 hospitalizations each year in the United States. Among these hospitalized patients, mortality approaches 10%. Many additional patients undergo outpatient evaluation, prompted by symptoms or signs suggestive of GI bleeding or by screening evidence of asymptomatic GI blood loss. The magnitude of the outpatient problem is harder to estimate, but researchers in the Netherlands reviewed several large population studies from Europe and Australia and estimate that rectal bleeding alone accounts for 8 of every 1000 visits to a general practice setting.

GI bleeding can be divided into three categories by mode of presentation: (1) overt upper GI bleeding, defined as proximal to the ligament of Treitz; (2) overt lower GI bleeding; and (3) occult GI bleeding. Relative frequency of the three categories of bleeding is unknown. Of overt bleeding episodes serious enough to require hospitalization, 80% originate in the upper tract and the remaining 20% in the lower tract. Table 59-1 lists the important causes within each category. Whereas the prevalence of some etiologies may differ between women and men, women are vulnerable to all important causes. In the following sections, general guidelines that apply to all patients precede a separate discussion of each mode of presentation.

GENERAL GUIDELINES FOR ALL PATIENTS

History

As for any major clinical problem, an episode of GI bleeding demands that a careful history be performed. Comorbid conditions must be identified because of their profound impact on prognosis. Most of the morbidity and mortality in GI bleeding occurs in older patients with significant comorbidity. Medications, either prescribed or over the counter, may either cause or exacerbate an episode of bleeding. Patients on systemic anticoagulation medication should be identified; however, unless they undergo excessive anticoagulation, an explanation for their bleeding should be vigorously sought; more than 80% have a significant bleeding lesion.

Physical Examination

The physical examination in a bleeding patient should first assess hemodynamic stability. Blood pressure and pulse should be taken in the supine position then repeated in the upright position unless supine readings already suggest significant volume depletion. Careful cardiovascular and pulmonary examinations should be performed. Any patient with postural change in blood pressure or pulse or any other sign of decreased vital tissue perfusion, such as a change in mental status, must be assumed to have acute volume depletion due to blood loss and managed accordingly. All patients should be examined for signs of a more generalized bleeding disorder such as telangiectases, ecchymoses, petechiae, or oral or nasal mucosal hemorrhage. Rectal examination with fecal occult blood testing (FOBT) should be performed in all patients.

Laboratory Studies

The extent of laboratory evaluation required depends on the severity of the bleeding episode. Patients whose bleeding episode is mild by history and who have no orthostatic change in vital signs or other evidence of hemodynamic instability require a complete blood count (CBC) to assess the magnitude and chronicity of blood loss. Whereas a fall in hematocrit may not be evident early in a bleeding episode, this initial value provides an important baseline for comparison as the patient is followed over time. If hypochromia and microcytosis are present, this suggests that blood loss has been chronic, at least in part. Coagulation studies should be ordered on all patients who are on anticoagulants or who have risk factors for clotting abnormality (eg, liver disease). Coagulation studies in otherwise healthy patients who are not on anticoagulants are rarely abnormal and add little to patient care. Other general laboratory testing should be individualized to document the presence and activity level of known or suspected contributing or comorbid conditions. For example, patients with liver or kidney disease need to have appropriate studies checked. Patients who have known ischemic heart disease or who are at high risk should have an electrocardiogram performed and, when possible, compared with an old tracing to determine if bleeding is causing acute myocardial ischemia.

Table 59-1. Important Etiologies of Gastrointestinal Bleeding

Overt Upper Gastrointestinal Bleeding
Peptic ulcer disease
Gastritis
Esophageal varices
Mallory-Weiss tear
Esophagitis
Gastric neoplasm
Angiodysplasia (patients with renal failure)
Overt Lower Gastrointestinal Bleeding
Hemorrhoids and other lesions of the anal canal
Neoplasms of the colon and rectum
Colonic vascular ectasias
Diverticulosis
Inflammatory bowel disease
Mesenteric vascular insufficiency
Meckel diverticulum
Occult Gastrointestinal Bleeding
Neoplasms of the colon and rectum
Peptic ulcer disease
Gastritis
Esophagitis

All patients with active hematemesis, heavy rectal bleeding, orthostasis, or other signs of hemodynamic instability require more extensive laboratory evaluation, including platelet count, prothrombin time, partial thromboplastin time, type and crossmatch, electrolytes, creatinine, and blood urea nitrogen.

Treatment

Before undergoing any diagnostic evaluation, all hemodynamically compromised patients must receive appropriate resuscitation with intravenous fluids and blood products. Failure to provide adequate resuscitation leads to most of the early mortality and morbidity in GI bleeding. Any unstable comorbidity also should be promptly identified and treated.

Treatment to control bleeding is discussed in the appropriate sections later. Discussion of the long-term management of the many potential causes of GI bleeding is beyond the scope of this chapter, and readers are referred to other chapters in this book or other resources.

Indications for Hospital Admission

All patients with active hematemesis, heavy rectal bleeding, orthostasis, or other evidence of hemodynamic instability should be immediately referred to an emergency department for stabilization and admission. For those whose condition does not stabilize quickly, intensive care unit admission is advisable. Patients with melena alone who are hemodynamically and medically stable can be cautiously managed as outpatients; however, since such patients have often had significant blood loss, admission may be advisable in older patients and those with significant comorbidity. As long as there is no evidence of volume depletion, outpatient management is entirely appropriate for patients with rectal bleeding that is mild by history and for those with occult GI blood loss.

Indications for Consultation

Urgent consultation by both a gastroenterologist and a general surgeon is indicated for all patients with active hematemesis, heavy rectal bleeding, or hemodynamic instability and for all patients with persistent bleeding despite aggressive medical therapy. All such patients require endoscopic investigation of either their upper or lower GI tract. Although most do not require surgery, those who do cannot be reliably identified at the time of presentation, and it is important to have a surgeon involved well before a decision about surgery has to be made.

A gastroenterologist should see the remaining patients whenever the primary care physician needs assistance regarding diagnosis or management. Patients whose bleeding is controlled medically require surgical consultation only if an underlying lesion requiring surgery is identified.

OVERT UPPER GASTROINTESTINAL BLEEDING

Patients with overt upper GI bleeding present with hematemesis, melena, or both. It is first important to establish that either manifestation is genuine. Bleeding in the nasal passages, oral cavity, and respiratory tree can lead to swallowing of blood with subsequent apparent hematemesis. Dark stools may be caused by the ingestion of iron or other substances.

True hematemesis occurs only with bleeding in the upper tract. Melena usually indicates upper GI bleeding, but can also be seen in patients with bleeding in the more distal small bowel or proximal colon. Non–upper GI causes of melena are sufficiently rare that patients presenting in this way should initially be presumed to have an upper source. Upper GI bleeding occurs less often in women, with a male predominance of up to 2 : 1. This probably reflects ulcer disease, the commonest cause of upper GI bleeding, which afflicts men twice as often as it does women.

Etiologies

Two large multicenter studies including more than 6200 patients with acute upper GI bleeding found that 40% to 50% had discrete ulcer disease of the stomach or duodenum, 20% to 30% had gastritis or gastric erosions, 10% to 15% had esophageal varices, 4% to 8% had Mallory-Weiss tears, 5% to 7% had esophagitis, and 2% to 4% had cancer. Only one of the studies provided information regarding patient gender; in that study, 750 of 2225 patients were women. No significant difference in etiology of bleeding between women and men was reported. Episodes of massive upper GI bleeding leading to hemodynamic instability were almost always due to ulcer disease, severe erosive gastritis, or esophageal varices. Among patients with renal failure, angiodysplasia in the upper GI tract is the leading cause of bleeding, followed by esophagitis.

History

Patients with overt upper GI bleeding should be carefully questioned regarding preexisting upper GI disease, especially ulcer disease or varices, and regarding risk factors for the common causes of upper GI bleeding. Esophageal varices are exceedingly rare in patients without historical or physical evidence suggesting chronic liver disease or portal hypertension. A history of repeated vomiting or retching followed by the abrupt onset of hematemesis suggests a Mallory-Weiss tear. Nonsteroidal antiinflammatory drugs increase the bleeding rate from both gastric and duodenal ulcers. Aspirin, even in doses as low as 300 mg a day, significantly increases the risk of upper GI bleeding. Corticosteroids taken alone do not increase the risk of upper GI bleeding, but taken in combination with nonsteroidal antiinflammatory drugs dramatically increase the risk.

In addition to providing clues to etiology and prognosis, history may be useful in assessing the severity and acuity of a bleeding episode. Hematemesis indicates significant, active bleeding. Acute postural symptoms such as dizziness or faintness suggest that bleeding has been rapid enough to cause intravascular volume depletion. Melena alone is less helpful in this regard and may occur with limited bleeding and persist for several days after active bleeding has stopped.

Physical Examination and Clinical Evaluation

Evidence of chronic liver disease or portal hypertension such as ascites, jaundice, or splenomegaly dramatically increases the likelihood of varices. Whereas a careful abdominal and general examination are important, these have not been useful in establishing the relative likelihood of causes other than varices.

A nasogastric tube should be passed in all patients with hematemesis or hemodynamic instability to document active or recent bleeding. Lavage should be performed on the stomach with body-temperature tap water until the aspirate is clear, then the tube can be removed. There is no evidence that continued lavage with any fluid at any temperature stops bleeding or prevents recurrence. A negative nasogastric aspirate finding does not rule out active bleeding, especially when the source is a duodenal ulcer.

Combining findings from physical examination with data from the history allows separation of patients with acute upper GI bleeding into groups with distinctly different risk of persistent bleeding or other poor outcomes. Clinical variables consistently associated with increased risk of further bleeding or other poor outcomes include the following: age older than 60 years, significant comorbidity, objective evidence of chronic liver disease, hypotension on presentation, and failure of clinical bleeding to stop promptly after presentation. Patients lacking any of these risk factors have a less than 5% probability of further bleeding, only a 2% probability of needing further surgery, and a less than 1% probability of death. As a patient accumulates risk factors, these probabilities increase; in patients with three or more risk factors, probability of further bleeding or other poor outcome exceeds 50%.

Diagnostic Evaluation

Esophagogastroduodenoscopy (hereafter referred to as endoscopy) is the most sensitive and specific diagnostic test for patients with upper GI hemorrhage. When performed within 12 hours of clinical bleeding, endoscopy demonstrates an actively bleeding lesion, a lesion with evidence of recent bleeding, or a single lesion compatible with the bleeding episode in 85% to 90% of patients. The remaining 10% to 15% of patients either have a negative study result or multiple nonbleeding lesions. The sensitivity of endoscopy, particularly for active bleeding, declines after 12 hours.

In addition to establishing a diagnosis in most patients, endoscopy provides important prognostic information in patients who are bleeding from ulcer disease or varices. Ulcer patients with active bleeding or "stigmata of recent hemorrhage," such as a visible vessel in the ulcer base, have a rebleeding risk of up to 50%; rebleeding risk is similarly high in patients with varices. Furthermore, endoscopy allows both biopsy and culture and thus may prove useful in guiding long-term management, particularly now that infection with *Helicobacter pylori* has emerged as an important, treatable cause of ulcer disease.

Barium contrast radiography, even using double-contrast techniques, has a sensitivity of only 50% to 70% and interferes with subsequent endoscopy or angiography. Diagnostic angiography and radionuclide imaging should be reserved for patients with active bleeding who are undiagnosed after endoscopy.

Even among patients admitted to the hospital for their bleeding episode, at least 75% stop bleeding promptly with only nonspecific supportive care and will never rebleed. Emergency endoscopy should be reserved for patients who have persistent bleeding or hemodynamic instability despite 1 to 2 hours of aggressive supportive therapy. For patients whose bleeding stops promptly, decision regarding both the need for and timing of endoscopy should be based on the patient's risk of rebleeding or poor outcome and on the importance of establishing a diagnosis as a guide to long-term management. Patients judged to be at moderate or high risk based on clinical criteria (see earlier) should undergo endoscopy at the first available elective opportunity. Diagnostic yield is highest if this is done within 12 to 24 hours of active bleeding. Among low-risk patients, use of endoscopy should be individualized. Young patients with a single self-limited episode of bleeding usually have minor acid peptic disease and often can be safely and effectively managed without a definitive diagnosis.

Treatment

Although benefit has been difficult to demonstrate in controlled trials, most experts advise the empirical use of a histamine$_2$ receptor antagonist in all patients with upper GI bleeding. Other therapies are directed at the 20% to 25% of patients whose bleeding does not stop spontaneously.

Endoscopic therapies have been extensively studied in patients with acute nonvariceal bleeding; a meta-analysis of 30 randomized clinical trials of endoscopic hemostatic treatment demonstrated decreased rates of further bleeding, surgery, and mortality among treated patients with ulcer disease who had either active bleeding or a nonbleeding visible vessel in the ulcer base. Patients with adherent clot or flat pigmented spots in the ulcer base did not benefit from endoscopic therapy.

Patients with persistent bleeding from varices have a poor prognosis. No form of therapy has been clearly demonstrated to reduce hospital mortality or prolong long-term survival. Nonetheless, several modalities show at least a trend toward better control of acute bleeding. Intravenous vasopressin lowers portal pressure in actively bleeding patients and may help control variceal bleeding; however, it is a potent vasoconstrictor in all vascular systems and must be used with great caution in elderly patients or those with known vascular disease. Somatostatin and its longer-acting analogue octreotide also decrease portal pressure but do not cause vasoconstriction elsewhere and thus may offer a safer alternative. Current studies suggest that somatostatin is at least as effective as vasopressin in controlling hemorrhage and has fewer complications. Patients who continue to bleed despite vasopressin or somatostatin should have endoscopic therapy attempted. Endoscopic injection sclerotherapy and endoscopic band ligation are equally effective in controlling acute bleeding; band ligation may have a lower complication rate.

The few patients whose upper GI bleeding is uncontrolled after these therapies have been tried require surgery or therapeutic angiography.

OVERT LOWER GASTROINTESTINAL BLEEDING

Etiologies

Hematochezia usually indicates bleeding in the colon, rectum, or anal canal, although distal small bowel diseases or even brisk upper GI bleeding also may lead to the passage of blood per rectum. Hemorrhoids and other lesions of the anal canal account for up to 80% of all episodes of hematochezia but are a rare cause of massive bleeding. Other common causes include neoplasms of the colon and rectum, colonic vascular ectasias, and diverticulosis; the latter two are particularly common in older patients. Less common but important etiologies include inflammatory bowel disease (IBD), mesenteric vascular insufficiency, and Meckel diverticulum. Endurance athletes, especially long-distance runners, may experience rectal bleeding during or after heavy exertion. Among women with lower GI bleeding, intestinal endometriosis should always be included in the differential diagnosis, although bleeding is an exceedingly rare complication of this disorder. Notice that intestinal endometriosis is seen in both premenopausal and postmenopausal women. Erosion of an abdominal ectopic pregnancy into large or small bowel also can present as overt, sometimes massive, lower GI bleeding.

History

Many patients with rectal bleeding do not report this to a physician unless directly asked. The study mentioned earlier, which found that 8 of 1000 visits to a general practitioner are for rectal bleeding, also found that when asked about it on a survey, 20% of the general population reported at least one episode of rectal bleeding within the last year. Primary care physicians must remember to ask about this important symptom and to inquire about prior history of other disorders of the anal canal or lower GI tract.

All patients should be questioned about risk factors for colon cancer. Risk is highest in those with hereditary polyposis, the cancer family syndrome, and ulcerative colitis of longer than 10 years' duration; it is moderately increased in patients with a prior history of colonic adenomas or cancer and those with a history of colon cancer in first-degree relatives. Women who have had ovarian, endometrial, or breast cancer also may be at increased risk.

Heavy rectal bleeding in an otherwise asymptomatic elderly patient suggests either diverticulosis or colonic vascular ectasia. History also may provide important clues to some of the less common causes of lower GI bleeding. A history of diarrhea, lower abdominal cramping, or tenesmus increases the likelihood of IBD, whereas patients with generalized vascular disease, congestive heart failure, or chronic atrial fibrillation have an increased risk of mesenteric vascular insufficiency. Patients with mesenteric vascular insufficiency also may complain of severe pain that seems out of proportion to findings on subsequent physical examination. Meckel diverticulum should be considered in a young patient with severe but otherwise asymptomatic lower GI hemorrhage.

Physical Examination and Clinical Evaluation

In many patients with lower GI bleeding, careful inspection and digital examination of the anorectal region may reveal either hemorrhoids or other disease of the anal canal. Unfortunately, patients who are bleeding from other sources often have coincident hemorrhoids, so the finding of an anorectal lesion, especially one that is not bleeding at the time of the examination, does not always obviate the need for further investigation. On the other hand, a patient younger than 40 years of age with a hemodynamically insignificant episode of rectal bleeding and hemorrhoids on examination has such a low likelihood of any other dangerous pathologic process that no further evaluation other than careful follow-up is necessary.

Physical examination may provide clues to other potential causes of lower GI bleeding. Colorectal cancer may produce a mass on rectal or abdominal examination. In patients with advanced disease, evidence of weight loss, lymphadenopathy, hepatomegaly, or other signs of metastatic disease may be present. Patients with active IBD often appear to be acutely ill, even when blood loss is minimal, may have significant tenderness on abdominal examination, and often are febrile during an acute exacerbation of their disease. Mesenteric vascular insufficiency may be associated with diminished peripheral pulses, bruits in the abdomen or elsewhere, atrial fibrillation, or signs of congestive heart failure. An association between colonic vascular ectasias and aortic stenosis has been observed, although the significance of this association is uncertain.

Diagnostic Evaluation

Patients whose history or physical examination suggests hemorrhoids or other disease of the anal canal should undergo prompt anoscopy. If the patient is young and the bleeding episode is trivial, positive findings on this examination obviate the need for further workup.

All older patients and all patients with more than small amounts of rectal bleeding require more thorough evaluation. Strategy depends on whether the patient is actively bleeding. Colonoscopy is the most sensitive and specific diagnostic procedure and should be employed in all patients who are not bleeding heavily at the time of evaluation. An electrolyte purgative should be administered to improve diagnostic yield.

Heavy bleeding (more than 1 mL/minute) obscures vision through the colonoscope and demands a different approach. If history or physical examination suggests colitis, it may be possible to establish this diagnosis with rigid or flexible sigmoidoscopy. Otherwise, either angiography or radionuclide imaging may be needed to establish the likely site of bleeding and guide further management. Because barium in the colon interferes with subsequent examination by colonoscopy or angiography, barium enema should not be performed in any patient with active or recent lower GI bleeding.

Because patients with massive upper GI bleeding can present with the passage of blood per rectum, evaluation of the upper GI tract needs to be considered in all patients with rectal bleeding and hemodynamic instability, particularly if history or physical examination suggests increased risk of ulcer disease, severe gastritis, or varices.

Treatment

Most episodes of lower GI bleeding stop spontaneously with only supportive care. Therapy for patients with persistent bleeding depends on the underlying lesion. Bleeding from colonic vascular ectasias can be controlled through the colonoscope with a variety of hemostatic modalities. Likewise, bleeding polyps can be cauterized or removed colonoscopically. Aggressive medical management controls bleeding in most patients with IBD. Surgery or angiographic therapy may be required when bleeding from diverticula or other sources fails to stop with supportive care.

OCCULT GASTROINTESTINAL BLEEDING

Positive fecal occult blood testing, either as part of a home screening program or detected during digital rectal examination, and unexplained iron deficiency anemia are the two most common presenting manifestations of occult GI bleeding. Efforts must be made to assure that either manifestation genuinely indicates GI blood loss. False-positive results on FOBT are reduced if patients avoid rare red meat, horseradish, cantaloupe, and uncooked fresh vegetables for 3 days before testing. Women with iron deficiency anemia should be carefully questioned about excessive menstrual or other vaginal blood loss.

Etiologies

Although evidence of occult GI blood loss can be found with bleeding anywhere in the GI tract, the most serious concern is colonic neoplasia. Controlled trials indicate that among asymptomatic patients older than 50 years of age found to have a positive result on FOBT, about 8% have a colon cancer and another 30% to 40% have an adenoma. A positive FOBT finding on digital rectal examination also is significant, particularly in older patients. Researchers at the University of South Alabama found that among 185 patients without GI complaints referred for colonoscopy because of a positive FOBT result on digital rectal examination, 51 (27%) had significant neoplasms (13 adenocarcinomas and 38 adenomatous polyps), whereas 59 (32%) had nonneoplastic lesions (33 hemorrhoids or fissures, 10 diverticula, 9 hyperplastic polyps, 4 nonbleeding vascular ectasias, 3 miscellaneous minor lesions). The remaining 75 patients had no lesions found on colonoscopy and presumably had bleeding outside of the colon or false-positive tests. The mean age of the study population was 59.4 years; 45% were women and 55% were men. The frequency of neoplastic and nonneoplastic colonic lesions was similar in women and men. No colonic neoplasms were found among the 23 patients who were younger than 45 years of age.

A recent study of 100 consecutive patients with unexplained iron deficiency anemia demonstrated an upper GI bleeding source in 37 patients and a lower GI source in 26; one patient had both upper and lower tract lesions. The distribution of upper GI lesions was similar to that seen in overt upper GI bleeding: 19 patients (51%) had discrete ulcer disease, 6 (16%) had gastritis, 6 (16%) had esophagitis, and 3 patients had vascular ectasia. Gastric cancer, portal hypertensive gastropathy, and gastric adenomatous polyp each occurred in one patient. In contrast, the prevalence rate of neoplastic disease among patients with a lower GI source was 62% (11 colon cancers and 5 polyps among 26 patients), which was much higher than in patients with overt rectal bleeding. Other lower GI sources included vascular ectasias (5 patients), colitis (2), cecal ulcers (2), and parasitic infection (1). Fifty-one patients in this study were women, 9 of whom were menstruating; none had a history of unusual or heavy flow.

History

Patients who have not previously reported risk factors or symptoms often do so when questioned directly after a positive FOBT result or when unexplained iron deficiency anemia is identified. In the previously mentioned study of 100 patients with unexplained iron deficiency anemia, 33 patients had symptoms specific to either the upper or lower GI tract. Among the 22 patients with upper GI symptoms, 17 had lesions found in the upper tract and none had lesions found in the colon. Conversely, among 11 patients with lower GI symptoms, 9 had lesions in the colon and none had lesions in the upper tract. Among the remaining 67 patients who were truly asymptomatic, 19 had upper tract lesions, 16 had colonic lesions, and 31 had no GI lesion discovered.

Because the gravest concern for patients with occult bleeding is colon cancer, patients should be questioned about risk factors (see "Overt Lower Gastrointestinal Bleeding") and about changes in stool caliber or obstructive symptoms. It is also important to ask about systemic evidence of malignant disease, such as weight loss or symptoms suggestive of metastases.

Physical Examination

Among the important causes of occult GI bleeding, only colorectal cancer is likely to be associated with distinctive physical findings. A mass may be detected on rectal or abdominal examination. Patients with more advanced disease may show signs of weight loss and may have hepatomegaly, lymphadenopathy, or other evidence of metastases.

Diagnostic Evaluation

When present, symptoms should be used to guide the initial evaluation in patients with occult GI bleeding. Endoscopy should be performed first in patients with upper GI symptoms and colonoscopy (or sigmoidoscopy plus air-contrast barium enema) first in patients with lower GI symptoms. If the initial study provides a convincing explanation for blood loss, appropriate treatment should be initiated and further workup done only if evidence of bleeding persists despite therapy. If the initial study result is negative, the alternative study should be performed. Caution should be exercised in accepting a minor upper GI lesion as the cause of bleeding, particularly if the patient is at increased risk of colon cancer.

Asymptomatic patients with occult GI bleeding should undergo colonoscopy first. If the colonoscopy finding is positive, no further evaluation is needed. If the colonoscopy result is negative and the patient has lost a sufficient blood volume to become iron deficient, upper endoscopy is probably indicated, although the yield of clinically important lesions is low. If the only evidence of occult blood loss was a positive FOBT finding without iron deficiency anemia and the colonoscopy finding is negative, close follow-up without upper endoscopy is sufficient.

CONSIDERATIONS IN PREGNANCY

Differential diagnosis of GI bleeding during pregnancy includes all causes already mentioned. Pregnancy does affect the relative frequency of some important causes. The incidence of esophagitis and hemorrhoids are increased in pregnancy, whereas ulcer disease seems to improve. Colon cancer, diverticulosis, and colonic vascular ectasias are distinctly unusual in women of childbearing age. The course of IBD during pregnancy is variable. Usually, if IBD is quiescent at the time of conception, it remains so throughout pregnancy. Conversely, if IBD is active at the time of conception, it tends to remain active or worsen. In patients with Crohn disease, exacerbations occur most commonly in the third trimester, whereas in ulcerative colitis they occur most commonly in the first trimester.

Careful judgment should be exercised before embarking on an extensive workup of GI bleeding during pregnancy. If symptoms of esophagitis are present in a woman with minor upper GI bleeding or guaiac-positive stool, empirical therapy is appropriate. Likewise, minor rectal bleeding associated with obvious hemorrhoids need not be further evaluated. On the other hand, major bleeding episodes require prompt control and evaluation because of the potentially devastating impact on both mother and fetus.

Upper GI bleeding severe enough to lead to hospitalization is rare in pregnancy. A study of 29,317 pregnancies over 7½ years at Robert Wood Johnson University Hospital (New Brunswick, NJ) and two affiliates found that only 13 patients were hospitalized with hematemesis and only one with melena. Of these, 9 underwent endoscopy: 4 had esophagitis, 2 had duodenal ulcer, 2 had Mallory-Weiss tear, and 1 had gastritis.

When needed, upper endoscopy seems to be reasonably safe throughout pregnancy. In the study just mentioned, 11 women underwent endoscopy for indications other than bleeding in addition to the 9 who were bleeding. Of the total of 20 women, 6 were in the first trimester, 8 were in the second trimester, and 6 were in the third trimester. There were no serious complications during or after the procedure, and labor was not induced in any case. Pregnancy outcome was known for 19 patients; in all cases, both mother and baby did well. Notice that the total number of patients who underwent endoscopy in this study was small; the procedure should still be done during pregnancy only when there are definite indications and even then with caution. All patients should be given supplemental oxygen and monitored by electrocardiography and pulse oximetry during the procedure.

Although women with cirrhosis become pregnant infrequently, maternal death rate in such patients is reported to range from 10% to 18%, and the most common cause of death is massive GI hemorrhage, usually from varices. In patients with definite varices, the risk of bleeding during pregnancy may be as high as 30% to 45%. Endoscopic injection sclerotherapy has been used both for emergent control of variceal bleeding during pregnancy and for prophylactic treatment of varices early in pregnancy or in cirrhotic patients who hope to become pregnant. The number of cases reported is small, but in experienced hands, the procedure seems to be safe and effective.

Persistent heavy rectal bleeding not caused by hemorrhoids fortunately is rare during pregnancy. When it does occur, etiologies found in younger patients such as IBD or Meckel diverticulum should be considered, as should abdominal ectopic pregnancy early in the first trimester. In rare cases where persistent hemorrhage requires diagnostic evaluation, flexible sigmoidoscopy probably should be done first since it is both simpler and safer than full colonoscopy, particularly in the later stages of pregnancy. Such cases would obviously require careful management by an expert team, including both an obstetrician and a gastroenterologist.

BIBLIOGRAPHY

Bordley DR. Acute upper gastrointestinal bleeding. In: Panzer RJ, Black ER, Griner PF, eds. Diagnostic strategies for common medical problems. Philadelphia: American College of Physicians, 1991.

Brint SL, DiPalma JA, Herrera JL. Is a hemoccult-positive rectal examination clinically significant? South Med J 1993;86:601.

Cappell MS, Sidhom O. A multicenter, multiyear study of the safety and clinical utility of esophagogastroduodenoscopy in 20 consecutive pregnant females with follow-up of fetal outcome. Am J Gastroenterol 1993;88:1900.

Cook DJ, Guyatt GH, Salena BJ, Laine LA. Endoscopic therapy for acute nonvariceal upper gastrointestinal hemorrhage: a meta-analysis. Gastroenterology 1992;102:139.

Fijten GH, Blijham GH, Knottnerus JA. Occurrence and clinical significance of overt blood loss per rectum in the general population and in medical practice. Br J Gen Pract 1994;44:320.

Friedman LS, Martin P. The problem of gastrointestinal bleeding. Gastroenterol Clin North Am 1993;22:717.

Goff JS. Gastroesophageal varices: pathogenesis and therapy of acute bleeding. Gastroenterol Clin North Am 1993;22:779.

Iwase H, Morise K, Kawase T, Horiuchi Y. Endoscopic injection sclerotherapy for esophageal varices during pregnancy. J Clin Gastroenterol 1994;18:80.

Korelitz BI. Inflammatory bowel disease during pregnancy. Gastroenterol Clin North Am 1992;21:827.

Laine L, Peterson WL. Bleeding peptic ulcer. N Engl J Med 1994;331:717.

Lieberman D. Gastrointestinal bleeding: initial management. Gastroenterol Clin North Am 1993;22:723.

Nattinger AB. Colon cancer screening and detection. In: Panzer RJ, Black ER, Griner PF, eds. Diagnostic strategies for common medical problems. Philadelphia: American College of Physicians, 1991.

Pajor A, Lehoczky D. Pregnancy in liver cirrhosis. Gynecol Obstet Invest 1994;38:45.

Richter JM. Occult gastrointestinal bleeding. Gastroenterol Clin North Am 1994;23:53.

Rockey DC, Cello JP. Evaluation of the gastrointestinal tract in patients with iron-deficiency anemia. N Engl J Med 1993;329:1691.

Primary Care for Women, edited by Phyllis C. Leppert and Fred M. Howard. Lippincott-Raven Publishers, Philadelphia © 1997.

60
Gastroesophageal Reflux Disease

KARIN J. DUNNIGAN

Gastroesophageal reflux disease (GERD) is one of the most common gastrointestinal disorders seen by the primary care physician. Nearly everyone experiences heartburn or acid regurgitation at some point. GERD encompasses a spectrum of disorders; the presenting symptoms and signs may vary widely. It is probably best defined as the presence of symptoms or tissue damage resulting from episodes of gastroesophageal reflux.

EPIDEMIOLOGY

At least 40% of people in the United States suffer from heartburn or acid regurgitation once a month or more. Between 5% and 10% of patients polled in a recent survey reported daily heartburn. It is estimated that over 25% of American adults ingest antacids more than twice a month. Most of these heavy users of antacids suffer from reflux, and many experience relief with this therapy.

GERD is often thought of as a disorder of advancing age. Indeed, persons over age 50 are much more likely to require medical attention for symptoms or complications of reflux than younger persons. However, GERD may occur in any age group, including young children. Although there is no reported difference in the rate of GERD between men and women, up to 75% of pregnant women experience heartburn. Males are more likely than females to be affected with some of the complications of GERD, such as esophagitis (2 : 1) or Barrett's esophagus (10 : 1). GERD occurs in all demographic groups.

Some patients with GERD develop local complications such as esophagitis, esophageal ulcer, stricture, or cancer. Fewer develop extraesophageal complications, including asthma, laryngitis, and pneumonitis. Worldwide, it is estimated that the evaluation and treatment of GERD is responsible for $2 to $3 billion per year in medical costs.

An iceberg model is often used to describe populations with GERD. The majority of persons with GERD make up the hidden base of the iceberg: they experience only mild symptoms and rarely seek medical care. Just below the surface is a smaller group whose symptoms are frequent and severe enough to require medical attention, although in this group complications are uncommon. The tip of the iceberg represents the small proportion of patients with GERD who have severe, chronic symptoms, commonly associated with complications such as esophagitis, stricture, bleeding, or cancer. They invariably seek and require medical care.

ETIOLOGY

GERD is a spectrum of disorders in which there is reflux of acid and other noxious substances from the stomach into the esophagus. This causes symptoms such as heartburn or acid regurgitation with or without associated damage to the esophageal mucosa. Nearly everyone has episodes of gastroesophageal reflux, usually after eating; they are considered a normal physiologic occurrence and are usually asymptomatic. When the contact between the gastric secretions and the esophageal mucosa is unusually long, however, GERD may develop.

Many factors affect whether someone develops GERD, including the antireflux barrier, esophageal clearance, the potency of refluxate, and esophageal mucosal defenses. Abnormalities in any one of these can lead to symptoms and signs of GERD (Fig. 60-1).

Reflux of gastric contents into the esophagus is usually prevented by barrier mechanisms. The most important antireflux barrier is the lower esophageal sphincter (LES). This ring of smooth muscle is 2.5 to 3.5 cm long and is located at the gastroesophageal junction, just below the diaphragm. (When a hiatus hernia is present, the gastroesophageal junction and the LES extend above the diaphragm.) The sphincter relaxes in response to swallowing a bolus of food, allowing the food to pass into the stomach. Once the food passes, the LES reverts back to a high enough pressure to prevent gastric contents from refluxing back into the esophagus.

Several factors—drugs, hormones, and foods—may affect the tone of the LES and lead to inappropriate relaxation (Table 60-1). This allows gastric contents to enter the esophagus more frequently or in greater amounts, exacerbating reflux in susceptible persons.

Several different medications may lead to a decrease in the LES pressure, including anticholinergic drugs, calcium channel blockers (particularly nifedipine), nitrates, α-adrenergic antagonists, β_2-adrenergic drugs, and methylxanthines, such as theophylline. Prostaglandins, dopamine, meperidine, diazepam, morphine, and barbiturates also may potentiate reflux with a decrease in the LES pressure. Angiotensin-converting enzyme inhibitors and cardioselective β_1-antagonists such as metoprolol have a similar effect.

Hormones may also affect the tone of the LES. Oral contraceptives and hormonal supplements decrease the LES pressure. This effect is probably related to the progesterone content of the drugs, although estrogen may also play a role. Heartburn is more common in the latter parts of the menstrual cycle and pregnancy. This effect is due at least partially to a hormonally related decrease in the sphincter pressure.

Many foods decrease LES pressure. Chocolate is a notorious promoter of reflux and probably adversely affects the sphincter because of its methylxanthine content. Carminatives such as spearmint and peppermint also relax the LES; onions may have a similar effect. Fatty foods are particularly effective in increasing esophageal acid exposure. This effect is related to two mechanisms induced by fat ingestion: reduction in the LES pressure and delayed gastric emptying. Although coffee has a bad reputation when it comes to GERD, its effect on the LES is unknown. Recent studies seem to indicate that coffee promotes GERD by direct irri-

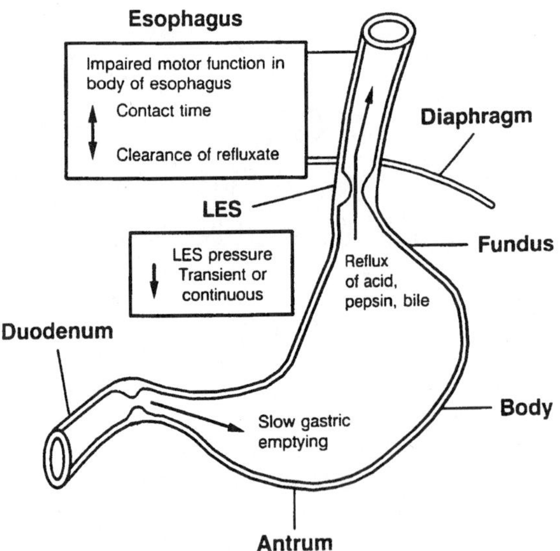

Figure 60-1. Mechanisms involved in the development of gastroesophageal reflux disease. (Adapted from Wolfe MM, Pathophysiology and clinical implications of gastroesophageal reflux disease. Practical Gastroenterology, 1994; 18:S10.)

tation of the esophageal mucosa and by increasing acid production, not by reducing LES pressure. Alcohol and nicotine both relax the LES and promote GERD.

Certain diseases are associated with a chronically diminished tone of the LES, including scleroderma and mixed connective tissue disease. GERD frequently complicates these systemic disorders and may be particularly severe.

Table 60-1. Factors Causing Diminished LES Pressure

Drugs
Anticholinergics
Calcium channel blockers
Nitrates
α-Adrenergic antagonists
β_2-Adrenergics
Methylxanthines
Prostaglandins
Meperidine
Diazepam
Morphine
Barbiturates
Angiotensin-converting enzyme inhibitors
Cardioselective β_1-antagonists
Oral contraceptives and hormonal supplements
Foods
Chocolate
Carminatives (spearmint and peppermint)
Onions
Fat
Alcohol
Nicotine
Systemic Disorders
Scleroderma
Mixed connective tissue disease
Pregnancy

Esophageal clearance—the ability of the esophagus to empty or neutralize gastric contents—is important in the prevention of GERD. Primary peristalsis is stimulated by swallowing, secondary peristalsis by esophageal distention. Together these clear much of the refluxed material; the rest is neutralized by swallowed saliva. Persons with GERD have prolonged esophageal clearance times. This is best illustrated in esophageal motor disorders such as scleroderma, where there is diminished peristaltic function, resulting in impaired esophageal clearance and GERD. An impaired flow of saliva affects the rate of neutralization of the refluxate. Salivary flow diminishes at night, making this a vulnerable time for GERD. Chronic xerostomia, seen in Sjögren syndrome, or diminished salivary flow due to cigarette smoking or the use of anticholinergic drugs promotes esophageal acid exposure.

The esophageal mucosal defense mechanisms, although not well understood, undoubtedly play an important role in the prevention of GERD. The esophagus has several defenses against cellular acidification, a process that leads to tissue injury. The superficial layer of squamous epithelium of the esophageal mucosa, the stratum corneum, is a "tight" epithelium that deters back-diffusion of hydrogen ions and other toxic substances into the mucosa. This defense can be overcome when a high concentration of hydrochloric acid is perfused into the esophageal lumen. Acidification of the surface cells occurs, they become ballooned and necrotic, and esophagitis results.

The potency of the material that refluxes into the esophagus also affects the development of GERD. Hydrogen is probably the final mediator of tissue injury within the esophagus, but other substances such as pepsin, bile, and food hyperosmolality may also play a role in causing injury. Most people with GERD have normal or perhaps slightly elevated basal levels of gastric acid secretion; only a few have gastric hypersecretion.

Foods promote reflux in several ways. Many affect the LES pressure, as noted above. Other foods, such as coffee, beer, and milk, are potent stimuli of gastric acid secretion. Still others may directly irritate the esophageal mucosa, such as orange juice, tomato drinks, and perhaps coffee.

Gastric and intraabdominal pressure increases may exceed the ability of even a normal LES to keep gastric contents within the stomach. For example, there is an association between morbid obesity and GERD. In obese people, the gastroesophageal pressure gradient, not the absolute LES pressure, determines reflux. Tight clothing, ascites, pregnancy, or obesity encourages reflux during sphincter relaxation, whatever the cause.

The role of hiatus hernia in GERD is controversial. At different times during the past 50 years, hiatus hernia has been thought to be either synonymous with GERD or an insignificant bystander. Current understanding suggests that hiatus hernia may well be a factor in the development of GERD. Along with the smooth muscle LES, the striated muscle crural diaphragm is a component of the antireflux barrier. In the setting of a hernia, the anatomic relation between the diaphragm and the LES is altered, potentially weakening the antireflux barrier. In addition, acid clearance by the esophagus may be impaired in the setting of a hiatus hernia.

Other factors may play a role in the development of GERD. Delayed gastric emptying as a result of mechanical, hormonal, or neurologic factors predisposes to more frequent episodes of reflux. Exercise, such as jogging, may induce reflux.

In summary, the consistent event in the development of GERD is the movement of gastric secretions from the stomach into the esophagus. If the refluxed material is particularly injurious, if peristalsis is impaired, if salivation is diminished, or if mucosal defenses are overcome, GERD occurs.

CLINICAL FEATURES

Symptoms

GERD encompasses a spectrum of symptoms (Table 60-2). The most common symptom, reported by over half of affected patients, is heartburn. Also called pyrosis, this is classically described as a burning sensation in the retrosternal area. It may radiate, wavelike, from the epigastrium up to the neck or, less commonly, into the back or the arms. Sometimes the discomfort is limited to the epigastric area or the throat.

Heartburn is an intermittent symptom, usually occurring within an hour after meals (particularly if they are large or high in fat), during exercise, or with bending or lying down. It is usually relieved quickly with antacids, although the effect may not last very long. Heartburn is thought to be caused by the stimulation of nerve endings in the esophageal epithelium by refluxed acid.

Heartburn may be associated with regurgitation, the return of gastric or esophageal contents into the pharynx. The fluid may be bitter or sour. It most commonly occurs when the person is lying down or bending over. Some are awakened at night by this. Vomiting is less common, is generally effortless, and is not associated with nausea or abdominal contractions when related to GERD.

Water brash is the spontaneous appearance of fluid in the mouth. It is secondary to the esophagosalivary reflex, the stimulation of salivary secretion that occurs with reflux. The fluid is described as salty or bland-tasting.

Dysphagia occurs in about one third of patients with GERD. This is a sensation that food is delayed as it moves from the pharynx to the stomach. Acid reflux with or without tissue damage may lead to intermittent motility disturbances of the esophagus that result in dysphagia. An abnormal sensory perception within the esophagus may play a role in this symptom. Progressive dysphagia in the setting of GERD suggests the development of a peptic or malignant stricture.

Odynophagia refers to pain with swallowing. The pain is usually localized to the retrosternal area and is an unusual complaint with uncomplicated GERD. Odynophagia invariably indicates a severe inflammatory process. It is more common in the setting of severe erosive or ulcerative esophagitis, infectious esophagitis, pill-induced esophagitis, or esophageal cancer.

Chest pain distinct from heartburn or odynophagia may occur as a result of GERD. It is the only symptom in 10% of patients with this disorder. The pain may be gripping or knife-like and usually occurs in the retrosternal area. The pain is not always related to swallowing, but may be triggered by the ingestion of very hot or cold liquids. It may radiate to the abdomen, back, neck, or arm, and it can be severe. It may be difficult to distinguish it from cardiac pain; in fact, over half of the patients with chest pain who have normal coronary angiograms probably have GERD as a cause of their symptoms. The cause of chest pain in people with GERD is unclear. It may be an extension of heartburn or secondary to acid-induced esophageal spasm.

Globus sensation is the almost constant perception of a lump, fullness, or tickle in the throat. It is unrelated to swallowing and is occasionally seen as a manifestation of GERD. The mechanism for this symptom is not well understood, although psychological factors may be important.

Table 60-2. Clinical Features of GERD

Heartburn: Most common symptom of GERD, experienced by over 75%
Regurgitation: Nearly as common as heartburn
Vomiting: "Effortless" when associated with GERD
Water brash: Increase in salivary flow; salty or bland-tasting
Dysphagia: Difficulty swallowing due to acid-induced dysmotility
Odynophagia: Painful swallowing; uncommon in uncomplicated GERD
Chest pain: May mimic cardiac pain
Globus sensation: Persistent lump or tickle in the throat
Hoarseness: Related to laryngeal inflammation from acid reflux
Cough: Manifestation of laryngeal or pulmonary disease from GERD
Asthma: 50% of adults with asthma have associated GERD
Pneumonia: Possible complication of GERD

Complications

The complications of GERD reflect the mucosal injury or esophagitis that occurs in some patients. Low-grade inflammation is often detected only histologically. More significant inflammation may be detected grossly at endoscopy. Red streaks or erosions extending proximally up the esophagus are the earliest changes. As the damage progresses, the injury becomes more confluent, eventually involving the entire circumference of the esophageal lumen. Edema, hyperemia, and friability of the mucosa may develop, with progression to deep ulceration. Histologic findings range from increased height of the papillae and basal cell hyperplasia as the earliest changes, to infiltration of the mucosa by acute and chronic inflammatory cells. The presence of columnar epithelium represents the metaplasia that occurs with chronic injury and is known as Barrett's esophagus.

Bleeding may occur from reflux-induced erosions or ulcerations of the esophageal mucosa. The bleeding is often insidious and can eventually lead to an iron deficiency anemia. Frank hemorrhage is rare and usually comes from an esophageal ulcer. Only 2% of patients with gross upper gastrointestinal bleeding are bleeding from the esophagus.

A stricture of the esophagus, a narrowing of the lumen, is a complication that results from longstanding ulceration of the esophageal mucosa. Continued mucosal damage with partial healing leads to fibrosis, and the lumen of the esophagus narrows. Strictures are more common in the elderly, in those with Barrett's esophagus, and in patients with scleroderma. Most patients who develop strictures have a history of heartburn, although perhaps 25% of patients present without a history suggestive of GERD. Certain drugs may increase a patient's tendency to develop strictures in the setting of GERD, including potassium tablets, doxycycline, quinidine, and nonsteroidal antiinflammatory drugs. The most common presenting symptom of a stricture is dysphagia. In the case of a reflux-induced stricture, the dysphagia is initially for solid food, particularly meat. If it is left untreated, patients may eventually have difficulty with soft foods and liquids as well. Reflux-induced strictures are usually short and located in the distal esophagus (Fig. 60-2).

The most severe histologic consequence of chronic GERD is Barrett's esophagus, in which squamous epithelium is replaced with metaplastic columnar epithelium. The columnar epithelium theoretically provides greater resistance to the injurious effects of refluxed acid. There are three histologic types of Barrett's epithelium: a specialized columnar epithelium similar to intestinal mucosa, a junctional type of epithelium resembling gastric cardia mucosa, and a gastric fundus type of epithelium containing parietal cells. Barrett's esophagus is defined as columnar epithelium extending more than 3 cm above the gastroesophageal junction. This metaplastic change may involve a small portion of the distal end of the esophagus or may involve the entire organ. Patients with Barrett's esophagus generally have severe GERD, although the symptoms are no different than in those without Barrett's esophagus. In fact, up to a third of patients with Barrett's esophagus have no symptoms of reflux. Perhaps the esophageal mucosa is relatively insensitive to pain in these patients.

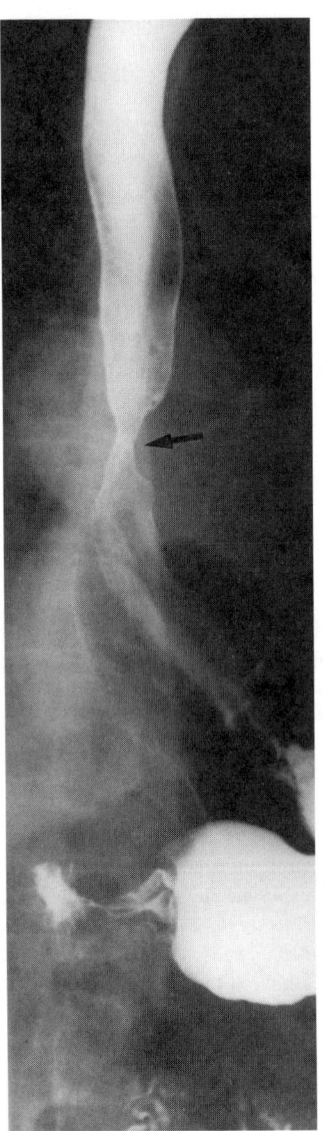

Figure 60-2. Barium esophagogram reveals a benign esophageal stricture *(arrow)*.

The frequency of Barrett's esophagus in the general population is unknown. In patients with GERD who undergo endoscopy, the prevalence is 5% to 12%. In patients with more severe GERD, such as those with strictures or scleroderma, Barrett's esophagus reportedly occurs in as many as 40%. Barrett's esophagus is more common in men than women (10 : 1).

The significance of Barrett's mucosa is its malignant potential, as the columnar epithelium is more likely to develop adenocarcinoma. The magnitude of this risk is reported to be a 30- to 50-fold increase when compared to the general population. Other factors that affect the risk are smoking, the extent of Barrett's esophagus, and the presence of dysplasia.

Extraesophageal Manifestations

Extraesophageal disorders that may develop as a result of GERD include signs and symptoms related to the oropharynx, larynx, and respiratory tract.

Several laryngeal symptoms are thought to have an association with GERD. Hoarseness, a persistent nonproductive cough, a sensation of pressure deep in the throat, and the need to clear the throat continually may indicate GERD-induced laryngeal disease. These otolaryngologic symptoms may be due to direct tissue injury by refluxed gastric contents. Classic symptoms of reflux or esophagitis are often minimal in these patients. Nocturnal reflux may be the key to the development of laryngeal disorders, perhaps related to a diminution of the upper esophageal sphincter tone at night. Acid might then be allowed to reach the level of the larynx.

GERD probably has a role in promoting asthma in some patients. Up to 50% of adult patients with asthma may have associated GERD. The exact mechanisms responsible for the pulmonary manifestations of reflux are not well understood. The two proposed mechanisms are recurrent microaspiration of gastric contents, with resultant acid-induced injury and bronchoconstriction, and vagally mediated reflex bronchoconstriction that occurs when acid refluxes into the esophagus. In many cases, the association may be more that of a shared risk factor, such as smoking. As is seen with laryngeal disease, many persons with asthma and GERD have minimal reflux symptoms or esophagitis. Symptoms that may suggest reflux-related asthma include onset of asthma at a late age, nocturnal cough or wheezing, asthma that is exacerbated after meals, exercise, or the supine position, and asthma that is exacerbated by bronchodilators. Theophylline and β-agonist therapy for asthma may reduce LES tone and potentiate reflux. The response to antireflux therapy, whether it be medical or surgical, is variable in asthmatics.

Recurrent pneumonia, bronchitis, and possibly pulmonary fibrosis have also been proposed to be complications of GERD.

NATURAL HISTORY

Little is known about the natural history of GERD. For example, it is not known how often GERD is an acute self-limited disease versus a chronic relapsing problem. There is no clear relation between symptoms and either the amount of reflux or the degree of mucosal injury within the esophagus.

A 3-year follow-up study of patients with endoscopically mild esophagitis indicated that only 5% progressed to a more severe type of esophagitis; 50% had no changes, and 45% spontaneously healed. On the other hand, those with more severe reflux esophagitis at the time of diagnosis have only about a 30% chance of improving; even with intensive medical therapy, relapses are common.

DIFFERENTIAL DIAGNOSIS

Several gastrointestinal and nongastrointestinal disorders may mimic GERD. Although symptoms of GERD are generally quite characteristic, it is sometimes necessary to distinguish them from those related to cholelithiasis, peptic ulcer, gastritis, infectious or pill esophagitis, dyspepsia, coronary artery disease, and esophageal motor disorders.

Although classic heartburn is unlikely to be confused with cardiac pain, some patients with GERD experience chest pain that is difficult to distinguish from angina or myocardial infarction. It may even radiate into the jaw or arms and be exacerbated by exertion. Because both GERD and coronary artery disease are disorders of middle-aged persons, some have symptoms of both and may have trouble distinguishing between the two. If chest pain is prominent, a cardiac evaluation should be performed before gastrointestinal studies.

Dyspepsia refers to a number of symptoms, including upper abdominal fullness, nausea, early satiety, anorexia, vomiting, belching, and heartburn. This constellation of symptoms is probably a disorder of gastric motility, with the heartburn related to secondary reflux. Standard antireflux treatment often helps the heartburn but not the other symptoms.

Pill and infectious esophagitis are usually associated with significant odynophagia, which is rare in uncomplicated GERD. Infectious esophagitis can be seen in immunocompromised persons and is commonly caused by the herpes simplex virus, cytomegalovirus, or *Candida albicans*. *Candida* is associated with a cheesy exudate on the surface of the mucosa of the esophagus; herpes and cytomegalovirus typically cause multiple punctate ulcerations. Pills of potassium chloride, quinidine, and tetracycline may cause single deep ulcers, usually at a level where the pill may transiently hang up, such as the aortic arch.

Most of the other disorders that could be clinically confused with GERD can be ruled in or out with upper endoscopy, an upper gastrointestinal series, and biliary ultrasonography.

DIAGNOSIS

The diagnosis of GERD may be established in several different ways. In most cases, a good history elicits symptoms that are consistent with GERD. Heartburn or regurgitation that occurs after meals and is relieved by antacids is the typical symptom of GERD. In most persons, no further diagnostic testing is required.

Further investigation is warranted in patients with complaints or findings suggestive of significant esophageal mucosal injury (eg, dysphagia, odynophagia, guaiac-positive stools, or anemia). Atypical symptoms or persistent problems despite therapy are also indications to pursue the diagnosis.

A barium esophagogram is often the first test used to investigate GERD. When a double-contrast technique is used, cases of moderate and severe esophagitis may be demonstrated, especially if ulcerations are present. However, mild esophagitis may be missed. The demonstration of reflux by this study has questionable significance and may not be seen in over half of patients with GERD. The barium esophagogram remains the initial examination of choice in a patient with dysphagia because of its ability to detect subtle strictures and assess esophageal peristaltic function.

Upper endoscopy is considered if studies to document GERD are required. Endoscopy provides direct visualization of the esophageal mucosa and has a high sensitivity and specificity in detecting mucosal injury. Endoscopic findings in patients with GERD include erythema, edema, friability, exudate, erosions, ulcerations, strictures, and Barrett's epithelium. Endoscopic biopsy is the most sensitive test to document tissue injury.

About one third of patients with GERD have no detectable esophagitis on endoscopy, even when they have severe symptoms. If endoscopy and endoscopic biopsy are normal, a Bernstein test may help confirm that the symptoms are acid-related. After positioning a nasogastric tube in the esophagus, normal saline and hydrochloric acid are infused separately. The reproduction of symptoms during acid but not saline infusion constitutes a positive test. This test is fairly sensitive in determining whether the symptoms are due to acid reflux. However, this test is negative in some patients with Barrett's esophagus, whose mucosa may be relatively insensitive to pain.

Twenty-four-hour esophageal pH monitoring remains the gold standard for detecting excess reflux and should be considered in patients who are unresponsive to acid-suppressive therapy or who have atypical symptoms. A small pH electrode is positioned in the lower esophagus, and the pH within the esophagus is measured continuously over 24 hours. The percentage of time that the pH in the lower esophagus is less than 4 is a good criterion for GERD, although there may be some overlap between normal persons and those with GERD. Patients with typical symptoms and verified esophagitis do not benefit from this study; patients who do not respond to therapy or who have atypical chest pain, pulmonary symptoms, or hoarseness may.

Esophageal manometric studies can measure the LES pressure and esophageal peristalsis but are of limited value in diagnosing GERD. The measurement of esophageal motility may be necessary, however, if disorders such as achalasia or scleroderma are to be ruled out. If a patient with GERD is being considered for surgical therapy, motility studies help verify the presence of effective peristalsis within the esophagus, which should be confirmed to avoid postoperative dysphagia.

TREATMENT

The goals of treatment of GERD are to control symptoms, to heal esophagitis, and to prevent relapse and complications.

Lifestyle Modifications

Lifestyle modifications should be part of the initial management in almost everyone with GERD, whether it is mild or severe. They include elevating the head of the bed about 6 to 8 inches, avoiding recumbency for 3 hours after meals, stopping smoking, decreasing fat intake, avoiding tight-fitting garments, restricting alcohol and chocolate intake, losing weight if necessary, and avoiding drugs that potentially decrease LES pressure (Table 60-

Table 60-3. Lifestyle Modifications for GERD

Elevate the head of the bed 6" to 8".
Avoid eating for 3 hours before retiring.
Stop smoking.
Reduce alcohol consumption.
Eat small meals.
Lose weight if necessary.
Avoid tight clothes.
Avoid dietary fat, chocolate, coffee (caffeinated and decaffeinated), tea, carminatives, cola.
Avoid drugs that decrease LES pressure.

3). These modifications promote the esophageal clearance of acid and minimize episodes of reflux. Many sufferers improve significantly after following these suggestions.

Pharmacologic Therapy

Antacids and Alginic Acid

The use of antacids and alginic acid is also considered in the initial therapy of GERD. Antacids increase gastric pH, deactivate pepsin, and may increase LES pressure through gastric alkalinization. Alginic acid forms a foamy layer on the surface of gastric secretions and creates a barrier between acid and the esophageal mucosa. Antacids and alginic acid have been shown to be more effective than placebo in relieving symptoms of GERD. In two open studies, combined antacid/alginic acid use led to an improvement in symptoms in 80% of subjects with GERD.

Histamine-2 Receptor Antagonists

Most patients with symptomatic GERD do well with lifestyle changes and intermittent antacid or alginic acid therapy. Those with persistent symptoms or a complication of GERD, however, generally require pharmacologic intervention. The histamine-2 receptor antagonists (H_2RAs) inhibit gastric acid secretion by blocking the histamine-2 receptors on the parietal cell. The H_2RAs marketed in the United States are cimetidine, ranitidine, famotidine, and nizatidine (Table 60-4). When gastric acid production is inhibited by these agents, the material refluxed from the stomach is less harmful to the esophageal mucosa.

Several clinical trials have investigated the efficacy of H_2RAs in GERD. The designs and results of these studies vary, but in general they indicate that 50% to 75% of persons with GERD have a significant reduction in symptoms after treatment with standard doses of H_2RA for 6 to 12 weeks. However, symptom resolution does not correlate well with the healing of esophagitis. Healing rates are inversely proportional to the severity of esophagitis, and higher, more frequent doses of H_2RAs than standard may be necessary in severe cases. In addition, healing is directly proportional to the length of treatment, and at least 12 weeks of therapy may be required to heal most cases of esophagitis.

H_2RAs are safe: the reported incidence of adverse reactions is about 4%. Cimetidine may bind reversibly to the cytochrome P-450 microsomal enzymes of the liver, resulting in drug interactions. Interactions may occur with theophylline, warfarin, phenytoin, and benzodiazepines, and caution should be used when cimetidine is combined with one of these drugs. Ranitidine may also bind to the cytochrome P-450 system, although with less affinity. This property has not been described with famotidine or nizatidine.

Other potential side effects include CNS disturbances (< 0.2%) and hepatotoxicity. Isolated cases of hematologic side effects have been noted. Cimetidine has weak antiandrogenic activity, and rare instances of gynecomastia, impotence, and hyperprolactinemia have been reported.

Table 60-4. Drugs for GERD

DRUG	POTENCY RELATIVE TO CIMETIDINE	STANDARD DOSE	SUPER-STANDARD DOSE
Cimetidine	1	400 Mg bid	400 Mg qid
Ranitidine	1.5–3.0	150 Mg bid	300 Mg bid
Famotidine	2.0–3.0	20 Mg bid	40 Mg bid
Nizatidine	1.5–3.0	150 Mg bid	300 Mg bid

Omeprazole

Omeprazole is a proton pump inhibitor. It inhibits the activity of H^+/K^+-ATPase, the final common step of acid secretion by the parietal cell. Omeprazole leads to a prolonged and profound inhibition of gastric acid production. It has a stronger inhibitory effect on acid secretion than the H_2RAs. As a result, it is considered the most effective medical therapy for controlling symptoms of GERD and for healing esophagitis. Studies have demonstrated its effectiveness when compared with placebo, as well as its superiority to cimetidine and ranitidine in the treatment of GERD (Fig. 60-3). Omeprazole has also been shown to be effective in the treatment of severe erosive esophagitis resistant to long-term, superstandard dose therapy with H_2RAs.

Omeprazole is safe, and side effects are rare. It may interact with the cytochrome P-450 system and inhibit the metabolism of certain drugs, including warfarin, phenytoin, and diazepam. The main safety concern has been its ability to produce hypergastrinemia and gastric carcinoid tumors in rats. Gastrin release is regulated by a negative feedback mechanism. A low intragastric pH inhibits gastrin secretion. Omeprazole, by its potent action and resultant hypochlorhydria, turns off this negative feedback and may cause elevations in serum gastrin. Gastrin has a trophic effect on the oxyntic mucosa, including the enterochromaffin-like (ECL) cells within the stomach, and a proliferation of the ECL cells may lead to the formation of carcinoid tumors. In humans, omeprazole 20 to 40 mg/day causes a two- to four-fold increase in serum gastrin levels, and short-term treatment with omeprazole for up to 6 months does not increase ECL cell numbers. However, caution must be used and a careful evaluation made of the risks and benefits of long-term use, as studies of its safety in this situation have yet to be done. It is reasonable to monitor gastrin levels in patients on long-term omeprazole.

Prokinetic Agents

Prokinetic drugs are often used in conjunction with acid suppression in the treatment of GERD. These agents may increase LES pressure, accelerate gastric emptying, and improve peristalsis within the esophagus.

Bethanechol, a cholinergic agonist, enhances LES pressure and increases the flow of saliva. When used in a dose of 25 mg four

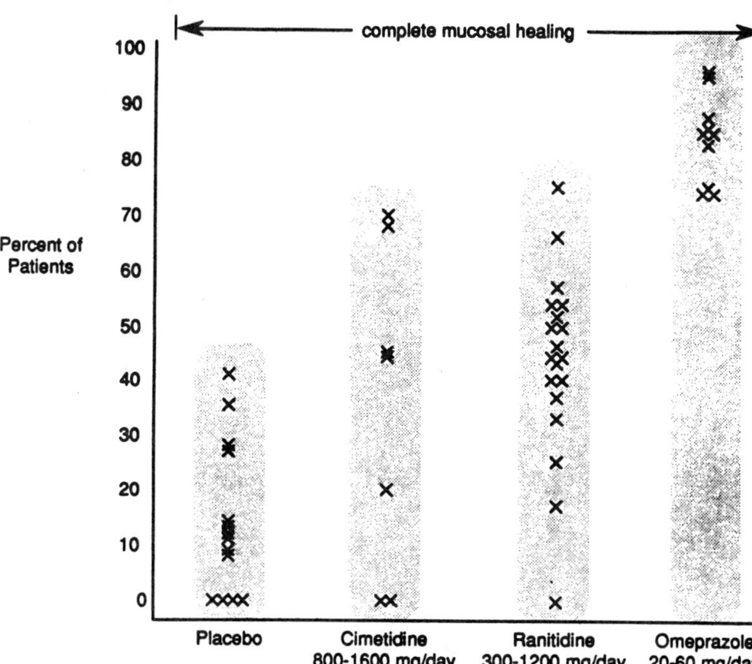

Figure 60-3. Summary of clinical trials: healing of esophagitis. Each x represents the percentage of patients healed in each treatment group of the clinical studies. (Sontag SJ, The medical management of reflux esophagitis: role of antacids and acid inhibition. Gastroenterol Clin North Am 1990; 19:683.)

times a day, bethanechol improves symptoms of GERD compared to placebo. Unfortunately, its usefulness is limited due to the high frequency of side effects such as flushing, blurry vision, abdominal cramps, and urinary frequency. It is contraindicated in patients with asthma, peptic ulcer, ischemic heart disease, or obstruction of the intestine or urinary tract. It is best used as an adjunct to some form of acid-suppressive therapy.

Metoclopramide, a central and peripheral dopamine antagonist and a cholinergic agonist, has effects similar to those of bethanechol in increasing LES pressure. Metoclopramide is effective in the symptomatic treatment of GERD when used alone, but it has not been consistently shown to heal esophagitis. Because this drug crosses the blood–brain barrier, CNS side effects such as drowsiness, agitation, and dyskinesia are frequent.

Cisapride releases acetylcholine at the myenteric plexus, increases the amplitude of esophageal peristalsis and LES pressure, and promotes gastric emptying. Several studies have supported its effectiveness as a single agent in the symptomatic relief of GERD and in the healing of esophagitis; when used in a dose of 10 mg three times a day, it was comparable to H_2RAs in standard doses. It also works synergistically with acid-suppressive agents. Side effects seem to be minimal; a transient increase in stool frequency is the most common.

Domperidone, a dopamine antagonist, may increase LES pressure. This experimental promotility drug has variable results in treating GERD. It crosses the blood–brain barrier less rapidly than metoclopramide and has fewer side effects.

Site-Protective Agents

Sucralfate, a salt of aluminum hydroxide and sucrose octasulfate, is often useful in the treatment of esophagitis. It works locally, binding to damaged epithelium, and possibly acts as a barrier to the noxious effects of acid and pepsin. Studies have not shown sucralfate to be uniformly effective in GERD, although patients with more severe mucosal disease may respond better, possibly because of greater retention of the drug in the damaged esophagus. Although its systemic absorption is minimal, sucralfate must be used cautiously if at all in patients with renal disease, where aluminum toxicity may occur.

Surgical Therapy

Surgical treatment should be considered in patients who fail to respond to standard medical therapy. The Nissen fundoplication, the Belsey Mark IV repair, and the Hill posterior gastropexy repair are the most common procedures performed. Each involves reduction of a hiatus hernia and the construction of a valve mechanism to reestablish competence of the LES. Results depend on careful patient selection and the surgeon's experience.

Maintenance Therapy

Many patients with GERD ultimately require long-term, perhaps lifetime therapy. Once esophagitis is healed, maintenance therapy is often required to prevent recurrence. The difficulty in maintaining remission is directly related to the degree of initial mucosal damage. The proper maintenance therapy varies from patient to patient, and there are no hard-and-fast rules. Low-dose H_2RAs are usually ineffective, and full doses may fail as well. Prokinetic agents may be beneficial. Omeprazole can maintain remission, but the proper dose and the agent's long-term safety are unknown.

DIAGNOSTIC AND THERAPEUTIC APPROACH

The patient with symptoms of GERD is best approached in a stepwise fashion (Fig. 60-4). Most patients who present with recurrent, uncomplicated heartburn should first be instructed in lifestyle modifications and the use of antacids or alginic acid. An empiric

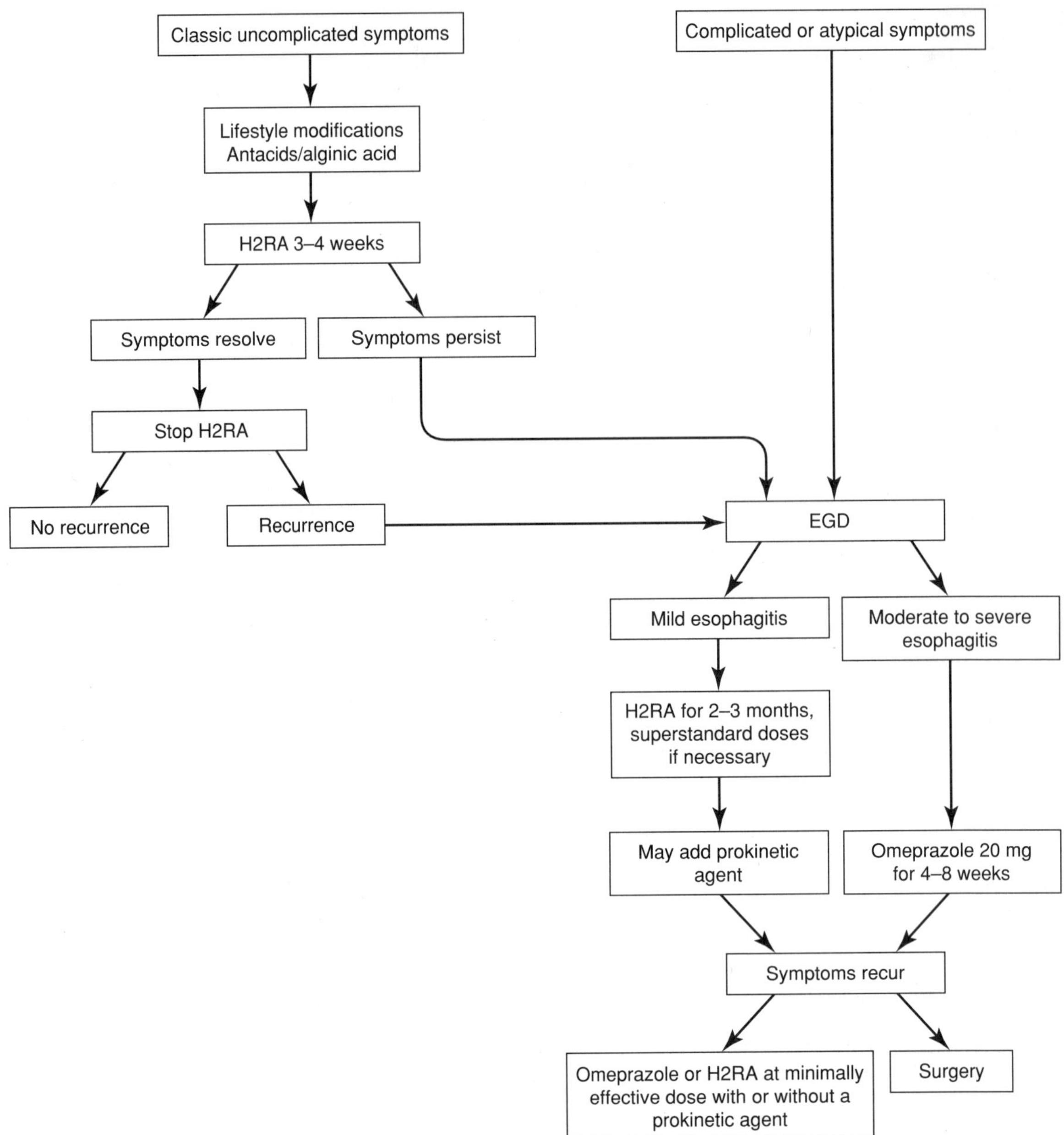

Figure 60-4. Management of gastroesophageal reflux disease.

course of an H_2RA in a standard dose for no longer than 3 to 4 weeks is also appropriate.

If the patient does not respond to these measures, if symptoms return after the H_2RA is stopped, or if the initial symptoms suggest complicated disease, the patient should be referred to a gastroenterologist. Upper endoscopy with esophageal mucosal biopsy is appropriate at this point: other diagnoses are ruled out and the extent of mucosal damage can be determined. If the patient does not have significant esophagitis, she is at low risk for major complications. Patients with severe esophagitis, characterized by erosions or ulcerations, are at relatively high risk for complications.

In the low-risk patient, the next step is to continue the H_2RA in standard doses for another 2 to 3 months. If symptoms had not responded to this initially, superstandard doses (see Table 60-4) should be given. A promotility agent, preferably cisapride 10 mg four times a day, can be added if symptoms persist. If this combination fails to suppress symptoms, the patient should be given omeprazole 20 mg/day for a month or two.

Once the drug or drugs have been stopped, the patient is monitored for recurrence of symptoms. If they recur quickly, continued acid suppression with either an H_2RA or omeprazole at the minimally effective dose is often needed. Because of the lack of data regarding the long-term safety of omeprazole, it must be used with caution and only when other drugs, including a combination of H_2RAs in superstandard doses with a prokinetic agent, have failed. Younger women with recurrent symptoms, facing a lifetime of taking drugs for GERD, may consider surgical therapy.

If endoscopy reveals evidence of severe esophagitis characterized by erosions or ulcerations, omeprazole 20 to 40 mg/day for a month or two should be given in an attempt to heal the mucosal disease. A promotility agent may be added if necessary. Because the relapse rate in patients with erosive esophagitis is as high as 90% at 12 months, maintenance therapy of some type is recommended to minimize the rate of relapse and to prevent complications. This may include H_2RAs in at least standard doses, with or without a promotility agent, or omeprazole 20 mg/day. As an alternative, younger women may opt for surgery. Patients should be encouraged to continue lifestyle modifications.

TREATMENT OF COMPLICATIONS

Stricture

Dilatation by bougienage is the most common approach to the treatment of esophageal strictures. About 40% of patients with a stricture respond to one dilatation. Strictures of the esophagus may recur, requiring periodic dilatations. This procedure is not risk-free, and the complication rate is about 0.5%. Therefore, it is important to emphasize routine nonpharmacologic measures to minimize the effects of GERD. The chronic use of omeprazole has been shown to be effective in reducing the need for repeated dilatations. It is premature to recommend the use of the proton pump inhibitor in all patients with strictures, but it is reasonable to consider its use in the patient who is difficult or risky to dilate and requires it frequently.

Barrett's Esophagus

Barrett's esophagus must be managed as both severe GERD and as a premalignant lesion. Aggressive medical therapy usually reduces symptoms and may prevent or reduce the development of strictures, but it is unknown if treatment reverses Barrett's epithelium. Several studies have shown a lack of progression of Barrett's epithelium with medical therapy, but documented regression has been limited to anecdotal reports. High-dose omeprazole is being studied for its effectiveness in reversing the metaplastic process. Surgery is recommended in severe cases, especially in young women. The role of surveillance for dysplasia and cancer in patients with Barrett's esophagus is not well defined, although large-scale screening programs are probably not cost-effective. Because those who have extensive Barrett's changes or high-grade dysplasia, especially those who drink or smoke, are considered to be at high risk, endoscopy with biopsy every 6 months to a year has been recommended. Low-risk patients may benefit from surveillance every 3 or 4 years. It has not been established whether early diagnosis will affect outcome.

Extraesophageal Complications

The management of the extraesophageal complications of GERD, particularly laryngeal, pharyngeal, and pulmonary diseases, includes aggressive treatment of reflux, often with omeprazole. The subsequent response of asthma, hoarseness, or cough to this therapy is usually the best evidence that the problem is a complication of GERD.

CONSIDERATIONS IN PREGNANCY

Pregnancy has a major effect on gastrointestinal motility and thus predisposes some women to developing GERD. Heartburn is reported in over 75% of pregnant women. Although it may occur during any trimester, heartburn most commonly develops at 5 months of gestation, becoming more pronounced as the pregnancy progresses. It is at its worst during the final months. Symptoms are usually mild, and only rarely do complications occur. In most cases, heartburn ceases soon after delivery. Subsequent pregnancies are often associated with recurrent GERD symptoms.

The etiology of GERD in pregnancy has been extensively studied. The LES pressure progressively diminishes during pregnancy, and by 36 weeks' gestation nearly all women have a low LES pressure (Fig. 60-5). This pressure returns to normal in the postpartum period. The decrease in pressure appears to be an effect of progesterone on the smooth muscle, although estrogen may be required for a priming effect. As the uterus enlarges, the increased intraabdominal pressure may further compromise an already weakened LES.

The diagnosis of pregnancy-related GERD is easily made from the history. The clinical features of GERD in pregnancy do not differ from those in general: heartburn and regurgitation are the predominant symptoms. Referral to a gastroenterologist and endoscopy are rarely needed and should be reserved for patients in whom the diagnosis is unclear or treatment is ineffective, or when

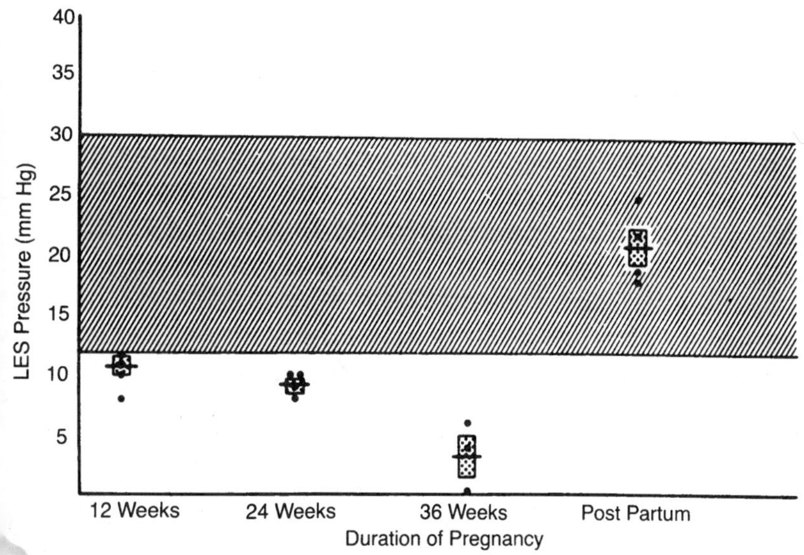

Figure 60-5. Lower esophageal sphincter pressure recorded in four volunteer women during pregnancy and the postpartum period. Lower esophageal sphincter pressure declined progressively during pregnancy but returned to normal in the postpartum period. (Van Thiel DH, et at. Heartburn of pregnancy. Gastroenterology 1997; 72:666.)

complications such as bleeding occur. When needed, endoscopy can be done safely during pregnancy, with standard monitoring techniques. Histologic esophagitis may be seen, but severe erosive esophagitis is rare. On occasion, 24-hour pH studies are needed to confirm the diagnosis. X-rays should be avoided.

Many pregnant women with reflux respond well to lifestyle modification. Small meals, not eating for several hours before retiring, avoiding stooping and bending, and elevating the head of the bed should be the initial recommendations. If pharmacologic intervention is required, it is reasonable to start with antacids or alginic acid, which are safe and effective in pregnancy; however, they may interfere with iron absorption. Sodium bicarbonate should be avoided, as it may cause a metabolic alkalosis and fluid overload in both mother and fetus. Sucralfate appears to be safe because of its limited systemic absorption and in one study was found to be better than placebo in treating heartburn in pregnancy.

If symptoms are refractory to nonsystemic therapy, an H_2RA may be required. This class of drug crosses the placenta and is secreted in breast milk. Animal studies do not reveal evidence of teratogenicity, and although the H_2RAs have not been studied prospectively in humans, anecdotal experience with cimetidine and ranitidine suggests that they are safe. Famotidine and nizatidine have few reports of any kind and probably should be avoided during pregnancy. Information is also limited in regard to omeprazole. High doses have been associated with fetal toxicity and pregnancy disruption in animals. Therefore, omeprazole should also be avoided during pregnancy.

The approach to the pregnant patient with GERD is similar to that in the general population. The diagnosis is usually made by a careful history. If symptoms are atypical or suggest complications such as bleeding or stricture formation, referral to a gastroenterologist for endoscopy or 24-hour pH studies is appropriate. Reassurance and lifestyle modifications are the first step in the therapy of uncomplicated GERD in pregnancy. If symptoms persist, antacids or alginic acid given after meals and at bedtime can be added. An alternative nonsystemic treatment is sucralfate 1 g three times a day given on an empty stomach. In severe or refractory cases, cimetidine 400 mg given after dinner can be used. In pregnancy, the least amount of medication needed to control symptoms should be used, and a once-a-day regimen is preferred.

BIBLIOGRAPHY

Baron TH, Richter JE. Gastroesophageal disease in pregnancy. Gastroenterol Clin North Am 1992;21:777.

DeVault KR, Castell DO. Current diagnosis and treatment of gastroesophageal reflux disease. Mayo Clin Proc 1994;69:867.

Kahrilas PJ, Hogan WJ. Gastroesophageal reflux disease. In: Sleisenger MH, Fordtran JS, eds. Gastrointestinal disease. Philadelphia: WB Saunders, 1993:378.

Pope CE. Acid-reflux disorders. N Engl J Med 1994;331:656.

Sontag SJ. The medical management of reflux esophagitis: role of antacids and acid inhibition. Gastroenterol Clin North Am 1990;19:683.

61

Peptic Ulcer Disease

JANET R. REISER

Primary Care for Women, edited by Phyllis C. Leppert and Fred M. Howard. Lippincott-Raven Publishers, Philadelphia

EPIDEMIOLOGY AND RISK FACTORS

Peptic ulcer disease (PUD) is a common problem, affecting up to 10% of all Americans at some point in their lives. Before this century, PUD was infrequently recognized. From the early 1900s onward, the rate of occurrence has steadily increased until the 1960s. Since then, the occurrence rate of uncomplicated duodenal ulcer (DU) and possibly gastric ulcer (GU) has declined. For complicated ulcers (PUD complicated by hemorrhage, perforation, or obstruction), the occurrence rate seems to be stable. Making definitive interpretations regarding ulcer prevalence is difficult since the method of detection has become markedly more sensitive with the use of endoscopy, and increased occurrences may represent only increased detection. Certain interesting trends, however, have become apparent. In the past, a male predominance of PUD was observed, with a male : female ratio of approximately 2 : 1. The ratio now approaches 1 : 1. This may represent a true increase among women with at least two possible explanations. First, many older women consume large amounts of nonsteroidal antiinflammatory drugs (NSAIDs). Complications from NSAID use increase with age in association with an increased rate of prescription; but age and female sex may be independent risk factors as well. Second, smoking rates are increasing in women whereas they are declining in men. An alternative explanation is that PUD in women is recognized more often. It may be that in the past, complaints of abdominal pain in female patients were less likely to be evaluated and were more likely to be considered as psychosomatic or irritable bowel complaints. Abdominal complaints also may have been misinterpreted as gynecologic in origin.

GU tends to occur in patients older than 50 years of age whereas DU tends to occur in younger patients. A seasonal variation may occur with higher rates of occurrence during the fall and spring.

Significant risk factors for PUD include use of NSAIDs, infection with *Helicobacter pylori*, and cigarette use. Family history is another notable risk factor. Although genetic susceptibility to PUD was initially hypothesized to be the causative mechanism, the recognition of *H. pylori* as an etiologic agent suggests that the familial predilection is attributable to exposure and infection with this organism, since person-to-person transmission can occur. Steroid use probably is a significant risk factor, but this remains controversial. Diet does not seem to play a major role in the pathogenesis of ulcers, although patients have strong beliefs about it. Personality type (ie, type A personality) by itself is not a risk factor for PUD. However, in patients with an ulcer diathesis, stress seems to contribute to the development of symptoms. Each of these risk factors are examined in more detail later in the chapter since there are important implications in counseling patients. Furthermore, patients have definite opinions about proper "ulcer diets" and often question physicians about this.

PATHOGENESIS

Peptic ulcer disease historically has been considered a disease of acid and pepsin secretion and decreased mucosal resistance. In the last 10 years, the discovery of infection with *H. pylori* has revolutionized this understanding. To some extent, treatment of DU needs to be considered as treatment of an infectious disease. *H. pylori* also is involved in the pathogenesis of GUs, although the evidence is less overwhelming.

The old dictum "no acid, no ulcer" generally remains true with regard to DU. Patients who are achlorhydric rarely develop DUs. Whereas acid secretion in patients with DUs may be low, normal, or elevated, most patients with DU are hypersecretors. However, there is considerable overlap with normal secretors, and acid hypersecretion is neither necessary nor sufficient to cause a DU. Breakdown of mucosal defenses also must occur. Figure 61-1 summarizes the current leading hypothesis for the pathogenesis of DU. (This is not the case with pathologic states of acid secretion such as Zollinger-Ellison syndrome in which the acid secretion is of such magnitude it overwhelms the mucosal defenses.)

Mucosal defenses against acid and other noxious agents (eg, bile, pepsin) include several mechanisms. Bicarbonate secreted by the duodenum and pancreas neutralizes acid. Mucus produced in the stomach and duodenum also protects the mucosa from the topical effects of pepsin and acid. The ability of the epithelial cell to limit back-diffusion of acid is a second line of defense against acid secretion. This is facilitated by the presence of tight junction barriers, membrane transport mechanisms to remove excess hydrogen, and antioxidants. Finally, normal mucosal blood flow is a third line of defense against acid secretion. Decreased mucosal blood flow may play a particularly important role in the pathogenesis of stress ulcers in critically ill patients.

Acid hypersecretion plays a less prominent role in the pathogenesis of GUs. Patients with GUs generally are not hypersecretors of acid and, in fact, have low to normal secretion of acid. Accordingly, the failure of cytoprotective mechanisms is a critical determinant in the development of a GU. NSAID use and *H. pylori* infection are the most common causes of GUs, and both are postulated to affect local mucosal factors. NSAIDs also cause DUs, but less frequently than GUs. In fact, NSAIDs are capable of wreaking havoc on the entire gastrointestinal (GI) tract; esophageal ulceration and stricture may occur, as well as small intestinal ulcers and probably colonic lesions.

Hypothesis: The Quintet of DU Pathogenesis??

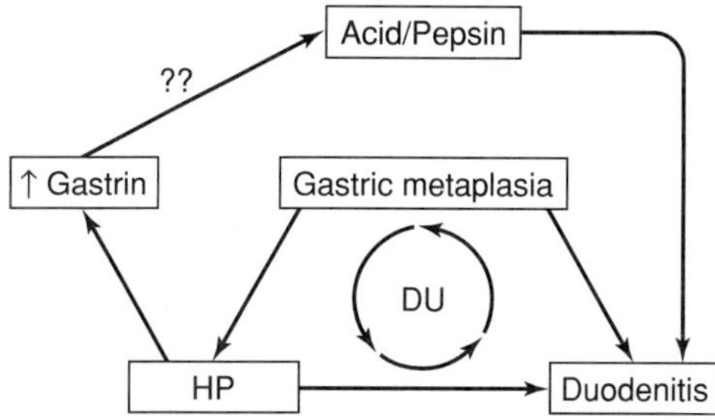

FIGURE 61-1. Hypothesis for the relation of acid hypersecretion with gastric metaplasia, duodenitis, and duodenal *H. pylori. DU,* duodenal ulcer; *HP, Helicobacter pylori.* (Sleisinger MH, Fordtran JS, Scharschmidt BF, Feldman M, Cello JP. Gastrointestinal Disease, 5th ed. Philadelphia: WB Saunders, 1993:586.)

The mechanism of action of NSAID gastropathy is twofold: there is a direct effect (NSAIDs are corrosive) on the mucosa, and a systemic effect via inhibition of prostaglandin synthesis. This is termed the *dual insult hypothesis*. Certain prostaglandins are protective in the GI tract by causing suppression of gastric acid secretion and by enhancing mucosal protective factors such as blood flow and bicarbonate and mucus production. NSAIDs decrease production of these protective prostaglandins. The toxicity of NSAIDs is dose related. There is a higher risk of developing an ulcer in patients who consume a greater number of pills, a higher dose per pill, or longer acting preparations. Although there are no clear indicators for which patients are most at risk for NSAID toxicity, several risk factors have been identified. These include history of ulcer, history of NSAID-induced abdominal pain, concomitant use of prednisone, and smoking. Interestingly, one might expect that active infection with *H. pylori* is a risk factor for developing NSAID gastropathy, but this has not been demonstrated and remains controversial. Addressing the known risk factors for the development of NSAID gastropathy has major implications for ulcer prophylaxis, which is discussed in the treatment section.

Aspirin is a type of nonsteroidal antiinflammatory drug, although not always regarded as one. Use of aspirin causes ulcers by the same mechanisms mentioned earlier. There is direct mucosal injury from the drug, which is a weak acid. Inhibition of prostaglandin production with subsequent loss of protective prostaglandins in the GI tract is the second pathway of injury. Enteric-coated aspirin causes less direct mucosal injury, but the effect on prostaglandins is the same, and thus the risk of ulcer formation is not eradicated. The nonacetylated salicylates (eg, choline magnesium trisalicylate [Trilisate], salsalate [Disalcid]) do not inhibit systemic production of prostaglandins and therefore cause ulcers less commonly, but ulcer formation may still occur. Unfortunately, these preparations are not as potent in controlling arthritis symptoms and, due to their lack of inhibition of platelet aggregation, cannot be used for prophylaxis against myocardial infarction.

The role of *H. pylori* infection in ulcer formation is a new and fascinating development. *H. pylori* is a gram-negative rod that lives only in gastric mucosa. It was first discovered in 1983 by a pathologist and a gastroenterologist who noted this previously unrecognized bacteria in the stomachs of virtually all patients with DUs. The flurry of research that followed this association has largely validated the hypothesis that *H. pylori* infection is a causative factor in ulcer development. *H. pylori* infection also is associated with GUs and is found in approximately 70% to 80% of patients with GUs. The route of infection seems to be fecal–oral. The prevalence is increased in patients from a lower socioeconomic background.

The pathogenesis is not clear but is speculated to be the following: Once the bacterium is swallowed into the stomach, it has a predilection to infect the antrum and to reside superficially near the mucus layer. *H. pylori* contains urease that changes the local pH, creating its own microenvironment. It also possesses adherence factors and a number of other virulence factors, including proteolytic enzymes and cytotoxins that seem to cause mucosal damage. Chronic active gastritis is the initial injury in the stomach.

This may be followed by the development of a GU. The development of chronic active gastritis has been demonstrated in two human volunteers (gastroenterologists!) who ingested *Helicobacter pylori*. The gastritis was cured by eradication of the organism. Resolving the chronic active gastritis in *H. pylori*–positive patients by eradicating the infection has been demonstrated in many clinical studies as well. In fact, *H. pylori* infection has been recognized as the most common cause of chronic active gastritis.

Since *H. pylori* lives only in gastric mucosa, it is curious that this infection also results in the development of DU (even more commonly than GU). The duodenal bulb is known to respond to an excessive acid load by developing gastric metaplasia. This is the development of gastric-type mucosa within the duodenal bulb and is a teleologic response since it allows the duodenal bulb to become more resistant to acid. (It is slightly analogous to the response of the esophagus to reflux. In some patients, gastric-type mucosa develops in the esophagus in response to excessive reflux. The new metaplastic tissue, Barrett's esophagus, is more acid resistant than the squamous mucosa of the esophagus.) Whereas the development of gastric metaplasia is an adaptive response and protects the duodenal bulb from acid injury, it also allows a suitable environment for *H. pylori* to colonize. This can result in active chronic duodenitis and, in some, the development of a DU.

Probably the strongest evidence that *H. pylori* is a pathogen in PUD is the effect on the natural history of PUD when the infection is eradicated. Although historically PUD has been considered to be a chronic disease with multiple recurrences and exacerbations, the rate of recurrence is sharply reduced when the bacterium is cleared. Traditionally, DUs, once healed, have had a 50% to 80% recurrence rate within 1 year. If *H. pylori* infection is eradicated, the recurrence rate falls sharply. In addition, in the case of refractory ulcers that fail to heal on H_2 blocker therapy, eradication of *H. pylori* infection sometimes facilitates healing.

Infection with *H. pylori* is also found in large numbers of patients without PUD. The prevalence varies with the region studied and is greater in developing countries, which have higher numbers of persons per household and less developed hygiene and sanitary practices. The incidence of infection increases with age. By 40 years of age, it is present in greater than 60% of persons in developing countries. In developed countries, the prevalence by 40 years of age ranges from 10% to 50%, depending on the population studied. The significance of this finding, based on current knowledge, is that the presence of *H. pylori* infection alone is not an indication to initiate antibiotic therapy.

More speculative at this point is the possible association between *H. pylori* infection and gastric carcinoma. Since gastric atrophy and intestinal metaplasia may occur in patients with chronic gastritis, it is theorized that increased cell turnover may predispose to the development of gastric carcinoma. Supporting evidence includes several serologic studies in banked serum showing an increased frequency of antibodies to *H. pylori* in patients who subsequently developed gastric carcinoma. Although neither necessary nor sufficient to cause gastric carcinoma, *H. pylori* infection may be a risk factor, along with other risk factors such as diet (ie, high intake of nitrosamines found in smoked foods, high ScH intake, and low intake of fresh fruits and vegetables containing antioxidants) and cigarette use. Further research is ongoing; the outcome will be of great interest.

Patients who use tobacco have a higher frequency of nonhealing ulcers and ulcer recurrence. Cigarettes have several effects on the GI tract, including decreasing mucosal blood flow, inhibiting duodenal and pancreatic production of bicarbonate, increasing acid secretion, increasing pepsinogen secretion, and decreasing gastric mucosal prostaglandin production.

Steroids are a controversial topic. Study results conflict on whether steroid use can cause ulcer formation. One recent meta-analysis found an increased ulcer risk with steroids use for more than 30 days or with a cumulative 1-g dose of prednisone. A more recent study found that the increased risk of PUD when using steroids was attributable to the effect of using steroids in conjunction with NSAIDs. Nonetheless, it is reasonable to place patients who are to receive long-term or high-dose steroids on prophylactic H_2 blockers, especially those who are also using aspirin or other NSAIDs concomitantly.

Many patients have the impression that dietary indiscretions can cause ulcers, and that a person with an active ulcer requires a special diet. This conception arises because the intake of certain foods, beverages, and spices may indeed cause dyspepsia. However, there is little evidence that specific foods cause, reactivate, or impede healing of PUD. From 1911 until the early 1970s, an ulcer diet consisting of milk, cream, and bland foods was advocated. Milk was thought to have a beneficial buffering effect because of its alkaline properties. However, use of milk has been questioned because it actually stimulates more acid secretion than it buffers. Nonetheless, milk intake may reduce acid-induced pain, and it seems unnecessary to discourage patients from drinking milk if it ameliorates their symptoms.

Endoscopic studies in which volunteers ingested spicy foods have had conflicting results. Some show the development of acute mucosal damage and some do not. Greasy foods may aggravate biliary symptoms but do not cause ulcer disease. Some evidence shows that a high fiber diet is protective against DU disease through mechanisms that are unclear. A study from India noted a higher rate of recurrence of DU in southern India, where there is a lower intake of fiber, as opposed to northern India. (Rice is a mainstay of diet in southern India). (However, it is now recognized that rice bran and rice oil are ulcerogenic substances if kept in prolonged storage.) A subsequent prospective study in Scandinavia showed that patients with healed DUs who were randomly assigned to a high fiber diet had a lower rate of DU recurrence. Thus, high fiber diets may play some beneficial role in prevention of DU disease.

Surprisingly, alcohol use has no association with gastritis or chronic peptic ulcer, although ingestion of high-proof ("hard liquor") beverages has been shown to cause acute erosions on endoscopic study and can cause acute epigastric pain in susceptible patients. However, these acute effects do not seem to cause any chronic effects. Patients commonly believe that coffee causes or perpetuates ulcers because it frequently causes dyspepsia, but this has not been borne out in rigorous studies. Esophageal manometry was performed in a group of patients who developed dyspepsia with coffee intake. Lower esophageal dysfunction (reflux) was observed after coffee intake in this group. Coffee stimulates acid secretion, but no more so than a variety of other beverages.

Stress is a complex issue. First, it would be helpful to clarify the different uses of this term. Stress ulcers arise in critically ill patients with multisystem failure, with mucosal ischemia as the presumed etiology. There are two subtypes of stress ulcer, both of which have a predilection for the stomach. The first subtype refers to deep ulcers where response to treatment is poor and mortality rates are high. The second subset of stress ulcers are superficial, and bleeding usually is controllable.

Stress is also used as a term to connote the role of personality type. Historically, PUD was one of the illnesses thought to be of psychosomatic origin, and a specific ulcer personality was described. Studies related PUD with a certain personality profile (ie, a dependent personality type), but subsequent review of these studies has found them to be poorly controlled and biased. There is no one personality type more likely to cause the development of an ulcer. (Interestingly, ulcerative colitis was another illness thought to be of psychosomatic origin, and "talking therapy" was its primary mode of therapy. When prednisone became available in the early 1950s with its excellent clinical responses, the psychosomatic school lost some of its legitimacy.)

Stress also refers to an acute condition causing mental or physical tension. In a patient with an ulcer diathesis, this type of stress probably contributes to the development of an ulcer. When listening to patients who develop an acute ulcer, many clearly attribute it to being under an acute stress with no other identifiable cause. There is an extremely complex interaction between the gut and the brain—the so-called brain–gut axis. Furthermore, there now appears to a neuroimmune axis, with an interaction between neural systems and the immune system clearly demonstrated in laboratory animals. A tantalizing but preliminary observation noted recently suggests that the site of action of H_2 blockers may not be solely in the parietal cell in the stomach, but also in the immune cells in the lamina propria of the stomach, providing possible further evidence along these lines.

Associated Illnesses

Illnesses associated with PUD include chronic obstructive pulmonary disease, cirrhosis, reflux esophagitis, and renal failure. Peptic ulcers occur in up to 30% of patients with chronic obstructive pulmonary disease. Conversely, in patients with PUD, the frequency of lung disease is increased two to three times above average. GU is more strongly associated with pulmonary disease than is DU, but the association has been observed with both. Cigarette use seems to be the common element in both diseases. Cirrhosis is associated with an increased frequency of DU and GU. The pathogenesis is unclear. Speculated reasons include decreased gastric mucosal prostaglandin production, decreased hepatic metabolism of GI hormones, and altered mucosal blood flow. The association of gastroesophageal reflux and PUD is attributed to hypersecretion of acid, although this remains controversial. In renal failure, the increased risk of PUD pertains to hemodialysis patients and to those who have undergone renal transplantation. The risk is greater for developing DU than GU. In dialysis patients, disordered calcium metabolism is thought to stimulate excessive acid secretion. In renal transplant recipients, the ulcers that develop appear to be a type of stress ulcer. Immunosuppression can lead to the development of viral ulcers, with cytomegalovirus being an important pathogen.

Uncommon Forms of Peptic Ulcer Disease

It is important to look for NSAID use and *H. pylori* infection when an ulcer is found, since the absence of these risk factors is significant and directs the workup toward less common etiologies. Other entities to consider include inflammatory bowel disease such as Crohn disease. Viral infections such as herpes simplex and cytomegalovirus can cause ulcers in immunosuppressed patients. Drug use such as crack cocaine can impair mucosal blood flow and cause ulcer formation. Acid hypersecretory syndromes also need to be considered and are of several types. Gastrinoma is an islet cell tumor of the pancreas, characterized by gastrin hypersecretion. This in turn stimulates excessive acid secretion; multiple ulcers and secretory diarrhea usually ensue. Multiple endocrine neoplasia-1 includes hyperparathyroidism, pituitary adenomas, and islet cell tumors of the pancreas. The most common islet cell tumor is a gastrinoma. Multiple endocrine neoplasia-2A usually includes medullary carcinoma of the thyroid, parathyroid hyperplasia, and pheochromocytoma. Systemic mastocytosis, characterized by infiltration of body tissues by mast cells, can be associated with hypersecretion of acid secondary to elevated serum histamine levels. DU may occur in up to 50% of patients. Increased histamine levels also cause development of ulcers in myeloproliferative disorders associated with basophilia.

CLINICAL PRESENTATION

Symptoms

Epigastric pain relieved by food is the classic presentation of DU. Other textbook features include pain occurring 1 to 3 hours after meals, nocturnal awakening secondary to pain, and a burning "hunger-like" quality to the pain. In contrast, classic GU symptoms include epigastric pain unrelieved by food or antacids, occurring soon after meals and more commonly in older patients.

Unfortunately, studies have found these symptoms to be neither sensitive nor specific predictors for PUD. Patients with nonulcerative dyspepsia may present with with classic symptoms of PUD, and patients with PUD may present with atypical symptoms. One study found that GU was relieved by food in almost 50% of patients. Some patients with PUD may present with symptoms typical of gastroparesis such as bloating or fullness. Others may present with belching and fatty food intolerance. Heartburn frequently occurs, probably because PUD often is associated with gastroesophageal reflux. Table 61-1 describes the symptoms experienced by patients with DUs, GUs, and nonulcerative dyspepsia.

Probably even more importantly, patients with ulcer disease may be asymptomatic until they present with complications such as bleeding. Persons particularly at risk for such "silent" presentations include the elderly and patients on NSAIDs. With aging, there is decreased cutaneous sensitivity and possibly also visceral sensitivity. It is unfortunate this group tends to present with complications since these patients frequently have comorbid illnesses and are less able to tolerate GI bleeding. Surgery may be required for penetration or obstruction, and patients in this age group are frequently suboptimal operative candidates.

Patients on NSAIDs often have asymptomatic ulcers on upper endoscopy performed for indications other than suspected PUD. It is postulated that patients using NSAIDs may present without pain because of the intrinsic analgesic effect of the medication, and have an increased propensity to bleed because of the effect of NSAIDs on platelet function. Thus, NSAID-associated ulcers may present incidentally, with pain or with complications. Not surprisingly, NSAID use in the elderly is associated with a higher rate of complications. Gastric outlet obstruction occurs in up to 10% of elderly patients on NSAIDs.

Table 61-1. Symptoms of Gastric and Duodenal Ulcers and Nonulcer Dyspepsia

SYMPTOM	GASTRIC ULCER (%)	DUODENAL ULCER (%)	NONULCER DYSPEPSIA (%)
Pain/discomfort*	100	100	100
Features of the pain:			
Primary pain			
Epigastric	67	61–86	52–73
Right hypochondrium	6	7–17	4
Left hypochondrium	6	3–5	5
Frequently severe	68	53	37
Within 30 min of food	20	5	32
Gnawing pain	13	16	6
Increased by food	24	10–40	45
Clusters (episodic)	16	56	35
Relieved by alkali	36–87	39–86	26–75
Food relief	2–48	20–63	4–32
Occurs at night	32–43	50–88	24–32
Not related to food or variable	22–53	21–49	22–65
Radiation to back	34	20–31	24–28
Increased appetite		19	
Anorexia	46–57	25–36	26–36
Weight loss	24–61	19–45	18–32
Nausea	54–70	49–59	43–60
Vomiting	38–73	25–57	26–34
Heartburn	19	27–59	28
Nondyspeptic symptoms	2	8	18
Fatty food intolerance		41–72	53
Bloating	55	49	52
Belching	48	59	60

Data combined from three series (refs. 440, 441, 442) for gastric ulcer, duodenal ulcer, and nonulcer dyspepsia.

*Patients were ascertained for these series by dyspepsia or upper abdominal pain presenting in a hospital setting. It is obvious that the symptom complexes are usually not specific.

(Soll AH. Gastric, duodenal and stress ulcer. In Sleisinger MH, Fordtran JS, Scharschmidt BF, Feldman M, Cello JP, eds. Gastrointestinal Disease, 5th ed. Philadelphia: WB Saunders, 1993:611.)

A patient who presents with a sudden change in a previously stable pattern of epigastric pain may be describing symptoms of ulcer complications. The development of pain radiating to the back, more intense pain, or more localized pain may signal a posterior penetration of the ulcer. Vomiting may indicating a gastric outlet obstruction. Dizziness or orthostatic symptoms may indicate GI bleeding. The development of melanotic (black) stools is a likely sign of GI hemorrhage, although patients also should be questioned about their consumption of bismuth subsalicylate (Pepto-Bismol) and iron supplements, both of which can cause darkening of the stools.

DIAGNOSIS

Although the physical examination of ulcer patients may reveal epigastric tenderness, this finding lacks sensitivity and specificity and has a low predictive value for PUD. Examination of the conjunctivae and nail beds may be helpful in looking for signs of anemia. Examination of the stool for color and occult blood may give information regarding GI bleeding. Evidence of any systemic diseases that may be associated with PUD, such as cirrhosis or pulmonary disease, should be sought.

Laboratory studies that may be helpful include complete blood cell count, serum creatinine, and serum calcium. A serum gastrin level should be checked in patients with multiple ulcers or those unresponsive to medical therapy. A newly marketed test, an enzyme-linked immunosorbent assay for IgG antibodies to *H. pylori*, seems to be of value, although its role in the workup is not well established. The difficulty with serologic testing for *H. pylori* lies in the interpretation of a positive titer. A positive titer is indicative of a past infection with *H. pylori* but does not necessarily indicate active infection. Furthermore, *H. pylori* infection is extremely common and in many patients causes no significant pathologic changes. It is difficult to definitively interpret a positive serologic finding when the actual disease in the GI tract is not known.

The next decision in evaluating dyspeptic patients is whether to proceed with further workup or treat empirically. In patients older than 40 years of age, the development of new dyspeptic symptoms should be further investigated. In patients younger than 40 years of age with uncomplicated dyspepsia (absence of weight loss, anemia, or GI bleeding), empiric therapy with H_2 receptor antagonists for a period of 4 to 8 weeks is reasonable. If there is no response to therapy or if the patient relapses after therapy is discontinued, additional investigation is warranted.

Further investigation requires some visualization of the upper GI tract. Options include an upper GI series (UGI) or an upper endoscopy. An UGI is less expensive and often more accessible to the primary care provider. Its sensitivity varies depending on the expertise of the radiologist, the ability of the patient to cooperate, and the specific techniques employed, such as air contrast and the use of paddles to compress and highlight the duodenal bulb. The size of the lesion also affects the sensitivity of the test, as ulcers less than 0.5 cm are difficult to reliably visualize. In good hands, 80% to 90% of DUs can be detected on UGI, and GUs are detected in 65% to 90% of patients. One of the disadvantages of UGI includes radiation exposure to the patient. Furthermore, it is not as sensitive as upper endoscopy, and small ulcers can be missed, even by the most experienced radiologist. Larger lesions can be missed by less experienced practitioners. If an abnormality is found and a biopsy is needed, a repeat examination with endoscopy is indicated, requiring two procedures. An UGI is unable to give any information regarding the presence of esophagitis, gastritis, or duodenitis unless it is severe, and it cannot provide information about the presence or absence of *H. pylori*. The sensitivity of an UGI is limited in the postoperative stomach or in a deformed duodenal bulb, whereas endoscopy is quite sensitive. Upper endoscopy is a more invasive procedure since the esophagus needs to be intubated with a small endoscope, and most patients require an intravenous catheter to receive conscious sedation. Once the endoscope is introduced, biopsies can be obtained and pathology samples obtained to exclude inflammation, carcinoma, and infection with *H. pylori*. The chief disadvantages of endoscopy are its cost and invasiveness.

The evaluation of GUs generally requires endoscopy to obtain biopsies of the ulcer to exclude carcinoma. Follow-up endoscopy to document healing also is required. If the initial diagnosis of GU is made on UGI and the ulcer is small and benign appearing, it is acceptable to treat and wait 6 to 12 weeks to perform the follow-up endoscopy to document healing. DUs generally do not require biopsy as the risk of carcinoma is extremely rare, but if there is any suspicion of other etiologies such as granulomatous disease or viral infection, mucosal biopsies are necessary.

In the author's experience, most patients do not express strong opinions regarding a preference for either procedure. Although patients are reticent to swallow the endoscope when the procedure is explained to them, the endoscope usually passes easily and the sedation reduces anxiety and discomfort. Sedation is not given before an UGI, and many patients find the ingestion of barium to be unpleasant. Compression paddles, if used, also may be uncomfortable. When there is a possibility that a second examination will be needed if an UGI is to be performed first, many patients prefer to proceed directly to endoscopy. Invariably, a few anxious patients find the idea of a tube too disquieting and prefer an UGI series.

Complications from either test are rare. The chief risks of upper endoscopy are medication or procedure related. Medication-related complications include respiratory depression and allergic reactions. Respiratory status usually is monitored with pulse oximetry. Severe allergic reactions to narcotics or benzodiazapines are extremely rare. The risk of anaphylaxis is more applicable in patients receiving antibiotics for endocarditis prophylaxis. Procedure-related complications include instrument injury from the endoscope. Perforation is the most feared result. Perforation usually is related to abnormal anatomy, either from postoperative changes or from diverticula, strictures, cancer, or deep ulcers. The rate of perforation is reported as 1 in 3300 examinations.

Detection of *H. pylori*

H. pylori infection can be detected in a variety of ways. Noninvasive testing includes serologic study and breath testing. Serologic study is commercially available. Its limitations have been discussed. Serologic study can be used to determine the effectiveness of eradication therapy. Antibody titers should fall by approximately 50% over 6 to 12 months if the bacteria have been successfully eradicated. Breath testing relies on the urease in the bacterium causing release of carbon dioxide from radiolabeled urea, which patients have swallowed into the stomach. It is sensitive and specific, but false-negative results occur if patients have been on recent antibiotics or omeprazole. It is not yet commercially available.

Invasive testing involves endoscopic biopsy. A rapid test can be performed, using a *Campylobacter*-like organism card. Biopsy specimens from the antrum are placed in pH-sensitive gel. The urease in the *H. pylori* causes the gel to turn color. Biopsies also provide an accurate histologic diagnosis, and Giemsa stains are used to detect the bacilli.

DIFFERENTIAL DIAGNOSIS

The differential diagnosis of dyspepsia is broad. As already noted, no features clearly differentiate PUD from other causes of dyspepsia. The most important diagnosis to exclude is gastric carcinoma since delay in making this diagnosis can be life threatening. Whereas advanced gastric carcinoma is usually incurable, early gastric carcinoma is treatable, with a 5-year survival rate exceeding 85%. Gastric or esophageal cancer is found in approximately 1% of all examinations done for dyspepsia. Gastric cancer is currently the sixth leading cause of cancer mortality in the United States. Early gastric cancer accounts for only a small percentage (approximately 6 per 10,000) of all gastric cancers diagnosed in the United States as opposed to Japan, where it accounts for up to 40% of cases. (Gastric cancer is fairly common in Japan, and mass screening programs are employed to detect early cases. Screening is cost effective because of the high prevalence of the disease.) Early gastric carcinoma is frequently asymptomatic or may present as intermittent peptic symptoms. Patients at increased risk for the development of gastric cancer include those with a family history, blacks, smokers, and possibly those who are positive for *H. pylori* infection. Gastric carcinoma should be excluded in patients older than 50 years of age presenting with new onset of dyspeptic symptoms.

Gastroesophageal reflux is a common cause of epigastric distress. Classically it presents with heartburn symptoms. It may present atypically, with the complaint of epigastric pain being most prominent. Conversely, up to 60% of patients with DU may complain of heartburn symptoms; DU and gastroesophageal reflux commonly coexist.

Motility disorders may cause epigastric pain. Motility disorders also are characterized by prominent complaints of distention, fullness, belching, and bloating. GI motility disorders may be idiopathic or may be seen in diabetics (diabetic gastroparesis), after gastric surgery, and in collagen vascular disease.

Drug-induced dyspepsia is important to consider since patients are commonly taking medications that may produce epigastric discomfort. The most common offenders are NSAIDs. Use of theophylline, digitalis, coffee, caffeine, alcohol, and cigarettes also can cause dyspeptic symptoms. Obtaining a careful drug history is helpful since discontinuing the offending agent may ameliorate symptoms.

Nonulcerative dyspepsia (NUD) refers to ulcer-like pain with no ulcer found on examination. The gastric and duodenal mucosa may be normal, or there may be antritis or antroduodenitis without an ulcer. It is unclear why antritis or antroduodenitis cause dyspepsia in some patients whereas others with this pathologic finding are entirely asymptomatic.

In patients with entirely normal findings, the term *functional dyspepsia* also applies. Functional dyspepsia also may present with associated irritable bowel symptoms such as an alternating bowel pattern, crampy abdominal pain before evacuation, and sensation of incomplete evacuation. Irritable bowel syndrome is seen most commonly in young, female patients.

Biliary colic most commonly presents with severe right upper quadrant pain, often with radiation to the right scapula. However, it sometimes presents atypically, with up to 25% of patients with gallstones having the initial complaint of epigastric pain. Ultrasonography of the right upper quadrant is helpful.

Other causes of dyspepsia include uncommon entities such as Crohn disease of the upper GI tract, lymphoma or sarcoidosis involving the upper GI tract, duodenal carcinoma, and rare infections such as gastric and duodenal tuberculosis or atypical *Mycobacterium* infection. Mesenteric ischemia sometimes presents as postprandial pain, and intestinal ischemia may result in ulcer formation. A more frequently seen problem is *Giardia* infection; this may present with upper abdominal discomfort usually accompanied by nausea, diarrhea, and anorexia. It is important to obtain a travel history and inquire into sources of drinking water.

Non-GI sources of abdominal pain such as pleurisy or an atypical presentation of myocardial ischemia also should be considered.

TREATMENT

Drugs to treat ulcer disease work by reducing or eliminating acid secretion or by augmenting mucosal protection against injurious agents.

H_2 Receptor Antagonists

The parietal cell is the acid-secreting cell of the stomach; it has three receptors: the histamine receptor, gastrin receptor, and acetylcholine receptor. H_2 receptor antagonists function by blocking H_2 receptors on the parietal cell, causing reduction in intracellular levels of cyclic AMP and consequently reduction of acid secretion. Four drugs are available for use in the United States: cimetidine (Tagamet), ranitidine (Zantac), famotidine (Pepcid), and nizatidine (Axid). The four drugs vary in relative potency, as demonstrated in Table 61-2. The drugs are safe and effective. The most data on long-term safety is on cimetidine since it has been available since 1978. No significant problems have been observed with long-term use, but its long-term safety has not been established with absolute certainty. Therefore, its use as a chronic maintenance drug has been limited by many physicians to patients with frequent symptomatic recurrences and to those with complicated ulcers. Efficacy and speed of ulcer healing varies slightly with different dosing regimens, depending largely on the degree of acid secretion inhibited. For DUs, healing on H_2 blockade is 78% at 4 weeks and 92% at 8 weeks. For GUs, healing is 63% at 4 weeks and 88% at 8 weeks.

Concomitant use of antacids decreases absorption of H_2 receptor antagonists by 10% to 20%. Therefore, patients using both antacids and H_2 receptor antagonists need to space the dosing by at least 1 hour. Cimetidine, and to a lesser degree, ranitidine, interact with the cytochrome P_{450} system, potentially inhibiting diazepam, warfarin (Coumadin), and phenytoin (Dilantin) metabolism. Cimetidine rarely has been reported to cause antiandrogen effects such as gynecomastia and impotence. However, these side effects are dose related, are generally reversible with cessation of therapy, and are probably less notable in female patients. Cimetidine has been associated with CNS side effects such as confusion, sedation, headaches, and agitation. Although cimetidine is more often associated with these CNS side effects than the other H_2 blockers, similar disturbances have been reported with the other drugs, and the early reports may represent only more use and recognition of associated side effects of cimetidine. All four drugs are eliminated by a

Table 61-2. H_2 Blockers

DRUG	SERUM HALF-LIFE	RELATIVE POTENCY	EQUIVALENT DOSE (MG)	STANDARD DAILY DOSE (MG)	MAINTENANCE DOSE (MG)
Cimetidine	1.5–2.3 h	1	600–800	800 hs (400 bid)	400 hs
Ranitidine	1.6–2.4 h	4–10	150	300 hs (150 bid)	150 hs
Nizatidine	2.5–4 h	20–50	20	300 hs (150 bid)	150 hs
Famotidine	1.1–1.6 h	4–10	150	40 hs (20 bid)	20 hs

H_2, histadine; hs, hour of sleep; bid, twice daily.

(Modified from Feldman M, Burton ME. Histamine$_2$-receptor antagonists: standard therapy for acid–peptic diseases. N Engl J Med 1990;323:1672.)

combination of hepatic metabolism and renal excretion. Dosing needs to be adjusted in the elderly, in neonates, and in patients with decreased creatinine clearance.

Omeprazole

Omeprazole (Prilosec) works by irreversibly inhibiting the H^+ pump of the parietal cell. Three receptors on the parietal cell initiate acid secretion, multiple events occur within the cell, and acid secretion occurs via the final common pathway, the H^+/K^+–ATPase pump. Acid suppression by omeprazole is potent because it affects this final stage of acid output. At a dose of 20 mg/day, it inhibits approximately 90% of acid secretion; at a dose of 40 mg/day, virtually 100% of acid secretion is inhibited.

For DU, the rate of healing on 20 mg/day of omeprazole is 90% to 100% at 4 weeks, which is accelerated compared with H_2 blocker therapy. For GU the rate of healing on 30 mg/day of omeprazole is approximately 70% at 4 weeks and 92% to 100% at 6 to 8 weeks. Overall, the rate of healing of GUs with omeprazole is only slightly higher than with H_2 receptor antagonists. Omeprazole at a high dose (40 mg/day) is advantageous in healing the refractory GU. (Other approaches, such as eradication of *H. pylori*, also are helpful in treating the refractory DU or GU and are discussed later.)

Omeprazole is similar to the H_2 receptor antagonists in having few side effects for routine short-term use. There is an interaction with the cytochrome P_{450} system, and the metabolism of warfarin, diazepam, and phenytoin is inhibited.

The potential for developing hypergastrinemia is a concern regarding long-term use of omeprazole. Gastrin is a hormone produced by G cells in the antral and duodenal mucosa. Gastrin acts directly on the parietal cell via the gastrin receptor to stimulate H^+ secretion. Elevated levels of H^+ inhibit gastrin release; low levels of H^+ stimulate gastrin release. Long-term use of omeprazole results in long periods of low H^+ output and chronically elevated gastrin levels. Aside from stimulating acid secretion, gastrin also can cause hyperplasia of enterochromaffin-like cells in the stomach and carcinoid tumors of the body of the stomach. In rats, high doses of omeprazole result in gastric carcinoid tumors. For these reasons, omeprazole should be used long term (more than 8 weeks) only for very clear indications. Monitoring serum gastrin levels probably is valuable. Referring such patients to a gastroenterologist is appropriate.

The consequence of rendering the stomach achlorhydric also has been raised as a potential problem associated with the use of omeprazole and H_2 receptor antagonists. When gastric acid secretion is inhibited, bacterial cell counts in the stomach increase, as do nitrosamine levels. This could result in an increased risk of developing GI infections and gastric cancer. With hypochlorhydria secondary to pernicious anemia, there is an increased risk of acquiring nontyphoid salmonellosis and cholera, as well as infection with *Giardia*, *Strongyloides*, and *Entamoeba histolytica*. However, in medically produced hypochlorhydria, this risk seems to be more theoretical than real. GI infections have been reported only rarely, and an increased risk of gastric carcinoma has not been demonstrated.

The role of omeprazole in PUD has not been clearly defined. It is highly efficacious in ulcer healing, but H_2 receptor antagonists are almost equally effective if continued for a sufficient length of time. Omeprazole is helpful in healing the refractory ulcer, but eradication of *H. pylori* is also effective in such cases. In patients who test negative for *H. pylori* infection with refractory ulcers, omeprazole offers a clear advantage over H_2 receptor antagonists. If a patient is admitted with a complication of PUD such as GI bleeding, omeprazole offers an advantage because it accelerates healing. Notice that the rate of recurrence of PUD is no less if the ulcer was healed with omeprazole as opposed to H_2 receptor antagonist therapy. Before the discovery of *H. pylori* infection, it was noted that bismuth was the only drug used in ulcer healing that reduced the rate of recurrence. This is probably because of its antibiotic properties and because *H. pylori* was being eradicated without clinicians fully understanding bismuth's mechanism of action.

Sucralfate

Sucralfate (Carafate) acts by augmenting mucosal protective factors. It is a complex salt of sucrose sulfate and aluminum hydroxide. Sucralfate is poorly soluble in water, resulting in little net absorption from the GI tract. The mechanism of action of sucralfate is not entirely understood, but several possible effects have been proposed. Sucralfate adsorbs to pepsin and seems to have significant antipeptic effects. It is site protective by providing a physical barrier between the contents of the lumen (such as acid, pepsin, and bile salts) and mucosal surfaces. Arachidonic acid metabolism is affected by sucralfate, and it seems to cause release of prostaglandins from the gastric mucosa. Sucralfate also increases bicarbonate output and thus aids in acid neutralization. Lastly, it seems to have beneficial effects on tissue growth, regeneration, and repair.

Since systemic absorption is minimal, side effects are few with this drug. Constipation is the most common problem, occurring in 1% to 3% of patients. In patients with renal insufficiency and especially those on dialysis, the concern of aluminum toxicity has been raised. (Increased levels of aluminum are found in the brains of patients with Alzheimer disease.)

Sucralfate significantly interferes with the absorption and bioavailability of several drugs, including ciprofloxacin, norfloxacin, theophylline, tetracycline, aminophylline, phenytoin, digoxin, and amyitryptyline. Patients who are on fluoroquinone antibiotics should not take sucralfate.

For healing of DU, sucralfate seems to be similar to cimetidine in efficacy. Seventy-three percent of DUs are healed at 4 weeks and 87% at 8 weeks of treatment. For maintenance therapy for DU, sucralfate is effective at a dosage of 1 g orally twice daily. Sucralfate currently is not approved by the Food and Drug Administration for treatment of GUs. However, in clinical studies its efficacy is equivalent to H_2 receptor antagonists.

In clinical practice, it is common to employ combination therapy using H_2 receptor antagonists plus sucralfate. Although this makes intuitive sense since the drugs act by different mechanisms, notice that no controlled trials demonstrate that this therapy is more effective than either drug as a single agent.

Potential but not yet confirmed advantages of sucralfate include treatment of PUD in smokers and prophylaxis of stress ulcers in intensive care unit (ICU) patients. Smoking is known to increase the chance of developing an ulcer and of causing ulcer recurrence. One researcher reports that the delayed healing in smokers treated with H_2 receptor antagonists is not observed with sucralfate. This has not been confirmed in other studies. Sucralfate does not seem to offer a clear advantage in smokers. The second possible advantage of using sucralfate versus acid blockers pertains to the potential problems associated with rendering the stomach achlorhydric and possibly increasing the rate of nosocomial pneumonia. This is of particular concern in the critically ill ICU patient, particularly those requiring mechanical ventilation. However, current evidence does not show that use of sucralfate as ulcer prophylaxis in the ICU setting is superior to H_2 receptor antagonists with regard to less frequent development of nosocomial pneumonia. The two drugs appear to be equivalent. There is evidence that nosocomial pneumonia occurs with antacids more frequently than with sucralfate.

Sucralfate seems to have a bacteriostatic effect against *H. pylori*. It suppresses but does not eradicate the organism.

Antacids

Antacids are an effective therapy in treating PUD, but the dosages required to achieve ulcer healing are such that patient compliance often becomes a problem. Generally, a dose of 1000 mEq/day is required, which usually means dosing seven times per day. Antacids are effective for control of pain while waiting for the H_2 receptor antagonist to heal the ulcer crater. In large doses, magnesium-containing preparations cause diarrhea, whereas aluminum-containing antacids tend to be constipating. Both should be avoided in patients with renal failure, although the aluminum salts are helpful in binding phosphate, which can be elevated significantly in this condition.

The mechanism by which antacids work appears not to be merely by buffering acid. Antacids also bind bile and pepsin. Furthermore, they seem to promote growth of normal mucosa and suppress (but not eradicate) *H. pylori*.

Antacids tend to bind to other medications. Dosing of H_2 receptor antagonists, as well as other medications, needs to be spaced at least 1 hour from ingestion of antacids. Adverse effects of antacids and other antiulcer medications are summarized in Table 61-3.

Misoprostol

Misoprostol (Cytotec), the first synthetic analogue of prostaglandin E_1 to become commercially available, is used in the treatment of NSAID-induced gastroduodenal ulcerations. NSAIDs cause injury by directly harming the gastroduodenal mucosa and by systemic inhibition of prostaglandins. Prostaglandins are protective to the GI tract.

Misoprostol has at least two mechanisms of action: it inhibits the basal and stimulated secretion of gastric acid; and it is also cytoprotective and inhibits gastric mucosal damage from irritants such as bile salts and NSAIDs. The mechanism of cytoprotection is not entirely clear but is possibly due to increased secretion of mucus and bicarbonate, increased mucosal blood flow, and increased cell proliferation (ie, healing) of the gastric mucosa.

The chief side effect of misoprostol is a dose-related diarrhea that is usually self-limiting. The recommended dose is 200 µg orally four times daily. At this dose, the frequency of diarrhea ranges from 13% to 39%. At a dose of 100 µg orally four times daily, the incidence rate of diarrhea ranges from 10% to 25%. For this reason, the author generally starts patients at 100 µg orally twice daily and increases the dose as tolerated.

Table 61-3. Adverse Effects from Antiulcer Therapy

	H_2 BLOCKERS	OMEPRAZOLE	SUCRALFATE	ANTACIDS
I. Toxic effects	*Hypochlorhydria:* Bacterial overgrowth; Hypergastrinemia; Altered absorption from alkalinization; Decreased absorption of divalent cations; Decreased B_{12} absorption			
II. Side effects	Antiandrogenic: cimetidine CNS reactions: headaches: immune modulation: cardiac conduction abnormalities: idiosyncratic hepatic injury: immune hypersensitivity reactions: thrombocytopenia: granulocytopenia		Aluminum absorption, phosphate depletion	
III. Drug interactions				
A. Absorption	Intraluminar alkalinization, inhibits absorption (e.g., ketoconazole)		*Intraluminal drug binding of:* Tetracycline, ciprofloxacin, isoniazid, chloroquine, warfarin, digoxin, phenytoin, quinidine, aspirin and other NSAIDs, cimetidine, ranitidine, ferrous sulfate, theophylline	
B. P_{450} mediated	*Cimetidine (>>ranitidine)* Warfarin, theophylline, phenytoin, diazepam, propranolol	Diazepam, warfarin, phenytoin		
C. Excretion	↓ Renal tubular excretion of procainamide			

H_2, histadine, NSAIDs, nonsteroidal antiinflammatory drugs.

(From Sleisinger MH, Fordtran JS, Scharschmidt BF, Feldman M, Cello JP. Gastrointestinal Disease, 5th ed. Philadelphia, WB Saunders, 1993:623.)

The other major side effect of mi8soprostol is stimulation of uterine contractions. In studies in women who were undergoing elective first-trimester abortions, misoprostol caused partial or complete abortion in 11% of subjects. Therefore, it is absolutely contraindicated in pregnancy or in any women of childbearing potential. Furthermore, patients should be advised of the abortifacient properties and be advised not to give the drug to others. (Misoprostol has reportedly been sold as an abortifacient in Brazil).

Use of misoprostol has been shown to prevent development of ulcers in patients on NSAIDs and to heal existing ulcers in patients using NSAIDs. Results with misoprostol need to be considered separately for gastric and DUs. The efficacy of misoprostol compared with the above-mentioned drugs also needs to be critically examined since misoprostol has a higher side effect profile. Lastly, the clinical relevance of endoscopic findings such as erosions, NSAID gastropathy, or asymptomatic ulcers, on which the rationale for misoprostol therapy has been based, also needs to be considered.

The literature is murky with regard to the question of ulcer prophylaxis. Studies with misoprostol have been endoscopic studies on relatively healthy subjects who require NSAIDs. Patients with a history of PUD generally have been excluded from the studies, although they are among the group with the highest likelihood of NSAID-induced problems and the group who may benefit the most from use of misoprostol. In the patients studied, endoscopic findings of gastropathy (superficial mucosal damage) or erosions are less in the misoprostol-treated groups, but no data prove that acute gastropathy or erosions are clinically significant. Gastropathy often does not cause symptoms and often resolves without further treatment, even with further NSAID exposure. Another large study assessed the cumulative rate of development of endoscopically defined GU and DU. Misoprostol reduced the frequency of development of both GU and DU. However, patients with a history of PUD were excluded. Furthermore, no data prove that these endoscopically defined ulcers would have had any clinical sequelae. Nonetheless, it is reasonable to conclude that misoprostol is effective in preventing the development of NSAID-associated ulcers. Additional studies have shown that misoprostol is more effective than H_2 antagonists or sucralfate in preventing NSAID-associated GUs.

For prophylaxis of DUs, misoprostol seems to be similar in efficacy to H_2 receptor antagonists and sucralfate. Several studies looking at cost–benefit analysis have addressed the question of whether routine treatment of NSAID users with misoprostol should be undertaken. However, since no studies have looked at clinically significant end points (hemorrhage or perforation), there are insufficient data to draw any conclusions. In the author's opinion, it is reasonable to use misoprostol in patients who have a history of GUs who need to begin NSAID therapy. If the patient has a history of a DU, it is probably advantageous to use another drug since the side effect profile will be better.

With regard to ulcer healing, misoprostol is efficacious, but no more so than other therapies. It is not recommended as a first-line therapy since its side effects are more frequent than those of other drugs. An additional question that arises is the role for misoprostol if the NSAID cannot be discontinued. Misoprostol is superior to placebo in ulcer healing with continued NSAID use, but it has not been compared with other antiulcer drugs. It seems reasonable to use dual therapy in such situations (ie, H_2 receptor antagonist or omeprazole plus misoprostol), but no data support this. The most effective way to heal an existing NSAID-induced ulcer is to discontinue the NSAID whenever possible.

Treatment of *H. pylori*

Treatment of *H. pylori* infection is indicated in patients who are infected with the bacteria and who have a gastric or DU. Other indications for therapy include (1) patients with active infection and a history of PUD but no active ulcer, who are thought to require maintenance antiulcer therapy, and (2) those with a history of a complicated or refractory ulcer. Whereas treatment of *H. pylori* infection does not completely eliminate the chance of ulcer recurrence, it reduces it significantly, from approximately 50% to 70% (on no maintenance) to approximately 20%. In the fragile or elderly patient in whom a recurrence could be life threatening, it is appropriate to both eradicate *H. pylori* and continue maintenance therapy with H_2 receptor antagonists if the initial presentation of the ulcer was complicated. Children with *H. pylori* infection should receive specific treatment because otherwise the infection is likely to be present for a lifetime. Patients with *H. pylori* infection and a family history of gastric carcinoma (in a first-degree relative) probably should be treated. The latter two recommendations are controversial, and there is not strong evidence to support them; nonetheless, based on our current knowledge of the infection, the author agrees with these recommendations.

Implicit in the treatment of *H. pylori* infection is that the presence of the organism has first been demonstrated in some way. Empiric treatment is not recommended. If a DU has been found on UGI, the subsequent detection of *H. pylori* infection by serologic testing probably is adequate and allows the patient to avoid more invasive testing.

It is also important to determine which patients do not require treatment. Patients with *H. pylori* infection who are asymptomatic or who have NUD do not require antibiotic therapy. Controlled trials of eradication of *H. pylori* infection in patients with NUD have failed to show any benefit.

A variety of treatment regimens are available to treat *H. pylori* infection (Table 61-4). The most used and successful is the triple regimen of metronidazole, tetracycline, and bismuth subsalicylate (Pepto-Bismol). Disadvantages of this regimen include the four-times-a-day dosing and the necessity of three drugs, which may reduce patient compliance. If an active ulcer is seen, it needs to be treated with any of the antiulcer drug regimens described earlier. The antibiotics can be taken concurrently with the antiulcer therapy or subsequent to it. The author usually prefers to treat the ulcer first, with H_2 receptor antagonists or omeprazole, and then to begin triple therapy after the ulcer is healed. Antibiotics have frequent GI side effects, and the author prefers not to use them with acute ulcers. Bismuth subsalicylate can darken the stool, thus making it uncertain whether active GI hemorrhage is present. (There appears to be evidence that treatment with antibiotics alone heals gastric and DUs and that acid suppression may not be necessary, but this evidence is preliminary and this mode of therapy currently cannot be recommended.) If a regimen such as omeprazole plus amoxicillin is used, efficacy seems to be better if the drugs are started at the same time. Omeprazole should be continued long enough to heal the ulcer (ie, at least 4 weeks). The dosing for omeprazole is 20 mg twice daily for the first 2 weeks then one time daily for the

Table 61-4. Eradication of *H. Pylori*

DRUGS*	DOSE	DURATION	% ERADICATION
Bismuth subsalicylate (Pepto-Bismol) }	2 tabs qid	×2 wk	
Metronidazole (Flagyl)	250 qid	×2 wk	80%–90%
Tetracycline	500 qid (can substitute amoxicillin 500 qid if tetracycline intolerant)	×2 wk	
Amoxicillin }	500 mg qid	×2 wk	50%–80%
Omeprazole (Prilosec)	40 mg qd		
Clarithromycin }	500 mg po tid	×2 wk	70%–80%
Omeprazole	40 mg po qd		

qid, four times daily; tabs, tablets; po, orally; tid, three times daily.

*Amoxicillin may be reused in treatment failures. Macrolides (erythromycin, azithromycin, and clarithromycin) inhibit *Helicobacter pylori,* but the bacterium has a propensity to develop resistance; therefore, patients should not be retreated with macrolide. Metronidazole is cidal but resistance occurs; if treatment fails, retreatment with triple regimen is controversial, but most advocate changing to a different regimen.

next 2 to 6 weeks. Amoxicillin is dosed at 500 mg orally four times a day for 2 weeks.

Antibiotic resistance, especially to metronidazole, has become an increasingly common problem. The author generally explains this to the patient and emphasizes the importance of complying fully with the regimen.

Ancillary Treatment of Peptic Ulcer Disease

As mentioned earlier, various modifications of diet and behavior certainly affect dyspepsia and the development and propagation of PUD. No foods or beverages cause ulcers, but certain foods can cause dyspeptic symptoms. Patients with acute ulcers should avoid any foods that cause pain and avoid consuming hard liquor. Patients may ingest coffee and spicy foods if consumption does not produce symptoms. Smoking should be discontinued. There is strong evidence that smoking propagates PUD and can make healing of the ulcer more difficult. Institution of a formal program, such as the use of nicotine patches or gum, or referral to a smoke enders program, is appropriate.

NSAIDs need to be discontinued whenever possible. Patients are frequently unaware of which drugs fall into this category. Specific instruction on this topic often is needed. If aspirin must be used, enteric-coated preparations are preferred.

Nonacetylated forms of acetylsalicylic acid (choline magnesium trisalicylate, salsalate) seem to cause less (but potentially still some) GI injury. If NSAIDs must be prescribed, lower doses lessen the chance of injury (in strength per pill, number of pills consumed, and use of shorter acting preparations).

Role of Surgery

Since the development of antiulcer pharmacology, surgical treatment of routine presentations of this disease has markedly decreased. Nevertheless, intractable disease, perforation, or the development of severe hemorrhage may necessitate surgical intervention. Interestingly, probably because of the widespread use of NSAIDs, the frequency of development of complicated PUD seems to be unchanged despite the availability of antiulcer pharmacology.

Pregnancy

Dyspeptic symptoms during pregnancy are common. As discussed earlier, symptoms are relatively unhelpful in differentiating PUD from other etiologies. This becomes even more unclear during pregnancy, when associated problems such as reflux and hyperemesis may arise. The actual incidence of PUD during pregnancy is not known since empiric therapy is usually given and workup is deferred unless absolutely necessary. However, the prevalence is probably no different than in any other population. There is no evidence that pregnancy changes the risk of developing PUD.

Treatment of dyspeptic symptoms first includes instituting dietary changes such as frequent small meals and avoidance of fatty or spicy foods. Cigarettes should be completely discontinued. Elevating the head of the bed and avoidance of late night meals is of value. Avoidance of foods that relax the lower esophageal sphincter, such as peppermint, coffee, alcohol, chocolate, and fatty foods, is appropriate.

Medical treatment includes antacid use as first-line therapy. Antacids seem to be safe, especially after the first trimester. Use of antacids during breast-feeding seems to be safe as well. Carafate has little systemic absorption and seems to be safe during pregnancy and breast-feeding. Cimetidine has been safely used by many pregnant women, but congenital defects have been reported in infants of women taking cimetidine, although no causal relationship has been shown. It is secreted into breast milk and should not be used unless absolutely necessary. Omeprazole has been demonstrated to cause toxicity in animal studies of rat embryos. Misoprostol has abortifacient properties and is absolutely contraindicated during pregnancy.

Patients who have refractory symptoms unresponsive to symptomatic measures or to medical therapy require further investigation, as do patients with GI hemorrhage. UGI should not be performed because of the radiation to the patient and the fetus; therefore, endoscopy is the diagnostic test of choice. If sedation can be avoided, it may be preferable, but meperidine and diazepam seem to be safe drugs if necessary. Endoscopy seems to be safe during pregnancy.

BIBLIOGRAPHY

Marshall BJ, Warren JR. Unidentified curved bacilla in gastric epithelium in active chronic gastritis. Lancet 1983;1:1273.

Megraud F, Lamoullatte H. *Helicobacter pylori* and duodenal ulcer: evidence suggesting causation. Dig Dis Sci 1992;37:769.

Peterson, Walter. *Helicobacter pylori* and peptic ulcer disease. N Engl J Med 1991;324:1043.

Fennerty MB. *Helicobacter pylori.* Arch Intern Med 1994; 154:721.

Parsonnet J, Friedman GB, Vandersteen DP, et al. *Helicobacter pylori* infection and the risk of gastric carcinoma. N Engl J Med 1991;325:1127.

Soll AH. Gastric, duodenal and stress ulcer. In Sleisenger MH, Fortren JS, Sharschmidt BF, et al, eds. Gastrointestinal disease, 5th ed, p 580. Philadelphia: WB Saunders, 1993.

Primary Care for Women, edited by Phyllis C. Leppert and Fred M. Howard. Lippincott-Raven Publishers, Philadelphia © 1997.

62
Acute Liver and Biliary Tract Disease

JANET R. REISER

The term *hepatocellular damage* refers to hepatocyte necrosis and the subsequent development of elevated transaminase levels. Transaminases include aspartate aminotransferase (AST, formerly known as serum glutamic oxaloacetic transaminase [SGOT]) and alanine aminotransferase (ALT, or serum glutamic pyruvic transaminase [SGPT]). Levels of transaminases are highest in patients with viral hepatitis or damage secondary to toxins. However, viral hepatitis can also present with a cholestatic pattern of liver injury. Serum transaminase values in the range of 200 to 300 mU/mL in patients with jaundice are nonspecific for hepatocellular injury and can occur when there is obstruction to bile flow from a stone or tumor.

Cholestatic liver injury refers to impaired bile formation or bile flow and is characterized by elevated alkaline phosphatase and conjugated bilirubin levels. This may be secondary to extrahepatic obstruction (most commonly from stones or a tumor) or due to intrahepatic causes. The latter can be subdivided into hepatocellular and canalicular dysfunction (viral, drug-induced, sepsis, other disorders) and diseases causing obliteration or obstruction of the intrahepatic ducts (eg, primary biliary cirrhosis, primary sclerosing cholangitis).

VIRAL HEPATITIS

Viral hepatitis includes hepatitis A, B, C, D, and E, as well as nonhepatitis viruses such as Epstein-Barr, cytomegalovirus, and herpes simplex. Hepatitis A through D appear to have the same clinical course in well-nourished pregnant patients as in nonpregnant patients; malnourished pregnant patients with acute viral hepatitis may have a worse prognosis. Hepatitis E has been reported to have up to a 20% mortality rate during pregnancy. Herpes simplex hepatitis has been associated with a worse prognosis in pregnant patients, but the use of acyclovir has greatly improved the outcome if the patient is diagnosed and treated promptly.

Hepatitis A

Hepatitis A (HAV) is highly contagious and its spread is enteric (fecal–oral). It tends to occur in developing countries where hygiene and sanitation practices are less developed. In such areas, patients tend to have anti-HAV antibodies by age 10. In developed countries, the disease occurs less often among children, but the prevalence of the antibody increases with age. In developed countries, certain groups are at increased risk for acquiring HAV infection, including travelers to areas where HAV is endemic and homosexuals who practice oral–anal contact.

The incubation period of HAV is fairly short, with a mean duration of 30 days. Viral shedding may occur before symptoms of acute illness develop. The virus is in both blood and stool for 2 to 3 weeks before the onset of jaundice and persists in the stool for 8 days or longer after the disease onset. Symptoms generally include nausea, vomiting, and fever, but patients sometimes present with mild symptoms or subclinically, during which time the infection may be recognized incidentally. Nonhepatic manifestations of acute viral hepatitis (ie, bone marrow abnormalities or arthralgias) generally do not occur with HAV. Enzyme levels are elevated for about 8 weeks. Mortality is less than 1%, although it may be higher in the elderly.

HAV is diagnosed by serologic testing for IgM antibodies to HAV (IgM antibodies usually persist for 6 months). The presence of IgG anti-HAV indicates past infection and immunity. Patients with HAV do not develop a chronic carrier state. Once antibodies are developed, they persist for life.

There is no evidence that HAV is more common or more severe during pregnancy. The neonate rarely acquires the disease, presumably because of transplacental delivery to the fetus of maternal anti-HAV antibodies.

Treatment of HAV is supportive. Patients are monitored for the development of fulminant hepatitis. Close contacts of the patient (household, sexual, day-care, institutions) should receive passive prophylaxis with HAV immune globulin as soon as possible (unless they have documented immunity to HAV), no later than 2 weeks after exposure. Preexposure prophylaxis for HAV is recommended for travelers going to areas where it is endemic. An active vaccine for HAV is available and may supplant some of the uses of passive vaccination.

Hepatitis B

Hepatitis B (HBV) virus is transmitted in blood and some body fluids. HBV surface antigen has been noted in semen, saliva, sweat, tears, and breast milk. The route of transmission is both percutaneous and nonpercutaneous exposure. Persons at high risk for percutaneous exposure include health care workers and intravenous drug abusers. Persons at risk for nonpercutaneous exposure include promiscuous heterosexuals and homosexuals.

HBV occurs after a mean incubation period of 80 days. It affects all ages. Symptoms commonly include nausea and vomiting and extrahepatic manifestations such as arthralgias. Jaundice is not uncommon. The mean duration of liver enzyme elevation is 4 months. Generally, the bilirubin level does not exceed 20 mg/dL. There is some correlation between the severity of the disease and the height of the bilirubin rise. Once the bilirubin level has peaked, it tends to decline by about 50% per week. Coagulation tests such as prothrombin time and partial thromboplastin time are normal in acute, uncomplicated viral hepatitis. A prolonged prothrombin time may suggest the incipient development of subacute hepatic necrosis or fulminant hepatitis. Fulminant hepatitis is manifested by the development of coagulopathy, with a prothrombin time more than 2 seconds above control, hypoglycemia, and encephalopathy. If the prothrombin time is elevated by more than 2 seconds above control, the patient should be closely monitored.

Mild anemia, mild leukopenia, and mild to moderate thrombocytopenia are common nonhepatic manifestations of acute HBV. Aplastic anemia is a serious but rare complication that tends to occur 9 weeks after the onset of hepatitis. About 200 cases of aplastic anemia have been reported in association with HBV. Severe hemolytic anemia has also been described. Polyarteritis nodosa also occurs in association with HBV. Glomerulonephritis may precede, coexist with, or follow acute HBV-induced hepatitis.

Unlike HAV, which resolves in almost all patients (fewer than 1% develop a fatal course) and does not involve the development of a carrier state, HBV can become chronic. Of the 300,000 cases of HBV reported to the Centers for Disease Control each year, about 10% develop chronic HBV.

HBV is diagnosed by drawing serology for hepatitis B surface antigen (HBsAg), hepatitis B core antibody (anti-HBc), and hepatitis B surface antibody (anti-HBs). With resolution of the illness, HBsAg disappears before anti-HBs appears. In this "window" period, anti-HBc is the only marker of infection. The presence of anti-HBs generally implies immunity to HBV. Chronic HBV is defined as persistence of HBsAg and lack of development of anti-HBs.

HBV is treated supportively, with monitoring for complications. Sexual contacts and persons who have had percutaneous or permucosal exposure to the patient should receive vaccination with HBV immune globulin (passive immunoprophylaxis) and HBV vaccine, unless they have immunity to HBV. Preexposure vaccination is recommended for persons with occupational risk, clients and staff in institutions, hemodialysis patients, populations in which HBV is endemic, and travelers to endemic areas.

Babies born to mothers who developed acute HBV infection during pregnancy should receive passive immunization. Acute HBV infection becomes chronic in 10% in adults, but the rate was about 90% in babies exposed perinatally before the use of passive and active immunization. With the use of combined HBV immune globulin and HBV vaccine, more than 90% of cases of HBV are prevented in infants. Acquisition of chronic HBV in infancy may lead to the development of cirrhosis and its complications, liver failure and hepatocellular cancer. These complications may develop as early as the teens and 20s, with a peak incidence in the fourth and fifth decades of life. In countries with a high prevalence of hepatoma (Southeast Asia, sub-Saharan Africa), an estimated 60% to 90% of cases are associated with HBV.

Hepatitis C

Hepatitis C (HCV), previously termed non-A, non-B hepatitis, is the most common cause of transfusion hepatitis. About 40% of patients with HCV are intravenous drug abusers. Sexual exposure is the route of transmission in about 6% of cases, blood transfusions are responsible for about 6% of cases, occupational blood exposure accounts for 2% of cases, household exposures are responsible for about 3% of cases, and hemodialysis accounts for 0.6% of cases. About 40% of patients have no clear route of transmission.

The clinical presentation is usually insidious. Nausea and vomiting are common; jaundice, fever, and arthralgias occur less often. The most common manifestation is subclinical, with asymptomatic transaminitis noted incidentally on routine screening of liver enzymes. Unlike HBV, in which about 10% of patients develop chronic hepatitis, about 50% of HCV patients develop chronic hepatitis.

Diagnosis is serologic. A recently developed ELISA tests for an antibody to a nonstructural peptide of HCV. False-positive results may occur in autoimmune liver disease. Detection of viral RNA by polymerase chain reaction is more accurate and will become commercially available in the future.

There is no active HCV vaccine, and passive vaccination is controversial. In needlestick exposures with known anti-HCV–positive blood, some authorities recommend passive prophylaxis with immune globulin, but its efficacy is equivocal.

Hepatitis D

Hepatitis D (HDV) occurs only as a coinfection with HBV or as a superinfection. Only patients who have HBV surface antigenemia can develop HDV. It generally presents with severe hepatitis, and the mortality rate is about 3%. Patients can develop a carrier state. HDV is highly infectious; transmission is percutaneous and sexual.

Diagnosis is made by serology. IgM anti-HDV connotes acute σ infection, and IgG anti-HDV connotes previous or chronic σ infection.

Hepatitis E

Hepatitis E (HEV) is similar to HAV in that it is transmitted by the fecal–oral route. Contaminated water is generally thought to be the source of infection. The mean incubation period is 40 days. Nausea, vomiting, fever, and jaundice are common. The duration of enzyme elevation tends to be short, as with HAV. The disease is generally mild, but in pregnancy mortality rates of up to 20% have been reported.

HEV is rare in the United States and has occurred in North America only in persons returning from endemic areas (south, east, and central Asia; northern, eastern, and western Africa). It has also been described in Mexico. This may become an issue when advising pregnant women with travel plans.

Diagnosis can be made by assaying for anti-HEV, but this is not commercially available.

Summary of Hepatitis A Through E

Illness tends to be mildest in HCV and is slightly more severe in HAV and HEV. It is more severe in HBV and most severe in HDV superinfection of HBV. The enteric viruses (HAV, HEV) do not progress to chronicity, but HBV, HCV, and HDV do so with varying frequencies. In pregnancy, acute maternal infection with HBV is of most concern; the baby needs routine vaccination for HBV and passive vaccination with HBV immune globulin.

Herpes Simplex Hepatitis

Herpes simplex hepatitis can be associated with a fulminant course during pregnancy, probably because of the immunocompromise associated with pregnancy. Patients usually present in the third trimester with upper respiratory infection symptoms and fever. There usually are vesicular lesions of the skin, perineum, or cervix. Patients do not usually have icterus, and the initial presentation of the liver disease may be hepatic coma. Transaminase levels are elevated, with values usually above 2000 mU/mL. There is often associated pneumonitis or encephalitis. Acyclovir has improved the mortality rates and should be given promptly once the diagnosis is recognized.

Cytomegaloviral Hepatitis

In the normal host, cytomegalovirus causes few symptoms, although some patients may develop an illness resembling mononucleosis or mild hepatitis, which subsequently resolves. Problems occur when the virus becomes reactivated in latent carriers who become immunosuppressed, such as AIDS patients and transplant recipients. In such patients, chronic hepatitis may occur.

Epstein-Barr Hepatitis

Epstein-Barr virus is the cause of infectious mononucleosis. Jaundice and hepatitis are seen as part of the clinical spectrum in up to 5% of cases. In older patients, mild hepatitis is occasionally the predominant feature.

BILIARY TRACT DISEASE

Gallstones are a common ultrasonographic finding, but most persons with gallstones (60% to 80%) are asymptomatic. Each year, about 1% to 2% of patients with gallstones develop symptoms. Because this rate is low, prophylactic cholecystectomy is not recommended for asymptomatic persons. Similarly, in diabetics, prophylactic cholecystectomy is no longer recommended if the gallstones remain asymptomatic. In patients with a porcelain gallbladder (calcified wall of the gallbladder), cholecystectomy is recommended because of the relatively high risk (about 25%) of malignancy.

Nonsurgical treatment of gallstones includes gallstone dissolution therapy and lithotripsy. Nonsurgical therapy is not used to treat gallstone complications, but it is used in selected patients to eliminate the gallstones. Nonsurgical therapy is effective only for cholesterol stones (80% of all gallstones). For dissolution therapy, the stones should be small (< 15 mm in diameter) and the cystic duct should be patent. The two drugs used to dissolve gallstones are chenodeoxycholic acid and ursodeoxycholic acid. Several months are required for dissolution. Extracorporeal shock wave lithotripsy uses fluid shock waves to fragment small radiolucent (cholesterol) stones. These therapies are best for patients who are unfit for surgery; cholecystectomy remains the optimal therapy in operative candidates.

Complications of cholelithiasis include cholecystitis, biliary colic (the most common), choledocholithiasis, acute cholangitis, and acute pancreatitis. Biliary pain is classically felt in the right upper quadrant or epigastrium, but it may also be felt in the left upper quadrant or toward the umbilicus. Pain usually is episodic, lasting 30 minutes to several hours, and resolves gradually. It may be accompanied by nausea or vomiting. Once a patient with gallstones experiences an episode of biliary colic, future episodes are likely. Such patients are also at risk for developing other complications of gallstone disease.

Acute Cholecystitis

Acute cholecystitis occurs when the cystic duct is obstructed by a stone or stones, causing acute inflammation of the gallbladder wall. Early in the disease, bacterial infection is not a causative factor, but as the inflammatory process continues for several days, patients may become superinfected and at risk for complications (eg, septicemia, empyema). Acute cholecystitis is associated with abdominal pain, tenderness, fever, and leukocytosis.

Clinical manifestations include abdominal pain similar to biliary colic, but this pain does not resolve. Fever is generally present (99° to 101°F).

The physical examination is notable for tenderness in the right upper quadrant. A palpable gallbladder may be present. The Murphy sign is characteristic (deep inspiration causes tenderness in the right subcostal area). Elderly or debilitated patients may have very few physical findings.

Laboratory values may show mild jaundice, but usually the bilirubin level is less than 4 mg/dL. Leukocytosis is typical, with a range of 12,000 to 16,000 polymorphonuclear leukocytes and an increase in band forms. The alkaline phosphatase level is typically elevated three to four times above normal, with elevations also noted in ALT and AST. The serum amylase level is usually normal; if it is elevated and the patient has nausea, vomiting, or abdominal pain radiating to the back, gallstone pancreatitis should be considered.

The diagnosis of acute cholecystitis is primarily clinical, but confirmatory studies are helpful. A kidney, ureter, and bladder x-ray study should be ordered. About 15% of gallstones are calcified and can be seen on plain X-rays, although this does not confirm the diagnosis of acute cholecystitis. However, plain films are important to exclude other conditions, such as a perforated viscus. Ultrasound is the test of choice for detecting gallstones, gallbladder sludge, dilated bile ducts, and gallbladder wall thickening. Radionuclide scanning, usually the DISIDA scan, is used to check the patency of the cystic duct. Radiolabeled material is injected intravenously. In a patient without obstruction, the radionuclide is excreted by the liver into the bile and then enters the gallbladder. However, if the cystic duct is not patent, the gallbladder fails to visualize. Aside from acute cholecystitis, other causes of nonvisualization of the gallbladder include a contracted gallbladder secondary to not eating; patients who are receiving hyperalimentation or who have undergone major surgery fall into this category.

Treatment of acute cholecystitis is cholecystectomy. Before surgery, most patients need intravascular fluid volume replacement. Antibiotic coverage of gram-negative aerobes and enterococci is usually necessary. Analgesia may be required. In patients who are severely ill with septic shock, antibiotic coverage should be broadened to include all enteric organisms, including anaerobes.

Biliary Tract Disease During Pregnancy

Females are more likely to develop gallstones, and this likelihood is even greater during pregnancy. Gallbladder volumes are higher during pregnancy, increasing the stagnancy of gallbladder bile. This may be due to progesterone's effect of reducing gallbladder motility. Also, the hormonal effects of pregnancy cause changes in the lithogenicity of bile. Biliary tract disease is second only to acute appendicitis as the most common surgical disease in pregnant women. Cholecystitis requiring cholecystectomy occurs in one to six per 10,000 pregnancies.

The clinical presentation of biliary tract disease during pregnancy is similar to that seen in nonpregnant patients, but the differential diagnosis is broader. The pain of acute appendicitis is more likely to be localized in the right upper quadrant because of the upward displacement of the abdominal viscera by the gravid uterus. Liver diseases unique to pregnancy (eg, preeclampsia, HELLP syndrome, acute fatty liver of pregnancy) must be considered. Ultrasound is the imaging procedure of choice.

Treatment of biliary colic includes analgesics and a low-fat diet. Acute cholecystitis often responds to parenteral antibiotics and intravenous hydration. Surgery can often be delayed until after delivery. However, refractory biliary colic, cholecystitis that does not respond to antibiotics, or severe gallstone pancreatitis may require cholecystectomy. Cholecystectomy is best performed during the second trimester. At this time, the uterus does not encroach on the surgical field and fetal organogenesis has been completed. An incidence of fetal loss of up to 5% has been reported in association with any abdominal surgery during the first trimester, whereas the outcome is generally good during the second trimester. Laparoscopic cholecystectomy was thought to be contraindicated during pregnancy, but its safe performance has been reported.

Bile acid dissolution therapy has rarely been used during pregnancy, as these substances cross the placenta. Extracorporeal biliary lithotripsy has not been used in pregnant patients.

DRUG-INDUCED ACUTE LIVER INJURY

Many drugs are hepatotoxins, with alcohol probably the most common offender. Most pregnant patients limit their consumption of prescription and nonprescription drugs and alcohol.

Oral contraceptives and estrogen replacement therapy cause cholestatic abnormalities on liver function tests. Almost all oral contraceptives are noted to cause subclinical impairment of sulfobromophthalein transport (sulfobromophthalein is an organic anion extracted from the blood by the liver and excreted into bile). However, only a few patients develop clinical jaundice. Cholestatic jaundice secondary to oral contraceptive use is manifested by pruritus, dark urine, and light stools. Liver biopsy shows a bland cholestatic process that resolves with discontinuation of the medication. There appears to be a familial predilection for the development of this syndrome.

Use of combined oral contraceptives appears to increase the risk of hepatic cell adenomas (benign hyperplastic epithelial tumors), presumably secondary to the estrogen effects. The risk increases with the duration of use and is elevated in women older than 30. The overall risk is estimated at 3.4 per 100,000 females. Complications that may arise from hepatic adenomas include rupture and hemorrhage, especially in adenomas more than 3 cm in diameter. Patients may present with abdominal pain or a palpable mass or with shock secondary to rupture and hemoperitoneum, or the disease may be discovered as an incidental finding on a liver sonogram. The increased estrogen levels associated with pregnancy may be associated with rapid growth of hepatic adenomas.

With discontinuation of the oral contraceptives, many hepatic adenomas regress, but some progress and new sites of tumor growth have been reported. It is unclear whether liver cell adenomas have a potential for malignant transformation. Given the concerns of rupture and possible malignant transformation, many authorities recommend the resection of large adenomas, especially before pregnancy.

FULMINANT HEPATIC FAILURE

Fulminant hepatic failure (FHF) is a serious condition involving massive necrosis of hepatocytes. Clinically, it is characterized by severely impaired liver function and hepatic encephalopathy. The encephalopathy occurs within 8 weeks of the onset of illness. FHF occurs in patients with no evidence of preexisting liver disease.

The etiologies of FHF (Table 62-1) include viral hepatitis, chemical-induced hepatitis, and miscellaneous causes. The most common cause of FHF is acute viral hepatitis; the second most common is drug-induced hepatitis, which includes idiosyncratic

Table 62-1. Causes of Fulminant Hepatic Failure

Causes
Acute Viral Hepatitis
Hepatitis A virus
Hepatitis B virus
Hepatitis C virus
Hepatitis D virus
Coinfection with HBV
Superinfection with HBV
Hepatitis E virus
Other viral agents
Chemical-Related Hepatitis
Idiosyncratic drug reactions
Acetaminophen toxicity
Amanita mushroom poisoning
Industrial poisons
Miscellaneous Causes
Reye syndrome
Wilson disease
Acute fatty liver of pregnancy
Budd-Chiari syndrome
Ischemia
Malignancy

drug reactions, dose-dependent effects, and exposure to toxic chemicals. Miscellaneous causes are much rarer.

Acute Viral Hepatitis

HBV is responsible for about 75% of cases of FHF. Overall, FHF occurs in less than 1% of cases of acute HBV. The survival rate in FHF from HBV is about 40%. FHF from HAV is rare and has a survival rate of about 66%. Death occurs in 0.01% to 0.1% of all cases of acute HAV. HCV causes up to 25% of cases of fulminant viral hepatitis. This infection has a reported survival rate of 10% to 20%, but full literature on FHF due to HCV is in evolution, as the assay for HCV became available only recently. HDV seems to be associated with a higher mortality rate than HBV. HEV is an enterically transmitted virus that has been responsible for outbreaks in developing countries. For unclear reasons, the mortality rate in pregnant women is very high (about 20%), but otherwise the disease is generally benign. FHF due to other viruses such as herpes simplex I and II, cytomegalovirus, Epstein-Barr virus, varicella zoster, and adenovirus is rare, but reports of fulminant hepatitis exist. Fulminant hepatitis appears to be more likely in immunosuppressed or pregnant patients.

Chemically Induced Hepatitis

Acetaminophen toxicity secondary to overdose from suicide attempts is a fairly common cause of FHF. An area of controversy is whether therapeutic doses of acetaminophen cause hepatocellular injury in certain patients. Acetaminophen is metabolized by the liver cytochrome P-450 enzyme system to a toxic metabolite that is then normally detoxified by conjugation with glutathione. If glutathione stores are depleted or if the glutathione detoxification system is saturated, as in chronic alcoholics or in patients on concomitant liver enzyme-inducing drugs, it may be possible to accumulate toxic metabolites of acetaminophen and develop subsequent hepatocellular injury even with therapeutic doses of acetaminophen.

The drugs most commonly causing idiosyncratic reactions include halothane anesthetics, isoniazid, anticonvulsants, and certain antidepressants. Lipid-lowering agents can cause a dose-related fulminant hepatitis. If hepatotoxicity is noted in patients taking these medications, the agent should be stopped promptly. Industrial exposure to chemicals such as carbon tetrachloride, 2-nitropropane, and trichloroethylene can cause FHF. Industrial and chemical exposures should be elicited as part of the history in evaluating patients with FHF.

Amanita mushroom poisoning is another cause of chemically induced hepatitis. Ingestion is usually followed by prolonged vomiting and diarrhea, with the development of hepatic failure 3 to 8 days after ingestion.

Miscellaneous Causes of Fulminant Hepatitis

Wilson disease usually presents with a picture of chronic liver disease but occasionally presents as FHF. It is important to recognize this entity. Patients are usually younger than age 20. Associated findings may include evidence of hemolytic anemia and renal insufficiency. Patients may have Kayser-Fleischer rings (deposits of copper in the cornea) noted on slit-lamp ophthalmologic examination. Aminotransferase elevations usually are less than ten times the upper limit of normal, in contrast to other causes of FHF.

Reye syndrome and acute fatty liver of pregnancy are the two most common causes of FHF characterized by microvesicular steatosis. Reye syndrome occurs in children, usually after an acute febrile illness such as influenza or varicella. It is usually associated with salicylate use. Patients develop malaise and irritability with vomiting. There may be subsequent improvement, or delirium and encephalopathy may develop. The physical examination is noteworthy for hepatomegaly. The transaminase level is usually elevated in the range of 500 units/L but can occasionally exceed 20,000 units/L. The bilirubin level is generally not elevated. The prothrombin time is usually prolonged within the range of 2 to 8 seconds but may be prolonged even more markedly. Hypoglycemia can be a significant problem.

Acute fatty liver of pregnancy, a condition of the third trimester, is discussed later in the section on liver diseases unique to pregnancy. It is associated with preeclampsia and is more common in nulliparous patients.

Budd-Chiari syndrome, another uncommon cause of FHF, is characterized by hepatic venous outflow obstruction. The syndrome is caused by thrombosis and occlusion of the major hepatic veins or by mass lesions of the major hepatic veins or inferior vena cava. Causes of this disorder include the conditions associated with vascular thrombosis such as polycythemia rubra vera, paroxysmal nocturnal hemoglobinuria, and other myeloproliferative disorders. Tumors such as renal cell carcinoma, hepatocellular carcinoma, Wilms tumor, and right atrial myxoma can also cause this syndrome. The use of oral contraceptives has been associated with this disorder. Budd-Chiari syndrome can occur during pregnancy but more often presents during the postpartum period. It is characterized by right upper quadrant pain, ascites, and hepatomegaly. If this disorder is suspected, hepatic vein patency should be evaluated using ultrasonography, computed tomography, or magnetic resonance imaging. Doppler analysis can be helpful in demonstrating abnormalities in the direction of flow in the hepatic veins.

Ischemia of the liver is a rare cause of FHF. It may be due to hypoperfusion from heart disease or shock, or to a tumor cell burden from hepatic metastases or lymphoproliferative malignancies.

Work-Up

Patients presenting with FHF should have hepatitis serologies for HAV, HBV, and HCV. Other viral infections should be considered, and an acetaminophen level should be ordered. A careful drug history of any prescription, over-the-counter, and herbal remedies should be obtained. Patients should be questioned specifically regarding ingestion of mushrooms and any industrial exposures. In patients less than age 20, Wilson disease should be considered and serum ceruloplasmin, serum copper, and 24-hour urinary copper excretion studies may be helpful. In a patient with associated renal insufficiency, however, it may be difficult to interpret urinary copper findings. Slit-lamp examination for Kayser-Fleischer rings can be helpful.

The degree of hepatic failure can be assessed with pH and prothrombin time. The degree of elevation of bilirubin correlates somewhat with the prognosis.

Medical Management

Consultation with a hepatologist is appropriate. The patient should be transferred to the intensive care unit of a medical center that has liver transplantation capacity. Patients should be transferred early; as soon as hepatic encephalopathy becomes evident, patients are at risk for subsequent cerebral edema. If the acetaminophen level is toxic, oral N-acetylcysteine is an effective treatment, especially if given within 8 to 10 hours after ingestion. However, it probably should be initiated as late as 36 to 72 hours after ingestion.

LIVER DISEASES UNIQUE TO PREGNANCY

Several liver diseases occur only in pregnancy (Table 62-2). Some liver function tests vary during pregnancy. Alkaline phosphatase is released from the placenta and progressively increases to twice the upper limits of normal during pregnancy. Cholesterol and triglycerides increase by two- and threefold respectively because of increased synthesis. Prothrombin time and AST and ALT levels are unchanged. Albumin is slightly decreased because of hemodilution.

Hyperemesis Gravidarum

Hyperemesis gravidarum (HG) is intractable nausea and vomiting during the first trimester. Although today it generally responds to supportive treatment, historically it was a significant cause of maternal death: in 1863, 46 deaths were reported from HG in one series.

Etiology

The etiology is unclear. A psychological etiology has been discussed but never proven. Hepatic dysfunction has been postulated as a causative factor, but liver abnormalities are not seen in all affected patients, and liver dysfunction is more likely to be a consequence rather than a cause of HG. Hyperthyroidism has been postulated, but there is little evidence to support this thesis. The hormonal changes associated with pregnancy have also been proposed as a cause of this disorder.

Clinical Presentation

HG is generally accompanied by loss of more than 5% of the prepregnancy body weight. There is associated dehydration. The incidence of this condition ranges from three to ten per 1000 pregnancies. Factors that appear to be associated with an increased risk for HG include high prepregnancy body weight, nulliparity, and twin gestation. Factors associated with a decreased risk include advanced maternal age and cigarette smoking.

Table 62-2. Causes of Increased Liver Function Tests During Pregnancy

DISEASE	SYMPTOMS	DIAGNOSTIC TEST	TIME OF ONSET	COMMENT
Viral hepatitis	Anorexia, nausea and vomiting, jaundice	Hepatitis A,B,C,D serology	Any trimester of pregnancy	Most common cause of jaundice in women of childbearing age. Herpes simplex hepatitis and hepatitis E are more often fulminant when occurring during pregnancy. Herpes simplex hepatitis responds to acyclovir therapy.
Gallstones	Right upper quadrant pain	Ultrasound of the RUQ	Any trimester of pregnancy	Medical therapy should be attempted. If surgery is required, second trimester is optimal time.
Hyperemesis gravidarum	Severe nausea and vomiting	Clinical diagnosis, exclude viral hepatitis and gallstones	First trimester	LFT abnormalities probably a consequence rather than a cause of the disease. Hepatic complications are mild; Wernicke encephalopathy can be severe and irreversible, must replete thiamine. Liver biopsy, if performed, shows central cholestasis and centrizonal vacuolization.
Intrahepatic cholestasis of pregnancy	Pruritus, jaundice	Clinical diagnosis, exclude viral hepatitis and gallstones	Classically occurs in third trimester but can occur any trimester	Second most common cause of jaundice during pregnancy. Supplemental vitamin K should be administered. Familial predilection.
HELLP syndrome	RUQ and epigastric pain, nausea, vomiting	Clinical diagnosis, hemolysis, low platelets, normal prothrombin time. Transaminases normal to >1000.	Third trimester	Patients should be considered to have severe preeclampsia and delivered promptly.
Acute fatty liver of pregnancy	RUQ and epigastric pain, nausea and vomiting, jaundice, liver failure	Clinical diagnosis, Prolonged prothrombin time, transaminases normal to >1000. May have associated DIC. Exclude other causes of fulminant hepatic failure.	Third trimester	Treatment is delivery. Intense supportive care is necessary in fulminant hepatic failure.

LFT, liver function tests; *RUQ,* right upper quadrant.

Physical Findings

Physical findings generally include orthostatic hypotension and decreased turgor of the skin, consistent with dehydration. Abdominal pain is usually absent and if present should prompt investigation of other causes of abdominal pain and vomiting, such as peptic ulcer disease. Excessive salivation (ptyalism) is frequently noted, but patients generally do not complain about it. Jaundice is sometimes noted. Hepatomegaly is sometimes evident on the physical examination.

Laboratory Studies

Laboratory findings are consistent with dehydration: significant ketonuria or ketonemia, elevated specific gravity of the urine, and increased blood urea nitrogen. An increased hematocrit associated with hemoconcentration may be seen. About 50% of patients have hepatic complications, including hyperbilirubinemia and elevated serum aminotransferase levels. Liver biopsy, if performed, may show central cholestasis and centrizonal vacuolization.

Treatment and Outcome

This disease generally responds well to supportive treatment. Intravenous fluid is the mainstay of therapy. Patients should be take nothing by mouth. In severe cases, total parenteral nutrition may be required. Rarely, termination of pregnancy may be necessary.

Adequate replacement of thiamine is important because the development of Wernicke encephalopathy has been described in this condition. Wernicke encephalopathy can be severe and irreversible.

Antiemetic drugs are another mainstay of therapy. Parenteral metoclopramide is generally effective. Caution should be used with chlorpromazine because of its tendency to cause cholestasis, especially in the presence of jaundice.

Although a psychological etiology has never been proven, a multidisciplinary approach that includes psychological support is often used.

It is unclear whether HG has any effect on the outcome of pregnancy, or whether there is an increased risk of fetal deformity.

Intrahepatic Cholestasis of Pregnancy

Intrahepatic cholestasis of pregnancy (ICP) is the second most common cause of jaundice in pregnancy, after viral hepatitis. It is responsible for about 20% of the cases of jaundice that occur during pregnancy. ICP is associated with a benign maternal outcome but paradoxically with a significant incidence of fetal injury during pregnancy.

Incidence

The incidence of this disease varies geographically. It reportedly occurs in about 1% to 3% of pregnancies in Scandinavia and 2% to 5% of those in Chile. It appears to be more common among Chileans of Indian descent than those of Caucasian descent. In other sites, the incidence is reported to be 0.003% to 0.5% of pregnancies. There appears to be a familial predilection.

Etiology

The etiology is not completely understood, but it appears to be attributable to an hepatic abnormality of estrogen metabolism. In patients predisposed to this condition, increased estrogen during pregnancy causes a cholestatic hepatitis. The role of estrogens was examined in a study in which healthy, nonpregnant women and men were given low doses of ethinyl estradiol. In patients with a past history of ICP or with a family history of ICP, this drug induced a fall in the clearance of sulfobromophthalein. The fall in clearance was significantly different in patients with a past history of ICP or in men with a family history of ICP than in matched controls. Thus, the inherent hepatic metabolic response may become stressed during pregnancy because of elevated levels of estrogens. A problem that is otherwise clinically insignificant may become evident only during periods of stress such as pregnancy, when estrogen levels become elevated. Administration of an oral contraceptive to susceptible patients may cause a similar cholestatic picture.

Clinical Presentation

This illness usually begins in the third trimester, although up to a third of patients present in the first trimester. The primary symptom is pruritus. Pruritus generally begins in the palms and soles but may extend to the legs, thighs, back, arms, breasts, and abdomen. It is sometimes followed by the development of anorexia, pain in the right upper quadrant, nausea, and vomiting. About 20% of patients develop jaundice, generally 2 to 4 weeks after the development of pruritus. Nonspecific symptoms such as malaise and anorexia may also develop, but if they are prominent complaints and if the jaundice is severe, the differential diagnosis must be extended to viral hepatitis and biliary tract disease. If symptoms occur near the end of pregnancy, acute fatty liver of pregnancy also must be considered.

The physical examination is notable for the absence of stigmata of chronic liver disease. Laboratory findings are consistent with a cholestatic picture. The total bilirubin level is usually less than 5 mg/dL. The alkaline phosphatase level is quite elevated because of the cholestatic injury as well as the normal placental production of alkaline phosphatase. The aminotransferase level is elevated two to ten times normal. Patients may have overt steatorrhea because of bile salt malabsorption. This may lead to malabsorption of fat-soluble vitamins and can lead to a prolonged prothrombin time.

HAV and HBV should be excluded, as well as biliary tract disease. If the patient has severe nausea and vomiting, anorexia, or any evidence of renal or hematologic insufficiency, other causes of jaundice must be evaluated, such as acute fatty liver of pregnancy or HELLP syndrome. The condition should resolve postpartum.

The sequelae are relatively few for the mother but may be significant for the fetus. Increased formation of cholesterol gallstones has been described in the mother, and patients are at increased risk for biliary tract disease. For the fetus, multiple problems may occur, including increased incidence of fetal wastage, stillbirth, and prematurity in up to 60% of cases. The reasons for this are unclear, but placental insufficiency due to placental permeability to maternal bile acids has been postulated. Maternal vitamin K deficiency can lead to neonatal intracranial hemorrhage. For these reasons, patients with ICP should be placed on prophylactic subcutaneous or oral vitamin K.

ICP tends to recur in subsequent pregnancies, especially in mothers who develop the icteric form of the disease. In this group, the recurrence rate is about 60% to 70%. It tends to resolve by 1 to 2 weeks postpartum. ICP is not an indication for routine induced premature delivery because it does not put the mother at increased risk for complications.

Treatment

Treatment is anecdotal. A low-fat diet and rest have been recommended. Cholestyramine has been tried because of its effectiveness in binding bile acids and estrogen, but it may cause malabsorption of fat-soluble vitamins and worsen the steatorrhea. Phenobarbital has been used to increase bile flow, but it may cause respiratory depression in the newborn. Oral ursodeoxycholic acid has been found anecdotally to alleviate pruritus and reduce serum levels of bile salts and alanine aminotransferase. However, more experience with this drug is necessary before any recommendation can be made.

Acute Fatty Liver of Pregnancy

Acute fatty liver of pregnancy (AFLP) is a rare condition characterized by fatty infiltration of the liver in the third trimester. Earlier estimates placed the incidence at one in 1 million pregnancies, but estimates now are about one in 13,000 pregnancies. This increasing frequency is most likely due to better recognition of this illness. About half the patients are primiparous, but AFLP can occur with any gestation.

Pathogenesis

The pathogenesis is unclear. Carnitine deficiency has been speculated, as has deficiency of long-chain 3-hydroxyacyl coenzyme A dehydrogenase. The latter is in the setting of a mother who is heterozygous for the disorder, with a homozygously affected fetus. AFLP may also be a manifestation of preeclampsia and eclampsia, as about half the patients who develop AFLP also have signs of this condition.

Clinical Presentation

The presentation is nonspecific. Symptoms may include fatigue, malaise, headache, or anorexia. Abdominal pain may be generalized, or it may be localized to the right upper quadrant. These symptoms may mimic biliary tract disease, acute pancreatitis, or gastroesophageal reflux. Jaundice is a relatively late finding.

On the physical examination, the patient appears ill. The liver size may be normal to small. Spider and palmar erythema may be observed, but these are normal findings during pregnancy. Neurologic findings such as confusion and asterixis may be present. Pruritus is unusual and should suggest ICP.

Laboratory Studies

Leukocytosis is common, with a white count usually exceeding 15,000 and occasionally as high as 50,000. The peripheral blood smear may demonstrate microangiopathic abnormalities such as schistocytes. Thrombocytopenia is common. There is often evidence of disseminated intravascular coagulation. Values consistent with disseminated intravascular coagulation include thrombocytopenia, microangiopathic hemolysis, coagulopathy with elevated prothrombin and activated partial thromboplastin times, reduced fibrinogen, and increased fibrin degradation products. Fibrinogen is normally elevated at the end of pregnancy, but because of consumption of fibrinogen its levels in this condition may be normal to below normal. If there is significant hepatic failure, hypoglycemia may ensue. Hyperammonemia may also occur. Liver function tests are generally only mildly elevated. Aminotransferases are in the range of 300 to 500 units (in contrast to viral hepatitis, in which transaminases usually exceed 1000). The total bilirubin level generally is less than 10.

Renal insufficiency is a common complication of AFLP. Findings include increased creatinine, blood urea nitrogen, and uric acid levels.

Diagnosis

The diagnosis is largely clinical. If a liver biopsy is performed, microvesicular fat is a pathognomonic finding, but often coagulopathy precludes this procedure. The diagnosis is often presumptive. It is important to exclude other etiologies such as a drug reaction or drug overdose, viral hepatitis, and HELLP syndrome. HELLP syndrome is not a cause of FHF, unlike AFLP. The prothrombin and activated partial thromboplastin times are normal in HELLP syndrome.

Treatment

Close fetal monitoring is necessary. Treatment is delivery of the baby. Usually there is improvement within 2 to 3 days of delivery. Treatment of the liver disease is supportive, including replacement of coagulation factors, close attention to mental status for evidence of encephalopathy, and close monitoring of serum glucose levels. If there is no improvement within 24 to 48 hours of delivery, transfer to a tertiary center that has liver transplantation capability should be considered.

Earlier reports described a 75% to 85% mortality rate, but the current mortality rate varies from 8% to 33%. This lower mortality rate is probably due to increased recognition of less severe cases of this disease, as well as better supportive care and better intensive care management. Fetal mortality varies from 14% to 66%. One case has been reported of orthotopic liver transplantation for a patient who did not improve after delivery.

HELLP Syndrome

HELLP syndrome is the liver disease associated with preeclampsia. Patients with HELLP syndrome are not always hypertensive (about 70% of patients in various series had elevated blood pressure). Consequently, many patients are often misdiagnosed as having other medical or surgical problems.

The acronym "HELLP syndrome" was coined in 1982: **H** for hemolysis, **EL** for elevated liver enzymes, and **LP** for low platelets. Hemolysis must be present (microangiopathic hemolytic anemia). Platelet counts are generally less than 100,000. Transaminases are modestly elevated to at least twice normal. LDH is above 600 mU/mL. Bilirubin is usually greater than 1.2 mg/dL.

Etiology

This syndrome is part of preeclampsia but can occur without hypertension. The cause of liver damage is unclear, but it has been suggested that fibrin deposition is the primary event. An alternate hypothesis is that segmental vasospasm occurs, leading to the hepatic injury and injury to other organs. Consequent to the vasospasm, there is initiation of platelet aggregation and fibrin deposition.

Clinical Presentation

The incidence of HELLP syndrome in preeclampsia is reportedly 2% to 12%. Patients with HELLP syndrome tend to be older and multiparous.

The patient usually complains of epigastric or right upper quadrant pain. Nausea and vomiting are common, as is a history of malaise. Patients usually have significant weight gain and generalized edema. Severe hypertension may not be present, although HELLP syndrome is though to indicate a severe form of preeclampsia.

Differential Diagnosis

The differential diagnosis includes other microangiopathic hemolytic disorders, including thrombotic thrombocytopenic purpura, and hemolytic-uremic syndrome.

Treatment

Patients with HELLP syndrome who are close to term should be considered preeclamptic and delivered promptly. This includes patients who are at or beyond 34 weeks' gestation, or if there is evidence of fetal lung maturity. Patients who are remote to term should be transferred to a tertiary care center for intensive fetal monitoring and for further assessment and stabilization of the maternal condition. Various modalities have been described to treat or reverse HELLP syndrome in patients remote from term, but none has been well studied. If the syndrome develops before 34 weeks' gestation and there is evidence of fetal or maternal jeopardy, delivery must be considered. Evaluation of fetal lung maturity is performed, with administration of steroids if there is immaturity. HELLP syndrome is not an indication for immediate delivery by cesarean section; patients who are presenting in labor can be allowed to deliver vaginally in the absence of any other obstetric contraindications.

Hepatic rupture is the most feared complication of preeclampsia and HELLP syndrome. Patients presenting in shock with evidence of ascites or pleural effusions or with shoulder pain should be evaluated by ultrasound or computed tomography of the liver to exclude subcapsular hematoma of the liver. Generally, rupture of the liver involves the right lobe. It is often preceded by the development of a hematoma. There may be several hours of severe epigastric pain that progresses to circulatory collapse. The finding of a ruptured subcapsular hematoma of the liver in a patient presenting in shock is an indication for laparotomy and aggressive blood product replacement. Even with appropriate treatment, mortality is over 50% for the mother and the fetus. If the hematoma has not ruptured and the patient is not hypotensive, this complication can be managed conservatively with close monitoring and visualization with serial computed tomography scans or ultrasound.

BIBLIOGRAPHY

Abell TL, Riely C. Hyperemesis gravidarum. In: Abell TL, Riely C, eds. Gastroenterology clinics of North America: gastrointestinal and liver problems in pregnancy. Philadelphia: WB Saunders, 1992.

Barton J, Sibai B. Care of the pregnancy complicated by HELLP syndrome. In: Abell TL, Riely C, eds. Gastroenterology clinics of North America: gastrointestinal and liver problems in pregnancy. Philadelphia: WB Saunders, 1992.

Bass N. An integrated approach to the diagnosis of jaundice. In: Kaplowitz N, ed. Liver and biliary diseases. Baltimore: Williams & Wilkins, 1992.

Douglas D, Rakela J. Fulminant hepatitis. In: Kaplowitz N, ed. Liver and biliary diseases. Baltimore: Williams & Wilkins, 1992.

Fagiuoli S, Wacker T, Ruthardt F, Van Thiel D. The liver and pregnancy. In: Karlstadt R, Surawicz C, Croitoru R, eds. Gastrointestinal disorders during pregnancy. Monograph, American College of Gastroenterology.

Mabie W. Acute fatty liver of pregnancy. In: Abell TL, Riely C, eds. Gastroenterology clinics of North America: gastrointestinal and liver problems in pregnancy. Philadelphia: WB Saunders, 1992.

Malet P. Complications of cholelithiasis. In: Kaplowitz N, ed. Liver and biliary diseases. Baltimore: Williams & Wilkins, 1992.

Mishra L, Seeff L. Viral hepatitis, A–E, complicating pregnancy. In: Abell TL, Riely C, eds. Gastroenterology clinics of North America: gastrointestinal and liver problems in pregnancy. Philadelphia: WB Saunders, 1992.

Reyes H. The spectrum of liver and gastrointestinal disease seen in cholestasis of pregnancy. In: Abell TL, Riely C, eds. Gastroenterology clinics of North America: gastrointestinal and liver problems in pregnancy. Philadelphia: WB Saunders, 1992.

Riely C. Liver diseases of pregnancy. In: Kaplowitz N, ed. Liver and biliary diseases. Baltimore: Williams & Wilkins, 1992.

Seeff LB. Acute viral hepatitis In: Kaplowitz N, ed. Liver and biliary diseases. Baltimore: Williams & Wilkins, 1992.

Primary Care for Women, edited by Phyllis C. Leppert and Fred M. Howard. Lippincott-Raven Publishers, Philadelphia © 1997.

63
Chronic Liver Disease

BETH SCHORR-LESNICK

Chronic liver disease is a diagnostic and management challenge for the primary care physician, especially since many patients are appearing for examination in an early, asymptomatic stage, their condition revealed only by minor abnormalities in screening liver function tests. Although specialty consultation should be obtained in the care of these patients at the onset, and also if complications of therapy or advanced disease arise, it is the primary care physician who provides long-term care and follow-up.

This chapter educates the practitioner about chronic liver diseases in general, with emphasis on diseases that are more prevalent in women, such as primary biliary cirrhosis and autoimmune hepatitis. It also discusses unique considerations in caring for pregnant patients with liver disease.

PRIMARY BILIARY CIRRHOSIS

Primary biliary cirrhosis is a chronic, progressive, immune-mediated cholestatic liver disease that results in the granulomatous inflammation and obliteration of the small and medium-sized intrahepatic bile ducts. It leads ultimately to fibrosis, cirrhosis, and liver failure. It occurs primarily in women between 40 and 50 years of age.

Etiology and Diagnosis

Patients may be recognized when asymptomatic, solely on the basis of an elevated alkaline phosphatase or hepatomegaly. Or, they may appear for treatment with insidious symptoms of fatigue and pruritus, followed by jaundice and hyperpigmentation of the skin, gastrointestinal bleeding, encephalopathy, or ascites. Nineteen percent present with hepatic decompensation. Ninety-five percent of patients have antimitochondrial antibodies (AMAs), a pathognomonic feature, usually greater than 1 : 40. These features, plus characteristic findings on liver biopsy, confirm the diagnosis. Xanthomatosis with hyperlipidemia, steatorrhea, hypergammaglobulinemia, osteoporosis, and thyroid dysfunction also may be seen. Surprisingly, there is no increased risk of death due to atherosclerosis.

Five percent of patients may have associated autoimmune disorders, pointing to an autoimmune etiology for the disease. These patients have a poor prognosis. Other features of prognostic significance include albumin, bilirubin, age of the patient, prothrombin time, hepatomegaly, and hepatic histologic features. The life span of the asymptomatic patient approaches that of the normal population. At the onset of symptoms, an average life span of 10 to 12 years can be predicted. The differential diagnosis includes common bile duct obstruction, primary sclerosing cholangitis, and autoimmune hepatitis.

Treatment

The management of the asymptomatic patient involves periodic liver function tests and monitoring for symptoms. Cholestyramine (8 g given two to four times daily), ursodeoxycholic acid, antihistamines, rifampin, metronidazole (Flagyl), or opioid antagonists may be useful for treating pruritus. Parenteral vitamins A, D, and K may reverse malabsorption. A calcium supplement of 800 to 1000 mg daily and vitamin D may be used to treat the associated hepatic osteodystrophy. Medium chain triglycerides may be helpful for steatorrhea.

Medical therapy for the underlying disorder generally has been problematic. Biochemical, clinical, and histologic improvements have been obtained with ursodeoxycholic acid (13 to 15 mg/kg/day and ranging from 600 to 1800 mg/day) in precirrhotic patients with virtually no toxicity. It is unclear if ursodeoxycholic acid has any effect on survival. And, unfortunately, some treated patients still progress to cirrhosis and its complications.

Primary biliary cirrhosis is the second most common indication in the United States for liver transplant. Patients should be referred for evaluation when their disease becomes progressive and refractory. The 5-year actuarial rate for survival after transplant is 70%. AMAs usually persist after transplantation. Recurrence of the disease in the new liver may occur. The patients who benefit the most from liver transplantation are those with a more favorable prognosis at the time of referral for transplantation. For this reason, long delays before referral are ill advised.

CHRONIC HEPATITIS (GENERAL)

Chronic hepatitis is defined by the persistence of abnormal liver test results for at least 6 months. Evaluation, management, and treatment of patients with chronic inflammation of the liver is an important task for the practitioner.

Etiology

Multiple causes of chronic hepatitis exist, but a specific cause can be found only in 10% to 20% of patients. Other than alcohol abuse, chronic viral infection is the major cause of chronic hepatitis. Hepatitis B and C are frequent causes and may result in cirrhosis. Autoimmune processes, which may be an ongoing reaction to the continued use of a therapeutic drug, and Wilson disease also should be considered.

Diagnosis

Primary biliary cirrhosis, primary sclerosing cholangitis, and nonalcoholic steatohepatitis all may mimic chronic hepatitis. Primary hemochromatosis and alpha$_1$-antitrypsin deficiency, although rare, also may resemble chronic hepatitis. A careful search for the specific cause of chronic hepatitis is critical because the natural history, prognosis, and treatment is dependent on the cause. Advances in diagnosis and the availability of effective therapy for many patients has heightened interest in these disorders. The etiology of chronic liver disease usually can be determined by clinical history, physical examination, and serologic tests for disease markers. Liver biopsy is used primarily to exclude granulomatous disease and to determine the presence, severity, and type of histologic injury for prognostic and therapeutic purposes.

AUTOIMMUNE CHRONIC ACTIVE HEPATITIS

Autoimmune hepatitis is a chronic, progressive, inflammatory disorder of the liver of unknown etiology that occurs predominantly in women. It is gratifying to the clinician to identify because the patient often responds considerably to immunosuppressive therapy. If untreated, it is an invariably fatal disease with a mortality rate of 90% in 10 years.

Diagnosis

Although many patients are diagnosed while asymptomatic, patients may complain of anorexia, malaise, arthralgia, myalgia, hirsutism, striae, acne, and, in young women, amenorrhea. In addition, associated autoimmune disorders are seen. Physical findings are nonspecific.

Laboratory Studies

Laboratory findings in autoimmune chronic active hepatitis (AICAH) include hyperglobulinemia, especially IgG higher than twice normal; antinuclear antibodies more than 1 : 40 in a homogeneous pattern; anti–smooth muscle antibody IgM more than 1 : 80; elevated aspartate aminotransferase greater than ten times normal; and alanine aminotransferase (ALT) more than five times normal. AMAs of more than 1 : 40 may be found in 10% to 30% of patients, but the differentiation of AICAH from primary biliary cirrhosis is rarely a clinically important problem. It has been postulated that an environmental factor, possibly viral in etiology, is required to trigger the disorder in genetically susceptible individuals. The demonstration of hepatitis C virus (HCV) antibodies in patients with autoimmune hepatitis suggests a possible etiologic agent.

Diagnosis

Differentiating AICAH from hepatitis C may be difficult, but diagnostic guidelines are elucidated in Table 63-1. Autoimmune hepatitis has been classified into several subgroups. These groups are described in Table 63-2.

Table 63-1. Differentiation Between Autoimmune Hepatitis and Hepatitis C

FEATURES	AUTOIMMUNE HEPATITIS	HEPATITIS C
Age	Young, middle aged	All
Sex	Female	Male and Female
Symptoms	Jaundice, fatigue	None
Association with autoimmune diseases	+	–
Transaminase levels	> 10 × NL	< 10 × NL
Contact with blood	–	+
Histologic findings	Plasma cell infiltrate, rosetting	Portal lymphoid aggregates, bile duct damage and loss, steatosis
Response to steroids	+	–

Treatment

Patients with type 2a disease who do not respond to steroids progress rapidly to cirrhosis and may require transplantation. Interferon therapy in these patients may result in an exacerbation of their disease. Type 2b disease probably represents true hepatitis C with secondary autoimmune phenomena. It responds to interferon. Studies suggest that type 3 is an unusual variant of type 1 disease rather than a unique independent subtype. Patients with cryptogenic chronic hepatitis actually may have autoimmune disease that has escaped detection by standard testing.

The treatment of choice for autoimmune hepatitis is prednisone, with or without azathioprine as a steroid-sparing agent. Therapy prolongs life, improves symptoms and blood chemistries, and decreases inflammation seen on biopsy. However, there is less evidence that progression to cirrhosis is slowed or prevented. The remission rate induced by initial therapy is 60% to 80%. A steroid response is demonstrated by a decrease in transaminase levels, bilirubin, and globulin levels and by improved clinical status of the patient within 1 to 3 months of treatment. Therapy should be continued for at least 1 to 2 years. Relapse occurs commonly after discontinuation of therapy, requiring repeated treatment or long-term maintenance therapy for most patients. Relapses may occur despite improvement in histologic features. Patients whose initial biopsy specimens show evidence of cirrhosis are more likely to relapse, and they have markedly decreased survival rates. Patients most likely to respond are those with active hepatitis, markedly elevated gamma globulins, and marked histologic inflammation. Histologic changes lag behind biochemical changes and titers of autoantibodies do not correlate with disease activity, making it difficult to use these parameters as indicators of response. HLA type may predict nonresponse to treatment. The longer it takes to obtain a remission, the less likely it is that lasting improvement will occur. Asymptomatic patients with mild histologic changes may simply be observed without therapy by monitoring progression of histologic changes on subsequent liver biopsy specimens. Initial treatment with a 20- to 60-mg dose of prednisone daily may be begun in all patients, with or without cirrhosis or fibrosis, who show severe histologic inflammatory changes. Alternatively, 50 mg of azathioprine per day may be given continuously *with* 30 mg of prednisone per day to achieve remission, with the prednisone dose tapered to 10 mg per day over 1 month once a response is seen. Maintenance therapy may be solely on prednisone or on 5 to 10 mg/day of prednisone and 50 to 150 mg (1 mg/kg/day) of azathioprine. If azathioprine maintenance alone is desired, 2 mg/kg body weight is required. Patients on long-term low-dose azathioprine should be monitored for thrombocytopenia and marrow suppression. These patients do not appear to have an increased frequency of lymphoma and other malignancies.

Despite therapy, however, progression to cirrhosis and its complications may occur. Surprisingly, hepatocellular carcinoma is

Table 63-2. Classification of Autoimmune Hepatitis

TYPE	HYPERGLOBULINEMIA	SEX	ANA	ASMA	ANTI-LKM1	ANTI-SLA	HCV AB	STEROID RESPONSE	INTERFERON RESPONSE
1 (classic)	+	F	+	+	–	–	–*	+	–
2a	–	F	–	–	+	–	–	+	–
2b	–	M	low titer	low titer	low titer	–	+	–	+†
3	+	F	–	–	–	+	–	+	–
Cryptogenic	+	F	–	–	–	–	–	+	–

ANA, antinuclear antibodies; *ASMA,* anti–smooth muscle antibody; *anti-LKM1,* anti–liver-kidney microsomal antibody; *anti-SLA,* anti-soluble liver antigen; *M,* male; *F,* female; *HCV* ab, hepatitis C antibody.

*False-positive results may occur.

†Approach with caution, perhaps only after failure of steroids.

rare in these patients. Patients who experience treatment failures are candidates for orthotopic liver transplantation. Recurrence is rare, and the 5-year survival rate after transplantation is 92%.

DRUG-INDUCED CHRONIC LIVER DISEASE

Etiology

Several therapeutic drugs are known to have potential for causing chronic active hepatitis (CAH). The liver disease may continue as long as the drug therapy is continued. Often improvement occurs after withdrawal of the suspected etiologic agent. Implicated drugs tend to be those that have been taken for prolonged periods. Most cases are in women.

Oxyphenisatin and nitrofurantoin have been implicated as causative agents in CAH, and symptoms resemble those seen in patients with AICAH. Methyldopa, once a commonly used antihypertensive, may cause severe hepatitis progressing to cirrhosis. Isoniazid and halothane also produce an illness that histologically resembles CAH.

Diagnosis

An eosinophilic infiltrate on liver biopsy specimen is helpful in suggesting a diagnosis, but one is not often found. Improvement may take days to weeks after drug withdrawal.

VIRAL HEPATITIS

General

Forty years ago, the predominant etiology for chronic hepatitis was thought to be autoimmune disorder. With the advent of serologic testing for hepatitis B and C, approximately 70% of all cases of chronic hepatitis have been identified as viral in origin. As more about the pathogenesis of these viruses is discovered, therapies are being developed to improve the treatment outcome of chronic viral hepatitis in certain patients.

Chronic alcohol abusers are predisposed to viral hepatitis, especially hepatitis C, potentiated by their life-style and perhaps by other unknown factors. Alcohol also appears to exacerbate persistent viral hepatitis. Conversely, concomitant viral infection may accelerate the progression of alcoholic liver disease (ALD). Patients with chronic hepatitis B or C should be told to markedly reduce their intake of alcohol.

Chronic Hepatitis B

Hepatitis B virus (HBV) is the most common cause of chronic hepatitis in Africa, Asia, the Middle East, and the Far East. It is the most common worldwide cause of viral-induced liver disease, producing around 300 million carriers.

Etiology

Transmission comprises perinatal, sexual, and parenteral routes.

Laboratory Studies

Hepatitis B is easily detected by assays for hepatitis B surface antigen (HBsAg), hepatitis B e antigen (HBeAg), or for HBV-DNA.

Diagnosis

Patients who progress to chronic hepatitis B are often those who have had a clinically silent acute infection. Generally, they are asymptomatic and have only elevated transaminase levels. These patients are susceptible to cirrhosis and its complications and, ultimately, to hepatocellular carcinoma, despite the seemingly clinical benign nature of their disease, making therapy desirable when appropriate. In others, hepatitis B may appear as acute hepatitis and may continue to destroy the liver. Immunosuppression and acquisition of the virus in the perinatal period or in childhood appears to increase the likelihood for progression to chronicity. Hepatitis B progresses to chronic infection in 2% to 5% of cases.

Prevention

Transmission can be prevented by screening and vaccination of high-risk groups, including male homosexuals, intravenous drug users, health care workers, immunosuppressed patients, persons from endemic areas, and household contacts and sexual partners of known HBsAg-positive persons. Universal testing for HBeAg of all pregnant women near delivery, as well as universal HBV vaccination of infants and children, has significantly decreased the risk of chronic hepatitis B. The height of transaminase levels correlates with the extent of active hepatic inflammation. A poor prognosis is suggested by a high and rising serum bilirubin level. Successful treatment with interferon, an antiviral and immunomodulatory agent, causes a flare-up of clinical hepatitis with activation of the immune system against the virus. Chronic hepatitis B develops when the host is unable to effectively eradicate the virus and rid the liver of all infected cells.

Treatment

Candidates for treatment with interferon are patients with hepatitis B whose transaminase levels are at least one and a half times normal (preferably greater than two to three times normal), patients who are HBeAg or HBV-DNA positive, and those with active inflammation found on liver biopsy. Contraindications to therapy include cytopenia, decompensated liver function due to cirrhosis, history of depression, autoimmune disorders, and advanced human immunodeficiency virus (HIV) infection.

The optimal dosing regimen for interferon is 5 million U given subcutaneously daily for 16 weeks. The goal of therapy is to halt viral replication, reduce infectivity, diminish inflammation, improve symptoms, and reduce the risk of hepatocellular carcinoma.

Measures of therapeutic success are an initial increase in transaminase levels within a few weeks to a few months, loss of HBeAg and HBV-DNA, and reduction in aminotransferase levels, which correlates well with histologic findings. HBsAg disappears in up to 30% of treated patients within months to years after successful therapy.

Response rates are 40% to 50%, and responses are usually lasting. Adults with low pretreatment HBV-DNA levels (< 200 pg/mL) and ALT over 100 U/L with active inflammation seen on liver biopsy are most likely to respond. The relapse rate is low at 10% to 15%, but these relapses occur within the first year.

Side effects of therapy include the following: (1) dose-related flu-like symptoms, which generally appear early, are self-limited, respond to acetaminophen, and rarely require dose adjustments; (2) neutropenia and thrombocytopenia requiring dose reduction; (3) depression and mood swings; (4) thyroid problems; and (5) exacerbation of underlying autoimmune processes. Thus, monitoring tests include complete blood cell count, platelet count, thyroid function tests, antinuclear antibodies, anti–smooth muscle antibodies, AMAs, transaminase levels, and hepatitis serologic studies.

Due to the tendency for reinfection in the transplanted liver, transplantation because of failure of medical therapy is not an option.

Chronic Hepatitis C

Hepatitis C virus is the most frequent cause of chronic hepatitis in the United States, Western Europe, and Japan and is the leading cause of hepatocellular carcinoma.

Etiology

Although the parenteral route of transmission has been established, the role of the sexual and perinatal route are not as clear. Forty percent to 50% of patients have no clearly defined source. Studies reveal that 70% of persons with a history of *any* intravenous drug abuse are infected with HCV, and over 80% of parenteral drug users have serologic evidence of past infection with hepatitis B or C. Although around 80% to 90% of cases of transfusion-associated hepatitis are due to hepatitis C, only 5% to 15% of hepatitis C cases have had a blood transfusion. Therefore, screening blood for transfusion has had little overall impact on the rate of HCV infection.

Diagnosis and Laboratory Tests

HCV may be recognized within 1 to 6 months of acute infection by an improved enzyme-linked immunosorbent assay for antibodies to the virus. A supplemental recombinant immunoblot assay is used for confirmation. Ribonucleic acid (RNA) testing for HCV is available as well. It may prove useful in the evaluation of acute and chronic hepatitis for predicting and assessing the effects of therapy. The presence of antibody does not confer protection, and any patient possessing the antibody should be considered to have a transmissible, possibly injurious, living virus.

Although most patients are asymptomatic, with incidental increases in transaminase levels noted on screening for blood transfusions or insurance examinations, some patients do have chronic fatigue and tender hepatomegaly. This diagnosis ought to be considered in the workup of a patient with chronic fatigue. One hundred fifty thousand cases of acute HCV infection occur each year in the United States. Chronicity occurs in 50% to 75% of cases, and 20% to 50% of these develop cirrhosis within 10 years of infection. Advancement in age and an asymptomatic acute infection are risk factors for progression to chronicity and cirrhosis. Occasionally, the diagnosis of chronic hepatitis C is made only after the appearance of hepatocellular carcinoma since symptoms sometimes do not appear until late in the course of the disease. One study shows a 10-year lag to the diagnosis of chronic hepatitis from the date of transfusion, 21 years to cirrhosis, and 29 years to hepatocellular carcinoma.

Diagnosis is made on the basis of raised transaminase levels and antibody to HCV, and is confirmed by recombinant immunoblot assay or quantitative HCV RNA. In addition, patients with any elevation in liver test results, hepatomegaly, or other signs of liver disease also should be screened for HCV. Unlike hepatitis B, the height of the transaminase levels is poorly correlated to the degree of histologic damage and the transaminase levels may fluctuate widely, even approaching normal values, throughout the course of the illness. The peak ALT is usually between 400 and 800 IU.

Treatment

Treatment is indicated in patients with transaminase levels more than one and a half times normal. In hepatitis C, transaminase levels fluctuate widely and may even normalize for a time, despite ongoing hepatic inflammation, histologic inflammation, and HCV RNA. Decisions about initiating treatment should be weighed against the relatively slow progression of the disease, the mild disease presence in some patients, the possible side effects, the cost of interferon, and any contraindications. The same is true of hepatitis B. Asymptomatic patients with HCV antibody, normal aminotransferase levels, and mild hepatic inflammation are not candidates for therapy. The extent of histologic injury alone, however, is not well correlated with therapeutic success.

Standard treatment of chronic hepatitis C is with 3 million U of interferon given subcutaneously three times per week for 24 weeks. The lower doses employed for hepatitis C, compared with hepatitis B, are associated with a lower incidence of side effects. HCV antibody disappears in less than half of cases with therapy, and no panel of markers is available to follow for HCV, as there is for HBV. Therefore, the therapeutic endpoints are normal transaminase levels and negative HCV RNA, usually within 12 weeks, and improved histologic features on liver biopsy. A rise in the transaminase levels, as seen with successful therapy of hepatitis B, should not occur.

The response rate to interferon in the successful treatment of chronic hepatitis C is about 40%. However, at least half of these patients relapse. Improved response rates may be seen with prolonged duration of therapy. HCV RNA levels are inversely related to the likelihood of therapeutic success. A test for these levels is available commercially. Despite the modest overall cure rate for hepatitis C, it is still useful to attempt therapy to prevent cirrhosis and reduce the risk of hepatocellular carcinoma.

Liver transplantation has been fairly successful in hepatitis C. Although reinfection of the graft can occur, the disease progresses more slowly than with hepatitis B and is often clinically insignificant.

NONALCOHOLIC STEATOHEPATITIS

Nonalcoholic steatohepatitis is a fatty, inflammatory condition of the liver, usually seen in obese women with persistently elevated transaminase levels. It is usually accompanied by hyperlipidemia or diabetes and is generally asymptomatic. Although this is usually a benign, reversible condition, some patients progress to cirrhosis. The best approach to therapy is to encourage weight loss, use lipid-lowering therapy, and control hyperglycemia.

ALCOHOL-INDUCED LIVER DISEASE

Preventive medicine is most important in ALD. The generalist is in an excellent position for early diagnosis, at a time when abstinence may allow complete healing. Abstinence at the time of cirrhosis does not necessarily cause the disease to regress, but may retard its progression.

Etiology

Approximately 5% of adults in the United States are chronic alcoholics. Twenty percent of them develop some form of liver disease, with 10% progressing to cirrhosis. This makes alcoholism the most common cause of liver disease in our society. Critical factors in the development of cirrhosis are the daily amount of alcohol consumed and the duration of consumption, rather than the type of beverage consumed. Daily ingestion of at least 6 cans of beer, 6 ounces of whiskey, or a quart of wine for at least 5 to 10 years may lead to cirrhosis.

Women are more susceptible than men to alcohol-induced liver disease with more modest levels of intake. Therefore, the clinician must have a higher index of suspicion for making this diagnosis in women.

Diagnosis

Frequent findings associated with chronic liver disease include the following: jaundice, palmar erythema, spider angiomas, parotid and lacrimal gland enlargement, clubbing of the fingers, splenomegaly, muscle wasting, Dupuytren contracture, ascites with or without peripheral edema, female escutcheon, gynecomastia, and testicular atrophy in men.

Laboratory Studies

Patients with ALD often have asymptomatic hepatomegaly and mild elevation of liver function tests. Aspartate aminotransferase often is more than twice the alanine aminotransferase. An elevated alkaline phosphatase, gamma glutamyl transferase, and an elevated mean corpuscular value also may be seen. These features are particularly helpful in identifying the occasional patient who denies alcohol intake on an initial interview. The findings may help direct further questioning in that area.

Chronic alcohol abusers display a variety of patterns of liver injury. The most common are steatohepatitis (or fatty liver), alcoholic hepatitis, and alcohol-induced cirrhosis. Patients with alcoholic cirrhosis are at increased risk for hepatocellular carcinoma. Chronic alcoholics seem to have an increased prevalence of both hepatitis B and C. The clinical significance of this is not known.

CIRRHOSIS

Etiology

Known etiologies of cirrhosis include the following: alcohol, viral, biliary obstruction, drugs, and inherited conditions, such as Wilson disease, hemochromatosis, and alpha$_1$-antitrypsin deficiency.

Diagnosis

The term *cirrhosis* indicates a pathologic diagnosis reflecting irreversible chronic injury and distortion of the hepatic parenchyma, including extensive fibrosis associated with the formation of regenerative nodules. This process is the final common pathway of many types of chronic liver injury. In more advanced disease, fibrosis and distorted vasculature cause portal hypertension, gastroesophageal varices, splenomegaly, ascites, and encephalopathy. The liver is usually shrunken, stigmata of chronic liver disease are often present, and the transaminase levels may be normal. Hypoalbuminemia and an elevated prothrombin time are common. Jaundice, edema, and metabolic abnormalities may be seen. In addition to expectant care of patients with asymptomatic cirrhosis and specific therapy directed at the underlying condition when appropriate, management of patients with cirrhosis is directed at the prevention and therapy of its complications. The principles of management are outlined in the following sections.

Hepatic Encephalopathy

Hepatic encephalopathy is a complex neuropsychiatric syndrome that complicates both acute and chronic liver disease and leads ultimately to impaired consciousness or coma. It is often caused by potentially reversible metabolic abnormalities. It is characterized predominantly by augmented neural inhibition, reflecting direct or indirect central nervous system exposure to substances poorly cleared by the damaged liver. Precipitating factors are excess dietary protein, upper gastrointestinal bleeding, constipation, dehydration (due to overdiuresis), hypoxia, anemia, shock, sedatives or hypnotics, azotemia, infection, and electrolyte abnormalities, particularly metabolic alkalosis.

Clinical Features

Clinical features include the following: disturbance of consciousness; impaired intellectual function; neuromuscular abnormalities, especially asterixis or a flapping tremor; electroencephalographic changes (slow waves); abnormalities in psychometric testing (number connection, five-pointed star, serial 7s); and fetor hepaticus (fruity odor to the breath).

Laboratory Tests

Laboratory tests are of moderate significance. Uremia and hypoglycemia should be ruled out, as well as precipitating factors such as hypokalemia and metabolic alkalosis. Abnormal liver tests and coagulation parameters reflect the underlying liver disease. Arterial plasma ammonia levels are increased in most patients with this syndrome, although they are nonspecific and correlate poorly with the stage of encephalopathy.

Treatment

Principles in treatment of hepatic encephalopathy are as follows: (1) correction or removal of precipitating factors; (2) reduction of absorption of nitrogenous substances from the intestinal tract; (3) reduction of increased portal systemic shunting of blood; and (4) reversal of contributing neuropathophysiologic events with drugs acting directly on the brain.

To minimize absorption of nitrogenous substances, protein restriction should be enforced with a 40 g vegetable protein diet. This high fiber diet eliminates nitrogenous wastes. The fiber also decreases transit time, reduces intraluminal pH, and increases fecal ammonia excretion.

Other modes of increasing nitrogen elimination include giving lactulose, neomycin, and metronidazole. Lactulose, given in a dose of 30 to 120 mL/day (titrated to two to four loose bowel movements per day) or as an enema, acidifies the gut to decrease ammonia absorption. It functions as a cathartic, decreasing intestinal transit time and decreasing the production and absorption of gamma-aminobutyric acid (GABA). Side effects include dehydration, hypernatremia, and nausea due to its hyperosmolarity and sweet taste. Patients must be well hydrated and have electrolytes checked frequently. Neomycin, given in an oral dose of 1 to 2 g four times a day, or metronidazole, 250 mg three to four times a day, should decontaminate the gut and decrease the production of ammonia from proteins and amino acids from urease-containing enteric bacteria. Neomycin also reduces production and absorption of GABA. It may, however, be ototoxic or nephrotoxic. Use of metronidazole may be limited because peripheral neuropathy may be a side effect. Zinc acetate in an oral dose of 600 mg/day may improve the activity of urea cycle enzymes and correct the zinc deficiency seen in alcoholics. The use of branched chain amino acids is controversial and not recommended as standard therapy.

Flumazenil, a benzodiazepine antagonist, reverses the neuropathophysiologic events contributing to encephalopathy by competing for binding to the benzodiazepine receptor. It rapidly and completely reverses the sedative and other neurologic effects of benzodiazepine receptor agonists, such as diazepam. Its benefit is transient, but it may be useful in differentiating hepatic encephalopathy from other encephalopathies. A positive response to treatment may indicate a potentially reversible encephalopathy and a more favorable prognosis, suggesting the need for more aggressive treatment of underlying liver failure. As such, the drug may provide a bridge to liver transplantation.

Ascites

Ascites, the accumulation of excessive fluid in the peritoneal cavity, is another complication of advanced cirrhosis and portal hypertension. Symptoms are increased portal pressure, hypoalbuminemia, and excessive retention of sodium and water. The spontaneous development of ascites in cirrhosis implies decompensated liver function and a significantly worse prognosis.

Clinical Features

Clinical features of ascites in include increasing abdominal girth with eventual shortness of breath due to elevation of the diaphragm. On physical examination, distention, periumbilical tympany, shifting dullness, or a fluid wave may be demonstrated when more than 1 L of fluid is present. Smaller amounts may be detected by pelvic ultrasound. With large accumulations of fluid, an everted umbilicus may occur.

Diagnosis

Diagnostic paracentesis is essential to confirm the cirrhotic etiology and exclude other causes or complications. Typical cirrhotic ascites is transudative. The most helpful indices are the cell count, cultures, and the protein and albumin. A polymorphonuclear count of more than 250 cells/μL suggests spontaneous bacterial peritonitis, and an ascitic fluid protein of less than 1 g/dL implies a predisposition to spontaneous bacterial peritonitis. The serum-to-ascites albumin gradient is used to distinguish between ascites due to portal hypertension and ascites due to other causes. Tuberculous peritonitis produces a mononuclear leukocytosis. Acid-fast bacillus stain, culture, or peritoneal biopsy help to confirm this diagnosis. Cytologic examination may aid in the diagnosis of peritoneal tumors.

Treatment

Standard therapy for portal hypertensive ascites is bedrest and 2 g sodium restriction, which is effective in 10% of patients, and diuretic therapy in the nonresponders. Fluid restriction should be employed only if the serum sodium is less than 125 mEq/L. Daily weights, fluid input and output, and urine and serum electrolytes must be obtained to monitor the effectiveness and possible complications of therapy. Complications of therapy may include electrolyte abnormalities, prerenal azotemia, hepatic encephalopathy, hepatorenal syndrome, and muscle cramps and gynecomastia due to spironolactone (Aldactone).

Initially, spironolactone in a dose of 100 mg/day is begun with or without 40 mg of furosemide (Lasix). Furosemide is added at the onset for a more rapid diuresis or if the urine sodium is low. The spironolactone is increased by 100 mg/day and the furosemide by 40 mg/day every 4 days if there is no treatment-induced complication and if weight loss is less than 0.45 kg (1 lb) each day. If the patient has peripheral edema, 0.9 to 1.35 kg (2 to 3 lb) each day can be diuresed. The goal is to achieve an increase in the urine sodium and ultimately to maintain patients with minimal or no ascites. If 400 g of spironolactone and 160 mg of furosemide per day is approached without adequate weight loss, the ascites is refractory. This occurs in about 4% of cases.

Large-volume paracentesis of 4 to 6 L/day should be employed in patients with refractory ascites, respiratory compromise, and impending rupture of an umbilical hernia due to tense ascites. It may also be used intermittently in nonazotemic patients and in those with peripheral edema. A plasma expander, such as salt-poor albumin, dextran 70, or hetastarch, also should be given for any paracenteses of more than 5 L and for patients without pedal edema. In these cases, 6 to 8 g of salt-poor albumin should be given per liter removed. Large-volume paracentesis shortens the hospital stay considerably but must be repeated periodically. Maintenance diuretics and a low sodium diet should be employed after the elimination of ascites by paracentesis to avoid reaccummulation.

Patients with refractory ascites may benefit from peritoneovenous shunts (Denver or LeVeen shunt). However, the usefulness of this technique is limited by a high complication rate. Portacaval shunts or transjugular intrahepatic portosystemic shunts may reduce ascites by lowering portal pressure and decreasing extravasation of fluid, but the reduction of hepatic blood flow is accompanied by hepatic encephalopathy in a significant number of patients.

Liver transplantation improves the overall 3- to 5-year survival rate of patients to 70% and should be considered in otherwise good candidates when they spontaneously develop ascites.

Esophagogastric Varices

Another sequela of portal hypertension is the development of portosystemic collateral circulation to bypass the high-pressure area in the liver. Major sites of collateral flow involve the veins around the gastroesophageal junction, the rectum, and the falciform ligament of the liver. Complications at these sites may include esophagogastric varices, hemorrhoids, or the development of caput medusae, respectively.

Bleeding from varices occurs in 30% of patients with cirrhosis and carries an immediate mortality rate of 50% to 60%. The bleeding is usually painless and massive, occurring generally in a patient with known chronic liver disease, a history of alcoholism or prior viral hepatitis, and often with stigmata of chronic liver disease or a coagulopathy.

Treatment

Initial therapy should always be fluid replacement and replacement of blood and blood products. Endoscopy is valuable once the patient is hemodynamically stable to identify varices as the source of the bleeding. Most commonly, injection sclerotherapy or, more recently, variceal ligation has been employed to halt acute bleeding and is successful in up to 90% of cases. Subsequent treatments fully eradicate the varices and prevent recurrent bleeding.

Along with therapeutic endoscopy, intravenous vasopressin and nitroglycerin or somatostatin may be of benefit in controlling acute bleeding. If unsuccessful, balloon tamponade may be attempted. Prophylactic sclerosis of nonbleeding varices is not indicated. Beta-adrenergic blocking agents, in a dose sufficient to reduce heart rate by 25%, although of no value in acute bleeding, may be of benefit prophylactically against first bleeding. Their usefulness in preventing recurrence of bleeding is unclear. If bleeding still recurs, portosystemic shunting may be successful. The major adverse effects of this procedure are hepatic encephalopathy and worsening hepatic function. The severity of liver disease before surgery is the most important prognostic indicator. The transjugular intrahepatic portosystemic shunt is attractive because it avoids surgery and may be an effective bridge to transplantation.

TRANSPLANTATION

A complete discussion of hepatic transplantation is beyond the scope of this chapter. However, for the primary care physician, the most essential information is to recognize the indications and contraindications for such a procedure as well as the timing, in order to know when to refer the patient. Most patients referred for transplantation have cirrhosis or fulminant hepatitis with little likelihood of spontaneous recovery and with progressive, irreversible liver injury.

The most common indications for liver transplantation in patients with chronic liver disease include refractory autoimmune hepatitis; chronic hepatitis C; drug-induced hepatitis; alcoholic cirrhosis, if the patient has become abstinent; alpha$_1$-antitrypsin deficiency; Wilson disease; primary biliary cirrhosis; sclerosing cholangitis; and vascular and metabolic disorders.

In patients with progressive, irreversible liver injury (due to the causes discussed earlier), variceal hemorrhage, uncontrolled ascites, spontaneous bacterial peritonitis, hepatic encephalopathy, hepatorenal syndrome, persistent coagulopathy with prothrombin time greater than 16 seconds, hepatic osteodystrophy, disabling fatigue, malnutrition, worsening jaundice, and recurrent cholangitis, prompt referral to a transplant center is necessary. Contraindications include most metastatic malignancies; HIV-positive serologic findings; active substance abuse within the last 6 months; uncontrolled extrahepatic sepsis; severe cardiac or pulmonary disease; and chronic hepatitis B, because it inevitably recurs.

CONSIDERATIONS IN PREGNANCY

The pregnant woman with chronic liver disease is a challenge to the clinician. Fortunately, the number of patients in this group is small. Pregnancy rarely occurs in patients with severe chronic liver disease because of diminished libido, diminished fertility, and early menopause. However, these patients, although less fertile, are often less vigilant about contraception because of irregular or infrequent menses, or because of misguided advice from their obstetrician-gynecologist or primary care physician to discontinue contraception, thereby enabling some of them to conceive. Consequently, the clinician should counsel women of childbearing age with liver disease *before* pregnancy occurs, with consideration of transplantation before conception, if appropriate, or of sterilization. In addition, the clinician should anticipate and plan for possible complications of the particular liver disease.

Most patients with mild disease can expect to have normal fertility and an uncomplicated pregnancy. Those with severe disease are at increased risk for complications of their liver disease, such as variceal bleeding. Also, patients with chronic liver disease are more likely to have premature deliveries, stillbirths, and infants with low birth weights. However, progression of liver disease is not usually seen.

Autoimmune Chronic Active Hepatitis and Pregnancy

Patients taking steroids or other immunosuppressive drugs for AICAH should be continued on these medications throughout pregnancy. Dosages of steroids need not be adjusted. Flare-ups of the disease during the pregnancy do not generally occur.

Chronic Viral Hepatitis and Pregnancy

No evidence suggests that hepatitis B or C worsens during pregnancy. In addition, chronic hepatitis B and C seem to have little effect on the progression of pregnancy unless advanced cirrhosis is present.

Chronic hepatitis B carriers are potentially infectious, with vertical transmission seen in up to 90% of infants, especially if the mother is HBeAg positive. Therefore, all pregnant women should be screened for HBeAg. Universal prophylaxis also has been recently recommended for all infants and children, with the addition of hyperimmune globulin in children of carriers. This is because of the shortcomings of identifying patients at risk by history alone, the high rate of vertical transmission, and the availability of effective methods for the prevention of maternal–fetal transmission.

In patients with chronic hepatitis C infection, the risk of transmission to the newborn may be as high as 13%. Infection with both HIV and HCV increases the risk of the fetus acquiring HCV infection to as high as 44%. Unfortunately, no available immunoglobulin or vaccine prevents vertical transmission, and it is unclear if giving immune serum globulin would be helpful. Long-term sequelae of this transmission are unknown. However, the pediatrician should be notified of the mother's condition so that appropriate follow-up of the newborn can be arranged. Cesarean delivery does not reduce the risk of transmission of either hepatitis B or C to the newborn.

Patients with chronic hepatitis due to hepatitis B and C who are being treated with interferon should be strongly warned against pregnancy, or adequate birth control measures should be ensured before initiation of therapy. Administering interferon to the already pregnant mother might diminish perinatal transmission to the newborn.

Cirrhosis, Variceal Hemorrhage, and Ascites in Pregnancy

Although, in general, cirrhosis detrimentally affects fetal outcome, some women with cirrhosis have delivered healthy infants. Variceal bleeding is the most feared complication in pregnant patients with cirrhosis. In fact, therapeutic abortion might be considered in patients with previous variceal hemorrhage who become pregnant because of the increased likelihood of hemorrhage in the peripartum period.

The management of bleeding varices in pregnant women is no different than in nonpregnant women, except that the use of vasopressin with or without nitroglycerin, somatostatin, or prophylactic beta-blockade have not been reported in pregnancy. Portosystemic shunt surgery and transjugular intrahepatic portosystemic shunts may be considered.

Ascites and hepatic encephalopathy occur in pregnancy with a frequency equal to the nonpregnant population and are treated in the same fashion.

Wilson Disease and Pregnancy

Wilson disease frequently occurs during the reproductive years. Treated patients generally have normal reproductive function and, therefore, normal pregnancies. Pregnancy should be viewed favorably, as the projected life span is nearly normal for most treated patients.

Ascites and variceal hemorrhage are common complications if cirrhosis is already established. When a patient presents with fulminant Wilson disease with resultant hemolytic anemia and renal failure, transplantation may be the only option.

Patients on penicillamine, trientine, or zinc therapy for Wilson disease should continue to receive these throughout the pregnancy, although these may be teratogenic. Zinc seems to be the safest of the options. The dosage can be reduced by half during pregnancy and the original dosage resumed after lactation. Discontinuation of therapy is associated with exacerbation of the disease.

BIBLIOGRAPHY

Aiza I, Perez GO, Schiff ER. Management of ascites in patients with chronic liver disease. Am J Gastroenterol 1994;89:1949.

Dienstag JL, Isselbacher KJ. Chronic hepatitis. Isselbacher KJ, Braunwald E, Wilson JD, Martin JB, Fauci AS, Kasper DL, eds. In: Harrison's principles of internal medicine, 13th ed. New York: McGraw-Hill,1994: 1338.

Gerbes AL. Medical treatment of ascites in cirrhosis. J Hepatol 1993;17(suppl 2):S4.

Johnson PJ, McFarlane IG. Chronic active hepatitis. Gut 1991;32(suppl)S63.

Krawitt EL. Autoimmune hepatitis: classification, heterogeneity and treatment. Am J Med 1994;96(suppl 1A):23S.

Lambiase L, Davis GL. Treatment of chronic hepatitis. Gastrointest Pharmacol 1992;21:659.

Lee WM. Pregnancy in patients with chronic liver disease. Gastroenterol Clin North Am 1992;21:889.

Maddrey WC. Chronic hepatitis. Dis Mon 1993;39:53.

Mistry P, Seymour CA. Primary biliary cirrhosis: from Thomas Addison to the 1990's. Q J Med 1992;82:185.

Neuberger J, Lombard M, Galbraith R. Primary biliary cirrhosis. Gut 1991;32(Suppl)S73.

Resnick RH. Management of varices in cirrhosis. Hosp Prac 1993;28:123.

Wilkinson ML. Diagnosis and management of liver disease in pregnancy. Adv Intern Med 1990;35:289.

Primary Care for Women, edited by Phyllis C. Leppert and Fred M. Howard. Lippincott-Raven Publishers, Philadelphia © 1997.

64
Gallstones and Cholecystitis

RAYMOND J. LANZAFAME

The gallbladder is a sac-like, pear-shaped, hollow organ that lies in the gallbladder fossa on the under-surface of the liver. The position of the gallbladder defines the anatomic boundary between the right and left lobes of the liver and the anatomic structures of the liver.

The gallbladder is innervated by sympathetic and parasympathetic nerve fibers. The sensation of pain is mediated by visceral sympathetic fibers, whereas the motor stimulus for gallbladder contraction is mediated by the vagus nerves and the celiac ganglion.

A primary function of the gallbladder is to concentrate bile by absorption of sodium and water. The gallbladder is capable of reducing hepatic bile volume by 80% to 90%. Reabsorption of gallbladder fluid is largely due to the transport of sodium.

Evidence suggests that bile flows in a continuous fashion, with some gallbladder emptying occurring constantly. The ingestion of food and release of cholecystokinin (CCK) are the major stimuli for gallbladder emptying. CCK release from the duodenum is induced most potently by fat. However, most foodstuffs stimulate CCK release. This latter fact explains why dietary control for symptomatic gallbladder disease is ineffective. Several other agents, including motilin, secretin, histamine, and prostaglandins, affect the contraction of the gallbladder.

Bile is a solution of water, organic lipids, and electrolytes secreted by hepatocytes. Bile salts, cholesterol, and phospholipids account for 80% of the dry weight of bile. Bile acids, cholesterol, and phospholipids are the major lipid components of bile. Most of the cholesterol found in bile is synthesized de novo in the liver rather than being attributable to absorption of dietary cholesterol. Lecithin accounts for over 90% of the phospholipids found in human bile. HMG-CoA reductase is the rate-limiting enzyme in the cholesterol production pathway and is inhibited by drugs that have been used as gallstone dissolution agents.

The hepatic synthesis of bile acids is regulated by a negative feedback mechanism via the enterohepatic circulation. This system is efficient, with approximately 95% of the hepatic synthesized bile acid pool being actively absorbed in the terminal ileum as conjugated bile acids or passively reabsorbed in the colon as deoxycholic or lithocholic acid produced as a result of enzymatic dehydroxylation by colonic bacteria.

Cholesterol is essentially insoluble in bile. However, in the presence of a sufficiently high concentration of bile acids, the bile acids form micelles. The incorporation of lecithin into the micelle allows the structures to absorb water, swell, and transport greater amounts of cholesterol. Unilamellar cholesterol–phospholipid vesicles are present in both hepatic and gallbladder bile. These latter structures also account for a significant portion of cholesterol transport. The concentrations of total bile acids and total lipids and the degree of cholesterol saturation determine the amount of cholesterol that is solubilized in micelles or vesicles. Evidence suggests that interference with the equilibrium between micelles and vesicles leads to crystal formation and, subsequently, to cholesterol gallstone formation.

In humans, gallstones are principally composed of cholesterol, with pigment stones occurring much less commonly. Pigmented gallstones are commonly found in patients with hemolytic disorders and liver cirrhosis. The formation of cholesterol stones is believed to result from cholesterol supersaturation in bile, accelerated cholesterol crystal nucleation, and impaired gallbladder motility. Gallstones tend to grow for the first 2 or 3 years, after which the growth tends to stabilize. Over 85% of gallstones are less than 2 cm diameter.

Approximately 10% to 15% of the adult population in the United States, or more than 20 million people, have gallstones. Estimates suggest that one million new patients are diagnosed annually. This incidence of cholelithiasis is consistent with the 10% to 20% prevalence rate observed in industrialized countries. The incidence of gallstones increases with age and is higher in women. Certain ethnic groups such as Pima Indians and Mexican Americans have a higher incidence of cholelithiasis, whereas black Africans with a high fiber diet rarely exhibit gallstones. Multiple pregnancies, obesity, rapid weight loss, and total parenteral nutrition have been associated with an increased incidence of gallstone formation.

Gallstones represent a frequent reason for hospitalization and represent the most common digestive disease, with an estimated annual cost of more than five billion dollars overall. Over 600,000 patients underwent cholecystectomy in 1991, and estimates suggest that the numbers of cholecystectomies performed in 1992 and 1993 were 20% to 30% higher due to the availability of laparoscopic cholecystectomy. Several factors have been suggested as the cause of the increase of cholecystectomies. However, the mechanism by which the patient with cholelithiasis is referred for surgical consultation remains poorly defined. Recent data from hospital discharge databases suggest that improved outcomes for patients undergoing cholecystectomy preceded the advent of laparoscopic cholecystectomy, as evidenced by decreased morbidity and mortality rates over the last 10 years. Some data suggest that patients are undergoing operation earlier in their clinical course, that laparoscopic cholecystectomy has resulted in fewer surgeries being performed for acute cholecystitis, and that serious sequelae of cholelithiasis and the frequency of emergency cholecystectomies is declining. Further study of these trends is warranted.

CLINICAL PRESENTATIONS AND FINDINGS

Patients with gallstone disease may present in a variety of ways. Many patients are asymptomatic, some present with atypical or nonspecific complaints, and others present with regular or episodic symptoms.

Biliary colic is the most common presentation. Pain lasts for more than 15 to 30 minutes and occurs postprandially. The pain is typically precipitated by a fatty or protein-rich meal (although CCK stimulation may occur with most foodstuffs) and occurs 30 to 60 minutes after eating. It may persist for several hours. The pain may be constant rather than spasmodic. It is usually located in the epigastrium or in the right hypochondrium with or without radiation to the back or the right shoulder. Nausea and emesis are frequently associated with attacks of biliary colic. The frequency of biliary colic is unpredictable but generally tends to increase in frequency and intensity over time.

Acute calculous cholecystitis usually presents with right upper quadrant abdominal pain. The pain is persistent and may radiate to the back of the epigastrium or the right shoulder. The onset and initial character of the pain are similar to that of biliary colic. However, the pain persists for more than 4 to 6 hours and may last for several days. The mechanism by which cholecystitis develops remains unclear but is usually associated with impaction of a gallstone in the infundibulum of the gallbladder or cystic duct occlusion. Progressive inflammation involves the parietal peritoneum, causing the patient to complain of more localized right upper quadrant abdominal pain. Many patients experience anorexia, nausea, vomiting, and low-grade fever. Nausea and emesis may occur in up to 86% of patients and fever (up to 38°C) is present in nearly half.

On physical examination, the patient may have a positive Murphy sign. Murphy sign is described as inspiratory arrest during deep palpation of the right upper quadrant. A palpable mass may be present in 20% to 30% of patients and is usually secondary to omentum overlying an inflamed gallbladder. Liver function tests and serum bilirubin may be elevated. Most patients have a mild leukocytosis in the 12,000 to 15,000 mL range. White blood cell counts in the 20,000 m/L range are suggestive of gangrenous cholecystitis, perforation of the gallbladder, or cholangitis. The differential diagnosis of acute cholecystitis includes acute appendicitis, perforated ulcer, acute pancreatitis, acute pyelonephritis, right lower lobe pneumonia, cholangitis, and acute myocardial infarction.

Gallstone pancreatitis occurs in approximately 15% of patients with symptomatic gallstone disease and may account for 30% to 70% of all cases of acute pancreatitis. Typical signs and symptoms of acute pancreatitis develop, often with highly elevated amylase and lipase levels with or without transient increases in the serum bilirubin and liver function tests. Although most patients have relatively mild courses, necrotizing pancreatitis may occur. Patients with documented biliary pancreatitis have a recurrence rate of 60% or more, with a variable frequency of episodes ranging from days to months. Whereas the management of these patients is controversial, most surgeons recommend cholecystectomy during the same hospital admission, once the chemical pancreatitis has resolved.

A variety of symptoms have been associated with biliary tract disease that are nonspecific for cholecystitis. These include fatty food intolerance, belching, postprandial bloating, dyspepsia, or diarrhea. These symptoms may be indicative of irritable bowel syndrome, peptic ulcer disease, or gastroesophageal reflux disease. Patients with these symptoms require diligent diagnostic workup before attributing these symptom constellations to gallstones alone.

IMAGING STUDIES

Plain abdominal roentgenograms are frequently obtained for patients with or without acute abdominal pain. This study can detect calcified gallstones, which occur in 5% to 20% of patients with cholelithiasis, but is of limited value. It may, however, detect gas bubbles in the gallbladder lumen or wall in cases of emphysematous cholecystitis. This condition is caused by gas-forming organisms such as *Escherichia coli* and *Clostridia*.

Ultrasonography represents the most commonly used diagnostic test for the detection of gallstones or acute cholecystitis. The sensitivity rate of ultrasonography ranges from 90% to 95%, and the specificity rate ranges from 70% to 90% for acute cholecystitis, based on which criteria are used to interpret the sonogram. The major criteria for analysis are the presence of gallstones and nonvisualization of the gallbladder. Other abnormalities, such as masses and the presence of dilated intrahepatic or extrahepatic biliary ducts, may be visualized with a skillfully performed examination. Several authors list criteria for the diagnosis of acute cholecystitis via ultrasonography. These include a greater than 5-mm thickening of the gallbladder wall, tenderness of the gallbladder when palpated during the examination, a rounded gallbladder shape, and pericholecystic fluid. The overall diagnostic accuracy of ultrasonography is 90% for the evaluation of the patient with suspected gallstones.

Oral cholecystography is a simple and cost-effective test for the diagnosis of gallstones and gallbladder function. These test was developed by Graham and Cole in 1924. A radiopaque iodine halogenated dye is ingested by the patient. Typically, the patient is given a double dose of contrast material. The material must be absorbed by the gastrointestinal tract, then extracted and excreted into the bile by the liver. A normally functioning gallbladder concentrates the dye, which opacifies the gallbladder on x-ray. The study result is positive when gallstones are visualized, as a filling defect in the gallbladder or the gallbladder does not opacify after a double dose of contrast. The diagnostic accuracy rate of this test is 95%, but the following limitations must be considered. The presence of hepatic dysfunction or hyperbilirubinemia beyond 1.4 to 2.0 mg/dL interferes with dye excretion. Also, failure to ingest the dye or failure of gut absorption results in a false-positive study result.

Biliary scintigraphy depends on the intravenous administration of one of several technetium 99–labeled iminodiacetic acid compounds. The radioisotope is cleared by the hepatocytes and is excreted into the bile. The test provides a function test for the liver, the extrahepatic bile ducts, and the gallbladder. It assesses the patency of the cystic duct and infers the presence of acute cholecystitis based on cystic duct obstruction (although cystic duct obstruction may be chronic). This test can be used in the jaundiced patient and may be useful in determining the level of biliary obstruction. The sequence of filling and emptying of the gallbladder relative to the release of contrast into the duodenum provides evidence for chronic cholecystitis or biliary dyskinesia.

Computed tomography has been used occasionally for evaluating the patient with suspected biliary tract disease. Although the computed tomography scan is useful in the evaluating the jaundiced patient as regards the nature and location of biliary obstruction and the status of the pancreas, it is not particularly sensitive for the identification of gallstones.

Magnetic resonance imaging also has been used for evaluating patients with abdominal complaints. However, its role in the evaluation of patients with hepatobiliary diseases remains unclear.

Both percutaneous transhepatic cholangiography and endoscopic retrograde cholangiopancreatography (ERCP) are used for the evaluation and management of the jaundiced patient. These procedures are discussed more fully in Chapter 68. Both procedures depend on the technical skill of the radiologist or interventional gastroenterologist and provide an actual anatomic road map. Preoperative ERCP and papillotomy has been successful in resolving jaundice due to gallstones or benign strictures related obstruction of the common bile duct. This may simplify patient management and allow laparoscopic cholecystectomy to be performed electively.

Stimulation tests of gallbladder function may be useful in managing patients with suspected biliary tract disease with no evidence of gallstones or sludge on conventional workup. These studies evaluate the ability of the gallbladder to empty after stimulation by the administration of a "fatty meal" or the intravenous injection of CCK. A gallbladder ejection fraction can be calculated, and a positive result occurs when the ejection fraction is less than 35%. These studies have been done using ultrasound, oral cholecystography, or biliary scintigraphy. Arguably, biliary scintigraphy with CCK stimulation may be the most convenient and accurate.

PATIENT MANAGEMENT (TREATMENT)

The management of patients with asymptomatic gallstones should be expectant and conservative. Most gallstones remain silent throughout life, with a 1% to 4% yearly incidence rate of developing symptoms or complications of gallstone disease. Approximately 10% of patients develop symptoms in the first 5 years after diagnosis, and approximately 20% develop symptoms by 20 years. Invariably, the asymptomatic patient develops symptoms well before a complication. Therefore, with few exceptions, the prophylactic treatment of asymptomatic patients cannot be justified. A problem, however, is the certainty with which one can verify that a patient is truly asymptomatic. Many patients with vague symptoms or a wide array of dyspeptic symptoms *may* benefit from elective cholecystectomy. The most prudent course of action, therefore, would be careful patient follow-up or surgical referral for counseling as to the care of the specific case.

This also applies to diabetic and elderly patients. However, higher morbidity and mortality rates occur in diabetic patients after emergency operations. Therefore, diabetic patients should be referred for elective cholecystectomy promptly when symptoms first occur. Considerable controversy exists regarding the need for elective cholecystectomy in the elderly patient with asymptomatic gallstones. Whereas comorbid conditions must be weighed individually, recent literature suggests that clinical observation, rather than routine surgery, is appropriate.

The issue of incidental cholecystectomy during nonbiliary abdominal surgery in the asymptomatic patient is another area of clinical debate. Although the evidence is clear that incidental cholecystectomy is not warranted in high-risk patients, such as those with portal hypertension or cirrhosis, patients with sickle cell anemia or other blood dyscrasia and children may pose diagnostic dilemmas in the future. Therefore, cholecystectomy may be justified. Immunosuppressed or pretransplantation patients, or patients who are isolated from medical care for long intervals, have sufficiently high morbidity and mortality from gallstone complications to warrant referral for consideration of elective cholecystectomy.

The risk of carcinoma of the gallbladder is higher in patients with gallstones, but it is only approximately 1 per 1000 patients per year. Therefore, prophylactic cholecystectomy for cancer prevention is not generally justifiable. Patients with a porcelain (calcified) gallbladder, with or without associated calculi, have a 25% incidence of gallbladder cancer and are an exception to this rule. Other exceptions include North and South American Indians, individuals with solitary biliary polyps greater than 1 cm in diameter, patients with gallstones greater than 3 cm in diameter, and those with anomalous junctions of the pancreaticobiliary junctions. These patients too have been reported to have an increased risk of gallbladder carcinoma relative to the general population with gallstones.

The need for treatment of the patient with symptoms is more straightforward. Once gallstone symptoms occur, they tend to recur in most patients, and complications develop in approximately 25% of patients within 10 to 20 years if left untreated. Thus, most symptomatic patients should be treated. Ninety percent to 95% of patients with typical biliary pain are cured after successful therapy. Patients with atypical pain, painless dyspepsia (ie, bloating, belching, and fatty food intolerance) have a lesser degree of successful symptom relief after therapy. These patients should have careful diagnostic testing to determine whether the symptoms are caused by irritable bowel syndrome, peptic ulcer disease, gastroesophageal reflux, or other disease processes.

NONSURGICAL APPROACHES

Some authors observe that nearly half of patients with symptoms referable to gallstones (followed for up to 20 years) experience stabilization or reduction of the severity of their symptoms. Some patients may even become asymptomatic. This has been used to justify nonsurgical management of gallbladder stones. Cholesterol gallstones account for nearly 80% of gallstones. These stones are amenable to dissolution by oral bile acid therapy, the combination of extracorporeal shock wave lithotripsy (ESWL) and oral bile acid therapy, or by direct instillation of cholesterol solvents into the gallbladder. These methods generally require a patent cystic duct and are contraindicated in patients with severe or recurrent biliary symptoms, as well as those with evidence of inflammation of the gallbladder. Patients with calcified stones similarly are not candidates for nonsurgical management. Patients with small stones (< 5 mm) are most likely to respond to dissolution therapy. The most commonly used oral agents are ursodeoxycholic acid and chenodeoxycholic acid, which may be used alone or in combination. Side effects of therapy include recurrent biliary pain, diarrhea (in approximately one third of patients treated), elevation of liver enzymes, and modest hypercholesterolemia. Although the clearance of stones from the gallbladder is successful in 50% of patients, the rate of stone recurrence approaches 50% within 6 months after the cessation of therapy. ESWL uses a variety of methods to fragment noncalcified calculi, ideally into fragments smaller than 3 mm. This therapy is most successful when combined with oral agents. However, combined ESWL and oral dissolution therapy is not more effective than oral agents alone regarding long-term stone clearance. Complications related to this therapy include cholestasis, pancreatitis, or cholecystitis in 3% to 5% of patients. Emergency cholecystectomy or sphincterotomy is required in 2% to 5% of treated patients. Biliary pain related to the passage of stone fragments occurs in 30% to 40% of patients in the first few months after therapy. Adverse effects to the surrounding tissues are usually minor, but include petechiae in 8% of patients and gross hematuria in approximately 4% of patients treated. ESWL therapy remains investigational in the United States.

Contact dissolution therapy is another nonsurgical option. Patients eligible for this approach are those with a gallbladder attached to the liver bed who have an open cystic duct and radiolucent stones. This procedure is invasive, requiring 10 to 15 hours of therapy and still has the drawback of stone recurrence. Several agents, including diethyl ether, mono-octanoin, and methyl tert-butyl ether (MTBE). This approach does not require a limitation on the maximum number of stones present within the gallbladder, as does ESWL. It, too, remains investigational.

Other investigational methods for stone removal include percutaneous approaches for stone extraction, including crushing of stones with a vortex creating impeller device or other direct extraction techniques. These techniques require a drainage catheter to be left in the gallbladder for several days.

As was noted earlier, although some authors believe that as many as 20% symptomatic patients are amenable to nonsurgical therapies, stone recurrence rates range from 30% to 50% and are highest in patients with multiple stones. The risk of development of acute symptoms during therapy and the incidence of biliary pain remain significant problems with these therapies. Therefore, these approaches generally are reserved for patients who refuse surgery or are not considered to be surgical candidates.

SURGICAL APPROACHES

The traditional approach to the management of symptomatic gallstones has been cholecystectomy, surgical removal of the gallbladder. Cholecystectomy is the most frequently performed elective surgical procedure in the United States, with over 600,000 cholecystectomies having been completed in 1992. Both open and laparoscopic approaches to cholecystectomy are safe when performed by properly trained, skilled surgeons. Studies document a progressive decline in the morbidity and mortality after cholecystectomy over the last 10 years. In addition, data suggest that the frequency of complications of gallstone disease may be declining, as evidenced by fewer emergency cholecystectomies and fewer cases of biliary sepsis and gangrenous or perforated cholecystitis.

The anatomic aftermath of cholecystectomy is identical with both surgical approaches, namely, the complete removal of the gallbladder and its contents. In both cases, the patient must be sufficiently fit to tolerate general anesthesia. The indications for cholecystectomy are identical, regardless of the approach.

Open cholecystectomy is usually accomplished via a right subcostal (Köcher) incision. The patient remains hospitalized from 2 to 5 days postoperatively and requires 4 to 8 weeks for full recovery. This approach affords the surgeon the opportunity to palpate and assess the common bile duct directly and facilitates exploration of the common bile duct and biliary enteric anastomosis, when indicated. However, patient disability and discomfort are dramatically more severe than with laparoscopic surgery. Patients treated laparoscopically typically remain hospitalized for less than 24 hours and are able to resume full normal activity in 2 to 10 days postoperatively.

Laparoscopic cholecystectomy has replaced open cholecystectomy for most patients with symptomatic gallstones. Patients must be able to tolerate general anesthesia and must be without serious cardiopulmonary diseases or comorbid conditions that preclude operation. The risks of surgery are similar to open cholecystectomy in experienced hands and include the following: infection or bleeding (1%), biliary ductal injury (0.1% to 0.2%), or biliary leak (0.1% to 1%). Large series note that the rate of conversion to open cholecystectomy is approximately 5% and that this typically occurs for uncontrolled hemorrhage, aberrant or difficult to delineate anatomy, or choledocholithiasis. Of these reasons for conversion, choledocholithiasis may be managed by ERCP or laparoscopically in selected patients when the appropriate equipment and skilled therapists are available. The decision to convert the procedure to open cholecystectomy should be considered to be sound surgical judgment rather than a complication of laparoscopy. Postoperative pulmonary complications such as atelectasis and pneumonia occur much less frequently after laparoscopic cholecystectomy compared with its open counterpart. Obese candidates may safely undergo laparoscopic cholecystectomy, providing that the instruments are capable of passing through the thick abdominal wall to reach the area of dissection. Patients with chronic obstructive pulmonary disease usually tolerate laparoscopic cholecystectomy. However, carbon dioxide used to insufflate the abdomen may cause hypercarbia and acidosis.

Patients not usually considered to be candidates for laparoscopic cholecystectomy include those with generalized peritonitis, septic shock or cholangitis, severe acute pancreatitis, end-stage cirrhosis of the liver with portal hypertension, severe coagulopathy unresponsive to treatment, known cancer of the gallbladder, and cholecystoenteric fistulas. The issue of laparoscopic cholecystectomy during pregnancy is discussed later.

GALLSTONES AND PREGNANCY

Cholecystitis represents a common condition during pregnancy. Acute cholecystitis is the second most frequent nonobstetric emergency of pregnancy after acute appendicitis. Acute cholecystitis occurs at a frequency of 1 to 6 per 10,000 pregnancies. Multiple pregnancies are associated with an increased risk of developing gallstones. Several studies suggest that biliary physiologic makeup is altered during pregnancy in such a way that cholesterol formation is promoted. Others document that both basal and residual gallbladder volumes are significantly higher during the second and third trimesters compared with the first trimester or nonpregnant women. These abnormalities of contractility resolve within the first postpartum week. Thus, pregnancy creates an environment in which gallbladder motility is inhibited and bile stasis occurs. Current speculation indicts progesterone as the most likely candidate for producing this defect because high concentrations of progesterone inhibit gastrointestinal smooth muscle contractibility in vitro. Physiologic changes of biliary lipid composition and kinetics during pregnancy create a lithogenic environment due to the following: an increased bile acid pool size, decreased enterohepatic circulation, a decreased percentage of chenodeoxycholic acid, an increased percentage of cholic acid, an increased secretion of cholesterol, and the stasis of bile in the gallbladder.

Symptomatic cholecystitis with severe episodes of pain are noted by several authors to be more common during the puerperium and in the early months postpartum than during pregnancy. The symptoms of biliary colic during pregnancy are similar to those of nonpregnant individuals. However, the differential diagnosis in pregnancy includes the following: acute viral hepatitis; acute alcoholic hepatitis; duodenal ulcer; acute pancreatitis; pulmonary embolus; right lower lobe pneumonia; acute myocardial infarction; acute appendicitis; acute fatty liver of pregnancy; preeclampsia; and the syndrome of hemolysis, elevated liver enzymes, and low platelets (HELLP syndrome). Acute appendicitis is four to five times more common than acute cholecystitis during pregnancy. The pain of acute appendicitis may localize to the right upper quadrant due to the cephalad shift of the abdominal viscera by the gravid uterus.

Traditional dogma suggests that episodes of biliary colic should be managed conservatively during pregnancy, if possible, with surgery being delayed until the postpartum period. Conservative management includes symptomatic measures for pain, such as analgesics, antispasmodics, fat-restricted diet, and intravenous hydration. The decision to perform cholecystectomy during pregnancy generally is based on repeated episodes of pain or the appearance of biliary complications such as choledocholithiasis or pancreatitis. Abdominal surgery of any type during the first trimester of pregnancy has been associated with fetal loss, and the rate with open cholecystectomy has been estimated to be as high as 5%. It is also believed that surgery later in pregnancy, during the second trimester, is safe and without risk of fetal mortality.

Laparoscopic cholecystectomy during pregnancy has been reported by several authors. Approximately 45 cases have been completed without fetal loss. Laparoscopic cholecystectomy was performed in most patients during the second trimester. However, four patients underwent operation during the first trimester and four underwent operation during the third trimester. Tocolytic agents have been used perioperatively in some cases. Laparoscopic cholecystectomy late in the third trimester may be hazardous due to the large size of the uterus, which increases the potential for iatrogenic fetal or maternal injury intraoperatively. Whereas additional clinical data are required, it seems that laparoscopic cholecystectomy is safe during pregnancy in the hands of the skilled laparoscopist.

SUMMARY

Gallstones are a common condition, affecting 10% to 20% of the population. Symptomatic cholelithiasis occurs in approximately 10% of patients with gallstones. Whereas asymptomatic patients do not require treatment, the symptomatic patient should be treated. Laparoscopic cholecystectomy has become the preferred management option for symptomatic patients who are candidates for general anesthesia. Laparoscopic cholecystectomy seems to be safe for the pregnant patient with intractable symptoms.

BIBLIOGRAPHY

Cheslyn-Curtis S, Lees WR, Hatfield AR, Russell RC. Percutaneous techniques for the management of symptomatic gallbladder stones. Dig Dis 1992;10:208.

Constantino GN, Vincent GJ, Mukalian GG, Kliefoth WL Jr. Laparoscopic cholecystectomy in pregnancy. J Laparoendoscopic Surg 1994;4:161.

Den Toom R, Terpstra OT. Incidence and prevention of gallbladder stones after non-operative treatment. Eur J Surg 1994;160:131.

Gallstones and laparoscopic cholecystectomy. NIH Consensus Statement 1992;10:1.

Gholson CF, Sittig K, McDonald JC. Recent advances in the management of gallstones. Am J Med Sci 1994;307:293.

Kadakia SC. Biliary tract emergencies: acute cholecystitis, acute cholangitis, and acute pancreatitis. Med Clin North Am 1993;77:1015.

Keating JJ, Corrigan OT, Chua A, et al. Non-surgical approaches to stones in the biliary tree. Dig Dis 1993;11:102.

Kloiber R, Molnar CP, Shaffer EA. Chronic biliary-type pain in the abscence of gallstones: the value of cholecystokinin cholescintigraphy. Am J Roentgenol 1992;159:509.

Lanzini A, Northfieid TC. Pharmacological treatment of gallstones: practical guidelines. Drugs 1994;47:458.

Perissat J, Huibregtac K, Keane FC, Russell RC, Neoptolemos JP. Management of bile duct stones in the era of laparoscopic cholecystectomy. Br J Surg 1994;81:799.

Rosenthal RA, Anderson DK. Surgery in the elderly: observations on the pathophysiology and treatment of cholelithiasis. Exp Gerontol 1993;28:459.

Roslyn J, Zinner MJ. Gallbladder and extrahepatic biliary system. In: Schwartz SI, Shires GT, Spencer FC, eds. Principles of surgery, 6th ed. New York: McGraw Hill 1994:1367.

Schoenfield LJ, Marks JW. Oral and contact dissolution of gallstones. Am J Surg 1993;165:427.

Soper NJ. Effect of nonbillary problems on laparoscopic cholecystectomy. Am J Surg 1993;165:522.

Strasberg SM, Clavien PA. Overview of therapeutic modalities for the treatment of gallstone diseases. Am J Surg 1993;165:420.

Talamini MA. Controversies in laparoscopic cholecystectomy: contraindications, cholangiography, pregnancy and avoidance of complications. Baillieres Clin Gastroenterol 1993;7:881.

Traverso LW. Clinical manifestations and impact of gallstone disease. Am J Surg 1993;165:405.

65
Pancreatitis

TARUN KOTHARI

Primary Care for Women, edited by Phyllis C. Leppert and Fred M. Howard. Lippincott-Raven Publishers, Philadelphia © 1997.

ACUTE PANCREATITIS

Acute pancreatitis is a common disorder. It is an inflammatory condition of the pancreas. Classic presentation consists of severe pain of the upper or middle part of the abdomen, or both, with radiation to the back. Pain is usually associated with nausea and vomiting, lasting for hours or days. Invariably, there is elevation of serum amylase and lipase.

History

Over 100 years ago, Reginald Fitz described acute pancreatitis for the first time. Opie connected gallstones with pancreatitis. Much later, alcohol became firmly established as an important causative factor. Over time, incidence of the disease has steadily increased. Incidence is now estimated to be 200 to 750 per million among men and 112 to 484 per million among women. The rising incidence is related both to increased alcohol use and to improved diagnostic ability.

Etiology

Causes of pancreatitis are numerous and varied (Table 65-1). Gallstones remain the most common cause of acute pancreatitis, accounting for approximately 45% of cases. Alcohol is the second most common cause, accounting for approximately 35% of cases, although this percentage varies from country to country and in different ethnic populations. Ten percent of the cases are miscellaneous, and in a final 10% of cases the etiology is unknown.

Regardless of cause, pathogenesis of acute pancreatitis remains unclear. There is usually peripancreatic fat necrosis, congestion of the gland, depletion of zymogen granules within the acini, or necrosis of the pancreas. A series of chemical events leads to premature release of inactive digestive enzymes. Each causative factor starts the process differently.

Three theories have been forwarded to explain gallstone pancreatitis: (1) common channel and bile reflux theory; (2) duodenal reflux theory, and (3) pancreatic ductal hypertension theory.

Precisely how alcohol causes pancreatitis remains unclear, as only 10% of alcoholics develop pancreatitis. Ethanol probably affects the pancreas with direct toxicity. The disease can present as a single acute episode or recurrent intermittent acute attacks, commonly called chronic relapsing pancreatitis. Attacks are usually temporally related to ethanol use.

Hypertriglyceridemia causes pancreatitis in 10% of patients. High triglyceride levels are found in 25% to 35% of patients. Elevated cholesterol levels are not associated with pancreatitis. When triglyceride levels rise above 1000 mg/dL, significant acute attacks occur. Type V lipid abnormality is most commonly found. The mechanism of the pancreatitis in hypertriglyceridemia remains unclear.

More than 85 drugs have been reported to cause acute pancreatitis. The drugs associated with the highest incidence are mercaptopurine (about 3% to 5%) and didanosine. Certain drugs, such as azathioprine, mercaptopurine, metronidazole, salicylates, and sulfa, cause pancreatitis by hypersensitivity reactions, whereas other drugs, like pentamidine, valproic acid, and didanosine, seem to cause injury by accumulation of toxic metabolites.

The initial clinical feature of 3% of patients with pancreatic carcinoma is acute pancreatitis. Of patients with acute pancreatitis, 1.3% are found to have pancreatic carcinoma. Therefore, endoscopic retrograde cholangiopancreatography (ERCP) should be carried out in all patients with so-called idiopathic pancreatitis, especially if episodes are multiple and patients are older than 40 years of age.

In about 10% of cases, the cause cannot be determined after diligent search, and they are labeled idiopathic.

Physical Examination and Clinical Findings

Presentation of acute pancreatitis includes epigastric or diffuse upper abdominal pain, which can be steady, dull, burning, or sharp and severe. The pain usually radiates to the back, chest, or flanks. Pain may persist for hours to days and usually requires strong narcotic analgesics for relief. It can be made worse by lying down, and better by sitting or curling up in bed, usually in a fetal position. Nausea, vomiting, and mild abdominal distention are associated with the acute episode in over 85% of patients. The degree of pain correlates strongly with the extent of pancreatic involvement.

Physical examination usually reveals an ill-appearing, anxious patient. The patient may be febrile. Deep palpation reveals tenderness in the upper abdomen, usually with voluntary guarding.

Table 65-1. Causes of Acute Pancreatitis

Obstructive	Gallstones and common bile duct stones, pancreatic or ampullary tumors, worms, pancreatic divisum, hypertensive sphincter
Toxins and Drugs	Alcohol, insecticides, azathioprine (Imuran), mercaptopurine, calcium, anticholinesterases, didanosine, estrogen, thiazides, furosemide, salicylates, valproic acid, metronidazole, pentamidine, tetracyclines, sulfa, ERCP contrast
Trauma	Blunt trauma to abdomen (commonly found in children), postoperative trauma, endoscopic sphincterotomy or manometry of sphincter of Oddi
Hypertriglyceridemia	
Infections	Ascariasis, clonorchiasis, mumps, rubella, HIV, Epstein-Barr virus, *Mycoplasma,* tuberculosis
Vascular	Ischemia, embolization, vasculitis, postabdominal aneurysm surgery, shock
Other	Idiopathic, congenital, hereditary

ERCP, endoscopic retrograde cholangiopancreatography; *HIV,* human immunodeficiency virus.

Severe pancreatitis is associated with elevated temperature, tachycardia, and hypotension. Hypovolemia may contribute to hypotension. Bowel sounds may be diminished or absent due to an ileus-like presentation related to pancreatitis. Flank ecchymosis (Grey Turner sign) or periumbilical ecchymosis (Cullen sign) may be observed in patients with severe hemorrhagic pancreatitis. Ascites is occasionally present or it may develop later in severe cases.

Laboratory and Imaging Studies

The diagnosis of acute pancreatitis is initially made by its clinical presentation with elevated serum amylase or lipase levels. The serum amylase level is the most reliable and most widely available laboratory test. Serum amylase begins to rise 2 to 12 hours after the onset of symptoms and stays elevated for up to 3 days. Increased levels may be due to increased release, increased absorption, or both. Sometimes patients with acute pancreatitis may have normal levels of amylase, particularly patients with alcoholic pancreatitis. Serum amylase levels correlate poorly with the severity of the disease. Levels tend to be higher in patients with acute biliary pancreatitis compared with those with alcohol-induced pancreatitis. Many conditions other than pancreatitis can cause hyperamylasemia. These are listed in Table 65-2. The lipase assay shows greater sensitivity and specificity in the diagnosis of acute pancreatitis. Lipase levels stay elevated for several days compared with amylase. Hence, they are a more useful indicator in patients who present several days after the onset of pain. Urinary amylase levels, or the urinary amylase and urinary creatinine clearance ratio, are no longer used for clinical diagnosis.

Other laboratory values such as leukocytosis, hyperglycemia, hypocalcemia, hypoalbuminemia, and hypoxia may be seen in acute pancreatitis. Liver function test abnormalities are observed more frequently in acute biliary pancreatitis. High sensitivity and specificity are seen if three or more biochemical parameters are elevated, including alanine aminotransferase (ALT), aspartate aminotransferase (AST), bilirubin, alkaline phosphatase, and gamma glutamyl transferase (GGT). When combined with ultrasound, gallstone pancreatitis can be diagnosed with 95% sensitivity and specificity.

Radiologic imaging studies play a helpful role in the diagnosis. Free air series may show sentinel loop (localized dilation and ileus of the duodenal loop), paralytic ileus of the small bowel, colon cut-off sign, ascites, pancreatic calcifications, and calcified gallstones. Chest x-ray may show pleural effusions and sometimes infiltrates in severe cases.

When biliary tract disease is suspected, radionuclide scanning, as with diisopropyl iminodiacetic acid (DISIDA), is useful. Ultrasound and computed tomography (CT) complement the information previously obtained. Ultrasound reliably demonstrates gallstones (sensitivity 98%, specificity 93%) and detects a dilated common bile duct system, with or without stones. A major drawback of ultrasound is its inability to identify pancreatic disease in patients with gas or in obese patients. CT is the best imaging modality available to assess acute pancreatitis. It is used in the following cases: (1) in diagnosis of acute pancreatitis; (2) to detect complications of acute pancreatitis, like phlegmon, pseudocysts, and abscess formation; and (3) to guide aspiration and drainage procedures. Patients with disease limited to the gland, as seen on an early CT scan, usually have a mild clinical course with no complications. Those with inflammatory extension outside of the gland into peripancreatic tissues, resulting in phlegmon, pancreatic necrosis, abscess, and hemorrhage, have a severe protracted course. Magnetic resonance imaging is less useful than CT in most

Table 65-2. Causes of Hyperamylasemia

Pancreatic Causes

Acute pancreatitis
Pseudocyst of pancreas
Carcinoma of pancreas
Plegmon and abcess
Post-ERCP contrast injection

Acute Abdominal Conditions

Perforated ulcer
Mesenteric infarction
Intestinal obstruction
Peritonitis
Ruptured ectopic pregnancy
Postsurgical

Other Causes

Renal failure
Acidosis
Macroamylasemia
Salivary gland diseases

ERCP, endoscopic retrograde cholangiopancreatography.

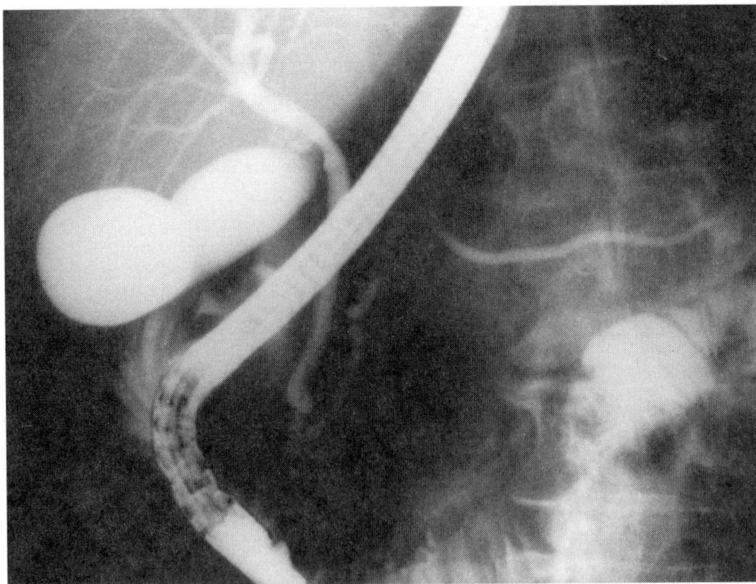

Figure 65-1. ERCP showing normal pancreatobiliary duct anatomy, including gallbladder.

cases of pancreatitis. Endoscopic retrograde cholangiopancreatography (ERCP) has a role in acute pancreatitis. It is most useful for delineating suspected biliary disease as the cause of acute pancreatitis (Figs. 65-1 and 65-2). Common bile duct stones can be removed during ERCP by papillotomy, which facilitates eventual laparoscopic cholecystectomy. ERCP also can be used for diagnosis of carcinoma of the pancreas appearing as acute pancreatitis and for placing endobiliary stents in appropriate ductal systems. Idiopathic pancreatitis should be diagnosed only after performing ERCP, as many occult causes can be found during the test, such as ultrasound-negative gallstones or common bile duct stones; obstruction of pancreatic duct by stricture, stones, or carcinoma; choledochocele; and pancreatic divisum (Figs. 65-3 through 65-5). Contrast injection during ERCP causes pancreatitis in 1% of cases. ERCP with sphincter of Oddi manometry can pinpoint select cases of hypertensive sphincter as a treatable cause of acute recurrent pancreatitis.

Treatment

The ability to assess the severity of the disease and to predict the prognosis is clearly useful to all clinicians. Pain severity, serum amylase levels, and the patient's general condition are not reliable predictors. Various clinical criteria have been designed. These include Banks clinical criteria, Ranson early prognostic signs, modified Ranson prognostic signs, Imerie prognostic criteria, and Apache II criteria. Commonly used combinations of clinical and laboratory data that can indicate severity of pancreatitis within the first 48 hours of admission are most useful (Table 65-3).

Acute pancreatitis can be complicated by either local or systemic events. Mortality increases if the disease is complicated by infection, sepsis, and pulmonary complications. Mortality is higher in children. Obesity has been considered a major risk factor for severe acute pancreatitis. Complications are summarized in Table 65-4.

The complications of acute pancreatitis may begin during the first week of hospitalization with multisystem organ failure involving the cardiovascular, pulmonary, and renal systems. Cardiovascular complications also may occur from bleeding or angina. Respiratory complications can be as mild as hypoxemia and pleural effusions, to as severe as pneumonia and adult respiratory distress syndrome. Renal failure occurs from hypotension, dehydration, and acute tubular necrosis. Sterile and infected pancreatic and peripancreatic necrotic tissues are seen in severe disease. It is

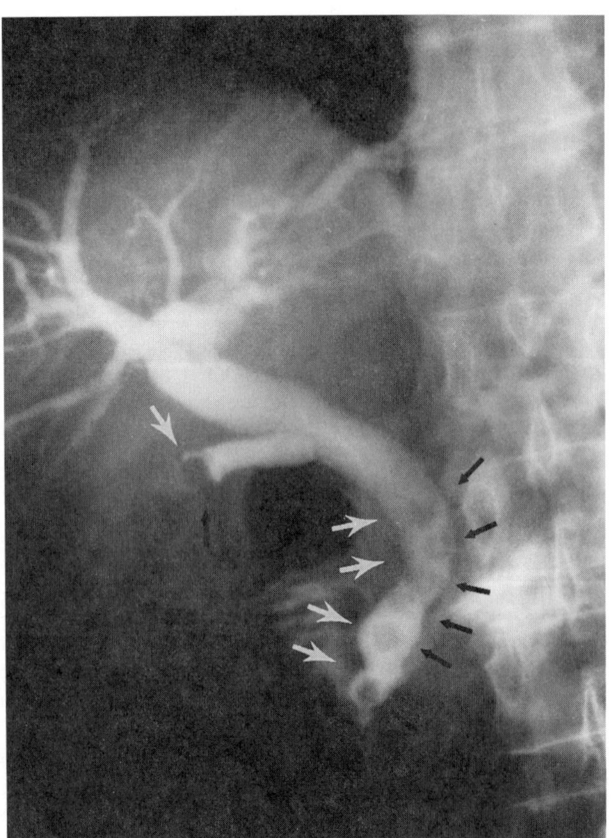

Figure 65-2. ERCP with contrast in common bile duct system, showing multiple common bile duct stones and obstructing cystic duct stone (arrows).

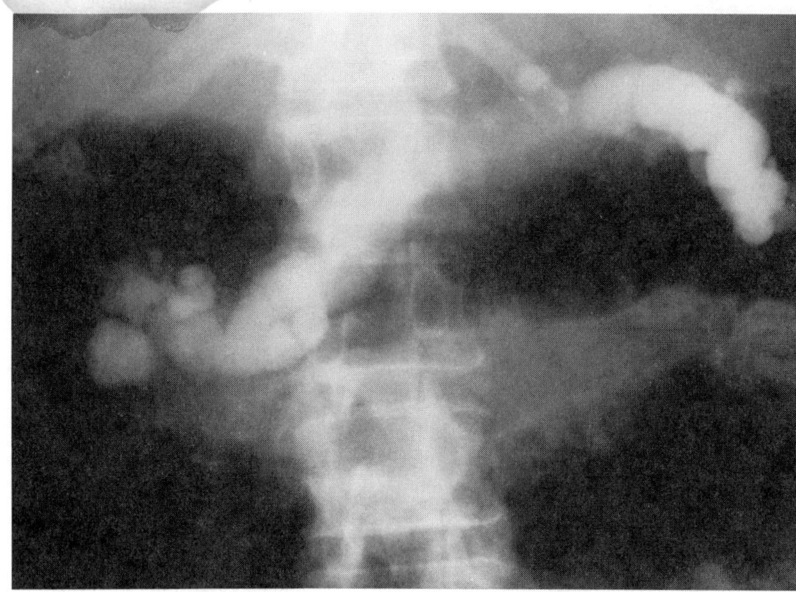

Figure 65-3. ERCP showing markedly dilated, irregular common pancreatic duct system indicative of severe chronic pancreatitis.

difficult to differentiate infected from noninfected necrotic tissue. CT-guided percutaneous aspiration of tissue may identify the two conditions.

Local complications may lead to pseudocysts, phlegmon, or abscesses. Pseudocysts may complicate 1% to 8% of acute pancreatitis cases, and abscesses may complicate 1% to 4% of cases. Appearance of a pancreatic mass on CT may be cystic or solid. Sterile cystic masses are pseudocysts, and infected ones are infected pseudocysts or necrotic abscesses.

Pancreatic ascites is the accumulation of ascitic fluid that occurs as a result of spontaneous decompression of a pseudocyst or direct leakage from pancreatic ductal disruption. The patient experiences increasing abdominal girth and varying degrees of abdominal pain. The diagnosis is based on the finding of an ascitic fluid amylase level in excess of serum amylase levels in an exudative ascites.

Treatment of acute pancreatitis continues to evolve. The mainstay of treatment remains largely supportive. Over 80% of patients have rapid resolution of this inflammatory process and a noncomplicated course. Patients with mild disease are treated by eliminating oral intake, instituting intravenous hydration, and providing frequent parenteral analgesia. Nasogastric suction is not indicated routinely, unless patients have recurrent emesis or ileus. Removal of factors that may have caused the attack, such as drugs or alcohol, is appropriate. Once pain and nausea have subsided and amylase levels have either normalized or significantly decreased, oral intake may begin with liquids and slowly advance to a solid, low fat diet.

The techniques and timing of surgical intervention in mild or severe acute pancreatitis have been clearly demonstrated. Cholecystectomy should be performed early after an attack of biliary pancreatitis to prevent recurrences, ideally during the same admission. If laparoscopic cholecystectomy is to be performed on a patient with suspected choledocholithiasis, preoperative ERCP with sphincterotomy and stone extraction is preferred to performing this procedure postoperatively or to evaluating the common bile duct with intraoperative cholangiogram. This avoids the risk of technical failure with ERCP postoperatively or subjecting the patient to both a laparoscopy and an open cholecystectomy.

Treatment of hyperlipidemic pancreatitis is given by decreasing the serum triglyceride levels to less than 500 mg/dL. Lipid-lowering agents, including appropriate diet therapy, are the main treatment. Large doses of pancreatic enzymes should be administered orally to alleviate abdominal pain symptoms. When triglyceride levels fall below 500 mg/dL, the pancreatic enzymes should be stopped and the patient continued on diet and drug therapy. This treatment is successful in over 85% of cases.

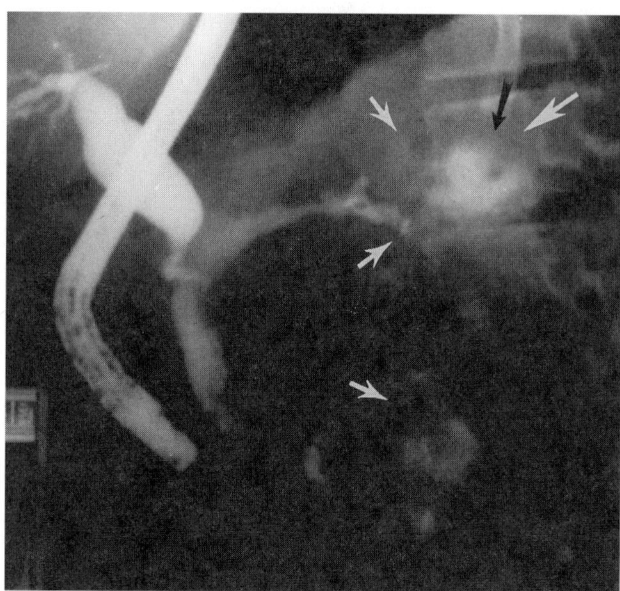

Figure 65-4. ERCP showing dilated, irregular common pancreatic duct system with large pancreatic pseudocyst arising from tail of the pancreas (*arrows*).

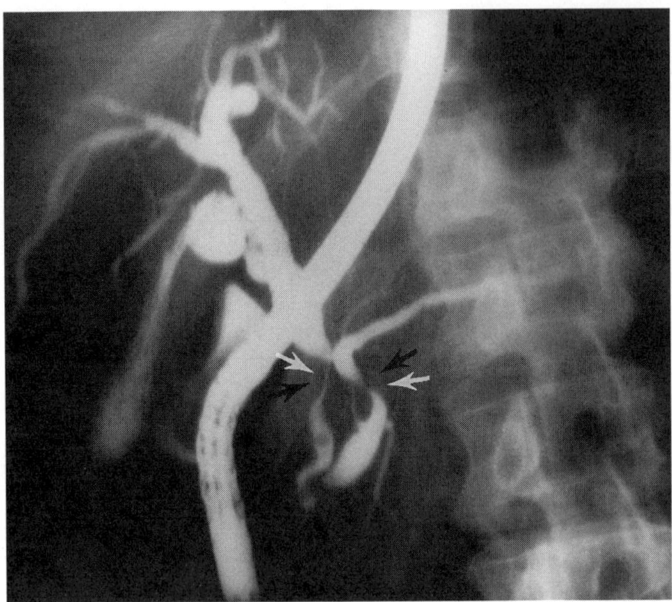

Figure 65-5. ERCP showing the double duct sign, classic for carcinoma of the pancreas, causing partial obstruction in distal common bile duct (*arrows.*)

Severe acute pancreatitis usually requires intensive management of cardiovascular, pulmonary, renal, and septic complications. The role of surgery has become important for the management of necrotizing pancreatitis. The most important single factor that determines poor outcome of patients with pancreatic necrosis is bacterial contamination. This is found in approximately 40% of patients. Prophylactic antibiotics have not played any useful role in the prevention of septic complications. Antibiotics are started in patients with spiking fevers awaiting surgical consultation and intervention. Traditionally indicated procedures include the following: exploration in patients with an acute abdomen; removal of impacted gallstones from the common bile duct, along with the gallbladder; drainage of pancreatic fluid collections; and debridement of necrotic tissue. Although interventional radiologists can drain an infected collection of fluid, surgical drainage usually is more successful. Various operations have been proposed, including pancreatic resection and necrosectomy with closed drainage, or open drainage with debridement. Peritoneal lavage for treatment of severe necrotizing pancreatitis is controversial and not commonly employed. Somatostatin as a treatment modality is equally controversial. Gastroenterology and surgical consultations should be requested early during the initial hospitalization.

Table 65-3. Ranson Criteria for Determining Severity of Pancreatitis

Signs on Admission	Age older than 55 y
	WBC > 16000 mm^3
	Serum glucose > 200 mg/dL
	Serum LDH > 350 IU/L
	AST > 250 IU/L
Signs During First 48 h	Fall in hematocrit >10%
	BUN rise > 5 mg%
	Serum calcium < 8 mg%
	Base deficit > 4 mEq/L
	Estimated fluid sequestration > 6 L
	Arterial PO_2 < 60 mm Hg
Predicted Mortality	2 or fewer signs, 1%
	3–4 signs, 15%
	5–6 signs, 40%
	> 6 signs, 100%

WBC, white blood cell count; *LDH,* lactate dehydrogenase; *BUN,* blood urea nitrogen; *AST,* aspartate aminotransferase;

Considerations in Pregnancy

Gallstone diseases and pancreatitis often are linked with pregnancy. There may be a strong suggestion that pregnancy is a potential predisposing factor. Seventy percent to 80% of gallstones in the United States are composed of at least 50% cholesterol. Pregnancy progesterone levels have been implicated in altering gallbladder motility and biliary lipid composition. Studies are too limited, and no firm conclusions can be derived. The symptoms of pancreatitis in pregnant patients tend to be similar to those in nonpregnant women. Differential diagnosis in pregnancy is varied. It includes acute viral hepatitis, acute alcoholic hepatitis, acute cholecystitis, duodenal ulcers, pulmonary embolism, pneumonia, acute appendicitis, acute fatty liver of pregnancy, and preeclampsia.

Ultrasound of the abdomen has greatly improved the ability to diagnose. Accuracy is not diminished by pregnancy. In difficult clinical situations, particularly late in pregnancy, radionuclide scanning also is helpful. There is general agreement that the occurrence of acute pancreatitis is more likely during the third trimester. Fetal loss may occur in 10% to 20% of cases of pancreatitis and pregnancy. Maternal mortality may reach 3% to 4% in severe cases. Pancreatis caused by drugs, hyperlipidemia, or idiopathic reasons behaves the same in pregnant patients as in nonpregnant

Table 65-4. Complications of Acute Pancreatitis

Local
Necrosis of sterile tissue or infected tissue
Pancreatic fluid collections forming pseudocysts or abscesses
Gastrointestinal hemorrhage from ulcers, varices, or gastritis
Splenic rupture or hematoma
Systemic
Shock
Coagulopathy
Respiratory failure
Acute renal failure
Hyperglycemia
Hypocalcemia
Subcutaneous nodules
Psychosis

patients. Measurement of amylase and lipase levels remain the cornerstone of diagnosis.

The management of patients with acute pancreatitis during pregnancy is supportive, just as it is for nonpregnant patients. Most patients with gallstone pancreatitis can be managed successfully with elective cholecystectomy after delivery. However, cholecystectomy can be safely done during pregnancy. Endoscopic papillotomy and removal of common bile duct stones can be accomplished with limited sedation and radiation exposure by experienced endoscopists. Metabolic causes are treated with drug and diet therapy. If alcohol or drugs are the cause of the pancreatitis, these should be eliminated.

CHRONIC PANCREATITIS

Chronic pancreatitis is a chronic inflammatory process of the pancreas that eventually destroys the gland and causes exocrine and endocrine dysfunction of the pancreas. The prevalence or incidence of this condition is unknown.

Etiology

The most common cause of chronic pancreatitis worldwide is excessive and prolonged alcohol ingestion. It accounts for over 75% of the cases. Other causes are hyperlipidemia, congenital predispositions, neoplasia, trauma, hyperparathyroidism, cystic fibrosis, and idiopathic. Gallstones do not cause chronic pancreatitis.

Physical Examination and Clinical Findings

Alcohol has direct toxicity to the acinar cells of the pancreas. It causes glandular inflammation, changes secretory function, increases enzyme production, and increases protein production, which eventually causes protein plugs. Calcification of the pancreas is a classic manifestation of chronic pancreatitis and is seen more often in alcoholic chronic pancreatitis than in the idiopathic or metabolic variety. Cancer of the pancreas, most often ductal in origin, can mimic the pain and glandular destruction of chronic pancreatitis. This condition must be ruled out before treating chronic pancreatitis, especially in patients older than 40 years of age. Chronic alcoholic pancreatitis is rare in patients older than 60 years of age.

Loss of acinar tissue causes loss of secretion, but most of the gland must be destroyed before clinical manifestation of pancreatic insufficiency occurs. Fat malabsorption occurs, with malabsorption of other nutrients and important vitamins. Vitamin B_{12} deficiency is common in chronic pancreatitis. Diabetes mellitus results from endocrine dysfunction and from deficient insulin and glucagon secretion.

Pain is usually the first and the main symptom. It is characterized by recurrent attacks of upper abdominal pain. These attacks progress in frequency until pancreatic fibrosis sets in. Painless chronic pancreatitis in alcoholics is rare, but it is common in chronic pancreatitis of nonalcoholic causes. Patients may present first with fat malabsorption, weight loss, or diabetes. Several theories are available to explain the cause of pain. Pseudocysts of the pancreas developing after a bout of acute pancreatitis may be a cause of abdominal pain. Significant pain relief is achieved in most of these patients after surgical drainage. This supports the cause-and-effect relationship between pancreatic hypertension and pain. There can also be increased vascular resistance and poor blood flow, which can cause ischemia within the gland. The ischemia causes abdominal pain. Intrapancreatic nerves also can be involved in the inflammatory process of chronic pancreatitis.

Family history of chronic pancreatitis and social history of chronic alcohol ingestion and smoking should be sought. The physical examination is usually unreliable because stigmata of chronic pancreatitis, such as malabsorption and weight loss, seldom exist until most of the gland is destroyed.

Laboratory and Imaging Studies

Stool examination for qualitative and quantitative fat loss is a sensitive test of chronic pancreatitis. The findings of neutral fat in the stool is suggestive of pancreatic disease. Muscle fibers can be found in the stool along with fat. A loss of more than 7 g of fecal fat per day on a challenge of 100 g of dietary fat is the most sensitive and specific test of chronic pancreatitis and pancreatic insufficiency.

Investigations ordered in patients with chronic pancreatitis must probe functional and structural components of this disorder. Both exocrine and endocrine functions should be measured. Serum amylase and lipase levels are usually normal, mildly elevated, or even lower in chronic pancreatitis compared with acute pancreatitis.

Several other tests are available to measure pancreatic insufficiency but are not widely used. These include serum trypsin levels, bentiromide screening test, hormone levels (cholecystokinin, secretin, cerulein), stimulation of pancreatic secretion with duodenal collection of juice, pancreatic polypeptide levels, fecal chymotrypsin, and triolein breath test.

Structural damage to the pancreas can be detected by radiographic studies. Plain abdominal films may detect pancreatic calcifications in about 20% of cases. Abdominal ultrasound, CT, and ERCP have been widely used as diagnostic imaging studies. Ultrasound has a 60% sensitivity whereas CT has a 75% sensitivity. ERCP may diagnose the condition in 85% of cases. It can also unearth ductal abnormalities, pancreatic stones, pancreatic pseudocysts, and pancreatic cancer (see Figs. 65-3 through 65-5). ERCP is also useful for collecting cytologic and biopsy specimens and, at the same time, therapeutic options like stent placement can be exercised. Fine-needle aspirate of the pancreas under ultrasound on CT guidance may assist the diagnosis, especially if malignant cells can be found. Magnetic resonance imaging of the pancreas is not well defined and is not used widely.

Treatment

Treatment goals in chronic pancreatitis include pain relief, correcting fat malabsorption and nutritional deficiencies, preventing complications, and eventually changing the clinical course of the disease. Oral pancreatic enzyme supplementation (trypsin and lipase) are the mainstay of the treatment program. Endocrine insufficiency, like diabetes, is treated with diet modifications and insulin therapy. Significant pain relief may be obtained by negative feedback inhibition from enzyme and hormonal therapy. The response rate is variable, because large ductal disease does not respond as well as small ductal disease. Supplemental enzyme therapy certainly reduces steatorrhea. Failure of this treatment should cause serious rethinking and rediagnosis.

Conventional pancreatic enzymes can be destroyed by gastric acids. Large doses given to deliver sufficient enzymes may cause side effects such as nausea, gas, bloating, and abdominal pain. Newer pancreatic enzyme supplements are especially coated to withstand gastric pH. They also contain enough trypsin and lipase to reduce the daily intake for better compliance. Creon and Pancrease of various strengths are now widely used. The former is an enteric-coated microtablet, and the latter has a timed-release formula.

Pain should not be managed by chronic narcotics. Addiction needs to be avoided, especially in alcoholics. Severe pain and weight loss may prompt prolonged hospitalization and parenteral nutrition. Celiac plexus block by topical anesthetics or neurotoxins has been reported to be successful for pain control. This is particularly useful in inoperable pancreatic carcinomas. Endoscopic therapy has been used to reduce interductal pressure. Promising results are being reported by placing stents through diseased pancreatic ducts for better drainage. Chronic pancreatitis from pancreatic divisum is being treated by placing stents through minor papilla.

Several different surgical options are available in suitable, selected chronic pancreatitis patients, encompassing various drainage procedures. Imaging studies, including CT and ERCP, are mandatory before surgery. When the pancreatic duct is dilated, lateral pancreaticojejunostomy, known as modified Puestow procedure, is the likely choice. It provides relief of symptoms in over 80% of patients. When the pancreatic duct is narrow or nondilated with chronic pancreatitis, pancreatic resections are considered. Various types of pancreatic resections have been designed, depending on the results of pancreatography studies. Diabetes is a likely result after total or subtotal pancreatectomy. These operations are difficult, hence, they should be done by experienced surgeons.

Patients with human immunodeficiency virus–positive serologic findings who have alcohol- or drug-induced chronic pancreatitis pose special management problems. Various other gastrointestinal manifestations of AIDS may be present with overlapping symptoms and signs. Conservative management is favored due to the overall poor prognosis of AIDS.

BIBLIOGRAPHY

Agarwal H, Pitchumoni CS, Sivaprasad AV. Evaluating tests for acute pancreatitis. Am J Gastroenterol 1990;85:356.

Calleja G, Barkin J. Acute pancreatitis. Med Clin North Am 1993;77:1037.

Hodgdon AK, Wolfson AB. Pancreatitis. Emerg Med Clin North Am 1990;8:873.

Holt S. Chronic pancreatitis. South Med J 1993;86:201.

Holt S. Management of chronic pancreatitis. Compr Ther 1994;20:24.

Malfertheiner P, Dominguez-Munoz JE, Bichler MW. Chronic pancreatitis: management of pain. Digestion 1994;55:29.

Meyer P, Calvien PA, Robert J, et al. Role of imaging techniques in the classification of acute pancreatitis. Dig Dis 1992;10:330.

Scott L. Gallstone disease and pancreatitis in pregnancy. Gastroenterol Clin North Am 1992;21:803.

Steinbert W. Predictors of severity of acute pancreatitis. Gastroenterol Clin North Am 1990;19:849.

Steinberg W, Tenner S. Acute pancreatitis. N Engl J Med 1994;330:1198.

Toskes P. Hyperlipidemic pancreatitis. Gastroenterol Clin North Am 1990;19:783.

Underwood TW, Faye CB. Drug-induced pancreatitis. Clin Pharmacol 1993;12:440.

Ventrucci M. Update on laboratory diagnosis and prognosis of acute pancreatitis. Dig Dis 1993;11:189.

66

Gastroenteritis and Diarrheal Diseases

MATTHEW R. MOOG
ASHOK N. SHAH

Primary Care for Women, edited by Phyllis C. Leppert and Fred M. Howard. Lippincott-Raven Publishers, Philadelphia © 1997.

INTRODUCTION

The term *gastroenteritis* describes a broad range of infectious and noninfectious disorders of the alimentary tract, primarily involving the stomach, small intestine, colon, and rectum. Gastroenteritis is typically a brief, self-limited disease that presents commonly in the primary care setting and does not usually require hospitalization. The most common symptom is diarrhea, but patients may also present with nausea, vomiting, dehydration, fever, bloody stools, anorexia, tenesmus, myalgias, and crampy abdominal pain. This discussion concentrates on infectious diarrhea, the most common of the gastroenteritides.

Oral rehydration is usually the only treatment needed for the management of infectious diarrhea, although persistent and severe cases may warrant intravenous fluids, antimotility agents, and antibiotic therapy. The primary risk in pregnancy is wasting of the fetus in utero and spontaneous abortion due to maternal dehydration and electrolyte imbalances. The bacterial, viral, and protozoal organisms which cause infectious diarrhea are not known to be teratogenic. Unfortunately, the toxicities of many antimicrobial agents to the mother, fetus, and newborn limit the number of options available in treating the pregnant patient.

ETIOLOGY

Bacterial Gastroenteritis

The severity of bacterial gastroenteritis depends on several host defense factors and the virulence of the organism. Hygiene is one of the most important of the host defenses because a large inoculum is required for the transmission of most pathogenic bacteria. Most enteric bacterial infections are acquired via the fecal-oral route and appear to be sensitive to the acidic environment of the stomach. Use of antacid therapy, H_2-receptor blockers, or an achlorhydric state from other causes may compromise this barrier. A decrease in intestinal transit time is another factor that may impair clearance of pathogens from the small bowel. Defective bowel motility can predispose to bacterial overgrowth and infection. Decreased transit time may also inhibit water and sodium reabsorption. The normal anaerobic bowel flora appear to have a protective effect that is reduced by abnormal bowel motility and previous antibiotic use. Immunity is also important to host defense, because passively acquired antibodies in the early neonate may be protective against many agents. Antibodies and other protective factors may pass to the newborn through breast-feeding.

The virulence of the pathogen may also determine the severity of the illness. Virulence may come from various toxins produced by enteric pathogens or from tissue invasion and destruction. For example, cholera can activate secretory mechanisms and lead to profuse, watery diarrhea through the action of enterotoxins. This may be mediated by the adenylate cyclase-cyclic AMP pathway. Enterotoxins may also stimulate emesis as well as inhibit water and sodium absorption. Cytotoxins are associated with the bloody, dysenteric stools produced in shigellosis, and are thought to aid in disruption and invasion of the bowel surface. Preformed neurotoxins, such as those from *Clostridium botulinum* and *Staphylococcus aureus,* may rapidly lead to neurologic symptoms including emesis, meningismus, paresthesias, paralysis, and even seizure activity. Various other properties may increase the virulence of a pathogen, including bowel wall adherence, attachment, and direct invasion.

Invasive Bacteria

Invasive enteric bacteria cause infection by mucosal penetration of the large bowel and terminal ileum. This leads to disruption of the mucosal surface and invasion of the lamina propria. These bacteria may cause diarrhea for several reasons, including toxin production, malabsorption from mucosal surface damage, and prostaglandin synthesis. The patient typically presents with bloody diarrhea that is mixed with pus and mucus, known as dysentery. This syndrome typically includes symptoms of lower abdominal and rectal pain or tenesmus. There is less stool output than found in the profuse, watery noninvasive diarrheas. Red blood cells and leukocytes are typically found on examination of the stool. Proctoscopic exam typically reveals rectal ulceration with a hemorrhagic, friable mucosal surface. In all cases of dysentery, narcotics and medications that impair intestinal motility are contraindicated due to the risks of abscess formation, toxic megacolon, and perforation.

Shigella sonnei causes most of the invasive bacterial diarrhea in the United States, estimated at up to 80% of known cases. More severe infections are seen in developing countries with the strains *Shigella dysenteriae* and *Shigella flexneri.* This disease tends to occur in the winter months in developed countries and the summer months in the tropics. It attacks children more often than adults and is easily spread from person to person with a very small inoculum. *Shigella* enterotoxin affects the small bowel, which causes watery diarrhea at first. *Shigella* bacillus then superficially invades the distal small intestine and colon producing clinical dysentery.

The incubation period of shigellosis is typically 3 days to over a week. Symptoms in uncomplicated cases may last for up to 12 days. The patient may initially complain of high fever, malaise, and headache, associated with severe abdominal cramps and watery diarrhea. After a few days, the complaints are of frequent episodes of small caliber, bloody stools, associated with severe rectal burning pains. This condition is always self-limited and bacteremia is rare, so transmission across the placenta to the fetus is unlikely. This infection may infrequently become chronic and relapsing.

The treatment of bacillary dysentery from *Shigella* includes oral rehydration and supportive measures, but antibiotic therapy may be warranted in moderate-to-severe cases. Ampicillin and trimethoprim-sulfamethoxazole have been used to treat this organism, but quinolone antibiotics such as ciprofloxacin or norfloxacin may be warranted in particularly resistant cases. Mild symptoms may persist for several days despite adequate antibiotic therapy, probably due to damage to the mucosa. In the pregnant patient with only mild symptoms, antibiotics should be avoided and supportive therapy given. Of the recommended antibiotics, ampicillin is the only one that has not shown significant risk to the developing fetus or breast-feeding neonate. It should be noted that Shigella has maintained high rates of resistance to this antibiotic.

Salmonellosis is caused by a group of hundreds of enteric bacilli that are typically gastrointestinal pathogens. They can be spread by food, water, or human waste, or transmitted via the fecal-oral route. Salmonellosis tends to occur in the first year of life and in the elderly. Unlike *Shigella,* this organism chiefly causes invasion of the ileum, which can lead to lymphatic invasion and bacteremia by penetration to the lamina propria. Hematogenous dissemination of *Salmonella* may present as several syndromes, including bacteremia with various localized infections and typhoidal or enteric fever that is seen with infection by *Salmonella typhi* and *Salmonella paratyphi* strains.

The typical case of *Salmonella* gastroenteritis requires an incubation time from 6 hours up to several days. The symptoms of nausea, vomiting, periumbilical cramps, diarrhea, and sometimes fever may last for up to 4 or 5 days. Salmonellosis most commonly presents as a mild syndrome with watery diarrhea, but stools may also have the gross appearance of dysentery. In the rare chronic carrier state, stool cultures may remain positive for over a year.

Most cases of salmonellosis should not be treated with antibiotics due to high rates of resistance. There has been no proven reduction in the duration of the diarrhea after antibiotics. Therapy is indicated only in the elderly or in patients with certain complicating conditions: immunosuppression, malignancies, cardiovascular abnormalities, prosthetics, or hemolytic anemia. Ampicillin or trimethoprim-sulfamethoxazole may be used if the particular strain shows susceptibility, but ciprofloxacin has been effective with low rates of resistance or relapse. Antibiotics may also be indicated in the pregnant patient with positive blood cultures, fever, or a septic appearance. If antibiotics are to be considered in this case, ampicillin or ceftriaxone are the drugs of choice. Sulfa drugs including trimethoprim-sulfamethoxazole can lead to jaundice in the fetus and the breast-fed newborn. Fluoroquinolones should also be avoided because of teratogenic effects.

The findings of persistent salmonellosis with bacteremia, fever, splenomegaly, abdominal pain, and delirium herald typhoid fever, which is caused by *S typhi* and several other strains. This condition is extremely rare with good sanitation, but may be spread by contaminated food and water. These organisms primarily attack the small intestine with immediate lymphatic penetration and bacteremia. Hematogenous dissemination may lead to localized infection at multiple distant organ sites. Further involvement of the bowel wall may lead to disruption of vessels and hemorrhage, or even intestinal perforation.

S typhi usually requires a 1- to 2-week incubation period, and can lead to a 4-week course that begins with headache, fever, and abdominal pain. These symptoms may be followed by splenomegaly and a characteristic rash. Delirium may be seen. Hematogenous spread may result in multiple organ infections. The carrier state is extremely common, because up to half of all typhoid patients may continue to shed viable organisms in the stool. Before the advent of antimicrobial therapy, untreated typhoid fever was associated with increased maternal deaths, spontaneous abortions, and premature deliveries. This infection still poses some risk of maternal-to-fetal transmission despite antibiotic therapy.

Resistance to many antibiotics has been found, so therapy should be guided by susceptibility data. The drugs of choice include ciprofloxacin, ceftriaxone, cefoperazone, and trimethoprim-sulfamethoxazole. A wide range of antibiotics have also been proven effective against sensitive organisms, including ampicillin, amoxicillin, and chloramphenicol. Steroids should be used only in cases of severe sepsis.

The most common strain of *Campylobacter* is *Campylobacter jejuni*, which is transmitted by the fecal-oral route in humans. It may be responsible for approximately 10% of all diarrheal illness in the United States. *Campylobacter* produces a colitis with a typical incubation time of 1 to 3 days. Cases commonly last 1 week but may continue past 2 weeks, and may have a relapsing course if incompletely treated. Patients may present with multiple constitutional complaints, followed by fevers and diarrhea that initially improve, then worsen. Symptoms of severe abdominal pain, tenesmus, and stools with blood and pus may occur. Vomiting is much less common with this infection.

Mild campylobacteriosis does not appear to benefit from antibiotics. Ciprofloxacin is of benefit in treating *Campylobacter*, although resistance has been found. Erythromycin has been effective in culture-proven cases when used within the first 3 days of the clinical presentation. Clindamycin, gentamicin, and doxycycline also have been shown to be effective alternatives. Pregnant women with IgA deficiency are at an increased risk of spontaneous abortion with this infection. Treatment of the pregnant patient with fluoroquinolones, aminoglycosides, and doxycycline poses risk of teratogenic side effects. Erythromycins, other than erythromycin estolate, and clindamycin appear to pose less risk if needed in serious cases.

Yersinia enterocolitica may cause a mild gastroenteritis but can also result in frank dysentery. This organism is more common in developed nations outside the United States, where it is seen in foodborne outbreaks. *Yersinia* causes inflammation and invasion of the mucosa and lamina propria, primarily within the ileum and colon. Some strains may also cause diarrheal symptoms by the elaboration of enterotoxin. This syndrome is quite variable and has been found to last from 24 hours up to several weeks. Most cases of yersiniosis present with typical symptoms of gastroenteritis, but nausea and vomiting are less common. *Yersinia bacteremia* occurs rarely in cases where patients have concurrent chronic diseases. Some cases may present in a manner very similar to acute appendicitis. This infection also has a rare association with migratory polyarthritis and erythema nodosum.

Antibiotics have not been shown to decrease the duration of the gastrointestinal symptoms, but may be indicated in particularly severe infections. In these cases, the drug of choice is a third-generation parenteral cephalosporin, combined with an antipseudomonal aminoglycoside. Doxycycline is an alternative, but amino glycosides are teratogenic.

Enteroinvasive *Escherichia coli* and enterohemorrhagic *E coli* represent two pathogenic forms of *E coli* that cause bloody diarrhea. Enteroinvasive *E coli* is relatively rare and difficult to isolate in the United States. Enterohemorrhagic *E coli* has typically been seen with foodborne outbreaks. This organism causes dysenteric stools with crampy abdominal pain, but no fever. Patients with this infection may present less commonly with hemolytic-uremic syndrome or thrombotic thrombocytopenic purpura. There is no clear evidence showing antibiotic therapy to be of benefit with these infections.

Noninvasive Bacteria

The noninvasive enteric bacteria colonize the upper small intestine without mucosal penetration or bacteremia. These organisms attach to the mucosal surface and elaborate a toxin that activates adenylate cyclase, producing cyclic AMP. This mechanism causes increased secretion of fluid and electrolytes, resulting in diarrhea. Clinically, these organisms cause midabdominal pain with a profuse, watery stool output. Alternatively, these organisms may cause disease by a process of altering the capacity of the villus to perform its normal absorptive function. Fecal blood and leukocytes are not generally seen with this noninflammatory diarrhea. The most common complication of this process is dehydration.

Several *E coli* strains, including enteropathogenic, enterotoxigenic, and enteroadherent subtypes, may cause a noninvasive infectious diarrhea. Enteropathogenic *E coli* attacks by adherence to the mucosal wall and causes cellular structural changes. It typically occurs as a watery diarrhea in newborns and children. Clinically, this disease may appear with fever and abdominal pain as well. Enterotoxigenic *E coli* causes colonization of the upper small bowel followed by the elaboration of toxins that activate the adenylate cyclase pathway and cause watery diarrhea. This infection is most common in children of underdeveloped nations, who may be the primary source of infection to adult travelers in the Third World. This strain appears to be the most common cause of traveler's diarrhea. The incubation period is 24 to 48 hours, and the clinical course is otherwise unremarkable. Enteroadherent *E coli* attaches to the mucosal surface and colonizes the upper small bowel. It is also found most commonly in young children in undeveloped nations. There is no conclusive evidence that the course of these self-limited conditions can be decreased with antibiotics.

S aureus is a common cause of food poisoning, second only to *Salmonella* in frequency. A large infectious dose of the staphylococcal endotoxin is required to cause a clinical case of gastroenteritis. This infection has an incubation period of 1 to 6 hours and is associated with significant nausea and vomiting, abdominal pain, and explosive, watery diarrhea. The typical duration of this disease is 8 to 24 hours. Intravenous fluids may be necessary in the pregnant patient because oral rehydration will likely be impossible. This disorder is self limited, and there is no effective antibiotic regimen.

Clostridium perfringens is the next most common cause of food poisoning syndromes after *Salmonella* and *Staphylococcus*. This organism must be ingested in a large dose, usually in improperly cooked meat, to cause infection. It is believed to be mediated by in vivo production of an enterotoxin that acts at the ileum, causing superficial damage to the mucosa. This infection is marked by abdominal cramps and loose stools typical of noninvasive diarrheas. Symptoms may begin from several hours to a day after the infected food is consumed and last 12 to 36 hours at most. Nausea, vomiting, and fever are not common features. No antibiotic treatment is typically indicated due to the short-lived nature of this illness. Oral rehydration is generally sufficient in the pregnant patient.

Aeromonas is typically spread by the consumption of contaminated water during the summer. This organism has been found to produce a chronic diarrheal syndrome in adults, lasting up to several weeks. Because of high rates of resistance, antibiotic therapy should only be considered in cases of culture-proven infection with chronic diarrhea.

Vibrio cholerae, the bacterium that causes cholera, is extremely rare in the United States and other developed nations. The organism is virulent and in some cases is known to cause death within several hours after infection. Symptoms may begin up to 72 hours after infection and last for 2 to 12 days. Cholera may present with symptoms of nausea, vomiting, and bloating that progress to massive volumes of explosive, watery diarrhea, dehydration, electrolyte abnormalities, and shock. The watery stool of cholera does not contain leukocytes or blood. Fever is not typically seen in this disease. Cholera can be treated with fluid replacement, correction of electrolyte abnormalities, and antibiotic therapy. Antibiotics used in this disease have included doxycycline, norfloxacin, and alternatively, trimethoprim-sulfamethoxazole. Special care should be taken in the treatment of pregnant women because all these agents have teratogenic potential.

Vibrio parahaemolyticus is rarely seen in the United States, except in coastal areas, but is more common in the Far East and Japan, where it is contracted by eating raw seafood. This organism causes illness by enterotoxin production as well as by tissue invasion. The incubation period varies from several hours to 2 days, and the typical duration of symptoms is 3 to 10 days. Symptoms are quite similar to those of cholera and may include headache and fever. Dysentery may also be seen, associated with proctitis from superficial ulceration. Antibiotics have not been shown to be of benefit in this short-lived infection, though doxycycline and fluoroquinolones have been used in severe cases.

Bacillus cereus is a rare cause of food-borne gastroenteritis that may appear as either a vomiting or diarrheal illness, depending on the particular toxin produced. No clear proof has demonstrated that human transmission is a factor in this disease, and strains of this bacteria have been found in many foods as extremely resistant spores. The vomiting syndrome has an incubation period of only 1 to 6 hours and lasts for 8 to 12 hours. It is self-limited and presents as vomiting with crampy abdominal pain. Diarrhea is less common. The incubation of the diarrheal illness, on the other hand, may require over 12 hours. Symptoms may last for 24 to 36 hours. The clinical syndrome is usually manifest by watery diarrhea, abdominal cramps, and, more rarely, vomiting. No treatment appears to be indicated.

Viral Gastroenteritis

Viral gastroenteritis is thought to cause up to 40% of the infectious diarrhea in the United States, while another 40% of cases have no clear cause. The etiologic agents in viral diarrhea include Norwalk virus, rotavirus, enteric adenovirus, calcivirus, and astrovirus. Norwalk virus is most clearly associated with food and waterborne outbreaks in adults, whereas the others are more common in children. No fecal leukocytes are typically found on stool exam. All viral gastroenteritides are treated symptomatically with therapy centering on oral rehydration. No teratogenicity has been associated with these viral infections.

Norwalk virus is responsible for up to 40% of the viral outbreaks found in communities and institutional settings in the United States. This infection is generally found only in older youths and adults, and is transmitted by the fecal-oral route. The virus primarily affects the epithelial cells on the surface of small intestinal villi. Changes in cellular morphology, as well as shortening of villous height, probably contribute to malabsorptive symptoms. Also, mucosal digestive enzyme activity is notably diminished, thus impairing absorption of several nutrients. This virus does not appear to cause intestinal fluid secretion by the adenylate cyclase mechanism.

Norwalk virus infection usually causes symptoms within 1 to 2 days. It may present as an acute syndrome of nausea, vomiting, diarrhea, fever, headache, and myalgias that lasts for up to 48 hours. Impaired gastric motility may result, as well as decreased absorption of basic fats and sugars for 1 to 2 weeks after infection. Patients may continue to excrete virus particles for up to 2 days after symptoms resolve.

Rotavirus is the major cause of viral gastroenteritis in children and appears to be responsible for over half of these cases. Most cases of rotaviral diarrhea occur up to 15 months of age, with less frequent and less severe cases seen in adults after contact with an infected child. This infection appears to have a predisposition for the colder months of winter and is most likely spread via the fecal-oral route. The microstructural changes which occur in the small intestine after rotaviral infection are very similar to those seen with Norwalk virus.

Symptoms begin 1 to 3 days after infection with this virus, with the onset of profuse vomiting. The infection typically lasts 1 week, although intestinal epithelial changes have been found to last for 8 weeks. The diagnosis may be made by assays for viral antigens in the stool. Antibodies are produced after infection with this virus and appear to be transferred across the placenta. Newborns appear to be protected by passively acquired maternal antibodies for 3 months after birth.

Enteric adenovirus is the second most common cause of gastroenteritis in children after rotavirus. It has a longer incubation period. This adenovirus is not associated with upper respiratory or coryza symptoms. The infection is typically found in children under 1 year of age and is rarely seen in adults. Diarrhea may appear over a week after infection and lasts 5 days to over 2 weeks. This symptom may be accompanied by vomiting and fever.

Calcivirus is an uncommon cause of pediatric infectious diarrhea, representing less than 3% of cases. This virus may also be transmitted to adults from infected children. Symptoms may appear within 72 hours of infection, with a clinical syndrome very similar to that of other viral gastroenteridites.

Astrovirus is found in infants and children up to age 7, as well as in the very elderly. The clinical syndrome is unremarkable, with a predominant symptom of loose, watery stools. It may appear up to 48 hours after infection and may last 3 days or longer.

DIARRHEAL SYNDROMES

Traveler's Diarrhea

Traveler's diarrhea is the predominant illness found among international travelers. Symptoms of traveler's diarrhea may be significant, but the mortality rate is extremely low. The highest risk of contracting this disease exists for international travelers to Africa, the Middle East, Latin America, and Southeast Asia. Less risk is found in travelers to Israel, the Caribbean, and Southern Europe. The highest rates of infection are seen in patients in their 20s, with decreased occurrence noted after age 55. The risk of contracting traveler's diarrhea increases substantially after 2 weeks of travel.

Traveler's diarrhea is typically spread by contaminated food and beverages. The highest risk is associated with improperly cooked meats, seafood, and vegetables. Local water, ice, fruits, and dairy products may also cause infection.

Bacterial sources may account for up to 80% of identified cases, although 40% of cases worldwide remain unidentified. Enterotoxigenic *E coli*, *Shigella*, *Aeromonas*, and *Salmonella* are the most common etiologic agents, typically found during the warm, rainy season. The drier, colder season brings an increase in campylobacteriosis. Viruses most commonly associated with traveller's diarrhea include Norwalk virus and rotavirus.

Traveler's diarrhea may present with as little as three loose stools within 24 hours, from 2 to 10 days after international travel, although cases have been reported up to a month later. The typical case lasts 1 to 5 days, with less than 1% requiring hospitalization. Watery, noninflammatory diarrhea may be found in association with abdominal cramps, gas, fatigue, tenesmus, and anorexia. Nausea, vomiting, and low-grade fevers are less common and occur in up to a third of traveler's diarrhea patients. Dysentery, which is present in up to 10% of cases, may suggest shigellosis.

Therapy for traveler's diarrhea includes rehydration, antisecretory and antimotility agents, and antibiotics. Oral rehydration is usually recommended as the best therapy, typically with a hypotonic, glucose-based solution. Antisecretory medications such as bismuth subsalicylate and loperamide have been found to decrease the frequency of diarrhea episodes by 50%. Antimotility agents are not recommended in cases with fever or dysentery.

Antibiotics should be used carefully in this syndrome, with particular attention to adverse drug effects. The bacterial causes of traveler's diarrhea carry a high degree of resistance, and antibiotics may select out more virulent organisms. Antibiotic therapy should be considered after several diarrheal stools are reported, or with continued symptoms after other measures have failed. Trimethoprim-sulfamethoxazole or a fluoroquinolone may reduce a typical course to only a few hours or a day. A single dose of norfloxacin or ciprofloxacin may be sufficient. Paralytic ileus and abdominal distension are possible complications when antimotility agents are combined with fluoroquinolone antibiotics.

Prophylactic therapy should be used only when there is a substantial risk of complications from infection. Antibiotics are contraindicated in pregnancy, and pregnant women should be treated with rehydration only. Nonprescription, nonabsorbed medications including attapulgite may be considered in noninflammatory cases.

Food Poisoning

The risk of contracting food-borne infectious gastroenteritis has increased in recent years because of the increase in meals consumed in mass-produced settings. International sources of foodstuffs also place a larger population at risk. The recent trend of ingesting raw meats, raw seafoods, and raw milk products has also led to an increased incidence of food poisoning.

Diagnosis of this infection must be confirmed with at least two similar cases within 72 hours and objective evidence of a common food source. Approximately two thirds of food poisoning cases have been traced to bacterial causes, but protozoal, parasitic, viral, and noninfectious agents have also been implicated. Nonmicrobial agents, including heavy metals, toxins, and chemical poisons, typically cause gastrointestinal symptoms within a few minutes and resolve 3 hours after the onset of emesis. Of the bacterial causes of foodborne gastroenteritis, *Salmonella* has been predominant, linked to about one third of cases of reported food poisoning.

Large-scale waterborne outbreaks of gastroenteritis have been traced most commonly to *Giardia lamblia*. This protozoal illness typically attacks small bowel mucosa without invasion, producing watery diarrhea with increasing abdominal pain, distention, and gas. Untreated giardiasis may present with symptoms of several weeks' duration. *Entamoeba histolytica* and *Cryptosporidium* have also been found in poorly filtered water wells. Amoebiasis usually causes hemorrhagic diarrhea associated with colonic tissue invasion. Bacterial, protozoal, and viral sources have also been found to cause outbreaks in swimming areas with inadequate sanitation.

In the evaluation of cases of suspected food poisoning, once the offending agent has been traced an educated differential diagnosis can be constructed based on the symptom complex and duration. The acute onset of upper gastrointestinal distress with nausea, vomiting, and watery diarrhea within a 6-hour period of consumption is suggestive of a preformed toxin. These cases of diarrhea are usually secondary to *S aureus* or *B cereus*. The nonmicrobial etiologies of acute gastrointestinal distress must also be considered with this brief syndrome.

The onset of watery, noninflammatory diarrhea with generalized abdominal pain or cramps, from 6 hours to 3 days after ingestion, suggests diseases with enterotoxin production in vivo. This may be due to *C perfringens*, enterotoxigenic *E coli*, the diarrheal syndrome of *B cereus*, *G lamblia*, *V cholerae*, and Norwalk virus. Vomiting may or may not result from these infectious agents. Inflammatory diarrhea associated with tenesmus, less stool output, and ulcerated rectal mucosa, found up to 5 days after ingestion, should increase suspicion of infection with the more invasive organisms.

Listeria is a rare cause of food poisoning syndromes and is notable for an extended incubation period of up to 6 weeks. This organism has a high rate of mortality compared with the more common pathogens. It tends to cause a more systemic syndrome with bacteremia, fever, and myalgias and has an increased incidence in pregnant or immunosuppressed patients. Findings of neurologic dysfunction on exam should be investigated for possible neurotoxin poisoning. The differential diagnosis includes seafood toxins, parasite toxins, *Clostridium botulinum* toxin, mushrooms, pesticides, and reactions to monosodium glutamate. All cases of suspected food poisoning must be reported to state and federal health agencies.

AIDS Diarrhea

Over half of all AIDS patients will present with diarrhea at some point in their illness, with much higher rates noted in less developed nations. The differential diagnosis is quite broad in these immunocompromised patients, and diarrhea may result with no apparent cause or from primary infection of the intestinal wall by the HIV organism itself. Viral gastroenteridites are thought to play a significant role, with cytomegalovirus among the most common pathogens in AIDS patients with diarrhea. The other common agents which cause infectious diarrhea in AIDS include cryptosporidium, microsporidium, *E histolytica*, *G lamblia*, *Salmonella*, *Campylobacter*, *Shigella*, *Clostridium difficile*, *Vibrio parahaemolyticus*, and mycobacteriae. AIDS patients may improve with antimicrobial therapy, but will likely have an extended course.

HISTORY, PHYSICAL EXAMINATION, AND CLINICAL FINDINGS

The primary care physician must employ a rational approach to the evaluation of infectious diarrhea, because routine testing and stool cultures do not present a cost-effective solution to this dilemma. Positive test results remain difficult to obtain, making an extensive workup of this self-limited disease difficult to justify in other than severe infections. No etiologic agent is identified in most cases. The following approach is recommended:

1. First, evaluate the time course of the patient's complaints and physical signs of volume depletion. If there are no signs of marked dehydration, begin simple oral rehydration and symptomatic therapy. Most cases of noninvasive diarrhea will be adequately treated with conservative management only.
2. Illness marked by symptoms of dysentery, severe abdominal pain, weight loss, tenesmus, or fever should be investigated further. A detailed history of recent antibiotic exposure, travel experience, eating habits or seafood ingestion, recent illnesses, sexual exposures, and immunosuppression is necessary. A stool smear for fecal leukocyte examination should be obtained. If blood and pus are not grossly apparent in the stool, microscopic evaluation of the stool may reveal an inflammatory etiology for the diarrhea.
3. A noninflammatory stool smear is suggestive of noninvasive bacterial organisms, *G lamblia*, cryptosporidium, and viral disease. Therapy in these cases is generally symptomatic because these illnesses will be of short duration. Further evaluation is warranted only if there is no resolution of symptoms.
4. The appearance of inflammatory cells in the stool smear is suggestive of invasive bacterial disease, *C difficile* enterocolitis, or *E histolytica*. Patients with suspected inflammatory diarrhea or recurrent illness should have routine culture, especially for *Salmonella*, *Shigella*, and *Campylobacter jejuni*. *C difficile* cytotoxin should also be checked in these cases if the patient has recently been on antibiotics. Blood cultures may be checked if the patient is febrile. Empiric antimicrobial therapy may have to be considered in these cases.
5. The presence of blood without discernible leukocytes may suggest infection with enterohemorrhagic *E coli* or with agents that disrupt cellular structure, including *E histolytica* and *C difficile*.
6. Diarrhea of greater than 1 week's duration should be evaluated with stool sampling for ova and parasites, especially when the patient has a history of recent travel or an immunocompromised state. Suspicion of parasitic infection should be evaluated with a stool wet-mount preparation for *G lamblia* and *E histolytica*. Antiparasitic therapy should be tailored to the particular agent in this case.
7. Direct visualization of the gastrointestinal tract with endoscopy or colonoscopy may be necessary in the face of recurrent symptoms and a negative workup. These procedures may distinguish between infectious diarrhea, malabsorption, and colitis from other causes.
8. Finally, noninfectious causes should be considered in cases of prolonged symptoms that do not respond to antibiotics.

TREATMENT

Treatment of infectious gastroenteritis involves rehydration, dietary changes, antimotility agents, and antibiotic therapy in selected situations. The noninvasive organisms, which tend to cause a large-volume diarrhea, lead to dehydration as the reabsorptive capacity of the large intestine is overcome by the fluid loss. The primary method of treatment is oral rehydration.

Oral rehydration is superior to intravenous replacement because this method incurs far fewer complications and can be employed in the outpatient setting. Glucose-containing solutions are best because they take advantage of the coupling of glucose with sodium and water absorption in the enterocytes. Rehydration solutions should approximate plasma electrolyte concentrations as closely as possible. Food-based rehydration solutions, containing various cereals and grains, may also help to decrease the amount of diarrheal stools.

Dietary changes that are recommended in cases of acute infectious gastroenteritis include avoidance of foods that may increase stool output. The most likely offenders include fatty, spicy, and high-fiber foods. Dairy products, alcohol, and caffeinated beverages may stimulate secretory mechanisms and increase stool output. The patient should be encouraged to consume juices, noncarbonated drinks, and soft foods.

Antimotility agents are believed to be effective in the treatment of noninvasive diarrhea but are not recommended in invasive disease or dysentery because of concern over prolonging or exacerbating the illness. These medications have several effects, including decreasing fluid losses, decreasing small intestinal motor activity, and decreasing transit time. Antimotility agents include opiates, loperamide, diphenoxylate, and bismuth subsalicylate. Opiates are believed to both decrease fluid output and increase mucosal fluid reabsorption. Loperamide has been found to bring about significant symptomatic improvement without the side effects of opiates. It works by decreasing intestinal motility and intestinal fluid secretion. It may also increase fluid and electrolyte absorption. Diphenoxylate may also be useful in reducing gut hyperperistalsis. Bismuth subsalicylate improves diarrhea for two reasons: the salicylate moiety has antisecretory effects and the bismuth moiety has antibacterial and antiinflammatory effects. Finally, this medication may reduce enterotoxin activity.

Antibiotics may be indicated in suspected invasive or parasitic diarrheal disease, especially with febrile dysentery. Other indications for antimicrobial therapy may include *C difficile*, traveller's diarrhea, and particularly severe cases of salmonellosis. In cases of noninvasive, watery diarrhea, antibiotic therapy is generally not warranted because these cases tend to be self-limited and show no symptomatic benefit from antibiotics. Antibiotic use is also limited by a high degree of antibiotic resistance among enteric bacteria.

CONSIDERATIONS IN PREGNANCY

Several antimicrobial drugs have potential risk of teratogenicity to the fetus, as well as damage to the breast-feeding newborn. These agents should be considered only in cases where the seriousness of the infection in the pregnant patient outweighs this risk to the fetus.

BIBLIOGRAPHY

Avery ME, Snyder JD. Oral therapy for acute diarrhea: the underused simple solution. N Engl J Med 1990;323:891.

Blacklow NR, Greenberg HB. Viral gastroenteritis. N Engl J Med 1991;325:252.

DuPont HL, Ericsson CD. Prevention and treatment of traveller's diarrhea. N Engl J Med 1993;328:1821.

Eron LJ. Gastrointestinal infections in the pregnant patient. In: Rustgi VK, Cooper JN, eds. Gastrointestinal and hepatic complications in pregnancy. New York: John Wiley & Sons, 1986:46.

Gorbach SL. Infectious diarrhea and bacterial food poisoning. In: Sleisenger MH, Fordtran JS, eds. Gastrointestinal disease: pathophysiology, diagnosis, management, 5th ed. Philadelphia: WB Saunders, 1993:1128.

Guerrant RL, Babak DA. Bacterial and protozoal gastroenteritis. N Engl J Med 1991;325:327.

Guerrant RL. Principles and syndromes of enteric infection. In: Mandell GL, Bennett JE, Dolin R, eds. Principles and practice of infectious diseases, 4th ed. New York: Churchill Livingstone, 1995:945.

Hedberg CW, Osterholm MT. Outbreaks of food-borne and water borne viral gastroenteritis. Clinical Microbiology Reviews 1993;6(3):199.

Park SI, Giannella RA. Approach to the adult patient with acute diarrhea. Gastroenterology Clinics of North America 1993;22(3):483.

Taterka JA, Cuff CF. Viral gastrointestinal infections. Gastroenterology Clinics of North America 1992;21(2):303.

Primary Care for Women, edited by Phyllis C. Leppert and Fred M. Howard. Lippincott-Raven Publishers, Philadelphia © 1997.

67

Inflammatory Bowel Disease

KARIN DUNNIGAN

The term *inflammatory bowel disease* (IBD) encompasses a group of chronic, relapsing disorders of the large and small intestine that includes ulcerative colitis and Crohn disease. The etiology of these diseases is poorly understood, although they may be immunologically mediated with genetic and environmental influences. The clinical and endoscopic features, histology, and response to therapy of ulcerative colitis and Crohn disease often differ, but similarities in geographic, racial, sex, and ethnic distribution and age of onset support the theory that these two disorders are related.

EPIDEMIOLOGY

Inflammatory bowel disease occurs throughout the world, although the incidence depends on geographic location. The high-incidence areas include the United Kingdom, North America, Scandinavia, and northern Europe. Among whites in northern Europe and North America, the incidence of ulcerative colitis ranges from two to 10 cases per 100,000 per year. The incidence of Crohn disease among this same population is one to six cases per 100,000 per year. In central and southern Europe and South Africa, IBD occurs less frequently, whereas in Asia, Africa, and South America it is rare. Jews have a higher incidence of both ulcerative colitis and Crohn disease, and the rates of both are higher in American and European Jews than in Israeli Jews. This evidence supports a genetic component in the etiology of IBD, but also demonstrates that environmental factors are important. In the United States, the incidence of both ulcerative colitis and Crohn disease in African-Americans is one fifth to one half that seen in the white population.

Although they may present at any age, both ulcerative colitis and Crohn disease primarily affect young adults from ages 15 to 35. There is a smaller secondary peak of incidence in the 55-to-65-year-old group. The incidence rates for men and woman are probably similar, although a few studies suggest that women may be more prone to develop some form of IBD. Ulcerative colitis and Crohn disease are found more often in higher socioeconomic populations.

At first glance, it appears as though the incidence of Crohn disease has risen dramatically in the past 30 years, whereas that of ulcerative colitis has changed little. The apparent increase in incidence of Crohn disease may be more representative of greater awareness and better diagnostic techniques. Most believe, however, that in areas such as northern Europe and the United States, where IBD is more common, the incidence of ulcerative colitis has plateaued and that of Crohn disease continues to rise.

One significant difference between those affected by these diseases is the relation of smoking. The incidence of smoking is less among patients with ulcerative colitis than in the general population; among those with Crohn disease, the incidence of smoking is as high, if not higher, than the general population.

About 10% to 20% of patients with IBD have a family member who has either ulcerative colitis or Crohn disease. Most of this association is among first-degree relatives. The incidence of IBD among first-degree relatives of patients with the disease is 30 to 100 times that of the general population. Relatives of patients with Crohn disease have a higher incidence of both Crohn disease and ulcerative colitis. The same holds true for relatives of those with ulcerative colitis. There have been only a few reports of affected, unrelated members of families, such as spouses and adopted children. This pattern suggests that ulcerative colitis and Crohn disease are related diseases and supports a genetic rather than environmental association. There is no clear mendelian pattern of inheritance in these disorders.

ETIOLOGY AND PATHOGENESIS

The etiologies of IBD remain unknown, although theories abound. The pathogenesis of these diseases is probably immunologically mediated, with significant genetic and environmental influences. It is unclear if these disorders are a result of an appropriate immunologic response to an injurious agent, or whether they are a result of an abnormal immune response to a common intraluminal antigen.

IBD is characterized by unrestrained inflammation. The lamina propria is infiltrated with lymphocytes, macrophages, and other cells of the immune system. The specific antigen that triggers the immune response is unknown. Various viruses and bacteria have been proposed as possible candidates. Several studies have looked at strains of *Escherichia coli* and cytomegalovirus as possible agents in ulcerative colitis, and *Mycobacterium paratuberculosis* or paramyxovirus as a cause of Crohn disease, but conclusive evidence is lacking. Potential dietary antigens, such as milk protein and sugar, have also been examined as possible triggers. Results of studies have been conflicting, and there has been no consistent finding relating the ingestion of particular foods to the development of IBD of either type.

Some evidence suggests that patients with IBD have either an impairment in down-regulation of inflammation or an alteration in mucosal host defense mechanisms. The normal intraluminal contents of the bowel can activate immune cells with subsequent tissue damage. Intact intestinal mucosal defenses, as well as normal immunoregulatory mechanisms, prevent this from occurring. Defects in epithelial defense mechanisms or in immunoregulation, possibly genetically determined, would allow normal intraluminal contents to lead to uncontrolled immune activation and subsequent tissue destruction.

Numerous substances that are mediators of inflammation have been identified, and many probably play a role in the clinical expression of IBD. Prostaglandins and leukotrienes, both products of the metabolism of arachidonic acid, have been found in increased amounts in the intestinal mucosa of patients with IBD, as have platelet activating factor and thromboxane A_2, interleukins, tissue necrosis factor, and interferon. In addition, neuropeptides, complement, bradykinin, reactive oxygen metabolites, and cleavage products of the coagulation factors may play a role in the development of IBD.

CLINICAL FEATURES

Ulcerative Colitis

Ulcerative colitis is an inflammatory disorder involving the rectum that extends proximally to involve a variable amount of colon. The inflammation in ulcerative colitis generally involves only the mucosa and submucosa. In its most limited distribution, ulcerative colitis may affect only the distal rectum; at its most extensive, the entire colon is involved. The clinical features of ulcerative colitis, including symptoms, physical findings, and laboratory data, reflect the extent and severity of the colonic inflammation. The common symptoms in ulcerative colitis are rectal bleeding, diarrhea, and abdominal pain.

Left-Sided Ulcerative Colitis

More than 70% of patients with ulcerative colitis have disease limited proximally by the splenic flexure. This is known as left-sided ulcerative colitis. Ulcerative proctitis and proctosigmoiditis are subsets of left-sided ulcerative colitis. When mucosal inflammation is confined to the rectum, it is known as ulcerative proctitis, a chronic and recurrent entity that is generally mild in both its presentation and clinical course. Ulcerative proctitis represents half of all patients with left-sided ulcerative colitis. Proctosigmoiditis includes those in whom the proximal extent of involvement by inflammation is within the sigmoid colon. Patients with limited distal disease, whether proctitis or proctosigmoiditis, often have similar clinical features.

The most common presenting complaint of distal ulcerative colitis is rectal bleeding, present in more than 90% of affected patients. The bleeding is persistent and usually small in volume. It may be passed alone, mixed with mucus or loose stool, or coating the outside of solid stool. The symptoms are often mistaken for hemorrhoidal bleeding.

Half of these patients develop bowel changes. This usually presents as loose stools or diarrhea, but a third of patients with distal ulcerative colitis complain of constipation.

Characteristically, ulcerative proctitis is painless: fewer than 10% of patients note mild lower abdominal pain, perirectal discomfort, or lower back pain. Systemic complaints, such as fatigue, malaise, weight loss, fever, or extraintestinal manifestations, are uncommon with proctitis, although they may be seen with more extensive left-sided disease.

Physical examination of the patient with distal ulcerative colitis is invariably unremarkable, except for the presence of blood or pus on rectal examination. Occasionally, rectal tenderness is present. Laboratory abnormalities are uncommon; a mild anemia or an elevation in the sedimentation rate is occasionally seen. Sigmoidoscopic examination reveals an inflamed mucosa, with the proximal extent of the disease being limited to the left side of the colon.

Although spontaneous remissions occur in about 20% of patients with distal disease, most patients have persistent or relapsing symptoms. The clinical course of ulcerative proctitis and proctosigmoiditis is usually benign. About 10% to 15% of patients progress from limited involvement to extensive ulcerative colitis, usually within 12 to 18 months of the initial presentation. It is important to differentiate patients with limited distal disease from those in whom the inflammation is more extensive, as there are implications in terms of therapy, prognosis, and risk of colon cancer.

Extensive Ulcerative Colitis

Patients with ulcerative colitis that extends proximal to the descending colon have extensive disease, often associated with more severe clinical features. In one study looking at the extent of ulcerative colitis at the time of presentation, 16% of patients had total colonic involvement. The onset of ulcerative colitis is characteristically insidious, progressing from an increase in stool frequency to bloody diarrhea over several weeks to months. When it presents more acutely, it may be difficult to distinguish from infectious colitis.

Rectal bleeding is the most common sign of this disorder, present in 80% to 90% of patients with ulcerative colitis. The bleeding may be free or mixed with a purulent exudate, or it may be associated with soft or liquid stool. Massive hemorrhage is unusual, occurring rarely in patients with severe inflammation.

Diarrhea is present in at least 80% of patients with extensive ulcerative colitis and occasionally occurs in the absence of rectal bleeding. The diarrhea is characteristically small in volume. It commonly follows meals, and in many cases occurs during the night.

Tenesmus, the sensation of incomplete evacuation, is common in ulcerative colitis.

Abdominal pain occurs in about half of the patients with ulcerative colitis. The pain is usually vague and may be localized to the left lower quadrant, the lower abdomen, or the lower back. Although usually not a prominent symptom, abdominal pain and cramping may be severe with severe attacks of ulcerative colitis.

Systemic symptoms such as anorexia, nausea, weight loss, and fever occur in about half of patients with ulcerative colitis, especially when severe in activity. Extraintestinal manifestations of ulcerative colitis are the predominant presenting symptom in some cases.

The physical examination in patients with ulcerative colitis often helps determine the severity and extent of the disease. Patients with limited left-sided disease and with mild or even moderate extensive disease often have a normal physical examination except for the rectal examination, which usually reveals the presence of blood. Patients with severe disease may have lost weight and may appear pale. Tachycardia reflects dehydration and toxicity. Fever may be present. Abdominal findings, which are usually absent in milder forms of this disease, are more significant when it is severe. Abdominal tenderness may be elicited over the affected colon. In more fulminant disease, the abdomen may be distended and tympanitic, with diminished bowel sounds. The presence of peritoneal signs suggest a complication such as toxic colitis or perforation.

The severity of ulcerative colitis usually corresponds to the extent of colonic involvement and may be classified by a scheme developed by Truelove and Witts in the mid-1950s. Mild disease is characterized by less than four stools daily, with or without blood, the absence of systemic symptoms such as fever or tachycardia, and a normal sedimentation rate. Patient with moderate disease have more than four stools per day but have no or few systemic symptoms. Severe disease results in more than six stools daily with blood, in addition to systemic symptoms such fever, tachycardia, and anemia and an elevated sedimentation rate. The severe category applies to only 10% to 15% of patients with limited distal disease but to more than half the patients whose colitis extends to at least the splenic flexure.

Close to two thirds of patients with ulcerative colitis have intermittent attacks of disease that may last from weeks to months. The length of remission varies from weeks to years. A rare patient has a single episode with no recurrences. Ten percent to 15% have a continuous course with persistent symptoms. The course of disease is at least in part determined by the extent of colonic involvement, and those with more extensive disease are more likely to have severe attacks. The mortality of ulcerative colitis has decreased dramatically since the introduction of corticosteroids and the use of maintenance therapy with sulfasalazine.

Crohn Disease

First described by Crohn, Ginsberg, and Oppenheimer in 1932, the clinical features of Crohn disease span a wide spectrum. Crohn disease may affect any portion of the gastrointestinal tract, from mouth to anus. It is characterized by transmural inflammation, and its clinical presentation reflects the part of the gastrointestinal tract that is involved.

There are three major patterns of involvement of Crohn disease. The first is disease of the ileum and proximal colon, a pattern seen in 40% of patients at presentation. Thirty percent of patients present with disease confined to the small intestine, most in the distal ileum. Crohn disease presents with disease confined to the colon in 25% of patients. About a third of the patients with colonic disease have segmental involvement, but most have pancolitis, a pattern that can be confused with ulcerative colitis. More proximal parts of the gastrointestinal tract, including the esophagus, stomach, duodenum, jejunum, and more proximal ileum, are involved less commonly. The anatomic location of Crohn disease is important as far as clinical features, prognosis, potential complications, and indications for surgery.

The common symptoms affecting 90% of patients with Crohn disease are diarrhea, abdominal pain, and weight loss. The character of each symptom varies with the location of the inflammation. The symptoms may initially be vague and intermittent, and the patient may go for months or years before the diagnosis is considered.

Diarrhea occurs in almost all patients. It is often gradual in onset and typically occurs after eating or at night. Small-volume diarrhea is characteristic of colonic disease and, with rectal involvement, may be associated with urgency and tenesmus. Small intestinal disease characteristically has larger-volume stools and is due to various mechanisms, including bacterial overgrowth and bile-salt malabsorption.

Abdominal pain is also present in almost all patients with Crohn disease. Postprandial crampy or colicky right lower quadrant or suprapubic pain is seen in patients with ileocolonic disease. It is often at least partially relieved with defecation and may represent partial obstruction of the intestinal lumen. Pain may also occur as a result of transmural inflammation and serosal involvement.

Rectal bleeding is not as common in Crohn disease as it is in ulcerative colitis, and is most often seen with colonic involvement. In contrast to ulcerative colitis, gross rectal bleeding is seen in only half the patients with extensive colitis. Massive hemorrhage is rare and is more common in colonic disease.

Crohn disease is often complicated by significant weight loss. This is due to a number of factors, including diminished intake related to anorexia or the exacerbation of symptoms by eating, and because of malabsorption due to small bowel disease.

Findings on physical examination in Crohn disease also reflect the disease location and severity. Abdominal tenderness is often present, and thickened bowel loops may be manifest by a mass or fullness, often in the right lower quadrant. There may be fistulous openings, induration, redness, and tenderness near the anus. When Crohn disease is active and severe, malnutrition and anemia may be present.

Laboratory findings in Crohn disease are nonspecific. Anemia due to blood loss, nutritional deficiencies, and chronic disease is often present. A mild leukocytosis is common, although a high white blood cell count is more suggestive of a septic complication such as an abscess. Hypoalbuminemia is seen with severe disease. An elevated sedimentation rate is particularly common with Crohn disease of the colon.

As with ulcerative colitis, the course of Crohn disease is characterized by remissions and exacerbations. Overall, about 70% of patients with Crohn disease eventually require surgery, and up to half of those operated on have recurrence of disease.

DIAGNOSIS

Ulcerative Colitis

The diagnosis of ulcerative colitis relies on the clinical history, examination of the stool for pathogens, and examination of the colonic mucosa by sigmoidoscopy or colonoscopy. The most common infections that mimic acute ulcerative colitis are *Shigella*, *Salmonella*, and *Campylobacter*. In addition, infection with *E coli* 0157 and amebiasis may present with bloody diarrhea. Appropriate stool examinations looking for these organisms are part of the evaluation of all patients who present with bloody diarrhea.

Sigmoidoscopy/Colonoscopy

Sigmoidoscopy should be performed if the clinical presentation suggests ulcerative colitis. The normal colonic mucosa is pink and glistening, with visible submucosal vessels within the rectum. The rectal valves and haustral folds in the sigmoid colon are sharp. In the early stages of ulcerative colitis, the rectal vascular pattern is obscured by edema and hyperemia. The valves and haustral folds become thick and blunted. With more severe inflammation, the mucosa becomes granular and friable so that it may bleed with minimal trauma from the endoscope. In more severe cases, the bleeding is spontaneous, exudate may coat the mucosa, and occasionally superficial ulcers are seen. Once remission is obtained, the mucosa may return to normal or may appear thinned and featureless. Pseudopolyps may be present in longstanding disease.

In ulcerative colitis, the inflammatory reaction is continuous and rectal involvement is characteristic. Therefore, colonoscopy is unnecessary for making the initial diagnosis, and in fact is contraindicated in the presence of severe inflammation. However, colonoscopy in ulcerative colitis is useful for determining the extent of the inflammation and for surveillance for cancer and assessment of strictures and polyps.

Histology

The histologic findings on mucosal biopsy from sigmoidoscopy are helpful in confirming the diagnosis of ulcerative colitis. The distinction between acute self-limited colitis (such as that seen with infections) and chronic ulcerative colitis is based on several histologic features, including crypt architecture, cellularity of the lamina propria, and distribution of the inflammation. Irregularly shaped, dilated, or branching crypts are a sign of chronic inflammation, are suggestive of ulcerative colitis, and are not seen in acute self-limited colitis. Ulcerative colitis is also characterized by an increase in mononuclear cells in the lamina propria; in acute colitis, the inflammatory infiltrate is primarily neutrophils. In ulcerative colitis, the distribution of inflammatory cells is the same in all areas of all specimens. Crypt abscesses are seen in both acute and chronic colitis.

X-Rays

A plain film of the abdomen in severe ulcerative colitis may show thickening of the bowel wall or colonic dilatation in the case of toxic dilatation. Double-contrast barium studies, which should not be done in the presence of severe inflammation because of the risk of perforation or exacerbation of colitis, may show a fine mucosal granularity that is continuous and circumferential. In longstanding ulcerative colitis, the colon may be straightened, with a loss of haustral markings. Computed tomographic scanning may show homogeneous thickening of the bowel wall, with proliferation of perirectal fat in some cases of ulcerative colitis.

In summary, the diagnosis of ulcerative colitis is based on the clinical presentation and sigmoidoscopic findings. Stool cultures and parasite examinations are negative, and the biopsy results should be characteristic. Evaluation of the extent of the disease by colonoscopy can be done on an elective basis.

Crohn Disease

The diagnosis of Crohn disease is based on several criteria, including the clinical presentation, endoscopic or radiologic findings, and histologic changes. The major diagnostic modalities used are endoscopy and contrast radiography. The study of choice depends in large part on the presentation, and in many patients more than one type of examination may be required to establish the diagnosis and the extent of involvement.

X-Rays

Contrast radiography is useful in defining the distribution of Crohn disease of the small bowel, and either small bowel follow-through or enteroclysis examinations can be used (Fig. 67-1). The earliest changes include a coarse villous pattern, hyperplasia of the lymphoid follicles, and aphthoid ulcers. As the disease progresses and extends transmurally, folds become thickened and distorted

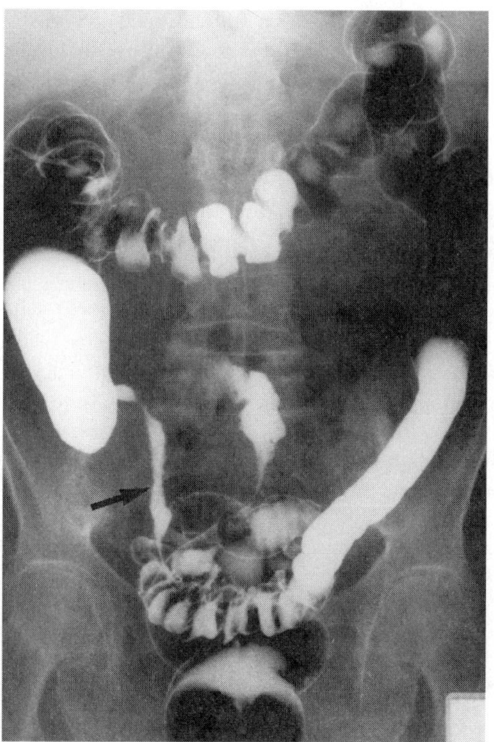

Figure 67-1. Narrowed, irregular segment of terminal ileum in Crohn disease (*arrow*).

and ulcers enlarge to take on a stellate or linear shape. In advanced Crohn disease, cobblestoning of the mucosa and large flat ulcers can be seen. Strictures of the small bowel, a common complication of this disease, can be observed with small bowel radiography. Fistulas originating in the small intestine are often outlined on small bowel x-rays.

A double-contrast barium enema may reveal similar changes in the colon in cases of Crohn colitis. The colon may be foreshortened. Radiographic studies may better define strictures and fistulas of the colon than does endoscopy.

Computed tomography is also often helpful in evaluating patients with Crohn disease. Bowel wall thickening may be seen, fistulas defined, and abscesses noted. Magnetic resonance imaging is thought to be superior in evaluating complex perineal fistulas.

Colonoscopy

Colonoscopy, with visualization of the colonic and terminal ileal mucosa, may reveal a broad spectrum of abnormalities in Crohn disease. In general, the endoscopic findings are focal, patchy, and distributed asymmetrically. This contrasts with the diffuse symmetric involvement with ulcerative colitis. The rectum may be normal, a feature that also helps differentiate Crohn disease from ulcerative colitis.

Scattered aphthoid erosions with surrounding normal mucosa are the earliest lesions noted in Crohn disease. Ulcerations, ranging from small to large and serpiginous, develop as the disease progresses. The ulcers may become deep with heaped-up borders. Between the ulcerations, the mucosa may appear nodular and elevated, creating a characteristic cobblestoned appearance. In severe disease, extensive ulceration may involve the entire circumference of the bowel.

Pseudopolyps may be seen, although less frequently than in ulcerative colitis. Strictures may develop, due primarily to fibrotic scarring. Fistulous openings are not always readily apparent, but when seen are surrounded by mucosal ulceration and inflammation.

If the ileum can be intubated, characteristic ulcerations of the mucosa may be noted. This study is important if radiographic findings are difficult to interpret.

Histology

The most important histologic feature of Crohn disease is the granuloma, found in both affected and seemingly unaffected mucosa. Granulomas are seen in only about 30% of patients with Crohn disease. Other histologic criteria supportive of Crohn disease are a discontinuity of the inflammatory infiltrate, transmural inflammation, and the presence of fissuring ulcers. Microscopic focality also is characteristic of Crohn disease. Unfortunately, endoscopic biopsies are superficial, and the limited material obtained may not be sufficient to detect the characteristic features of Crohn disease.

COMPLICATIONS OF INFLAMMATORY BOWEL DISEASE

Fistulas

The fistula is one of the most common complications of Crohn disease. Fistulas represent the extension of transmural inflammation into adjacent or distant organs. Internal fistulas are communications between the bowel and another viscus. They originate in an area of active inflammation. Enteroenteric fistulas, such as ileoileal and ileocecal fistulas, are the most common. Ileosigmoid, cologastric, and coloduodenal fistulas are also seen in Crohn disease. Enterourinary and enterogenital fistulas are less common.

External fistulas usually begin in the ileum or colon and terminate on the skin. They may develop postoperatively and pass through surgical scars, or occur spontaneously due to progression of inflammation.

Management of fistulas depends on their location and the symptoms they cause. Many are associated with few symptoms and can be managed with drugs such as metronidazole or immunosuppressants. Others may lead to significant problems and require surgery.

Perineal Disease

Perineal disease may be a prominent clinical feature of Crohn disease. Perineal disease occurs most commonly in patients with Crohn disease of the ileum and colon and is one of the most potentially physically and psychologically disabling complications of IBD. Seen in about a third of patients, these lesions include edematous skin tags around the anus, fissures and ulcers in the anal canal, fistulas from anus to perineum or vagina, and abscesses.

Abscess

Like fistulas, the abscesses seen in Crohn disease are related to the transmural extension of inflammation through the bowel wall. Abscesses occur in about 15% of patients with Crohn disease and commonly present with abdominal pain and fever. Treatment includes antibiotics, drainage of the abscess, and at times resection of the involved segment of bowel.

Toxic Megacolon

Acute toxic inflammation of the colon with dilatation may occur in both ulcerative colitis and Crohn disease. It is one of the most serious complications of IBD and may be life-threatening: mortality rates are reported as high as 20%. Dilatation of the colon is invariably associated with a deterioration in the patient's clinical status, with severe abdominal pain, high fever, tachycardia, and obtundation. Plain films of the abdomen show colonic dilatation, usually maximal in the transverse colon (Fig. 67-2). The pathophysiology of toxic dilatation is unknown but may relate to an alteration in colonic motility secondary to massive inflammation. Certain risk factors may predispose a patient to develop toxic dilatation, including antimotility agents, diagnostic procedures such as barium enema or colonoscopy, and electrolyte abnormalities.

Intensive medical therapy with intravenous fluids, nasogastric suction, antibiotics, and corticosteroids is indicated in cases of toxic dilatation. Clinical deterioration or failure to improve in 24 to 48 hours is an indication for surgery.

Perforation

Perforation of the colon may occur in the setting of toxic dilatation, although it may also occur in severe IBD without dilatation. Free perforation occurs almost exclusively in ulcerative colitis and is rare in Crohn disease. This complication is more likely to occur during an initial attack of ulcerative colitis. Most perforations occur

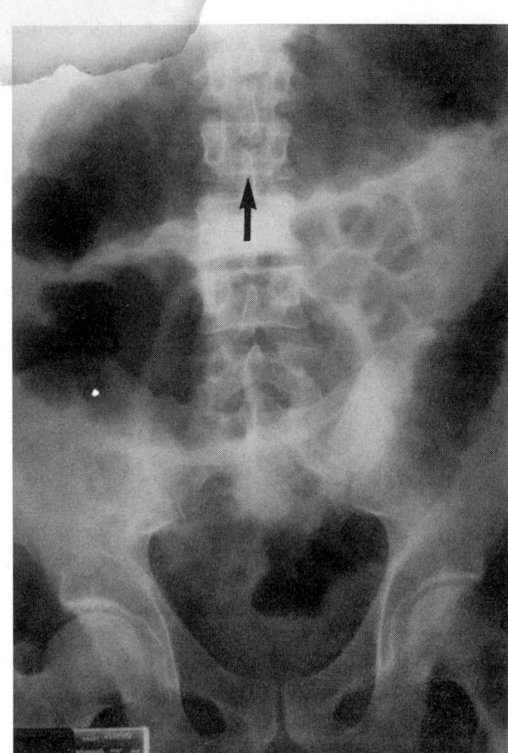

Figure 67-2. Dilated transverse colon in toxic megacolon of ulcerative colitis (*arrow*).

in the left colon. Free perforation of the small intestine, particularly of the terminal ileum, may complicate severe Crohn disease.

Obstruction

Obstruction, especially of the small intestine, occurs more frequently in Crohn disease and is one of the most common indications for surgery. It is a rarer complication of ulcerative colitis. Obstruction may result from stricture formation due to progressive scarring, carcinoma of the large or small bowel, a giant pseudopolyp, postoperative adhesions, or potentially reversible edema and inflammation of the bowel.

Cancer

Patients with ulcerative colitis have a markedly increased risk of developing colon cancer when compared to the general population. The actual magnitude of this risk is unknown, but the overall annual incidence of colon cancer in patients with longstanding ulcerative colitis may be 0.5% to 1.0%. The risk of cancer becomes significant 8 to 10 years after diagnosis and increases exponentially with time. This risk is higher with extensive disease than with left-sided colitis. Limited proctitis does not have a significant association with cancer. The severity of the inflammation does not appear to affect the risk of developing cancer.

Patients with Crohn disease are also at risk for developing cancer, although probably less so than those with ulcerative colitis. Patients with colonic Crohn disease are at higher risk. As with ulcerative colitis, disease duration is a significant factor in cancer risk.

Most authorities agree that ulcerative colitis patients with disease proximal to the descending colon that has been present for at least 8 years should undergo regular colonoscopic surveillance for dysplasia, a precancerous change. The presence of high-grade dysplasia or carcinoma is an indication for colectomy. Patients with extensive Crohn colitis of a similar duration may also benefit from a surveillance program.

Extraintestinal Manifestations

A number of extraintestinal manifestations are associated with IBD and may be responsible for a significant degree of morbidity. These conditions may be the presenting symptom, overshadowing the bowel complaints, and may be more difficult to control than the bowel disease. Up to a third of patients with IBD develop at least one extraintestinal manifestation. The most frequently affected sites are the joints, skin, eyes, and hepatobiliary system. Most occur with both Crohn disease and ulcerative colitis. The pathogenesis of extraintestinal manifestations remains unclear.

Musculoskeletal Manifestations

One of the most common extraintestinal manifestations is arthritis, which occurs in about 25% of patients with IBD. Peripheral arthritis accounts for 75% of all types of arthritis seen. Most commonly it presents with involvement of a single large joint. Less commonly, multiple joints are affected, usually in an asymmetric fashion. Joint aspirates are sterile, radiologic changes are infrequent, and residual deformity is rare. Rheumatoid factor is negative. The activity of this form of arthritis usually parallels that of the underlying bowel disease. Successful treatment of the bowel disease generally results in improvement of the arthritis.

Twenty-five percent of patients with arthritic manifestations have central arthritis. Sacroiliitis and ankylosing spondylitis may run a course independent of the underlying bowel disease, and treatment of the bowel disease does not influence the progress of central arthritis. It is more common in ulcerative colitis. Ninety percent of patients with ankylosing spondylitis are positive for HLA B-27.

Dermatologic Manifestations

Skin lesions are also common and have been reported to occur in up to 15% of patients with IBD. The most frequent skin lesion seen is erythema nodosum, which is most common in Crohn disease involving the colon. It is the most common extraintestinal manifestation seen in children. The development of erythema nodosum typically correlates with bowel disease activity and improves with treatment of the bowel disease.

Pyoderma gangrenosum occurs in up to 5% of patients with ulcerative colitis; it occurs less frequently in Crohn disease. This is considered by many to be the most severe skin lesion associated with IBD. Unlike erythema nodosum, the course of pyoderma gangrenosum does not always parallel that of the underlying bowel disease, and there are reports of this lesion developing many years after colectomy for ulcerative colitis.

Metastatic Crohn disease is defined as a granulomatous dermatitis occurring at a site remote from the gastrointestinal tract - in a patient with Crohn disease. It may occur during both quiescent and active periods of intestinal disease, and may remit and relapse spontaneously. Treatment is as with the underlying bowel disease.

Cutaneous vasculitis, cutaneous polyarteritis nodosa, and cutaneous granulomatous vasculitis have all been described in Crohn disease.

Ocular Manifestations

Several inflammatory lesions of the eye have been associated with IBD, including conjunctivitis, episcleritis, and uveitis. Anterior uveitis (iritis) is the most feared ocular lesion due to the potential for loss of sight. Uveitis commonly occurs during an exacerbation of bowel disease activity. Treatment includes local corticosteroids and treatment of the underlying bowel disease.

Hepatobiliary Manifestations

A broad spectrum of hepatobiliary complications is associated with IBD, constituting some of the most significant extraintestinal manifestations. Pericholangitis is the most common hepatic disorder associated with IBD. It is equally frequent in ulcerative colitis and Crohn disease. It is usually a benign disorder, although the lesion may progress to cirrhosis.

Steatosis is seen in about 50% of patients with IBD. It may result from malnutrition or toxicity and is reversible with clinical improvement of the bowel disease.

Primary sclerosing cholangitis occurs in 1% to 5% of patients with IBD and is more commonly associated with ulcerative colitis. This chronic, fibrosing inflammatory disorder involves the intrahepatic and extrahepatic bile ducts. The diagnosis is usually made by endoscopic retrograde cholangiopancreatography (ERCP), which demonstrates diffusely distributed multifocal strictures associated with irregularity and tortuosity of the ducts. There appears to be no association of sclerosing cholangitis with the activity, severity, or duration of the bowel disease. It may precede the bowel disease, and colectomy does not prevent its later development.

Adenocarcinoma of the bile duct occurs more frequently in patients with ulcerative colitis than in the general population. Sclerosing cholangitis may precede the development of cancer.

Chronic active hepatitis, granulomatous hepatitis, and hepatic amyloidosis have all been described in IBD.

DIFFERENTIAL DIAGNOSIS OF INFLAMMATORY BOWEL DISEASE

The clinical features of ulcerative colitis and Crohn disease may be similar. In some circumstances (eg, planning the most appropriate surgical procedure), it is important to make the distinction between the two (Table 67-1). Diarrhea is common in both entities but is more likely to be bloody in ulcerative colitis. Abdominal pain, particularly when severe, suggests Crohn disease. Right lower quadrant tenderness and mass are also more characteristic of Crohn disease. Fistulas, abscesses, strictures, and perianal involvement also support a diagnosis of Crohn disease. Endoscopic features may also help to differentiate between the two. Rectal involvement, a continuous distribution of inflammation, and disease limited to the mucosa of the colon are more characteristic of ulcerative colitis. Crohn colitis may spare the rectum, and its inflammation is often discontinuous, with "skip areas." Deep ulcers with discrete margins and aphthoid ulcers are seen in Crohn disease. Small bowel involvement signifies Crohn disease, as does transmural inflammation.

About 5% to 10% of cases of chronic colitis cannot be characterized as either Crohn disease or ulcerative colitis by clinical, endoscopic, radiographic, or histologic criteria. Patients in this category are said to have indeterminate colitis.

Recent-onset IBD must be distinguished from infectious colitis. The clinical features of *Shigella*, *Salmonella*, amebiasis, and *Campylobacter* may be similar to those of ulcerative colitis. Infections with *Campylobacter* and *Shigella* may produce endoscopic findings indistinguishable from those of ulcerative colitis. The endoscopic appearance of amebiasis usually consists of small, discrete ulcers covered with a yellow exudate, most commonly found in the cecum and the ascending colon. Stool cultures and serology for amebiasis help make the distinction between infectious colitis and IBD. *Clostridium difficile* colitis, related to antibiotic use, can be ruled out with the appropriate toxin assay.

Ischemia of the colon should be considered in an elderly patient who presents with abdominal pain and rectal bleeding. Mucosal edema, erythema, and discrete ulcers may be seen on colonoscopy. Ischemia rarely involves the rectum. Ischemic colitis may be difficult to distinguish from Crohn disease, except that it usually resolves spontaneously within a few weeks.

Other infections, including *Yersinia*, giardiasis, tuberculosis, and chlamydia may mimic Crohn disease. Tuberculosis commonly affects the ileum and cecum and may present without coexistent pulmonary disease. Giardiasis causes prolonged diarrhea, crampy abdominal pain, and weight loss. Stool examination or duodenal aspirate may identify this parasite. *Yersinia* infection presents with diarrhea and abdominal pain, which may localize to the right lower quadrant.

Anal intercourse in homosexual men predisposes them to sexually transmitted proctitis, which may resemble ulcerative proctitis. *Neisseria gonorrhoeae*, chlamydia, herpes simplex, and *Treponema pallidum* are all potential organisms that cause proctitis. In patients with AIDS, chronic diarrhea and abdominal pain are commonly seen and may be a result of infection with *Cryptosporidium*, *Isospora*, or *Mycobacterium avium-intracellulare*, all of which cause pathology in the small intestine. Colitis in these patients may result from infection by herpes and cytomegalovirus.

Diverticulitis tends to be an acute problem but may also resemble Crohn disease, presenting with abdominal pain, fever, diarrhea, and rectal bleeding. Acute appendicitis may be difficult to distinguish from the initial presentation of Crohn disease involving the ileum.

Patients who have undergone radiation therapy for intraabdominal or pelvic cancer may develop proctitis or colitis. The clinical features of radiation colitis are similar to those of ulcerative colitis or Crohn colitis. Telangiectasias of the rectal mucosa, which may be present in the late stage of radiation colitis, and a history of radiation therapy support the diagnosis.

Irritable bowel syndrome is characterized by chronic abdominal pain and diarrhea. Occasionally, it is difficult to distinguish this entity from mild Crohn disease, although systemic symptoms such as fever and weight loss are more suggestive of Crohn disease. These two diseases may coexist.

Intestinal lymphoma may mimic Crohn disease and present with fever, weight loss, diarrhea, and abdominal pain. Lymphoma is often more extensive in its involvement of the bowel than Crohn disease.

Collagenous colitis, commonly seen in middle-aged women, is characterized by watery diarrhea. Histologic examination of the mucosa reveals a thick collagen deposition in the subepithelial layer. The etiology is unknown.

Table 67-1. Inflammatory Bowel Disease Differential Diagnosis

CROHN DISEASE	ULCERATIVE COLITIS
Epidemiology	**Epidemiology**
Incidence is 1–6 cases/100,000	Incidence is 2–10 cases/100,000
Incidence rising	Incidence has plateaued
Higher incidence in Jews	Higher incidence in Jews
Peak incidence 15–35 years	Peak incidence 15–35 years
Secondary peak 55–65 years	Secondary peak 55–65 years
Incidence in whites > African-Americans	Incidence in whites > African-Americans
Incidence smoking > general population	Incidence smoking < general population
Anatomic Distribution	**Anatomic Distribution**
Small bowel: 30–40%	Rectum/rectosigmoid: 30–40%
Small and large bowel: 40–55%	Extension above sigmoid: 40%
Large bowel: 15–25%	Entire colon: 20%
Perianal: 5–40%	Perianal: rare
Mouth, esophagus, and stomach/duodenum: less common	Rectum invariably affected
90% with small bowel disease have terminal ileum affected	Continuous distribution of inflammation
Rectum often unaffected	
"Skip areas" common	
Clinical Features	**Clinical Features**
Symptoms	*Symptoms*
Abdominal pain: often in right lower quadrant; crampy or colicky; partially relieved by defecation	Rectal bleeding: present in > 90%
Diarrhea: postprandial or nocturnal; caused by, bacterial overgrowth, bile-salt malabsorption or decreased water absorption	Diarrhea: present in at least 80% of those with extensive colitis and in at least 50% of those with colitis
Rectal bleeding: in 50% with extensive colonic disease	Constipation: seen in a third of patients with distal colitis
Weight loss: secondary to malabsorption or diminished intake	Tenesmus: sensation of incomplete evacuation; common
Anorexia, nausea, and fever	Abdominal pain: vague and localized to left lower quadrant, lower abdomen or back
	Anorexia, weight loss, fever: occur in 50%; associated with severe activity

continued

MEDICAL MANAGEMENT

The mainstays of medical therapy for IBD have remained unchanged for decades. However, the development of new agents, better analogs of old agents, and improved modes of drug delivery offer great promise for future therapy.

5-Aminosalicylates

Sulfasalazine was developed in the late 1930s for the treatment of rheumatoid arthritis. Because the etiology of rheumatoid arthritis was thought to be bacterial, it was logical to combine an antibacterial agent (sulfapyridine) and an antiinflammatory agent (5-aminosalicylic acid) for use in the treatment of this disorder. Patients who had enteric arthritis and were treated with this new drug had improvement not only in their arthritis but also in their IBD. Sulfasalazine remains a highly valued agent for the management of IBD. It is effective in the treatment of acute ulcerative colitis of mild to moderate severity, as well as in the maintenance of remission of this entity. Its benefits in Crohn disease have been harder to define but are probably real, especially when the colon is involved. It may reduce the frequency of postoperative recurrence of Crohn disease.

5-aminosalicylic acid (5-ASA) is the active moiety in sulfasalazine. Sulfapyridine has little or no clinical effect, acting simply as the vehicle for the delivery of 5-ASA to the colon. Once there, bacterial azo-reductases cleave the azo-bond linking the sulfapyridine and the 5-ASA molecules. The sulfapyridine is subsequently absorbed and eventually excreted in the urine. The 5-ASA

Table 67-1. *(Continued)*

CROHN DISEASE	ULCERATIVE COLITIS
Physical findings	**Physical findings**
Findings reflect disease location and severity	Blood present on rectal exam
Abdominal tenderness often in right lower quadrant	Pallor, weight loss
Abdominal mass often in right lower quadrant	Tachycardia or fever reflect severe disease
Perineal disease: fistulas, induration, erythema, tenderness	Abdominal tenderness is uncommon except in severe inflammation
Signs of malnutrition	Perineal disease rare
Sigmoidoscopy/Colonoscopy	**Sigmoidoscopy/Colonoscopy**
Patchy, focal, asymmetric inflammation	Continuous distribution of inflammation
Rectum often normal	Rectum involved
Ulcerations may become deep	Superficial ulcers
Cobblestoning	Loss of submucosal vascular pattern; granularity and friability
Pseudopolyps less common	Pseudopolyps
Radiography	**Radiography**
Small bowel x-rays: define distribution; wide range of abnormalities Barium enema: defines distribution; images strictures and fistulas	Barium enema: fine mucosal granularity, straightening; loss of haustral markings
CT scan: bowel wall thickening; fistulas; abscesses	CT scan: homogeneous bowel wall thickening and proliferation of perirectal fat
MRI: complex perineal fistulas best evaluated	
Histology	**Histology**
Cryptitis and crypt abscesses	Cryptitis and crypt abscesses
Granulomas seen in 30%	No granulomas
Discontinuous inflammatory infiltrate	Continuous inflammatory infiltrate
Transmural inflammation	Mucosal inflammation
Fissuring ulcers	
Complications	**Complications**
Fistulas: most common complication; internal and external	Toxic megacolon: mortality 20%
Perineal disease	Perforation of colon
Abscesses	Obstruction is rare
Toxic megacolon	Carcinoma of colon
Free perforation of colon or small bowel is rare	Hemorrhage
Obstruction: common indication for surgery	
Carcinoma: less common than in ulcerative colitis	

remains within the lumen of the large intestine, where it has several actions that may attenuate colonic inflammation. It is a potent inhibitor of prostaglandin synthetase and 5-lipoxygenase, with reduced production of prostaglandins and leukotrienes. It may also block the chemotactic activity of bacterial peptides and be a scavenger of oxygen free radicals.

The efficacy of sulfasalazine is dose-related. For the treatment of acute disease, the patient should be given 4 g/day in divided doses. A response can be expected within 1 or 2 weeks, although occasionally 3 or 4 weeks of therapy are required before symptoms respond. The recommended dose for maintenance of remission is 2 g/day, although higher doses may be required. The drug should be taken indefinitely.

The incidence of side effects in patients treated with sulfasalazine is high. About half of the patients who take this drug experience an adverse effect, most of which are due to sulfapyridine. Side effects are of two types: dose-related, which are thought to be related to serum sulfapyridine levels, and hypersensitivity reactions. The first group includes headache, nausea, vomiting, abdominal discomfort, and low-grade hemolysis. Because sulfapyridine is metabolized by acetylation, slow acetylators have a higher rate of dose-related side effects. The incidence of these effects increases with doses of 4 g/day or more. Dose-related side effects usually develop within the first few weeks of therapy and disappear when the drug has been reduced or discontinued.

The hypersensitivity reactions include rash, fever, aplastic anemia, agranulocytosis, and autoimmune hemolysis. These are often more severe than the dose-related effects and are not related to the dose, acetylator status, or serum sulfapyridine levels. Agranulocytosis is probably the most common fatal side effect. Complete blood counts should be closely monitored in patients on this drug. Sulfasalazine may interfere with folate absorption from the small bowel.

To minimize some of the dose-related side effects, sulfasalazine can be given in an enteric-coated form and in gradually increasing doses, reaching the goal dose in 1 or 2 weeks. Taking it with food also improves tolerance.

By removing the sulfapyridine moiety, 5-ASA can be given in much higher doses with the potential for improved therapy and fewer side effects. Several preparations of 5-ASA are available in the United States, including mesalamine (Asacol, Pentasa, Rowasa) and olsalazine (Dipentum). Asacol is 5-ASA coated with Eudragit-S, designed to be released at pH 7.0 in the ileum or cecum. Pentasa is 5-ASA packaged in ethylcellulose-coated beads for slow release in the small bowel and colon. Dipentum consists of two molecules of 5-ASA linked by a diazo bond. The bond is cleaved by bacteria in the colon, liberating two molecules of 5-ASA.

Like sulfasalazine, the 5-ASA preparations are effective in the treatment of mild to moderate ulcerative colitis and in maintaining remission. The optimal dosing has not been determined, but their minimal toxicity allows higher and therefore potentially more effective doses to be given.

There is increasing evidence that the 5-ASA compounds are effective in the treatment of mild to moderate Crohn disease and in the maintenance of remission. Optimistic results have been obtained with Pentasa in both small and large bowel disease. In addition, more and more data have accumulated that these agents are effective in the postoperative prevention of recurrence.

The oral 5-ASA drugs have the advantage of being tolerated by 80% to 90% of patients who are allergic to or intolerant of sulfasalazine. Although no study has proven them to be clinically superior to sulfasalazine in equivalent doses, the safety of these drugs is one of their main advantages. In addition, these aminosalicylates offer the opportunity to deliver more drug to areas of disease than is possible or safe with sulfasalazine. The experience with high doses, especially over prolonged periods, is limited, however, and further studies are needed to support their safety.

The potential for nephrotoxicity is the major concern in high-dose therapy. Chronic interstitial nephritis has been described in animals. Rare cases of acute allergic nephritis and nephrosis attributed to mesalamine in humans have been seen. Renal function should be monitored in patients on long-term, high-dose 5-ASA therapy. Pancreatitis, pericarditis, pulmonitis, and hepatitis have been reported as well. Olsalazine is associated with a secretory diarrhea in about 10% of patients.

Topical 5-ASA, given as a suppository or an enema, is available (Rowasa) and has proven to be extremely effective in the control of distal colitis and proctitis. Topical 5-ASA is also effective in patients unresponsive to topical corticosteroids. Distribution of the enema has been shown to be as high as the splenic flexure.

In most patients with mild to moderate ulcerative colitis or Crohn disease, it is reasonable to start with sulfasalazine. It is an effective drug when tolerated and costs less than the newer 5-ASA preparations. The latter should be reserved for patients intolerant of sulfasalazine. The dosing of these newer agents is variable and should be individualized. Because higher doses of 5-ASA are more effective, it may be the drug of choice in patients unresponsive or only partially responsive to sulfasalazine. In patients with mild to moderate proctitis or left-sided ulcerative colitis, topical therapy with Rowasa is the initial treatment of choice.

Corticosteroids

Systemic and local corticosteroids are highly useful in patients with acute ulcerative colitis or Crohn disease of moderate to severe degree. Their usefulness is limited by the side effects associated with high doses and long-term use. In addition, corticosteroids have not been shown to be beneficial in the maintenance of remission or the prevention of postoperative recurrence in IBD.

The most promising new steroid is budesonide, a highly potent and rapidly metabolized agent. It has been demonstrated to be beneficial when administered as an enema for distal colitis, where it has low systemic bioavailability. Trials in Canada and Europe suggest both acute and maintenance benefit from a controlled ileal release formulation of budesonide in Crohn disease. Not yet available in the United States, budesonide does not appear to be more effective than conventional corticosteroid preparations but may have fewer side effects. Its ultimate benefit may be in maintenance of long-term remission of IBD without toxicity, although this remains to be proven.

Azathioprine and 6-Mercaptopurine

Both 6-mercaptopurine and azathioprine are beneficial in ulcerative colitis and Crohn disease through their steroid-sparing effect, their efficacy in refractory patients and in maintaining remission, and their benefit in fistulous disease. The widespread use of these immune-modulating agents has demonstrated their safety.

These drugs show efficacy in two thirds to three quarters of patients with Crohn disease. Although they appear to work best in colonic disease, they can be beneficial in ileitis and ileocolitis. Relapse is prevented in 80% to 90% of patients when one of these drugs is maintained. They close or decrease the activity of fistulas, both internal and perianal.

The response rate to these drugs in patients with ulcerative colitis refractory to 5-ASA and steroids is 80%, and relapse is prevented in 75% of these particular patients. They should probably not be used in the patient with longstanding ulcerative colitis who is at high risk for cancer and has persistently active disease; surgery may be a better choice.

The toxicity of these two drugs is low. Early effects include pancreatitis and hepatitis (3%), classic allergic reactions (2%), and mild bone marrow suppression (2%), all of which are rapidly reversible when the drug is stopped. Long-term data suggest that there is no increase in the incidence of superinfections or neoplasms in these patients.

The onset of action of azathioprine and 6-mercaptopurine is slow and averages 4 to 6 months.

Cyclosporine A

Cyclosporine A is produced by the soil fungus *Tolypocladium inflatum gams*. It interrupts the cellular immune response by blocking the production of interleukin-2 by T-helper lymphocytes. It also indirectly inhibits B-cell function by blocking the production of B-cell activating factors and interferon by T-helper cells. The actual effect of cyclosporine A on the immune system in IBD is unknown.

Cyclosporine A has been proposed as an alternative to azathioprine or 6-mercaptopurine for refractory IBD, as its onset of action is rapid. Several controlled and uncontrolled studies have concluded that high-dose cyclosporine A is effective in severe ulcerative colitis and inflammatory and fistulous Crohn disease. Because it must be used in relatively high and potentially toxic doses to achieve efficacy in IBD, it probably has no role in long-term therapy. Cyclosporine A may ultimately be best used as a rapid-acting therapy in acutely ill ulcerative colitis patients who fail intravenous corticosteroids as a bridge to other, safer, long-term agents that may have a slow onset of action or lower efficacy. The side effects include profound immunosuppression, seizures, hypertension, and nephrotoxicity.

Methotrexate

Methotrexate has antiinflammatory properties, and a few controlled trials have supported the effectiveness of parenteral methotrexate in the treatment of IBD, where it may improve symptoms, reduce steroid requirements, and maintain remission. The mechanism by which methotrexate suppresses inflammation is unknown. Side effects are common, even with low doses. The role of methotrexate in the treatment of these diseases is not yet well defined, and further randomized trials and long-term experience are necessary before it can be recommended.

Lipoxygenase Inhibitors

Leukotriene B4 has been identified as a mediator of colonic inflammation. Zileuton inhibits the 5-lipoxygenase pathway, reducing the production of leukotriene B4. Unfortunately, it has not been shown to be consistently effective in clinical trials in treating IBD. More potent inhibitors of the 5-lipoxygenase pathway are under investigation.

Diversion of mediators away from the 5-lipoxygenase pathway to less proinflammatory derivatives has been accomplished by administration of high concentrations of omega-3 fatty acids (fish oils). The fishy odor limits their usefulness.

Antibiotics

Antibiotics are important in the management of septic complications of IBD and as primary therapy for Crohn colitis and perianal disease. Accepted indications for the use of antibiotics include the treatment of abscesses, bacterial overgrowth, and toxic colitis with or without megacolon. The goal of therapy in these situations is to decrease extraluminal tissue invasion. This requires a combination of agents active against both aerobic and anaerobic organisms—for example, metronidazole and ciprofloxacin, metronidazole and a second-generation cephalosporin, or metronidazole, ampicillin, and gentamicin.

When using antibiotics as primary therapy, the goal is to suppress the activity of Crohn disease. The best-studied antibiotic is metronidazole. This drug has been found to be as effective as sulfasalazine and superior to placebo in several well-designed studies of patients with Crohn disease. It appears to be more effective in colonic disease than small bowel disease. In patients who do not respond to sulfasalazine or 5-ASA, metronidazole 250 mg three or four times a day may be effective.

High-dose metronidazole is widely used for perianal complications of Crohn disease. Long-term therapy is usually necessary, as this drug has a slow onset of action, and relapses are the norm when it is stopped.

The side effects of metronidazole may limit its use, especially in long-term situations. Metallic taste, dark urine, alcohol sensitivity, nausea, and anorexia are relatively common. Peripheral neuropathy is the most severe common complication. It is less likely to occur if the dose is maintained at less than 10 mg/kg/day. About half the patients who develop neuropathy while on this drug improve when it is stopped.

Tobacco

Smokers are less likely to have ulcerative colitis, and the onset of colitis is often associated with the cessation of smoking. Resumption of smoking may reduce symptoms. The opposite appears to be true for Crohn disease. Nicotine has been shown to inhibit thromboxane synthetase, cyclooxygenase, and lipoxygenase. It also stimulates colonic mucus production.

One study concluded that the addition of transdermal nicotine to standard maintenance therapy improved symptoms in left-sided ulcerative colitis as compared to placebo. There was a relatively frequent intolerance to therapy in this study, including headaches and sleep disturbances. In addition, transdermal nicotine is expensive. Further studies defining an optimal dose and the safety of this drug are required.

SURGICAL MANAGEMENT

Ulcerative Colitis

Despite advances in medical therapy, 20% to 30% of patients with ulcerative colitis require surgery. The most common indication is failure of medical therapy. Other indications include dysplasia, carcinoma, complications of medical therapy, or complications of the disease such as toxic dilatation, perforation, or occasionally intractable extraintestinal manifestations. Surgical techniques have improved, and elective options include total proctocolectomy with end ileostomy, total abdominal colectomy with ileoproctostomy, continent ileostomy, and ileoanal pouch.

Crohn Disease

Seventy percent of patients with Crohn disease require one or more operations. The indications for surgery in this disease differ from those in ulcerative colitis because ulcerative colitis is cured with a proctocolectomy, whereas Crohn disease is not amenable to surgical cure. The rate of symptomatic recurrence after resection approaches 40% within 5 years and 60% by 10 years. Surgery for Crohn disease is therefore best reserved for treatment of symptoms and complications uncontrolled by medical therapy. Recurrent or persistent intestinal obstruction is the most common reason to operate. Certain fistulas and abscesses may also require surgical intervention. Toxic colitis, massive hemorrhage, and small intestinal carcinoma are rare complications of Crohn disease that may require surgery.

CONSIDERATIONS IN PREGNANCY

As IBD affects women primarily during their reproductive years, there are concerns regarding the effects of these diseases and the drugs used to treat them on fertility and pregnancy outcome. Conversely, there are also concerns about the potential exacerbation of IBD during pregnancy. Most women with ulcerative colitis and Crohn disease can conceive safely and complete a normal full-term pregnancy.

Fertility

Patients with both ulcerative colitis and Crohn disease in remission have the same fertility as the general population. Fertility in women with ulcerative colitis, even when active, approaches normal rates. In active Crohn disease, however, fertility may be compromised. The primary reason for this decrease in fertility is the debilitated state of the patient when the disease is active—malnutrition, diarrhea, fever, and perineal disease may all play a role. Male patients treated with sulfasalazine may have impaired sperm motility and oligospermia. This effect is reversible once the drug is stopped. Problems with male fertility are not seen with the newer 5-ASA agents.

Effect of IBD on Pregnancy

Women with inactive ulcerative colitis have an excellent chance to complete a full-term pregnancy, with rates reported to be 90%. The rate of stillbirths, spontaneous abortions, and congenital abnormalities are similar to those in the general population. However, patients whose colitis is active are less likely to complete a pregnancy successfully.

The same observations have been noted in Crohn disease. Women with inactive disease have successful pregnancies about 85% of the time. However, there is an increase in abnormal outcomes, such as spontaneous abortions, when Crohn disease is active at the time of conception or during pregnancy.

Patients can be reassured that once conception has occurred, with quiescent disease the pregnancy outcome seems to be similar to that seen in the general population. However, patients with moderate to severely active disease should be discouraged from becoming pregnant. It makes sense to counsel patients with IBD to plan conception during a time when the woman's disease is inactive, as there may be a better prognosis.

Patients with proctocolectomy and ileostomy are at no added risk during pregnancy, although there may be local problems with the ileostomy from increasing abdominal pressure. Vaginal delivery is routine except in Crohn disease with extensive perineal or perianal disease. The safety of episiotomy in Crohn disease has not been systematically studied. This is a significant issue, due to the concern that an episiotomy may lead to the development of new-onset or activate previous perineal Crohn disease.

Effect of Pregnancy on IBD

About a third of patients with inactive ulcerative colitis relapse during pregnancy, a rate similar to that seen in nonpregnant persons. The relapse rate appears to be highest in the first trimester. If the colitis is active at the time of conception, activity worsens in almost half of patients. Recent data suggest that if ulcerative colitis flares during pregnancy and is adequately controlled with drugs, the prognosis approaches that seen in patients whose disease remains quiescent. Fulminant colitis in pregnancy is rare and is associated with an increase in fetal mortality. The course of ulcerative colitis in subsequent pregnancies cannot be predicted by activity in prior pregnancies.

Relapse rates of Crohn disease in pregnancy are also similar to those in the general population, about 25%. If activity is present at the time of conception, one third of patients worsen during pregnancy, one third continue unchanged, and one third improve.

Medical Management During Pregnancy and Lactation

Active IBD should be aggressively treated during pregnancy, as the disease activity has a more deleterious effect than drug therapy on the fetal outcome. Sulfasalazine may be administered with relative safety in pregnant and lactating women and should be continued or started when disease activity requires that the drug be used. Bilirubin displacement by sulfapyridine is minimal, and neonatal jaundice is not increased. Folate supplementation should be provided to minimize the risk of folate deficiency. There are some data on the newer 5-ASA compounds and their use in pregnancy and lactation, and they also appear to be safe.

Retrospective human data support the safety of corticosteroids in pregnancy, and because active IBD is more harmful to the fetus than steroids, they should be used when required to treat significant activity of IBD. The relative risk for fetal malformations in women treated with corticosteroids is no different from nonsteroid-treated pregnancies or the general population. The major obstetric concerns for patients on corticosteroid therapy are abnormal glucose metabolism and enhanced calcium excretion. Glucose values should be closely monitored and sufficient calcium supplementation provided. Neonatal adrenal suppression is rare. The safety of breastfeeding when steroids are being administered in high doses or for long periods has not been studied, and their safety is uncertain.

Metronidazole crosses the placenta, and limited data are available on its use in pregnancy. It is mildly fetotoxic and teratogenic in mice. It is generally recommended that metronidazole be avoided during pregnancy. Methotrexate is contraindicated in pregnancy.

Azathioprine and 6-mercaptopurine both cross the placenta and have been reported to cause fetal abnormalities in animals. In transplant patients on either drug, congenital abnormalities occur in about 4%. In the limited experience with these drugs in IBD and pregnancy, there has been no statistically significant incidence of prematurity, spontaneous abortions, or congenital abnormalities. However, most authorities recommend that these drugs be stopped 3 months before conception.

Cyclosporine should not be used during pregnancy.

Surgical Management During Pregnancy

Surgery for IBD in pregnancy is indicated for significant complications or life-threatening conditions. The indications for emergency surgery in ulcerative colitis are the same whether the patient is pregnant or not. Surgery for Crohn disease should be performed only if medical measures have been ineffectual. If possible, each case should be managed by a team including a gastroenterologist, surgeon, obstetrician, and neonatologist.

Diagnostic Studies During Pregnancy

Gastrointestinal endoscopy may often be considered during pregnancy. Occasionally a patient presents with a problem that requires a prompt diagnosis, and endoscopy may be required. No studies have examined the safety of these diagnostic techniques, but in cases of suspected or worsening IBD, endoscopy may be a reasonable alternative to conventional x-rays. However, endoscopic procedures should be considered only when the findings have a potentially significant influence on management. Attention should be paid to careful observation of maternal blood pressure and fetal monitoring depending on gestational age.

X-ray studies should be avoided except in life-threatening situations. Prenatal exposure of less than 2 rads has not been associated with adverse effects on the fetus.

Nutritional Support During Pregnancy

IBD may adversely affect maternal nutrition, leading to anemia, intrauterine growth retardation, and preeclampsia. In the average patient, an additional 300 to 500 kcal/day are needed during pregnancy. When nutrition is impaired due to IBD, the patient may require enteral or total parenteral nutrition. Indications for nutritional support in patients with IBD may include prepregnancy malnutrition, excessive weight loss during pregnancy, or suboptimal weight gain in the third trimester.

Genetic Counseling

The risk that a child will develop IBD when one parent has it is 8.9%. The risk increases to 34% when both parents are affected.

Summary

Most patients with IBD can successfully conceive and complete a normal pregnancy. Patients with Crohn disease or ulcerative colitis should be advised to conceive when their disease is quiescent. They should be reassured that, when necessary, sulfasalazine, other 5-ASA compounds, and corticosteroids are safe and appropriate to use during pregnancy. Diagnostic studies should be avoided if possible.

BIBLIOGRAPHY

Burakoff R, Opper F. Pregnancy and nursing. In: Peppercorn MA, ed. Gastroenterology clinics of North America. Philadelphia:WB Saunders, 1995:689.

Gitnick G, ed. Inflammatory bowel disease: diagnosis and treatment. New York: Igaku-Shoin, 1991.

Kornbluth A, Salomon P, Sachar D. Crohn disease. In: Gastrointestinal disease. Philadelphia: WB Saunders, 1993:1270.

Peppercorn MA. Advances in drug therapy for inflammatory bowel disease. Ann Intern Med 1990;112:50.

Present DH, Hanan IM. Pregnancy and inflammatory bowel disease. In: Karlstadt RG, Surawicz CM, Croitoru R, eds. Gastrointestinal disorders during pregnancy. Monograph, American College of Gastroenterology, 1994.

Sartor RB, Lichtman SN. Mechanisms of systemic inflammation associated with intestinal injury. In: Targan SR, Shanahan F, eds. Inflammatory bowel disease from bench to bedside. Baltimore: Williams & Wilkins, 1994:210.

Woolrich AJ, DaSilva MD, Korelitz BI. Surveillance in the routine management of ulcerative colitis. Gastroenterology 1992;103:431.

Primary Care for Women, edited by Phyllis C. Leppert and Fred M. Howard. Lippincott-Raven Publishers, Philadelphia © 1997.

68

Irritable Bowel Disease

PAUL S. DZIWIS

Irritable bowel syndrome (IBS) is an intriguing entity that has confounded clinicians and scientists for over a century. This three-word phrase has represented a hodgepodge of gastrointestinal disorders that potentially can be distressing to patients. These patients, in turn, often are difficult to manage. However, it need not necessarily be this way if one approaches this entity with a solid definition, an appropriate workup, and a compassionate attitude. Much has been learned recently about IBS due to improved techniques in evaluating the small and large intestines.

IBS has been known by as many as 35 different names. These names include spastic colitis, neurogenic mucous colitis, mucous colitis, membranous enteritis, membranous colitis, and nervous colitis. However, it is crucial to stress that there is no colitis present, that is, there is no inflammation of the colon either grossly or microscopically. Nor is this entity confined to just the large bowel; IBS also involves the small intestine. Therefore, these names should be forever discarded and replaced with the description *irritable bowel syndrome*.

Because IBS is a syndrome, it requires the presence of a constellation of symptoms. In 1978, Manning published the following criteria to identify patients with IBS: (1) abdominal pain relieved by a bowel movement; (2) more frequent stools with onset of pain; (3) looser stools with onset of pain; or (4) abdominal distention evident by tighter clothing or by visible distention. This classification has held up remarkably well. The more criteria present, the more likely the patient has IBS. However, in some studies, the sensitivity of these criteria has been questioned and criticized as being as low as 42%.

In the early 1990s, the International Congress of Gastroenterology published strict criteria to identify patients with IBS. These criteria, known as the Rome criteria, are listed in Table 68-1

IBS is considered a functional disorder, which means, by definition, that no structural or biochemical abnormalities are present to explain the symptoms. It is one of several functional digestive disorders. Others affect the esophagus, stomach, and biliary system. Categorization as a functional disorder does not imply that

Table 68-1. Rome Criteria

Diagnostic criteria

At least 3 mo continuous or recurrent symptoms of:

1. Abdominal pain or discomfort that is:
   (a) relieved with defecation
   (b) and/or associated with a change in frequency of stool
   (c) and/or associated with a change in consistency of stool

and

2. Two or more of the following, at least a quarter of occasions or days;
   (a) altered stool frequency*
   (b) altered stool form (lumpy/hard or loose/watery stool)
   (c) altered stool passage (straining, urgency, or feeling of incomplete evacuation)
   (d) passage of mucus
   (e) bloating or feeling of abdominal distention

*For research purposes "altered" is defined as > 3 bowel movements/day or < 3 bowel movements/wk.

(Thompson WG. Functional bowel disease and functional abdominal pain. Gastroenterol Int 1992; 5:77.)

IBS is a psychiatric disorder, although symptoms can be influenced by psychological factors and stressful situations.

This syndrome is common. It affects 15% of Western and Chinese populations. It accounts for 3 million visits a year to primary care providers, leading to 2 million medical prescriptions. Approximately 25% to 50% of all referrals to gastroenterologists are related to this diagnosis. However, most patients with IBS do not consult a physician; only 20% to 25% do so.

In Western countries, there are approximately three females for every one male affected with IBS. However, this is not true in India and Sri Lanka, where more men seem to be affected. Reportedly, it is more acceptable for men than for women in these countries to describe somatic symptoms. Symptoms begin before 35 years of age in 50% of patients. Forty percent of patients are 35 to 50 years of age.

IBS is more common in the white population by a 5 : 1 margin. Jewish people also tend to have a higher incidence compared with the non-Jewish population. IBS has been noted to be the second most common reason for absenteeism from work. The common cold is number one.

ETIOLOGY

The pathophysiologic mechanism causing IBS is not completely understood and likely is multifactorial. Initially, IBS was thought of as primarily a psychiatric disorder. It is true that approximately 70% to 80% of clinic patients with the diagnosis of IBS have abnormal psychiatric profiles involving somatization, hypochondriasis, and major depression. However, it seems that IBS patients who do not seek medical advice have similar psychiatric profiles compared with a controlled population. Therefore, other possible mechanisms to explain IBS must exist. Studies also reveal that 50% of patients report onset of symptoms during a stressful period of their life and exacerbation of these symptoms with stressful events. However, data suggest that the symptoms of psychological stress have nothing to do with the *development* of IBS. They do, however, influence the decision to *consult* a physician. This has been termed the "self-selection" hypothesis.

During the last few decades, much has been learned about the bowel that helps understand the pathophysiologic mechanism behind IBS. Both abnormal motor function and abnormal visceral perception have been studied.

In the 1970s, a cyclic basal myoelectric rhythm of the colon was described. This rhythm also is referred to as the slow-wave frequency. Contraction of the colon occurs when spiked potentials are superimposed on the basal electrical rhythm. Normal healthy individuals typically have a dominant frequency (90% of the time) of six cycles per minute. Patients with IBS more commonly have a frequency of slow waves at three cycles per minute. However, this slower rhythm does not seem to be specific for IBS. Psychoneurosis is one diagnosis that seems to have a similar rhythm.

Patients with IBS also seem to have slower changes in motor activity in response to anger, pain, psychological stress, hormonal stimulation, and balloon distention. Unfortunately, it is difficult to consistently demonstrate a direct association between the specific changes in colonic motility and symptoms of IBS. Therefore, much remains to be known about colonic motility in IBS.

In the 1980s, alterations in small bowel motility were described in IBS patients. Normal motility of the small bowel in a healthy subject has been studied well. It is characterized by the migrating motor complex that occurs cyclically every 60 to 120 minutes in the *fasting* state. There are four phases. Phase 1 is motor quiescence. Phase 2 involves irregular intermittent contractions that increase in frequency and amplitude over a 30-minute period. Phase 3 is marked by a brief sequence of uninterrupted rhythmic contractions lasting 5 to 15 minutes. This allows propagation of contractions and sweeps food out of the stomach. This phase is commonly referred to as the "housekeeper" phase. Phase 4 represents the short period of time between the active phase 3 and the inactive phase 1. In the *fed* state, small bowel motility is characterized by a pattern of continuous irregular contractions.

There are two specific motor patterns seen more commonly in IBS patients compared with controls. Both occur during phase 2 of the migrating motor complex. The first involves continuous irregular bursts of contractions called discreet clustered contractions (DCCs), presumed to be propulsive. The second is a pattern characterized by prolonged (greater than 12 seconds), large-amplitude, rapidly propagating contractions (PPCs). These are associated with propulsion of luminal contents. Although normal subjects can have DDCs and PPCs, individuals with IBS seem to have increased pain and sensitivity to these patterns. Kellow and colleagues report that 61% of intermittent PPCs were associated with pain in IBS patients compared with only 17% of controlled subjects. There also seems to be increased motor activity in the small bowel of IBS patients in response to fatty meals and hormonal stimulation.

Increased visceral sensitivity seems to be more prominent in patients with IBS. These patients commonly complain of excess bloating and gas. Studies have shown, however, that these patients do not have elevated amounts of intestinal gas. Rather, they have abnormal pain at a given volume of gas. Ritchie and colleagues in the early 1970s inflated balloons in the rectums of patients. These patients exhibited pain at a much lower interstitial wall tension than normal patients. This increased anal–rectal sensitivity may explain the symptoms of pain before bowel movements and the sense of incomplete evacuations often cited by IBS patients.

IBS patients also may have a heightened sensitivity to other types of painful stimuli *outside* of the gastrointestinal tract. Studies, however, do not support this. Tolerance for hand immersion in ice water is the same as in normal patients.

The physiologic makeup of the bowel obviously is a complicated subject. Multiple control mechanisms are at work, including the central nervous system, autonomic nervous system, enteric nervous system, and hormonal input. Peptides such as vasoactive intestinal polypeptide, substance P, cholecystokinin, and enkephalins are found in the gut and brain and seem to have integrative activities.

DIFFERENTIAL DIAGNOSIS AND HISTORY

Irritable bowel syndrome is a diagnosis of exclusion. Unfortunately, there is no one simple physical finding, blood test, or x-ray that unquestionably confirms the diagnosis. Certain features, however, support the diagnosis. Therefore, a good solid history is indispensable (Table 68-2)

Symptoms generally start in late adolescence or early adulthood and uncommonly begin late in life. The abdominal pain often is poorly localized but most frequently occurs in the middle or lower abdominal region. The most common site is the left lower quadrant, although many patients have two or more sites of pain.

Table 68-2. Significant Clinical Features

Supporting the Diagnosis (more reliable features)
Lower abdominal pain
Precipitated by meals
Relieved by defecation
Does not awaken the patient
Small stools (constipated or diarrheal)
Chronic symptoms, consistent in pattern but variable in severity
Symptoms correlated with periods of stress
Against the Diagnosis
Onset in old age
Steady progressive course
Frequent awakening by symptoms
Fever
Weight loss not attributable to depression
Rectal bleeding other than fissures or hemorrhoids
Steatorrhea
Compatible With the Diagnosis
Extreme pain
Nausea and vomiting
Other upper GI symptoms (found in 25–50%)
Inability to correlate symptoms with stress
Rectal bleeding from hemorrhoids or fissures (found in 20%)

(From Schuster M. Diagnostic evaluation of the irritable bowel syndrome. Gastroenterol Clin North Am 1991;20:273.)

Descriptions of the pain may include crampy, burning, dull, sharp, steady, bloating, and knife-like. The pain typically does not radiate. It is commonly precipitated by meals and relieved by defecation. Stools can be described either as diarrhea or constipation. It is important to have the patient describe exactly what she means by diarrhea or constipation. Many people believe that if they do not have a daily bowel movement, they have constipation. In reality, normal stool frequency is from three times a day to every 3 days.

In IBS, if the patient complains of diarrhea, the volume is small. A stool volume greater than 200 mL/day suggests a different diagnosis. Both the pain and diarrhea resolve during sleeping. It is important to make the distinction between being awakened by pain and diarrhea versus being awakened for other reasons and noticing pain and the need to evacuate. If the patient has a true secretory cause for the diarrhea, she would be awakened from a sound sleep with diarrhea. If the diarrhea continues during a 24-hour fasting state, this would be evidence against IBS and in favor of a secretory cause. However, maintaining a true 24-hour fast on an outpatient basis is difficult.

Stools may be pencil thin, which has been attributed to rectal sigmoid spasm. Typically in patients with diarrhea, the patient states that the initial stool is formed. Subsequent stools are increasingly loose and eventually are liquid. Patients with constipation, typically have small, "pellet-like" stools resulting from spasm.

Rectal bleeding suggests another diagnosis unless related to hemorrhoids or a fissure from straining. Weight loss is important to address. This is unusual in a patient with IBS unless there is concomitant depression. As mentioned earlier, bloating, belching, and flatus all are commonly present in IBS patients.

These symptoms are chronic, although variable in severity. Steady progressing pain suggests another entity. The patient who knows exactly the date of onset of symptoms usually does not have IBS. Rather, the onset of symptoms in IBS is gradual and vague.

In history-taking, a detailed dietary history, travel history, and medication history are necessary. The patient should make a diary of the quality and quantity of food and drink consumed during symptomatic periods. Records for at least 7 days should be kept. Notice if the patient is a binge eater as well as when she eats.

Lactose intolerance symptoms can mimic IBS or at least contribute to IBS. About 40% of patients with IBS also have lactose intolerance. Lactose is present in a wide variety of foods and, therefore, it is critical that labels be read to eliminate this sugar from the diet. A patient can be formally tested with a hydrogen breath test if there is any question of intolerance to milk products. The breath test is much more sensitive than the blood test. Lactose intolerance affects 90% of Asians and Africans and up to 50% of southern Europeans.

Sorbitol, which is a common sweetening agent used in "sugar-free" and other dietetic foods, also may contribute to symptoms. Normally, at least 90% of ingested sorbitol is absorbed in the small intestine by passive diffusion in which no enzyme in required. Ingestion of more than 30 g of sorbitol has been known to cause osmotic diarrhea. Some individuals tolerate much less (approximately 10 g). Ten grams of sorbitol is present in four to five sugar-free mints (some varieties). A study by Jain and colleagues suggests that severe sorbitol intolerance was found in 32% of blacks and 4% of whites.

Fructose also can cause significant abdominal distress. This sugar occurs naturally in fruits but also is added to a variety of processed foods. Symptoms seem to be related to the fermentation effect of colonic bacteria and malabsorbed carbohydrates. The combination of sorbitol and fructose can contribute to diarrhea and, therefore, should be eliminated from the diet on a trial basis.

Caffeinated products, including coffee, tea, and cola, carbonated products, and gas-producing foods, also may contribute to symptoms of bloating. Common gas-producing foods include broccoli, cabbage, Brussels sprouts, asparagus, cauliflower, and beans. Smoking, chewing gum, and eating quickly also seem to cause more swallowed air, resulting in increased gas and bloating. Excessive alcohol consumption may lead to increased rectal urgency.

A list of all current and past medications, both prescribed and over the counter, is necessary. Multiple medications alter bowel motility and exacerbate symptoms. The patient also may be taking a laxative and not realizing that this is contributing to her symptoms. Antacids containing magnesium or aluminum can cause diarrhea or constipation, respectively.

A detailed surgical history, especially any abdominal surgery, needs to be obtained. Adhesions may cause symptoms that mimic IBS. A good social history involving questions related to sexual and physical abuse is mandatory (Table 68-3). Drossman and colleagues report that 44% of patients with functional gastrointestinal disorders have a history of sexual or physical abuse in childhood or later in life. (All but one of the physically abused patients had been sexually abused also.) Patients are unlikely to volunteer this information unless specifically asked.

An accurate record of family history with regard to inflammatory bowel disease, colon cancer, or malabsorption states such as sprue is important. Therefore, the importance of history-taking cannot be stressed enough. By far, this is more important than the physical examination.

PHYSICAL EXAMINATION AND CLINICAL FINDINGS

On physical examination, IBS patients typically appear tense and may have tachycardia and hypertension. Some tenderness may be elicited on abdominal examination. However, if tympanitic bowel sounds, rebound tenderness, or board-like rigidity are present, an obstruction or an acute abdomen should be suspected and a surgeon consulted immediately. A fever also is worrisome because this goes against the diagnosis of IBS. Rectal and pelvic examinations are performed to assess for masses or anal disease (hemorrhoids, fissures) that could explain symptoms.

LABORATORY AND IMAGING STUDIES

A set core of blood and stool tests must be checked (Table 68-4). A complete blood cell count with differential, chemistry profile, and sedimentation rate is suggested. To rule out infection with *Giardia* and other parasites, stool should be sent for the ova-and-parasite (O & P) test three times.

The stool should be checked for occult blood; results should be negative in IBS patients. A methylene blue stain looking for white blood cells (WBCs) also should be performed. The presence of large numbers of WBCs is diagnostic of inflammation. A Sudan stain on a stool specimen to look for fat also is suggested. This is performed by adding 2 drops of acetic acid, 2 drops of Sudan III, and 95% alcohol to a slide. The slide is gently heated to boiling. Normally, only a few small red-staining fat globules are seen. In severe steatorrhea, many large fat globules are seen. Stools should be checked for *Clostridium difficile* toxin if there has been recent (last 6 weeks) antibiotic exposure.

A proctosigmoidoscopy with biopsy should be performed on patients younger than 40 years of age. Although grossly the mucosa may appear normal, biopsy may reveal microscopic or collagenous colitis, diagnoses that could account for the patient's symptoms. For patients older than 40 years of age, a barium enema plus flexible sigmoidoscopy or a full colonoscopy may be necessary. A colonic neoplasm needs to be ruled out. The insufflation of air during the examination often reproduces IBS symptoms. Notice that IBS may coexist with other bowel problems that are not mutually exclusive.

TREATMENT

The treatment of IBS is variable because this entity suggests a heterogeneous group. However, once the diagnosis is strongly considered, based on a detailed history, physical examination, and blood work, Camilleri and Prather from the Mayo Clinic suggest that patients be sorted into one of three major subclassifications,

Table 68-3. History of Abuse in Patients With Functional or Organic Diagnoses*

VARIABLE	PATIENTS WITH FUNCTIONAL DIAGNOSES	PATIENTS WITH ORGANIC DIAGNOSES	ODDS RATIO (95% CI)
	n/N (%)		
Sexual abuse			
Sexual exposure	29/74 (39)	29/124 (23)	1.90 (1.00–3.67)
Threat of sex	30/75 (40)	28/124 (23)	2.25 (1.17–4.29)
Touched patient	28/75 (37)	34/124 (27)	1.37 (0.72–2.62)
Patient touched other	13/73 (18)	18/124 (15)	1.23 (0.55–2.74)
Rape or incest	23/75 (31)	22/125 (18)	2.08 (1.03–4.21)
Any sexual abuse	40/75 (53)	47/126 (37)	1.71 (0.93–3.12)
Physical abuse (often)	9/70 (13)	2/123 (2)	11.39 (2.22–58.48)

*After controlling for age, race, and marital status with logistic regression.

(From Drossman DA, Leserman J, Nechman G, et al. Sexual and physical abuse in women with functional or organic gastrointestinal disorders. Ann Intern Med 1990;113:830.)

Table 68-4. Significant Laboratory Features

TEST	CONDITION INVESTIGATED
CBC	Anemia, inflammation
ESR	Inflammation
Differential	Eosinophilia (parasites)
	Monocytosis (Tbc)
	Toxic granulation (Inflammation)
Stools × 3 for O&P	Amoeba, *Giardia,* others
Proctosigmoidoscopy with	Structural lesions or inflammation
Microscopic exam of mucus in warm saline	Amoebiasis
Methylene blue stain of stool	Leukocytes (inflammation)
Occult blood test	Inflammation, tumor
Lactose tolerance test or 2-wk lactose-free diet	Lactose intolerance
Laboratory Features Against the Diagnosis	
Elevated ESR	
Leukocytosis	
Blood, pus, or fat in stool	
Stool volume > 200 mL/d	
Persistence of diarrhea after 48-h fast (indicates secretory diarrhea)	
Manometry failing to show spastic response to rectal distention	

ESR, erythrocyte sedimentation rate; *O&P,* ova and parasites.
(From Schuster M. Diagnostic evaluation of the irritable bowel syndrome. Gastroenterol Clin North Am 1991;20:274.)

depending on which symptom is dominant (Fig. 68-1). The three symptom groups are (1) abdominal pain, gas, and bloating; (2) constipation predominant; and (3) diarrhea predominant. The extent of the symptoms—mild, moderate, or severe—also should be considered. The key word in treatment is *individualization,* depending on the group to which the patient belongs.

The concept of "optimal management" is controversial. There are no well-designed placebo-controlled studies providing convincing evidence that one particular therapy is effective in all patients. This results partly from the high placebo response rate (70%) and partly from lumping all patients together rather than sorting patients by symptoms. Even with the classifications just mentioned, many patients do not fall clearly into any one of these groups but, rather, fall into an overlap group.

If the patient's symptoms predominantly involve bloating and abdominal pain, the initial workup is normal, and dietary modifications are not helpful, a flat plate of the abdomen during the acute onset of symptoms is recommended. If the etiology is related to a small bowel obstruction, the x-rays should reveal bowel distention and air fluid levels. If the x-ray is negative, a trial of an antispasmodic is suggested, assuming the patient is not pregnant. No currently available antispasmodic has consistently proven efficacy. Commonly used antispasmodics include dicyclomine (Bentyl), hyoscyamine (Levsin), Donnatal, and Librax. It is important to start treatment at a low dose and then increase it gradually. Unfortunately, sometimes efficacy is obtained only after a level at which side effects are more common. Potential side effects include urinary retention, xerostomia, and mydriasis, due to the anticholinergic properties of these medications. These side effects should be discussed with the patient beforehand. The timing of the dosing also is crucial. Because many patients have postprandial symptoms, it is wise to give each of these medications 30 minutes before meals. If a sublingual preparation is prescribed, it can be given at the time that the discomfort begins. In patients with predominantly gas and bloating symptoms, Beano (a D-galactosidase) or a simethicone preparation (Gas X, Phazyme) also can be tried. If the patient remains symptomatic, a small bowel follow-through should be performed.

If the symptom is predominantly constipation and the result of the initial workup is negative, a trial of increased roughage should be undertaken. Psyllium should be encouraged. Some patients have increased gas once fiber is consumed, and about 15% cannot tolerate fiber at all. Therefore, it is recommended that fiber be increased incrementally and taken with a meal, usually breakfast. Sometimes tap water enemas during the "break-in" of progressive fiber supplements are helpful. If necessary, a stool softener or osmotic laxative also can be used temporarily. An insufficient dose of fiber is a frequent cause of failure. Chronic use of stimulant laxatives should be discouraged.

If the constipation persists, further investigation is warranted. A colonic transit test using radiopaque markers with x-rays taken on days 4 and 7 after ingestion of 20 markers is performed. Anorectal manometry, tests of rectal sensation and expulsion, and assessment of pelvis for descent are sometimes necessary. These tests require referral to a specialized gastrointestinal center. There may be a role for prokinetic agents in constipation. Cisapride (Propulsid) has been shown to increase small bowel transit and may be helpful, although data to support its indiscriminate use are

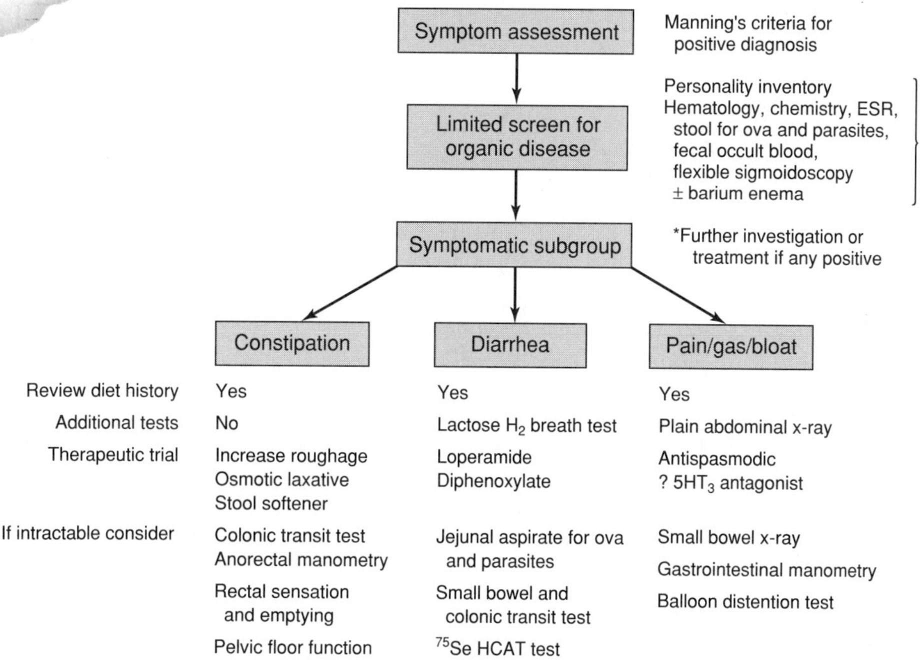

Figure 68-1. Strategy for evaluation of subgroups of patients with the irritable bowel syndrome. Note the stepwise series of evaluations guided by the symptom complex (Manning's criteria), by exclusion of organic disease, and by focusing on the major systems for subsequent testing. *ESR*, erythrocyte sedimentation rate; *$5HT_3$*, 5-hydroxytryptamine; *lactose H_2*, lactose hydrogen; *^{75}Se HCAT*, selenium-75 homocholic acid taurine. (Compiled from Camilleri M, Prather CM. The irritable bowel syndrome: mechanisms and a practical approach to management. Ann Inter Med 1992;116:1001.)

not overwhelming. Cisapride seems to work by facilitating acetylcholine release from the myenteric plexus. Metoclopramide (Reglan) is not recommended because, although it is a prokinetic agent, it does not act on the large intestines.

Tricyclic antidepressants may aggravate constipation because of their anticholinergic side effects. Therefore, they should be avoided.

Diarrhea-predominant patients are the third group. Loperamide (Imodium) is the most commonly used agent and is available over the counter. The prescribed dose is as much as 2 to 4 mg four times a day for a maximum of 16 mg/day. It decreases intestinal transit time, enhancing intestinal water absorption and strengthening rectal sphincter tone. It does not cross the blood–brain barrier, although other agents do (Lomotil, codeine). Patients with IBS often are sensitive to antidiarrheal agents. Sometimes a single dose causes constipation. Preferably, a soluble dietary fiber (psyllium, pectin, oat bran) should be tried before using the loperamide. A low fat diet with smaller meals also may help. Tricyclic anti-depressants can alleviate diarrhea and associated pain in a certain proportion of patients. This is thought to be due to their anticholinergic properties.

There is an entity called idiopathic bile acid catharsis in which bile acid entering the colon irritates the large bowel, causing functional diarrhea. A trial of cholestyramine (up to 4 g every 6 hours) is warranted. There is a high false-negative rate (up to 25%) and an appreciable false-positive rate with cholestyramine use. In specialized centers, bile acid malabsorption can be assessed by the ^{75}Se HCAT test.

Lastly, some researchers suggest that ondansetron, a serotonin receptor antagonist ($5HT_3$), may be useful in slowing colonic transit time. However, it is not approved by the Food and Drug Administration for this indication.

Although there are prescription medications for treating IBS, their use is not necessary in all individuals and, at times, may be counterproductive. Drugs have side effects. Also, a high initial placebo effect causes patients to continue medication indefinitely when, in fact, these medications are not effective. Drossman and Thompson in 1992 stressed that the foundation of treatment involves confidence in the diagnosis and a strong physician–patient relationship. IBS is a chronic disorder and, therefore, good communication is the key component. It is helpful to explain to the patient that IBS is a real disorder in which the intestine is especially sensitive to stimuli. It is necessary to determine the patient's understanding of the illness and her concerns because some patients believe they may have cancer. It is definitely worthwhile to tell the patient that IBS does not lead to cancer, require surgery, or shorten life expectancy. The patient's expectations for improvement must be elicited. Her involvement in the treatment plan is important, but limits must be set, especially if the patient is asking for narcotics.

There are some alternative therapies that are being tested for IBS, including relaxation response training, hypnosis, biofeedback, and psychotherapy. Family counseling also may be helpful if family dysfunction is responsible for symptom exacerbation. Guthrie reports that factors favoring a good response to psychotherapy include patients with predominantly diarrhea and pain, the association with IBS of overt psychiatric symptoms, intermittent pain exacerbated by stress, short duration of bowel complaints, and few

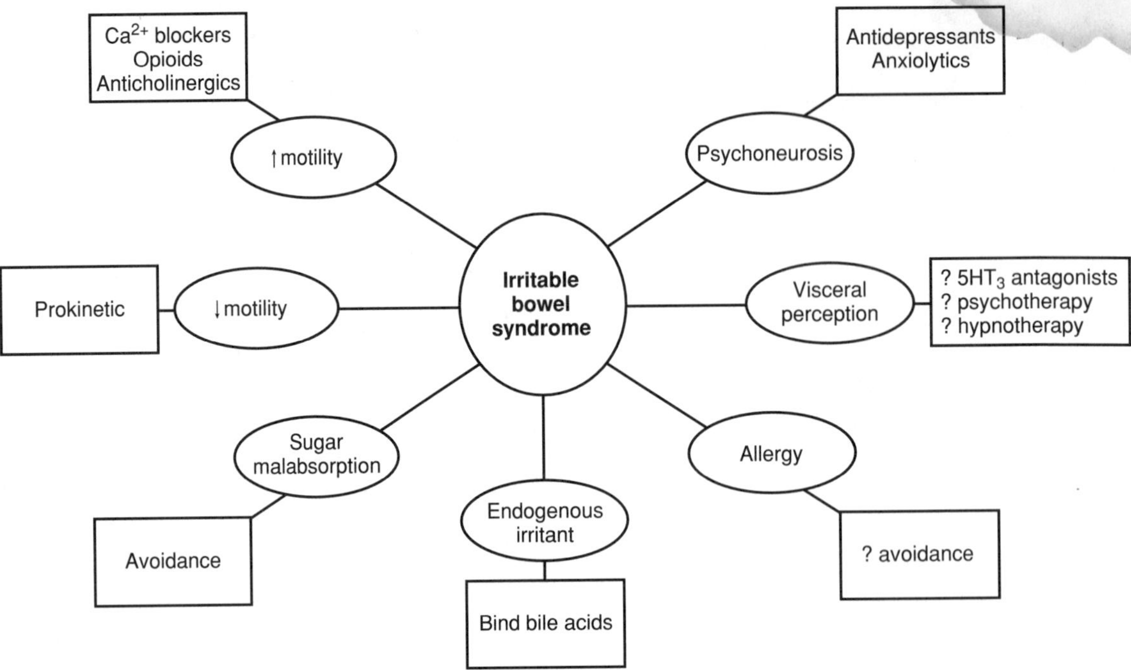

Figure 68-2. Targeting therapy for the irritable bowel syndrome. Examples of strategies aimed at correction of putative dysfunctions in the syndrome. Ca^{++}, calcium (channel); $5HT_3$, 5–hydroxytryptamine. (From Camilleri M, Prather CM. The irritable bowel syndrome: mechanisms and a practical approach to management. Ann Intern Med 1992;116:1001.)

sites of abdominal pain. Patients with constant abdominal pain do poorly with psychotherapy or hypnotherapy.

In the evaluation of pelvic pain, IBS needs to be ruled out. Statistics reveal that 21% of IBS patients and 14% of patients with functional bowel disease aged 18 to 40 years have undergone hysterectomies. This is significantly higher than the national average of 5.5%.

CONSIDERATIONS IN PREGNANCY

Irritable bowel syndrome in pregnancy has not been specifically studied. On the other hand, there is evidence for exacerbation of IBS during menses (Fig. 68-3). In 1990, Whitehead and colleagues stated that menstruation was associated with one or more bowel symptoms in 34 patients who denied previous symptoms of IBS or functional bowel disorders. These symptoms included increased diarrhea in 19%, increased gas in 14%, or increased constipation in 11%. Patients who already had IBS were significantly more likely to experience exacerbations of each of these bowel symptoms, but especially increased bowel gas. The physiologic basis for these bowel symptoms has not been established clearly. One possible etiology is progesterone. However, controlled studies fail to show a difference in gastrointestinal transit time between the luteal and follicular phases of the menstrual cycle. This rules out progesterone as the cause of menses-related bowel symptoms.

On the other hand, bowel symptoms do seem to worsen during the first day of menses, when there are elevated levels of certain prostaglandins (E_2 and F_2) in menstrual fluid. These prostaglandins are known to be powerful stimulants of contractile activity in the colon. Prostaglandins are rapidly metabolized. Therefore, it is not known whether these prostaglandins released in the uterus and carried by the circulation to gastrointestinal smooth muscle are sufficient enough to stimulate contractions of the colon. Research into whether prostaglandin antagonists would be helpful in IBS patients with menstrual exacerbation has been suggested.

Treatment for pregnant patients with IBS is limited with regard to medications because of possible teratogenic effects. Conservative management is the rule, involving a high fiber diet and eliminating lactose, sorbitol, fructose, caffeine, and gas-producing foods. Exercising regularly, eating smaller meals, and increasing

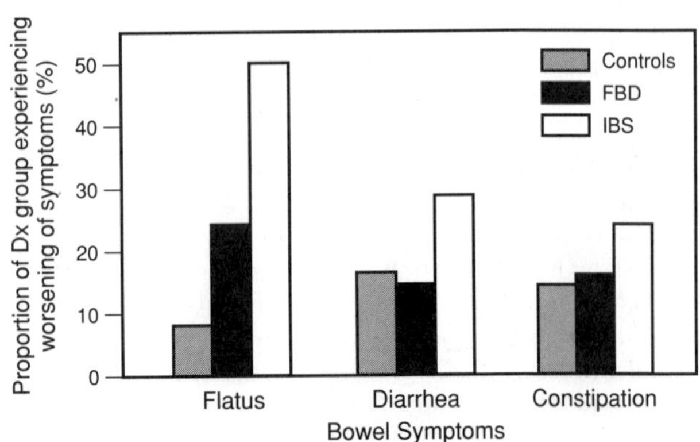

Figure 68-3. Irritable bowel syndrome (IBS) exacerbates the bowel symptoms experienced by women during menstruation. *Dx*, diagnosis; *FBD*, functional bowel disorder. (From Sparberg M. Roundtable conference on IBS: Part II. Practical Gastroentrol 1993:6.)

water intake should be suggested by the primary care provider. Adequate time for meals in quiet surroundings can be therapeutic. Setting aside a time to defecate is advised. The urge to defecate should never be ignored.

CONCLUSION

Much progress has been made in defining, evaluating, and treating IBS patients. However, there is a group of patients with severe symptoms who do not respond to therapies. These are the individuals who need to be referred to a gastroenterologist with expertise in IBS.

Obviously, many unanswered questions remain. As we approach the 21st century, hopefully there will be more and more answers.

BIBLIOGRAPHY

Camilleri M, Prather CM. The irritable bowel syndrome: mechanisms and a practical approach to management. Ann Intern Med 1992;116:1001.

Drossman DA, Leserman J, Nachman G, et al. Sexual and physical abuse in women with functional or organic gastrointestinal disorders. Ann Intern Med 1990;113:828.

Drossman DA, Thompson WG. The irritable bowel syndrome: review and a graduated multicomponent treatment approach. Ann Intern Med 1992;116:1009.

Guthrie E, Creed F, Dawson D, Tomenson B. A controlled trial of psychological treatment for the irritable bowel syndrome. Gastroenterology 1991;100:450.

Jain NK, Rosenberg DB, Ulahannan MJ, Glasser MJ, Pitchumoni CS. Sorbitol intolerance in adults. Am J Gastroenterol 1985;80:678.

Kellow JE, Gill RC, Wingate DL. Prolonged ambulant recordings of bowel motility demonstrate abnormalities in the irritable bowel syndrome. Gastroenterology 1990;98:1208.

Kellow JE, Phillips SF. Altered small bowel motility in irritable bowel syndrome is correlated with symptoms. Gastroenterology 1987;92:1885.

Manning AP, Thompson WG, Heaton KW, Morris AF. Towards positive diagnosis of the irritable bowel. Br Med J 1978; 2:653.

Owens DM, Nelson DK, Talley NJ. The irritable bowel syndrome: long-term prognosis and the physician–patient interaction. Ann Intern Med 1995;122:107.

Prior A, Whorwell PJ. Gynaecological consultation in patients with the irritable bowel syndrome. Gut 1989;30:996.

Schuster MM. Diagnostic evaluation of the irritable bowel syndrome. Gastroenterol Clin North Am 1991; Vol 20.

Snape WJ, Carlson GM, Cohen S. Colonic myoelectric activity in the irritable bowel syndrome. Gastroenterology 1976;70:326.

Sparberg M. Round table conference on IBS. Part II. Pract Gastroenterol 1993;Feb:6.

Talley NJ, Zinsmeister AR, VanDyke C, Melton LJ. Epidemiology of colonic symptoms and the irritable bowel syndrome. Gastroenterology 1991;101:927.

Thompson WG. Functional bowel disease and functional abdominal pain. Gastroenterol Int 1992;5:75.

Whitehead WE, Cheskin LJ, Heller BR, et al. Evidence for exacerbation of irritable bowel syndrome during menses. Gastroenterology 1990;-98:1485.

Whitehead WE, Holtkotter B, Enck P, et al. Tolerance for rectosigmoid distention in irritable bowel syndrome. Gastroenterology 1990;-98:1187.

Whorwell PJ, Prior A, Faragher EB. Controlled trial of hypnotherapy in the treatment of severe refractory irritable bowel syndrome. Lancet 1984;2:1232.

Primary Care for Women, edited by Phyllis C. Leppert and Fred M. Howard. Lippincott-Raven Publishers, Philadelphia © 1997.

69

Diverticular Disease

EDWARD G. FLICKINGER

Diverticular disease is a spectrum of diseases related to diverticulosis coli that may be acquired over one's lifetime. It has achieved clinical significance only during the twentieth century in economically developed Western societies. With the introduction of the roller process for milling wheat flour during the 1880s, dietary patterns rapidly changed, resulting in a widespread increase in the consumption of refined white flour. Conversely, the overall intake of fiber as bran decreased. This abrupt environmental dietary change is now universally accepted as the explanation for the dramatic increase in the prevalence of colonic diverticula within our population during this century. Diverticular disease has subsequently become the most common colonic malady of modern times for Western civilization.

Although the actual prevalence of diverticulosis coli is not known, it increases almost linearly with age. Before 1900, diverticula were thought to occur in less than 5% of the population and rarely produced clinical symptoms. It is now estimated that nearly one third of the population will have developed diverticula by the sixth decade and two thirds by the eighth decade. Earlier in the century, there was a definite male predominance in the distribution of diverticular disease, but this gender difference has completely disappeared.

Whereas diverticula usually remain entirely asymptomatic, they may produce a wide variety of clinical presentations, ranging from mild abdominal discomfort and bowel irregularity to potentially life-threatening complications of acute inflammation, abscess formation, free perforation, obstruction, and bleeding. Because physicians frequently must assess abdominal complaints in women of all ages, it is imperative to consider diverticular disease in the differential diagnosis.

ETIOLOGY

The decrease in consumption of dietary fiber produces a corresponding decrease in stool bulk. Consequently, higher intraluminal colonic pressures must be generated to ensure fecal transit. Two conditions must be present physiologically for diverticula to develop: (1) a pressure gradient between the bowel lumen and the serosal surface, and (2) relative areas of weakness in the colonic wall caused by disordered colonic motility. Colonic manometry has confirmed band-like or segmental high pressure areas with slow waves cycling 12 to 18 times per minute. Within these high pressure segments, a pulsion-type diverticulum may develop through naturally occurring anatomic weak points where nutrient vessels penetrate the two antimesenteric taeniae. It is actually a pseudodiverticulum because the wall is composed of only the mucosal layer, lacking a true muscularis and serosa. This dietary explanation is well supported by additional observations that diverticular disease is distinctly rare among both lower socioeconomic populations, in whom dietary fiber intake remains high, and self-imposed vegetarians.

Diverticula rarely occur in the rectum where the taeniae actually coalesce into a complete longitudinal muscular layer. They develop most commonly in the sigmoid colon and decrease in frequency in the more proximal colon. Cecal diverticula are uncommon, and when present, are usually true diverticula and believed to be of congenital origin. They are of little clinical significance.

Symptoms may occur only after a diverticulum has developed. Colonic contents (seeds, pits, or other indigestible or partially digestible material) may become trapped in a narrow-mouthed diverticulum, ultimately producing a localized inflammatory reaction. Alternatively, nutrient colonic vessels may erode at the site of the diverticulum, producing painless colonic bleeding. When symptoms develop, the sigmoid colon is involved more than 90% of the time. More than 50% of the time, the sigmoid is the only portion of the bowel involved. Ninety percent of all operations for diverticular inflammation involve the sigmoid.

Up to 20 g of bran may be required daily to provide adequate fiber to prevent diverticula from developing or for ameliorating symptoms once they have occurred. Whole-meal breads, fruits, vegetables, and cereals are the most common source of dietary fiber. However, commercially available bran cereals vary widely in actual fiber content, so one should always read package labels carefully. Psyllium seeds (Metamucil) absorb up to 15 mL of water per gram of fiber compared with actual bran, which absorbs only 3 mL of water per gram. Not surprisingly, psyllium often is recommended along with other dietary measures as the basis of diverticular disease prevention and treatment.

HISTORY

Most individuals with diverticulosis coli are asymptomatic and are identified only at the time of either a screening barium enema or colonoscopy. Because this condition is acquired over a lifetime, symptomatic patients usually are middle aged or older. This is not to say that younger people cannot experience symptoms of diverticular disease; just less commonly so. However, if patients do present with symptoms before 40 years of age, there is growing evidence that this form of diverticular disease may be more aggressive, with more than 60% eventually requiring surgery.

Most symptomatic patients initially complain of intermittent abdominal pains, often of a cramping nature. They also may have either bowel irregularity or actual constipation. These symptoms are relatively common and may be difficult to distinguish from irritable bowel syndrome. However, once the patient is identified as having diverticulosis coli, nearly all of them can be managed medically with dietary counseling and fiber supplementation. It may actually be advantageous to simply add fiber (most easily and cheaply in the form of bran cereals) to the diets of all people older than 50 years of age. The desired result is a softer, bulky stool that can be passed without straining. The actual amount of fiber required to achieve this result is subject to individual variation.

Whereas the symptoms mentioned earlier are relatively common and may predate the onset of acute diverticulitis, some patients present with an acute inflammatory process involving a single diverticulum as their first symptom. When the narrowed neck of the diverticulum becomes obstructed by fecal material, bacterial overgrowth occurs, ultimately creating localized inflammation. At this point, the patient usually complains of more significant abdominal pain and may suffer from nausea and vomiting. A low-grade fever is common. Such patients require specific medical attention and may need to be hospitalized. Should the inflammation extend to involve the parietal peritoneum, signs of peritoneal irritation are elicited on physical examination. As a consequence, the patient may develop abdominal distention secondary to either a paralytic ileus or a relative mechanical obstruction at the site of the inflammatory process. Should the process continue to exacerbate or progress to a contained perforation, either a fullness or a discreet mass may be palpated in the area overlying the involved bowel segment (usually the sigmoid colon). A bimanual pelvic and rectal examination (although uncomfortable to the patient) can further delineate the extent of the acute process. Most episodes of diverticulitis respond to medical therapy, precluding the need for surgery. The patient should continue to follow dietary restrictions and fiber supplementation, but the possibility always exists for recurrent bouts of diverticulitis to occur. Usually, the same bowel segment is involved and the clinical presentation is similar to the initial bout. Sometimes both the patient and her physician recognize early signs of diverticulitis and make immediate dietary adjustments to prevent the development of full-blown symptoms.

In rare situations, an inflamed diverticulum may rupture freely into the abdominal cavity, producing pneumoperitoneum, signs of diffuse peritonitis, and an unstable clinical condition requiring rapid resuscitation and emergent surgical intervention.

If a patient recuperates from a particularly virulent attack of diverticulitis or has experienced numerous recurrent episodes of diverticulitis, the involved segment of bowel (usually the sigmoid colon) may become chronically narrowed, producing either a further alteration in bowel function or frank colonic obstruction. Clinically, this may be difficult to differentiate from an obstructing colonic malignancy. If the involved bowel is contiguous with either the urinary bladder or vagina, a chronic colovesical or colovaginal fistula may develop, causing symptoms that require surgical intervention.

A final form of clinical presentation does not involve an acute or chronic inflammatory process. As previously noted, the pseudodiverticula of diverticulosis coli occur at the site of anatomic penetration of nutrient vessels through the bowel wall. Should one of these nutrient vessels erode or simply rupture, painless lower intestinal bleeding ensues. The location of the leaking vessel and the rate of bleeding determine the patient's clinical course. The bleeding episode may be insignificant and self-limited or may be exsanguinating and life-threatening. Passed blood may be bright red, but more commonly is maroon. Although it may be relatively easy to diagnose diverticular disease as the pathologic process causing such a bleed, it may be extremely difficult, if not impossible, to actually localize which particular diverticulum in one of several possible locations is the one actually producing the bleed.

PHYSICAL EXAMINATION AND CLINICAL FINDINGS

For the patient experiencing only abdominal cramps and constipation, the physical examination is unremarkable, and only the patient's age may suggest the possibility of diverticulosis coli. Once inflammation arises within a diverticular sac, the physical findings usually reflect both the extent and location of the process. When the inflammatory process is locally extensive or a contained abscess has developed, a tender abdominal mass may be present, usually in the left lower quadrant. A pelvic and rectal examination should be performed to define the mass. Whereas such a mass does not necessarily confirm diverticulitis as the underlying cause, the suspicion is clearly raised. Further diagnostic studies are required to differentiate it from a locally perforated neoplasm. A spiking fever usually occurs once an abscess has developed.

When the patient presents with colonic obstruction secondary to a scarred and narrowed colon, abdominal distention may preclude palpation of any underlying mass that may be present. Lack of a mass clearly does not rule out the possibility of chronic diverticular disease. If a fistula has developed, the patient may present with recurrent urinary tract infections, pneumaturia, fecaluria, or perhaps chronic perineal soilage from vaginal involvement.

If the patient presents with bleeding from diverticulosis coli, it is likely that no unusual physical findings will be present whatsoever, and the patient may not have any antecedent history suggestive of diverticular disease.

LABORATORY AND IMAGING STUDIES

Usually, the patient's age and clinical symptoms (left lower quadrant pain) suggest the possibility of diverticular disease. Treatment should not be delayed, particularly if fever and leukocytosis are already present. A mass or peritoneal irritation need not be present to institute therapy. If the episode represents a recurrence of previously documented diverticular disease, one can probably be fairly certain of the current diagnosis. If diverticulosis coli has not been confirmed previously, the following diagnostic workup should be considered.

Plain abdominal x-rays are rarely, if ever, diagnostic but may show the presence of an ileus, with either localized or diffuse bowel distention. The presence of pneumoperitoneum confirms the need for emergent surgical intervention without actually confirming diverticular disease as the exact source of the patient's problem. If a patient has had a previous barium enema, residual barium sometimes remains in colonic diverticula for extended periods of time. A complete blood cell count, serum amylase, pregnancy test, and urinalysis also should be obtained early in the clinical course to rule out other potential diagnostic possibilities.

A rigid proctoscopic or flexible sigmoidoscopic examination may be helpful in documenting the presence of sigmoid diverticula. However, the patient's lower abdominal and pelvic tenderness may be so severe as to preclude them as useful diagnostic tests. Ultrasonic examination of the symptomatic area is useful only if a mass (ie, abscess) is already present. An emergent barium enema usually is not necessary, and most radiologists suggest delaying it until the risk of perforation from the pressure of an infused column of barium has diminished after several days of treatment. A computed tomography (CT) scan (preferably with intraluminal water-soluble contrast) is generally accepted as the diagnostic procedure of choice in the acute setting because it provides clearer delineation of the colonic wall and pericolonic tissue planes. Obviously, minimal inflammation can be missed, even by a CT scan. Colonoscopy becomes more valuable in documenting the presence of diverticulosis coli after acute symptoms have waned. A delayed contrast study or colonoscopy also can rule out other causes of the acute illness.

If the patient presents with evidence of a colovesical fistula, then a cystogram, cystoscopy, flexible sigmoidoscopy, and contrast evaluation of the distal colon and rectum all may be appropriate to define the etiology and to rule out a malignant source. Obviously, if the patient presents with symptoms of a colovaginal fistula, then a proctosigmoidoscopy and a speculum examination of the vagina should be performed.

If the patient presents with bleeding diverticulosis coli, then one can attempt localization of the bleeding vessel by either a nuclear bleeding scan or, preferably, by selective angiography of the inferior and superior mesenteric arteries. However, these studies are helpful only if the patient is actually bleeding at the time that the procedure is performed. The patient must be bleeding at a rate of 0.5 to 1.0 mL/minute for the angiogram to demonstrate contrast extravasation. Colonoscopy may readily document the presence of diverticulosis coli, but usually it is nearly useless in localizing the actual bleeding site because blood is everywhere throughout the colon.

TREATMENT

Preventive

Because diverticulosis coli is so common in Western society, it is probably worthwhile for all patients (men and women, regardless of age) to develop good dietary habits at a young age that may prevent the later development of diverticula and their complications. This includes the drinking of at least three glasses of water per day and the consumption of natural grain breads, fruits with a high fiber content, and leafy vegetables. The diet may be supplemented with additional fiber in the form of bran or psyllium as the patient gets older and may naturally be predisposed to symptoms of constipation. As noted previously, diverticula are extremely rare among vegetarians who partake of this type of diet regularly. As in other situations, prevention is far more effective than later treatment.

Acute Diverticulitis

When an acute episode of diverticulitis develops, the patient should be admitted to a hospital with the immediate institution of bowel rest. If the patient shows signs of ileus or partial mechanical obstruction, a nasogastric tube should be placed for comfort and decompression. Intravenous fluids should be administered along with broad-spectrum parenteral antibiotics. This may be either single-agent or combination therapy, consisting of drugs known to be effective against common enteric organisms (both aerobes and anaerobes). The combination of clindamycin plus an aminoglycoside is frequently effective. A narcotic may be necessary to provide adequate pain control. This regimen usually provides symptomatic relief within several days. The patient may start on a clear liquid diet soon thereafter and gradually advance as tolerated to the standard high fiber diet outlined earlier. Foods containing small seeds, kernels, pits, and other poorly digested particulate matter should be avoided. The patient should then adhere to this diet indefinitely.

Intravenous antibiotics usually may be discontinued after 7 to 10 days. A course of oral antibiotics may be prescribed if mild clinical symptoms persist. Less than 20% of patients experiencing an attack of acute diverticulitis require surgery. If the abdominal pain and fever do not subside, one should begin to suspect that a complication of diverticular disease has occurred, and additional workup is then indicated.

Perforated Diverticulitis

Patients who develop a contained or walled-off perforation require further evaluation and additional therapeutic intervention. If the abscess is localized, it may be accessible for either ultrasonic or CT-guided percutaneous drainage. This option may postpone the need for emergent surgical intervention and allow for a later single-staged resection of the involved bowel with primary colonic anastomosis, thus precluding the need for a temporary diverting colostomy. However, percutaneous drainage may not be technically possible because of the location of the abscess, or the extent of drainage obtained via this method may be insufficient to provide adequate resolution of the acute symptoms. When surgery is required in the acute setting, it usually is inappropriate, if not impossible, to perform a single-stage colon resection and primary anastomosis because of the risks associated with such contaminated cases. However, if the colon can be adequately prepared preoperatively and the perforation is entirely contained within the mesentery of the involved bowel segment, then, on rare occasions, this surgical option—including complete removal of the contained abscess—might be considered. Usually the procedure of choice is to resect the diseased bowel and create a temporary proximal diverting colostomy. This distal bowel segment (assuming adequate length) may be brought up to the abdominal wall as a mucus fistula or simply closed over in the lower abdomen or pelvis as a Hartmann pouch. This form of therapy eventually necessitates a later operative procedure to close the colostomy, thereby reestablishing colorectal continuity. Rarely is it necessary or appropriate to simply drain the abscess and perform a proximal colostomy (leaving the diseased bowel in situ), unless the patient's condition does not permit more extensive resection.

Antibiotics should be continued until evidence of infection has resolved. Enteral nutrition may be started with return of colostomy function. If the patient's course is complicated and prolonged, then total parenteral nutrition should be instituted. Once the patient has totally recuperated from such an operation (usually several months), colostomy closure may be considered.

An acute free perforation requires aggressive preoperative resuscitation and emergency laparotomy. The usual procedure is resection of the perforated bowel and proximal colostomy with irrigation of the abdominal cavity and drainage of any residual infected cavities. Once stabilized postoperatively, the patient may be managed in the same manner as described earlier.

Bleeding Diverticulosis Coli

Most patients with diverticular bleeding stop spontaneously and do not bleed again. For patients who continue to bleed and have their bleeding site confirmed angiographically, a trial of selective intraarterial vasopressin (initial rate of 0.2 U/minute) infusion is indicated. If the patient continues to bleed despite vasopressin infusion or if the site of bleeding cannot be identified, emergency surgery is indicated. If intraoperative evaluation fails to isolate the bleeding to either the right or left side of the colon, then an emergency abdominal colectomy with ileorectal anastomosis should be performed. The bleeding itself will have prepared the colon more than adequately to allow safe performance of an ileorectal anastomosis.

CONSIDERATIONS IN PREGNANCY

Because diverticular disease primarily afflicts postmenopausal women, rarely, if ever, does it complicate pregnancy. However, if patients of childbearing age do develop symptomatic diverticulitis, they should be managed just like anyone else. Both the patient and her physician should not be surprised if her course is of an aggressive nature, and she will likely require surgical intervention at some future time. If diverticulitis (or one of its complications) does develop during pregnancy, the patient should be treated aggressively. Obviously, if surgery is required, the risk to the pregnancy is significant and the patient's obstetrician should be closely involved in the patient's care.

BIBLIOGRAPHY

Casstille TA, Cohn I Jr. Diverticulosis and diverticulitis of the large intestine. In: Moody FG, ed. Surgical treatment of digestive disease. Chicago: Year Book Medical Publishers, 1986:647.

Hackford AW, Veidenheimer MC. Diverticular disease of the colon: current concepts and management. Surg Clin North Am 1985;65:347.

Morris J, Stellato TA, Haaga JR, Lieberman J. The utility of computed tomography in colonic diverticulitis. Ann Surg 1986;204:128.

Ouriel K, Schwartz SI. Diverticular disease in the young patient. Surg Gynecol Obstet 1983;156:1.

Painter NS. Diverticular disease of the colon: the first of the Western diseases shown to be due to a deficiency of dietary fibre. South Afr Med J 1982;61:1016.

Stabil BE, Puccio E, vanSonnenberg E, Neff CC. Preoperative percutaneous drainage of diverticular abscesses. Am J Surg 1990;159:99.z

Primary Care for Women, edited by Phyllis C. Leppert and Fred M. Howard. Lippincott-Raven Publishers, Philadelphia © 1997.

70

Constipation

MICHAEL BARRETT
STEPHEN M. RAUH

An interview inquiring into the basic health of a patient in the primary care setting would be incomplete without asking about the patient's bowel habit. "Normal" bowel function is considered a prerequisite for good health in the minds of nearly everyone. Therefore, constipation is a serious issue for patients who feel they suffer from it.

Constipation is only a symptom, and thus it is subjectively determined by the patient. The best definition of constipation is that it is a subjective term describing difficulty in defecation, either infrequent passage of small, hard stools or difficulty with straining at defecation. Because of its subjective nature, there is no agreement as to the scientific definition of constipation. Definitions vary from any patient who strains at defecation and does not have at least one stool per day to a patient who strains at stools 25% of the time or has fewer than three stools per week.

Although this ambiguity makes the scientific study of constipation difficult and sometimes confusing, in the primary clinical care of patients the issue is clear: a patient's complaint of constipation needs investigation to determine the nature and severity of the problem. Once this is known, if the patient's bowel habits are not out of the realm of normal, education may be all that is necessary, as reassurance removes significant anxiety. If the investigation reveals gastrointestinal tract dysfunction, further evaluation is required to determine the nature of the problem and to provide appropriate therapy.

The epidemiology of constipation varies based on the definition used and on whether constipation is self-reported or measured in a clinical research center. Most researchers have estimated that the incidence of constipation in the United States is 2% to 3% in the general adult population; the incidence increases to 20% to 30% in persons age 70 and older. Females are twice as likely to be affected by constipation as males. When the colonic transit time is evaluated in constipated patients, females are much more likely to have delayed transit than males.

Many studies have shown an increased incidence of abdominal pain and constipation in children who are victims of sexual abuse. An increased incidence of sexual abuse has also been observed in women evaluated at a tertiary care gastroenterology center for functional gastrointestinal disorders (having no organic cause). Therefore, sexual abuse must be considered in the evaluation of patients with chronic idiopathic constipation.

ETIOLOGY

The etiology of constipation can be broken down into extracolonic and colonic causes. The extracolonic causes include various metabolic, endocrine, and neurologic disorders. Drug therapies that decrease colonic motility also cause constipation. Some have proposed that the higher incidence of constipation in women is secondary to hormonal imbalances: some clinical data have supported this theory, but it has not gained widespread acceptance.

The colonic causes are divided into structural and functional causes. The structural group includes obstructive processes and intestinal aganglionosis (ie, Hirschsprung disease). The functional causes cannot be explained anatomically.

Metabolic abnormalities associated with constipation include uremia, hypokalemia, porphyria, sporadic primary amyloidosis (causing a neuropathy), diabetes, and hypercalcemia. Endocrine disorders associated with constipation include hypothyroidism, pseudohypoparathyroidism, pheochromocytoma, glucagon-producing tumors, and disorders that lead to hypercalcemia (eg, primary hyperparathyroidism, milk-alkali syndrome, disseminated bony metastasis). Neurologic causes of constipation include lesions of the central and peripheral nervous systems. Central lesions include cerebral tumors, injury secondary to cerebrovascular accident, Parkinson disease, and multiple sclerosis. The peripheral nervous system disorder most commonly seen with constipation is autonomic neuropathy.

Many medications are associated with constipation. The most commonly recognized are narcotic analgesics and various muscle relaxants. Many other drugs are sometimes implicated, including calcium and aluminum antacids, diuretics, medications used to treat parkinsonism, antidepressants, monoamine oxidase inhibitors, iron supplements, anticholinergics, and calcium channel blockers. Chronic laxative abuse has been thought to cause local injury to the innervation of the colon and subsequent dysmotility and constipation.

The structural causes of colonic dysmotility include obstructive processes and intrinsic neurologic problems. Obstructive etiologies include extraluminal obstructions (tumors, chronic volvulus, various hernias) and luminal obstructive processes of the colon and rectum (various tumors and benign structures secondary to inflammatory diseases or following surgical reconstruction). Descending perineum syndrome and rectocele can also lead to constipation. Lesions of the anal canal, including stenosis, anterior ectopic anus, anal fissures, and mucosal prolapse, can all play a role in constipation. Hemorrhoids are not a cause of constipation, although some argue that hemorrhoids can be worsened by chronic constipation.

The functional causes of colonic constipation are divided into two categories: colonic dysmotility and anorectal (defecatory) dysfunction. Colonic dysmotility involves slow colonic transit times and constipation. Its mechanism is unknown but thought to be secondary to muscular, neurologic, or even psychological problems. Colonic dysmotility may be generalized throughout the colon or segmental. Patients may also have anorectal problems, but usually they are not seen concurrently.

Anorectal dysfunction is a cause of functional obstruction and great difficulty in defecation. For defecation to proceed smoothly, there must be coordination between the rectum and the anus. As the rectum contracts to expel the stool, the anus must relax to open the rectal outlet and allow passage of the fecal mass. Failure of this coordination leads to anorectal dysfunction and constipation. Failure of the rectum to contract is known as rectal inertia; failure of the anus to relax is called outlet obstruction. Anismus describes the failure of the anal sphincters to relax; anorectal dyssynergia is used to indicate increased anal contraction during defecation. Rectal outlet obstruction is therefore a failure of the normal rectoanal inhibitory reflex.

HISTORY

A good history provides the foundation for all further evaluation and therapy. Because constipation is a symptom, an accurate description of the problem from the patient's point of view is crucial. For instance, is the chief complaint frequent straining at stools, but with a normal number of bowel movements? Is infrequent defecation the greatest concern? Accurate documentation of the patient's typical bowel habits (eg, timing, frequency, amount of time spent straining, usual result) is required. The nature of the stool (eg, hard or soft, small or large, brown or bloody or melanotic) should be determined. Many patients can be reassured that their bowel habits are actually normal, resolving their anxiety.

One of the most important points in the history is the onset of constipation. If it has been since birth, a congenital abnormality or Hirschsprung disease should be considered. If the patient is middle-aged and the symptoms are chronic (> 2 years), it is less likely that significant pathology is to blame. However, if the onset was less than 2 years before presentation, the risk of a partially obstructing colonic malignancy is increased.

The patient's diet and use of medications are also important. Particularly important is the amount and source of fiber in the diet. A list of the patient's medications should be reviewed, with potential constipating agents noted. If the patient has been treating her constipation with dietary changes or medications, this should also be carefully reviewed.

Finally, given the increased incidence of sexual abuse in females with functional gastrointestinal disorders, a history of abuse should be carefully elicited by sensitive questioning.

PHYSICAL EXAMINATION AND CLINICAL FINDINGS

The physical examination is as important as the history. A complete examination is required, as other medical problems may be related to or causing the constipation. In particular, stigmata of systemic diseases (eg, hypothyroidism) or metabolic abnormalities should be noted.

Examination of the abdomen should note the presence or absence of bowel sounds, along with their level of activity. Palpable masses are an important finding, indicating a possible near-obstructing lesion. Lower quadrant tenderness may indicate an ongoing inflammatory process such as diverticulitis. In thin patients, hard stool can be palpated in the colon.

Hernias are often a cause of partial obstruction and can present with the complaint of constipation. A good hernia examination must be done to rule out these abdominal wall defects. Femoral hernias are more common in women than in men: special attention must be paid to this area in women because it is the most often overlooked hernia.

The anorectal examination may be the most important part of the examination, but because it is usually unpleasant for the patient and the physician, it is often given less than the required attention and time. Digital examination of the anus and rectum is done to rule out mass lesions and to assess the content of the rectal vault. Fecal impaction can quickly convince the physician of the diagnosis of constipation.

The digital examination also can give a good assessment of basic anorectal coordination. The patient is asked to bear down as if to strain against stool, and the physician notes the behavior of the internal and external anal sphincters. If the normal anorectal reflex is present, straining leads to anal sphincter relaxation. If the patient contracts the anal sphincters instead, a diagnosis of anismus can be considered. The digital examination also reveals the function of the pelvic floor in defecatory activity and may be useful in helping to make the diagnosis of descending perineum syndrome.

Examination of the anus by direct visualization and anoscopy should be part of the initial examination. The external examination can reveal evidence of an ectopic external anus, which is associated with outlet obstruction. The presence of anal fissures should also be noted. Anal fissures cause enough pain and swelling that patients refrain from defecating, causing a functional outlet obstruction and hardening of the stools, which worsens the problem.

Gross examination of the anus may show it to be patulous and lax. It may also show evidence of local trauma such as abrasions or multiple fissures. Both of these signs have been linked to sexual abuse and may lead to direct questioning.

A complete examination includes a pelvic examination as well. Rectocele should be ruled out. The breasts should also be examined, as several studies have indicated a possible link between constipation and breast disease.

Sigmoidoscopy, preferably flexible, should be included in the initial office work-up of constipation (particularly constipation of recent onset). Flexible sigmoidoscopy can assess the descending colon, sigmoid colon, and rectum for evidence of neoplastic lesions and diverticular disease. Melanosis coli, a dark pigmentation of the colorectal mucosa, is associated with significant laxative use.

LABORATORY AND IMAGING STUDIES

The laboratory and imaging studies used in the evaluation of constipation in the primary care setting are relatively few and simple. However, for patients who fail routine management and have no identifiable anatomic pathology, the number of studies used for evaluation increases greatly, as does their complexity.

Laboratory studies useful in the evaluation of patients with constipation include serum chemistries (important to rule out hypercalcemia and uremia) and thyroid function tests. A blood count with red blood cell volume is done to rule out a microcytic anemia.

Studies of the gastrointestinal tract can be divided into anatomic and functional studies. Anatomic studies address mechanical obstructions, pseudo-obstruction, and histologic disease (agangliosis [Hirschsprung disease]). They are indicated in the initial evaluation of all patients older than age 30 who are presenting with new onset of symptoms (< 2 years) if unexplained by other causes. Anatomic studies are also indicated if gross or occult rectal blood is found during a routine examination or by history. These studies can be either colonoscopic or radiographic. Total colonoscopy allows direct visualization and tissue biopsy. Barium enema is also a suitable study, offering a similar sensitivity but less specificity due to the inability to gather histologic data. When megacolon or megarectum is suspected by history, the barium enema is the better examination.

If no anatomic cause of constipation is discovered and the patient has failed conventional therapy, a diagnosis of chronic idiopathic constipation is made and further study is in order. Colonic motility is first examined, and the most widely used study for this purpose is the radiologic marker transit study. Twenty to thirty radiopaque markers are ingested, and their passage through the colon is monitored by serial abdominal flat plates. An abnormal transit time is greater than 72 hours. Serial abdominal films may give an idea of segmental transit variations. If specific segmental transit data are necessary, electromyographic testing is required, with intraluminal probes passed from the anus to the cecum. This shows abnormalities in the passage of the electrical pacemaker wave and can show segmental differences. However, this test is performed only in the most specialized centers. The marker transit test remains a safe, reliable, and reproducible measure of colonic transit time and is sufficient to rule out colonic dysmotility.

The complex nature of the anatomy and function of the pelvic floor and anus is reflected in the number and diversity of studies designed to describe and quantify their integrated function. These studies are indicated in chronic idiopathic constipation when anatomic disorders and colonic dysmotility have been ruled out. Each tertiary referral center has an accepted series of tests, but a few of the more commonly used tests are described below.

Anorectal manometry is done using a manometer placed through the anus and into the rectum. It gives resting, straining, and squeeze pressures from the rectal and anal canals, allowing assessment of the normal rectoanal inhibitory response. The compliance of the rectum can also be determined, with a high compliance associated with an increased risk of megarectum.

Electromyography can evaluate pudendal nerve activity in the puborectalis muscle and the anal sphincter during straining. This can allow documentation of abnormal, continued electrical activity in the anal sphincter during straining, making the diagnosis of anismus.

The balloon expulsion test is a simple test that measures the ability of the pelvic floor to generate enough pressure to expel stool. A balloon is inserted into the rectum and filled with 80 mL of warm water. The patient's ability to expel the balloon is tested without and with the addition of weight to the balloon. Normal patients spontaneously pass the balloon. Some patients with defecatory disorders cannot expel the balloon spontaneously or require a significant amount of weight to be added to expel the balloon.

TREATMENT

The most important part of treatment lies in the initial evaluation. If a patient who complains of constipation is found to have normal bowel habits, simple teaching and reassurance may solve the problem. Once the history and physical examination are completed, screening laboratory tests and an endoscopic examination or a contrast study are done. If these are negative, a treatment plan can be formulated. If the patient uses laxatives, a trial without them is important to assess baseline bowel function.

The next intervention should deal with toilet training and bowel habit. Patients should be encouraged not to suppress the urge to defecate, because doing so promotes constipation. Patients should try to defecate after a specific meal, establishing a routine. Increased activity is also important, as physically active people tend to experience less constipation than sedentary types.

Dietary adjustment is the next intervention to make. An increase in dietary fiber to 20 to 30 g/day often eliminates constipation. This can usually be accomplished by eating raw fruits and vegetables, along with whole-meal breads and breakfast cereals. Increased dietary fiber results in increased water retention and subsequently increased stool weight. This usually provides larger and softer stools, which are more easily passed. Many people find it difficult to attain this goal for dietary fiber. Adding 20 g of wheat bran to the daily diet guarantees sufficient dietary fiber.

If the patient finds dietary adjustments too difficult or distasteful, bulking agents can be added instead of natural fiber. These include psyllium (plantago seed), methylcellulose, malt soup extract, and polycarbophil. A total of 4 to 12 g/day significantly increases stool bulk. For most patients seen in routine practice, the addition of a bulking agent leads to the resolution of constipation, but for some organic causes of constipation (obstruction or megacolon/megarectum), bulking agents actually worsen the symptoms.

Numerous other laxative preparations exist, but their use should be confined to short-term trials in an effort to clean out the bowel. Long-term use is almost never indicated and is considered dangerous to the health of the colon. Osmotic laxatives include both the salts and the nonabsorbed sugars. The salt (or saline laxatives) include magnesium citrate, magnesium hydroxide (milk of magnesia), magnesium sulfate, and the sodium phosphates. The nonabsorbed sugars include lactulose, lactitol, sorbitol, and mannitol. The salts provide an osmotic load that leads to increased water retention in the colon and subsequently in the stool. The nonabsorbed sugars provide an osmotic load and are also metabolized in the gut lumen to form short-chain fatty acids. The overall effect is increased water retention, with subsequent increased bulk and softness of the stools. The salts and the nonabsorbed sugars are harmless when used in moderation, but long-term, frequent use is unwarranted without further work-up of the etiology of the constipation.

Emollient laxatives work by increasing the mixture of fatty and aqueous substances in the stool. These are detergents such as docusate sodium and are sometimes referred to as stool softeners. Although they are probably not harmful, their benefit is dubious and has not been proven in clinical studies.

Lubricant laxatives generally rely on mineral oil in some form and can be taken orally or as a retention enema. Routine use can result in decreased absorption of the fat-soluble vitamins and subsequent problems. Oral washout solutions such as polyethylene glycol are used in some centers routinely with success; 250 to 500 mL can be given orally at night.

Stimulant laxatives work by stimulating the smooth muscle of the colon to contract and by causing increased secretory activity in the colon. These include bisacodyl, cascara sagrada, castor oil, phenolphthalein, and senna. Stimulant laxatives are highly effective in the short term but have no role in the long-term management of constipation.

Although no studies have shown a clear benefit to the use of prokinetic agents such as cisapride, these agents should theoretically be useful in treating constipation. The work that has been done has shown decreased laxative consumption in patients on cisapride but no complete responses to cisapride alone.

If no response to simple behavioral and dietary changes is noted, the addition of supplemental bran fiber or bulking agents should be tried. Most patients respond to this, but some (probably < 1%) fail this trial and are then classified as having intractable constipation. Further work-up by a specialist is in order. This evaluation involves the assessment of colonic motility and pelvic floor function and must be done in an organized fashion for best results. Even with a complete evaluation, a cause for constipation is found in only about 30% of these patients. Figure 70-1 outlines a plan for this evaluation, with the treatment options listed as the final steps.

The colonic transit time is determined, usually by a radiopaque marker study. If the transit time is normal and the patient has no symptoms of defecatory dysfunction (eg, excessive straining, digital disimpaction), a trial with bulking agents or a colonic cleansing agent is made. If this fails, a psychological evaluation may be helpful in further assessment of these patients with no functional abnormalities.

If the colonic transit time is clearly increased, the patient should be evaluated for evidence of pelvic floor dysfunction. An acceptable evaluation of the pelvic floor could include anorectal manometry, anorectal electromyographic studies, or a balloon expulsion test, alone or in combination. If this work-up is negative, a similar conservative trial of bulking or cleansing agents should be attempted. A psychological evaluation should also be done, making every effort to manage the problem conservatively. If after 2 to 3 months no improvement is noted, surgical intervention is in order.

Surgical therapy for intractable constipation is applicable only for patients with documented slow colonic transit times who have failed conservative management and are cleared by psychological evaluation. The operation of choice is a subtotal colectomy with ileorectostomy. In skilled hands, this operation has a low morbidity and mortality; results have shown most patients having three or four stools per day for the first 2 years and two stools per day after this. Recurrence rates of constipation are very low. With appropriate patient selection, excellent results can be expected.

If the colonic transit time is prolonged and pelvic floor function studies show an abnormality, the pelvic floor problem should be addressed first. If it is a simple mechanical problem such as a mucosal or rectal prolapse, a tumor, or a rectocele, resection or repair should be performed. If pelvic floor dysfunction is diagnosed, a psychological evaluation should be completed, followed by a therapeutic trial of biofeedback. Biofeedback has a success rate of up to 70% in the resolution of pelvic floor dyssynergy (anismus). If constipation persists and is then thought to be secondary to slow colonic transit, conservative therapy should be attempted. If this fails, the patient can be treated with subtotal colectomy with ileorectal anastomosis.

Patients with normal colonic transit times but some element of pelvic floor dysfunction can be treated for the pelvic floor dysfunction with biofeedback; in most cases, symptoms resolve. Those who fail should continue with conservative management

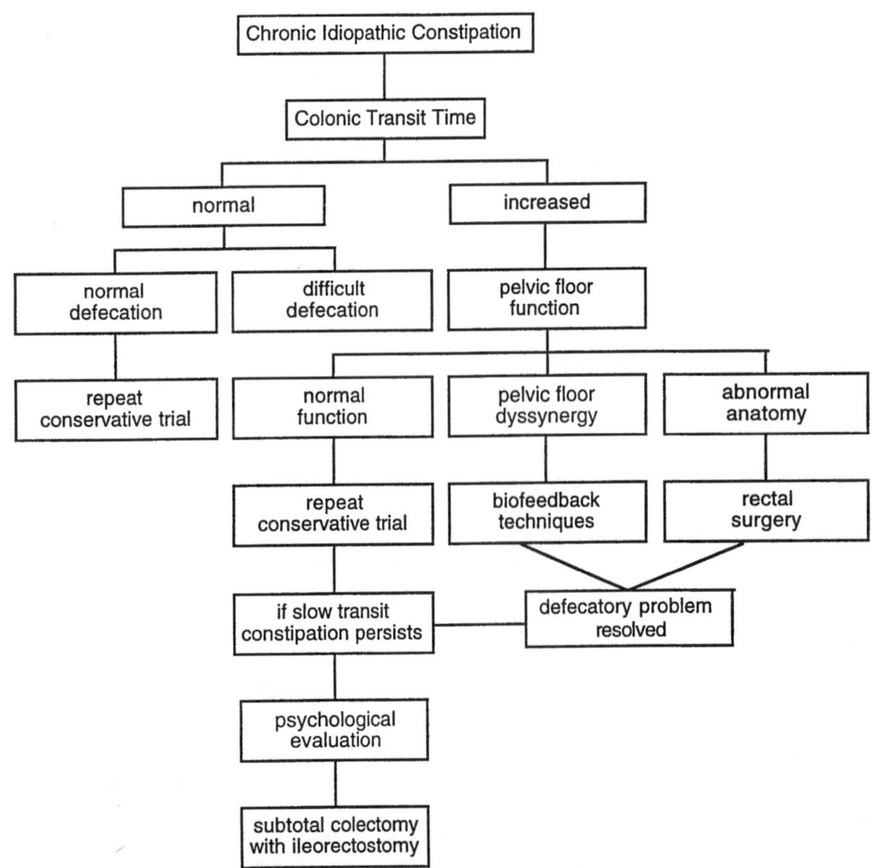

Figure 70-1. Work-up and treatment of chronic idiopathic constipation.

and undergo psychological evaluation. In patients with severe anorectal dysfunction who fail biofeedback and suffer so severely from their constipation that their quality of life is destroyed, surgical intervention with creation of an ileostomy remains an option and should be considered.

The evaluation and treatment of patients with intractable constipation must be done carefully, with strict adherence to the plan and careful interpretation of test results. If patients with slow colonic transit or pelvic floor dysfunction are carefully selected, surgical intervention or biofeedback has a high likelihood of success. An integrated approach is important in these patients; patients with psychological problems underlying constipation nearly always fail surgery and should be excluded from this treatment option.

CONSIDERATIONS IN PREGNANCY

The prevalence of constipation in pregnancy is unclear: some studies show an increase and others show no difference or a decrease. A few gastrointestinal motility studies have shown an increase in gastrointestinal transit times during the second and third trimesters. This is associated with elevated levels of progesterone and decreased levels of motilin, a stimulant hormone. Mechanical factors may play a role in constipation in pregnancy, with the pelvic floor musculature placed under great strain. Pressure of the fetal head against the rectum may also play a role.

The evaluation of pregnant patients complaining of constipation should be done in the same manner as in nonpregnant patients. A careful history is taken and a physical examination performed. If an obstructing lesion is suspected, evaluation of the rectum and colon by endoscopy is performed rather than using a radiologic procedure. Thyroid function tests are performed to rule out hypothyroidism, and the serum calcium level is checked.

Treatment begins with patient education and behavioral changes that may lead to more regular bowel habits. Dietary fiber and liquid intake is maximized. Bulking agents can then be added to maintain regularity; these are safe in pregnancy. Emollient laxatives such as docusate sodium (Colace) are used extensively in pregnancy, with no reported adverse effects. Lubricant laxatives such as mineral oil can be effective but should not be used routinely, as they lead to decreased maternal absorption of the fat-soluble vitamins. This has reportedly caused neonatal hypoprothrombinemia, which resulted in hemorrhage. Stimulant laxatives may cause abdominal cramping and have been associated with premature labor. Saline hyperosmotic agents are effective but may result in maternal sodium retention.

Because the pelvic floor musculature plays an important role in constipation, strengthening and protection of the pelvic floor may be helpful. Biofeedback-assisted Kegel exercises have been show to increase the number of bowel movements each week. These are performed routinely and on a long-term basis for the best chance of success.

BIBLIOGRAPHY

Camilleri M, Thompson WG, Fleshman JW, Pemberton JH. Clinical management of intractable constipation. Ann Intern Med 1994;121:520.

Devroede G. Constipation. In: Sleisenger MH, Fordtran JS, Scharschmidt BF, Feldman M, Cello JP, eds. Gastrointestinal disease: pathophysiology, diagnosis, and management, 5th ed. Philadelphia: WB Saunders, 1993:837.

Drossman DA, Leserman J, Nachman G, et al. Sexual and physical abuse in women with functional or organic gastrointestinal disorders. Ann Intern Med 1990;113:828.

Drossman DA, Zhiming L, Andruzzi E, et al. U.S. Householder survey of functional gastrointestinal disorders: prevalence, sociodemography, health impact. Digest Dis Sci 1993;38:1569.

Lennard-Jones JE. Clinical management of constipation. Pharmacology 1993;47(suppl 1):216.

Pemberton JH, Rath DM, Ilstrup DM. Evaluation and surgical treatment of severe chronic constipation. Ann Surg 1991;214:403.

Shafik A. Constipation: pathogenesis and management. Drugs 1993;-45(4):528.

Talley NJ, Weaver AL, Zinsmeister AR, Melton LJ. Functional constipation and outlet delay: a population-based study. Gastroenterology 1993;105:781.

West L, Warren J, Cutts T. Diagnosis and management of irritable bowel syndrome, constipation, and diarrhea in pregnancy. Gastroenterol Clin North Am 1992;21:793.

Primary Care for Women, edited by Phyllis C. Leppert and Fred M. Howard. Lippincott-Raven Publishers, Philadelphia © 1997.

71

Colorectal Cancer

MARTIN BROWER

Colorectal cancer is a major health concern for women. The National Cancer Institute estimates that 67,500 new colorectal cancers occurred in American women in 1995, resulting in 28,100 deaths—more than the number of deaths caused by all gynecologic malignancies combined. Colorectal cancer is the third most common fatal malignancy in American women, after lung cancer and breast cancer.

Colorectal cancer is primarily a disease of the middle-aged and the elderly. Fewer than 10% of cases are diagnosed before 50 years of age. The median age of American women with newly diagnosed colorectal cancer is 73 years.

About half of all colorectal cancer in American women arises in the left colon: approximately 24% in the rectum and 25% in the sigmoid colon. The other half arise more proximally. More cases of colon cancer occur in women than in men, but rectal cancer has a slight male preponderance.

ETIOLOGY

Certain genetic syndromes predispose to colorectal cancer. Virtually all patients with familial polyposis, an autosomal dominant trait, develop colorectal cancer before 50 years of age. Gardner syndrome is a variant of familial polyposis associated with osteomas of the jaw and skull, soft tissue tumors such as desmoids, and upper intestinal polyps and malignancies. Turcot syndrome is an association of familial polyposis with malignant brain tumors.

Peutz-Jeghers syndrome combines distinctive mucocutaneous pigmentation with hamartomatous polyposis and intestinal cancer. Colon cancer risk also is increased in patients with familial juvenile polyposis.

The hereditary nonpolyposis colorectal cancer (HNPCC) syndromes, with autosomal dominant inherited susceptibility to early onset colorectal cancer in the absence of diffuse colonic polyposis, are more common than familial polyposis. In type I HNPCC, the familial susceptibility to neoplasia is limited to colorectal cancer. Patients with type II HNPCC have an increased susceptibility to extracolonic neoplasms, including ovarian and endometrial cancers.

A personal or family history of breast or endometrial cancer is associated with increased risk for colorectal cancer and vice versa. Individuals with one sibling or parent with colorectal cancer have almost twice the lifetime risk of colorectal cancer as control patients. The risk is particularly great if an affected relative was younger than 45 years of age at diagnosis, or if more than one first-degree relative had the disease.

Patients with inflammatory bowel disease are at increased risk for colorectal cancer. In one population-based study, the incidence of colorectal cancer was increased over fivefold in patients with ulcerative colitis. The risk is highest in patients with pancolitis, and particularly in those diagnosed with pancolitis before 15 years of age. The risk of developing colorectal cancer within 35 years of the diagnosis of juvenile pancolitis exceeds 40%. Patients with ulcerative proctitis, left-sided colitis, or Crohn colitis also are at increased risk, but their risk is only two to three times that of the general population.

Extensive study of the epidemiology of colorectal cancer has revealed a remarkable range of colorectal cancer death rate around the world. The annual age-adjusted death rate from colorectal cancer per 100,000 women varies from 3.1 in Mexico to 20.5 in New Zealand. If the annual U.S. death rate (11.4 per 100,000 women) could be reduced to the rate in Mexico, over three quarters of the deaths of American women from colorectal cancer would be averted.

In 1971, the noted British physician Sir Denis Burkitt proposed that the rarity of colorectal cancer in Africa and other underdeveloped countries might be related to diet. Specifically, he proposed that the low fat and high fiber diets in third-world countries reduce the incidence of colorectal cancer. In 1990, a landmark study of 88,751 American woman provided strong support for Burkitt's hypothesis. Women with the highest intake of animal fat had an 89% greater risk of colorectal cancer than women with the lowest animal fat intake. Women who ate red meat every day had a risk of colorectal cancer 2fi times that of women who ate red meat less than once a month.

Colorectal cancer incidence is high in populations with a low intake of dietary fiber. High fiber diets common in underdeveloped nations may decrease the risk of colorectal cancer by diluting the concentration of carcinogens in the feces and by shortening stool transit time through the bowel, minimizing the contact of stool carcinogens with the bowel wall. Colorectal cancer also seems to be high in populations with low dietary calcium intake.

The link between fat and fiber in the diet and colorectal cancer incidence has not been established unequivocally. Decades may elapse between exposure to carcinogens and the development of cancer; colorectal cancer in a 70-year-old woman may more closely reflect what she ate as a teenager than her current diet. Vitamin supplements and short-term dietary manipulations have not been shown to reduce the incidence of colorectal cancer or of adenomas. Nonetheless, the epidemiologic links between fat and fiber and colorectal cancer incidence make it prudent to comply with the National Cancer Institute's dietary guidelines: reduce fat content to 30% or less of calories, increase fiber intake to 20 to 30 g/day, and include vegetables and fruits in the daily diet.

Regular exercise reduces the incidence of colorectal cancer, perhaps by shortening stool transit time. Regular use of aspirin or other nonsteroidal antiinflammatory agents also may reduce the incidence of colorectal cancer, perhaps by reducing bowel inflammation caused by stool carcinogens.

Alcohol seems to increase the risk of colorectal cancer. A recent study added colon cancer to the long list of neoplasms that are associated with cigarette smoking, but only after a long latency period. Men who were smokers more than 35 years ago have almost twice the risk of colon cancer compared with those who were nonsmokers at that time. This association between remote smoking and colorectal cancer risk further supports the concept that decades may elapse between carcinogen exposure and the development of colorectal cancer. Table 71-1 lists major risk factors, both inherited and acquired, for colorectal cancer.

Most cases of colorectal cancer originate as adenomas. Adenomas less than 1 cm in diameter are rarely malignant, but the incidence of malignancy increases with increasing size. The progression of adenomas to frank malignancy is usually slow, requiring many years.

The progression of a neoplasm from a small adenoma to a frankly invasive adenocarcinoma with metastatic potential is accompanied by a series of genetic alterations. Vogelstein and col-

Table 71-1. Major Risk Factors for Colorectal Cancer

CLASSIFICATION	RISK FACTOR
Genetic polyposis syndromes	Familial polyposis
	Gardner syndrome
	Turcot syndrome
	Peutz-Jeghers syndrome
	Familial juvenile polyposis
Genetic nonpolyposis syndromes	Hereditary nonpolyposis
	Colorectal cancer, type I and II
	Personal history of breast or endometrial cancer
	Family history of colorectal cancer
Concurrent Illness	Ulcerative colitis
	Crohn colitis
Environment and diet	High animal fat intake
	Low dietary fiber intake
	Lack of exercise
	Low calcium and vitamin D intake
	Alcohol use
	Smoking

leagues at Johns Hopkins University have demonstrated that an accumulation of *multiple* genetic changes is necessary for colorectal cancer development. They showed that deletions of portions of chromosomes 5, 17, and 18 are frequent in colorectal cancers. The gene responsible for familial adenomatous polyposis, *APC*, is located on chromosome 5, and is frequently abnormal in patients with sporadic colon cancer. Deletion of the *p53* tumor suppressor gene is associated with changes on chromosome 17, and loss of the gene *DCC* ("deleted in colon cancer") is associated with changes on chromosome 18. Mutations in the k-*ras* oncogene also are frequent in advanced colon cancer. Typically, small adenomas possess only a few of these genetic alterations, but as the adenomas become dysplastic and then frankly malignant, more genetic lesions occur.

Recently, the study of colorectal cancer led to the discovery of a novel class of genes that cause cancer when mutated—genes that control DNA mismatch repair. Mutations in these genes, including *hMSH2* on human chromosome 2 and *hMLH1* on human chromosome 3, are common both in the HNPCC syndromes and in sporadic colorectal cancer.

CLINICAL PRESENTATION

A change in bowel habit (constipation or diarrhea) and rectal bleeding are the most common symptoms of colorectal cancer. Because of the narrower lumen and the solid nature of the bowel contents in the left colon and rectum, change in bowel habit is more often a sign of left-sided cancer. Patients with left-sided colon cancer sometimes report tenesmus or a sense of incomplete evacuation. The caliber of the stool may be reduced. Bright red rectal bleeding is frequently caused by hemorrhoids, but rectal bleeding must be thoroughly investigated with sigmoidoscopy, barium enema, or both. Mucus discharge may be a sign of villous adenoma or carcinoma.

Colon cancers, particularly in the right bowel, often present with fatigue caused by anemia. Postmenopausal women with iron deficiency anemia must be investigated for the possibility of gastrointestinal malignancy as the source of blood loss.

In advanced cases, patients present with weakness, generalized malaise, anorexia, or weight loss. Patients may notice a palpable abdominal mass. There may be abdominal pain from intermittent obstruction or intussusception, or back pain from malignant retroperitoneal adenopathy. Patients may present acutely with symptoms of bowel perforation or obstruction. Colon cancer can mimic acute diverticulitis in its clinical presentation.

CLINICAL FINDINGS

Physical examination of patients with suspected colorectal cancer should focus on the liver, abdomen, and rectum. Women should have pelvic and breast examinations because of the known association of colorectal cancer with breast and gynecologic malignancies. Patients with evidence of ascites, liver or lymph node metastases, or palpable abdominal masses on physical examination should undergo computed tomographic (CT) scanning of the abdomen and pelvis. Those without evidence for advanced disease can proceed to sigmoidoscopy, colonoscopy, or barium enema for diagnosis.

A normal physical examination and a negative finding on a stool test for occult blood do not exclude colorectal cancer. In the presence of symptoms, sigmoidoscopy, barium enema, or colonoscopy are indicated to exclude malignancy. Approximately 30% of patients with documented colorectal cancer have negative findings on stool tests for occult blood.

LABORATORY AND IMAGING STUDIES

Most patients believed to have colorectal cancer should undergo sigmoidoscopy followed by a double-contrast barium enema. If a lesion suspicious for malignancy is found, most patients undergo colonoscopic or sigmoidoscopic biopsy to achieve a tissue diagnosis. However, a classic appearance of cancer on barium enema ("apple core" lesion) is sufficient to warrant operative intervention. Large polyps (> 3 to 5 cm) also require surgical intervention, as malignancy cannot be excluded, even with colonoscopic biopsy of such lesions.

Most malignancies of the colon and rectum are adenocarcinomas, but lymphoma, melanoma, small cell carcinoma, carcinoid tumor, and sarcomas of the bowel do occur. Carcinomas of the anus frequently are squamous cell tumors. The management of these unusual types of colorectal cancer is beyond the scope of this chapter.

Because patients with colorectal cancer are at risk for synchronous colon cancers or adenomas, patients should have colonoscopy of their entire bowel. Unless there is an obstructing lesion or there is an emergent need for operative intervention, this is performed preoperatively.

Before surgery, patients should have a complete blood count (CBC), liver and kidney function tests, and a chest x-ray. Some surgeons obtain a preoperative CT scan of the abdomen and pelvis in all patients with colon cancer, but most only order a CT scan in patients believed to have advanced disease by physical or laboratory examination. In patients with rectal cancer, preoperative rectal ultrasound and pelvic CT provide invaluable information regarding the anatomic location of the tumor and the extent of surgery likely to be required.

Carcinoembryonic antigen (CEA) is a serum glycoprotein elevated in most patients with advanced colorectal cancer. Unfortunately, it is not sufficiently sensitive or specific for use in screening. CEA is not a specific test for colorectal cancer; elevated levels of this tumor marker are frequent in many other forms of malignancy. Only 25% of patients with early colorectal cancer have CEA levels over 5 ng/mL compared with 45% of patients with lymph node metastases and 65% of patients with metastatic disease.

SCREENING

The American Cancer Society's screening guidelines for colorectal cancer are listed in Table 71-2.

A landmark case–control study of screening sigmoidoscopy from the Kaiser Permanente Health Maintenance Organization was published in 1992. A 70% reduction in the risk of death from left-sided colorectal cancer was seen in individuals who had undergone rigid sigmoidoscopy at any time in the previous 10 years. Because most colorectal cancers grow slowly as adenomas before the development of frank malignancy, marked reduction in death rates can be achieved with screening as infrequently as every 3 to 5 years. Screening sigmoidoscopy does not detect right-sided colon cancers. However, half of all colorectal cancers can be reached by the 35-cm flexible sigmoidoscope. The presence of adenomatous polyps detected by sigmoidoscopy is a marker for increased risk of

Table 71-2. American Cancer Society Recommendations for the Early Detection of Colorectal Cancer in Asymptomatic People*

TEST OR PROCEDURE	AGE	FREQUENCY
Sigmoidoscopy, preferably flexible	50 y and older	Every 3–5 y
Fecal occult blood test	50 y and older	Every year
Digital rectal examination	40 y and older	Every year

*Persons at higher risk for colorectal cancer, such as with inflammatory bowel disease, familial polyposis syndromes, family history or colon cancer, or personal history of breast, endometrial, or ovarian cancer may need more intense screening.

cancer throughout the large bowel. Patients found to have left-sided adenomas on sigmoidoscopy should undergo colonoscopy to rule out right-sided neoplasia.

Fecal occult blood screening also is recommended by most authorities. Typically, six stool samples are tested for occult blood using Hemoccult while the patient is on a diet without red meat, nonsteroidal antiinflammatory drugs, or peroxidase-containing vegetables such as broccoli, turnip, or cauliflower. (All of these substances can cause false-positive guaiac results in stools). Vitamin C, which can cause false-negative guaiac results, also should be avoided. If a positive sample is found, the patient undergoes screening colonoscopy.

Recent results from a randomized prospective study of 46,551 participants support routine fecal occult blood screening. Annual stool guaiac testing with colonoscopic follow-up for positive results reduced colorectal cancer mortality by 33%—82 deaths over 13 years from colorectal cancer in the group screened annually—compared with 121 deaths in the control group. However, 38% of the screened patients underwent colonoscopy over the 13-year period, indicating that stool guaiac testing has a high false-positive rate for colorectal neoplasia.

Researchers are trying to find more sensitive, more specific, and less invasive techniques to screen for colorectal cancer. Analyzing DNA in the stool for genetic changes characteristic of colorectal malignancy is one promising technique that may simplify early detection of this cancer. Genetic screening of family members of patients with polyposis or carcinoma will be available shortly, permitting early identification of people who have inherited mutations in genes such as *APC*, associated with familial adenomatous polyposis, and the human DNA-mismatch–repair genes associated with HNPCC. Such patients would then undergo intensive screening at an early age to reduce colorectal cancer mortality.

TREATMENT

The primary treatment of colorectal cancer is surgery. Surgeons perform a right hemicolectomy for cancers of the cecum and ascending colon; for cancers of the descending or proximal sigmoid colon, the surgical procedure a left hemicolectomy. Surgeons perform a low anterior resection for distal sigmoid and proximal rectal lesions. In each case, the surgeon must achieve an adequate margin and resect regional lymph nodes. Patients who present with perforation or obstruction frequently require creation of a temporary colostomy at the time of surgery. A total or subtotal colectomy may be necessary for patients with multiple lesions or with cancer in the setting of inflammatory bowel disease or familial cancer syndromes.

Patients usually are admitted to the hospital 1 day before colon cancer surgery to receive a bowel-cleansing regimen consisting of systemic and oral nonabsorbable antibiotics. It is technically feasible to perform a colectomy for cancer with laparoscopic techniques, but long-term follow-up of patients undergoing laparoscopic resection of colon cancer is not available. Most surgeons rely on standard open surgical techniques.

Rectal cancers are usually treated with abdominoperineal resection requiring a permanent colostomy. Fortunately, with modern surgical stapling techniques, colostomy is necessary only for the lowest lying rectal cancers. The pelvis in women is wider than in men, so sphincter-sparing surgery is technically easier in women. Only cancers located within 6 to 8 cm of the anal verge require a permanent colostomy. Many patients with rectal cancer require postoperative radiation therapy. To prevent radiation injury, the small bowel should be excluded from the pelvis at the time of surgery using a sling or mesh.

Small rectal cancers that do not penetrate the bowel wall can be managed with wide excision or with endocavitary irradiation. It is not known if long-term survival with these conservative treatments is equivalent to that achieved with abdominoperineal resection. Large rectal cancers sometimes are unresectable due to fixation to the pelvic wall. Preoperative irradiation may render these tumors operable.

In the United States, standard therapy for operable rectal cancer is initial surgical resection, followed by postoperative chemotherapy and radiation therapy in high-risk patients. However, some physicians use preoperative radiation therapy (or radiation therapy plus chemotherapy) followed by surgery in the treatment of operable rectal cancer. Randomized studies are underway comparing these two approaches.

The abdomen must be thoroughly explored at the time of surgery. If a surgeon finds a lesion that may be a metastatic focus, a biopsy must be performed to obtain tissue confirmation of metastatic disease.

Some surgeons routinely perform prophylactic oophorectomy at the time of colectomy for colorectal cancer in postmenopausal women. The ovary is a frequent metastatic site of colorectal cancer in women, and often an ovarian metastasis is the first detected site of recurrence. Unfortunately, an ovarian metastasis is usually a harbinger of widely disseminated disease, and it is unlikely that oophorectomy at the time of colectomy prevents recurrence elsewhere or improves survival. On the other hand, oophorectomy in postmenopausal women undergoing colectomy does have the advantage of almost eliminating the risk of ovarian cancer.

After surgery, patients with colorectal carcinoma are assigned a surgical stage. In the United States, the Astler-Coller modifica-

Table 71-3. Commonly Used Staging Classifications for Invasive Colorectal Cancer

ASTLER-COLLER MODIFICATION OF DUKES CLASSIFICATION	TNM STAGING	DEFINITION
Modified Dukes A	Stage I: T1, N0, M0	Primary tumor invades no deeper than submucosa; negative lymph nodes; no metastases
Modified Dukes B1	Stage I: T2, N0, M0	Primary tumor invades into but not through the muscularis propia; negative lymph nodes; no metastases
Modified Dukes B2	Stage II: T3, N0, M0, T4, N0, M0	Primary tumor invades through the muscularis propia; negative lymph nodes; no metastases
Modified Dukes C	Stage III: Any T, N1 to 3, M0	Positive lymph nodes; no distant metastases
Modified Dukes D	Stage IV: Any T, any N, M1	Distant metastases

tion of the Dukes classification and the TNM staging system are most commonly employed (Table 71-3, Fig. 71-1).

After curative resection of modified Dukes A (T1, N0, M0) or B1 (T2, N0, M0) colon or rectal cancer, no chemotherapy or radiation therapy is needed. Some oncologists administer postoperative chemotherapy to selected patients after curative resection of modified Dukes B2 (T3, N0, M0) colon cancer whom they deem at high risk for recurrence, but randomized studies do not support the routine use of adjuvant treatment in Dukes B2 disease outside of clinical trials.

In a major advance in the management of colorectal cancer, randomized studies published in 1990 and 1991 proved that postoperative therapy dramatically improves the survival of patients after curative resection of Dukes C (node-positive) colon cancer and Dukes B2 and C rectal cancer. Patients with colon cancer are treated with chemotherapy; those with rectal cancer (below the peritoneal reflection) receive combined modality therapy (chemotherapy and radiation therapy). Radiation therapy is used because rectal cancer has a much higher propensity for symptomatic local recurrence within the pelvis.

The postoperative adjuvant treatment of colon cancer combines injections of the chemotherapy drug 5-fluorouracil (5-FU) with tablets of levamisole, an antihelminthic drug with immunostimulatory properties. The National Intergroup Study demonstrated that a year of treatment with 5-FU and levamisole in patients with Dukes C colon cancer reduces the rate of recurrence by 41% and the death rate by 33% (Fig. 71- 2). Similar reduction in recurrence and death rates are achieved with combined modality chemotherapy and radiation therapy after resection of Dukes B2 and C rectal cancers.

Patients with Dukes D disease (distant metastases) are not curable except in rare patients with one or two liver or lung lesions that can be resected surgically. Five-year survival rates as high as 25% have been reported in patients who undergo resection of solitary liver or lung metastases. Unfortunately, most patients with metastatic disease do not have resectable disease. The most common sites of metastases are the liver, the peritoneum, the lungs, and the retroperitoneum. Bone and brain metastases are occasionally seen.

Radiation therapy can be employed to palliate incurable patients with metastatic colorectal cancer with bone or brain recurrences. Locally recurrent rectal cancer is a particularly troublesome problem that can often be palliated with radiation.

Cryosurgery is a novel technique that is increasingly being used in the palliative management of metastatic colorectal cancer to the liver. Patients who are not suitable for resection of liver metastases but who have a limited number of lesions less than 3 to 5 cm in diameter can have metastatic deposits frozen intraoperatively using ultrasound guidance. Cryosurgery requires laparotomy and is associated with complications including bile leak, myoglobinuria with transient renal failure, and hepatic cracking with associated hemorrhage. Long-term survival results after cryosurgery are not available.

Chemotherapy is the most commonly employed treatment for patients with unresectable colorectal cancer. For the last three decades, 5-FU has been the mainstay of palliative chemotherapy for this disease. The combination of 5-FU with leucovorin (folinic acid) is slightly superior to 5-FU alone in the management of metastatic colorectal cancer. Two thirds of treated patients have symptomatic improvement with chemotherapy. In about one third of treated patients, the tumor shrinks by at least 50% (partial

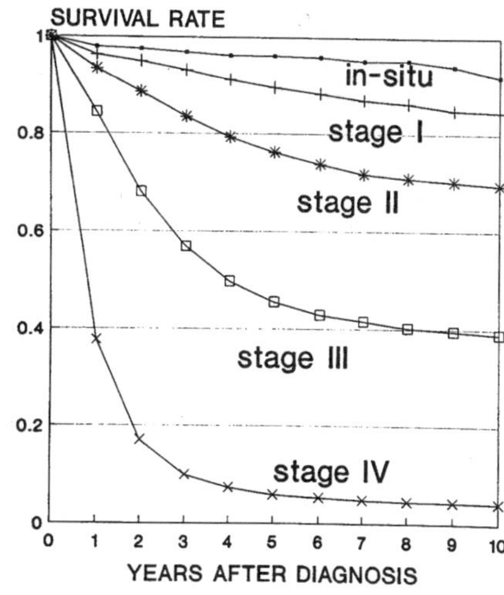

FIGURE 71-1. Relative survival rates of patients with colorectal cancer according to the stage of the diease, based on 111,110 patients staged between 1973 and 1987. (From American Joint Committee on Cancer, Handbook for staging of cancer, 4th ed. Philadelphia: JB Lippincott, 1993:98.)

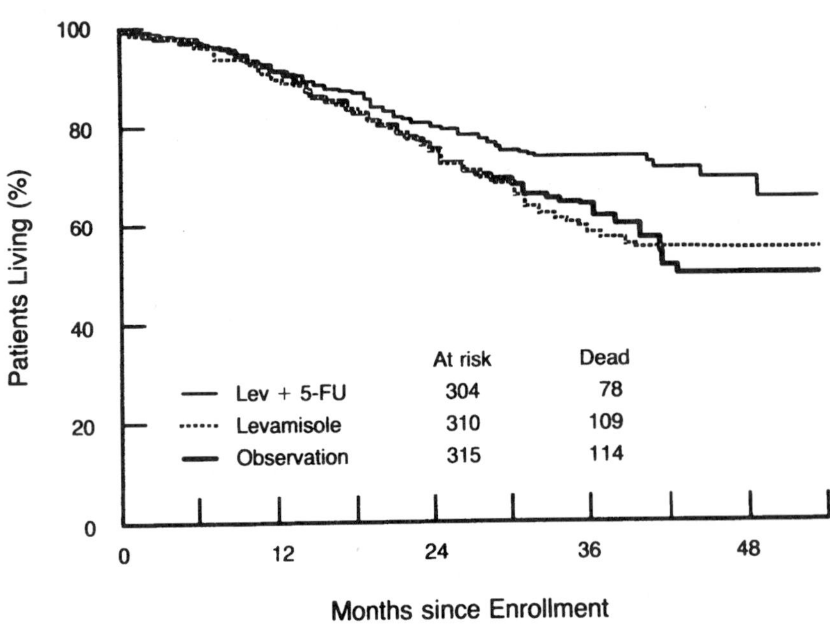

FIGURE 71-2. Survival of patients treated with levamisole and 5-fluorouracil, levamisole alone, or observation after resection of node-positive (Dukes C) colon cancer. (Moertel CG, Fleming TR, MacDonald JS, et al. Levamisole and fluorouracil for adjuvant therapy of resected colon carcinoma. N Engl J Med 1990;322:352.)

response), and another one-third of patients have stable disease. Toxicities of 5-FU–based chemotherapy include mild nausea and hair loss. Life-threatening diarrhea, granulocytopenia, and severe mucositis can occur, particularly in elderly patients.

Unfortunately, the typical duration of response is under 1 year. Although some patients with metastatic colorectal cancer have a remarkably indolent course, most patients die within two 2 years after diagnosis.

Not all patients with unresectable metastatic colorectal cancer should receive immediate treatment with chemotherapy. Patients who are asymptomatic with minimal tumor burden sometimes have a symptom-free period of several months or years and can be treated with chemotherapy when they become symptomatic or show evidence for rapid tumor progression. Patients with markedly impaired performance status, active infections, or other severe comorbid medical problems rarely benefit from chemotherapy.

Decades of research have failed to find any chemotherapy for advanced colorectal cancer that is clearly superior to 5-FU and leucovorin. There has been great interest for decades in regional chemotherapy for unresectable liver metastases using hepatic arterial infusions of chemotherapy. Although response rates with hepatic arterial chemotherapy are somewhat higher than with standard chemotherapy, studies have not demonstrated a consistent survival benefit. Biologic response modifiers such as interferon and interleukin-2 have minimal activity in this disease.

It is extremely rare for second-line chemotherapy drugs to benefit patients with tumors refractory to standard 5-FU and leucovorin therapy. Researchers are continuing to test other agents that may have activity in this disease.

FOLLOW-UP OF PATIENTS WITH COLORECTAL CANCER

Hundreds of thousands of American women are alive today after curative resection of colorectal cancer. How should the primary care physician follow these patients?

Patients with resected colorectal cancer are at risk for development of new cancers. Physicians and patients should follow American Cancer Society screening guidelines for breast and gynecologic malignancy. In addition, patients should undergo stool testing for occult blood at least once annually and undergo colonoscopy every 2 to 3 years to exclude new adenomas or cancers. The goal is to find new cancers at an early stage when they are amenable to surgical cure.

Patients with resected colorectal cancer also are at risk for recurrence. There are rare instances in which recurrent or metastatic colorectal cancer can be treated surgically for cure. Suture line recurrences, solitary lung metastases, or one (or occasionally up to four) liver metastases can be resected in selected patients. Of all tests available to detect tumor recurrence, the most sensitive is the CEA determination, which becomes elevated before any clinical signs or symptoms of cancer recurrence in up to two thirds of patients with metastatic disease. Therefore, many physicians follow patients with previous colorectal cancer aggressively with history and physical examination and CEA determination every 3 months for 5 years postoperatively.

Recently, the effectiveness of intensive CEA follow-up has been questioned. Few patients with metastatic or recurrent colorectal cancer are surgically curable. The "early" detection of asymptomatic incurable cancer is not clinically useful. False-positive CEA elevations are common. Cancer cures attributable to CEA monitoring are infrequent. Certainly, CEA monitoring in frail elderly patients who are not candidates for major salvage surgery is not warranted. Regardless of whether CEA monitoring is employed, patients should be seen by a physician every 3 to 6 months.

CONSIDERATIONS IN PREGNANCY

Because colorectal cancer is a disease of the middle-aged and the elderly, pregnancy in patients with colon cancer is rare. Only 29 cases were reported in a recent review of the world literature. Diagnosis of colorectal cancer in pregnant women is frequently delayed because symptoms such as nausea, abdominal pain, and constipation are often attributed to the pregnancy. Persistent anemia, failure to gain weight appropriately, or a palpable mass may be clues to the presence of cancer. As in all patients, rectal bleeding in pregnant woman cannot be assumed to be hemorrhoidal in origin. One must particularly consider the diagnosis of colorectal cancer in pregnant women with predisposing factors such as familial cancer syndromes or inflammatory bowel disease.

If localized colorectal cancer is diagnosed during the first two trimesters of pregnancy, surgical therapy for the cancer can proceed and the fetus can be left in utero. If colorectal cancer is discovered in the last trimester, cancer surgery can be delayed until fetal lung maturation, at which time a cesarean section can be performed at the time of the cancer surgery.

BIBLIOGRAPHY

American Cancer Society National Conference on Colorectal Cancer. Cancer 1992;70:1205.

Heise RH, Van Winter JT, Wilson TO, Ogburn PL. Colonic cancer during pregnancy: case report and review of the literature. Mayo Clin Proc 1992;67:1180.

Levin B, Murphy GP. Revision in American Cancer Society recommendations for the early detection of colorectal cancer. Ca 1992;42:296.

Kane MJ. Colorectal cancer. Semin Oncol 1991;18:315.

Krook JE, Moertel CG, Gunderson LL, et al. Effective surgical adjuvant therapy for high-risk rectal carcinoma. N Engl J Med 1991;324:709.

Mandel JS, Bond JH, Church TR, et al. Reducing mortality from colorectal cancer by screening for fecal occult blood. N Engl J Med 1993;328:1365.

Moertel CG. Chemotherapy for colorectal cancer. N Engl J Med 1994;330:1136.

Moertel CG, Fleming TR, Macdonald JS, Haller DG, Laurie JA, Tangen C. An evaluation of the CEA test for monitoring patients with resected colon cancer. JAMA 1993;270:943.

Moertel CG, Fleming TR, MacDonald JS, et al. Levamisole and fluorouracil for adjuvant therapy of resected colon carcinoma. N Engl J Med 1990;322:352.

Ransohoff DF, Lang CA. Sigmoidoscopic screening in the 1990s. JAMA 1993;269:1278.

Selby JV, Friedman GD, Quesenberry CP, Weiss NS. A case–control study of screening sigmoidoscopy and mortality from colorectal cancer. N Engl J Med 1992;326:653.

Willett WC, Stampfer MJ, Colditz GA, Rosner BA, Speizer FE. Relation of meat, fat, and fiber intake to the risk of colon cancer in a prospective study among women. N Engl J Med 1990;323:1664.

Primary Care for Women, edited by Phyllis C. Leppert and Fred M. Howard. Lippincott-Raven Publishers, Philadelphia © 1997.

72
Fecal Incontinence

KATHLEEN MARTIN

Fecal incontinence is the second most common cause of institutionalization of the elderly and by some estimates consumes one third of the annual budget used to care for the institutionalized elderly. As the number of elderly mushrooms, we will need to learn how to manage this socially incapacitating problem. As with all problems suffered by the elderly, we would like to learn what we can do in terms of preventive strategies to minimize its occurrence.

The precise incidence of fecal incontinence is unknown, partly because we do not specifically ask our patients the question. Fecal incontinence has such a negative social stigma that patients are reluctant to discuss it. Double incontinence—both fecal and urinary incontinence—may be 12 times more common than fecal incontinence alone.

Our understanding and treatment of this entity are in their infancy. This chapter attempts to describe the current state of knowledge, realizing that recognition and ongoing research in this area are paramount.

PATHOPHYSIOLOGY

Multiple factors come into play in maintaining fecal continence, including stool volume and consistency, transit time, rectal distensibility, anal sphincter integrity and function, anorectal sensation, intact anorectal reflexes, and intact mental status. Derangement of any of these aspects can lead to the unintentional loss of feces or flatus.

Diarrheal states caused by infection, inflammatory disease, short gut syndrome, laxative abuse, or radiation enteritis can result in fecal incontinence. This can occur despite a mechanically and neurologically intact anorectal complex. Medical interventions that decrease the fecal bolus and make the stool formed have a favorable impact on these patients.

Colonic transit time may affect fecal continence in two different ways, depending on whether transit time is increased or decreased. For example, decreased physical activity prolongs transit time. This places the patient at increased risk of constipation, stool impaction, and subsequent spurious overflow incontinence. Alternatively, the patient may suffer from a rapid transit time, as in short gut syndrome. This patient may benefit from decreasing stool quantity with a low-fiber diet and decreasing bowel motility with opioid derivative agents.

Rectal distensibility and compliance are decreased by age, radiation, tumor, and scarring after surgery, resulting in rectal urgency at lower rectal volumes.

The principal mechanism of fecal continence is provided by the internal anal sphincter (IAS), which contributes 85% of the resting anal pressure. It is innervated largely by the sympathetic system via the hypogastric plexus. The IAS relaxes reflexively when the rectum is distended via the rectoanal sphincter inhibitory reflex. The external anal sphincter (EAS) provides 15% of the resting anal pressure and is innervated by the inferior rectal branch of the pudendal nerve. The EAS is a striated, voluntary muscle, as is the puborectalis. Tonic activity of the EAS and the puborectalis is maintained by a sacral spinal loop reflex. The IAS is an extension of the inner circular smooth muscle of the rectum. Delancey has found that the IAS makes up 54% of the thickness of the anal sphincter complex.

The entire sphincter complex is 1.8 cm thick and about 3 cm long. Patients may have a defect in the EAS/IAS complex secondary to obstetric injury. Alternatively, age and hormonal deprivation secondary to menopause may lead to sphincter atrophy.

The puborectalis, which is part of the levator ani complex (see Chap. 33), also participates in maintaining fecal continence by maintaining the anorectal angle. The degree to which this angle contributes to the continence mechanism is unclear. The puborectalis is innervated by S3 and 4 motor roots. The anorectal angle is normally about 90° at rest and becomes more obtuse during defecation as the puborectalis relaxes. There is, however, a large overlap in continent and incontinent patients; therefore, the importance of this angle is in contention.

Anorectal sensation is important in allowing a patient to differentiate solid, liquid, and gas in the rectum. Receptors in the proximal anal canal, and especially along the dentate line, are thought to be active in discerning the nature of rectal contents by a poorly understood mechanism of sampling. Equally important are the stretch receptors in the levator ani that stimulate the rectoanal sphincter inhibitory reflex. This reflex links the rectal compartment to the anal compartment, causing initial relaxation of the IAS to allow rectal content sampling and concurrent contraction of the EAS to preserve continence. This reflex creates the urge to defecate or pass flatus. The volume of the fecal bolus that is required to stimulate the reflex and the ability to distinguish among gas, liquid, and solid affects the ability to maintain continence. Intussusception and rectal prolapse can chronically stimulate the anorectal sphincter inhibitory reflex and can lead to fecal incontinence. Decreased rectal sensation has been noted in patients with diabetes, megarectum, and fecal impaction.

Fecal continence relies on an intact cerebrospinal–end organ connection; interruption at any level can lead to dysfunction. The differential includes congenital malformations (eg, meningomyelocele, spina bifida), multiple sclerosis, dementia, cerebrovascular accidents, diabetes mellitus, and spinal cord injury. The end organ in this regard is really multifaceted, in that it requires the coordinated efforts of the IAS, EAS, and levator ani.

Pelvic floor denervation may play a pivotal role in the etiology of fecal incontinence and may explain why incontinence is more prevalent in women. Stretch and crush injuries of the pudendal nerve have been documented to occur during vaginal delivery. The pudendal nerve is especially vulnerable to stretch injury secondary to its relatively fixed position for part of its course in Alcock's canal. Studies are ongoing as to the impact vaginal delivery has on the pelvic floor and how the obstetrician or midwife may be able to minimize that impact.

Probably as important, if not more so, is the pudendal nerve injury incurred by chronic straining with defecation. Thirty percent to 60% of patients with fecal incontinence have a long history of excessive straining to defecate. Over the long term, this can lead to injury of the pudendal nerves, resulting in perineal descent syndrome. Perineal descent is characterized by complete laxity of the levator ani, resulting in the anus being level with the perineum rather than in its usual position of being pulled into the gluteal fold. Perineal descent has been found in 50% of constipated women. It is an intriguing idea that we could prevent the development of incontinence just by discussing bowel habits and modifying behaviors.

Mental status is a factor in maintaining continence in that, all other factors being normal, defecation is a volitional event. In the demented patient who has no motivation to maintain continence, the solutions largely involve maintaining some degree of hygiene. Care should be taken, however, to ensure that the patient's sensorium is not clouded by polypharmacy or other metabolic conditions.

Several age-related changes hinder the fecal continence mechanism. The resting and maximum anal sphincter pressures are reduced. A smaller fecal bolus is necessary to stimulate the rectoanal inhibitory reflex. The size and compliance of the rectal ampulla are reduced with age as well.

The most common cause of fecal incontinence in the institutionalized elderly is fecal impaction. Complications of impaction include intestinal obstruction, urinary retention, and overflow fecal incontinence with diarrhea. Fecal impaction leads to changes in anorectal physiology involving impaired rectal sensation that results in increased fecal boluses to elicit the urge to defecate. An empty rectum does not necessarily rule out impaction; an abdominal x-ray may reveal significant fecal retention.

Because a major risk factor in the development of fecal incontinence is thought to be chronic excessive straining with bowel movements, the management of constipation is pertinent. The definition of constipation would at first seem too basic to mention. However, what the clinician defines as constipation may not necessarily correlate with the patient's conception. The definition of constipation is slightly elusive, but most clinicians would agree that a bowel movement less frequently than every third day would define this condition. The patient, however, may describe herself as constipated if she has small, hard stools every day or if she feels that she incompletely defecates. Others may strain daily with their bowel movements and describe this as constipation. Clearly, this straightforward clinical entity becomes more complicated on closer inspection.

Constipation is thought to be more common in the elderly. One study found that 75% of nursing home patients use laxatives. The incidence of constipation in the hospitalized geriatric population is estimated to be 10% to 25% and increases to 50% of nursing home residents. Many elderly patients use laxatives regularly despite the fact that they may have multiple stools per day. This may be in part secondary to an old belief that regular purgation is healthy. The elderly often suffer from depression and confusion, which may lead to preoccupation with somatic functions and result in the exaggeration of symptoms. It is important to recognize this behavioral overlay and counsel the patient accordingly.

Risk factors for the development of constipation include physical inactivity (increases colonic transit time), inadequate caloric and fiber intake, dehydration, certain medications (eg, analgesics, anticholinergics, iron supplements), functional limitations (immobility, inadequate toilet arrangements), dementia, endocrine disorders (eg, hypothyroidism), and colonic obstruction secondary to tumors or diverticulitis. Therefore, whether a patient strains because she is constipated or because she perceives herself as being constipated, the end result may be pelvic floor dysfunction.

Fecal obstruction by tumor, rectovaginal or colovaginal fistulas, and congenital anorectal malformation are other causes of fecal incontinence. Rectovaginal fistulas are most often seen after episiotomy breakdown of a third- or fourth-degree repair. They also can be seen in inflammatory bowel disease. Colovaginal fistulas are usually seen in posthysterectomy patients with diverticulitis.

PATIENT INTERVIEW

The patient interview must be direct and specific to obtain information that is the key to determining the etiology of fecal incontinence. It is important to document the patient's chief complaint regarding fecal incontinence in her own words. This helps clarify the quality-of-life issues relative to this condition that most concern the patient.

First, the clinician should ascertain the nature of the patient's incontinence—that is, whether it is mucus, fecal seepage, flatus, or liquid or solid stool. The patient should be asked when it began—for instance, after surgery, vaginal delivery, or trauma, when starting a new medication, or with recent travel. The clinician should ask specific details about the nature of her bowel habits: How often does she have a bowel movement? What is the consistency of her stools? Does she strain to have a bowel movement? Has anything changed recently in regard to these bowel habits? How often does she experience fecal incontinence? Does anything seem temporally related to the incontinent episode? Does she experience any numbness, tingling, or radiation of pain that might suggest a neurologic cause? Does she experience pain with defecation? This may suggest an abscess, fistula, or hemorrhoids. Does she notice perianal itching or burning? This is seen commonly with pruritus ani, a perianal dermatitis caused by overwashing of the area. Often this can weep and soil the underwear, but it really is not fecal soiling or incontinence. Does she notice a bulge? If so, the clinician should consider hemorrhoids, rectal prolapse, or tumor. Does she note rectal bleeding? If she complains of vaginal pressure or the need to replace a vaginal bulge to accomplish a bowel movement, the clinician should consider genital prolapse. Does she note rectal pressure or tenesmus that may suggest proctitis? Does she have concomitant abdominal pain suggestive of diverticulitis or inflammatory bowel disease? In addition, the clinician should ask how she has handled her symptoms up to this point.

Once a thorough review of symptoms has been completed, a full medical history is obtained. The clinician should inquire about laxative use, previous surgery, urinary incontinence, a family history of colorectal cancer, and the patient's obstetric history, including the size of her largest baby and any history of operative vaginal delivery or a complicated episiotomy.

PHYSICAL EXAMINATION

The clinician can assess the patient's mobility as she walks into the office and her mental status as the interview is carried out. These two factors are crucial to devising an evaluation and treatment plan.

The examination includes a careful abdominal examination, specifically looking for masses or tenderness. The pelvic examination starts with close inspection of the perianum, perineum, and vulva, looking for scars, tumors, prolapse, perineal descent, and anal tone (does the anus appear to be gaping?). Evidence of pruritus ani is sought. The examination of the pelvic floor is described in Chapter 33. The bimanual examination includes an assessment of pubococcygeal tone. The sacral reflex arc can be assessed by eliciting the bulbocavernosus reflex or perianal wink (see Chap. 80). The sensory S2, 3, and 4 dermatomes and lower extremity reflexes should be thoroughly assessed.

Rectal examination includes assessment of the tone of the EAS and levator ani. The anorectal angle resulting from the puborectalis muscle is palpated (Fig. 72-1). The patient is asked to squeeze her anus tightly so the clinician can assess resting and squeeze pressure. The clinician should be able to appreciate the rectum being pulled forward during the squeeze maneuver, indicating an intact neuromuscular unit. The levator tone should be evaluated separately from that of the anal sphincter complex. The clinician should look for diastasis of the levator ani, a common finding in genital prolapse. It can be appreciated as a widening of the space between the paired levator muscles (by transvaginal palpation of the levator muscles). The levators are located at about 5 and 7 o'clock and are extensions of the pubococcygeus. How wide the levator hiatus should be is unknown; however, with experience it becomes easier to distinguish the abnormal patient. IAS tone, which is tonically contracted, is also evaluated. The entire length of the anal sphincter complex is 3 to 5 cm, well within reach of the clinician's fingertips. The dentate line, where abscesses often occur, should be palpated. The clinician should palpate circumferentially for the presence of hemorrhoids. In addition, a rectovaginal examination should be performed as described in Chapter 33. Anoscopy is performed to rule out hemorrhoids. During anoscopy, the patient is asked to strain; this causes the internal hemorrhoids to dilate and improves detection. A rigid sigmoidoscopy can be done to look for masses and occult rectal prolapse and intussusception. The scope should be placed to a distance of about 10 to 15 cm, specifically looking for abnormal vasculature, tumors, and polyps. Occult prolapse can be difficult to elicit. Detection can be improved by giving the patient an enema, having her evacuate, and then repeating the rigid sigmoidoscopy. The scope is slowly removed while asking the patient to strain.

WORK-UP

The tests done to evaluate anorectal function include manometry, electromyography of the EAS and puborectalis muscle, evaluation of pudendal nerve terminal motor latency, anal sphincter ultrasound, and defecography.

Anal manometry is a method of measuring anal canal pressures. Fluid- or air-filled catheters are placed in the rectum and pressure measurements are taken. Parameters of interest include resting and squeeze anal pressures, inhibition reflex, and anal functional length. The strength of the anal sphincter complex and the volume needed to induce the inhibitory reflex can be assessed. More importantly, the clinician can ascertain if the patient senses the volume needed to induce the inhibitory reflex.

Needle electromyography of the EAS and puborectalis muscle looks for evidence of denervation, nerve regeneration, the chronology of the lesion, and muscle disease. Basically, the needle picks up motor unit action potentials from the muscle fibers and summates the activity from all the action potentials innervated by that single axon. The motor unit action potential exhibits different phases and durations in different disease states, and these patterns are read and interpreted by the neurologist. This test effectively identifies neuropathy if present. The needle studies have the disadvantage of being uncomfortable.

The pudendal nerve can be evaluated by measuring the pudendal nerve terminal motor latency. This is done by stimulating the pudendal nerve at the ischial spine and measuring the latency time to contraction of the EAS. For the patient, it is like having a prolonged rectal examination. The contraction of the EAS feels odd for the patient but is not perceived as pain. This test assesses whether pudendal neuropathy is present.

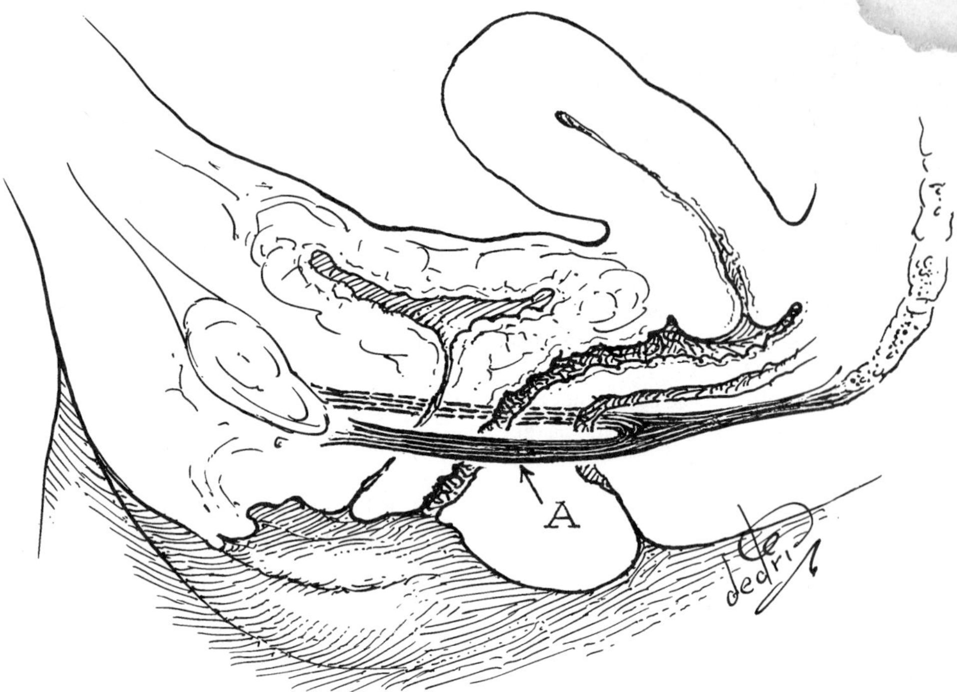

Figure 72-1. The vaginal axis. Notice the almost horizontal upper vagina and rectum lying on and parallel to the levator plate. The latter is formed by fusion of the pubococcygeal muscles (A) posterior to the rectum. The anterior limit of the point of fusion is the margin of the genital hiatus, immediately posterior to the rectum. (Nichols DH, Milley PS. Clinical anatomy of the vulva, vagina, lower pelvis, and perineum. In: Scirra J, Droegemuller W, eds. Gynecology and obstetrics. Philadelphia: JB Lippincott, 1993:4.)

Anal sphincter ultrasound is a fairly new modality used to evaluate the intactness of the anal sphincter complex. Atrophy of the complex may be appreciated as well.

Defecography is a radiologic study that evaluates the pelvic floor at rest, with Valsalva, and during defecation. It is most informative when contrast is placed in the bladder, vagina, and rectum and orally to picture all elements involved with the dynamic process of pelvic floor function. The clinician can identify pelvic floor descent, genital prolapse (including rectocele, cystocele, and enterocele), the anorectal angle, and the presence of resting incontinence. This study may be helpful in identifying intussusception in a patient without overt rectal prolapse. Defecography can identify defecation disorders such as tenesmus, in which the EAS and puborectalis muscle paradoxically contract during defecation. Special note is made of the anorectal angle.

Colonic transit time is measured by having the patient ingest radiopaque beads and then taking temporally spaced x-rays to measure the transit of the beads through the gastrointestinal tract.

MEDICAL MANAGEMENT

The general principle in the medical management of fecal incontinence is to reduce the threat from intestinal contents while maximizing the efficiency of the sphincter complex. In a patient with fecal incontinence secondary to diarrhea, the clinician must determine the etiology of the diarrhea and treat the patient accordingly. Causes of diarrhea include infection, inflammatory bowel disease, diverticular disease, and decreased colonic transit time. The latter can be treated with opiate derivatives such as loperamide. The treatment of the former diseases is described in Chapter 66. Another reason for diarrhea is overzealous laxative use, which is easily handled by discontinuation.

The active management of constipation is important to avoid the fecal impaction so often seen in nursing homes. The mainstay of treatment is to increase physical activity, which in itself increases bowel peristalsis. Adding fiber to the diet increases stool bulk, decreases colonic transit time, and therefore increases the frequency of defecation. However, patients who suffer from constipation secondary to megacolon or megarectum are better managed by decreasing stool volume with a fiber-restricted diet and by timed evacuation. These patients also benefit from enemas once or twice a week.

Keeping the patient with constipation well hydrated is of additional benefit. Laxatives and enemas should be used judiciously. Chronic use of stimulant laxatives (eg, castor oil, phenolphthalein, bisacodyl, cascara, senna, and casanthranol) should be discouraged. However, these are ingredients in many over-the-counter preparations, and many patients are reluctant to eliminate them totally. Overuse of these agents can result in abdominal cramping, fluid and electrolyte disturbances, and malabsorption syndromes, but use of these agents once or twice a week should not do any harm.

A better choice for treatment of constipation is lactulose or sorbitol. Sorbitol is more cost-effective and can be given orally in a dose of 120 mL of 25% solution. Its onset of action is 24 to 48 hours. It has the side effect of abdominal bloating. Docusate salts, another alternative, are given in doses of up to 200 mg/day and have an onset of action of 24 to 72 hours. Mineral oil should be avoided due to the risk of aspiration lipid pneumonia and deficiency of fat-soluble vitamins if taken regularly. Stool softeners are indicated only in patients with hard stools and are usually not helpful in patients with constipation.

Complications of chronic constipation include fecal impaction and excessive straining with defecation. In the elderly, this excessive straining can lead to transient ischemic attacks and syncope secondary to their compromised cerebrovascular and cardiovascular systems.

Management of fecal impaction includes saline, water, or phosphate enemas, along with polyethylene glycol and electrolyte solutions to cleanse the colon completely. Soap-sud enemas should be avoided due to the mucosal damage they can cause. Daily enemas are continued for 5 to 6 weeks, allowing the sensation in the rectum to normalize; thereafter, enemas are given once or twice a week. Patients who suffer from fecal impaction develop impaired rectal sensation so that they require larger fecal boluses to elicit the urge to defecate. For this reason, regular enemas are probably required long term to prevent recurrent episodes of impaction in these patients. Patients also benefit by restricting dietary fiber, thereby decreasing the amount of stool formed.

Patients with rectal prolapse benefit from surgical intervention. Medical management should be offered only to patients who are very poor operative risks. Nonoperative management involves steps to improve colonic transport and treatment of constipation. However, these are remedial measures only and provide nominal benefit to the patient with fecal incontinence secondary to rectal prolapse. The advancing rectal prolapse acts as a fecal bolus activating the rectoanal inhibitory reflex, thereby decreasing anal canal pressure. These patients also have shorter anal sphincter complexes and decreased anal sensation. Although surgery is the mainstay of treatment, the recurrence risk after surgery is high. The most successful approaches have been transabdominal rather than transperineal.

Physical therapy, including biofeedback and electrical stimulation, has achieved rates of improvement of up to 80% in fecal continence. Candidates for such treatment must be motivated and able to comprehend and follow instructions.

Patients who have fecal incontinence on a neurologic basis and or secondary to a decreased rectal reservoir benefit from planned defecation using laxatives and suppositories. Fiber restriction should be instituted to decrease stool volume and opiate derivatives should be given to prolong transit time. The management scheme should include enemas given once or twice a week to prevent fecal impaction.

A patient who has fecal incontinence secondary to a nonintact anal sphincter or fistula should be referred to a urogynecologist or colorectal surgeon for repair. Patients who are refractory to medical management or who have severe incontinence should also be referred to a surgeon. Patients who have a fistula secondary to inflammatory bowel disease tend to heal poorly after surgery, and the recurrence rate is high.

SUMMARY

Fecal incontinence is a socially debilitating disease that is multifactorial and still not completely understood. Even though our understanding of its pathophysiology is primitive, there are many interventions we can offer these patients, not the least of which is an empathetic ear and the courage to broach the question.

BIBLIOGRAPHY

Bartolo DC. Gastroenterological options in faecal incontinence. Annales De Chirurgie 1991;45:590.

Berkelmans I, et al. Perineal descent at defecography in women with straining at stool. 1995;7:75.

Caputo RM, Benson JT. Idiopathic fecal incontinence. Curr Opin Obstet Gynecol 1992;4:565.

Hallan RI, George B, Williams NS. Anal sphincter function: fecal incontinence and its treatment. Surg Ann 1993;25:85.

Madoff RD, Williams JG, Caushaj PF. Fecal incontinence. N Engl J Med 1992;326:1002.

Toglia MR, Delancey JO. Anal incontinence and the obstetrician-gynecologist. Obstet Gynecol 1994;84:731.

Wald A. Constipation and fecal incontinence in the elderly. Semin Gastro Disease 1994;5:179.

Primary Care for Women, edited by Phyllis C. Leppert and Fred M. Howard. Lippincott-Raven Publishers, Philadelphia © 1997.

73

Hemorrhoids

STEPHEN M. RAUH
TIMOTHY SIEGEL

Despite the remarkable prevalence of hemorrhoids in the United States, they remain one of the maladies most misunderstood by both patients and clinicians. Hemorrhoids affect about 5% of the general population of the United States at any given time; about 50% of people over age 50 are eventually affected. Patients who present with perianal complaints often attribute them to hemorrhoids, but the differential diagnosis includes fissure, abscess, fistula in ano, warts, hypertrophied anal papillae, rectal prolapse, prolapsing rectal polyp, and most importantly anorectal neoplasms. Not all pains in the rectum are due to hemorrhoids. Clinicians who are aware of these myriad conditions, and their own capabilities or limitations in regard to treatment, have many grateful patients.

Hemorrhoids are normally present in healthy persons and consist of highly vascularized, fibromuscular cushions that line the upper anal canal. These cushions are supported by muscles that arise partly from the internal sphincter and partly from the conjoined longitudinal muscles. They may be important in anal continence, cushioning the anal canal and supporting its mucosal lining during defecation.

Pathologically, the term "hemorrhoid" describes the downward displacement of these anal cushions during defecation, causing dilatation of small venules. With time, the supporting tissue to the cushions deteriorates, leading to increased distention of the venules, bleeding, and prolapse.

External hemorrhoids are located below the dentate line (squamocolumnar junction) and are covered by sensate, modified squamous epithelium. Internal hemorrhoids arise from above the dentate line and are covered by relatively insensitive columnar epithelium.

ETIOLOGY

Hemorrhoids are mainly a condition of the Western world and its low-fiber, high-fat diet. Chronic constipation and straining with defecation are thought to be important in their pathogenesis. Straining causes engorgement and secondary prolapse of the hemorrhoidal vascular cushions. With persistent straining, blood vessels become progressively dilated and the submucosal tissue loses its normal attachment to the underlying sphincter, eventually resulting in bleeding or prolapse. People with hemorrhoids tend to have higher resting anal sphincter pressures, as measured by anal manometry.

CLINICAL SYMPTOMS

External and internal hemorrhoids are further classified based on the associated clinical problems. External hemorrhoids may become acute (painful, swollen, and often thrombosed) or remain chronic (hemorrhoidal tags). They may be irritating, causing difficulty with hygiene, pruritus, or discomfort, but they often go unnoticed by patients.

Internal hemorrhoids are ubiquitous and typically asymptomatic; when symptomatic, patients have various complaints. Internal hemorrhoids are classified based on the presenting symptomatology: painless bleeding with defecation but no prolapse (first degree), prolapse with defecation and spontaneous reduction with or without bleeding (second degree), prolapse requiring manual reduction (third degree), and irreducible or incarcerated prolapse (fourth degree).

Bleeding is commonly bright red, minimal in quantity, and associated with straining. The blood is seen on the toilet paper and in the bowl. Blood may show on the surface of stool, but blood mixed in stool is uncommon. With chronic internal hemorrhoid prolapse, the exposed rectal mucosa can cause perianal irritation and mucofecal staining of underclothes. Pain is rare with internal hemorrhoids and is usually attributable to a coincident external hemorrhoid component, an anal fissure, or rarely internal hemorrhoid thrombosis.

Hemorrhoids and rectal bleeding may be coincidental, so all adults, regardless of age, should be evaluated for a colorectal neoplasm or inflammation before bleeding can be safely attributed to hemorrhoidal disease.

CLINICAL FINDINGS

The regional examination includes inspection of the perianal skin, digital rectal examination, anoscopy, and sigmoidoscopy. Inspection of the perianal skin (spreading of the buttocks enough to expose the anal verge) demonstrates many helpful findings, including irritation, discharge of pus, mucus, or feces, anal tags, and external hemorrhoids. This often leads the examiner to diagnose other anal conditions that the patient has attributed to hemorrhoids, including chronic pruritus ani, anal fistula, fissure, or anal Crohn disease. The "sentinel tag" associated with an anal fissure is just external to the painful fissure and may appear to the inexperienced examiner to be an external hemorrhoid; however, it is unrelated to the pain or treatment.

A symptomatic thrombosed external hemorrhoid contains sufficient clot to cause purplish-blue discoloration beneath the epidermis. The pain is due to tensing of the very sensitive anal skin. Occasionally the natural history of the process causes breakdown of the overlying skin, allowing partial extrusion of the clot. This is associated with the appearance of dark blood from the clot or fresh blood from skin edges or hemorrhoidal veins.

The digital rectal examination is more useful to exclude other pathology (eg, neoplasm, fissure) than to diagnose internal hemorrhoids, which are not readily palpable. Paradoxically, extreme tenderness on the digital examination (when there are minimal findings on inspection of the perianal skin) is rarely due to hemorrhoid disease; instead, it suggests a severe fissure or occult abscess and should be managed by a colorectal surgeon.

Anoscopy requires practice and patience, but the direct visualization of the anal canal and distal rectum that it allows is mandatory in the complete evaluation of anorectal disease. This is the most useful evaluation for internal hemorrhoids. No patient preparation is required. Various instruments are available, and the practitioner should evaluate several and choose the variety most useful to him or her.

When the patient complains of intermittent prolapsing tissue that is not evident on inspection and anoscopy, the patient can be asked to strain (Valsalva maneuver) on the toilet. The patient bends forward to allow the examiner to observe the perineum. This helps demonstrate prolapse and allows the clinician to differentiate between severe hemorrhoids and true rectal prolapse.

Patients with anorectal bleeding (fresh blood per rectum not mixed with stool) must have at least the rectum and sigmoid colon examined. Rigid sigmoidoscopy is the minimum test required and is appropriate for younger patients. Flexible sigmoidoscopy, with its significantly longer reach, is becoming more available and is recommended for those at risk for neoplasm (eg, those over age 40).

More proximal evaluation of the large intestine, such as a barium enema x-ray or colonoscopy, should not be routinely used when the clinical picture strongly suggests hemorrhoidal bleeding. These examinations are costly and overused in the setting of anorectal disease. They should be reserved for clinical situations suggesting colonic disease, such as altered bowel function, dark blood mixed with stool, fecal occult blood, and any bleeding unexplained or unsolved by anorectal investigation and treatment.

TREATMENT

The first line of therapy for patients with hemorrhoids is dietary manipulation. The goal is to avoid constipation and straining with defecation. The practitioner should outline a therapeutic fiber diet (20 to 30 g/day) with increased fluid intake (six to eight glasses of water daily). Fiber supplementation with psyllium or methylcellulose provides bulk and is universally available. For many patients, the benefits of a therapeutic fiber diet (even with supplemental fiber products) are lifelong, with virtually no adverse effects except cost. This dietary recommendation is also consistent with other primary care objectives regarding cardiovascular disease and cancer prevention. It is convenient to give the patient written guidelines that she can refer to after leaving the office. Patients should be encouraged to avoid prolonged attempts at defecation and should not defer the urge to defecate.

Treatment also includes dispelling the myths associated with hemorrhoids. This affliction is not related to the patient's sex, to any specific activity or occupation, or to any of the myriad of lay concepts (eg, standing on concrete). Treatment goals should include allowing the patient to resume desired activities that she may associate with symptoms, including work, sports, travel, and childbirth.

Persistent symptoms should trigger further treatment or, in the case of bleeding, further investigation. Return visits should be encouraged. Use of a specialist is indicated when symptoms are refractory or unexplained. Colorectal surgeons have the most comprehensive training and experience in the treatment of hemorrhoids and offer "one-stop shopping" for the diagnosis and management of hemorrhoids and all anorectal disease. If a colorectal surgeon is unavailable, the expertise of a general surgeon or gastroenterologist is required when the primary care team exhausts its resources.

Patients who fail to respond to simple measures or who have severe or disabling symptoms should be offered interventional therapy. Almost all interventional therapy for hemorrhoids, even conventional hemorrhoid surgery, can be performed on an outpatient basis for all but a few patients. The vast majority of patients are handled with office modalities, including excision of thrombosed hemorrhoids, elastic band ligation, infrared photocoagulation, or minor surgical excisions. Some therapies have lost popularity in the United States (eg, sclerotherapy, cryotherapy, anal dilatation, electrocoagulation, laser ablation) and need not be discussed further. All operative treatment requires local anesthesia and the availability of an assistant, minor surgical instruments, sutures, and the like.

Thrombosed external hemorrhoids are a common and vexing problem for primary care providers. The first decision is whether operative or nonoperative therapy is indicated. If symptoms are disabling (interfering with sleep, work, or bowel function), and particularly if pain is escalating, operative intervention is best. Excision is preferred rather than incision and drainage (lancing). The latter often is incomplete due to the multiple loculated clots, and the patient has persistent or increased pain if not all the clots are treated. Incision is associated with more delayed recurrence than excision. However, incision and drainage can be useful in alleviating the acute pain and is simpler to perform, rarely requiring suturing.

When the pain from an external thrombosis is resolving, a decision to incise or excise must be balanced carefully against the likelihood that the intervention will be more uncomfortable than the resolving thrombosis. Warm soaks or occasionally ice therapy are comforting. Topical anesthetic/steroid preparations abound but rarely meet the patient's expectations. Suppositories are not indicated in the treatment of external hemorrhoids. When choosing an oral analgesic, side effects such as constipation and antiplatelet activity should be considered.

Elastic band ligation has been performed safely since 1954. It is best for first-, second-, and many third-degree hemorrhoids. The technique is a brief office procedure performed through an anoscope. It requires no anesthesia and is associated with minimal discomfort or disability. Specially designed instruments grasp the hemorrhoid and apply the band to its base. The captured tissue necroses and passes, and the local inflammatory reaction leads to beneficial scarring and fixation of the surrounding hemorrhoidal mass. One or more hemorrhoid areas can be banded at a single session, but discomfort increases with multiple bandings. Usually patients with multiple hemorrhoids requiring banding return at 4- to 6-week intervals for further treatment. There is an 80% success rate for elastic band ligation of internal hemorrhoids.

Elastic band ligation can be used only on internal hemorrhoids, so common tags, external hemorrhoids, or mixed (internal/external) complexes cannot be treated this way. This is because the relatively insensate columnar epithelium covers internal hemorrhoids, allowing the slower strangling process of the bands to proceed without much interference to the patient's usual activity. Conversely, the transitional and squamous epithelium covering external hemorrhoids (distal to the dentate line) is exquisitely sensitive and makes rubber banding intolerable.

Complications of banding are rare. They include bleeding, pain, ring breakage, external thrombosis, and sepsis. Hemorrhage requiring urgent intervention occurs in 1% to 4% of patients. It can occur up to 3 weeks after banding and is associated with antiplatelet medications or a focus of sepsis at the site. It often requires suture ligation, cauterization, or hospitalization. Severe pain at the time of the procedure indicates placement too distally (involving sensitive anoderm) and is treated by immediate removal of the band. Breakage or slippage results in incomplete treatment of that area; dietary management helps prevent this complication. Postligation sepsis is extremely rare but is life-threatening. It presents with a delayed onset of pain, fever, and urinary retention and is treated with antibiotics and urgent debridement. Any practitioner performing interventional hemorrhoid treatment should be prepared to recognize and manage these complications.

Infrared photocoagulation is mainly used for bleeding, nonprolapsing hemorrhoids. It can be used alone or in combination with other techniques such as banding. The tip of the coagulation probe, passed through an anoscope, focuses infrared irradiation on the hemorrhoid tissue. The infrared energy is converted to heat, resulting in protein coagulation about 3 mm deep and the formation of a small ulcer. The resulting fixation and decreased blood flow effectively treat the area.

Over 80% of patients respond to nonsurgical or office treatment. Those needing further intervention are offered surgical hemorrhoidectomy. This is reserved for patients with large, prolapsing hemorrhoids, incarcerated prolapsed hemorrhoids (an emergency), combined internal/external hemorrhoids, or hemorrhoids associated with other anorectal pathology. The procedure of choice is the Ferguson hemorrhoidectomy. Local or regional anesthesia is used, and a hospital stay is not mandatory. Both the internal and external components are excised using an elliptic incision. Absorbable sutures are used. One to four incisions are made, based on the involved areas, typically the right anterior, right posterior, and left lateral quadrants.

Unlike many other hemorrhoid interventions, hemorrhoidectomy results in significant discomfort and temporary disability. Complications include urinary retention (4% to 30%), hemorrhage (1% to 3%), fecal impaction (2% to 5%), anal stenosis or weakness (< 1%), and sepsis (< 1%). Recurrence of symptoms occurs in less than 10% of patients and usually responds to office treatment. The use of lasers does not significantly alter the results of surgical treatment.

CONSIDERATIONS IN PREGNANCY

Any situation (including pregnancy) that increases abdominal pressure can increase the incidence of symptomatic hemorrhoids. During pregnancy, hormonal changes can cause increased vascularity and softening in the skin, muscles, and abundant connective tissue of the perineum; this may predispose to hemorrhoid problems. Labor and delivery can result in symptoms even in women with no prior hemorrhoid history.

Symptomatic pregnant women are offered noninterventional therapy until after delivery and then are treated according to standard guidelines. Pregnant and postpartum women with severe symptoms who have not responded to conservative measures can safely undergo hemorrhoidectomy at any time. Local anesthesia is preferred. Surgery is reserved for patients with disabling pain or persistent or severe bleeding. Only symptomatic areas are excised. There is a slightly increased risk of complications in this setting.

BIBLIOGRAPHY

Mazier WP. Hemorrhoids, fissures, and pruritus ani. Surg Clin North Am 1994:74:1277.

Mazier WP, Wolkomir AF. Hemorrhoids. Sem Colon Rectal Surg 1990;1:4.

Saleehy RG Jr et al. Hemorrhoidectomy during pregnancy: risk or relief? Dis Colon Rectum 1991;34:260.

Smith LE. Hemorrhoids. In: Fazio VW, ed. Current therapy in colon and rectal surgery. Philadelphia: BC Decker, 1990:9.

Primary Care for Women, edited by Phyllis C. Leppert and Fred M. Howard. Lippincott-Raven Publishers, Philadelphia © 1997.

VIII

Urinary Tract Problems

74

Urinary Tract Infections

JEANNE E. GROVE

One of the most common types of infection seen by primary care physicians who care for women continues to be urinary tract infection (UTI). Acute UTIs are more common in women than in men. It has been estimated that 25% to 35% of women between ages 20 and 40 have had the diagnosis of UTI at least once. Acute uncomplicated UTI in young women accounts for more than 5 million physician office visits per year. Recurrence occurs in about 20% of women. UTI is the most common infectious disease of the elderly. Fifteen percent to 20% of elderly women incur bacteriuria when living in the community and 30% to 50% when hospitalized. UTI continues to be a major health problem and accounts for considerable morbidity and health care costs.

Bacteriuria is the presence of bacteria in the urine. To ascertain the presence of infection in the urinary tract, bacteriuria in a midstream urine sample, suprapubic aspiration of urine, or urethral catheterization of urine must be obtained. The standard for bacteriuria in the past has been 10^5 bacteria/mL or more. This standard implies that infection must be seriously considered in the presence of 10^5 bacteria/mL. More recently, it has been recognized that patients with lower urinary tract symptoms and 10^2 to 10^4 bacteria/mL may have true bacterial infection. However, asymptomatic patients continue to be evaluated by the standard of 10^5 bacteria/mL.

UTIs are divided into lower and upper infections. Lower UTIs are characterized by dysuria, frequency, suprapubic pain, and urgency. Isolated lower tract infections are benign and self-limited, especially when only cystitis is considered. *Cystitis* is the clinical syndrome caused by bacteria and accompanied by the symptoms outlined above. However, these symptoms may be related to lower urinary tract inflammation involving the urethra only; the term *cystourethritis* is thus preferred. The clinical entity of urethritis is now referred to as frequency/dysuria or urethral syndrome because it may be the result of bacterial (eg, gonococcal urethritis) or nonbacterial (eg, chlamydia urethritis) causes. Upper UTI (eg, acute pyelonephritis) is more ominous with respect to systemic disease and long-term morbidity and mortality. Acute pyelonephritis is flank pain with or without fever and chills; it is often associated with dysuria, urgency, and frequency and is accompanied by significant bacteriuria (10^5 bacteria/mL or more) and acute infection in the kidney. The symptoms of lower tract and upper tract infections may overlap, especially when both processes are occurring concomitantly, but the clinical picture is usually clear.

Recurrent UTIs fall into two categories—reinfection and relapses. A recurrence of bacteriuria with a different microorganism is a reinfection. Most recurrent lower tract infections represent ascending reinfections with a different microorganism. It is important to clarify that the patient has a reinfection. Less frequently, reinfection occurs with the same microorganism, which may have persisted in the vagina or feces. Persistence in the urinary tract of the organism that was present before therapy was started is a relapse.

PATHOGENESIS

The most common pathway of infection in the urinary tract is the ascending route. Hematogenous and lymphatic pathways also have been implicated as routes of UTI, but both are uncommon. Initiation of the ascent of bacteria occurs in the urethra. The short length of the female urethra, together with the tendency to periurethral contamination with pathogenic bacteria, may explain why UTIs are more common in females than in males. The urethra is a sterile organ except for the distal portion. The female urethra appears particularly susceptible to colonization with colonic gram-negative bacilli due to its proximity to the anus, its short length (about 4 cm), and its termination beneath the labia. Migration of organisms from the urethra to the bladder is facilitated by sexual intercourse and diaphragm and spermicide use.

The incidence of UTI in ambulatory patients who have required straight catheterization of the bladder is about 1%. Patients with indwelling catheters with open drainage systems may develop UTIs within 3 or 4 days of initiation. Cultures of the periurethral and rectal areas have revealed an excellent correlation with the organisms subsequently found to be the cause of the UTI in catheterized patients. This evidence supports the suggestion that the ascending route is the most common pathway of infection in the urinary tract.

Although young women are susceptible to UTIs, the urinary tract is actually highly resistant to infection. Bacteria placed in the bladder, under normal circumstances, are cleared rapidly by the flushing and dilutional effects of voiding and the direct antibacterial properties of urine and the bladder mucosa. Bacterial growth is also inhibited by the high urea concentration, acidity, and high osmolality of the urine. Mucosal cells producing organic acids, along with local antibody responses and polymorphonuclear leukocytes in the bladder wall, appear to destroy bacteria that remain in the bladder mucosa after urination. When bacteria enter the urinary tract, UTI results only if the appropriate interaction occurs between the bacterial virulence factors, inoculum size, and adequacy of the host defense mechanism. The anatomic level of the UTI is also determined by these factors. Recurrent UTI is primarily a failure of normal host defense mechanisms rather than microbial characteristics.

The three major elements researchers believe determine the virulence of pathogenic bacteria are adhesions, hemolysis, and aerobactin. Most commonly, these characteristics are found in *Escherichia coli* strains. Adhesion was documented in 50% of patients with cystitis and 70% of patients with pyelonephritis. *E coli* isolates from patients with pyelonephritis usually have virulence factors not usually present in ordinary fecal isolates. These factors include fimbriae (adhesions), which are surface organelles that mediate attachment to specific receptors on the epithelial cells of the vagina. At least four different types of adhesions have been described: type I fimbriae, type II fimbriae, the P adhesion, and diffuse adhesion. Related to *E coli*'s avidity for iron are the other two major elements believed to determine the virulence of pathogenic bacteria: hemolysins, which degrade red cells, and aerobactin, a siderophore that enhances iron uptake.

The most effective host defense mechanisms are the turnover of epithelial cells and the flushing effect of voiding. Researchers have reviewed tissue factors that are secreted from the lower urinary tract that should prevent bacteria from adhering to its mucosal membranes. These factors include oligosaccharides, uromucoids (Tamm-Horsfall proteins), immunoglobulins (IgG, IgA, and secretory IgA), and bladder mucopolysaccharides, which have the potential to inhibit or prevent attachment or to detach bacteria from the mucosal surface. The urothelial mucosal cells that produce these factors are deficient in women prone to UTIs, especially recurrent infections.

MICROBIOLOGIC CRITERIA FOR CONFIRMING INFECTION

The most precise method for diagnosing infection is microscopic examination of the urine. The criterion for the assessment of UTI is the quantitative analysis of urinary bacteria. As noted earlier, patients with 10^5 bacteria/mL or more were previously considered to have true bacteriuria. This diagnostic criteria was found to be insufficiently sensitive for clinical applications because more than half of the women with acute symptomatic coliform infection had bacterial counts below this level. A value that provides good sensitivity, specificity, and predictability is 10^2 bacteria/mL. Photometry and bioluminescence are used to detect bacteriuria. These methods provide a sensitive measure of bacterial counts, but in detecting levels of 10^2 to 10^4/mL they are unsatisfactory. Physicians commonly treat patients with dysuria empirically based on symptoms and forego pretreatment urinalysis in symptomatic patients.

URINARY PATHOGENS AND URINARY TRACT INFECTIONS

Several endogenous factors help inhibit bacterial growth: high urine osmolality, urea concentration, organic acid concentration, and a low pH. The etiology of acute uncomplicated UTI rarely implicates more than one bacterial species. The presence of multiple organisms in a urine sample often reflects a contaminated specimen, unless the patient is at risk for a complicated UTI. Isolation of organisms usually residing as normal flora on the distal urethra and skin suggests contamination (eg, *Staphylococcus epidermidis*, diphtheroids, lactobacilli, *Gardnerella vaginalis*, and anerobes).

Facultative anaerobes, usually originating from the flora of the bowel, cause most infections. Flora of the vagina or perineal skin in females (eg, group B streptococci, *S epidermidis*, and *Candida albicans*) are other pathogens that may cause infection.

The most common urinary pathogen, *E coli*, accounts for about 70% to 85% of all community-acquired UTIs. Other enteric gram-negative bacteria (eg, *Proteus*, *Klebsiella*, and *Staphylococcus saprophyticus*) are less commonly responsible for community-acquired UTIs. *S saprophyticus*, a coagulase-negative nonhemolytic coccus and part of the flora of the skin and vaginal vault, is the second most common causative agent, producing about 10% to 20% of UTIs in young women.

E coli accounts for half the UTIs in hospitalized patients. Other urinary pathogens in hospitalized patients include *Klebsiella*, *Enterobacter*, *Citrobacter*, *Serratia*, *Pseudomonas aeruginosa*, *Providencia*, enterococci, and *S epidermidis*. Fungal infections are almost exclusively incurred by hospitalized patients. Fungi, especially *Candida* spp, usually infect the urinary tract of patients with indwelling catheters who have received antimicrobial therapy. Other urinary pathogens associated with UTIs in the hospital in association with instrumentation and catheterization are *G vaginalis*, lactobacilli, *Mycoplasma* spp including *Ureaplasma urealyticum*, and *S epidermidis*. Group B streptococcal infections are found predominantly in diabetic patients. Noninstrumented patients usually incur *Streptococcus faecalis*.

Sexually transmitted urethritis may involve pathogens such as *Chlamydia trachomatis*, *Neisseria gonorrhoeae*, and herpes simplex virus. Vaginitis caused by *Trichomonas vaginalis* and *Candida* spp may mimic acute urethritis or urinary tract infection.

Asymptomatic bacteriuria, present in 4% to 7% of pregnant women, develops into acute pyelonephritis in an estimated 20% to 40% of cases. Besides pyelonephritis, asymptomatic bacteriuria during pregnancy is also associated with preterm labor and low-birth-weight infants. Microbes present in the urethra and bladder presumably ascend the ureters into the renal collecting systems, ultimately invading susceptible tissue and inciting an inflammatory response. The bacteria responsible for most cases of pyelonephritis are primarily the aerobic inhabitants of the lower female genital tract. Members of the Enterobacteriaceae, such as *E coli*, *Klebsiella pneumoniae*, and *Proteus mirabilis*, are the most commonly recovered, as well as some other gram-negative bacteria such as *Enterobacter, Citrobacter*, and gram-positive organisms (eg, group B streptococcus).

Lower genital tract bacteria colonize the lower urinary tract through various mechanisms, including adhesion to the uroepithelium mediated by fimbriae on the bacterial cell wall. Upper tract accessibility is facilitated during pregnancy by urinary stasis and upper urinary tract dilation as a result of mechanical obstruction by the enlarging uterus and the engorged pelvic vasculature. The smooth muscle relaxation effects of progesterone also promote bacterial access to the upper tract. Upper tract dilation is more pronounced in women with pyelonephritis in pregnancy.

In the elderly, unlike in younger women, the pathogenesis of UTI is related to abnormal bladder function, bladder outlet obstruction, vaginal and urethral atrophy, use of long-term indwelling catheters, and puddling related to bed rest. The organisms causing infection in the elderly relate to the ecology of the patient's environment. Many have a greater variety of pathogenic organisms, especially women living in nursing homes and in particular those with permanent indwelling catheters. Many of these organisms may be antibiotic-resistant.

As mentioned before, the development of an infection and its outcome are determined by the interactions of the virulence of the bacteria and the host defense mechanisms. Some urinary pathogens are relatively opportunistic and avirulent and thus can induce UTI only when natural host defense mechanisms are compromised. Other organisms can cause infection and invade the lower or upper urinary tract in the absence of obstruction, other structural abnormalities, or urinary tract catheterization.

CLINICAL FINDINGS

Depending on the patient's age, the location of the infection, and concomitant urologic disease, symptomatology varies. Neonates and children less than 2 years old present with vomiting, fever, and failure to thrive. Clinical signs and symptoms in adults with UTI include frequency, dysuria, small amounts of urine, urgency, hematuria, low back pain, or suprapubic pain. Low-grade fever may accompany lower tract infection. Lower tract infections in the elderly are usually asymptomatic. The usual symptoms of lower tract infections (eg, frequency, dysuria, hesitancy, and incontinence) are present in many noninfected elderly patients and therefore are nonspecific.

Classically, upper tract infections present with the triad of fever (38°C, often with chills and rigors), costovertebral angle or flank tenderness or pain, and lower tract symptoms. In moderate to severe cases of acute pyelonephritis, the temperature may be high (40°C), with intermittent spikes. If vomiting and insensible water loss have caused significant dehydration, the patient may be weak and may appear debilitated. Clinical hypotension may ensue and rarely progresses to overt septic shock. Lower tract symptoms are the only presentation in 10% to 50% of patients with concomitant upper tract infections. The elderly and neurologically impaired often have atypical clinical presentations. Symptoms may include appetite reduction, decreased social interaction and personal hygiene, changes in mentation, abdominal pain, incontinence, urgency, and nocturia.

Patients may present without symptoms but still have a lower or upper tract infection. Asymptomatic bacteria has been observed in up to 50% of catheterized, hospitalized patients. The most common source of bacteremia produced by gram-negative bacilli is UTI. In the presence of an indwelling catheter, bacteremia may occur with no urinary symptoms.

DIAGNOSIS

The initial step in the laboratory diagnosis of UTI is microscopic examination of the urine for leukocytes. In symptomatic women, urinalysis is the most accurate method for predicting bacteriuria. The periurethral and urethral areas are difficult to sterilize; therefore, frequent contamination of the urine specimen occurs. As a result, the presence of bacteria on urinalysis is not used as a single criterion for the diagnosis of UTI. The method of urine collection affects the results; the three acceptable methods for urine collection include midstream clean-catch, catheterization, and suprapubic aspiration. A urine specimen is obtained by one of these methods. A drop of unspun urine is examined, as well as the sediment from a specimen obtained by centrifugation for 5 minutes at 2000 rpm.

The urine sample is examined for the presence of leukocytes. Each leukocyte seen in a centrifuged specimen under high power represents about five to ten cells/mm^3 of urine. The upper limit of normal has been stated to be ten to 50 white blood cells/mm^3. A clean-catch midstream urine specimen with five to ten leukocytes per high-power field in the sediment is thus considered the upper limit of normal, as this represents 50 to 100 cells/mm^3.

This method has been criticized primarily because of the varying volumes used for suspension after centrifugation. Others have relied on quantitative leukocyte counts in a standard counting chamber with unspun urine.

There is a striking association between pyuria and bacteriuria. In a symptomatic adult, pyuria is associated with infection, but in children this is not as predictable. The elderly are usually asymptomatic but have pyuria. Therefore, patients with or without pyuria may or may not have infection.

Occasionally, microscopic or sometimes gross hematuria is seen in a patient with UTI. Red blood cells may reflect other disorders such as calculi, tumor, vasculitis, glomerulonephritis, or renal tuberculosis. White cell casts in the presence of an acute infectious process are strong evidence for pyelonephritis, but the absence of white cell casts does not rule out upper tract infection. White cells can also be seen in renal disease in the absence of infection.

A common but not universal finding in UTI is proteinuria. Patients with UTI usually excrete less than 2 g of protein in 24 hours; excretion of 3 g or more suggests glomerular disease.

Another useful test in the presumptive diagnosis of UTI is the microscopic examination of a specimen for bacteria. The ability to identify bacteria in the urine depends on whether the specimen has been centrifuged and on whether it has been stained with methylene blue or Gram stain. The presence of at least one bacterium per oil-immersion field in a midstream clean-catch uncentrifuged urine specimen correlates with 10^5 bacteria/mL of urine or more. In a stained sedimented specimen, the absence of bacteria in several fields indicates the probability of less than 10^4 bacteria/mL. Gram stain of urine smears is a rapid, accurate, and inexpensive way to detect greater than 10^5 bacteria/mL, with a 94% sensitivity, greater than 70% specificity, and a negative predictive value of 99%. However, low-count bacterial infection of the lower tract may be associated with a negative Gram stain.

The introduction of dipstick and automated techniques of screening urine for potential infection has brought questions about the accuracy of these newer methods and how they compare with traditional microscopic examination of the urine. Direct microscopy and Gram stain of urine have reasonable specificity for infection but are somewhat insensitive, especially to lower levels of bacteriuria. Both tests are difficult to standardize in terms of volume of urine tested, centrifugation time, number of microscopic fields examined, and experience of the technician. Comparison of accuracy and cost of the technique of leukocyte esterase or nitrite reductase dipsticks with Gram stain revealed that Gram stain had superior sensitivity and specificity. However, the estimated cost of the Gram stain was $1.94 per test, compared with 33 to 48 cents for dipstick methods. Urine microscopy remains the most accurate rapid test for UTI. However, in the office setting where a laboratory is not readily available, other rapid tests having slightly lower sensitivity and specificity may be appropriate. An extensive metanalysis of 51 published articles concluded that if leukocyte esterase or nitrite strip dipsticks revealed a positive result, they should be interpreted as a positive screen. However, a negative dipstick test, according to this analysis, cannot exclude the diagnosis of UTI in patients with a high likelihood of infection. As noted earlier, up to half of UTIs in women with acute dysuria are characterized by growth of 10^2 to 10^4 bacteria/mL in midstream cultures, and all rapid urine tests are relatively insensitive to detecting these lower levels of bacteriuria.

Traditionally, rapid urine tests done in the office have been used only for screening patients who may require a urine culture. More recently, some authorities have recognized that a urine culture is not necessary in all patients with a suspected UTI. Some researchers recommend that patients with definite symptoms of an uncomplicated lower tract infection and a positive screening test do not need to incur the expense of a pretreatment culture because the probability that the diagnosis is correct is high (usually 80% to 90%). Also, the urine culture results are usually not available until after the patient has already received adequate treatment. The same researchers also do not recommend posttreatment follow-up cultures in such patients unless the symptoms persist. Women with complicating factors should have urine cultures done.

Under routine testing conditions, up to 15% of uncomplicated UTIs yield negative culture results. Organisms such as *C trachomatis*, *U urealyticum*, or *Mycoplasma hominis* should be considered when cultures are negative. Because pathogenic etiologies of UTI in the elderly are less predictable, urine cultures should guide antibiotic therapy in this population. Cultures should also be obtained when symptoms of upper tract infection are present or if a complicated infection is suspected.

TREATMENT

The initial approach to the management of UTIs in women includes antibiotic therapy, administration of a high fluid volume to flush the system, and if needed the administration of urinary tract analgesics. Symptomatic patients, as well as asymptomatic patients with high urine bacteria counts, should have therapeutic intervention. The elimination of bacteria from the urinary tract is the objective of treatment. The foundation of treatment for UTIs is antibiotic therapy. Antibiotic therapy usually produces symptomatic relief (clinical cure), but bacteriuria may persist. Appropriately chosen antibiotics relieve the symptoms shortly after therapy commences. Frequently, phenazopyridine hydrochloride is prescribed to relieve the symptom of burning. However, it should not be used more than 2 days because it may mask the symptoms of UTI progression. Patients with renal dysfunction should not use phenazopyridine because the incidence of adverse effects is greater in this population.

Infection severity and epidemiologic factors (eg, age, institutionalization, underlying disease, and history of UTI) influence the choice of drug and the duration of treatment. The optimal antibiotic is one that achieves high urinary concentrations (above the infecting organism's minimum inhibitory concentration); has both gram-positive and gram-negative antimicrobial activity; has little potential for promoting bacterial resistance; has minimal effect on the anaerobic flora and microaerophilic normal flora but eradicates aerobic gram-negative rods from the fecal and vaginal flora; has a long half-life (which facilitates long dosing intervals); has acceptable patient tolerance and adverse effect profile; and is inexpensive.

In hospitalized patients, enterococci account for about 15% of UTIs. Aminopenicillins alone (ampicillin or amoxicillin) may be sufficient if the infection is confined to the bladder. However, if there is renal tissue involvement (and this may be difficult to diagnose), the combination of gentamicin and ampicillin may be required. The goal is a high urine concentration of aminoglycosides; therefore, serum concentrations may be kept low (40 to 50 ug/mL and 3 to 5 ug/mL, respectively). Vancomycin should be used in patients allergic to penicillin.

In pregnant women and elderly patients, asymptomatic bacteriuria is a serious threat. The potential adverse effects of bacteriuria on the mother (eg, persistent bacteriuria, symptomatic UTI, and acute and chronic pyelonephritis) and fetus (eg, increased frequency of preterm delivery, low birth weight, and fetal infection) must be minimized with appropriate antibiotic therapy. The most appropriate management in the elderly patient is controversial. As mentioned before, elderly patients with bacteriuria are often asymptomatic, and there are no guidelines to identify patients likely to benefit from therapy. Prevention of subsequent infections with treatment has not been established. Commonly, there are increased adverse reactions, the development of resistance, and early recurrence. Patients with spinal cord injuries also experience early recurrence and therefore are treated only if bacteria counts of 10^2 colony-forming units (cfu)/mL or more are associated with symptoms.

Antimicrobial Therapy

The characteristics of the antimicrobial agent and the location and etiology of the infection must be considered when selecting a therapeutic agent. Previously, sulfonamides and aminopenicillins were used to treat initial episodes of UTI in young women. However, more recently the relatively frequent resistance to these agents has lessened their use. Resistance rates to ampicillin of 25% have been reported in studies evaluating the susceptibility patterns of uropathogens cultured from patients with nonnosocomial UTIs. Trimethoprim with or without a sulfonamide, amoxicillin/clavulanate, cephalosporins, fluoroquinolones, and nitrofurantoin are the agents of choice.

β-Lactamase resistance has been addressed with the development of clavulanate potassium, an irreversible competitive inhibitor of this enzyme. Clavulanate protects the β-lactam ring of amoxicillin—thus, when used in combination with amoxicillin, a synergistic bactericidal effect results that expands the spectrum of activity of amoxicillin against many strains of β-lactamase-producing bacteria that are resistant to amoxicillin alone. UTIs caused by *E coli*, *Klebsiella* spp, *Enterobacter* spp., or *P mirabilis* have been treated effectively with this combination.

Three generations of oral cephalosporins have been used in the treatment of UTIs. The spectrum of activity of these agents varies. First-generation cephalosporins are more active against gram-positive organisms; third-generation cephalosporins are more active against gram-negative organisms. There is no oral cephalosporin with significant activity against enterococci and *Pseudomonas* spp. Cefixime has poor activity in vitro against *S saprophyticus*. The long half-life of ceftriaxone, a parenteral third-generation cephalosporin with an extended spectrum of activity, allows once-a-day dosing.

The fluoroquinolones are a group of antibacterial agents that are structurally related to the prototype quinolone, nalidixic acid. The antibacterial spectrum and potency of this class of drugs have been broadened by the fluorination of the quinolone ring. Fluoroquinolones are effective in vitro against both gram-positive and gram-negative organisms, including *S saprophyticus* and, in the case of ciprofloxacin, *P aeruginosa*. Dosing on once- or twice-daily basis is sufficient. They have been shown to be effective in both complicated and uncomplicated UTIs.

Nitrofurantoin, a nitrofuran-derivative antibacterial agent, is active against most gram-negative bacteria and enterococci but is inactive against *Proteus* and *Pseudomonas* spp. Nitrofurantoin achieves rapid high concentrations in the urine because it is readily absorbed in the gastrointestinal tract. It does not promote the emergence of resistant bacteria in fecal flora and therefore is effective as a chronic prophylactic agent in recurrent infections.

Definition of Response to Therapy

The response of UTIs to antibiotic therapy can be assessed clinically and microbiologically. The clinical goal is the resolution of symptoms. There are four patterns of microbiologic response of bacteriuria to antimicrobial therapy: cure, persistence, relapse, and reinfection. Within 48 hours after initiation of an antimicrobial agent, the quantitative bacterial counts in urine should decrease, provided the microorganism is sensitive in vitro. It is unlikely that continued therapy will be successful if titers do not decrease within this time. Cure is defined as negative urine cultures achieved while the patient is on the therapy and during the 1 to 2 weeks of the follow-up period. Persistence means either significant bacteriuria after 48 hours of treatment or the presence of low numbers of the infecting organism in the urine after 48 hours. Drug resistance, subtherapeutic urinary antibiotic concentrations, or the presence of a bacterial nidus within the soft tissue or calculi may cause persistence. A relapse of UTI with symptoms can be the result of persistence.

Therapy is considered to have failed if the asymptomatic patient has 10^5 cfu/mL of uropathogen, or if the symptomatic patient has 10^3 cfu/mL and pyuria occurring 5 to 9 days or 4 to 6 weeks after therapy.

Relapses and reinfections are differentiated on the basis of the second isolate identified. Relapse results when the original infecting organism persists in the urinary tract. Within 1 to 2 weeks after antibiotic treatment, a relapse can occur. Relapse may be associated with renal infection and structural abnormalities of the urinary tract. Women with acute UTIs experience frequent relapses (about 20%), accounting for a great deal of morbidity, increased health care costs, and time lost from work. Reinfection, sometimes called superinfection, usually occurs after initial sterilization of the urine. It involves either a different bacterial species or a different serotype of the same species (usually *E coli*), or the same serotype. It is attributed to contamination by fecal flora and occurs in 2% to 10% of patients. Superinfection can also occur during the treatment of a UTI. This is sometimes defined as the presence of a new organism resistant to the antibiotic.

Treatment of Acute Uncomplicated Lower Urinary Tract Infections

Traditional therapy—oral antimicrobial agents prescribed for 7 to 14 days—is successful in more than 80% of uncomplicated infections in women. The causative organisms, on initial exposure, are susceptible to most antibiotics with gram-negative activity, including nitrofurantoin, trimethoprim–sulfamethoxazole (TMP/SMX) (in a 1:5 ratio), and first-generation cephalosporins. There are minimal resistance problems with initial exposure to nitrofurantoin and TMP/SMX. The cost of these drugs is acceptable to most patients. A creatinine clearance above 40 mL/min is necessary to achieve a concentration of nitrofurantoin in the urine appropriate for adequate bactericidal activity. Because of decreased renal elimination, serum concentrations are increased, resulting in increased toxicity in patients with renal dysfunction.

Table 74-1 lists the dosage, side effects, and precautions for common antibiotics used in UTIs. Tetracycline is generally not prescribed because of the possibility of developing plasmid-mediated resistance in gram-negative organisms. Doxycycline is occasionally used because less bacterial resistance develops and good urine concentrations are achieved; it is given twice daily. Resistance rates of 25% to 35% have been reported for *E coli* with the use of ampicillin or sulfonamide. The high resistance rate reported for sulfonamide is overcome with the use of TMP/SMX. Other alternatives are the cephalosporins and amoxicillin/clavulanic acid, provided the organism does not produce cephalosporins or type I β-lactamase.

Fluoroquinolones are impressive in the treatment of UTIs. Their greatest advantage is improved patient tolerance compared to TMP/SMX. However, higher doses of amifloxacin and fleroxacin have resulted in some adverse experiences. They are useful in a range of clinical situations but should not be considered first-line treatment because of their cost and the emergence of resistant isolates. Quinolones should be considered in complicated UTIs, in a patient allergic to a conventional agent, or in a patient whose infection is caused by gram-negative bacilli with multiple resistance, or if the toxicity of alternate therapy is greater.

Short-Course Therapy

Due to its effectiveness, improved compliance, lower cost, reduced emergence of resistant bacteria, and fewer adverse reactions, short-course therapy has become the treatment of choice for uncomplicated lower tract infections. The rationale for the use of short-course therapy is that lower tract infection is a superficial mucosal infection only.

The regimens range from a single dose to multiple doses for up to 3 to 5 days. These regimens should be limited to young, nonpregnant women presenting with symptoms of less than 7 days in duration who have insignificant urinary infection histories. Patients must be willing and able to come for follow-up. Longer treatment regimens should be prescribed for post-menopausal women. Follow-up is necessary. Relapse after a short or full course of therapy should be treated with a 2-week course of therapy.

Only antibiotics with documented efficacy should be considered for single-dose therapy (Table 74-2). High urinary concentrations for at least 12 to 24 hours are essential. Cure rates have been reported to be 61% to 100%. The organism involved influences the success of these therapies. For instance, *E coli* seems to

Table 74-1 Dosage and Side Effects of Oral Antibiotics Commonly Used in the Treatment of Urinary Tract Infections in Young Women

DRUG	DOSAGE		SIDE EFFECTS AND PRECAUTIONS
	Treatment	*Prophylaxis*	
Amoxicillin/clavulanate potassium	250 mg/125 mg every 8 h		Gastrointestinal, rash, *Candida* vaginitis
Cephalosporins			
Cefaclor	250–500 mg every 8 h		Cross-reactivity in 20% of patients with a history of anaphylactic reactions to penicillin, *Candida* vaginitis
Cefixime	400 mg once a day		
Cefuroxime	250–500 mg every 12 h		
Ceftriaxone	1–2g daily IM		
Cephalexin	250 mg every 6 h or 500 mg every 12 h		
Fluoroquinolones			
Ciprofloxacin	250–500 mg every 12 h		Gastrointestinal, dizziness, headache; contraindicated in children or pregnancy because induces cartilage erosion in young animals; *Candida* vaginitis
Norfloxacin	400 mg every 12 h		
Ofloxacin	400 mg every 12 h		
Lomefloxacin	400 mg once a day		
Nitrofurantoin	50–100 mg every 6 h	50–100 mg daily	Nausea, vomiting, neuropathy, pulmonary hypersensitivity reactions
Trimethoprim	100 mg every 12 h or 200 mg every day	100 mg at bedtime	Rash occurring 7 to 14 days after initiation of therapy; gastrointestinal
Trimethoprim/sulfamethoxazole	160 mg/800 mg twice a day	40–80 mg/ 200–400 mg every day or three times/week	Rash, gastrointestinal, fatal hypersensitivity reactions (ie, Stevens-Johnson syndrome)

(Sravani A. Treatment of urinary tract infections in young women. American Urology Association Update Series, Lesson 6. 1993;12:42. Reproduced by permission.)

be eradicated more effectively than *S saprophyticus* (however, the differing pathogenic strains of *E coli* must be considered).

In a review of 28 trials, single-dose treatment was found to be less effective than 3- or 5-day or longer treatment courses in eradicating bacteriuria. Extending the single-dose regimen to multiple doses (3 to 5 days) appears to be superior. β-Lactams are more effective when given for 5 days or more, compared with TMP/SMX given for 3 days. No benefits are achieved by increasing treatment with TMP/SMX to 5 days or greater. Adverse reactions occur more frequently when the length of cephalosporin treatment time is increased. However, when penicillins and norfloxacin are given for 3 days, the incidence of adverse reactions does not increase. When treatment is given for more than 3 days, adverse reactions increase markedly overall. Three-day regimens of the fluoroquinolones demonstrate excellent bacterial eradication (95% to 97%). A 3- to 5-day course of therapy serves as a reasonable alternative to single-dose therapy for acute lower tract infection. If relapse occurs or if symptoms and bacteriuria persist after treatment, renal parenchymal involvement, bacterial resistance, or underlying urologic anomalies may be present. Short-course treatment may serve as a screening mechanism for more serious renal disease.

Follow-Up Culture

The need for a follow-up culture after treatment of an uncomplicated lower tract infection is controversial. If done, the post-treatment urine culture should be collected 1 to 2 weeks after discontinuing therapy, primarily to detect relapses. It is prudent to obtain a urine sample for culture and sensitivity in all women with a UTI; the exception is a young, nonpregnant woman who remains asymptomatic after therapy.

Treatment of Uncomplicated Upper Urinary Tract Infections/Pyelonephritis

Because pyelonephritis may result in serious complications such as renal scarring, immediate treatment with a broad-spectrum antibiotic should be initiated. Some believe that intravenous antibiotic therapy and hospitalization are necessary, but the more general consensus is that not all patients need intravenous antibiotic therapy, especially those who are minimally symptomatic. The goal is to achieve high urinary, serum, and tissue levels of antibiotic. Because more than 30% of strains causing acute pyelonephritis are ampicillin-resistant, an appropriate alternative is a quinolone antibiotic.

In patients who require parenteral therapy, empiric treatment should be based on the findings of the urine Gram stain. Acceptable agents include the second- or third-generation cephalosporins, TMP/SMX, fluoroquinolones, and broad-spectrum penicillins. When the patient becomes afebrile and can tolerate oral hydration and medication, parenteral therapy can be stopped and oral therapy begun. The fluoroquinolones and TMP/SMX are optimal broad-

Table 74-2. Single-dose Oral Antibiotic Treatment Options for Urinary Tract Infections in Women

DRUG	DOSE
Amoxicillin	3 g
Cefaclor	2 g
Cefadroxil	1 g
Cefuroxime	1000 mg
Cephalexin	3 g
Ciprofloxacin	250 mg, 500 mg
Enoxacin	600 mg
Fleroxacin	200 mg, 400 mg
Nitrofurantoin	400 mg
Norfloxacin	400 mg, 800 mg
Ofloxacin	200 mg, 400 mg
Sulfisoxazole	2 g
TMP/SMX	2 double-strength tablets
Trimethoprim	400 mg

TMP/SMX, trimethoprim/sulfamethoxazole in a 1:5 ratio by weight.
(Hatton J, Hughes M, Raymond C. Management of bacterial urinary infections in adults. Ann Pharmacother 1994;28:1264. Reproduced by permission.)

spectrum agents. However, Faro (1992) compared the efficacy of the quinolones with TMP/SMX and found greater bacterial cure with the quinolones than with TMP/SMX. Oral therapy should last 10 to 14 days. To diagnose a relapse, follow-up cultures are recommended. Evaluation of the upper tract for suppurative foci, calculi, or urologic disease should ensue if the patient remains febrile after 72 hours of treatment or if relapse occurs. With a relapse, treatment should continue for 6 weeks if no complicating factors are discovered.

Treatment of Complicated Urinary Tract Infections

Host factors such as a structural or functional abnormality of the urinary tract can complicate a UTI. The choice of antibiotic and the duration of treatment are affected when a UTI ascends to the kidney. Therapy may include parenteral antibiotics until the patient is afebrile for 12 to 24 hours; therapy is usually required for at least 14 days. Empiric therapy must consider the setting and medical history of the patient, as well as coverage for suspected gram-negative organisms.

Catheterization is an independent risk factor for UTI. Patients who develop bacteriuria from temporary catheterization (eg, postoperatively) should receive antibiotic therapy before and for 24 hours after the catheter is removed. Others recommend antibiotic therapy only before and once or twice postoperatively. Asymptomatic patients less than 65 years old may be given a single dose of two double-strength TMP/SMX tablets to prevent UTI after catheterization. Cultures at 1 week and 1 month after catheter removal are recommended. When *P mirabilis* is isolated, a full course of antibiotic therapy is prescribed; *P mirabilis* can cause renal calculi and catheter encrustations, thus establishing a nidus of infection. With permanent catheter placement, bacteriuria is prevented by intermittent use of antibiotics, but with eventual isolation of resistant organisms. Thus, treatment of bacteriuria in patients with permanent catheters is indicated only if the patient is immunocompromised or if the threat of sepsis is evident. If treatment is initiated, the catheter should be replaced.

Complicated UTIs require aggressive management with antibiotic therapy and prolonged treatment for 2 to 6 weeks. Patients who are debilitated, such as those in hospitals or nursing homes or those with spinal cord injuries, often acquire infections with more resistant gram-negative rods. The isolates from the urine of these patients are usually *Enterobacter cloacae* and *P aeruginosa*, microorganisms with a propensity to acquire resistance rapidly to many antibiotics. Broad-spectrum antibiotics are indicated if risk factors are present. Until the organism is identified and susceptibilities are known, reasonable empiric choices include antipseudomonal β-lactams (mezlocillin, piperacillin, ticarcillin, ceftazidime, ceftriaxone, cefotaxime), imipenem/cilastatin, aztreonam, aminoglycosides, and quinolones.

Often, atypical symptoms lead to delayed diagnosis and increase the risk of urosepsis. Broad-spectrum antibiotics should be included in the initial regimens. In high-risk populations, it is challenging to dose aminoglycosides empirically: the reduced muscle mass interferes with the interpretation of serum creatinine, and aminoglycoside concentrations are often higher than predicted. These patients have recurrent complicated UTIs, and thus repeated exposure to aminoglycosides may increase the risk for toxicity. Most studies reveal good to excellent cure rates with the quinolones, which were consistently more effective than the comparison drugs in complicated UTIs.

Treatment of Urinary Tract Infections in the Elderly

With increasing age, the prevalence of UTI increases, reaching over 50% for institutionalized patients of either sex. Asymptomatic and symptomatic bacteriuria present a risk factor for bacteremia, sepsis, and increased mortality (especially for elderly women). Bacteriuria in the elderly is a complex problem. UTI is more difficult to treat, and its pathogenesis is related to abnormal bladder function, bladder outlet obstruction, vaginal and urethral atrophy, use of long-term indwelling catheters, and puddling related to bed rest. Bacteriuria is usually asymptomatic, and there is no indication for the treatment of asymptomatic bacteriuria except before invasive genitourinary procedures. Antimicrobial adverse effects and the emergence of resistant organisms, as well as the inability to prevent subsequent symptomatic episodes, form the rationale for not treating asymptomatic bacteriuria in elderly patients.

Recurrent bacterial infection in the elderly may be related to poor hygiene, particularly associated with fecal and urinary incontinence. Admission of elderly patients for gram-negative bacteremia secondary to acute pyelonephritis is common. These patients can be treated effectively, resulting in a 97% survival rate.

CONSIDERATIONS IN PREGNANCY

Dilation of the ureters and renal pelves begins in the first trimester and progresses to term, allowing bacteria in the bladder to reach the upper tract. This makes pregnant women more susceptible to UTI and subsequent acute pyelonephritis. Asymptomatic bacteriuria occurs in 4% to 7% of pregnancies. Pyelonephritis occurs in 20% to 40% of pregnant women with untreated bacteriuria. One in 3000 pregnant women with pyelonephritis develops end-stage renal disease if untreated.

Bacteriuria during pregnancy is associated with an increased incidence of adverse effects for the mother (persistent bacteriuria, symptomatic UTI, acute and chronic pyelonephritis, and probably anemia) and fetus (increased frequency of premature delivery, low birth weight, fetal infection, and risk of perinatal death). The fetal adverse effects are reported to be up to three times more common in the bacteriuric woman than in a nonbacteriuric one.

Whether symptomatic or asymptomatic, it is imperative to treat bacteriuria in pregnancy. Quantitative urine cultures should be performed at the initial prenatal visit. Asymptomatic bacteriuria noted on two consecutive urine specimens should be treated with an agent to which the organism is susceptible.

E coli is responsible for about 80% of all community-acquired UTIs in pregnancy. Other pathogens, such as *K pneumoniae*, *P mirabilis*, and *Enterococcus faecalis*, are also common. Aminopenicillins, cephalosporins, nitrofurantoin, and TMP-SMX in single-dose or 3-day regimens can be used in the treatment of bacteriuria. Sulfonamides should not be used in the third trimester because of possible kernicterus in the neonate. Quinolones are not used in pregnancy because studies in immature animals report cartilage erosion.

The single-dose cure rate of amoxicillin in pregnancy is about 80%. If the organism is susceptible to amoxicillin, a 3-g single dose should be prescribed in the asymptomatic pregnant patient. If single-dose therapy fails, treatment for 14 days for presumed renal infection is required.

In the symptomatic pregnant patient with UTI, if the organism is susceptible, amoxicillin 500 mg three times daily for 3 days is recommended. If there is no improvement, even though the organism is susceptible to the agent, the patient should be retreated for 14 days. If resistant pathogens do not allow improvement, the pregnant patient should be retreated for 3 days with an antibiotic to which the organism is susceptible.

Acute pyelonephritis in the pregnant patient is treated by hospitalization and parenteral antibiotics. Repeat cultures every 4 to 6 weeks during pregnancy should be performed.

RECURRENT URINARY TRACT INFECTIONS

UTIs recur in about 20% of the patients. The three primary causes of recurrent UTI are persistence of the organism in the urine during therapy; relapse caused by reemergence of the original infecting organism because of a failure to eradicate it from renal tissue; and reinfection caused by the entry of new organisms into the bladder from the fecal/perineal reservoir. In these patients, there is usually no anatomic or functional cause of infection. Relapses occur whether single-dose or longer courses of therapy are prescribed. Most women who have had a 10- to 14-day regimen of antibiotic treatment without successful eradication of the infection are cured by 6 weeks of treatment, unless a pathologic condition of the upper urinary tract underlies the infection.

Therapeutic options shown to be effective in the management of recurrent UTIs include continuous low-dose oral antimicrobial prophylaxis, intermittent self-treatment, and postcoital prophylaxis. Women who experience two or more symptomatic UTIs over a 6-month period or three or more episodes over a 12-month period should begin prophylaxis, after any existing infection has been eradicated.

In patients with chronic or recurrent infections, continuous long-term therapy is useful. Continuous prophylaxis with daily or thrice-weekly doses of TMP-SMX, nitrofurantoin, or trimethoprim have been effective in controlling more than 90% of recurrences. Most authorities recommend a 6-month trial, after which the patient is recultured. Some patients require 2 or more years of antibiotic therapy. Postcoital prophylaxis with TMP-SMX (40 mg/200 mg), nitrofurantoin, or cephalexin should be used in women whose infections are temporally related to sexual intercourse. Reliable women who are uncomfortable taking antimicrobials over an extended period may self-treat with single-dose or 3-day antimicrobial therapy when they experience symptoms.

Adverse effects of the antimicrobial agents used to treat recurrent UTI include gastrointestinal, hepatic, renal, neurologic, hematologic, and dermatologic symptoms and complications. The quinolones are generally safe and tolerated well. Temafloxacin was recently removed from the market because of reports that it caused fetal allergic reactions, hemolytic anemia, and renal failure.

BIBLIOGRAPHY

Andriole VT. Urinary tract infections in the 90s: pathogenesis and management. Infection 1992;20(suppl 4):S251.

Bailey RR. Management of lower urinary tract infections. Drugs 1993;(suppl 3):139.

Bergman A. Urinary tract infections in women. Curr Opin Obstet Gynecol 1991;3:541.

Bump RC. Urinary tract infection in women: current role of single-dose therapy. J Reprod Med 1990;35:785.

Cunningham FG, Lucas MJ. Urinary tract infections complicating pregnancy. Bailliere's Clin Obstet Gynecol 1994;8:353.

Elder NC. Acute urinary tract infection in women. What kind of antibiotic therapy is optimal? Postgrad Med 1992;92:159.

Faro S. New considerations in treatment of urinary tract infections in adults. Urology 1992;39:1.

Fihn SD. Lower urinary tract infections in women. Curr Opin Obstet Gynecol 1992;4:571.

Gleckman RA. Urinary tract infection. Clin Geriatr Med 1992;8:793.

Hatton J, Hughes M, Raymond CH. Management of bacterial urinary tract infection in adults. Ann Pharmacother 1994;28:1274.

Kiningham RB. Asymptomatic bacteriuria in pregnancy. Am Family Phys 1993;47:1232.

Neu HC. Urinary tract infections. Am J Med 1992;92:63S.

Nicolle LE. Prophylaxis: recurrent urinary tract infection in women. Infection 1992;20(suppl 3):S203.

Norrby SR. Evaluation of antibiotics for treatment of urinary tract infections. J Antimicrob Chemother 1994;33(suppl A):43.

Sable CA, Scheld WM. Fluoroquinolones: how to use (but not overuse) these antibiotics. Geriatrics 1993;48:41.

Sobel JD, Kaye D. Urinary tract infections. In: Mandell GL, Douglass RG, Bennett JE, eds. Principles and practice of infectious diseases, 2d ed. New York: John Wiley & Sons, 1990:582.

Sravani A. Advances in the understanding and treatment of urinary tract infections in young women. Urology 1991;36:503.

Sravani A. Treatment of urinary tract infections in young women. American Urology Association Update Series 1993;12:42.

Sravani A, Bischoff W. Antibiotic therapy for urinary tract infections. Am J Med 1992;92:95S.

Stamm WE. Criteria for the diagnosis of urinary tract infection and for the assessment of therapeutic effectiveness. Infection 1992;20(suppl 3):S151; discussion S160.

Vercaigne LM, Zhanel GG. Recommended treatment for urinary tract infection in pregnancy. Ann Pharmacother 1994;28:248.

Weissenbacher ER, Reisenberger K. Uncomplicated urinary tract infections in pregnant and non-pregnant women. Curr Opin Obstet Gynecol 1993;5:513.

Primary Care for Women, edited by Phyllis C. Leppert and Fred M. Howard. Lippincott-Raven Publishers, Philadelphia © 1997.

75
Urethral Syndrome

FRED M. HOWARD

Acute urethral syndrome (AUS) is defined as less than 3 weeks of painful and frequent urination, with a voided urine that is sterile or has fewer than 100,000 microorganisms/mL. Chronic urethral syndrome (CUS) is similarly defined by dysuria and frequency but has associated pelvic pain, suprapubic pain, dyspareunia, or urinary urgency. Symptoms of CUS are persistent or recurrent rather than acute. AUS and CUS appear to be quite different diseases, with no specific relation to one another: AUS does not precede, precipitate, or predispose to CUS. A specific infectious etiology for AUS can generally be determined and cure effected with antibiotic therapy. Urine cultures are sterile with CUS, and usually no specific etiology is found. Despite many recommended therapies, cure is often difficult to obtain.

Dysuria and frequency account for more than 5 million office visits per year in the United States. About 40% of women with acute dysuria and frequency have AUS, whereas 60% have cystitis (defined as bacteriuria of 100,000 or more bacteria/mL of urine). The prevalence of CUS is unknown.

ETIOLOGY

The urethra plays an important role in the prevention of ascending bacterial infection. Normally in the distal urethra there are an average of six to eight species of bacteria, but in the proximal urethra there are none. The midurethra has a high-pressure zone that functions as a mechanical barrier to bacterial ascent. Additionally, the posterior urethral glands produce mucus that serves as a barrier by trapping bacteria and by activity of immunoglobulin A.

Many cases of AUS represent an early stage of ascending urinary tract infection. At least 30% to 50% of women with untreated AUS subsequently develop cystitis. Also, at the time of diagnosis of AUS about 50% of women have bacteria in the bladder, but at concentrations of 10,000/mL or less.

Usually the cause of AUS is infectious. In one third to one half of cases, a uropathogen is isolated from the urine, most often *Escherichia coli*, but occasionally other uropathogens such as *Staphylococcus saprophyticus*. In contrast to cystitis, bacterial growth is fewer than 100,000 colonies/mL (usually 10,000/mL or less) and is often of mixed bacterial species. Organisms other than common uropathogens also cause AUS: in particular, *Neisseria gonorrhoeae* and *Chlamydia trachomatis* account for 25% or more of cases. Chlamydia seems to cause AUS more commonly than does gonorrhea. Whether genital *Mycoplasma* have a role in the etiology of AUS is controversial. Current evidence suggests that *Ureaplasma urealyticum* may have a role, but there is no evidence that *Mycoplasma hominis* is associated with AUS. In most series, *E coli* and *C trachomatis* are the most common infectious agents found with AUS.

The etiology of CUS is unknown. Cultures are uniformly negative, but there is evidence that at least in some cases infection may have an underlying role. Evidence of chronic inflammation or infection is suggested by the progressive structural and inflammatory changes that are sometimes found histologically in the periurethral glands. However, these structural and inflammatory changes are not always present, suggesting that even if chronic infection has a role, it is not the only etiology.

In many cases of CUS, urethral spasm and irritability of the external urethral sphincter can be urodynamically demonstrated. Both the smooth and skeletal muscles of the urethra are involved in this spasticity. Concomitant pelvic floor spasm or tension may also occur. Several voiding abnormalities may result: high resting urethral tone, increased mean and maximal urethral closure pressures, inability to relax the urethra voluntarily, incomplete funneling of the bladder neck, distal urethral narrowing, and intermittent urinary flow patterns. These changes account for many of the symptoms of CUS, particularly dysuria, frequency, and postcoital voiding dysfunction. Pain may occur due to urethral spasticity and coincident stimulation of the pelvic muscle spindles with increased pelvic floor tension. Increased pelvic floor tension may result in pelvic muscular dysfunction and dyspareunia. Prolonged spasticity and increased tone may produce periurethral, urethral, or levator ani muscle fatigue, with resultant chronic pelvic pain. However, none of this addresses the underlying cause of the urethral spasticity and irritability. As suggested above, it may be due to inflammation or chronic infection in some cases. Biopsychosocial factors influence the course of the disease and could have an etiologic role. Another hypothesis is that due to anatomic, physiologic, or psychological factors, some women are susceptible to repetitive urethral trauma with intercourse, and this plays the causative role in establishing urethral syndrome and producing its symptoms. In clinical practice, usually no etiology can be determined.

DIFFERENTIAL DIAGNOSIS

Acute Urethral Syndrome

The most common causes of acute dysuria or frequency are AUS, cystitis, pyelonephritis, vaginitis, and herpetic infection (Table 75-1). Cystitis or pyelonephritis accounts for 50% of cases, AUS for 40%, and vaginitis or herpes for 10%.

Conventionally, a urine culture that grows one organism at a concentration of 100,000 bacterial colonies/mL confirms the diagnosis of cystitis in patients with dysuria or frequency. Patients with similar symptoms but cultures showing fewer uropathogens are not diagnosed with cystitis, but may be diagnosed with AUS or assumed not to have an infectious cause of their symptoms. How-

Table 75-1. Differential Diagnoses of Acute and Chronic Urethral Syndromes

Acute Urethral Syndrome
Cystitis
Vaginitis
Herpes genitalis
Pyelonephritis
Chronic Urethral Syndrome
Chronic or recurrent cystitis
Interstitial cystitis
Irritable bladder syndrome
Urethral diverticulum

ever, this distinction may be more arbitrary than substantial. This definition of cystitis is based on the work of Kass; however, that work used the criteria of 100,000 bacteria/mL to distinguish women with pyelonephritis from women who were asymptomatic or had contaminated urine cultures, and did not study women with only lower tract symptoms. There is evidence that the presence of 100 or more bacteria/mL of midstream urine is the most sensitive and specific diagnostic criterion of cystitis. Thus, many women diagnosed with AUS due to low bacterial counts have cystitis. Cystourethritis or urethrocystitis may be more appropriate diagnostic labels in these cases.

Vaginitis may also cause dysuria and dyspareunia, but a careful history usually identifies some differences. Dysuria associated with vaginitis is external, with burning as the urine contacts the external genitalia. Dyspareunia due to vaginitis is generalized in vulvovaginal location rather than localized anteriorly at the vagina underlying the urethra and bladder base, as it is with urethral syndrome. Finally, with vaginitis there is almost always vulvovaginal pruritus, a symptom not present with urethral syndrome.

Chronic Urethral Syndrome

CUS is generally a diagnosis of exclusion, requiring a high index of suspicion in women with suggestive symptoms (Table 75-2). Because it is often misdiagnosed as chronic or recurrent urinary tract infection, it is important that urine cultures be obtained before repeated antibiotic therapy. Such cultures show at least 100 colonies/mL of a uropathogen in cystitis or AUS but are negative in CUS. Repeated empiric antibiotic treatment of women with CUS may delay accurate diagnosis and make subsequent therapy difficult.

Irritable bladder syndrome and interstitial cystitis present with chronic irritative urinary tract symptoms similar to those of CUS. Dysuria is rarely present with either of the former syndromes but is common with CUS. Irritable bladder syndrome and interstitial cystitis usually present with nocturia and pain on bladder filling, symptoms not common with urethral syndrome. Nocturia, when present with urethral syndrome (or cystitis), is usually early nighttime frequency related to sensory dysfunction of the urethra or bladder. In contrast, the nocturia of interstitial cystitis is due to a limited bladder capacity that causes consistent voiding throughout the night. Pain with interstitial cystitis is usually suprapubic, may radiate to the low back or groin, and is often relieved by voiding. Dyspareunia is common with interstitial cystitis, irritable bladder syndrome, and CUS. Tenderness of the urethra and bladder base is usually found with urethral syndrome but is infrequent with irritable bladder or interstitial cystitis. Cystoscopic findings are normal with irritable bladder syndrome and urethral syndrome; glomerulations or Hunner's ulcer is found with interstitial cystitis.

Urethral diverticula sometimes present with similar symptoms to urethral syndrome, including dyspareunia, pelvic pain, urgency, and frequency. Usually urethral diverticula can be diagnosed by the presence of a suburethral tender mass or by visualization with urethroscopy or cystourethrography.

CLINICAL PRESENTATION

The classic symptoms of AUS and CUS are urinary urgency, frequency, and dysuria. Patients with AUS may also complain of low back pain, suprapubic pain, dyspareunia, or gross hematuria. Symptoms are usually of sudden onset when the syndrome is due to uropathogens, but less so when due to chlamydia or gonorrhea.

Other symptoms of CUS include postvoiding fullness and incomplete voiding, urge or stress incontinence, voiding difficulties (especially postcoitally), suprapubic pain, low back pain, pelvic pain, or vaginal pain (see Table 75-2). Dyspareunia is common with CUS and generally localizes to the anterior vagina. Coitus also often causes voiding dysfunction, burning dysuria, or urgency. A history of treatment of recurrent urinary tract infections without documentation of positive cultures is typical with CUS. Nocturia may be present with either AUS or CUS but is usually limited to the early nighttime.

PHYSICAL EXAMINATION

A pelvic examination is essential in the evaluation of both acute and chronic urethritis. In distinction to findings in males, women with AUS due to *N gonorrhoeae* or *C trachomatis* rarely have a frank urethral discharge. However, gentle massage of the urethra may yield a discharge, suggesting gonococcal or chlamydial infection. Inspection of the cervix for mucopurulent cervicitis may also suggest a chlamydial infection.

Palpation should start with a gentle, single-finger evaluation of the vulva and vagina, including palpation of the urethra, trigone, and bladder base. Tenderness of the anterior vagina at the urethra

Table 75-2. Symptoms of Patients With Chronic Urethral Syndrome

DOMINANT SYMPTOMS	PERCENT
Frequency	65
Dysuria	60
Urgency	60
Dyspareunia	45
Postcoital voiding dysfunction	45
Postvoiding fullness	40
Nocturia	40
Abdominal pain	35
Suprapubic pain	25
Incontinence	25
Vulvodynia	25

and bladder base is almost always present with CUS. The tenderness elicited classically mimics the patient's pain with coitus. Pubococcygeal muscle tenderness is often present. Suprapubic tenderness is occasionally found with AUS but is not a consistent finding. The rest of the pelvic examination is usually normal, with absence of uterine or adnexal tenderness.

Endoscopic and urodynamic evaluations are useful in women with suspected CUS. In many of these patients, urethroscopy shows erythema, exudate, cystic dilation of the periurethral glands, and inflammatory fronds throughout the urethra. It may also demonstrate incomplete funneling of the bladder neck and distal urethral narrowing. In women with pelvic pain as part of their symptom complex, urethroscopy invariably reproduces the pain symptoms. Passing a urethral catheter may often produce similar excessive pain. Cystoscopy is normal. As previously noted, urodynamic evaluations may show voiding abnormalities, including a high resting urethral tone, increased mean and maximal urethral closure pressures, inability to relax the urethra voluntarily, and intermittent urinary flow patterns.

LABORATORY STUDIES

A microscopic examination of a midstream urine sample for leukocytes and bacteria is basic. In uncentrifuged urine, a finding of one or more bacteria per oil immersion field correlates with 100,000 or more bacteria/mL, whereas the absence of bacteria in several oil immersion fields suggests a bacterial count of 10,000 or less/mL. Pyuria may be evaluated by direct hemocytometer counts of leukocytes in uncentrifuged urine. If centrifuged urine is to be examined, it is prepared by centrifuging 10 mL of urine, with resuspension of the resultant sediment in 1 mL of urine. In centrifuged urine, a finding of five to 10 leukocytes per high-power field (×400) suggests pyuria; a finding of 100 or more bacteria per high-power field is consistent with 100,000 or more bacteria/mL.

Urine cultures are indicated, as well as cultures or antigen tests of the urethra and cervix for gonorrhea and chlamydia. Traditional midstream urine specimen cultures, however, may have limited usefulness in diagnosing AUS. For example, in patients with AUS, when cultures are directly taken of bladder urine via transurethral catheterization or suprapubic aspiration, more than 50% are positive for uropathogens, but at concentrations of less than 100,000 bacteria/mL. In such cases, when a single bacterial species is isolated from the bladder urine at less than 1000 organisms/mL, midstream specimens are positive for the organism isolated from the bladder in less than half of cases. Furthermore, even when the organism is present in the midstream urine culture, it is mixed with one to four other bacterial species. Thus, in cases of AUS due to common uropathogens, midstream urine cultures are often nondiagnostic.

Biochemical urine tests are useful for diagnosing cystitis but are not well studied for usefulness in diagnosing AUS. A positive nitrite test correlates with bacteriuria of 100,000 or more/mL. A positive leukocyte esterase test implies pyuria of eight or more leukocytes/mm^3. Pyuria strongly correlates with recovery of uropathogens from the bladder (but, as discussed above, not necessarily from a midstream specimen). Women with bacteria cultured from the bladder, even at low concentrations, usually have pyuria. Seventy percent of women with AUS show pyuria, and 90% of those with pyuria have cultures positive for uropathogens in the bladder (< 100,000 organisms/mL) or for chlamydia or gonorrhea from the urethra or cervix.

As women with chlamydial or gonococcal urethral infections tend to have pyuria, evaluations for chlamydia and gonorrhea should be done in patients with sterile pyuria. Chlamydia appears to cause AUS more often than does gonorrhea. More than two thirds of women with pyuria and sterile urine have chlamydia. Conversely, it is uncommon for women with chlamydial urethritis not to have pyuria and a negative urine culture. Only 5% of women with symptoms of AUS without pyuria have chlamydia. Thus, the practitioner must take cultures for gonorrhea and cultures, direct immunofluorescence, or enzyme-linked immunoassays for chlamydia from the cervix and urethra of women with pyuria without bacteriuria who are considered at risk for sexually transmitted disease or who have mucopurulent cervicitis. Gram stain of any cervical discharge may be useful, particularly if gram-negative intracellular diplococci suggestive of gonorrhea are seen.

Urodynamic studies may be useful in patients with CUS (Table 75-3). These studies can identify patients with abnormal voiding patterns due to dyssynergic voiding. Voiding and electromyographic studies reveal prolonged or intermittent voiding patterns and hyperactivity of the pelvic floor or external urethral sphincter. Mean urinary flow rates are notably decreased (< 15 mL/sec; normal is > 15 mL/sec) and mean flow times are increased (35 to 80 sec; normal is < 30 sec). Maximal urethral closure pressure is twice normal in women with CUS (105 cm H_2O, compared to controls of 50 cm H_2O). Despite the common symptom of incomplete emptying, women with CUS do not have increased residual volume. Detrusor instability is usually not found by regular or provocative cystometry. Not all patients with clinical evidence of CUS have urodynamic abnormalities.

Radiographic studies are not generally indicated in the evaluation of AUS or CUS. However, to rule out urethral diverticula in the differential diagnosis of CUS, radiographic urethrography is sometimes useful.

TREATMENT

Acute Urethral Syndrome

For cystitis, single-dose and three-day antibiotic regimens are effective (Table 75-4). These regimens are probably also effective

Table 75-3. Urodynamic Findings With Chronic Urethral Syndrome

TEST	CHRONIC URETHRAL SYNDROME	NORMAL
Mean urinary flow rate	< 15 mL/sec	> 15 mL/sec
Mean flow time	35–80 sec	< 30 sec
Maximum urethral closure pressure	105 cm H_2O	50 cm H_2O
Residual volume	< 50 mL	< 50 mL

Table 75-4. Treatment Regimens for Acute Urethral Syndrome

Uropathogens
Trimethoprim–sulfamethoxazole double strength, two tablets
Trimethoprim–sulfamethoxazole double strength, one twice a day for 3 days
Amoxicillin–clavulanic acid, 250 mg three times a day for 3 days
Norfloxacin, 400 mg twice a day for 3 days
Ciprofloxacin, 500 mg twice a day for 3 days
Chlamydia
Doxycycline, 100 mg twice a day for 7 days
Azithromycin, 1 g orally in a single dose
Ofloxacin, 300 mg orally twice a day for 7 days
Erythromycin, 500 mg four times a day for 7 days
Tetracycline, 500 mg four times a day for 7 days
Gonorrhea
Ceftriaxone 250 mg intramuscularly
Cefixime 400 mg orally
Ciprofloxacin 500 mg orally
Ofloxacin 400 mg orally
Plus one of the above regimens for chlamydia.

when AUS is due to common uropathogens such as *E coli*. However, they have not been well studied for AUS. Common short-therapy regimens for cystitis are listed in Table 75-4. Primary treatment with sulfonamides, ampicillin, or amoxicillin is not usually recommended due to *E coli* resistance.

These regimens are not effective when AUS is due to gonorrhea or chlamydia (see Table 75-4). Chlamydia may be treated with the regimens shown in Table 75-4.

Gonorrhea is treated with ceftriaxone 250 mg intramuscularly plus one of the above regimens for chlamydia. Recently, the Centers for Disease Control and Prevention have also included cefixime, ciprofloxacin, or ofloxacin as possible single-dose treatments for uncomplicated gonorrheal infections (see Table 75-4). They have also suggested that all patients with gonorrhea be given follow-up treatment with a regimen effective against chlamydia, as up to 40% of patients with gonorrhea also have chlamydia.

Doxycycline is a good choice for empiric treatment pending cultures, as it has been well studied in a randomized, placebo-controlled, blinded study and showed efficacy for AUS due to either uropathogens or chlamydia (Table 75-5).

Women with acute dysuria and frequency but without bacteriuria, positive cultures, or pyuria do not benefit from antibiotic therapy. Resolution of symptoms occurs in more than 70% of such women and is not hastened by antibiotic therapy. Half of the women with AUS treated with placebo show a clinical response, with resolution of symptoms (see Table 75-5).

Chronic Urethral Syndrome

Numerous treatments are used for CUS, including antibiotics, bladder neck opening, internal urethrotomy, urethral dilation, local steroid injections, estrogens, tranquilizers, and psychiatric therapy. Often the choice of treatment is based on tradition or empiric trial and error. Specific treatment based on a defined potential etiology seems most appropriate, but often no such etiology can be found.

A common and reasonable initial treatment for women with CUS is suppression with antibiotics (eg, nitrofurantoin or tetracycline), urethral dilation, or both. Dilations usually are to 36 to 38 French, done three times at biweekly intervals. There is some evidence that these treatments are effective, both individually and combined. However, they probably work best in cases that show urethroscopic evidence of urethral inflammation. Antibiotics probably work via eradication of chronic, occult bacterial infection. Urethral dilations open obstructed and inflamed periurethral glands, allowing drainage of inflammatory exudate and bacteria. Urethral dilation also increases peak and mean urine flow rates, but these changes are not seen with antibiotic treatment alone.

In cases of CUS with urodynamic studies showing evidence of external urethral sphincter spasm, diazepam at 2 to 6 mg/day for 2 to 5 months has been effective. Phenoxybenzamine hydrochloride, 10 to 40 mg/day, is an effective alternative. Smooth muscle relaxants such as prazosin or dibenzyline, used alone or combined with a skeletal muscle relaxant such as diazepam, can also be used in patients with urethral muscle spasm. As the external urethral

Table 75-5. Results of a Randomized, Placebo-controlled Trial of Treatment of Acute Urethral Syndrome With Doxycycline

	DOXYCYCLINE (N = 32)	PLACEBO (N = 30)	P VALUE
Clinical Cure			
Bladder bacteria	11/12	4/10	.016
Sterile pyuria	10/10	3/9	.003
No pyuria	7/10	8/11	.63
All cases	28/32	15/30	.002
Microbiologic Cure			
E coli/S saprophyticus	11/12	3/10	.005
C trachomatis	4/4	0/3	.03
Resolution of Pyuria			
Bacteria in urine	8/12	3/10	.09
Sterile urine	9/10	2/9	.005

sphincter is innervated by the pudendal nerve, pudendal nerve block has also been used with some success.

Behavioral modification may also be helpful in patients with urethral sphincter spasm. Monitored relaxation and contraction of the pelvic floor (levator muscles) may lead to reestablishment of voluntary control of the urethral sphincter and cessation of involuntary spasm. Establishing a regular voiding schedule is also helpful in this approach.

Surgical treatments for CUS have not been adequately evaluated. Surgical therapies are best done in research protocols and are not advised for widespread use. Many women with CUS are misdiagnosed and undergo unneeded surgical evaluation or treatment. For example, in one case series, 25% of patients had undergone total abdominal hysterectomy and bilateral salpingo-oophorectomy, 25% diagnostic laparoscopy, and about 12% ovarian cystectomy before the diagnosis of CUS was established.

CONSIDERATIONS IN PREGNANCY

Pregnancy symptoms themselves are unlikely to lead to a misdiagnosis of AUS or CUS. Pregnancy causes frequency of urination, but not the other symptoms of either syndrome. Conversely, pregnancy has little effect on the symptoms of AUS or CUS. Pregnant women with symptoms suggestive of either should be evaluated as previously described.

Treatment options are affected by pregnancy—in particular, doxycycline and tetracycline are contraindicated. Erythromycin is substituted for these antibiotics in the treatment regimens for chlamydial or gonococcal infection. The use of trimethoprim–sulfamethoxazole is debatable during pregnancy, so alternatives are preferable when available. Nitrofurantoin appears safe except for concerns about fetal hemolytic anemia if used near delivery. Endoscopic and radiologic evaluations should be avoided during pregnancy, especially if other than local anesthesia is required. Delay of such testing until after delivery is unlikely to worsen the prognosis.

BIBLIOGRAPHY

Barbalias GA, Meares EM. Female urethral syndrome: clinical and urodynamic perspectives. Urology 1984;23:208.

Bergman A, Karram M, Bhatia NN. Urethral syndrome: a comparison of different treatment modalities. J Reprod Med 1989;34:157.

Stamm WE, Running K, McKevitt M, Counts GW, Turck M, Holmes KK. Treatment of the AUS. N Engl J Med 1981;304:956.

Stamm WE, Wagner KF, Amsel R, et al. Causes of the AUS in women. N Engl J Med 1980;303:409.

Summit RL. Urogynecologic causes of chronic pelvic pain. Obstet Gynecol Clin North Am 1993;20:685.

Summit RL, Ling FW. Urethral syndrome presenting as chronic pelvic pain. J Psychom Obstet Gynaecol 1991;12(suppl):77.

Primary Care for Women, edited by Phyllis C. Leppert and Fred M. Howard. Lippincott-Raven Publishers, Philadelphia © 1997.

76

Nephrolithiasis

STEPHEN M. SILVER
RICHARD H. STERNS

Each year, half a million Americans suffer from symptoms related to kidney stones. About 5% of women and 10% of men are affected during their lifetime. In the last 10 years, significant advances have been made in the surgical treatment of nephrolithiasis. However, even in this "age of lithotripsy," a preventive program remains the mainstay of therapy. Such a program requires a dedicated effort from both the primary physician and the patient. This chapter reviews the etiology and treatment of renal stone disease, emphasizing issues of special relevance to women.

ETIOLOGIES OF KIDNEY STONES

Kidney stones are considerably less common in women than in men. Stone disease in women is more likely to be associated with specific conditions such as hyperparathyroidism, medullary sponge kidney, and urinary tract infection. Table 76-1summarizes the incidence of the most common causes of nephrolithiasis.

Calcium Stones

Calcium stones represent about 75% to 85% of renal stones in North Americans. Most are composed of calcium oxalate, or a mixture of calcium oxalate and calcium phosphate. Calcium phosphate stones (composed of apatite, or less commonly, brushite) are less common, and their presence suggests an unusual cause (eg, renal tubular acidosis [RTA], primary hyperparathyroidism, or milk-alkali syndrome). Calcium stones form when the urinary concentration of calcium salts is too high (because of increased rates of excretion or decreased urine volume), when inhibitors of calcium precipitation like citrate or magnesium are deficient, or when anatomic abnormalities are present.

Metabolic Abnormalities in Patients With Calcium Stones

Hypercalciuria. Daily excretion of more than 4 mg of calcium per kg body weight (250 mg in the average woman) is defined as hypercalciuria. About 60% of patients who form calcium stones are hypercalciuric. Hypercalciuria usually is idiopathic, but primary hyperparathyroidism is an important cause of calcium stones, particularly in middle-aged and older women. RTA and sarcoidosis are much rarer causes. Idiopathic hypercalciuria is incompletely understood. Increased intestinal calcium absorption and increased bone resorption are responsible to varying degrees in patients with the disorder. In clinical practice, usually it is not necessary to distinguish the responsible pathogenic mechanism. Diets high in sodium, protein, or both exacerbate idiopathic hypercalciuria. However, calcium supplements given to prevent

Table 76-1. Major Causes of Nephrolithiasis

STONE TYPE AND ETIOLOGY (% OF ALL STONES)	OCCURRENCE OF SPECIFIC ETIOLOGY (ALONE OR WITH OTHER CAUSES) (%)	F:M RATIO
Calcium Stones (80%)		1:2
Primary		
Hypercalciuria	60	1:2
Hyperuricemia	20	1:4
Hyperoxaluria	20	1:1
Hypocitraturia	20	1:1
Idiopathic	10	1:2
Secondary		
Medullary sponge kidney	20	1:2
Hyperparathyroidism	5	10:3
Distal renal tubular acidosis	1	1:1
Enteric hyperoxaluria	1	1:1
Primary hyperoxaluria	< 1	
Other hypercalciuric states	< 1	
Milk alkali syndrome		
Immobilization		
Sarcoid		
Vitamin D intoxication		
Malignancy		
Hyperthyroidism		
Uric Acid Stones (5–10%)		
Gout	50	1:3
Idiopathic	50	1:1
Other	< 1	
Myeloproliferative disorders		
Enzyme defect		
Enteric		
Cystine (1%)		1:1
Struvite (10–15%)		5:1

osteoporosis do not seem to increase the risk of renal stones. In healthy premenopausal women, calcium supplementation increases urinary calcium excretion only during the first 2 to 3 weeks of treatment. In postmenopausal women without a previous history of stone disease, calcium supplementation increases urine calcium even less. In patients with a strong family history of active stone disease (who may hyperabsorb dietary calcium), measurement of urinary calcium excretion may be indicated before and after calcium supplementation.

Hyperoxaluria. Mild hyperoxaluria (45 to 90 mg/24 hours), alone or in combination with other abnormalities, is found in up to 20% of calcium stone formers. Oxalic acid is an end product of protein metabolism. Daily intake varies widely, from 100 to 1000 mg, of which less than 10% is absorbed from the intestine. Thus, normal urine oxalate excretion is 10 to 40 mg/day. Urine calcium is five times as high as urine oxalate; thus, milligram for milligram, an increase in oxalate excretion has a much greater impact on the solubility product of calcium oxalate than does an increase in calcium excretion. Oxalate binds with calcium in the intestinal lumen to form an insoluble and nonabsorbable salt. Thus, low calcium intake may paradoxically predispose to calcium oxalate stones by making oxalate more available for absorption. As is discussed later in the chapter, intestinal fat malabsorption (eg, in Crohn disease or after ileal surgery) causes hyperoxaluria by a similar mechanism. High vitamin C intake in susceptible individuals also can increase oxalate absorption.

Hypocitraturia. Citrate is a product of the Krebs cycle. In the urine, it combines with calcium to form a soluble complex, making calcium less available to combine with oxalate. Urinary citrate excretion is decreased in up to 20% of patients with idiopathic calcium nephrolithiasis. A high ratio of the concentrations of calcium to citrate in the urine is one of the strongest predictors of calcium stone disease. Acidosis (eg, via diarrhea or RTA) and hypokalemia decrease citrate excretion. Thus, hypokalemia caused by thiazides may neutralize their effectiveness in preventing stone formation. Urinary citrate is higher in premenopausal women than in men. During pregnancy, urine citrate excretion increases, offsetting the increase in urinary calcium excretion.

Hyperuricosuria. Increased uric acid excretion is found in about 20% of patients with calcium stones, predominantly men, and generally has been attributed to increased dietary intake of purines. Uric acid crystals may act as a nucleus for calcium oxalate precipitation or may bind natural inhibitors of stone formation. The best evidence linking hyperuricosuria to calcium stone formation was provided by one controlled study showing that treatment of hyperuricosuric patients with allopurinol decreased the recurrence rate of calcium stones. Uncontrolled studies indicate that treatment of patients with hyperuricemia and calcium stone disease with potassium citrate also may prevent stone recurrence.

Specific Disease States in Patients With Calcium Stones

Primary Hyperparathyroidism. Hyperparathyroidism should be strongly considered in women with renal stones. Calcium phosphate stones and aggressive recurrent nephrolithiasis with bilateral renal involvement should increase suspicion of the disease. High or high-normal serum calcium is usually present in hyperparathyroidism but the elevation may be subtle: the true upper limit of normal serum calcium in women (10.1 mg/dL) is slightly lower than in men. The differential diagnosis of hypercalcemia with calcium nephrolithiasis includes sarcoidosis, vitamin D intoxication, use of lithium or thiazides, and malignancy.

Renal Tubular Acidosis. Calcium nephrolithiasis often complicates distal (type I) RTA, which is characterized by a nonanion gap acidosis and a persistently elevated urine pH (> 5.3 in a morning urine). Causes of RTA in adults include autoimmune disorders (particularly Sjögren syndrome), myeloma, or drugs such as lithium. A high urine pH in the presence of hypercalciuria promotes calcium phosphate precipitation. The excretion of citrate, which inhibits crystallization, is characteristically low (< 150 mg/day) in distal RTA, contributing to nephrolithiasis. Patients with an "incomplete" form of distal RTA are not systemically acidotic, but have defective urinary acidification and low urinary citrate excretion; like patients with "complete" RTA, they commonly present with calcium phosphate stones or nephrocalcinosis. Urinary citrate excretion should be measured if RTA is suspected.

Medullary Sponge Kidney. Medullary sponge kidney is a common condition that is present in up to 30% of women with calcium stones. It is characterized by obstruction and small cystic dilation of the collecting ducts at the papillary tips. The diagnosis is made by intravenous pyelogram, which demonstrates characteristic linear densities extending from the papillary tips. Medullary sponge kidney, in contrast to polycystic kidney disease and medullary cystic disease, is benign and does not result in proteinuria or renal insufficiency. The clinical manifestations include calcium stones, hematuria, and urinary tract infection. The stones (usually calcium oxalate or calcium phosphate) form within the cysts and commonly appear radiographically as nephrocalcinosis. It should not be assumed that the anatomic abnormalities are the sole cause of the stones. Hypercalciuria, for unknown reasons, is frequently present and should be treated.

Enteric Hyperoxaluria. Small bowel malabsorption, due to resection or disease, leads to a number of metabolic abnormalities that predispose to nephrolithiasis. Malabsorption leads to increased levels of fatty acids and bile salts in the gut lumen. Intestinal calcium is bound in soaps and unavailable for insoluble calcium oxalate complex formation. As a result, free oxalate is hyperabsorbed in the colon, predisposing to hyperoxaluria and calcium oxalate stones. Poorly absorbed bile salts also stimulate increased colonic absorption of oxalate. The metabolic acidosis associated with diarrhea decreases urinary citrate excretion, another factor predisposing to calcium stones. Decreased levels of urinary magnesium, caused by magnesium malabsorption from the gut, also may promote calcium oxalate precipitation because magnesium chelates oxalate. Finally, decreased urine volume, caused by dehydration, promotes all forms of stone formation.

Infection Stones

Urinary tract infection may result in formation of struvite stones, which account for up to 15% of urinary calculi. They are much more common in women than in men. Struvite stones, which consist of magnesium, and ammonium phosphate, are associated with urease-producing bacteria. Urease breaks down urinary urea to ammonia, which alkalinizes the urine (decreasing the solubility of phosphate) and combines with water to form ammonium. Bacteria that produce urease include Proteus (most common), Serratia, Klebsiella, Staphylococcus, Ureaplasma urealyticum (an anaerobic mycoplasma), and Pseudomonas.

Struvite stones consist of either pure struvite or struvite in combination with calcium. Women (who typically have lower rates of calcium excretion and a lower incidence of calcium stones than men) usually form pure struvite stones. Predisposing conditions to recurrent urinary tract infection and struvite stones include urinary tract instrumentation, neurogenic bladder, or a structural abnormality of the urinary tract, for example, ureteral stricture, urinary diversion, or congenital conditions such as horseshoe kidneys. Patients with pure struvite stones commonly present with staghorn calculi that extend to the renal pelvis and to the calices and are too large to pass spontaneously. They result in bleeding, obstruction, or further infection and require urologic intervention.

Uric Acid Stones

Uric acid stones, which are less common in women than in men, account for about 10% of the urinary calculi diagnosed in the United States. Risk factors for uric acid stones include increased uric acid excretion, low urine volume, and, most importantly, low urine pH. The urine pH of patients with uric acid stones is lower than that of calcium stone formers, and an increase of the urine pH from 6 to 7 increases the solubility of uric acid tenfold. About half of patients with uric acid stones have a history of gouty arthropathy. Other risk factors include increased intake of protein (which contains purines and amino acids that result in an acid urine) and acidotic states such as chronic diarrhea. Young adults with high uric acid excretion and urolithiasis may have a partial enzyme defect of purine metabolism, and a detailed family history and screening is indicated. Initial treatment is directed at increasing urinary volume and pH and decreasing dietary intake of purines.

Cystine Stones

Cystine, a disulfide of cysteine, is excreted in the urine in large amounts in patients with cystinuria—an autosomal recessive defect in the ability to reabsorb cystine and three other amino acids in the proximal tubule of the kidney and in the jejunum. The poor urinary solubility of cystine leads to nephrolithiasis, the only clinical manifestation of cystinuria. The stones are radiopaque, although less so than calcium stones, and must be at least 4 mm before being visualized on a plain x-ray of the abdomen. Stones commonly form in a bilateral obstructive staghorn configuration, and end-stage renal disease may result.

Medications and Vitamins

Medications may cause renal stones, but they do so rarely. Acyclovir, sulfa drugs, and triamterene have limited solubility in urine and may precipitate. Acetazolamide alkalinizes the urine and promotes calcium phosphate precipitation. Vitamin C promotes hyperoxaluria, and vitamins A and D increase calcium excretion. As discussed earlier, calcium supplements are not an important cause of kidney stones.

CLINICAL MANIFESTATIONS

Asymptomatic

Nephrocalcinosis typically occurs when calcium stones, which form in the renal papillae, remain in the renal medulla and are demonstrated by multiple papillary calcifications on radiographic studies. The presence of nephrocalcinosis (which is usually asymptomatic) is common in distal RTA, hyperparathyroidism, and medullary sponge kidney. Renal stones from other causes form in the renal pelvis and may be detected in asymptomatic patients by radiographic studies done for other reasons. In one study of asymptomatic patients whose stones were discovered incidentally, about half became symptomatic within 5 years and often required a procedure such as extracorporeal lithotripsy. Most of the patients who became symptomatic had a previous history of stone disease. In those without such a history, the risk of a clinically apparent stone-related episode was low. Struvite, cystine, and uric acid stones that are discovered incidentally may become too large to enter the bladder and grow to form staghorn calculi that fill the renal pelvis and calices.

Hematuria

Renal stone disease, along with renal infection, neoplasms, and cysts, are the most common causes of isolated microscopic hematuria. The hematuria associated with nephrolithiasis is usually accompanied by pain. In addition, hematuria and loin pain have been associated with hypercalciuria and hyperuricosuria, even in the absence of renal stones. Measurement of these urinary constituents should be considered in patients with isolated hematuria of unknown cause.

Renal Colic

An obstructing or partially obstructing stone in the upper ureter or renal pelvis is typically associated with severe flank or upper abdominal pain lasting for minutes to hours, often with nausea and vomiting. In contrast to the patient with peritoneal irritation, the patient with renal colic typically is restless and writhing in pain. Obstruction in the middle or lower segment of the ureter commonly causes pain that radiates to the inguinal ligament and to the labia and urethra. A stone lodged in the lower ureter, within the bladder wall, may cause dysuria and frequency and thus be mistaken for cystitis or urethritis. Patients with kidney stones sometimes have low-grade intermittent pain, which may be mistaken for musculoskeletal discomfort, and may chronically pass "gravel."

ACUTE EVALUATION AND TREATMENT OF NEPHROLITHIASIS

For the most part, urinary calculi present with severe symptoms well known to most clinicians but do not require immediate surgical management. The history and physical examination should be directed to ruling out other causes of the presenting symptoms and assessing for evidence of infection and sepsis. Laboratory evaluation should include urinalysis, measurement of serum electrolytes, blood urea nitrogen and creatinine, and a complete blood count. Plain x-rays by themselves have a low sensitivity and specificity. An intravenous pyelogram is preferred because it defines the degree of obstruction, the size of the stone, and the presence of anatomic abnormalities such as medullary sponge kidney more effectively. Hydronephrosis is expected in symptomatic patients. Renal ultrasound can detect stones 4 mm or more in diameter and is useful when contrast media is contraindicated, for follow-up of hydronephrosis and uric acid stones (which are radiolucent), in children, and during pregnancy. Infusion of hypotonic solution (eg, one half normal saline) provides volume repletion and encourages urine flow.

Evidence of systemic infection, a stone that is completely obstructing, or intractable pain require hospital admission and urologic consultation. Hydronephrosis on initial evaluation is not necessarily an indication for intervention. However, persistent hydronephrosis on follow-up examination requires intervention, even if the patient's symptoms are improved and the size of the stone seems small enough to pass spontaneously. The same applies to patients with recurrent pain and emergency room visits, even for a small stone. Hematuria is rarely severe enough to warrant intervention in the absence of other indications. Stones smaller than 4 mm have about an 80% likelihood of passing, but few stones larger than 7 mm do so. In general, intervention is appropriate in patients with ureteral stones larger than 4 to 5 mm.

Extracorporeal Shock Wave Lithotripsy

In extracorporeal shock wave lithotripsy (ESWL), a recently developed technique, shock waves generated from a source outside of the body are directed at a curved reflector that focuses the reflected waves on the stone. The stone is localized with either ultrasound or fluoroscopy. Because the waves are of low frequency, they do not to dampen and pass through water and body tissue. Minimal sedation is required unless stents are placed. Patients usually return to normal activity in 1 to 2 days.

About 70% of stones may be treated with ESWL. It is the preferred treatment for most stones in the proximal ureter and many in the mid and distal ureter; stones can be pushed up the ureter with a stent to bring them into the field of ESWL, but this requires cystoscopy and anesthesia. Most calcium, uric acid, and struvite stones break up easily with this technique, but cystine stones fragment poorly. The most consistent success with ESWL is with stones 2.0 cm or smaller, yielding a stone-free rate of about 90%. As the size of the stone increases, multiple ESWL treatments may be necessary, and the risk of obstruction from a stone fragment increases. Stones 3.0 cm or larger generally are treated with percutaneous techniques.

Absolute contraindications to ESWL include bleeding diathesis and pregnancy. Renal artery calcifications and aortic aneurysms should be out of the path of ESWL. Severe obesity or orthopedic deformity may be limitations. Patients with dual-chamber cardiac pacemakers require reprogramming to ventricular pacing only during ESWL. Postlithotripsy fever is common, and passage of stone fragments after ESWL may be painful and may require further intervention with ureteroscopy (see later). Uncommon acute sequelae include gastrointestinal bleeding and pancreatitis.

Radiographic studies have demonstrated renal injury (hematoma, kidney swelling) in most patients after ESWL that resolves after several weeks. Nephrotic-range proteinuria has been reported. The long-term effects on renal function after ESWL, however, have not been fully assessed. Hypertension may be associated with ESWL in a small number of patients, and it may be advisable to check the blood pressure 3 to 4 months after ESWL.

An important concern is the possible mutagenic effects and decrease in fertility in women receiving fluoroscopy and ESWL to the distal ureter. Animal studies and a single limited retrospective study did not demonstrate such effects, but treatment of distal stones with ESWL remains controversial in women of childbearing age.

Percutaneous Nephrolithotomy

Stones may be removed directly from the kidney and ureter with this technique. Under fluoroscopic guidance, a guide wire is placed through the kidney and down the ureter, a nephrostomy tube is placed, and a nephroscope is inserted into the collecting system. Stones may be removed intact, but ultrasonic lithotripsy to fragment the stone is usually required. The procedure is more invasive than ESWL and requires general anesthesia and several days of hospitalization. Its major indications include proximal ureteral stones that have failed ESWL, cystine stones, stones within the kidney that are larger than 2 to 3 cm, or in dependent or dilated calices. A combination of ESWL and percutaneous techniques may be needed, especially in the setting of staghorn calculi due to struvite stones.

Ureteroscopy

Stones also can be approached from below, with a flexible or rigid ureteroscope placed through the urethra and bladder and into the ureter. Initially, only small distal stones could be removed with basket techniques, but using intraureteral lithotripsy allows large stones, located throughout the ureter or renal pelvis, to be approached with this technique. Regional or general anesthesia is required for ureteroscopy, but it can be performed on an outpatient basis or with a one-night stay in the hospital. Its major indications in stone disease include lower ureteral calculi in settings where ESWL has failed or in conjunction with ESWL to remove stone fragments.

Table 76-2. Evaluation and Prevention After the First Stone

History

Stone history
- Previous radiologic evaluation
- Calculi passed or removed
- Stone analysis
- Family history
- Symptoms: pain, dysuria, grossly bloody urine

Associated conditions
- Urinary tract infection and instrumentation
- Gout
- Inflammatory bowel disease
- Sarcoidosis
- Renal tubular acidosis
- Malignancy

Medications associated with renal stones
- Triamterene
- Acyclovir
- Acetazolamide
- Vitamins C, A, D
- Sulfonamides

Diet
- Dairy products, meat/protein, soft drinks, alcohol, calcium supplementation
- Oxalate-containing foods: spinach, nuts, chocolate, rhubarb
- Water intake: amount and pattern

Lab

Urinalysis: for pH, crystals, evidence of infection

Calcium concentration (×2), renal function, electrolytes, phosphate, uric acid

Intravenous pyelogram and flat plate of abdomen

Stone analysis

General Preventive Measures

2–2.5 L urine output/d (6–8 glasses of water/d)

0.8–1 g/kg lean body weight protein (vegetable > animal) < 3g sodium, low oxalate diet

PREVENTION OF NEPHROLITHIASIS

All patients with a history of nephrolithiasis should undergo a full history and physical examination, as well as limited laboratory and radiologic examination (Table 76-2). Initial evaluation is simplified if a stone has been retrieved: uric acid, struvite, and cystine stones suggest specific diagnoses, and stones that are primarily calcium phosphate suggest RTA, primary hyperparathyroidism, or infection. Considerable disagreement exists over whether patients that have passed a single stone require an extensive metabolic evaluation. Some advocate a full evaluation after just one episode of nephrolithiasis, reasoning that an episode of renal colic is debilitating and that lithotripsy, if required, is invasive, expensive, and has some morbidity. On the other hand, the chance of forming a second stone is relatively low: about 15% at 1 year, 40% at 5 years, and 50% at 10 years. In addition, potential side effects of thiazides and allopurinol, the major drugs used to treat the specific metabolic abnormalities that cause kidney stones, are significant. Currently, most authorities recommend that a full metabolic evaluation be deferred for first-time calcium oxalate stone formers, or for patients after one episode of renal colic without a stone for analysis. However, such patients should be treated aggressively with general dietary intervention, as described later.

Indications for full evaluation after a first stone are listed in Table 76-3. Urine collections performed on an inpatient do not reflect the patient's normal metabolic state; collections should be performed during the patient's normal activity at least 4 weeks after hospital discharge. On the basis of the collections, treatment can be directed at improving the factors that predispose the patient to nephrolithiasis. A full metabolic evaluation includes two 24-hour urine collections for calcium, uric acid, oxalate, citrate, sodium, urea, and creatinine. In one of these collections, cystine should be measured. Table 76-4 lists values for excretion of these metabolites. Many laboratories require separate collection for citrate in a preacidified container; a single collection for citrate is acceptable if this is the case. Creatinine excretion is measured to assess the accuracy of the collections. Serial follow-up collections, 6 to 8 weeks after the initial evaluation, monitor response to treatment and patient compliance with diet. If only calcium excretion is being followed, the measurement of a urinary calcium to creatinine ratio may be a reliable alternative to 24-hour urine collections: the ratio, multiplied by 1100, approximates the amount of calcium excreted per day in milligrams.

Table 76-3. Indications for Full Metabolic Evaluation of Nephrolithiasis

Recurrent stone formation
Women age less than 30
Osteoporosis, pathologic fracture
Urate stones or gout
Struvite stones
Urinary tract infection
Cystine stones
Medullary sponge kidney
Positive family history
Intestinal disease

Table 76-4. 24-Hour Urinary Excretion of Several Metabolites

SOLUTE	MEN	WOMEN
Calcium (upper limits of normal)		
mg/24 h	300	250
mg/g creatinine	140	140
mg/kg body wt	4	4
Uric acid (upper limits of normal)		
mg/24 h	800	750
Citrate (mg/24 h)		
Average excretion	600	700
Lower limits of normal	280	320
Renal tubular acidosis	< 150	< 150
Oxalate (range of normal)		
mg/24 h	20–40	20–40
Cystine (upper limits of normal)		
mg/24 h	400	400
Creatinine		
mg/kg body wt/d	20–25	15–20

As is discussed later, dietary sodium and protein intake may be important in stone formation and can be estimated from urinary excretion. Sodium in urine collections is expressed in milliequivalents; multiplying this value by 23 (the molecular weight of sodium) yields the sodium excretion in milligrams per 24 hours and closely estimates sodium intake. This measure can be used to follow compliance with a low sodium diet (2 to 4 g/day). Urea is the major by-product of protein metabolism and also may be collected to assess protein intake:

$$\text{Dietary protein intake (g/day)} = 6.25\,(\text{UUN} + [\text{body wt (kg)} \times .03])$$

where UUN is urine urea nitrogen excretion in grams per day.

The Primary Role of Diet

Dietary intervention, the primary tool for preventing kidney stones in most patients, is underused. Aggressively applied, it prevents most recurrences after the first stone episode. In fact, a good deal of the full metabolic evaluation described earlier is devoted to assessing dietary compliance. The enthusiasm of the physician, and involvement of a dietitian, are key elements in the success of dietary treatment. Dietary factors are discussed in the following paragraphs.

Fluid Intake

Increased fluid intake is possibly the most effective nonpharmacologic therapy for renal stones. Adding water to the urine decreases the concentrations of calcium, phosphate, oxalate, and uric acid, making crystal formation less likely. A reasonable goal should be a urine output of at least 2 L/day. The most important aspect of fluid therapy is to prescribe it as one would a medication: for example, two 240-mL (8-oz) glasses of water with each meal, and one in between meals, or, to fill a container with 2.5 to 3 L and finish it by the end of the day. Many patients prefer soft drinks to water, but soft drinks acidified with phosphoric acid have been associated with an increased risk of stone formation and should be avoided.

Sodium

The volume expansion associated with a high sodium intake inhibits sodium and calcium reabsorption in the proximal tubule, significantly increasing calcium excretion. Increasing sodium intake from 80 mEq (2 g) to 200 mEq (4.5 g) led to a 40% increase in calcium excretion in one study of patients with idiopathic hypercalciuria. A 2-g sodium diet is achievable but stringent; a reasonable compromise would be to recommend a 3 g or lower sodium intake.

Protein

Metabolism of sulfur-containing amino acids in animal protein generates acid that predisposes to stone formation. An acid load increases urine calcium excretion and decreases citrate excretion. The acid generated by a high protein diet also lowers urine pH, predisposing to uric acid stones. Vegetable protein has less of an effect on stone formation because its metabolism generates less acid than animal protein. A 60 g (or about 0.8 g/kg lean body weight) protein diet, consisting predominantly of vegetable protein, is recommended.

Oxalate

A high dietary oxalate intake can markedly increase the tendency to calcium oxalate stone formation. Foods with high oxalate content include leafy green vegetables, chocolate, tea, peanuts, spinach, and rhubarb.

Calcium

It seems logical that increased calcium intake exacerbates renal stone disease in patients with calcium stones, especially because many hypercalciuric patients are "hyperabsorbers" of calcium. However, the opposite appears to be the case. A recent prospective study showed that men with a high dietary calcium intake had about half the chance of developing symptomatic nephrolithiasis than those with low intake. Calcium supplements did not, in contrast, appear to influence the risk of forming stones. This paradox may be due to the ability of calcium to bind oxalate in the gut and prevent its absorption and excretion. Although calcium excretion did rise with an increased calcium intake, the relative saturation of calcium oxalate fell by 20% to 25%. Similar data are not available in women. However, the time-honored recommendation of a reduced calcium diet with calcium nephrolithiasis should be abandoned. It may predispose to both further stone formation and osteoporosis in women. Although the optimal dietary calcium intake in patients with calcium stones is unknown, at least a moderate intake (two to three dairy servings per day) should be encouraged. Women with calcium oxalate nephrolithiasis need not necessarily stop calcium supplements given to prevent osteoporosis. Collection of urine both on and off supplements may be helpful to determine their contribution to the stone disease.

MEDICAL THERAPY

Calcium Stones

Idiopathic Calcium Stones

If dietary measures have failed, that is, patients have recurrent stone formation as evidenced by colic or radiographic progression, treatment can be tailored to the abnormalities found in the 24-hour urine collection. The collection may reveal that fluid intake is inadequate or that sodium or protein intake is excessive, and the patient can be further counseled in this regard.

If hypercalciuria is present, addition of a thiazide diuretic, for example, 25 mg of hydrochlorothiazide twice a day, may be added. Thiazide diuretics enhance calcium reabsorption in the distal tubule of the nephron; the effect can be nullified by excess sodium intake. The use of a divided dose is most effective. A reasonable goal is a 25% to 50% reduction in calcium excretion; response to therapy can be monitored by spot urine testing for the calcium to creatinine ratio. If the desired response to thiazide does not occur, the dose may be increased to 50 mg twice a day. However, typical metabolic side effects of thiazides, including hypokalemia, hyperuricemia, glucose intolerance, and lipid abnormalities may be common at this dosage. Hypokalemia should be treated with potassium citrate, 20 to 60 mEq/day, instead of potassium chloride. Potassium citrate alkalinizes the urine, and in the presence of hypercalciuria, a urine pH above 7 may promote the formation of calcium phosphate stones. Thus, urine pH should be checked if high doses of potassium citrate are prescribed. A potential benefit of thiazide diuretics, especially in women, is maintenance of calcium balance by a decrease in calcium loss in the urine and prevention of osteoporosis.

Orthophosphate, which binds calcium in the gut, has been used to treat calcium stones. However, this agent has potential for causing both negative calcium balance and increased oxalate excretion in the urine and generally should be avoided.

If hyperuricosuria is identified in the evaluation of recurrent calcium oxalate stones, an attempt should first be made to reduce dietary purine intake. If this is unsuccessful, allopurinol (300 mg/day) may be instituted. An alternative treatment, especially in patients with lower urinary citrate levels and mild hyperuricemia, is alkalinization of the urine with potassium citrate in a dose of 30 to 60 mEq/day in two to three doses. By raising urinary pH to about 6 to 6.5, urate-induced calcium oxalate crystallization may be reduced. In a subset of patients with calcium oxalate nephrolithiasis, no metabolic abnormality can be found. In this group, treatment with both thiazide diuretics and allopurinol may reduce stone recurrence.

Renal Tubular Acidosis

Continued maintenance of a high urine output is crucial. In addition, electrolyte replacement should include potassium, sodium, and alkali. The adult patient with type I RTA usually requires 1 to 2 mEq/kg body weight of base a day in three to four divided doses, which can be given as a preparation of sodium potassium citrate (eg, Polycitra, which contains 2 mEq potassium, 1 mEq sodium, and 2 mEq base/mL). Normalization of plasma bicarbonate does not necessarily ensure adequacy of treatment. Indeed, nephrolithiasis is the major clinical manifestation in patients with "incomplete" RTA and a normal serum bicarbonate. In addition to correction of serum bicarbonate, urinary citrate excretion should be monitored and brought into the low-normal range.

Enteric Urolithiasis

Patients with enteric urolithiasis, as discussed earlier, may have multiple metabolic abnormalities that require treatment. General recommendations include frequent ingestion of fluids, during and between meals, to ensure a large urine volume. Dietary oxalate and fat should be restricted, and calcium intake should be increased to 1 to 1.5 g/day unless hypercalciuria is present. Correction of hypomagnesemia should be attempted but may be limited by exacerbation of diarrhea. Acidosis should be treated with potassium citrate until serum bicarbonate and urinary citrate excretion are corrected. If there is evidence of uric acid stones, the urine pH should be increased to 6.5 and allopurinol treatment may be necessary (see later).

Hyperparathyroidism

Surgical repair usually corrects hypercalcemia and prevents further stone formation.

Urate Stones

In patients with clinical gout (tophi, gouty arthritis), hyperuricemia, or both, urate stones can be treated with allopurinol. In patients without these characteristics and with uric acid excretion of less than 1000 mg/day, alkalinization of the urine to a pH of 6.5 to 7 with potassium citrate often results in dissolution of urate stones. Urine pH should be monitored by the patient with nitrazine paper, and pH values above 7 should be avoided because of the risk of calcium phosphate stones. In patients with excretion of more than 1000 mg of uric acid/day who are unresponsive to alkali and fluid intake, allopurinol is indicated.

Struvite (Infection) Stones

Struvite stones, especially common in women, are characterized by aggressive stone growth. Treatment of urinary tract infection with appropriate antibiotics is necessary. However, this may not affect stone growth because bacteria sequestered within stones, resistant to treatment, continue to produce urease and alkalinize the urine. Use of acetohexamic acid, a urease inhibitor, may retard or even reverse stone growth but has been associated with deep vein thrombosis, and its long-term safety and effectiveness are not clear.

Without invasive urologic intervention, struvite stones will grow in at least half of patients until nephrectomy is required. Debulking of the stone with ESWL alone may be possible if it is smaller than 2 to 3 cm. If the stone is larger than this, however, percutaneous lithotripsy, nephrolithotomy, or both are required, followed by ESWL to eliminate smaller fragments. It is crucial that these fragments are removed because remaining fragments larger than 5 mm predict a high rate of recurrence. Computed tomography without contrast, superior to ultrasound, can detect fragments of 1 mm or larger. The interventions are followed by a 2- to 4-week course of antibiotics, possibly with potassium citrate if smaller fragments remain. Periodic follow-up, initially every 3 to 6 months, is required to ensure lack of stone growth and sterile urine.

Cystine Stones

The major goal of treatment for cystinuria is to increase urine output to at least 3 L/day and decrease the concentration of cystine to less than its solubility limit of 1 to 2 mmol/L. Limiting protein intake also may be helpful. The solubility of cystine can be enhanced by alkalinization of the urine to a pH of about 7 with potassium citrate. However, patients may excrete as much as 15 mmol/day, making even a urine output of more than 4 L/day ineffective. Such patients can be treated with penicillamine (1 to 2 g/day), which forms a soluble salt with cystine and prevents formation of cystine stones. This agent, however, is associated with side effects that include nephrotic syndrome, dermatitis, and pancytopenia.

SPECIAL CONSIDERATIONS IN PREGNANCY

During gestation, urinary calcium excretion increases twofold to threefold and a uric acid excretion also increases slightly. However, possibly because of a concurrent increase in citrate excretion, nephrolithiasis is no more common in pregnancy than in nonpregnant women. Complications of stone disease during pregnancy can be severe, and are associated with a high incidence of preterm births. Most stones are diagnosed during the second or third trimester. The diagnosis should be considered in pregnant women with abdominal or flank pain, or hematuria. It should also be considered if bacteriuria and urinary tract infection have not resolved after treatment with an appropriate antibiotic.

Establishing a firm diagnosis of nephrolithiasis is important, in part because empirical treatment for stones may be disastrous if another abdominal process is missed. Ultrasonography, although not as reliable as in the nonpregnant state, may be diagnostic in one half to two thirds of cases and should always be attempted initially. Modified excretory urography (0.4 to 1 rad) is then indicated if significant management decisions hinge on the results, but even this low level of radiation late in gestation may increase the risk of childhood malignancy. Promising diagnostic techniques that may decrease the need for exposure to radiation include use of Doppler ultrasound and vaginal ultrasound probe.

About 50% to 80% of stones in pregnancy pass spontaneously with supportive care that includes hydration and analgesia. Epidural anesthesia has been reported to augment the passage of calculi, possibly by decreasing ureteral spasm. Indications for invasive intervention include declining renal function, intractable pain, obstruction of a solitary kidney, infection proximal to an obstructing stone, and colic that precipitates premature labor.

Percutaneous nephrostomy, internal ureteral stent placement, and ureteroscopy are the major alternatives for definitive treatment of renal stone disease in pregnancy. Cystoscopic placement of an internal stent is generally recommended as the initial approach. X-ray guidance, which is relatively contraindicated early in pregnancy, usually is used in placement. However, avoidance of x-ray exposure by ultrasound placement of stents has been well described. If a stent cannot be placed or an abscess is present that cannot be drained by a stent, a percutaneous nephrostomy is inserted. This can be performed with local anesthesia and ultrasound guidance. In a septic patient, percutaneous nephrostomy may be preferable to stent placement to ensure drainage. The use of ureteroscopic stone removal as an alternative to percutaneous nephrostomy is controversial. Definitive treatment with ESWL or percutaneous stone removal should be deferred until after pregnancy. Crust tends to form on both internal stents and percutaneous nephrostomy tubes, mandating their replacement every 6 to 8 weeks; adequate hydration is essential to maintain patency.

BIBLIOGRAPHY

Coe FL, Parks JH, Asplin JR. The pathogenesis and treatment of kidney stones. N Engl J Med 1992;327:1141;

Consensus Development Panel, National Institutes of Health. Prevention and treatment of kidney stones. JAMA 1988;260:977.

Curhan GC, Willett WC, Rimm EB, Stampfer MJ. A prospective study of dietary calcium and other nutrients and the risk of symptomatic kidney stones. N Engl J Med 1993;328:833.

Kurtzman NA (ed). Medical and surgical management of nephrolithiasis. Semin Nephrol 1990;10(1).

Levy FL, Adams-Huet B, Pak CYC. Ambulatory evaluation of nephrolithiasis: an update of a 1980 protocol. Am J Med 1995;98:50.

Loughlin KR. Management of urologic problems during pregnancy. Urology 1994;44:159.

Pak CYC. Etiology and treatment of urolithiasis. Am J Kidney Dis 1991;18:624.

Parks JH, Coe FL. A urinary calcium–citrate index for the evaluation of nephrolithiasis. Kidney Int 1986;30:85.

Uribarri J, Oh MS, Carroll HJ. The first kidney stone. Ann Intern Med 1989;111:1006.

Primary Care for Women, edited by Phyllis C. Leppert and Fred M. Howard. Lippincott-Raven Publishers, Philadelphia © 1997.

77

Chronic Renal Disease

EDWARD C. CLARK AND
RICHARD H. STERNS

Chronic renal disease results from a variety of pathologic entities, all of which are characterized by an irreversible reduction in glomerular filtration rate. *End-stage renal disease* (ESRD) refers to a total or near-total loss of renal function necessitating renal replacement therapy; *chronic renal insufficiency* refers to lesser degrees of irreversible renal injury. As of 1991, 178,000 people in the United States were being treated for ESRD. The incidence of ESRD has been increasing at approximately 8.8% per year since 1982. It seems likely that there are considerably more patients with lesser degrees of renal insufficiency. Differences in the incidence of ESRD exist between racial groups and the sexes, with African Americans and Native Americans having an approximately fourfold higher incidence of ESRD than whites (Table 77-1). Overall, males with ESRD slightly outnumber females; this is due, however, pri-

Table 77-1. Age, Gender and Race Distribution of Major Causes of ESRD

DISEASE	MEDIAN AGE	% FEMALE	EACH RACE'S TOTAL ESRD (%)			
			White	*African American*	*Asian*	*Native American*
Diabetes mellitus	61	52.6	34	32.5	36.8	63.9
Hypertension	68	42	25.2	37.9	23.0	11.9
Glomerulonephritis	54	38.1	13.6	10.2	20.0	9.7
Collagen vascular disease	41	73.3	2.0	2.2	3.0	1.4
Cystic kidney disease	54	46.6	3.9	1.1	2.3	1.8
Interstitial nephritis	63	53.7	3.7	1.5	3.0	1.9
Obstructive nephropathy	68	27.5	2.5	1.1	1.4	1.3

(From the United States Renal Data System 1994 Annual Data Report. Pub. No. PB95105003. Bethesda, MD: The National Institutes of Health, National Institute of Diabetes and Digestive and Kidney Diseases.)

marily to a predominance of males in the white population with ESRD. Among Native Americans, females predominate, whereas in African Americans ESRD is evenly distributed between sexes. The etiology of ESRD also demonstrates some racial differences. Overall, diabetes mellitus is the most common cause of ESRD, particularly among Native Americans. Hypertensive nephrosclerosis is the most common etiology among African Americans.

The primary care physician plays a central role in the identification of chronic renal disease and, when possible, determination of a specific etiology. Long-term management of the multisystem complications of chronic renal insufficiency is also frequently overseen by the primary care physician. Referral to a nephrologist is appropriate when there is uncertainty regarding the etiology and appropriate therapy of chronic renal disease or when renal replacement therapy is indicated.

ETIOLOGY

Etiologies of end-stage renal disease are categorized as either systemic diseases with renal involvement or primary renal diseases (Table 77-2). The most common etiologies of chronic renal disease in the United States are discussed in the following sections.

Diabetes Mellitus

In the United States, end-stage diabetic nephropathy is steadily increasing in incidence and currently represents one third of all patients with ESRD. Considerably more data exist regarding the natural history and clinical course for insulin-dependent diabetes mellitus (IDDM) than are available for non–insulin-dependent diabetes mellitus (NIDDM). In IDDM, about 30% to 40% of patients ultimately develop nephropathy. This usually occurs after 10 or more years of diabetes and is manifest as persistent proteinuria, hypertension, and declining renal function. Microalbuminuria, defined as urinary albumin excretion at a rate below what is detectable by conventional laboratory tests, predicts eventual progression to overt diabetic nephropathy. Once persistent proteinuria is present, renal function slowly and inexorably declines, resulting in ESRD in approximately 7 to 10 years. The degree of proteinuria can vary significantly, ranging from 0.5 g to 20 g per day. In those with overt nephropathy, associated diabetic complications such as retinopathy, neuropathy, and cardiovascular disease are very common.

The cumulative incidence of nephropathy in NIDDM is in the range of 10% to 20% for whites, but is somewhat higher for African Americans and some Native American tribes. The reasons underlying these racial differences are not well understood. As in IDDM, overt nephropathy is heralded by the development of persistent proteinuria, hypertension, and renal insufficiency. Progression to ESRD follows a time course roughly similar to that of IDDM. Evaluation of renal disease in patients with NIDDM is more complicated than with IDDM because these patients tend to be older with more complex medical problems.

Studies of the pathogenic mechanisms underlying the development of diabetic nephropathy have focused on the role of functional changes such as hyperfiltration and renal hypertrophy, and ultrastructural changes such as thickening of the glomerular basement membrane and mesangial expansion. Whether sustained hyperglycemia alone or other aspects of the diabetic milieu are responsible for these changes is not yet known.

Hypertension

Arterial hypertension is both a common etiology and a consequence of chronic renal disease. About 25% of all patients with ESRD carry a diagnosis of hypertensive nephrosclerosis. This group of patients includes those with nephrosclerosis due to essential hypertension, those with malignant-phase essential hypertension, and those with renovascular disease. Hypertensive nephrosclerosis is predominantly a disease of African Americans, perhaps due to the greater incidence of malignant-phase hypertension in this group.

Essential Hypertension

Patients in whom no specific or reversible etiology of hypertension can be determined are categorized as having primary or essential hypertension. Impaired-pressure induced sodium excretion and abnormally increased vasopressor tone have been proposed as pathophysiologic factors causing essential hypertension. Epidemiologic data further suggest an important role for both genetic and environmental factors. Hypertensive nephrosclerosis in patients with essential hypertension is usually seen in those with inadequately controlled diastolic hypertension or recurrent episodes of accelerated hypertension. The clinical course of hyper-

Table 77-2. Etiology of ESRD

DISEASE	TOTAL ESRD (%)
Systemic Disease with Renal Involvement	
Diabetes mellitus	33.8
Hypertension	28.3
Autoimmune/collagen vascular disease	
Systemic lupus erythematosus	1.3
Goodpasture syndrome	0.3
Wegener's granulomatosis	0.2
Scleroderma	0.2
Hemolytic uremic syndrome/TTP	0.2
Polyarteritis	< 0.1
Henoch-Schönlein purpura	< 0.1
Hereditary disease	
Autosomal dominant polycystic kidney disease	3.0
Autosomal recessive polycystic kidney disease	< 0.1
Sickle cell disease	< 0.1
Alport syndrome	0.3
Fabry's disease	< 0.1
Cystinosis	<0.1
Hyperoxaluria	< 0.1
Dysproteinemia	
Multiple myeloma/light chain nephropathy	0.8
Amyloidosis	0.3
HIV-related nephropathy	0.3
Primary Renal Disease	
Glomerulonephritis	
Membranous nephropathy	0.4
Membranoproliferative glomerulonephritis	0.3
Focal glomerulosclerosis	1.4
IgA nephropathy	10.0
Interstitial renal disease	
Analgesic nephropathy	0.8
All other interstitial disease	2.2
Obstructive nephropathy	2.0
ESRD of unknown cause	11.8

(From the United States Renal Data System 1994 Annual Data Report. Pub. No. PB95105003. Bethesda, MD: The National Institutes of Health, National Institute of Diabetes and Digestive and Kidney Diseases.)

tensive nephrosclerosis is variable, related to the severity of hypertension and effectiveness of control.

Accelerated Malignant Hypertension

Accelerated malignant hypertension is a hypertensive emergency. It is usually seen with diastolic blood pressures > 140 mm Hg and is associated with evidence of rapidly progressing end-organ injury. Organ pathology seen in this setting may include rapidly worsening renal insufficiency, grade III or IV hypertensive retinopathy, encephalopathy, intracranial hemorrhage, acute myocardial infarction or left ventricular failure, and acute aortic dissection. End-organ injury in this syndrome results from an autoregulatory failure of resistance vessels, which allows transmission of the markedly elevated arterial pressure to the microvasculature. Before effective antihypertensive therapy became available, prognosis in malignant hypertension was dismal, with a 1-year mortality higher than 90%. Prompt recognition and effective treatment of malignant hypertension has greatly improved the outcome in these patients. Control of blood pressure in this setting may initially be associated with worsening of renal function. However, with sustained blood pressure control, renal function tends to improve over a period of weeks. Over the long term, however, many of these patients ultimately develop ESRD. Accelerated malignant hypertension most commonly represents an aggressive phase of underlying essential hypertension; it can also be seen, however, as a consequence of renovascular disease, acute glomerulonephritis, primary aldosteronism, pheochromocytoma, primary intracranial hemorrhage, or intoxication with a drug such as cocaine.

Renovascular Disease

Hemodynamically significant stenosis of one or both renal arteries results in renin-mediated hypertension. Chronic renal insufficiency develops when there is significant narrowing of both renal arteries, resulting in ischemic renal injury or the development of hypertensive nephrosclerosis in the nonstenotic kidney. The exact incidence of renovascular disease and its contribution to ESRD is not known, but it appears to be increasing. About two thirds of renovascular disease is atherosclerotic in origin; the remaining one third is due to fibromuscular dysplasia. Atherosclerotic disease is most commonly seen in men over the age of 55 years, whereas fibromuscular disease is predominantly a disease of younger woman aged 15 to 40 years. Clinical clues suggesting the presence of renovascular disease include the presence of a systolic and diastolic abdominal bruit, the development of hypertension before the age of 30 years or over the age of 60 years, acceleration of previously well-controlled hypertension, and hypertension with associated renal insufficiency. A variety of screening procedures have been evaluated for the detection of renovascular disease, including captopril nuclear renography, Doppler ultrasonography of the renal arteries, magnetic resonance angiography, and intravenous digital subtraction angiography. The sensitivity and specificity of these tests vary from center to center and may be operator-dependent (eg, Doppler ultrasonography). Most experts consider hypertensive or rapid sequence intravenous pyelography an outmoded and insensitive screening study.

A form of renovascular disease seen with increasing frequency is cholesterol embolization. This is typically seen in patients with severe atherosclerotic disease following invasive vascular procedures such as arteriography, coronary artery bypass grafting, or repair of an abdominal aortic aneurysm. It is caused by the disruption of cholesterol plaque with subsequent showering of the microvasculature with cholesterol particles. Clinically this may be manifest as livido reticularis seen primarily in the lower extremities, abdominal pain due to ischemic bowel or pancreatitis, stroke, or a sudden decrease in renal function. Less commonly, cholesterol embolization can occur spontaneously without vascular manipulation.

Glomerulonephritis

Glomerulonephritis may be seen as a primary renal disease limited to the kidney or as the renal manifestation of a variety of systemic diseases. When all forms of glomerulonephritis are grouped together, they constitute the third most common cause of ESRD (see Table 77-1). Injury to the glomerulus and in particular the glomerular basement membrane by inflammatory and hemodynamic factors results in the characteristic clinical and histologic findings in glomerulonephritis. These include proteinuria and hematuria, both of which are consequences of a disrupted glomerular filtration barrier.

The nephrotic syndrome is characterized by heavy proteinuria (> 3.5 g/day), hypoproteinemia, hyperlipidemia, and edema. The presence of oval fat bodies in the urine sediment is diagnostic of the nephrotic syndrome. In the nephritic syndrome, the urine sediment is more typically characterized by hematuria, often with red cell casts, but more modest degrees of proteinuria. Due to their transit through the glomerular basement membrane and renal tubules, red cells of glomerular origin are frequently dysmorphic in appearance. It is important to remember, however, that hematuria is overall more commonly the result of lower urinary tract pathology, which, in most cases, must first be excluded. Strong clues that hematuria is of glomerular origin are the presence of dysmorphic red cells, cellular casts, and proteinuria. The most commonly encountered types of primary and secondary glomerulonephritis are reviewed in the following sections.

Primary Glomerulopathies

Membranous Glomerulonephritis. Membranous glomerulonephritis (MGN) is the most common etiology of the nephrotic syndrome in adults, typically presenting as the gradual onset of proteinuria and edema. Urinary protein losses can be quite variable in this disorder, exceeding 20 g/day in some patients, but less than 1 g/day in others. Membranous glomerulonephritis is most commonly idiopathic, but may also result from a variety of infections (eg, hepatitis B, *Plasmodium malariae*, syphilis), drugs (eg, gold, captopril, penicillamine), or autoimmune disorders such as systemic lupus erythematosus (SLE). Primarily in patients over the age of 50, there is an association between membranous glomerulonephritis and the presence of malignancy. Screening examinations for occult malignancy are indicated in such patients. The urine sediment in MGN is typically bland, only rarely containing gross hematuria or red cell casts. On renal biopsy, the characteristic histologic findings are the presence of thickening of the glomerular basement membrane on light microscopy and the presence of subepithelial electron-dense deposits seen on electron microscopy.

The variable clinical course of this disorder complicates treatment. Spontaneous remission of proteinuria may occur in as many as 25% of patients, with 10-year renal survival rates varying between 50% and 90%. Clinical characteristics associated with a more favorable prognosis include female gender, normotension, younger age, and proteinuria below the nephrotic range.

Minimal Change Disease. Minimal change disease (MCD), also known as lipoid nephrosis and nil lesion, derives its name from the absence of any identifiable glomerular abnormality on light microscopy. Electron microscopy reveals fusion of epithelial cell foot processes—a nonspecific finding seen in all forms of nephrotic syndrome. Diagnosis is therefore one of exclusion. MCD is the most common cause of nephrotic syndrome in children, accounting for 90% of nephrotic syndrome in children under the age of 4 and 50% in those under the age of 10. In adults, however, the incidence is much lower, causing approximately 15% of all cases of the nephrotic syndrome. Onset of proteinuria is typically sudden and may follow a viral illness. Proteinuria can be massive, occasionally in excess of 20 g/day with associated anasarca. The urine sediment is typically bland with heavy albuminuria, oval fat bodies, and occasionally microscopic hematuria. Gross hematuria and red cell casts are rare.

As with membranous glomerulonephritis, MCD is most commonly idiopathic; however, it can be associated with malignancies such as Hodgkin disease or T-cell lymphomas, and drugs, most commonly nonsteroidal anti-inflammatory agents. As discussed below, response to corticosteroid therapy is very good in children, but in adults is less dramatic and may take more prolonged courses of therapy.

Focal and Segmental Glomerulosclerosis. Focal and segmental glomerulosclerosis (FSGS) is a pathologic entity that derives its name from the presence of sclerotic lesions involving some glomeruli but leaving others uninvolved (focal), and affecting only portions of a given glomerulus (segmental). As with minimal change nephropathy, FSGS comprises approximately 15% of nephrotic syndrome in adults. FSGS is most commonly an idiopathic disease, but can be seen in association with a variety of other disorders including reflux nephropathy, HIV infection, sickle cell disease, morbid obesity, cyanotic heart disease, and heroin nephropathy. Some authors postulate that FSGS in certain patients may be a progressive form of minimal change disease seen in those patients who failed to achieve a long-term response to corticosteroid therapy. FSGS is seen more commonly in African Americans than in whites and is the predominant cause of nephrotic syndrome in obese patients. The clinical course of FSGS is unfavorable, with most patients progressing to end-stage renal disease. This, however, may take up to 20 years from the time of initial presentation. In a subset of patients with FSGS, the clinical course is very rapid, with progression to ESRD in 2 to 3 years. This form of FSGS, called malignant focal sclerosis, tends to recur rapidly in transplanted kidneys.

Membranoproliferative Glomerulonephritis. Membranoproliferative glomerulonephritis (MPGN) is characterized histologically by the combination of thickening of glomerular capillary walls and mesangial hypercellularity. Pathologists identify two varieties. Type I, thought to be due to immune complex deposition, is characterized by immunofluorescence staining for complement fragments and immunoglobulins in capillary walls and mesangial areas. In type II MPGN, also known as dense deposit disease, continuous electron-dense deposits are seen in the glomerular basement membrane by electron microscopy. Of these two varieties, type I is much more common, accounting for approximately 10% of nephrotic syndrome in children and adults. Clinical manifestations are variable, with either a nephrotic or nephritic urine sediment being possible. At presentation, many patients have hypertension and renal insufficiency. MPGN usually follows a slow, unremitting course with approximately half of patients progressing to ESRD in 10 years. Characteristic laboratory findings include hypocomplementemia, which in some instances is due to the presence of circulating nephritic factors. These factors are autoantibodies that bind to convertases of the complement pathways, thereby preventing their degradation and promoting continued complement activation. Although usually idiopathic, MPGN may result from hepatitis B or C viral infection, cryoglobulinemia, chronic bacterial infection, SLE, or complement deficiency states. MPGN has a propensity to recur in transplanted kidneys.

IgA Nephropathy. Both in the United States and worldwide, IgA nephropathy is the most common cause of glomerulonephritis. It can be seen in association with Henoch-Schönlein purpura or chronic liver disease, or as an isolated glomerulonephritis. Diagnostic histologic findings are immunofluorescent staining for IgA, predominantly in the mesangial areas. Electron microscopy usually demonstrates electron-dense deposits correlating to areas of IgA immunostaining. The clinical presentation is extremely variable, including isolated microscopic hematuria with or without proteinuria, chronic glomerulonephritis, rapidly progressive glomerulonephritis, or the nephrotic syndrome.

Both the initial presentation with hematuria and subsequent exacerbations often occur following upper respiratory tract infection. IgA nephropathy was previously considered a benign entity; it has become clear, however, that some patients do develop progressive renal insufficiency. In those who develop chronic renal insufficiency, it tends to be a very slow process, with approximately 20% of patients reaching ESRD after 40 years. Factors associated with a less favorable prognosis are the nephrotic syndrome, glomerular crescents on biopsy, and sustained hypertension. IgA nephropathy often recurs in transplanted allografts, but this should not prevent renal transplantation because it does not usually cause progressive loss of allograft function.

Glomerulopathies Associated With Systemic Disease

Postinfectious Glomerulonephritis. Although most commonly seen following streptococcal infection, postinfectious glomerulonephritis can also be seen in association with a variety of other infections, such as visceral abscesses, osteomyelitis, bacterial endocarditis, or infection of ventriculovascular shunts. The most common postinfectious glomerulonephritis is an immune complex–mediated disease resulting from pharyngitis or impetigo due to Group A streptococci. The risk of developing glomerulonephritis is slightly greater following impetigo than with pharyngitis. This is a disease primarily of children, but it does occur in adults.

Typically, patients with poststreptococcal glomerulonephritis present with hematuria, edema, flank pain, and sometimes with hypertension and signs of volume overload. A renal biopsy during the acute phase of the illness usually demonstrates an acute, diffuse glomerulonephritis with neutrophils visible within glomerular capillary lumens. In the vast majority of patients, these glomerular lesions slowly resolve, although occasionally with some focal residual scarring. Persistent microscopic hematuria or low-grade proteinuria may be present for many months. The long-term prognosis in children is excellent, with chronic renal insufficiency only rarely encountered. In adults, however, the prognosis may be less benign.

Systemic Lupus Erythematosus. Systemic lupus erythematosus (SLE) is a disorder predominantly affecting women, with a female-to-male ratio of 2 : 1. It is seen most commonly in younger patients, with the peak incidence between 15 and 40 years of age. Approximately half of all patients have clinical evidence of glomerulonephritis at the time of diagnosis with SLE, and an additional 25% have clinically apparent renal involvement at some point during their course. Even if clinical signs of renal involvement are absent, histologic evidence of lupus nephritis can be seen in 95% of all patients who meet the diagnostic clinical criteria for SLE. The presenting manifestations of lupus nephritis are variable and include microscopic or gross hematuria, low-grade proteinuria, nephrotic syndrome, and rapidly progressive glomerulonephritis. Hypertension is present in roughly half of all patients.

Lupus nephritis results from glomerular deposition of circulating immune complexes thought to be composed of DNA, anti-DNA, and complement fragments. The various histologic patterns seen with lupus nephritis have been categorized by the World Health Organization as follows:

- Class I—no identifiable lesion
- Class II—mesangial glomerulonephritis
- Class III—focal proliferative glomerulonephritis
- Class IV—diffuse proliferative glomerulonephritis
- Class V—membranous glomerulopathy.
- Class VI—sclerosing nephropathy.

Histologic classification is of significant prognostic and therapeutic value. Patients with diffuse proliferative glomerulonephritis (Class IV) have a less favorable prognosis, whereas a more benign course is seen in patients with Class I and II disease. The prognosis in Class V disease is less clear.

Antiglomerular Basement Membrane-Mediated Glomerulonephritis. Antiglomerular basement membrane-mediated glomerulonephritis is characterized by rapidly progressive glomerulonephritis and the demonstration of circulating autoantibodies to constituents of the glomerular basement membrane (GBM). Immunofluorescent microscopy shows linear deposition of IgG along the GBM, and light microscopy usually reveals glomerular crescents and variable degrees of segmental glomerular necrosis. In Goodpasture's disease, anti–GBM-associated glomerulonephritis is seen in conjunction with alveolar hemorrhage. This syndrome affects predominantly men. There is a bimodal age distribution, with peaks in the 3rd and 6th decades of life. Before glomerulonephritis is diagnosed, many patients complain of nonspecific symptoms such as weight loss or malaise for up to several months. Glomerulonephritis in this syndrome generally follows a rapidly progressive course to end-stage renal disease. Up to 75% of patients may have associated pulmonary involvement. Alveolar hemorrhage is most common in patients with an associated pulmonary insult such as respiratory tract infection, toxin exposure or cigarette smoking.

ANCA-Associated Diseases. Over recent years, several pathologic entities previously thought to be distinct have been shown to be associated with autoantibodies directed against components of neutrophil cytoplasm—termed anti-neutrophil cytoplasmic antibodies (ANCA). These pathologic entities include Wegener's granulomatosis, microscopic polyarteritis nodosa, leukocytoclastic angiitis, and the pauci-immune variety of rapidly progressive glomerulonephritis. Two general classes of ANCA have been identified. These are *c-ANCA* and *p-ANCA,* correlating to the *cytoplasmic* or *perinuclear* immunostaining pattern of neutrophils by these autoantibodies. In general, p-ANCA is more commonly seen in those with disease limited to the kidney, whereas those with more systemic disease tend to have c-ANCA. It has recently been established that most c-ANCA are directed against proteinase 3, whereas p-ANCA are specific for myeloperoxidase. Most patients present with a prodrome of constitutional symptoms including fever, arthralgias, weight loss, or anorexia. Renal involvement is manifest by hypertension, renal insufficiency, proteinuria, and hematuria, frequently with red cell casts. Roughly half of patients with ANCA-associated glomerulonephritis have respiratory tract involvement. This may be manifest as pulmonary hemorrhage, sinusitis, or otitis media. Histologic examination of the kidney in these patients is notable for segmental necrotizing glomerulonephritis with crescent formation. Immunofluorescent studies are typically negative; thus the term *pauci-immune glomerulonephritis* has been applied to this entity. Most patients tend to be older, with a peak incidence in the 5th and 6th decades of life. Before the availability of more effective supportive and immunosuppressive therapy, these patients followed a rapidly progressive course resulting in a very high incidence of ESRD or death.

Dysproteinemia-Associated Renal Disease. A variety of renal lesions may result from the pathologic production of monoclonal proteins by plasma cells. In many patients, overt multiple myeloma is present, whereas in others there is an apparent plasma cell proliferative process as indicated by the production of monoclonal proteins, but no pathologically identifiable neoplasia. Primary amyloidosis (AL) is the result of deposition within the glomerulus of immunoglobulin light chains that form amyloid fibrils. These deposits stain positively with Congo red. With primary amyloidosis, there is frequently cardiac involvement manifest as a restrictive cardiomyopathy and neural involvement characterized by peripheral neuropathy or carpal tunnel syndrome. The prognosis in primary amyloidosis is poor, with most patients succumbing to cardiac disease. Light chain deposition disease, which is characterized histologically by nodular nephrosclerosis similar to that seen in diabetic nephropathy, is also caused by deposition of light chains within the glomerulus. Patients with both of these entities typically present with the nephrotic syndrome. Other renal lesions associated with multiple myeloma include acute renal failure due to tubular obstruction from paraprotein casts and hypercalcemic nephropathy. Secondary amyloidosis (AA) is seen in chronic inflammatory diseases such as rheumatoid arthritis, inflammatory bowel disease, chronic cutaneous abscesses due to parenteral drug abuse, and familial Mediterranean fever. Amyloid fibrils in this disorder deposit in the kidney and other organs and result from production of serum amyloid A, a protein produced by the liver as an acute phase reactant in inflammatory states.

Human Immunodeficiency Virus–Associated Nephropathy. As our experience with human immunodeficiency virus (HIV) infection increases, renal complications of this infection are seen with greater frequency. The exact incidence of renal complications of HIV infection is not well known; however, approximately 1% of military recruits who test seropositive for HIV infection have urinary abnormalities. A variety of glomerular lesions have been reported in association with HIV infection, including membranous nephropathy, minimal change disease, focal and segmental glomerulosclerosis, membranoproliferative glomerulonephritis, and mesangial proliferative glomerulonephritis. The clinical presentation most frequently encountered is rapid onset of the nephrotic syndrome, frequently with very heavy proteinuria, large echogenic kidneys by ultrasonography, and the rapid progression to ESRD, usually within 6 months from the onset of proteinuria. African American heterosexual males with a history of intravenous drug abuse make up the majority of these patients. This disorder therefore bears some demographic similarity to heroin nephropathy; it differs markedly, however, in that it progresses much more rapidly to ESRD. Pathologically, HIV nephropathy is most commonly characterized by focal and segmental glomerulosclerosis with the presence of tubuloreticular inclusions in vascular endothelium.

Congenital or Inherited Renal Disease

Autosomal Dominant Polycystic Kidney Disease. Autosomal dominant polycystic kidney disease (AKPKD), affecting approximately 500,000 Americans, is one of the most common inherited disorders in the United States. As its name indicates, it is inherited in an autosomal dominant fashion and therefore affects males and females equally. It is characterized by the presence of numerous and progressively enlarging cysts in both kidneys. The exact incidence and prevalence of this disorder are not known, however, because only approximately one half of all affected patients progress to ESRD. Many affected persons therefore never manifest clinical signs or symptoms of ADPKD. Their disease is discovered incidentally during evaluation for some other problem or at postmortem examination. Cysts apparently arise from renal tubules, but the mechanism by which this happens remains unknown. The mechanism by which these cysts produce renal insufficiency is not clear either, but it may be related to compression of adjacent nephronal structures by enlarging cysts. Those who progress to ESRD generally do so in the 5th through 7th decades of life. Two varieties of this disorder, ADPKD-1 and ADPKD-2, have been differentiated based on the chromosomal location of the genetic defect. Approximately 10% of affected patients have no known family history of ADPKD, perhaps representing spontaneous mutations. Renal insufficiency develops very slowly in these patients and correlates with increasing cyst and kidney size. Hypertension often accompanies the development of renal insufficiency. The rate at which renal insufficiency develops in patients with ADPKD, however, is extremely variable and, as noted earlier, approximately half of all patients never progress to ESRD.

Pathologically, ADPKD is characterized by the progressive enlargement of numerous cysts throughout both kidneys (Fig. 77-1). Roughly 90% of all affected patients have ultrasonically identifiable cysts by age 30 years. In many patients, however, cysts can be identified by ultrasonography or CT scanning at a much younger age and have even been visualized in utero.

In addition to hypertension and renal insufficiency, there are several other renal complications of ADPKD. These include bleeding into cysts, cyst infection, and urinary calculi. These episodes present with abdominal pain and can present a significant management problem. ADPKD is also associated with a number of extrarenal manifestations, including colonic diverticulosis, cardiac valvular abnormalities, hepatic cysts (see Fig. 77-1), inguinal hernias, and, most importantly, intracranial aneurysms.

Other Cystic Diseases. Autosomal recessive polycystic kidney disease is rarer than ADPKD and usually progresses to ESRD in childhood. Medullary cystic disease, also quite rare, is divided into recessive and dominant forms. Both present early in life, with the usual clinical course being eventual progression to ESRD. Medullary cystic disease should not be confused with medullary sponge kidney (MSK), a disorder characterized by dilated intramedullary collecting ducts. MSK is often complicated by urolithiasis and hypercalciuria, but otherwise follows a benign course.

Sickle Cell Nephropathy. In the United States, approximately 4% of all patients with sickle cell anemia eventually develop ESRD.

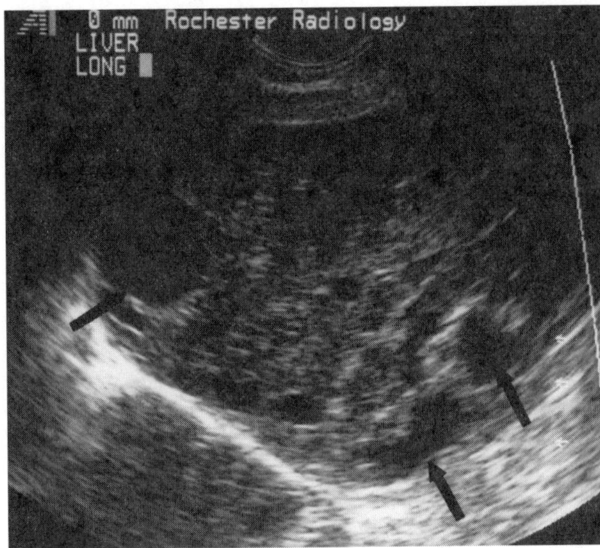

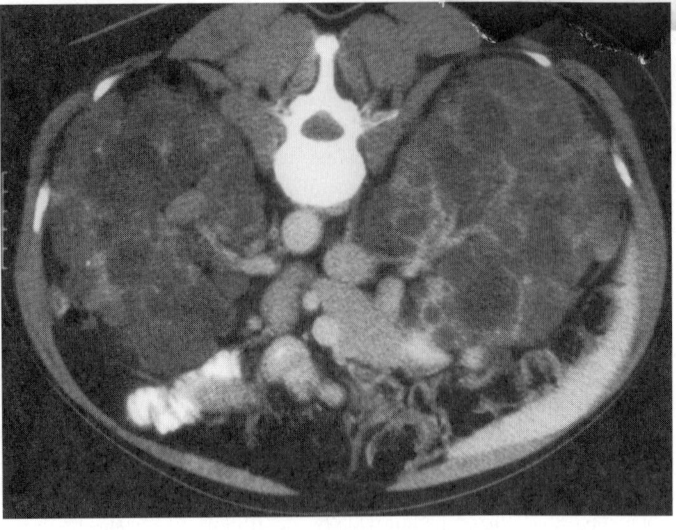

Figure 77-1. *(**A**)* Abdominal ultrasound of an asymptomatic 37-year-old woman with ADPKD. The arrow to the left indicates a large hepatic cyst, and the two arrows to the right identify two renal cortical cysts. The patient's blood pressure, urinalysis and renal function were normal. *(**B**)* Abdominal CT scan of a 58-year-old man with massive renal enlargement and advanced renal insufficiency from ADPKD.

These patients usually present with hypertension and proteinuria, with focal and segmental glomerulosclerosis seen histologically. In patients with sickle cell trait, medullary ischemia can result in hematuria and impaired urinary concentration, but rarely leads to ESRD.

Hereditary Nephritis (Alport's Syndrome) Hereditary nephritis (Alport's syndrome) is an inherited renal disease with a gene frequency of approximately 1 in 5000. In most affected families it has an X-linked transmission. Underlying this disorder is the absence of a component of type IV collagen from the glomerular basement membrane. This molecular defect is likely responsible for the frayed appearance and segmental thinning of the glomerular basement membrane as seen by electron microscopy. Patients typically present with microscopic or gross hematuria and modest degrees of proteinuria. Women with hereditary nephritis follow a more benign course, perhaps due to inactivation of one X chromosome per cell (the Lyon hypothesis). Approximately 20% of affected women develop ESRD, but usually after age 50 years. Affected males invariably progress to ESRD. Extrarenal manifestations of hereditary nephritis include sensorineural hearing loss, ocular abnormalities, and leiomyomata of the gastrointestinal or genitourinary tract.

Vesicoureteral Reflux. Vesicioureteral reflux (VUR) usually presents in childhood in association with urinary tract infection. Progressive renal insufficiency from severe VUR represents a serious problem in children and accounts for approximately 10% of ESRD in the pediatric population. The mechanism by which VUR results in progressive renal insufficiency remains unknown. Also controversial is the role of coexisting bacterial infection in causing renal injury in this disorder. The severity of VUR is graded 1 through 5 based on findings on voiding cystourethrography. In grade 1, urine reflux is into the distal ureter but with no dilatation of the urinary tract, whereas in grade 5, urine reflux is into the renal calices, with marked dilatation of the entire urinary tract. Progressive renal insufficiency is usually associated with hypertension and proteinuria.

Analgesic Nephropathy. Chronic use of a variety of analgesic preparations, including salicylates, acetaminophen, and nonsteroidal anti-inflammatory drugs, results in chronic interstitial nephritis. In some countries, this is a significant problem responsible for as much as 10% to 20% of all cases of ESRD. In the United States, it is seen less commonly and accounts for approximately 1% of all patients with ESRD. Cumulative intake of approximately 1 to 2 kg of analgesics over several years is usually required before this syndrome develops. It is seen more commonly in women and frequently is associated with some chronic pain syndrome such as headaches or rheumatoid or degenerative arthritis. Histologically, chronic interstitial nephritis, interstitial fibrosis, and papillary necrosis are seen. Progression to ESRD usually follows a very slow course over several decades. Transitional cell carcinomas of the urinary tract are associated with analgesic nephropathy.

CLINICAL SYMPTOMS AND SIGNS

Renal disease may manifest itself in a variety of ways. In many patients, renal disease is identified only incidentally after the performance of a routine urinalysis, blood chemistries, or blood pressure monitoring. Many other patients present in the advanced stages of chronic renal disease with nonspecific complaints such as fatigue, anorexia, and lethargy. Still others do not seek medical attention until overt uremia is present, manifest by anorexia, nausea, vomiting, slowed mentation, neuromuscular irritability, and serositis such as pericarditis or pleuritis.

When attempting to elicit a history suggestive of chronic renal disease, the physician should focus questioning on the presence of a previous history of renal disease, a family history of renal disease (eg, ADPKD, hereditary nephritis), and the presence of any systemic illness that may have associated renal involvement (eg, diabetes mellitus, SLE, vasculitis). Questions identifying specific symptoms and signs directly related to kidney disease should also be pursued. For example, patients with glomerular disease often present with complaints of edema or hematuria. A comprehensive past medical history is also very important in the evaluation of chronic renal disease. This should include any previous surgical or angiographic procedures and a medication history, with particular reference to nonsteroidal anti-inflammatory agents. The etiology of chronic renal disease can often be determined from a careful history. In patients with longstanding diabetes mellitus complicated by retinopathy, proteinuric renal disease is most likely diabetic in origin. Longstanding essential hypertension, particularly if poorly controlled and in African Americans, suggests hypertensive nephrosclerosis. Renal insufficiency associated with new-onset or accelerated hypertension in a patient with known atherosclerotic vascular disease suggests the diagnosis of renovascular disease. Constitutional or rheumatologic symptoms such as fever, arthritis, arthralgias, skin rashes, or weight loss may point to a diagnosis of systemic lupus, vasculitis, or malignancy-associated glomerulopathy. Nocturia due to impaired urinary concentrating ability is also a common but nonspecific presenting complaint. History of recurrent urinary tract infections may suggest underlying vesicoureteral reflux, whereas urinary hesitancy and frequency may indicate bladder neck obstruction. A detailed social history is also important, with specific reference to risk factors for transmission of HIV and exposure to environmental nephrotoxins such as lead.

A careful physical examination also plays a crucial role in the evaluation of patients with chronic renal disease. Blood pressure should be measured. An assessment of volume status is made by examining orthostatic blood pressures and jugular venous pressure. Peripheral edema and pulmonary congestion can reveal the presence of chronic renal disease. Depending on the nature of their renal disease, patients may present volume overloaded, euvolemic, or volume depleted. In patients presenting with advanced renal failure, the uremic syndrome may be present. On physical examination, this may be characterized by slowed mentation or confusion, neuromuscular irritability manifest by clonus, asterixis or hyperreflexia, and the presence of uremic pleuritis or pericarditis with friction rubs. Uremic pericarditis may be associated with signs and symptoms of pericardial tamponade. Abdominal bruits or an abdominal aortic aneurysm raise the possibility of renovascular disease, whereas the presence of palpably enlarged kidneys might suggest ADPKD.

LABORATORY AND IMAGING EVALUATION

Laboratory studies and imaging procedures play an important role in the evaluation of patients with chronic renal disease. An overall scheme to the work-up of renal insufficiency is given in Figure 77-2. The goal of these studies is to identify in as minimally invasive a manner as possible the etiology of the patient's renal disease. In this attempt, special emphasis is given to treatable and potentially reversible forms of chronic renal disease. Once renal disease is identified, the first task of the clinician is to determine its duration. This information can best be obtained from the patient's medical history and previous laboratory studies revealing azotemia or urinary abnormalities. Imaging studies also play an important role in assessing the chronicity of renal disease.

The initial laboratory diagnosis of chronic renal disease is made by the elevation in serum creatinine and blood urea nitrogen, indicating a decrease in glomerular filtration rate, or the presence of urinary abnormalities such as hematuria, proteinuria, or pyuria. The measurement of glomerular filtration rate is an important step in assessing the severity of chronic renal disease. In the clinical setting, glomerular filtration rate is usually estimated by the clearance of creatinine calculated from the 24-hour urinary excretion of creatinine and the serum creatinine according to the formula in Figure 77-3*A*. The utility of creatinine as a filtration marker can be improved by the administration of cimetidine during the period of urine collection and blood sampling. Cimetidine blocks the tubular secretion of creatinine, thereby causing its clearance to be due almost completely to glomerular filtration. Radioisotopic methods for measuring glomerular filtration rate with a single injection of ^{125}I iothalamate have also been standardized. This method, however, is not available in all centers. In patients with a stable serum creatinine, the formula of Cockroft and Gault given in Figure 77-3*B* can be used to estimate creatinine clearance.

Careful examination of the urine sediment by dipstick and microscopy also plays a major role in the initial evaluation of

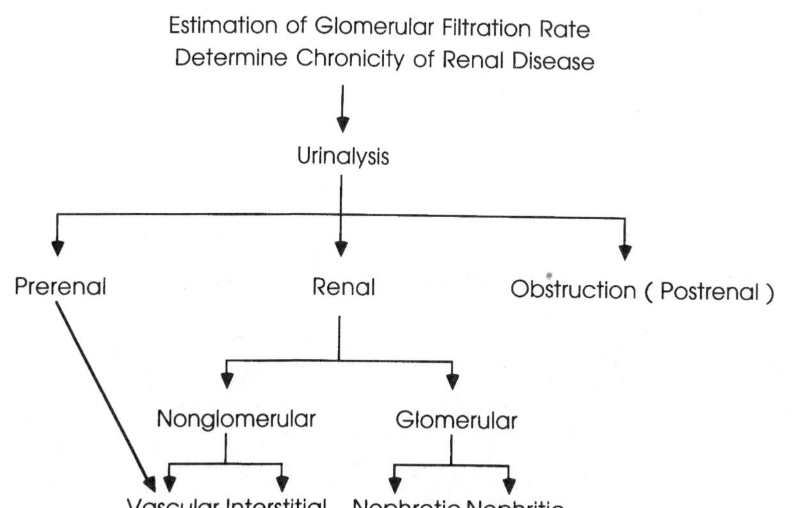

Figure 77-2. Systematic approach to diagnosing the etiology of chronic renal disease. (Rose BD. Pathophysiology of renal disease, 2nd ed. New York: McGraw-Hill Book Company, 1987.)

A

$$C_{Cr}\,(\text{ml/min}) = \frac{U_{Cr}\,(\text{mg/ml}) \times U_{Volume}\,(\text{ml/1440 min})}{P_{Cr}\,(\text{mg/ml})}$$

B

$$C_{Cr}\,(\text{ml/min}) = \frac{[140 - \text{age(years)}] \times \text{weight (kg)}}{P_{Cr}\,(\text{mg/dl}) \times 72} \times 0.85 \text{ (for women)}$$

Figure 77-3. (***A***) Formula for determination of creatinine clearance from plasma creatinine and 24-hour urinary excretion of creatinine. (***B***) Cockroft and Gault's formula for estimation of creatinine clearance.

Table 77-3. Classification of Renal Disease Based on Urinary Findings

URINARY FINDING	ETIOLOGY
Heavy proteinuria (>3.5 g/day), lipiduria	Nephrotic syndrome
Hematuria, red blood cell casts, proteinuria	Nephritic syndrome
Pyuria, low-grade proteinuria (<1.5 g/day), granular or waxy casts	Tubulointerstitial disease, obstruction
Normal or near-normal: low-grade proteinuria, hyaline casts	Prerenal disease, renovascular disease, obstruction

(Adapted from Rose BD. Pathophysiology of renal disease, 2nd ed. New York: Mc-Graw Hill, 1987.)

chronic renal disease. The presence of proteinuria, hematuria, pyuria, or cellular casts can significantly narrow the diagnosis of chronic renal disease. The presence of proteinuria should be assessed both by dipstick, which measures albuminuria, and sulfosalicylic acid, which identifies any form of urinary protein. Classification of renal disease based on urinary findings is given in Table 77-3.

Serum Chemistries and Serologic Evaluation

Depending on the type and severity of chronic renal disease present, abnormalities in a variety of serum chemistries may be present. With mild to moderate renal insufficiency (serum creatinine < 2.5 mg/dL), serum electrolytes and other chemistries may remain normal. With advanced renal insufficiency, abnormalities most commonly encountered include hyperkalemia, metabolic acidosis, anemia, and secondary hyperparathyroidism with hypocalcemia, hyperphosphatemia, and an elevated alkaline phosphatase. Diabetics in particular are prone to hyperkalemia because of relative insulin deficiency and the presence in some of type IV renal tubular acidosis. Hypoalbuminemia and hypogammaglobulinemia may be present in heavily nephrotic patients. Serologic studies also play an important role in the evaluation of glomerular disease. The use of these studies should be tailored to the diagnostic possibility suggested by the patient's clinical presentation and urinary findings. Table 77-4 correlates laboratory findings with diagnostic possibilities.

Imaging Studies

A variety of imaging techniques that assess both renal structure and function are available. These greatly assist in diagnosing chronic renal disease and identifying its etiology. The most commonly employed imaging studies are discussed, with a review of each procedure's utility, in the following sections. General goals in imaging evaluation of patients with renal disease are to employ as noninvasive a test as possible, to avoid intravenous contrast where possible, and to avoid radiation exposure in pregnancy and to gonads in younger patients.

Plain Abdominal X-Ray

Plain abdominal x-ray (KUB) provides limited information but can be helpful in identifying nephrocalcinosis and urolithiasis.

Table 77-4. Laboratory Diagnosis of Renal Disease

SEROLOGIC FINDING	DIAGNOSTIC POSSIBILITIES
Hypocomplementemia	SLE, MPGN (C3 nephritic factor), postinfectious glomerulonephritis, cryoglobulinemia
Antinuclear antibodies	SLE
Elevated anti-streptococcal antibodies	Poststreptococcal glomerulonephritis
Elevated IgA level (IgA-fibronectin aggregates)	IgA nephropathy
Hepatitis B surface antigen	MGN, MPGN, systemic vasculitis
Hepatitis C antibody	MPGN
HIV antibody	HIV-associated nephropathy
Cryoglobulinemia	MPGN
ANCA	ANCA-associated glomerulonephritis
Anti-GBM antibodies	Goodpasture's syndrome, anti-GBM glomerulonephritis
Monoclonal paraproteinemia	Multiple myeloma, amyloidosis

Occasionally it gives a gross estimate of renal size. Tomography improves the sensitivity of this study.

Intravenous Pyelography

Intravenous pyelography (IVP) provides a great deal of information about both urinary tract structure and function. It visualizes the entire urinary tract and also provides qualitative information regarding renal function. It is the initial study of choice in patients with suspected urolithiasis, renal trauma, or urinary tract tumors. In patients with advanced renal disease, however, renal concentration and clearance contrast may be significantly delayed, thereby preventing adequate visualization of the urinary tract. Rapid sequence or hypertensive IVPs are a relatively insensitive screening test for renovascular disease.

Ultrasonography

Renal ultrasonography has numerous advantages. It provides good visualization of renal parenchyma, is noninvasive, requires no preparation, and does not employ intravenous contrast. It is particularly useful during pregnancy, when avoiding radiation exposure is obviously of major concern. Ultrasonography, however, has the disadvantage of not providing information about renal function, and the quality of images can be affected by the skill of the operator and patient factors such as cooperation or obesity. This procedure is particularly helpful in evaluating suspected urinary tract obstruction, renal cysts, renal tumors, and stones. It also plays an important role in assessing the chronicity of renal disease. Indices of chronicity by ultrasound examination include small kidney size ($<$ 9 cm in an adult), cortical thinning, and increased parenchymal echogenicity. The safety and reliability of percutaneous renal biopsy has been improved when performed under ultrasound guidance.

Doppler renal flow study of the renal arteries is an important addition to renal ultrasound examinations. In skilled hands, the sensitivity of this technique in detecting renal artery stenosis has been reported to be 90% or greater. This technique has also been used to study renal venous flow when renal vein thrombosis is suspected clinically. As with routine ultrasonography, patient obesity can significantly impair the quality of this study.

Retrograde Ureteropyelography

Retrograde ureteropyelography is an invasive cystoscopic procedure performed by the urologist. It is the definitive study in ruling out urinary tract obstruction. When there is a strong clinical suspicion of obstruction and other imaging studies fail to demonstrate any obstruction, retrograde pyelography may be necessary. Other indications include better evaluation of urinary tract tumors, particularly ureteral tumors, urinary tract bleeding with a normal IVP, and ureteral strictures. This technique can also be employed in patients who require visualization of the entire urinary tract but are allergic to intravenous contrast.

Computed Tomography

Computed tomography (CT) is increasingly employed for evaluating renal structure and function. Its main advantages are its high resolution and detailed cross-sectional views of the kidney. Its primary utility is in the evaluation of renal tumors and cysts, but it is also helpful in identifying urinary tract obstruction and abscess formation. Use of intravenous contrast is frequently necessary to fully evaluate the possibility of renal cell carcinoma. Intravenous contrast also provides a qualitative assessment of renal function and can diagnose vascular disorders such as segmental renal infarction. CT guidance is also used in fine needle aspiration of renal masses for diagnostic purposes.

Magnetic Resonance Imaging

Magnetic resonance imaging is used primarily to further evaluate renal neoplasms or in patients who are allergic to radiocontrast material. Magnetic resonance angiography is an evolving technique that shows significant promise in evaluating renal artery stenosis.

Angiography

Visualization of the renal arterial system is best achieved by an arterial approach using digital subtraction techniques. This procedure employs smaller catheters and a smaller quantity of contrast media than conventional arteriography and therefore reduces complications. Images produced by digital subtraction following the IV bolus administration of radiocontrast are frequently of inadequate quality. Indications for renal angiography include suspected renal artery stenosis, renal vasculitis, and, less commonly, evaluation of renal mass. Complications of angiography include hematoma at the arterial puncture site, cholesterol embolization, contrast nephropathy, and radiocontrast allergy.

Nuclear Renography

A variety of radiopharmaceuticals that allow assessment of renal function are available. Because of poor imaging resolution, these are usually poor studies of renal anatomy, however. [^{99}TC] DTPA is most commonly used as a measure of glomerular filtration, whereas [^{131}I] iodohippuran is used to estimate renal perfusion. The principal utility of these studies is to measure right vs. left kidney function to evaluate suspected renovascular disease. The sensitivity of the nuclear renogram in detecting unilateral renal artery stenosis can be improved to approximately 85% if it is performed after administration of captopril. Gallium 67 citrate– or indium 111–labeled leukocytes may be helpful in the evaluation of renal inflammatory disorders such as perinephric abscess and acute interstitial nephritis.

Voiding Cystourethrogram

Voiding cystourethrogram (VCUG) involves urethral or suprapubic catheterization of the bladder and instillation of radiocontrast material. Images are then taken during voiding to determine the presence and severity of vesicoureteric reflux. In some centers, VCUGs can be performed using radioisotopes, thereby minimizing gonadal radiation exposure.

Approach to Urinary Abnormalities

Proteinuria

Once proteinuria is identified, the clinician must determine the quantity of proteinuria present and the type of protein excreted. Most commonly, the quantity of proteinuria is determined by the amount of protein present in a 24-hour urine collection. This procedure allows separation of those patients with significant proteinuria from glomerular disease from those with benign or transient proteinuria due to exercise, postural change, or fever. In an adult, protein excretion exceeding 150 mg/day is considered abnormal. An alternative method of quantitating protein excretion is to use the urinary protein-to-creatinine ratio. The ratio of protein concentration in mg/dL divided by the urinary creatinine concentration in mg/dL closely approximates the 24-hour protein excretion in grams. This method can be particularly useful in children and elderly patients for whom 24-hour collections are impractical. Protein excretion in excess of 1 g/day strongly suggests glomerular disease and in excess of 3.5 g/day indicates that the nephrotic syndrome is present. Benign orthostatic proteinuria can be assessed by performing two separate urine collections—one covering 16 hours during normal daytime activities and the second following 8-hour overnight recumbency. Total 24-hour excretion in this condition is less than 150 mg/day.

The initial step in determining the type of protein excreted is examination of the urine with sulfosalicylic acid. The presence of positive reaction to sulfosalicylic acid with a negative dipstick suggests the presence of nonalbumin proteins. This is most commonly seen in multiple myeloma and is the result of excretion of large quantities of immunoglobulin light chains. To definitively identify the type of protein excreted, urine immunoelectrophoresis identifies any monoclonal protein present.

Hematuria

The discovery of hematuria on urinalysis is relatively common. The initial step in its evaluation is to search for other urinary findings suggestive of glomerular disease such as proteinuria or casts. Hematuria in the setting of proteinuria and red blood cell casts constitutes a nephritic urine sediment and is seen in a variety of glomerulonephritides. Urinary tract infection is also an important initial consideration and should be assessed by examination of the urine for pyuria and bacteriuria, along with a urine culture. If there is no evidence for glomerular disease in the urine sediment, the hematuria is most likely of urologic origin; overall, hematuria is most commonly of urologic origin. The list of diagnostic possibilities is sizable and includes carcinoma of the bladder, ureters or kidney; urolithiasis; prostatitis; cystic renal disease; trauma; vascular malformations; and interstitial cystitis. Benign hematuria of glomerular origin is also a possibility and is seen following strenuous exercise and in thin basement membrane disease. Evaluation of persistent hematuria in the absence of evidence for glomerular disease should include intravenous pyelography and referral to a urologist for cystoscopy.

TREATMENT

Numerous advances have been made in our ability to treat chronic renal disease and its complications, thereby greatly improving the quality of life of these patients. As discussed in the following sections, treatment of these patients addresses the following issues: (1) treatment of the primary renal disease; (2) treatment aimed at slowing the progression of chronic renal disease; (3) treatment of extrarenal complications of chronic renal disease; and (4) renal replacement therapy in patients with ESRD.

Progression of Chronic Renal Disease

In many patients with established chronic renal disease, renal function slowly and inexorably declines to ESRD. This can occur regardless of the initial renal disease and even if the initial disease has become quiescent. The pathophysiologic mechanisms responsible for this progressive loss of renal function are summarized in Figure 77-4. With reduced renal functional mass, the remaining nephrons undergo a variety of hemodynamic and metabolic adaptations. Although these adaptations serve the purpose of maintaining glomerular filtration in the short term, they may prove maladaptive in the long term, by promoting further renal injury. Glomerular adaptations include increased plasma flow and filtration rates per remaining nephron with resultant glomerular hypertension. Altered permeability of the glomerular basement membrane leads to increased traffic of plasma proteins into the mesangium and activation of immune cells. Compensatory hypertrophy of nephrons is also associated with progressive renal injury. Tubular adaptations include accelerated rates of ammoniagenesis per nephron, increased production of reactive oxygen species, and interstitial deposition of calcium phosphate resulting from hyperphosphatemia. All of these factors promote progressive glomerulosclerosis and tubulointerstitial fibrosis, thereby perpetuating a cycle of progressive injury.

Although no treatments exist that arrest progression of chronic renal disease, it is possible to slow it. This is best achieved with rigid control of hypertension and, to a lesser extent, with dietary protein restriction. Treatment of hypertension with angiotensin-converting enzyme inhibitors may offer additional benefit in slowing progression over conventional antihypertensive medications. This appears to be particularly true in diabetic patients and may be

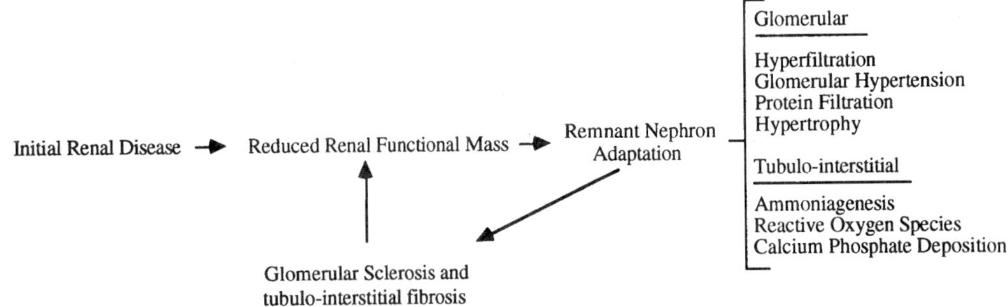

Figure 77-4. Proposed pathophysiologic mechanisms responsible for progression of chronic renal failure.

related to the ability of these agents to more effectively lower glomerular pressures. The efficacy of dietary protein restriction in slowing progression is more controversial. A recent large multicenter study, the Modification of Diet in Renal Disease Trial, did not show significant benefit of a low protein (0.58 g protein/kg body weight/day) in patients with an initial glomerular filtration rate below 25 mL/min. Use of very-low-protein diets (0.28 g/kg body weight/day) with ketoacid supplements also failed to demonstrate any clear-cut benefit. Smaller, earlier studies, however, did seem to demonstrate some benefit from very-low-protein diets and ketoacid supplementation. This remains a controversial area among nephrologists, and definitive recommendations are therefore difficult to make.

Treatment of Initial Renal Disease

Diabetic Nephropathy

In addition to slowing progression of disease as noted earlier, several other interventions are worth considering in diabetics. Most studies of the treatment of diabetic nephropathy deal with IDDM, with less known about NIDDM. It is increasingly clear that strict metabolic control may at least delay the development of complications such as microalbuminuria, nephropathy, and retinopathy. Preliminary evidence indicates that pancreas transplantation also may delay the onset of nephropathy. Use of angiotensin-converting enzyme inhibitors (ACEI) has also been found to be beneficial even in normotensive diabetics with proteinuria. Diabetics with renal insufficiency who are treated with ACEI must be followed closely for the development of hyperkalemia. This can frequently be prevented by concomitant use of a loop diuretic. Other diabetic complications that may impair renal function are the development of renovascular disease and functional urinary tract obstruction resulting from autonomic neuropathy involving the bladder.

Glomerulonephritis

The decision of whether to treat primary or secondary glomerulonephritides is frequently complicated and in most cases merits referral to a nephrologist. Potential toxicities of immunosuppressive therapy coupled with the marginal response to therapy of many of these disorders warrants referral in most cases.

Hypertensive Nephrosclerosis

Little can be done for hypertensive nephrosclerosis other than control of hypertension and possibly dietary protein restriction. The possibility of underlying renovascular or glomerular disease should be excluded.

Renovascular Disease

Once a hemodynamically significant lesion has been identified angiographically, revascularization can be achieved by either balloon angioplasty or surgical bypass. Balloon angioplasty is most effective in the fibromuscular lesions and in non-ostial atherosclerotic lesions. Roughly one third of patients who respond to angioplasty will eventually restenose. Angioplasty is ineffective and carries a risk of atheroembolic complications when it is attempted for ostial lesions in patients with significant aortic atherosclerotic plaque. Deployment of vascular stents to maintain patency of a stenotic renal artery is a procedure increasingly used in many centers. The most commonly employed surgical techniques are hepatorenal, splenorenal, or aortorenal bypass procedures.

Autosomal Dominant Polycystic Kidney Disease

Treatment in autosomal dominant polycystic kidney disease is geared toward slowing progressive renal insufficiency by blood pressure control and dietary protein restriction.

Vesicoureteral Reflux

Uncertainty exists among nephrologists, urologists, and pediatricians regarding the appropriate management of vesicoureteral reflux. Infants and children should be screened for VUR with their first urinary tract infection. Preadolescent siblings of affected children also should be screened because up to 50% of them will have abnormalities on VCUG. Bacteriuria should be treated aggressively with antibiotics, and some patients may require long-term suppressive therapy. A point of controversy in managing this problem is the appropriate role of antireflux surgery. It does not benefit patients with established renal insufficiency, hypertension, or persistent proteinuria. If surgery is to be effective, therefore, it must be instituted early. The issue is complicated by the fact that VUR resolves in many children as their urinary tracts mature. Referral for a urologic opinion is appropriate.

Extrarenal Complications of Chronic Renal Disease and ESRD

Chronic renal disease and ESRD produce numerous derangements in the function of many other organ systems. The more prominent complications and their treatment are reviewed in the following paragraphs.

Fluid and Electrolyte Disturbances

Volume overload caused by impaired salt and water excretion is best treated with loop diuretics, frequently in high dosages. Addition of metolazone significantly augments the diuretic response to a loop diuretic. Dietary sodium restriction also plays an important role in controlling volume overload in these patients. Hyperkalemia can also be managed with loop diuretics. Administration of sodium bicarbonate (2 to 4 g/day) also assists in the management of hyperkalemia by treating metabolic acidosis, which is frequently present, and also helps to prevent diuretic-induced volume depletion. Metabolic acidosis may alternatively be treated with sodium citrate solution (Bicitra) 10 to 30 mL four times daily.

Hematologic Abnormalities

Progressive anemia due to diminished renal production of erythropoietin is an almost universal finding in patients with advanced renal disease. The availability of recombinant erythropoietin has greatly aided in the management of patients with advanced renal disease, with significant improvement in their quality of life and sense of well-being. In predialysis patients, erythropoietin administration is usually started once the hematocrit is below 30 and the serum creatinine is greater than 3.0 mg/dL. Initial dosing is approximately 50 U/kg subcutaneously twice per week. Once the patient is on dialysis, it can be given intravenously with each dialysis treatment. Target hematocrits must be individualized for each patient based on symptoms and the presence of coronary disease. Iron stores must be monitored frequently and supplemented as needed.

Coagulopathy due to abnormal platelet function is a frequent finding in advanced ESRD. This is best treated emergently with desmopressin acetate (0.3 μg/kg by slow intravenous infusion) or administration of a cryoprecipitate. More effective dialysis and conjugated estrogens have also been shown to improve platelet function in this setting.

Renal Osteodystrophy

A variety of metabolic bone disorders are associated with chronic renal disease, including (1) secondary hyperparathyroidism and osteitis fibrosa, (2) aluminum-induced osteomalacia, (3) adynamic bone disease, and (4) dialysis-related amyloidosis. Secondary hyperparathyroidism results from diminished renal production of 1,25-dihydroxyvitamin D_3 coupled with phosphate retention. This is best treated by lowering the serum phosphorus with a phosphate-restricted diet and orally administered phosphate binders. Calcium-containing phosphate binders such as calcium carbonate and calcium acetate are most effective and should be administered with meals. Administration of exogenous calcitriol also plays an important role in treating secondary hyperparathyroidism by elevating serum calcium and suppressing parathyroid hormone secretion. Patients treated with calcitriol must be followed closely for the development of hypercalcemia. Dialysis patients with severe secondary hyperparathyroidism refractory to medical therapy may require parathyroidectomy.

Aluminum bone disease results from aluminum ingestion, usually in the form of aluminum-containing phosphate binders. If present, this can be treated by chelation with deferoxamine.

Adynamic bone disease is a poorly understood form of osteomalacia seen in dialysis patients. It may be the result of aluminum intoxication or of long-standing suppression of parathyroid hormone secretion by calcitriol administration.

Bone disease resulting from dialysis-related amyloid is due to bone deposition of ß2 microglobulin. ß2 microglobulin is a low-molecular-weight protein that is poorly cleared by dialysis and therefore accumulates to high levels in these patients. Carpal tunnel syndrome is a common complication of this disorder.

Endocrine Abnormalities

Approximately 50% of premenopausal women with ESRD are amenorrheic, and an even greater percentage are anovulatory. Infertility, therefore, is a common problem among premenopausal women maintained on dialysis. This appears to be the result of a combination of factors, including hyperprolactinemia and impaired positive feedback of estrogens on pituitary gonadotropin release. Prolactin levels are rarely in excess of 100 ng/mL, and elevations of greater magnitude should prompt evaluation for pituitary adenoma.

Other endocrinopathies encountered with ESRD include insulin resistance, which may be the result of secondary hyperparathyroidism. Total serum levels of T_4 and T_3 may be low in ESRD due to displacement from protein binding sites. Free levels of T_3 and T_4 are normal. An elevation in serum TSH is a reliable indication of hypothyroidism in these patients.

Renal Replacement Therapy

Patients with advanced renal insufficiency should be referred to a nephrologist for renal replacement therapy well in advance of their developing uremic symptoms. This allows adequate time for patient counseling, decision-making, and planning for the modality of renal replacement therapy best suited for each patient. Discussion of the advantages and disadvantages of peritoneal dialysis, hemodialysis, and renal transplantation is beyond the scope of this chapter. In general, younger, more active patients who wish to take a more active role in their own care do better with peritoneal dialysis or renal transplantation. Chronic hemodialysis is attractive to some patients because it requires less active participation on their part. It has the disadvantage of needing to maintain long-term vascular access.

CONSIDERATIONS IN PREGNANCY

Physiologic Changes with Pregnancy

Renal function undergoes dramatic changes during normal pregnancy. These include an increase of approximately 30% to 40% increase in plasma volume with roughly 50% increases in renal plasma flow and glomerular filtration rate. As a result of this increased GFR, serum creatinine falls to an average value of 0.7 mg/dL and BUN to 9 mg/dL. Blood pressure also normally falls early in pregnancy and during the second trimester averages 105/60 mm Hg. Kidney size increases by 1 to 1.5 cm due to hyperperfusion. Under the influence of very high plasma levels of progesterone, ureters and renal calices dilate, producing the so-called hydronephrosis of pregnancy. Although this does not result in urinary tract obstruction, sluggish urine flow through the dilated collecting system may promote the development of bacteriuria. Electrolyte changes during pregnancy include a mild respiratory alkalosis due to the effect of progesterone and a reduction in plasma sodium concentration by approximately 5 mEq/L due to resetting of the hypothalamic osmostat.

Identifying renal disease in pregnancy must take into account the above physiologic changes. For example, a blood pressure of 140/90 might be considered normal in many adults, but is clearly an elevated value in the pregnant patient. Serum creatinine and BUN values must also be judged against what should normally be found during pregnancy.

Chronic Renal Disease in Pregnancy

Pregnancy in women with chronic renal disease poses a difficult management problem, most appropriately referred to centers specializing in high-risk obstetric care. The two basic problems encountered are the role of chronic renal disease in affecting maternal and fetal outcome and the role of pregnancy in accelerating underlying chronic renal disease. Maternal morbidity is primarily affected by the increased risk of preeclampsia in women with underlying chronic renal disease, hypertension, or both. Fetal outcome is also adversely affected, with increased risks of preterm delivery and intrauterine growth retardation seen even with mild chronic renal disease (serum creatinine < 1.4 mg/dL). Overall fetal survival in these patients is approximately 95%. In women with more advanced renal disease, the clinical course of pregnancy is frequently complicated, with fetal survival as low as 50% to 75%. Pregnancy in women with ESRD on dialysis is rare, occurring in approximately 1% of all female dialysis patients of childbearing age. Management of these patients is complicated by worsening hypertension and anemia, and children are usually born prematurely and small for gestational age. The overall success rate of pregnancies in dialysis patients averages 50%.

The effect of pregnancy on the course of underlying chronic renal disease remains somewhat controversial. In patients with only mild renal insufficiency (serum creatinine < 1.4 mg/dL), there may be a transient increase in serum creatinine and worsening hypertension during pregnancy. Following delivery, however, renal function generally returns to baseline levels. In those with proteinuric renal disease, the quantity of urine protein excretion commonly increases over the course of pregnancy. In patients with more advanced renal disease (serum creatinine >1.4 mg/dL) the course is less clear. There may be an acceleration in the progressive loss of renal function induced by pregnancy in these patients. Inadequate control of hypertension may play an important role in the acceleration of renal disease in these patients. Protein-restricted diets should be avoided in pregnancy. Particular problems are presented by pregnant patients with underlying renal insufficiency due to insulin-dependent diabetes mellitus and systemic lupus erythematosus. Difficulty with metabolic control in the diabetic and flares of lupus activity in the patient with lupus can significantly complicate the course of these pregnancies.

Following successful renal transplantation, fertility is restored. Pregnancy in these patients may be complicated by accelerated hypertension, worsening renal disease, or graft rejection. In pregnancies that survive past the first trimester, overall pregnancy success rate is 92%. Azathioprine and cyclosporine are generally well tolerated, but may be associated with growth retardation.

A particularly difficult problem in managing pregnant patients with renal disease is accurately diagnosing preeclampsia in the setting of underlying renal disease. Many of the clinical and biochemical markers of preeclampsia, such as hypertension, proteinuria, renal insufficiency, and hyperuricemia, can all be seen with chronic renal disease alone. These patients therefore merit very close monitoring. The development of hyperreflexia strongly suggests preeclampsia, as this is only seen in chronic renal disease when the uremic syndrome is present. Other biochemical features of preeclampsia, such as elevation in liver enzymes, coagulopathy, thrombocytopenia, or microangiopathy, are relatively late signs.

Management

Prompt recognition and treatment of hypertension plays a vital role in the management of these patients. Blood pressure values higher than 140/85 mm Hg are clearly abnormal, and adverse fetal outcomes are associated with blood pressures above 125/75 mm Hg. Conservative management of hypertension consists of bed rest and avoidance of tobacco and alcohol. Dietary salt restriction should be avoided. In patients who are hypercoagulable from the nephrotic syndrome, prolonged bed rest increases their risk of venous thromboembolism. A variety of antihypertensive agents have proven effective and safe in managing hypertension in pregnancy when pharmacologic therapy is necessary. First-line agents include alpha methyldopa, hydralazine, or beta blockers. Experience with calcium channel blockers is limited. Alpha methyldopa, which remains the first-line drug of choice, may be started at 250 mg 3 to 4 times daily and increased to a maximum daily dose of 2 g. In hypertensive emergencies, intravenous labetalol is the drug of choice. Antihypertensive agents to be avoided include all angiotensin-converting enzyme inhibitors, reserpine, sodium nitroprusside, ganglion blocking agents, and clonidine. Judicious use of diuretics may be necessary in the volume-expanded hypertensive patient with chronic renal disease. In patients with renal insufficiency, magnesium sulfate must be used cautiously in the treatment of preeclampsia. Impaired renal excretion of magnesium can lead to dangerous hypermagnesemia and respiratory muscle paralysis in these patients. Alternative anti-seizure medications such as benzodiazepines should be considered in this situation.

Both peritoneal dialysis and hemodialysis have been used successfully in pregnant patients with ESRD. A special attempt should be made to provide efficient dialysis, keeping the BUN below 50 mg/dL. In those patients who progress to ESRD while pregnant, dialysis is generally initiated earlier than for the non-pregnant patient in an attempt to avoid any complications of the uremic syndrome.

BIBLIOGRAPHY

Daugirdas JT, Ing TS. Handbook of dialysis, 2nd ed. Boston: Little, Brown, 1994.

Davison JM. Dialysis, transplantation, and pregnancy. Am J Kidney Dis 1992;17:127.

Gabow PA. Polycystic kidney disease: clues to pathogenesis. Kidney Int 1991;40:989.

Greenberg A, Cheung AK, Coffman TM, et al. Primer on kidney diseases. San Diego, CA; Academic Press, 1994.

Hayslett JP. Maternal and fetal complications in pregnant women with systemic lupus erythematosus. Am J Kidney Dis 1991;17:123.

Jungers P, Houillier P, Forget D, Henry-Amar M. Specific controversies concerning the natural history of renal disease in pregnancy. Am J Kidney Dis 1991;17:116.

Kaplan NM. Clinical Hypertension, 5th ed. Baltimore: Williams & Wilkins, 1990.

Kasiske BL, Kalil RSN, Ma JZ, et al. Effect of antihypertensive therapy on the kidney in patients with diabetes: A meta-regression analysis. Ann Intern Med 1993;118:129.

Klahr S, Schreiner G, Ichikawa I. The progression of renal disease. N Engl J Med 1988;318:1657.

Knochel JP, Breyer JA, Cronin RE, et al. Medical knowledge self-assessment program in the subspecialty of nephrology and hypertension. Philadelphia:American College of Physicians, 1994.

Reece EA, Coustan DR, Hayslett JP, et al. Diabetic nephropathy: Pregnancy performance and fetomaternal outcome. Am J Obstet Gynecol 1988;159:56.

Rose BD. Pathophysiology of renal disease, 2nd ed. New York: McGraw-Hill, 1987.

Schrier RW, Gottschalk CW. Diseases of the kidney, 5th ed, vol 1. Little, Brown and Company, 1993.

Renal Data System. USRDS 1994 annual data report. Pub PB 95105003. Bethesda, MD: The National Institutes of Health, National Institute of Diabetes and Digestive and Kidney Diseases, July 1994.

Woodward JR, Rushton HG. Reflux nephropathy. Pediatr Clin North Am 1987;34:1349.

Primary Care for Women, edited by Phyllis C. Leppert and Fred M. Howard. Lippincott-Raven Publishers, Philadelphia © 1997.

78

Acute Renal Failure

AARON SPITAL
J. GARY ABUELO
RICHARD H. STERNS

Acute renal failure may be defined as a sudden fall in the glomerular filtration rate (GFR). Such a sudden loss of renal function, which occurs in up to 5% of hospitalized patients, can be a devastating event. Because the kidneys perform many vital functions, including maintenance of the proper volume and composition of body fluids, loss of renal function predisposes to serious fluid and electrolyte disorders and also may lead to dysfunction of many organ systems throughout the body. Thus, it is not surprising that acute renal failure causes significant morbidity and, at least when acquired in the hospital, is associated with a sixfold to eightfold increase in mortality.

The development of acute renal failure is usually brought to the physician's attention in one of three ways: (1) by an increasing blood urea nitrogen (BUN) or serum creatinine concentration; (2) by a fall in urine output; or, less commonly, (3) by a complication of the sudden loss of renal function, such as hyperkalemia or volume overload.

A rising serum creatinine concentration is the most reliable indicator of declining renal function. Creatinine is derived from muscle creatine and is removed from the blood primarily by glomerular filtration. Because creatinine is produced at a fairly constant rate proportional to muscle mass, acute changes in its serum level usually reflect changes in GFR, with a rise in creatinine concentration indicating a fall in GFR (Fig. 78-1). Rare exceptions may occur when interfering substances such as acetoacetate and cefoxitin spuriously raise the measured creatinine concentration, or when the normal small amount of tubular creatinine secretion is inhibited by drugs such as trimethoprim or cimetidine. In such cases, there may be a small increase in the serum creatinine without a fall in the GFR.

In general, the more rapid the increase in serum creatinine, the more severe the decrease in GFR. It is also important to understand that the serum creatinine concentration cannot be used to estimate the GFR in a nonsteady state. For example, if renal blood flow (RBF) is suddenly interrupted, the GFR drops to zero, but until creatinine has had time to accumulate, the serum creatinine remains normal. This concept has important implications for drug dosing in acute renal failure.

Although the BUN also correlates inversely with GFR, it is a less reliable indicator of renal function than is the serum creatinine. Urea is not only filtered, but it is also reabsorbed by the tubules at a rate which is directly proportional to water reabsorption. Therefore, in addition to the GFR, the state of hydration affects the efficiency of urea excretion (ie, its clearance) and hence the steady state serum level. For example, with dehydration, the BUN often is elevated out of proportion to the creatinine. Furthermore, in contrast to creatinine, which is produced at a fairly constant rate, the production of urea varies with the rate of protein metabolism. Thus, during ingestion of large amounts of protein, during hypercatabolism secondary to illness or steroids, or when there is blood in the gastrointestinal tract, the BUN may be elevated without a proportional fall in the GFR.

Urine volume is not a reliable marker of renal function. Whereas oliguria (< 400 to 500 mL of urine per day) does indicate that renal function is impaired, *the absence of oliguria does not mean that renal function is normal*. In fact, some estimates suggest that most cases of acute renal failure are nonoliguric, with the urine output remaining in the normal range.

DIFFERENTIAL DIAGNOSIS

When acute renal failure occurs, it is important to identify the etiology, because appropriate treatment varies according to the cause. However, frequently the kidneys have received multiple insults, and it is not always possible to identify one as being most important. Nevertheless, it is useful to divide acute renal failure into three major etiologic categories (Table 78-1): (1) prerenal azotemia, (2) renal azotemia, and (3) postrenal azotemia. (Azotemia refers to the retention of nitrogenous compounds in the blood, which results from decreased excretion secondary to impaired renal function.)

Prerenal Azotemia

Prerenal azotemia is probably the most common form of acute renal failure. It is defined as renal failure that develops as a consequence of reduced perfusion of otherwise healthy kidneys. This may result from absolute volume depletion (eg, from hemorrhage, urinary or gastrointestinal fluid loss), effective volume depletion (eg, congestive heart failure or pericardial tamponade), renal vasoconstriction despite systemic vasodilation (eg, liver disease or sepsis), or obstruction of the renal arteries (eg, bilateral renal artery stenosis). The hallmark of prerenal azotemia is its reversibility with restoration of normal renal perfusion.

Although the glomerular capillary pressure is an important determinant of GFR, a major reduction in renal perfusion pressure is required before the GFR falls in healthy people. This is because autoregulation maintains the GFR and RBF relatively constant over a wide range of perfusion pressures, until the mean arterial pressure falls below about 80 mm Hg; at this point, RBF and GFR decline precipitously with further decreases in blood pressure (Fig. 78-2). However, in patients with hypertensive, diabetic, or atherosclerotic vascular disease, the ability to autoregulate may be markedly impaired, predisposing such

Table 78-1 Differential Diagnosis of Acute Renal Failure

Prerenal Azotemia

- Absolute volume depletion
  - Hemorrhage
  - GI losses
    - Vomiting
    - Diarrhea
    - Fistulas
  - Renal losses
    - Diuretic drugs
    - Osmotic diuresis
    - Salt-wasting
  - Third spacing
- Effective volume depletion
  - Cardiac dysfunction
    - Heart failure
    - Arrhythmias
    - Valvular dysfunction
    - Pericardial tamponade
    - Pulmonary embolism
  - Peripheral vasodilatation
    - Sepsis
    - Liver failure
    - Antihypertensive drugs
  - Renal vascular obstruction
    - Renal artery stenosis, thrombosis
    - Renal artery embolism
    - Dissecting aneurysm
  - Impaired autoregulation
    - NSAIDs
    - ACE inhibitors
    - Hypercalcemia

Postrenal Azotemia

See Table 78-2

Renal Azotemia

- Glomerulonephritis
  - RPGN
  - Lupus nephritis
  - Goodpasture syndrome
  - Poststreptococcal
  - Endocarditis
- Vascular disorders
  - Vasculitis
  - TTP
  - Scleroderma
  - Malignant hypertension
  - Cholesterol emboli
- Tubulointerstitial disorders
  - ATN
    - Ischemia
    - Nephrotoxins
      - Aminoglycosides
      - Radiocontrast agents
      - Heavy metals
      - Amphotericin
      - Cisplatin
      - Foscarnet
    - Pigment induced
      - Myoglobinuria
      - Hemoglobinuria
  - Acute interstitial nephritis
    - Drugs
    - Infection
    - Systemic disease
    - Idiopathic
  - Tubular obstruction
    - Uric acid nephropathy
    - Ethylene glycol intoxication
    - Methotrexate
    - Acyclovir
  - Neoplastic disorders
    - Lymphomatous infiltration
    - Myeloma kidney

ACE, angiotensin converting enzyme; *ATN,* acute tubular necrosis; *GI,* gastrointestinal; *NSAIDs,* nonsteroidal antiinflammatory drugs; *RPGN,* rapidly progressive glomerulonephritis; *TTP,* thrombotic thrombocytopenic purpura.

individuals to prerenal azotemia, even during small reductions in perfusion pressure.

When cardiac output is low, either because of hypovolemia or heart disease, blood pressure is maintained by high levels of systemically active vasoconstricting substances (eg, angiotensin II and catecholamines). These vasoconstrictors also increase the resistance to blood flow in the kidney. If unopposed, this effect decreases RBF and GFR. Because renal vasoconstriction is mitigated by vasodilatory prostaglandins, the administration of nonsteroidal antiinflammatory drugs (NSAIDs), which block prostaglandin synthesis, can dramatically reduce RBF and GFR in patients with impaired tissue perfusion.

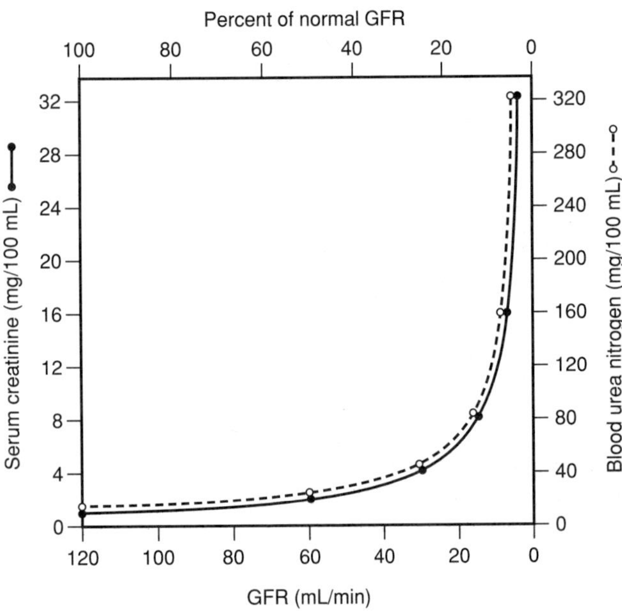

Figure 78-1. Relationship of the serum creatinine and blood urea nitrogen to the glomerular filtration rate (GFR). (Kassirer JP. N Engl J Med 1971;285:385.)

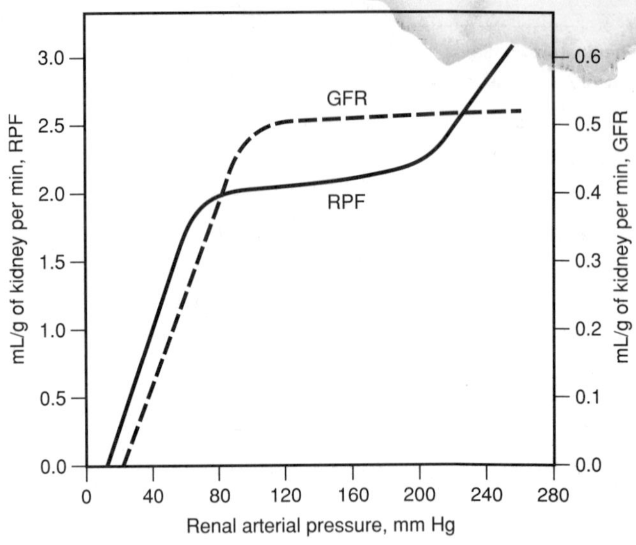

Figure 78-2. Autoregulation of glomerular filtration rate (GFR) and renal blood flow (RBF) in the dog. (Rose BD. Renal circulation and glomerular filtration rate. In: Clinical physiology of acid–base and electrolyte disorders. New York:McGraw-Hill, 1984.)

Angiotensin converting enzyme (ACE) inhibitors also can reduce the GFR when renal perfusion is compromised, as in bilateral renal artery stenosis or severe congestive heart failure. In these conditions, maintenance of the GFR becomes partially dependent on angiotensin II, which constricts glomerular efferent arterioles and thereby preserves glomerular capillary hydrostatic pressure.

Postrenal Azotemia

Postrenal azotemia refers to renal failure that develops as a consequence of obstruction to urine flow from otherwise healthy kidneys. Obstruction increases the pressure in the renal tubules and Bowman space, thereby opposing glomerular filtration. Like prerenal azotemia, if recognized and treated promptly, postrenal azotemia is completely reversible. Whereas some authors include in this category intrarenal obstruction, for example, from precipitation of uric acid or light chains within the tubules, we restrict the term postrenal azotemia to mean obstruction occurring outside the kidney. This may develop anywhere along the urinary tract (Table 78-2). However, because most people have two kidneys and because a healthy kidney can compensate in large part for the loss of its mate, obstruction must involve both collecting systems to cause a marked change in overall renal function. Therefore, when the serum creatinine is more than mildly elevated due to upper tract obstruction (ie, above the bladder), this implies that either both ureters are involved or that the patient had only one healthy kidney. On the other hand, lower urinary tract obstruction (eg, of the urethra or bladder trigone) requires only one localized anatomic process to interrupt the entire flow of urine, thereby causing renal failure. In catheterized patients, an unusual cause of such lower tract obstruction is an obstructed Foley catheter.

It is a common misconception that when acute renal failure is caused by obstruction, the urine flow is always low. This is only true when obstruction is complete. With partial obstruction, the patient usually is not oliguric. Therefore, postrenal azotemia may present with virtually any urine volume, including anuria (ie, no urine), oliguria, normal, or even high urine flow. Rarely, when obstruction is intermittent, there may even be alternating polyuria and anuria.

Renal Azotemia

Renal azotemia refers to the development of renal dysfunction secondary to pathologic processes developing within the kidney itself. It is useful to further subdivide these processes according to the primary structure affected: (1) glomerulonephritis, which may be primary (eg, poststreptococcal or rapidly progressive) or secondary to a systemic disease (eg, systemic lupus erythematosus [SLE] or endocarditis); (2) vascular disorders (eg, vasculitis, malignant hypertension, thrombotic thrombocytopenic purpura [TTP], and cholesterol embolization); (3) interstitial nephritis, which is most commonly due to a hypersensitivity reaction to certain drugs but also may be seen occasionally in some systemic diseases (eg, SLE, sarcoidosis), infections, and rarely as an idiopathic process; and (4) tubular disorders, which include acute tubular necrosis (ATN) and intratubular obstruction (eg, from precipitation of uric acid, oxalate, light chains, methotrexate, and acyclovir). These categories are not mutually exclusive, and often several structures are involved simultaneously. Notice that uncomplicated urinary tract infection is not on this list because it does not cause renal failure.

ATN is the most common cause of intrinsic acute renal failure in hospitalized patients. The term ATN actually is a misnomer because histologic evidence of tubular necrosis is sparse and limited primarily to the late proximal tubule and loop of Henle. These parts of the nephron are located in the medulla, where the PO_2 is normally low. The thick ascending limb of Henle loop is particularly susceptible to hypoxic injury because its cells have the highest metabolic rate of any tubular cells.

TABLE 78-2. Causes of Postrenal Azotemia in Women

Ureteral
Intraluminal
Stones
Sloughed papillae
Diabetes mellitus
Sickle cell disease
Analgesic nephropathy
Blood clots
Fungus balls
Ureteral malignancy
Extraluminal
Retroperitoneal or pelvic malignancy
Lymphoma
Colonic
Cervical
Ovarian
Retroperitoneal abscess, hematoma, or fibrosis
Pelvic abscess
Surgical injury
Endometriosis
Pregnancy
Uterine prolapse
Aneurysm
Bladder
Carcinoma
Neurogenic bladder
Diabetes mellitus
Spinal cord injury and disease
Anticholinergic drugs
Narcotics
Ganglionic blockers
Urethra
Carcinoma
Stones
Obstructed urethral catheter

ATN usually develops in the setting of serious illness or injury or postoperatively, and is caused by one or more of the following: (1) ischemic injury; (2) pigmenturia (ie, myoglobinuria or hemoglobinuria) resulting from rhabdomyolysis or massive intravascular hemolysis; or (3) nephrotoxins. Ischemic ATN is probably the commonest form of severe hospital-acquired acute renal failure. It usually develops within 24 hours of a readily identifiable event that severely compromises renal perfusion, such as a hypotensive episode.

The two most common causes of nephrotoxic acute renal failure in hospitalized patients are aminoglycosides and radiocontrast agents. Aminoglycoside nephrotoxicity develops in about 10% of patients receiving a full course of therapy, and usually requires at least several days of drug administration. It may occur even when aminoglycoside levels are maintained within the recommended therapeutic range. When renal failure does occur, it is usually nonoliguric and manifested by a slowly rising serum creatinine. Radiocontrast-induced acute renal failure presents as a rising serum creatinine beginning within 24 to 48 hours of the procedure. Diabetics with baseline renal insufficiency are at greatest risk, but even in these patients, only a minority develop clinically important renal failure.

Why the GFR falls in ATN is not certain. Theories include tubular obstruction secondary to cellular debris, back-leak of filtrate through damaged tubules, reduced renal blood flow secondary to vasoconstriction (perhaps mediated by tubuloglomerular feedback), and a reduction in the permeability of the glomerular filtration barrier.

In contrast to prerenal and postrenal azotemia, there is no established intervention that rapidly reverses ATN. Nevertheless, it is important to eliminate causative factors, because if the patient does not die from the underlying disease and if further renal insults are avoided, renal function usually returns to normal. Despite good supportive care, the serum creatinine frequently continues to rise at a rate proportional to the degree of renal injury; the maximum increase is 2 to 3 mg/dL/day.

Community Versus Hospital-Acquired Acute Renal Failure

Prerenal azotemia is common in both inpatient and outpatient settings; however, postrenal azotemia, glomerulonephritis, and certain nephrotoxins (such as NSAIDs and ethylene glycol) are much more common among community-acquired cases, whereas ATN caused by ischemia, surgery, or aminoglycosides is primarily a disorder of hospitalized patients. Therefore, when trying to identify the origin of acute renal failure, it is worthwhile considering whether it developed inside or outside of the hospital.

The Importance of Searching for Treatable Reversible Causes

When evaluating a patient with acute renal failure, it is important to search carefully for causes that are treatable and reversible. In such cases, prompt, appropriate intervention will improve renal function and may prevent permanent renal damage. The most important examples include prerenal azotemia from volume depletion or sepsis, urinary tract obstruction, and renal failure caused by NSAIDs, ACE inhibitors, and aminoglycosides.

CLINICAL MANIFESTATIONS

In patients with acute renal failure, a variety of signs and symptoms may be encountered. These usually result from either the underlying pathologic process causing renal dysfunction or from the complications of renal failure.

Signs and Symptoms of the Causative Process

Although rarely diagnostic, signs and symptoms may suggest the pathologic process causing acute renal failure. For example, symptoms of voiding difficulty and flank pain may accompany urinary tract obstruction. Flank pain also may be seen with renal infarction, renal vein thrombosis, or inflammatory processes affecting the kidneys, such as glomerulonephritis or interstitial nephritis. Gross hematuria also suggests several possibilities, including glomerulonephritis, nephrolithiasis, papillary necrosis, or an obstructing malignancy. A history of a seizure or trauma raises the possibility of rhabdomyolysis and myoglobinuric renal failure, whereas vomiting, diarrhea or diuresis points to volume depletion and prerenal azotemia. Fever, skin rash, and eosinophilia are typical of drug-induced acute interstitial nephritis. A declining urine output is a nonspecific indicator of renal dysfunction.

Sometimes, acute renal failure is caused by a systemic disease. In such cases, the manifestations of the underlying process may dominate the clinical picture. For example, joint pains and skin rashes are common in patients with lupus nephritis; bone pain, anemia, and hypercalcemia suggest multiple myeloma; fever, anemia, and heart murmurs point to endocarditis (which can cause glomerulonephritis); focal digital ischemia and livedo reticularis are typical of cholesterol embolization; general malaise, joint pains, palpable purpura, and sinusitis suggest vasculitis; hemoptysis is frequent in Goodpasture syndrome; jaundice and ascites suggest hepatorenal syndrome; and thrombocytopenic nonpalpable purpura is characteristic of patients with TTP.

Complications of Acute Renal Failure

Numerous complications may punctuate the course of acute renal failure and result in a variety of signs and symptoms (Table 78-3). Continued intake of sodium and water in the face of impaired excretory capacity causes volume overload, which may result in peripheral and pulmonary edema. If more free water is taken in than is lost through renal and nonrenal routes, hyponatremia ensues. Hyperkalemia is an ever-present danger, particularly in oliguric patients, and may be precipitated by endogenous (eg, secondary to tissue injury, as may occur in rhabdomyolysis or bowel necrosis) or exogenous sources of potassium; hyperkalemia may cause serious cardiac arrhythmias and, when severe, even cardiac arrest. High anion gap metabolic acidosis is common and results from an impaired ability to excrete the daily acid load; compensatory hyperventilation may be manifested by Kussmaul respirations and dyspnea. Hypocalcemia and hyperphosphatemia also are frequently seen.

Neurologic complications of severe azotemia include altered personality, confusion, asterixis, myoclonus, seizures, and coma. Anorexia, nausea, and vomiting are classic gastrointestinal symptoms of renal failure, and gastrointestinal hemorrhage also may occur. Uremic pericarditis, increased susceptibility to infection, anemia, and a bleeding diathesis (secondary to platelet dysfunction) are other common complications.

Table 78-3. Potential Complications of Acute Renal Failure

Electrolyte
Hyperkalemia
Hyponatremia
Metabolic acidosis
Hypocalcemia
Hyperphosphatemia
Hypermagnesemia
Cardiopulmonary
Pulmonary edema
Pericarditis
Arrhythmias
Gastrointestinal
Nausea
Vomiting
Anorexia
Hemorrhage
Hematologic
Anemia
Platelet dysfunction
Neurologic
Confusion
Obtundation
Asterixis
Myoclonus
Seizures
Dialytic
Infections
Urinary
Pulmonary
Wound
Bacteremia
Drug toxicity

EVALUATION OF THE PATIENT WITH ACUTE RENAL FAILURE

When approaching a patient with an elevated serum creatinine concentration, the first step is to rapidly exclude life-threatening complications that require urgent treatment, such as hyperkalemia and pulmonary edema. Once this is accomplished, the first diagnostic issue to address is whether the elevation in creatinine is acute or chronic. The most reliable way to answer this question is to review previous laboratory data. When old creatinine values are unavailable, the serum creatinine should be checked daily for several days, because the resulting picture indicates whether renal function is stable or changing. However, even a stable elevation of serum creatinine may be the result of a relatively new process. In such cases, an assessment of kidney size (eg, by ultrasonography) may be helpful, because small kidneys are indicative of chronic disease.

Whenever the duration of renal failure remains in doubt, one should always assume that the process is new because acute renal failure is frequently treatable and reversible, whereas chronic renal failure is not. Furthermore, when a patient with known chronic renal disease develops a rising serum creatinine, one should not automatically assume that this is secondary to progression of the underlying disease; such patients are more susceptible to additional renal insults than are healthy individuals, and therefore the physician must exclude a superimposed new process.

After concluding that acute renal failure is present, the next step is to try to determine the cause. In general, outpatients should be evaluated in the hospital because of the danger of complications, unless renal failure is mild and easily correctable (eg, worsening prerenal azotemia secondary to excessive diuresis in a patient with heart failure).

History and Physical Examination

The evaluation should begin with a careful history and physical examination directed particularly toward finding reversible processes that require intervention. Therefore, the physician should search for clues pointing to prerenal azotemia (eg, diarrhea, vomiting, diuresis, bleeding, or heart failure), postrenal azotemia (eg, flank pain, gross hematuria, voiding difficulty, or a history of pelvic malignancy or urinary stones), or drug-induced acute interstitial nephritis (eg, fever and skin rash). Nephrotoxins (eg, aminoglycosides, NSAIDs, or ACE inhibitors) and symptoms of treatable systemic diseases that often involve the kidneys (eg, SLE, endocarditis, and multiple myeloma) also should be sought.

In hospitalized patients, it is important to search the medical record for hypotensive and septic episodes, surgical procedures, and angiographic or other radiocontrast studies, particularly on the day before the serum creatinine began to rise. If available, changes in weight and imbalances in input and output should be noted. A complete review of medications (including over-the-counter drugs) is critical. Finally, the physician should always be aware of the patient's previous medical history, asking specifically about diabetes mellitus, cardiovascular disease, and intravenous drug abuse.

The physical examination is also directed toward uncovering treatable problems. A careful assessment of the volume status is critical for diagnosing prerenal azotemia and for recognizing volume overload. Proper assessment of volume status requires examining the patient, including measurement of orthostatic changes in pulse and blood pressure, and cannot be estimated from laboratory data alone. For example, the urine sodium concentration and osmolality are similar in all prerenal states, whether caused by absolute or effective volume depletion (eg, from heart failure).

The patient also should be examined for the presence of fever, skin coolness and rashes, generalized and focal cyanosis, livedo reticularis, hypertensive retinopathy, cardiac murmurs, flank and muscle tenderness, bruits, diminished pulses, and a palpable distended bladder. Rectal and pelvic examinations can be helpful in identifying diseases that can cause obstruction.

Table 78-4 Diagnostic Studies in the Evaluation of Acute Renal Failure

Routine blood tests
BUN, creatinine
Glucose
Electrolytes
Calcium, phosphorus
Protein, albumin
Uric acid
LDH, bilirubin
CBC, differential
Selected blood tests
Arterial blood gases
Blood cultures
ANA
ANCA
ASLO titer, streptozyme test
Anti-GBM antibody
Cryoglobulins
Complement
Protein electrophoresis
CPK
Osmolality
Magnesium
Routine urine tests
Urinalysis
Selected urine tests
Hansel stain (eosinophils)
Sodium, osmolality, creatinine
Protein electrophoresis
Uric acid
Renal Ultrasonography
Radionuclide renography
Chest x-ray
Electrocardiogram

ANA, antinuclear antibody; *ANCA,* antineutrophil cytoplasmic antibody; *anti-GBM,* anti–glomerular basement membrane; *ASLO,* antistreptolysin-O; *BUN,* blood urea nitrogen; *CBC,* complete blood cell count; *CPK,* creatine phosphokinase; *LDH,* lactate dehydrogenase.

Laboratory Studies

All patients should have a standard biochemical profile and a complete blood cell count (Table 78-4), because these may help pinpoint the etiology of acute renal failure and identify complications. For example, an increase in the BUN-to-creatinine ratio suggests prerenal azotemia. A low platelet count associated with hemolytic anemia raises the question of TTP. Eosinophilia suggests acute interstitial nephritis or cholesterol embolization. An isolated elevation of lactate dehydrogenase may be due to renal infarction or hemolysis (as seen in TTP), whereas an elevated creatinine phosphokinase points to rhabdomyolysis and myoglobinuric renal failure. An extremely high uric acid level in a patient with a hematologic malignancy suggests uric acid nephropathy. Hypercalcemia, or even an inappropriately normal serum calcium, may be a clue to the presence of malignancy (including multiple myeloma) or the milk-alkali syndrome.

Blood cultures should be obtained in febrile patients to exclude endocarditis and sepsis. A serologic screen (including antinuclear antibody (ANA), complement, and antineutrophil cytoplasmic antibody (ANCA) levels) is indicated when renal involvement secondary to SLE or vasculitis is suspected. In elderly patients with

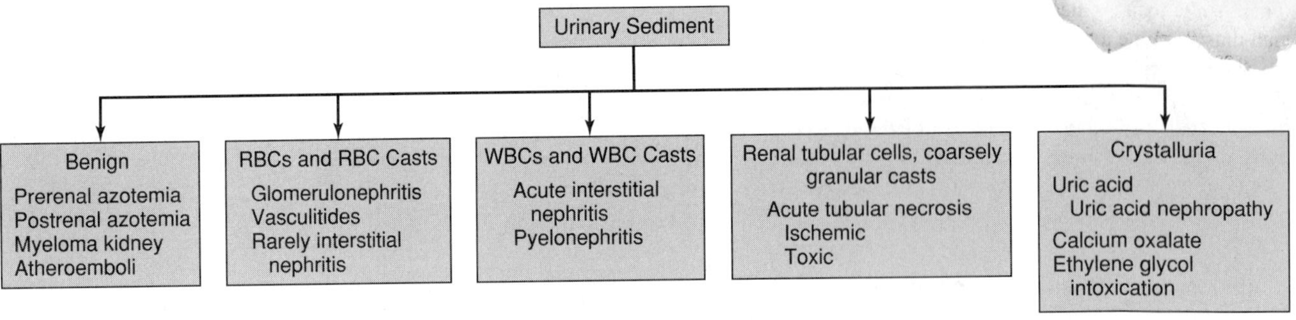

Figure 78-3. Use of the urinary sediment to help localize the cause of acute renal failure. *RBC*, red blood cell; *WBC*, white blood cell.

unexplained acute renal failure, urine and serum protein electrophoresis should be obtained to exclude unsuspected multiple myeloma.

Urinalysis

A careful urinalysis can be of enormous help in determining the cause of acute renal failure (Fig. 78-3). A normal urinalysis suggests prerenal and postrenal azotemia, although hyaline casts are common in the former and hematuria and crystalluria may be seen in the latter. When azotemia is due to intrinsic renal disease, the urine sediment is usually abnormal, but may be benign in renal failure caused by myeloma, hypercalcemia, or cholesterol embolization. Hematuria, proteinuria, and red blood cell casts point to acute glomerulonephritis, whereas white blood cells (especially eosinophils) and while white blood cell casts suggest acute interstitial nephritis. Renal tubular cells and brown granular casts suggest ATN. Calcium oxalate crystals raise the possibility of ethylene glycol intoxication, whereas uric acid crystals may be seen in acute uric acid nephropathy and in uric acid nephrolithiasis. Urine that is dipstick positive for blood but contains few or no red blood cells, suggests myoglobinuria or hemoglobinuria.

Renal Imaging

In all patients with unexplained acute renal failure, urinary tract obstruction must be excluded, because this is a treatable reversible condition. Renal ultrasonography has emerged as the screening procedure of choice because it has been shown to be highly sensitive and specific for the detection of obstruction. However, this technique does not detect obstruction directly, but rather, its usual consequence: dilatation of the collecting system. Rarely, urinary tract obstruction may not cause dilatation (eg, when the ureters are encased by fibrosis or malignancy). In these unusual cases, renal ultrasonography may give false-negative results. Therefore, when the index of suspicion is high, despite normal findings on ultrasonography, other diagnostic approaches must be considered, including retrograde and antegrade pyelography.

Renal ultrasonography also provides a reliable estimate of renal size. This may be helpful when the duration of renal failure is uncertain. Marked asymmetry suggests unilateral obstruction or renovascular disease.

A radionuclide renal scan provides an estimate of renal blood flow and shows whether perfusion is homogeneous. This study may be useful to screen for suspected renal infarction or bilateral renal artery thrombosis.

Urinary Indices

On occasion, it may be difficult to distinguish prerenal azotemia from ATN. In such cases, urinary indices measured on a "spot" urine specimen may be helpful (Table 78-5). Prerenal azotemia is characterized by a concentrated, sodium-free urine, whereas in ATN the urine is isosmotic and contains sodium. However, there is overlap between these groups, especially when other factors affecting urinary concentrating ability and sodium excretion are at play (eg, recent diuretic use). Overlap may be reduced, although not eliminated, by calculating the fractional excretion of filtered sodium (FeNa):

$$\text{FeNa} = \frac{(\text{U/P})_{\text{Na}}}{(\text{U/P})_{\text{Cr}}} \times 100\%$$

where U and P are the urine and plasma concentrations, respectively, of sodium (Na) and creatinine (Cr).

Urine Volume

Whereas the urine volume generally is not helpful diagnostically, total anuria is unusual and suggests complete urinary tract obstruction, bilateral renal artery occlusion, shock, or cortical necrosis. Alternating anuria and polyuria suggests intermittent obstruction.

Role of Renal Biopsy

Renal biopsy should be considered when the origin of acute renal failure remains unclear after a thorough investigation. Renal biopsy also should be considered in patients with a presentation

Table 78-5 Urinary Indices in Acute Renal Failure

INDEX	PRERENAL	ATN
U_{osm} (mOsm/kg H_2O)	> 500	< 350
U_{Na} (mEq/L)	< 20	> 40
FeNa (%)	< 1	> 1

ATN, acute tubular necrosis: *FeNa,* fractional excretion of filtered sodium; U_{Na}, urinary sodium concentration; U_{osm}, urinary osmolality.

suggestive of rapidly progressive glomerulonephritis, which may occur as an idiopathic process or secondary to a variety of systemic diseases, because this disorder may be reversible with appropriate treatment.

PREVENTION

Be aware of risk factors for the development of acute renal failure. Such knowledge allows the physician to implement preventive strategies and to identify patients who need to be monitored closely so that if renal failure does occur, it will be detected and managed early, before life-threatening complications occur. Important risk factors include the following:

- Reduced renal perfusion (eg, secondary to volume depletion, heart failure, major surgery, or sepsis)
- Exposure to nephrotoxins (eg, aminoglycosides, radiocontrast agents in diabetics with renal dysfunction, cisplatin, amphotericin, NSAIDs in patients with decreased perfusion, and ACE inhibitors in patients with bilateral renal artery stenosis)
- Treatment of hematologic malignancies
- Extensive muscle injury
- Diffuse vascular disease
- Preexisting renal dysfunction

Debilitated elderly patients also seem to be at higher risk than those who are younger and in better physical condition.

The following are general principles of prevention: (1) optimize renal perfusion by avoiding or correcting absolute volume depletion, treating heart failure, and eliminating systemic infection; (2) avoid nephrotoxic agents whenever possible, using them only when a safer alternative does not exist; and (3) always consider whether the potential benefits of any planned invasive procedure, such as vascular surgery or angiography, outweigh the renal (and other) risks.

Observations from uncontrolled studies suggest that in some settings, more specific preventive measures may be of value. Examples include the use of allopurinol, saline, and possibly bicarbonate before chemotherapy of certain hematologic malignancies; mannitol, bicarbonate, and saline in patients with rhabdomyolysis; mannitol and saline before amphotericin, or vascular or biliary surgery; and volume expansion with saline alone before and after administration of radiocontrast agents.

TREATMENT

The goals of treatment of acute renal failure include (1) facilitation of recovery of renal function; (2) correction of established complications; and (3) avoidance of new complications.

Facilitation of renal recovery can be readily achieved when acute renal failure is caused by reversible factors that are identified and appropriately treated. For example, prerenal azotemia can be repaired by restoring renal perfusion, postrenal azotemia by relieving urinary obstruction, and certain types of nephrotoxic renal failure reverse with removal of the offending agent. Renal involvement in some systemic diseases also may be treatable. Even when dealing with established ATN, renal hypoperfusion and nephrotoxic insults should be avoided because these may interfere with recovery. Good general supportive care, including prevention and eradication of infection and provision of adequate nutrition, also is extremely important. With regard to the latter, remember that acute renal failure is a catabolic state, and therefore the need for calories and nutrients is increased.

The role of diuretics in established oliguric ATN is uncertain. When administered early in the course, mannitol and high doses of loop diuretics frequently lead to an increase in urine flow and may convert some oliguric patients to nonoliguric ones. There is also some evidence that low-dose dopamine, combined with furosemide, can increase urine output in patients resistant to furosemide alone. However, it is not known if such an induced increase in urine flow improves prognosis. Although it appears that "responders" have a lower mortality than do "nonresponders," it is possible that a response to diuretics merely identifies patients with intrinsically less severe disease. Nevertheless, because it is easier to manage nonoliguric patients, it is reasonable to try a single large dose of furosemide (160 to 240 mg over 40 to 60 minutes), alone or in combination with low-dose dopamine, early in the course of ATN. If there is no response, these agents should be discontinued.

There is no evidence that continuous "renal-dose dopamine" is of value in established ATN. Furthermore, dopamine is not benign. Therefore, continuous infusions of dopamine are not recommended for treating acute renal failure in the absence of hypotension. Other potentially therapeutic agents under active investigation include atrial natriuretic peptide, calcium channel blockers, prostaglandin analogues, adenine nucleotides, growth factors, and scavengers of oxygen free radicals.

Potential complications of acute renal failure have been discussed earlier. Perhaps the most lethal is hyperkalemia. To avoid this, the plasma potassium (and other electrolytes) should be monitored at least daily and potassium intake should be restricted. However, severe hyperkalemia may develop despite exogenous potassium restriction because of cellular potassium release from injured tissue and hypercatabolism. Life-threatening hyperkalemia, defined as a plasma potassium concentration greater than 6.5 mEq/L or electrocardiographic changes beyond peaked T waves (eg, loss of P waves, widened QRS complexes), requires immediate treatment with intravenous calcium gluconate, glucose and insulin, and sometimes bicarbonate (Table 78-6). Inhaled β_2 agonists also can rapidly lower the plasma potassium in some patients. However, these treatments do not eliminate excess potassium from the body. Potassium removal is vital and can be accomplished in most patients with oral or rectal sodium polystyrene sulfonate (Kayexalate). Forty grams of this cation exchange resin given orally (in sorbitol) every 2 to 3 hours is usually highly effective. In the unusual cases where this approach is unsuccessful, hemodialysis is required, which rapidly removes potassium from the body.

Volume overload and hyponatremia should be avoided by limiting sodium and water intake to match output. Remember that large amounts of fluid often are given during the administration of drugs and must be taken into account. When volume overload occurs in oliguric patients or when large volumes of fluid are required to provide nutrition, fluid removal by dialysis or newer ultrafiltration techniques is required. Daily weights are extremely helpful in assessing changes in volume status.

Acid-base status and calcium and phosphate levels also should be monitored regularly. Metabolic acidosis, although common, is usually not severe enough to require specific therapy. Indeed, aggressive correction of acidemia in hypocalcemic patients may

Table 78-6. Therapy for Hyperkalemia

DRUG	DOSE	ONSET OF ACTION
Calcium gluconate	10–30 mL of 10% solution	Few minutes
$NaHCO_3$	44–132 mEq	15–30 min
Glucose and insulin	Glucose: 25–50 g/h by continuous IV drip	15–30 min
	Regular insulin: 5 U IV q 15 min	
Sodium polystyrene sulfonate (Kayexalate)	Enema (50–100 g)	60 min
	Oral (40 g)	120 min

$NaHCO_3$, sodium bicarbonate; *IV*, intravenous; *q*, every.

(Tannen RL. Potassium disorders. In: Kokko,Tannen, eds. Fluids and electrolytes. Philadelphia: WB Saunders, 1986.)

precipitate tetany by decreasing the ionized calcium concentration. In patients having oral intake, hypocalcemia and hyperphosphatemia can usually be controlled with calcium carbonate (eg, Tums); this agent limits phosphorus absorption in the intestine while providing supplemental calcium. Magnesium-containing antacids should be avoided because magnesium excretion is impaired in renal failure.

The dosage of medications that are excreted by the kidneys must be adjusted appropriately in acute renal failure. As previously discussed, when the serum creatinine is rapidly increasing, it cannot be used to estimate the GFR. In such cases, it is best to assume that the GFR is less than 10 mL/minute and dose medications accordingly, following drug levels when possible. If the serum creatinine stabilizes, the GFR for women can be estimated from the following formula:

$$\frac{(140 - \text{age}) \times \text{Weight (kg)}}{72 \times \text{Screatinine}} \times 0.85$$

(To calculate the GFR for men, do not multiply by 0.85.) When prescribing narcotics, meperidine should not be used because its metabolites accumulate in renal failure and can cause seizures.

Because infection remains the leading cause of death in acute renal failure, unnecessary instrumentation is to be avoided. Foley catheters are not useful in nonobstructed oligoanuric patients and also should be avoided in nonoliguric patients who are awake and able to void normally.

It is also important to check the bleeding time before performing invasive procedures such as renal biopsy or surgery, or in the presence of refractory hemorrhage. If prolonged, the bleeding time may be shortened by intravenous DDAVP (0.3 μg/kg given over 30 minutes in 50 mL of normal saline). The role of erythropoietin in the management of anemia in acute renal failure has not been established, although it seems reasonable to use this agent when renal function does not improve quickly.

When acute renal failure is severe and prolonged, dialysis or another extracorporeal cleansing technique (eg, continuous hemodiafiltration) usually becomes necessary. In general, to avoid complications, dialysis should be instituted prophylactically to maintain the BUN and creatinine concentrations below 100 mg/dL and 10 mg/dL, respectively. There is no evidence that more intensive dialysis improves prognosis. Emergent indications for dialysis include refractory hyperkalemia, pulmonary edema, and, possibly, uremic seizures. Other less urgent indications include metabolic acidosis, pericarditis, and uremic symptoms.

After relief of urinary tract obstruction or during the diuretic phase of recovering ATN, most patients simply excrete any excess sodium and water previously retained. Rarely, patients develop a severe concentrating defect and sodium wasting. The resulting inappropriate losses must be replaced to avoid volume depletion and hypernatremia.

PROGNOSIS

Despite advances in supportive and dialytic care, hospital-acquired oliguric ATN remains a deadly disease, with an overall mortality rate of about 50%. However, most treated patients who die do so not because of acute renal failure per se, but rather because of severe underlying illness or the development of major complications. Indeed, one of the most important prognostic factors is the number of other organ systems that fail. For example, in patients with isolated acute renal failure, the mortality rate may be less than 10%; however, if three or more additional organs fail, the mortality rate approaches 100%. The development of respiratory failure and sepsis are particularly ominous.

Other prognostic markers include the urine output and the severity of renal failure. The mortality rate of nonoliguric patients (25%) is only about half that of oliguric patients (50%), perhaps because nonoliguric renal failure indicates milder renal injury and generally correlates with less severe underlying disease. Indeed, in some studies of ATN, mortality correlates directly with the severity of renal failure. Not surprisingly, readily treatable forms of acute renal failure, such as prerenal and postrenal azotemia, and those caused by nephrotoxins have a much better prognosis than does ischemic ATN.

Most patients who survive recover normal or nearly normal renal function after a variable period of time. Patients with easily correctable causes, such as prerenal or postrenal azotemia, recover quickly after appropriate therapy. Patients with ATN will usually require longer to regain function, typically about 1 to 3 weeks.

ACUTE RENAL FAILURE IN PREGNANCY

Acute renal failure is distinctly uncommon in pregnant women, who are generally young and healthy. Nevertheless, to facilitate recognition of the rare cases which do occur, the physician should be aware of the normal renal physiologic changes that take place during pregnancy, and of the unique conditions that may cause renal failure in this setting.

Physiologic Changes in Renal Function and Blood Pressure During Pregnancy

During normal pregnancy, a reduction in systemic vascular resistance leads to a rise in cardiac output and a fall in diastolic blood pressure of about 10 to 15 mm Hg. Near term, the blood pressure rises again toward prepregnancy levels. An increase in diastolic blood pressure of more than 15 mm Hg or in systolic pressure of more than 30 mm Hg from values earlier in pregnancy, or a blood pressure greater than or equal to 140/90 mm Hg defines hypertension.

The renal plasma flow and GFR gradually increase to about 50% above prepregnancy levels by the second trimester, and these increases are sustained until delivery. As a result, the BUN and serum creatinine concentrations fall to mean values of 9 and 0.5 mg/dL, respectively, with 15 and 0.8 mg/dL being the upper limits of normal. Urinary protein excretion also increases in pregnancy, so that 250 to 300 mg/day (rather than 150 mg) is the upper limit of normal. In response to hormonal changes and perhaps uterine compression, the urinary collecting system dilates during pregnancy and remains so for up to 12 weeks postpartum; this physiologic response complicates noninvasive radiologic evaluation of possible urinary tract obstruction.

Causes of Renal Failure in Pregnancy

Whereas gravid women may develop any of the forms of acute renal failure previously discussed, these are much less common than those that only occur during and soon after pregnancy, such as ATN secondary to ischemia from uterine hemorrhage and idiopathic postpartum renal failure. Table 78-7 lists these and other less common causes of acute renal failure unique to gestation.

Hyperemesis gravidarum is a condition characterized by idiopathic intractable vomiting occurring during the second and third months of pregnancy. Volume depletion may result and induce prerenal azotemia. Treatment usually includes hospitalization, metoclopramide, fluid, electrolyte and vitamin replacement, and, in some cases, parenteral nutrition.

The gravid uterus, particularly when overdistended by polyhydramnios or multiple gestations, may obstruct the ureters and cause postrenal azotemia. Treatment options include delivery, drainage of polyhydramnios, bypassing the obstruction with ureteral catheters, or placing a percutaneous nephrostomy tube.

Preeclampsia is a syndrome unique to pregnancy characterized by the development of hypertension, edema, and proteinuria occurring after the 20th week of gestation. Renal insufficiency with a mild increase in serum creatinine is common. The characteristic pathologic finding in the kidneys is swelling of glomerular endothelial cells. Whereas preeclampsia is probably the most common cause of renal dysfunction in pregnancy, the serum creatinine rarely exceeds 1.3 mg/dL in the absence of other complications.

Acute fatty liver of pregnancy is a rare condition that develops late in the third trimester or early puerperium. Patients present with abdominal pain and vomiting and then develop jaundice, mildly elevated liver enzymes, and disseminated intravascular coagulation. Renal failure, which is usually mild, may complicate the course and is probably due to a variant of the hepatorenal syndrome.

The syndrome of *h*emolysis, *e*levated *l*iver function test results, and a *l*ow *p*latelet count (HELLP syndrome) is a severe variant of preeclampsia. It can cause acute renal failure, usually in association with other severe complications such as abruptio placenta and convulsions. In contrast to acute fatty liver of pregnancy, evidence of disseminated intravascular coagulation is usually absent in uncomplicated HELLP syndrome.

Ischemic ATN may develop after severe hypotension or during the course of sepsis. Thus, pregnant women with puerperal sepsis, septic abortion, amniotic fluid embolism, abruptio placenta, or other causes of uterine hemorrhage are at risk. Acute pyelonephritis rarely causes renal failure, perhaps because of associated sepsis.

Idiopathic postpartum renal failure (also known as postpartum hemolytic-uremic syndrome) occurs one day to several weeks after delivery and is characterized by azotemia, severe hypertension, microangiopathic hemolytic anemia, and thrombocytopenia, often with clinical bleeding. A prodrome of vomiting, diarrhea, or respiratory symptoms may occur. Hematuria and proteinuria usually are present. The value of therapy, which may include corticosteroids, antiplatelet agents, plasma exchange, and control of hypertension, is uncertain, and most patients who survive have persistent renal failure.

Renal cortical necrosis is caused by thrombosis of the small arteries, afferent arterioles, and glomerular capillaries in the cortex; the medulla is spared. Perhaps because pregnancy is a hypercoagulable state, in the past the most common settings for cortical necrosis were complications of pregnancy, including abruptio placenta or other uterine hemorrhage, puerperal sepsis, septic abortion, preeclampsia, or prolonged intrauterine death. Extensive cortical necrosis is one of the few conditions that cause anuria; prolonged oliguria and bloody urine also may be seen. Fortunately, this disorder has become unusual in developed countries with modern obstetric care.

Table 78-7. Causes of Acute Renal Failure in Pregnancy

Prerenal Azotemia
Hyperemesis gravidarum
Uterine hemorrhage
? Acute fatty liver
Postrenal Azotemia
Ureteral compression by the gravid uterus
Renal Azotemia
Cortical necrosis
Abruptio placenta
Puerperal sepsis
Septic abortion
Severe preeclampsia
Intrauterine death
Acute tubular necrosis
Uterine hemorrhage
Sepsis
Amniotic fluid embolism
Preeclampsia
HELLP Syndrome
Postpartum HUS

HELLP, hemolysis, elevated liver function test results, and low platelet count; *HUS,* hemolytic-uremic syndrome.

Evaluation of Acute Renal Failure in Pregnancy

The approach to new azotemia in the gravid woman follows the same general guidelines outlined earlier. However, because mild hydronephrosis is normal in pregnancy, urinary obstruction can be detected by ultrasonography only when the collecting system is more dilated than anticipated for the stage of gestation. Intravenous pyelography generally is not performed during pregnancy to avoid exposure to ionizing radiation. In questionable cases, a trial of urinary drainage may be necessary to see if renal function improves. When renal failure occurs in the third trimester or puerperium, liver function tests, a complete blood cell count and platelet count, red cell morphologic study, and coagulation tests should be obtained. A serum uric acid level that is elevated out of proportion to the degree of renal failure can be a clue to preeclampsia. Renal biopsy is rarely indicated during pregnancy, but, if absolutely necessary, may be performed safely in the first two trimesters.

Differential Diagnosis

When prerenal azotemia occurs during pregnancy, the physician must consider hyperemesis gravidarum and uterine bleeding in addition to the other causes outlined earlier. When renal failure occurs in the third trimester, preeclampsia, the HELLP syndrome, and acute fatty liver of pregnancy are concerns. Thrombocytopenia and microangiopathic hemolytic anemia developing during the first weeks after delivery suggest idiopathic postpartum hemolytic-uremic syndrome. Whereas renal failure that follows a period of severe hypotension usually indicates ATN, lack of recovery after several weeks raises the possibility of cortical necrosis, which can be demonstrated with contrast-enhanced computed tomography.

Management and Prognosis

The same principles of treatment outlined earlier apply to pregnant women. Additional caution must be used when prescribing medications, because the safety of many drugs has not been established in pregnancy and some are known to be dangerous. For example, ACE inhibitors are contraindicated because they may cause developmental problems in the fetus and neonatal renal failure.

General indications for dialysis also apply to pregnant women. Either peritoneal or hemodialysis may be used. However, early dialysis is recommended because of the assumption that minimizing the uremic environment reduces the risk of adverse events for both the mother and fetus. Therefore, the authors suggest starting dialysis when the BUN rises above 60 mg/dL and that dialysis be performed as needed to maintain the BUN at or below 50 to 60 mg/dL. The well-being of the fetus must be monitored closely.

Specific treatment of hyperemesis gravidarum, obstruction by the gravid uterus, and postpartum renal failure have been discussed. Renal failure caused by preeclampsia, the HELLP syndrome, or acute fatty liver should be managed with early delivery.

The prognosis of acute renal failure depends more on the precipitating process than on the severity of azotemia. Prerenal and postrenal azotemia are completely reversible with appropriate therapy. Renal dysfunction caused by preeclampsia, the HELLP syndrome, and acute fatty liver usually improves after delivery if the patient survives. On the other hand, renal cortical necrosis often causes permanent renal injury; but, because the process is frequently patchy, there may be some improvement over time. Finally, severe postpartum hemolytic-uremic syndrome usually causes irreversible renal failure and the need for permanent renal replacement therapy.

BIBLIOGRAPHY

Agmon Y, Brezis M. Acute renal failure: a multi-factorial syndrome. Contrib Nephrol 1993;102:23.

Alkhunaizi AM, Schrier RW. New perspectives. Management of acute renal failure: New perspectives. Am J Kidney Dis 1996;28:315.

Anderson RJ. Prevention and management of acute renal failure. Hosp Pract 1993;28:61.

Badr KF, Ichikawa I. Prerenal failure: a deleterious shift from renal compensation to decompensation. N Engl J Med 1988;319:623.

Barrett BJ, Parfrey PS. Prevention of nephrotoxicity induced by radiocontrast agents. N Engl J Med 1994;331:1449.

Barri YM, Al-Furayh O, Qunibi WY, Rahman F. Pregnancy in women on regular hemodialysis. Dialysis Transplant 1991;20:652.

Bidani A, Churchill PC. Acute renal failure. Dis Mon 1989;35:57.

Brady HR, Singer GG. Acute renal failure. Lancet 1995;346:1533.

Dixon BS, Anderson RJ. Nonoliguric acute renal failure. Am J Kidney Dis 1985;6:71.

DuBose TD, Molony DA, Verani R, McDonald GA. Nephrotoxicity of nonsteroidal anti-inflammatory drugs. Lancet 1994;344:515.

Hayslett JP. Postpartum renal failure. N Engl J Med 1985;312:1556.

Hou SH, Bushinsky DA, Wish JB, Cohen JJ, Harrington JT. Hospital-acquired renal insufficiency: a prospective study. Am J Med 1983;74:243.

Kassirer JP. Clinical evaluation of kidney function: glomerular function. N Engl J Med 1971;285:385.

Kaufman J, Dhakal M, Patel B, Hamburger R. Community-acquired acute renal failure. Am J Kidney Dis 1991;17:191.

Krane NK. Acute renal failure in pregnancy. Arch Intern Med 1988;148:2347.

Lieberthal W, Levinsky NG. Treatment of acute tubular necrosis. Semin Nephrol 1990;10:571.

Maikranz P, Katz AI. Acute renal failure in pregnancy. Obstet Gynecol Clin North Am 1991;18:333.

Martinez-Maldonado M, Kumjian DA. Acute renal failure due to urinary tract obstruction. Med Clin North Am 1990;74:919.

Miller TR, Anderson RJ, Linas SL, et al. Urinary diagnostic indices in acute renal failure. Ann Intern Med 1978;89:47.

Shusterman N, Strom BL, Murray TG, Morrison G, West SL, Maislin G. Risk factors and outcome of hospital-acquired acute renal failure. 1987;83:65.

Sibai BM, Ramadan MK. Acute renal failure in pregnancies complicated by hemolysis, elevated liver enzymes, and low platelets. Am J Obstet Gynecol 1993;168:1682.

Sirmon MD, Kirkpatrick WG. Acute renal failure: what to do until the nephrologist comes. Postgrad Med 1990;87:55.

Thadhani R, Pascual M, Bonventre JV. Acute renal failure. N Engl J Med 1996;334:1448.

Thompson BT, Cockrill BA. Renal-dose dopamine: a siren song? Lancet 1994;344:7.

Turney JH. Acute renal failure: some progress? N Engl J Med 1994;331:1372.

Turney JH, Ellis CM, Parsons FM. Obstetric acute renal failure 1956–1987. Br J Obstet Gynaecol 1989;96:679.

Primary Care for Women, edited by Phyllis C. Leppert and Fred M. Howard. Lippincott-Raven Publishers, Philadelphia © 1997.

79
Interstitial Cystitis

FRED M. HOWARD

The definition and diagnostic criteria of interstitial cystitis are controversial and unclear, but most commonly interstitial cystitis is defined by the following triad: (1) irritative voiding symptoms; (2) absence of objective evidence of another disease that could cause the symptoms; and (3) a characteristic cystoscopic appearance of the bladder. The typical irritative voiding symptoms are frequency, urgency, and nocturia. Several other diseases, particularly urinary tract infections and urethral syndrome, may cause similar symptoms and must be excluded. Cystoscopy is essential to diagnosis, showing characteristic petechial, submucosal hemorrhages (termed "glomerulations") on a second filling of the bladder. Linear cracking and Hunner's ulcer, named for Hunner, who first described interstitial cystitis in 1914, also may be noted but are not always present. Pelvic pain is often present with interstitial cystitis, but it is not a consistent symptom and is not necessary to make the diagnosis.

Interstitial cystitis occurs predominantly in women aged 30 to 59 years. The disease seems to be unrelated to menopausal status, occurring both premenopausally and postmenopausally. The incidence is not known, but is estimated at 36 cases per 100,000 women in the United States and 18 cases per 100,000 women in Finland.

ETIOLOGY

The etiology of interstitial cystitis is unknown. More than one disease may be encompassed in the syndrome. Current thinking suggests that patients with interstitial cystitis have defects in the glycosaminoglycan layer of the bladder wall, although there is no evidence that the glycosaminoglycan is intrinsically defective or abnormal. The glycosaminoglycans of the bladder surface are hydrophilic polysaccharides that form a layer of micelles of water on the bladder epithelium. This micellar layer acts as a barrier between the transitional epithelial cells and urine. It is hypothesized that a defect in this layer allows "leaking" of the epithelium, resulting in a dysfunctional epithelium with excessive permeability. This causes exposure of the transitional epithelium and muscularis to noxious substances in the urine. Such leaking of urinary constituents into the bladder wall might explain the nonspecific inflammatory reaction characteristically found in the submucosa and muscularis of bladder biopsy specimens of patients with interstitial cystitis. However, this is only a partial explanation, possibly explaining the end-effect mechanism. It does not address the mechanism by which the permeability or leakiness of the glycosaminoglycan layer occurs.

An autoimmune cause of this leakiness seems possible. Several researchers have demonstrated an increased number of mast cells in the bladder wall of patients with interstitial cystitis, which is consistent with a potential autoimmune process. Other proposed mechanisms include viral infection, toxin exposure, or other inflammatory mediators.

The physiologic causes of pain with interstitial cystitis also are not clear. Algesic substances released by the inflammatory reaction of the bladder wall may cause nociceptor stimulation of visceral neural pathways. In some patients, chronic inflammation results in a contracted bladder of limited capacity that may cause pain, as well as urgency and frequency. Such chronic visceral pain may result in spasm of the pelvic floor muscles (levator ani syndrome) with resultant pelvic pain.

DIFFERENTIAL DIAGNOSIS

Frequency, urgency, nocturia, and pelvic pain may be associated with several other diagnoses. Acute, recurrent, or chronic infections of the urinary tract especially must be considered. A urine culture showing 100,000 or more bacterial colonies of one organism confirms cystitis. Infections of the urethra may show similar culture results, but more commonly show either lower colony counts or negative bacterial culture results. A positive result from a chlamydial antigen screening test of the urethra, Skene's glands, or cervix suggests chlamydial urethritis. Gonococcal urethritis also must be considered and appropriate culture specimens for *Neisseria gonorrhoeae* be taken from the urethra, Skene's glands, and cervix. Tuberculous cystitis also is a possibility, particularly with aseptic pyuria. A positive tuberculin skin test result and chest x-ray findings of tubercular disease support this diagnosis. However, urine cultures and stains for acid-fast bacilli, as well as histologic findings on bladder biopsy consistent with tubercular cystitis, are needed to confirm the diagnosis.

Bladder tumors, including carcinoma in situ, may present with similar symptoms. Because of this possibility, urine cytologic studies and cystoscopically directed bladder biopsies generally should be performed as part of the diagnostic workup. A bladder tumor also may be suggested by the presence of microscopic hematuria.

Chronic urethral syndrome also manifests symptoms similar to those of interstitial cystitis. Culture results are negative with both, but with chronic urethral syndrome there is usually marked tenderness to palpation of the anterior vaginal wall under the urethra and to passage of a catheter or cystourethroscope. Neither of these symptoms occurs with interstitial cystitis.

Another syndrome, probably best termed irritable bladder, has symptoms that are nearly identical to interstitial cystitis, but cystoscopy and bladder histologic findings are normal. The etiology of irritable bladder also is not known, but probably results from a source of bladder irritation that causes increased pelvic muscle activity. This muscle activity causes pelvic pressure with a strong desire to void when there is little urine in the bladder. Subsequent urination is dysfunctional because the bladder volume is insuffi-

Table 79-1. Medications for Irritable Bladder Syndrome

MEDICATION	DOSE
Anticholinergics/antispasmodics	
Flavoxate hydrochloride	100–200 mg q 6–8 h
Hyoscyamine sulfate	0.125–0.30 mg q 6–8 h
Oxybutynin chloride	5 mg q 6–12 h
Smooth muscle relaxants	
Phenoxybenzamine hydrochloride	10–20 mg q 8–12 h
Prazosin hydrochloride	1–5 mg q 8–12 h
Terazosin hydrochloride	1–5 mg qd
Skeletal muscle relaxants	
Carisoprodol	350 mg q 6–8 h
Cyclobenzeprine	10 mg q 8–12 h
Methocarbamol	500–1000 mg q 6–8 h
Diazepam	2–10 mg q 6–12 h
Analgesics/others	
Phenazopyridine	200 mg q 8 h
Ketorulac tromethamine	10 mg q 6 h
Naproxen sodium	275–550 mg q 6–12 h
Ibuprofen	200–800 mg q 6–8 h
Amitryptilline	25–75 mg qd

cient to trigger normal reflex coordinated micturition via detrusor contraction and simultaneous outlet relaxation. Urination is accomplished by straining, producing pain, hesitancy, and an intermittent stream. This may cause further bladder irritation, producing a "vicious cycle" of urgency, frequency, and pain. The original cause of bladder irritation is undoubtedly varied, including such things as acute cystitis, coital trauma, or sexual abuse, but this usually cannot be discerned at the time of clinical presentation. Treatment for irritable bladder is similar to the behavior modification and autodilation methods for interstitial cystitis, subsequently discussed under the section entitled "Treatment." Additionally, water consumption should be increased and dietary bladder irritants should be avoided (coffee, tea, carbonated beverages, citrus, cranberry juice, tomato juice and sauces, and alcohol). Treatment with warm baths and local heat, relaxation training, biofeedback, or physical therapy may be helpful. Symptomatic, medical therapy for irritable bladder syndrome is sometimes indicated. Antispasmodics, smooth and skeletal muscle relaxants, and analgesic or nonspecific medications such as those listed in Table 79-1 may be empirically tried. Narcotic medications should be avoided in treating irritable bladder. Again, cystoscopic findings distinguish irritable bladder from interstitial cystitis.

Infections (particularly tubercular or fungal), certain toxins (eg, cyclophosphamide or formalin), radiation cystitis, neoplasms (especially carcinoma in situ), and overdistention of a defunctionalized bladder may mimic cystoscopic "glomerulations." These diagnoses may be distinguished from interstitial cystitis by history or by histologic findings.

In summary, the differential diagnosis of interstitial cystitis is not always easy. In a sense, it is a diagnosis of exclusion, being a disease of variable symptoms, of unknown etiology, possibly of heterogeneous causation, and with no specific marker (except Hunner's ulcer, a finding generally not present).

CLINICAL SYMPTOMS

Unremitting frequency and urgency of urination are the characteristic symptoms of interstitial cystitis. Dysuria is not a characteristic symptom, but the urgency and frequency experienced is so severe that these women commonly give histories of recurrent treatment for urinary tract infections. Typically there is a history of 3 to 7 years of symptoms before the diagnosis is established. Nocturia, with voiding three or more times per night, is also a characteristic and troublesome symptom. Incontinence does not generally occur.

Pelvic pain, although not as universal a symptom of interstitial cystitis as urgency, frequency, and nocturia, occurs in more than one half of women with interstitial cystitis. Typically, the pain is suprapubic and may radiate to the low back or the groin. Most of the women with chronic pelvic pain associated with interstitial cystitis also have dyspareunia. In many patients, pain increases with bladder filling and decreases after voiding.

The symptoms of interstitial cystitis generally worsen over the first several years after onset, eventually reaching a relatively stable level of intensity. However, it is usual for the intensity of symptoms to vary. About 10% of women have spontaneous resolution of symptoms.

Obviously, a thorough clinical history relating to the urinary tract needs to be taken from these women. This is crucial for planning an efficient and accurate diagnostic evaluation. It may also be useful in subsequent therapeutic interventions. For patients whose symptoms suggest interstitial cystitis, the history should include specific questions about the number of times the patient voids during the day at her best and at her worst. It should also include the number of voidings during the night, both at best and worst. The patient should be asked to estimate the volumes voided at urination, both daytime and nighttime. Finally, the patient should be asked to recall her voiding habits before the onset of irritative bladder symptoms.

CLINICAL FINDINGS

The physical examination in women with interstitial cystitis usually yields normal results. Some may have anterior vaginal wall tenderness under the trigone, but this is inconsistent.

Cystometric evaluation reveals decreased bladder capacity and compliance in most women with interstitial cystitis. In fact, decreased bladder capacity is sometimes used as a diagnostic criterion. If bladder capacity is measured without general or spinal anesthesia, it is less than 600 mL. Significant pain and urgency occur with such volumes. In fact, if a patient tolerates bladder volumes of 600 to 700 mL without severe pain and urgency, then the diagnosis of interstitial cystitis is unlikely.

Cystoscopy is an essential part of the diagnostic evaluation. Because significant bladder distention is needed and is painful in women with interstitial cystitis, general or spinal anesthesia should be used. Cystoscopy is performed in a standardized manner for the best diagnostic results without confusing artifactual findings. After urethroscopy is completed, the bladder is not allowed to collapse around the cystoscope because this may traumatize the bladder mucosa and cause iatrogenic artifacts. The bladder is distended to

70 to 80 cm H_2O for 1 minute or more. This may require compression of the urethra by upward digital compression of the anterior vaginal wall against the urethroscope to prevent leakage. Although the risk is low, it is possible to rupture the bladder during this distention. Findings during the first filling are usually normal, although occasionally faint trabeculation may be observed. When maximal capacity is reached, the volume is noted and the irrigant drained. The terminal portion of this drainage may be blood tinged. When this protocol is followed, mean cystoscopic bladder capacity in patients with interstitial cystitis is 545 mL, with a range of 150 to 950 mL. The bladder is refilled, and examination reveals splotchy submucosal hemorrhages throughout the bladder of the patient with interstitial cystitis. These hemorrhages are called glomerulations. Glomerulations do not occur in a normal bladder. Rarely, Hunner's ulcer may be seen and, when noted, is diagnostic. Patients with markedly decreased bladder capacities are more likely to show Hunner's ulcer. Bladder biopsies are usually indicated and are discussed subsequently.

Any infection needs to have been cleared for several weeks before cystoscopy, not only because of concerns of reinfection, but also because current or recent infection may cause cystoscopic findings similar to those of interstitial cystitis.

LABORATORY STUDIES

Urinary frequency and urgency also are symptoms of urinary tract infection, necessitating urinalysis and urine culture. A history of recurrent urinary tract infections and improvement with antibiotic therapy (usually without culture-positive documentation) does not negate the need for urinalysis and culture. Empiric antibiotic therapy should not be done in these patients because it only delays the diagnosis and further confuses the patient. A patient without infection, but with such a history, may respond to antibiotic treatment as a result of the placebo effect or of the increased fluid intake, which is usually recommended with the antibiotics (dilute urine is less irritating to the bladder). After the antibiotic course is completed, fluid intake usually returns to its low pretreatment level, with recurrence of full-blown symptoms.

Urinalysis results generally are normal with interstitial cystitis. About 20% of patients have 5 to 10 white blood cells per high-power microscopic field and less than 10% have greater than 10 white blood cells per high-power field. Urine and urethral culture findings should be negative. In patients with persistent symptoms after appropriate antibiotic treatment for a positive urine culture finding, cystoscopy should be considered for evaluation of possible interstitial cystitis. However, as previously observed, infection must be cleared for several weeks before the cystoscopic diagnosis of interstitial cystitis because infection may cause bladder changes similar to glomerulations. Less than 10% of women with interstitial cystitis have greater than 5 red blood cells per high-power field in a urinalysis. In the occasional patient with hematuria, urine cytologic testing is essential. Some suggest that urine cytologic studies are advisable in all patients before the diagnosis of interstitial cystitis. If the patient has a history of smoking, then urine cytologic study should be done. Of course, cytologic findings should be negative in patients with interstitial cystitis.

Radiographic studies are mostly useful to rule out other conditions but not to specifically confirm the diagnosis of interstitial cystitis. In selected patients, intravenous pyelography, voiding or static cystography, skeletal and pelvic x-rays, sonography, or computed tomography may be indicated. These study results should be normal with interstitial cystitis.

Ongoing research suggests a potential usefulness of antinuclear antibodies, eosinophil cationic protein, histamine metabolites, epidermal growth factor, and glycosaminoglycan layer components assays, but evidence is insufficient to warrant routine clinical use of any of these determinations.

Biopsies at the time of cystoscopic diagnosis are generally advised to rule out carcinoma or carcinoma in situ. Also, the histologic finding of increased mast cells (special fixation and staining required) has been reported to be useful for confirmation of interstitial cystitis. Nonspecific inflammation in the bladder submucosa and muscularis, as well as vasodilation and edema in the submucosa, are characteristic but not pathognomonic of interstitial cystitis.

TREATMENT

Treatment can be a frustrating experience for both the patient and her physician, because none of the currently available therapies are curative. Significant biopsychosocial consequences are not surprising, considering the patient is told she has a disease of unknown cause with no known cure and with potentially incapacitating consequences. Such consequences may be compounded by the triviality sometimes accorded her urinary symptoms by family, physicians, and friends. Because of such issues, it is crucial that the physician educate and involve the patient fully, as well as the patient's family when possible or appropriate. Interstitial cystitis tends to be a relapsing disease, even after seemingly successful treatment. The woman must be educated about this characteristic of the disease both before treatment is instituted and after successful treatment is finished. Subsequent acceptance of the need for possible retreatment may be made easier by such education. However, this need not be presented in such a negative way that only hopelessness is conveyed. The real possibility of long periods of remission after successful treatment, especially with active patient participation in behavioral modification, can be optimistically presented without any deceit on the physician's part. Some of the self-help measures can be initiated before cystoscopic diagnosis. The appendix contains an example of a handout of some self-interventions that the patient can initiate either before or after diagnosis.

The mainstay of urologic treatment of interstitial cystitis for more than 50 years has been hydrodistention of the bladder. This procedure can be performed at the time of diagnostic cystoscopy if general or spinal anesthesia is used. After diagnostic evaluation is completed, the bladder is filled to maximal capacity at 100 cm H_2O for 2 minutes. The risk of bladder rupture with this procedure is less than 15%. Patients complain of increased pain immediately postoperatively, and it is generally several weeks until they notice a remission of symptoms. About 50% of patients have a successful response to hydrodistention (Table 79-2) Remission generally lasts for 6 to 10 months, with a gradual recurrence of symptoms in most patients. After recurrence, retreatment with hydrodistention has a greatly diminished success rate. The mechanism of action of hydrodistention is not known. Speculation is that one or both of the following mechanisms may apply: (1) the dysfunctional epithelium is damaged and regeneration of normal epithelium is stimulated, or (2) there is significant nerve damage with resultant denervation. Regardless of the actual mechanism, hydrodistention is a reasonable initial therapy. It has a good (albeit temporary) response rate,

TABLE 79-2. Therapy of Interstitial Cystitis

METHOD	SUCCESS RATE
Hydrodistention of bladder	50% (60–10 months)
Autodilation	80–85% (selected patients)
Dimethylsulfoxide, 50%, intravesical	40–50%
Heparin, intravesical	40–50%
Heparin, subcutaneous	30–35%
Pentosanpolysulfate, oral	40–50%
Nonsteroidal antiinflammatory drugs	—
Oxychlorosene, 0.4%, intravesical	—
TENS unit	—
Nd:YAG laser	—
Cystectomy and diversion	—

TENS, transcutaneous electrical nerve stimulation.

it is fairly easy and safe to perform, and it can be done at the time of the diagnostic cystoscopy.

Another useful treatment, as long as the patient does not have severe pain, is autodilation (see Table 79-2). This is a behavioral modification modality whereby the patient increases her bladder capacity through gradually increasing the intervals between voidings. With this technique, the patient keeps a diary of times and volumes of urination, of fluid intake, of pain intensity, and of any suspected factors that might effect symptoms (eg, menses, sexual activity, or stress). The patient and physician review the initial diary to establish baseline severity of symptoms and set concrete treatment goals. Specific goals need to be set and followed. The goals must be aimed toward a slow, gradual progression. If the patient attempts to progress too rapidly, failure is inevitable. An initial increase of voiding intervals of no more than 15 minutes should be attempted. After about a month of successfully increasing the minimum voiding interval by 15 minutes, the minimum interval should be increased again. Generally, it is reasonable to try to increase the voiding interval by 15 minutes each month until a minimum interval of 3 to 4 hours is attained. The patient should continue to keep her diary throughout this treatment. This assists with compliance, adherence, motivation, and monitoring of her progress. Monthly physician visits are also helpful for the same reasons. Remission rates of 80% to 85% have been obtained with this treatment. However, relapse of symptoms is likely if the patient is not vigilant with the training. Success with autodilation is limited to patients with mild or controllable pain.

Dimethylsulfoxide (DMSO, Rimso-50) is the only drug with a U.S. Federal Drug Administration (FDA)–approved indication for interstitial cystitis. DMSO is a product of the wood pulp industry, a derivative of lignin. It is a superb solvent, being miscible with water, lipids, and organic agents. DMSO has several pharmacologic properties that led to interest in its use for interstitial cystitis: (1) membrane penetration without membrane damage; (2) enhancement of drug absorption (eg steroids); (3) antiinflammatory activity; (4) topical analgesic activity via interruption of conduction in peripheral nerves; (5) promotion of collagen breakdown or dissolution via weakening of cross-linking; (6) muscle relaxation; (7) bacteriostasis; (8) vasodilation; and (9) enhancement of mast cell histamine release. All but the last of these pharmacologic properties are potential mechanisms by which DMSO might decrease symptoms in interstitial cystitis. In contrast, the DMSO effect on mast cells could account for the initial transient worsening of symptoms in some patients with interstitial cystitis undergoing DMSO treatment.

DMSO has low systemic toxicity. It is primarily excreted via the renal system as unchanged DMSO and dimethylsulfone. A small percentage is excreted via the respiratory system as dimethylsulfide. Dimethylsulfide accounts for the garlic-like taste and breath odor after DMSO treatment. Some early animal studies raised concerns of lenticular opacities, but this has never been reported with therapeutic doses or human use. DMSO has been reported to be teratogenic in animal studies, so its use in pregnancy is contraindicated.

Initial attempts to use DMSO were transdermal, but results were mediocre. This led to trials of intravesical administration, which gave more promising results and led to FDA approval. Intravesical treatment can be done as an office procedure. It is best to perform a urinalysis before treatments to exclude bacteriuria. Additionally, DMSO treatment should not be done in the 3 to 4 weeks after bladder biopsies to avoid excessive absorption via the unhealed biopsy sites. The urethra may be anesthetized with 2% lidocaine topically. Sometimes the treatment is painful, so analgesics preoperatively may be beneficial. Some also suggest vesical nerve block via subvesical injection of 10 to 20 mL of 1% lidocaine (Fig. 79-1), but definitive evidence has not been presented that this improves comfort during the procedure or enhances the therapeutic response. A small urethral catheter (8 to 12 French) is inserted and the bladder emptied. A 50 mL-volume of 50% DMSO (Rimso-50) is instilled, and the catheter removed. The patient waits 15 to 30 minutes before voiding. Treatments are usually repeated four to eight times at 1- to 2-week intervals. As mentioned earlier, some patients find this treatment painful, so in these patients a pretreatment dose of ibuprofen, naproxen sodium, or ketorolac tromethamine might be considered. Some patients complain of significant irritation and burning of the urethra with DMSO treatment. This can be diminished by leaving the catheter in and clamped for the 15 to 30 minutes of treatment, then emptying the DMSO via the catheter before removal. Painful bladder spasms occur in about 10% of patients, and these may be treated with anticholinergics or belladonna and opium suppositories. All patients notice a garlic-like odor of breath and taste in the mouth for 24 to 48 hours after DMSO treatment. This can be personally and socially unpleasant for the patient, so each patient needs to be counseled about this side effect. Commonly, symptoms worsen transiently after the first treatment, so success cannot be determined until more than two treatments are done. In addition to subjective evidence of decreased symptoms, objective evidence of significantly increased bladder capacity (> 100-mL increase) has been demonstrated. Unfortunately, DMSO treatments result only in remission of disease, not cure. At least 30% to 60% of patients relapse within the first year after successful treatment. Compounding this, retreatment with DMSO after relapse of symptoms is less effective, and many patients ultimately become resistant to DMSO treatment.

Other therapies for interstitial cystitis have been less extensively studied than hydrodistention, autodilation, and DMSO. Additionally, none of the other drug therapies have FDA approval

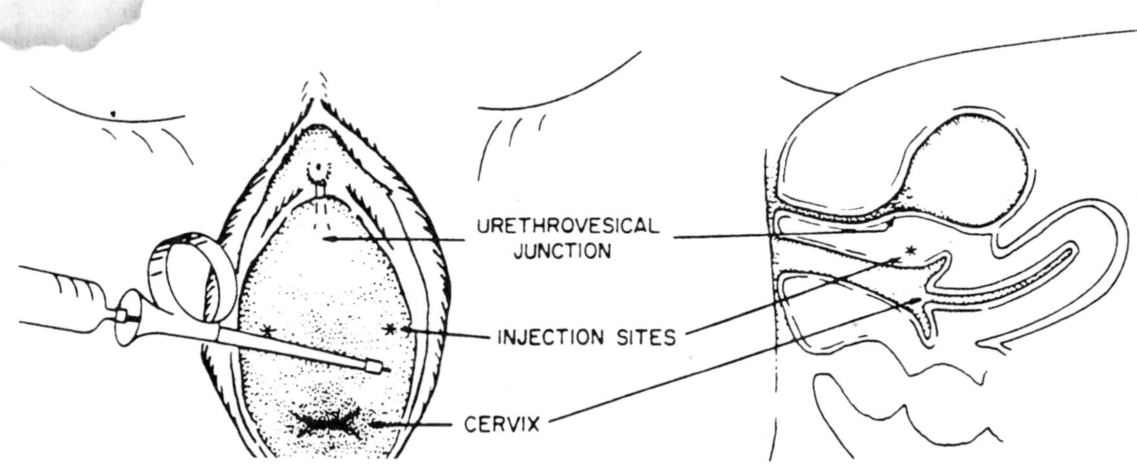

Figure 79-1. Sites for vesical neural block for DMSO treatment of interstitial cystitis shown from front and side views. (From Sand PK, Bowen LW, Ostergard DR, Bent A, Panganiban R. Cryosurgery versus dilation and massage for the treatment of recurrent urethral syndrome. J Reprod Med, 1989;34:499.)

for treating interstitial cystitis. Although this does not preclude their use, it does mean that patients should be appropriately counseled as to the "investigational" nature of the treatment.

Heparin has been used both subcutaneously and intravesically. Both of these modalities have the advantage that the patient can be taught self-administration. Given subcutaneously, the usual dose is 2500 to 5000 U three times per week. Although anticoagulation is unlikely with this dose, it is still advisable to check several partial thromboplastin times over the first 3 weeks of treatment. Response rates with subcutaneous heparin are no higher than one in three (see Table 79-2). In patients with a clinical response, this treatment should not be continued more than 8 to 10 weeks because chronic heparin use may cause osteoporosis and hair loss. In a patient with a good response but with recurrence after a full course of therapy, retreatment may be tried if the patient has been off heparin for at least 3 months.

Intravesical heparin has been slightly more effective than subcutaneous heparin, with about 40% to 50% of patients responding. Three to five times per week, 10,000 U of heparin in 10 mL of sterile water are instilled into the bladder via a small urethral catheter (8 to 12 French). The patient can be taught to do this herself. She needs to retain the heparin without voiding for at least 1 hour. Heparin is not significantly absorbed into the circulation from the bladder, so partial thromboplastin time assays are not needed. A prophylactic antibiotic dose with each treatment is recommended.

Sodium pentosan polysulfate (PPS) is a polyanionic analogue of heparin that has been used to treat interstitial cystitis. It may be administered orally. Reported results of its effectiveness have been mixed, but at least one placebo-controlled, double-blinded study showed a 50% response rate compared with the placebo response rate of 23%. PPS dosage in this study was 100 mg orally three times a day. It is not FDA approved, but it is currently available on a compassionate or protocol basis.

The exact modes of action of heparin and PPS are not known. However, both are complex sulfated polysaccharides and are extremely hydrophilic. Because of this, when bound to the surface epithelium, they are capable of forming or enhancing the layer of micelles of water over the epithelium. Thus, at least theoretically, they may improve the barrier and antiadherence activity of the endogenous glycosaminoglycan layer of the bladder epithelium.

Other nonsurgical treatments for interstitial cystitis have been reported, but evidence of their effectiveness is scant. Transcutaneous electrical nerve stimulation (TENS) therapy has been used for pain control with 20% to 60% improvement after 6 or more weeks of use. Tricyclic antidepressants, particularly amitriptyline, have been used, but little objective data are available on their effectiveness. Evidence from their usefulness with other chronic pain syndromes implies at least some effectiveness for pain symptoms.

Approximately 5% of patients have unresponsive, intractable, incapacitating symptoms that justify surgical treatment. Such patients usually have small capacity bladders (< 400 mL), void 18 to 20 times per day, and have severe, uncontrolled pain. Cystectomy, urethrectomy, and continent diversion with a Koch or Indiana pouch has been the most successful and acceptable surgical treatment. However, in one series of such patients, 2 of 15 developed subsequent pouch pain.

A less aggressive surgical approach, with some degree of success, is neodymium (Nd):YAG laser ablation of the bladder lining. Of 39 patients (33 women) treated with the Nd:YAG laser, 30 had an initial response. More than 50% had subsequent recurrence of symptoms and required retreatment. Additionally, two of the patients had small bowel perforations caused by unrecognized laser injury, both of whom presented with the complications several days after laser irradiation. Obviously, Nd:YAG laser treatment must be considered experimental and should be done under study or protocol conditions by surgeons experienced with use of the Nd:YAG laser.

In summary, the mainstays of current treatment for interstitial cystitis are hydrodistention, autodilation, and DMSO. Individually, these treatments generally achieve 40% to 60% remission rates. The effectiveness of combining these modalities has not been well studied. More research on the effectiveness of treatment for interstitial cystitis is needed, but such research is difficult to perform. Because the major clinical characteristics of interstitial cystitis are subjective symptoms, it is crucial that measurements such as visual or verbal analogue pain ratings, voiding intervals, voided volumes, and visual or verbal analogue ratings of urgency be used. Also, placebo-controlled studies are needed because studies show placebo response rates of 10% to 25% in interstitial cystitis patients.

BIBLIOGRAPHY

Gillenwater JY, Wein AJ. Summary of the National Institute of Arthritis, Diabetes, Digestive and Kidney Disease workshop on interstitial cystitis. National Institutes of Health, Bethesda, Maryland, August 28–29, 1987. J Urol 1988;140:203.

Hanno PM, Buehler J, Wein AJ. Use of amitriptyline in the treatment of intersitial cystitis. J Urol 1989;141:846.

Hanno P, Levin RM, Monson C, et al. Diagnosis of interstitial cystitis. J Urol 1990;143:278.

Messing EM. The diagnosis of interstitial cystitis. Urology 1987;(suppl)29:4.

Parsons CL. Sodium pentosanpolysulfate treatment of intersitital cystitis: an update. Urology 1987;(suppl)29:14.

Parsons CL, Koprowski PF. Intersititial cystitis: successful management by increasing urinary voiding intervals. Urology 1991;38:207.

Perez-Marrero R, Emerson LE, Feltis JT. A controlled study of dimethyl sulfoxide in intersititial cystitis. J Urol 1988;140:36.

Ramahi AJ, Richardson DA. A practical approach to the painful bladder syndrome. J Reprod Med 1990;35:805.

Sant GR. Intravesical 50% dimethyl sulfoxide (RIMSO-50) in the treatment of intersitital cystitis. Urology 1987;(suppl)29:17.

Shanberg AM, Malloy T. Treatment of intersitial cystitis with neodymium:YAG laser. Urology 1987;(suppl)29:31.

APPENDIX
SELF-HELP FOR PATIENTS WITH IRRITABLE BLADDER SYMPTOMS

There are things that can be done to help relieve irritative bladder symptoms of frequency, urgency, or pain on urination. These symptoms may have several different causes, including bacterial infection, substances in the urine causing irritation, or intrinsic bladder problems such as interstitial cystitis or tumors. Antibiotics are indicated only for bacterial infections, so a urine culture should be taken before starting any antibiotic, unless the physician specifically advises otherwise.

At the first signs of discomfort or urgency, fluid intake should be increased. Some have found that starting with 480 mL (16 oz) of water mixed with 1 teaspoon of baking soda helps to relieve symptoms. The patient should continue drinking 40-mL (8 oz) of plain water every 20 minutes over the next several hours. This dilution of urine or "flushing out" the bladder occasionally relieves symptoms completely. If not, it is okay to use acetaminophen or ibuprofen for pain relief. Bladder analgesics such as pyridium also may help and do not alter the results of a subsequent urine culture. If the increased fluid intake does not relieve symptoms completely, the physician should be called to arrange for a urine culture. This may be obtained via a midstream voided specimen or may require a catheterization for accurate culture results.

Some patients with chronic or current irritative bladder problems find that specific foods or beverages cause flare-ups or contribute to their symptoms. Some of the more common dietary irritants are as follows:

Alcoholic beverages
Apples and apple juice
Cantaloupe
Carbonated drinks
Chili and similar spicy foods
Citrus fruit
Chocolate
Coffee
Cranberries and cranberry juice
Grapes
Guava
Peaches
Pineapple
Plums
Strawberries
Sugar
Tea
Tomatoes and tomato juice
Vitamin B complex
Vinegar

To discover if any of these foods contribute to symptoms, the patient can follow an elimination diet with add-back of one food or beverage at a time. In other words, all of the above foods and beverages, or only the ones suspected of flaring symptoms, should be eliminated for at least 10 days. This may bring marked relief of symptoms in some cases. The patient may then begin to add the eliminated foods back to the diet only one at a time, every 10 to 14 days. If symptoms return, this suggests that the specific food or beverage is an irritant and is best avoided. The patient may find that foods or beverages other than those listed above contribute to symptoms.

80
Urinary Incontinence

KATHLEEN MARTIN

Primary Care for Women, edited by Phyllis C. Leppert and Fred M. Howard. Lippincott-Raven Publishers, Philadelphia © 1997.

The problem of urinary incontinence in women has become increasingly recognized by the medical community. In the past, underreporting of this condition was common due to embarrassment or the belief that this phenomenon was an unavoidable result of aging. Even now specific medical training in this area is deficient. What makes incontinence clinically elusive is that the patient does not expire or even become outwardly ill from its presence. However, its social impact and quality-of-life issues can be devastating. For instance, a major factor in determining whether an elderly patient should be institutionalized is whether she can maintain continence. The cost in medical dollars is well above the $10 billion per annum estimate made in 1988. The prevalence in the general female population is 10% to 25% by some estimates and increases to greater than 50% in the institutionalized elderly. It has been estimated that up to 40% of sanitary napkins are purchased for urinary incontinence.

The problems encountered by these patients affect every aspect of their lives. The emotional aspects of incontinence, including embarrassment, anxiety, and fear of bedwetting, are obvious; the interference with sexual function and enjoyment, dealing with urine odors, difficulty performing household chores, hindrance with employment, limitation of physical exercise, added cost of sanitary pads, and ruined clothes are other problems. The improvement in quality of life that can be made with fairly simple interventions is highly rewarding, but the clinician must ask the right questions.

This chapter reviews the basic principles and physiology of bladder storage and micturition and highlights their relevance to the strategies involved in the diagnosis and treatment of urinary incontinence. Treatment options include behavioral, pharmacologic, and physical therapy options as well as surgery.

PREDISPOSING FACTORS

As important as it is to understand how to diagnose a disease process, it is even more important to understand the predisposing factors so that it can be prevented. Women have a natural "defect" in their pelvic floor, the vagina. Then, when they reach menopause, the hormones that help maintain the integrity and health of the pelvic floor disappear. The trauma of childbirth and the hormone deprivation that accompanies aging explain why women suffer from urinary incontinence more than men.

Other factors come into play as well. Collagen accounts for the intrinsic strength and character of the endopelvic fascia. The endopelvic fascia is the supportive latticework that becomes the uterosacral and cardinal ligaments to support the uterus and the pubourethral and pubovesical ligaments to support the urethra and bladder. These collagen fibers may be congenitally weak or may become weak from chronic stress secondary to a chronic cough or heavy lifting, or from glycosylation due to diabetes. This weakness allows the bladder to descend from its normal intraabdominal position and allows disparate forces to act on the dome of the bladder versus the bladder neck. The bladder neck is no longer under the same pressure as the dome, and therefore stress incontinence may occur.

The primary care provider can have an impressive impact in preventing development of urinary incontinence. Women whose jobs require them to lift heavy objects (eg, waitresses, nurses, or factory workers) must understand the importance of strengthening their pelvic floor by regular Kegel exercises. Chronic coughers (eg, smokers or asthmatics) should be encouraged to quit smoking and be compliant with their medications to decrease the chronic strain on the pelvic floor. Women with diabetes must understand the importance of good control, as the disease can also contribute to incontinence. Weight control is important: obesity, along with all its other health risks, adds chronic stress to the pelvic floor. Good posture is important, as poor posture changes the vectors of force applied to the pelvis, increasing the vector to the levator ani and decreasing the force vector to the pubic bone. On the physical examination, the clinician may note excessive striae that are suggestive of congenitally weakened collagen.

The pelvic floor is made up of a "hammock" of muscles, the levator ani. The name refers to their role in elevating the anus. This muscle complex extends from the pubic bone to the sacrum and coccyx. It is composed of two muscle groups, the pubovisceral muscle group and the iliococcygeus. It is important to understand the anatomy and function of the levator muscles to be able to teach the patient how to flex these muscles and perform Kegel exercises. Kegel exercises are named after the gynecologist who popularized them in Hollywood in the 1950s, initially to improve sexual satisfaction. Only later did he find that it had the additional benefit of improving urinary continence. Kegel exercises are discussed further below. The clinician should evaluate the patient throughout her life as to how well she can perform the exercises. Patients should be encouraged to do Kegel exercises because they help maintain pelvic floor strength and perhaps minimize future pelvic floor weakness and its attendant effects on continence.

The complex issue of hormone replacement therapy is not discussed in detail here, but the tissues of the pelvic floor, as well as those of the bladder, urethra, and vagina, are rich in estrogen and progesterone receptors. The withdrawal of hormonal support after menopause results in atrophy and thinning of these tissues, thereby compromising their function. Discussion of this aspect of hormone replacement therapy with the patient is important.

Another aspect of bladder health is bowel health. Over the long term, constipation and chronic straining with bowel movements have a significant impact on pelvic floor health. The parasympathetic and sympathetic plexus of nerves envelops the bladder and bowel in a filmy sheet. When the rectosigmoid is chronically distended by constipation, this triggers stimuli throughout the neural network, thereby affecting bladder function as well. It is not surprising to see patients in the urodynamic suite who also complain of irritable bowel symptoms. It is therefore important to teach patients that having a bowel movement every 3 to 4 days is not normal and that chronic straining has serious implications on the future development of genital prolapse.

The neurology of urine storage and micturition requires multiple reflex pathways; these pathways in turn require intact cortical, spinal, and autonomic coordination. Therefore, a CNS or spinal injury or pathology can affect these reflex arcs. Patients with disk disease, diabetic peripheral neuropathy, strokes, vitamin B_{12} deficiency, multiple sclerosis, or meningomyelocele, to name a few, are at risk for interruption of one or more of these pathways, resulting in urinary incontinence.

The elderly are especially at risk for transient causes of incontinence. These include delirium, infection, atrophy, severe depression, restricted mobility, stool impaction, and polypharmacy. Once these conditions are reversed or eliminated with the proper therapeutic interventions, cure of the incontinence results.

ANATOMY

A detailed discussion of female pelvic anatomy can be found in Chapter 33. Here, a few concepts are highlighted. Inasmuch as genuine stress incontinence can be partly explained by the descent of the bladder neck and its hypermobility at times of increased abdominal pressure, it is important to understand the supports to the bladder, bladder neck, and urethra. The endopelvic fascia is a tissue made up of collagen, elastin, and smooth muscle that condenses in the pelvis into what we have termed ligaments. (This is a misnomer, but the terminology is established.) This fascia stretches and breaks and allows the bladder and the bladder neck to descend. The abdominal pressure that normally affects the bladder neck and bladder equally now transmits only to the bladder. This pushes the urine out, and thus stress incontinence is demonstrated.

An equally important part is the integrity and strength of the urethra and its support. The proximal urethra is supported not only by these condensations of endopelvic fascia but also inferiorly by the anterior vaginal wall. The anterior vaginal wall is supported by its attachments to the levator ani and to the arcus tendineus along the pelvic sidewall. Thus, several scenarios can lead to the so-called "dropped bladder," including a defect in the endopelvic fascia condensations, a defect in the attachments of the vagina to the levator ani or arcus tendineus, or a lax levator ani hammock.

In addition to the support of the proximal urethra by the above mechanisms, the integrity of the urethral sphincter mechanism is important. The urethral sphincter is made up of two components: the internal and external sphincters. The internal sphincter is made up of smooth muscle and is an extension of the detrusor muscle at the bladder base. The internal sphincter is primarily responsible for continence. The external sphincter is striated and composed of three components: the sphincter urethrae, the compressor urethrae, and the urethrovaginal sphincter. The compressor urethrae and urethrovaginal sphincter, formerly called the deep transverse perineal muscle, are located on the ventral aspect of the urethra at the distal third. The sphincter urethrae surrounds the proximal two thirds of the urethra. The external sphincter functions as a backup for the internal sphincter and helps maintain continence in acute situations. However, if the internal sphincter is deficient, the external system fails during a stress event such as a cough. The proximal aspect of the urethra, therefore, is the most important functionally, as it is the location of the internal sphincter. It extends into the proximal 20% of the urethra. The external sphincter extends from 20% to 80% of the rest of the urethra.

Another important aspect of urethral anatomy is the submucosal vasculature, which helps in coapting the urethral lumen to effect a proper seal. This vasculature becomes thin during menopause, leading to dysfunction and incontinence.

The normal female urethra is about 4 cm long, and the normal location for the bladder neck is posterior to the lower third of the pubic bone.

NEUROUROLOGY

This chapter is not intended to describe the many complex reflex arcs and pathways that allow proper storage and planned disposal of bladder contents. Indeed, it is unnecessary to understand these complexities to apply the fundamentals of neurourology in the clinical setting. A useful mnemonic is that an intact **S**ympathetic system is necessary to **S**tay **S**ocial (storage) and an intact **P**arasympathetic system to void (pee). The sympathetic system allows for storage of urine via three mechanisms: it increases bladder accommodation via β-adrenergic receptors in the bladder, it increases outlet resistance via α-adrenergic receptors in the bladder neck, and it inhibits bladder contractions by blocking parasympathetic transmission. The sympathetic nerves arise in T10-L2 and travel to the bladder via the hypogastric plexus. The parasympathetic system causes bladder contractions via S2-4 and the pelvic plexus. The primary mediators are cholinergic. There are only muscarinic receptors in the bladder, which can be blocked by atropine. The parasympathetic and sympathetic plexuses merge into the inferior hypogastric plexuses of Frankenhauer and from there innervate all the pelvic organs, including the rectum and bladder.

Bladder and urethral sensations are governed by the complex interplay of reflexes mediated by the hypogastric and pelvic plexuses and also by pudendal nerve afferents. These impulses ultimately are processed in the cortex, superior frontal gyrus (bladder), and the paracentral lobule (sphincter).

The external urethral sphincter, external anal sphincter, and perineum are supplied by the pudendal nerve. The proximal sphincter is innervated by the pelvic plexus. The levator ani are innervated both by the pudendal nerve and a direct branch from S2-3-4.

The pudendal nerve is the nerve most in jeopardy during childbirth (Fig. 80-1). The pudendal nerve arises from S2-3-4 and passes between the coccygeus and piriformis muscles. From there it exits the pelvis through the greater sciatic foramen and reenters through the lesser sciatic foramen. The nerve then joins the puden-

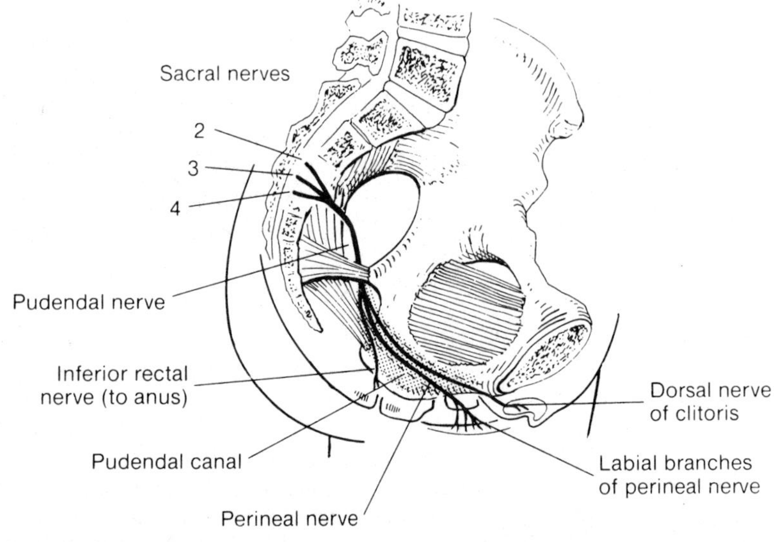

Figure 80-1. Course and branches of the pudendal nerve in the female pelvis. Shaded area represents section of nerve sometimes damaged with childbirth. (Walters MD, Karram MM. Clinical urogynecology. St. Louis: Mosby Yearbook, p. 159.)

dal vessels as it courses along the lateral aspect of the ischiorectal fossa in a tunnel created by the obturator fascia (Alcock's canal). It then dives into the urogenital diaphragm and divides into its branches (inferior hemorrhoidal and perineal). Its relatively fixed position in Alcock's canal allows it to be stretched during labor as the pelvic floor descends. This stretching of the nerve can lead to neuropathy that manifests as urinary or fecal incontinence or the inability to contract the pubococcygeus, as in a Kegel exercise.

CLASSIFICATION

Urinary incontinence can be described by symptomatology, such as stress or urge incontinence. This designation implies that no formal urodynamic evaluation has occurred and is a descriptive diagnosis only. The major diagnostic categories are listed in Table 80-1. Genuine stress incontinence, detrusor instability, mixed incontinence, and a subcategory of genuine stress incontinence called intrinsic sphincter deficiency are based on objective urodynamic criteria. Overflow incontinence can be diagnosed without formal urodynamics, but its etiology may be better defined by this study.

Genuine stress incontinence (GSI) is the objective loss of urine in the presence of increased abdominal pressure without a detrusor contraction (Fig. 80-2). This is a urodynamic diagnosis and cannot be made based on the symptoms or physical examination alone. Classically, the patient gives a history of urine loss with a cough or sneeze not accompanied by urgency. The cause of GSI is descent of the bladder neck during increased abdominal pressure. Although surgical remedies have historically been championed as the primary treatment, nonsurgical interventions have a role to play as well.

Detrusor instability is the loss of urine secondary to a rise in vesical pressure alone. Subtracted multichannel urodynamic testing allows concurrent recording of the abdominal and vesical pressures to gain a subtracted pressure curve that represents detrusor pressure (Fig. 80-3). This entity should be distinguished from detrusor hyperreflexia, which is detrusor instability secondary to a neurologic cause. Possible neurologic causes of detrusor hyperreflexia include stroke, multiple sclerosis, Parkinson disease, and meningomyelocele. Causes of detrusor instability include inflammation secondary to cystitis, urethritis, stones, tumor, suture, postoperative edema, and drugs (eg, parasympathomimetics such as bethanechol) (Table 80-2). The most common cause of detrusor instability is idiopathic.

Mixed incontinence occurs when both GSI and detrusor instability are demonstrated on urodynamic evaluation.

Intrinsic sphincter deficiency is the term used to describe a weakened internal urethral sphincter. There are several ways to assess the adequacy of the internal urethral sphincter. At cystoscopy, the bladder neck can be visualized; if it is wide open, this is evidence for intrinsic sphincter deficiency. On urodynamic testing, the abdominal leak point pressures and maximal urethral closure pressures can be measured; in intrinsic sphincter deficiency, the former should be less than 60 cm H_2O and the latter less than 20 cm H_2O. It is important to identify these patients because they do poorly with the conventional procedures used to treat GSI.

Table 80-1. The Major Diagnostic Categories of Urinary Incontinence

Based on Urodynamic Criteria
Genuine stress incontinence
Intrinsic sphincter deficiency
Detrusor instability
Mixed incontinence
Urodynamic Criteria Not Essential
Overflow incontinence

Table 80-2. Causes of Detrusor Instability and Detrusor Hyperreflexia.

Detrusor Instability
Inflammation
Cystitis
Urethritis
Calculi
Tumor
Suture
Postoperative edema
Pharmacologic
Idiopathic
Detrusor Hyperreflexia
Stroke
Multiple sclerosis
Parkinson disease
Meningomyelocele

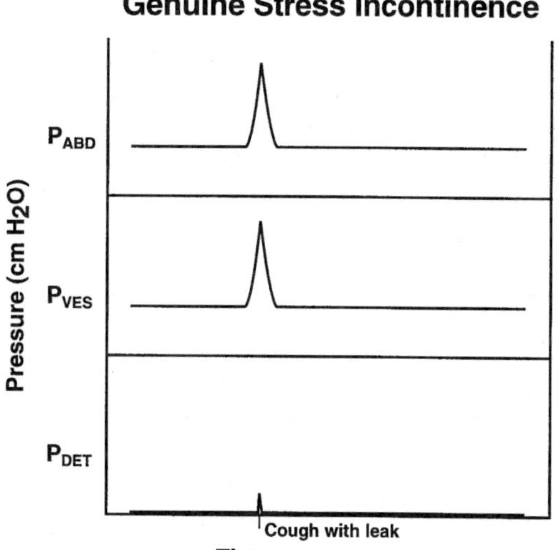

Figure 80-2. Genuine stress incontinence.

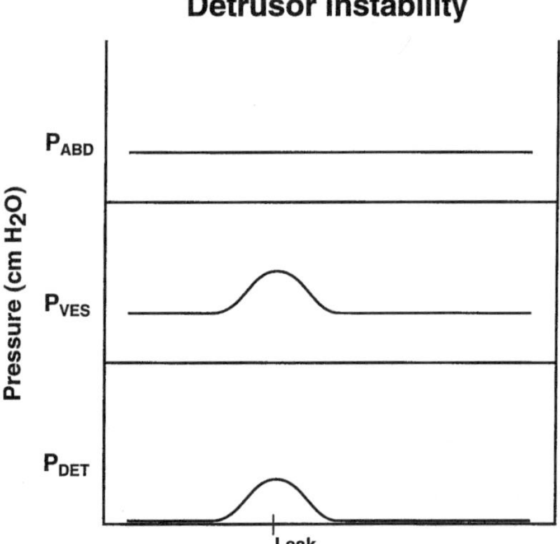

Figure 80-3. Detrusor instability.

Overflow incontinence is the loss of urine secondary to an overly full bladder. The diagnosis does not require urodynamics, but such testing may identify functional aspects of the bladder that may help direct therapy. For instance, a patient may have complaints of difficulty passing her stream as well as constant urinary dribbling. The clinician may hope to find a large prolapse that may explain a functional obstruction as the cause of what sounds like an outlet obstruction. If there is no evidence of prolapse, the clinician must consider the diagnosis of urogenital fistula. Postvoiding residual volumes should be checked and in this case might be 200 mL on multiple evaluations. At this juncture there are several possibilities: the most likely is an underactive detrusor, which can be demonstrated during a pressure void study. In this scenario, the clinician must also consider neurologic etiologies. A neurologic examination and possibly a pelvic floor nerve study can be done to clarify the issue.

PATIENT INTERVIEW

The interview is probably the most important aspect of the entire evaluation. If the clinician does not specifically ask about urine leakage, this malady will not be found. Simply asking the patient whether she has a bladder problem is not sufficient. The patient is usually incredibly embarrassed about this and does not volunteer the information. As word gets out that there is treatment for this problem, primary care providers may well see this problem mushroom in their practices. The patient should also be asked directly about fecal incontinence (see Chap. 72).

A thorough urogynecologic review of symptoms is long (Fig. 80-4). It is simpler to have the patient answer the questions at home and bring the questionnaire with her to the office. Some of the key points warrant further discussion. Are the symptoms largely stress- or urge-related, or both? How long has she had this problem, and how severe is it for her? This again highlights the subjectivity and quality-of-life issues that characterize urinary incontinence: for some women, the need for a light pad with aerobic exercise is intolerable, whereas for others the wearing of daily pads for leaking seems manageable. What is the frequency of her daytime voids and the number of episodes of nocturia? Normal figures are eight and one, respectively. How long is the interval between voids? Normal is 3 to 4 hours. What is her fluid intake? Most women with incontinence usually live in a slightly dehydrated state, as they try to minimize their incontinent episodes by minimizing their fluid intake. This has the secondary effect of constipation, which leads to straining with bowel movements and more stress to the pelvic floor. Also, concentrated urine can be irritating to the bladder, making urgency symptoms worse. Does she consume caffeinated beverages or chocolate? Caffeine is a bladder irritant and a diuretic.

To get a better picture of daily intake, urine output, frequency, and number of incontinent episodes, a voiding diary is invaluable (Fig. 80-5). The patient is asked to keep such a diary for 24 to 48 hours and bring it with her on her next visit. This helps the clinician gauge the severity of the incontinence. Again, this is a quality-of-life issue that has no gold standard of measurement except that of the patient. The diary also helps follow progress as different therapeutic modalities are applied. The clinician can also assess whether excessive intake is part of the problem.

Patients with detrusor instability often relate that the sound or sight of water stimulates their urge to void, that they cannot stop their stream once started, and that they have an urgent desire to void, with leakage before reaching the toilet.

The clinician should specifically ask about the regularity of bowel movements and straining to defecate. Is manual replacement of a "bulge" required to defecate or urinate? Does the patient strain to void? Symptoms of voiding difficulty include hesitancy, slow stream, a feeling of incomplete emptying, and postvoid dribbling. Voiding difficulty may be caused by obstruction created by a large prolapse or may be secondary to an underactive detrusor. Urodynamic study is necessary to differentiate the two.

Sexual activity is common in the elderly and not so elderly. Inquiries as to whether there are problems with intercourse or orgasm should be discussed in a sensitive but forthright manner. Alterations in bowel or sexual function may signify pelvic autonomic/somatic dysfunction.

Infectious or calculi etiologies may be suggested by a history of pain with urination, flank pain, or hematuria. Renal and bladder cancers also present with hematuria, and a high index of suspicion should always be present in a heavy smoker or one who has been exposed to aniline dyes.

A full medical, neurologic, surgical, obstetric, and gynecologic history must be obtained. Especially pertinent aspects of the medical history include a history of asthma (increased abdominal pressure), renal disease, diabetes mellitus, poliomyelitis, stroke, arthritis, radiculopathies, sciatica, multiple sclerosis, syphilis, and vitamin B_{12} deficiency. Pertinent previous surgery includes hysterectomy (especially if done for previous prolapse), bladder repair, and urethral dilatation. Obstetric history should include any history of prolonged labor or surgical delivery, complicated episiotomy, and the weight of the largest baby. Menopausal status is also important.

Obesity is also important. Thirty percent of Americans are overweight, and the medical community must address this issue by

Urogynecology History Questionnaire

	Circle	
1. Do you leak urine when you cough, sneeze, or laugh?	Y	N
1A. If yes, does it come out in a spurt, dribble or constant stream?	Y	N
2. Did you have bedwetting problems beyond age 5?	Y	N
3. Have you wet the bed in the past year?	Y	N
4. Do you ever have such an uncomfortably strong need to urinate that if you don't reach the toilet you will leak?	Y	N
4A. If yes, do you ever leak before you reach the toilet?	Y	N
5. How many times during the day do you urinate? ________________		
6. How many times at night do you get up to void? ________________		
7. Do you develop an urgent need to void when you are nervous, under stress, or in a hurry?	Y	N
8. Do you develop a urgent need to void when you hear water running, prepare to bathe, or in cold weather?	Y	N
9. Do you leak urine for no apparent reason at all?	Y	N
10. Do you leak urine with intercourse?	Y	N
11. Do you drink coffee, tea, or cola drinks, or eat chocolate? (Circle all that apply)	Y	N
12. Do you find it hard to begin urinating?	Y	N
13. Do you have a slow urinary stream?	Y	N
14. Do you strain to pass urine?	Y	N
15. After urination, do you have dribbling or a sense that your bladder is still full?	Y	N
16. When passing urine, can you usually stop the flow?	Y	N
17. Have you ever had a bladder infection?	Y	N
17A. If yes, how many?____________ Any in past year?	Y	N
18. Is your urine ever bloody?	Y	N
19. Are you troubled by pain or discomfort when you urinate?	Y	N
20. Have you ever had bladder/pelvic surgery?	Y	N
21. Have you ever been treated with urethral dilatation?	Y	N
21A. If yes, did it help?	Y	N

(continued)

Figure 80-4. Urogynecology history questionnaire.

Urogynecology History Questionnaire *(Continued)*

	Circle
22. Did your urine problem start during or just after pregnancy?	Y N
23. Did your urine problem start after an operation?	Y N
Which type? ______________________	
24. List all your medications (including vitamins, aspirin): ______________________ ______________________	
25. Did your urine problems start after radiation therapy?	Y N
26. Have you ever been treated for: kidney or bladder disease	Y N
kidney stones	Y N
kidney or bladder tumors	Y N
kidney or bladder injuries	Y N
27. Did menopause make urine loss worse?	Y N
28. Do you have problems with constipation or irregular bowel movements?	Y N
29. Have you ever had brain, spinal, or back surgery?	Y N
(Circle all that apply)	
30. Have you ever been treated for: Paralysis	Y N
Polio	Y N
Multiple sclerosis	Y N
Stroke	Y N
Diabetes mellitus	Y N
Back pain	Y N
Syphilis	Y N
31. Do you need to wear a pad because of leaking?	Y N
31A. If yes, during the day only?	Y N
all the time?	Y N
32. How often do you leak in 24 hours? ______________________	
33. How long have you had a problem with leaking? ______________________	
34. Does anyone else in the family have a similar problem with leaking?	Y N
35. Did/does anyone in your family have problems with bedwetting?	Y N

Figure 80-4. (*Continued*) Urogynecology history questionnaire.

gentle consultation with the patient and by example. Aside from the obvious chronic increase in abdominal pressure that may predispose to urogenital prolapse, the additional strain on the skeleton leads to degenerative joint disease and subsequent disk disease, which can lead to neuropathy of the pelvic floor.

Medications can affect bladder function. Diuretics are probably the major offenders, but prazosin and other α-antagonists used for hypertension can cause urinary incontinence. α-Agonists found in many over-the-counter cold medications, as well as the anticholinergic effects of antidepressants, can lead to urinary retention and overflow incontinence. Sedative/hypnotic drugs can cloud the sensorium of a frail elderly patient and may lead to incontinence. The clinician must obtain a full list of medications and carefully evaluate their impact on the patient's continence.

PHYSICAL EXAMINATION

Observing the patient walking into the examination room immediately reveals any mobility problems that may make the bathroom inaccessible. Examination of the abdomen may reveal multiple striae, which may indicate a congenital weakness of collagen. All abdominal scars should be accounted for. Lower extremity edema should be noted. Patients who suffer from congestive heart failure routinely third-space fluid in their lower extremities during the day, only to be in the bathroom all night as this fluid is mobilized. Pelvic or abdominal masses should be looked for and ruled out. Genital atrophy should be assessed and treated if present. A thorough pelvic examination should be performed, including a full assessment of pelvic floor prolapse (see Chap. 33). The urethra and bladder base should be carefully palpated for tenderness and masses, which may lead one to suspect the presence of a diverticulum. A clean-catch urine specimen should be evaluated by urinalysis and culture to rule out infection and hematuria.

A neurologic examination, including the bulbocavernosus reflex, sensory evaluation of the S2-3-4 dermatomes, and lower extremity reflexes, should be performed. The bulbocavernosus reflex tests the intactness of the sacral reflex arcs. It can be elicited by gently touching just lateral to the clitoris with a cotton-tipped applicator and observing contraction of the external anal sphincter. Alternatively, the so-called anal wink can be elicited by gently touching just laterally to the external anal sphincter and observing the contraction of the anal sphincter. This should be done at the beginning of the examination, as this reflex accommodates to touch and is less likely to be elicited later in the examination. This reflex is absent in about 15% of normal patients. Also important is the assessment of external anal sphincter tone during the rectovaginal examination.

At this point, if the patient still has a full bladder, the clinician can look for stress incontinence by asking the patient to perform the Valsalva maneuver or to cough and observing for urine loss. If no urine loss is documented in the lithotomy position, the patient should be asked to stand and again to cough.

For an adequate bimanual examination, the patient must empty her bladder. The physician will be drier and the patient more likely to bear down vigorously during the evaluation of the pelvic floor if she has emptied her bladder. After the patient empties her bladder, the clinician can measure a postvoiding residual volume to assess the efficiency of bladder emptying. Normal postvoiding residual values have not been well defined, but most would agree that less than 50 mL is normal and more than 200 mL is abnormal.

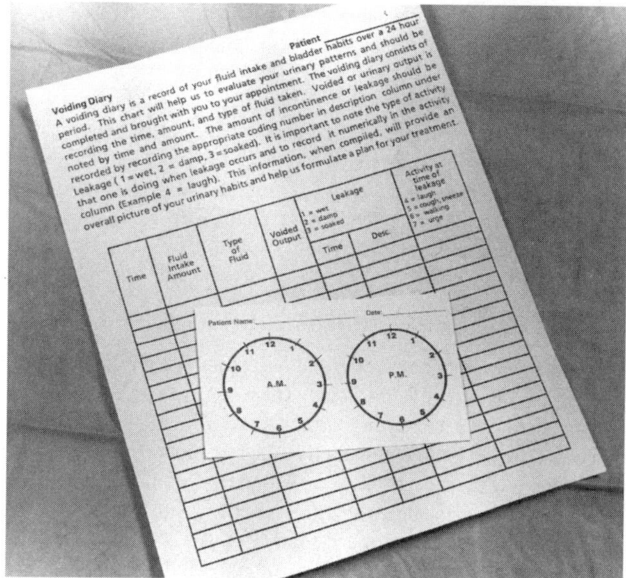

Figure 80-5. Voiding diary.

The patient's ability to contract her levator ani can be evaluated by asking her to squeeze the clinician's fingers with her vagina. The response can be graded as absent, poor, fair, or good.

The mobility of the bladder neck can be assessed by placing a sterile plastic cotton-tipped applicator soaked with 2% lidocaine jelly into the urethra. The patient is instructed to bear down as hard as possible, and the deflection of the cotton-tipped applicator is measured using an instrument designed to measure angles, such as a goniometer with a leveler to keep the clinician oriented to the horizontal. Hypermobility has not been exactly defined, but most studies consider greater than 20° to 30° of movement of the cotton-tipped applicator to be hypermobility (or > 1 cm of movement of the bladder neck by ultrasound measurement). The tip of the applicator must be placed at the bladder neck; otherwise, inaccurate results are obtained. This is why the so-called "Q-tip test" has been received poorly by researchers. In most patients, one can easily feel when the applicator has passed from the urethra into the bladder, and in these patients the test can provide an estimate of bladder neck mobility.

The assessment of bladder neck mobility is important in determining the type of surgical procedure to be performed. Many investigators are still evaluating this technique, and in this age of diminishing medical dollars it behooves investigators to find the least expensive technique. To evaluate every patient with videofluoroscopy would be exorbitant.

In very incontinent patients, the vulva is often excoriated by the constant dampness. Frequent pad changes and the use of Desitin ointment and cornstarch are immediate interventions. However, for many elderly women, frequent changes of sanitary pads are prohibitively expensive.

Patients with vulvar atrophy and incontinence should be treated with estrogen, except those in whom its use is contraindicated. The urogenital tissues are extremely sensitive to estrogen deprivation and become thin, with a diminished blood supply. This leads to less turgor in the tissues around the bladder neck and proximal urethra, resulting in poor luminal coaptation and an increased risk of incontinence. Many elderly women are averse to taking yet another medication by mouth but often agree to vaginal estrogen. Many different regimens have been espoused, but none has been well studied for effectiveness. One that anecdotally seems beneficial is 1 to 2 g per vagina once or twice a week at bedtime. Vaginal estrogen is well absorbed, and therefore care must be taken not to give a dose that would be equivalent to unopposed estrogen in the patient who still has a uterus.

URODYNAMIC TESTING

The question of who needs urodynamic testing is a poignant one in this age of cost-effective medicine. There has been much debate as to how predictive the symptom of stress incontinence is of the diagnosis of GSI and how predictive the symptom of urge incontinence is of detrusor instability. Jensen and colleagues (1994) reviewed 29 articles addressing this question, with a total of 6000 patients. They found that the symptom of stress urinary incontinence as a predictor of GSI had a sensitivity of 90.6%, a specificity of 51.1%, a positive predictive value of 74.9%, and a negative predictive value of 77.1%. Similarly, the symptom of urge incontinence correlated with the diagnosis of detrusor instability with a sensitivity of 73.5%, a specificity of 55.2%, a positive predictive value of 56.1%, and a negative predictive value of 72.8%.

Clearly, urodynamic testing has a role in elucidating the etiology of urinary incontinence. Most would agree that urodynamic testing is indicated if a surgical intervention is planned, if the patient has failed previous surgery, if the clinical picture is unclear, and if the patient has failed a medical therapeutic trial. More than in many tests, however, the results are dependent on the skill of the clinician performing the test. This is especially true when studying a patient with significant prolapse. The key to performing accurate studies is to reproduce in the laboratory the symptoms that occur at home.

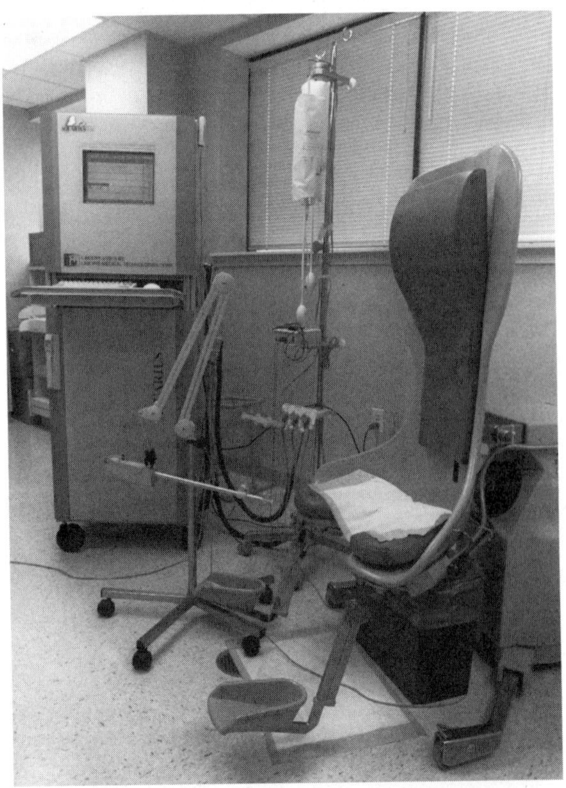

Figure 80-6. Typical urodynamic laboratory.

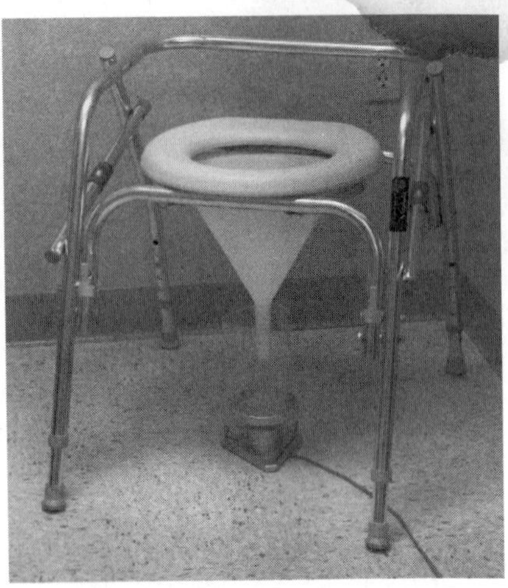

Figure 80-7. Commode linked to electrical device to perform uroflow.

The urodynamic examination allows identification and quantification of the in vivo process of urine storage and micturition. Figure 80-6 shows a typical urodynamic laboratory set up with a birthing chair and urodynamic software used in data processing. Details about urodynamic testing are beyond the interest of most primary care physicians, but it is helpful to know what information to expect when a patient is sent for such testing. The evaluation typically consists of a uroflow, cystometrogram, urethral pressure profile, and pressure-voiding study.

The uroflow is a straightforward test in which the patient is asked to void on a commode that is linked to an electrical device that can measure time versus volume and thereby assess urine flow patterns (Fig. 80-7). This is largely a screening tool for voiding dysfunction. A normal uroflow pattern is shown in Figure 80-8. An

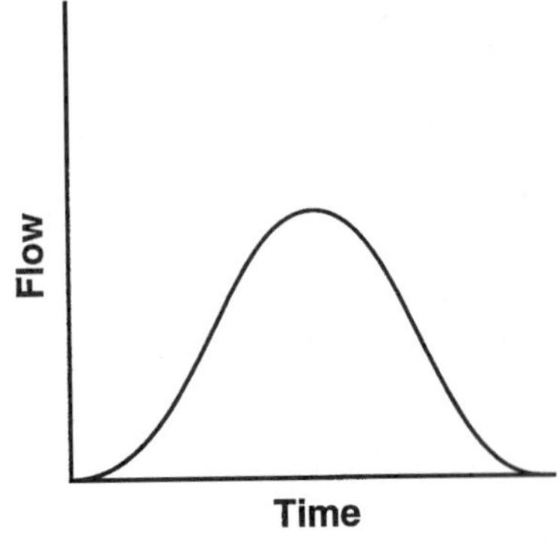

Figure 80-8. Normal uroflow pattern.

intermittent or prolonged uroflow pattern suggests a voiding disorder but cannot be further elucidated without the pressure-flow study.

The other tests are performed by placing a pressure transducer catheter (either microtip or water) into the vagina to measure abdominal pressure and a double-sensor catheter in the urethra and bladder. By subtracting the abdominal pressure from the vesical pressure, the true bladder (ie, detrusor) pressure can be measured while filling the bladder with sterile saline or water.

The cystometrogram is performed with the catheters in place, with the goal of differentiating GSI from detrusor instability. The patient is asked to cough or perform the Valsalva maneuver at different times during the bladder filling, and it is noted whether she leaks urine with such provocation. If she leaks at the exact moment of increased abdominal pressure without a concomitant rise in detrusor pressure, then she has GSI (see Fig. 80-2). If, on the other hand, she leaks without an increase in abdominal pressure, but instead the detrusor pressure rises, this represents detrusor instability (see Fig. 80-3). During the bladder filling phase, the patient is asked to state when she would first start looking for a bathroom (volume of first sensation; normal is 100 to 200 mL), when she would definitely be looking for a bathroom (functional bladder capacity; normal is 350 to 500 mL), and when she can no longer take any more fluid without great discomfort (maximal bladder capacity; normal is 500 to 600 mL). These estimates of normal reflect this author's experience and have not been rigorously studied.

During the filling phase, bladder compliance can also be assessed. As the bladder fills, the change in pressure should be minimal. Several abdominal leak point pressures are measured during this segment of the examination. Abdominal leak point pressures are one of the parameters used in assessing intrinsic urethral sphincter function.

Urethral Pressure Profile

Pressure (cm H2O)

P_{URA}

P_{VES}

P_{UCP}

Time (Length)

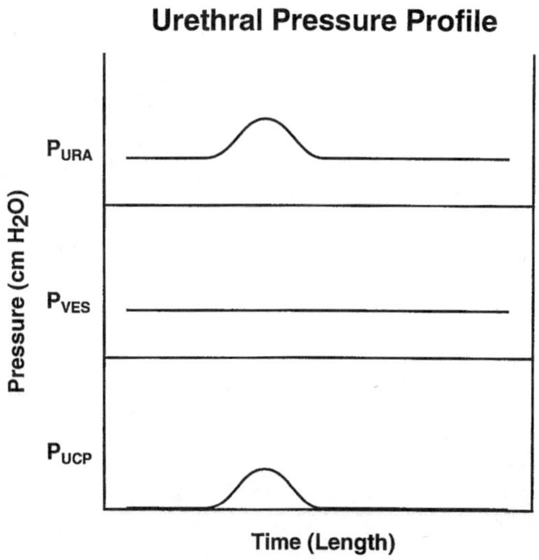

Urethral Pressure = P_{URA}

Vesical Pressure = P_{VES}

Urethral Closure Pressure = $P_{UCP} = (P_{URA} - P_{VES})$

Figure 80-9. Urethral pressure profile.

The urethral pressure profile is performed by pulling the urethral catheter along the length of the urethra and measuring the urethral closure pressures along its length (Fig. 80-9). A maximum urethral closure pressure of less than 20 cm H_2O is another parameter that suggests intrinsic sphincter deficiency. This test can also measure the functional urethral length, the length of the urethra that maintains a pressure above that of the bladder (normal, > 2.5 cm.)

Finally, the patient is instructed to void with the catheters in place, and a pressure-void study is performed to assess the voiding mechanism. A normal voiding mechanism involves urethral relaxation with detrusor pressure elevation (Fig. 80-10). Especially in the elderly, a prolonged uroflow pattern can be found with no functional outlet obstruction from prolapse. Usually these patients are found to have underactive detrusor contractions, which can be documented during this examination.

MEDICAL MANAGEMENT

Genuine Stress Incontinence

Nonsurgical interventions can be instituted for GSI. Some studies suggest that two thirds of patients can avoid surgery with medical management alone. In a patient who, by history and physical

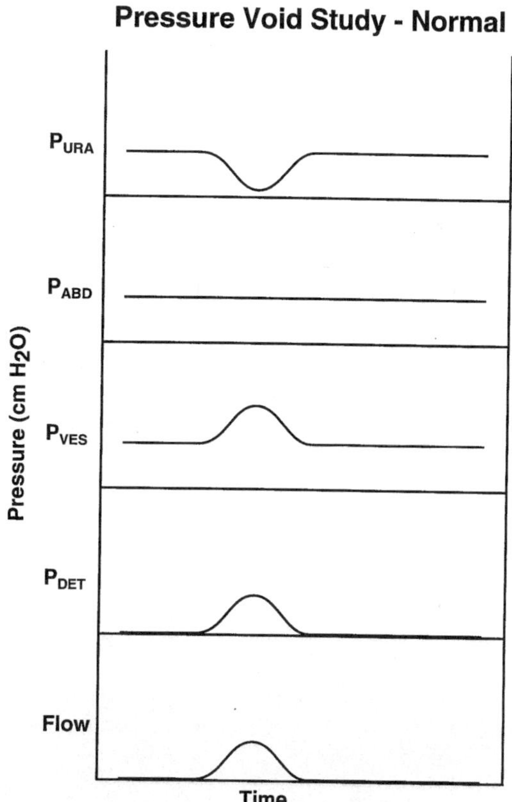

Note that the urethral pressure drops just prior to the rise in detrusor pressure. Abdominal pressure is unchanged throughout.

Figure 80-10. Pressure void study—normal.

examination, appears to have simple stress incontinence, these simple therapeutic modalities can be tried before urodynamic evaluation and diagnosis. In the menopausal patient, the first intervention is oral or vaginal estrogen replacement, assuming no contraindications exist. The patient's ability to perform Kegel exercises should be assessed, and she should be instructed to perform this exercise at least 45 times a day. The clinician can explain that the levator ani muscles act as a hammock to hold up the bladder, vagina, and rectum. For a patient with a large prolapse, performing Kegel exercises does not cure the prolapse but helps strengthen the pelvic floor and may forestall worsening of the condition. In addition, if the patient learns to perform Kegel exercises efficiently, she may be able to prevent leakage by doing so when she is in a leak-type situation (eg, coughing). Patients who cannot perform a Kegel may benefit from physical therapy.

Because caffeine is a bladder irritant and a diuretic, incontinent patients should avoid it. Caffeine need not be eliminated, however, in a patient without urge symptoms who has been shown to have GSI alone.

α-Agonists such as phenylpropanolamine (found in drugs such as Entex, Ornade, and Tavist-D) help stimulate the bladder neck. Imipramine also has α-adrenergic effects. In addition, continence rings, fitted in similar fashion to a pessary, may be effective. The newest version, a device called Introl, is made of silicone and has prongs that are fitted on either side of the bladder neck. This has shown promise, but the $300 price tag may prove prohibitive to many patients.

Detrusor Instability

In a patient who has urge incontinence or documented detrusor instability, estrogen therapy is again important. Elimination of caffeine is imperative. A trial of the various anticholinergic and antispasmodic agents should be applied (Table 80-3). The patient can be started on oxybutynin chloride (Ditropan) 2.5 mg twice a day, increased as necessary. It is important to inquire about narrow angle glaucoma, as anticholinergic therapy is contraindicated in these patients. The most common complaints when starting anticholinergic therapy are a dry mouth and, less commonly, somnolence. Many drug trials have shown up to a 50% placebo effect. The key elements of starting such therapy are to titrate the doses slowly and to give each drug a 6-week trial if possible.

Table 80-3. Commonly Used Drugs for Urinary Incontinence

Estrogen
Anticholinergics (caveat: glaucoma)
Propantheline bromide (Pro-Banthine) 15 mg tid or qid
Antispasmodics
Oxybutynin chloride (Ditropan) 5–10 mg tid (available as suspension; also anticholinergic effects)
Flavoxate (Urispas) 100–200 mg tid or qid
Dicyclomine (Antispas) 10–20 mg tid or qid (less effective than Ditropan; use when Ditropan's side effects are intolerable)
Antidepressants
Imipramine 10 mg tid–50 mg bid/25 mg tid (α-adrenergic and anticholinergic effects)
Anesthetics
Phenazopyridine (Pyridium) 200 mg tid ×2–3 days only
Antiseptic/Parasympatholytic
Urised
α-Blockers
Terazosin 1 mg qd up to 5 mg/d; increase dose over 3-week period
Prazosin
Phenoxybenzamine (Dibensiline) 10 mg bid up to 40 mg tid, incr qod (caveat: orthostatic hypotension; indication: retention)
α-Antagonists
Phenylpropanolamine (Entex, Ornade, Tavist-D) 50 mg bid
Indication: GSI/temporary intermittent use only secondary to small risk of seizures and strokes
Parasympathomimetics
Bethanechol (Urecholine); indication: hypotonic bladder

Most patients with detrusor instability have frequency, and this can be abated to a large extent by initiating, in concert with starting medication, a behavioral modification technique called bladder drill training. The patient is instructed to determine the longest interval she can wait between voids without risking an urge incontinence

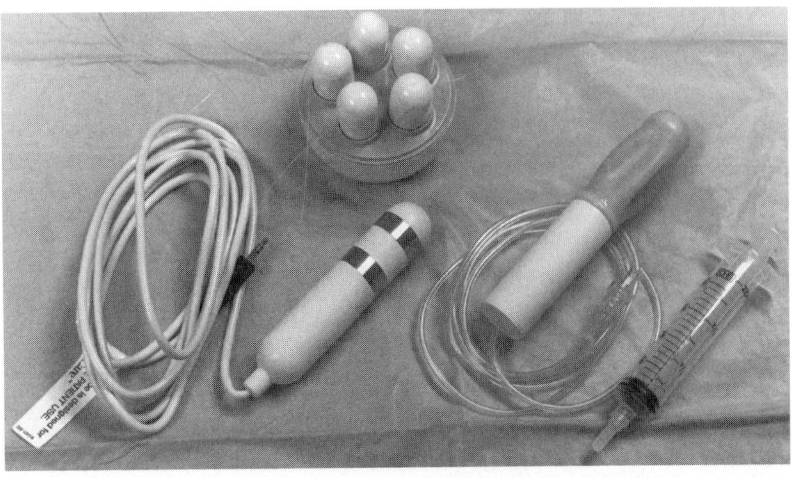

Figure 80-11. Vaginal cones, vaginal sensors for electrical stimulation and biofeedback.

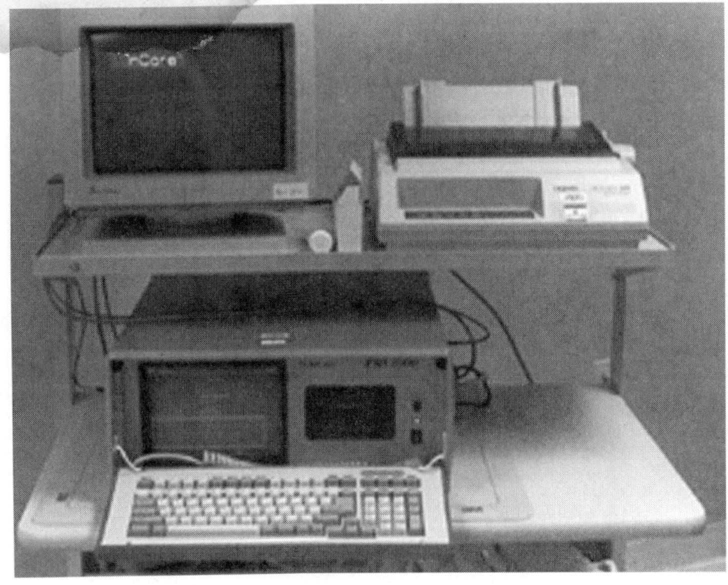

Figure 80-12. Biofeedback monitor to enhance pelvic floor function.

episode. She is then instructed to void on this initial schedule, then to increase the interval by 15 to 30 minutes every week or two. For example, if a patient states she voids every hour during the day, then this is the interval that is initiated. She then increases this interval, with a goal interval being every 3 to 4 hours. If her bladder insists on her voiding sooner, she is instructed to attempt to dismiss the urge by performing a strong Kegel. By flexing the levator ani, it is theorized that a reflex arc is interrupted, allowing the bladder to relax. It is therefore important to teach these patients proper Kegel technique. If the patient fails medication, she is a candidate for electrical stimulation. The patient's progress can be followed with urologs and bladder drill "clock" cards, as shown in Figure 80-5.

PHYSIOTHERAPY OF THE PELVIC FLOOR

When patients cannot perform Kegels or fail medications for detrusor instability, physical therapy interventions can be of help. These techniques include vaginal cones, biofeedback, and electrical stimulation.

Biofeedback is performed by placing a sensor in the vagina and having the patient isolate her levator ani by visual cues from a screen. Biofeedback strengthens the levator ani, thereby maintaining the bladder neck in a favorable position during stress, as well as strengthening the periurethral striated muscle, assisting in luminal coaptation.

Electrical stimulation is also done via the vagina (Fig. 80-11). This is theorized to work in several ways. It may improve reinnervation of partly denervated pelvic floor muscles by promoting growth of the surviving motor axons. It also stimulates reflex inhibition of the detrusor muscle. Some suggest that it may restore normal urethral and bladder reflexes, although this is unproved. Numerous studies show the efficacy of this technique. A 1994 study reviewed 52 patients in a prospective randomized fashion and found that electrical stimulation cured or improved 62% of them. A 1993 study showed this treatment to be effective in 71% of patients with GSI and 70% of patients with detrusor instability. When compared with the cumulative 5-year surgery success rate of 75%, these numbers are respectable. Another author found that biofeedback improved 66% of GSI patients and 33% of those with detrusor instability. Remembering that the fundamental issue is one of quality of life, these modalities clearly are beneficial.

Figure 80-12 shows a typical set-up, with screens to allow feedback to the patient as she is undergoing this therapy.

Vaginal cones, shown in Figure 80-11, are graduated weights that the patient holds in the vagina for 15 minutes twice daily. She is fitted with the heaviest weight she can hold. As she masters one weight, she progresses to the next higher level. Once she reaches the heaviest cone, she begins to do these exercises while doing increased levels of activity. Again, she is followed by urologs. A patient who cannot volitionally stop her urine flow by performing a Kegel exercise or one who has no palpable Kegel ability is probably not a good candidate for this therapy.

Patients are no longer instructed to perform Kegels only when they are voiding, as this practice can actually instigate voiding dysfunction. The patient may occasionally test the strength of her Kegel during a void, but this should not be a routine practice.

SUMMARY

The 1992 U.S. Department of Health and Human Services Clinical Practice Guideline stated, "As a general rule, the least invasive and least dangerous procedure that is appropriate for the patient should be the first choice. . . . For many forms of urinary incontinence, behavioral techniques meet these criteria." When these modalities fail or when the patient has concomitant symptomatic prolapse, surgery is clearly in order. The clinician should present all the options to the patient and help her decide which treatment is best for her.

BIBLIOGRAPHY

Bent A. Etiology and management of detrusor instability and mixed incontinence. Obstet Gynecol Clin North Am 1989;16:853.

Clinical practice guideline: urinary incontinence in adults. US Dept. of Health and Human Services, 1992.

Jensen JK, Nielsen FR, Ostergard DR. The role of patient history in the diagnosis of urinary incontinence. Obstet Gynecol 1994;83:904.

Parulkar BG, Barrett DM. Urinary incontinence in adults. Surg Clin North Am 1988;68:945.

Resnick NM. Diagnosis and treatment of incontinence in the institutionalized elderly. Seminars in urology 1989;7:117.

Thiede HA. The prevalence of urogynecologic disorders. Obstet Gynecol Clin North Am 1989;16:709.

Walters MD, Realini JP. The evaluation and treatment of urinary incontinence in women: a primary care approach. J Am Board Family Practice 1992;5:289.

Primary Care for Women, edited by Phyllis C. Leppert and Fred M. Howard. Lippincott-Raven Publishers, Philadelphia © 1997.

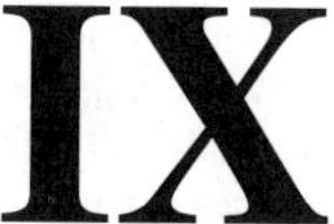

Immunologic and Infectious Diseases

81

Allergies

PHYLLIS C. LEPPERT

It is estimated that at least 20%, and perhaps more, of the United States population may be allergic to one substance or another. In developed countries, allergies account for a sizable amount of illness and medical expense. Because the allergic response is not a typical health problem in developing countries where parasitic disease is common, and because in both circumstances the individual affected produces high quantities of immunoglobulin E (IgE), a hypothesis has been suggested to account for allergies. This hypothesis states that the IgE response was initially evolved to help humans cope with parasites. Therefore, any person with the genetic trait that allowed an effective attack to be mounted against parasitic disease had a survival advantage. These people would live longer and produce more offspring. As a result, this parasite defense system developed as a common system. In individuals who no longer encounter parasites, this IgE system is free to react to other substances, such as ragweed pollen. However, animal studies of this hypothesis are inconclusive. Nevertheless, allergic conditions remain a phenomenon of the developed world.

Asthma and its sequelae are thought to be responsible for 1% of all health care costs in the United States. Most allergic individuals have allergic rhinitis or asthma. However, food allergies occur in many children and in some adults as well. Others are allergic to drugs, such as penicillin. Some individuals have local and systemic reactions to insect stings. In certain situations, allergic reactions may be fatal.

ETIOLOGY

Allergy is due to a misdirected immune response. Different allergens initiate distinct symptoms as they react with the immune system at different body sites. For instance, in the upper airways, the response leads to sneezing and nasal congestion: the symptoms of allergic rhinitis. In the lower smaller airways, bronchial constriction and airway obstruction cause wheezing and a sensation of air hunger: the signs of asthma. In the gastrointestinal tract, allergens cause nausea, abdominal cramps, diarrhea, and vomiting. They also cause atopic dermatitis. Allergens that enter the systemic circulation can induce anaphylaxis. This response, if severe, can cause death.

The allergic response is a complex chain of molecular and cellular interactions. Allergens cause a biphasic response that is IgE dependent. The allergic response is universally initiated by the activation of the mast cells by IgE. During the active phase of the allergic response, IgE bound to the membranes of basophils and mast cells cross-links with the allergen. This is followed by the release of vasoactive mediators (histamine, proteases, proteoglycans), leukocyte chemotactic factors, and cytokines. These released substances cause the clinical manifestations of the acute phase of the allergic reaction. The late-phase response (LPR) is associated with an infiltration of inflammatory cells and is important in the pathogenesis of chronic allergic disease. The cell membrane lipid breakdown product of leukotrienes C_4, D_4, E_4, prostaglandin D_2, and platelet-activating factor have potent proinflammatory effects that contribute to allergic reactions. They contribute to the increased vascular permeability, vasodilation, bronchial smooth muscle contraction, and increased mucus production. These leukotrienes also cause increased chemotaxis of eosinophils, neutrophils, and mononuclear cells.

The cross-linking of IgE on mast cells and basophils initiates the synthesis and release of many cytokines, such as interleukin (IL)-1, IL-3, IL-4, IL-5, IL-6, granulocyte macrophage colony-stimulating factor, and tumor necrosis factor-α. These cytokines contribute to late-phase allergic responses. They also regulate IgE synthesis, promote eosinophil differentiation and survival, and help sustain chronic allergic inflammation. They affect leukocyte effector function and the expression of cellular adhesion molecules.

The synthesis of IgE is induced by two signals. The first signal is delivered by IL-4 and allows B cells to synthesize IgE in the presence of a second signal. Second signals are the physical contact with T cells, a number of B-cell activators, including Epstein-Barr virus infection. It has recently been found that T_H1 cells, which secrete interferon $_{\delta}$ (IFN-$_{\delta}$), are IgE-suppressor cells. However, IL-4–secreting T_H2 cells are IgE-helper cells.

In persons with atopic dermatitis, it is suggested that an imbalance of IL-4 and IFN-δ promotes IgE secretion. Also, persons with a large number of Th2 cells secrete increased IgE. Table 81-1 lists some of the substances released from activated mast cells and basophils that contribute to the allergic reaction.

When an allergic individual is exposed to an allergen, an immediate reaction occurs, caused by the acute degranulation of mast cells. The onset typically occurs within 15 to 60 minutes of the exposure and then subsides within 30 to 90 minutes. At such times, elevated plasma histamine and mast cell–derived tryptase is measurable.

The LPR occurs 3 to 4 hours after the acute phase has subsided. It is characterized by an infiltration of eosinophils, mononuclear cells, and some neutrophils. The neutrophils and eosinophils peak at 6 to 8 hours. Then, in 24 to 48 hours after the single-allergen challenge, the infiltration of cells is made up mostly of T cells, monocytes, and macrophages. The local deposition of eosinophil basic protein of the LPR contributes to the respiratory epithelial damage of asthma. During this LPR, leukocyte adhesion molecules occur. It is also known that persons with asthma and atopic dermatitis have autoantibodies to IgE, which contributes to the tissue inflammation of chronic asthma. Allergic diseases, such as asthma, allergic rhinitis, and atopic dermatitis, therefore, are chronic inflammatory diseases.

CLINICAL PICTURE

Asthma

Acute asthma occurs because of reversible airway obstruction and airway hyperresponsiveness. Inflammation of the airway is thought to be the primary mechanism responsible for these pathologic responses. The lungs of asthmatics become hyperinflated because tenacious viscous mucus plugs the airway. Bronchial epithelium becomes desquamated. When the lungs of asthmatics are studied at autopsy, edema, basement membrane thickening, smooth muscle cell hyperplasia, and hypertrophy are seen. Mast cells, T lymphocytes, and eosinophils are seen in the subepithelium, and neutrophil elastase is present, especially near areas of epithelial damage. It is thought currently that airway obstruction results more from bronchial wall edema and mucous plugs than from contraction of bronchial smooth muscle.

Allergic Rhinitis

Allergic rhinitis gives a clinical picture of sneezing, rhinorrhea, and nasal irritation. There is submucosal edema and an infiltration of eosinophils and granulocytes. Allergic rhinitis occurs during seasonal exposure to specific allergens. Nasal epithelial mast cell proliferation occurs with increased basophils and eosinophils. Mast cells are present initially predominately in the submucosa. However, after 4 to 5 days of exposure to a specific pollen, mast cells appear on the surface of the nasal epithelium. Following this, mast cell numbers increase. Eosinophils also increase during seasonal exposure. The number of nasal eosinophils and basophils correlates well with the symptomatologic profile.

Atopic Dermatitis

Atopic dermatitis produces symptoms of pruritus and dry skin. Acute lesions display edema and an inflammatory infiltrate of T lymphocytes, which are predominately CD4 cells. Usually, normal numbers of mast cells are present but few basophils, neutrophils, or eosinophils. Chronic lesions become lichenified, and these lesions exhibit an increased number of granulated mast cells, monocyte macrophages. Langerhans cells, and lymphocytes. Atopic dermatitis is a disease of children and is found in the flexor surfaces of extremities and on scalp surfaces.

The allergic diseases of allergic rhinitis, asthma, and atopic dermatitis are chronic inflammatory problems. They have a course characterized by flare-ups and remissions. The interaction of the allergen with the immune system is complex. A vicious cycle of allergen exposure leading to inflammation and tissue destruction occurs with each exacerbation of the allergic disease, making the clinical situation worse.

Table 81-1. Mediators of Allergic Reactions

CHEMICAL	ACTIVITY	SYMPTOMS
Mediators From Granules		
Histamine	Constricts bronchial airways	Wheezing; difficulty breathing
	Dilates blood vessels	Local redness at sites of allergen delivery; if dilatation is widespread, it can contribute to a lethal drop in blood pressure (shock)
	Stimulates nerve endings	Itching and pain in skin
	Stimulates secretion of mucus in airways	Congestion of airways
Platelet-activating factor	Constricts bronchial airways	Same as for histamine
	Dilates blood vessels	Same as for histamine
Lipid Mediators		
Leukotrienes	Constrict bronchial airways	Same as for histamine
	Increase permeability of small blood vessels	Same as for histamine
Prostaglandin D	Constricts bronchial airways	Same as for histamine

(Lichtenstein LM. Allergy and the immune system. Sci Am 1993;269:116.)

Food Allergy

The clinical picture of food allergy runs the gamut from systemic anaphylaxis through asthma, urticaria, and rhinitis to atopic dermatitis. Foods that usually cause IgE-mediated allergic reactions are eggs, cow's milk, nuts, wheat, soy, white fish, and shellfish. Edema and pruritus of lips and oral mucosa, palate, and pharynx occur. There may be a history of nausea, vomiting, bloating, flatulence, diarrhea, and abdominal pain. In some food allergies, blood may be lost in the stool. Protein-losing enteropathy and eosinophilic gastroenteritis may occur as a response to food allergies. Systemic anaphylaxis occurs, but is rare.

About 1% of all infants are allergic to cow's milk. β-Lactoglobulin is thought to be the most allergenic of the milk proteins, but other proteins, such as casein and whey proteins and α-lactalbumin are allergenic as well. These allergies are IgE mediated. Symptoms include anaphylaxis, urticaria, eczema, rhinitis, and asthma. Several studies suggest that breast-feeding prevents milk allergy. Treatment consists of the use of partially hydrolyzed formulas such as Good Start, which is not available in the United States, and Nutramigen, which is available in the United States. Soy-based formulas have been shown to provoke allergic reactions and are not recommended.

It is important for the primary care provider to know the difference between food intolerance and a food allergy mediated by IgE. Examples of food intolerance are lactose intolerance due to lactase deficiency leading to diarrhea, bloating, abdominal pain, and flatulence. Sulfites used as a preservative may cause asthma in certain persons. Monosodium glutamate in an individual with an intolerance to it causes headache, chest and facial flushing, and a general burning feeling. These conditions are not food allergies, however.

Insect Stings

As much as 4% of the population of the United States is thought to be allergic to the venom of stinging insects such as bees, fire ants, and wasps. The venom of stinging insects contains phospholipases, hyaluronidases, and other antigens that directly affect vascular tone and permeability. Individuals who are allergic to insect stings are at high risk for systemic allergic reactions or anaphylaxis on recurrent stings, because venom diffuses easily into the blood circulation and, therefore, reaches mast cells in multiple body locations.

Anaphylaxis

Anaphylaxis is a true medical emergency. It starts as a general reaction that then evolves rapidly to respiratory or circulatory collapse, or both. Early symptoms often are a marked exacerbation of allergic symptoms such as nasal, pharyngeal, and ocular itching. There is a flushing of the face and a tightness in the throat. These signs and symptoms are accompanied by a tachycardia. *Tachycardia does not occur in a vasovagal event.* Be alert, however, to the fact that tachycardia will not occur in true anaphylaxis in persons on beta-blockers. Other early symptoms are bronchospasm, urticaria or other rash, and angioedema. Individuals with anaphylaxis have a feeling of impending doom. Sometimes diarrhea, cramps, vomiting, and urinary urgency occur. Hypotension and then cardiac arrhythmia occur, followed by cardiovascular collapse. Dilatation of large blood vessels contribute to shock. There is an extreme drop in blood pressure. Seizure can occur due to the severe hypotension. If appropriate measures are not taken, death can occur within minutes.

Penicillin Allergy

Reaction to penicillin is uncommon, occurring in 2% to 5% of individuals. These reactions include anaphylaxis and other immediate forms of allergic response, such as angioneurotic edema and severe urticaria. The LPR is characterized by morbilliform eruptions, serum sickness, and urticaria. A fever may occur and is drug related. In addition, hemolytic anemia may occur due to the interaction of antibody, penicillin, and red blood cells. Allergic reactions to all penicillin derivatives have been reported. The incidence of cross-allergenicity between penicillin and cephalosporin is relatively low. Cephalosporin has been administered to individuals with prior penicillin reactions without incidence. Cephalosporins should not, however, be given to a person with a documented immediate reaction to penicillin. Drug allergy history for any drug, including penicillin, should be recorded in an easily observed place on the person's medical record.

HISTORY AND PHYSICAL EXAMINATION

Many individuals assume allergic causes for illnesses after exposure to certain foods, pollens, or dust, when, in fact, their disease has other causes. Seasonal incidence of symptoms is not always helpful in making the diagnosis. Allergies and infections are both acute and chronic. Allergy season often coincides with outbreaks of viral respiratory infection.

A carefully obtained family history may suggest the diagnosis. Children who have two parents with allergies have between a 65% to 75% chance of having significant allergies themselves, whereas those with one parent with allergies have a 35% chance of having allergies. If an individual has allergic siblings, then her chances of allergic conditions increase. Often, respiratory infections spread through families, and reinfection is common. This cyclical nature of illness can be helpful in determining an infectious etiology of the illness.

Individuals with asthma have wheezing on examination of the lung fields during an attack. Care needs to be applied, because often asthmatics with severe bronchospasm have little wheezing due to almost complete absence of air movement in and out of the airways. As the individuals begin to improve and spasm is relieved, wheezing begins. The inexperienced physician may believe the condition is getting worse, when, in fact, it is improving.

The primary care provider must look for signs of allergy, such as allergic "shiners" or the "allergic salute." The latter manifests as a nasal crease on the tip of the nose. An open-mouthed facies is common in patients with allergic rhinitis and in those with eczema. A word of caution: food allergies do not cause hyperactivity in children. Also, allergies are not due to "environmental illness." Some practitioners subscribe to "clinical ecology," which has no scientific basis.

The physician must observe the color of the nasal mucosa. It is usually pinkish blue in the case of allergic illness and red in the case of infection. The nasal mucous is clear, thin, and watery in allergy, but thick and purulent in infection. For persons with allergic rhinitis, the otolaryngologist examines the nasal vault with a fiberoptic endoscope to observe the mucosa and to obtain exudate for analysis.

The skin surfaces should be carefully examined for evidence of eczema, urticaria, and erythema. Individuals with food allergies have abdominal distention and bloating. In severe situations such as celiac sprue, colonoscopy or sigmoidoscopy for biopsy is necessary for diagnosis.

Signs and symptoms of vasovagal events and anaphylaxis are outlined in Table 81-2.

LABORATORY TESTING

The goal of all laboratory evaluations of individuals with a history that suggests allergy is to document the following two aspects of disease: (1) to discover that IgE-mediated degranulation of mast cells and basophils are causing the symptoms, and (2) to identify the nature of the allergens.

Two types of testing for in vivo diagnosis usually are used by allergists. One is provocation or challenge testing and the other is skin testing. The provocation test is the administration of the potential allergen in a clinically relevant situation to see if the symptoms appear. Skin testing involves injecting the skin with small amounts of the suspected allergen to determine if the wheal-and-flare reaction triggered by mast cells occurs. This testing only determines if IgE antibodies specific to the allergen are present on skin mast cells and does not duplicate the clinical setting.

Two types of provocation or challenge tests are used. The oral challenge test documents food allergy. This test, done in an office setting, is either a double-blind placebo-controlled provocation or an open challenge. Drug allergies and allergies to food additives and preservatives are tested by challenge tests as well.

The inhalation challenge test is helpful in determining respiratory allergies. This provocation testing may be a natural challenge, or it may use "whole allergic material" such as pollen grains. A natural challenge test is useful to assess the response to allergen exposure at home or work. The peak expiratory flow rate is measured at the place of possible exposure and away from it. This test is clinically relevant. Inhalation challenges using other than natural exposure may not be clinically relevant.

Skin testing is conducted either by the epidermal or epicutaneous method and the intradermal method. Whereas epidermal testing is easy and rapid, intradermal testing is more sensitive and reproducible. Appropriate positive and negative controls must be used.

Table 81-2. Signs and Symptoms of Vasovagal Events and Anaphylaxis

SIGNS	VVE	ANAPHYLAXIS
Skin color/temperature	Pale/cool	Red/warm
Sweating	Absent	May be present
Itching, rash, or edema	Absent	May be present
Respiratory distress	Absent	May be present
Pulse	Slow	Rapid
Blood pressure	Normal	Low
Emotions	Variable	Feeling of doom

VVE, vasovagal event.

(Modified from Gordon BR. Prevention and Management of office allergy emergencies. Otolaryngol Clin North Am 1992;25:119.)

Table 81-3. Recommended Basic Emergency Supplies*

1. Cot, or examination table with ability to put patient into Trendelenburg position
2. Monitoring equipment: sphygmomanometer, stethoscope, ECG monitor, defibrillator, and pulse oximeter, if distant from facility with such equipment
3. Tourniquets
4. Epinephrine 1:1000 (1 mg/mL). This is the most important drug. At the first suggestion of trouble, give epinephrine. Prefilled 0.3-mL dual-dose syringes are available commercially.
5. O_2 and ventilation support. O_2 is the second key agent. Hypoxemia triggers cardiovascular collapse in anaphylaxis.
6. Intravenous supplies: IV catheters, 16–18 gauge syringes, needles, alcohol wipes, connecting tubing, IV fluids, tape, second tourniquet, IV pole
7. Suction and catheter
8. Albuterol (Ventolin or Proventil) inhalers
9. Ipratropium (Atrovent) inhaler
10. Dopamine (Intropin)
11. Phentolamine (Regitine)
12. Nitroglycerin sublingual tablets
13. Lidocaine: the drug of choice for ventricular cardiac arrhythmia.
14. Atropine: the drug for bradycardia and heart block
15. Antihistamine
16. Corticosteroid, such as IV methylprednisolone or dexamethasone
17. Heparin
18. Magnesium sulfate
19. Vitamin C
20. Index cards containing clear, brief description of how to mix each drug, the dose and frequency, and route

ECG, electrocardiogram; *IV*, intravenous; O_2, oxygen.

*Personnel should periodically check the kit for any missing or outdated items. Staff also should have periodic emergency drills.

(Gordon BR. Prevention and management of office allergy emergencies. Otolaryngol Clin North Am 1992;25:119.)

In addition, histamine and mast cell tryptase may be measured in serum of persons with allergic symptoms. Histamine also is detectable in urine. This measurement, however, demonstrates when the clinical symptoms result from degranulation of mast cells or basophils, but does not prove that the degranulation was the result of an allergy.

Elevated levels of IgE are associated with the presence of allergies, but normal levels are not. These levels are not good screens for allergies. Atopic persons can have relatively normal levels of IgE. Elevations are also found in patients with parasitic infections, allergic bronchopulmonary aspergillosis, immunodeficiency diseases, and some malignancies.

IgE-specific antibodies may be detected by allergosorbent tests. These tests are not as sensitive as allergy skin tests. They are difficult to interpret and are semiquantitative.

Results of tests for allergy must be evaluated as one part of the total clinical picture of history and physical examination. The physician administering the test should have a thorough understanding of the pathophysiologic mechanisms of allergic diseases. Clinical acumen is more important than testing.

Table 81-4. Allergy Emergency Evaluation and Treatment: Sample Protocol

Initial Evaluation of Possible Allergic Reaction

Whenever observation indicates a possible allergic reaction:

1. Cease administration of allergenic extracts.
2. Record symptoms.
3. Record vital signs: pulse, blood pressure, respiratory rate, skin color/temperature/moisture.
4. Quickly assess type of reaction.
5. Consult other clinicians within office.

Office Treatment for Allergic Reactions

Once specific reaction type is established, carry out appropriate treatment:

1. *Vasovagal Reaction*
   Lower head, loosen clothing.
   Confirm diagnosis.
   Give low-flow oxygen by mask.
   Teach and reassure patient after reaction.
2. Immediate or Delayed *Local Reaction*
   Check injection technique.
   Consider antihistamine before each injection.
   Reduce dose if bothersome reactions continue.
   Teach and reassure patient after reaction.
3. Immediate or Delayed *Large Local Reaction*
   Confirm that there is no general reaction.
   Reduce next dose, then consider slow readvancement.
   For repeat large local reactions, retest allergen sensitivities.
   Teach and reassure patient after reaction.
4. Immediate or Delayed *General Reaction*
   Mild Reaction
   Lower head, loosening clothing.
   Confirm diagnosis.
   Notify supervisor physician.
   Give oral H_1 antihistamine.
   Severe Reaction (Suspect Anaphylaxis)
   If respiratory symptoms, low-flow oxygen by mask.
   If bronchospasm occurs, give albuterol inhaler, 2 puffs.
   If symptoms are severe, give epinephrine 1:1000, give 0.3–0.5 mL SC or IM (adult; notice precautions),
   or epinephrine 1:1000, 0.2 mL SC or IM (elderly or on beta-blocker),
   or epinephrine 1:1000, 0.5 mL SC or IM (on MAO inhibitor),
   or epinephrine 1:1000, 0.01 mg/kg, up to 0.3 mL SC or IM (child).
   Consider oral or IM corticosteroid to abort late-phase reaction.
   Reevaluate future treatment; plan nurse–physician conference.
   Teach and reassure patient after reaction
   If symptoms progress, change diagnosis to anaphylaxis.
5. *Anaphylaxis*
   Lower head, loosen clothing.
   Apply tourniquet above allergen injection site.
   Confirm diagnosis.
   Give epinephrine 1:1000, 0.3–0.5 mL SC or IM (adult; notice precautions),
   or epinephrine 1:1000, 0.2 mL SC or IM (elderly or on beta-blocker),
   or epinephrine 1:1000, 0.05 mL SC or IM (on MAO inhibitor),
   or epinephrine 1:1000, 0.01 mg/kg, up to 0.3 mL SC or IM (child).
   Consider local injection of epinephrine 1:1000 around antigen entry site.
   If severe hypotension (shock) *is present,* give epinephrine 1:10,000, 0.5–1 mg in 10 mL; for children, give transtracheal or intralingual injection IM, 0.1 mg/kg in 5 mL
   Call for help
   Notify supervisor physician; call for crash cart, defibrillator, suction machine, oximeter.
   Call ambulance.
   Assign duties to team; begin recording symptoms, vital signs, personnel response, and treatment.
   If angina occurs, nitroglycerin 0.4 mg SL, every 3 min to relief or to 3 doses maximum; repeat every 30 minutes.
   Give 100% oxygen by mask; if oximeter is available, adjust to keep oxygen saturation above 90%.
   If bronchospasm occurs, give albuterol inhaler, 2 puffs; repeat if not effective.
   If bronchospasm continues, give ipratropium inhaler, 15 to 30 puffs.
   If respiratory distress *occurs,* begin artificial ventilation, intubation or cricothyrotomy, suction
   If no pulse, begin CPR.
   Monitor on electrocardiogram machine as soon as available.
   Consider second dose of epinephrine; continue to repeat at least every 5–10 min until satisfactory clinical improvment occurs; give subsequent doses, depending on clinical need.
   Check, loosen tourniquet every 5 min.
   Establish venous access.
   If bronchospasm continues, administer IV magnesium sulfate, 1–4 g over 20 min with reflex monitoring.
   If hypotension occurs, administer IV fluid, up to 1000 mL every 20 minutes; start second IV.
   If hypotension persists, start IV dopamine drip at 2 μg/kg/min; increase as needed.
   If hypotension persists, administer IV colloid solution at wide open setting.
   If hypertension occurs, give phentolamine 5–10 mg IV; repeat as often as needed.
   If ventricular ectopy present, give lidocaine bolus 1 mg/kg IV, then 0.5 mg/kg every 1–10 min until ectopy is controlled, or to 3 mg/kg maximum; start IV drip.
   Give IV H_1 antihistamine: diphenhydramine, 50–100 mg.
   Give IV H_2 antihistamine: ranitidine, 50 mg, or cimetidine, 300 mg (over 5 min).
   Give IV corticosteroid: dexamethasone, 20 mg, or methylprednisolone, 40 mg.
   If shock occurs, increase corticosteroid (dexamethasone up to 1 mg/kg, methylprednisolone up to 30 mg/kg).
   Consider IV heparin 10,000 units (notice precautions).
   Consider IV vitamin C, 2 g.
   If respiratory obstruction requires CPR or ventilation but lungs cannot deflate, add external end-inspiratory thoracic compressions (requires two persons).
   Transport via ambulance to hospital as soon as possible; communicate with emergency room physician; consider cardiology consultation.
   Debrief personnel, complete records, replenish supplies.

CPR, cardiopulmonary resuscitation; *IM,* intramuscularly; *IV,* intravenous. *MAO,* monoamine oxidase; *SC,* subcutaneously;
(Gordon BR. Prevention and management of office allergy emergencies. Otolaryngol Clin North Am 1992;25:119.)

Certain problems exist with the allergy testing methods available to primary care physicians through commercial laboratories: (1) the tests are available to and evaluated by physicians who may not be adequately educated in their appropriate use and interpretation; (2) the testing, which is done in laboratories away from the environment of the person with the symptoms, is used to make recommendations about therapy and changes in the patient's environment by physicians who do not know the patient personally; and (3) internal and external quality control is difficult to monitor and assess. Therefore, the prudent primary care provider is well advised to refer individuals with suspected allergy to a physician with expertise in allergic disease.

TREATMENT

Severe forms of allergic reactions, such as anaphylaxis, need immediate treatment. Persons with known allergies to bee stings should likewise be prepared for emergency treatment. Such persons should wear a tag indicating these allergies. Avoidance measures should be discussed with allergic individuals. When walking in open areas or woods, they need to be alert to insect nests. Protective clothing such as long pants, appropriate socks, and high shoes with pant legs tucked in are helpful measures. Persons should be careful where they sit or step when in outdoor areas. An emergency epinephrine kit or syringe should be prescribed for all persons with a history of a systemic allergic reaction to insects. Proper instruction in how to self-administer the epinephrine should be given to the individual, or to the parent in the case of a young child. Because a number of studies have shown consistently that insect venom immunotherapy reduces the risk of reactions in about 5% of sting victims, and that after such therapy the reactions that do occur are milder, venom immunotherapy is recommended. The only exception to this is that children with only skin reactions to insect stings are at low risk of developing a systemic reaction. Their risk is reportedly less than 10% and, thus, immunotherapy is not recommended. Persons with other serious allergies such as to drugs should also wear Medi-Alert tags.

First- and second-generation antihistamines are competitive antagonists with histamine at H_1 receptors in various target organs. They are used prophylactically to prevent allergic symptoms and allergic rhinitis. The treatment of asthma is discussed in Chapter 54. Treatment of atopic dermatitis is discussed in Chapter 135.

Emergency Treatment

Every physician's office, even if it is in a hospital, must be prepared to effectively treat the first critical minutes of emergency care in the case of a systemic allergic reaction. All staff should be trained and be current in basic cardiopulmonary resuscitation. The major error in treating patients with anaphylaxis, a systemic reaction, is the failure to institute cardiopulmonary resuscitation when the individual has no effective cardiac output. Physicians might wish to have training in advanced cardiac life support. The goal of emergency treatment is to stabilize the affected person until hospital transfer. Thus, the role of office staff and the primary physician is to diagnose the problem quickly, initiate prompt, appropriate treatment, and stabilize the individual so that transportation to the hospital can be expedited. This is necessary because successfully treated anaphylaxis may relapse hours later into a refractory late-phase reaction that can include angioedema, pulmonary edema, gastrointestinal hemorrhage, pulmonary hemorrhage, and severe persistent bronchospasm.

Table 81-3 lists recommended basic emergency supplies. Table 81-4 outlines emergency evaluation and treatment.

CONSIDERATIONS IN PREGNANCY

It is often difficult to predict how atopic dermatitis will behave during pregnancy. Some women appear to have worsening of symptoms, others appear to improve.

Asthma, as mentioned in Chapter 54, may worsen slightly in one third of women with prior asthma, remain unchanged in one third, and improve in one third. Pregnant women with asthma should be followed carefully with early pharmacologic intervention during any exacerbation.

All pharmacologic drugs used to treat asthma are appropriate in pregnancy except, perhaps, epinephrine. Use of this drug in pregnancy remains controversial. Those who use it in pregnancy say that it is endogenous. It is available and is readily metabolized. Furthermore, there are no apparent long-term sequelae in the fetus. Physicians who do not use it point out that epinephrine has been linked to decreased uterine blood flow and congenital malformations. These studies have been questioned by many careful experts in maternal–fetal medicine. A leading text in the field, however, states that epinephrine probably should be avoided in the first trimester.

In general, however, it is safe to conclude that the treatment of allergies in pregnant women is similar to that in nonpregnant women.

BIBLIOGRAPHY

Borish L, Joseph BZ. Inflammation and the allergic response: clinical allergy. Med Clin North Am 1992;76:765.

Bush RK. The role of allergens in asthma. Chest 1992;101:378S.

Busse WW. Role of antihistamines in allergic disease. Ann Allergy 1994;72:371.

Clinton MJ, Niederma MS, Matthay RA. Maternal pulmonary disorders complicating pregnancy. In: Reece EA, Hobbins JC, Mahoney MT, Petrie RH, eds. Medicine of the fetus and mother. Philadelphia: JB Lippincott, 1992:955.

Galant SP. Treatment and prevention of milk allergy. West J Med 1993;158:612.

Gordon BR. Prevention and management of office allergy emergencies. Otolaryngol Clin North Am 1992;25:119.

Horak F. Seasonal allergic rhinitis: newer treatment approaches. Drugs 1993;45:518.

Jarvis WT. Allergy-related quackery. NY State J Med 1993;93:100.

Leung DY. Mechanisms of the human allergic response: clinical implications. Pediatr Clin North Am 1994;41:727.

Lichtenstein LM. Allergy and the immune system. Sci Am 1993;269:116.

Mabry RL. Allergic and infective rhinosinusitis: differential diagnosis and interrelationship. Otolaryngol Head Neck Surg 1994;111:335.

Marks DR, Marks LM. Food allergy: manifestations, evaluation, and management. Postgrad Med 1993;93:191.

Moffitt JE, Yates AB, Stafford CT. Allergy to insect stings: a need for improved preventive management. Postgrad Med 1993;93:197.

Smith TF. Allergy testing in clinical practice. Ann Allergy 1992;68:293.

Spector SL. The role of allergy in sinusitis in adults. J Allergy Clin Immunol 1992;90:518.

Szefler SJ. Anti-inflammatory drugs in the treatment of allergic disease. Med Clin North Am 1992;76:953.

Primary Care for Women, edited by Phyllis C. Leppert and Fred M. Howard. Lippincott-Raven Publishers, Philadelphia © 1997.

82
Systemic Lupus Erythematosus

CHRISTOPHER T. RITCHLIN

Systemic lupus erythematosus (SLE) is a chronic autoimmune disorder characterized by wide diversity in clinical presentation and course. The disease is cyclical, with unpredictable flares and remissions, and disease severity ranges from fatigue, arthralgia, and a photosensitive rash to life-threatening major organ involvement. The diagnosis usually is based on information obtained from the history and physical findings combined with results from a number of serologic tests. Criteria have been developed to identify patients for clinical studies, but they also are useful to the practicing physician (Table 82-1). It is important that the primary physician caring for women be familiar with the cardinal signs and symptoms of SLE because it occurs primarily in female patients and is associated with a number of complications in the pregnant patient.

SLE has been described in all age groups but is most common between the ages of 13 to 40 years. Approximately 90% of the patients are female. In the older age groups, the female predominance lessens considerably. The disease is three times more common in Asians and African Americans, with an annual incidence that varies from 6 per 100,000 in whites to 35 per 100,000 cases in blacks. The concordance rate for SLE in identical twins is approximately 30%, and the likelihood that first-degree relatives of an affected patient will develop SLE is about 5%.

ETIOLOGY AND DIFFERENTIAL DIAGNOSIS

The cause of SLE is unknown, but the epidemiologic and scientific data suggest a complex interplay between genetic and environmental factors, with the weight of each of these varying from patient to patient. The fundamental defects seem to include a loss of tolerance to self-antigens and excessive B-cell activity. This results in the overproduction of autoantibodies that alter cell function and formation of immune complexes that deposit in various tissues and stimulate an inflammatory response. SLE has been associated with the human leukocyte antigens (HLA) DR2 and DR3 and with deficiencies in complement proteins, particularly C2 and C4. Environmental agents associated with the onset of SLE include various drugs, ultraviolet light, and infections.

SLE mimics several other disorders. Prominent among these are subacute bacterial endocarditis, septicemia, sarcoidosis, tuberculosis, Lyme arthritis, and the acquired immunodeficiency syndrome. The disease often is initially diagnosed as rheumatoid arthritis. Differentiation from other autoimmune disorders, such as scleroderma, Sjögren syndrome, polymyositis–dermatomyositis, and mixed connective tissue disease, is based on characteristic clinical features and distinctive serologic study results.

HISTORY

The clinical manifestations of SLE are varied and often subtle, so the physician must take a complete history and maintain a high index of suspicion. Table 82-2 lists a series of questions that aid in making the diagnosis. Constitutional complaints are common and include fatigue, fevers (usually less than 39°C [102°F]), and weight loss. Fatigue often is extreme, resembling that seen in fibromyalgia or chronic fatigue syndrome.

Nearly all patients complain of arthralgia or arthritis. The small joints of the hands, wrists, and knees are often painful, stiff, and swollen, particularly in the morning. Muscle aches and weakness also are frequent complaints. Skin involvement often presents as a malar blush or peripheral rash that is variable in appearance, generally nonscarring, and often induced by sunlight. Most patients complain of photosensitivity described as either a rash or an overall sense of not feeling well after sun exposure. Mouth ulcers tend to be painless, which differentiates them from canker sores. Transient hair loss is common during active disease.

It is essential to determine from the history if major organs such as the lung, heart, or CNS are affected in patients believed to have SLE. Pleuritic chest pain may represent pleural or pericardial inflammation. Dyspnea may be the result of pneumonitis, pleural or pericardial effusion, congestive heart failure, or pulmonary emboli. Neuropsychiatric symptoms range from mild, including mood lability, poorly localized headaches, difficulty concentrating, to more severe, arising from frank psychosis, depression, seizures, strokes, or cranial neuropathy.

PHYSICAL EXAMINATION

Low-grade fever often is associated with a lupus flare, and tachycardia may be the result of increased temperature, anxiety, anemia, or volume depletion. Tachypnea may reflect pulmonary or cardiac involvement. Elevated blood pressure may be idiopathic in origin but often is related to underlying inflammatory kidney disease.

Acute skin lesions are variable in appearance and location. The typical butterfly rash is a nonpapular raised erythema over the cheeks and nose with sparing of the nasolabial folds. Maculopapular erythematous eruptions are frequently observed, and these can be triggered by sunlight or medications, especially sulfa drugs and penicillin derivatives. Urticaria and angioedema, bullae, palpable purpura, and livedo reticularis are less common skin eruptions. Painless mucosal ulcerations arise on the hard and soft palate but also are seen in the upper respiratory tract, nasal septum, and the vagina. Alopecia usually is diffuse, and hair loss is transient if scarring discoid lesions are not present.

The arthritis of SLE typically presents with symmetric swelling in the small joints of the hands, wrists, and knees. In general, the

Table 82-1. The 1982 Revised Criteria for Classification of Systemic Lupus Erythematosus*

CRITERION	DEFINITION
1. Malar rash	Fixed erythema, flat or raised, over the malar eminences, tending to spare the nasolabial folds
2. Discoid rash	Erythematous raised patches with adherent keratolic scaling and follicular plugging; atrophic scarring may occur in older lesions
3. Photosensitivity	Skin rash as a result of unusual reaction to sunlight, by patient history or physician observation
4. Oral ulcers	Oral or nasopharyngeal ulceration, usually painless, observed by a physician
5. Arthritis	Nonerosive arthritis involving two or more peripheral joints, characterized by tenderness, swelling or effusion
6. Serositis	a. Pleuritis—convincing history of pleuritic pain or rub or heard by a physician or evidence of pleural effusion, or b. Pericarditis—documented by electrocardiogram or rub or evidence of pericardial effusion
7. Renal disorder	a. Persistent proteinuria 0.5 g/d or 3+ if quantitation not performed, or b. Cellular casts—may be red blood cell, hemoglobin, granular, tubular, or mixed
8. Neurologic disorder	a. Seizures—in the absence of offending drugs or known metabolic derangements, e.g., uremia, ketoacidosis, or electrolyte imbalance, or b. Psychosis—in the absence of offending drugs or known metabolic derangements, e.g., uremia, ketoacidosis, or electrolyte imbalance
9. Hematologic disorder	a. Hemolytic anemia—with reticulocytosis, or b. Leukopenia—$<4.0\times10^9$/L (4000/mm3) total on occasions, or c Lymphopenia—$<1.5\times10^9$/L (1500/mm3) on $\geq$ 2 ocasions, or d. Thrombocytopenia—<100x109/L (x103/mm3) in the absence of offending drugs
10. Immunologic disorder	a. Positive lupus erythematosus cell preparation, or b. Anti-DNA antibody to native DNA in abnormal titer, or c. Anti-Sm—presence of antibody to Sm nuclear antigen, or d. False-positive serologic test for syphilis known to be positive for at least 6 mo and confirmed by negative *Treponema pallidum* immobilization or flourescent treponemal antibody absorption test
11. Antinuclear antibody	An abnormal titer of antinuclear antibody by immunoflourescence or an equivalent assay at any point in the absence of drugs known to be associated with drug-induced lupus erythematosus syndrome

Sm, Smith antigen.

*The proposed classification is based on 11 criteria. To identify patients in clinical studies, a person shall be said to have systemic lupus erythematosus if any 4 or more of the 11 criteria are present serially or simultaneously, during any interval of observation.

(Condemi JJ. The autoimmune diseases. JAMA 1992; 286:2882.)

arthritis is nonerosive, but reducible deformities resembling rheumatoid arthritis do occur as a result of tendon inflammation. Patients can develop proximal muscle weakness secondary to an inflammatory myositis, but this is usually not severe. Osteonecrosis must be considered in any SLE patient on corticosteroids who presents with acute monarticular joint pain, especially in the hip, shoulder, or knee.

Serositis is a frequent manifestation of SLE and can involve the pleura, pericardium, or peritoneum. Physical findings pointing to pleural involvement include tachypnea, diminished breath sounds with dullness, or a pleural rub. Pericarditis should be suspected if heart sounds are distant or a rub is present along the left sternal border. Pulsus paradoxus indicates possible cardiac tamponade, a rare complication. Severe and diffuse abdominal pain with rebound tenderness may occur secondary to serositis, mesenteric vasculitis, or a ruptured viscus.

Nervous system involvement in SLE can be broken down into neurologic (involvement of the central nervous system, cranial, and peripheral nerves) and psychiatric (organic brain syndrome with delirium and dementia, psychosis, and major depression). Presenting signs are remarkably diverse, and most patients have a combination of neurologic and psychiatric manifestations. Grand mal seizures, headaches, often migrainous in quality, and strokes can occur in the setting of a lupus flare or as an isolated event. Cranial neuropathies usually involve the second, third, and fifth nerves, presenting as field cuts, ptosis, or tic douloureux. Neuropsychiatric signs and symptoms may be secondary to metabolic abnormalities or infection and not a lupus flare. Making this distinction early is important because treatment approaches may vary dramatically.

CLINICAL SUBSETS OF SLE

There are many subsets of SLE that do not follow the more classic pattern. Presentation in elderly patients is characterized by a predominance of pleuropericarditis and equal incidence in males and females. Drug-induced lupus has been associated with several medications, but the strongest associations are with procainamide, hydralazine, isoniazid, chlorpromazine, and methyldopa. Autoantibodies generally are restricted to histone antigens in drug-induced lupus. Major organ involvement and low complement levels are unusual, and activity is usually limited to the skin, joints, and pleuropericardia. Subacute cutaneous lupus occurs in patients with anti-Ro antibodies. They often develop a photosensitive eruption

Table 82-2. Key Questions in Evaluating Patients for Systemic Lupus Erythematosus

1. Are your joints painful, swollen, or stiff?
2. Are you sensitive to the sun (not sunburn)?
3. Have you noticed painless sores in your mouth?
4. Have you ever been told that you have low blood counts?
5. Have you ever had protein or cells in your urine?
6. Have you ever had pleurisy or pain on deep breathing lasting more than a few days?
7. Do you have frequent headaches, difficulty concentrating, or memory loss?
8. Have you ever had a persistent facial rash?
9. Have you had periods of rapid hair loss?
10. Do your hands change colors or become uncomfortable in the cold?

(Modified from Shur PH. Clinical features of SLE. In: Kelly WN Jr, Harris ED Jr, Ruddy S, Sledge CB, eds. Textbook of rheumatology, 4th ed. Philadelphia: WB Saunders, 1993:1017.)

that can be papulosquamous or annular; systemic disease tends to be mild. Patients with discoid lesions have a scarring hypopigmented rash, but antinuclear antibody (ANA) positivity and systemic involvement are rare. Patients with mixed connective tissue disease usually have high titers of antibodies against ribonuclear protein associated with sausage digits and Raynaud phenomenon. They also may have features of SLE, myositis, Sjögren syndrome, or scleroderma. In these patients, lung involvement with pulmonary hypertension and interstitial inflammation is more common than lupus nephritis.

Antiphospholipid antibodies are present in about 25% of patients with SLE. These antibodies have been associated with arterial and venous thrombosis, thrombocytopenia, livedo reticularis, and premature fetal death. The mechanisms responsible for thrombosis are not understood, although several studies demonstrate that these antibodies interact with phospholipid binding proteins such as β_2-glycoprotein, prothrombin, and proteins C and S. These phospholipid-binding proteins are composed of a group of molecules that seem to have anticoagulant functions under physiologic conditions. Antiphospholipid antibodies can be detected by the presence of elevated titers of anticardiolipin antibodies or a positive lupus anticoagulant assay. Both tests should be ordered because many patients have positive results in only one of the assays, reflecting the heterogeneous nature of these antibodies. Patients who develop thrombosis in a major blood vessel are fully anticoagulated with warfarin (Coumadin; international normalized ratio > 3.0), often for life. Subcutaneous heparin and low-dose aspirin can improve pregnancy outcome in patients with recurrent fetal loss. An antiphospholipid antibody syndrome with clinical features similar to those observed in patients with SLE can occur in patients without an underlying autoimmune disorder.

LABORATORY AND IMAGING STUDIES

The production of antibodies to an array of autoantigens is a hallmark of SLE. Some of the more common autoantibodies are listed in Table 82-3. The fluorescent antinuclear test is a good screening test with a sensitivity approaching 99%, but often is positive in other autoimmune diseases. The higher the titer of the fluorescent antinuclear test (> 1 : 160), the more likely it is that an associated autoimmune disorder is present. Antibodies to double-stranded DNA (dsDNA) and Smith antigen (Sm) are highly specific, so they are useful in confirming a diagnosis of SLE. Antibodies to Ro, La, and ribonuclear protein help to identify clinical subsets of SLE (see earlier).

Several laboratory measures are useful in monitoring disease activity in SLE, but baselines and patterns must be established and followed in each individual patient. For example, falling complement levels and rising titers of antibodies to dsDNA may indicate an impending flare of lupus nephritis in one patient, but may not be associated with any end-organ disease in another. In general, laboratory measures used to follow disease activity are C3 and C4 levels, titers of dsDNA antibodies, erythrocyte sedimentation rate, complete blood cell count, and urinalysis. Changing titers of antinuclear antibodies do not correlate with disease activity.

Patients with SLE can have a number of hematologic abnormalities, including anemia secondary to chronic disease, hemolysis that is Coombs positive, and iron deficiency secondary to gastric or menstrual blood loss. Low white cell counts, predominantly lymphopenia, is a frequent occurrence. Mild thrombocytopenia is common, although thrombocytopenic purpura with platelet counts less than 20,000/mm3 can be the initial presentation of SLE. Routine urinalysis should be obtained on initial evaluation and in routine follow-up, looking for proteinuria, cellular casts, and cellular elements, all indicative of inflammatory renal disease. The use and timing of renal biopsy is controversial, but renal histopathologic examination can be helpful in determining the extent of disease activity and confirming the diagnosis of membranous or proliferative renal disease before initiation of immunosuppressive therapy. Radiographs of affected joints should be reviewed for the presence

Table 82-3. Autoantibodies in Systemic Lupus Erythematosus

AUTOANTIGEN	PREVALENCE (%)	COMMENT
Histone	70	Predominant autoantigen in DIL
Double-stranded DNA	40	Associated with kidney disease
Sm	30	Highly specific for SLE
RNP	30	High titers associated with MCTD
SSA/Ro	35	Associated with subacute cutaneous SLE, neonatal lupus
SSB/La	15	

DIL, drug-induced lupus; *MCTD,* mixed connective tissue disease; *RNP,* ribonuclear protein; *SLE,* systemic lupus erythematosus; *Sm,* Smith antigen.

of erosions, which would favor an inflammatory arthritis over SLE. Imaging studies, including computed tomography (CT) scan or ultrasound, can help in differentiating an inflamed viscus from lupus serositis. Head CT scans are particularly useful for detecting infarcts or hemorrhage in patients presenting with focal findings, but magnetic resonance (MR) imaging scans are more sensitive for detecting small cortical or subcortical infarctions. Electroencephalography (EEG) and quantitative electroencephalography (QEEG) can help to confirm an organic etiology in patients with various neuropsychiatric features, and quantitative electroencephalography can be used to monitor response to therapy. Aseptic necrosis of the hip or other joints can be visualized on bone scan, MR imaging, or CT scan before it is visible on plain radiographs. Other nonspecific laboratory abnormalities encountered frequently in SLE are hypergammaglobulinemia, positive rheumatoid factor, false-positive VDRL, and circulating cryoglobulins.

Table 82-4. Major and Nonmajor Organ Activity in Systemic Lupus Erythematosus

MAJOR ORGAN*	NONMAJOR ORGAN†
Glomerulonephritis	Arthritis
Central nervous system disease	Mouth ulcers
Myositis/myocarditis/valvulitis	Pleurisy
Pneumonitis	Pericarditis
Severe hemolytic anemia	Alopecia
Vasculitis of major organs	Fatigue
	Fever
	Hepatitis

*Treatment includes high-dose steroids (1 mg/kg/day or higher), and often immunosuppressive drugs are added for additional activity and to minimize long-term corticosteroid side effects.

†Generally does not require high-dose corticosteroids.

TREATMENT

The most important initial step in the treatment of a patient newly diagnosed with SLE is education and reassurance. The diagnosis of a chronic autoimmune disease is stressful, and patients often have fearful misconceptions about the disease and prognosis. Emphasis on the disease variability, while underscoring that most patients live a normal life span, helps to alleviate anxiety. Informing family members of the more common manifestations of disease activity and pointing out that patients with SLE often feel much worse than they appear can be helpful. Lifestyle modifications, such as obtaining adequate rest and exercise, along with stress reduction should be emphasized. The help of a counselor, nutritionist, and physical or occupational therapist may be beneficial. Patients should be advised to avoid sunlight, estrogens in premenopausal patients, and sulfa drugs because they may trigger a lupus flare. Estrogens are usually not withheld from postmenopausal women with established SLE, although in a recent prospective cohort study, use of these drugs was associated with an increased risk of developing SLE.

In any patient with SLE, determination that a presenting symptom or sign is a manifestation of disease activity can be extremely difficult. For example, in the patient who develops a fever, infection must be excluded. A rising creatinine may be secondary to uncontrolled hypertension or radiocontrast dye and not active lupus. However, once it has been determined that the problem represents an exacerbation of SLE, treatment can be guided by the presence or absence of major organ involvement (Table 82-4).

One of the major pitfalls in treating patients with SLE is inappropriate use of corticosteroids for patients with non-major organ disease. Patients with arthritis, myalgia, and pleurisy often respond to the use of a nonsteroidal antiinflammatory drug (NSAID). Plaquenil provides additional antiinflammatory activity and is particularly beneficial for treatment of serositis, as well as joint and skin disease. This drug also lowers the frequency of disease flares in patients who take it chronically. Occasionally, patients with more severe pleurisy or pericarditis require corticosteroids in the range of 20 to 30 mg/day for a short period. High-dose corticosteroids are the cornerstone of treatment in patients presenting with major organ disease. Initial doses are administered at 1 mg/kg/day in divided doses, with consolidation to a single morning dose in 1 to 2 weeks, tapering to an alternate day regimen in 4 to 8 weeks. Use of high-dose steroids for more than 6 weeks increases the risk of infection, diabetes mellitus, aseptic necrosis of the hip, and steroid myopathy.

Occasionally, patients with major organ or life-threatening disease, such as rapidly progressive glomerulonephritis or hemorrhagic pneumonitis, are treated with pulse doses of corticosteroids at 1 g of methylprednisolone/day for 3 days. Intravenous cyclophosphamide is effective for patients with proliferative nephritis and in CNS disease resistant to other therapies. Seizures often respond to anticonvulsants with or without corticosteroids. Plasmapheresis is of unproven benefit but is often administered for life-threatening major organ disease.

CONSIDERATIONS IN PREGNANCY

Most patients with SLE can become pregnant and have successful outcomes. It had previously been thought that SLE activity increased during pregnancy, but more recent studies reach different conclusions. In patients who do flare during pregnancy, renal and hematologic involvement tends to be more common than arthritis. Pregnant SLE patients also are more likely to have problems with preeclampsia, hypertension, diabetes mellitus, and urinary tract infections than controls. Less common manifestations in the pre- and postpartum period include uterine rupture, bilateral retinal detachments, deep venous thrombosis in patients with antiphospholipid antibodies, and the maternal syndrome of hemolysis, elevated liver enzymes, and low platelet count (HELLP syndrome).

The major events responsible for adverse fetal outcomes are fetal loss and preterm labor. Fetal loss occurs in both the first and second trimesters, but those in the second trimester are more strongly associated with elevated levels of anticardiolipin antibodies. Preterm birth can result from early labor, fetal distress, premature rupture of membranes, preeclamptic toxemia, and oligohydramnios. These complications are more common in patients with active lupus.

Neonatal SLE is a syndrome mediated by transplacental passage of maternal antibodies to Ro/La antigens that can manifest in utero or at birth. Infants with neonatal SLE can have thrombocytopenia, leukopenia, hepatosplenomegaly, and cutaneous lesions that typically resolve by 6 months of age without therapy. More serious complications include myocarditis, endocardial fibrosis, and congenital complete heart block. Congenital complete heart block can occur after the 16th week of gestation and is detected by a drop in fetal heart rate. Permanent pacemakers are often required in these newborns soon after birth. Interestingly, mothers of affected infants are frequently asymptomatic before and during the pregnancy, so autoimmune disease is not suspected. A significant percentage develop SLE (usually mild) or Sjögren syndrome later in life.

It is advisable that patients with SLE not conceive at a time when the disease is active. Mothers who develop active SLE during pregnancy or are in the midst of a flare when they become pregnant often require prednisone. Prednisone is metabolized by the placenta and does not pose a major risk to the fetus, but the drug increases the risk of diabetes, hypertension, and preeclampsia in the mother. It is recommended that women who have recurrent fetal loss and elevated antiphospholipid antibodies receive treatment with subcutaneous heparin (10,000 U twice daily) and low-dose aspirin throughout the pregnancy. Some physicians continue this therapy for 6 weeks postpartum. This therapy has improved pregnancy outcome. Hydroxychloroquine and azathioprine can be continued in the pregnant patient if they are required to control lupus activity, but methotrexate, cyclophosphamide, and NSAIDs should be discontinued because of possible adverse effects on the fetus.

Pregnant patients with SLE should be considered high risk, and close cooperation between the obstetrician and rheumatologist maximizes the possibility of a positive outcome. Generally, patients are followed monthly during the first two trimesters by both physicians and more frequently thereafter. Some groups start biophysical profiles and umbilical artery analysis after the 26th week of gestation. Mothers who have anti-Ro antibodies should have serial four-chamber echocardiograms beginning in the 18th week of pregnancy. If fetal heart block or myocarditis is detected early, plasmapheresis can be effective in some cases if initiated early. Differentiating preeclampsia from a flare can be difficult, but falling complement levels or elevated complement split products are more strongly associated with active SLE.

PROGNOSIS

Patients with SLE have an excellent prognosis with a 10-year survival rate of 90%, and most patients live a normal life span. Patients with major organ disease, particularly involving the CNS and kidney, have a poorer prognosis with infection, CNS lupus, and coronary artery disease responsible for most deaths. Survival has increased dramatically over the last 40 years secondary to the early and widespread use of glucocorticoids, renal dialysis, antibiotics, and antihypertensive agents.

BIBLIOGRAPHY

Condemi JJ. The autoimmune diseases. JAMA 1992;286:2882

Feinglass EJ, Arnett FC, Dorsch CA, Zizic TM, Stevens MB. Neuropsychiatric manifestations of systemic lupus erythematosus: diagnosis, clinical spectrum and relationship to other features of the disease. Medicine 1976;55:323

Ginzler EM, Diamond HS, Weiner M, et al. A multicenter study of outcome in systemic lupus erythematosus. I. Entry variables as predictors of prognosis. Arthritis Rheum 1982;25:601

Kamashta M, Cuadrado MJ, Mujic F, Taub N, Hurt B, Highes RV. The management of thrombosis in the antiphospholipid antibody syndrome. N Engl J Med 1995;332:993

Lockshin MD. Antiphospholipid antibody syndrome. Rheum Dis Clin North Am 1994;20:45

Petri M. Systemic lupus erythematosus and pregnancy. Rheum Dis Clin North Am 1994;20:87

Ritchlin CT, Chabot RJ, Alper K, et al. Quantitative electroencephalography: a new approach to the diagnosis of cerebral dysfunction in systemic lupus erythematosus. Arthritis Rheum 1992;35:1330

Sanchez-Guerrero J, Liang MH, Karlson EW, Hunter DJ, Colditz GA. Postmenopausal estrogen therapy and the risk for developing systemic lupus erythematosus. 1995;Ann Intern Med 122:430

Schur PH. Clinical features of SLE. In Kelley WN Jr, Harris ED Jr, Ruddy S, Sledge CB, eds. Textbook of rheumatology, 4th ed. Philadelphia: WB Saunders, 1993:1017.

Steinberg AD. Systemic lupus erythematosus. Ann Intern Med 1991;115:548

Steinberg AD. The treatment of lupus nephritis. Kidney Int 1986;30:769

Waltuck J, Buyon JP. Autoantibody-associated congenital heart block: outcome in mothers and children. Ann Intern Med 1994;120:554

Primary Care for Women, edited by Phyllis C. Leppert and Fred M. Howard. Lippincott-Raven Publishers, Philadelphia © 1997.

83

Sarcoidosis

GARY W. WAHL

Sarcoidosis is a multisystem disorder of unknown cause, pathologically characterized by nonnecrotizing granuloma. Although any organ system can be involved, the lung and mediastinal lymph nodes are the most prominent sites of involvement. Young adults are most frequently affected, but sarcoidosis has also been diagnosed in small children and in octogenarians. The incidence of sarcoidosis varies significantly among ethnic and geographic groups. In the United States, approximately 11 per 100,000 individuals are affected, but African Americans (particularly women) have a rate of 20 per 100,000, almost ten times that of whites. African blacks have incidence rates estimated at 2 to 4 per 100,000. The majority of patients has an uneventful spontaneous remission. However, many patients have significant symptoms while the condition is active that require careful monitoring to determine need for therapy.

ETIOLOGY

Sarcoidosis is characterized by nonnecrotizing granulomas that can involve any organ. The best current evidence suggests that still unknown antigens stimulate circulating macrophages and lymphocytes to release cytokines. In the lung, a lymphocytic alveolitis that is composed of "killer" (CD4) lymphocytes is stimulated. This inflammatory process usually abates spontaneously within 6 to 24 months, but in some individuals, the process results in the proliferation of fibroblasts with extensive formation of fibrosis in the involved organ.

The causative antigen is unknown, and it is possible that sarcoidosis is a common injury response to several different triggers. Stimuli considered in the past have included infection with tuberculosis, fungi, viruses, and retroviruses; exposure to pine pollens, a variety of chemicals, and drugs; and autoimmune or genetic factors. In some studies, nearly one third of lymph nodes involved with sarcoid have DNA sequences in common with *Mycobacterium tuberculosis*, but other investigators have observed much lower rates.

Although noncaseating granuloma are the pathologic hallmark of sarcoidosis, they are not specific. Nearly identical lesions can be seen with beryllium exposure, tuberculosis, leprosy, hypersensitivity pneumonitis, Crohn disease, primary biliary cirrhosis, fungal infection, and local sarcoid reaction, which occurs in lymph nodes draining neoplastic or chronically inflamed regions. Because the symptoms of sarcoidosis are also nonspecific, the diagnosis is often one of exclusion.

HISTORY

Sarcoidosis can present asymptomatically, with systemic symptoms of fever, malaise, and weight loss or with a history reflecting dysfunction of the organ system involved. In Japan, where the incidence of sarcoidosis is only about 1 in 100,000, 60% of patients are discovered on routine chest x-ray. In contrast, over 90% of African American women with sarcoid present with symptoms. Table 83-1 reviews the most common complaints, by organ system, at initial presentation.

Pulmonary involvement occurs pathologically in 90% of all patients and is the most frequent cause of symptoms. Dyspnea with exertion, dry cough, and vague substernal chest pain is seen alone or in combination with other symptoms in over one third of patients. Occasionally the chest pain is severe and mimics cardiac pain. Severe cough associated with wheezing can occur when there is extensive airway involvement. This presentation is often first mistakenly diagnosed as asthma. Hemoptysis (sometimes with cavitation of lung on x-ray), pleural effusion, and pneumothorax have all been described but are rare and prompt a careful investigation for an alternative diagnosis.

Presentation with nonspecific constitutional symptoms such as fever, weight loss, fatigue, anorexia, and even chills and night sweats occurs in about one third of patients. The association of constitutional symptoms, particularly fever, with erythema nodosum of the lower legs and bilateral hilar adenopathy syndrome (Löfgren syndrome) in a young adult is a common presentation with an excellent prognosis.

About 20% of American patients are discovered when a routine chest x-ray is performed. Most commonly, these patients have bilateral hilar adenopathy alone, but some may show evidence of pulmonary fibrosis.

Table 83-1. Presenting Symptoms in Sarcoidosis

PRESENTING SYMPTOM	AFRICAN AMERICANS (%)	WHITE AMERICANS (%)
Respiratory	30–50	30–50
Asymptomatic	5–15	10–25
Skin involvement	20–30	3–10
Constitutional signs	5–30	10–40
Erythema nodosum	2–5	7–10
Ocular	5–15	2–5

One fourth of patients present with dermatologic complaints. Waxy maculopapular lesions and nodules on the extremities are the most common skin findings. Erythema nodosum (as part of Löfgren syndrome) is particularly common in white and Hispanic populations, particularly in young women. Lupus pernio is a violaceous lesion that occurs on the nose, cheeks, ears, and lips. It is a relatively specific finding for sarcoidosis.

Ocular findings occur in 20% of patients at some point in the course of sarcoidosis, but only in a small percentage at presentation. Granulomatous uveitis is the most common finding. The acute inflammation results in a red, frequently painful eye. This often clears spontaneously, but chronic uveitis (which may be painless) may lead to glaucoma, cataract formation, adhesion between the iris and lens, and even blindness. Conjunctival follicles, lacrimal gland enlargement, and keratoconjunctivitis sicca are also seen in this population. Most patients diagnosed with sarcoidosis should have formal ophthalmologic evaluation with slit-lamp examination.

Although 25% of patients have granuloma in the heart, symptomatic presentation with cardiac disease is rare. Abnormal conduction is the most common finding—it is sometimes associated with palpitations, but this is usually asymptomatic. Complete heart block with syncope and even sudden death has been described. Rarely, fibrotic replacement of myocardium can result in congestive heart failure.

Fewer than 5% of patients develop symptomatic neurologic involvement, but identification is important. Cranial nerve involvement, particularly cranial nerve VII (Bell's palsy), is the most common abnormality. A predilection of the inflammatory process toward involving the base of the brain probably explains the development of these palsies as well as rarely seen episodes of aseptic meningitis, hydrocephalus, hypophyseal replacement, and pituitary dysfunction. Peripheral neuropathy and symptoms of space-occupying lesions may result from granulomatous inflammation in strategic locations.

Enlargement of cervical, supraclavicular, epitrochlear, or axillary nodes is fairly common, occurring in 10% to 50% of patients. The spleen is rarely enlarged. Granulomatous involvement of the liver is common, but only rarely causes tenderness, cirrhosis, or jaundice. Among the 10% to 15% of patients with hypercalcemia, a small percentage develops kidney stones as a manifestation of the disease. One fifth of patients may develop arthralgia as a result of involvement of the joint capsule. Upper airway involvement has been reported to result in nasal obstruction and sinusitis.

LABORATORY AND IMAGING STUDIES

The diagnosis of sarcoid is based on clinical presentation, observation over time, and exclusion of other causes for the findings. Several laboratory and x-ray findings support the diagnosis, but none is specific. Biopsy demonstrating noncaseating granuloma is frequently used when the alternative diagnoses cannot be excluded with less invasive methods.

The chest x-ray is central to diagnosis and management in most patients. A staging system describes findings that correlate with lung function and prognosis. About 10% of patients have normal x-rays—stage 0 sarcoidosis. Stage I disease, bilateral hilar and mediastinal adenopathy with no evidence of lung parenchyma involvement, is seen in 35% to 45% of patients at presentation. Stage II sarcoidosis consists of bilateral hilar and mediastinal adenopathy along with parenchymal lung disease. The pulmonary involvement usually appears as a reticular pattern diffusely in the lung, but occasionally is seen as multiple small nodules. Twenty percent of patients have stage III disease, diffuse lung involvement without adenopathy. There may be cystic changes associated with this more advanced involvement. Longitudinal studies have shown that patients with progressive disease evolve from stage I to stage III. Although computed tomography (CT) of the chest demonstrates more adenopathy and parenchymal involvement than can be visualized by conventional chest x-rays, these findings have not helped clinically in the management of patients. The principal use of chest CT has been to exclude other diagnostic possibilities, most notably lung cancer.

In stage I, lung function is usually normal, and over 80% of patients resolve completely or remain permanently stable. Stage II patients have mild lung dysfunction and 60% to 80% remain stable or resolve. In Stage III, lung function is much more disturbed, and 40% to 50% of patients have progressive disease.

When abnormal pulmonary function studies demonstrate a restrictive pattern, patients with extensive airway involvement may demonstrate an obstructive pattern, but generally they have no response to inhaled bronchodilators like that seen in asthma patients. The diffusion capacity for carbon monoxide tends to be reduced, but not usually to extreme levels. Exercise-induced hypoxemia may occur when pulmonary involvement is severe.

There is no specific blood test to identify sarcoidosis. Anemia, leukopenia, lymphocytopenia, eosinophilia, thrombocytopenia, hypergammaglobulinemia, an increased erythrocyte sedimentation rate, hypercalcemia, and hypercalcuria may all be seen. Serologies for collagen vascular diseases show no abnormalities. Gallium scan and analysis of bronchoalveolar lavage fluid have been of some research interest, but have not proved specific enough to be helpful in diagnostic or management decisions. The Kveim-Sitzbach test—injection of carefully processed splenic material followed by biopsy of the injection site—is only of historic interest because the reagent is no longer available.

The circulating level of angiotensin converting enzyme (ACE) is elevated in two thirds of patients with sarcoidosis. However, numerous conditions including several in the differential diagnosis also increase the ACE level (Table 83-2). Although the role of ACE as a diagnostic tool is limited, some feel the ACE level is useful in following disease activity.

When alternative diagnoses cannot be excluded, confirmatory biopsy is often required. Transbronchial biopsy of the lung through a fiberoptic bronchoscope is the most commonly performed procedure.

Table 83-2. Conditions Associated With Elevation of Angiotension Converting Enzyme Level

Likely Alternative Diagnoses	Unlikely Alternative Diagnoses
Asbestosis	Diabetes mellitus
Berylliosis	Gaucher disease
Coccidioidomycosis	Hyperthyroidism
Granulomatous hepatitis	Adult respiratory distress syndrome
Hypersensitivity pneumonitis	Inflammatory bowel disease
Lymphoma	Leprosy
Miliary tuberculosis	Liver cirrhosis
Pulmonary neoplasm	
Silicosis	

It carries a low morbidity and is diagnostic in 60% of patients when there is no lung abnormality on chest x-ray and in nearly 90% of patients when interstitial infiltrates are present (stages II and III). When there are visible skin lesions, palpable lymph nodes, or granular abnormalities of the conjunctiva, biopsy of these areas has a very high yield. Liver biopsy results are positive in most patients, particularly in those with abnormal liver function but the procedure carries significant risk. Scalene lymph node biopsy or mediastinoscopy has very high yields but at significant expense and some risk. Open lung biopsy should almost never be required to diagnose sarcoid.

Some authorities feel biopsy should be performed on all patients before treatment is instituted, but this is controversial. Many patients do not require biopsy. Patients with bilateral hilar adenopathy who are asymptomatic or have erythema nodosum and arthralgia virtually always have sarcoidosis. In a large series of patients with bilateral hilar adenopathy, up to 20% had lymphoma, but all lymphoma patients have significant symptoms. Similarly, the small percentage of patients with lung cancer were symptomatic. Those with fungal or tuberculous causes had fever or purulent sputum. All patients in these series who were asymptomatic had sarcoidosis.

TREATMENT

The decision to treat sarcoidosis generally involves consultation. Corticosteroids are effective in treating sarcoidosis, but are indicated in only a minority of patients. The majority of patients remain stable or resolve spontaneously, and although steroids clearly accelerate recovery, there is no strong evidence that they affect long-term outcome. Obviously, the benefits of treatment must be balanced against the potentially serious side effects that 3 to 12 months' use of systemic steroids may cause.

The most important factor affecting the decision to treat with systemic steroids is the presence of symptoms. Asymptomatic patients with normal lung function and stage I radiographic changes should not be treated. If they have constitutional symptoms, arthralgias, or erythema nodosum, nonsteroidal antiinflammatory medications are usually effective. Sometimes short courses (5 to 10 days) of prednisone are needed to "carry" a patient through a difficult period. Stable patients are typically monitored with pulmonary function at 3 months, and 1 year, and usually with pulmonary function 6 to 12 months after presentation.

Respiratory symptoms, particularly if progressive (cough, dyspnea, significant chest pain), usually are treated. Asymptomatic patients with involvement of the lung (stage II and III) observed on x-rays are frequently treated, and, if not, are very closely followed for evidence of progressive pulmonary fibrosis. Patients with moderate or severe abnormalities of lung function, even if asymptomatic, should be treated.

Ocular, neurologic, cardiac, and upper airway involvement are indications for systemic treatment. Patients with asymptomatic hepatic involvement with normal liver function need not receive therapy, but must be monitored frequently for deterioration.

The optimal dose and duration of therapy is not known. Most patients respond to 30 to 40 mg/day of prednisone, and this dose is usually reduced to 10 to 15 mg/day after 4 to 8 weeks. Alternate day steroids are probably effective in the maintenance phase, although there are concerns about decreased compliance with these regimens. Therapy is generally continued for 3 to 6 months. Perhaps one fifth of patients with a good response to steroids have recurrence when therapy is tapered or discontinued, and in these patients long-term treatment may be required. Inhaled steroids are sometimes effective in patients with airway symptoms (ie, cough, wheeze) but no other indication for therapy. Plaquenil has been anecdotally reported to benefit skin lesions of sarcoidosis. There is no wide experience with steroid-sparing drugs such as methotrexate, cyclophosphamide, or azothiaprine, which have had limited success in other forms of interstitial lung disease.

Fortunately, the majority of patients never require therapy, and most who do require it respond. Recurrence after complete resolution and successful withdrawal of steroids (if used in treatment) is unusual.

CONSIDERATIONS IN PREGNANCY

Sarcoidosis does not affect fertility or pregnancy. The placenta has not been observed to be involved with sarcoid granulomas. Several studies of over 100 pregnancies in patients with sarcoidosis demonstrated no increase in cesarean section rates or in maternal or fetal difficulties, and pregnancy does not appear to affect disease activity in the mother. About 10% to 20% of patients have progression of their sarcoidosis during pregnancy, similar to the rate expected in a nonpregnant population. Indications for treatment are said to be unchanged during pregnancy, although realistically there is a tendency to wait until delivery if symptoms are not severe.

BIBLIOGRAPHY

Chesnutt AN. Enigmas in sarcoidosis. West J Med 1995;162:519.

Izumi T. Sarcoidosis: pulmonary and critical care medicine, vol 2. St Louis: Mosby–Year Book, 1992.

Johns CJ. Sarcoidosis: pulmonary diseases and disorders, vol 1. 2nd ed. New York: McGraw-Hill, 1988.

King TE. Restrictive lung disease in pregnancy. Clin Chest Med 1992;13:607.

Sharma OP. Pulmonary sarcoidosis and corticosteroids. Am Rev Respir Dis 1993;147:1598.

Weissler JC. Southwestern Internal Medicine Conference: sarcoidosis—immunology and clinical management. Am J Med Sci 1994;307:233.

Winterbauer RH, Moores KD. A clinical interpretation of bilateral hilar adenopathy. Ann Intern Med 1973;78:65.

Primary Care for Women, edited by Phyllis C. Leppert and Fred M. Howard. Lippincott-Raven Publishers, Philadelphia © 1997.

84

AIDS in Women

JOHN LAMBERT

Following the initial description of acquired immunodeficiency syndrome (AIDS) in 1981, a rapid succession of discoveries led to the identification of the causative virus in 1983 and 1984, with the development of a serologic screening test for the presence of human immunodeficiency virus (HIV) in 1985. A few isolated cases of HIV–AIDS were documented before 1981, as far back as the 1960s and 1970s, which were not recognized at the time. Review of pathologic specimens on these individuals revealed evidence of HIV infection and complications of AIDS. Transmission of HIV occurs in a few distinctive settings: through sexual contact; the sharing of contaminated needles; receiving infected blood or blood products; through infected organs or tissue transplants; and from mother to infant during gestation or delivery. Since 1985 in the United States, blood, blood products, and other tissues have been screened with the HIV antibody test and virtually eliminated the chance of an individual becoming infected from transfusions or transplantation. No epidemiologic evidence exists to implicate mosquitoes or nonsexual transmission such as touching, sneezing, talking, handshaking, or use of eating and drinking utensils, although much speculation about these modes of transmission inappropriately and inaccurately circulates from time to time in the lay press.

ETIOLOGY

Biology of Infection

HIV is a retrovirus with an RNA genome and an outer lipid envelope. The virus is 100 nm in diameter. The term *retrovirus* describes a virus that contains reverse transcriptase, a viral enzyme that permits DNA to be copied from RNA. The copying direction is the reverse of cellular transcriptase, which copies RNA from DNA. The RNA genome codes for genes, and these genes produce proteins that represent different components of the virus, including outer coat and internal structural proteins, that, when assembled, represent infectious virus. The retrovirus is part of a group of lentiviruses (slow viruses) that are cell associated, cause chronic infection and immunologic damage over variable periods of time, and infect multiple animal species. Many of the lentiviruses have oncogenic potential. HIV is able to gain entry into cells by means of attachment to a T4 receptor found on the surface of many cell populations. Several different cells in the body contain this receptor, including monocytes, macrophages, colorectal cells, neuronal cells, glial cells, Langerhans-dendritic cells, follicular dendritic cells, and the circulating lymphocyte (the CD4/T4 cell), also known as the helper-inducer T lymphocyte. Thus, many tissues are infected by HIV, not just the circulating T4 lymphocyte cells. The T4 cells are central to the normal function of the immune system. They stimulate the maturation of B cells to plasma cells, which then secrete antibodies. They stimulate the maturation of T8 cells (suppressor-cytotoxic lymphocytes), which kill cells infected with HIV and other pathogens. They suppress further growth of T4 and T8 cells when infection is controlled. They also proliferate into memory clones, which recognize and destroy pathogens to which the clones have previously been exposed.

Transmission of HIV

The most infectious bodily secretions are blood and semen or seminal fluid, although HIV has been identified in other bodily secretions, including vaginal fluid, cerebrospinal fluid (CSF), breast milk, saliva, and tears. Infants can be infected from breastfeeding; colostrum in milk of HIV-infected mothers has been shown to contain infected cells. Male-to-female transmission is more efficient compared with female-to-male transmission. This probably explains the relative infectivity of semen in vaginal secretions. Not all individuals exposed to HIV become infected; this may be due to a difference in the virulence of HIV isolates, the amount of virus, the host immune response, or some combination of these factors. It is also likely that other environmental cofactors influence infection. After exposure and infection with HIV, many individuals have an acute febrile illness, resembling influenza or mononucleosis, often accompanied with rash, although individuals may be totally asymptomatic during the acute seroconversion period. Once an individual becomes infected with the virus, it can take a decade or longer for the infection to manifest itself as disease. During this asymptomatic period, individuals are infectious and may transmit the virus. Over a period of years during the incubation of HIV, the classic abnormality described is a progressive decrease in the number of T4 lymphocytes. As a result of both quantitative and qualitative defects in the immune system, individuals are prone to a number of infections that ultimately result in severe damage to the immune system and serious morbidity and mortality. During this time, individuals advance through the stages of HIV infection and disease, which is discussed in later sections.

EPIDEMIOLOGY

Dimensions of the AIDS Epidemic

In the mid-1990s, AIDS has surpassed unintentional injury as the leading cause of death in male Americans between 25 and 44 years of age. For women in the same age group, AIDS ranks fourth behind unintentional injury, breast cancer, and heart disease. By the end of the 1990s, it will likely be the leading cause of death in women in this age group. Accurate statistics on the dimensions of the HIV–AIDS epidemic are difficult to obtain. Lack of consistent mandatory reporting, reporting of only AIDS cases and not all cases of HIV infection, and fear of discrimination from HIV disclosure, have made assessment of the pandemic in the United States and worldwide difficult. The World Health Organization estimates that in the first decade of the HIV–AIDS epidemic, there were about 500,000 cases of AIDS in women and children, most of which have been unrecognized. Worldwide during 1994, an estimated 4 million new cases of HIV infection occurred—nearly 10,000 a day. During the 1990s, it is estimated that 3 million women and children will die of HIV–AIDS. Until recently, little attention has been paid to the special problems of women with HIV, including mothers and their children. This may be due to the fact that in the United States, the epidemic initially affected young and middle-aged men, primarily in certain urban centers. However, in the second decade of the epidemic, there has been a slow but steady increase in heterosexual populations infected with HIV, both young and middle aged. In addition to the increasing HIV incidence among these sexually active populations in urban areas, spread to rural areas has also been noted. HIV case rates have increased in the southern United States in the last few years, from 1.6 to 2.0 per 1000. In all of the United States, case rates of AIDS in 1994 have had striking ethnicity trends, with increasing representation of minority populations; rates were as follows: (cases per 1000 population) white 21, African-American 129, Hispanic 8, American Indian 16. Worldwide, the AIDS epidemic is a heterosexual disease with equal representation of men and women. Because of the population initially affected in North America, the statistics still represent AIDS as primarily a disease of men, in almost a 10 : 1 male–female ratio. However, the statistics on HIV infection, although not as well documented, indicate that over the next decade, women will become infected in a similar proportion to those in third-world countries, approaching a 1 : 1 male–female ratio.

The following factors are associated with an increased risk of HIV infection in women: using intravenous (IV) drugs, being the sexual partner of an at-risk individual (bisexual men or IV drug users), and having received transfused blood products between 1978 and March 1985. The use of crack cocaine is associated with hypersexual behavior, such as exchanging sex for drugs, thus exposing the women to several male sexual partners who are at high risk for HIV infection. Most other mood-altering drugs, including alcohol, are associated with changes in behavior that can cause an increased likelihood of exposure to HIV. Historically, most of the women in the United States who acquired HIV were IV drug users themselves, but recent statistics indicate that over half of women in the United States are being reported to have acquired HIV by heterosexual means. The rate among men and women in some communities (eg, Armed Service recruits, inner city residents, and Job Corps applicants) demonstrates a pattern resembling that of the African HIV epidemic with equal representation of both sexes.

The efficiency of heterosexual transmission of HIV between women and men has not been fully characterized. Another sexually transmitted disease (STD), gonorrhea, has an efficiency approximating 25% after a single male contact with an infected female, and nearly 90% for transmission by infected males to female partners. HIV transmission is much less efficient. The extremely long incubation period of HIV disease also hinders specific inferences about the relative efficiencies of transmission. Estimates for each sexual contact range from more than 3 per 100 for the most efficient transmitters in certain male homosexual cohort studies, to less than 1 in 1000 contacts in serodiscordant heterosexual partners. Certain studies report that over a 2- to 5-year period of regular unprotected sexual exposure, the male-to-female and female-to-male transmission rate of HIV is 17.5%; over longer time periods (5 to 10 years), this percentage is likely to increase. Cofactors that affect transmission include sex during menstruation, anal sex, traumatic sex, number of sexual contacts, contraceptive practices, other STDs including genital ulcer disease, and the infectiousness of the HIV-infected partner. Persons with more advanced infection, as determined by clinical and laboratory parameters, have been shown to be more likely to transmit HIV to their sexual partners, which is consistent with an increasing viral burden. Multiple sexually transmitted infections have been associated with HIV infection, although some of the associations may not be causal. Genital ulcer disease seems to be an independent factor that increases the efficiency of HIV transmission. Ulcerative diseases, which include syphilis and infection with herpes and *Hemophilus ducreyi*, are thought to be potent facilitators of transmission, resulting in direct access of HIV to mucosal tissues, lymphatic drainage, and systemic leukocytes. Nonulcerative STDs may produce increased inflammatory exudates, resulting in enhanced HIV transmission. The presence of genital warts has not been clearly associated with HIV infection. Menstruation introduces an average of 80 mL of blood into the genital tract over a 3- to 5-day period; this blood contains HIV-infected cells and cell-free virus. Levels of cell-free virus in peripheral blood fluctuate widely during the course of infection and disease, with higher titers of virus and increased likelihood of efficient transmission during both the acute seroconversion phase and late stages of HIV infection. Other factors that affect the menstrual cycle and flow (eg, contraceptive use, menopause, hysterectomy, pregnancy and parturition, age, general health) may modulate levels of HIV in cervicovaginal secretions. Cervical pH may have significant effect on titers of infectious HIV since HIV is inhibited by low pH concentrations. Certain conditions raise vaginal pH close to neutral and might be associated with increased titers of HIV in the female genital tract, including blood in the vagina, vaginosis, menopause, intercourse, and the use of certain contraceptives. Thus, there are certain unique features of HIV in women that have not been adequately addressed until recently.

AIDS in Women

Several studies from recently established cohorts of HIV-infected women have revealed some interesting findings. First, HIV-infected women are more likely to die without an AIDS-defining condition than are HIV-infected men. The reason women are at higher risk for early death is not clear, but it has been suggested that an important factor may be the poor access to, or use of, health care resources in this group. Other factors include the frequency of domestic violence and lack of social support for these women.

Early clinical manifestations of HIV also are different in women than in men. In many women, the initial manifestations may involve the genital tract, most commonly vulvovaginal candidiasis, pelvic inflammatory disease, genital warts, and cervical disease. Anecdotal studies describe a high prevalence of oligomenorrhea and amenorrhea in these women; however, these studies do not control for drug use. The most commonly acquired opportunistic infection (OI) in this group of women was *Pneumocystis carinii* pneumonia (PCP); however, women were more predisposed to *Candida* esophagitis, recurrent bacterial pneumonias, sinusitis, mycobacterial infections, and wasting syndrome. Women had less frequent episodes of the AIDS-related cancer, Kaposi sarcoma. Additionally, when men and women were compared in these cohorts in terms of survival and OIs, the women were younger, more likely to be African-American or Hispanic, more likely to report a history of injectable drug use, and had higher T4 lymphocyte counts than the men.

Other issues specific to women involve the impact of this disease on their societal and familial roles. The woman's role in her family may prevent her from being able to seek treatment for herself. She may be the last in line in a family with multiple HIV-infected members to receive treatment. Additionally, a clear link exists between drug use and HIV infection in women. Society has made policies that discriminate against women using drugs, and this may prevent women seeking care because of fear of losing their children. There continues to be a need to develop prevention, intervention, and treatment programs that involve women and consider their social and economic situations. This chapter reviews the diagnosis and treatment of HIV infection, with special attention to features unique to women and their unborn children.

DIFFERENTIAL DIAGNOSIS

Human Response to HIV

One of the body's capabilities is to recognize and to try to eliminate what is foreign by making antibodies (humoral immunity) or by priming cells to recognize the offending target (cellular immunity). The enzyme immunosorbent assay (ELISA) antibody test, which has been available since 1985 and is currently used to screen for HIV infection, detects antibodies to HIV in the serum of infected individuals. The ELISA has high sensitivity but may lack specificity. Nonspecific antibody reactions can occur against other non-HIV proteins, as is known to happen with syphilis and other infections, resulting in false-positive reactions. False-positive ELISA reactions against HIV can occur in individuals with certain genetic types (more frequently observed in multiparous women and multiply transfused women), and in the setting of severe alcoholic liver disease, hematologic malignancies, lymphoma, renal transplant, chronic renal failure, passively acquired antibody (ie, contained in hepatitis B immunoglobulin), acute DNA viral infections, and HIV-2 infection. Since antibody tests do not detect viral antigens in the patient's blood, it may give false-negative results in those early in acute HIV infection, who have not developed antibody, or in severely immunocompromised individuals not capable of developing an antibody response. In primary HIV infection, the time interval from infection to the appearance of antibody is generally 4 to 12 weeks, although the interval may be longer. Thus, sequential ELISA tests may be necessary to account for this "window period." Other causes of false-negative ELISA reactions to HIV include malignancy, blood replacement transfusion, bone marrow transplantation, and B-cell dysfunction.

Several different confirmatory tests are more expensive but more specific than the ELISA, and are done after a positive screening from an ELISA test. These include the Western blot (WB), radioimmunoprecipitation, and immunofluorescence assays. The WB tests whether a patient's serum reacts with different HIV proteins, including the outer coat and inner parts of HIV, which in total make up the virus. Multiple bands on the WB indicate multiple antibody responses to different proteins of HIV. This test is helpful in confirming the diagnosis of HIV, with a positive predictive value of 99.5% in both low- and high-risk populations. Individuals infected with HIV have WB bands to multiple HIV proteins, and algorithms have been established that require the criteria of two different WB bands as positive to confirm HIV infection. Occasionally, individuals in the acute seroconversion period have just one positive WB band, and uninfected individuals may have one band positive on WB. Other causes of false-positive WB reactions include cross-reactivity with normal human ribonucleoproteins, other human retroviruses besides HIV-1, antibodies to human cellular antigens, and globulins produced during polyclonal gammopathy. Sequential ELISA and WB assays may be necessary in equivocal infection and in suspected false-positive or false-negative reactions. The standard for diagnosis of HIV infection is to repeat the tests every 3 to 6 months after each new exposure. Confusing serologic results warrant subspecialty consultation.

Other tests that do not the depend on antibody tests include a number of antigen detection techniques. Antigen detection techniques eliminate the need to depend on the antibody results to make the diagnosis of HIV infection. These include viral antigen capture of the viral p24 antigen with monoclonal antibody, in situ hybridization to detect HIV viral DNA or RNA products (ie, polymerase chain reaction [PCR]), and tissue culture of HIV from blood or other body fluids. Being able to isolate HIV from body fluids or detecting HIV by special technology such as PCR is especially helpful in atypical cases of HIV infection in the window period (before the immune system has produced antibody after a recent infection) and in the newborn period. When a mother is HIV infected, she passively transfers her antibody to her baby's circulation, resulting in HIV antibody tests that cannot separate maternally acquired antibody from the antibody produced by the baby in response to the baby being infected with HIV. A positive HIV antibody test result is not considered reliable until 18 months of age in infants for diagnostic purposes, since maternal HIV antibody may take up to 18 months after birth to decay and be eliminated from the infant's system. Direct detection of HIV in blood and tissues can assist in the early diagnosis of HIV in infants and children, with most antigen assays being able to conclusively rule in or rule out HIV infection by 3 to 6 months of life. However, because of the concerns for false-positive and false-negative results, and the consequences of a wrong diagnosis, multiple antigen and antibody tests over a scheduled time period should be performed to at least 18 months of age.

PRESENTATION OF HIV AND INFECTIOUS COMPLICATIONS

HIV gradually destroys the T4 helper lymphocyte population, which is critical to the proper functioning of the cellular and humoral immune system. Lack of these cells, both qualitatively in early HIV infection, and, later, quantitatively in symptomatic HIV disease, predisposes the patient to a host of parasitic, viral, fungal, and bacterial infections. Diagnosis of HIV infection depends on obtaining an HIV antibody test in an individual at high risk for HIV. However, high-risk criteria that have been established to screen pregnant women detect less than 50% of those infected with HIV. Thus, some argue for universal HIV testing of all pregnant women. Currently, however, this is not being done consistently. Table 84-1 is a guide to identify those at higher risk for acquisition of HIV-1 infection. Once an individual is infected with HIV, the infectious complications can be best predicted and evaluated by understanding the natural history of HIV infection and the risk of different infectious agents at the different stages of immune suppression.

Table 84-1. Candidates for HIV Testing in a Primary Care/Obstetric–Gynecologic Setting

Social and Sexual History
Injecting drug users who share needles
Sexual partners of injecting drug users who share needles, of bisexual men, or of HIV-positive men
Transfusion recipients of blood or blood products (1978–1986)
Current or previous multiple sexual partners
Area of origin for patient or partner is country where the incidence of HIV is high
Clinical History
Unexplained persistent constitutional symptoms
Recurrent vulvovaginal candidiasis
History of, or current, sexually transmitted diseases such as syphilis, chancroid, gonorrhea, or herpes simplex virus
Presence of tuberculosis or any illness for which an HIV-positive test result might affect the recommended diagnostic evaluation, treatment, or follow-up
Recurrent bacterial pneumonia
Herpes zoster infection
Laboratory Tests
Serologic evidence of hepatitis B and C markers
Autoimmune thrombocytopenic purpura
Condyloma or dysplasia on Pap smear

HIV, human immunodeficiency virus.

Natural History and Classification

Several different classifications exist, with patients commonly being classified as having AIDS based on criteria established by the Centers for Disease Control and Prevention (CDC). Most of these complications are seen in the setting of long-standing, advanced HIV infection. However, the simplest description of HIV and its interaction with its host can be better understood by classifying patients in the following stages: (1) the acute retroviral syndrome; (2) the clinically latent period (asymptomatic, with or without persistent generalized lymphadenopathy); (3) early symptomatic HIV infection (previously called AIDS-related complex); (4) AIDS (which includes indicator conditions established by the CDC in 1987 and was updated in 1993 to include a CD4 cell count $< 200/\text{mm}^3$); and (5) advanced HIV infection defined as CD4 cell count less than $50/\text{mm}^3$. Table 84-2 provides a summary of these classifications.

Acute Retroviral Syndrome

Symptomatic primary HIV infection has been reported to occur in up to 30% to 70% of cases. The time of symptoms from exposure is typically 2 to 4 weeks but may be longer. Typical symptoms found in most symptomatic cases include fever, myalgia, lymphadenopathy, pharyngitis, and an erythematous maculopapular rash. Less common symptoms include mucocutaneous ulcerations, diarrhea, nausea and vomiting, hepatosplenomegaly, and oral candidiasis, occurring in 10% to 30%. Neurologic features can include peripheral neuropathy, meningoencephalitis, facial palsy, cognitive impairment, and psychosis. Individuals also can seroconvert without symptoms.

Asymptomatic Infection

During the asymptomatic infection period, the patient is generally asymptomatic and has no remarkable findings on physical examination except for enlarged lymph nodes and persistent generalized lymphadenopathy, defined as enlarged lymph nodes involving two noncontiguous sites other than the inguinal nodes. While the patient is asymptomatic, immune damage takes place at the level of the lymph tissue and causes progressive damage, despite the fact that the viral burden in peripheral blood is relatively low. With time, it is hypothesized that HIV escapes the control of the immune surveillance of the lymph tissue and freely circulates in the peripheral blood, which contributes to the symptoms of HIV infection.

Early Symptomatic HIV infection

Early symptomatic HIV infection includes complications that are not necessarily AIDS-indicator conditions, but are more common and more severe because of the coexistence of HIV infection. Examples include oral candidiasis; vaginal candidiasis that is persistent, frequent, or difficult to manage; cervical dysplasia; cervical cancer; constitutional symptoms; and idiopathic thrombocytopenic purpura.

AIDS

The original definition of AIDS used conditions that were found in the setting of severe immunosuppression, especially defective cell-mediated immunity. It has been recognized that infections mediated primarily by the humoral immune system and complications in women and heterosexual populations were not adequately represented in the original case definition of AIDS. Three additions were included: recurrent bacterial pneumonia, invasive cervical cancer, and pulmonary tuberculosis (TB). Additionally, patients with a CD4 cell count less than 200/mm^3 are now given the diagnosis of AIDS. Previously, the CD4 count was not used in the case definition of AIDS.

Table 84-2. Indicator Conditions in Case Definition of AIDS (Adults)*

All HIV Seropositive Adults With CD4 < 200/mm^3
Candidiasis of esophagus, trachea, bronchi, or lungs
Cervical cancer, invasive†‡
Coccidioidomycosis, extrapulmonary†
Cryptococcosis, extrapulmonary
Cryptosporidiosis with diarrhea > 1 mo
Cytomegalovirus of any organ other than liver, spleen, or lymph nodes
Herpes simplex with mucocutaneous ulcer > 1 mo or bronchitis, pneumonitis, esophagitis
Histoplasmosis, extrapulmonary†
HIV-associated dementia†: disabling cognitive or motor dysfunction interfering with occupation or activities of daily living
HIV-associated wasting†: involuntary weight loss > 10% of baseline plus chronic diarrhea (≥ 2 loose stools/d ≥ 30 d) or chronic weakness and documented enigmatic fever ≥30 d
Isoporosis with diarrhea > 1 mo†
Kaposi sarcoma in patient younger than 60 y (or older than 60 y†)
Lymphoma of brain in patient younger than 60 y (or older than 60 y†)
Lymphoma, non-Hodgkin of B-cell or unknown immunologic phenotype and histologic features showing small, noncleaved lymphoma or immunoblastic sarcoma
Mycobacterium avium or *Mycobacterium kansasii,* disseminated
Mycobacterium tuberculosis, disseminated†
M tuberculosis, pulmonary†,‡
Nocardiosis†
Pneumocystis carinii pneumonia
Pneumonia, recurrent–bacterial (≥ 2 episodes in 12 mo)†,‡
Progressive multifocal leukoencephalopathy
Salmonella septicemia (nontyphoid), recurrent†
Strongyloidosis, extraintestinal
Toxoplasmosis of internal organ
Wasting syndrome due to HIV (as defined above: HIV-associated wasting)

HIV, human immunodeficiency virus.

*Includes original AIDS case definition established in 1987 plus revision in 1993.

†Requires positive HIV serologic findings.

‡Added in the revised case definition 1993.

Advanced HIV Infection

Patients with CD4 cell counts less than 50/mm^3 have a median survival of 1 to 1½ years. Most patients who die of HIV-related complications such as multiple OIs, AIDS-related malignancies, and other infectious complications of immunosuppression are in this CD4 count stratum.

Progression of HIV Infection and Disease

The median rate of progression from infection to the development of an AIDS-defining diagnosis, in the absence of treatment, is approximately 10 years. The most rapid rate of progression from initial infection to death was 26 weeks from AIDS, as recorded in a case from a cohort of gay men residing in San Francisco. As a rule, 0% of HIV infected individuals develop an AIDS-defining diagnosis at 1 year, 3% at 3 years, 12% at 5 years, 36% at 8 years, 53% in 10 years, and 68% at 14 years. Mean survival time after a CD4 count of 200/mm^3 is 38 to 40 months, and 12 to 18 months for those with CD4 counts less than 50/mm^3. A certain group of infected individuals have been recently recognized who are remarkably stabile and remain asymptomatic with CD4 counts in a normal range for 7 to 10 years following infection with HIV. These individuals have been referred to as "long-term survivors" and may represent as many as 20% of all those infected with HIV. Whether this is related to the host immune system or the infecting virus, or some combination of these factors, is not clear. It has been estimated in the San Francisco Cohort that 10% to 17% of gay men will remain asymptomatic for 20 years or longer. Other factors may lead to a change in this natural history, including antiviral therapy and prophylactic antibiotics, which may lengthen survival; and other comorbid conditions such as IV drug use and alcohol use. It is unlikely that an inner city woman embroiled in the drug and sexual behavior and other social issues will be a long-term survivor, unless many of these nonmedical issues, which often coexist with HIV, are also addressed.

HISTORY

All patients benefit from preventive health and health maintenance measures, regardless of their HIV status. Screening of individuals at risk for HIV allows assessment of the immunologic status of these individuals. Initial assessment should include a comprehensive medical evaluation, with the goal of appropriate monitoring and initiation of antiretroviral therapy and antibiotic prophylaxis of OIs, if indicated. Careful review of the major organ systems affected by HIV often discloses treatable, symptomatic disease in apparently asymptomatic individuals. Fever can simply be a nonspecific marker of advancing HIV disease, or may represent an undiagnosed occult infection or malignancy. A careful history of common infections that are found to coexist with HIV, including hepatitis B and C, syphilis, herpes simplex, herpes zoster, and TB, may assist in appropriate evaluation and treatment. Table 84-3 summarizes a recommended baseline evaluation for newly diagnosed HIV-infected individuals. Undiagnosed HIV infection may be determined by offering HIV testing in those with certain sentinel comorbid infections. Patients should be asked if they know, or they think they know, when they were exposed to HIV, since approximately 50% of individuals progress to AIDS within 10 years of seroconversion. Staging HIV disease may provide prognostic and treatment direction.

Table 84-3. Baseline Laboratory Assessment of HIV-1–Infected Patients

T-lymphocyte subsets
CBC with differential and platelets
Electrolytes, urea nitrogen, creatinine, liver function tests
ESR and LDH
VDRL or RPR
Hepatitis B surface antigen and hepatitis B surface antibody
Hepatitis C antibody
Toxoplasma IgG titer
PPD and two DTH controls
Chest radiograph
Gynecologic examination:
Pelvic
Test for gonorrhea, chlamydia
Papanicolaou smear
Wet mount examination of vaginal secretions

CBC, complete blood count; *DTH,* delayed type hypersensitivity; *ESR,* erythrocyte sedimentation rate; *LDM,* lactate dehydrogenase; *PPD,* purified protein derivative; *RPR,* rapid plasma reagin.

A complete medical history should be performed with special attention to the following:

- Constitutional symptoms: fever, weight loss, fatigue, night sweats
- Pulmonary symptoms: cough, shortness of breath
- Gastrointestinal: diarrhea, loose stools, odynophagia, sore throat
- Prior infections: pneumonia, sinusitis, other bacterial infections
- Hepatitis and TB exposure
- Sexual history
- Gynecologic–obstetric history: menstrual history, STDs, abnormal findings on Pap smear, pelvic infections (including candidiasis, genital warts)
- Alcohol and drug use history
- Neurologic: headaches, seizure disorders, visual disturbances
- Dermatologic: skin rashes, skin lesions, genital ulcers
- Allergies: complications with sulfa drugs is especially common
- Transfusion history
- Underlying medical conditions and comorbid factors
- Travel to an HIV-endemic country.

A thorough history assists in the detection of newly diagnosed HIV infection and in the evaluation of the status of those already infected with HIV.

PHYSICAL EXAMINATION

A baseline physical examination assists with the diagnosis of HIV infection and estimates prognosis of those already infected. Certain HIV-associated conditions, including oral candidiasis, oral hairy leukoplakia, folliculitis, unexplained weight loss, and fevers, are all associated with advancing immunodeficiency and a worsening prognosis in terms of future morbidity and mortality. Certain common manifestations of HIV disease, early and late, can be anticipated and prevented by appropriate evaluation, including periodic complete and focused physical examinations.

On completion of an initial comprehensive physical examination, all individuals, regardless of sex or risk factor, should have routine follow-up examinations. At each subsequent visit, a focused examination should evaluate the patient for fevers, weight loss, and examine the mouth for evidence of complications that may harbinger the onset of progressive immunodeficiency. A more complete examination of other organ systems affected commonly by HIV, including the lymph system, skin, and abdomen, should be performed at least twice annually. Other routine preventive examinations, performed in consultation with appropriate specialists, include ophthalmologic examinations at periodic intervals and pelvic and Pap smear every 6 to 12 months. Modifications in the frequency of these evaluations is determined by the immune status of the individual and the finding of abnormalities at routine screening visits. With regard to Pap smear evaluation, more aggressive testing is justified by the reporting of increased rates (eight- to tenfold) of cervical dysplasia in this population. Results of Pap smears requiring further evaluation and treatment are outlined in Table 84-4. The Pap smear has a diagnostic yield of close to 90% in the presence of cervical malignancy and premalignancy in HIV-negative women; however, some reports in HIV-positive women have revealed a high rate of false-negative Pap smears. If abnormalities are found, treatment options include cryotherapy, loop excision, and laser conization. The highest cure rates are from conization. Treatment failures for cervical intraepithelial neoplasia are higher in HIV-positive women than their uninfected counterparts, with higher recurrences in the more immunocompromised women.

Abnormalities on general examination that may require further evaluation and follow-up include the following: weight change; general muscular status; adenopathy; eye examination revealing exudates consistent with cytomegalovirus (CMV) retinitis, toxoplasmosis, or syphilis; oral abnormalities including herpes simplex lesions, oral leukoplakia, candidiasis, aphthous ulcers, and Kaposi sarcoma; skin abnormalities including seborrheic dermatitis, psoriasis, molluscum contagiosum, and Kaposi sarcoma; and mental status changes. Pelvic and genitourinary examination may detect abnormalities on routine Pap smear (as mentioned earlier), and genital and perianal lesions including ulcerative disease, molluscum, condylomata, and other nonulcerative STDs. Genital ulcerative disease may represent herpes genitalis, syphilis, chancroid, lymphogranuloma venereum, granuloma inguinale, or noninfectious or invasive lesions. Molluscum and condyloma appear as nonulcerative genital lesions. A rectal examination may reveal a mass lesion, commonly due to malignancies, infectious agents, or both.

LABORATORY AND IMAGING STUDIES

Guidelines for HIV testing and interpretation of these results are discussed in "Differential Diagnosis." Once an individual is diagnosed as HIV infected, routine laboratory evaluation should be performed as part of preventive health care. Further evaluation may be warranted based on the results of the preventive evaluation.

HIV Serology

Remember that a form for informed consent is required by state law in 41 states and recommended in others without this requirement. HIV serologic testing is considered as invasive due to the potential consequences in terms of discrimination in insurance, employment, health care, and personal relationships. Pretest and

Table 84-4. General Guidelines Based on Pap Smear and Results of Colposcopy with Biopsy

Atypia	Repeat Pap smear every 6 mo and colposcopy annually
Low-grade squamous intraepithelial lesions (CIN 1)	Follow with Pap and colposcopy every 4–6 mo or treat with loop excision
High-grade squamous intraepithelial lesions (CIN 2 or 3)	Treat with loop excision or conization (see above)
Carcinoma in situ	Loop excision or conization (see above)
Invasive carcinoma	Surgery or radiation therapy

CIN, cervical intraepithelial neoplasia.

posttest counseling is required as part of this testing. Certain states waive the requirement of informed consent and pretest and posttest counseling. All donors of blood or organs have mandatory testing to permit the testing of the source in cases of exposure to health care workers.

Clinical Laboratory Testing

HIV infection and disease has protean manifestations, and most organ systems can be affected. Additionally, several other medical conditions can be associated with a person's risk behavior, such as STDs and chronic renal failure or liver disease associated with drug and alcohol use.

Complete Blood Cell Count and Differential

A complete blood cell count is a standard laboratory test and is especially important in HIV because anemia, leukopenia, lymphopenia, and thrombocytopenia are common complications. This test should be performed annually, and more frequently in the setting of abnormalities consistent with marrow suppression, in those receiving marrow suppressing drugs, and in those with marginal cell counts.

Lymphocytes Markers

The best studied prognostic studies involve the absolute T4 cell count, the percentage of T4 cells, and the T4-to-T8 ratio. A decrease in each of these indexes is strongly associated with progression to AIDS in seropositive persons. CD4 counts are used as guidelines for initiating antiretroviral therapy and initiating antibiotic prophylaxis, including those of prevention of PCP (Table 84-5). Recommendations for the frequencies of monitoring CD4 counts have been established; they should be monitored at a minimum of every 6 months, and more frequently with declining CD4 counts, at the time of initiation of therapy, and when there is high risk of certain OIs. Some clinicians stop monitoring CD4 counts below $50/mm^3$. Normal values for most laboratories have a mean of 800 to $1050/mm^3$ with a range representing two standard deviations of approximately 500 to $1400/mm^3$. Factors that influence CD4 counts include laboratory-to-laboratory variation, seasonal and diurnal variation, certain intercurrent illnesses, and corticosteroids. Lowest daily changes are at 12:30 PM, and peak values are at 8:00 PM. Thus, lymphocyte markers should be measured at a consistent time of day in an individual, and should be performed at a time that minimizes confounding factors, that is, not during an acute illness.

Serologic Testing for Other Infections

Serologic testing for hepatitis viruses (eg, hepatitis B and C, and, potentially, others) are indicated because the risk factors for HIV also apply to these viruses. The specific test depends on the clinical situation and can be used to assess immunity, the need for vaccination, or reexposure to the hepatitis virus.

Toxoplasmosis serologic testing (IgG) assists in the differential diagnosis of complications involving the central nervous system (CNS), should be tested at baseline evaluation, and need not be repeated. Syphilis serologic testing is indicated to screen for latent syphilis, to assess response to therapy, and to evaluate new exposure to this STD. Both false-positive and false-negative VDRL and rapid plasma reagin (RPR) serologic types have been reported in patients with HIV infection, but these are rare. Syphilis tests should be performed annually, and abnormal serologic results may require consultative advice.

Serum Chemistry Panel

A serum chemistry panel (ie, SMA-12, SMA-21) is commonly performed in the initial evaluation of HIV infection due to the high rate of hepatitis in patients at risk for HIV, the need for baseline values in patients who likely have multisystem disease, and to assess the ability to tolerate treatment with potentially hepatotoxic agents. A chemistry panel also screens for renal and nutritional disease.

Screening for Fungal Diseases

Cryptococcus neoformans is the fourth most common OI in persons with AIDS. However, the cryptococcal antigen test, although a reliable marker of acute disease, is not useful as a

Table 84-5. Recommendations for T-Lymphocyte Monitoring

CD4* (CELL COUNTS/MM^3)	MANAGEMENT	REPEAT TESTING
>600	No intervention indicated	Every 6 mo
500–600	Antiretroviral treatment may be indicated soon; closer surveillance needed	Every 3 mo
300–500	Antiretroviral treatment recommended by most experts	Every 6 mo
200–300	Antiretroviral treatment indicated soon; closer surveillance needed	Every 3 mo
<200	PCP prophylaxis and antiretroviral treatment indicated	Optional

PCP, Pneumocystis carinii pneumonia.

*Normal CD4 counts: range, 400–1400 cells/mm^3; mean, 800–1050 mm^3.

screening test in the asymptomatic patient. The presence of fungal pathogens in blood or tissue specimens implies invasive disease, but obtaining superficial cultures of most fungi and yeast from mucocutaneous surfaces implies only colonization.

Chest X-Ray

A routine CXR is recommended, in part to detect asymptomatic TB. Additionally, it is a baseline for patients who eventually have a high frequency of pulmonary disease; in those with advanced disease, the x-ray may detect otherwise unrecognized infectious and anatomic abnormalities. This test should be repeated as clinically indicated.

PPD Skin Testing

The CDC recommends annual testing with a purified protein derivative (PPD; Mantoux, 5TU units) run in parallel with an anergy panel, using two skin test reagents chosen from among *Candida*, tetanus, and mumps. The criterion for a positive PPD test for individuals with HIV infection is 5 mm of induration, versus 10 or 15 mm in non-HIV infected populations. Anergy, described as a lack of induration on any recommended skin test, is found in approximately 25% of those with T4 counts over 600, and in 75% of those with counts less than 200. Annual screening with the PPD is recommended if the initial test result is negative and the patient is *not* anergic. If the PPD result is negative and there is a family history of exposure, a history of being PPD positive, or a history of prior or recent exposure to a contact person, the CXR should be obtained for further evaluation of pulmonary TB.

Sexually Transmitted Disease Cultures

All women should be screened for gonorrhea and chlamydia, even if asymptomatic. All symptomatic men should have cultures performed. All patients with positive culture results should be treated.

Gynecologic Examination

The CDC recommends evaluation with pelvic examination and Pap smear at initial evaluation, a repeat 6 months later and, then annually if the results are normal. Women with HIV infection have more aggressive cervical dysplasia and cancer (as previously discussed) and more frequent mucocutaneous *Candida* infections. As part of gynecologic evaluation, routine pregnancy testing, counseling, and referral (prenatal care, family planning services, safer sex counseling) may be appropriate.

Surrogate Markers for Evaluation of HIV Infection

In the future, we will likely be less dependent on HIV antibody tests and CD4 counts for evaluating and monitoring HIV infection. PCR, which detects HIV genetic material in an HIV-infected patient's cells, is available and is useful in the diagnosis of HIV infection in infants and in adults in the window period of acute seroconversion. Several other laboratory assays correlate with HIV disease progression; these include β_2-microglobulin, neopterin, p24 antigen, acid-dissociated p24 antigen, p24 antibody, erythrocyte sedimentation rate, soluble interleukin-2 receptors, and measures of HIV viral load. These assays are not recommended in most clinical situations. They often are expensive, not well standardized, and still are considered research tools.

TREATMENT

Treatment of HIV infection involves using the knowledge gained from the previous sections regarding an individual's level of immunosuppression, attempting to diagnose individuals early in the stages of HIV infection, preventing further spread of HIV, treatment of HIV infection and disease with available antiretroviral agents, prophylaxis of OIs, and treatment and long-term suppression of already established infections.

Primary caregivers are gaining experience in caring for their HIV-infected patients. If one takes the view of HIV as a chronic infection with a long latency period, similar to other diseases such as diabetes mellitus, it logically follows that patients should be managed by the primary caregiver for many years with appropriate comanagement or consultative assistance from the appropriate subspecialists. However, factors other than logic enter into the unwillingness of many caretakers to care for HIV-infected individuals.

Predicting Complications of HIV

Certain rules of thumb can assist the clinician in caring for HIV-infected individuals. The degree of immunosuppression assists the clinician in generating a differential diagnosis (Table 84-6). For example, cough in an immunocompetent HIV-infected individual is more likely to represent a bronchitis or a sinusitis rather than an AIDS-defining pneumonia such as PCP. With HIV, multiple different infections may be occurring simultaneously. It is common to have a patient with fever and to have multiple causative etiologies for this fever. The source of the infection in HIV individuals is usually endogenous; most AIDS-defining infections represent reactivation of organisms that are already present in these individuals (ie, toxoplasmosis, herpes simplex virus [HSV], varicella zoster virus [VZV]); exceptions to this rule include TB and salmonellosis.

With advanced disease, most infections are more difficult to treat and often present with unusual manifestations. Once the infection has been controlled, it may require lifelong maintenance therapy for suppression and prevention of reactivation of the same infection, which may never be totally eradicated by the initial therapy. Certain infections have epidemiologic and geographic predilection; TB is more common in inner city populations; other infections, including histoplasmosis and coccidioidomycosis (fungal infections seen with advanced HIV infection) are directly related to their prevalence in geographic areas where these patients live or have traveled.

Thus, it is important to evaluate and stage the patient's HIV status, remembering the correlation between HIV-associated complications in relation to CD4 cell counts. In the setting of early HIV infection, HIV-infected individuals have problems similar to their HIV-negative counterparts, except they may have more frequent bacterial infections. Thus, a recently infected individual with high CD4 cell counts with fever and cough should have the appropriate clinical evaluation and initiation of therapy, determined by the clinical diagnosis. Workup for OIs, which are seen primarily in advanced HIV disease, are not appropriate at this time. Sinusitis, otitis, pharyngitis, bronchitis, and bacterial pneumonia are more

Table 84-6. Correlation of Complications with CD4 Cell Counts

CD4 CELL COUNT	INFECTIONS	NONINFECTIOUS*
>500/mm^3	Acute retroviral syndrome	Persistent generalized lymphadenopathy (PGL)
	Candidal vaginitis	Guillain-Barré syndrome
	Syphilis	Polymyositis
	Otitis/sinusitis	Aseptic meningitis
	Folliculitis	Cervical intraepithelial neoplasia
200–500/mm^3	Pneumococcal and other bacterial pneumonia	Cervical cancer
	Pulmonary TB	Kaposi sarcoma
	Herpes zoster infection	Anemia
	Thrush	Mononeuritis multiplex
	Candidal esophagitis	Idiopathic thrombocytopenic purpura
	Cryptosporidiosis, self-limited	
<200/mm^3	*Pneumocystis carinii* pneumonia	Wasting
	Disseminated or chronic herpes simplex	Peripheral neuropathy
	Toxoplasmosis	HIV-associated dementia
	Cryptococcosis	CNS lymphoma
	CMV retinitis	Cardiomyopathy
	Disseminated histoplasmosis and coccidioidomycosis	
	Cryptosporidiosis, chronic	
	Microsporidiosis	
	Miliary/extrapulmonary TB	
<50/mm^3	Disseminated CMV (eye, lung, GI)	Multisystem malignancies
	Disseminated *Mycobacterium avium complex*	
	Gram-negative sepsis	
	Hospital-acquired infections	

CMV, cytomegalovirus; *CNS,* central nervous system; *GI,* gastrointestinal; *HIV,* human immunodeficiency virus; *TB,* tuberculosis.

*Some conditions listed as "Noninfectious" may be associated with transmissible microbes: lymphomas, cervical cancer, cervical intraepithelial neoplasia, and Kaposi sarcoma.

common diagnoses in this setting. Other infections that are more common in the setting of high CD4 cell counts include syphilis and pulmonary TB.

Individuals with lower T-cell counts, in the range of 200 to 500, continue to be predisposed to recurrent bacterial infections, and these infections may be more refractory to treatment and tend to be recurrent. Pulmonary TB, herpes zoster, mucocutaneous candidiasis, *Candida* esophagitis, and cryptosporidiosis can be seen in this setting.

Noninfectious problems commonly seen in this range of immunodeficiency include cervical intraepithelial neoplasia, cervical cancer, Kaposi sarcoma, and idiopathic thrombocytopenic purpura.

With a T-cell count less than 200, PCP is classically seen. A wide range of infectious and noninfectious complications start to be seen in this stratum. When T4 cells are less than 50, infection with disseminated CMV, *Mycobacterium avium-intracellulare* complex (MAC), and disseminated fungus are more common, as well as CNS toxoplasmosis and lymphomas. With end-stage HIV infection—often in the setting of multiple organ damage, bone marrow suppression, neutropenia, poor skin integrity, leaky mucosal surfaces, and central venous catheter use—a wide spectrum of community-acquired, nosocomial, and OIs are common. Patients with end-stage HIV infection often die from terminal infection with multiple pathogens, including gram-negative bacteremia, sepsis, and pneumonia. Thus, the clinician must use clinical skills and laboratory evaluation to guide evaluation and treatment (Table 84-7).

CLASSIC OPPORTUNISTIC INFECTIONS

Whereas it is important to have knowledge of the classic OIs that occur in AIDS (which represent complications of end-stage immunodeficiency), earlier in the immunodeficiency of HIV infection, the primary caretakers will diagnose many other atypical, complicated, and difficult-to-treat infections, before their patients present with AIDS-defining conditions.

Pneumocystis carinii Pneumonia

P carinii pneumonia is the most common, serious, yet treatable serious OI seen in AIDS. Before the availability of PCP prophylaxis, more AIDS patients died of this infection than any other. With the initiation of primary and secondary antibiotic prophylaxis, there have been less deaths due to PCP. *P carinii* is a ubiquitous organism. Disease is commonly a consequence of reactivation of the organism, acquired through the respiratory tract early in life. PCP is strictly an

Table 84-7. Common Manifestations of HIV Disease

EARLY	LATE
Constitutional	**Constitutional**
Fatigue	Bacterial sepsis
Generalized lymphadenopathy	Cytomegalovirus infection
	Disseminated *Mycobacterium avium* complex infection
	Extrapulmonary tuberculosis
	Histoplasmosis
	HIV-related fever
	HIV wasting syndrome
Hematologic	**Pulmonary**
Anemia	Recurrent bacterial pneumonia
Thrombocytopenia	Recurrent *Pneumocystis* pneumonia
Leukopenia	Typical or atypical tuberculosis
Dermatologic	**Neurologic**
Folliculitis	AIDS dementia complex
herpes simplex and zoster	Cerebral toxoplasmosis
Seborrheic dermatitis	Cryptococcal meningitis
	CNS lymphoma
	Neurosyphilis
	Peripheral neuropathy
	Progressive multifocal leukoencephalopathy
Oral	**Gastrointestinal**
Aphthous ulcerations	*Cryptosporidium* and *Isospora enteritis*
Candidiasis	Esophageal candidiasis
Oral hairy leukoplakia	HIV enteropathy
Herpes simplex	
Necrotizing gingivitis	
Genital	**Ocular**
Candidiasis	Cytomegalovirus retinitis
Anogenital herpes simplex infection	Syphilitic retinitis/papillitis
Severe pelvic inflammatory disease	
Syphilis	
Pulmonary	**Renal**
Bacterial pneumonia	HIV nephropathy
Pneumocystis carinii pneumonia	
Pulmonary tuberculosis	

AIDS, acquired immunodeficiency syndrome; *CNS,* central nervous system; *HIV,* human immunodeficiency virus.

opportunistic pathogen, requiring moderate immunosuppression to cause disease (CD4 < 200/mm^3). Common presenting symptoms include fever, progressive shortness of breath, and nonproductive cough. A purulent sputum, if present, is usually due to other common bacterial upper respiratory or pulmonary infections, including TB. Symptoms may be mild in early cases and signs are nonspecific, and diagnosis may be made by a combination of CXR, arterial blood gas or oximetry determination, and evaluation of induced pulmonary specimens for detection of PCP organisms by special staining techniques. The CXR, which may be normal in 5% of patients with PCP, usually shows diffuse peripheral or basilar interstitial infiltrates; less commonly, upper lobe infiltrates, alveolar consolidation, bullae formation, cavitation, and pneumothorax (especially in the setting of prophylaxis with inhaled pentamidine), and even unilateral lobar infiltrates may be present. The diagnosis is fairly straightforward in the setting of an individual with CD4 less than 200/mm^3, an abnormal finding on CXR, hypoxemia, and detection of *P carinii* cysts in pulmonary secretions. If induced sputum does not detect the cysts, bronchoscopy and lavage may be necessary. Treatment requires specialist consultation, and standard therapies include trimethoprim-sulfamethoxazole (TMP-SMX), pentamidine, atovaquone, and others, which are often initiated in hospital and continued as an outpatient to complete 21 days of therapy. Corticosteroids are added with serious cases; pulmonary mechanical ventilation may be required when patients cannot be oxygenated by Ventimask. Without prophylaxis, after full-course treatment, PCP commonly recurs within a year. Even with prophylaxis, breakthrough infections are common in the setting of advanced immunosuppression, and it is common for AIDS patients to have two or more episodes of PCP before their deaths.

Cytomegalovirus Infections

Most CMV infection in AIDS patients represents reactivation of an infection acquired at a younger age. With advanced immunosuppression, patients may become viremic and disseminate CMV to multiple tissue sites. CMV isolated from superficial sites (ie, urine) does not necessarily imply tissue level infection. Most common sites of infection, seen in the setting of advanced immunosuppression, include the eye, gastrointestinal tract, lung, and liver. CMV retinitis is diagnosed on ophthalmologic examination and by the presence of fluffy yellow-to-white infiltrates, and often areas of hemorrhage. Diagnosis of retinitis requires the consultative advice of an experienced ophthalmologist who must differentiate the findings from CMV, syphilis, toxoplasmosis, and other infectious causes of retinitis. Histopathologic evidence of CMV involvement in the tissue obtained by biopsy (ie, liver, lung, gastrointestinal tract) is required to make the diagnosis and initiate therapy (except for CMV retinitis). Approved drugs active against CMV include ganciclovir and foscarnet. These agents must be monitored by a specialist, as they are relatively toxic agents. CMV infections require lifelong therapy; the antiviral agents are virustatic and not virucidal, so that even with appropriate therapy, the disease process eventually progresses to death, often in 6 to 12 months.

Herpes Simplex and Zoster Infections

Both HSV and VZV infections are common and occur at all stages of immunosuppression. With more advanced HIV disease, they are more difficult to treat and more likely to recur. These infections are often due to reactivation of infections acquired earlier in life, with varicella being commonly contracted in childhood and HSV acquired as a STD in young adulthood. Treatment of acute or recurrent HSV requires either oral or parenteral acyclovir, depending on the severity of disease. Treatment of HSV shortens the duration of lesion formation but does not prevent recurrences. Prophylactic acyclovir is necessary in the setting of multiple recurrences (three to six per year). Severe mucocutaneous, anorectal, and disseminated herpes simplex infections generally require more aggressive and long-term therapy, and those who do not respond to standard therapy may be found to harbor acyclovir-resistant HSV and require IV foscarnet for successful treatment. VZV usually causes dermatomal zoster (shingles), which is treated with acyclovir. Involvement of facial dermatomes can result in ocular disease and loss of vision.

Esophagitis

Patients with esophagitis often complain of dysphagia. The most common cause is *Candida* species, although occasionally CMV, herpes simplex, and aphthous ulcers can cause similar problems. Presumed *Candida* esophagitis should be treated with a systemic antifungal agent, such as fluconazole or ketoconazole. Response to treatment is considered a diagnostic test, and patients usually improve within a week; maintenance systematic therapy beyond full treatment is often necessary; alternatively, maintenance with topical agents such as nystatin suspension or clotrimazole troches may be satisfactory. Endoscopy is required for those who do not respond to therapy, to rule other infectious and noninfectious causes. Treatment for CMV and HSV is the same as for the treatment of herpes virus infections in other locations, with IV ganciclovir used to treat CMV and acyclovir to treat HSV. Aphthous ulcers often respond to prednisone.

Toxoplasmic Encephalitis

Toxoplasma gondii is a protozoan parasite that causes disease in advanced stages of immunosuppression. Disease usually occurs as a result of reactivation of prior infection. Infection is more common in developing countries and in areas where undercooked meat is eaten, such as France. CNS toxoplasmosis usually occurs in patients with T4 cell counts less than 50. The most common presentation is altered mental status, dementia, fever, and focal neurologic signs, including seizures. Other etiologies include HIV encephalopathy, cryptococcal meningitis, fungal infections, tuberculoma, and lymphoma. Approximately 20% to 47% of HIV-infected patients with anti-*Toxoplasma* IgG antibodies eventually develop toxoplasmosis. *Toxoplasma* antibody titers are positive about 85% of the time at the beginning of the acute illness. Diagnosis is assisted by magnetic resonance imaging or computed tomography scan. Solitary mass lesions in the presence of a negative *Toxoplasma* titers often require biopsy for definitive diagnosis since CNS lymphoma is also common. First-line therapy against *Toxoplasma* encephalitis requires pyrimethamine and sulfadiazine, which requires 6 to 8 weeks of acute treatment, and then lifelong suppressive therapy.

Mycobacterium avium-intracellulare Complex

Mycobacterium avium-intracellulare complex is a ubiquitous pathogen of low virulence, requiring advanced immunosuppression to cause disease. Infection occurs from digesting organisms in water and food; respiratory-caused infections rarely occur. MAC disease occurs commonly in patients with less than 50 to 100 T4 cells. Involvement of almost any organ system can occur, and MAC can be found in biopsy specimens, bone marrow aspirates, and blood and pulmonary specimens. Clinical presentation includes fever, night sweats, diarrhea, weight loss, wasting, and abdominal pain secondary to visceral inflammation. Since this infection is commonly seen with end-stage AIDS, it is often hard to attribute symptoms specifically to this infection. Therapy consists of a combination of antituberculous agents, such as rifabutin, clarithromycin, ethambutol, clofazimine, or amikacin. Treatment of symptomatic MAC can improve the patient's quality of life, but this must be balanced with the toxicity of the drugs used.

Mycobacterium tuberculosis

Mycobacterium tuberculosis is a highly virulent organism, more prevalent in ethnic minorities, injection drug users, and in populations with lower social economic status. Disease most often represents reactivation of latent infection but can represent newly acquired infection. This organism must be considered at all stages of immunosuppression with HIV, and when an acid-fast organism is identified on sputum stain, anti-TB therapy should be initiated pending culture results, which may take for 6 to 8 weeks until the final report is available. In addition to pulmonary TB, HIV patients are more likely to have extrapulmonary or disseminated disease. Granulomas usually are not seen on histopathologic study. TB skin test results are often negative in patients with advanced disease. Standard drugs are isoniazid (INH) and rifampin (pyrazinamide and streptomycin or ethambutol may be added) for 9 months; most individuals respond, but some with delayed recovery should be treated for 9 months beyond negative cultures for acid-fast bacteria; additionally, those refractory to standard therapy should be evaluated for multidrug-resistent TB.

Cryptococcal Meningitis

Patients commonly present with fever, photophobia, stiff neck, and headache. However, there may be no meningeal signs and symptoms or inflammatory exudate, yet the *Cryptococcus* organism can be isolated from the CSF. In more than 90% of cases, the serum cryptococcal antigen test result is positive, and a definitive diagnosis is made by the antigen test on the CSF or by the presence of organisms in the CSF. Blood cultures may yield positive findings, and there may be disseminated disease without CNS involvement. Treatment is with IV amphotericin B, followed by oral fluconazole. After acute treatment, chronic suppressive therapy of fluconazole is necessary to prevent relapse.

AIDS-Related Kaposi Sarcoma

AIDS-related Kaposi sarcoma presents as nodular, pigmented skin lesions with red–violet coloring; they are not limited to one area of the skin and can occur internally in the mouth, lungs, and the gastrointestinal tract. This is the most common neoplasm in persons with AIDS. Kaposi sarcoma is much more common in homosexual men, is less frequently seen in minorities, and less common in women and children. Recently, it has been found to be associated with a newly described herpesvirus.

Other Infections and Complications

In certain populations, salmonellosis is common, requiring suppressive therapy with antimicrobial agent because of the high rate of recurrence; shigellosis is occasionally seen. Disseminated histoplasmosis and coccidioidomycosis occur in endemic areas, *Cryptosporidium* and *Isospora belli* are causes of chronic diarrhea. A neurologic disease, called progressive multifocal leukoencephalopathy (PML), which presents with limb weakness and mental status deterioration, is caused by a papovavirus (J.C. virus). Lymphomas, both CNS and non-CNS, appear to be associated with the Epstein-Barr virus.

DISEASE PREVENTION

Adults with HIV infection should receive an annual influenza vaccine, an initial pneumococcal vaccination, (repeated every 6 years) and hepatitis B vaccination if indicated (those with negative serologic findings). There are no specific recommendations for the use of *Haemophilus influenzae* B vaccine, although recent evidence indicates an increased risk of invasive *Haemophilus* flu disease in HIV-infected adults. Pregnancy does not change the recommendations for pneumococcal, influenza, or hepatitis B vaccine. Tetanus boosters should be administered every 10 years and as clinically indicated. Measles vaccine should be given to HIV-infected adults who work in a health care setting or attend a post-high school institution, if they were born after 1957, and if they have no serologic evidence of prior measles. Live vaccines (yellow fever, live oral polio, and live typhoid vaccines) are to be avoided in persons with HIV infection.

Antibiotic Prophylaxis

All patients who are PPD positive and do not have active disease should receive 1 year of isoniazid, 300 mg, and pyridoxine (BL), 50 mg daily, since the chance of reactivation of TB in this population approaches 8% annually. PCP prophylaxis is initiated with CD4 cell counts less than 200 or a history of prior PCP. Treatment options include TMP-SMX tablet daily or three times weekly, or, as an alternative, dapsone 50 to 100 mg/day, or aerosolized pentamidine, 300 mg once monthly. Twenty percent to 50% of HIV-infected individuals cannot tolerate sulfa drugs because of drug allergy. Recommended prophylaxis for MAC infection is oral rifabutin, 300 mg per day, to be given to those with CD4 counts less than 75/mm^3 and a history of AIDS-related opportunistic diseases, or CD4 less than 50/mm^3. Clarithromycin is an alternative, with doses of 500 mg to 1 g/day suggested. Deep fungal prophylaxis has not been proven to be beneficial, but many clinicians initiate treatment with oral fluconazole, 50 to 200 mg daily. Fluconazole, 200 mg, in patients with T cells less than 50 is effective prophylaxis against cryptococcal meningitis. Individuals who take TMP-SMX for PCP prophylaxis have been shown to have less frequent toxoplasmic infections of the CNS. Those who cannot tolerate sulfa or those with positive *Toxoplasma* serologic findings are often prescribed dapsone, 50 mg orally daily and pyrimethamine, 50 mg orally weekly. This form of prophylaxis is still considered experimental, and when used, should be offered to those with T cells less than 100 and positive *Toxoplasma* serologic findings. Primary prophylaxis for CMV, although not formally recommended, is commonly given to patients with a CD4 count less than 50 to 100/mm^3 or positive CMV IgG, in the form of oral ganciclovir, 1 g orally three times daily. Acyclovir is not effective for CMV. Acyclovir is effective prophylaxis of recurrent HSV in a dose of 200 mg orally three times daily or 400 mg orally twice daily.

Immune Globulins

After measles exposure, all symptomatic HIV-infected persons should receive measles immune globulin (IMIG), O.5 mL/kg, up to a total dose of 15 mL intramuscularly. Before travel to underdeveloped countries or after exposure to hepatitis from a close personal contact or sex partner, immune serum globulin should be administered in a dose of 0.02 mL/kg intramuscularly. IV immune globulin (IVIG) is used to treat idiopathic thrombocytopenic purpura. Indications for therapy include platelet count less than 30,000, bleeding, or the need to increase platelet counts before surgery. Regimen options include IVIG, 400 mg/kg/day for 2 to 5 consecutive days, or 1 g/kg for up to three doses; this is often followed by maintenance treatment with repeat dosing every 2 weeks and as needed.

Hyperimmune Globulins

Varicella zoster immune globulin is indicated for treatment of the susceptible adult host after significant exposure to chicken pox or zoster (shingles). Individuals without detectable varicella antibody are susceptible to infection, and a regimen of 125 U/kg, up to 625 U intramuscularly, should be administered after significant exposure. Significant exposures include a household contact, close indoor contact for greater than 1 hour, sharing the same hospital room, or prolonged face-to-face contact. Hepatitis B immune globulin (HBIG) should be administered after needle stick or sexual contact with a person who is surface antigen positive (HBsAg). A regimen of HBIG of 0.06 mL/kg is administered and is followed by the hepatitis B vaccine series. CMV immune globulin has been proven to be of benefit for prophylaxis of renal and liver transplant recipients, but studies have not been done in HIV-infected patients to evaluate the efficacy in this setting.

TREATMENT OF HIV INFECTION

The first available antiretroviral agent, zidovudine (also known as ZDV or Retrovir), demonstrates a strong survival benefit in the first clinical trial in AIDS patients. Since this time, other clinical trials in asymptomatic individuals have not reproduced clinical benefit. The best evidence of clinical benefit of ZDV has been demonstrated in a study giving this agent to HIV pregnant women, where there was substantially reduced rates of HIV transmission from mother to infant. None of the newer antiretroviral agents, which are in the same class of agents as ZDV (nucleoside analogues) have been shown to be superior to ZDV as initial single-drug therapy of HIV infection. Didanosine (ddI or Videx) has shown delayed progression to the endpoints of AIDS or death when given to patients previously taking AZT. Zalcitabine (ddC or HIVID) appears to be as good or better when given to patients who have been on long-term ZDV therapy. The more recently approved drug, stavudine (D4T or Zerit) is licensed to be used in patients intolerant to other antiretroviral agents. The doses of these drugs and most common side effects are summarized in Table 84-8. Several agents currently are under study, especially agents of different classes of antiretrovirals. These include nonnucleoside analogues, tat inhibitors, and protease inhibitors. It is likely that future therapies will consist of multiple combinations of different classes of antiretrovirals to maximize the antiviral effect by damaging HIV at multiple steps of its replication cycle. This will, in theory, limit the development of drug resistance and minimize the side effects of the combined agents. The CD4 count continues to be the standard test to stage HIV infection and provide guidelines for initiation of antiviral therapy and prophylaxis for opportunistic pathogens.

CONSIDERATIONS IN PREGNANCY

Both pregnancy and HIV infection are immunosuppressive conditions. During pregnancy, the T lymphocyte helper-suppressor ratio falls and cell-mediated immunity is diminished. There were initial concerns that pregnancy and HIV infection might synergistically depress maternal immune function, but large prospective studies have failed to identify any evidence of accelerated HIV disease in pregnancy. Although impairment of cell-mediated immunity occurs during pregnancy, this has not been associated with adverse clinical outcomes.

T4 Cells and Pregnancy

Alterations and impairment of cell-mediated immunity and decrease in the number and proportion of T4 lymphocytes have been reported in normal pregnancies without HIV infection. In pregnancies complicated by HIV infection, a progressive decrease in T4 cells is found, peaking in the third trimester. Whether this decline occurs because of HIV or pregnancy, or is a function of pregnancy-related hemodilution is not clear. Other reports reveal that immunologic changes seen in HIV-positive pregnant women parallel their HIV-negative counterparts, except that the T4 decline is 10% to 20% greater among the seropositive women, and T4 does not return to prepregnancy levels. The T4 cells of HIV-negative women rebound to their prepregnancy levels. Other factors that may contribute to the immunosuppression of pregnancy include increased levels of total steroids and other hormones, including human chorionic gonadotropin, α-fetoprotein, and α_2-glycoprotein.

Prevention of Perinatal Transmission

Estimates of the frequency of mother-to-infant transmission of HIV range from 10% to 50%. Factors associated with an increased risk of transmission (Table 84-9]) include advanced maternal HIV stage; high maternal viral load; maternal immunodeficiency with decreased percentage of T4-positive lymphocytes; the presence of p24 antigen; complications of pregnancy such as preterm labor; and obstetric events during labor and delivery, including long duration of labor, duration of rupture of membranes, mode of delivery, chorioamnionitis, and maternal blood exposure. Studies reveal that treating asymptomatic HIV-infected pregnant women whose T cells are over 200 with ZDV and giving continuous IV ZDV dur-

Table 84-8. Currently Licensed Antiretroviral Drugs

DRUG	DOSE	TOXICITY
Zidovudine (ZDV, Retrovir)	Usual: 200 mg po tid Low: 100 mg po tid HIV encephalopathy: 600–1500 mg/d in divided doses	Transient headache, GI upset, insomnia. Hematologic: anemia; neutropenia (common); thrombocytopenia (rare). Myositis, hepatic dysfunction (rare).
Didanosine (ddI, Videx)	Tablets (must be taken two at a time with each dose): Usual: 200 mg po bid <50 kg: 125 mg po bid Sachets (dissolve powder in water): Usual: <50 kg	GI upset, diarrhea, peripheral neuropathy, pancreatitis
Zalcitabine (ddC, Hivid)	Usual: 0.75 mg po tid <40 kg: 0.375 mg po tid	Stomatitis, rash, peripheral neuropathy, rarely pancreatitis
Stavudine (d4T, Zerit)	Usual: 40 mg bid <60 kg: 30 mg bid	Peripheral neuropathy, hepatitic toxicity, rarely pancreatitis

Table 84-9. Factors That May Increase the Risk of Vertical Transmission of HIV Infection

RISK FACTORS	MECHANISM
History of previous child with AIDS	Higher viral inoculum and decreased immunocompetence in mother
Overt AIDS in mother	Higher viral inoculum and decreased immunocompetence in mother
Preterm delivery	Decreased immunocompetence in neonate
Decreased maternal CD4 count	Impaired maternal defenses; decreased placental transfer of viral-specific antibody
p24 Antigenemia in mother	Higher viral inoculum and greater infectivity in mother
Firstborn twin	Greater exposure to infected maternal blood and genital tract secretions

ing labor, followed by treatment of the newborn with ZDV for 6 weeks (Table 84-10), reduces the risk of transmission from 26% in the placebo group to 8% in the ZDV-treated group. Based on this study, all HIV-infected pregnant women and their infants, regardless of T-cell count, are encouraged to take ZDV. A number of other approaches are being studied in experimental clinical trials to interrupt perinatal transmission. These include cesarean section studies, microbicidal cervicovaginal lavage with chlorhexidine, the use of AIDS vaccines, and the use of anti-HIV immunoglobulin products as a passive interruption strategy.

Invasive Obstetrical Procedures

During labor and delivery, every effort must be made to avoid instrumentation that would increase the fetal exposure to infected maternal blood and secretions. Specifically, if possible, fetal membranes should be left intact until delivery. Application of fetal scalp electrodes and scalp pH sampling should be avoided. Chorionic villus sampling and percutaneous umbilical blood sampling should not be performed if alternatives are available. Amniocentesis should be performed with caution, especially sampling through an anterior placenta, although there is not clear evidence that this procedure has led to increased transmission of HIV in the infant whose mother underwent this procedure. Universal precautions should be used by all health care workers. Delee suctioning should not be performed; a mucous trap should be attached to wall suction.

Postpartum Care

The mother should be advised to avoid any contact between her body fluids and any open area on the skin or mucous membranes of the neonate. She should also adopt appropriate sexual practices to prevent the spread of infection to her partners. The transmission of HIV by breast-feeding is plausible because HIV has been cultured from breast milk. Transmission from mother to infant via breast-feeding has been documented in women who have high levels of viremia during primary HIV infection, or in cases when inflammatory conditions exist (ie, mastitis). Some studies estimate that the additional risk of transmission through breast-feeding is approximately 14%, although estimates vary widely (1% to 14%). It is unclear whether maternal antiretroviral therapy could decrease the risk of breast-feeding–related transmission. In industrialized countries, where adequate infant nutrition can be achieved safely through the use of infant formulas, breast-feeding by HIV-infected women is discouraged.

The best way to avoid perinatal HIV infection is to prevent pregnancy in HIV-infected women. Thus, efforts should be made after delivery to counsel the women on family planning and birth control methods.

Table 84-10. Zidovudine Regimen Used in AIDS Clinical Trials Group Protocol 076 and Recommended by the U.S. Public Health Service for Use in HIV-Infected Pregnant Women and Their Newborns

Oral administration of ZDV 100 mg 5 times daily, initiated at 14–34 w of gestation and continued throughout pregnancy
During labor, intravenous administration of ZDV in a 1-h loading dose of 2 mg/kg of body weight at a rate of 1 mg/kg/h, followed by a continuous infusion of 1 mg/kg/h until delivery
Oral administration to the newborn (ZVD syrup: 2 mg/kg every 6 h) for the first 6 w of life, beginning 8–12 h after birth

ZDV, zidovudine.

Psychological Factors

HIV-infected individuals, especially those with advancing immunosuppression, should be counseled about preparing a living will to address such issues as do-not-resuscitate status, respirator support, power of attorney, child custody, and a will for the dispersal of assets. Patients should also be evaluated for benefits such as Medical Assistance, Social Security, and home services, if appropriate. This often requires suggestion and referral by the primary caretaker to arrange for appropriate involvement by a case manager or social worker.

Family-centered mental health counseling needs to be offered to these individuals, since HIV is associated with psychological and social stresses that add to the problems caused by HIV disease. Appropriate counseling should be offered and assistance offered to facilitate the individual coping with HIV stage-specific issues, such as new diagnosis, starting therapy, OIs, and concerns about death and dying. The issues become even more complicated with HIV-infected women who have additional family and child issues.

Our thinking about HIV infection and AIDS has changed dramatically over the last decade, as we come to grips with recognizing HIV as a STD that can affect any sexually active individual. Many myths remain regarding HIV as an infectious disease. These myths are mired in prejudice, politics, and fear. As HIV infects and affects women and children, there is an increasing need to better understand some of the unique issues of HIV infection and AIDS in this population. Most primary care physicians, many of them unknowingly, are already caring for patients who are a part of this "silent epidemic."

BIBLIOGRAPHY

Bartlett J. Medical management of HIV infection. Glennview, IL: Physicians & Scientists Publishing, 1994.

Brettle RP, Leen CL. The natural history of HIV and AIDS in women. AIDS 1991;5:1283.

Castro KG, Ward JW, Slutsker L, Buehler JW, Jaffe HW, Berkelman RL. 1993 Revised classification system for HIV infection & expanded surveillance case definition for AIDS among adolescents and adults. MMWR 1992;41:1.

Chin J. Current and future dimensions of the HIV/AIDS pandemic in women and children. Lancet 1990;336:221.

Duff P. Human immunodeficiency virus infection in pregnancy. Semin Perinatol 1993;17:379.

Hankins CA, Handley MA. HIV disease and AIDS in women: current knowledge and a research agenda. J AIDS 1992;5:957.

Jewett JF, Hecht FM. Preventive health care for adults with HIV infection. JAMA 1993;269:1144.

Kessler H. Clinical consensus on the management of HIV infection and disease. J AIDS 1994;7:S1.

Meinick SL, Sherer R, Louis TA, et al. Survival and disease progression according to gender of patients with HIV infection. JAMA 1994;272: 1915.

Minkoff H, DeHovitz JA, Duerr A. HIV infection in women. New York: Raven Press, 1995.

Morlat P, Parneix P, Douard D, et al. Women and HIV infection: a cohort study of 483 HIV-infected women in Bordeaux, France, 1985–1991: the Groupe d'Epidemiologie Clinique du SIDA en Aquitaine. AIDS 1992;6:1187.

Nanda D, Minkoff HL. Pregnancy and women at risk for HIV infection. Prim Care 1992;19:157.

Rompalo AM, Anderson JR, Quinn TC. Reproductive tract infections and their management in women infected with the human immunodeficiency virus. Infect Dis Clin Pract 1992;1:277.

Stratton P, Alexander NJ. Heterosexual spread of HIV infection. In: Smith P, ed. Reproductive medicine review. Manchester, England: Hodder and Stoughton Publishers, 1994.

Stratton P, Ciacco KH. Cervical neoplasia in the patient with HIV infection. Curr Opin Obstet Gynecol 1994;6:86.

Stratton P, Mofenson LM, Willoughby AD. Human immunodeficiency virus infection in pregnant women under care at AIDS clinical trials centers in the United States. Obstet Gynecol 1992;79:364:368.

von Overbeck J, Egger M, Smith GD, et al. Survival in HIV infection: do sex and category of transmission matter? AIDS 1994;8:1307.

Primary Care for Women, edited by Phyllis C. Leppert and Fred M. Howard. Lippincott-Raven Publishers, Philadelphia © 1997.

85

Sexually Transmitted Diseases

PATRICIA A. COURY-DONIGER

EPIDEMIOLOGY

Sexually transmitted diseases (STDs) are epidemic in the United States, with higher incidences than in most other developed countries. Approximately 12 million cases of STDs occur annually, the majority in persons aged 15 through 35 years. The epidemiology of individual STDs is also changing. In the past, gonorrhea and syphilis were the only known STDs. In the United States, public health control programs were implemented and the incidence of these infections had actually been decreasing. In recent years, other STDs have been recognized such as chlamydia and a new group of chronic, viral STDs—genital herpes, human papilloma virus (HPV), and human immunodeficiency virus (HIV). These STDs have shown significant increases in incidence over the past decade.

MEDICAL SEQUELAE

Women and children suffer disproportionate risks of morbidity and mortality related to STDs and HIV. Women, especially teenagers, are more easily infected with STDs and are much more likely to develop complications of these infections. STDs in women can lead to ectopic pregnancy, infertility, poor pregnancy outcomes, and cervical cancer. Each year, approximately 5000 women in the United States die as the result of invasive cervical cancer. Many STDs can be perinatally transmitted, resulting in birth defects, mental retardation, and fetal and infant death. HIV, which is often sexually transmitted to women, is now the leading cause of death of young women in the United States. The inner-city, poor populations with high representation of racial and ethnic minorities are also at disproportionate risk of experiencing higher rates of STDs and complications.

STD SCREENING

Episodic diagnosis and treatment of symptomatic STDs is no longer adequate because many STDs and HIV are asymptomatic but transmissable. Primary care providers must assume more responsibility for routine STD and HIV screening of sexually active young adolescents and young adults. More effective strategies for preventive education and counseling to promote healthy behaviors are also needed.

RELATIONSHIP OF STDS AND HIV

There is increasing recognition of the many relationships between STDs and HIV. It has become clear that many risk factors and behaviors that can lead to infection with various STDs are also responsible for the heterosexual transmission of HIV in women. For example, the exchange of sex for drugs increases a woman's risk of syphilis, chancroid, and HIV. Women with genital ulcer diseases such as syphilis and herpes as well as microscopic ulcerations of the cervix due to gonorrhea or chlamydia are more likely to be infected with HIV. This is presumably due to decreased genital mucosal immunity as a result of chronic or recurrent STDs. It is increasingly common for women to be co-infected with various STDs and HIV. The natural history of HIV produces immunologic responses that can affect the clinical course of STDs, resulting in greater difficulty in diagnosis and treatment.

Populations with high STD rates are also at disproportionate risk of HIV, and heterosexual transmission of HIV is occurring at high rates within this population. STDs are now seen as modifiable risk factors for the heterosexual spread of HIV in women. For these reasons, it is recommended that HIV counseling and testing be routinely offered to all sexually active women seen in any primary care setting. It is also recommended that women with STDs be encouraged to consent to HIV testing to optimize the efficacy of their STD treatment. Primary care providers should realize that many women with STDs have multiple infections. All women presenting with any STD should receive complete clinical evaluation and testing for other STDs and HIV.

SEXUALLY TRANSMITTED DISEASE SYNDROMES IN WOMEN

Vaginitis

Etiology

The three most common types of infectious vaginitis are Trichomonas vaginitis, candidal vulvovaginitis, and bacterial vaginosis. Trichomonas vaginitis is caused by a protozoal organism, *Trichomonas vaginalis*. Candidal vaginitis is the result of overgrowth of a fungal organism, *Candida albicans*, in the vaginal mucosa. Some non-albicans yeast species such as *Candida tropicalis* and *Torulopsis glabrata* have been demonstrated to cause a small proportion of vaginal yeast infections. Bacterial vaginosis is the result of an overgrowth of a characteristic group of bacteria, including *Gardnerella vaginalis, Mycoplasma hominis,* and anaerobic species that replace the normal flora of the vagina, predominantly *Lactobacillus acidophilus.* The bacteria do not actually infect the squamous epithelial mucous membrane layer of the vagina, but adhere to the surface of the squamous cells, resulting in a vaginosis and not a vaginitis condition.

Clinical Presentation

The histories of women with infectious vaginitis are highly variable; many are totally asymptomatic. Mild symptoms include increased vaginal discharge with abnormal color and odor. More severe symptoms usually result when a vulvitis component occurs and include itching, external dysuria, and dyspareunia. Predisposing factors for candidiasis include recent antibiotic therapy, oral contraceptive use, menstruation, diabetes mellitus, corticosteroid use, and, more recently, HIV infection.

Because bacterial vaginosis does not result in an inflammatory response, women with this condition are often asymptomatic or mildly symptomatic with an increased vaginal discharge and a fishy odor that is often most noticed after sexual intercourse. The odor is the result of an increased amount of amines in the discharge which are the byproduct of the metabolism of the anaerobic bacteria characteristic of this condition. On examination, a thin, whitish, homogenous discharge is often seen adhering to the mucous membrane surfaces of the vagina and vulva. There is usually little erythema or edema.

Trichomonas vaginalis and *Candida vaginalis* directly infect the squamous epithelial mucus membrane layer of the vagina and vulva. Thus, trichomoniasis and candidiasis can cause similar symptoms of severe itching, external dysuria, vulvar swelling, and dyspareunia. On examination, vulvar edema with excoriation may be seen along with marked erythema of the vaginal mucosa. The discharge of trichomoniasis, however, is often more profuse, frothy, greenish-yellow in color, and foul smelling, whereas candidiasis is characterized by a thick, white, curd-like vaginal discharge that can be seen adhering to the vaginal mucosal surfaces. Women with acute, symptomatic trichomoniasis who remain untreated may become totally asymptomatic but have chronic infection.

Clinical Criteria for Diagnosis

Because the symptomatology of vaginitis is so wide ranging and nonspecific, the diagnosis rests mainly on physical examination, microscopic examination of the vaginal discharge (vaginal wet smear), and determination of its pH (normal range 4.0–4.5). Because bacterial vaginosis is a polymicrobial syndrome rather than the result of a single, etiologic microbe, clinical criteria have been establi to aid in the diagnosis. These include the presence of character "clue cells" on a vaginal wet smear, a positive "whiff" test, the ob vation of thin, homogenous discharge on examination, and a pH greater than 5.0. Any three out of four of these criteria establishes the diagnosis. Candidiasis and trichomoniasis are diagnosed primarily on the basis of the vaginal wet smear.

Laboratory Testing

A specimen is collected for the vaginal wet smear by swabbing the vaginal mucosal surfaces with a cotton-tipped swab that is then placed in a test tube containing a small amount of normal saline. In the office laboratory, a wet smear is made by placing a few drops of the saline mixture on one slide and placing a coverslip over the material. A second slide is prepared in the same manner with the addition of a few drops of 10% KOH (potassium hydroxide) to the mixture. The presence or absence of an amine (fishy) odor is noted immediately (whiff test); then the slide is saved for later examination for yeast organisms. The wet smear is examined under the 40× objective of the microscope.

Normal findings on a wet smear include squamous epithelial cells with clear cytoplasm and linear borders, a few white blood cells (WBCs), and a predominance of large rods, *Lactobacillus acidophilus.* In bacterial vaginosis, characteristic clue cells can be seen along with a marked absence of *Lactobacillus* spp. and few white blood cells. Clue cells are squamous epithelial cells that have become covered with a variety of smaller, coccobacilli bacteria that give the cytoplasm of the cells a stippled appearance and cause the cell borders to appear irregular. *Trichomonas vaginalis* can be seen as a single-celled, protozoal organism approximately the same size as a white blood cell, but with a flagellum. The flagellum can be seen undulating, producing a characteristic motility of the trichomonad. Candidal vaginalis can be seen either as budding yeast cells in the vaginal wet smear or in its pseudohyphae form on the KOH slide. The pseudohyphae are larger, filamentous structures that enmesh and can be best seen using the 10× objective. In both of these conditions, there are increased number of white blood cells in the smear.

Trichomonas vaginalis can be cultured using a selective Diamond's medium. The culture has higher sensitivity than the wet smear, but is generally not commercially available. Yeast organisms can be cultured using Nickerson's media. This is not generally helpful in detecting *Candida albicans,* however, because this organism can be part of normal vaginal flora. However, if non-albicans species are suspected, culture is often more reliable than wet smear.

Management

Treatment of bacterial vaginosis, *Trichomonas vaginitis,* and candidal vulvovaginitis is given in Table 85-1.

Patient Education and Counseling

Sexual partners of women with trichomoniasis should be examined and screened for STDs and HIV. There is no reliable test to detect trichomonads in the male. Regular partners are presumed to be carriers and are treated presumptively with metronidazole 2 g stat. Recurrence of trichomoniasis should not occur unless there is reinfection from an untreated partner or a new sexual contact.

Although the characteristic group of bacteria that result in bacterial vaginosis are thought to be sexually transmitted, it is not the presence of these bacteria but their overgrowth that results in the clinical syndrome. Host factors that have not yet been identified play a role.

Table 85-1. Treatment of Vaginosis and Vaginitis

Treatment of Bacterial Vaginosis:
Recommended
Metronidazole 500 mg po BID for 7 days
Alternatives
Metronidazole 2 g po STAT
or
Clindamycin 300 mg po BID for 7 days
or
Clindamycin cream 2%, one applicator intravaginally at bedtime for 7 days
or
Metronidazole gel, 0.75%, one applicator intravaginally BID × 5 days
Treatment of Trichomonas Vaginitis
Metronidazole 2 g po STAT
or
Metronidazole 500 mg po BID for 7 days
Treatment of Candidal Vulvovaginitis
Butoconazole 2% cream intravaginally for 3 days
or
Clotrimazole 1% cream intravaginally for 7–14 days
or
Clotrimazole 100 mg vaginal tablet for 7 days
or
Clotrimazole 100 mg vaginal tablet, two tablets for 3 days
or
Clotrimazole 500 mg vaginal tablet, one tablet STAT
or
Miconazole 2% cream intravaginally for 7 days
or
Miconazole 200 mg vaginal suppository, one supp. for 3 days
or
Miconazole 100 mg vaginal suppository, one supp. for 7 days
or
Terconazole 0.4% cream intravaginally for 7 days
or
Terconazole 0.8% cream intravaginally for 3 days
or
Terconazole 80 mg suppository, 1 supp. for 3 days

Therefore, male sexual partners of women with bacterial vaginosis should be examined and screened for STDs and HIV, but not routinely treated. Recurrence of bacterial vaginosis without reinfection can occur.

Candidiasis results from overgrowth of the *Candida albicans* organism. Again, host factors including decreased cellular immunity, inadequate *Lactobacillus* colonization, and increased glucose levels play a role in recurrence of this condition. *Candida albicans* is not sexually transmitted and treatment of the male sexual partner is not recommended. Recurrences are common, and suppressive, anti-fungal regimens should be considered for some women.

Urethritis

Etiology

Although urethritis has been recognized as an STD in males for several decades, only recently have there been attempts to define this syndrome in women. The most common sexually transmitted organisms causing urethritis in women are *Chlamydia trachomatis, Neisseria gonorrhoeae,* and herpes simplex virus. These organisms also cause cervicitis and urethritis, and both syndromes may be present simultaneously. *Candida albicans* and *Trichomonas vaginalis* can cause a vulvitis with irritation of the urethral meatus, but are not considered causes of urethritis. Cystitis is usually caused by *Escherichia coli, Proteus* spp., and *Staphylococcus saprophyticus,* which are not sexually transmitted agents.

Clinical Presentation

The hallmark symptom of urethritis is dysuria, which is usually gradual in onset and intermittent. Women may complain of increased vaginal discharge if the cervix is also infected. Vulvitis usually results in a complaint of burning of the vulva that is exacerbated by the passage of urine over the inflamed tissue, referred to as external dysuria. Dysuria as the result of a cystitis usually has an abrupt onset and is more severe and continuous. Symptoms of gross hematuria, urgency, and bladder tenderness often help to distinguish cystitis from urethritis. All sexually active young women with dysuria or other urinary symptoms should receive a full genitourinary evaluation for urethritis, vaginitis, and cervicitis as well as cystitis. This includes a speculum examination with close examination for urethral discharge, vulvar lesions or inflammation, signs of vaginitis, and mucopurulent endocervical discharge.

Clinical Criteria for Diagnosis

In men, the microscopic observation of more than 5 polymorphonuclear cells (PMNs) per high-powered field (1000×) in a gram-stained specimen of urethral discharge establishes the diagnosis of urethritis. At this time, no such simple criterion exist for women, and the diagnosis is made by consideration of the history, physical examination findings, and laboratory test results. Vulvovaginitis due to candidiasis or trichomoniasis should be ruled out. Clinical findings of herpetic lesions of the vulva or cervix and mucopurulent endocervical discharge support a diagnosis of urethritis. The condition of sterile pyuria, defined as increased numbers of WBCs on urinalysis with a urine culture that shows no bacterial growth, is the best clinical criterion to support the diagnosis of urethritis in a woman.

Laboratory Testing

Laboratory studies should include urinalysis of a clean-catch urine specimen, a wet smear of vaginal discharge, a Gram stain of endocervical discharge, and specific testing for chlamydia and gonorrhea from urethral as well as cervical samples. A urine culture should be ordered if cystitis is suspected.

Management

Treatment for the presumptive diagnosis of acute urethral syndrome in women is doxycycline 100 mg by mouth twice a day for 7 to 10 days.

Patient Education and Counseling

Sexual partners should receive a complete STD/HIV evaluation and testing. Testing should include a urethral Gram stain for urethritis and specific tests for gonorrhea and chlamydia. Treatment for chlamydia or gonorrhea should be provided empirically if tests in the woman are positive.

Cervicitis

Etiology

The most common recognized causes of infectious, clinically recognizable cervicitis are *Chlamydia trachomatis, Neisseria gonorrhoeae,* and herpes simplex virus. These organisms can also cause urethritis, pelvic inflammatory disease, and proctitis in women.

Clinical Presentation

A familiarity with the normal anatomy and physiology of the cervix is necessary before an adequate assessment can be done. The cervix is composed of two main parts, (1) the exocervix, which is contiguous with the vagina, and (2) the endocervix, which is the lower part of the uterus. The exocervix is often covered by squamous epithelial cells, which are the same flat, nonsecretory cells that line the vaginal walls. Squamous epithelial tissue appears clinically as pink, smooth tissue. The endocervix includes the endocervical canal, which is lined with columnar epithelium. This tissue appears brick red in color, is more papillary, and secretes specific types of mucus in response to ovarian hormonal stimulation. The area where the squamous epithelium meets the columnar epithelium is called the transformation zone. A process called squamous metaplasia, which occurs continuously at the transformation zone, results in columnar epithelium being transformed into squamous epithelium over time.

In prepubescent girls, the endocervix, exocervix, and much of the vaginal walls are lined with columnar epithelial tissue. For this reason, prepubescent girls can develop gonococcal vaginitis and chlamydial vaginitis. As the girl enters puberty, ovarian production of estrogen and progesterone supports a change of vaginal pH from alkaline to acidic. The acidic pH begins the squamous metaplastic process and the gradual replacement of the columnar tissue with squamous epithelium.

By the end of puberty, most women have only squamous epithelium lining the vagina, but have areas of columnar epithelium still visible on the exocervix. This is clinically referred to as cervical ectopy and is evidence of an immature transformation zone. As women age reproductively, squamous metaplasia continues until the columnar tissue is located only in the endocervical canal and the entire exocervix is covered with squamous epithelium , resulting in a mature transformation zone.

Cervical ectopy is not abnormal, but does result in increased risk of certain STDs. *Neisseria gonorrhoeae* and *Chlamydia trachomatis* infect columnar epithelium and not squamous epithelium. Women with an immature transformation zone are at higher risk for gonococcal and chlamydial infection because the ectopy on the exocervix provides more extensive exposure to potentially infectious semen in the vagina. Women with ectopy also experience an increased amount of normal discharge.

Normal cervical discharge varies with the phases of the menstrual cycle. In the preovulatory phase, which is predominantly estrogenic, the cervical discharge is clear, stretchy, slippery, and lubricative. This is known as fertile mucus or Spinnbarkeit mucus. In the postovulatory phase, the progesterone hormone, which is produced by the corpus luteum of the ruptured ovarian follicle, dominates. Progesterone-influenced cervical discharge is white, thicker, more dense, and not stretchy. This is known as infertile or barrier mucus because it does not facilitate sperm transport. Cervical mucus mixed with squamous epithelial cells from the vaginal walls and *Lactobacillus* spp. of normal bacteria in the vagina creates the fluid that women experience as vaginal discharge.

This background understanding of vaginal and cervical anatomy and physiology serves as the basis for assessment of lower genital tract infections. After the speculum is inserted, the first step is to identify areas of squamous and columnar epithelium and assess each tissue for signs of infection. Clinical signs of infected epithelial tissue include erythema, hyperedema, friability, and abnormal discharge. Candidiasis and trichomoniasis of the vagina can extend to the squamous epithelium on the exocervix and result in an exocervicitis. In these cases, the clinical appearance of a red cervix is the result of erythematous changes of the squamous epithelium. The STD syndrome of cervicitis is an infection of the columnar epithelium which is really an endocervicitis in women with a mature transformation zone. In younger women with ectopy, the part of the exocervix containing columnar epithelium will also show signs of infection. In women with ectopy, the visual inspection of the exocervix is relevant to the diagnosis of cervicitis because the columnar epithelium can be directly assessed. In women without ectopy, the clinician has to rely on an assessment of the endocervical discharge, rather than the appearance of the exocervix.

Clinical Criteria for Diagnosis

Most women with cervicitis are asymptomatic. Some may notice an increase or a change in their vaginal discharge. Occasionally, spotting after intercourse may result from increased friability of cervical ectopy. Many women with cervicitis also have urethritis from coinfection with the same organism. The dysuria they experience from the urethritis may be their only symptom of cervical infection. Therefore, clinical criteria for the diagnosis of cervicitis do not rely on the presence of symptoms.

The following criteria can be used presumptively for the clinical diagnosis of mucopurulent cervicitis caused by gonorrhea or chlamydia:

- The observation of mucopurulent discharge from the endocervical os or areas of ectopy
- Demonstration of increased amounts of white blood cells in cervical discharge
- Observation of clinical signs of erythema, hyperedema, or friability in areas of ectopy on the exocervix or at the cervical os.

Cervicitis due to genital herpes infection usually produces a number of shallow, ulcerative, necrotic lesions on the exocervix. Clear vesicles that are often highly diagnostic for genital herpes when seen on the external genitalia are not seen on the cervix. A profuse, more watery cervical discharge can often be observed. This diagnosis must be confirmed by laboratory tests. It is estimated that up to 20% of women who develop genital herpes simplex infections have cervical involvement only without external lesions.

Laboratory Testing

A Gram stain of endocervical discharge can be used to confirm a clinical impression of mucopurulent endocervical discharge. An increased number of white blood cells is quantitated as 10 PMNs per high-powered field using an oil immersion lens with a magnification of 1000×. Cervical tests for gonorrhea and chlamydia should also be performed. For gonorrhea, endocervical culture is still the gold standard, with 85% to 90% sensitivity, 100% specificity, and low cost. Newer tests developed for gonorrhea that use ELISA and DNA probes are not as sensitive and specific and add cost. The chlamydial organism is more likely to lose viability during transport so that chlamydial cultures are impractical in many settings due to lower sensitivity and higher cost. Newer chlamydia tests including ELISA, direct fluorescent Antibody (DFA), and DNA probes are currently being widely used. However, the sensitivities of all of these newer, rapid diagnostic tests range from only 70% to 80%. This means that women with mucopurulent endocervicitis should be presumptively treated for chlamydia even if the chlamydia test is negative.

If necrotic, ulcerative areas are seen on the exocervix, a culture for herpes simplex virus should be obtained directly from the lesions. Herpes simplex can be isolated from over 80% of cervical samples taken from women with primary genital herpes infections.

Management

Women who meet the criteria for mucopurulent cervicitis should be treated presumptively for *Chlamydia trachomatis.* In populations with a high prevalence of *Neisseria gonorrhoeae,* combination therapy should be given (Table 85-2).

Patient Education and Counseling

Women with mucopurulent cervicitis must be advised that their infection may be due to gonorrhea or chlamydia even though approximately 40% of women with this syndrome do not have positive tests for gonorrhea or chlamydia. Lack of sensitivity of chlamdyia testing may be partially responsible, but all of the infectious causes of mucopurulent cervicitis are not known at this time. This condition, like urethritis, is only beginning to be understood and defined through research. Therefore, women with mucopurulent cervicitis should be advised to complete treatment even if their tests are negative. Women with herpetic cervicitis need extensive education and counseling (refer to the section on Genital Herpes).

Treatment of the Sexual Partner

Women who are treated for mucopurulent cervicitis should refer their partners for a complete STD/HIV evaluation and testing, even if they have no symptoms. Men should be specifically assessed for urethritis, tested for gonorrhea and chlamydia, and treated with a regimen effective against *Chlamydia trachomatis* even if all test are negative.

Table 85-2. Treatment of Cervicitis

Treatment of Mucopurulent Cervicitis (Chlamydia Coverage)
Doxycycline 100 mg po BID × 7 days
or
Azithromycin 1000 mg STAT po
or
Ofloxacin 300 mg po BID × 7 days
For Pregnant Women
Erythromycin base 500 mg po QID × 7 days
or
Erythromycin base 250 mg po QID × 14 days
or
Erythromycin ethyl succinate 800 mg po × 7 days
or
Erythromycin ethyl succinate 400 mg po × 14 days
or
Amoxicillin 300 mg po BID × 7–10 days
Gonorrhea Treatment for Cervicitis in Women
Cefixime 400 mg po STAT
or
Ceftriaxone 125 mg IM STAT
or
Ofloxacin 400 mg po STAT
or
Ciprofloxacin 500 mg po STAT
For Pregnant Women
Cefixime 400 mg po STAT
or
Ceftriaxone 125 mg IM STAT
For Pregnant Women Who Are Allergic to Penicillin
Spectinomycin 2 g IM STAT

Pelvic Inflammatory Disease

Etiology

Pelvic inflammatory disease (PID) is a term used to describe any combination of upper genital tract infections, including endometritis (uterus), salpingitis (fallopian tubes), and oophoritis (ovaries). PID disease can be an acute, first episode, recurrent, or chronic. These infections result from ascending organisms of the lower genital tract (ie, vagina and cervix). The mechanism by which normal flora of the vagina and cervix are prevented from ascending is not known. However, certain bacterial pathogens, such as *Neisseria gonorrhoeae, Chlamydia trachomatis,* and *Mycoplasma hominis* are known to circumvent these mechanisms and cause first-episode pelvic inflammatory disease. Other bacteria, particularly anaerobic species, such as *Bacteroides* spp. or *Peptostreptococcus* spp. also ascend from the lower genital tract, resulting in a polymicrobial infection. Once a woman has experienced an initial episode of PID, she is at increased risk of recurrent or chronic disease, even without reinfection with a sexually transmitted pathogen.

This section addresses only acute, first-episode PID, which is considered sexually transmitted unless there is a history of recent surgery or instrumentation.

Clinical Presentation

Women with PID usually give a history of lower abdominal pain. The pain may be mild and intermittent, increasing slowly over a period of weeks or severe and debilitating with an abrupt onset of a few hours or days. Women with endometritis may complain of increased vaginal discharge and intermenstrual bleeding and have uterine tenderness only on bimanual examination. Other symptoms of PID include dyspareunia, dysuria, and menometrorrhagia. In women with more severe pain, systemic symptoms such as fever, nausea, and vomiting may be present. All young, sexually active women who present with lower abdominal pain must be tested for STDs and evaluated for PID with a thorough speculum and bimanual examination.

Differential Diagnosis

The clinical diagnosis of PID is challenging, partially because of the difficulties in adequately palpating upper reproductive tract structures in some women. Traditionally, the clinical diagnosis of PID has not correlated well with the results of microbiologic sampling of the endometrium and fallopian tubes. In Sweden, laparascopic evaluations for PID are done routinely on an outpatient basis and increase the accuracy of the diagnosis. However, in the United States there is reliance on clinical criteria for the presumptive diagnosis and treatment of PID. The clinician should maintain a strong awareness of the likelihood of misdiagnosis and reexamine women with PID within 48 to 72 hours of initial treatment. Ovarian cysts, normal ovulation, ectopic pregnancy, appendicitis, and other intra-abdominal and pelvic conditions must be considered when making the diagnosis.

Diagnostic criteria for the presumptive diagnosis of PID include the following:

- Recent history of lower abdominal pain
- Pain reproduced by palpation of endometrium and/or fallopian tubes
- Cervical motion tenderness
- Evidence of lower genital tract infection.

Systemic signs such as elevated temperature, elevated ESR, and leukocytosis increase the specificity of the diagnosis but are not found in many cases of PID.

Laboratory Testing

Women with suspected PID should have a vaginal wet smear and an endocervical Gram stain to identify vaginitis or cervicitis. In addition, tests for chlamydia and gonorrhea should be taken from the cervix. Clinicians must recognize that studies have demonstrated that correlations between the results of cervical sampling and fallopian tube sampling in cases of PID are poor. Therefore, a negative cervical test result for gonorrhea or chlamydia does not rule out the possibility of sexually transmitted PID. In addition, there is no commercially available test for *Mycoplasma hominis,* which is another sexually transmitted pathogen.

Management

Because PID is a polymicrobial syndrome and the results of cervical sampling are not highly predictive of microbiologic etiology, all women with PID must be treated with a regimen that covers all the major STD pathogens as well as the facultative anaerobic bacteria.

There is controversy over the use of outpatient versus inpatient treatment regimens. Some infertility experts feel that all women who desire future pregnancies should be hospitalized for PID management. Minimally, adolescents, patients with nausea and vomiting, and cases involving an adnexal mass should be hospitalized for treatment. In addition, women who do not show significant improvement within 48 to 72 hours should be hospitalized for further evaluation and treatment (Table 85-3).

Women treated for PID on an outpatient basis should be advised to rest for at least 2 to 3 days until the pain has subsided.

Table 85-3. Treatment for Pelvic Inflammatory Disease

Outpatient Treatment for the Presumptive Diagnosis of PID
Ceftriaxone 250 mg IM STAT

followed by

Doxycycline 100 mg po BID × 14 d

or

Ofloxacin 400 mg po BID × 14 d

plus

Either Metronidazole 500 mg BID × 14 d

or

Clindamycin 450 mg po QID × 14 d

Inpatient Treatment for PID
Cefoxitin 2 g IV every 6 hours or Cefotetan 2 g IV every 12 h

plus

Doxycycline 100 mg IV or orally every 12 h

or

Clindamycin 900 mg IV every 8 h

plus

Gentamicin loading dose IV or IM (2 mg/kg) followed by a maintenance dose (1.5 mg/kg) every 8 h

Sexual intercourse should be avoided for at least 2 weeks. An IUD, if present, should be removed at the time of initial treatment.

Patient Education and Counseling

Women with PID need to be educated about their potential risk of infertility even in cases with mild symptoms. Ways to reduce this risk, including full compliance with treatment and avoidance of reinfection, should be explained. Lack of laboratory proof of a sexually transmitted infection can be frustrating and confusing for both patients and clinicians. Patients should be counseled about the presumptiveness of the diagnosis in relation to the serious medical sequelae of ectopic pregnancy or infertility if treatment is withheld.

Treatment of the Sexual Partner

Multiple studies have shown that the majority of male sexual partners of women with PID are asymptomatic. They are often carriers of gonorrhea or chlamydia or have asymptomatic urethritis. Therefore, all male sexual partners of women with PID must have a complete STD/HIV evaluation including specific tests for gonorrhea, chlamydia, and urethritis. However, even if all the tests are negative, the male partner should still be treated with a regimen effective for uncomplicated gonorrhea and chlamydia.

SEXUALLY TRANSMITTED GENITAL AND DERMATOLOGIC LESIONS IN WOMEN

Syphilis

Etiology

Syphilis is a disease caused by the bacterial spirochete *Treponema pallidum.* This organism is sexually transmitted through intimate contact of mucous membrane surfaces. The latest heterosexual epidemic of syphilis in the United States began in 1986.

Table 85-4. Treatment of Syphilis

Early Syphilis (<1 y)
Penicillin G benzathine 2.4 million U IM × 1
Alternate treatment for penicillin allergy: Doxycyline 100 mg BID × 14 d
Treatment for Late Syphilis (>1 y)
Penicillin G benzathine 2.4 million units IM × 3, at weekly intervals
Alternate treatment for penicillin allergy: Doxycyline 100 mg BID × 28 d

Clinical Presentation

With much individual variation, most patients with untreated syphilis pass through distinct stages. Early syphilis, defined as syphilis of less than 1 year's duration, is further divided into four clinical stages—incubating, primary, secondary, and early latent.

Incubating syphilis is the stage between infection with *T. pallidum* and appearance of the first clinical symptom, which takes from 10 to 90 days. Primary syphilis is characterized by the appearance of one or more cutaneous or mucous membrane ulcers known as chancres. These lesions, which are relatively painless, heal without scarring within 2 to 3 weeks. Painless, unilateral, inguinal lymphadenopathy is usually also present. Secondary syphilis is a systemic infection resulting from the dissemination of replicated *T. pallidum* from the original chancre to the lymphatic system and bloodstream. This dissemination produces a significant antibody response resulting in a wide range of clinical signs and symptoms, from generalized lymphadenopathy and a rash to highly infectious condylomata lata and mucous membrane patches. Secondary manifestations typically persist for 2 to 12 weeks, then spontaneously resolve. Early latent stage occurs from the time of spontaneous resolution of secondary signs and symptoms until about 1 year after the original time of infection.

Late syphilis, also known as syphilis of greater than 1 year's duration, is divided into two additional stages—late latent stage and tertiary stage. Late latent stage occurs from the end of early latent stage until such time as symptoms reappear, usually after 15 to 20 years of untreated infection. At that time approximately 30% of patients develop tertiary stage syphilis characterized by neurologic, cardiovascular, or bone deformation.

Differential Diagnosis

Staging is a clinical judgment made by considering the patient's medical and sexual history, physical examination, serologic tests, and epidemiologic investigation. Patients with primary and secondary syphilis have distinct clinical signs and symptoms that simplify staging. Distinguishing early latent from late latent disease is more challenging because such signs and symptoms are absent. Clinical staging must be completed before management decisions and accurate treatment can occur.

In general, patients with early syphilis are highly infectious through sexual or perinatal transmission and so are managed as priority cases by public health control programs. After 1 year, patients with untreated syphilis are no longer considered sexually communicable. However, perinatal transmission resulting in congenital syphilis can still occur. Epidemiologic investigation of sexual partners within the past year helps in differentiating early infectious syphilis from late noninfectious syphilis.

Syphilis has often been called the "great pretender" because the wide range of clinical signs and symptoms present during some stages can mimic so many other diseases. Primary stage chancres can be confused with genital herpes, chancroid, and Behçet's lesions. The rash of secondary syphilis appears similar to pityriasis rosea; the condylomata lata lesions look like venereal warts. The clinician must maintain a high index of suspicion for syphilis in sexually active persons under the age of 40, especially if genital lesions, unexplained rash, lymphadenopathy, and alopecia are present.

Laboratory Testing

A successful culture system to isolate *T. pallidum* has not been developed, so clinicians must rely on direct microscopy and serologic antibody testing to aid in the diagnosis of syphilis. The sensitivity and specificity of each type of test varies with the stage of disease.

Microscopy tests include the dark field examination and a newer, DFA for *T. pallidum* test that is like a fluorescent dark field. These tests can be used only if mucous membrane lesions are present and are most helpful in primary syphilis when serology tests are not yet reliable. With adequate specimen collection, *T. pallidum* spirochetes can be seen, resulting in the most definitive diagnosis. Because most patients are seen in later stages, the clinical value of these tests is limited.

Serology testing for syphilis involves the use of two different types of antibody tests. Nontreponemal serology tests (non–T-STS) measure antilipid antibodies produced by the host and so are not specific for treponemal antibody.

Non–T-STS are sensitive and inexpensive and so are effective for screening. In addition, the degree of reactivity is reported quantitatively, giving a numerical titer result. Non–T-STS titers correspond to the patient's clinical course and can be used to assist in clinical staging and to assess adequacy of response to treatment.

All current direct, treponemal serologic tests (T-STS) use antigens of *T. pallidum* and detect specific antibody. For this reason, the T-STS have higher specificity and are used to confirm a diagnosis of syphilis.

Management

In general, patients with reactive screening non–T-STS and reactive T-STS, with no history of syphilis, are considered new cases to be staged and treated. If the patient has clinical signs of primary or secondary syphilis or can give a reliable history of symptoms consistent with primary or secondary stage within the past year, early syphilis can be diagnosed. If a patient has a negative serologic tests for syphilis on record within the past year or is found to be the sexual partner of someone with an early case of syphilis, a presumptive diagnosis of early latent syphilis can be made. Patients who do not meet any of these criteria are diagnosed as cases of unknown duration and are treated for late latent syphilis.

For patients with reactive serology and a history of previous syphilis treatment, attempts should be made to contact the local health department in the area where the patient received treatment. Most county and state health departments maintain syphilis registries of all patients treated for syphilis. The syphilis registry can be used to verify treatment and thus avoid unnecessary retreatment in old cases of syphilis. This is particularly problematic for the many women treated in their early reproductive years, as the question of retreatment is raised at subsequent prenatal visits. They often are treated repeatedly and unnecessarily (Table 85-4).

Patient Education and Counseling

Patients must understand that the syphilis serology tests are antibody tests and so will remain positive even after treatment. Their serology titer should be explained at the time of treatment, as should the need to have repeat syphilis tests at specified intervals for 1 year to ensure adequate treatment. Successful treatment is usually defined as a fourfold or two-dilution decrease in titer within 3 to 6 months of treatment. Patients should be told their titers may remain at low levels (serofast) indefinitely after successful treatment. All patients with syphilis should be counseled and offered HIV testing. Persons coinfected with HIV and syphilis may follow a different clinical course and may need additional treatment.

Treatment of the Sexual Partner

All sexual partners of women with reactive syphilis serology should receive a complete STD/HIV evaluation and testing. Sexual partners exposed to a woman with early syphilis within the previous 90 days are offered prophylactic treatment for incubating syphilis, even if their serologic tests are negative. Because patients with late syphilis are not sexually communicable, male partners of women diagnosed with late, latent infection do not need treatment if their own tests are negative.

Chancroid

Etiology

Chancroid is a disease caused by a bacterial bacillus named *Haemophilus ducreyii.* This organism is transmitted by direct, intimate contact with infected mucous membrane surfaces. Usually, these bacteria colonize squamous epithelium in the genital region; however, female prostitutes have been found to maintain colonization in their pharynxes and to be able to transmit the disease through oral genital sexual contact. Chancroid was very uncommon in the United States in recent years until 1986. Cases of chancroid have been linked to cocaine use and the exchange of sex for drugs. Since 1990, cases of chancroid have again decreased significantly.

Clinical Presentation

The incubation time for chancroid is very short, usually 4 to 7 days. After that time, the patient usually notices a painful bump on the genitals that is often described as a pimple. The lesion quickly becomes larger and more painful, then ulcerates. Unilateral, painful, inguinal lymphadenopathy develops in about 50% of cases.

Examination reveals a painful ulcer with a "dirty" necrotic-appearing base and sharp, excavated edges. The exudate is yellowish and purulent, and secondary lesions due to autoinoculation from opposing mucous membrane surfaces are common in women. Ulcers are usually present around the introitus and on the surfaces of the labia minora. If unilateral lymphadenopathy is present, a characteristic inguinal bubo is formed that is pathognomonic for chancroid. The nodes become suppurative and a soft, fluctuant mass that is exquisitely painful can develop. The skin overlying the bubo becomes erythematous and hot to the touch. If untreated, the bubo can spontaneously rupture through the surface of the skin and drain purulent material.

Laboratory Testing

A culture for *Haemophilus ducreyii* has been developed but requires a selective medium (ie, New York City medium) that is not available in most areas. Culture results can also take more than 1 week and thus are not helpful in the initial management decisions. A Gram stain of exudate from the ulcers can demonstrate a predominance of small, gram-negative coccobacilli that are suggestive of *Haemophilus ducreyii.* However, the ulcers are often secondarily infected or contaminated with many other bacteria, resulting in difficulty in collecting an adequate specimen for Gram stain.

Other causes of genital ulcer disease must be ruled out. An HSV culture should be obtained and a dark-field test, and RPR,FTA should be ordered to rule out syphilis.

Differential Diagnosis

Chancroid is often a diagnosis of exclusion. Women with a history of STD risk behavior who present with painful genital ulcer disease and demonstrate no laboratory evidence of syphilis or herpes should be presumptively treated for chancroid.

Management

The ulcers respond very quickly to antibiotic therapy and usually heal with no scarring. If an inguinal bubo is present, however, antibiotic therapy alone is not adequate treatment. An inguinal bubo should be aspirated by introducing a large-bore needle (14-gauge) through adjacent, intact skin that has been locally anesthetized. Often 15 to 20 mL of purulent exudate can be aspirated (Table 85-5).

Patient Education and Counseling

Women should be told that this is a sexually transmitted disease and the result of sexual contact within the previous 2 weeks. They should be counseled about the association between cocaine use and chancroid and the relationship between genital ulcer disease and HIV infection. They should be encouraged to refer their sexual partners for treatment.

Treatment of the Sexual Partner

Sexual partners of women with chancroid should receive a full STD/HIV evaluation and testing. They should be treated empirically with a regimen effective for chancroid.

Genital Herpes

Etiology

There are two recognized types of herpes simplex virus, HSV-1 and HSV-2. HSV-1 most often infects the mucous membranes of the mouth and is usually acquired nonsexually during childhood. This oral herpes infection is commonly known as cold sores or

Table 85-5. Treatment of Chancroid

Ceftriaxone 250 mg IM STAT
or
Azithromycin 1000 mg po STAT
or
Erythromycin 500 mg po QID × 7 d

fever blisters. HSV-2 usually infects the genital mucous membranes and is acquired in adolescence or young adulthood as the result of sexual behavior. However, either type can infect either mucous membrane site. In recent years, oral–genital sexual techniques have become more common. This has resulted in up to 30% of cases of genital herpes being caused by HSV-1. Likewise, about 30% of new cases of oral herpes result from HSV-2 infection.

Young adults must be taught that cold sores are herpes simplex viral infections and oral–genital sex with a person with a cold sore can result in a genital herpes infection. Although HSV-1 can infect the genital area, it results in few recurrent outbreaks so that most recurrent genital herpes is due to HSV-2.

Clinical Presentation

There is a wide range of clinical manifestations of genital herpes, from multiple, painful ulcers to atypical, minor lesions to asymptomatic shedding. An initial genital herpes infection in a woman who has never had oral herpes is called a primary outbreak.

Primary infections are usually the most severe. Women present complaining of severe vulvar pain and dysuria. On examination, multiple, small, clear vesicles and shallow ulcers can be seen covering the vulva and exocervix. The ulcers have a pink base, clear and watery exudate, and an erythematous border. In primary infection, painful, unilateral, inguinal lymphadenopathy is present and systemic signs and symptoms of viremia such as fever, headache, myalgias, photophobia, and meningismus may also be present. Women with primary genital herpes lesions of the cervix may also have signs and symptoms of PID. Without treatment, resolution of the infection takes about 3 weeks. During this time, all genital ulcers spontaneously heal and the HSV establishes latency in the sacral ganglia. At variable intervals, recurrences occur that result in a new outbreak of vesicular and ulcerative lesions.

An initial genital herpes infection of a woman with a previous history of oral herpes is called a first-episode genital infection. The clinical presentation of first-episode genital HSV and recurrent genital HSV is similar, with mild symptoms of genital pain and dysuria. On examination, a smaller number of vesicles and ulcers can be seen localized to a smaller area of the vulva. Inguinal lymphadenopathy or systemic signs or symptoms of viremia are absent. Lesions heal spontaneously in 3 to 7 days.

Sometimes genital herpes lesions are atypical and appear as a single erythematous papule or very shallow fissures with erythema in the perineal area. In addition, many women with genital herpes demonstrate asymptomatic shedding of HSV from the cervix or vulva with no visible lesions. Women who are asymptomatically shedding HSV represent a major potential source of transmission to infants and sexual partners. Men with genital HSV also demonstrate asymptomatic shedding and represent a major potential source of transmission to their sexual partners.

Laboratory Testing

The HSV culture has been the gold standard test for herpes. The sensitivity varies with the moistness of the lesions, but is generally 90% within the first 3 to 5 days of an outbreak. A specimen is obtained by collecting cellular material from the base of the ulcers. This is best done using a small, sterile, urethral type Dacron-tipped swab. Results usually take 7 days, so presumptive treatment may be initiated before culture results come back. The biggest limitation of the HSV culture is that it can be used only when there are visible lesions.

Newer, rapid diagnostic tests for HSV have been developed using ELISA or DFA techniques. The sensitivities of these tests have been disappointingly low, however—in the range of 70% to 80% compared to culture. Therefore, these tests are being used only in areas where culture is not available. Sometimes the cytopathic effect of HSV can be seen as squamous epithelial giant cells on a Pap smear specimen. Cytologists report this as "evidence suggestive of HSV." The accuracy of this report depends largely on the experience of the cytologist but is considered presumptive and not definitive for genital herpes.

Type-specific HSV antibody serology tests have been developed using Western blot and immunodot techniques, which are highly sensitive and specific. These tests have been used by researchers to conduct large-scale seroprevalence surveys in various populations. Many studies have now shown that the prevalence of HSV-2 begins to increase in persons aged 15 to 19 years and then peaks at ages 30 to 35 years at approximately 20%. In studies of women with positive HSV-2 antibody, only about one third know they have genital herpes. Researchers recommend the use of these tests for screening purposes to detect greater numbers of cases of genital herpes. They are not yet commercially available.

Differential Diagnosis

The history and physical examination are often sufficient to permit the clinical diagnosis of genital herpes. However, due to the psychological impact of a diagnosis of genital herpes and the future obstetric implications, women who present with painful vesicles or ulcers of the genitals should be cultured for HSV. In addition, clinicians should maintain a high index of suspicion and culture all genital lesions with a pattern of recurrence, even if they appear atypical for genital herpes. Syphilis, chancroid, and candidiasis must be ruled out.

Management

Women with primary genital herpes should be treated with oral acyclovir. This significantly reduces viral shedding and promotes healing so the infection usually resolves completely within 5 to 7 days of treatment. Systemic viremia symptoms and dysuria that result from HSV infection of the urethra also resolve quickly with treatment. Initially, acyclovir was given FDA approval in ointment form. The oral capsules were approved a few years later. There is no clinical, safety, or economic benefit of using the ointment rather than the oral therapy.

Women with recurrent outbreaks who desire oral therapy should be taught to self-administer the treatment within 24 hours of noticing a new lesion. This maximizes the clinical benefit of acyclovir for recurrences. Many recurrences do not require acyclovir treatment because they are mild and resolve spontaneously in a few days.

Acyclovir can also be given daily to suppress recurrences. Although women taking suppressive therapy have significantly fewer recurrences, they may still demonstrate asymptomatic shedding and need to use barriers to prevent transmission. Suppressive therapy is best reserved for women whose pattern of recurrence is so frequent that their lives and coping abilities are disrupted. Suppressive therapy has been proven safe and effective (Table 85-6).

Patient Education and Counseling

Women with genital herpes need extensive education and counseling about genital herpes to facilitate a healthy emotional adjust-

Table 85-6. Treatment for Genital Herpes

Primary Genital Herpes
Acyclovir 200 mg po 5 times a day × 7–10 d

Recurrent Genital Herpes
Acyclovir 200 mg po 5 times a day × 5 d

or

Acyclovir 400 mg po TID × 5 days

or

Acyclovir 800 mg PO BID × 5 days

Daily Suppressive Therapy
Acyclovir 200 mg po 2 to 5 times a day

or

Acyclovir 400 mg po BID

ment. Women with this diagnosis experience the standard emotional stages of adjustment to any chronic illness—denial, anger, depression, and acceptance. Many women benefit from a short-term counseling program to enhance their acceptance of this chronic, sexually transmitted disease. Self-help support groups for women with genital herpes are available in many cities in the United States.

Most women newly diagnosed with genital herpes have numerous questions about transmission. Patients should be advised that even though they are most communicable to a sexual partner when they have active lesions, it is possible to transmit the virus even when no visible lesions are present. It is estimated that asymptomatic shedding is responsible for transmission in approximately 30% of new cases. Decisions about using barrier methods to prevent transmission resulting from asymptomatic shedding should be made by the woman and her sexual partner.

Treatment of the Sexual Partner

The sexual partner should be referred for a complete STD/HIV evaluation and testing. The absence of herpes lesions or any history of genital lesions does not rule out the diagnosis of genital herpes. Currently, however, there is no way to detect carriers of genital herpes who may asymptomatically shed intermittently. In the future, the type-specific serology tests may be useful for evaluating sexual partners.

Genital Warts

Etiology

Genital warts are exophytic papules caused by specific subtypes of human papilloma virus (HPV). HPV subtypes 6 and 11 cause most exophytic warts and are benign. Other HPV subtypes that may infect the genital area are types 16, 18, 31, 33, and 35, which have been strongly associated with genital dysplasia and carcinoma. These types are often associated with subclinical infection, but can be found in exophytic lesions. Genital warts are transmitted by direct sexual contact with infected skin or mucous membranes.

Clinical Presentation

The average incubation period before lesions appear is 2 to 3 months. Many women with warts do not notice the lesions, resulting in long delays in diagnosis. Occasionally women complain of symptoms of itching and tenderness of the tissue around the lesions. Genital warts usually appear as whitish, pinkish, or brownish sold papules with a characteristic verraceous, cauliflower-like surface. The surface of the papules often feels firm and granular. Genital warts often appear at the fourchette and adjacent labial surfaces and may spread to other parts of the vulva and perineal areas. Lesions can also infect the exocervix and appear exophytic or as whitish, flat lesions (flat condylomata).

Differential Diagnosis

The diagnosis is often made by visual inspection of the characteristic verraceous, exophytic papules. These papules must be distinguished from molluscum lesion, skin tags, hymenal tags, moles, and prominent sebaceous glands. A clinical manifestation of secondary syphilis previously described as condylomata lata mimics the appearance of genital warts and should be considered in the differential diagnosis.

Laboratory Testing

Atypical papules or flat lesions may require a biopsy to identify the cytopathic effect of HPV in epithelial tissue. A Pap smear may be used to identify a typical halo appearance around the nuclei of squamous epithelial cells which is reported as "koilocytic atypia suggestive of HPV infection." Newer DNA probes have been developed to identify specific subtypes of HPV from cervical samples. The clinical significance and, thus, the clinical use of the probes has not been confirmed. A screening serologic test for syphilis should be done.

Management

The goal of treatment is removal of the exophytic lesions and is, in a sense, cosmetic. No therapy has been shown to eradicate HPV infection. Host immune factors are responsible for inactivation of this infection. Some experts feel that treating the wart lesions may reduce communicability and prevent new areas of squamous tissue from becoming infected, but this has not been proved. After successful treatment of the lesions, recurrences can occur, usually as the result of reactivation of the subclinical HPV infection. If left untreated, genital warts may spontaneously resolve, remain unchanged, or grow and spread to adjacent areas. For this reason, treatment of lesions is usually recommended (Table 85-7).

Table 85-7. Treatment of External Genital Warts

1. Cryotherapy with liquid nitrogen or cryoprobe.
2. Podofilox 0.5% solution for self-treatment. Clients are advised to apply podofilox to warts twice a day for 3 days, followed by 4 days of no therapy. This cycle can be repeated as necessary for a total of 4 cycles. (This is not indicated for pregnant women).
3. Podophyllin 10%–20%, in compound tincture of benzoin. Limited areas are covered with the solution and the client is advised to wash the solution off thoroughly in 1 to 4 hours. This may be repeated weekly for up to 6 weeks. (This is not indicated for pregnant women).
4. Trichloracetic acid (TCA) 80%–90%. Apply only to warts, not necessary to wash off. Repeat weekly for up to 6 weeks. (Can be used for pregnant women).
5. Electrodesiccation or electrocautery.

Patient Education and Counseling

Educating and counseling women about genital wart infections is particularly frustrating because of the lack of definitive research about many commonly asked questions about communicability, sexual transmission risks, and risks of subsequent carcinoma. It is most important to stress that treatment of the warts does not result in eradication of the HPV infection.

The period of communicability following treatment of the lesions is unknown. Condom use is recommended at least until there is no evidence of active infection for 6 months in the woman or her sexual partner. At this time, it is assumed the host immune response has inhibited viral replication. However, the client must be advised that recurrences may occur throughout her life. Experts speculate that HPV infection may persist in a dormant state and become infectious intermittently. Many women with genital warts can benefit from HPV support groups, which have formed in many cities around the country.

Treatment of the Sexual Partner

The sexual partner should be examined for genital warts and have a complete STD/HIV evaluation and testing. The partner may demonstrate exophytic warts, but many are subclinically infected with HPV and have no visible lesions. No practical screening tests for subclinical HPV are available for male partners. Condom use is recommended, but, again, the period of communicability is unknown.

Molluscum Contagiosum

Etiology

Molluscum contagiosum is a benign condition of the skin and mucous membranes characterized by multiple papular lesions. This condition is caused by infection with the molluscum contagiosum virus (MCV), which is a member of the poxvirus family. Molluscum contagiosum, like herpes simplex virus, can be spread by both sexual and nonsexual routes of transmission. Children often develop this skin infection on the face, trunk, and extremities as the result of direct skin-to-skin contact or fomites. In adults, lower abdominal, thigh, groin, and genital lesions are common and are thought to result from direct skin-to-skin contact during sexual activity.

Clinical Presentation

The incubation period for molluscum lesions to appear is approximately 2 to 3 months. Lesions develop as smooth, pinkish papules that slowly enlarge over a period of weeks. At this time the papules are approximately 10 to 15 mm in diameter with a shiny, pearly surface. At maturity, the papules demonstrate a highly characteristic central umbilication from which a caseous, whitish "pearl" can be expressed. This pearl is the viral body, and its removal will result in resolution of the papule. Most women with molluscum papules are asymptomatic and unaware of the infection. Molluscum papules commonly occur in the groin areas frequently shaved by some women. Because of this distribution, many women who do notice the papules attribute them to shaving irritation.

Recently, atypical appearing and unusually large numbers of molluscum lesions have been described in persons infected with HIV, suggesting a role of host immunity in the control of MCV infection and its level of clinical expression.

Differential Diagnosis

Molluscum papules are often confused with venereal warts and diagnosed and treated inappropriately. The diagnosis is usually made by visual inspection and the identification of pink, fleshy papules, often umbilicated, from which a pearl can be expressed.

HPV lesions, as previously described, are solid papules with a verraceous surface.

Laboratory Testing

The only definitive diagnostic test for molluscum contagiosum is a biopsy of the papule. The material is histologically examined to identify enlarged epithelial cells with intracytoplasmic molluscum bodies which are pathognomonic. Biopsies are reserved for atypical lesions. Women with unusually large numbers or atypically appearing molluscum papules should be offered HIV counseling and testing.

Management

Molluscum infections are generally self-limited; individual lesions usually resolve spontaneously within 3 months and stop recurring in approximately 2 years. Decisions to use various treatments that may result in scarring must be made on an individualized basis. Treatment strategies are similar to those used for HPV lesions, eradication of lesions by mechanical or chemical destruction techniques. Treatments do not eradicate MCV, however, and recurrences of lesions are common until there is an adequate host immune response.

Treatment of molluscum contagiosum includes removal of each papule by skin curettage, application of trichloracetic acid and liquid nitrogen, and "coring" of lesions by expressing the pearl.

Patient Education and Counseling

The female client should be told that molluscum papules are the result of a benign viral infection of the skin that may be the result of nonsexual or sexual contact. They should be clearly distinguished from venereal warts and HPV infection. The client should be aware that there are no known complications of this infection and that there is usually spontaneous resolution without treatment of the papules.

Treatment of the Sexual Partner

Sexual partners should be referred for inspection for molluscum lesions as well as a complete STD/HIV evaluation and testing.

Scabies

Etiology

Scabies is an infestation of the itch mite, *Sarcoptes scabiei.* This infestation can occur nonsexually through household contact and skin-to-skin contact or sexually as the result of prolonged skin-to-skin contact during sexual activity. The female mite burrows into the epidermal layer of the skin and, within hours, begins depositing eggs. The eggs hatch to form adult mites in 10 days.

Clinical Presentation

The symptoms of scabies result from a sensitization reaction that develops in the human host over a period of several weeks. The most classic symptom of scabies is itching, particularly nocturnal itching. In addition, pruritic papules can be seen in a characteristic distribution in warm, moist areas of the skin. Distribution sites include finger webs, wrists, elbows, axillary folds, the beltline of the trunk, gluteal folds, and the genital area. The papules have usually been scratched severely, resulting in crusted excoriations.

Differential Diagnosis

Diagnosis is usually made by the clinical history and visual inspection. A history of itching that is severe, worsens at night, and involves more than one household member or a sexual partner is highly suggestive of scabies. The clinical appearance of papules with excoriation and crusting appearing in classic distribution sites strengthens the diagnosis. Burrows may be seen on the skin, appearing as short, wavy, dirty-appearing fine lines formed by the burrowing and egg-laying of the female mite. These burrows are pathognomic for scabies. Secondary infection or an eczematous reactions can complicate the clinical appearance.

Laboratory Testing

The most common test used is a skin scraping technique .The most recent, unexcoriated papule is located. Mineral oil is placed on the skin, which is then scraped vigorously with a sterile scalpel blade to dislodge the papule or burrow. The material is then placed on a slide and examined for microscopic evidence of the mite or fecal pellets containing the eggs. A burrow ink test (BIT) is sometimes used in which a fresh papule is rubbed with ink from a fountain pen. The ink is then wiped off the surface of the papule with an alcohol pad. In the BIT-positive lesion, the ink soaks down into the track of the mite burrow and forms a dark, zigzagging fine line. In complicated cases, a skin punch biopsy may be needed.

Management

Treatment is directed at killing the mites. Signs and symptoms are caused by a sensitization reaction, however, and so may persist for a few weeks after successful treatment. This results in overtreatment when clients are not properly educated and are self treating.

Treatment of scabies includes permethrin cream 5% applied to all areas of the body from the neck down and washed off after 8 to 14 hours or lindane 1%, 1 oz of lotion or 30 g of cream applied thinly to all areas of the body from the neck down and washed off after 8 hours. (Lindane is not recommended for pregnant women or children.)

Patient Education and Counseling

Clothing and bedding should be washed and dried on the hot cycles. All household members or a sexual partner should be treated at the same time. Clients especially need to understand that the itching and papules may persist for a week or two after treatment.

Treatment of the Sexual Partner

The regular sexual partner should be treated even if there are no signs or symptoms of scabies. The incubation period for an initial scabies infestation can be several weeks.

Pubic Lice

Etiology

Pubic lice, commonly called crabs, are caused by an infestation of *Phthirus pubis*. (This is a different species from those that cause head lice or body lice.)

Clinical Presentation

The pubic louse is approximately 1 mm in length and wider at the abdomen, giving it the appearance of a crab. The pubic louse attaches itself to the base of a pubic hair follicle and buries its mouthparts under the skin where it feeds on the host's blood. Adult pubic lice can be seen as reddish brown spots at the base of the hair follicles. Eggs are deposited in cylindrical structures (nits) that are attached to the shaft of the pubic hair. The nits can be seen as whitish flakes that cannot be easily dislodged from the hair shaft. The eggs hatch within 5 to 10 days. Symptoms include itching of the skin in the pubic hair region and bluish or reddish spots on the affected skin.

Differential Diagnosis

The diagnosis is made by clinical history and careful inspection of the pubic region for adult lice and nits. Often the adult louse may need to be dislodged from the base of the hair follicle with the blunt end of a wooden applicator. The legs can usually be seen moving.

Laboratory Testing

Confirmation of adult lice or nits can be made by microscopic assessment of samples using the 10× objective of a standard microscope.

Management

The ideal treatment kills both the adult lice and the eggs. All clothing and bedding should be washed and dried using the hot cycles. Recommended treatment is permethrin 1% creme rinse applied to affected area and washed off after 10 minutes or lindane 1% shampoo applied for 4 minutes and then washed off. (This treatment is not recommended for pregnant women or children).

Patient Education and Counseling

The female client should be given proper treatment instructions and advised to wash her clothing and bedding at the same time as administering the treatment.

Treatment of the Sexual Partner

The regular sexual partner should be treated simultaneously even if asymptomatic to avoid reinfestation.

BIBLIOGRAPHY

Cates W Jr, Whittington WL. Checking out the new STD tests. Contemporary OBGYN 1984;23:135.

Centers for Disease Control, U.S. Dept. of Health and Human Services. 1993 Sexually transmitted diseases treatment guidelines. MMWR 1993:42(RR-14):1.

Centers for Disease Control. Recommendations for the prevention and management of *Chlamydia trachomatis* infections. Morbidity and Mortality Weekly Report 1993;42(RR-12).

Coury-Doniger PA. Syphilis: managing patients with reactive serologic tests. STD Bulletin 1993;12.

Edlin BR, Irwin KL, Faroque S, et al. Intersecting epidemics—crack cocaine. use and HIV infection among inner-city young adults. N Engl J Med 1994;331:1422.

De Vincenzi I. A longitudinal study of human immunodeficiency virus transmission by heterosexual partners. N Engl J Med 1994;331:341.

Gilchrist MJR, Rauh JL. Office microscopic examination for sexually transmitted diseases: a tool to lower costs. J Adolesc Health Care 1985; 6:311.

Handsfield HH. Color atlas and synopsis of sexually transmitted diseases. New York: McGraw-Hill, 1992.

Holmes KK, Cates W, Lemon S, Stamm W. Sexually transmitted diseases, 2nd ed. New York: McGraw-Hill, 1990.

Hook E III, Marra CM. Acquired syphilis in adults. N Engl J Med 1992;326:1060.

Koutsky LA. The frequency of unrecognized type 2 herpes simplex virus infection among women. Sex Transm Dis 1989;17:90.

Larsen SA. A manual of tests for syphilis. Washington, DC: American Public Health Association, 1990.

Martin DH (ed). Sexually transmitted diseases. Med Clin North Am 1990;74:1339.

Mertz GJ. Frequency of acquisition of first-episode genital infection with herpes simplex virus from symptomatic and asymptomatic source contacts. Sex Transm Dis 1984;12:33.

Paavonen J, Stamm WE. Lower genital tract infections in women. Infect Dis Clin North Am 1987;1:179.

Stamm WE. The practitioner's handbook for the management of STDs. Seattle: HSCER Distribution, University of Washington, 1988.

Stamm WE. Dysuria: establishing a diagnostic protocol. Contemporary OBGYN, October 1988:81.

Sweet RL, Gibbs RS. Infectious diseases of the female genital tract, 2nd edition. Baltimore: Williams & Wilkins, 1990.

Thomason JL, Gelbart SM, Broekhuizen FF. Advances in the understanding of bacterial vaginosis. J Reprod Med 1989;34:581.

Wasserheit JN. "Epidemiological synergy: interrelationships between human immunodeficiency virus infection and other sexually transmitted diseases. Sex Transm Dis 1992;19:61.

Wasserheit JN. Pelvic inflammatory disease and infertility. Maryland Medical Journal 1987;36:58.

Wasserheit JN, Aral AS, Holmes K, Hitchcock P (eds). Research issues in human behavior and sexually transmitted diseases in the AIDS era. Washington, DC: American Society for Microbiology, 1991.

Wentworth B, Judson FN (eds). Laboratory methods for the diagnosis of sexually transmitted diseases, 2nd ed. Washington, DC: American Public Health Association, 1991.

Wisdom A. Color atlas of sexually transmitted diseases. Chicago: Year Book Medical Publishers, 1989.

Primary Care for Women, edited by Phyllis C. Leppert and Fred M. Howard. Lippincott-Raven Publishers, Philadelphia © 1997.

86

Pelvic Inflammatory Disease

FRED M. HOWARD

Pelvic inflammatory disease (PID) is an infection of the upper genital tract that may involve any or all of the following sites: endometrium (endometritis); myometrium (myometritis); uterine serosa and broad ligament (parametritis); fallopian tube (salpingitis); ovary (oophoritis); and pelvic peritoneum (peritonitis). The infectious process most commonly implied by the diagnosis of PID is acute salpingitis, and in clinical practice these two terms are used interchangeably. Salpingitis may, in fact, be the more appropriate term, because it is infection of the oviducts that accounts for the most characteristic symptoms, signs, and sequelae of PID.

Chronic PID is a term largely abandoned that refers to either recurrent episodes of acute PID or to the adnexal adhesions and damage (eg, hydrosalpinges) secondary to PID. These latter long-term sequelae are bacteriologically sterile. Although tuberculosis or actinomycosis may cause chronic infection, the common causes of PID do not cause chronic infection.

PID is a serious infection, in both personal and public health costs. There are about one million cases per year in the United States, with estimated direct and indirect costs of $3.5 billion. Each year, PID accounts for approximately 2.5 million physician visits, 300,000 hospital admissions, and 150,000 surgical procedures. It carries a significant risk of serious sequelae—infertility, ectopic pregnancy, and chronic pelvic pain. Twenty percent of women with a single episode of severe PID may have infertility due to tubal damage. The number of episodes of PID also influences the odds of developing tubal infertility (Table 86-1). The risk of subsequent ectopic pregnancy is increased at least sixfold after PID. The chance of developing chronic pelvic pain is increased fourfold after PID.

ETIOLOGY

Most often PID is a polymicrobial infection with organisms that ascend from the vagina and cervix to the endometrium and endosalpinx. The most commonly isolated organisms are listed in Table 86-2. The type and number of species vary, depending on the patient population and the stage of the disease when the cultures are obtained. In the early stages, gonorrhea, chlamydia, and aerobic organisms tend to predominate. Later in the course of the disease, anaerobic bacteria tend to predominate.

The exact mechanisms by which organisms ascend from the vagina and cervix to the upper genital tract are not known, but epidemiologic risk factors suggest several conditions that weaken the cervical barrier. Cervical infection with gonorrhea is a major risk factor for PID; 15% of women with gonococcal cervicitis subsequently develop PID. Chlamydial cervicitis is also a major risk factor. In the United States, these two organisms coexist in the same patient up to 40% of the time. These sexually transmitted organisms appear to have an etiologic role in 30% to 60% of cases of PID in the United States. Thus factors that increase the chance of acquiring either of these organisms also increase the chance of acquiring PID. Beginning intercourse at a young age, having multiple sexual partners, living in an area with a high prevalence of sexually transmitted diseases, and not using contraception are examples of these risk factors.

Unfortunately, sexual activity at a young age also appears to be an independent risk factor for PID and not just a marker for risk of sexually transmitted diseases. A sexually active adolescent has a 1 in 8 risk of developing PID, compared to a 1 in 80 risk for a woman over 25 years of age. Although sexual and contraceptive practices contribute to this difference, some of it is due to the increased predilection of chlamydia and gonorrhea to ascend to the upper tract in younger women. The reasons for this are not known. Because another risk factor for ascent is previous PID, the increased risk in these young women also puts them at risk for an increased chance of recurrent infections.

Contraceptive use, excluding the intrauterine device (IUD), tends to decrease the risk of PID. Oral contraceptives decrease the risk of PID by 70%, and barrier methods decrease the risk by 60%. The effect of oral contraceptives is thought to be due to thicker cer-

Table 86-1. The Association of Tubal Infertility and the Number of Episodes ofPelvic Inflammatory Disease

NO. OF EPISODES OF PID	TUBAL INFERTILITY, %
1	8
2	20
≥3	40

PID, pelvic inflammatory disease.

vical mucus and to decreased duration of menstrual flow. The barrier contraceptives' effect is thought to be due to their function as both mechanical and chemical barriers. IUD use, on the other hand, may increase the risk of PID two- to four-fold. This increased risk is probably related to the iatrogenic invasion of the cervix and endometrial cavity at the time of insertion and possibly to the string communicating between the vagina and endometrial cavity. The methodologies of many of the studies regarding IUD risk have been criticized, and the magnitude of any risk is still a subject of debate.

Vaginal douching is also a risk factor for PID, apparently increasing the likelihood of infectious ascent. Women who douche frequently have a risk of PID that is three- to fourfold greater than that of women who douche less than once a month.

Although tubal sterilization may a priori be predicted to serve a protective role against ascending infection and salpingitis, PID is not as uncommon after sterilization as previously thought. In reported series, the signs and symptoms are not changed by prior tubal sterilization. The mean time interval from sterilization until an episode of PID is about 4 years.

Etiologies for PID other than ascending infection from the vagina and cervix are less common (Table 86-3). *Hematogenous spread* probably accounts for most cases of tuberculous PID, an uncommon disease in the United States. *Direct extension* to the upper genital tract may occur with appendicitis or diverticulitis. *Iatrogenic* cases may occur after surgical or diagnostic procedures such as hysteroscopy, hysterosalpingography, endometrial biopsy, or IUD insertion. Iatrogenic PID may be more likely in the presence of chlamydial or gonococcal cervicitis, or in women with a history of prior PID.

Table 86-2. Common Microorganisms Isolated From the Fallopian Tubes of Women With Pelvic Inflammatory Disease

Sexually Transmitted
Chlamydia trachomatis
Neisseria gonorrhoeae
Mycoplasma hominis

Aerobic or Facultative
Streptococcus species
Staphylococcus species
Haemophilus species
Escherichia coli

Anaerobic
Bacteroides species
Peptococcus species
Peptostreptococcus species
Clostridium species
Actinomyces species

Table 86-3. Etiologic Mechanisms of Pelvic Inflammatory Disease

Ascent of cervical and vaginal microorganisms
Hematogenous spread of infection
Direct contiguous spread of infection
Iatrogenic introduction of infection

DIFFERENTIAL DIAGNOSES

The clinical diagnosis of PID is often difficult. Numerous other diagnoses may be confused with PID and vice versa (Tables 86-4 and 86-5). Often the only way to clearly differentiate PID from other causes of pelvic pain is laparoscopic evaluation. There are no pathognomonic signs or symptoms of PID.

Pain with *appendicitis* is usually unilateral at the right lower quadrant at some point in its clinical course, whereas PID is unilateral in less than 10% of cases. Other presenting signs and symptoms may be quite similar.

With *endometriosis*, there is usually a chronic history of pain and dysmenorrhea, in distinction to the acute onset of PID. Not uncommonly, however, several prior episodes of acute exacerbation of pain of endometriosis may be diagnosed as PID. A history of repetitive episodes of PID is a reasonable indication for laparoscopic evaluation.

A *hemorrhagic corpus luteum cyst* may be suggested by acute onset and rapid resolution of pain, by the presence of a palpable unilateral mass, by sonographic evidence of a characteristic ovarian cyst and increased peritoneal fluid, and by the absence of physical or laboratory evidence of infection.

Adnexal torsion usually presents with unilateral pain that is intermittently acutely severe. However, it may present with severe, persistent, diffuse pain that is not clinically distinguishable from PID. Sonography may show a unilateral complex mass that appears inconsistent with an abscess, suggesting torsion. Emergent surgery is indicated if adnexal torsion is suspected rather than PID.

Ectopic pregnancy, not PID, should be the initial clinical diagnosis with a positive pregnancy test. With currently available sensitive tests for serum b-hCG, it is rare to have a negative pregnancy test in cases of ectopic pregnancy. PID may occur in pregnancy, but it is extremely rare and should be considered only after ectopic pregnancy and *septic abortion* have been definitively excluded.

Table 86-4. Laparoscopic Diagnoses in Women in Whom the Clinical Diagnosis Pelvic Inflammatory Disease Was Incorrectly Made

LAPAROSCOPIC DIAGNOSIS	PERCENTAGE
Acute appendicitis	24
Endometriosis	16
Corpus luteum bleeding	12
Ectopic pregnancy	11
Pelvic adhesions only	7
Benign ovarian tumor	7
Chronic salpingitis	6
Miscellaneous	15
Total	100

Table 86-5. Incorrect Preoperative Clinical Diagnoses in 91 Women Diagnosed With Pelvic Inflammatory Disease at the Time of Surgery

INCORRECT CLINICAL DIAGNOSIS	NUMBER (%)
Ovarian tumor	20 (22)
Acute appendicitis	18 (20)
Ectopic pregnancy	16 (18)
Chronic salpingitis	10 (11)
Acute peritonitis	6 (7)
Endometriosis	5 (5)
Uterine myoma	5 (5)
Uncharacteristic pelvic pain	5 (5)
Miscellaneous	6 (7)
Total	91 (100)

Complications of *leiomyomata* may present with pain and low-grade fever similar to PID. Pain is usually not diffuse, but localizes to the myoma. Sonography may confirm the myomas or suggest degeneration of a leiomyoma that accounts for the acute symptoms.

Clear-cut differentiation of PID from other causes of acute abdominopelvic pain not infrequently requires laparoscopic evaluation.

CLINICAL SYMPTOMS

Women with PID may present with a wide range of symptoms and symptom severity. Some cases of chlamydial salpingitis appear to be almost silent, causing little if any pain or discomfort. Other patients present with a life-threatening illness due to overwhelming sepsis. In between these extremes, where the majority of PID patients are, is a wide range of possible presentations.

More than 90% of women with PID present with diffuse lower abdominal pain. Usually the pain is constant and dull, although it may become crampy and be accentuated by physical activity or coitus. The duration is usually 7 days or less at the time the patient presents. Rarely—less than 10% of the time—is the pain localized or unilateral.

Increased vaginal discharge is a common, albeit nonspecific, complaint. About one half of women with PID have this symptom. Close questioning usually reveals that it is yellow or yellow-green, consistent with purulence. Irregular vaginal bleeding is also relatively common; it is reported by about 40% of women with PID.

Fever or chills is reported by 40% to 50% of women with PID. Urinary urgency or frequency is reported by about 20%. Emesis occurs in only about 10% and is usually a later symptom due to severe disease and peritonitis.

Questions regarding historical risk factors may also aid in diagnosing PID. A well-documented history of previous PID is consistent with reinfection. A history of sexually transmitted disease, especially gonorrhea or chlamydia, is consistent with increased risk of PID. A history of multiple sexual partners, no use of barrier or oral contraceptives, use of an IUD, or frequent douching may also support a risk of PID. Recent surgical or invasive procedures, such as pregnancy termination or dilatation and curettage are also consistent with increased risk.

A small percentage, about 5% to 10% of women with PID, have pain in the right upper quadrant, sometimes with a pleuritic quality. This is due to perihepatic inflammation, the so-called Fitz-Hugh-Curtis syndrome. This results from transperitoneal or vascular dissemination of chlamydia or gonorrhea to the liver area. Chlamydia is believed to cause the majority of cases.

CLINICAL FINDINGS

Clinical criteria for the diagnosis of salpingitis have been proposed that take into account the recognized problems of both underdiagnosis and overdiagnosis (Table 86-6). Abdominal examination reveals direct abdominal tenderness, particularly at the lower abdomen. Rebound tenderness may also be present, but is not consistently found. Bowel sounds are usually normal, although they may be decreased or even absent with a severe infection complicated by peritonitis. Pelvic examination reveals cervical and uterine tenderness to movement, and adnexal tenderness to palpation. These three areas of tenderness—abdominal, cervical and uterine, and adnexal—are considered essential if a clinical diagnosis of salpingitis is to be entertained. More than 90% of women with PID have these findings. Sometimes an indiscreet adnexal fullness is found, representing inflammation, edema, and adhesions. In cases complicated by an adnexal abscess, a mass may be palpable, but often tenderness is too great to allow an adequate examination in these patients. It is estimated that 10% of women with PID have adnexal abscess formation.

About 40% of patients with PID have a temperature of ≥ 38°C.

The 5% to 10% of women with Fitz-Hugh-Curtis syndrome also have tenderness on palpation of the abdominal right upper quadrant and liver.

LABORATORY AND IMAGING FINDINGS

As noted in Table 86-6, in addition to the findings of abdominal, cervicouterine, and adnexal tenderness, at least one laboratory or imaging study must be abnormal to make a clinical diagnosis of PID if the patient is afebrile and has no palpable pelvic mass. Basic laboratory studies for suspected PID include complete blood count, Gram stain of the endocervix, gonococcal cultures, chlamydia testing, and a sensitive pregnancy test. Leukocytosis is present in about 60% of women with PID. Positivity of Gram stains, gonococcal cultures, and chlamydia tests varies widely, ranging from 5% to 85%. The finding of either gonorrhea or chlamydia at the endocervix does not prove that either is the primary or only pathogen in the upper genital tract. Pregnancy testing is mandatory,

Table 86-6. Clinical Criteria for the Diagnosis of Salpingitis

Necessary criteria
Abdominal tenderness, with or without rebound tenderness
Tenderness with motion of cervix and uterus
Adnexal tenderness

Plus one or more of the following criteria
Gram stain of endocervix positive for gram-negative, intracellular diplococci
Fever (>38°C)
Leukocytosis (>10,000)
Purulent material from peritoneal cavity by culdocentesis or laparoscopy
Pelvic abscess or inflammatory complex on bimanual examination or by sonography

because ectopic pregnancy represents a life-threatening disease and is still occasionally misdiagnosed as PID.

Other laboratory tests are determined by the patient's clinical signs and symptoms. Sedimentation rates have traditionally be done both for diagnosis and follow-up of PID. They are elevated in about 85% of cases and are sometimes helpful. A urinalysis and urine culture may be necessary to rule out urinary tract infection. Electrolytes may be important in seriously ill patients with emesis. Liver function tests may be needed in patients with right upper quadrant pain and tenderness. Chest x-rays and gallbladder ultrasound may also occasionally be needed in these cases.

In patients with a palpable mass or those with such tenderness that an adequate examination cannot be performed, a pelvic ultrasound may be indicated. This may allow the diagnosis or confirmation of an adnexal abscess.

Culdocentesis may be done to obtain specimens for staining and culture. However, in many women with PID this is a very painful procedure that contributes little to clinical management.

Currently the gold standard for diagnosis of PID is direct visualization of the upper genital tract with laparoscopy. Characteristic findings allow accurate diagnosis and grading (Table 86-7). Numerous published series have shown that laparoscopy greatly improves the accuracy of diagnosis. For example, a review of 1552 reported cases revealed that laparoscopy showed the clinical diagnosis to be correct in only 958 (62%) of patients. Other diagnoses were present in 271 (17%) of patients and there were normal findings in 323 (21%) of the patients. In addition to improving the accuracy of diagnosis, laparoscopy also allows collection of specimens for bacteriologic cultures and antibiotic sensitivity testing. It has been suggested that all women suspected of having PID should undergo laparoscopy for definitive diagnosis. However, due to concerns about cost and about potential complications, most women in the United States with suspected PID do not undergo laparoscopy. Clearly, in cases in which the diagnosis is uncertain or in which response to therapy is inappropriate, laparoscopy is indicated.

TREATMENT

After diagnosing PID, two specific decisions need to be made regarding treatment. The first is whether to treat the patient in the hospital or as an outpatient. The second is what antibiotics to use. These decisions are interconnected because the decision to treat as an outpatient usually limits the choice of antibiotics.

There is not a clear consensus on which to base a decision regarding hospital versus outpatient therapy. In an ideal world it would probably be best to treat all patients with in-hospital parenteral therapy, but this is not an option in the United States. Evidence suggests that failure rates with outpatient oral antibiotic treatment are 10% to 20%, compared to 5% to 10% failure rates with inpatient intravenous antibiotics. Trying to predict those women most likely to fail oral antibiotic treatment is problematic and thus there are varying opinions about indications for hospitalization (Table 86-8).

The decision of which antibiotics to use is almost always an empiric one; specific cultures of the upper reproductive tract are not usually obtained. Antibiotic protocols for PID should cover a wide range of organisms, including gonorrhea, chlamydia, anaerobic bacteria, gram-negative aerobic rods, and gram-positive cocci (see Table 86-2). The regimens recommended by the Centers for Disease Control and Prevention (CDC) are most commonly used (Table 86-9). Inpatient *regimen A* is cefoxitin 2 g intravenously every 6 hours or cefotetan 2 g every 12 hours plus doxycycline 100 mg orally or intravenously every 12 hours. With this regimen, other cephalosporins such as ceftizoxime, cefotaxime, and ceftriaxone that cover gonorrhea, other gram-negative aerobes, and anaerobes may be substituted for cefoxitin or cefotetan. Inpatient *regimen B* is clindamycin 900 mg intravenously every 8 hours plus gentamicin at a loading dose of 2 mg/kg body weight followed by a maintenance dose of 1.5 mg/kg every 8 hours.

With either of the inpatient regimens, intravenous antibiotics are continued for at least 48 hours after the patient clinically improves. After discontinuation of the intravenous regimen, doxycycline 100 mg orally every 12 hours should be continued for 10 to 14 days total. An alternative oral regimen is clindamycin 450 mg orally 4 times a day for 10 to 14 days. Even though clindamycin has shown effectiveness against chlamydia, if chlamydia is documented or strongly suspected, then doxycycline is the drug of choice.

Ampicillin or sulbactam plus doxycycline, as well as ofloxacin plus clindamycin or metronidazole, are alternate regimens that may be considered, but have not been as widely used as the previously discussed regimens. Evidence is insufficient to support the use of any single agent regimen for inpatient treatment.

Outpatient regimens traditionally recommended by the CDC initiate therapy with a parenteral antibiotic to cover gonorrhea: cefoxitin 2 g intramuscularly plus probenecid 1 g orally or ceftriaxone 250 mg intramuscularly or an equivalent third-generation cephalosporin. This is followed by an antibiotic to treat chlamydia—the CDC recommendation is doxycycline 100 mg orally 2 times a day for 10 to 14 days. The CDC has added an alternative regimen that avoids parenteral antibiotics: ofloxacin 400 mg orally two times a day for 14 days plus either clindamycin 450 mg orally

Table 86-7. Grading of Severity of Pelvic Inflammatory Disease by Laparoscopic Visualization

Mild	Erythema, edema, no spontaneous purulent exudate,* tube freely movable
Moderate	Gross purulent material evident, erythema and edema more marked, tubes may not be freely movable and fimbrial stoma may not be patent
Severe	Pyosalpinx or inflammatory complex, or abscess†

*The tubes may require manipulation to produce purulent exudate.
†The size of any pelvic abscess should be measured.

Table 86-8. Some Possible Indications for Hospital Treatment of Patients With Pelvic Inflammatory Disease

Nulliparity
Adolescence
Tuboovarian abscess or complex
Pregnancy
Nausea and vomiting
Upper abdominal peritoneal signs
IUD
HIV
Uncertain diagnosis
Inability to comply with or follow an outpatient regimen
Unable to arrange 72-h follow-up
Inadequate response to outpatient therapy

HIV, human immunodeficiency virus; *IUD,* intrauterine device.

Table 86-9. Inpatient Antibiotic Regimens Recommended by the Centers for Disease Control for the Treatment of Pelvic Inflammatory Disease

Regimen A

Cefoxitin 2 g IV q 6h or cefotetan 2 g IV q12 h PLUS doxycycline 100 mg IV or PO q 12h

(This regimen should be continued for at least 48 h after the patient demonstrates substantial clinical improvement)

THEN

Doxycycline 100 mg PO bid for a total of 14 d.

Regimen B

Clindamycin 900 mg IV q 8h PLUS gentamicin 2 mg/kg loading then 1.5 mg/kg q 8h

(This regimen should be continued for at least 48 h after the patient demonstrates substantial clinical improvement)

THEN

Doxycycline 100 mg PO bid or clindamycin 450 mg PO qid for a total of 14 d.

Alternative Regimens

Ampicillin or sulbactam 3 g IV q 6h *PLUS* doxycycline 100 mg IV or PO q 12h

Ofloxacin 400 mg IV q 12h *plus* either clindamycin or metronidazole

four times a day for 14 days or metronidazole 500 mg orally two times a day for 14 days.

Assurance of follow-up to document clinical response within 72 hours is important with outpatient treatment. If response is inadequate after 72 hours then hospitalization for parenteral therapy is recommended.

If response to inpatient treatment is inadequate after 72 to 96 hours of parenteral antibiotics, laparoscopy should be considered. This may confirm a different diagnosis or may demonstrate a tuboovarian abscess. Of course, it may be argued that all women with suspected PID should undergo diagnostic laparoscopy.

Extirpative surgical therapy is rarely necessary with current antibiotic regimens. In some patients with pelvic abscesses, medical therapy may not be successful, however, and drainage may be needed. Rarely is salpingectomy or salpingoophorectomy mandatory. Percutaneous drainage with CT or ultrasound guidance or laparoscopic drainage has been done successfully in unresponsive cases of tuboovarian abscesses, and these approaches may be preferable to laparotomy when feasible. It is vital that any surgical treatment be as conservative as possible. With the advent of assisted reproductive technology, pregnancy is possible even in women with only a uterus. Therefore a hysterectomy should not automatically be done even if it is necessary to remove both adnexa. The patient must be clearly counseled as to her options regarding future fertility.

CONSIDERATIONS IN PREGNANCY

PID is not common in pregnant women. In any pregnant woman in whom the diagnosis of PID is considered, septic abortion or ectopic pregnancy must be definitively ruled out. Both represent life-threatening diseases that, with current therapies, include mandatory termination of the pregnancy—by curettage with septic abortion and via abdominal surgery or methotrexate therapy with ectopic pregnancy.

When it occurs during pregnancy, PID tends to be a first-trimester infection, although some cases have been reported later in pregnancy. Its presenting symptoms and signs are similar to those in nonpregnant women (see Table 86-7). Abdominopelvic pain and tenderness, cervical tenderness, and adnexal tenderness are generally present. About half of the patients present with low-grade fevers. Causative organisms are the same as those in nonpregnant women (see Table 86-2) and the etiologies are probably similar, including ascending infection prior to 12 weeks gestation (see Table 86-3). Fetal wastage approaches 50% in pregnancies complicated by PID. Aggressive early medical treatment may improve this poor prognosis.

Inpatient parenteral antibiotic treatment is strongly recommended in any pregnant woman with PID. Of the inpatient regimens previously discussed, gentamicin-clindamycin is preferred, because doxycycline is contraindicated during pregnancy. In clinical practice, erythromycin is substituted for doxycycline for ongoing outpatient treatment after hospital discharge, but little evidence is available to ensure its effectiveness in PID.

BIBLIOGRAPHY

Blanchard AC, Pastorek JG, Weeks T. Pelvic inflammatory disease during pregnancy. South Med J 1987;80:1363.

Green MM, Vicario SJ, Sanfilippo JS, Lochhead SA. Acute pelvic inflammatory disease after surgical sterilization. Ann Emerg Med 1991;20:344.

Hager WD, Eschenbach DA, Spence MR, Sweet RL. Criteria for diagnosis and grading of salpingitis. Obstet Gynecol 1983;61:113.

Livengood CH, Hill GB, Addison WA. Pelvic inflammatory disease: findings during inpatient treatment of clinically severe, laparoscopy-documented disease. Am J Obstet Gynecol 1992;166:519.

McCormack WM. Pelvic inflammatory disease. N Engl J Med 1994;330:115.

MMWR 1993;42.

Primary Care for Women, edited by Phyllis C. Leppert and Fred M. Howard. Lippincott-Raven Publishers, Philadelphia © 1997.

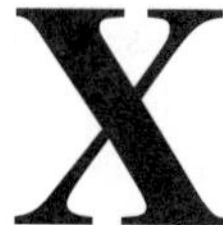

Hematologic and Oncologic Problems

87

Anemia

PETER A. KOUIDES

Anemia is not a disease in itself—it is the end-laboratory abnormality of numerous disease processes. Informing a patient only that she is anemic is not sufficient. It is incumbent on the physician to then logically proceed with additional laboratory testing to determine the underlying disease. This, of course, enables the physician to go beyond measures such as a red blood cell (RBC) transfusion or iron replacement in the hope of permanently correcting the anemic state. This chapter focuses more on diagnosis than on therapy.

What is the extent of the clinical problem of anemia? To answer this question, anemia must first be defined. In general terms, anemia is a reduction in the circulating red cell mass. In practical terms, anemia is defined by a reduction in the hematocrit, which is the percentage of red cells that make up the circulating blood volume or a reduction in the hemoglobin measured in g/dL. Obviously, the hematocrit goes hand in hand with the hemoglobin concentration and both are spuriously elevated in the case of dehydration. The hematocrit (as well as the hemoglobin) is a continuous laboratory variable, and the normal range depends on several factors including age, gender, and altitude:

- *Gender.* The World Health Organization criteria for anemia based on hemoglobin concentration use a cutoff of < 13 g/dL for adult men, < 12 g/dL for menstruating women, and < 11 g/dL for pregnant women. The difference in gender has been explained in part because of higher androgen levels in men, which stimulate RBC production.
- *Age.* The definition of anemia should be adjusted downward by roughly 1 g/dL in elderly men, ie, < 12 g/dL, and probably also in elderly women, ie, < 11 g/dL. The difference related to age may be due to both normal senescence of hematopoietic cells and, in the case of men, decreased androgen secretion. There is also the possibility of a higher incidence of underlying occult illnesses in the older population.
- *Altitude.* A higher altitude is associated with a higher normal range.

Disregarding all of these variables, the prevalence of anemia in the United States is up to 33% in the hospital setting

Two laboratory values other than hemoglobin and hematocrit that are indispensable in the evaluation of anemia are the mean cell volume (MCV) and the reticulocyte count. The MCV is the average size of the red cell, which is derived from the automated complete blood cell (CBC) count. The normal range is from 80 to 100 femtoliters (fL). Disorders deficient in hemoglobin understandably result in a decreased MCV (< 80 fL), ie, microcytosis, whereas disorders with an elevated MCV (< 100 fL), ie, macrocytosis, often reflect an inability of the red cell to fully mature because of a block in deoxyribonucleic acid (DNA) synthesis secondary to depletion of vitamin B_{12} or folate. Anemia associated with a normal MCV (normocytic RBCs) can reflect a systemic or marrow process that is inhibiting all phases of red cell development, thus resulting in decreased production with a normal RBC size. Occasionally a normocytic or macrocytic anemia is due to normal red cell production in the setting of acute blood loss or red cell destruction (hemolysis). This can be determined by the reticulocyte count. The reticulocyte count is the percentage of RBCs that stain as reticulated (having cytoplasmic inclusions of ribosomal and protein aggregates) cells by a supravital stain. An additional stain must be requested for this, ie, a specific test for the reticulocyte count apart from the automated CBC count. These young cells are larger than the older red cells. Consequently, their increase in the peripheral blood can increase the MCV from its baseline. The reticulocyte percentage must be corrected for the presence of anemia because it is spuriously elevated when the absolute number of RBCs is reduced and because reticulocytes released under clinical stress conditions have a longer life span than normal reticulocytes. The laboratory typically reports the reticulocyte count corrected for those reasons. Alternatively, the uncorrected percentage of reticulocytes can be multiplied by the RBC count—a value exceeding 100×10^9/L is consistent with acute blood loss or a hemolytic process.

ETIOLOGY AND DIFFERENTIAL DIAGNOSIS

Two very important points to remember about the pathophysiology of anemia are that a reduced red cell mass can be from essentially only two mechanisms—one central in terms of decreased production of the red cell mass, and the other peripheral in terms of increased destruction of the red cell mass or acute blood loss. The initial step in evaluating an anemic patient is to check the reticulocyte count. If the anemia is from decreased production, the reticulocyte count is normal or decreased. It is increased if the anemia is due to destruction or acute blood loss, that is, the response of a normal marrow to peripheral destruction or loss of the red cell mass wherein more of the "young," larger red cells are released—those red cells that still have ongoing protein synthesis and thus stain as reticulocytes. Figure 87-1 outlines the differential diagnosis of anemia, placing 25 to 30 conditions under the category of a decreased reticulocyte count (decreased production) and another ~25 conditions under the category of an increased reticulocyte count (increased destruction).

Anemias of Decreased Production—The Microcytic Anemias

Statistically, there are only a handful of anemias to consider that can be associated with a reduced MCV (wherein the reticulocyte count is reduced). The common pathway leading to decreased red cell production with small (ie, microcytic) red cells is a decrease in hemoglobin production:

Indirectly in terms of a decrease in iron

- Iron deficiency anemia, wherein there is an absolute decrease in iron, typically from gastrointestinal (GI) or menstrual blood loss
- Anemia of "chronic disease," wherein there is a decrease in free iron available for red cell production, one explanation being that the activated white cells of inflammation release a protein, lactoferrin, that binds to the iron. This reduces the iron available for hemoglobin synthesis and may be a mechanism for the anemia.

Directly in terms of a decrease in hemoglobin production despite available iron

- Thalassemia, an inherited defect in the gene coding for the α- or β-hemoglobin chains leads to decreased hemoglobin production
- Heavy metal poisoning such as lead poisoning, aluminum toxicity, or zinc excess with subsequent copper deficiency. These metals probably effect heme biosynthesis, thereby leading to decreased hemoglobin production.
- Sideroblastic anemia, the congenital form in particular, is characterized by a genetic defect in one of the enzymes involved in heme biosynthesis. The acquired form (often normocytic or macrocytic) can be secondary to alcohol or to antituberculous drugs.

Anemias of Decreased Production—The Normocytic Anemias

The peripheral blood smear can be very helpful in patients with a reduced reticulocyte count and a normal MCV. One reason may be that the anemia has more than one etiology, ie, it is a mixed anemia with one etiology a microcytic process such as iron deficiency, and another etiology a macrocytic process such as B_{12} deficiency that, in terms of the MCV, would then average out to a normal MCV.

A mixed anemia aside, the causes of a normocytic anemia can be broken down into either diseases within the bone marrow or diseases outside of the bone marrow such as inflammation or failure of the kidney, liver, or the endocrine organs. These disorders secondarily suppress red cell production of normal-sized red cells. It is worth making the distinction between a disease of the bone marrow and a disease outside of the bone marrow because once diseases outside the bone marrow are ruled out, a bone marrow examination should be considered.

Anemias secondary to diseases outside the bone marrow suppressing red cell production include the following:

- Anemia of renal failure, which is a major cause of a normocytic anemia. The kidney produces a growth hormone, erythropoietin, that is essential for normal red cell production. When the creatinine clearance decreases below ~40 mL/min, production of this hormone by the kidney begins to decrease, leading to the development of anemia.
- Anemia of chronic liver disease from multiple causes such as hypersplenism, variceal bleeding
- Anemia of endocrine failure (Addison disease, hypopituitarism, thyroid disease—usually hypothyroidism) can also lead to anemia because these various hormones (eg, androgens) usually have a stimulatory role in red-blood cell production.
- Anemia of chronic disease can be microcytic, as previously mentioned, but is often normocytic. Although anemia of chronic disease is the historic term for this condition, it is probably more helpful to refer to this as the "anemia of inflammation." It is not the disease itself that can cause anemia but the inflammatory component of the disease (as with chronic infection, collagen vascular disease, or malignancy) that accounts for the anemia by suppressing red cell production—in part from inflammatory cytokines such as interleukin-1, γ-interferon, and tumor necrosis factor, and in part by impairing iron utilization as previously mentioned.

The diseases that can cause a normocytic anemia that necessitates a bone marrow examination can be characterized further on the basis of the cellularity of the bone marrow specimen. If the bone marrow specimen shows more than the normal number of cells present in the marrow, ie, if it is hypercellular, then invariably the disease is a malignant process (though occasionally it can be a granulomatous infection), either a solid tumor metastasis to the bone marrow (termed "myelophthisic" anemia) or a malignant process of the hematopoietic or lymphatic system—acute or chronic lymphocytic or myelogenous leukemia, myelodysplastic syndrome (pre-leukemia), lymphoma, myeloma, or myeloid metaplasia with myelofibrosis. These infiltrating diseases crowd out normal red cell production and usually white cell and platelet production as well. One exception that may not present initially with associated platelet or white cell aberrations is the myelodysplastic syndrome (MDS); it can present as an isolated anemia. Furthermore, in several studies of hospitalized patients, after iron deficiency anemia, anemia from acute blood loss, anemia from renal failure, and anemia of chronic disease are ruled out, MDS is the next most likely diagnosis, particularly in the elderly patient. Thus, this condition deserves consideration in any anemic elderly patient but often such consideration is not made because MDS is a very difficult condition to understand, let alone diagnose. Part of the difficulty is that it is not a benign dysplastic disorder but a neoplastic disorder. It is a clonal disorder of hematopoiesis as in the case of the other primary hematologic malignant diseases previously mentioned, such as acute or chronic leukemia, lymphoma, and myeloma. In MDS, a clone at the level of the normal developing stem cell is present within the marrow. Over time it slowly expands, crowding out normal red cell and platelet production. In itself it does produce red cells, white cells, and platelets but not as

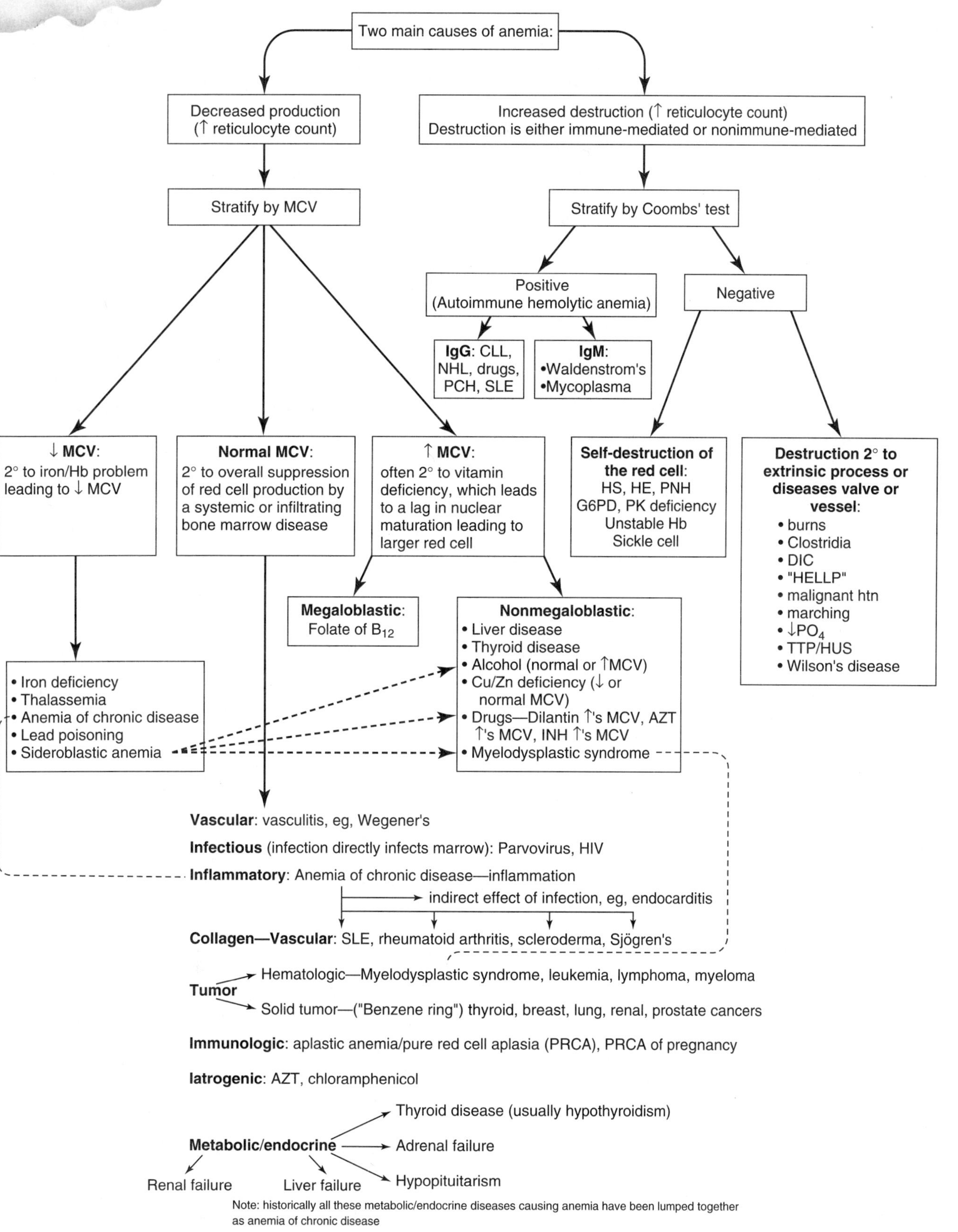

Figure 87-1. Differential diagnosis of anemia — "physiology leads to pathology approach to anemia." One anemia can be in more than one category, as shown with dotted lines.

effectively, hence the term "ineffective hematopoiesis." The morphologic manifestation is abnormal-appearing cells termed "dysplastic." Two implications are that (1) the initial laboratory manifestation will be a cytopenia, which typically involves the red cell series first, ie, as an isolated anemia, and that (2) the red cells, white cells, and platelets produced are not entirely normal because they arise from an abnormal clone. Hence, these patients may be prone in part to infection and bleeding because of respective white cell and platelet dysfunction. Infection is a major cause of death from MDS. Transformation to leukemia is the second most likely cause of death from MDS because the low-grade clonal expansion of the abnormal stem cell can lead in time to further genetic mutations and ultimately be clinically manifest as acute leukemia.

A hypocellular marrow that is associated only with a decrease in the cells of the erythroid lineage and not with the white cell- or platelet-producing lineage is termed pure red blood cell aplasia (PRCA). If it is associated with the absence of cells in all three lineages, it is termed "aplastic anemia," a very serious condition that can be either idiopathic (though typically thought to be immunologic) or secondary. Secondary causes of PRCA include collagen vascular disease, drug-induced (azathioprine, chloramphenicol, phenytoin, procainamide) disorders, lymphoproliferative disorders (particularly chronic lymphocytic leukemia or large granular lymphocyte leukemia), pregnancy, thymoma, and viral infections (Parvovirus B19, hepatitis). Collagen vascular diseases, drugs, chemicals such as benzene, and viral infections have also been associated with aplastic anemia.

Anemias of Decreased Production With Increased MCV—The Macrocytic Anemias

The six or seven causes of a macrocytic anemia can be easily subdivided into those causes secondary to vitamin B_{12} or folate deficiency (pathologically termed "megaloblastic") versus the other causes (nonmegaloblastic). Typically the MCV is markedly increased in vitamin deficiency (> 115 fL), whereas the macrocytosis of the non–vitamin deficiency states (alcohol use, chronic liver disease, drugs, hypothyroidism, MDS) typically is milder—in the 100- to 110-fL range.

The usual cause of folate deficiency is dietary. In the case of B_{12} deficiency, there are several causes that can be remembered best by understanding the physiology of B_{12} metabolism. The initial step is the dietary intake of B_{12}, thus, strict vegetarianism over a 10- to 15-year period can be a cause. The B_{12} then is liberated into a free form in the stomach by its acidic environment, hence H_2 blocker use can be a cause. The stomach also produces a protein called "intrinsic factor," which is responsible for the absorption of B_{12}. Major loss of stomach tissue as in the case of a total or partial gastrectomy can be causative, as can be pernicious anemia (PA), the specific autoimmune-mediated destruction of the intrinsic factor-producing parietal cells. While B_{12} is liberated by the acidic environment in the stomach and then passes through the jejunum, further release of its bound form by pancreatic enzymes occur, therefore, chronic pancreatic insufficiency can be a cause of deficiency. Also, bacterial overgrowth from blind loops or diverticula or fish tapeworm in the jejunum compete with the host for the B_{12}. Absorption takes place in the presence of intrinsic factor in the terminal ileum. Malabsorption (that can also cause folate deficiency) can be from numerous causes such as Crohn disease, Whipple disease, tropical sprue, celiac disease, radiation ileitis, and infiltrative diseases such as lymphoma or scleroderma.

The non–vitamin deficiency macrocytic anemias often are misdiagnosed initially as B_{12} or folate deficiency. A patient with a macrocytic anemia with a borderline low vitamin level may be started on folate or B_{12} injections without any further consideration for confirming the underlying cause of either folate or B_{12} deficiency. The clinician may observe after several months that the anemia is not responding to the vitamin supplementation.

Finally, certain drugs, particularly chemotherapy drugs, as well as the antiretroviral drug, azidothymidine, can cause a macrocytic anemia, typically a macrocytosis without much of an anemia. Chemotherapy drugs can increase the MCV significantly in the range of B_{12} or folate deficiency. Two other drugs to mention under the heading of macrocytic anemia are phenytoin and sulfasalazine, which can interfere with folate absorption.

Anemia of Increased Destruction—The Hemolytic Anemias

The anemias of increased destruction do not occur as frequently as those of decreased production, although they include several that necessitate long-term primary care, such as sickle cell anemia and hereditary spherocytosis. The two major categories of hemolytic anemias are immune-mediated and non–immune-mediated anemias.

Immune Mediated Hemolytic Anemias—Autoimmune Hemolytic Anemias

The autoantibody causing the hemolysis can be either an IgG (warm) or, less commonly, an IgM (cold). IgG-mediated hemolysis occurs via phagocytosis by splenic macrophages (extravascular hemolysis) engulfing part of the IgG-coated red cell membrane with each successive pass through the spleen wherein the red cell may re-seal each time, resulting in a spherical-shaped cell—a spherocyte. On the other hand, IgM-mediated hemolysis occurs in the intravascular compartment because this antibody is capable of fixing complement at a temperature < 37°C and lysing the red cell without the help of the splenic macrophages. Making the distinction between extravascular and intravascular hemolysis has implications in terms of diagnosis and therapy. The indices of hemolysis (the red cell breakdown products lactate dehydrogenase [LDH], serum glutamic-oxaloacetic transaminase [SGOT], hemoglobin) are more pronounced for the same degree of hemolysis in cold autoimmune hemolytic anemias (AIHA) compared to warm AIHA. In the latter, these products are absorbed within the spleen without much spillover into the plasma. Splenectomy would also have a therapeutic role in warm AIHA in contrast to cold AIHA.

In about 50% of cases of IgG- or IgM-mediated AIHA, an underlying cause is observed such as a lymphoproliferative disorder (chronic lymphocytic leukemia [CLL], lymphoma, Waldenstrom [IgM] macroglobulinemia), infection (usually the antibody is an IgM as in *Mycoplasma pneumoniae* or Epstein-Barr virus infection, rarely it is IgG and termed "paroxysmal cold hemoglobinuria," related to syphilis or certain viral infections), collagen vascular disease (lupus), delayed transfusion reaction, or drugs (IgG autoantibodies secondary to drugs such as quinidine, procainamide, penicillin, or Aldomet).

Non–Immune-Mediated Hemolytic Anemias

Non–immune-mediated hemolytic anemias can be further subdivided into intrinsic red cell defects or processes extrinsic to the red cell that are responsible for red cell destruction. In the case of non–immune-mediated hemolysis secondary to an intrinsic red cell defect (ie, the red cell is fragile), these conditions can be thought of in terms of their localization in relation to the various components of the red cell.

Disorders Involving the Red Cell Membrane. Disorders involving the red cell membrane include congenital disorders characterized by certain red cell shape changes. Hereditary spherocytosis (HS) is more common than hereditary elliptocytosis or hereditary stomatocytosis. HS is usually an autosomal dominant disorder. The explanation for the change in the red cell from its normal discoid appearance to a spherical shape is usually because of a deficiency in spectrin. This protein is like a girder holding up a canopy. In hereditary spherocytosis, there is a genetic deficiency in the production of this protein or the proteins that maintain this girder (eg, ankyrin, band 3 protein) and so in turn the canopy collapses, leading to a decrease in the surface to volume ratio. This spherical property (morphologically expressed as a spherocyte) confers a susceptibility to sequestration and destruction in the spleen. An acquired membrane disorder is paroxysmal nocturnal hemoglobinuria (PNH). This hemolytic disorder is secondary to a deficiency in a glycolipid anchor of the membrane that leads to a loss of several proteins on the red cell membrane including a group of proteins that inhibits complement-mediated lysis of the red cell. This lysis is favored by an acidic environment, hence the classic description of red urine upon morning awakening because of the relative acidosis that ensues during sleep from hypoventilation.

Disorders of the Cytoplasm. Disorders of the cytoplasm, eg, congenital deficiency of the glucose-6-phosphate dehydrogenase (G6PD) enzyme or one of the approximately 15 other red cell enzymes can lead to a decrease in the normal reducing power (ie, the level of NADH/NADPH is depleted) of the red cell and subsequent increased susceptibility to hemolysis in the setting of oxidative stress.

Disorders of Hemoglobin Structure. Sickle cell anemia is the classic example of a disorder of hemoglobin structure. Its genetic basis is a one-nucleotide mutation, which then codes for a different amino acid in the β-chain of the hemoglobin molecule. It is that one amino acid alone that changes the structural quality of the hemoglobin protein into one that can polymerize under hypoxic or acidic conditions with subsequent hemolysis or entrapment of the irreversibly sickled red cell. The latter leads to vasoocclusion and ischemic pain. Far less common hemoglobin disorders that can be associated with hemolytic anemia are the unstable hemoglobins and the toxic hemoglobinopathies. The unstable hemoglobins are congenital disorders in which the hemoglobin molecules are susceptible to oxidative denaturation leading to the conversion of hemoglobin to methemoglobin. Hemoglobin is also susceptible to oxidative denaturation if an agent (eg, dapsone, sulfasalazine, chloroquine) is ingested that can directly oxidize it or if a congenital deficiency of the enzyme methemoglobin reductase is present.

Disorders Outside the Red Cell. The last group of non– immune-mediated hemolytic anemias are those from a process extrinsic to the red cell. In these disorders, the red cell is normal but becomes an innocent bystander. Red cell destruction can be either from an infectious agent (Bartonella, babesiosis, or clostridia as in the classic setting of sepsis after an illegal abortion), trauma (marathon running—march hemoglobinuria or foot-strike hemolysis), metabolic perturbation (hypophosphatemia), or an abnormal heart valve or vessel (microangiopathic hemolysis) causing red cell fragmentation. In the case of a fragmentation-hemolysis anemia, patients with prosthetic valves, particularly mechanical valves in the aortic position, are at greatest risk for hemolysis. Hemolysis secondary to abnormal vessels occurs in the setting of any process that can decrease the lumen of the vessel in the microcirculation. The red cell must be able to bend through the microcirculation where the capillary diameter can be less than the diameter of the red cell. If the lumen is further narrowed by an inflammatory process, as in the case of vasculitis, eclampsia, or malignant hypertension, or if the narrowing is because of the development of intravascular thrombi, as seen in hemolytic uremic syndrome, thrombotic thrombocytopenic purpura, or disseminated intravascular coagulation, red cell fragmentation and hemolytic anemia may ensue. Examination of the peripheral blood shows red cells that have been injured because the passage through this narrow lumen leads to the appearance of fragmented red cells (schistocytes).

HISTORY

The following information may help when the history is taken:

- History of present illness. The classic common symptoms are fatigue, shortness of breath particularly with exertion, lightheadedness or dizziness, tinnitus, and palpitations. Less common complaints include a whirring or humming sensation in the head (probably from rapid blood flow through the cranial arteries), loss of libido, inability to concentrate, change in mood, and change in sleep pattern. The onset of symptoms is acute if the cause is acute blood loss or hemolysis, although mild hemolytic disorders like HS can be associated with a gradual onset of symptoms. History that can suggest a specific diagnosis should also be sought:
- Craving (pica) for substances such as ice (pagophagia) or substances not usually ingested such as venetian blind dust (coniophagia) or toothpicks (xylophagia) should suggest iron deficiency. Over 50 substances have been cataloged in the medical literature.
- History of acute blood loss or recent blood donation
- History of scleral icterus would suggest a hemolytic disorder such as HS.
- History of vegetarianism, paresthesia, ataxia, or cognitive changes suggests B_{12} deficiency.
- History of GI complaints suggests blood loss and iron deficiency; a history of GI disease such as sprue or Crohn disease suggests folate or B_{12} deficiency.
- Past medical history. Particularly if the patient has a normocytic anemia, a history for an inflammatory condition (collagen vascular disease, malignancy, or chronic infection) or organ failure (renal, liver, adrenal, pituitary, thyroid) should be sought. A history of gallstones suggests a chronic hemolytic disorder such as HS.
- Family history. The patient should be asked about family members with any of the congenital anemias—thalassemia, sideroblastic anemia, HS, sickle cell anemia, or G6PD deficiency.
- Social history. Alcohol use can be associated with anemia of liver disease, sideroblastic anemia, or GI blood loss.
- Medication use. Certain drugs are associated with certain subsets of anemia (primarily hemolytic anemia or production defects) as mentioned earlier in the section on etiology and differential diagnosis. Iron deficiency anemia can be secondary to nonsteroidal drug-induced gastritis.

PHYSICAL EXAMINATION

The physical examination covers the following areas:

- *Vital signs*. Tachycardia and bounding pulse pressure are nonspecific findings.
- *HEENT*. The word anemia is derived from a Greek word meaning "without blood," so obviously a pale appearance is typical. In people with dark pigmentation, this often is not readily apparent, so an additional helpful laboratory finding is obtained by examining the conjunctivae. The sclera should also be examined for icterus, which suggests a hemolytic disorder. Retinal hemorrhages can be associated with severe anemia or anemia with thrombocytopenia as in acute leukemia.
- *Lymph nodes*. Palpable nodes should increase suspicion for lymphoma or CLL associated with AIHA or for a solid tumor malignancy associated with anemia of chronic disease or a myelophthisic anemia.
- *Cardiopulmonary*. A systolic ejection murmur may be present and an S_3 can be noted if the anemia has led to cardiac failure.
- *Abdomen*. Splenomegaly suggests HS, lymphoma, hypersplenism, or warm AIHA.
- *Rectal*. Stool testing for occult blood should be a mandatory part of the physical examination given the fact that iron deficiency caused by blood loss is the most common cause of anemia.
- *Extremities*. Peripheral edema may be a nonspecific finding.
- *Skin and integument*. Progressive iron deficiency or B_{12} anemia also leads to deficiency of iron or B_{12} in the normal epithelial tissues. Iron and B_{12} are needed as cofactors for certain enzymes that maintain normal cellular functions, and their deficiency can account for spooning of the nails (koilonychia) seen occasionally in very chronic iron deficiency, breakdown of the epithelium at the juncture of the lips (cheilosis), and loss of the normal fissura of the tongue (glossitis) seen primarily in B_{12} deficiency. B_{12} deficiency can also be associated with vitiligo if the cause of the deficiency is PA.
- *Neurologic*. Testing for position sense, vibration, and ataxia should be done because B_{12} deficiency can lead demyelination as well as anemia. It has been reported that patients with B_{12} deficiency can first present with such neurologic signs and symptoms prior to the development of a macrocytic anemia.

LABORATORY STUDIES

1. Note on the hemogram whether the hematocrit is decreased; if it is, then look at the MCV because statistically the most common causes of anemia are those that decrease the MCV by reducing the amount of hemoglobin directly, as in thalassemia, or indirectly, as in iron deficiency.
2. Examine the peripheral blood smear (laboratory technicians are usually helpful and willing to assist) and obtain a reticulocyte count in further consideration of anemias of decreased production or increased destruction.

The associated morphologic abnormalities noted in the peripheral blood smear are shown in Table 87-1. They are often recorded as part of the CBC and differential. Figure 87-2 outlines additional laboratory tests that allow the cause to be precisely pinpointed from about 50 conditions capable of causing anemia.¯

Laboratory Evaluation of the Microcytic Anemias

Tests for iron deficiency should be done first in this subset. If old records can be located and long-standing microcytosis is noted for > 1 year or from childhood, then one could possibly first do a hemoglobin (Hb) electrophoresis in thinking of β-thalassemia trait and the characteristic pattern of an increase in the minor adult hemoglobin (HbA_2) and the fetal hemoglobin (HbF). α-Thalassemia, however, cannot be diagnosed by electrophoresis. That diagnosis depends on finding other family members with a similar microcytic anemia or on studies of globin synthesis in peripheral blood reticulocytes or gene-mapping techniques. If both iron studies and Hb electrophoresis and family history for α-thalassemia are nonrevealing, then the anemia of chronic disease should be considered. There should be adequate clinical or laboratory evidence for inflammation, and the serum ferritin must be elevated (although coincidental iron deficiency can lower the level to the 20- to 100-ng/mL range). Next, a free erythrocyte protoporphyrin level should be measured for consideration of lead poisoning if there is an appropriate clinical setting. If the diagnosis remains in doubt, a bone marrow examination should be done. The diagnosis of sideroblastic anemia may be established if red cell precursors in the bone marrow stain for deposits of iron in a perinuclear pattern.

Table 87-1. Peripheral Blood Cell Abnormalities in Relation to Categories of Anemia

MICROCYTIC ANEMIA	NORMOCYTIC ANEMIA	MACROCYTIC ANEMIA	COOMBS NEGATIVE HEMOLYTIC ANEMIA	COOMBS POSITIVE HEMOLYTIC ANEMIA
Hypochromia in Fe deficiency, thalassemia	*Burr cells (echinocytes)* in renal failure	*Macroovalocytes, hypersegmented WBCs*, B_{12} or folate deficiency	*Spherocytes* in HS *Elliptocytes* in HE	*Spherocytes* in warm AIHA
Target cells in thalassemia	*Spur cells (acanthocytes)* and/or *target cells* in liver disease		*Bite cells* in G6PD deficiency	*Rouleaux* in AIHA 2° to cold-reacting antibodies, eg, mycoplasma, Waldenstrom
Basophilic stippling in lead toxicity	*Basophilic stippling, Pelger-Huet-like cells, (hypolobulated WBC), giant or agranular platelets* all dysplastic features that are occasionally seen in MDS *Tear drop cells* in myeloid metaplasia with myelofibrosis		*Red-cell fragments (schistocytes)* in TTP/HUS, DIC, preeclampsia, malignant hypertension, prosthetic valve related hemolysis *sickled cells*, as in sickle cell anemia	

AIHA, autoimmune hemolytic anemia; *DIC*, disseminated intravascular coagulation; *Fe*, iron; *G6PD*, glucose-6-phosphate dehydrogenase; *HE*, hereditary elliptocytosis; *HS*, hereditary spherocytosis; *MDS*, myelodysplastic syndrome; *TTP/HUS*, thrombotic thrombocytopenic purpura/hemolytic uremic syndrome; *WBC*, white blood cell.

The iron tests usually done to diagnose iron deficiency anemia include serum iron, the total iron binding capacity (TIBC), percentage of transferrin saturation (serum iron divided by the TIBC), and the serum ferritin. The typical pattern is a reduced serum iron, increased TIBC, decreased transferrin saturation, and reduced serum ferritin. Hematologists are often asked by general practitioners whether they need to do all these tests or whether they can just order one test such as a serum iron or a serum ferritin. If the patient does not have any other ongoing medical condition—particularly one that can be inflammatory such as malignancy, infection, or collagen vascular disease—it is probably adequate just to check the serum ferritin. What is clearly insufficient is just to draw the serum iron. It can vary widely over a day, based on a recent meal, for example. It can be low in the anemia of chronic disease despite normal or increased body iron. It is also insufficient for the clinician to begin iron replacement therapy without further studies to find the actual cause of the iron deficiency. Again, the common theme that arises here is that anemia, in this case iron deficiency anemia, is not a disease in itself. In women with microcytic anemia seemingly out of proportion to menses (ie, a hematocrit < 36%), a GI lesion must be considered, but if the history is of very heavy menses in the setting of a hematocrit < 36%, it might be reasonable to first give iron and see if the hematocrit normalizes and remains stable before embarking on a GI work-up. There are no critical studies on which to base firm recommendations regarding this situation.

Laboratory Evaluation of the Normocytic Anemias

The first step that should be taken in this category is to look at the white blood cell (WBC) count and platelet count (PC) recorded with the hematocrit on the CBC. If the WBC or PC or both are abnormal, a bone marrow examination probably should be done next. If only anemia is present, the peripheral blood should be reviewed to rule out a mixed anemia, iron deficiency plus folate, or B_{12} deficiency wherein the MCV averages out. Before the peripheral blood smear is looked at for evidence of the elliptical or hypochromic cells of iron deficiency mixed with the large oval red cells and hypersegmented neutrophils of B_{12} or folate deficiency, a clue can be found in the red cell distribution width (RDW) that is reported on the CBC. In such a mixed anemia, it should be increased. After ruling out a mixed anemia, the next step should be obtaining serum chemistries (liver function tests, serum creatinine with an erythropoietin level to confirm anemia of renal failure if the creatinine is increased) followed by endocrine testing (such as thyroid-stimulating hormone) as well as iron studies because anemia of chronic disease can present with normocytic indices. Finally, a bone marrow examination should be done if all the previous serum studies are within normal limits (WNL). Even if the WBC and PC are WNL, a myelodysplastic syndrome can present as an isolated anemia as previously mentioned. A bone marrow aspirate in consideration of MDS:

- Has more cells than a peripheral blood sample to examine for the characteristic morphologic abnormalities (dysplasia) of this disorder
- Could be sent also for cytogenetic analysis because up to half of the cases have a confirmatory cytogenetic abnormality
- Can be examined for the percent of blasts for purposes of prognosis. Marrows with increased percent of blasts portend a worse prognosis as the percentage reflects a higher probability of progression to acute leukemia.

Laboratory Evaluation of a Macrocytic Anemia

A serum vitamin B_{12} and serum folate level should be drawn. In the case of folate, the RBC folate level is more sensitive than the serum levels, but for practical reasons, most laboratories first do a serum folate level. A hemolytic anemia or GI bleed should be considered because the associated increased reticulocyte count also increases the MCV, albeit mildly. The clinician should at the very least ask the hematology laboratory to review the peripheral blood smear for the characteristic macroovalocytes and hypersegmented polymorphonuclear (PMN) leukocytes. It is often said that the presence of just one 6-lobed PMN or 5% of 5-lobed PMNs is consistent with the diagnosis of B_{12} or folate deficiency. If these findings are absent, the causes of a falsely low B_{12} level must be considered: multiple myeloma, oral contraceptive intake, folate deficiency, and pregnancy. If these causes are absent, then serology supportive for pernicious anemia can be drawn (an antiintrinsic factor antibody, antiparietal cell antibody). Historically, a Schilling test was first done, but this is done less frequently although a recent study showed an alarmingly poor positive predictive value of 20% for a low B_{12} value.

If both folate and B_{12} levels are normal, a TSH level evaluates for hypothyroidism and serum chemistries assess liver disease, either of which can be the cause of macrocytic anemia. Again, it is emphasized that non–vitamin deficiency-related microcytic anemias have only a mild macrocytosis (100 to 110 fL) compared to the marked macrocytosis (< 115 fL) of B_{12} or folate deficiency. MDS can present as a macrocytic anemia, therefore, a bone marrow examination should be done after ruling out the above causes of a macrocytic anemia.

Laboratory Evaluation of a Hemolytic Anemia

If the anemic patient's reticulocyte count, as mentioned previously, is increased, a hemolytic work-up should commence, starting with a direct Coombs test. Its sensitivity is ~ 90%. Reviewing the peripheral blood smear for spherocytes is helpful. They are still seen in that ~ 10% subset of AIHA with a negative direct Coombs test. The direct Coombs test involves adding a mixture of antibodies—IgG (gamma Coombs reagent) and complement (non-gamma reagent)—that react to the red cell suspension. In autoimmune hemolytic anemia, reaction with a mixture of these reagents leads to agglutination of the red cells, which is viewed as a positive test. The gamma and non-gamma reagents are then reacted with the patient's red cells separately. If it is an autoimmune hemolytic anemia from the production of IgG (warm-acting) antibody, the gamma reagent and usually the non-gamma reagent as well give a positive test for agglutination. Less commonly, the patient has a hemolytic anemia not because of the production of an IgG antibody but because of the production of an IgM (cold-reacting) antibody. In such a case, the gamma Coombs test is negative but the non-gamma Coombs test is positive.

Because of the frequent association of AIHA with a lymphoproliferative disorder, particularly in the older patient, some hematologists often proceed with a bone marrow examination to rule out a lymphoproliferative disorder. Serologies for EBV or *Mycoplasma* infection are reasonable in the setting of cold AIHA if there is a consistent history.

If the Coombs test is negative, it is imperative to review the peripheral blood smear. The presence of spherocytes suggests hereditary spherocytosis (besides a false-negative direct Coombs test). An osmotic fragility test would be the confirmatory test in HS. If there

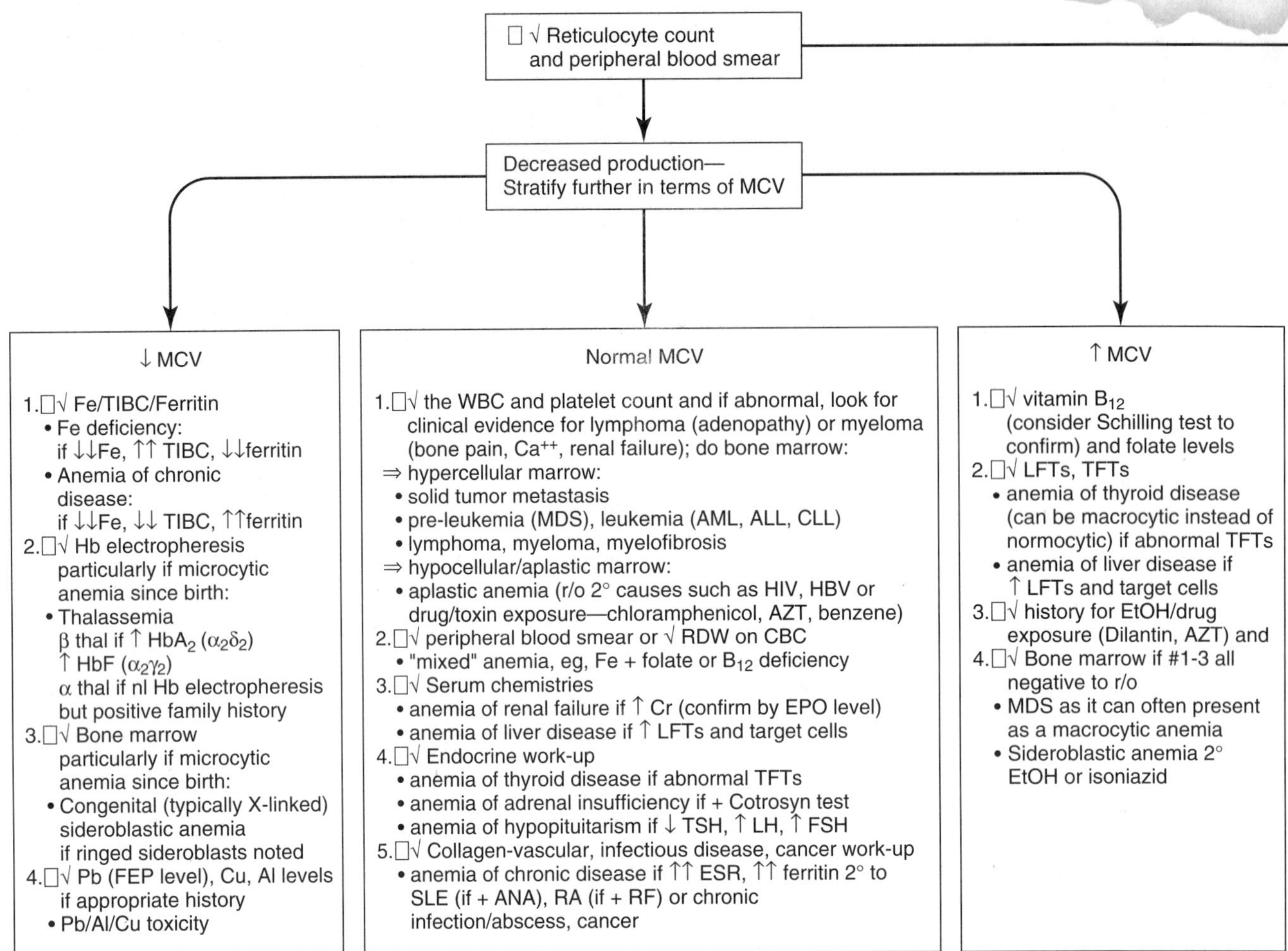

Figure 87–2. Laboratory evaluation of anemia starting from the mean cell volume and reticulocyte count.

are no spherocytes, paroxysmal nocturnal hemoglobinuria should be another membrane disorder to consider. A sucrose water hemolysis or acidified Ham test may be diagnostic particularly if the patient has pancytopenia, unexplained thrombosis, or recurrent abdominal pain. If there are sickled cells, a Hb electrophoresis should be done. If there are "bite" cells or if the previous tests are negative, a Heinz body test should be done. This would be positive in the setting of oxidative denaturation leading to hemolysis either from a RBC enzyme deficiency such as G6PD deficiency (G6PD screen should be done to confirm), an unstable hemoglobin, or methemoglobin reductase deficiency. An isopropanol instability test or the heat instability test establishes the presence of an unstable hemoglobin.

If fragmented or torn red cells are noted, the various causes of a microangiopathic anemia should be considered, including the hemolytic uremic syndrome (HUS) or thrombotic thrombocytopenic purpura (TTP). The presence of fragmented red cells in a patient with a prosthetic valve should prompt a transesophageal echocardiogram to rule out valve dysfunction.

In either a Coombs positive or Coombs negative hemolytic anemia, serum chemistries to gauge the severity of the hemolysis should also be drawn as outlined in Table 87-2. In intravascular hemolysis, ie, the Coombs negative hemolytic anemias, the LDH, SGOT, and indirect bilirubin are higher and the serum haptoglobin lower than in the extravascular hemolysis, ie, Coombs positive hemolytic anemias.

MANAGEMENT AND TREATMENT

Treatment of anemia involves treating the underlying cause.

Iron Deficiency Anemia

For iron deficiency anemia, 50 mg of elemental iron (325 mg in the sulfate form) is prescribed three to four times per day with a maximal absorption occurring 2 hours after a meal when there is a less acidic environment. An adequate response is a rise in the hemoglobin by > 2 g/dL in 2 to 3 weeks. A common clinical problem related to iron therapy is GI symptoms, including constipation. An attempt can be made to switch to the ferrous gluconate formula 300 mg orally three times per day, although unfortunately it is not associated with as much free elemental iron. Also, trying iron sulfate in the elixir form may help the intolerance if the main problem is swallowing pills. An occasional patient cannot tolerate any oral formulation of iron and therefore is a candidate for weekly intramuscular (IM) iron. A maximum of 100 mg at one time can be given once a week. Often the iron deficit is

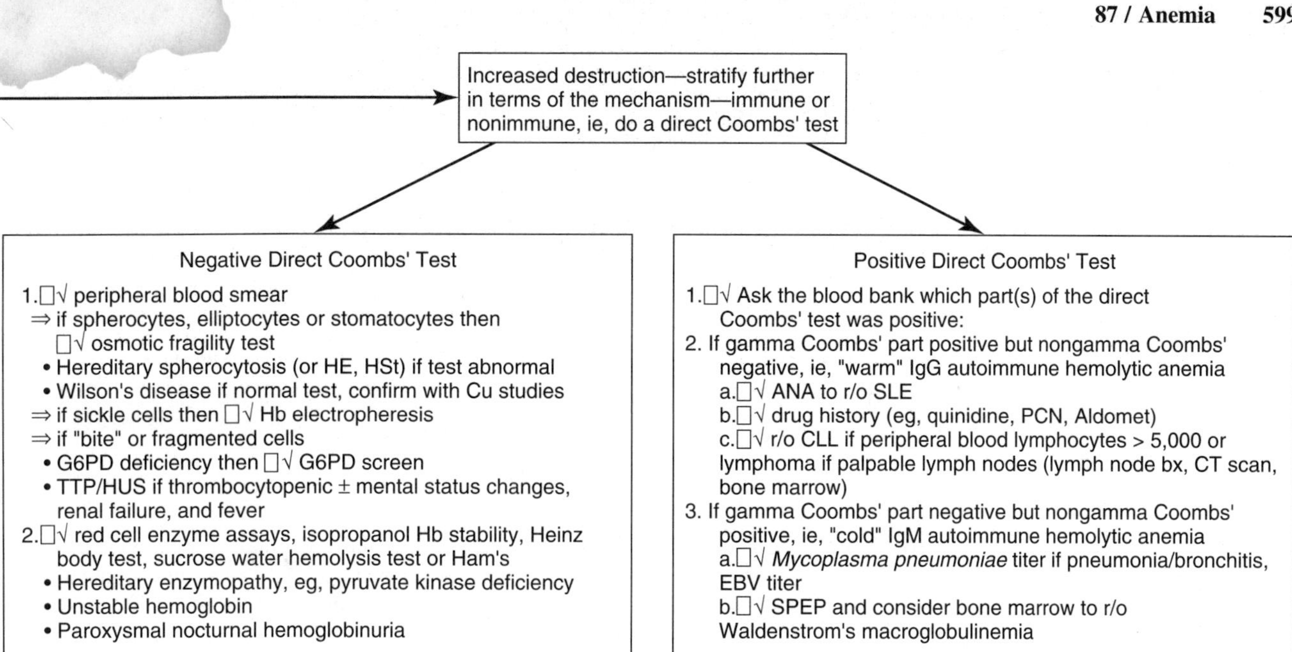

Figure 87–2. (Continued.)

about 1000 mg or more, so there is the inconvenience of numerous visits and the discomfort of the injection. Alternatively, the total iron deficit can be calculated and given as intravenous (IV) iron dextran (Imferon) over 4 hours. The total deficit is calculated as follows:

$$\text{mg of iron} = 0.3 \times \text{weight (lb)} \times \left(100 - \frac{\text{Hb} \times 100}{14.8}\right)$$

The risk of anaphylaxis is about 1 in 1000 patients, so a test dose is advised, but anaphylaxis is idiosyncratic.

Thalassemia

Management of thalassemia requires regular red cell transfusions for thalassemia major to maintain normal growth and development. This is at the price of iron overload, which develops after 10 to 20 units of RBCs. Such patients invariably need iron chelation with the subcutaneous (SQ) iron chelator desferrioxamine. There has been expanding use of allogeneic bone marrow transplantation for thalassemia major primarily in Europe. No specific therapy is needed for thalassemia trait although, because the diagnosis of α-thalassemia trait is one of exclusion and can masquerade as iron deficiency, iron should not be empirically prescribed for a microcytic anemia.

Anemia of Renal Failure

The successful use of erythropoietin in the correction of the anemia of renal failure has heralded a major advance—the use of the recombinant hematopoietic growth factors for hematologic disorders. Erythropoietin is given SQ 1 to 3 times a week. The usual starting dose is 50 units/kg SQ. The anemia of renal failure is corrected in most dialysis-dependent patients. In those not yet requiring dialysis and with still some endogenous erythropoietin production, lower or less frequent dosing may be sufficient.

Myelodysplastic Syndrome

Because myelodysplastic syndrome is a clonal bone marrow disorder that originates in the stem cell, no chemotherapy can permanently eradicate the clone with restoration of normal hematopoiesis. Furthermore, because this is a condition primarily of older patients, the emphasis is on supportive care: transfusing red cells as necessary and treating infections with antibiotics. If there are recurrent infections, a trial with granulocyte colony stimulating factor (G-CSF) or granulocyte-macrophage colony–stimulating factor (GM-CSF) can be effective in increasing the WBC. About one fifth of patients respond to SQ erythropoietin.

Pure Red Cell Aplasia or Aplastic Anemia

Pure red cell aplasia or aplastic anemia is a presumed immunologic disorder that may respond to treatment with steroids and cyclosporine plus antithymocyte globulin. If there is a sibling who is histocompatible and the patient is under 50 to 60 years of age, then an allogeneic bone marrow transplant is preferable.

Anemias of Decreased Production—Macrocytic Anemia

Vitamin B_{12} deficiency requires life-long repletion unless the patient has B_{12} deficiency from decreased gastric secretion secondary to H_2 blockers. The route is usually IM, but the SQ route is just as effective. Some clinicians have even tried oral vitamin B_{12}. This is not as efficacious as the parenteral route because the majority of B_{12}-deficient patients have impaired absorption either directly because of bowel disease or indirectly through the lack of intrinsic

Table 87-2. Laboratory Features of Extra- and Intravascular Hemolysis

	EXTRAVASCULAR HEMOLYSIS	INTRAVASCULAR HEMOLYSIS	
	Warm AIHA (eg, autoantibody is IgG)	Cold AIHA (eg, autoantibody is IgM)	Nonimmune hemolytic anemia (eg, HS, PNH, G6PD deficiency, Sickle cell dz, TTP/HUS)
Direct Coombs test	⊕ gamma Coombs/ ± non-gamma Coombs	–gamma Coombs/ ⊕ non-gamma Coombs	—
LDH	N or ↑	↑↑↑	↑↑↑
Haptoglobin	N or ↓	↓↓	↓↓
Urine hemosiderin	—	Occasionally ⊕	Occasionally ⊕

AIHA, autoimmune hemolytic anemia; *Dz,* disease; *G6PD,* glucose-6-phosphate dehydrogenase; *HS,* hereditary spherocytosis; *IgG,* immunoglobulin G; *IgM,* immunoglobulin M; *LDH,* lactate dehydrogenase; *PNH,* paroxysmal nocturnal nemuglobinuria; *TTP/HUS,* thrombotic thrombocytopenic purpura/hemolytic uremic syndrome.

factor. Initially, treatment is given at 1 mg/d IM SQ for 1 week, then twice a week for 1 week, then weekly for a month, and then monthly indefinitely. In the case of folate deficiency, 1 to 5 mg of oral folate per day is advised. It is important to note the potential dangers of administering folate if vitamin B_{12} deficiency have not been ruled out. The folate replacement may correct the hematologic abnormality as the folate bypasses the B_{12} deficiency within the bone marrow but it does *not* correct the neurologic deficit, which typically gets worse on folate.

Autoimmune Hemolytic Anemia

In the case of AIHA, the mainstay of therapy is corticosteroids at a dose of 1 to 2 mg/kg/d of prednisone. One third of patients do not achieve a durable remission and so the next step is splenectomy. If that fails, trials of immunosuppressive agents such as azathioprine, cyclosporine, or intravenous IgG have met with varying success. In cases of severe anemia, plasmapheresis may be tried. Generally it works poorly for an IgG-mediated autoimmune hemolytic anemia as opposed to an IgM because much of the IgG antibody is in the extravascular space.

Sickle Cell Anemia

Management of patients with sickle cell anemia could warrant a whole book in itself. The mainstay of treatment for vasoocclusive crisis has been supportive and includes a combination of hydration, oxygenation, and pain management. Partial exchange transfusion (eg, phlebotomize 500 mL whole blood, then infuse 300 mL normal saline, then phlebotomize another 500 mL whole blood followed by two to three units packed RBC transfusion) to reduce the HbS to < 30% is indicated in the approximately 25% of patients who develop stroke and the approximately 30% who develop vasoocclusion in the lungs (acute chest syndrome) and occasionally preoperatively. Unfortunately, generally there has been no benefit in exchange transfusion for the most common complication of sickle cell disease—vasoocclusive pain crisis. Painful crisis that necessitates a hospitalization is best managed with continuous-infusion morphine with dose adjustment by the patient (patient-controlled analgesia) as opposed to the historic practice of administering either morphine or meperidine (Demerol) IM on an as needed basis.

Recently, prospective studies have shown benefit from the use of agents to reduce the frequency of vasoocclusion by raising the level of fetal hemoglobin. An example is hydroxyurea, which actually is a chemotherapy drug. Based on an approximately 50% reduction in vasoocclusive episodes in a recent National Institutes of Health (NIH)-sponsored double-blind placebo-controlled randomized trial of hydroxyurea, an NIH Clinic Alert has been issued informing clinicians who care for these patients that hydroxyurea may have a considerable beneficial impact. However, the potential long-term toxicity is not known. Because this is a drug that inhibits enzymes in the bone marrow cells, there has been some concern, mostly theoretical, that it could lead to stem cell injury and the development of secondary leukemia. At this point, without long-term toxicity follow-up, it is difficult to advocate hydroxyurea for all patients with sickle cell anemia but certainly it appears to be indicated for patients whose quality of life has been significantly impaired because of recurrent vasoocclusive crises.

Theoretically, sickle cell anemia could be prevented through the use of genetic screening. In the United States, the gene frequency for sickle cell anemia among African Americans is quite high, roughly 8%. As such, statistically there is a 1 in 12 chance that an African American will have a single gene defect, ie, sickle cell trait, and, in turn, there is 1 in 640 chance that two such patients who marry and have a child with sickle cell anemia. Prenatal screening can be done by chorionic villus sampling or amniocentesis.

Patients with sickle cell trait are not anemic. Furthermore, they rarely have any complication of vasoocclusion except for three relatively unusual situations: (1) strenuous exercise at high altitudes, which has been associated with sudden death; (2) acute papillary necrosis, which can be associated with sickle cell trait because the acidic hypoxic environment of the renal collection system can favor sickling; and (3) pain from vasoocclusion, which can develop in joints with underlying inflammation such as rheumatoid arthritis.

Toxic Hemoglobinopathy

The use of methylene blue, 1 to 2 mg/kg IV, is effective in reducing methemoglobin to hemoglobin.

Anemia Secondary to Valve or Microangiopathic Hemolysis

The therapy for TTP or HUS involves plasmapheresis and in the case of TTP, it has reduced mortality from > 80% to ~ 20%.

CONSIDERATIONS IN PREGNANCY

In general terms, RBC transfusions are advised if the hematocrit is < 25% in the third trimester.

Iron Deficiency Anemia

Iron deficiency is very common in pregnancy. In socioeconomically disadvantaged patients, the prevalence reaches 50%; it is up to 80% in developing countries. A recent U.S. task force has not advised universal iron supplementation in pregnant patients because it is not certain that iron supplementation clearly favorably effects infant or maternal morbidity and mortality. However, the standard of care has been to prescribe 30 to 60 mg of elemental iron daily.

Folate Deficiency

Folate deficiency can be an endemic cause of anemia in certain areas in the world where folate supplements are not prescribed routinely. Its presence can also obscure the diagnosis of associated iron deficiency because the combination of these two could lead to normal MCV.

Pure Red Cell Aplasia and Aplastic Anemia

There are about 30 reports of pure red cell aplasia and aplastic anemia in pregnancy. In a laboratory model, ferrets that are in estrus can develop AA, which suggests that excess estrogen can inhibit red cell production.

Autoimmune Hemolytic Anemia

Autoimmue hemolytic anemia can present during pregnancy because autoimmune diseases are relatively common among young women. Management is the same as in non-pregnant patients, initially with corticosteroids.

Sickle Cell Anemia

The management of sickle cell disease in pregnancy is controversial. Specifically, it is not clear if all patients should undergo prophylactic red cell exchange transfusion to reduce the percentage of HbS. Close supportive care is mandatory because of the increased incidence of sickling complications in pregnancy such as acute chest syndrome and stroke as well as other complications such as preeclampsia and urinary tract infections with sepsis. Even with close management, fetal outcome is impaired with increased rates of prematurity, decreased birth weight, and 30% risk of fetal wastage. High-dose folate supplementation (5 mg per day) is indicated to prevent megaloblastic arrest of maternal red cell production because folate requirements increase further due to the needs of the fetus.

BIBLIOGRAPHY

Howard RJ, Lillis C, Tuck SM. Contraceptives, counselling, and pregnancy in women with sickle cell disease. Br Med J 1993;306:1735.

Miller WM. Anemia in women ages 20 to 89 years: rationale and tools for differential diagnosis. Clin Ther 1993;15:192.

US Preventive Services Task Force. Routine iron supplementation during pregnancy: Policy statement. JAMA 1993;270:2846.

Welborn JL, Meyers FJ. A three-point approach to anemia. Postgrad Med 1991;89:179.

Williams MD, Wheby MS. Anemia in pregnancy. Med Clin North Am 1992;76:631.

Primary Care for Women, edited by Phyllis C. Leppert and Fred M. Howard. Lippincott-Raven Publishers, Philadelphia © 1997.

88

Bleeding Disorders in Women

RONALD L. SHAM

The diagnostic approach to women with easy bruising or a suspected bleeding disorder includes a careful history and physical examination as well as a laboratory investigation. The history should elucidate whether or not a bleeding disorder exists and help determine possible causes. The physical examination should be comprehensive to identify systemic illness, yet also focused to evaluate clinical evidence of bleeding. The laboratory investigation should initially include only screening blood work; more specific diagnostic tests should be considered once the screening tests and clinical findings are reviewed. This chapter provides a framework for evaluating patients with suspected bleeding disorders or bruising and is organized in two sections: (1) a general approach to bleeding disorders discussed as abnormalities of coagulation factors, platelets, and disorders related to blood vessels and supporting tissues and (2) bleeding disorders associated with pregnancy. Emphasis is placed on bleeding problems seen in an ambulatory setting, and the complex coagulopathies seen in hospitalized patients are mentioned only briefly.

DIFFERENTIAL DIAGNOSIS AND APPROACH TO BLEEDING DISORDERS

Women with suspected bleeding disorders are frequently seen by their primary care physician for evaluation of easy bruising, menorrhagia, mild bleeding symptoms, or abnormal coagulation or platelet studies. These patients are distinct from patients with severe hemostatic abnormalities such as advanced liver disease or severe thrombocytopenia, and they do not require aggressive treatment or hospitalization. With the exception of specific bleeding disorders seen in pregnancy, focus here is on patients who are otherwise well clinically and are seen in an out-patient setting. Women with clinically recognized bleeding generally have either congenital hemostatic defects, acquired abnormalities due to medications or coexisting medical problems, or bruising related to vascular abnormalities. There is often a subgroup in whom no diagnosis can be established. The more common bleeding disorders are discussed in this chapter; disorders that are uncommon or rare are listed in the summary tables.

Disorders of Plasma Coagulation Factors

Disorders of blood coagulation are either congenital or acquired, and may result in clinically significant bleeding or occasionally only abnormalities in laboratory studies (Table 88-1). Congenital deficiencies are usually caused by a deficiency of a single coagulation factor, with the exception of von Willebrand disease, which involves both platelet dysfunction and deficiency of factor VIII. Hemophilia A (factor VIII deficiency) and B (factor IX deficiency) are extremely rare in women, although daughters of men with hemophilia are obligate carriers. A history of bleeding in male relatives is common, and specific assays for factor VIII and IX are needed and may reveal borderline low values in carrier women and a normal partial thromboplastin time (aPTT). Occasionally, more sophisticated genetic testing is necessary to determine carrier status. This becomes an issue when women in families with hemophilia are considering having children, because their sons have a 50% chance of having hemophilia. Factor XI deficiency is a less common deficiency overall than VIII and IX, but due to its autosomal inheritance can be seen in women and may present with mild bleeding. Bleeding due to congenital deficiency of other coagulation factors is extremely rare.

von Willebrand disease is one of the most common congenital bleeding disorders, estimated to be present in 1% of the population. Affected patients often have easy bruising or mucosal bleeding, and commonly present with heavy menstrual bleeding at menarche. This may be an unrecognized and underdiagnosed cause of menorrhagia in women. The screening laboratory data often show a prolonged bleeding time and aPTT. The diagnosis can be confirmed with specific assays for ristocetin cofactor activity, von Willebrand antigen, and factor VIII coagulant activity. It is well recognized that there is significant day-to-day variability in von Willebrand factor levels affecting both screening tests and specific assays, therefore the evaluation for von Willebrand disease often needs to be performed on more than one occasion if the clinical suspicion is high. Patients with von Willebrand disease usually have affected family members with similar degrees of hemostatic impairment. Affected patients usually have their bleeding complications managed by a hematologist and, depending on their clinical history, receive either DDAVP, cryoprecipitate, or clotting factor concentrates.

The most frequent acquired disorders of blood coagulation include vitamin K deficiency, warfarin therapy, liver disease, and coagulation inhibitors. The acquired inhibitors are due to antibodies which are reactive with specific coagulation factors, most commonly factor VIII. They usually cause severe bleeding, leading the patient to seek medical care, but can cause mild symptoms if residual factor levels are greater than 5%. Many cases are idiopathic, but inhibitors are often associated with autoimmune disease, medications, the peripartum state, and malignancy. The association of acquired inhibitors with pregnancy and autoimmune diseases makes this a notable problem in women despite the relative rarity of inhibitors seen in clinical practice. These inhibitors must be distinguished clinically and in the laboratory from the "lupus anticoagulant," which does not cause bleeding. Factor inhibitors almost always cause a prolongation of the aPTT or PT, may cause severe bleeding, and often require hospitalization for management.

Vitamin K is a necessary cofactor for synthesis of functional factors II, VII, IX, and X. Deficiency can be seen based on diet, but is often secondary to intrinsic gastrointestinal tract disease and malabsorption, or can be seen in association with the use of antibiotics, which decrease the production of vitamin K by intestinal bacteria. Vitamin K deficiency can occur within a few weeks and should be suspected in the appropriate clinical setting in the presence of a prolonged prothrombin time (PT). Vitamin K deficiency can usually be corrected with subcutaneous vitamin K.

Liver disease is a frequent cause of an acquired bleeding disorder with a complex pathogenesis including decreased synthesis of coagulation factors, decreased clearance of activated coagulation factors, accelerated fibrinolysis, and abnormal platelet function. Patients with coagulopathy secondary to liver disease often have clinical manifestations of portal hypertension to support the diagnosis, although this may not be the case in acute severe liver dysfunction. Both PT and the aPTT may be prolonged, and there are often decreases in fibrinogen, increased fibrin(ogen) degradation products, a prolonged bleeding time, and decreased platelets, particularly in patients with splenomegaly.

The last acquired disorder of coagulation to be discussed is that associated with amyloidosis. Amyloid fibrils can cause increased vascular fragility, which results in easy bruising. In addition, the amyloid protein can absorb factor X, resulting in an acquired coagulopathy that may further contribute to the bleeding disorder seen with amyloidosis.

Disorders of Platelets

Disorders of platelets may be quantitative or qualitative, and congenital or acquired (Table 88-2). Thrombocytopenia and thrombocytosis can be associated with bleeding and are diagnosed easily by obtaining a platelet count. Thrombocytopenia is much more common, but patients with thrombocytosis due to myeloproliferative diseases such as essential thrombocythemia can have bleeding in the setting of an elevated platelet count. Bleeding may either be

Table 88-1. Coagulation Disorders

Congenital Disorders	Acquired Disorders	Pregnancy-Associated Disorders
Mild hemophilia (factor VIII, IX, XI deficiency)	Circulating anticoagulants	Disseminated intravascular coagulation
von Willebrand disease	Vitamin K deficiency	Acute fatty liver
Dysfibrinogenemia	Liver disease	
Factor XIII deficiency	Amyloid-factor X deficiency	
α-2-plasmin inhibitor deficiency	Dysproteinemia	
Plasminogen activator inhibitor-1 deficiency	Myeloproliferative disorders	
	Warfarin therapy	

Table 88-2. Platelet Abnormalities

Qualitative Congenital Abnormalities	Qualitative Acquired Abnormalities	Pregnancy-Associated Abnormalities
Bernard-Soulier syndrome	Medications	Gestational thrombocytopenia
Glanzmann thrombasthenia	Uremia	HELLP syndrome
Storage pool disease	Liver disease	Eclampsia
Signal transduction abnormalities	Myeloproliferative disease	Immune thrombocytopenia
Receptor abnormalities	Dysproteinemia	
Wiskott-Aldrich syndrome	Acquired storage pool disease	
May-Hegglin anomaly	Attention deficit disorder	
Thrombocytopenia with absent radius	Szechwan purpura	
Hermansky-Pudlak syndrome	Antiplatelet antibodies	
Chediak-Higashi syndrome		
Platelet factor 3 deficiency—Scott syndrome		
	Quantitative Acquired Abnormalities	
	Thrombocytopenia	
	Thrombocytopenia with myeloproliferative disease	

HELLP, hemolysis, elevated liver enzymes, and low platelets.

a presenting feature or develop during the course of the illness. A variety of abnormalities in platelet function have been identified in these patients that contribute to bleeding and, in some patients, contribute to thrombotic complications. However, some patients have a normal bleeding time and normal platelet function tests and still show evidence of a hemostatic defect. Secondary thrombocytosis, such as that seen with inflammation, malignancy, or iron deficiency, is not associated with bleeding and needs to be distinguished from primary (essential) thrombocythemia. Because iron deficiency is common in women and can result in secondary thrombocytosis, this distinction is particularly notable in them.

Thrombocytopenia is a relatively common problem in women. The severity of bleeding due to thrombocytopenia is inversely correlated with the platelet count, with severe bleeding below 20,000/mL. Mild thrombocytopenia with a platelet count over 100,000/mL is typically asymptomatic, but mild bleeding and bruising is often seen with intermediate degrees of thrombocytopenia. The differential diagnosis of thrombocytopenia includes disorders due to decreased production and increased destruction of platelets. Disorders associated with decreased platelet production include congenital abnormalities, drug toxicity, thrombocytopenia due to infiltrative marrow replacement, and aplastic anemia. The congenital abnormalities are rare and include Wiskott-Aldrich syndrome, thrombocytopenia with absent radius, and the May-Hegglin anomaly. Drugs that are frequently associated with decreased platelet production include alcohol, thiazide diuretics, and estrogens, but a large number of drugs have been associated with thrombocytopenia occasionally. Lists of these drugs can be found in many hematology textbooks. Marrow infiltration with malignancy or infectious processes can cause thrombocytopenia, and deficiency of vitamin B_{12} or folate may also cause decreased platelet production.

Thrombocytopenia caused by accelerated platelet destruction is often immune mediated, and is either idiopathic or secondary to a drug or medical disorder. There are many disorders associated with immune dysregulation, and there are a number of conditions associated with pregnancy that result in thrombocytopenia, which the author discusses later. The evaluation of thrombocytopenia is dictated by the severity and by the presence of other clinical findings. The history should include a thorough review of both prescription and over-the-counter medications because of their frequent association with thrombocytopenia. Quinine is a common over-the-counter medication that is frequently taken for leg cramps and can cause immune thrombocytopenia. The evaluation should also focus on identifying autoimmune or collagen vascular disease, lymphoma, and human immunodeficiency virus (HIV) infection, which may be associated with immune thrombocytopenia. Many collagen vascular diseases such as lupus are relatively common in women, and HIV infection, which historically has been more common in men, is being recognized frequently in women and therefore should be considered when evaluating women with thrombocytopenia. HIV infection may cause thrombocytopenia through both immune mechanisms and direct marrow suppression, and may be the first clinical sign of HIV infection. HIV-associated immune thrombocytopenia may occur early in the infection, whereas HIV-associated bone marrow suppression tends to occur with more advanced disease. Treatment with antiretroviral drugs may improve HIV-associated thrombocytopenia. In summary, both primary and secondary immune thrombocytopenia are common in women. A number of treatment options exist including steroids, intravenous gamma globulin, splenectomy, danazol, cytotoxic drugs, and therapy of any underlying disease. These patients should be managed with the assistance of a hematologist.

Qualitative platelet disorders include both common and rare diseases. The congenital disorders are a heterogeneous group, often detected during childhood, and generally require specialized laboratory tests and a hematologist for diagnosis. They are caused by intrinsic abnormalities in platelet biology resulting in abnormal function and present with bleeding patterns similar to that seen in patients with thrombocytopenia. These disorders are discussed only briefly. Bernard-Soulier syndrome is associated with mild thrombocytopenia, giant platelets, and a prolonged bleeding time. Platelet aggregation studies show an impaired response to ristocetin due to an abnormality in the glycoprotein Ib-IX complex. Patients with Glanzmann thrombasthenia may have mild or severe bleeding, and platelet aggregation is impaired in response to epinephrine, ADP, and collagen due to an abnormality in glycoprotein IIb-IIIa, the primary platelet fibrinogen receptor. Platelet storage pool disorders result in abnormal platelet function and mild-to-moderate bleeding due to abnormalities in α-granules, dense granules, or both. Defects in platelet membrane receptors or in specific enzymes required for intracellular signal transduction constitute a heterogeneous group of congenital disorders of platelet function in patients with bleeding disorders.

In contrast to the rare congenital disorders, acquired disorders of platelet function are commonly seen in medical practice. Drugs are the most common cause of qualitative platelet dysfunction. Aspirin acetylates the enzyme cyclooxygenase, thereby inhibiting the platelet release reaction and resulting in a prolonged bleeding time and abnormal in vitro platelet aggregation. The effect is irreversible, and all circulating platelets are affected by the single administration of aspirin in low dose, resulting in abnormal platelet function and a hemostatic defect that persists until sufficient new platelets are released into the circulation, typically 4 to 6 days. The hemostatic defect is mild but may be important in the presence of an additional abnormality such as von Willebrand disease. The use of aspirin in prevention of arterial thrombotic disease has increased during the last decade, making aspirin a common cause of acquired platelet dysfunction. Other common medications that may result in platelet dysfunction include penicillin antibiotics, phosphodiesterase inhibitors, and nonsteroidal antiinflammatory drugs. These medications differ from aspirin because the effects of these drugs on platelet function are reversible, last only as long as the drug is present, and improve with discontinuation of the medication.

A variety of medical illnesses are associated with acquired platelet disorders, the most common being uremia and severe liver disease. The exact pathogenesis of the platelet dysfunction in uremia is unknown, but it is postulated that abnormal interactions of von Willebrand factor and the subendothelium play an important role. Although there is no direct correlation with blood urea nitrogen (BUN) or creatinine, bleeding tends to worsen as renal failure worsens and is commonly present in patients on dialysis. Patients with liver disease may have qualitative platelet abnormalities and coexisting acquired coagulation abnormalities that complicate the hemostatic defect. Abnormal platelet function can occur in myeloproliferative disorders and acute myelogenous leukemia and is associated with multiple functional defects. Patients with dysproteinemia such as multiple myeloma may manifest mild bleeding on the basis of paraprotein interference with platelet function. The platelet dysfunction improves with treatment of the underlying disorder.

Disorders of Blood Vessels

A number of vascular and connective tissue disorders have abnormalities in platelet function, coagulation, or fibrinolysis and are associated with mild bleeding and easy bruising (Table 88-3). Bleeding may be caused by increased transmural pressure, decreased mechanical integrity, or direct damage to the vessel wall. Bleeding associated with increased transmural pressure is typically petechial and mild. It occurs acutely on the upper body with childbirth, severe coughing, or vomiting or more chronically with chronic venous stasis of the lower extremities. Decreased integrity of the supporting tissue of blood vessels is seen in a variety of disorders causing purpura. Elderly women may develop senile purpura characterized by reddish purple lesions on the extensor surface of the forearms and hands, which are due to progressive decreases in collagen, elastin, and other proteins that occur with aging. Because this minor bleeding does not elicit an inflammatory response, senile purpura can persist chronically without reabsorption-induced color change. Patients with either exogenous or endogenous corticosteroid excess develop purpura, which appear similar to senile purpura. Steroid purpura is caused by loss of connective tissue and thinning of the epidermis making cutaneous vessels more fragile.

Vitamin C deficiency (scurvy) causes perifollicular purpura with corkscrew hairs; although rare, more extensive bleeding with severe deficiency or with trauma can be manifest in patients. Bleeding results from weakened skin connective tissue caused by defects in collagen synthesis, which is dependent on ascorbic acid for the conversion of proline to hydroxyproline. Patients with collagen disorders such as Ehlers-Danlos syndrome may have easy bruising and are recognized by clinical manifestations such as increased elasticity of the skin, joint hyperextension, pectus excavatum, and high arched palate. Other collagen disorders such as Marfan syndrome, pseudoxanthoma elasticum, and osteogenesis imperfecta may also be associated with easy bruising and are recognized by clinical features. Hemorrhagic skin lesions termed "pinch purpura" can occur in patients with amyloid. These lesions are caused by increased vascular fragility due to amyloid infiltration of vessel walls. Patients with amyloid may also develop petechiae due to increased transmural pressure as seen with the Valsalva maneuver or after sigmoidoscopy.

Easy bruising is reported considerably more often in women than men. Probably the most common diagnosis in women with easy bruising is purpura simplex. Its pathophysiology is poorly understood, but it is likely that there is hormonal sensitivity because bruising often varies with the menstrual cycle. Patients

Table 88-3. Disorders of Blood Vessels

Abnormal Vessel Wall and Supporting Tissue	**Increased Transmural Pressure**
Trauma—physical abuse	Valsalva-delivery
Senile purpura	Vasculitis (including allergic purpura)
Steroid purpura (endogenous and exogenous)	Amyloidosis
Pseudoxanthoma elasticum	Factitious
Marfan syndrome	Cryoglobulinemia, cryofibrinogenemia, dysproteinemia
Osteogenesis imperfecta	Psychogenic purpura (autoerythrocyte and DNA sensitivity)
Purpura simplex	Pigmented purpuric eruptions (Schamberg disease and others)
Hereditary hemorrhagic telangiectasia	Purpura associated with infection

with purpura simplex develop bruises that are often primarily a cosmetic concern, and these patients are not at risk for more significant bleeding. They occasionally have an extensive work-up that is unrevealing. Hemorrhagic manifestations may occur with vasculitis of diverse causes including hypersensitivity (anaphylactoid purpura) vasculitis, cryoglobulinemia, and the vasculitis associated with immunologic diseases such as systemic lupus or rheumatoid arthritis. These disorders should be considered in the appropriate clinical setting. Hereditary hemorrhagic telangiectasia (Rendu-Olser-Weber disease) causes mucocutaneous telangiectasia and bleeding, which often worsens with age and may be associated with abnormalities in von Willebrand protein that may contribute to the hemorrhagic diathesis. Other causes of easy bruising include psychogenic purpura (autoerythrocyte and deoxyribonucleic acid [DNA] sensitivity), factitious purpura, and purpura associated with trauma. Purpura associated with trauma may be a manifestation of physical abuse and warrant more detailed questioning. Questions regarding possible physical abuse should be asked in a supportive environment. This evaluation may require repeat visits until a level of comfort is established.

DIAGNOSTIC APPROACH TO SUSPECTED BLEEDING DISORDERS

History

A careful history is the most important element in the initial evaluation of a patient with a possible bleeding disorder. It serves to both establish the degree of clinical suspicion for a bleeding disorder and also to provide clues to a specific diagnosis (Table 88-4). The history should establish the duration of the suspected bleeding disorder and also identify the sites and severity of bleeding and any inciting circumstances. It is often difficult to determine if the bleeding described is beyond the normal range, particularly when evaluating easy bruising. Some types of bleeding such as hemoptysis, hematemesis, hematuria, hematochezia, and melena are clearly pathologic but usually have anatomic causes, and the adequacy of prior diagnostic evaluation including endoscopy and imaging studies should be evaluated. Hemarthrosis is always abnormal and indicates a severe hemorrhagic disorder in the absence of trauma. It is often difficult to determine whether or not a bleeding disorder exists when evaluating what may be normal bleeding such as that occurring with menses or childbirth, surgical bleeding, or bleeding with trauma. Because some blood loss is normal in these circumstances, and because many patients consider themselves to be easy bleeders, it is often difficult to evaluate the seriousness of this bleeding. It is important to have an appreciation of the range of normal bleeding and to recognize the considerable reporting differences between patients. Objective assessment regarding the severity of bleeding can be obtained from information regarding the need for transfusions, reoperation, and development of iron deficiency anemia. Abnormal bleeding that is frequently seen in normal individuals without a bleeding disorder includes gingival bleeding, epistaxis, and skin bruising. It is important to determine the frequency and circumstances of such bleeding and its association with local problems such as gingivitis, nasal infection and allergy, and trauma.

The history may provide clues to a specific diagnosis. A history of lifelong bleeding suggests a congenital disorder, and if the parents are available to interview, they may be able to provide information regarding childhood bleeding with dental eruptions, falls, minor injuries, and tonsillectomy. The family history is of critical importance and should be reviewed in detail. This sometimes requires more than one visit because the patient may need to discuss the family history further with relatives. If bleeding is of recent onset, questions regarding concurrent pregnancy, medical illnesses, and medications become important. A thorough medication history should include specific questions regarding aspirin and other medications that cause qualitative platelet dysfunction as well as drugs that could result in thrombocytopenia such as quinine and other over-the-counter medications that are frequently overlooked by patients. It is useful to review prior hemostatic challenges such as childbirth, menses, dental extractions, lacerations, fractures, and minor surgery. This information may allow the physician to date the onset of an acquired bleeding disorder.

Table 88-4. Approach to Patients with a Suspected Bleeding Disorder

INITIAL EVALUATION
History
1. Is there evidence for a bleeding disorder?
a. Bleeding that is always abnormal—hemarthrosis, GI, GU bleeding
b. Abnormal bleeding in a normal patient—epistaxis, bruising, gingival bleeding
c. Expected bleeding—may be abnormal quantity—menses, childbirth, surgery
2. What are the possible causes of bleeding?
a. Lifelong and family history—suspect congenital, need childhood history
b. Recent onset—suspect acquired bleeding, review medication, systemic diseases
Physical
1. Comprehensive search for systemic disease
Renal, hepatic, collagen vascular disease
2. Focused for signs of bleeding, bruising
Petechiae, purpura, ecchymosis size, location
Laboratory Tests
CBC with differential—blood smear review
PT, aPTT, bleeding time
Serum chemistries—liver and kidney function, serum globulins
FURTHER EVALUATION
Abnormal Screening Test Present
Evaluate for systemic disease, platelet or coagulation disorder
Normal Screening Tests
1. Low clinical suspicion
Evaluate for von Willebrand disease
2. High clinical suspicion
Evaluate for von Willebrand disease and other rare disorders

Physical

A complete physical examination should be performed when evaluating a patient for a suspected bleeding disorder. The physical examination is useful in uncovering evidence of a systemic disease. The examination should also carefully evaluate any evidence of bleeding or bruising, examining the skin for petechiae and purpura and noting the location and distribution of lesions. The pattern and physical characteristics of the bruises may also be important, particularly in cases of suspected physical abuse. The nose and mouth should be examined in patients complaining of epistaxis or gingival bleeding. More severe gastrointestinal or genitourinary bleeding requires diagnostic imaging tests in addition to the physical examination.

Laboratory Evaluation

Laboratory tests that are required in nearly all patients include a complete blood count with differential, platelet count, review of the peripheral blood smear, PT, aPTT, and bleeding time. Serum chemistries should be checked and may provide evidence of hepatic disease, renal dysfunction, or dysproteinemia. The extent of the further evaluation depends on the results of the initial findings. If the history and physical examination suggest the presence of a specific systemic disorder, this possibility should be pursued. In pregnant patients, there is a different spectrum of potential hemostatic disorders that needs to be pursued. These disorders are discussed later. Similarly, abnormal screening laboratory tests dictate further evaluation of specific coagulation or platelet disorders, or systemic illness. Patients with a significant bleeding disorder usually have abnormal findings noted on the initial evaluation, which lead to a specific diagnosis. There are, however, patients in whom no abnormalities are identified in the initial evaluation. The evaluation of these patients, with normal screening studies, poses a diagnostic challenge and raises the question, How far should I go? This is difficult to answer; clinical guidelines follow.

Patients who are not on medication and who have no coexisting medical conditions may have a primary bleeding disorder. von Willebrand disease has a relatively high frequency in the population and shows temporal variability in clinical severity and laboratory findings. Consequently, a normal aPTT and bleeding time may be found in mildly affected individuals. In many cases, it is necessary to repeat these tests and to obtain specialized tests such as assays for factor VIII, von Willebrand antigen, and ristocetin cofactor activity. These assays may need to be checked on more than one occasion if the clinical suspicion is high. The other causes of mild bleeding disorders are rare in the absence of clear abnormalities on the initial history, physical examination, and screening laboratory tests. It is inappropriate to pursue extensive laboratory evaluations in all patients who complain of easy bruising or have a equivocal history of mild bleeding. It is at this juncture that clinical judgment governs the decision regarding more extensive evaluation. If the clinical suspicion of a bleeding disorder is low initially and the screening studies are unremarkable, the patient should be reassured that it is very unlikely there is a significant bleeding disorder and advised that further evaluation would be required only in the presence of significant symptoms in the future. Women with a negative laboratory evaluation who have bruises in areas suggestive of physical abuse should be questioned further about this possibility.

If the initial clinical suspicion of a bleeding disorder is high, based on the history and findings on physical examination, a more extensive laboratory evaluation is indicated. Rare disorders do occur, and in these individuals where a high clinical suspicion exists, the full range of possibilities should be systematically pursued. Many of these rare disorders are listed in Tables 88-1 through 88-3, and if such a disorder is suspected, hematology consultation would be appropriate. Mild coagulation factor deficiencies can occur with a normal aPTT or PT, and specific factor assays may be required. Deficiencies of the fibrinolytic inhibitors, α_2 plasmin inhibitor, and plasminogen activator inhibitor type 1 do not affect screening coagulation tests, and specific assays are needed to detect these deficiencies. Severe factor XIII deficiency can be identified using a qualitative screening test. Most cases of dysfibrinogenemia result in a prolongation of the thrombin time. Specialized assays used to determine the presence of platelet functional abnormalities are also available. Finally, laboratory evaluation of family members is often useful, particularly if there is a suggestive family history.

BLEEDING DISORDERS ASSOCIATED WITH PREGNANCY

Many of the bleeding disorders already discussed may occur in pregnant women, may require treatment during pregnancy, or may be altered by pregnancy. In addition, there are a number of bleeding disorders that develop in women only during pregnancy. Some of these disorders are clinically mild and diagnosed in the outpatient setting, whereas others have a more abrupt clinical presentation and often require hospitalization for management. Bleeding disorders that arise during pregnancy are by definition acquired processes and can be categorized as platelet abnormalities, coagulation abnormalities, or disorders in which both are present.

Platelet abnormalities that arise during pregnancy often require the same initial diagnostic approach as those in the nonpregnant patient. Management, however, has the additional concerns about the successful completion of the pregnancy and the health of the fetus. Pregnancy is not associated with acquired qualitative platelet disorders; however, preexisting disorders may pose management problems, but in general they are approached as discussed previously. An acquired quantitative platelet abnormality, ie, thrombocytopenia, is a more common problem during pregnancy. The normal range of platelet counts should not be altered by pregnancy, therefore, low values warrant further evaluation. Thrombocytopenia in the 100,000 to 150,000 range that is new during the course of the pregnancy is most likely due to gestational thrombocytopenia. This is often a diagnosis of exclusion because platelet counts prior to the pregnancy may not be available. Distinguishing gestational thrombocytopenia from chronic immune thrombocytopenia (ITP) may be difficult due to the frequent occurrence of ITP in women of childbearing age. Hematology consultation may be advisable. Gestational thrombocytopenia is usually self-limiting and not harmful to the mother or fetus, does not require treatment or alter the course of the pregnancy, and usually resolves postpartum.

Immune thrombocytopenia differs from gestational thrombocytopenia because it may require therapy during pregnancy and occasionally results in maternal or fetal complications. If the thrombocytopenia is severe, ITP is a more likely diagnosis and can be treated with steroids or intravenous immunoglobulin; splenectomy can be performed during pregnancy if necessary. The fetus may be at risk for thrombocytopenia due to transplacental passage of maternal antibody, and in certain cases, fetal scalp vein sampling or percutaneous umbilical blood sampling can be performed to determine fetal platelet counts. Controversy regarding which pregnant patients with ITP require cesarean section persists and therefore decisions about vaginal delivery must be individualized.

There are a number of acute disorders that result in thrombocytopenia in pregnant women, usually in the setting of other clinical and laboratory evidence of a systemic illness. These include disseminated intravascular coagulation (DIC), thrombotic thrombocytopenic purpura (TTP) and hemolytic uremic syndrome (HUS), coagulopathy associated with preeclampsia and eclampsia, acute fatty liver of pregnancy, and the HELLP syndrome (hemolysis, elevated liver enzymes, and low platelets). Women with these problems cannot be managed in an outpatient setting and should be hospitalized by their obstetricians and managed with the assistance of a hematologist. These disorders are discussed briefly.

DIC that occurs during pregnancy is usually secondary to intrauterine fetal death or associated with another complication of delivery or abortion. Tissue thromboplastin derived from the dead fetus may result in DIC, which usually resolves with delivery of the fetus and placenta. Placental abruption and amniotic fluid embolism may result in DIC in the peripartum period and are managed with delivery of the fetus and placenta and other supportive measures used for managing DIC in nonpregnant patients. Lastly, DIC may be a factor in the coagulopathy associated with eclampsia and may be involved in the pathogenesis of eclampsia.

The pathogenesis of eclampsia is unknown but is felt to involve aberrant interactions between platelets and endothelial cells. Patients may develop a consumptive coagulopathy with greater effects on platelets than on coagulation factors. There are two additional syndromes that occur near term that share some clinical features with the hemostatic defects associated with eclampsia: acute fatty liver of pregnancy and the HELLP syndrome. These disorders can result in potentially devastating complications for the mother and fetus, including death, but usually improve with the delivery of the fetus. In summary, there are a number of hemostatic disorders that may affect women during pregnancy. Mild disorders such as gestational thrombocytopenia and ITP require careful observation and occasional intervention. Severe hemostatic defects may be life threatening and require hospitalization and hematology consultation.

BIBLIOGRAPHY

Bick RL. Platelet function defects: a clinical review. Semin Thromb Hemost 1992;18:167.

Burrows RF, Kelton JG. Fetal thrombocytopenia and its relation to maternal thrombocytopenia. N Engl J Med 1993;329:1463.

Burrows RF, Kelton JG. Thrombocytopenia at delivery: a prospective survey of 6715 deliveries. Am J Obst Gynecol 1990;162:731.

Deykin D. Uremic bleeding. Kidney Int 1983;24:698.

Lackner H, Karpatkin S. On the "easy bruising" syndrome with normal platelet count: a study of 75 patients. Ann Intern Med 1975;83:190.

McCrae KR, Samuels P, Schreiber AD. Pregnancy-associated thrombocytopenia: pathogenesis and management. Blood 1992;80:2697.

Rao AK. Congenital disorders of platelet function. Hematol Oncol Clin North Am 1990;4:65.

Ratnoff OD. Disordered hemostasis in hepatic disease. In: Schiff L, Schiff ER, eds. Diseases of the liver. 6th ed. Philadelphia: JB Lippincott 1987:187.

Ruggeri ZM, Zimmerman TS. Review: von Willebrand factor and von Willebrand disease. Blood 1987;70:895.

Sham RL, Francis CW. Evaluation of mild bleeding disorders and easy bruising. Blood Rev 1994;8:98.

Primary Care for Women, edited by Phyllis C. Leppert and Fred M. Howard. Lippincott-Raven Publishers, Philadelphia © 1997.

89

Venous Thromboembolism

JOHN P. OLSON

Venous thromboembolism is a focus of clinical interest and research. New diagnostic procedures and antithrombotic agents, newly defined hypercoagulable states, and a better understanding of the optimal use of diagnostic procedures and treatments have been the result. Despite 50 years of experience with antithrombotic agents, only in the last decade have serious efforts been undertaken to plan studies, evaluate evidence, and develop a consensus regarding the optimal use of heparin and warfarin. The American College of Chest Physicians 1995 Consensus Conference on Antithrombotic Therapy provides state-of-the-art treatment guidelines for virtually the entire spectrum of venous and arterial thromboembolic disease. This chapter focuses on venous thromboembolism (VTE)—deep venous thrombosis (DVT) and pulmonary embolism (PE)—with emphasis on risk factors, diagnostic approaches, prophylaxis, therapy, and special considerations in the pregnant patient.

Thrombosis of the deep venous system of the lower limbs, with its potential for the disabling, dangerous sequelae of PE and chronic venous insufficiency, develops in about 300,000 people yearly in the United States, roughly one case per 1000 population. This is a major cause of morbidity and mortality in adults and occurs with increased frequency in association with pregnancy. Physicians responsible for the primary care of women often are involved in the diagnosis, treatment, and prevention of this common condition.

ETIOLOGY AND RISK FACTORS

A complex, finely balanced system maintains blood fluidity but ensures protective hemostasis when the vascular system is disrupted. The importance of the triad of blood flow (stasis), vessel wall (endothelial injury), and blood constituents (hypercoagulability) in pathologic clotting was noted by Virchow in 1860; many details have been added since. Several risk factors for VTE have been identified (Table 89-1), and low-, moderate-, and high-risk groups have been defined (Table 89-2). This stratification of risk has led to recommendations for parallel stratification in the intensity of prophylactic measures.

Any VTE event signals a hypercoagulable state: the normal balance between blood flow and protective local hemostasis has

Table 89-1. Risk Factors for Venous Thromboembolism

PREEXISTING CONDITIONS	NEW EVENTS
Age >40	Major surgery
Obesity	Malignancy
Varicose veins	Heart failure or infarction
History of VTE	Hip or leg fracture
High-dose estrogens (OCs)	Other multiple trauma
Thrombophilia (see Table 89-3)	Immobilization >5 d
	Lower limb paralysis
	Pregnancy and puerperium

shifted and pathologic thrombosis has occurred as a result. The diagnosis of a hypercoagulable state, often termed "thrombophilia," usually denotes more specific inherited or acquired disorders that are strongly associated with pathologic thrombosis, often in otherwise healthy people (Table 89-3) They can often be detected by specific laboratory tests.

Natural anticoagulants inhibit and localize the hemostatic function of activated natural procoagulants. Inherited alterations in this natural anticoagulation system—primary hypercoagulable states—have been identified over the past 30 years (Table 89-4). Deficiencies of antithrombin III, protein C, and protein S are found in 5% of unselected patients and 15% to 20% of familial cases of VTE. Some rare inherited variants of fibrinogen (dysfibrinogenemia) make the fibrin clot resistant to fibrinolysis. A common inherited variant of factor V (factor V Leiden) that renders activated factor V resistant to activated protein C (APC resistance) was identified in 1994. One of these five alterations in the natural anticoagulant system is found in about 25% of unselected patients and up to 70% with familial VTE. APC resistance is responsible for about 20% and 50%, respectively, and the heterozygous state of this common disorder is found in 3% to 5% of the normal population.

The high frequency of the gene for APC resistance means that it is an additional prothrombotic factor in some patients with other risk factors, such as immobilization, pregnancy, oral contraceptive (OC) use, or protein C deficiency. For example, inheritance of both protein C deficiency and APC resistance is the cause for a remarkable variation in the frequency of thrombotic events in different protein C-deficient kindreds and in the risk of VTE for OC users. This reinforces the fact that pathologic thrombosis usually is a multifactorial process secondary to a variable cascade of disturbances in blood flow, endothelial integrity, and blood coagulability. The high frequency of heterozygous APC resistance has led to suggestions that pregnant women or OC users should be screened for this disorder.

In contrast to inherited bleeding disorders, the inherited alterations in the natural anticoagulant system produce an increased venous thrombotic risk in the heterozygous state. Homozygous persons have severe venous thrombotic disorders early in life (ATIII, protein C and S deficiency) or a somewhat increased lifelong risk (APC resistance). The relation to arterial thromboembolism is weak or equivocal.

Assays for alterations in the natural anticoagulant system are readily available. Testing is most likely to be helpful in patients with positive family histories, recurrent events, age less than 45 years, thrombosis in unusual sites (eg, mesenteric or cerebral venous systems), or progressive thrombosis despite adequate anticoagulation. Assays are unreliable or difficult to interpret when patients are on anticoagulants, so blood samples should be drawn before anticoagulants are started or 1 to 2 weeks after they have been discontinued. Meanwhile, family studies can be done.

The antiphospholipid syndrome is an autoimmune disorder that may be associated with unexplained and recurrent thromboembolism. Either the arterial or venous system may be affected.

Table 89-2. Risk Groups and Incidence of Venous Thromboembolism*

RISK GROUP	CALF DVT (%)	PROXIMAL DVT (%)	SYMPTOMATIC PE (%)
Low	<10	<1	0.2
Moderate	10–40	1–10	1–8
High	40–80	10–30	5–10
	Common Clinical Settings		
Low risk	Major surgery lasting <1 hr; age < 40; no other risk factors†		
	Hospitalized medical patients without other risk factors†		
Moderate risk	Major surgery; age >40 or other risk factors†		
	Major trauma, burns		
	Major medical illness and other risk factors†		
	History of previous VTE or thrombophilia in combination with pregnancy, minor illness, surgery, or trauma		
	Stroke with lower limb paralysis		
High risk	Fracture or major orthopedic surgery involving lower extremity		
	Major cancer surgery, abdomen or pelvis		
	Major surgery, trauma, or illness and history of VTE or thrombophilia		
	Lower limb paralysis due to acute spinal cord injury		

*Without prophylaxis.

†See Tables 89-1 and 89-3.

(Modified from Dalen JE. When can treatment be withheld in patients with suspected pulmonary embolism? Arch Intern Med 1993;153:1415, and Weinmann EE, Salzman EW. Deep vein thrombosis. N Engl J Med 1994;331:1630.)

Table 89-3. Common Hypercoagulable States (Thrombophilia)

Inherited alterations in the natural anticoagulant system
Variant factor V (factor V Leiden)—resistance to activated protein C
Antithrombin III deficiency
Protein C deficiency
Protein S deficiency
Variant fibrinogen (dysfibrinogenemia)—resistance to fibrinolysis
Antiphospholipid syndrome
Nephrotic syndrome
Paroxysmal nocturnal hemoglobinuria

Patients may have other clinical manifestations, including systemic lupus or lupus-like syndromes, recurrent fetal loss, a prolonged activated partial thromboplastin time (APTT), or thrombocytopenia. Autoantibodies are present that are active in vitro against thromboplastin reagents—the "lupus anticoagulant"—and against other phospholipids such as cardiolipins. The term "lupus anticoagulant" is a misnomer: most patients do not have lupus. The anticoagulant effect is an in vitro phenomenon that actually correlates with an increased risk of thrombosis. Assays for both the lupus anticoagulant and anticardiolipin antibodies should be ordered. In about two thirds of patients, only one test is positive.

OCs have been associated with an increased frequency of VTE and other cardiovascular occlusive disorders. The estrogen concentration is considered to be most relevant. In a 1994 report, the FDA Fertility and Maternal Health Drugs Advisory Committee found that over 90% of OC users take preparations with a low dose of estrogen (20 to 40 μg). The rate of VTE is 4 per 10,000 compared with 7 per 10,000 for high-dose preparations (50 μg). The risk of cerebral thromboembolism is increased 1.8 times for low-dose users and 2.9 times for high-dose users over the rate in women who do not use OCs. The rate of VTE in age-matched women who do not use OCs is about three per 10,000. Therefore, the lower-dose formulations are preferable, particularly in women age 40 or older or those with other risk factors. Replacement doses of estrogen used after menopause have no or only an equivocal increased risk of VTE.

The association between VTE and malignancy was described by Trousseau in 1865, and this relation, particularly with mucin-producing adenocarcinomas of the gastrointestinal and genitourinary tracts and the lung, has been confirmed. There is a two- to threefold increased risk of an occult malignancy when VTE does not appear to be secondary to some other risk factor. About one in 20 patients with idiopathic VTE develops evidence of a malignancy, usually within 6 to 12 months; those with recurrent idiopathic VTE have a substantially higher risk, in the range of about one chance in six. The value of screening is uncertain. It is unclear, for example, that expensive, invasive screening studies (eg, upper and lower gastrointestinal endoscopy) would provide an early diagnosis and contribute to improved survival or life quality. Mammography, chest x-ray, serum carcinoembryonic antigen, pelvic examination, and pelvic ultrasound studies should be considered for women with idiopathic VTE. A high index of suspicion, with focus on suggestive symptoms or signs, is indicated. Occasional patients with malignancies develop other manifestations of an intense hypercoagulable state. These include recurrent VTE while still on therapeutic doses of warfarin or soon after stopping anticoagulation, subacute or chronic disseminated intravascular coagulation, and nonbacterial endocarditis with arterial embolism.

Table 89-4. Natural Procoagulants and Their Specific Natural Anticoagulant Inhibitor

XII_a, XI_a, IX_a, X_a, thrombin	Antithrombin III
VIII_a, V_a	Protein C and protein S
Fibrinogen	Plasminogen
Platelets	Prostacyclin

In summary, there are some well-described, easily recognized risk factors for VTE and others that are occult but readily identified with laboratory tests. Usually it is possible to select patients with apparently idiopathic VTE for additional studies to detect the antiphospholipid syndrome, inherited alterations in the natural anticoagulant system, and occult malignancy. Prophylactic measures can be used when risks are defined; this is the preferable and cost-effective approach to VTE.

DIAGNOSIS

Classical findings characterize the history and physical examination in DVT and PE. Pain and swelling of a lower limb, combined with chest pain and dyspnea, make DVT and PE highly likely. However, these regional symptoms and signs have several other possible causes. The history and examination may provide important supportive evidence, such as recent immobilization or trauma, chronic venous insufficiency, a pleural friction rub, or a past or family history of VTE. However, the clinical suspicion of VTE is often proven incorrect. Accumulated data from the use of venograms, pulmonary angiograms, and noninvasive impedance plethysmography, duplex ultrasonography, and ventilation/perfusion (V/Q) scanning provide good evidence for the following statements.

When DVT is suspected, only 50% of venograms are positive. Therefore, there is a false-positive rate of 50% for a diagnosis based on clinical impression, and some venous imaging study is necessary. When PE is suspected, only 20% to 50% of pulmonary angiograms are positive. Therefore, there is a false-positive rate of 50% to 80% for a diagnosis based on clinical impression, and, again, some pulmonary vascular imaging study is necessary.

When PE is proven by pulmonary angiograms, the legs are asymptomatic 50% of the time but are positive by venography 70% of the time. Therefore, silent but clinically significant DVTs are common, and the lack of leg symptoms is not helpful in the differential diagnosis of chest symptoms.

When DVT is proven by venography, a V/Q scan is positive and indicates a high probability for PE in 40% to 50% of patients despite the lack of chest symptoms or of clinical suspicion of PE. Therefore, silent pulmonary emboli are common, and a diagnosis of DVT does not fully describe the clinical situation. The lack of chest symptoms does not justify a more leisurely diagnostic evaluation of suspected DVT, nor less urgency in starting therapy when DVT is confirmed or strongly suspected.

LABORATORY AND IMAGING STUDIES

Venography and pulmonary angiography are the gold standards for detecting DVT and PE, respectively. The reliability of clinical assessment and noninvasive studies is judged in comparison to these two invasive imaging techniques. However, they are labor-intensive, technically demanding, uncomfortable, require intra-

Table 89-5. V/Q Scan and Pulmonary Emboli When Validated by Pulmonary Angiogram

V/Q SCAN: PROBABILITY FOR PE	% WITH PE AND THIS SCAN RESULT	% WITHOUT PE AND THIS SCAN RESULT	% WITH THIS SCAN AND PROVEN PE	% WITH THIS SCAN AND PE IF CLINICAL SUSPICION IS HIGH	% WITH THIS SCAN AND PE IF CLINICAL SUSPICION IS LOW
High	40	<5	85	95	55
Intermediate	40	45	30	65	15
Low	20	40	25	40	5
Normal	<5	10	<1	—	—

venous contrast media and radiation, and often are not readily available. There is a small risk of provoking venous thrombosis with venography and of cardiopulmonary morbidity and death with pulmonary angiography.

Impedance plethysmography is a noninvasive technique for measuring changes in electrical conductivity in the calf when a thigh cuff is inflated and deflated. It is an easily repeated, portable technique but is somewhat less reliable than venography or duplex ultrasonography.

Duplex ultrasonography is somewhat more sensitive and specific than impedance plethysmography. The duplex technique weds direct imaging and compressibility of a vein to the Doppler assessment of blood flow; the addition of color Doppler provides "triplex" ultrasonography. Venous compressibility is the most reliable and useful parameter, however.

These noninvasive techniques are considerably less reliable than venography for visualizing calf vein and incompletely occlusive thrombi, for distinguishing residual venous alterations secondary to old thrombi from new thrombi, and for evaluating asymptomatic high-risk patients. Isolated calf vein thrombi and small nonocclusive thrombi are not likely to be the source of clinically significant emboli. However, thrombi may enlarge and extend, so repeat noninvasive studies every 2 to 4 days are advisable in suspicious or high-risk situations or when isolated calf thrombi are identified. Repeatedly negative duplex ultrasonography, either alone or as a supplement to impedance plethysmography, is a safe and reliable way of excluding clinically significant VTE in symptomatic patients.

V/Q scanning uses radioisotopes to identify areas of the lung that are ventilated but not perfused (ventilation/perfusion mismatch). Comparisons between the findings of V/Q scans and pulmonary angiograms in the same patients have led to criteria for describing V/Q scan results as normal or high, intermediate, or low probability for PE. Table 89-5 provides data from over 1000 patients evaluated with both V/Q scans and angiograms. Most patients with PE do not have high-probability scans; indeed, up to 20% have low-probability scans. A normal V/Q scan rules out significant PE. Abnormal V/Q scans are common (about 90%) in patients without PE who have cardiopulmonary symptoms. A high-probability V/Q scan, combined with strong clinical suspicion, indicates the presence of PE correctly more than 95% of the time; this is an indication for treatment. A low-probability V/Q scan, combined with a low level of clinical suspicion, indicates the absence of PE correctly more than 95% of the time. However, a low-probability V/Q scan may provide a dangerous false sense of security: 20% of patients with PE have this result, and when this scan result is combined with a high clinical suspicion, about 40% have PE.

There are extensive data comparing venography with impedance plethysmography and duplex ultrasonography, and pulmonary angiography with V/Q scans for the diagnosis of DVT and PE, respectively. Analyses of these data have led to the formulation of the following diagnostic strategies for the optimal use of these techniques in various clinical settings. The local availability of tests and interpretive expertise must be considered, of course. For most patients with suspected VTE, the results of noninvasive studies are sufficient to guide treatment decisions; also, the level of clinical suspicion is important and should be integrated with the results of noninvasive tests. The predictive value of the results declines substantially when they disagree with clinical judgment, and additional imaging studies are indicated in that event. "Clinical judgment" here is not well defined, but clinical findings and the number of risk factors are important components.

For suspected DVT, when the initial noninvasive study (duplex ultrasonography or impedance plethysmography) is normal, do not anticoagulate; repeat the test two or three times over 10 to 14 days if clinical suspicion persists. If the study becomes abnormal, anticoagulate; if it remains normal, do not anticoagulate, but perform venography if clinical suspicion is high. If the initial noninvasive study is abnormal, venography should be done if there is a previous abnormal study or a history of DVT; if there is no past history, anticoagulate unless clinical suspicion is low. Then do duplex ultrasonography (if impedance plethysmography was done first) or venography.

For suspected PE, if the initial V/Q scan is normal, do not anticoagulate. If it is a high-probability scan and clinical suspicion is low, or if there was a previous PE, consider pulmonary angiography or serial duplex ultrasonography or impedance plethysmography. If clinical suspicion is not low, anticoagulate. If the scan is of low probability and clinical suspicion is low, do not anticoagulate. If clinical suspicion is high and if cardiopulmonary compromise is present, consider anticoagulation, pulmonary angiography, or serial duplex ultrasonography or impedance plethysmography. If clinical suspicion is high and cardiopulmonary compromise is absent, perform a serial duplex ultrasonography or impedance plethysmography. If the scan is of intermediate probability, the level of clinical suspicion is less helpful. If cardiopulmonary compromise is present, consider anticoagulation, pulmonary angiography, or serial duplex ultrasonography or impedance plethysmography. If cardiopulmonary compromise is absent, perform pulmonary angiography or serial duplex ultrasonography or impedance plethysmography.

THERAPEUTIC CONSIDERATIONS

Options for Prophylaxis and Treatment

Effective nonpharmacologic measures include early ambulation, graduated compression stockings, intermittent external pneumatic compression (IPC) boots, and venous interruption. These are useful prophylactically, although venous interruption is generally used in high-risk patients who have failed or have major contraindications for antithrombotic therapy. Percutaneous transvenous placement of a vena cava filter has replaced other techniques of venous interruption. The procedure is safe and very effective in reducing the incidence of PE, but not that of DVT. IPC boots can enhance or serve as a substitute for prophylactic antithrombotic therapy in some moderate- and high-risk patients. Correct placement and monitoring by experienced personnel are critical, as deficiencies in placement and function of IPC boots have been found in 20% to 50% of patients.

There are several agents and regimens for effective pharmacologic therapy, depending on the intensity of VTE.

Aspirin produces an antithrombotic effect by interfering with the prostaglandin pathways necessary for platelet aggregation. It is less effective as a prophylactic agent in VTE than in arterial thromboembolism and is not as effective in preventing VTE as other antithrombotic regimens. However, a recent metanalysis found a reduction in VTE events of roughly 50% with prophylactic aspirin. This suggests a useful role in moderate- or high-risk patients after hospital discharge or in combination with low-dose heparin in hospitalized patients. Dose requirements are not well established in VTE, but in other settings 160 to 325 mg/day usually is as effective as higher doses, and gastrointestinal injury is less likely. The effect of a single dose lasts for the lifetime of exposed platelets and gradually wanes, as about 10% of platelets are replaced each day. The drug crosses the placenta but appears safe in low doses during the second and third trimesters. Fetopathic effects are uncertain and controversial during the first trimester.

Ticlopidine is an antiplatelet drug useful for prophylaxis in arterial thromboembolism when aspirin is ineffective or not tolerated. There are insufficient trials to assess a role in VTE. Side effects include diarrhea, rash, and neutropenia.

Warfarin is a vitamin K antagonist whose effect is mediated by a reduction in the activity of clotting factors II, VII, IX, and X. The natural anticoagulants protein C and S are also reduced. The development of full antithrombotic effect does not occur until after the third day of administration, although the prothrombin time (PT) may be prolonged earlier. This apparent anomaly is due to differences in the half-lives of the affected clotting factors, which vary from 6 hours for factor VII to 72 hours for factor II (prothrombin). The antithrombotic effect, in contrast to the effect on the PT, requires a decrease in all four factors. This is the main reason why heparin and warfarin should be given in combination during the first 5 days of treatment of active VTE and why large loading doses of warfarin should be avoided.

Thromboplastin reagents used in performing the PT differ in their sensitivity to a reduction of clotting factor activity. Monitoring of anticoagulation and adjustments in warfarin doses based only on the PT in seconds or the ratio between the patient's and the control PT may be unreliable, especially if different laboratories or different thromboplastic reagents are involved. Most laboratories report PTs in terms of the international normalized ratio (INR). This ratio is based on the sensitivity of the specific thromboplastin reagent in comparison with the international WHO standard. An INR between 2 and 3 represents therapeutic levels of anticoagulation in VTE.

When warfarin is used prophylactically in high-risk surgical patients, it can be started as a low dose 7 to 10 days preoperatively, with a target INR of 1.5. Alternatively, it can be started the night before surgery in the usual dose of 5 to 10 mg. The postoperative target is an INR of 2 to 3.

A very low fixed dosage of warfarin (1 mg/day) reduces the occurrence of VTE related to arterial and venous catheters and probably in breast cancer patients receiving chemotherapy. Trials in combination with low-dose aspirin for prophylaxis in other clinical settings are underway. Warfarin crosses the placenta, is fetopathic, and should be avoided during pregnancy. Safety in the third trimester is controversial.

Standard unfractionated heparin has an immediate anticoagulant effect mediated by the markedly increased activity of the natural anticoagulant antithrombin III when complexed with heparin. This inhibitory activity is directed at multiple activated clotting factors; activated factors II, IX, and X are most important in the treatment or prevention of VTE. Heparin is given intravenously or subcutaneously. It has a variable but short half-life (1 to 2 hr) and a variable but low bioavailability due to extensive protein binding. Frequent monitoring of the APTT is required. The full therapeutic effect of heparin requires concentrations of 0.2 to 0.4 U/mL plasma and prolongation of the APTT to about 1.5 to 2.5 times the control APTT. Assay systems vary in sensitivity to heparin-induced alterations in clotting factor activity; each laboratory should determine the therapeutic range of APTT.

In the treatment of active VTE or as a substitute for long-term warfarin anticoagulation, heparin can be given by a continuous intravenous route or in a subcutaneous dosage every 12 hours. In the intravenous regimen, 5000 to 10,000 U (or 80 U/kg bolus) is given at an initial infusion rate of 1200 to 1300 U or 18 U/kg/hour. Rapid achievement of a therapeutic APTT is critical. The infusion rate should be adjusted to maintain the APTT at more than 1.5 times and less than three times the control level. The average 24-hour requirement is 32,000 U, but 25% of patients require more than 35,000 U/24 hours (1670 U/hour). In the subcutaneous high-dose regimen, 5000 to 10,000 U (or 80 U/kg bolus) is given intravenously for immediate effect. The initial 20,000 U dosage is given subcutaneously every 12 hours. The APTT is measured 6 hours after the injection, and the dosage is then adjusted to achieve an APTT more than 1.5 times and less than three times the control level at 6 hours after each injection. After a stable therapeutic level is achieved, the dose requirements are stable, and the frequency of APTT monitoring can be reduced to weekly or less often.

Prophylactic heparin can be given at a fixed low dose of 5000 U subcutaneously every 8 to 12 hours or as an adjusted low dose of heparin subcutaneously every 12 hours. In the former, the APTT is prolonged very little but inhibition of activated factor X is pronounced. The former is effective in most moderate- or high-risk clinical settings. In the latter, the dosage is adjusted to achieve an APTT in the upper-normal range 6 hours after the injection. It is effective in the more intense hypercoagulable state occurring after hip surgery.

Low-molecular-weight heparins (LMWH) include several commercial preparations that have a mean molecular weight of 4500 (compared with 15,000 for standard unfractionated heparin). Mainly because of less nonspecific protein binding, LMWHs have several properties that make them an attractive alternative to heparin. The more predictable anticoagulant response makes monitoring usually unnecessary. LMWHs offer better bioavailability at low doses. Their longer half-life permits dosing once or twice daily. LMWHs have an equivalent or superior antithrombotic effect, coupled with evidence of decreased bleeding and thrombocytopenia. Several preparations have been used successfully in Europe for therapy and prophylaxis. As of July 1996, the FDA has approved two LMWH preparations for prophylaxis following hip, knee, or abdominal surgery and expanded indications are expected.

Thrombolytic therapy, unlike heparin or warfarin (Coumadin), attacks established VTE disease directly by lysing recent thrombi. Courses of therapy are short and must be followed by heparin and coumadin anticoagulation. Three effective products and regimens have been established for VTE: streptokinase (250,000 IU as a loading dose followed by 100,000 IU/hour for 24 hours), urokinase (4400 IU/kg as a loading dose followed by 4400 IU/kg/hour for 12 to 24 hours), and recombinant tissue plasminogen activator (100 mg as a continuous intravenous infusion over 2 hours). These agents are effective and are indicated in massive life- or limb-threatening VTE. They may produce better outcomes in respect to preserving venous function in the lower extremities and the vascular bed in the lungs in patients with VTE. However, the added cost, the increased risk of major bleeding, and uncertainty about important clinical benefits have limited their use.

Prophylaxis

All treatments for VTE except thrombolytic drugs and surgical thrombectomy are prophylactic. They are used either to prevent the initial clot or to prevent the extension and embolization of an existing venous clot. The intensity of the antithrombotic regimen should be tailored to the clinical setting.

Most hospitalized patients receive some planned VTE prophylaxis, which may range from early ambulation and leg exercises to insertion of a vena cava filter for those who fail or have a contraindication to pharmacologic antithrombotic therapy. The choice of prophylactic options depends on the level of risk for VTE (see Tables 89-1 and 89-2). In occasional patients, the choices are limited by unusual bleeding risks or other idiosyncrasies.

The risks for the most clinically significant proximal DVT range from less than 1% in young patients undergoing minor surgery to as high as 30% in older patients undergoing hip surgery. Multiple risk factors are often present in the same patient, and there is a rough association between the number of risk factors and the frequency of VTE. A focused history and a physical examination are necessary to assess the risks accurately and to select optimal prophylaxis. Only a minority of moderate- and high-risk patients in either teaching or nonteaching hospitals (about 45% and 20%, respectively) receive optimal prophylactic therapy, that which reduces the VTE risk to baseline or low-risk incidence. This goal can be achieved for most moderate- and high-risk patients.

Low-risk patients may benefit from leg exercises, early ambulation, or graduated compression stockings. Clinically significant VTE is rare.

Moderate-risk patients make up a large fraction of hospitalized medical and surgical patients. Proximal DVT and PE occur in up to 10% and 5%, respectively, of patients who do not receive prophylaxis. In addition to nonpharmacologic measures, these patients should receive specific antithrombotic therapy, usually with subcutaneous low-dose heparin (5000 U every 12 hours). IPC boots also are effective and are indicated in neurosurgical or other patients with a high bleeding risk.

A large minority of high-risk patients develop proximal DVT; up to 5% develop fatal PE if they do not receive adequate prophylaxis. Most patients should receive low-dose heparin (5000 U every 8 hours) or LMWH. Patients with hip fractures or prosthetic replacement require more intense prophylaxis with LMWH, adjusted-dose heparin, or perioperative warfarin. IPC boots give added protection in many high-risk patients. Patients at very high risk who also have a high bleeding risk, a protracted high risk for thrombosis, or a documented failure of antithrombotic therapy should be considered for transvenous placement of a vena cava filter.

Treatment of Established VTE

The following guidelines for anticoagulation with continuous intravenous heparin and warfarin provide a step-by-step approach and the rationale for each step. They can be used to generate orders or to develop a standardized order sheet for the initial anticoagulation of inpatients. They have been used successfully at Rochester General Hospital since 1992. (See box, Treatment for Venous Thromboembolism.)

Complications of Antithrombotic Therapy

Bleeding is the chief complication. Prophylactic heparin regimens in surgical patients are associated with a small increase in wound hematomas but no increase in major bleeding. The risk of bleeding with warfarin is related to the dose intensity. The incidence is about 4% for major bleeding with an INR of 2 to 3 but increases four- to fivefold to about 20% with more intense therapy (INR 3 to 4.5). The increased rate of heparin-related bleeding is less dramatic with more intensive therapy than with warfarin. The rate of major bleeding for the usual 5- to 7-day course of heparin is about 4%.

Several risk factors for bleeding have been identified: the intensity of anticoagulant therapy, chronic use of aspirin or other nonsteroidal antiinflammatory drugs, alcohol abuse, major comorbid disorders, and advanced age. The risk of bleeding increases with the number of risk factors and may occur in up to 25% of patients with multiple risks. Bleeding complications can be reduced in high-risk patients by more frequent assessment of anticoagulant intensity (PT, APTT); tightened control, selecting an intensity in the lower therapeutic range (INR 2 to 2.5 and APTT ratio of 1.5 to 2); and minimizing invasive procedures and exposure to antiplatelet drugs.

Many drugs, foods high in vitamin K, and intercurrent illness may alter vitamin K and warfarin metabolism. Elderly hospitalized patients with multiple comorbid disorders and a long medication list often are very sensitive to warfarin. Intercurrent illness, particularly when associated with decreased food intake and the use of broad-spectrum antibiotics, often results in increased sensitivity also. The PT should be checked one to three times a week during any change in health or medication until a stable, therapeutic PT is reestablished.

Thrombocytopenia develops in 25 to 50 per 1000 patients receiving full therapeutic doses of heparin and a smaller fraction of patients exposed to low-dose heparin or LMWH. It is usually mild and asymptomatic, but four per 1000 patients or up to 25% of those with thrombocytopenia also develop arterial or venous thromboembolism. The decline in platelet counts is mediated by an immune reaction involving platelets, heparin, and an antibody. The thrombotic process is not completely understood but is related to platelet aggregation and perhaps heparin inactivation. Thrombocytopenia develops an average of 10 days after heparin is started but can develop during the first day if there has been previous expo-

Treatment for Venous Thromboembolism

Diagnosis Suspected

- Baseline APTT, PT, platelet count
  - Baseline studies are important for future reference and to screen for coagulation disorders prior to treatment.
- Consider heparin 5–10,000 U IV bolus
  - Prevents progression if VTE disease is highly likely while diagnostic tests are being done.
- Diagnostic imaging studies
  - Diagnostic studies are necessary because a diagnosis based on clinical findings is wrong >50% of the time.

Diagnosis Confirmed

- *Heparin*
  - The goal is to achieve and maintain a heparin level of 0.2–0.4 U/m, which corresponds to an APTT >1.5 x and < 3 x the mean control value.
  - *5,000 U (or 80 U/kg) IV bolus* loading dose followed by
    - Usual effective dose. A *higher loading dose* of heparin (7500–10,000 U) may be required to achieve a therapeutic APTT in patients with massive DVT or large pulmonary emboli. A *lower loading dose* (2500–4000 U) may be adequate to achieve a therapeutic APTT in some patients with thrombocytopenia or low body weight. The response can be assessed by measuring the APTT 1 h after the bolus and again at 3–4 hours. A weight-based heparin dosing nomogram may provide more consistent therapeutic control.
  - *30–40,000 U/24 h* (1250-1650 U/h or 30–40 mL/h) of usual 20,000 U/500 mL solution by continuous IV infusion. (Initial infusion rate is 18 U/kg using *weight-based regimen*)
    - Most patients will maintain a therapeutic APTT at 30,000 U/24 h but up to 25% will require over 35,000 U/24 h. These doses are considerably higher than the frequent initial order for 25 mL/h (1000 U/h or 24,000 U/24 h) which is usually insufficient.
- *APTT Monitoring of Heparin*
  - Monitoring is necessary so that heparin infusion can be adjusted and a safe, effective APTT range established. This minimizes the risk of recurrent thromboembolism (15–20% risk) or of bleeding (~5% risk) when the APTT is <1.5 x or >3 x control respectively.
  - *4 hours* after the bolus
  - *Every 6 hours* until a stable therapeutic PTT is obtained
  - At least once daily for the duration of heparin administration
    - The half life of 5000 U of IV heparin bolus is 1 to 2 hours. After 4 hours the APTT value is due to the heparin infusion.
- *Heparin Dose Adjustments*
  - Staged incremental adjustments minimize wide swings in APTT. The lack of a standardized approach is a major cause of therapeutic failure. The nomogram below is modified from Coleman, Hirsh, Marder and Salzman. (The therapeutic range may differ in other laboratories).

APTT (SEC.)	REBOLUS (UNITS)	HOLD INFUSION (MIN.)	RATE CHANGE* (ML/H)	REPEAT APTT
<50	5000	0	+3	6 h
50-59	0	0	+3	6 h
60-85	0	0	0	next a.m.
86-95	0	0	-2	next a.m.
96-120	0	30	-2	6 h
>120	0	60	-4	6 h

*1 mL/h = 40 units/h

- Monitor *hematocrit* and *platelet count* q 2-3 days while on heparin.
  - This monitors for occult bleeding and for the occurrence of heparin-induced thrombocytopenia.
- *Warfarin*
  - Start warfarin on day 1 or 2 of heparin infusion. Continue both agents for 4–5 days then d/c heparin if PT is therapeutic with INR of 2–3.
    - This is safe and effective, and the most cost-effective approach.
  - Warfarin 10 mg initially and 5–10 mg next day. Then adjust daily dose to achieve INR of 2–3. The next day's dose should be held or reduced by 50% if > 3 sec rise in PT occurs.
    - Large loading doses are hazardous due to rapid decrease in protein C and factor VII. The frequently written order of 10 mg warfarin daily x 3 days is often excessive in hospitalized patients with comorbid disorders or advanced age.
  - Check PT 4 hours after heparin discontinued. Monitor daily until PT stable in therapeutic range.
    - To ensure the PT prolongation is due to warfarin rather than heparin effect at the time of switch over to warfarin alone.
  - Continue warfarin for a minimum of 3 months.
    - Optimum duration is uncertain but 3 months is recommended for initial VTE and longer or indefinitely for active risk factors or recurrence.

sure to heparin. It usually remits within 3 to 5 days after heparin is discontinued. Treatment requires immediate discontinuation of heparin not because of the thrombocytopenia itself but because of the life- and limb-threatening thrombotic risk. Control of the original VTE process may be obtained with coumadin, aspirin, intravenous dextran or, occasionally, a vena cava filter. The defibrinating agent ancrod, low-molecular-weight heparinoids (but not LMWH) and the antithrombin argatroban are investigational drugs that have been used successfully in this difficult situation.

The anticoagulation effect can be reversed as rapidly as necessary for both heparin and warfarin. Often an excessive effect can be corrected by reducing or holding the dose of these agents. Intravenous heparin has a half life of 1 to 2 hours, so the effect is gone within 4 hours of discontinuation. However, subcutaneous heparin may prolong the APTT for up to 24 hours after the last dose. Warfarin has a half life of 36 to 42 hours, so a decline in the PT may be delayed for 2 or more days after the last dose.

Protamine binds to and neutralizes circulating heparin immediately, and 1 mg of protamine neutralizes about 100 U of heparin. Protamine should be given intravenously at a rate of 1 to 2 mg/min in a sufficient dose to neutralize the amount of heparin administered over the previous 30 minutes. For examples, for an infusion rate of 1300 U/hour, the protamine dose would be about 6.5 mg. The APTT can be checked immediately and 2 hours after the protamine infusion. The choices with warfarin include low-dose vitamin K (0.5 to 1.0 mg subcutaneously or by a slow intravenous infusion) or fresh-frozen plasma (three to four units). Vitamin K produces a decline in the PT within 6 to 8 hours. Doses higher than 1 to 2 mg may make the patient resistant to warfarin for a week or more. Fresh-frozen plasma has an immediate effect but may need to be repeated because of the long half-life of warfarin.

CONSIDERATIONS IN PREGNANCY

Pregnancy is associated with a multifactorial hypercoagulable state characterized by an increased risk of VTE (two to four cases per 1000 pregnancies). About 75% to 85% of these events occur in the first 1 to 4 weeks of the puerperium, and the rate during pregnancy does not appear to be more than expected. PE caused about two deaths/100,000 live births and was responsible for 15% to 20% of the maternal deaths in the United States in the 1980s, despite a 50% decrease since the 1970s. The risks of recurrent VTE or of an initial VTE in patients with other risk factors are increased throughout pregnancy and are sufficient to justify prophylactic heparinization in selected patients. Table 89-6 lists factors common in pregnancy that increase the risk of VTE.

Table 89-6. Risk Factors for Venous Thromboembolism in Pregnancy

	PERCENT OF PREGNANCIES WITH VTE	RELATIVE RISK
Normal pregnancy	0.2–0.4	1×
Inherited defects of natural anticoagulants*	25–60	80–200×
Previous VTE*	4–12	20–60×
Age >40	2–4	10×
Cesarean section	1–6	3–16×
African-American	1	3–4×

*Prophylaxis recommended throughout pregnancy.

The differential diagnosis of VTE is pregnancy is complicated by the leg edema and discomfort that are common in the third trimester. Often this is due to external compression of the common iliac veins by the gravid uterus. Earlier in pregnancy, such physical findings are more commonly due to venous thrombi.

When VTE is suspected, the selection of diagnostic tests should follow the same general approach as in nonpregnant patients. Noninvasive studies should be used initially, with invasive venography or pulmonary angiography used to resolve uncertainties. Pregnancy introduces concern about radiation exposure of the fetus and also induces changes in the mother that affect interpretation of the studies. There is no radiation exposure with impedance plethysmography or duplex ultrasonography. In late pregnancy, the former may be falsely positive because of external venous compression from the gravid uterus. Retesting in the lateral decubitus position may result in a negative test. A persistently positive impedance plethysmogram in late pregnancy should be evaluated further with duplex ultrasonography or venography. The iliac vessels cannot be evaluated reliably with duplex ultrasound, particularly in late pregnancy. Isolated proximal femoral or iliac venous thrombosis does occur in late pregnancy and therefore could be missed by ultrasound. Impedance plethysmography or unilateral venography is indicated if the clinical suspicion is high.

Unilateral venography without abdominal shielding exposes the fetus to about 300 mrads compared with less than 50 mrads with limited venography and abdominal shielding. The latter technique, however, does not visualize the proximal thigh or iliac veins. A V/Q scan exposes the fetus to less than 55 mrads. This can be reduced by decreasing the dose of isotope used in the perfusion scan, canceling the ventilation study if the perfusion scan is normal, and having the patient void promptly after completion of the study. Pulmonary angiography can be done with abdominal shielding, fewer exposures, and a brachial route. These modifications reduce the fetal radiation exposure from about 400 to less than 50 mrads. It should be possible to perform an evaluation that is adequate (to avoid unnecessary anticoagulation and also to avoid missing a critical diagnosis) with no increased teratogenic risk and no or a minimally increased oncogenic risk to the fetus.

The use of antithrombotic drugs in pregnancy is complicated by the potential for increased maternal bleeding and for bleeding or teratogenic risk to the fetus. Standard unfractionated heparin and LMWH do not pass the placenta and do not appear to cause fetal damage. Warfarin and related anticoagulants reach the fetal circulation, and fetal malformations—warfarin embryopathy and CNS deficits—occur in up to 25% of exposures. Although exposure during the last half of the first trimester is most hazardous, there is evidence of adverse effects resulting from exposures in the second and third trimesters as well. Therefore, warfarin should be avoided during pregnancy. Aspirin passes the placenta, and its safety in the first trimester is controversial. Low doses (< 150 mg/day) appear to be safe when used in the second and third trimesters and are not associated with increased maternal bleeding.

Long-term heparin therapy during pregnancy may be associated with osteopenia and compression fractures. The risks with LMWH may be less. The changes appear to be reversible. The prophylactic value of calcium supplements has not been assessed adequately.

The American College of Chest Physicians consensus conference on antithrombotic therapy updated recommendations for the use of these agents in pregnant patients in 1995:

- A history of previous VTE or thrombophilia is an indication for low-dose heparin (5000 U every 12 hours subcutaneously) throughout pregnancy and for at least 4 weeks postpartum.
- VTE during the current pregnancy is an indication for heparin throughout pregnancy, followed by warfarin for at least the first 4 to 6 weeks of the puerperium. Heparin in full intravenous doses should be given for at least the first 5 days, followed by subcutaneous heparin every 12 hours at a dose sufficient to achieve an APTT 1.5 to 2.5 times the control value 6 hours after the injection. The required 24-hour dose of heparin is about 10% higher by the subcutaneous than the continuous intravenous route. Heparin should be discontinued 24 hours before delivery because of the prolonged effect of subcutaneous heparin on the APTT. Protamine can be used if necessary also. Therapeutic doses of intravenous heparin and warfarin should be started immediately after delivery. The heparin requirement is often reduced by 30% postpartum. Both agents should be continued together for at least 5 days, and then warfarin alone should be administered for at least 4 to 6 weeks. Warfarin is not contraindicated in mothers who are breast-feeding.
- Pregnant patients requiring long-term anticoagulation (eg, previous multiple VTE events or the presence of prosthetic heart valves) should be switched to full therapeutic doses of subcutaneous heparin (as defined above) early in the first trimester to avoid potential fetal damage from warfarin. If the pregnancy is planned, then heparin can be started at that time or, alternatively, after serial weekly pregnancy tests become positive.
- Recommendations for pregnant patients with antiphospholipid antibodies are in evolution. The therapeutic recommendations may include aspirin, steroids, or low-dose or full-dose heparin, depending on the clinical situation. Consultation with a rheumatologist or hematologist is advised.

Subcutaneous LMWH is an attractive alternative to subcutaneous standard unfractionated heparin during pregnancy, and there is substantial literature on its use in Europe. As noted earlier, it has a predictable weight-based dose and requires little or no monitoring. It has not been approved for this use in the United States.

BIBLIOGRAPHY

Antiplatelet Trialists' Collaboration. Collaborative overview of randomized trials of antiplatelet therapy—III: Reduction in venous thromboses and pulmonary embolism by antiplatelet prophylaxis among surgical and medical patients. Brit Med J 1994;308:235.

Chong BH. Heparin-induced thrombocytopenia. Brit J Haematol 1995;89:431.

Colman RW, Hirsh J, Marder VJ, Salzman EW, eds. Hemostasis and thrombosis: basic principles and clinical practice, 3d ed. Philadelphia: JB Lippincott, 1993.

Dahlbäck B. Inherited thrombophilia: resistance to activated protein C as a pathogenic factor of venous thromboembolism. Blood 1995;85:607.

Dalen JE. When can treatment be withheld in patients with suspected pulmonary embolism? Arch Intern Med 1993;153:1415.

Dolen JE, Hirsh J, eds. Fourth ACCP consensus conference on antithrombotic therapy. Chest 1995;108(Suppl. 1):225S–522S.

Fejgin MD, Lourwood DL. Low-molecular-weight heparins and their use in obstetrics and gynecology. Obstet Gynecol Surv 1994;49:424.

Goldhaber SZ. Contemporary pulmonary embolism thrombolysis. Chest 1995;107(Suppl 1):45.

Kelly MA, Carson JL, Palevsky HI, Schwartz JS. Diagnosing pulmonary embolism: new facts and strategies. Ann Intern Med 1991;114:300.

Lockshin MD. Which patients with antiphospholipid antibody should be treated and how? Rheum Dis Clin North Am 1993;19:235.

PIOPED Investigators. Value of the ventilation/perfusion scan in acute pulmonary embolism. Results of the prospective investigation of pulmonary embolism diagnosis (PIOPED). JAMA 1990;263:2753.

Prins MH, Lensing AW, Hirsh J. Idiopathic deep venous thrombosis. Is a search for malignant disease justified? Arch Intern Med 1994;154:1310.

Rutherford SE, Phelan JP. Deep venous thrombosis and pulmonary embolism in pregnancy. Obstet Gynecol Clin North Am 1991;18:345.

Weinmann EE, Salzman EW. Deep vein thrombosis. N Engl J Med 1994;331:1630.

Wheeler HB, Hirsh J, Wells P, Anderson FA Jr. Diagnostic tests for deep vein thrombosis. Clinical usefulness depends on probability of disease. Arch Intern Med 1994;154:1921.

Primary Care for Women, edited by Phyllis C. Leppert and Fred M. Howard. Lippincott-Raven Publishers, Philadelphia © 1997.

90

Hematologic Malignancies

PRADYUMNA D. PHATAK

The hematologic malignancies are a heterogenous group of disorders that arise from malignant transformation of hematopoietic cells. The malignant cells proliferate in the bone marrow or lymphoid tissues or both, where they eventually result in impairment of normal hematopoiesis, immune dysfunction, or lymph node enlargement. Disorders in which the neoplastic cells originate in the bone marrow and often circulate in the peripheral blood are termed "leukemias." Disorders that arise in lymphoid tissue and primarily cause lymph node enlargement and hepatosplenomegaly are termed "lymphomas." Although the broad topic of hematologic malignancies also includes the plasma cell dyscrasias, the discussion in this chapter is restricted to the common forms of leukemia and lymphoma. As a group, these disorders tend to be quite widespread at presentation and are generally responsive to chemotherapeutic agents and radiation therapy. In general, the management of these disorders is best left to individuals accustomed to dealing with the intricacies of their treatment. Referral to a subspecialist is probably appropriate when one of these conditions is suspected or diagnosed.

CLASSIFICATION

Leukemias

The leukemias can be classified based on their cell of origin and clinical course.

Myeloid

The myeloid leukemias can be acute or chronic.

- *Acute.* Acute myelogenous leukemia (AML) results in a proliferation of primitive myeloid cells (myeloblasts). Particularly in elderly patients, this malignancy can sometimes evolve from another clonal hematopoietic disorder, most commonly myelodysplastic syndrome. Several subtypes of AML have been described, based largely on the presumed lineage of the myeloblast. Table 90-1 lists the commonly used classification of AML.
- *Chronic.* Chronic myelogenous leukemia (CML) belongs to the myeloproliferative group of disorders in which both proliferation and maturation of myeloid cells occur. Thus, intermediate myeloid cells such as myelocytes and metamyelocytes predominate in the blood of patients with CML.

Lymphoid

Proliferation of lymphoid cells in the bone marrow and lymphoid tissues with malignant cells appearing in the blood results in the lymphoid leukemias.

- *Acute.* In acute lymphoblastic leukemia (ALL) the predominant neoplastic cell is a primitive lymphoid cell (lymphoblast). Three subtypes (L1–L3) have been described based on the morphology of the lymphoblast. ALL may be derived from B- or T-lymphocyte precursors.
- *Chronic.* In chronic lymphocytic leukemia (CLL), mature lymphocytes predominate. This neoplasm is usually derived from B lymphocytes but sometimes can be from T-lymphocytes as well.

Lymphomas

These consist of Hodgkin disease and non-Hodgkin's lymphomas.

Hodgkin's Disease

The diagnosis of Hodgkin's disease depends on the pathologic examination of an involved lymph node. Lymph node architecture is effaced by a mixture of cells including lymphocytes, histiocytes, plasma cells, and eosinophils. The pathognomonic feature is the presence of Reed-Sternberg cells, which typically contain two or more large vesicular nuclei, each with a prominent nucleolus. Although the presence of Reed-Sternberg cells is necessary for the diagnosis of Hodgkin's disease, it is not sufficient; Reed-Sternberg–like cells may rarely be seen in non-Hodgkin's lymphomas and solid tumors and even in viral infections.The Reed-Sternberg cell and its variants are believed to be the neoplastic cells of Hodgkin's disease. The relative paucity of neoplastic cells in involved tissues makes Hodgkin's disease unique among neoplastic disorders. The origin of the neoplastic cell continues to be debated. Its immunophenotype can have features of B cells, T cells, or occasionally histiocytes, suggesting either an aberrant lineage or the ability to mature along either lymphoid or histiocytic cell lines. Hodgkin's disease has been classified into four subtypes based on pathologic features as outlined in Table 90-2.

Table 90-1. Subtypes of Acute Myelogenous Leukemia

FAB TYPE	COMMON NAME	UNIQUE FEATURES
M1	Myeloid without maturation	
M2	Myeloid with maturation	t(8,21) in 10%
M3	Acute promyelocytic	DIC is common; response to retinoic acid
M4	Myelomonocytic	
M5	Monocytic	Gum and skin infiltrates
M6	Erythroleukemia	
M7	Megakaryoblastic leukemia	

Non-Hodgkin's Lymphomas

These are malignant disorders that arise from lymphocytes or lymphoid precursor cells. The term non-Hodgkin's lymphoma encompasses a wide spectrum of disorders that have been classified differently over the years. The working formulation that groups these neoplasms into three major categories is the most clinically useful way to classify them. Table 90-3 lists the types of non-Hodgkin's lymphoma using the working formulation and the older but still widely used Rappaport classification.

ETIOLOGY

The etiology of leukemia is not known but both genetic and environmental factors have been implicated. A familial tendency to develop leukemia has occasionally been noted and some congenital disorders such as Down syndrome are associated with an increased risk of leukemia. Exposure to radiation has been associated with an increased risk of developing both AML and CML and possibly ALL as well.

Hodgkin's disease occurs in a bimodal age distribution, and causative environmental factors have been strongly implicated, particularly in younger patients. Non-Hodgkin's lymphomas occur with increased frequency in immunosuppressed individuals including those with acquired immunodeficiency syndrome (AIDS). Viruses have also been implicated in the pathogenesis of certain types of non-Hodgkin's lymphoma such as Epstein-Barr virus in Burkitt lymphoma.

HISTORY

Acute Leukemias

The acute leukemias, AML and ALL, share many clinical features. Characteristically, the initial presentation is acute with symptoms for weeks to a few months. About one fourth of patients with AML, particularly elderly patients, may have underlying myelodysplastic syndromes with associated cytopenia for many months prior to the diagnosis. The presenting symptoms of the acute leukemias usually relate to the ensuing cytopenia with weakness, fatigue, and shortness of breath due to anemia, bleeding at various sites due to thrombocytopenia, and infections due to neu-

Table 90-2. Subtypes of Hodgkin Disease

SUBTYPE	FREQUENCY (%)
Lymphocyte predominance	5%
Nodular sclerosis	50%
Mixed cellularity	40%
Lymphocyte depletion	5%

Table 90-3. Histologic Classification of Non-Hodgkin's Lymphoma

WORKING FORMULATION	RAPPAPORT CLASSIFICATION
Low grade	
A Small lymphocytic cell	Diffuse well differentiated lymphocytic (DWDL)
B Follicular small cleaved cell	Nodular poorly differentiated lymphocytic (NPDL)
C Follicular mixed, small cleaved and large cell	Nodular mixed (NM)
Intermediate grade	
D Follicular large cell	Nodular histiocytic (NH)
E Diffuse small cleaved cell	Diffuse poorly differentiated lymphocytic (DPDL)
F Diffuse mixed, small cleaved and large cell	Diffuse mixed (DM)
G Diffuse large cell	Diffuse histiocytic (DH)
High grade	
H Large cell immunoblastic	Diffuse histiocytic
I Lymphoblastic	Diffuse lymphoblastic (LL)
J Small noncleaved cell; Burkitt	Diffuse undifferentiated (DUL)

tropenia. Occasionally patients with marked leukocytosis can present with symptoms of leukostasis such as visual blurring and shortness of breath. Rarely, pressure symptoms due to soft tissue masses of leukemia cells (chloroma), symptoms due to meningeal infiltration, or metabolic derangements due to tumor lysis syndrome can be presenting features.

Chronic Leukemias

The chronic leukemias have a more indolent presentation. CML may present with systemic symptoms such as fever and night sweats or be incidentally detected as splenomegaly or leukocytosis. CLL is most often detected as an incidental lymphocytosis.

Hodgkin's Disease

Patients with Hodgkin's disease usually present with painless lymphadenopathy that may or may not be accompanied by systemic symptoms including fevers, night sweats, weight loss, malaise, and pruritus. Adenopathy most often involves cervical and mediastinal lymph node groups with occasional contiguous involvement of paraaortic and inguinal nodes. Only a minority of patients have liver, spleen, bone marrow, or lung involvement at the time of diagnosis. Rarely, Hodgkin's disease presents in an extralymphatic site such as bone, breast, gastrointestinal tract, or endocrine gland.

Non-Hodgkin's Lymphomas

Two thirds of patients with non-Hodgkin's lymphomas present with painless lymphadenopathy. Systemic symptoms are less common than in Hodgkin's disease. Other features that distinguish non-Hodgkin's lymphoma from Hodgkin's disease include involvement of Waldeyer's ring, and frequency of extranodal presentations. Patients with low grade non-Hodgkin's lymphoma as described previously tend to have a more indolent presentation whereas aggressive non-Hodgkin's lymphoma can present with rapidly enlarging masses, systemic symptoms, or central nervous system involvement.

CLINICAL FINDINGS

The clinical findings in the acute leukemias usually relate to the accompanying cytopenia. Pallor is common and petechiae and ecchymoses often occur. Occasionally, splenomegaly is palpable. The monocytic variant is more likely to present with signs of tissue infiltration such as gum hypertrophy.

CML usually presents with splenomegaly. In CLL, both splenomegaly and lymphadenopathy can occur. Hodgkin's disease and non-Hodgkin's lymphoma often result in palpable lymphadenopathy or organomegaly.

A common dilemma facing the primary care provider is the approach to the work-up of an enlarged lymph node. Most experts agree that biopsy should be performed on a firm lymph node that measures more than 1 cm, is not associated with an apparent infection, and persists more than 4 to 6 weeks. In an asymptomatic patient in whom enlarged lymph nodes are incidentally found, a period of observation is often reasonable. When the patient detects the enlarged lymph node, more urgent biopsy is usually required. Factors to consider in making the decision to biopsy include size and number of the enlarged lymph nodes, age of the patient, and the coexistence of symptoms.

LABORATORY AND IMAGING STUDIES

Acute Leukemias

Diagnosis of the acute leukemias requires examination of the bone marrow. Usually, involvement is extensive by the time clinical presentation occurs. The distinction between the various types of acute leukemia can be made on morphologic grounds and with the appropriate use of cytochemical stains. Immunofluorescent staining followed by flow cytometric analysis is being increasingly used in this setting to assist with the differential diagnosis. From a management standpoint, it is very important to distinguish myeloid from lymphoid forms of acute leukemia whereas distinction of various subtypes is less important. In addition to tests required to make the diagnosis, the initial evaluation of patients with acute leukemia should include a chemistry profile to look for hyperuricemia, renal dysfunction, and other metabolic signs of tumor lysis because these may require urgent attention. A complete blood count is required to assess the presence of cytopenia and the need for transfusions.

Chronic Myelogenous Leukemia

The diagnosis of CML can often be suspected upon the examination of the peripheral blood smear. A moderate to marked leukocytosis is usually seen with the whole range of myeloid precursors being present, often referred to as a "garden party appearance." There is a predominance of intermediate myeloid cells including myelocytes and metamyelocytes. This type of blood morphology is sometimes seen in reactive states and is referred to as a leukemoid reaction. Features that distinguish CML from a leukemoid reaction include degree of leukocytosis (usually $< 50{,}000/mm^3$ in leukemoid reactions), leukocyte alkaline phosphatase score (usually very low in CML), and the presence in most cases of CML of a unique cytogenetic abnormality, t(9,22), called the "Philadelphia chromosome." The bone marrow in CML is usually hypercellular with predominance of myeloid precursors.

Chronic Lymphocytic Leukemia

CLL can often be diagnosed by the presence of lymphocytosis in the absence of an apparent infection. Morphologically, the peripheral blood lymphocytes are well differentiated and normal appearing. They tend to be fragile leading to the frequent occurrence of "smudge cells" on the peripheral blood smear. Immunofluorescence staining with flow cytometric analysis can reveal the diagnostic predominance of B cells that often have a surface antigen called CD5 and have either kappa or lambda light chains but not both reflecting clonality. The bone marrow examination can reveal varying degrees of diffuse or nodular lymphocytosis. Physical examination and x-ray evaluation may reveal varying degrees of lymphadenopathy or hepatosplenomegaly. A complete blood count may reveal varying degrees of cytopenia. Three broad stages of CLL have been defined that are of prognostic value. These are outlined in Table 90-4.

It is important to recognize that patients with CLL can develop immune hemolytic anemia or immune thrombocytopenia at any stage of the disease. The occurrence of immune cytopenia does not influence staging.

Lymphoma

The diagnosis of Hodgkin's disease or non-Hodgkin's lymphoma is usually based on the pathologic examination of an enlarged lymph node. After a pathologic diagnosis is established, further clinical, radiologic, and laboratory evaluation is directed toward defining the extent of the disease. This process is called clinical staging and is essential for selection of the most appropriate therapy.

The initial evaluation includes a careful history and physical examination with particular attention to lymph node–bearing areas, complete blood count, screening blood chemistries, and chest x-ray. Abnormal blood studies are common but not helpful in indicating stage or prognosis. If the chest x-ray is suspicious for mediastinal node involvement, computed tomography (CT) of the chest is indicated. An iliac crest bone marrow biopsy may reveal bone marrow involvement.

An abdominal CT scan is performed to assess retroperitoneal and iliac lymph node involvement and to image the liver and spleen. Lymphangiography may demonstrate abnormal retroperitoneal nodes even if the CT scan does not reveal adenopathy. The lymphangiogram allows assessment of nodal architecture as well as nodal size, and may indicate defects suggestive of involvement in nodes of normal size. CT scanning, on the other hand, allows visualization of upper paraaortic, porta hepatis, mesenteric, and splenic hilar nodes, which are not demonstrated by lymphangiography. The two techniques are therefore complementary, and in many centers a negative CT is routinely followed by a lymphangiogram.

Table 90-4. Staging of Chronic Lymphocytic Leukemia

STAGE	CLINICAL FEATURES	MEDIAN SURVIVAL
A	Lymphocytosis alone or with involvement of <3 lymph node groups	>10 y
B	Involvement of >3 lymph node groups	~5 y
C	Anemia or thrombocytopenia	~2 y

The use of a widely accepted, standardized staging system is extremely important in comparing results of treatment and predicting prognosis. The staging system for lymphomas is as follows:

- *Stage I.* Involvement of a single lymph node region (I) or localized involvement of a single extralymphatic organ or site (IE)
- *Stage II.* Involvement of two or more lymph node regions on the same side of the diaphragm (II) or localized involvement of a single associated extralymphatic organ or site and its regional lymph nodes on the same side of the diaphragm (IIE)
- *Stage III.* Involvement of lymph node regions on both sides of the diaphragm (III), which may also be accompanied by localized involvement of an associated extralymphatic organ or site (IIIE), or by involvement of the spleen (IIIS) or both (IIISE). Stage III1 indicates involvement of upper abdominal lymphatic structures: spleen, porta hepatis nodes, celiac nodes, or splenic hilar nodes. Stage III2 includes involved nodes in the paraaortic, iliac, mesenteric, or inguinal areas with or without involvement of the upper abdominal lymphatic structures.
- *Stage IV.* Disseminated (multifocal) involvement of one or more extralymphatic organs with or without associated lymph node involvement, or isolated extralymphatic organ involvement with distant (nonregional) nodal involvement.

If systemic symptoms of unexplained weight loss in excess of 10% of body weight, fever, or night sweats are present, the letter B is added to the stage. The letter A denotes absence of systemic symptoms.

In the case of Hodgkin's disease, staging laparotomy should be considered after the clinical staging evaluation described is complete. The purpose of staging laparotomy is to detect disease in retroperitoneal nodes, spleen, or liver that has not been identified by the clinical staging procedures and to confirm the presence of Hodgkin's disease in radiologically abnormal nodes visualized by CT or lymphangiogram. Laparotomy is indicated if its findings influence the choice of therapy. However, if the finding of occult abdominal or retroperitoneal disease would not influence the choice of therapy, then laparotomy should be omitted. In general, laparotomy is most often required in patients with clinical stage IA and IIA disease, and occasionally in patients with clinical stage IIIA disease. Patients with stage IIIB or IV disease require chemotherapy regardless of laparotomy findings; therefore the procedure would be superfluous in this group.

Most series report that laparotomy results in a change in the clinical stage in about 30% to 40% of patients, with most changes in the direction of increasing stage (ie, from stage I or II to stage III or IV). Reliance on clinical stage in these patients would result in undertreatment and high risk of subdiaphragmatic recurrence. The minority whose clinical stage is decreased by laparotomy are spared the toxicity of inappropriate overtreatment based on clinical stage.

Staging laparotomy is usually not required in non-Hodgkin's lymphomas because the results do not critically influence the therapeutic decision.

TREATMENT

When the diagnosis of a hematologic malignancy is made, it is important to evaluate the patient for other underlying medical conditions. A therapeutic decision needs to be individualized weighing the intensity of the planned treatment regimen against the age and general condition of the patient. Older patients or those with significant underlying disease processes might not be appropriate candidates for intensive chemotherapy.

Acute Leukemias

The management of acute leukemias involves the use of intense myeloablative chemotherapy with intent to cure. The initial phase of treatment called "remission induction chemotherapy" is the most important phase. Intensive systemic chemotherapy is administered with the goal of reducing the leukemic cell burden below the level of detection. Because the chemotherapy drugs used have little selectivity for leukemic cells over their normal bone marrow counterparts, therapy is usually accompanied by the development of severe myelosuppression prior to achieving a complete remission. The two most active drugs used in AML are cytosine arabinoside and daunorubicin. The combination of these agents results in a complete remission rate of 60% to 80%. The therapy in ALL may be less intense, particularly in children. Prednisone and vincristine are an important component of the chemotherapy used for ALL (particularly in children). In adults with ALL, additional intense chemotherapy that includes an anthracycline is also typically used. Induction therapy usually results in myeloablation over the course of 5 to 7 days. This is followed in 3 to 4 weeks by recovery of the normal marrow components. Supportive care during this time is a critical part of the management and usually involves long-term hospitalization. Blood product support is usually needed as is the appropriate management of intercurrent infections. It is generally advisable to use platelet transfusions to maintain the count over 15 to 20,000/mL. During the neutropenic phase, patients are at risk of developing potentially life-threatening infections. A fever in this setting requires prompt evaluation and often empiric therapy. Fungal infections are a common cause of morbidity and mortality in this setting and the appropriate institution of empiric antifungal therapy is crucial to achieving a favorable outcome.

Involvement of the central nervous system requires special attention because most chemotherapy regimens do not cross the blood brain-barrier. Prophylactic central nervous system therapy is usually indicated in ALL because occult involvement of the central nervous system is common. Certain subtypes of AML such as the monocytic variants have an increased tendency for central nervous system involvement as well.

If remission induction therapy does not result in a complete remission, the prognosis is grave. Once a complete remission is achieved it should be immediately followed by consolidation chemotherapy in order to achieve the best possible chance of a long-term remission. This therapy is also usually as intense as the initial induction treatment. In addition, the management of ALL typically involves lower dose maintenance therapy for several months.

These forms of consolidation and maintenance chemotherapy have been replaced in part since the early 1980s by bone marrow transplantation. Unfortunately, allogeneic bone marrow transplantation is a relatively risky procedure with high mortality and morbidity rates particularly in older individuals. Most centers exclude patients over 55 years of age from their allogeneic bone marrow transplant programs. Moreover, only about 30% of individuals have an HLA-matched sibling donor available. There is some controversy in the literature as to whether every patient under 55 years of age who has an HLA-matched sibling donor should automatically receive an allogeneic bone marrow transplant in first remission. Some centers reserve this technique for individuals who have disease relapses.

Modern-day intensive induction chemotherapy regimens followed by consolidation chemotherapy or bone marrow transplantation result in long-term cure rates in the order of 20% to 30% in patients with AML. Children with ALL have a better prognosis, with about 90% cure rates with chemotherapy alone. Adults with ALL have a prognosis similar to that of adults with AML.

Chronic Myelogenous Leukemia

The management of CML differs considerably from that of the acute leukemias. The disease course is characterized by an initial chronic phase in which most patients initially present. During this phase, mild oral chemotherapy using agents such as hydroxyurea and busulfan is usually sufficient to control the leukocytosis and associated symptoms. Unfortunately, these patients almost universally transform, in a median of 3.5 to 4 years, to an accelerated phase followed by blastic transformation. Once this occurs, the disease is almost uniformly fatal. The only curative therapy available is allogeneic bone marrow transplantation. This procedure is much more effective when performed in the chronic phase rather than after blastic transformation. Patients under 55 to 60 years of age who have HLA-matched sibling donors should be offered bone marrow transplantation early in the course of their disease. Individuals who do not have matched sibling donors should be offered the possibility of a matched unrelated bone marrow transplant. Because this procedure involves considerable risk of morbidity and mortality, the decision to proceed is a more difficult one, particularly in older patients.

Chronic Lymphocytic Leukemia

CLL is a slowly progressive neoplasm and the goals of therapy differ considerably from those noted previously. No curative therapy is currently available. On the other hand, patients with this disorder can enjoy long survival rates often with few symptoms. Therapy is indicated when symptoms occur or the disease is associated with significant cytopenia. Immune cytopenia are managed using steroids or splenectomy in a manner analogous to that used in these disorders when they occur in the absence of CLL. Cytoreductive therapy usually consists of oral alkylating agents, chlorambucil being most commonly used. The goal is to reduce the leukemic cell burden enough to relieve symptoms, shrink symptomatic lymphadenopathy and organomegaly, and relieve cytopenia.

Hodgkin's Disease

The treatment of Hodgkin's disease has improved dramatically in the past 30 years, illustrating the value of coordinated interdisciplinary cooperation consisting of meticulous pathologic classification, careful clinical and surgical staging, and a team approach to therapy by medical oncologists and radiation therapists. Prior to the development of modern radiotherapy and cytotoxic chemotherapy, the median survival of patients with Hodgkin's disease was about 2 years. Most patients with localized disease are cured with radiation therapy, and a majority of those with disseminated disease are cured with combination chemotherapy or combined modality treatment.

Current investigational efforts are directed toward finding treatment programs that maximize remission rates and durations and at the same time minimizing immediate and long-term complications. Application of these principles has led to the following general guidelines for treatment:

- *Stage IA, IIA*. Radiation therapy (40 to 45 Gy) delivered to areas of known involvement as well as adjacent lymph node areas at risk to contain occult disease (extended field irradiation)
- *Stage IIB*. Often treated with both radiation therapy and combination chemotherapy because of a high failure rate following radiation alone
- *Stage IIIA*. Controversial. Recommendations include radiotherapy alone, chemotherapy alone, and combined modality therapy.
- *Stage IIIB, IV*. Combination chemotherapy, primarily. Low-dose radiation to bulky sites of involvement is sometimes used for consolidation, particularly in patients with nodular sclerosis.

Over the years, several effective chemotherapy regimens have evolved for the treatment of Hodgkin's disease. The two most widely used regimens, MOPP and ABVD, are shown in Table 90-5. The development of MOPP chemotherapy by DeVita and associates in the 1960s marked the beginning of curative chemotherapy for advanced Hodgkin's disease. Since that time, several groups of investigators have attempted to improve on the results obtained using MOPP. One approach has been to use variations of the MOPP regimen. Another approach is to use different non–cross-resistant regimens such as the ABVD regimen of Bonadonna and colleagues. More recently, combinations of MOPP and ABVD-like regimens have been used.

Non-Hodgkin's Lymphomas

The management of non-Hodgkin's lymphoma starts with accurate pathologic classification, discussed earlier, and staging. As in the case of the other hematologic malignancies, assessment of the general health of the patient and coexistent illnesses is necessary to determine potential complications from therapy.

In general terms, the indolent lymphomas have a relatively benign clinical course and therapy is unlikely to be curative. The prototype pathologic subtype is the nodular, poorly differentiated lymphocytic lymphoma. The goal of treatment in the indolent lymphomas is to achieve palliation of symptoms. If the patient is asymptomatic, observation without therapeutic intervention may be appropriate. If symptoms are due to regional lymph node enlargement, local radiation therapy may provide relief. For more generalized disease, systemic chemotherapy is often useful. Alkylating agents such as chlorambucil and cyclophosphamide are often used, sometimes in combination with prednisone and, occasionally, vincristine.

The intermediate to aggressive non-Hodgkin's lymphomas are more likely to be symptomatic at presentation and have a rapidly fatal course if left untreated. On the other hand, a substantial proportion of these patients can be cured using combination chemotherapy. The prototype intermediate grade lymphoma is diffuse large cell lymphoma. Standard chemotherapy for this disease includes a combination of cyclophosphamide, doxorubicin, vincristine, and prednisone (CHOP). Of these patients, 50% to 60% achieve complete remission and about half of the remissions are sustained long term. More intensive chemotherapy regimens have been used in recent years but randomized trials have not proven these to be superior to the standard CHOP regimen. The more aggressive lymphomas such as Burkitt lymphoma and lymphoblastic lymphoma are treated with aggressive chemotherapy regimens similar to that used in ALL.

In patients with intermediate to aggressive non-Hodgkin's lymphomas that fail to respond or relapse after initial combination chemotherapy, salvage chemotherapy regimens have been used with limited success and little chance of sustained remission. Autologous and allogeneic bone marrow transplantation offer the only realistic chance of long-term disease control in this situation and are being increasingly used for this indication, particularly in younger patients.

Table 90-5. Chemotherapy for Hodgkin Disease

AGENT	DOSE
MOPP regimen*	
Nitrogen mustard	6 mg/m^2 IV days 1 and 8
Vincristine	1.4 mg/m^2 IV days 1 and 8
Procarbazine	100 mg/m^2 PO days 1–14
Prednisone†	40 mg/m^2 PO days 1–14
ABVD regimen*	
Adriamycin	25 mg/m^2 IV days 1 and 15
Bleomycin	10 mg/m^2 IV days 1 and 15
Vinblastine	6 mg/m^2 IV days 1 and 15
Dacarbazine	375 mg/m^2 IV days 1 and 15

*Repeat cycles every 28 days, minimum of 6 cycles.
†Cycles 1 and 4 only.

Long-Term Sequelae of Therapy

Long-term survivors after chemotherapy or radiation therapy or both are prone to certain complications that primary care practitioners should be aware of. These complications have been best studied in Hodgkin's disease survivors. Potential complications of radiotherapy include hypothyroidism, pericarditis, pneumonitis, spinal cord injury, infertility, and rarely damage to bone, liver, or kidney. Radiation to the mediastinum increases future risk of coronary atherosclerosis. Chemotherapy with MOPP and its variants produces permanent sterility in almost all men and many young women. ABVD has a lower likelihood of leading to sterility, but the use of doxorubicin and radiation to the heart may cause cardiomyopathy, and increased risk of pulmonary damage occurs in patients treated with both bleomycin and chest irradiation. Greater myelotoxicity is observed in patients receiving combined modality therapy also. Second malignancies, especially AML and non-Hodgkin's lymphomas, pose a substantial risk for patients treated with combined modality therapy or chemotherapy alone.

CONSIDERATIONS IN PREGNANCY

The occurrence of hematologic malignancies during pregnancy poses a particularly challenging therapeutic decision. Staging x-ray is contraindicated, at least relatively. The administration of chemotherapeutic agents during the first trimester is known to be teratogenic. A recent review of acute leukemia during pregnancy revealed a higher incidence of spontaneous abortion and premature delivery when leukemia was diagnosed and treated during the first or second trimester.

Factors to be considered when making therapeutic decisions during pregnancy include:

- The nature of the hematologic malignancy. In the aggressive neoplasms such as the acute leukemias, treatment is urgently needed. In the more indolent disorders such as the indolent lymphomas, treatment can sometimes be deferred until after delivery.
- The stage of pregnancy. In the first trimester, the teratogenic risk of chemotherapy is high and it may be appropriate to terminate the pregnancy. In the second and third trimester, teratogenic effects are less likely and it may also be more feasible to delay therapy until after delivery.
- Patient preference. A detailed discussion with the patient about the prognosis of the malignancy is necessary to enable her to make an informed decision regarding the risks and benefits of chemotherapy, postponement of therapy, and continuation of the pregnancy.

The ultimate decision should involve close collaboration between hematologist/oncologist, radiation oncologist, obstetrician, primary care physician, and the patient.

BIBLIOGRAPHY

Allen HH, Nisker JA. Cancer in pregnancy: therapeutic guidelines. New York: Futura, 1986.

Armitage JO. Bone marrow transplantation in the treatment of patients with lymphoma. Blood 1989;73:1749.

Armitage JO. Treatment of non-Hodgkin's lymphoma. N Engl J Med 1993;328:1023.

Champlin R, Gale RP. Acute lymphoblastic leukemia: recent advances in biology and therapy. Blood 1989;73:2051.

Coltman CA Jr, ed. Introduction: Hodgkin's disease 1990. Semin Oncol 1990;17:641.

Foon KA, Gale RP. Therapy of acute myelogenous leukemia. Blood Rev 1992;6:15.

Foon KA, Rai KR, Gale RP. Chronic lymphocytic leukemia: new insights into biology and therapy. Ann Intern Med 1990;113:525.

Hehlmann R. Chronic myelogenous leukemia: recent developments in prognostic evaluation and chemotherapy. Leukemia 1992;6(Suppl 3):110S.

Mandelli F, ed. Therapy of acute leukemias. Leukemia 1992;6:1.

Stone RM, Mayer RJ. Treatment of the newly diagnosed adult with de novo acute myeloid leukemia. Hematol Oncol Clin North Am 1993;7:47.

Primary Care for Women, edited by Phyllis C. Leppert and Fred M. Howard. Lippincott-Raven Publishers, Philadelphia © 1997.

91

Introduction to Chemotherapy

JOANNA M. CAIN

The use of chemotherapy to treat malignancy is always directed at a potential or verified metastatic disease process. Localized cancers are generally treated with radiation, surgical extirpation, or both. Chemotherapy is being combined with radiation and surgery for localized tumors when there is either the high potential of metastases (as in breast cancer) or the local response is enhanced by its use as a radiation sensitizer. The principles guiding the use of chemotherapy are outlined by Skipper and colleagues. In short, chemotherapeutic drugs kill a constant fraction of cancer cells regardless of size of the tumor (first-order kinetics); therefore, smaller tumors are more curable than large tumors. Second, resistance can emerge during treatment, or be present de novo, which has led to the preference for multiagent chemotherapy as a means to address different populations of cancer cells. The choice of drugs used in combination chemotherapy must each be at least partially effective when used alone for the cancer treated. It also is theoretically important to combine drugs that act in different parts of the cell cycle or cell division, with the hope that the resistance mechanism for one agent may be different than the other. Given the theoretic advantage of combining drugs that have different mechanisms and targets of action (with the presumed avoidance of cross-resistance), the major chemotherapeutic drugs are reviewed by mechanisms. The largest group focuses on affecting the nucleic acids of cancer cells by alkylation, strand scission, and intercalation.

CHEMOTHERAPEUTIC DRUGS

Alkylating Agents

Alkylating agents were the first class of chemotherapeutic drugs developed with nitrogen mustard, introduced in the 1940s and still used for lymphoma therapy—the for bearer of this class of drugs. The most commonly used agents are cisplatin and carboplatin, both of which do their work by cross-linking DNA strands. The platinum class of alkylating agents are unique in that they are the only heavy-metal compound in common use for chemotherapy. Drugs in this class with their likely toxicities and therapeutic targets are outlined in Table 91-1.

Antitumor Antibiotics

Antitumor antibiotics are, in many ways, a subset of the drugs that attack the nucleic acids. They work either by intercalation or by strand scission (bleomycin). One class of these agents, the anthracyclines, are the agents in this class (doxorubicin and daunomycin) that are most commonly used for solid tumors, particularly breast and lung, as well as for leukemias. The anthracyclines also have the unique side effect of cardiotoxicity, both an acute syndrome that is not dose dependent and a cumulative cardiomyopathy directly related to the overall dosage.

Enzyme Inhibitors

The point of affecting the output of different enzymatic processes of the cell is simply to have fewer building blocks available for DNA synthesis and eventual division. The different agents specifically block different pathways. 5-fluorouracil, widely used for gastrointestinal malignancies, specifically inhibits thymidylate synthetase. Methotrexate, used for gestational trophoblastic disease and now for some ectopic pregnancies, inhibits dihydrofolate reductase. Cytosine arabinoside, used for hematologic malignancies, inhibits DNA polymerase. Often these agents are combined with the normal product of a blocked metabolic path, such as leucovorin (5-formyl tetrahydrofolate), to either "rescue" normal cells

Table 91-1. Chemotherapeutic Drugs

CLASS	SELECTED DRUG	MOST FREQUENT SIDE EFFECTS	USED COMMONLY FOR
Alkylating (nucleic acid)	Cisplatin	Nausea, vomiting, nephrotoxicity (Mg, Ca wasting) ototoxicity, neurotoxicity	Ovarian, lung, endometrial
	Carboplatin	Milder symptoms than cisplatin	Ovarian, lung, endometrial
	Cyclophosphamide	Hemorrhagic cystitis, myelosuppression	Ovarian, breast, others
	Etoposide	Nausea, myelosuppression, neuropathy (especially combined with vincristine)	Lung, ovarian, lymphoma, testicular
Antibiotics (nucleic acid)	Bleomycin	Pulmonary fibrosis, fever, skin pigmentation, hypersensitivity	Cervix, germ cell malignancies
	Actinomycin d	Mucositis, stomatitis, diarrhea, myelosuppression, "radiation recall"	Germ cell, gestational trophoblastic disease
	Doxorubicin	Cardiac toxicity, skin necrosis with extravasation, myelosuppression	Breast cancer, sarcoma
Enzymes	Cytosine arabinoside	Nausea, myelosuppression, stomatitis, hepatotoxicity	Leukemia
	5-fluorouracil	Nausea, myelosuppression, hand and foot syndrome when combined with leucovorin	Colon, breast, ovarian cancers
	Hydroxyurea	Myelotoxicity	Leukemia
	Methotrexate	Mucositis, myelosuppression, nephrotoxicity at high doses	Gestational trophoblastic disease
Mitotic spindle	Vincristine and vinblastine	Neuropathy (vincristine), myelosuppression (vinblastine)	Leukemia, lymphoma, pediatrics
	Paclitaxel	Hypersensitivity, neutropenia	Ovarian, breast, others?

when large doses are given or to propel the cell systems toward a blocked path, as when it is used with 5-fluorouracil.

Mitotic Spindle Agents

These agents affect the function of the mitotic spindle in various ways, inhibiting division. Vincristine, vinblastine, and paclitaxel are the common agents of this group in widest use.

HORMONAL THERAPIES

Hormonal therapies are generally considered cytostatic rather than cytotoxic, because they do not directly cause the death of cells. The most commonly used agents are tamoxifen and progestational agents.

SIDE EFFECTS AND REACTIONS

Side Effects of Chemotherapy Agents

The major facets of chemotherapy of concern to the primary care provider are the side effects that they may be called on to identify and treat. These are not specifically associated with the class of drug, but rather the individual profile of each drug. Therapy for the common side effects and the consequences for further chemotherapy are outlined here.

Hypersensitivity Reactions

For some drugs, such as paclitaxel, the potential for hypersensitivity is high enough that all patients receive prophylaxis. For others it is idiosyncratic and related to mode of delivery. Major drugs with associated hypersensitivity include L-asparaginase, cisplatin, etoposide, and the anthracycline antibiotics. Treatment of the reaction is usually acute with treatment for hypotension as well as H_1- and H_2-receptor antagonists (hydroxyzine, cimetidine). Retreatment with the drug is generally contraindicated when severe hypotension is encountered. However, milder reactions may be alleviated by substituting analogs, if possible, or pretreatment with prednisone, H1 and H2 when this particular agent is important to the success of the cancer therapy.

Skin Reactions

Drug extravasation can have direct and dramatic effects on the skin as well as tendons and subcutaneous tissues. The major treatment is avoidance by careful administration techniques, particularly for doxorubicin, with blood return and free flow of fluids demonstrated before injection. Management of an area following a recognized extravasation varies; removal of fluid from the area, if possible, is the first option. Injection of substances into the skin to lessen the toxicity has also been proposed but the agent to be used is different for each agent. Most pharmacies mixing chemotherapy-class drugs would have a list of these agents. Ultimately, some of these extravasations may be severe enough to require skin debridement and grafting.

Skin burning can be initiated by a radiation-association effect, regardless of the timing of the radiation versus the drug (called after radiation recall), and by sunlight. The most significant reactions occur with actinomycin d, although doxorubicin, 5-fluorouracil, and hydroxyurea can initiate such a reaction. Major sunburns can occur in patients receiving methotrexate, 5-fluorouracil, and the Vinca alkaloids who do not protect themselves from sun exposure.

Finally, other skin side effects such as pigmentation increase, or tanning in areas of trauma (like in areas of scratching) and nail changes occur with different agents. Some of the skin changes are permanent; therefore, care should be taken at all times in the maintenance of skin integrity.

Oral Lesions

Mucositis and subsequent poor nutrition can occur with many chemotherapeutic agents. Management of the oral lesions is critical to maintenance of comfort and nutrition. Unfortunately, lesions that are initiated by chemotherapy have a natural course and there is no specific therapy to shorten that time course. Differentiation from herpetic outbreaks is critical, as is monitoring for secondary infections, both of which can be directly treated. Oral hygiene maintenance with saline mouth-rinsing and use of gentle tooth cleansing (foam brush) is key. A guideline to help during this period of treatment is commonsense avoidance of spicy, acidic, rough, very hot, or very cold foods. For pain, local anesthetic agents such as viscous Xylocaine or various mixtures that can be used before eating as well as in between meals may be helpful. Use of nutritional liquid supplements often is critical to the maintenance of nutrition during this time.

Chemotherapy-Related Nausea and Vomiting

Many of these chemotherapeutic regimens are highly emetic, which has spawned a wide variety of therapies over time. For many patients there are two components to the nausea: anticipatory and chemical. The anticipatory nausea is characterized by nausea (and, frequently, vomiting) that occurs before any drug is given and that is fairly frequent when previous emetic therapy has been given. This type of nausea is best treated with anxiolytic agents such as lorazepam added to the planned regimen prior to the timing of the anticipatory nausea. If, for example, the nausea occurs before leaving the house for treatment, then therapy should begin 30 minutes before leaving the house.

Treatment for chemotherapy-induced nausea and vomiting has progressed significantly over the years, with major new drug classes developed for control, particularly serotonin antagonists. Most chemotherapy regimens include metoclopramide, ondansetron, or granisetron. Both metoclopramide and ondansetron can be given orally. For sustained nausea following chemotherapy, continued oral medication should be planned and is very effective. Electrolytes and nutritional indices are indicated with anorexia and nausea related to chemotherapy.

Nephrotoxicity

An awareness of the nephrotoxicity of different agents is of importance in the long-term care of patients who have received chemotherapeutic agents. Whereas some of the complications, such as the rapid release of uric acid in the treatment of rapidly proliferating tumors (eg, lymphomas and leukemias) with subsequent hyperuricemic nephropathy are immediate effects of chemotherapy, some of the other sequelae are permanent. Most patients receiving directly nephrotoxic drugs (eg, streptozotocin or cisplatin) are followed by evaluation of creatinine clearances to decrease the risk at retreatment. However, some nephrotoxicity, such as that related to nitrosoureas (carmustine [BCNU], semustine [meCCNU]) may not appear for several months to years following chemotherapy. This is particularly true of doses of BCNU and meCCNU given > 1500 mg/m^2.

The nephropathy is induced by inorganic platinum coordination complexes, particularly cisplatin. This nephropathy is related to tubular necrosis, but is particularly focused on hypomagnesemia and hypocalcemia secondary to urinary magnesium wasting. The obvious outcome of unmonitored loss is seizure and tetany. Monitoring and replacement of patients' electrolytes may be an important preventative strategy for long-term primary care of these patients.

Neutropenia and Anemia

The majority of neutropenia and anemia associated with chemotherapy occurs 7 to 21 days after a dose of chemotherapy. Much of this is anticipated and the development of various cytokines to stimulate the production of white and red cells has significantly decreased admissions for neutropenia. A few guiding principles for evaluation of therapy with granulocyte colony stimulating factor (gCSF) are appropriate, however. First, the 3 days immediately following administration of gCSF, white cell counts climb rapidly into multiples of 10,000 in some cases. This does not mean that the gCSF should be stopped, because it represents demargination of white cells. Second, in combination chemotherapy, the expected nadir of white blood cells may be different for the several drugs, so treatment should cover the expected nadir of all drugs.

SUMMARY

Chemotherapy includes a wide variety of injectable agents that modify the growth of cancer cells. Because new agents are available all the time, it is prudent to keep track of the major acute and chronic toxicities of these agents. Neutropenia and bone marrow suppression are the most consistent of these acute side effects. However, everything from the dermis to the kidney can have long-term sequelae from these agents and, thus, requires the attention of the primary care provider.

BIBLIOGRAPHY

Clavel M, Bonneterre J, d'Allens H, Paillarse JM. Oral ondansetron in the prevention of chemotherapy-induced emesis in breast cancer patients. Eur J Cancer 1995;31A:15.

Cohen IJ, Zehavi N, Buchwald I, et al. Oral ondansetron: an effective ambulatory complement to intravenous ondansetron in the control of chemotherapy-induced nausea and vomiting in children. Pediatr Hematol Oncol 1995;12:67.

Greenberger PA, Patterson R, Simon R, Lieberman P, Wallace W. Pretreatment of high risk patients requiring radiographic contrast media studies. J Allergy Clin Immunol 1981;67:185.

Hayes FA, Green AA, Senzer N, Pratt CB. Tetany: a complication of cis-dichlorodiammineplatinum (II) therapy. Cancer Treat Rep 1979;63:547.

Ignoffo RJ, Friedman MA. Therapy of local toxicities caused by extravasation of cancer chemotherapeutic drugs. Cancer Treat Rev 1980;7:17.

Lenaz L, Page JA. Cardiotoxicity of adriamycin and related anthracyclines. Cancer Treat Rev 1976;3:111.

Malik IA, Khan WA, Qazilbash M, Ata E, Butt A, Khan MA. Clinical efficacy of lorazepam in prophylaxis of anticipatory, acute, and delayed nausea and vomiting induced by high doses of cisplatin: a prospective randomized trial. Am J Clin Oncol 1995;18:170.

Morstyn G, Foote M, Perkins D, Vincent M. The clinical utility of granulocyte colony-stimulating factor: early achievements and future promise. Stem Cells 1994;12:213.

Rieger PT, Haeuber D. A new approach to managing chemotherapy-related anemia: nursing implications of epoetin alfa. Oncol Nurs Forum 1995;22:71.

Schacht RG, Feiner HD, Gallo GR, Lieberman A, Baldwin DS. Nephrotoxicity of nitrosoureas. Cancer 1981;48:1328.

Skipper HE, Schabel FM, Jr, Wilcox WS. Experimental evaluation of potential anticancer agents on the criteria and kinetics associated with "curability" of experimental leukemia. Cancer Chemother Rep 1964;35:11.

Stewart A, McQuade B, Cronje JD, et al. Ondansetron compared with granisetron in the prophylaxis of cyclophosphamide-induced emesis in outpatients: a multicentre, double blind, double-dummy, randomised, parallel-group study. Emesis Study Group for Ondansetron and Granisetron in Breast Cancer Patients. Oncology 1995;52:202.

Tsavaris NB, Tsaroucha-Noutsou E, Karvounis N, Bacoyannis C, Pagou M, Kosmidis P. Comparison of different schedules of ondansetron (GR 38032F) administration during cisplatin-based chemotherapy: a randomized trial. Chemotherapy 1995;41:70.

Valeriote FA, Edelstein MB. The role of cell kinetics in cancer chemotherapy. Semin Oncol 1977;4:217.

Vose JM, Armitage JO. Clinical applications of hematopoietic growth factors. J Clin Oncol 1995;13:1023.

Williams LT, O'Dwyer JL. Guidelines for oral hygiene, denture care, and nutrition inpatients with oral complications. In: Peterson DE, Sonis ST, eds. Oral complications of cancer chemotherapy. Baltimore: Kluwer, 1983.

Yarker YE, McTavish D. Granisetron: an update of its therapeutic use in nausea and vomiting induced by antineoplastic therapy. Drugs 1994;48:761.

Primary Care for Women, edited by Phyllis C. Leppert and Fred M. Howard. Lippincott-Raven Publishers, Philadelphia © 1997.

92

Principles of Radiation Therapy

JOANNA M. CAIN

Simply stated, the benefit of radiation therapy for cancer is based on the tissue damage inflicted by the absorption of radiation energy in the tissue. The extent of that damage depends on the emitted energy of the photons, now usually emitted from linear accelerators and betatrons. Higher energy, in general, penetrates more deeply into the tissue being treated, whereas lower energy penetrates only superficially. The dose intensity delivered by a source to adjacent tissues or to personnel is governed by the inverse square law: the radiation intensity varies inversely as the square of the distance from the source; therefore, the best way to avoid radiation exposure or lessen toxicity is by increasing distance from the source (as well as limiting the time of exposure to a source). This phenomenon is also the reason why an implanted radiation source rapidly loses its intensity as distance from it increases. The amount of radiation at different points beyond the source are often described in isodose curves.

The general pattern of radiation therapy uses fractionated doses on the average of 200 cGy/d to accomplish the final dosage. This allows for differential killing of the cancers, with some repair of normal tissues in the field. The complications of radiation therapy depend primarily on the involvement of normal tissue in the radiated field. Multiple adaptations of treatment have developed to decrease these side effects, including computer targeting of the tumor, rotation, shrinking of the field to be treated later, normal tissue shielding, and the use of brachytherapy or interstitial implants to direct higher doses to only the tissue of interest (eg, breast or cervix). Most of the interstitial and brachytherapy implants have removable sources that can be loaded after (afterloaded) to decrease the exposure of staff to radiation sources. If there is any problem with the care of the patient, these sources can be removed rapidly.

Occasionally, patients receive radiation from isotopes in suspension (phosphorus isotope 32 [p32]) that have been used for intraperitoneal treatment of ovarian carcinoma and mesothelioma. This form of radiation has a short half-life (14 days) and has an effective penetration of only millimeters, thus not causing a major concern for exposure to caregivers. However, the surface dose is high and predisposes women to a high incidence of bowel complications, including obstruction and fistula. Other isotopes (eg, ^{125}I) are occasionally implanted in internal tissues, but also give very little exposure beyond several centimeters. Again, this presents little exposure risk for caregivers, but if a patient should die during the decay period of the isotope, removal at autopsy is required for radiation safety. Clearly, the presence of either of these isotopes would warn against close and extended personal contact (holding a child on the patient's lap, for example) until at least the half-time of these isotopes is passed.

RADIATION COMPLICATIONS

Side effects during radiation therapy include skin burning or tanning, local mucositis with concurrent nausea, and bowel mucositis with diarrhea. The majority of these side effects are easily controllable with local skin care (Silvadene or antibiotic ointment is often useful) and oral therapy for nausea and diarrhea (eg, Lomotil). Pelvic radiation may be associated with a mild cystitis and vaginal mucositis, also treated conservatively. These resolve after the therapy is completed.

LATE COMPLICATIONS

Over a longer term of follow-up, radiation induces intense fibrosis in many tissues. Only 20% to 30% of patients have some of the major long-term complications mentioned here, but it is worthwhile to identify their association with the radiation that the woman has received earlier and the unique problems in treatment that represents. For women who received radiation as a child (generally, when under 2 years of age), there are multiple potential late effects. These include: bone deformity, endocrine deficiency (depending on site), and atrophic skin changes; 7% develop second malignancies.

In the subcutaneous tissue that has received a high local dose (head, neck, or groin radiation), there is often a woody, indurated feeling to the tissue that can be permanent. In the lung, there is variable fibrosis with restrictive lung disease secondary to that. In the liver, if hepatic irradiation is used for total body irradiation or whole abdomen radiation, the result can be a radiation hepatitis that acts initially like venoocclusive disease with anicteric ascites appearing 2 to 4 months after radiation.

The bowel syndromes associated with radiation vary. Thirty per cent of patients have continued increases in gastrointestinal (GI) motility that require medication and diet adjustment. Lactase is often insufficient in these patients with significant mucosal radiation damage, and avoidance of milk products may significantly improve diarrhea. Also, avoidance of cruciferous vegetables and other foods associated with increased gut motility can benefit these patients. All patients continue to have diminished local microvascular function in the areas exposed to radiation with concurrent diminished reparative function. This would predict that the risk for GI complications are cumulative over time. In fact, this is true from esophageal to rectal syndromes associated with late effects of GI radiation.

The late effects on the esophagus include dysmotility and benign stricture formation, gastric ulceration, bowel bleeding, frequency, fistula formation, and obstruction. Unfortunately, the same pathophysiology that predisposes to these lesions predisposes to failure of healing after surgical intervention, so the risk of complications with surgery in an irradiated field is quite high. Attempts to control bleeding locally or affect these side effects medically is always the first line of therapy.

Urinary tract side effects follow the same pattern, with hemorrhagic cystitis and ureteral and urethral strictures being the more serious late complications. Also, because of the fibrosis and edema, significant contracture of the bladder can result, for which surgical repair can be especially challenging and which sometimes requires replacement of function with a conduit. The use of hyperbaric oxygen therapy has been proposed for many of these abnormalities of repair in radiated fields, because the delivery of adequate oxygen is essential to normal reparative function. For hemorrhagic cystitis as well as for nonhealing ulcers or surgical wounds in a radiated field, the use of hyperbaric oxygen can improve healing.

Radiation is curative therapy for a number of cancers, but it is not without side effects. The unique feature of radiation side effects is the duration of risk, with late-term risks that are significant. Second surgeries, diagnostic procedures, and so forth in the radiation field are associated with increased risks for poor wound healing and, depending on the organ involved, with increased risks for fistula formation.

BIBLIOGRAPHY

Cascinu S. Drug therapy in diarrheal diseases in oncology/hematology patients. Crit Rev Oncol Hematol 1995;18:37.

Coia LR, Myerson RJ, Tepper JE. Late effects of radiation therapy on the gastrointestinal tract. Int J Radiat Oncol Biol Phys 1995;31:1213.

Kroll SS, Woo SY, Santin A, et al. Long-term effects of radiotherapy administered in childhood for the treatment of malignant diseases. Ann Sur Oncol 1994;1:473.

Lawrence TS, Robertson JM, Anscher MS, Jirtle RL, Ensminger WD, Fajardo LF. Hepatic toxicity resulting from cancer treatment. Int J Radiat Oncol Biol Phys 1995;31:1237.

Lee HC, Liu CS, Chiao C, Lin SN. Hyperbaric oxygen therapy in hemorrhagic radiation cystitis: a report of 20 cases. Undersea Hyperb Med 1994;21:321.

Letschert JG, Lebesque JV, Aleman BM, et al. The volume effect in radiation-related late small bowel complications: results of a clinical study of the EORTC in patients treated for rectal carcinoma. Radiother Oncol 1994;32:116.

McIntyre JF, Eifel PJ, Levenback C, Oswald MJ. Ureteral stricture as a late complication of radiotherapy for stage IB carcinoma of the uterine cervix. Cancer 1995;75:836.

XI

Musculoskeletal Problems

Primary Care for Women, edited by Phyllis C. Leppert and Fred M. Howard. Lippincott-Raven Publishers, Philadelphia © 1997.

93

Evaluation of the Patient With Musculoskeletal Symptoms

CHRISTOPHER T. RITCHLIN

HISTORY

The initial phase of the patient interview should be directed toward determining if the musculoskeletal symptom is emanating from an articular, periarticular, or extraarticular site (Fig. 93-1). Articular structures include the juxtaarticular bone and underlying cartilage, the lining layer or synovium, and other integral structures such as the menisci and joint capsule. Articular pain is usually well localized to the involved joint and exacerbated by weight bearing; movement results in predictable abnormalities in function. The major periarticular sites are tendons, ligaments, and bursa. Pain of periarticular origin can be diffuse or very localized but in general it tends to be adjacent to the joint, and function is preserved. Pain from extraarticular structures such as bone, muscle, nerves, fascia, subcutaneous tissue, and skin is usually diffuse and not localized to the joint. The nature of the pain varies according to which tissue is involved. Neuropathic pain has a burning or lancinating quality often in a radicular pattern whereas muscle pain is often described as a diffuse aching sensation.

Determining whether extraarticular complaints are localized or systemic helps in the formulation of a differential diagnosis. Focal conditions include tennis elbow, trochanteric bursitis, muscle strain, and nerve entrapment syndromes. Generalized nonarticular pain suggests fibromyalgia, polymyositis, polymyalgia rheumatica, or a peripheral neuropathy.

Articular symptoms can arise from one joint (monarthritis) or more than one joint (polyarthritis) and may be secondary to inflammatory or noninflammatory processes. Inflammatory arthritis is associated with erythema, warmth, pain, and swelling in the joint. Systemic features such as morning stiffness, fatigue, low-grade fever, and generalized weakness are frequently present. A reasonable differential diagnosis can be determined based on the anatomic site of origin, number of joints involved, and the presence or absence of inflammation (Tables 93-1 and 93-2). The possibilities can be narrowed further by considering the patient's age, sex, race, and family history. Systemic connective tissue diseases such as polymyositis, systemic lupus erythematosus, and Reiter syndrome are observed in younger patients whereas osteoarthritis, polymyalgia rheumatica, and ischemic necrosis are more prevalent in patients over 50 years of age. Systemic lupus erythematosus (SLE) and sarcoidosis are more common in blacks whereas polymyalgia rheumatica and giant cell arteritis are rare in these patients. Women make up a much higher percentage of patients with SLE, rheumatoid arthritis, and fibromyalgia whereas spondyloarthropathies and gout are more common in men. Disorders that tend to aggregate in families include rheumatoid arthritis, ankylosing spondylitis, psoriatic arthritis, and some forms osteoarthritis.

The pattern of joint involvement and mode of onset can provide valuable clues. Migratory arthritis is seen in subacute bacterial endocarditis, disseminated gonorrhea, early Lyme disease, and acute rheumatic fever. Progressive involvement of the small joints of the hands and feet over time is typical for rheumatoid and psoriatic arthritis and SLE, whereas intermittent symptoms are suggestive of crystalline arthritis (gout or pseudogout), erosive osteoarthritis, or a foreign body in the joint. Rheumatoid arthritis, SLE, and the spondyloarthropathies tend to be insidious in onset. A sudden onset of inflammatory arthritis is more consistent with infection, crystalline arthritis, or a hypersensitivity reaction.

Extraarticular symptoms in the skin, eyes, mucous membranes, and major organs suggest the presence of an underlying inflammatory arthropathy or autoimmune disorder. Characteristic skin eruptions are observed in SLE, psoriatic arthritis, sarcoidosis, Reiter syndrome, and vasculitis. Eye involvement is a frequent occurrence in Reiter syndrome, Sjögren syndrome, and sarcoidosis. Painless oral ulcers are seen in patients with SLE; however, with Behçet disease and inflammatory bowel disease, they are painful. Cardiopulmonary symptoms are not uncommon in SLE, rheumatoid arthritis, and sarcoidosis. Cold-induced vasospasm or Raynaud phenomenon suggest SLE, scleroderma, or mixed connective tissue disease. Disorders of cognition can occur in SLE or Lyme disease whereas peripheral neuropathies can be associated with a number of disorders including rheumatoid arthritis, SLE, Lyme disease, vasculitis, and sarcoidosis.

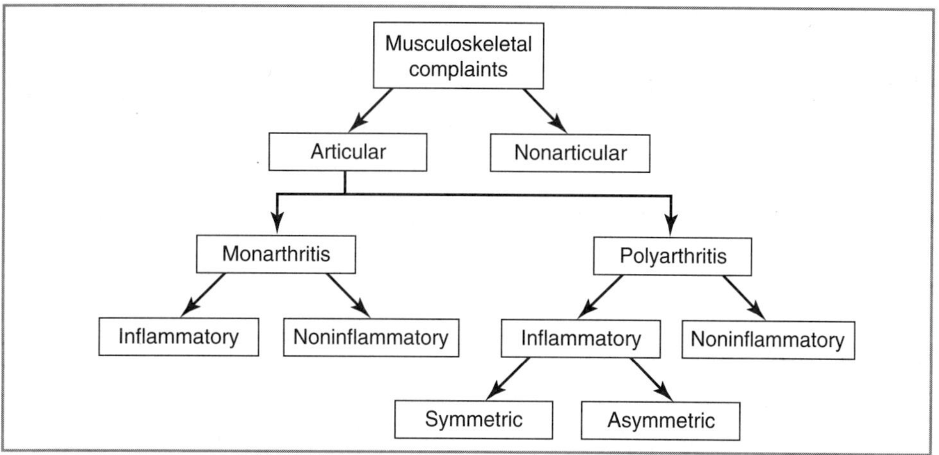

Figure 93-1. Approach to the patient with musculoskeletal symptoms. (Adapted from Zvaifler H. Evaluation of joint complaints. In: Stein JH, ed. Stein internal medicine, 4th ed. St. Louis: Mosby-Year Book, 1994.)

PHYSICAL EXAMINATION

The physical examination is an extension of the history and is guided by the same principal questions:

- Is this articular or nonarticular involvement?
- Is the process inflammatory or noninflammatory, diffuse or focal?
- What is the pattern of involvement and is there evidence of extraarticular disease?

The examination should be performed in an orderly sequence of inspection, palpation, and evaluation of range of motion or—more simply stated—look, feel, and move.

Inspection of joints and periarticular structures for swelling, erythema, or deformities should help to localize the anatomic site of pain. Deformities can arise as a result of subluxation, ankylosis, synovitis, contracture, bony enlargement, or ligamentous inflammation. Close scrutiny of extraarticular sites can also provide important information. Characteristic skin lesions including the malar rash of SLE, papulosquamous lesions in psoriasis and Reiter syndrome, and erythema nodosum associated with sarcoidosis and inflammatory bowel disease provide important clues. Eye findings such as iritis and conjunctivitis may be indicators of an underlying spondyloarthropathy, and dry eyes and mucous membranes are important features of Sjögren syndrome. Aphthous ulcers occur in Behçet disease and inflammatory bowel disease in contrast to the erythematous lesions seen in SLE. Extensor nodules usually indicate rheumatoid arthritis but can also be seen in SLE and acute rheumatic fever.

Table 93-1. Causes of Monoarthritis

Inflammatory	
Infection	Bacterial, fungal, Lyme, viral (hepatitis B, HIV, parvovirus)
Crystal	Gout, pseudogout
Noninflammatory	
Osteoarthritis	
Ischemic necrosis	
Trauma	

Palpation of the joint reveals the presence or absence of synovial thickening, crepitus, tenderness, or warmth. Determining specific areas of tenderness can help to distinguish bursal inflammation from synovitis or tendinitis. Special attention should be focused on the extent and distribution of synovial swelling, tenderness, and warmth.

The movement of a joint through active and passive range of motion can be very useful to the clinician. The patient is asked to imitate the examiner in the movement of the joint through all ranges of motion. If the complete range cannot be attained, the examiner moves the joint passively. Normal passive and abnormal active range of motion is observed in patients with muscle, ligament, or tendon abnormalities. When active and passive range of motion are equally diminished, suspect a block in the joint such as frozen shoulder or synovitis. Reproduction of a distinctive pattern of pain and limitation in a joint subjected to resisted movement helps to identify focal areas of tissue inflammation. For example, pain in the shoulder induced by resisted abduction of this joint arises from the supraspinatus muscle, whereas the pain of biceps tendinitis is increased following resisted supination of the forearm.

The distribution of objective joint findings helps in identifying etiology. Involvement of the axial skeleton (spine, hips, and shoulders) occurs in the spondyloarthropathies (ankylosing spondylitis, Reiter syndrome, psoriatic arthritis, and enteropathic arthritis). A useful maneuver to assess lumbar mobility is Schober's test. A mark is made in the mid-back area at the level of the posterior iliac spine while the patient is standing. A second mark is placed 10 cm above the first and the patient bends forward maximally. The two marks should be separated by at least 15 cm. Expansion less than this amount is suggestive of a spondyloarthropathy.

When examining the peripheral skeleton, the small joints of the hands and feet deserve special attention. Symmetric swelling of the metacarpophalangeal (MCP) and proximal interphalangeal (PIP) joints suggest rheumatoid arthritis (RA) or SLE. Distal interphalangeal (DIP) pain and swelling are associated with osteoarthritis or psoriatic arthritis. Diffuse swelling of a finger or toe (sausage digit or dactylitis) is commonly observed with the spondyloarthropathies, particularly psoriatic arthritis and Reiter syn-

Table 93-2. Causes of Polyarthritis

Inflammatory
Peripheral with axial involvement
- Ankylosing spondylitis, Reiter syndrome, enteropathic arthritis, psoriatic arthritis

Peripheral asymmetric
- Psoriatic arthritis, polyarticular gout, acute rheumatic fever, bacterial endocarditis, sarcoidosis

Peripheral symmetric
- Rheumatoid arthritis, SLE, hepatitis B, serum sickness

Noninflammatory
Osteoarthritis

Hemochromatosis

Acromegaly

Amyloidosis

SLE, systemic lupus erythematosus.

drome. A careful examination of the knees for signs of inflammation, decreased range of motion, locking, and crepitus should be carried out. Detection of a knee effusion can be very helpful because this joint can be readily aspirated.

Performance of a complete neurologic examination including testing motor and sensory function in the peripheral extremities is essential. Neuropathic and myopathic processes can mimic joint pain and also frequently accompany the different forms of inflammatory arthritis.

LABORATORY AND IMAGING STUDIES

Most patients with musculoskeletal problems can be diagnosed by a careful history and physical examination. Laboratory studies help to confirm clinical impressions and can provide measures of disease extent and severity. Patients with acute onset of inflammatory joint pain, with symptoms lasting more than 6 weeks, or with systemic symptoms often require more extensive evaluation.

Routine blood counts, urinalysis, and blood chemistries should be performed in all patients suspected of having a systemic inflammatory or infectious disease. The erythrocyte sedimentation rate (ESR) can help to differentiate inflammatory from noninflammatory musculoskeletal disorders but the test is nonspecific and has not proven useful as a screening test. Westergren ESR > 100 mm/h is generally seen in only systemic inflammatory, infectious, or neoplastic disease. The C-reactive protein (CRP) rises and falls quickly in response to inflammation and, unlike the ESR, is not influenced by anemia or elevated gamma globulins. Uric acid levels are usually elevated in patients with acute gout. Tests for antinuclear antibodies (ANA) and rheumatoid factor (RF) should be ordered in patients suspected of having SLE, rheumatoid arthritis, or a connective tissue disease (scleroderma, polymyositis, mixed connective tissue disease), but these tests are not specific and can lead to improper diagnosis if not placed in clinical context (see Chaps. 82 and 94).

Synovial fluid analysis is mandatory in patients who present with acute monarticular arthritis or polyarthritis with fever. Sending the fluid for a white blood cell count, Gram stain, culture, and sensitivity and crystal analysis helps to differentiate noninflammatory from inflammatory effusions and confirm the existence of crystalline or infectious arthritis (Table 93-3). If only a few drops of synovial fluid is withdrawn, preference should be given to Gram stain and culture in order to exclude an infectious etiology.

Plain x-rays are frequently normal in early inflammatory arthritis although joint effusions and soft tissue swelling are often present. X-rays are important to exclude a fracture or foreign body. Special views of the sacroiliac joints can confirm the diagnosis of a spondyloarthropathy, and calcification of joint cartilage seen on plain x-rays of the knees, wrists, and symphysis pubis is a characteristic feature of calcium pyrophosphate deposition disease (CPPD). It is important to point out that the majority of patients over 60 years of age have degenerative changes of sclerosis, joint space narrowing, and osteophytes on x-rays and these findings frequently do not correlate with symptoms. Therefore, degenerative changes on an x-ray film may not explain the cause of a particular musculoskeletal complaint in this population.

Radionuclide scintigraphy (bone scan) provides information about distribution and extent of an arthropathy but is nonspecific, thereby providing little information regarding etiology. Magnetic resonance imaging (MRI) provides clear images of the cervical and lumbar spine and is useful in defining architecture in peripheral joints especially when looking for a mechanical problem such as a rotator cuff tear in the shoulder or a degenerated meniscus in the knee. Computed tomography (CT) can also be used in the assessment of the axial spine but imaging of the peripheral joints is limited by relatively poor contrast resolution when compared to MRI.

CONSIDERATIONS IN PREGNANCY

A majority of patients develop musculoskeletal symptoms at some point during pregnancy. Generally these problems are transient but in some cases short-term and even permanent disability can occur. The

Table 93-3. Synovial Fluid Analysis

TYPE	APPEARANCE	CELL COUNT (WBCS/UL)	ETIOLOGY
Normal	Clear	<200	Physiologic
Noninflammatory	Clear yellow	200–5000	Osteoarthritis, trauma
Inflammatory	Cloudy yellow	5000–50,000 >60% pmns	Crystalline, rheumatoid arthritis, SLE, seronegative arthritis*
Septic	Purulent	>50,000 >85% pmns	Infection (occasionally crystalline)
Hemorrhagic	Bloody	RBCs predominant	Trauma, coagulopathy, sickle cell anemia

*Seronegative arthritis—psoriatic and enteropathic arthritis, ankylosing spondylitis, enteropathic arthritis.

Pmns, polymorphonuclear leukocytes; *SLE,* systemic lupus erythematosus.

clinician needs to be aware of those conditions that are associated with pregnancy because simple interventions often provide dramatic relief. Patients presenting with hip pain in the third trimester require prompt and thorough evaluation because two conditions affecting this joint, osteonecrosis of the femoral head and transient osteoporosis of the hip, can result in joint destruction, pain, and immobility.

Hormonal and mechanical alterations occurring during pregnancy can have profound effects on musculoskeletal structures. The release of the hormone relaxin causes increased mobility and widening of the sacroiliac joints and symphysis pubis at the same time that the enlarging uterus is placing increasing strain on the lumbar spine and sacroiliac region. Progressive edema of the upper extremities can compress adjacent joint structures including nerves and tendons, and changes in nutritional requirements can result in deficiencies of important vitamins and minerals. Knowledge of these changes, combined with attention to anatomy and disturbed function, helps in making the proper diagnosis.

Low back pain is a frequent complaint and this problem increases in frequency with parity and maternal age. The initial pain and tenderness are usually localized to the sacroiliac joints but often progress to involve the lower lumbar region, with radiation to the back of the thigh. Fibromyalgia and a herniated disk can also cause low back pain, but these entities should be readily diagnosed by history and physical examination.

Fibromyalgia is often described as diffuse muscle aching and fatigue with diagnostic tender points on examination. The pain from a herniated disk is referred to the lower extremities and may be associated with focal weakness and loss of deep tendon reflexes in a radicular distribution.

Generalized edema can compress nerves and tendons in the wrist, resulting in carpal tunnel syndrome and de Quervain tenosynovitis. Carpal tunnel syndrome most often presents as nocturnal numbness, tingling, and pain in the hand during the second and third trimester of pregnancy. These symptoms can be induced by having the patient flex both wrists (Phalen's sign) or by tapping over the median nerve with a reflex hammer (Tinel's sign). Symptoms improve with nocturnal wrist splints and almost always completely resolve after delivery. DeQuervain tenosynovitis presents as pain at the base of the thumb that migrates to the hand or forearm. The extensor pollicis brevis and abductor pollicis longus tendons run in a common sheath adjacent to the styloid process. Synovitis arises secondary to friction (presumably triggered by edema) between the tendon sheath and styloid process. On examination there is tenderness over the radial styloid, frequently accompanied by crepitus. Finkelstein's test, passive ulnar deviation of the wrist with the thumb flexed over the palm, usually reproduces the pain. Unlike carpal tunnel syndrome, de Quervain tenosynovitis tends to manifest postpartum.

Hip pain in a pregnant patient requires careful evaluation. Frequently the pain emanates from the outer aspect of the hip over the greater trochanter and radiates down the outer aspect of the thigh. This pattern of discomfort is most commonly caused by trochanteric bursitis and not by any problems intrinsic to the hip joint. The pain can be induced by palpating over the site of the bursa and is not increased by passive or active movement of the hip. True hip pain often is located in the groin and radiates into the thigh. Hip pain in the third trimester may be secondary to osteonecrosis or transient osteoporosis of the femoral head. In both conditions, internal rotation of the hip and weight bearing elicit pain.

In most patients, musculoskeletal problems can be diagnosed by history and physical examination. Patients with persistent severe low back pain, progressive neurologic symptoms in a radicular pattern, or hip pain may require imaging studies. Plain x-rays should be avoided in the first trimester because of possible adverse fetal effects. X-rays are often normal in the early phases of osteonecrosis and in lumbar disk disease. MRI provides detailed anatomic images of the spine and presumably does not pose a threat to the fetus, although long-term follow-up studies are not available.

BIBLIOGRAPHY

Hoppenfield S. Physical examination of the spine and extremities. New York: Appleton-Century-Crofts, 1976.

Liang MH, Sturrock RD. Evaluation of musculoskeletal symptoms. In: Klippel JH, Dieppe PA, eds. Rheumatology. St Louis: Mosby, 1994.

Polley HF, Hunder GG. Rheumatological interviewing and physical examination of the joints, 2d ed. Philadelphia: WB Saunders, 1978.

Schumacher HR, Dlippel JH, Koopman WJ, eds. Primer on the rheumatic diseases, 16th ed. Atlanta: Arthritis Foundation, 1993.

Zvaifler N. Evaluation of joint complaints. In: Stein JH, ed. Stein internal medicine, 4th ed. St Louis: Mosby, 1994.

Primary Care for Women, edited by Phyllis C. Leppert and Fred M. Howard. Lippincott-Raven Publishers, Philadelphia © 1997.

94

Inflammatory Arthritis

CHARLENE B. VARNIS

Inflammatory arthritis occurs in a number of rheumatologic diseases. Rheumatoid arthritis (RA) is the most common of these. It is a chronic polyarticular and systemic inflammatory disease affecting women two to three times more than men, with a peak incidence in women in the fourth through sixth decades. Inflammatory arthritis is also a manifestation of the seronegative spondyloarthropathies, which include ankylosing spondylitis, Reiter syndrome, reactive arthritis, and arthritis associated with inflammatory bowel disease (IBD). This group of diseases can be distinguished from RA by the absence of rheumatoid factor and variable involvement of the sacroiliac joints (sacroiliitis) and spine (spondylitis). Enthesitis (inflammation of tendons and ligament insertions on bone) and dactylitis (inflammation of joints and soft tissues of a digit resulting in a "sausage" appearance) also differentiate these disorders from RA. The seronegative spondyloarthropathies also share an association with the class I major histocompatibility antigen HLA-B27 (Table 94-1).

RHEUMATOID ARTHRITIS

RA occurs in a worldwide distribution affecting all races and ethnic groups. In the United States, RA incidence is 0.3% to 1.5%, with a predilection among women. There is a genetic susceptibility for developing the disorder, with familial clusters of cases seen.

Table 94-1. HLA-B27 Associations Among the Spondyloarthropathies

DISORDER	HLA-B27 FREQUENCY, %
Ankylosing spondylitis	90
Reactive arthritis (including Reiter syndrome)	60–80
Psoriatic arthritis with spondylitis*	50
IBD with spondylitis*	50

*There is no significant increased HLA-B27 frequency with peripheral arthritis.
HLA, human leukocyte antigen; *IBD,* inflammatory bowel disease.
(Adapted from Taurog JD. Seronegative spondyloarthropathies. In: Schumacher HR Jr, ed. Primer on the rheumatic diseases, 10th ed. Atlanta: Arthritis Foundation, 1993:152.)

This is further supported by a concordance rate of 15.2% in monozygotic twins compared with a rate of 3.6% in dizygotic twins. The rather low monozygotic twin concordance rate suggests that environmental factors play a major role in development of RA. The genetic susceptibility is associated with the class II histocompatibility gene product HLA-DR4. The HLA-DR4 antigen confers a fourfold risk of developing RA in the Caucasian population, with some variation in certain other ethnic groups. In some populations, an additional HLA antigen, DR1, may be associated with risk of developing the disease.

The etiology of RA is unknown, although there has been a long-standing interest in the potential role of infectious agents. No organism has been identified as the etiologic agent. The primary site involved in the disease process is the synovial lining of diarthrodial joints, usually a thin layer of tissue, only one to three cell layers thick with no basement membrane, which becomes chronically inflamed and thickened in RA.

Little is known about the initial stage of RA because tissue at this early stage is not readily available. It is likely that the inflammatory response is triggered by the presence of some antigen that reaches the synovial tissue via the circulation, initiating inflammatory response mediated by CD4+ T lymphocytes. Cytokines, which are potent inflammatory mediators, are released by cells at the site of inflammation. Interleukin-1 and tumor necrosis factor alpha are cytokines that are important in driving both acute and chronic inflammation in RA.

The inflammatory response progresses with synovial proliferation, edema, and new blood vessel formation. The resulting proliferative synovium, or pannus, releases damaging enzymes into the joint that degrade the structural components of cartilage and bone. The earliest damage is found at bare areas of bone located at the margins of joints, where the synovium directly attaches. Pannus can be seen invading this area of the joint microscopically, an area that corresponds to locations of erosions visible on x-rays.

Clinical Features

Rheumatoid arthritis is a systemic disease that initially presents with articular involvement. Often the onset of arthritis is accompanied by constitutional symptoms such as fatigue and malaise, reflecting the systemic nature of the disorder. In 55% to 70% of patients, onset is insidious joint pain and stiffness, developing over weeks to months. The typical pattern of joint involvement is symmetric polyarticular involvement of small joints of the hands, wrists, and feet. Stiffness lasting more than 30 minutes is significant for inflammatory involvement. Such stiffness is most marked after prolonged inactivity, particularly upon awakening. Stiffness lessens with movement and use of the affected joints. It is important to recognize that in 8% to 15% of patients, RA can present with acute pain and swelling developing over a few days. An intermediate onset of symptoms over days to weeks occurs in 15% to 20% of patients.

The metacarpophalangeal (MCP) and proximal interphalangeal (PIP) joints of the hands can be involved, almost always sparing the distal interphalangeal (DIP) joints. Stiffness and pain often precede observable swelling. In the feet, metatarsophalangeal (MTP) joint involvement results in pain in the forefoot, particularly when the patient walks without shoes. Persistence of joint swelling caused by synovitis has a number of consequences. Muscular atrophy occurs. Affected joints can develop contractures or decreased range of motion. Deformities of the hands often develop. Ulnar deviation at the MCP joints is common and can progress to ulnar subluxation, which significantly impairs hand function, limiting the ability to grasp and to extend the fingers. Periarticular inflammation involving tendons that have synovial sheaths occurs. Flexor tenosynovitis of the hands contributes to finger pain and impairment, often associated with tendon nodules and trigger finger symptoms. Another periarticular site of inflammation is the extensor carpi ulnaris tendon; inflammation of this tendon leads to pain and swelling at the ulnar styloid. Volar subluxation of the MCPs also causes functional limitation. Swan-neck (DIP flexion with PIP hyperextension) and boutonnière (DIP hyperextension with PIP flexion) deformities can also impair finger and hand function. Pannus present at the extensor tendons of the fingers can cause extensor tendon rupture. Inability to extend the finger should lead to considering the possibility of tendon rupture as the cause. Hand surgery can usually correct the abnormality. Foot deformities can be clinically significant and debilitating for the patient. The mechanics of the foot become affected by loss of the metatarsal arch, severe hallux valgus, and plantar subluxation of MTP joints leading to cock-up toe deformities.

Large joints of the extremities can be involved, including knees, talar and subtalar joints, shoulders, and elbows. When the knee joint is involved, synovial fluid may enter the gastrocnemius-semitendinosus bursa by a communication that is present in a large percentage of people. Accumulation of fluid here is known as a popliteal or Baker's cyst and may produce the symptom of popliteal fullness. When the knee is subjected to forces that can raise the intraarticular pressure, the cyst can rupture. A rupture usually leads to calf pain and swelling that mimic a deep venous thrombosis. After several days, ecchymosis can be seen in dependent portions of the leg, usually at the ankle below the malleoli.

Neck pain and stiffness result from involvement of synovial tissue at the atlantoaxial articulation of the cervical spine. The destructive changes that result can lead to instability of the joint and the risk of subluxation and spinal cord compression. Patients with RA who require intubation for general anesthesia should have the neck assessed with x-rays that include flexion and extension views to document possible instability of C1–C2. This should be done to identify risk for subluxation before any manipulation of the neck is performed, such as during oral intubation.

The clinician should be aware that complaints of hoarseness in the RA patient may signify involvement of the cricoarytenoid joint. If movement of the cricoarytenoid is impaired as a result of rheumatoid inflammation, lung aspiration can occur. When superimposed upper respiratory infection occurs, a potentially life-threatening complication of disease in this joint is upper airway obstruction.

Disease in RA is not restricted to the joints. A variety of extraarticular manifestations in RA reflect the systemic nature of the disease. Involvement at extraarticular sites can be clinically significant in a large number of patients. It is important to perform a systems review to identify possible extraarticular involvement.

Rheumatoid nodules are seen in 30% to 40% of patients with classic RA, usually occurring in subcutaneous locations. The extensor surface of the elbow is the most common site. Nodules can occur at pressure sites such as scalp, sacrum, and heels. The nodules are rarely painful but, depending on location, can cause mechanical interference with function. Deep nodules can develop in internal organs; sites favored are serosal surfaces of the lungs and heart as well as the lung parenchyma.

Nervous system involvement often presents as entrapment syndromes caused by synovitis resulting in median, ulnar, and posterior tibial neuropathies. The simultaneous occurrence of several isolated mononeuropathies, known as mononeuritis multiplex, may occur as a manifestation of rheumatoid vasculitis. Rare cases of peripheral polyneuropathy have been reported. Pulmonary involvement includes pleural effusions, parenchymal rheumatoid nodules, and diffuse interstitial pulmonary fibrosis. Pericarditis is the most common cardiac manifestation. Nodular disease or nonspecific myocarditis occasionally occurs, leading to conduction abnormalities.

The eye can be affected by keratoconjunctivitis sicca with symptoms of dryness, foreign-body sensation, burning, or thick discharge. Inflammatory lesions of the eye may also occur, including episcleritis, scleritis, keratitis, and corneal ulceration. A painful eye should alert the physician to obtain prompt ophthalmologic evaluation, because scleritis or corneal inflammation with or without ulceration can progress rapidly and lead to complications including perforation.

Clinically apparent vasculitis is a rare complication, usually seen in patients with long-standing seropositive disease. It occurs in men and women equally. Cutaneous lesions are the most common manifestation of rheumatoid vasculitis. The skin can be involved by nail edge infarcts and vasculitic ulcers. Constitutional symptoms such as weight loss can be seen. Mononeuritis multiplex is the classic neurologic manifestation. The heart and lungs occasionally can be involved. Uncommonly, vasculitic involvement of the gastrointestinal tract occurs.

Felty syndrome occurs in patients with long-standing deforming RA who have seropositive nodular disease. Leukopenia and splenomegaly complete the syndrome. Neutropenia of less than $100/mm^3$ correlates with increased bacterial infections in these patients. They may also have skin ulcerations and thrombocytopenia, and the syndrome can be present without active synovitis.

Laboratory and Imaging Studies

In the evaluation of a patient suspected of having RA, several laboratory studies help provide data to assist in diagnosis. Rheumatoid factor is positive in 75% of patients. However, it must be recognized that the rheumatoid factor is found not only in RA but also in other autoimmune diseases such as primary Sjögren syndrome, certain chronic bacterial infections, a number of viral diseases, and several other idiopathic inflammatory diseases such as sarcoidosis. The presence of rheumatoid factor in the sera of patients with RA is associated with more aggressive joint disease and a greater frequency of extraarticular manifestations.

Antinuclear antibodies (ANA) can be present in patients with RA. It is important to recognize this because many practitioners use commercial laboratory “arthritis panels” to obtain rheumatoid factor measurements. The ANA is often included on these panels. Studies report a wide range in the frequency of ANA positivity in RA—14% to 60%. It is more common to have ANA positivity in RA when the rheumatoid factor is also positive, and ANA are more likely to be positive in the setting of Sjögren syndrome. The rheumatoid factor and ANA can be present in a number of these arthritides, an important consideration in evaluating the patient. To reach a correct diagnosis, the results of the tests must be put in the context of a carefully obtained history and physical examination.

The erythrocyte sedimentation rate (ESR) is a test that reflects inflammatory activity. It is not a specific test, being elevated in a large variety of disorders including other inflammatory arthritides and chronic and acute infections, chronic renal failure and end-stage renal disease, chronic hepatic disease, and malignancy, as well as after surgery; mild elevation in ESR is also seen during pregnancy. ESR is usually elevated in active RA, often correlating with disease activity. Several hematologic abnormalities frequently occur. An anemia of chronic inflammation is often present. In active disease, a mild thrombocytosis and leukocytosis can be found.

X-ray studies, particularly of hands, wrists, and feet, can have characteristic findings. In early disease, x-rays may be normal. Decalcification of bone adjacent to the joints (juxtaarticular osteopenia) occurs, joint spaces narrow diffusely, and erosions starting at joint margins may be present.

Diagnosis of RA is based on clinical history and presentation, laboratory evaluation, and x-ray abnormalities. The American Rheumatism Association 1987 revised criteria may be helpful in guiding diagnosis, but are most applicable to the defining of populations for scientific studies (Table 94-2).

Treatment

RA is associated with significant morbidity, disability, and early mortality. The clinical course of RA is variable. Approximately 10% of patients develop progressive unrelenting disease, while 70% experience multiple cycles of intermittent exacerba-

Table 94-2. Classification Criteria for Rheumatoid Arthritis*

Morning stiffness ≥ 1 h duration
Arthritis involving ≥ 3 joint locations
Arthritis of hand joints (wrist, MCP, or PIP)
Symmetric arthritis
Rheumatoid nodules
Elevated serum rheumatoid factor
X-ray abnormalities (well-defined juxtaarticular osteopenia or bony erosions)

*The first four criteria must be present at least 6 weeks. A diagnosis of rheumatoid arthritis if four of the seven criteria are present.

MCP, metacarpophalangeal; *PIP,* proximal interphalangeal.

(Adapted from Arnett FC, Edworthy SM, Block DA, et al. The American Rheumatism Association 1987 revised criteria for the classification of rheumatoid arthritis. Arthritis Rheum 1988;31:315)

tions, each lasting months to years, often against a background of ongoing smoldering joint involvement. The remaining 20% may have a single episode of joint involvement lasting several years, followed by remission lasting at least a year.

Treatment of RA has become more aggressive, with a trend to move away from the treatment pyramid previously advocated as a guide to therapy. In that treatment model, a stepped approach to treatment was followed. Initial treatment was with nonsteroidal antiinflammatory drugs (NSAIDs). Later, when these failed, a second-tier agent, such as the antimalarials and gold, was tried. Only with failure of these or discontinuation because of their side effects, were drugs like methotrexate and azathioprine employed. The addition of second- or third-tier agents was often reserved for patients who developed erosive changes that were observed on x-rays.

This approach has been challenged as more experience is gained with disease outcome treated with the traditional regimen. Evidence indicates that the first 2 years of disease is the time when most of the damage occurs and when disability progresses most rapidly. Waiting for erosions to appear while the physician progresses through the traditional treatment pyramid may delay effective treatment during the very time its implementation is most appropriate. The therapeutic goal is to control inflammation as soon as possible, and this requires more aggressive use of medications in treating the disease. Second- and third-tier drugs, known as the slow-acting antirheumatic drugs (SAARDs), are started much earlier in the course of the arthritis in an attempt to achieve this goal. Some rheumatologists advocate using a combination of these agents at the outset.

Salicylates and NSAIDs continue to be used to manage acute inflammatory symptoms. Aspirin is a salicylate that has been a mainstay of therapy as an antiinflammatory for years. It is inexpensive and effective when given in appropriate antiinflammatory doses. Aspirin has several disadvantages: it requires frequent dosing, many patients have significant gastrointestinal intolerance to it, and it can cause tinnitus. This side effect usually correlates to supratherapeutic serum salicylate levels, but in the elderly often occurs at lower serum levels. In early RA, a starting aspirin dose of 3.6 g/day in four divided doses is suggested. If tolerated, it may be increased to 4.2 g/day. Enteric-coated preparations may avoid some of the gastric intolerance experienced by some patients. However, they do not alter the risk of ulceration or bleeding from aspirin. Slow-release preparations that reduce the frequency of dosing are also available, but are more expensive.

Commonly, patients are treated with NSAIDs. Many NSAIDs require less frequent dosing than does aspirin and often are tolerated better. One cannot predict which drug will have the best therapeutic effect in a given patient; likewise, it is not possible to predict which NSAID a patient will not tolerate. If one NSAID is not effective in a given patient, another one should be tried. Often, switching to an NSAID from a different chemical class can be helpful. The NSAID should be continued for at least 3 weeks before changing because of lack of effect. A variety of toxicities can result from use of these drugs, including gastric mucosal injury and potential ulceration. Renal toxicity can occur with decreased creatinine clearance and is more commonly seen in the elderly and in patients with any condition that leads to decreased renal perfusion. The nonacetylated salicylates such as choline magnesium trisalicylate and salsalate have less gastrointestinal toxicity, do not affect platelet function, and may be useful in patients with aspirin-sensitive asthma. Serum salicylate levels can be followed, with dose adjusted accordingly.

Corticosteroids have potent antiinflammatory effects and, when used in low doses equivalent to 10 mg prednisone or less daily, can be a helpful adjunct in RA treatment, particularly in controlling inflammation while beginning treatment with an SAARD. A corticosteroid is usually given as a single daily dose. Alternate day therapy does not usually provide enough control of symptoms, especially on the day no corticosteroid is given. Even at low doses, patients can experience accelerated loss of bone density, adrenal suppression, hypertension, hyperglycemia, mild fluid retention, or redistribution of body fat. Other side effects that are probably rare at the lower dose regimens are avascular necrosis, increased infection risk, and cataracts. When tapering corticosteroids, very gradual dose reductions are better tolerated, with less chance of worsening symptoms precipitated by the taper. Intraarticular corticosteroids are often effective when inflammation is limited to one or two joints. It must be emphasized, however, that joint aspiration should be performed with Gram stain analysis and cultures to exclude the possibility of a septic arthritis. This is particularly important in the patient who has no other evidence of active joint inflammation or disease symptoms.

An SAARD should be considered in any patient with active inflammation or with factors indicating poor prognosis including female gender, rheumatoid factor positivity, early erosions, nodules, and other extraarticular involvement. In general, these drugs take a considerable amount of time to have maximum affect and this time varies depending on the particular drug. Patients should be counseled about this so they do not become discouraged prematurely. Drugs in this category include hydroxychloroquine, methotrexate, auranofin (oral gold), injectable gold, sulfasalazine, D-penicillamine, and azathioprine. A recent metaanalysis found efficacy among methotrexate, injectable gold, D-penicillamine, and sulfasalazine to be similar. The analysis found oral gold was less effective than other drugs and injectable gold had greater toxicity leading to more frequent discontinuation of therapy.

Hydroxychloroquine is generally well tolerated, but has a delayed onset of action of 3 to 6 months with a response occurring in 40% to 60% of patients. Potential side effects include dermatitis, nausea, headache, blurred vision, myopathy, and hemolytic anemia. The drug can concentrate in the pigment layers of the retina. This can lead to retinal damage. With the current doses used, 400 mg/day, the incidence of retinopathy is no more than 0.5%. The earliest changes in the retina are asymptomatic, but can be detected by careful ophthalmologic examination. A baseline eye examination should be obtained before starting the medication, and every 6 months thereafter. If any signs of retinal toxicity are seen, hydroxychloroquine should be discontinued.

Sulfasalazine was originally developed to treat RA, but it has not been approved by the Food and Drug Administration for this indication as of this writing. However, it is used by many rheumatologists for the treatment of RA as well as other forms of inflammatory arthritis. The usual starting dose is 500 to 1000 mg/day, gradually increasing to 2 or 3 g/day, with onset of action in 6 to 8 weeks. Side effects include gastrointestinal upset, rash, drug-induced hepatitis, bone marrow suppression, agranulocytosis, and hemolytic anemia. A baseline glucose-6-phosphate dehydrogenase (G6PDH) is suggested prior to starting sulfasalazine, to identify patients at risk for developing severe hemolysis. A complete blood cell (CBC) count is followed every 2 weeks for the first 4 to 8 weeks, once a month for 6 months, and then once every 2 to 3 months. Liver function tests should be checked every 6 to 8 weeks.

Methotrexate has become an important treatment for RA, favored by many as the SAARD of choice in patients with active, aggressive inflammation early in the course of the disease. It has a significant antiinflammatory effect, with the most rapid onset of action of the SAARDs. Usually response is seen within 3 to 4 weeks of starting therapy. Methotrexate is given as a single dose once a week. The usual starting dose is 5 mg to 7.5 mg/wk, gradually increasing by 2.5-mg increments at 4- to 6-week intervals, depending on response. The goal is to treat with the lowest effective dose. Responses to 7.5 mg to 15 mg/wk are common. Occasionally higher doses are used, with greater chance of side effects and greater potential for immunosuppression. Stomatitis, nausea, vomiting, bone marrow suppression, hepatotoxicity with fibrosis and cirrhosis, lung hypersensitivity reactions, and teratogenesis are toxicities of the drug. Supplementation with 1 mg folic acid daily is helpful in preventing the stomatitis and nausea without affecting efficacy. The risk of methotrexate-related hepatic fibrosis and cirrhosis may be increased by alcohol abuse. Patients are advised to abstain from alcohol use while taking methotrexate. The presence of fatty liver seen in patients with obesity and diabetes may increase the risk as well. Reduction of the dose is required in mild renal insufficiency, and the drug should not be used in patients with renal failure or on dialysis. The use of trimethoprim-sulfamethoxazole antibiotics can be synergistic in causing toxicity, including severe bone marrow suppression. Baseline CBC count, liver function tests, and hepatitis B and C serologies should be obtained prior to treatment. Laboratory monitoring during therapy should include CBC count every 2 to 4 weeks for the first 1 to 4 months, then every 4 to 6 weeks. Liver function tests should be followed every 4 to 8 weeks.

Gold compounds were used extensively in treatment of RA before methotrexate became a favored choice. They remain an alternative for patients who fail other treatments or do not tolerate them. Oral gold is felt to be less efficacious than the other SAARDs and is being used less in treatment of this disease. Intramuscular gold compounds were found to be effective in 60% to 80% of patients, with onset of effect taking 3 to 6 months. Unfortunately, there is a high rate of side effects, and 35% of patients discontinue use as a result. Rash and stomatitis are the most common side effects. Other serious side effects include immune complex–mediated membranous glomerulonephritis, leukopenia, thrombocytopenia, and rare instances of aplastic anemia. The drug is administered in test doses of 10 mg the first week, 25 mg the second, and then a treatment schedule of 25 mg to 50 mg is given weekly. A CBC count and urinalysis are monitored weekly, usually prior to the next injection. Liver function tests should be done every 1 to 3 months. Two injectable preparations are available, aurothiomalate and aurothioglucose. Administration of aurothiomalate may be accompanied by a nitritoid reaction—flushing and transient hypotension—just after the injection. Switching to the other preparation may circumvent this. Once a clinical response is seen, the dosing schedule can be decreased to every other week, and ultimately to once a month if symptoms remain controlled.

D-penicillamine has been shown to have efficacy similar to that of intramuscular gold and azathioprine, but has a significant number of side effects including leukopenia, thrombocytopenia, rash, and proteinuria. Use of D-penicillamine can lead to a disease resembling lupus, polymyositis, myasthenia gravis, or Goodpasture syndrome. These toxicities lead to a withdrawal rate from treatment with the drug of 30% to 60%, limiting its usefulness. Dosing starts at 125 mg to 250 mg daily, taken on an empty stomach, and is slowly increased at 8-week intervals to no more than a total dose of 750 mg/day. As doses are increased, there is a higher incidence of side effects. Onset of response to the medication is delayed at least 3 months. Once a response is seen, the dose may be gradually decreased by 125 mg each day to determine the lowest effective dose.

Azathioprine is an immunosuppressive drug that has been shown to be an effective agent in treating RA. It is usually reserved for use in patients who have not responded to other therapies. There may be a risk of lymphoreticular neoplasm with long-term use, although the risk may not be greater than that caused by the disease itself. Immunosuppression, myelosuppression, hepatotoxicity, nausea, gastrointestinal intolerance, and macrocytic anemia are side effects of the drug. Concomitant use of allopurinol or angiotension converting enzyme inhibitors and renal insufficiency are risk factors for myelosuppression. The dosing initially is 1.0 mg/kg/day. A maximum dose of 2.0 mg/kg/day should not be exceeded. CBC count monitoring is imperative, and white blood cell count should not be allowed to fall below 3000 cells/mm^3. A response may begin after 12 weeks of treatment.

Medications are an important part of the treatment of patients with RA; however, other important aspects of treatment should not be overlooked. The patient should be educated about the disease, emphasizing differences from the more common osteoarthritis and highlighting the fluctuating nature of the disease. The systemic features of RA, including fatigue, should be explained and advice regarding structuring rest periods in the course of the day can be helpful. Physical and occupational therapists can teach the patient proper techniques in joint protection and exercise that maintain range of motion and strength. Joint protection techniques are designed to teach the patient how to continue performing daily activities while minimizing the stress to affected joints. Occupational therapists can fabricate splints that are useful in resting actively inflamed joints and also provide patients with adaptive equipment.

Patients often inquire about the role of diet in their disease, particularly with the rising interest in holistic medical practices. There is little evidence to suggest that diet plays a definitive role in the development or treatment of RA. Case reports have appeared in the literature that suggest corn, milk products, or tartrazine exacerbate symptoms of RA, but controlled trials attempting to document this have shown no difference between treatment groups. Despite the lack of scientific evidence to support the beneficial role of any specific dietary intervention, many books and articles in the popular press advocate specific dietary regimens. Some of these eliminate entire food groups, which can further worsen nutritional status in persons who are catabolic as a result of ongoing inflammation. The clinician should be aware of this, and counsel the patient accordingly.

Considerations in Pregnancy

Rheumatoid arthritis generally improves during pregnancy, but it is common to see the arthritis flare postpartum, particularly in lactating women. High levels of prolactin may play a role in the inflammatory response.

Pregnancy in a patient under treatment for RA raises concerns regarding the safety of the medications during gestation. Aspirin and NSAIDs cross the placenta and have been associated with prolongation of gestation and labor, more pronounced maternal anemia, intrapartum blood loss, and possible premature closure of the ductus arteriosus. Maternal indomethacin use has been associated with reduction in urine production in the fetus and oligohydramnios. Maternal aspirin use is associated with increased cutaneous and intracranial bleeding in preterm and low-birth-weight infants. Because of these concerns, discontinuing high-dose aspirin at least 2 weeks before delivery is prudent. NSAIDs are not found in high concentrations in breast milk, but their use in the nursing mother is not recommended. Aspirin in the neonate can lead to metabolic acidosis, altered pulmonary circulation, and bleeding, and therefore should not be used by nursing mothers.

There is variable experience with the use of SAARDs during pregnancy. The use of antimalarial drugs such as hydroxychloroquine is controversial. Chloroquine and hydroxychloroquine can cross the placenta. Case reports of ototoxicity and chromosomal damage in the fetus lead most practitioners to try to avoid use of this drug in the pregnant RA patient. If the patient conceives, the medication can be discontinued. Sulfasalazine has been used for treatment of IBD during pregnancy and found to be safe to use during both pregnancy and lactation. Folic acid supplementation should be given when the patient is treated with this medication. Although adverse effects have been reported with the use of azathioprine, the literature describes a small series of organ transplantation patients who have had successful pregnancies while using azathioprine. However, the use is best reserved for patients with severe rheumatic disease that the safer agents do not control. Methotrexate is teratogenic and is associated with increased spontaneous abortion. It is contraindicated for use during pregnancy, and sexually active women of reproductive age should be using effective contraception while on this drug. Only trace amounts are found in breast milk. The drug may be an option to consider for low dose treatment in lactating women who require additional medication for a severe flare, but adequate data are lacking regarding the effect of even trace amounts on infant health. If the flare can be controlled with corticosteroids, methotrexate is best avoided. The use of gold salts in animals shows the drugs to be teratogenic. The human data are not based on long-term studies, and relatively few patients have been evaluated. Reports of congenital anomalies are rare, but the potential toxicities of the drug lead most rheumatologists to avoid treatment with gold salts in pregnancy and lactation.

Corticosteroids given in low to moderate doses (10 to 20 mg prednisone or the equivalent) are generally safe during pregnancy. They have not been found to cause a significant increase in miscarriage, fetal mortality, prematurity, or congenital anomaly. Maternal prednisone use has been associated with gestational hypertension and diabetes, although this is probably of greater concern in patients with other rheumatic disorders that require treatment with high dose steroids. Adrenal suppression in the neonate occurs rarely, but can occur with high maternal corticosteroid doses, and the neonate should be monitored for this possibility. There is differential placental passage of the various forms of corticosteroids. Prednisone and prednisolone are metabolized in the placenta and have the lowest passage rate and are the preferred choice for maternal treatment. Alternatively, dexamethasone has a high placental passage rate to the fetus. Minimal excretion of prednisone in breast milk is at maternal doses of 20 mg or less and appears safe in lactation at these doses. Intraarticular steroids are an excellent choice of treatment for the RA patient suffering a flare in one or two joints while pregnant. There is relatively low systemic absorption of the steroid and such administration can be very effective in treating the joint flare.

SERONEGATIVE SPONDYLOARTHROPATHIES

Psoriatic Arthritis

Psoriatic arthritis is an inflammatory arthropathy that occurs in approximately 5% to 10% of persons with psoriasis. It occurs with approximately the same frequency in men and women. Although joint disease follows the onset of skin involvement, it can precede psoriasis in up to 21% of incidences, and joint involvement can present concurrently with the initial onset of skin disease in up to 11%. The skin involvement may be subtle, with only isolated nail findings of onychodystrophy or pitting, or skin with small plaques in areas that are difficult to observe such as scalp, intergluteal fold, and umbilicus.

The etiology is unknown, but studies of families and twins suggest a genetic predisposition with a high concordance rate in monozygotic twins. First-degree relatives of persons with psoriasis or psoriatic arthritis have a much higher chance of developing the skin or joint disease than that expected in the general population. Class I major histocompatibility antigens are found associated with psoriatic arthritis including HLA-B7, HLA-Cw6, and HLA-B17, in contrast to the class II HLA-DR4 association seen in RA. The class I major histocompatibility complex association suggests that CD4+ T lymphocytes are not mediators of the disease. This is further supported by the observation in human immunodeficiency virus (HIV) infection that, with decline of $CD4^+$ T-cell count, psoriatic skin and joint disease become very aggressive. Guttate psoriasis, consisting of widespread small lesions, can be precipitated by streptococcal upper airway infection, suggesting a possible role of bacteria or bacterial antigens in the pathogenesis.

Several patterns of joint involvement can be seen. The most common, seen in 40% to 60% of patients, is a polyarticular pattern that sometimes can be difficult to distinguish from RA, although appearance on x-rays may provide clues. An oligoarticular pattern (three or fewer joints in an asymmetric distribution), often with DIP or flexor tendon involvement and dactylitis, is seen. Sacroiliitis with or without spondylitis occurs in 20% to 40% of patients, with a predominance in men. DIP inflammation, usually associated with psoriatic nail changes, and arthritis mutilans, a deforming variant that affects the hands, occur much less commonly. Joint trauma may precipitate an inflammatory flare, likened to the Koebner phenomenon seen in psoriatic skin disease, wherein new lesions appear at skin injury sites. Extraarticular involvement is uncommon. Inflammatory eye involvement can occur with conjunctivitis in up to 20% of patients and iritis in 7%. The iritis is not seen in women, with most cases being reported in men with deforming arthritis.

Most patients do not develop the severe dysfunction that occurs in patients with RA, but a small percentage of patients have progressive joint disease that leads to significant impairment. A poorer prognosis is indicated by younger age at onset, extensive skin involvement, polyarticular involvement, lack of the expected clinical response to NSAIDs, and association with HIV infection.

Reiter Syndrome and Reactive Arthritis

Classically, Reiter syndrome is a triad of conjunctivitis, urethritis, and arthritis. It may present as an incomplete Reiter syndrome when it lacks the eye or genitourinary manifestations. The term "reactive arthritis" describes patients with joint manifestations in the absence of other features of the triad. Young people are most commonly affected, with equal frequency in men and women. A sterile, inflammatory arthritis occurs after an infection at a remote site, usually enteric or genitourinary. Enteric infections with *Shigella*, *Salmonella*, *Yersinia*, and *Campylobacter* and venereal infections with *Chlamydia* can be precipitants. However, a triggering infection cannot always be identified. Enthesitis such as Achilles tendinitis and plantar fasciitis may be prominent features. Eye, mucocutaneous, and systemic manifestations can occur.

A genetic susceptibility for the disease exists, with familial clustering seen. There is a strong association with the presence of the class I major histocompatibility antigen HLA-B27. Bacterial antigens from species known to trigger the disease have been recovered from synovial fluid. This has led to speculation that persistence of these antigens, with dissemination to articular and other sites, can initiate an inflammatory response. HLA-B27 may modulate the immune response allowing for persistence of bacterial antigen by impaired clearance.

Medical care is usually sought because of joint pain. Careful history is necessary to help identify a preceding illness or other symptoms the patient may not associate with the joint pain. Symptoms of enteric or urogenital infection may have been present a few days before or weeks before, with symptoms often being mild or unnoticed. Women with cervicitis may be asymptomatic. The disease occurs with varying severity. Systemic symptoms such as malaise, fatigue, and fever can be quite prominent in acute disease. An asymmetric oligoarthritis and enthesitis commonly occur. Mucocutaneous manifestations include keratoderma blennorrhagicum, a pustular or hyperkeratotic rash on the palms and soles that is sometimes difficult to distinguish from psoriasis. Circinate balanitis is a similar rash occurring on the glans penis in men. There is no corresponding genital rash in women. Oral ulcerations may appear on the palate, tongue, and buccal mucosa. Urethritis may present as a sterile mucopurulent urethral discharge, a symptom that may go unrecognized in women. Eye involvement includes conjunctivitis, resulting in a red-appearing eye with mild irritation and sterile discharge, and is typically self limited. Acute anterior uveitis presents with eye redness, pain, and photophobia and should be evaluated by an ophthalmologist. Uveitis can be recurrent and if not properly treated can lead to permanent visual damage.

In the majority of patients, inflammation resolves completely but the duration of symptoms can vary from a few days up to 1 year. However, recurrences are often seen and can be triggered by new infections or stress. A chronic course may develop in 20% to 50% of patients, with persisting inflammatory musculoskeletal manifestations.

Arthritis Associated With Inflammatory Bowel Disease

Peripheral arthritis, sacroiliitis, and spondylitis are extraintestinal manifestations of Crohn disease and ulcerative colitis. Men and women are affected equally. Asymmetric oligoarthritis and enthesitis may occur, often in the lower extremity. Flare of peripheral arthritis often correlates with active bowel disease. Spine and sacroiliac inflammation progress independently from the bowel disease. New joint inflammation in a patient with known IBD that has been quiescent may herald increased bowel disease activity that is not yet clinically evident.

Ankylosing Spondylitis

Ankylosing spondylitis has the strongest association with HLA-B27 of any arthropathy. It occurs in men three times more frequently than in women and the disease may progress more slowly in women. The major symptom is insidious onset inflammatory back pain that is worse with prolonged inactivity and improved with exercise or movement. The diagnosis should not be considered unless the symptoms have been present for at least 3 months. In severe cases, the pain awakens the person from sleep. Pain in the sacroiliac region may be misinterpreted as hip pain. Involvement of the thoracic spine and enthesitis at costosternal areas can produce chest pain and lead to limited chest wall expansion. Peripheral oligoarthritis occurs in 20% of patients.

Extraarticular manifestations include uveitis, pulmonary fibrosis, apical bullous lung disease, restrictive disease from decreased excursion, and inflammation of the aortic root occasionally leading to aortic insufficiency.

Initially examination may be relatively normal, but later findings include lumbar spine and sacroiliac region tenderness, loss of lumbar flexion, flattening of the lumbar lordosis, decreased chest expansion, limited movement of hips and shoulders, and evidence of peripheral joint inflammation.

Laboratory and Imaging Studies in Spondyloarthropathies

There are no specific laboratory tests for the spondyloarthropathies. Rheumatoid factor is negative. In psoriatic arthritis and ankylosing spondylitis, an elevated ESR and mild anemia may be present, but are often normal. In acute reactive arthritis, the ESR is usually markedly elevated and can normalize in later, chronic stage disease. At the acute onset, a mild leukocytosis and anemia may be present. Urinalysis should be included to assess for sterile pyuria due to urethritis.

An arthrocentesis should be performed whenever possible to obtain synovial fluid for cell counts, Gram stain and culture, and crystal examination. Such measures help assess for other entities in the differential diagnosis. In suspected Reiter syndrome or reactive arthritis, cultures of throat, feces, and urogenital tract may help identify the triggering organism as well as identify other infections such as gonorrhea, which when disseminated can have a similar presentation. In the event of negative cultures, one may consider obtaining serologic tests for the possible causative organisms known to precipitate the disease.

Evidence on x-ray of sacroiliitis includes a widened appearance and cortical irregularity of the sacroiliac joint due to erosions. Increased sclerosis is present adjacent to the joint, and ankylosis (fusion) occurs in more advanced disease. These findings are usually bilateral in ankylosing spondylitis, but often unilateral in reactive arthritis and psoriatic arthritis. Plain x-rays may be normal in early spondylitis. Later, "squaring" of the vertebral body, resulting from ossification of the anterior longitudinal ligament with loss of the normal anterior concavity, can be observed. Ligamentous ossification results in syndesmophyte formation, and bony fusion of apophyseal joints is sometimes seen. In psoriatic arthritis and Reiter syndrome, the syndesmophytes are usually very large and asymmetric.

In psoriatic arthritis, x-rays may show no abnormalities in early involvement. The juxtaarticular osteopenia observed in x-rays in RA is not present. Any of the interphalangeal joints including DIP joints, which are usually spared in RA, can fuse or develop destructive changes with erosion of the distal aspect of the phalanx and bony proliferation of the adjacent phalanx at its proximal aspect. When this change is very advanced, a "pencil-in-cup" deformity is seen in x-rays. Resorption of the distal tufts of the fingers is sometimes observed.

Treatment of the Spondyloarthropathies

The mainstay of treatment is the NSAIDs, with indomethacin favored by some as the NSAID of choice. Worsening of psoriasis has rarely been reported to occur with NSAIDs. They may cause exacerbation of gastrointestinal symptoms in IBD, and nonacetylated salicylates may be the preferred choice in these patients. When inflammatory symptoms in psoriatic arthritis, IBD-associated arthritis, and ankylosing spondylitis do not respond to NSAIDs alone, sulfasalazine is an effective treatment. There is some evidence that it may control psoriasis.

In psoriatic arthritis, other SAARDs are sometimes used. Hydroxychloroquine is likely effective in treating the articular involvement in psoriatic arthritis, although its use is controversial because several studies have suggested that skin disease may worsen in some patients. Methotrexate is an effective treatment for aggressive psoriatic joint and skin involvement in the absence of immunodeficiency or contraindications such as liver disease and alcohol abuse. Gold compounds have been shown to be effective for peripheral arthritis and are an alternative treatment to consider for patients who are not candidates for methotrexate and have not responded to other medications. Flare of skin disease and photosensitive reactions have been reported with the use of gold compounds in patients with psoriasis.

Intraarticular steroids remain an alternative to treat a single inflamed joint if infection is ruled out. In Reiter syndrome and reactive arthritis, moderate doses (20 to 40 mg/day prednisone) of systemic steroids are occasionally used to treat patients with multiple joint involvement found to be refractory to antiinflammatory doses of NSAIDs. Systemic steroids are not effective for sacroiliac or spine inflammation. The potential role of long-term antibiotic therapy for reactive arthritis is under investigation.

Patient education is an important part of treatment, particularly when spondylitis is prominent. The patient needs to become informed about the disease, the importance of proper posture, and the possible complications of the disease. Physical therapy is an important adjunct to provide patient training in flexibility and spine extension. Proper posture training encourages a position of function, if the disease progresses to fusion.

Considerations in Pregnancy

The same attention has not been given to pregnancy in the spondyloarthropathies as in RA. The numbers in studies are relatively small, but from the information available, it appears there is a different response in ankylosing spondylitis from those women who go through pregnancy with psoriatic arthritis.

In patients with ankylosing spondylitis, symptoms do not seem to improve, and in some patients, low back pain, stiffness, and enthesopathic symptoms may be exacerbated in pregnancy. In patients with psoriatic arthritis, there was improvement during the gestation, with most women experiencing a reappearance of symptoms during the first 10 weeks postpartum. Neither ankylosing spondylitis nor psoriatic arthritis appeared to affect pregnancy outcome, including mode of delivery. Medications used to treat these forms of arthritis are mentioned in the earlier review of medications in pregnancy and lactation in this chapter.

BIBLIOGRAPHY

American College of Rheumatology Ad Hoc Committee on Clinical Guidelines. Guidelines for monitoring drug therapy in rheumatoid arthritis. Arthritis Rheum 1996;39:723.

American College of Rheumatology Ad Hoc Committee on Clinical Guidelines. Guidelines for RA management. Arthritis Rheum 1996;39:713.

Arend WP, Dayer JM. Inhibition of the production and effects of interleukin-1 and tumor necrosis factor alpha in rheumatoid arthritis. Arthritis Rheum 1995;38:151.

Arnett FC, Edworthy SM, Block DA, et al. The American Rheumatism Association 1987 revised criteria for the classification of rheumatoid arthritis. Arthritis Rheum 1988;31:315.

Bennett, RM. Psoriatic arthritis. In: McCarty DJ, Koopman WJ, eds. Arthritis and allied conditions: a textbook of rheumatology, 12th ed. Philadelphia: Lea & Febiger, 1993;1079.

Borigini MJ, Paulus HE. Rheumatoid arthritis. In: Weisman MH, Weinblatt ME, eds. Treatment of the rheumatic diseases. Philadelphia: WB Saunders, 1995;31.

Caldwell JR, Furst DE. The efficacy and safety of low-dose corticosteroids for rheumatoid arthritis. Semin Arthritis Rheum 1991;21:1.

Harris ED Jr. Clinical features of rheumatoid arthritis. In: Kelley WN Jr, Harris ED Jr, Ruddy S, Sledge CB, eds. Textbook of rheumatology, 4th ed. Philadelphia: WB Saunders, 1993;874.

Jimenez-Balderas FJ, Mintz G. Ankylosing spondylitis: clinical course in women and men. J Rheum 1993;20:2069.

Khan MA, van der Linden SM. Ankylosing spondylitis and other spondyloarthropathies. Rheum Dis Clin N Am 1990;16:551.

Ostensen M. The effect of pregnancy on ankylosing spondylitis, psoriatic arthritis and juvenile rheumatoid arthritis. Am J Reprod Immunol 1992;28:235.

Ostensen M. Treatment with immunosuppressive and disease modifying drugs during pregnancy and lactation. Am J Reprod Immunol 1992;28:148.

Silman AJ. Epidemiology of rheumatoid arthritis. APMIS 1994;102:721.

Taurog JD. Seronegative spondyloarthropathies. In: Schumacher HR Jr, ed. Primer on the rheumatic diseases, 10th ed. Atlanta: Arthritis Foundation, 1993:152.

van de Laar MA, van der Korst JK. Rheumatoid arthritis, food, and allergy. Semin Arthritis Rheum 1991;21:12.

Wilske KR, Healey LA. Remodeling the pyramid: a concept whose time has come. J Rheum 1989;16:565.

Primary Care for Women, edited by Phyllis C. Leppert and Fred M. Howard. Lippincott-Raven Publishers, Philadelphia © 1997.

95

Crystal-Induced Arthritis: Gout and Calcium Pyrophosphate Deposition Disease

C. DOUGLAS ANGEVINE

Since the introduction of polarized light microscopy in the 1960s, several types of specific crystal-induced arthropathies have been identified. This has enabled physicians to promptly make a precise diagnosis and initiate appropriate therapy. The most common forms of crystal-induced arthritis, gout and calcium pyrophosphate deposition disease (CPDD), are the focus of this chapter.

ETIOLOGY AND DIFFERENTIAL DIAGNOSIS

Gout is a disease that in most instances is the result of persistent hyperuricemia over several years that may present clinically in a variety of ways; the most common initial presentation is acute arthritis. The mechanisms of hyperuricemia include decreased renal excretion of uric acid, increased endogenous uric acid production, or a combination of these factors. The decreased renal excretion and the increased production of uric acid may be on a primary or secondary basis. The majority of patients with primary gout have a hereditary defect in their ability to excrete uric acid as the cause of their hyperuricemia. There is a small group of patients with primary gout who have specific enzyme abnormalities (ie, a mild form of 5-phosphoribosyl 1-pyrophosphate synthetase superactivity and partial hypoxanthine-guanine phosphoribosyltransferase deficiency: both enzymes are produced from X-linked genes) as the mechanism of their hyperuricemia. In the hyperuricemic population, there are individuals whose elevated uric acid, whether due to underexcretion or overproduction, is on a secondary basis. Examples would be chronic renal disease and diuretic therapy for underexcretors, and myeloproliferative disease and psoriasis for overproduction. Generally, individuals in the primary categories develop the manifestations of gout at an earlier age and have more aggressive disease than individuals with hyperuricemia on a secondary basis. Some individuals, however, have significant hyperuricemia for many years and never suffer any consequences.

For hyperuricemic individuals who do experience arthritis, this is initiated by the presence of uric acid crystals in the synovial fluid. This may occur from the release of uric acid crystals from intraarticular deposits or precipitation of the crystals from a supersaturated state in synovial fluid. Factors that may trigger the release or precipitation of crystals include joint trauma, stress, excessive alcohol intake, dehydration, and rapid change of the serum uric acid level.

The urate crystals' presence in synovial fluid attract polymorphonuclear leukocytes that phagocytotize the crystals. This initiates lysosomal disruption, causing a local inflammatory reaction that involves several inflammatory mediators (eg, bradykinin, complement, kallikrein). There may also be systemic release of interleukins and tumor necrosis factor causing fever, leukocytosis, and elevation of the sedimentation rate.

In CPDD, it is the calcium pyrophosphate dihydrate (CPPD) crystal that is responsible for the articular manifestations of the disease. Individuals with CPDD may be classified in several subgroups: idiopathic, hereditary, posttraumatic, or associated with a metabolic disease. The hereditary form of CPDD is an autosomal dominant pattern.

There is no routine laboratory test for inorganic pyrophosphate levels but the plasma or urinary excretion levels are not increased in individuals with CPDD. The CPPD crystals are deposited in articular cartilage, synovium, tendons, and ligaments. It is the shedding of CPPD crystals into the joint space that attracts polymorphonuclear neutrophil leukocytes (PMNs) into the joint space, resulting in lysosomal enzyme release and an acute inflammatory reaction similar to that described for gout.

The arthritis, in both conditions, may be monarticular or polyarticular in its presentation. Early in the course of these diseases, the presentation is more apt to be monarticular. In view of this, the major differential diagnostic considerations are septic arthritis, psoriatic arthritis, osteoarthritis, Reiter syndrome, injury, and cellulitis. If the presentation is polyarticular, an infectious etiology is still a major diagnostic consideration as well as a seronegative spondyloarthropathy, and psoriatic arthritis if the joint involvement is asymmetrical or rheumatoid arthritis, with a symmetrical pattern of joint involvement.

HISTORY

Both gout and CPDD have several clinical stages, the initial presentation usually being an acute inflammatory arthritis involving a single joint of a lower extremity, although it may involve a small hand joint or wrist; occasionally the initial presentation may be polyarticular. After the initial episode, there may be a period of several years with few if any episodes of arthritis. Then the episodes of arthritis recur and often progress to a chronic progressive pattern with continuous synovitis, development of tophi, and ultimate joint destruction. Acute crystal arthritis may progress from mild joint "twinges" to acute joint pain, swelling, and tenderness with marked erythema in a few hours. Frequently, onset begins at night and the patient is awakened with an attack. Chills and fever may occur. If untreated, the episode usually resolves in 7 to 10 days. Often there is desquamation of the skin about the involved joint. The attacks of acute arthritis are frequently associated with trauma to the joint, a stressful event such as a medical or surgical illness, or excessive alcohol consumption.

In the general population, gout is perhaps the second most common form of inflammatory arthritis. Until about the age of 50 years gout is diagnosed primarily in men. In men older than 30 years of age, gout is the most common inflammatory arthritis. Gout is rare in premenopausal women but the incidence increases as they enter menopause and increase their testosterone to estradiol ratio, which is associated with hyperuricemia. Also, as women enter middle age they frequently require medications such as thiazide diuretics that may cause hyperuricemia. CPDD is usually first recognized in individuals in their fifth and sixth decades with no sexual preponderance. In the population of individuals in their mid-80s, an incidence of CPDD as high as 30% to 60% has been reported.

The chronic forms of gout and CPDD are characterized by generalized and often symmetrical arthritis, therefore, it may be misdiagnosed and treated as rheumatoid arthritis or osteoarthritis. Chronic gout is associated with soft tissue, bone and joint deposition of uric acid crystals causing tophi with bone and joint destruction if not recognized and appropriately treated. CPDD in the chronic state is capable of causing a very destructive degenerative arthritis of shoulders, hips, and knees.

Acute and chronic gout may be associated with uric acid renal stone formation. Obesity, diabetes mellitus, hyperlipidemia, hypertension, and atherosclerosis are frequently present in patients with gout. CPDD is strongly associated with hyperparathyroidism, hemochromatosis, hypomagnesemia, and aging. Likely associated conditions include osteoarthritis, amyloidosis, Bartter syndrome, hypermobility, and hypocalciuric hypercalcemia.

PHYSICAL EXAMINATION AND CLINICAL FINDINGS

In the acute stage of gout and CPDD, the significant finding on examination is the acute arthritis usually of a single joint. The involved joint is typically very swollen and tender with warmth and erythema. Even limited active or passive range of motion is extremely painful. With a polyarticular presentation, there is usually asymmetrical joint involvement. Fever may be documented and patients may report chills prior to or at onset of the arthritis. After the acute attack resolves, the involved joint returns to its baseline state.

As crystal disease progresses to the chronic phase, the joints become chronically swollen and tender and deformities may begin to develop that interfere with joint function and the performance of daily activities. Frequently, the joint involvement is polyarticular and symmetrical. In chronic gout, tophaceous deposits frequently develop. Common sites are the helix of the ear, olecranon bursae, tendons, and bone. There are individuals, particularly in the elderly population, with extensive tophi who have no history of acute or chronic arthritis. Individuals who are hyperexcretors of uric acid frequently experience recurrent episodes of renal stones.

LABORATORY AND IMAGING STUDIES

Hyperuricemia in most laboratories is a serum level of greater than 6.0 mg/dL for women and 7.0 mg/dL for men. Documented hyperuricemia in patients with acute or chronic arthritis raises the question of gout. However, a definite diagnosis requires the demonstration of intracellular uric acid crystals in synovial fluid of an involved joint. During an acute attack of gout, the joint fluid can be very cloudy and even purulent in appearance with a cell count that is very high. Joint fluid white blood cell (WBC) counts range from 20,000 to 100,000 cells/mm^3 with the predominant cells being PMNs. Cell counts of 50,000 or greater should make one suspect that the joint might be infected. There have been cases of gout and septic arthritis simultaneously in a joint. At the time of arthrocentesis, fluid samples should be sent for cell count with differential, Gram stain, culture, and sensitivity and crystal analysis. For crystal analysis, a drop or two of the fluid from the syringe or a red top tube is placed on a slide with a coverslip and examined with a polarizing microscope at 10× or 40× magnification. If the fluid obtained is relatively clear with a low cell count, it is helpful to centrifuge the fluid and examine the pellet of cells obtained for crystals. With the polarizing lens in place, the urate crystals are strongly birefringent, generally intracellular, thin, and longer than the diameter of the WBC that has phagocytozed the crystal. Most polarizing scopes have a red plate filter that enables the examiner to differentiate uric acid and CPPD crystals by color identity. Uric acid crystals are yellow if parallel to the axis of the red plate and blue if perpendicular to the axis. Although in most instances uric acid crystals are present in the joint fluid at the time of the attack, there are situations in which early in the attack crystals may not be present but are identified when a subsequent arthrocentesis is performed when the attack is more established. The presence of uric acid crystals has been noted in synovial fluid of asymptomatic joints. Uric acid crystals may be identified in tophi by opening the skin with a small needle and examining the chalky material obtained under the polarizing scope. Gout may cause an acute olecranon bursitis and fluid from the bursa may contain uric acid crystals. These findings are presumptive evidence for the diagnosis of gout. To make a definitive diagnosis intracellular crystals must be identified in the synovial fluid during active arthritis.

As in gout, it is the presence of intracellular CPPD crystals in joint fluid during an attack of arthritis that makes possible a definite diagnosis of CPDD. Joint fluid obtained should be analyzed in the same manner as detailed previously. CPPD crystals are smaller than uric acid crystals, rhomboid in shape, frequently paired, intracellular, and harder to identify because of their size, as well as being less refringent under the polarizing microscope than uric acid crystals. CPPD crystals, when viewed with the red plate in place, have a color identity opposite that of uric acid crystals. When parallel to the axis of the red plate, CPPD crystals are blue and when perpendicular to the axis of the red plate they are yellow in color.

Because individuals with gout and CPDD may have associated conditions as noted earlier, appropriate laboratory testing is necessary to determine if any such conditions are present. Recommended screening studies include serum calcium, phosphorus, alkaline phosphatase, magnesium, thyroid-stimulating hormone (TSH), ferritin, iron, and total iron binding.

X-rays in the early stages of gout are frequently negative aside from soft tissue swelling of the involved joint during an acute attack. As the disease progresses small punched-out lesions are noted in bone adjacent to the joint. These are small tophi. If untreated they become more numerous, increase in size, and may break through the bone cortex and cause adjacent soft tissue deposition of tophaceous material with swelling. Uric acid renal stones may be a complication of gout. Pure uric acid stones are radiolucent and are not detected on routine abdominal x-rays.

X-ray findings in CPDD are frequently present prior to the first attack of arthritis and would be indication to perform appropriate screening tests to determine if associated treatable conditions are present. Plain joint films reveal stippling of the articular cartilage (the most specific finding), periarticular soft tissue calcification, and joint line spur formation. Calcification of the meniscus of the knees may be present, but this is not specific for CPDD—it may occur with aging or trauma.

For screening purposes for CPDD, x-rays of the hands, including the wrists and knees, give the highest yield of positive findings. As the disease progresses the involved joints develop progressive degenerative changes and in some cases marked destruction that may necessitate surgical joint replacement.

Joint imaging studies or bone scan add little diagnostic information in these conditions and thus are not routinely indicated.

TREATMENT

There is treatment for all the stages of gout that in most instances is very effective and well tolerated. Goals of therapy are rapid resolution of the acute episode of arthritis, prevention of frequent recurrent attacks of arthritis that ultimately may lead to a destructive arthropathy, and prevention of the formation of tophi or renal stones. In view of the potential toxicity of the medications used in treatment, it is important to review with the patient any history of gastrointestinal, hematologic, hepatobiliary, or renal disorders before starting these medications. Pretreatment laboratory studies should include: complete blood count, blood urea nitrogen (BUN), creatinine, urinalysis, 24-hour urine collection for total protein and creatinine clearance, and baseline liver function tests. During each phase of therapy the patient should be informed not only of the possible side effects, but also the role that each drug has in the treatment program.

Nonsteroidal antiinflammatory drugs (NSAIDs), colchicine, corticosteroids, and adrenocorticotrophin hormone (ACTH) are effective agents for the treatment of the acute attack of gouty arthritis and are effective for treatment of chronic gout. If the diagnosis of gout is established shortly after onset of symptoms these agents should be effective in significantly reducing joint pain, swelling, and tenderness in 24 to 48 hours, followed by complete resolution of symptoms in 5 to 7 days.

Colchicine is effective in treating acute attacks of gout and preventing recurrent attacks when administered prophylactically. For acute attacks colchicine is most effective when administered early (within 12 hours) after the onset of symptoms. It may be administered orally or intravenously. Oral dosing guidelines are: 1 tablet (0.5 or 0.6 mg) orally every hour until the symptoms begin to improve, side effects (nausea, vomiting, abdominal pain, or diarrhea) occur, or a total dose of 6 mg has been reached. Any one, or combination of, these events is an indication for stopping colchicine. Although 90% of individuals treated with colchicine within 12 hours of the onset of their attack have an excellent response to treatment, 50% experience significant gastrointestinal side effects. IV colchicine therapy for an acute attack avoids the gastrointestinal toxicity of the oral preparation. An initial dose of 2 mg is usual with an additional 1 mg dose every 6 to 12 hours. A total IV dose of 4 mg should not be exceeded when treating an acute attack. When colchicine is administered by the IV route each dose should be diluted in 20 to 30 cc of normal saline and given over 15 to 30 minutes. Failure to do this may cause a localized thrombophlebitis. If the infusion should infiltrate, it may cause sloughing of the skin and subcutaneous tissue. For individuals with glomerular filtration less than 50 mL/min it is advisable to reduce the oral colchicine by 50% and not administer the drug IV. In treatment of an acute attack it is recommended that a combination of IV and oral therapy not be used. If colchicine is not effective changing to an NSAID or corticosteroid therapy is indicated.

In administering colchicine prophylactically, to prevent recurrent attacks of arthritis or when uric acid reduction therapy is initiated, dosing is less complicated and there are fewer side effects. The prophylactic dose is 0.5- or 0.6-mg tablets once or twice a day. This is usually quite effective and well tolerated. However, some individuals with chronic renal disease even on this low dose may develop a neuromyopathy. Patients unable to tolerate colchicine, in any dose, may be treated prophylactically with a low dose of an NSAID such as indomethacin 25 mg once or twice a day.

All NSAIDs are allegedly effective in the treatment of gouty arthritis. However, most physicians select 2 or 3 drugs in the class to become familiar with and use on a regular basis. Treatment is initiated at the usual recommended dosage and continued until the joint symptoms have completely resolved. If an attack is well established (greater than 24 hours' duration) NSAIDs are more effective than colchicine. The usual side effects of this group of drugs are rash, gastrointestinal irritation, and renal side effects. The latter are secondary to inhibition of intrarenal prostaglandin production, which may induce significant sodium retention resulting in edema or hypertension.

If there are contraindications to the use of NSAIDs or full dose colchicine, ACTH may be given in short courses to treat an acute attack of crystalline synovitis with good results. For an acute attack, prednisone 20 to 40 mg/d for 3 to 4 days gradually tapering off over 7 to 14 days or ACTH 40 to 80 units IM initially followed by 40 units every 6 to 12 hours for several days is effective therapy. Often it is helpful to start the patient on a low maintenance dose of colchicine (0.5 or 0.6 mg once or twice a day) during the last few days of steroid treatment to prevent a recurrent episode of acute arthritis when the steroid therapy is discontinued. A single dose of an intraarticular steroid frequently brings about a dramatic response. Prior to using any form of steroid therapy, the clinician must be certain that the patient does not have a concurrent septic arthritis in the affected joint.

Individuals with intermittent episodes of gouty arthritis and persistent hyperuricemia over several years may develop chronic arthritis, tophi, and occasionally uric acid renal stones. As mentioned, low-dose NSAID or colchicine may reduce the frequency of the attacks of arthritis. Other beneficial measures include weight reduction, avoiding excessive alcohol, limiting dietary purine intake, and discontinuing drugs that cause hyperuricemia, if possible. If these efforts fail to control the arthritis, specific drug treatment to reduce the serum uric acid level may be necessary. The agents most frequently used are probenecid and allopurinol. When therapy is initiated with either drug the patient's renal function should be evaluated with baseline studies to include: urinalysis, BUN, serum creatinine and 24-hour urine collection for creatinine clearance and uric acid excretion.

Probenecid is a uricosuric agent. Its mechanism of action is to inhibit renal tubular reabsorption of uric acid. Thus it is indicated in individuals who are hypoexcretors of urinary uric acid (< 800 mg/24 h on an unrestricted diet), with a glomerular filtration rate (GFR) of > 50 to 60 mL/min who have no history of kidney stones. The initial dose is 500 mg/d that, if tolerated, is gradually increased to 1 g BID. Patients on probenecid should maintain a fluid intake of at least 2L/d and should not take compounds containing salicylates. The goal of therapy is to maintain a serum uric acid of 6.0 mg/dL or less.

The most common side effects of probenecid are rash and gastrointestinal distress. Certainly formation of uric acid stones is a major concern. If that should occur in spite of appropriate therapeutic measures, then changing to allopurinol therapy would be indicated. If there should be a contraindication to the use of allopurinol, administration of probenecid with sodium bicarbonate or potassium citrate to maintain a urinary pH of 6.0 or higher might be helpful in preventing recurrent stone formation. Uricosuric agents frequently are not effective in individuals over 60 to 65 years of age because of the decrease in GFR that occurs with aging. When probenecid therapy is started patients often begin to experience acute attacks of gout. To prevent this, in addition to the probenecid, the patient is started on a low dose of colchicine or an NSAID. After 6 months if the patient's serum uric acid is 6.0 mg/dL or less and there have been no attacks of gout, the prophylactic cover drug may be discontinued and probenecid continued.

Allopurinol is a xanthine oxidase inhibitor and thus prevents the metabolism of hypoxanthine to xanthine and xanthine to uric acid. This lowers the serum and urinary uric acid levels. Because hypoxanthine and xanthine are far more soluble than uric acid, they do not cause crystalline arthritis or renal stone formation. The use of allopurinol is indicated for patients with urate overproduction or with urate nephrolithiasis or who have contraindications for the use of a uricosuric agent. The usual starting dose is 300 mg/d that may be administered as a single daily dose. If renal function is decreased (GFR < 50 mL/min), a lower dose of allopurinol (≤ 100 mg/d) is indicated to prevent high blood levels of the drug, which would significantly increase the risk of side effects. When allopurinol is started, patients should also be started on a low dose of an NSAID or colchicine to prevent acute attacks of arthritis which are commonly seen with the initiation of allopurinol alone. If after 6 months of combined therapy the uric acid level is in the normal range and there have been no episodes of arthritis, the NSAID or colchicine may be discontinued and allopurinol continued.

Common side effects of allopurinol include a pruritic erythematous papular rash, headaches, gastrointestinal upset, and abnormal liver function tests. There is also a syndrome of allopurinol hypersensitivity. This is characterized by toxic symptoms that may include urticarial rash, fever, eosinophilia, leukocytosis, granulomatous hepatitis, toxic epidermal necrolysis, interstitial nephritis, and renal failure. For individuals allergic to allopurinol but who have a critical need to take the medication, cautious desensitization regimens have been successful.

Physicians using urate-lowering drugs need to be aware of the interaction with other medications. Probenecid inhibits urinary excretion of indomethacin, acetazolamide, penicillins, and dapsone. When allopurinol and ampicillin are given simultaneously there is a high incidence of allergic skin rashes. Occasionally, patients with severe tophaceous gout are treated with combined allopurinol and probenecid therapy. Because allopurinol may increase the half-life of probenecid and probenecid accelerates the excretion of allopurinol, it may be necessary to increase the dose of allopurinol and decrease the dose of probenecid used.

A frequent therapeutic issue is the question of what treatment, if any, is indicated for individuals with asymptomatic hyperuricemia. Physicians vary in their approach to this problem. In general the risk of gout, tophi formation, renal stone formation,or urate nephropathy is low and thus in most individuals no treatment of the hyperuricemia is indicated until one or more of these events occurs. However, studies have shown that a serum uric acid greater than 11 mg/dL is associated with a 24-hour urinary uric excretion of greater than 1000 mg and that individuals with urate excretion levels greater than 1000 mg/24 h have an increased risk of forming uric acid stones or developing a uric acid nephropathy. Thus a baseline 24-hour urinary uric acid level is helpful in identifying individuals at risk who require careful follow-up and initiation of immediate treatment if there is evidence of decreasing renal function.

Treatment of CPDD is less complicated than the treatment of gout. For acute attacks of arthritis, NSAIDs, colchicine, ACTH, and oral and intraarticular steroids are quite effective. For the chronic arthropathy NSAIDs and low-dose maintenance colchicine are usually effective. There is no medication that effectively removes the CPPD crystal depositions from joints and soft tissue. In addition to treating the arthritis it is necessary to treat appropriately any of the associated conditions that are identified. Unfortunately, however, treatment of the associated condition has no effect on the CPPD crystal depositions.

CONSIDERATIONS IN PREGNANCY

During normal pregnancy the maternal serum uric acid level normally decreases until about the 24th week; at that time until 12 weeks postpartum there is an increase in the serum urate level. If the pregnancy is complicated by preeclampsia or toxemia, due to the reduction of urate renal clearance, the serum uric acid level is further elevated. The highest perinatal mortality occurs when the serum urate is significantly elevated (> 6.0 mg/dL) and associated with diastolic hypertension of greater than 110 mm Hg.

The transient increase in the serum uric acid level during normal labor is probably due to a decrease in urate renal clearance and perhaps increased urate production. This increase persists for only a day or two postpartum.

The occurrence of the acute arthritis of gout or CPDD is rarely if ever seen with pregnancy. If a case were documented appropriate treatment would be oral prednisone, ACTH, or intraarticular steroid injection.

BIBLIOGRAPHY

Agudelo CA. Crystal deposition disease. In: Weisman MH, Weinblatt ME, eds. Treatment of the rheumatic diseases: companion to the textbook of rhematology. Philadelphia: WB Saunders, 1995:271.

Kelley WN, Schumacher HR. Gout. In: Kelley WN Jr, Harris ED, Ruddy S, Sledge CB, eds. Textbook of rheumatology, 2 vols. 4th ed. Philadelphia: WB Saunders, 1993:1291.

McCarty DJ. Calcium pyrophosphate crystal deposition disease. In: Schumacher HR Jr, ed. Primer on the rheumatic diseases. 10th ed. Atlanta: Arthritis Foundation, 1993:219.

Moskowitz RW. Diseases associated with the deposition of calcium pyrophosphate of hydroxyapatite. In: Kelley WN Jr, Harris ED, Ruddy S, Sledge CB, eds. Textbook of rheumatology. 2 vols. 4th ed. Philadelphia, WB Saunders, 1993:1337.

Ryan LM, McCarty DJ. Calcium pyrophosphate crystal deposition disease; pseudogout; articular chondrocalcinosis. In: McCarty DJ, Koopman WJ, eds. Arthritis and allied conditions: a textbook of rheumatology. 2 vols. 12th ed. Baltimore: Williams & Wilkins, 1992:1835.

Terkeltaub RA. Pathogenesis and treatment of crystal-induced inflammation. In: McCarty DJ, Koopman WJ, eds. Arthritis and allied conditions: a textbook of rheumatology. 2 vols. 12th ed. Baltimore: Williams & Wilkins, 1992:1819.

Terkeltaub RA, Tate GA, Schumacher HR, Pratt PW, Ball GV. Gout. In: Schumacher HR Jr, ed. Primer on the rheumatic diseases. Vol 2. 10th ed. Atlanta: Arthritis Foundation, 1993:209.

Wyngaarden JB. Gout. In: Wyngaarden JB, Smith LH, Bennett JC, eds. Cecil textbook of medicine. Vol 2. 19th ed. Philadelphia: WB Saunders, 1992:1107.

Primary Care for Women, edited by Phyllis C. Leppert and Fred M. Howard. Lippincott-Raven Publishers, Philadelphia © 1997.

96

Osteoarthritis

DAVID A. CARRIER

Osteoarthritis, also known as degenerative joint disease and osteoarthrosis, refers to a noninflammatory type of arthritis. It is the most common joint disease seen by orthopedists and rheumatologists, and the prevalence increases with age: radiographic evidence of osteoarthritis is present in more than 80% of people older than age 75. The high prevalence of osteoarthritis and the medical care sought by patients makes osteoarthritis a significant factor in overall health care costs.

Epidemiologically, women are twice as likely to develop osteoarthritis in the knee than men, and black women are twice as likely as white women. The prevalence of hip osteoarthritis is lower in Chinese, South African blacks, East Indians, and Native Americans than in Caucasians. It is uncommon for osteoarthritis to be a problem during pregnancy, as it is generally a disease that affects women after their reproductive years.

ETIOLOGY

Osteoarthritis has been classified into primary, or idiopathic, and secondary groups depending on the absence or presence of an etiologic factor (Table 96-1). Both the idiopathic and secondary forms probably result from multifactorial conditions; the causes of the idiopathic form are unidentified.

The leading risk factor for developing primary osteoarthritis is increasing age. Despite the high prevalence of radiographic evidence of osteoarthritis in older people, fewer than half of these patients are symptomatic. Genetics probably plays a role in the development of osteoarthritis, as having family members with osteoarthritis increases the risk.

Obesity increases the risk primarily for osteoarthritis of the knee, whereas hip arthritis is not as strongly associated with obesity. A weight loss of 5 kg can halve the risk of developing symptomatic knee osteoarthritis. Obese patients are thought to have increased subchondral bone density in response to higher bone stresses, and this leads to osteoarthritis. The denser subchondral bone is less shock-absorbing than normal or osteoporotic bone, leading to increased wear on the cartilage and causing osteoarthritis.

Joint trauma is a well-recognized risk factor for osteoarthritis. Displaced intraarticular fractures often lead to arthritis with varying degrees of severity. Injuries that result in joint malalignment or that alter the mechanical function of the joint can generate an uneven distribution of joint forces, with resultant increased articular wear in areas of higher stress. Osteoarthritis is prone to develop in surgical removal of injured knee menisci and unstable knees secondary to ligamentous insufficiency. Direct injury to the articular cartilage also can lead to osteoarthritis, particularly because the ability of articular cartilage to repair itself is poor.

It is debatable whether long-term repetitive use of joints (eg, long-distance running) can lead to osteoarthritis. Athletic repetitive use generally is not associated with osteoarthritis unless there are other predisposing factors. Occupational repetitive activities in laborers or assembly line workers, however, can increase the risk of osteoarthritis in susceptible people.

PATHOPHYSIOLOGY

The primary joint damage in osteoarthritis occurs at the weight-bearing portions of the joint. Initially, the articular cartilage swells as the water content increases secondary to damage to its collagen framework. Proteoglycan synthesis increases in an attempt to repair the damaged cartilage, but degeneration persists and overwhelms such repair attempts. As the disease progresses, the joint cartilage thins and becomes soft, resulting in fibrillation and fissuring of the cartilage surface. The damaged cartilage can ultimately wear through, exposing underlying bone. Fibrocartilaginous repair tissue is formed, but its ability to function as an articular surface is inferior to that of the native hyaline cartilage.

In addition to the cartilage loss, bone changes occur, including subchondral appositional bone growth, eburnation of bone exposed by worn cartilage, microfractures, and formation bone cysts as a consequence of localized osteonecrosis. One of the hallmark changes of osteoarthritis is the growth of cartilage and bone at the joint margins, leading to osteophytes. As a result of the cartilage and bone damage, joint deformity and malalignment can develop. Synovitis can also be seen in osteoarthritis.

DIAGNOSIS

The diagnosis of osteoarthritis is based on the entire clinical picture, including the history, physical examination, and radiographic evidence. It is distinguished from other arthritides in that it generally affects older patients; a history of prior joint injury or deformity may be elicited; the larger weight-bearing joints, spine, and fingers are often affected; and there are classic radiographic signs of diminished joint space with associated bone sclerosis and osteophyte formation. Laboratory tests are not needed to make the diagnosis but are useful in atypical cases to rule out inflammatory types of arthritis.

HISTORY

Osteoarthritis is characterized by a progression of signs and symptoms. Pain, usually the presenting symptom, is described as worse with activity and relieved by rest. In more advanced stages of the disease, night pain can occur and can interfere with sleep. Joint stiffness can occur, especially after immobility. It is important to screen for arthritis in joints other than just the one being evaluated as the chief complaint. The risk factors listed in Table 96-1 should also be reviewed to elucidate possible etiologies for the arthritis.

Table 96-1. Classification of Osteoarthritis

Primary (idiopathic)
Localized (single joint)
Generalized (multiple joints)
Secondary
Trauma
Acute (intraarticular fractures)
Chronic (slipped capital femoral epiphysis)
Congenital/developmental
Developmental dysplasia of the hip
Perthes disease
Bone dysplasias (multiple epiphyseal dysplasia)
Metabolic
Alkaptonuria
Wilson disease
Hemochromatosis
Crystalline arthropathy (gout, CPPD)
Septic arthritis
Other
Neuropathic arthropathy
Osteonecrosis
Hemophilic
Acromegalic
Paget disease

PHYSICAL EXAMINATION

Because osteoarthritis is a progressive disease, the physical examination of the patient can change with time. Initially, only pain may be present, noted mostly at the extremes of motion of the affected joint. As the symptoms increase with time, range of motion may become limited, with resultant joint contractures. Mild to moderate joint swelling secondary to low-grade synovitis and joint effusions may be detected. Later stages of the disease demonstrate joint enlargement secondary to osteophytes, angular deformity, and sometimes joint instability. Atrophy of muscles controlling affected joints can also occur.

Arthritis in the digits can be manifested by pain, swelling, decreased range of motion, and bone spurs described as Heberden (distal interphalangeal joint) and Bouchard (proximal interphalangeal joint) nodes. Mucoid cysts can also occur at these joints. The basal joint of the thumb (carpometacarpal) and the pantrapezial joints are also prone to osteoarthritis, particularly in women; this can lead to decreased grip strength.

Osteoarthritis in the knee demonstrates classic signs, particularly pain and decreased range of motion, as well as palpable and audible crepitus with range of motion. Large osteophytes on the distal femoral flares can be palpated and create a visual deformity. Knee malalignment, particularly bowleggedness, can occur when one knee compartment is affected more than the other. Just the patellofemoral joint can be affected, elicited by peripatellar tenderness.

Osteoarthritis in the hip usually causes pain that localizes to the groin, but pain can also be felt in the knee and buttocks. Hip flexion contractures can lead to a bent-over gait, and limitations in internal and external rotation can also be detected.

Posttraumatic osteoarthritis in the ankle is not uncommon and is manifested by pain and limited motion. The great toe metatarsophalangeal joint is another common site for osteoarthritis, causing pain while walking and sometimes shoe-fitting problems.

Osteoarthritis in the spine can affect the intervertebral joints anteriorly and the facet joints posteriorly. The lower lumbar spine is most commonly affected, but the cervical spine is also susceptible. Advanced disease can lead to compression of isolated nerve roots, leading to radiculopathy, or complete spinal stenosis can develop, causing spinal cord impingement in the cervical spine or diffuse nerve root compression in the lumbar spine. Symptoms of neurogenic claudication and possibly the cauda equina syndrome can result.

IMAGING STUDIES

Plain radiographs are usually the only imaging study needed to diagnose osteoarthritis. They are insensitive for detecting mild to moderate thinning of the articular cartilage, but in knees the sensitivity can be improved by obtaining weight-bearing anteroposterior views, particularly with the knees partially flexed. Hallmark radiographic changes include a narrowed joint space secondary to progressive car-

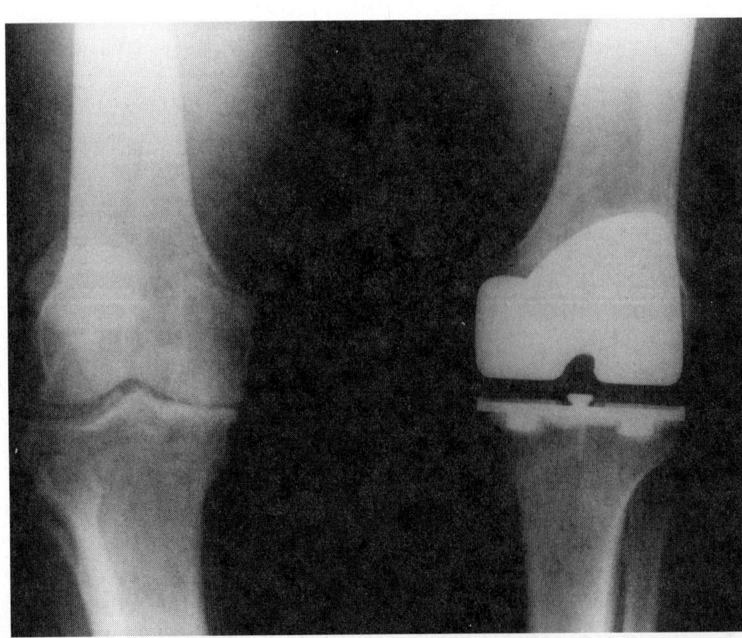

Figure 96-1. Osteoarthritis in the knee and total replacement. The right knee demonstrates medial joint space narrowing, tibial subchondral sclerosis and osteophyte formation, and associated varus deformity. The left knee has undergone total knee replacement using metal femoral and tibial components with a polyethylene tibial spacer between the metal components.

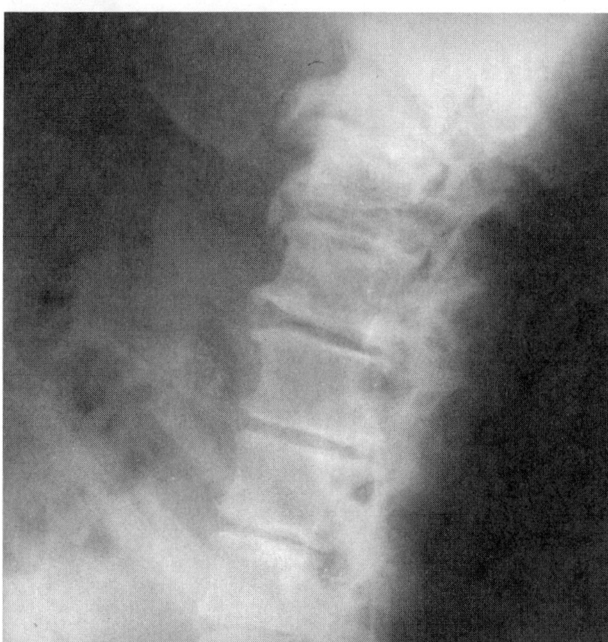

Figure 96-2. Osteoarthritis of the lumbar spine. This radiograph demonstrates severe osteoarthritis of the lumbar spine with diminished intervertebral joint spaces, anterior osteophytes, and sclerosis and osteophyte formation around the posterior facet joints.

tilage loss, subchondral sclerosis, and new bone formation, or osteophytes, at the periphery of joints (Figs. 96-1 through 96-4).

Computed tomography and magnetic resonance imaging (MRI) techniques are generally not used for imaging osteoarthritic joints. As MRI technology advances, however, it may become more sensitive in detecting early arthritic changes, supporting uncertain diagnoses of osteoarthritis. MRI is particularly useful in the hip to rule out osteonecrosis of the femoral head; this is important because early treatment can prevent the development of severe secondary osteoarthritis. MRI is often used to detect meniscal damage in knees, the symptoms of which sometimes mimic those of early osteoarthritis.

TREATMENT

Physical Therapy

Physical therapy is important for maintaining joint range of motion and reducing the loss of strength in supporting muscles. Application of heat through warm pads or baths can facilitate gains in joint range of motion; ice therapy can help during acute flares. Reducing stress on affected joints decreases joint pain. Weight loss and assistive devices such as a cane can be used to reduce the stress on the weight-bearing joints of the lower extremity. Non–weight-bearing exercises such as bicycling or swimming are preferable to running or aerobics. For lumbar spine arthritis, flexibility and abdominal strengthening exercises are emphasized.

Drug Therapy

Nonsteroidal antiinflammatory drugs (NSAIDs) are the first-line treatment for osteoarthritis because they reduce joint inflammation and relieve pain. A regular NSAID regimen can be therapeutic by preventing increased inflammation associated with activity. A major side effect, however, is gastrointestinal upset, prohibiting many patients from taking them. In addition to NSAIDs, analgesics such as acetaminophen, with or without a narcotic, can offer added pain relief, particularly when pain interferes with sleep.

The intraarticular injection of corticosteroids is often a second-line tool for osteoarthritis. The total number of injections should be limited, so they are best reserved for episodes of acute inflammation and pain. Too many injections can accelerate articular cartilage deterioration, and inadvertent injection into adjacent tendons or ligaments can lead to their atrophy and failure.

Referral to Specialist

Referral to a specialist is appropriate when the diagnosis of osteoarthritis is uncertain or when the disease has not responded well

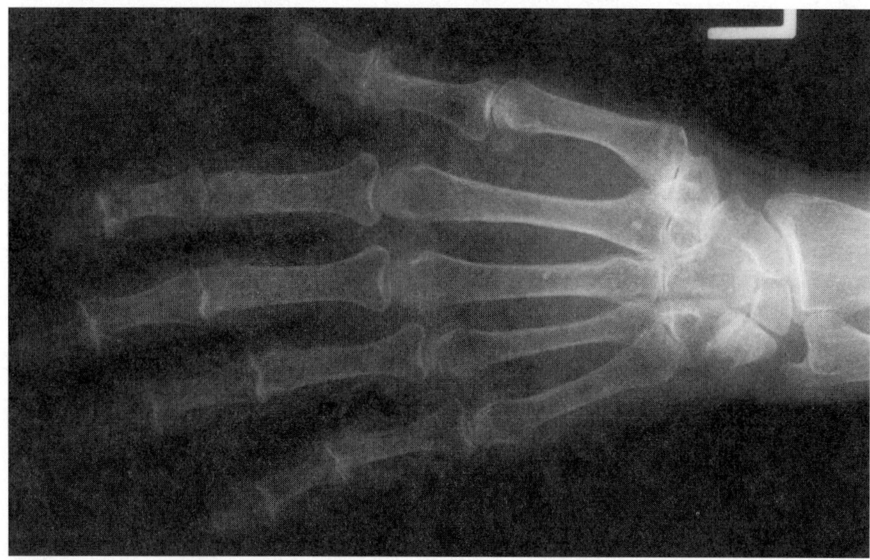

Figure 96-3. Osteoarthritis of the hand. Loss of joint space and subchondral sclerosis are seen in the interphalangeal joints of all digits. There is also joint space narrowing in the basal joint (carpometacarpal joint) of thumb.

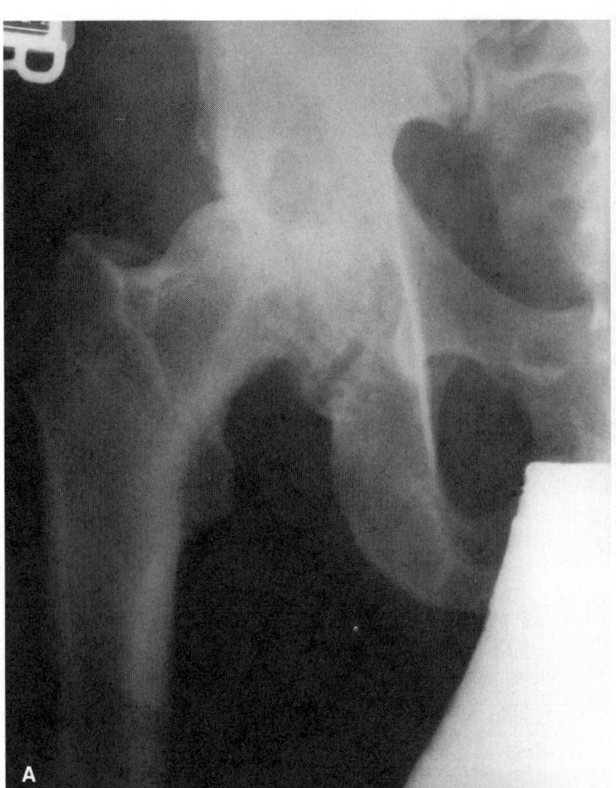

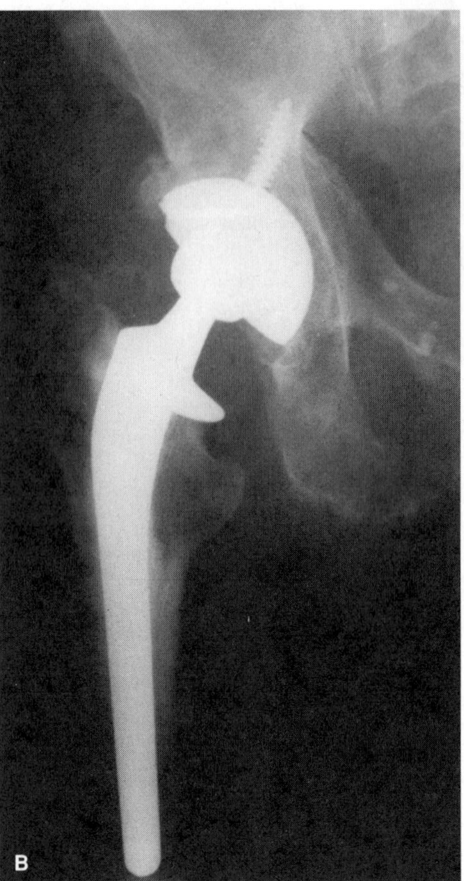

Figure 96-4. Pre- and postoperative radiographs of hip osteoarthritis. (***A***) Absent joint space and subchondral cyst formation in the weightbearing portion of the acetabulum and femoral head. (***B***) Total hip replacement.

to initial NSAID treatment. Intraarticular injections of the knee are often competently performed by the primary care physician, but injections of smaller joints (eg, those of the hand) are sometimes better left to specialists more familiar with the anatomy. When nonoperative measures have failed and the patient is significantly impaired by her symptoms, referral to a surgeon is indicated.

Surgery

Surgery in osteoarthritis is both preventive and therapeutic. Early treatment of developmental hip dysplasia, for example, can prevent the long-term complication of hip arthritis. In an anterior cruciate ligament-deficient knee in a younger person, ligamentous reconstruction may protect the patient from developing secondary osteoarthritis. Preservation of torn menisci is important in preventing future arthritis, so repair of torn menisci, when possible, rather than resection has become the preferred technique. Appropriate management of fractures, which sometimes requires surgically reconstructing fractured articular surfaces, can prevent posttraumatic osteoarthritis.

With advances in surgical technology, more options are becoming available to patients and surgeons for the treatment of osteoarthritis. Arthroscopic irrigation and debridement of damaged articular surfaces in the knee can provide up to 5 years of relief in as many as 80% of patients with osteoarthritis. Arthroscopy also allows direct visualization of the articular cartilage, which helps determine the stage and course of the disease and also provides information for planning future surgical options.

In middle-aged patients with angular deformity of the knee, realignment osteotomies of the proximal tibia or distal femur can redistribute stresses in the knee joint to healthier areas of articular cartilage. Satisfactory results beyond 10 years have been achieved with these osteotomies. Intertrochanteric osteotomies about the hip, which are more popular in Europe than the United States, have alleviated arthritic hip symptoms by unclear mechanisms.

Joint replacement has become the mainstay of treatment for patients with advanced osteoarthritis. Replacement of the articular surfaces of the hip, knee, and shoulder with metal and polyethylene components has been tremendously successful. Satisfactory results beyond 20 years of follow-up for hips and 15 years for knees have been reported. More conservative replacement of only the affected portions of the knee joint is also possible with unicompartmental components. Excellent results have also been achieved in the basal joint of the thumb with ligament reconstruction and joint replacement with interposition of rolled-up tendon.

Fusion of affected joints is another surgical alternative, particularly in the distal interphalangeal joints and affected levels of the spine. Fusion is a more durable alternative in hips and knees than replacement and is often favored in younger, high-demand patients.

BIBLIOGRAPHY

Crenshaw AH, ed. Campbell's operative orthopaedics, 8th ed. St. Louis: Mosby, 1992.

Evarts CM, ed. Surgery of the musculoskeletal system. New York: Churchill-Livingstone, 1983.

Frymoyer JW, ed. Orthopaedic knowledge update 4: home study syllabus, 1st ed. Illinois: American Academy of Orthopaedic Surgeons, 1993:93.

Kelley WN, Harris ED, Ruddy S, et al. Textbook of rheumatology, 3d ed. Philadelphia: WB Saunders, 1989:1469.

Schumacher HR, Klippel JH, Koopman WJ, eds. Primer on the rheumatic diseases, 10th ed. Georgia: Arthritis Foundation, 1993:184.

Primary Care for Women, edited by Phyllis C. Leppert and Fred M. Howard. Lippincott-Raven Publishers, Philadelphia © 1997.

97
Osteoporosis

MARIE E. AYDELOTTE

Osteoporosis is a disease of epidemic proportions, with major public health significance. Its prevention and treatment must be carefully considered in women of all ages, and medical practitioners must be aware of the risks and benefits of available therapies.

Osteoporosis is defined as a decrease in bone mass due to microarchitectural deterioration causing increased susceptibility to fracture. Although the composition of bone mineral and matrix is normal, trabecular thinning occurs, with resultant fragility. Osteopenia is the condition of bone mass reduction prior to fracture; of note, radiographic evidence of osteopenia indicates at least 30% loss of bone mineral. Osteomalacia refers to abnormal mineralization of bone with normal matrix (often due to vitamin D deficiency).

Osteoporosis is heterogeneous, and can be characterized as primary (basic etiology unknown, no underlying disease) or secondary (attributable to an inherited or acquired abnormality or disease) (Table 97-1). In turn, primary osteoporosis is classified as Type I, which results from estrogen loss during the 8 to 10 years after menopause, or Type II, which relates to calcium and vitamin D deficiency in persons of either sex after age 70. Other lifestyle and genetic factors also play a role in the pathogenesis of primary osteoporosis.

EPIDEMIOLOGY

Age-related bone loss occurs in all individuals once they have passed the third decade, when bone mass peaks. Multiple factors, including hormonal, genetic, nutritional, and lifestyle influences, impact on the development of primary osteoporosis. The disease is found throughout the world, although fracture incidence varies markedly, with the highest rates in developed countries such as the United States, Scandinavia, and New Zealand, and the lowest in rural Africa. Incidence is greater in urban than in rural populations, and is increased in Caucasian and Asian ethnic groups compared with persons of African heritage.

The morbidity, mortality, and cost associated with osteoporotic fractures are significant. In the United States, osteoporosis affects more than 25 million persons and is present in 1 in 4 women over the age of 65. About 1 in 10 women currently aged 35 will have a hip fracture later in life. Underlying osteoporosis contributes to over 1.3 million fractures annually, including at least 250,000 hip fractures, 500,000 spinal fractures, and 240,000 wrist fractures. Costs, including those due to lost productivity, hospital care, and nursing care, are in excess of 10 billion dollars each year. Hip fracture, in particular, is associated with high morbidity, in that half of those who suffer a hip fracture will need short- or long-term nursing home care and half will subsequently require assistive devices for mobility. There is also a striking 5% to 20% excess mortality in the year after a hip fracture.

With demographic shifts leading to the "graying" of the United States population, some authors have projected that direct and indirect costs of osteoporotic fractures may reach 60 billion dollars annually by the year 2020.

CALCIUM AND BONE PHYSIOLOGY

Before a complete discussion of etiologic factors can occur, calcium and bone metabolism must be briefly reviewed. Changes that occur with aging should also be understood.

The major organs involved in calcium balance are the small intestine, kidney, and bone (Fig. 97-1). Optimal calcium intake in premenopausal women is around 1000 mg per day, of which 20% to 40% is absorbed in the gut. Vitamin D is a major factor influencing the rate of calcium absorption. With aging, several problems may occur that affect this step in maintaining calcium balance. Efficiency of calcium absorption is decreased, in part due to lower circulating vitamin D levels. This causes mild hypocalcemia, triggering an increase in parathyroid hormone (PTH) levels and subsequent bone resorption: the "age-related" (Type II, or non–estrogen-dependent) osteoporosis syndrome (Fig. 97-2). Other factors that can affect calcium absorption include inadequate intake, possibly related to an acquired lactase deficiency, and diminished gastric acid, which is required to solubilize calcium and permit its absorption.

The kidney filters and reabsorbs calcium, and is not normally a major site of calcium excretion at any age. Calcium resorption is coupled to sodium transport, and is regulated to a lesser extent by PTH levels.

Bone is a unique organ in that it has a structural function as well as being the body's major calcium repository. Cortical bone, located in long bone diaphyses, is the major source of structural support. Cancellous bone, located in long bone metaphyses, vertebrae, and flat bones, has a higher surface-to-volume ratio and is the primary site of calcium mobilization. The major concept in bone physiology is that bone is a dynamic tissue made of a variety of cells that constantly form and resorb bone in response to stimuli, including systemic and local hormones as well as physical stress.

Table 97-1. Common Causes of Secondary Osteoporosis

Hyperparathyroidism
Cushing Disease
Hyperthyroidism
Multiple myeloma
Anorexia nervosa
Athletic amenorrhea
Chronic renal failure
Chronic liver failure
Immobility
Alcoholism
Medications (see Table 97-3)

The balance between formation and resorption reflects calcium balance and determines skeletal health.

Young adults maintain this balance. With aging, multiple factors, including estrogen deficiency, calcium malabsorption, decrease in vitamin D levels, and lack of weight-bearing exercise can conspire to cause a net loss of bone that can become significant over time.

Several hormones are important to maintain calcium balance. Parathyroid hormone, secreted by the parathyroid gland, plays a major role in increasing serum calcium levels in response to hypocalcemia. It acts by increasing renal calcium reabsorption, by increasing conversion of vitamin D to its active form, and by stimulating osteoclasts to mobilize calcium from bone.

Vitamin D acts at multiple sites to influence calcium metabolism. The vitamin is produced in the skin by exposure to ultraviolet light; the other major source is from dairy products supplemented with vitamin D. Standard multivitamins also contain vitamin D. Vitamin D is hydroxylated in the liver to its storage form, 25-hydroxy D, then is again hydroxylated in the kidney to the active form, 1,25-dihydroxy D. Major target organs of the active vitamin are the small intestine, bone, and parathyroid. As discussed previously, vitamin D facilitates calcium absorption from the gut, which in turn promotes bone formation. However, when PTH is present, vitamin D may also enhance its action.

Vitamin D deficiency is common in older persons, and may be due to several factors including lack of sunlight exposure, poor dietary intake of vitamin D, and decreased formation of the active hormone in the kidney.

Estrogen has a complex effect on bone in women. In general terms, its presence stimulates bone formation and prevents net bone loss. During the 8 to 10 years after menopause, estrogen deficiency causes increased bone resorption with mobilization of calcium, which is then excreted (Fig. 97-3). In the postmenopausal state, mild hypercalcemia leads to suppression of PTH and vitamin D levels. This contrasts with age-related osteoporosis, where PTH is elevated, though vitamin D is not. After about 10 years, the rate of bone loss slows. Although administration of exogenous estrogen can eliminate this phase of rapid bone resorption, the loss begins as soon as the estrogen is stopped.

RISK FACTORS FOR OSTEOPOROSIS

Risk factors for osteoporosis include hormonal, genetic, and lifestyle influences (Table 97-2). Estrogen deficiency from any etiology plays a major role in the development of the disease. Age-related decreases in calcium absorption and vitamin D production are also important, as discussed in the preceding section.

Multiple "lifestyle" factors affect the likelihood of osteoporosis. The achievement of a high peak bone mass in the third decade of life is important, and depends on optimal calcium intake throughout the preceding years, as well as on genetic factors. Weight-bearing exercise is receiving increasing attention as a preventive strategy. Both alcohol and tobacco use increase the incidence of osteoporosis. Excessive dietary protein causes obligate urinary calcium loss and should be avoided. Multiple medications may cause bone loss; these include corticosteroids, anticonvulsants, heparin, and excessive amounts of thyroid hormone (Table 97-3).

Genetic factors influence osteoporosis primarily by their effects on the development of peak bone density. Women with a positive family history or with slight stature are more likely to develop the disease. As noted previously, osteoporosis is most common in women of European or Asian descent.

CLINICAL EVALUATION

Clinical evaluation of the peri- and post-menopausal woman should include the information summarized in Table 97-4. The history includes information on lifestyle and genetic factors which influence the development of osteoporosis. Assessment of cardiovascular risk

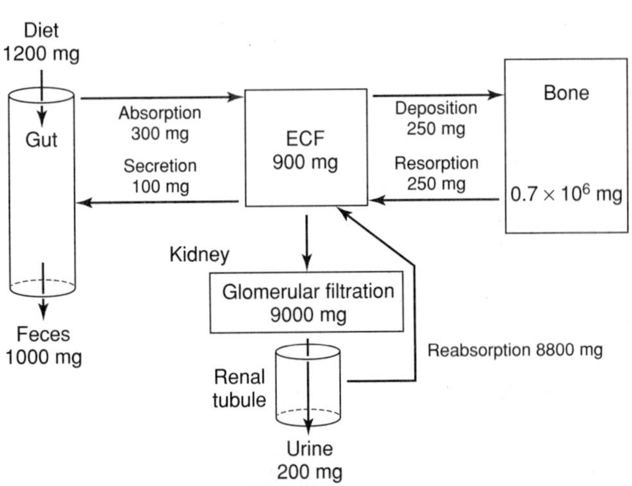

Figure 97-1. Model of calcium metabolism. The principal organs (small intestine, kidney, and bone) involved in mass calcium transport and the approximate daily flux rates of calcium between the compartments in young normal women. The size of the compartments are given in milligrams, and the daily flux rates are indicated next to the corresponding arrows. (Baylink DJ, Jennings JC. Calcium and bone homeostasis and changes with aging. In: Hazzard WR, Bierman EL, Blass JP, et al, eds. Principles of geriatric medicine. New York: McGraw-Hill, 1994.)

↓Vitamin D → Calcium malabsorption → Small ↓ serum Ca → ↑PTH → ↑Bone resorption

Figure 97-2. Type II "age related" osteoporosis.

is relevant to decisions about the use of estrogen replacement therapy. Personal and family history of malignancy can also influence this choice. The focus of the physical examination is the exclusion of secondary causes of osteoporosis, as well as the assessment of coronary heart disease risk. Laboratory testing in women without fracture may be minimal; in those with established osteoporosis, a more thorough evaluation is recommended. In the latter group, testing may help to rule out disease of the thyroid or parathyroid as well as the presence of secondary osteoporoses. A 24-hour urine collection helps assess the adequacy of calcium intake and rules out excessive calcium loss in the urine (idiopathic calciuria).

There are currently several noninvasive techniques by which bone mass can be quantitated. The most frequently used are dual-photon absorptiometry (DPA), dual-energy absorptiometry (DEXA) and quantitative computerized tomography (CT). Bone density at a high-risk site (hip or spine) is estimated; results are compared with age-matched controls. Of note, CT delivers significantly more radiation exposure than DPA or DEXA. The indications for bone mass measurement remain somewhat controversial. It is generally agreed that mass screening of perimenopausal women is unjustified. The cost of these techniques is significant (in the $100 to $300 range) and is in many cases not reimbursed by insurers. In a perimenopausal woman with risk factors for cardiovascular disease or osteoporosis, or in a woman with a hysterectomy, a favorable risk-benefit ratio for estrogen treatment may be present and further testing would be unnecessary. Groups in whom testing may be useful include women with a lower risk for osteoporosis or CVD, to assess the potential benefit of estrogen use; women with a higher risk but who are equivocal about estrogen therapy; and women with conditions often associated with bone loss, such as anorexia nervosa, athletic amenorrhea, or steroid use. Bone densitometry may also be useful to follow response to therapy, such as during research protocols. Future trends in the "risk stratification" of perimenopausal women include the increased use of biochemical markers of bone turnover to supplement bone mineral density and historical data.

PREVENTION AND TREATMENT

Lifestyle Factors

Although the diagnosis of osteoporosis is definitive only with the occurrence of fracture, women of any age should be concerned with osteoporosis prevention. Avoidance of smoking and heavy alcohol use, as well as an ongoing exercise program, should be encouraged. Current recommendations for calcium intake are summarized in Table 97-5. Calcium may be obtained from the diet or from supplements; some common preparations are listed in Table 97-6.

Vitamin D supplements of 600 to 800 IU per day are recommended for women after the age of 60.

Fall Prevention

Although significant loss of bone mass is extremely common in older women, some affected individuals never experience fracture. Falls are an important immediate contributor to osteoporosis morbidity and mortality. Falls are common in community-dwelling older persons; although some are minor, over 90% of hip fractures are the result of a fall. Counseling older women about fall prevention is an appropriate strategy for the health care provider.

Falls are multifactorial in etiology; a full discussion is presented in Chapter 11. Some risk factors for falls include sensory loss (visual and hearing), disorders of gait and balance, foot deformities, and medication use. In particular, medications that cause volume depletion, orthostatic hypotension, or sedation should be used with caution or not at all. The use of four or more medications has been found to be an independent risk factor for falling.

Assessment of the home environment is also beneficial. Uneven floor surfaces (steps or throw rugs), poor lighting, and lack of bathroom safety devices (grab bars, non-skid mats) may all contribute to fall risk.

Estrogen Replacement Therapy

Estrogen replacement is the mainstay of treatment in preventing rapid bone loss at menopause. Despite its common use over the past fifty years, estrogen therapy has never been evaluated in a large-scale randomized, controlled trial. This weakens the epidemiologic data regarding both the beneficial and adverse effects of estrogen, and makes some of its putative associations (eg, with breast cancer) difficult to interpret.

Estrogen is primarily an antiresorptive agent, and is usually started before significant bone loss has occurred. Estrogen use is clearly linked to a decreased risk of hip fracture, in the range of 25% risk reduction overall. However, duration of use is an important variable; the fracture rate is even lower in women who have used estrogen for a prolonged period (7 to 10 years or more), and, conversely, returns to baseline 6 or more years after stopping therapy. Thus, the optimal duration of therapy to prevent osteoporotic fracture is unknown.

Postmenopausal estrogen replacement dramatically decreases the incidence of coronary heart disease (CHD), the leading cause of death in older women. The mechanism for this effect is not completely known: estrogen favorably affects lipoproteins, decreases platelet adhesiveness, and also directly affects vascular tone. The magnitude of the risk reduction is around 50%, with a more beneficial effect in women with known CHD, and with increasing duration of therapy. From a public health standpoint, estrogen use has more impact on CHD mortality than on osteoporosis-related mortality in older women, since more women die of CHD. For this rea-

Type I Estrogen-dependent Osteoporosis

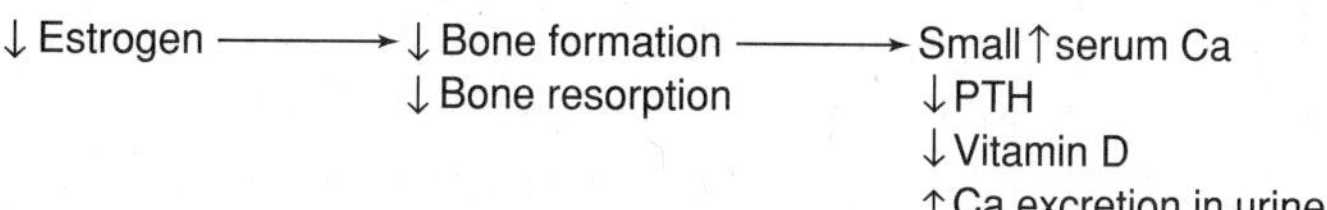

Figure 97-3. Type I "estrogen-dependent" osteoporosis.

Table 97-2. Risk Factors for Osteoporosis

Estrogen deficiency
Natural or surgical menopause
Anorexia nervosa
Athletic amenorrhea
Age-related calcium malabsorption
Inadequate calcium intake
Inactivity
Alcohol use
Tobacco use
Excessive dietary protein
Genetic factors

son, decisions about estrogen use in older women must include assessment of cardiovascular risk as well as risk of osteoporosis. Since CHD tends to be chronic and progressive, with death at a median age of 74 years, optimal duration of estrogen use is once more an issue. In the past, controversy has existed regarding the potential for thrombosis when estrogen is used in patients after myocardial infarction. A recent 3-year randomized controlled trial has shown a decrease in fibrinogen levels with estrogen use, which suggests that estrogen may be safely used in this setting, although long-term follow-up is needed. The same trial reported that a favorable effect on serum lipoproteins occurred even when progestins were added to the estrogen regimen.

The data on breast cancer risk and estrogen use are confusing and conflicting. Some gaps include few studies on estrogen plus progestin regimens, and the lack of large randomized, controlled trials. Most studies concur that short-term estrogen use (less than 5 to 7 years) is not associated with an increase in breast cancer risk. Some data show that long-term therapy (more than 8 years) may be associated with a 20% to 30% increase in breast cancer incidence, though others do not report this finding. There has been no definitive report of an increased breast cancer mortality in estrogen users.

Use of unopposed estrogen is clearly associated with an increased risk of endometrial cancer; this risk is eliminated by the addition of a progestin to the regimen. Gallbladder disease occurs about twice as often in women who receive estrogen. Recent data disclose that estrogen use does not cause elevation of blood pressure.

Overall, decisions about estrogen use must be made by individualized assessment of a woman's risk for osteoporosis, CHD, and breast cancer. Estrogen use should be considered in all women, particularly if there is a history of hysterectomy or risk factors for CHD. In women with personal or family history of breast cancer, the risk of long-term estrogen therapy is unclear, until long-term follow-up from ongoing trials is available. Current recommendations for hormone replacement regimens and surveillance strategies are presented in Tables 97-7 and 97-8.

Table 97-3. Medications Associated with Bone Loss

Corticosteroids
Heparin (long-term use)
Excessive thyroid hormone
Diphenylhydantoin (Dilantin)
Barbiturates

Table 97-4. Clinical Evaluation of the Peri- and Post-Menopausal Woman

History
Age at menopause
Menopausal symptoms?
Calcium intake
Exercise
Smoking
Alcohol use

Past medical history
Cardiovascular risk factors—hypertension, diabetes mellitus, hypercholesterolemia, hypertriglyceridemia
Secondary causes of osteoporosis
Malignancy of breast, uterus, ovary
Medication use

Family history
Osteoporosis
Cardiovascular disease
Malignancy of breast, uterus, ovary

Physical exam
Height, weight
Blood pressure, heart rate
Thyroid
Presence of vertebral fracture
Evidence of other systemic disease

Laboratory data—women without fracture
?Calcium, phosphorus, alkaline phosphatase
?TSH
Cardiovascular risk—lipid profile

Laboratory data—women with fracture
Calcium, phosphorus, alkaline phosphatase
PTH
TSH, T4
Serum protein electrophoresis
Complete blood count
Vitamin D level
Consider 24-hour urine for calcium/creatinine
Cardiovascular risk—lipid profile

Further testing
Bone densitometry

Calcitonin

Calcitonin is an inhibitor of bone resorption. It is a safe and well-tolerated medication that may be administered intranasally or by subcutaneous injection. Calcitonin is an effective osteoporosis treatment; resistance to its effects may occur within 12 to 24 months,

Table 97-5. Optimal Calcium Intake

AGE	ELEMENTAL CALCIUM IN MG PER DAY
11–24 y	1200–1500
25–50 y	1000
>50 (postmenopausal)	
On estrogen	1000
Not on estrogen	1500
Pregnant or nursing	1200–1500

(National Institutes of Health Consensus Panel, 1994.)

Table 97-6. Common Calcium Supplements

PREPARATION	MG OF ELEMENTAL CA PER G OF CA SALT	DOSE TO PROVIDE 1000 MG OF ELEMENTAL CA PER DAY
Ca carbonate*	400 mg/g	4 650 mg tabs/day
Ca citrate†	211 mg/g	5 950 mg tabs/day

*Needs low pH to dissolve; take with meals.
†Dissolves independent of pH; use in achlorhydric patients.

however. Calcitonin has analgesic properties, which make it a treatment of choice for painful vertebral compression fractures. The recommended dosage of synthetic salmon calcitonin is 200 IU intranasaly per day in one nostril, alternating nostrils daily. The dosage for subcutaneous administration is in the range of 50 to 100 IU daily or every other day. Duration of use in the setting of an acute vertebal fracture is usually 1 to 4 weeks.

Bisphosphonates

Bisphosphonates are antiresorptive agents that show great promise for the treatment of osteoporosis. They have been used for the treatment of Paget disease and hypercalcemia of malignancy for more than a decade. Alendronate has recently been approved for osteoporosis treatment; this medication is more effective and has fewer side effects than others in its class. Alendronate is taken once daily with water, at least 30 minutes before eating or drinking. With all anti-resorptive agents, adequate calcium and vitamin D supplementation is essential.

Other Agents

Sodium fluoride acts by stimulating bone formation and is approved for use in osteoporosis in several European countries, but not, at present, in the United States. Previous trials of fluoride use reported an increase in bone mass, but no reduction in fracture rate and a significant percentage of side effects. More recently, much lower doses of slow-release fluoride plus calcium supplementation have been shown to increase bone mass and reduce vertebral compression fractures, with minimal side effects. The low cost and wide availability of this product make fluoride an attractive option if these results are borne out.

Anabolic steroids also act to increase bone formation, but produce adverse effects including elevation of hepatic enzymes, adverse effects on serum lipids, and virilization. They are not recommended for general use.

Table 97-7. Hormone Replacement Regimens

Unopposed estrogen
0.625 mg oral conjugated estrogen (Premarin) or equivalent daily

Oral route preferred (topical preparations lose effect on lipids)

Estrogen and Progestin
Oral conjugated estrogen (Premarin) 0.625 mg daily plus medroxyprogesterone acetate (Provera) 5–10 mg for 10–14 days each month

Oral conjugated estrogen (Premarin) 0.625 mg daily plus medroxyprogesterone acetate (Provera) 2.5 mg daily

Table 97-8. Surveillance of Women on Hormone Replacement Therapy

Women on unopposed estrogen
Women with or without hysterectomy:

- Breast self-exam monthly
- Clinical breast exam annually
- Mammography annually

Women with intact uterus:

- Pelvic exam at onset of therapy
- Endometrial biopsy at onset of therapy
- Evaluation of any episode of vaginal bleeding unless recently evaluated (within 6 months)
- Endometrial biopsy annually

Women on Estrogen plus Progestin
Pelvic exam at onset of therapy

For women on cyclic therapy:

- Further evaluation only if bleeding occurs during non-progestin part of cycle

For women on continuous therapy:

- If bleeding is heavy or prolonged, or persists more than 10 months after therapy begun

For all women:

- Monthly breast self-exam
- Annual clinical breast exam
- Annual mammography

BIBLIOGRAPHY

Allen SH. Primary Osteoporosis: methods to combat bone loss that accompanies aging. Postgrad Med 1993;93(8):43.

Aloia JF, Vaswani A, Yeh JK, et al. Calcium supplementation with and without hormone replacement therapy to prevent postmenopausal bone loss. Ann Intern Med 1994;120(2):97.

American College of Physicians. Guidelines for counseling postmenopausal women about preventive hormone therapy. Ann Intern Med 1992;117(12):1038.

Baylink DJ, Jennings JC. Calcium and bone homeostasis and changes with aging. In: Hazzard WR, Bierman EL, Blass JP, et al, eds. Principles of Geriatric Medicine and Gerontology, 3rd ed. New York: McGraw-Hill, 1994:879.

Chapuy MC, Arlot ME, Duboeuf F, et al. Vitamin D3 and calcium to prevent hip fractures in elderly women. N Engl J Med 1992;327(23):1637.

Chapuy MC, Chapuy P, Meunier PJ. Calcium and Vitamin D Supplements: effects on Calcium Metabolism in Elderly People. Am J Clin Nutr 1987;46:324.

Chesnut CH III. Osteoporosis. In: Hazzard WR, Bierman EL, Blass JP, et al, eds. Principles of Geriatric Medicine and Gerontology, 3rd ed. New York: McGraw-Hill, 1994:897.

Consensus Development Conference: Diagnosis, prophylaxis, and treatment of osteoporosis. Am J Med 1993;94:646.

Felson DT, Zhang Y, Hannan MT, Kiel DP, Wilson PW, Anderson JJ. The effect of postmenopausal estrogen therapy on bone density in elderly women. N Engl J Med 1993;329(16):1141.

Grady D, Rubin SM, Petitti DB, et al. Hormone therapy to prevent disease and prolong life in postmenopausal women. Ann Intern Med 1992;117(12):1016.

Healy B. PEPI in perspective—good answers spawn pressing questions (editorial). JAMA 1995;273(3):240.

Heaney RP. Fluoride and osteoporosis (editorial). Ann Intern Med 1994;120(8):689.

Henrich JB. The postmenopausal estrogen/breast cancer controversy. JAMA 1992;268(14):1900.

Hodes RJ. Osteoporosis: emerging research strategies aim at bone biology, risk factors, interventions. J Am Geriatr Soc 1995;43(1):75.

Nelson ME, Fiatarone MA, Morganti CM, Trice I, Greenberg RA, Evans WJ. Effects of high-intensity strength training on multiple risk factors for osteoporotic fractures. A randomized control trial. JAMA 1994;272(24):1909.

NIH Consensus Conference. Optimal calcium intake. JAMA 1994; 272(24):1942.

Pak CY, Sakhaee K, Piziak V, et al. Slow-release sodium fluoride in the management of postmenopausal osteoporosis. A randomized control trial. Ann Intern Med 1994;120(8):625.

Prince RL, Smith M, Dick IM, et al. Prevention of postmenopausal osteoporosis. N Engl J Med 1991;325(17):1189.

Steinberg KK, Thacker SB, Smith J, et al. A meta-analysis of the effect of estrogen replacement therapy on the risk of breast cancer. JAMA 1991;265(15):1985.

Storm T, Thamsborg G, Steiniche T, Genant HK, Sorenson OH. Effect of intermittent cyclical etidronate therapy on bone mass and fracture rate in women with postmenopausal osteoporosis. N Engl J Med 1990; 322(18):1265.

Tilyard M, Spears GFS, Thomson J, Dovey S. Treatment of postmenopausal osteoporosis with calcitriol or calcium. N Engl J Med 1992;326(6):357.

The Writing Group for the PEPI Trial. Effects of estrogen or estrogen/progestin regimens on heart disease risk factors in postmenopausal women. JAMA 1995;273(3):199.

Primary Care for Women, edited by Phyllis C. Leppert and Fred M. Howard. Lippincott-Raven Publishers, Philadelphia © 1997.

98

Hip Fracture

MARIE E. AYDELOTTE

Hip fracture is a dreaded cause of disability and death in older women. The public health importance of this condition is enormous, due its prevalence, severity, and great financial cost. Following is a description of the clinical aspects of hip fracture, as well as risk factors and preventive strategies.

EPIDEMIOLOGY

Hip fracture is primarily a disease of the elderly, and is related to multiple risk factors, including osteoporosis and falls. In women, incidence increases exponentially after menopause. By 80 years of age, 1 in 7 women suffers a hip fracture; by 90 years of age, this figure rises to 1 in 3. Rates of hip fracture appear to be increasing. Some of this rise is explained by the aging of the population. Overall, 75% of all hip fractures occur in women and 25% in men; the ratio becomes more equal with advancing age. Caucasian women generally have higher rates of hip fracture than Hispanic, Asian, or African-American women. In 1988, over 250,000 hip fractures occurred. At that time, direct and indirect costs of fracture, including hospital and nursing home expenses and lost time at work, totalled over 6 billion dollars.

Disability after hip fracture is a common and greatly feared complication. Up to 50% of patients require short- or long-term nursing home care; more than one-third are able to ambulate only with an assistive device (cane or walker).

Mortality is also increased for 6 to 12 months after fracture. The in-hospital death rate may vary from 5% to 15%, with higher rates in more debilitated persons. After 1 year, mortality rates may be as high as 15% to 30% in older persons who were previously community dwelling. This represents a significant excess in mortality over that expected from age alone. In general, mortality is highest in the first 4 months after fracture, in the oldest patients, and in persons with concomitant medical illness.

PATHOPHYSIOLOGY AND RISK FACTORS

Overview

Hip fracture is a complex disease, which has been described as "Gompertzian" in its epidemiology. Benjamin Gompertz, a British actuary living in the 18th century, discovered that mortality rates increase exponentially with aging. The term Gompertzian has evolved to describe diseases for which almost everyone in a population is at risk and which begin early in life and progress silently until becoming clinically apparent late in life. At that time, their incidence rises exponentially. These diseases have multiple risk factors and are thus more difficult to prevent or treat.

Osteoporosis and falls are major contributors to the risk of hip fracture, but the relationship is complex. Elderly women with severe osteoporosis have only about a 2% annual risk of hip fracture; many never experience a fracture. Although 90% of hip fractures are preceded by a fall, only 2% of falls result in hip fracture in this age group. Both of these risk factors, low bone density and falls, increase with advancing age, but, even taken together, they cannot explain the exponential rise in hip fracture incidence.

Current hypotheses about hip fracture (Cummings and Nevitt) place risk factors into a cascade leading to the endpoint of fracture (Fig. 98-1). These interrelated factors are discussed later.

Falls

Because the vast majority of hip fractures are preceded by falls, fall prevention may be an effective strategy. Orientation of the fall is important: impact directly on the hip (occurring in about one fourth of all falls) is more likely to cause fracture. Falls occurring while standing still or walking slowly may be more likely to impact the hip. A more rapid gait may result in a fall onto outstretched arms with a distal radial (Colles') fracture. It is important to real-

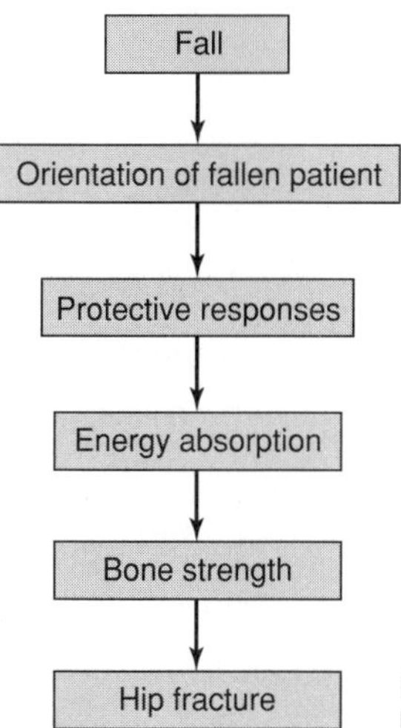

Figure 98-1. Cascade of risk factors leading to hip fracture.

ize that not all risk factors for falls are risk factors for falls resulting in hip fracture. Fall risk factors shown to increase fracture risk include visual impairment, neuromuscular disease, and psychotropic medication (Table 98-1). Environmental hazards, such as steps, poor lighting, and slippery pavement may also contribute to falls resulting in fracture.

Protective Responses and Energy Absorption

Factors relating to protective responses and energy absorption have been less well characterized than those causing falls and osteoporosis. Elderly persons may have slow or ineffective postural responses after falling, related in some cases to slowed reaction time or decreased muscle strength. Psychotropic medications and alcohol, which are known to increase fall risk, may act at this step. Soft tissues such as skin, adipose tissue, and muscle have significant capacity to absorb the energy of an impact. Women with lean body habitus or loss of muscle mass may have less ability to absorb energy related to falls and may be predisposed to fracture. External hip padding, though bulky, can halve the rate of fracture. The type of impact surface also affects the amount of potential energy transmitted to the faller.

Bone Strength

Osteoporosis is an important contributor to hip fracture (Table 98-2). Virtually all older women with hip fracture have advanced osteoporosis, although the reverse is not true. The fact that some women with low bone density never break a hip is best explained by the Gompertzian view: many risk factors must converge to cause a single end result.

Table 98-1. Risk Factors for Falls Resulting in Hip Fracture

Visual impairment
Neuromuscular disease
Stroke
Parkinson disease
Other gait or mobility disorder
Psychotropic drug use
Long-acting benzodiazepines
Narcotics
Antidepressants
Antipsychotics

Table 98-2. Risk Factors for Hip Fracture Related to Decreased Bone Mass

Advancing age
Female sex
Caucasian race
Immobility
Lean body habitus
Bilateral oophorectomy
Smoking
Heavy alcohol use
Hyperthyroidism
Corticosteroid therapy
Other causes of secondary osteoporosis (see Chapter 97)

Advanced age, female gender, and white race are strongly associated with both osteoporosis and with hip fracture. Lifestyle factors, including smoking, alcohol use, calcium intake, and physical activity are also important. Conditions such as hyperthyroidism, oophorectomy, and corticosteroid use increase fracture risk by increasing the likelihood of osteoporosis.

In persons with inadequate intake, calcium and vitamin D supplementation may be moderately protective in preventing hip fracture. Estrogen therapy greatly decreases hip fracture risk. Recent data estimate a risk reduction of 50% with either unopposed estrogen or an estrogen-progestin regimen. The benefit of estrogen wanes rapidly after cessation of therapy. Other medications useful in the treatment of osteoporosis have also become available. Osteoporosis is discussed in greater detail in Chapter 97.

TYPES OF HIP FRACTURE

Hip fractures are generally classified according to their anatomic location. There are three major categories of proximal femoral fracture: subcapital (femoral neck), intertrochanteric, and subtrochanteric fractures (Fig. 98-2). Approximately one third of fractures are subcapital; the remainder are intertrochanteric or subtrochanteric. Each fracture possesses unique attributes and prognostic features, which are outlined in Table 98-3.

Subcapital fractures occur within the joint capsule. They are classified according to the degree of displacement and the degree of comminution (fragmentation). A common staging system, the Garden classification, defines stage I as incomplete fracture with impaction (crushing together or invagination of opposing surfaces), and stage II as a nondisplaced fracture. Garden stages III and IV involve significant displacement or comminution or both, and can be associated with disruption of the blood supply to the proximal bone fragment. Joint hematomas and necrosis of the femoral head are common complications, especially if nailing techniques are used. For this reason, replacement of the femoral head and neck (hemiarthroplasty) is sometimes used instead of nailing in stage III and IV subcapital fractures. The Austin-Moore implant is a common unipolar prosthesis (Fig. 98-3). Frailer patients may benefit from this technique, because it allows almost immediate ambulation and eliminates the need for a second operation for a failed pinning procedure. However, internal fixation of stage III and IV fractures is still the preferred procedure in many cases.

Intertrochanteric fractures result from a greater degree of bony stress, and occur in older patients who have advanced osteoporo-

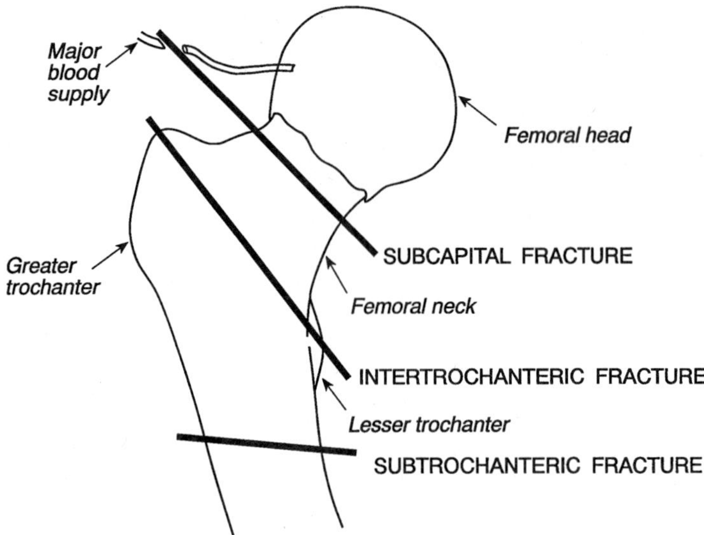

Figure 98-2. Types of hip fracture.

sis. The mortality rate is twice that of subcapital fracture (16% versus 8% at 3 months). This may relate to the greater blood loss from the fracture, the more extensive surgery required, and the frailer underlying medical condition of the patient. Intertrochanteric fractures are classified according to anatomic location (proximal to distal) and degree of comminution. Treatment is generally open reduction with fixation using a sliding compression screw with side plate assembly (Fig. 98-4).

Occasional patients who were previously debilitated and nonambulatory may be considered for nonoperative treatment, ie, traction alone. However, the outcome in these patients is poor (35% mortality) and may be partially attributable to the prolonged period of immobilization required. Surgery may also help to reduce pain. The decision for nonoperative treatment must be made carefully, on an individual basis, and with close attention to the quality of nursing care.

Subtrochanteric fractures occur between the lesser trochanter and the isthmus of the diaphysis. Again, classification is by anatomic location, degree of displacement, and degree of comminution. Configuration of fracture lines (eg, transverse, spiral) is also important. Treatment is open reduction with the choice of fixation device (compression screw, medullary nailing) dictated by type of fracture. Due to high mechanical stresses in this region, fracture nonunion and implant failure may be late complications. Nonoperative treatment is an option for a minority of previously bedridden patients; most studies have not demonstrated satisfactory outcomes.

CLINICAL EVALUATION

History

Most hip fractures occur in community-dwelling elderly women. A prior history of functional impairment often exists, such as trouble with independent mobility, bathing, or stair-climbing. Multiple chronic medical illnesses are common, and medication effects may be contributory. The majority of hip fractures occur after a fall, usually caused by an environmental hazard. However, an acute medical illness such as infection, cardiac ischemia, or adverse drug effect should be sought for as a precipitating factor. Ten percent to 20% of fractures are the result of a syncopal event. This history should trigger an evaluation for causes of syncope, including cardiac and neurologic disease. Postural hypotension from a variety of etiologies may lead to syncope.

Early medical complications from hip fracture may occur, even in women who were previously healthy. These complications

Table 98-3. Characteristics of Types of Hip Fracture

TYPE	DESCRIPTION	TREATMENT	WEIGHT BEARING
Subcapital (femoral neck) nondisplaced	Intracapsular	Closed reduction, pinning	Usually immediate
Subcapital (femoral neck) displaced	Intracapsular Hematoma or necrosis of femoral head may result	Pinning, or femoral head prosthetic replacement	Protected weight bearing for 2–3 mo
Intertrochanteric	Older, frailer patients Often comminuted fracture Higher mortality	Open reduction Dynamic compression screw or intramedullary rod	Usually immediate
Subtrochanteric	High stress area— Can have nonunion or implant failure	Open reduction compression screw, nail and rod techniques	Protected weight bearing until healed

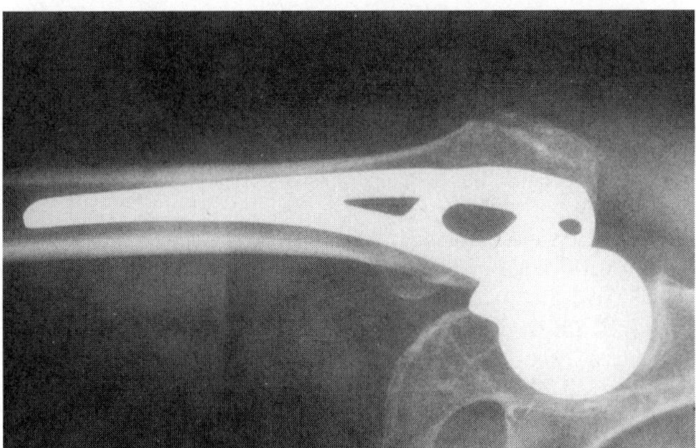

Figure 98-3. Hemiarthroplasty using Austin Moore prosthesis for repair of subcapital hip fracture.

include rapid blood loss into the fracture site, dehydration, electrolyte imbalance, and even rhabdomyolysis if there is prolonged immobility. For these reasons, surgical repair of hip fracture is often postponed at least 24 hours so that a thorough medical evaluation may take place.

Physical Examination

Patients with hip fracture are usually in severe discomfort and are unable to arise if they have fallen. Palpation or movement of the joint is painful. Muscle spasm and guarding are usually present. The classic physical finding is fixed external rotation, with shortening of the affected leg, but this sign is not always present. The diagnosis is confirmed by x-ray.

A complete examination should be performed to search for evidence of acute illness. Laboratory testing is also important. General guidelines for clinical evaluation are presented in Table 98-4

TREATMENT AND RECOVERY

The importance of preoperative medical evaluation in patients with hip fracture has already been emphasized. In addition to the workup outlined in Table 98-4, consultation with an internist or subspecialist may be helpful. Choice of anesthesia must be individualized; there are no data demonstrating the superiority of either regional or general anesthesia. Although a full discussion of operative techniques is beyond the scope of this chapter, an overview was presented under Types of Hip Fracture.

Table 98-4. Clinical Evaluation of Suspected Hip Fracture

History
Prior level of function (mobility, bathing, climbing stairs)
Chronic medical illnesses
Medications
Alcohol use
Falls
Environmental hazards
Syncopal events
Review of systems: Cardiac, neurologic symptoms Symptoms of infection (especially urinary and respiratory tract)
Physical Examination
Vital signs
Skin, mucous membranes
Cardiac
Pulmonary
Musculoskeletal: Spasm, guarding, external rotation, shortening of affected leg
Diagnostic Testing
X-ray of hip
Laboratory testing: Complete blood count with differential, blood chemistries, creatine kinase, urinalysis and culture, chest x-ray, electrocardiogram

Prevention of postoperative complications is an important part of the care of hip fracture patients. Deep venous thrombosis (DVT) prophylaxis (usually with warfarin) should be standard treatment. Without prophylaxis, 30% of patients experience proximal (above the knee) DVT, and up to 5% of these die of a pulmonary embolus. Medical illnesses are common complications in the postoperative period. Delirium occurs at some point in up to one half of hip fracture patients, some of whom may have underlying dementia. Reversible causes of delirium include infection, pain, electrolyte imbalance, or adverse medication effects (eg, from narcotics, sedatives, or histamine blockers). Other common medical complications include cardiac arrhythmia and congestive heart failure, urinary tract infection, pneumonia, and depression.

As previously noted, mortality is increased in the months after hip fracture. Serious medical illness and persistent delirium are the most important predictors of mortality. Advanced age alone is not a predictor of death, although male sex and African-American background are associated with a poor outcome. The reason for these findings is unclear, but may relate to the burden of medical illness.

In patients who survive the immediate postoperative period, the major predictors of recovery include good prefracture social, physical, and cognitive function and the absence of depression. Early diagnosis and treatment of depression, which occurs in at least one half of all hip fracture patients, is of the utmost importance.

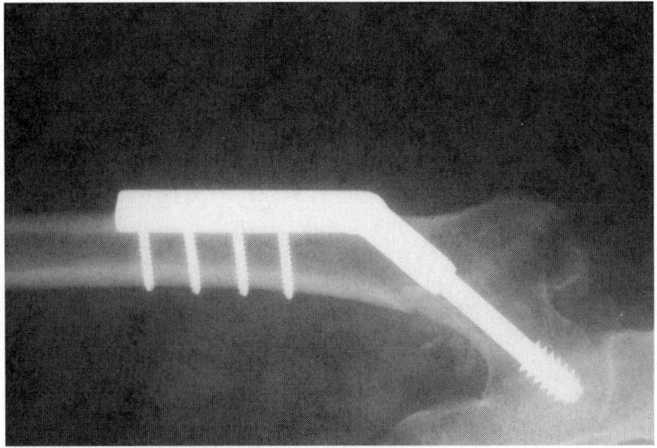

Figure 98-4. Compression screw and side-plate assembly used for repair of intertrochanteric hip fracture.

Virtually all hip fracture patients benefit from intensive rehabilitation, which should be initiated immediately after surgery.

Table 98-5. Strategies for Hip Fracture Prevention

1. Osteoporosis prevention (see also Chapter 97)
   - Weight-bearing exercise
   - Establish optimal intake of calcium, vitamin D, protein, and calories
   - Avoid smoking or heavy alcohol use
   - Treat causes of secondary osteoporosis
   - Use postmenopausal estrogen
   - Consider for established disease, antiresorptive or positive bone-forming agents (calcitonin, bisphosphonates)
2. Fall prevention (see also Chapter 11)
   - Diagnose and treat visual impairment
   - Make environmental assessment for fall hazards
   - Adjust or minimize medication, especially psychotropic agents
   - Consider external hip protectors in frequent fallers

Although current surgical techniques allow early weight bearing, joint range of motion is limited and muscle strength may be suboptimal. Physical and occupational therapists assist with strengthening and stretching exercises, balance training, and teaching of techniques to achieve independence in daily activities. Recovery of ability to ambulate usually stabilizes after 6 months, although the oldest patients may continue to improve for 1 year or more. Only one third of patients regain their prefracture level of mobility. One half of hip fracture patients require short-term nursing home care; around 20% reside in a nursing home for more than 1 year. A team approach involving the patient, family, orthopedist, primary care physician, nurse, rehabilitation staff, and social worker is the best way to optimize patient outcome. Whether disposition involves discharge to home, rehabilitation facility, or nursing home, the best predictor of functional outcome is the quality of the available rehabilitation services.

CONCLUSION

Hip fracture is a cause of significant morbidity and mortality in older women. The disease has a complex epidemiology, with an exponential rise in fracture rates in the last decades of life. A hip fracture should be viewed as the result of the interaction of multiple risk factors over time. Strategies to decrease the likelihood of hip fracture should focus on osteoporosis prevention and minimization of fall risk (Table 98-5).

Outcome after hip fracture has improved with newer surgical techniques that include preoperative medical stabilization, early weight bearing, and DVT prophylaxis. Mortality after fracture is still increased, especially in patients with concomitant medical illness. Factors that favorably influence recovery include early treatment of medical illness and depression. High-quality rehabilitative services play a major role in enhancing functional recovery after hip fracture.

BIBLIOGRAPHY

Bonar SK, Tinetti ME, Speechley M, Cooney LM. Factors associated with short-versus long-term skilled nursing facility placement among community-living hip fracture patients. J Am Geriatr Soc 1990;38:1139.

Campion EW, Jette AM, Cleary PD, Harris BA. Hip fracture: a prospective study of hospital course, complications, and costs. J Gen Intern Med 1987;2:78.

Ceder L, Svensson K, Thorngren KG. Statistical prediction of rehabilitation in elderly patients with hip fractures. Clin Orthop Relat Res 1980;152:185.

Cummings SR, Nevitt MC. A hypothesis: the causes of hip fractures. J Gerontol 1989;44:M107.

Farnworth MG, Kenny P, Shiell A. The costs and effects of early discharge in the management of fractured hip. Age Ageing 1994;23:190.

Fisher ES, Baron JA, Malenka DJ, et al. Hip fracture incidence and mortality in New England. Epidemiology 1991;2:116.

Gerety MB, Soderholm-Difatte V, Winograd CH. Impact of prospective payment and discharge location on the outcome of hip fracture. J Gen Intern Med 1989;4:388.

Greenspan SL, Myers ER, Maitland LA, Resnick NM, Hayes WC. Fall severity and bone mineral density as risk factors for hip fracture in ambulatory elderly. JAMA 1994;271:128.

Grisso JA, Kaplan F. Hip fractures. In: Hazzard WR, et al, eds. Principles of geriatric medicine and gerontology. New York: McGraw-Hill 1994:1321.

Grisso JA, Kelsey JL, Strom BL, et al. Risk factors for falls as a cause of hip fracture in women: The Northeast Hip Fracture Study Group. N Engl J Med 1991;324:1326.

Jette AM, Harris BA, Cleary PD, Campion EW. Functional recovery after hip fracture. Arch Phys Med Rehabil 1987;68:735.

Judge JO, Lewis CG. Hip fractures. In: Calkins E, Ford AB, Katz PR, eds. Practice of geriatrics. 2nd ed. Philadelphia: WB Saunders 1992:411.

Kelsey JL, Hoffman S. Risk factors for hip fracture. (Editorial) N Engl J Med 1987;316:404.

Kenzora JE, McCarthy RE, Lowell JD, Sledge CB. Hip fracture mortality—relation to age, treatment, preoperative illness, time of surgery, and complications. Clin Orthop Relat Res 1984;186:45.

Lauritzen JB, McNair PA, Lund B. Risk factors for hip fractures: a review. (Review) Dan Med Bull 1993;40:479.

Lyon LJ, Nevins MA. Management of hip fractures in nursing home patients: to treat or not to treat? J Amer Geriatr Soc 1984;32:391.

Melton LJ III. A "gompertzian" view of osteoporosis. (Editorial) Calcif Tissue Int 1990;46:285.

Mossey JM, Mutran E, Knott K, Craik R. Determinants of recovery 12 months after hip fracture: the importance of psychosocial factors. Am J Public Health 1989;79:279.

Palmer RM, Saywell RM, Zollinger TW, et al. The impact of the prospective payment system on the treatment of hip fractures in the elderly. Arch Intern Med 1989;149:2237.

Ray WA, Griffin MR, Baugh DK. Mortality following hip fracture before and after implementation of the prospective payment system. Arch Intern Med 1990;150:2109.

Russell TA. Fractures of hip and pelvis. In: Crenshaw AH, ed. Campbell's operative orthopedics. St Louis: Mosby–Yearbook 1992:895.

Thorngren KG, Ceder L, Svensson K. Predicting results of rehabilitation after hip fracture: a ten-year follow-up study. Clin Orthop Relat Res 1993;287:76.

van der Sluijs JA, Walenkamp GH. How predictable is rehabilitation after hip fracture? a prospective study of 134 patients. Acta Orthop Scand 1991;62:567.

Primary Care for Women, edited by Phyllis C. Leppert and Fred M. Howard. Lippincott-Raven Publishers, Philadelphia © 1997.

99
Carpal Tunnel Syndrome

RICHARD A. LEWIS

Carpal tunnel syndrome (CTS) is a common cause of hand pain. Because it occurs frequently, it is often diagnosed as the reason for any hand pain. However, recognition of the clinical features of CTS will make the diagnosis clear and a logical treatment regimen can be carried out. The public has a higher awareness of CTS due to many articles written in the lay press and in specialty magazines about CTS and repetitive stress disorders. Hardly a month goes by where a computer magazine or a sports subspecialty periodical does not have a few tips on how to avoid developing CTS. Engineers and designers are redesigning everything from keyboards to coffee cups to try to protect the public from the development of CTS.

Workman's compensation cases, more than ever before, are being filed for CTS that has developed as a result of the repetitive trauma of daily activities at work, rather than during a specific accident on the job. These claimants can't tell when they where hurt, only that they developed symptoms while doing their job every day. Of course, people use their hands in repetitive ways every day of their lives, so the competent producing cause of these, perhaps, work-related CTSs are hotly debated by third-party payers.

Primary care physicians need to be able to make the diagnosis of CTS correctly. They may choose to treat it conservatively at first, and will be successful in alleviating symptoms for many patients. The primary care practitioner needs to refer these patients to a specialist for diagnostic confirmation and surgical decompression if there is a failure to respond to conservative treatment. It is unnecessary to refer every mild CTS to a surgeon. However, one needs to remember that chronic nerve compression will eventually do irreversible damage to a nerve and complete recovery of a compressed nerve may be impossible if "conservative therapy" is allowed to continue too long, without any noted clinical improvement.

ETIOLOGY

The carpal canal is a tunnel that is surrounded by unyielding rigid tissues. With its rigid bony walls and floor and its tight roof, made up of the transverse carpal ligament, there is little extra room. It is the anatomy of the carpal canal the explains the pathophysiology of CTS. Any variant that further compromises the space within the carpal canal will increase the pressure within the canal. The structure most sensitive to crowding in the canal is the median nerve. The ulnar nerve lies outside of the carpal tunnel, but is subject to its own compressive neuropathy in its canal of Guyon.

Various etiologies can compromise the carpal canal, and any of these etiologies can produce CTS. For example, a ganglion within the carpal canal or an abnormal distal muscle belly on a finger flexor can reduce space in the canal by its presence. These are rare causes of carpal tunnel. The flexor tendons are surrounded by tenosynovium in the carpal canal. Any condition that causes swelling of this tenosynovium around the flexors in the canal can compromise and crowd the median nerve. This would include the collagen vascular diseases, such as rheumatoid arthritis, as well as nonspecific arthritides. The repetitive-use syndromes may cause CTS on this basis by producing a low-grade chronic tenosynovitis that crowds the median nerve with a persistent low-grade swelling in a space that cannot accommodate.

From an understanding of the pathophysiology, it is clear that anything that crowds the nerve can produce CTS. This includes edema and swelling in the wrist due to such diverse conditions as trauma, hypothyroidism, or lymphedema after radical axillary node dissection. Pregnancy, oral contraceptives, pre-eclampsia, and nursing have all been implicated in an increased incidence of CTS due to fluid retention.

The other feature of this canal is that it seems to be further encroached upon by wrist position. Holding the wrist in the flexed position further squeezes the median nerve on its way to the hand, thereby increasing the symptoms of CTS. This is the basis of the Phalen test (see Physical Examination and Clinical Findings).

One must understand that the median nerve supplies sensation to the thumb, the index finger, the long finger, and the radial half of the ring finger on their respective volar aspects (Fig. 99-1). This is the classic common distribution; however, variation does occur. The splitting of the ring finger by the ulnar and median nerves can move either way as a variant, thus making the ring finger all ulnar nerve or all median nerve in some individuals. The median nerve does not supply the back of the hand and one should question the diagnosis of CTS in a patient with numbness over the back of the hand in radial nerve territory. The median nerve can supply the dorsum of the thumb, the index finger, the long finger, and the radial half of the ring finger, but only distal to the proximal interphalangeal joint. The identification of diminished sensory acumen in the anatomical distribution of the median nerve is the hallmark of the condition known as CTS. If diminished sensation is present outside of that distribution than one must suspect another or an additional disorder. It is common to have diminished sensation in the ulnar and the median distribution based on compression neuropathies of both nerves. The ulnar nerve can be compressed at the elbow or wrist, or in both locations. Diminished sensation should not be present in the volar forearm, but pain in the forearm is, in my experience, a common complaint.

The distal motor branch of the median nerve, distal to the carpal canal, supplies the short thumb muscles of the thenar eminence. A severe CTS will have weakness of thumb abduction and thenar atrophy. This is a late sign of CTS. Once weakness and atrophy have developed the need for surgical decompression becomes more critical. One should not treat this type of advanced stage of CTS with conservative therapy without obtaining a neurological and a surgical consult.

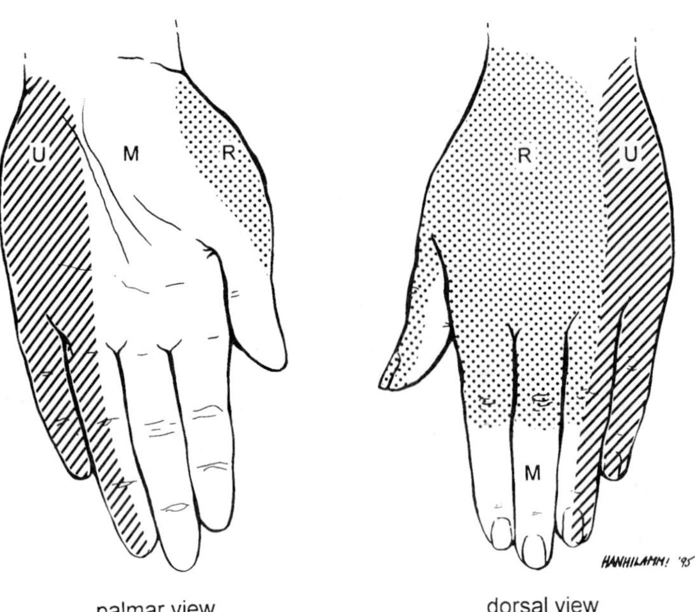

Figure 99-1. Classical sensory nerve innervation pattern of the hand.

DIFFERENTIAL DIAGNOSIS

The differential diagnosis of CTS includes everything that causes peripheral neuropathy, including metabolic causes, toxic agents, drug reactions, and infections. Other causes of hand pain that are in the differential are brachial plexus irritation from a Pancoast tumor in the lung apex, or the far more common cervical radiculopathy. Median nerve compression anywhere above the carpal canal (eg, at the pronator level) can also look like CTS. An acute compartment syndrome is a surgical emergency and has some features of CTS. Both conditions cause numbness in the median nerve distribution, but the similarity stops there. The acute compartment syndrome has severe pain and swelling in the volar forearm. Passive extension of the index and thumb cause severe pain; the forearm feels tight. It is usually of acute onset after trauma or drug overdose, or after lying on the forearm for hours. If this is suspected get immediate help, in minutes if possible. Irreversible changes occur in the nerve after 8 hours of increased pressure. The pressure can be monitored if there is a question of a low-grade compartment syndrome.

HISTORY

In CTS the patient usually complains of pain. Some patients will describe the classical sensory distribution. Most will not make it so easy for the clinician. Numbness means different things to various people and you should define it as "diminished feeling" for the patient before accepting their complaint of numbness.

Awakening at night with pain and numbness is a common classic symptom of CTS. This is believed to be due to the dropping of the wrist into flexion during sleep thus further compressing an already compromised median nerve.

One need to ask the duration of symptoms, the onset, what makes it worse, and what makes it better. The character and distribution of the symptoms are essential. Also, since CTS is so often bilateral, one need to ask about the opposite extremity and record if the patient is right or left hand dominant.

Many patients complain of pain and paresthesias with repetitive activity such as writing. Cramps in the forearm are *not* a feature of CTS. Nor is carpal spasm and involuntary wrist flexion. If these symptoms are present than a neurologist, preferably one with experience in the movement disorders, should be consulted to rule out a focal dystonia known as "writer's cramp".

PHYSICAL EXAMINATION AND CLINICAL FINDINGS

The positive Tinel sign is the product of paresthesias in the distal distribution of a nerve by light tapping over the nerve. A positive Tinel sign indicates irritation, or disturbed physiology, of the nerve. For the test to be positive in CTS the patient needs to complain of tingling in the median enervated fingers not at the sight of the tapping.

The Phalen test involves holding the wrist flexed over a period of 30 to 40 seconds. This position will provoke symptoms in patients with a tight carpal tunnel. This test reproduces the symptom of awakening with numbness at night due to the flexed wrist.

A direct compression test has been described where pain and paresthesias are reproduced by direct pressure over the carpal canal. The examiner holds the patients hand palm up in neutral and presses firmly with his thumb over the patients carpal canal just distal to the wrist flexion crease. A positive test is, again, the production of paresthesias in the median nerve innervated fingers.

These tests all require a cooperative patient and are presumptive tests based on the patient's responses. The sensory testing exam is somewhat more subjective and demands a cooperative, alert patient. For sensory testing the most reproducible and useful technique is the two-point tactile exam. Light and firm pressure or temperature are not nearly as useful. One can do two-point tactile testing with a simple rebent paper clip. Simply bend the clip like a long letter "U" and measure the distance between the points with a millimeter rule. One then asks the patient to close their eyes and to respond if they feel one point or two points. Gradually decrease the distance between the points until the patient fails to feel the two points and responds with "one" when touched by two. Usually, in a normal distal median nerve the two-point discrimination will be at least 4 mm. Much greater failures to discriminate of 7 or 8 mm indicate nerve dysfunction. Severe impairment of 14 mm or greater is barely protective sensation and a sign of severe dysfunction. Vary the test by deliberate touch with one point or no touch to assure the patient is being honest in their responses. Testing of at least the distal radial volar side of the index finger should be done as this is an autonomous area for the median nerve. That is an area that should not have any variants or crossover with the other nerves in the hand. Testing of the distal volar aspect of all of the fingers can be quickly done and recorded. This serves to establish the diagnosis as well as to monitor improvement or worsening of the condition. There are simple two-point testers such as cardiologist or cartographer dividers that work at least as well as a paper clip. The instrument should not be sharp as touch and not pain is being tested. The bent paper clip works well and the patient is less frightened that they will be stuck by the examiner.

All of the above physical exams and findings are related to sensory abnormality in CTS. The motor branch distal to the tunnel supplies the short muscles of the thenar eminence. The way to test for weakness of these median-supplied muscles is to check the strength of thumb palmar abduction. The hand is held palm up and the patient is told to lift the thumb up from the plane of the palm. The examiner can resist this motion with light downward pressure on the radial aspect of the distal thumb. At the same time one can see and feel the shape of the thenar muscles. This is when the examiner can identify weakness or atrophy and flattening of the thenar muscles, in more severe cases. Atrophy is usually a late feature after years of symptoms.

The carpal tunnel syndrome does not weaken any of the muscles in the arm or forearm. If true weakness of wrist motors or long finger motors are detected, another diagnosis should be considered.

LABORATORY AND IMAGING STUDIES

Simple imaging studies such as plain x-rays should always be done to evaluate a hand and wrist suspected of having CTS; in CTS, they are expected to be negative. They may, however, reveal a secondary condition that is causing the compression of the median nerve in the carpal canal. An x-ray may be the first sign of rheumatoid arthritis or of a post-traumatic osteoarthritis with collapse of the normal bony architecture.

Most x-ray facilities can take a carpal tunnel view in which the wrist is dorsiflexed and the x-ray beam travels through the carpal tunnel in line with the nerve. I find this view most useful in cases of trauma when there is a fracture of a carpal bone. The local swelling can cause this type of traumatic CTS.

Electrodiagnostics are the most useful way to follow a patient with CTS. These studies can confirm your clinical impression as well as help you to monitor improvement or worsening of the nerve's status. Electrodiagnostics may show improvement or worsening sooner than the patient's clinical change is noted. A patient

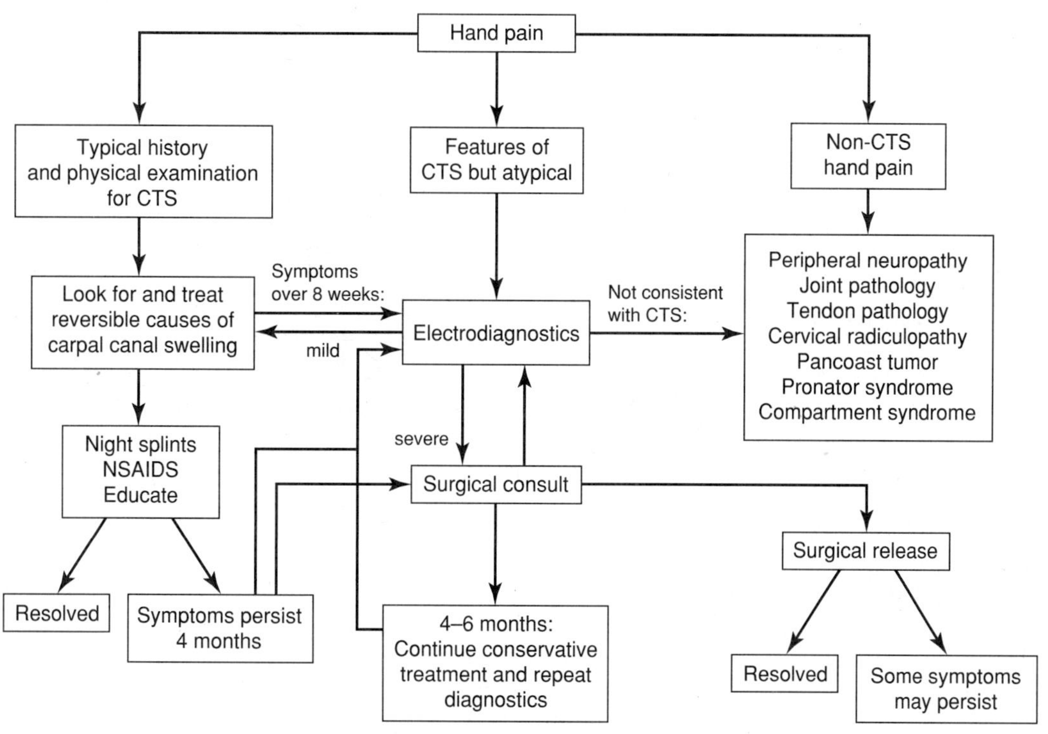

Figure 99-2. Suggested treatment algorithm for carpal tunnel syndrome.

on conservative therapy may appear unchanged while serial electrodiagnostics may show improvement of the nerve's status. They are useful, therefore, as a means of monitoring the response to treatment and in making decisions about changing treatment. Early on the studies can demonstrate subtle diminished velocity of conduction through the carpal canal. In late or more severe cases these studies can report denervation of the thenar muscles and development of potentially irreversible changes in the nerve. Knowing a good source of nerve conduction testing is critical to your management of this condition. Some neurologists have subspecialty training in electrodiagnostics, while, in some communities, these studies are done by hand specialists or physical medicine specialists. The resources in one's own community must be evaluated.

TREATMENT

The treatment of CTS makes sense when one understands the pathophysiology (Fig. 99-2). A careful history will reveal what activities of the hand and wrist may be contributing to the syndrome. Repetitive activities that increase symptoms should be discontinued. The patient is educated to work with the wrist in a neutral or slight dorsiflexion of the wrist to avoid flexion and crowding the canal. A rigid padded wrist splint is used at night to avoid the wrist dropping and awakening the patient with pain. This can be used in the day time as well as part of educating the patient on the ideal hand position. Any causes of hand swelling that are treatable should be searched for and treated. This includes ruling out thyroid disease.

Nonsteroidal antiinflammatories are useful to reduce swelling in the adjacent tenosynovium, provided they are well-tolerated and do not contribute to the generalized edema in the arm.

A carpal tunnel associated with severe tenosynovitis may require a hand dressing to immobilize and rest the entire hand. This needs to be seen by a hand surgeon to rule out a compartment syndrome and to decide if acute decompression is indicated as opposed to immobilization and elevation.

Clinicians differ on the usefulness of injection into the carpal canal with steroids to reduce swelling. Some feel it unwise to inject into a closed space and add pressure to the already compromised nerve. Others feel they can cure many a carpal tunnel with this technique. Inadvertent injection into the nerve itself can be a catastrophic problem. It is best left to the consultant to make this decision.

A baseline electrodiagnostics study is helpful in deciding which carpal tunnels are mild enough to treat nonoperatively. It is also useful to evaluate improvement or worsening.

Surgical decompression by simple division of the transverse carpal ligament is the definitive treatment for CTS. The structure is surprisingly thick and wide (about 2 cm from the volar flexion crease into the hand). The operation is done by orthopedic surgeons, neurosurgeons, plastic surgeons, and general surgeons. Recently, attempts have been made to bring arthroscopic technology to the field to perform this release. This is still hotly debated among specialists because of the potential disastrous risk to the motor branch of the nerve, especially as one begins to climb the learning curve to master the technique. The gold standard is still the simple 15-minute open division of the transverse carpal ligament with direct visualization of the nerve.

CONSIDERATIONS IN PREGNANCY

Next to backache, carpal tunnel is the most common complaint during pregnancy. It is often bilateral and presents with the typical pain, tingling, and night pain. The basis of this carpal tunnel is probably due to swelling in the carpal canal. It occurs more commonly in patients with finger swelling and in patients with preeclampsia and hypertension. Diuretics may be useful to reduce swelling. The nice thing about this form of carpal tunnel is that almost all of them resolve within weeks of delivery. Patients may be susceptible to recurrence with subsequent pregnancy or later in life. Still, some CTSs in pregnancy defy conservative treatment and interfere enough with function that a surgical release may be needed. This can be done with regional or local blocks.

An increased incidence is also reported in nursing mothers who did not have symptoms during pregnancy. This has been blamed on the fluid retention affects of prolactin. I might also suggest that some of these post-partum CTSs are related to the way the mother supports or carries the baby. I saw a patient with CTS that had a colicky baby that she carried and tapped constantly day and night. Certainly a full-time repetitive activity.

BIBLIOGRAPHY

Ekman-Ordeberg G, Salgeback S, Ordeberg G. Carpal tunnel syndrome in pregnancy. A prospective study. Acta Obstet Gynecol Scand 1987;66:233.

Greene DP. Operative hand surgery. New York: Churchill Livingstone, 1991.

Heckman JD, Rhett S. Current concepts review. Musculoskeletal considerations in pregnancy. J Bone Joint Surg 1994;76A:1720.

Nygaard IE, Saltzman CL, Whitehouse MB, Hankin FM. Hand problems in pregnancy. Am Fam Physician 1989;39:123.

Omer GE, Spinner M. Management of peripheral nerve problems. Philadelphia: WB Saunders, 1980.

Sabour MS, Fadel HE. The carpal tunnel syndrome—a new complication ascribed to the "pill." Am J Obstet Gynecol 1970;107:1265.

Snell NJ, Coysh HL, Snell BJ. Carpal tunnel syndrome presenting in the puerperium. Practioner 1980;224:191.

Wand JS. Carpal tunnel syndrome in pregnancy and lactation. J Hand Surg 1990;15B:93.

100

Neck and Back Pain

ROBERT H. CARRIER

Primary Care for Women, edited by Phyllis C. Leppert and Fred M. Howard. Lippincott-Raven Publishers, Philadelphia © 1997.

Back and neck pain has many different origins that are difficult to sort out, and the pain often is protracted and refractory to therapy. The fact that litigation is common in patients with spinal pain contributes to the difficulty. However, every effort should be made to determine the origin of the pain, because the etiology is paramount to effective treatment.

ETIOLOGY

Neck and back pain is so pervasive that the symptoms are often passed off as "back strain," "pinched nerve," or similar nonspecific diagnoses. The axiom "If you don't think of the diagnosis, you won't look for it, and if you don't look for it, you won't find it" is particularly pertinent. However, most cases of back and neck pain cease spontaneously with simple conservative treatment, so an extensive work-up for etiology is often not indicated.

The most common sources of neck and back pain are musculoskeletal or neurologic in origin. However, occasionally neck and back pain can be related to intrathoracic, intracranial, abdominal, or visceral pathology. Cardiac pain, problems with the great vessels, or pulmonary problems can produce radiating pain into the neck. Likewise, intracerebral pathology such as tumors, vascular disease, or lesions of the spinal nerves can cause neck pain. Various intraabdominal problems can also produce back pain. Duodenal ulcers not uncommonly produce back pain. Leaking aortic aneurysms can produce back pain, often radiating into the perineum. Kidney stones are well-known producers of back pain, typically radiating to the perineum or groin. In fact, almost any intraabdominal problem, particularly those that are retroperitoneal, can cause back pain. Malignancy can present as spinal pain. A complete test of all the causes of back and neck pain could include most of the ailments known to beset humans (Table 100-1).

HISTORY AND DIAGNOSTIC EVALUATION

The history is paramount in the initial evaluation. Neck or back trauma requires immediate attention. Numbness or weakness in the extremities must be promptly investigated. Atraumatic neck or back pain requires a complete history to evaluate the various potential etiologic factors. Past history is also important. Have these symptoms ever been present before? Has anyone in the patient's family had similar problems? Is litigation or worker's compensation involved? How long have the symptoms been present? Are they continuous or episodic? What aggravates and alleviates them? All these questions guide the examiner into the appropriate physical examination and further work-up.

It is helpful to have a diagnostic protocol for the initial evaluation of patients with neck and back pain. One way of approaching the work-up can be based on the duration of symptoms and their relation to injury: acute (up to 5 days from onset of symptoms), subacute (presenting to the physician 5 to 30 days after onset of symptoms), and chronic (30 days or more after onset of symptoms). These categories are artificial and may overlap.

Table 100-1. Etiologic Factors in Neck and Back Pain

Vascular
Occlusive
Aneurysmal
Neoplastic
Primary
Metastatic
Intervertebral disc
Muscular
Ligamentous
Neurologic
CNS
Peripheral
Visceral
Kidney stones
Gastrointestinal tract
Metabolic (eg, gout)

Acute

Trauma

Pain Requiring Immediate Transport to Hospital. Great care must be taken to immobilize the spine on a back board with "one piece" or sliding motion to get the patient on the back board at the scene. The neck is immobilized with sand bags. No twisting of the neck, flexion, or extension is allowed. If a helmet or headgear is on, it is left in place until after x-rays are taken.

In the emergency department, the usual attention is paid to airway, bleeding, and circulation. After the patient is stabilized, a careful neurologic evaluation is done and recorded for baseline reference. X-rays of the spine are then taken. In the neck, a single lateral view is done with the patient recumbent and in the supine position. If they are abnormal, immediate orthopedic or neurosurgical consultation is sought before proceeding further. If the x-rays and the neurologic examination are normal, a routine cervical spine series is done with careful flexion/extension lateral views, with the patient doing the flexion/extension and stopping when symptoms develop. In the thoracic and lumbar spine, routine x-rays alone are done with the patient recumbent before further studies are obtained.

Pain Not Requiring Immediate Transport to Hospital. A routine history is taken, a physical examination performed, and an x-ray taken. Patient-controlled flexion/extension lateral views are indicated. If neurologic symptoms or signs are present, prompt orthopedic or neurosurgical referral is indicated.

Nontraumatic

A routine history is taken and a physical examination, including a neurologic evaluation, is performed. X-rays are indicated unless the symptoms are minor.

Subacute

A routine history is taken, a physical examination is performed, and x-rays are obtained. If there are definite symptoms or signs of anatomic distribution of pain into the lower or upper extremities, a magnetic resonance imaging (MRI) scan of the cervical spine or an MRI or computed tomography (CT) scan of the lumbar spine is indicated (CT is less expensive). MRI or CT scanning is unnecessary with simple localized pain or nonanatomic pain in the legs.

Chronic Pain

The evaluation is the same as for subacute injuries, but the clinician should be more prone to use CT or MRI scans. Orthopedic or neurologic consultation is commonly indicated.

PHYSICAL EXAMINATION AND CLINICAL FINDINGS

The physical examination is guided by the history and is as complete as necessary to arrive at an accurate diagnosis. Sometimes a thorough, complete physical examination is needed in diagnostic puzzles; in other circumstances, a localized examination is all that is needed. The clinician should always remember that neck and back pain has many etiologies. Knowledge of anatomy helps guide the physical examination.

Objective findings are particularly significant because spinal pain often presents with symptoms that cannot be substantiated objectively. Examples of objective findings include muscle spasm (includes all large joints, upper and lower extremities); loss of motion (may be due simply to pain, which is subjective); muscle weakness or atrophy; and abnormal results on the neurologic examination (eg, sensory deficit; abnormal Babinski sign, clonus; abnormal deep tendon reflexes; abnormal cremasteric or perianal reflexes; positive straight-leg raise test; positive femoral stretch test). The straight-leg raising test can be done with the patient sitting on the edge of the examining table and straightening the knee or with the patient recumbent. It is positive if there is pain in the buttock or the back with the straight-leg lift, not pain in the hamstring area. Doing the test in two positions helps evaluate litigious patients who have learned proper responses to various tests. The femoral stretch test, done with the patient prone and the knee lifted off the table, tests the femoral nerve or L2,3 nerve roots with pain in the front of the thigh.

Vascular deficit is sought by checking the pulses in the feet and the popliteal and femoral arteries and by observing for an abdominal aneurysm.

ANATOMIC CONSIDERATIONS

As Last points out, the examination findings must be localized to a specific anatomic area for proper diagnosis and treatment. The anatomy of the spine is complex, but the only anatomy the primary care physician needs to know can be outlined in the sensory distribution diagrams known to all and the segmental innervation of muscles and joints (Fig. 100-1).

Most muscles are supplied from two adjacent spinal segments. Muscles sharing a common primary action on a joint are all supplied by the same (usually two) segments. Their opponents sharing

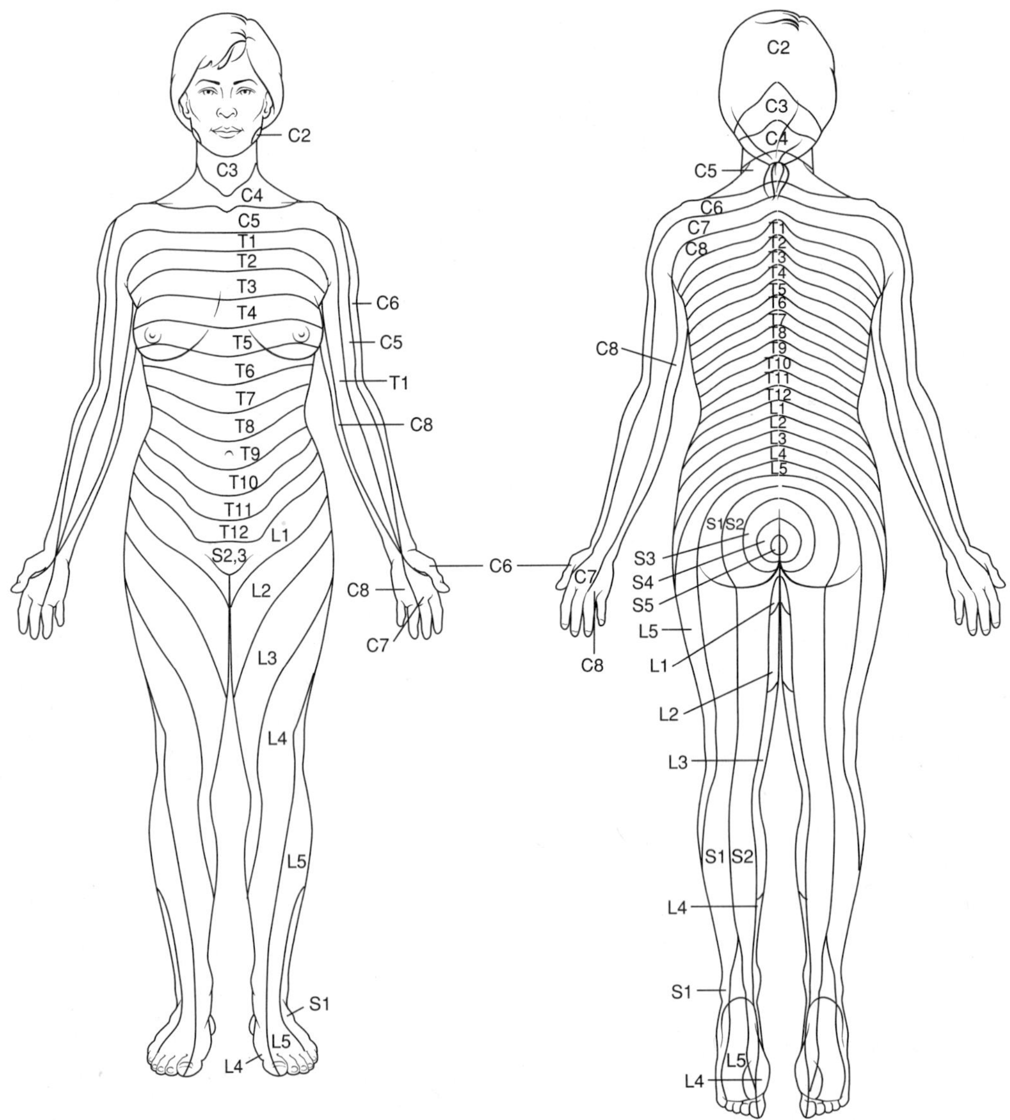

Figure 100-1. Dermal Segmentation. Despite schematic demarcation, in actuality there is considerable overlap between nerve supply of adjacent segments. (Redrawn from Netter FH, Brass AM, Dingle RV, eds. The CIBA collection of medical illustrations, Part I, Vol. I, Section VI, Plate 16, CIBA, 1983.)

the opposite action are likewise supplied by (usually two) segments, and these segments usually run in numeric sequence with the former. In other words, there are spinal centers for joint motion, and these spinal centers tend to occupy four continuous segments in the cord. The upper two segments innovate one motion, the lower two segments the opposite motion. For example, the hip center is L2, L3, L4, and L5. The knee center, one joint distal, has its center one joint distal—namely, L3, L4, L5, and S1. This is shown in Table 100-2 for the lower extremity and is illustrated in Figure 100-2. A similar arrangement occurs in the upper extremity, except that joint movements are controlled unisegmentally. By noting the area of loss of sensation or motion, it becomes easy to extrapolate back to the spinal segments involved to determine the anatomic location of the suspected lesion.

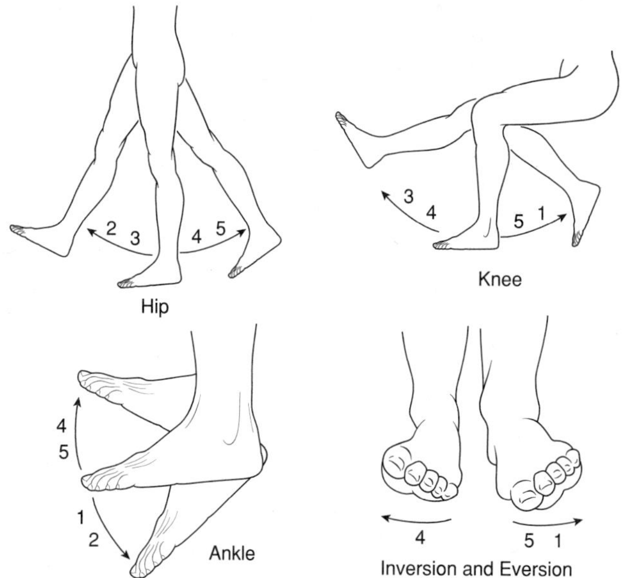

Figure 100-2. The segmental innervation of the movements of the lower limb. (Last RJ. Anatomy: regional and applied, 2nd ed. Boston: Little, Brown, 1959:38.)

LABORATORY AND IMAGING STUDIES

If, after an appropriate history and physical examination are done, the diagnosis is unclear and the severity of symptoms warrants further work-up, then laboratory and imaging studies are indicated. However, the routine use of these studies before the history and physical examination are done should be condemned. They are often unnecessary and produce discomfort and exposure when lesser measures will suffice.

Laboratory studies include a complete blood count and analysis for rheumatoid factor and antinuclear antibodies. Routine laboratory studies are often used for screening to rule in or out many problems. The sedimentation rate is useful as a screening test; if normal, it rules out major malignancy, infection, or inflammatory arthritis. A lupus erythematosus (LE) preparation is done to evaluate possible inflammatory arthritis or connective tissue disease; if positive, it may lead to more sophisticated studies.

If in doubt as to the best imaging study for a particular anatomic area, the radiologist should be consulted. Routine x-rays should always be done before ordering more expensive and sophisticated studies. Generally, CT is better than MRI in evaluating cortical bone, but MRI is better at imaging soft tissues and marrow. MRI is better for the cervical spine and probably the thoracic spine, but there is no uniformity of opinion on the best study for the lumbar spine.

TREATMENT

Patients with back or neck pain can be divided into two categories: those with known, demonstrable, objective findings and diagnosis, and those without a definitive diagnosis substantiated by objective findings.

Patients in the first category are treated as their condition requires: fractures require appropriate treatment by an orthopedic surgeon, ulcers by an internist, vascular lesions by a vascular surgeon, ruptured discs by a neurologic surgeon, and so forth.

Patients in the second category, unfortunately, are far more common. They are often labeled as having neck or back spasm, neck or back sprain, pinched nerve, myositis, arthritis, and other nonspecific diagnoses. They form a large group of patients and are a formidable treatment challenge. In these patients, the physician must continue to search for a positive diagnosis. Labeling the patient as having "pain of unknown origin" without persistent attempts to determine the etiology may rob her of proper treatment. Conservative treatment is indicated in almost all these patients. Analgesics should be given, appropriate to the severity of pain. The patient should apply heat or ice, whichever feels better; there is no scientific rationale for one being better than other except in acute trauma, where ice is preferable. Modified activity should be prescribed. Bed rest should be used sparingly. Patients recover more quickly with less functional deficit if they remain ambulatory with light activity and early return to work. In 1994, the federal Agency for Health Care Policy released guidelines for treatment of low back pain showing that acute surgery is rarely indicated and that manipulative treatment is of some benefit. There was no support for injections, lasers, or acupuncture.

Table 100-2. Segmental Innervation of the Movement of the Lower Limb

HIP	KNEE	ANKLE
2, 3 } Flex	3, 4 } Extend	4, 5 } Dorsiflex
4, 5 } Extend	5, S1 } Flex	S1, S2 } Plantar-flex

(Last RJ. Anatomy: regional and applied, 2d ed. Boston: Little, Brown & Co., 1959:37.)

Physical Therapy

A brief (3 to 9 weeks) trial of physical therapy is useful, but prolonged treatment is rarely indicated. Manipulation is of some benefit, so long as a good medical work-up shows no anatomic problems that would be injured by manipulation. Cervical traction is often helpful in the neck for degenerative disc disease and can be

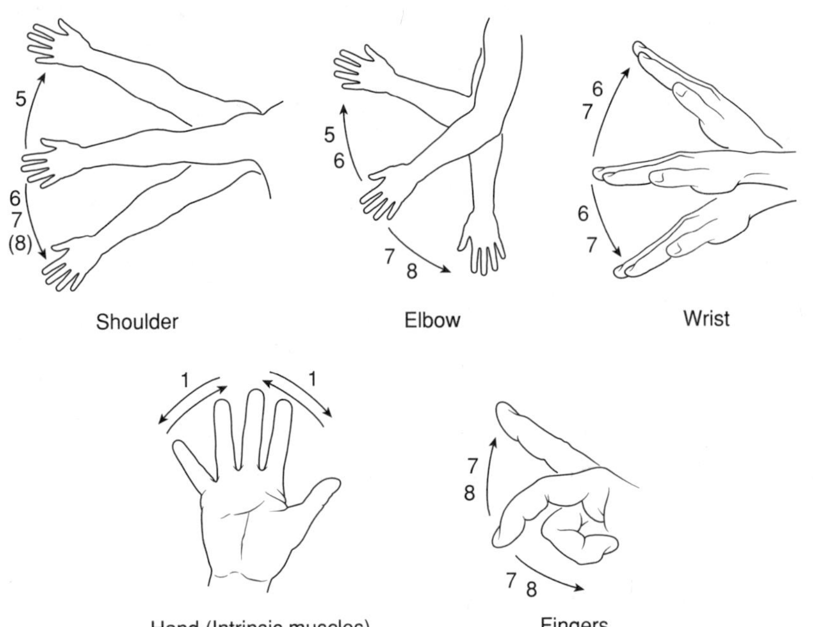

Figure 100-3. The segmental innervation of the movements of the upper limb. (Last RI, Anatomy: regional and applied, 2nd ed. Boston: Little, Brown, 1959:39.)

used at home. It is less helpful in low back pain. Ultrasound, hot packs, and infrared lamps are sometimes helpful symptomatically, but prolonged use is not indicated. Massage is of brief symptomatic help only. In transcutaneous electrical nerve stimulation, patient-controlled electrical impulses are used to block pain receptors. This modality is expensive and scientifically unproven, but some patients find it helpful. Iontophoresis is the passage of steroids through the skin with electrical impulses; there is no scientific evidence of benefit. A back exercise program is helpful.

CONSIDERATIONS IN PREGNANCY

Spinal problems in pregnancy are due to hormonal and mechanical factors. The hormone relaxin increases the mobility and produces widening of the sacroiliac syndesmosis and the pubic symphysis. The increasing size of the fetus produces significant mechanical effects on the lumbar spine. Lumbar lordosis is greatly aggravated by the gravid uterus, throwing increased strain on the supporting ligaments and joints of the low back. Hormonal effects also play a role. Between 50% and 75% of pregnant women experience low back pain during pregnancy. Women who have had low back pain before pregnancy are more prone to have back pain during pregnancy. Pain radiating into the thighs later in pregnancy is common as the sacroiliac joints widen, but true ruptured discs are uncommon. The pain is usually aggravated by prolonged standing and relieved by lying down. Pain in the upper back or neck is not increased over that found in nonpregnant women. Women in good physical condition before pregnancy are less prone to develop back symptoms.

X-rays should be avoided completely in the first trimester, except in unusual circumstances, and used sparingly in the later months. The use of MRI would seem safe if indicated, but there are no good studies to document its safety in pregnancy.

Back pain can usually be relieved by modified activity, specific exercises such as pelvic rocking, periods of recumbency, and back support. A simple lumbosacral corset often helps, although sometimes a more sophisticated lower abdominal support that transfers uterine weight to the shoulders is necessary. Surgery is contraindicated unless a herniated disc is producing significant neurologic deficit or bowel or bladder incontinence.

Medication for back pain in pregnancy should be limited to acetaminophen. Aspirin and nonsteroidal antiinflammatory agents in the doses required to alleviate musculoskeletal back pain are relatively contraindicated in pregnancy, as their prostaglandin inhibition may increase the risk of intracranial bleeding and they have been associated with improper timing of closure of the ductus arteriosus in the fetus.

Back and neck pain due to rheumatoid arthritis often improves with pregnancy; ankylosing spondylitis may worsen.

If back pain persists beyond 6 weeks postpartum, a diagnostic evaluation should be undertaken, as previously outlined.

BIBLIOGRAPHY

Heckman JD, Sassard R. Musculoskeletal considerations in pregnancy. J Bone Joint Surg 1994;76(A):1720.

Keim HA, Kirkaldy-Willis WH. Low back pain. Annual Clinical Symposia, Summit, NJ: Ciba-Geigy Corp. 1980;32.

Last RJ. Anatomy: regional and applied, 2d ed. Boston: Little, Brown & Co., 1959.

Netter FH, Brass A, Dingle RV, eds. The CIBA collection of medical illustrations, vol. I: Nervous system; pt. I: Anatomy and physiology. Summit, NJ: Ciba-Geigy Corp.

Primary Care for Women, edited by Phyllis C. Leppert and Fred M. Howard. Lippincott-Raven Publishers, Philadelphia © 1997.

101
Hip Pain

CHRISTOPHER W. OLCOTT

Hip pain in women includes a wide array of both traumatic and nontraumatic disorders. In the evaluation of a woman with hip pain, a thorough history must be accompanied by a complete musculoskeletal exam, not limited to the hip, and judicious use of x-rays. Importantly, hip pain resulting from hip pathology must be differentiated from that of lumbosacral, retroperitoneal, or vascular origin.

In the evaluation of hip pain it is imperative to understand the type, location and duration of pain, as well as any exacerbating or alleviating factors. Some common questions include: did the hip pain follow a traumatic episode (eg, a fall) or a recent illness? What are the associated symptoms? Night pain? Are assistive devices (eg, cane, walker) necessary for ambulation? Any limp? What is the distance the patient is able to walk? Morning stiffness? Other joint involvement? Use of drugs or steroids?

HISTORY AND PHYSICAL EXAMINATION

While hip pain may signal actual hip pathology, it may be referred from the lumbar spine (eg, spinal stenosis, herniated lumbar disc). Hip pain can be either focal or diffuse, and often presents with pain, limp, and stiffness. For example, pain laterally over the greater trochanter may arise from trochanteric bursitis, while groin pain is more indicative of hip joint pathology. Even though hip pain may radiate to the knee it seldom extends below the knee, unlike radicular pain or claudication.

Examination of the hip must include evaluation of the entire musculoskeletal system. Observe the patient's gait and posture. For example, a Trendelenberg gait indicates abductor muscle weakness or more general hip pathology. In Trendelenberg gait the patient's pelvis drops on the side opposite the weight-bearing limb and the trunk often shifts to this contralateral side. In other words, the pelvis of a patient with weak abductors (ie, gluteus medius, gluteus minimus) will sag to the contralateral side when asked to stand on the affected limb. This drop of the pelvis on the unsupported side indicates weak abductors in the weight-bearing limb. An antalgic gait or painful limp represents an attempt to put less weight on the affected lower extremity. In other words, a patient with a painful hip will demonstrate a short stance phase on the affected side and quickly transfer her weight to the opposite, noninvolved side. An antalgic gait is often accompanied by visible signs of pain, for example facial grimacing when weight-bearing on the affected side. Pelvic obliquity, often a sign of spinal pathology (eg, scoliosis) or leg length discrepancy, is determined by checking the level of the iliac crests while the patient stands upright.

Next examine the patient supine. Inspect the affected limb for atrophy or abnormal rotation and flexion. Palpate the anterior superior iliac spine (ASIS), greater trochanter, and surrounding musculature. Measure leg lengths by extending a tape measure from the ASIS to the ipsilateral medial malleolus of the ankle. Evaluate and compare range of motion of both hips and record degrees of flexion, extension, internal and external rotation, abduction, and adduction. Women often have increased femoral anteversion and, therefore, greater internal rotation as compared to men. The Thomas Test allows for evaluation of a hip flexion contracture which may lead to either limb length inequality or decreased range of motion. The Thomas test is performed with the patient supine. The examiner brings both knees to the patient's chest to reduce lumbar lordosis and then passively extends one leg while the patient clutches the other to the chest. A hip flexion contracture is demonstrated by an inability to passively extend one leg to lie flat on the table, and can be calculated by measuring the angle formed by the examining table and leg. The Patrick Test produces pain and is very specific for pain originating in the hip joint. To perform the Patrick Test, have the patient lie supine and flex, abduct, and externally rotate the involved hip so that the foot lies on the opposite knee. Pain in this position is indicative of hip joint pathology. Anesthetic injection of the hip joint often helps to differentiate mechanical pain of hip pathology from the referred pain of lumbosacral disease, but is a procedure performed, often under fluoroscopic guidance, by the orthopaedist. In traumatic situations, simple rotation or gentle axial compression of the hip, followed by radiographic examination, will most likely demonstrate the etiology of the pain that is the hip fracture.

RADIOGRAPHY

Pain and symptoms localizing to the hip warrant at least plain x-rays. Most often an anteroposterior (AP) pelvis and tube lateral view of the hip are adequate. However, an AP view centered on the hip may show more detail, especially in cases of nondisplaced hip fractures. Arthrography is helpful in cases of possible septic arthritis or infected prosthetic hip replacement. Magnetic resonance imaging (MRI) and computed tomography (CT) scans have limited roles and are used almost exclusively in cases of fractures not evident on plain films, complex fractures of the acetabulum, early avascular necrosis, tumors, and loose bodies.

ETIOLOGY

Traumatic disorders of the hip represent one of the most common causes of hip pain. While hip fractures are three times more common in elderly women, hip fractures in young and middle-aged women are usually secondary to high energy trauma (eg, motor vehicle accident). In addition to high-energy trauma, young, active women may suffer a stress fracture of the femoral neck from repetitive activity.

In women over the age of 65 the increased incidence of fractures about the hip is due to osteoporosis; black women, however, have a much lower rate of hip fractures. Fractures about the hip include: femoral head and neck fractures, intertrochanteric fractures, subtrochanteric fractures, acetabular fractures, and pubic rami fractures. While most require operative stabilization, the latter two may often be treated nonoperatively.

While there are many nontraumatic causes of hip pain in women, the most common include: osteoarthritis, inflammatory arthropathies (eg, rheumatoid arthritis, ankylosing spondylitis), seronegative spondyloarthropathies (eg, psoriatic arthritis, Reiter syndrome, crystal-induced arthritides), connective tissue disorders (eg, systemic lupus erythematosus, and scleroderma), and avascular necrosis of the femoral head. In general, osteoarthritis is a mild inflammatory disorder of cartilage while rheumatoid arthritis is a systemic inflammatory disorder of synovium and seronegative spondyloarthropathies, characterized by inflammation at tendon insertions and large joint destruction.

Osteoarthritis of the hip may result from congenital, traumatic, or metabolic disorders. Symptoms include dull, aching pain, often localized to the groin or buttocks, with radiation to the knee or lumbar spine. Weight-bearing aggravates the pain while rest occasionally relieves it. Signs include an antalgic or painful gait, limp, loss of motion, muscle atrophy, and spasm. X-rays show joint space narrowing (especially superolaterally), subchondral sclerosis and cyst formation, and osteophytes.

Hip pain secondary to rheumatoid arthritis presents with morning stiffness, which improves with exercise, and associated joint involvement (eg, hands). X-rays usually show concentric joint narrowing, osteopenia, subchondral cysts, and protrusio acetabuli in advanced cases. Interestingly, other causes of hip pain in the rheumatoid include trochanteric bursitis, contractures, lipid nodules, and synovial cysts.

In patients with seronegative arthropathies, hip pain is often bilateral and an AP pelvis x-ray may demonstrate sacroiliac joint sclerosis, concentric joint space narrowing, subchondral sclerosis, and erosions. Also, periostitis or cortical reaction at entheses (tendon insertion into bone) is a hallmark. Pregnant women with rheumatoid arthritis often enjoy decreased symptoms during pregnancy while those with seronegative spondyloarthropathies suffer an exacerbation of symptoms.

Of the crystal-induced arthritides, pseudogout exceeds gout in terms of hip involvement. Hip pain associated with pseudogout is usually chronic in nature and x-rays show abnormal calcifications (see Chap. 95). Gouty attacks of the hip joint are rare, but x-rays may show sclerosis and small erosions.

In connective tissue disorders, hip pain often arises from avascular necrosis secondary to high-dose corticosteroids.

Avascular necrosis (AVN) of the femoral head is another common cause of hip pain in women. Avascular necrosis includes a predictable cascade of events from pain and microscopic cell death to sclerosis and collapse of the femoral head. Etiologies include post-traumatic causes, excessive steroid administration, alcohol intake, sickle cell disease, Caisson disease, smoking, pregnancy, and idiopathic causes. Symptoms mimic those of osteoarthritis, but plain x-rays may be normal. MRI is extremely helpful in diagnosing AVN in the early stages when treatment such as hip aspiration, core decompression, or vascularized fibular graft may halt the cascade of events leading to advanced degenerative disease. Pregnant women have increased risk of AVN of the femoral head. While the exact etiology is unknown, theories point to the third trimester increase in cortisol to greater than three times normal. Symptoms in the third trimester include deep groin pain with radiation to the knee or back. Often the disorder is misdiagnosed, attributing the pain to pelvic instability.

Other causes of hip pain in women include infection, and bone and soft-tissue tumors. A septic hip usually results from the hematogenous spread from another source, especially in women who are immunosuppressed, suffer from chronic diseases, or have a concomitant infection. Symptoms are usually limited to one hip and are associated with fever, chills, or both, and other constitutional symptoms. Importantly, elderly women often present with more nonspecific complaints. On physical exam the leg is held flexed, abducted, and slightly externally rotated to decrease the pressure within the hip capsule. Motion is markedly limited. Laboratory values often show leukocytosis with a left shift and an elevated sedimentation rate. X-rays, in the early stages, may show capsular distention but usually are unremarkable. Capsular distention can be evaluated radiographically on an AP view of the pelvis or hip by measuring the distance from the medial side of the femoral head to the "teardrop" of the pelvis and comparing this value to the opposite side. Late findings include bony changes, such as subchondral sclerosis and joint space narrowing, and erosions or cysts. Diagnosis requires joint aspiration, and treatment involves arthrotomy and thorough irrigation and debridement.

Neoplasms around the hip include metastasis (especially from lung, breast, and kidney), primary bone tumors, and soft-tissue tumors. The hallmark of night pain often points toward an underlying neoplastic process. Hip pain that prompts radiographic evaluation, which demonstrates either a bony lesion or soft-tissue mass, should also prompt referral to an orthopaedist and an organized, thorough work-up.

Finally, hip pain in women can be attributed to one of the most common metabolic disorders—osteoporosis. Osteoporosis refers to decreased bone mass and is divided into two types. Type I, or postmenopausal, is secondary to decreased estrogen production and increased bone resorption. Type II, or age-related, is due to decreased bone formation. More than one half of women over the age of 50 have radiographically detectable osteoporosis. Osteoporosis is a major cause of morbidity and mortality in women over the age of 65 because of increased susceptibility to hip fracture.

CONSIDERATIONS IN PREGNANCY

Transient osteoporosis of the hip is a rare disorder seen in pregnant women. Like AVN of the femoral head during pregnancy, transient osteoporosis presents during the third trimester and is characterized by pain and decreased range of motion. The pain is worse with weight-bearing. X-rays show unilateral or bilateral osteopenia with a normal joint space. Accurate diagnosis is essential as continued weight-bearing can lead to fracture of the femoral neck and resultant disastrous consequences, for example AVN and degenerative joint disease. Treatment includes protective weight-bearing until symptoms resolve.

Widening of the symphysis pubis is another potentially painful condition during pregnancy. Hormonal changes, such as an increase in relaxin from the corpus luteum, lead to ligamentous laxity at the sacroiliac joints and pubic symphysis. Often radiographic examination during the first trimester will demonstrate widening of the pubic symphysis. This widening may gradually increase until term, but almost always resolves postpartum and rarely requires surgical intervention.

In conclusion, while the cause of hip pain in women includes a multitude of etiologies, a correct diagnosis usually results from a complete history and physical, in conjunction with specific lab tests and x-rays.

BIBLIOGRAPHY

Heckman JD, Sassard R. Musculoskeletal considerations in pregnancy. J Bone Joint Surg 1994;76A:1723.

Steinberg ME, ed. The hip and its disorders. Philadelphia: WB Saunders, 1991:56, 75, 502, 527, 589, 623, 648.

Primary Care for Women, edited by Phyllis C. Leppert and Fred M. Howard. Lippincott-Raven Publishers, Philadelphia © 1997.

102
Knee Pain

ROBERT CARRIER

The remarkable thing about knees is that they function as well as they do. There is no bony stability, as there is in the hip or elbow. Knee stability depends entirely on the soft tissues around the knee, so that integrity of these supporting structures is essential for good knee function. Hence, a basic knowledge of knee anatomy is essential for understanding the pathophysiology of knee function.

LIGAMENTS

The knee is a simple hinge joint allowing a range of motion in flexion and extension only. Stability is provided by the muscular and ligamentous units crossing the knee joint.

In simple terms, mediolateral stability is provided by the medial and lateral collateral ligaments. The medial collateral ligament arises from the medial femoral condyle and has a deep portion that is strong and bridges the tibia and femur close to the knee joint. The superficial medial collateral ligament fans out distally to attach 4 to 5 cm below the tibial joint line, so it is significant if tenderness is felt in this area after a knee injury. The lateral collateral ligament, which arises from a small area on the lateral femoral condyle, is a round, discrete, and palpable ligament attaching to the fibular head. The capsular attachments to the femur and tibia augment these ligaments. A thickening in the posteromedial portion is called the posterior oblique ligament and in the posterolateral portion is called the arcuate complex.

Anteroposterior stability is the primary responsibility of the cruciate ligaments. The anterior cruciate ligament arises from the anteromedial portion of the tibia and rotates posterolateral to insert on the posterior aspect of the lateral femoral condyle. The posterior cruciate ligament crosses the anterior cruciate ligament posteriorly, arising from the back of the tibial plateau and inserting on the medial femoral condyle. The anterior cruciate ligament stabilizes the tibia from anterior excursion; the posterior cruciate ligament stabilizes the tibia from posterior displacement.

The musculotendinous units crossing the knee are also critical to knee function. Anteriorly, the quadriceps muscle (a cluster of four muscles: rectus femoris, vastus medialis, lateralis, and intermedius) provides knee extension as it passes into the quadriceps tendon at the superior pole of the patella and the patellar ligament from the distal pole of the patella to the tibial tubercle. The aponeurotic expansion of the quadriceps mechanism fans out across the front of the knee to attach to the tibial joint margins across the anterior half of the knee. Medially, the pes anserinus ("goose's foot"), consisting of the sartorius, gracilis, and semitendinosus, attaches to the medial tibial metaphysis about 3 to 4 cm below the joint line in front of the medial collateral ligament. Just proximal to the insertion of these muscles is the anserine bursa, which sometimes becomes inflamed. Posteriorly, the hamstring tendons provide knee flexion and limit knee extension. Medially, the semitendinosus attaches with the pes anserinus; the semitendinosus attaches to the back of the tibia. Laterally, the biceps femoris muscle attaches to the fibular head and the back of the tibia. The medial and lateral heads of the gastrocnemius muscle arise from the postfemoral condyles and also play a role in knee function.

ETIOLOGY

Traumatic knee pain can be either acute or chronic. Acute trauma refers to a specific injury that causes the symptoms; the injury usually occurs less than 2 weeks before the presentation for treatment. Chronic trauma refers to repetitive injuries to the knee or to symptoms produced by injuries that occurred longer than 2 weeks before presentation.

Arthritic pain may have many different etiologies, but degenerative arthritis is by far the most common. Infection is the source of arthritis that presents most acutely and requires the most urgent care. Systemic forms of arthritis, such as rheumatoid arthritis, or collagen vascular diseases are also fairly common. Gout and pseudogout, crystalline arthropathies, must also be considered.

Developmental knee pain can be due to malalignment of limbs from congenital or metabolic abnormalities of growth or prior trauma. Patellar malalignment, a major cause of knee pain in adolescents, can be related to a congenital malalignment of the quadriceps mechanism.

Neoplasia, both benign and malignant, must be considered in the diagnosis of knee pain.

Hip disease not uncommonly radiates to the knee and must be considered in knee pain that is not obviously caused by problems with the knee. Likewise, spinal abnormalities can produce radicular pain radiating into the knee; this must also be ruled out in puzzling knee pain.

HISTORY

The first question relates to trauma. With trauma, the problem of injury to the ligaments, meniscus, muscle-tendon units, and neurovascular structures arises. Without trauma, all the other causes of knee pain can be present. How acute was the onset of pain? Are other joints involved? Are there systemic symptoms of illness? Is there a history of prior joint involvement? Is there a family history of joint pain? Is the pain constant or episodic?

PHYSICAL EXAMINATION AND CLINICAL FINDINGS

The knee examination after fracture involves primarily the affected knee, but in the absence of trauma the examination must also include, at a minimum, the other knee and adjacent joints. If the diagnosis is uncertain, a general physical examination is necessary. Both lower extremities must be bare so that the clinician can compare the affected leg with the other extremity and can evaluate the effect of the knee pain on the muscles, nerves, vascular supply, and other joints of the limb. A sturdy table is needed so that the patient can be completely flat and relaxed; the examiner must be able to move on both sides to evaluate each limb separately. More diagnostic mistakes are made by not following these simple precepts—in other words, by not looking—than any other cause.

In acute trauma, an x-ray of the involved part must be taken after initial evaluation of the circulation, sensation, and motion of the limb to evaluate possible fracture. Fracture examination and management is outside the scope of this chapter (see Chap. 103). If knee pain is due to an acute fracture, the knee should be immobilized with splints. Careful assessment of the skin and the motor, sensory, and circulatory function of the part distal should be made and recorded for future reference.

The specific examination of the knee first involves asking the patient to do what she can voluntarily. This allows evaluation of the acute function of the knee and the degree of pain involved. Then a gentle examination can be performed. Can the patient do an active straight leg raise? If not, there may be an injury to the quadriceps mechanism. Can she flex the knee voluntarily? The range of active motion is recorded for future reference, and the appearance of the knee and entire lower extremity is compared to the opposite side. Is there muscle wasting? In which muscles? Is the part visibly swollen or hot? What is the appearance of the foot and ankle? What is the vascular supply? Are the feet involved in the source of knee pain?

Next, the knee is felt and the amount of swelling and the temperature of the part are assessed. An intraarticular effusion bulges well above the patella; simple prepatellar bursitis, which is extraarticular, swells anterior to the patella. This is crucial in evaluating infections about the knee, as an intraarticular effusion is much more serious than prepatellar bursitis. Cultures are important, but a needle should never be inserted through an area of cellulitis into the knee above the patella. Aspiration of a prepatellar bursa, with the patella between the needle and the knee joint, is of low risk for contaminating the knee.

Examination of the ligaments is important, particularly after trauma. Stress of the collateral ligaments is done with the knee at 0° extension and with the knee flexed at 30°. Points of tenderness about the knee are helpful in determining the site of the ligamentous tear. The superficial part of the medial collateral ligament attaches 4 to 5 cm distal to the medal joint line.

The anterior cruciate ligament is injured more often in female athletes than in males in the same sport. It is best evaluated with the Lachman sign, in which anterior displacement of the tibia on the femur is measured with the knee flexed at 30° and compared with the other knee. Normal knee laxity varies from person to person. The "drawer sign" is elicited with the foot stabilized on the table and the knee flexed 90°. Anterior displacement of the tibia on the femur is measured. This is not as reliable as the Lachman sign in evaluating knee instability. Another reliable sign of anterior cruciate ligament insufficiency is the lateral pivot shift: valgus stress is applied across the knee with the foot interiorly rotated, the knee is moved from 90° to 0° slowly, and a shift of the tibia slipping forward on the femur is felt. Posterior cruciate instability is best assessed with the knee bent 90° and the foot either on the examination table or held by the examiner with the hip flexed 90°. Posterior sag of the tibia on the femur is observed compared with the other side.

Examination of the hip, ankle, and foot on both sides is important. The range of motion is recorded and compared. Any pain with

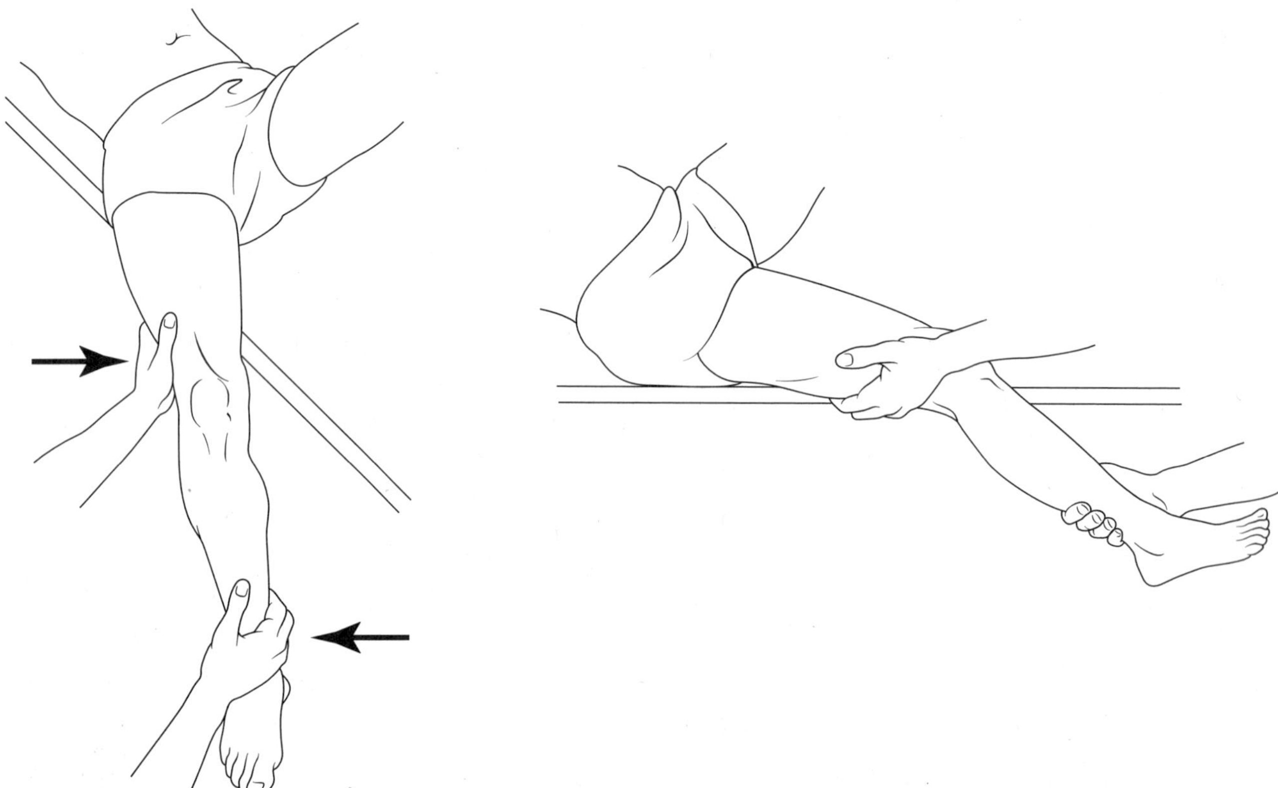

Figure 102-1. Abduction stress test (see text). (From AH Crenshaw. Campbell's Operative Orthopedics. 7th ed., Vol. 3. St. Louis, Mosby. 1987, p. 1537. Redrawn from Hughston JC, Andrews JR, Cross MJ, Moschi A. J Bone Joint Surg 58-A:159, 1976.)

motion of other joints is noted. Pain in and about the hip joint can cause radiating pain into the knee, which may be the presenting source of pain. Internal rotation of the hips should always be done, as this maneuver almost always causes pain if the source of the problem is intraarticular hip pain.

The neurologic examination is often helpful because the quadriceps muscle is innervated by the three myotomes L2, L3, and L4; sensation over the front of the knee is from L2 and L3. Pain can radiate to the knee from the hip. Reflex testing and a sensory examination can be added to the previously examined muscle function.

LABORATORY AND IMAGING STUDIES

Routine knee x-rays are almost always done first. Magnetic resonance imaging and computed tomography are seldom needed, and it is a waste of resources to order them initially. Magnetic resonance imaging is the standard for evaluating ligaments or menisci in the knee, but a routine history, physical examination, and x-rays usually are all that is necessary on an initial examination. Arthrography is seldom used anymore.

Laboratory studies also should start with the simple and proceed to the complex. A knee aspiration in cases with an effusion is helpful. The sample is checked for appearance and sent for culture and sensitivities, cell count, differential, an examination for gouty crystals (urate) and pseudogout (calcium pyrophosphate) crystals, and glucose determination. A Gram stain is added in cases of suspected infection.

A complete blood count and sedimentation rate are done next. The sedimentation rate, although nonspecific, is helpful when normal, as it suggests that there is no systemic illness associated with the knee pain.

Routine laboratory tests are helpful for screening for possible systemic disease and hyperuricemia. Urinalysis is done for the same reasons. Studies of rheumatoid factor, an antinuclear factor LE preparation, can be added as indicated.

TREATMENT

Treatment, of course, depends on the diagnosis. There are four conditions that are urgent and require prompt treatment. With vascular insufficiency due to a knee problem, a dislocated knee comes most readily to mind and almost always requires an arteriogram. With a worsening neurologic deficit distal to the knee, the first step in alleviating neurovascular insufficiency is to reduce the fracture or dislocation. This often goes a long way to relieving the problem and can often be done promptly in the emergency department. Patients with open fractures or lacerations into the joint should be taken to the operating room within 6 hours of injury for cleaning and debridement. In septic arthritis, the enzymes from some organisms can destroy articular cartilage within 12 to 24 hours. Thus, this requires prompt drainage and antibiotic administration.

CONSIDERATIONS IN PREGNANCY

The increased weight of pregnancy tends to aggravate preexisting conditions. Patellar malalignment problems causing anterior knee pain about the patella are common in young women. Hence, if a pregnant patient has any history of prior knee pain of this nature, she should avoid squatting, kneeling, or excessive stair-climbing while carrying extra weight.

BIBLIOGRAPHY

Beck JL, Wildermuth BP. The female athlete's knee. Clin Sports Med 1985;4:345.

Estok PJ, Rudy EB. Marathon running: comparison of physician and psychosocial risks for men and women. Research in Nursing & Health 1987;10:79.

Gray J, Taunton JE, McKenzie DC, et al. A survey of injuries to the anterior cruciate ligament of the knee in female basketball players. Int J Sports Med 1985;6:314.

Hutchinson RM, Ireland ML. Knee injuries in female athletes. Sports Med 1995;19:288.

Knapik JJ, Bauman CL, Jones BH, et al. Preseason strength and flexibility imbalances associated with athletic injuries in female collegiate athletes. Am J Sports Med 1991;19:76.

Sailors ME, Keskula DR, Perrin DH. Effect of running on anterior knee laxity in collegiate-level female athletes after anterior cruciate ligament reconstruction. J Orthop Sports Phys Therapy 1995;21:233.

Sakai H, Tanaka S, Kurosawa H, Masujima A. The effect of exercise on anterior knee laxity in female basketball players. Int J Sports Med 1992;13:552.

Primary Care for Women, edited by Phyllis C. Leppert and Fred M. Howard. Lippincott-Raven Publishers, Philadelphia © 1997.

103

Principles of Fracture Diagnosis and Care

RICHARD A. LEWIS

The primary care physician is often the first line of defense for patients with acute fractures. Many fractures require minimal care and do well while the practitioner watches the healing process. However, fracture care is also fraught with pitfalls: the unwary physician can be trapped in a situation that compromises the result and creates permanent deformity or dysfunction. Liberal use of orthopedic consultation is recommended, and it should be done early rather than late, when the course of treatment may be irreversible.

The injury should be viewed as part of a whole, not just as a limb with a broken bone. It is common to see a patient with a devastating ligamentous injury leave the emergency department with only an elastic bandage and a report that there are no fractures. The same is true in the ankle: a patient with a grade 3 ligamentous injury that should be treated in a cast is told she has a sprain and should use crutches until it feels better. Awareness of the soft tissues means thoroughly assessing the neurovascular status of the limb as close to the time of injury as possible and repeating the evaluation at every follow-up visit, especially if a circumferential dressing is part of the treatment.

Heat should never be part of the treatment of an acute fracture. Cold and elevation are safe and reduce pain and the need for analgesics.

The primary care practitioner must also avoid considering a fracture affecting a small bone to be a small problem. A small "chip" fracture in the hand, if treated in the wrong position of immobilization, may require late surgery that might have been avoided by early correct treatment. A boutonnière deformity of a finger, a notorious deformity to correct late, might not have occurred with extension splinting. Splinting a metacarpophalangeal joint in extension may lead to the development of a contracture that interferes with normal daily function. However, learning some simple principles of fracture care allows the primary care physician to manage many of these simple fractures with excellent outcomes.

ETIOLOGY AND DIFFERENTIAL DIAGNOSIS

The etiology of most fractures is trauma in the form of outside energy. The bone and surrounding tissues receive an input of kinetic energy, which is then dissipated in the bone and surrounding soft tissue. The magnitude, duration, direction, and rate of loading affect the bone and determine if it will fracture. The fracture and soft-tissue injury are the result of energy release in the tissues. Sometimes, the injury results when an object strikes the tissue; at other times, the injury results when the kinetic energy of the body in motion strikes an object, as in a fall.

The severity of the injury is related to the amount of energy. Energy is the capacity to do work (work = force × distance). Force is a push or a pull that when applied to a free body tends to accelerate or deform (force = mass × acceleration). A high-velocity rifle can do a lot more damage to bone and soft tissue than a .22-caliber handgun: a larger bullet and a faster muzzle velocity create more force. One is much less likely to survive a head-on encounter with an 18-wheeled truck (more mass) than with a motorcycle. In a fall, the height of the fall alters the velocity of the impact and thus the severity of the energy discharge.

The same mechanism of injury and the same amount of energy dissipated in the tissues produce different injuries in persons of different ages because of the relative strength and elasticity of the tissues at different ages. Much more energy is required to produce the same bone displacement in a Colles wrist fracture in a 20-year-old man than in a 70-year-old woman. Thus, more energy is dissipated into the surrounding soft tissues, causing more damage and tissue destruction in the 20-year-old. As another example, a knee is struck on the lateral aspect, forcing it into valgus. In a youngster with an open growth plate, a fracture may occur through the growth plate. In a woman in her 20s, the medial collateral ligament may tear. In a woman in the sixth decade of life, the bone is weaker than the ligaments, and a lateral tibial plateau fracture is probable. Understanding the role kinetic energy plays, coupled with the weakening of the skeleton with aging, explains why older women have such a high incidence of wrist and shoulder fractures from mild falls.

Stress fractures and pathologic fractures have no antecedent history of acute kinetic loading. In stress fractures, kinetic loading occurs over a period of time in a pattern greater than what the patient is accustomed to. In pathologic fractures, the weakened state of the abnormal bone allows fracture to occur within the range of physiologic kinetic loading.

Healthy bone can support loads because its design allows it to support compressive loads and shear and tension stresses. When bone fails, a fracture occurs. Compression fractures occur when the bone fails in compressive loading. Avulsion fractures are a form of failure in tension loading. Fractures with shear loading create simple or complex fracture patterns, depending on the speed and direction of loading.

HISTORY

The history of an injury is essential for understanding the forces exerted on the tissues. It helps the physician understand the direction of bone displacement and determine which side of the bone might have torn periosteum and which side is intact. This information is essential in selecting the position of immobilization that will provide the most stability. For example, in a simple Colles fracture, where the history of the fall is an impact on the outstretched palm,

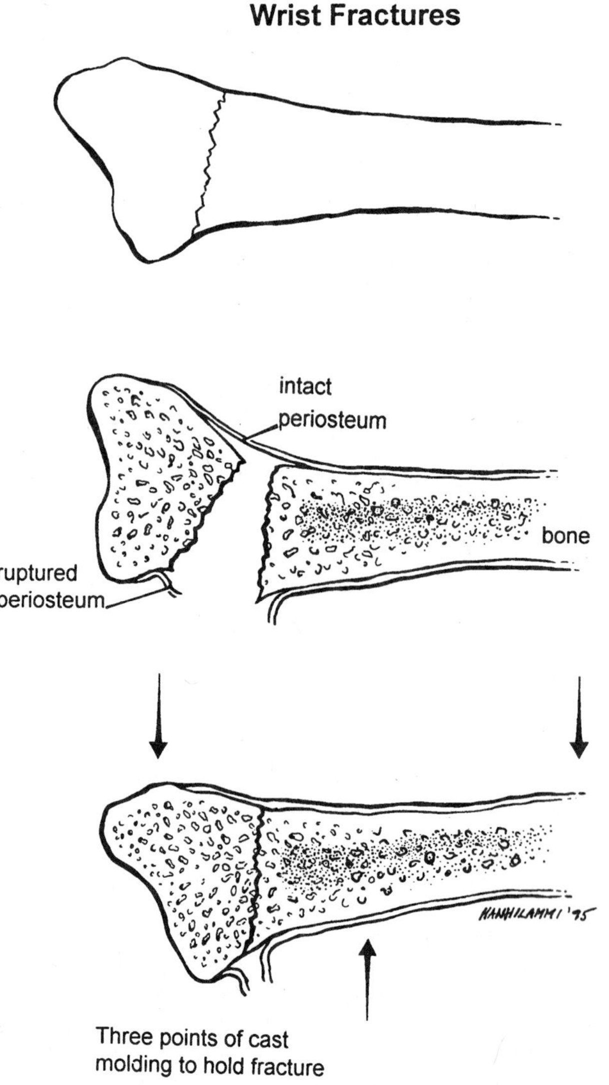

Figure 103-1. Anatomy of a simple fracture and how a cast holds it stable.

the distal fracture fragment tends to displace dorsally, with tearing of the volar periosteum. The best position for immobilization is opposite to the direction of displacement, so in this case reduction in flexion provides the most stability by using the intact hinge of periosteum dorsally to stabilize the fracture fragments (Fig. 103-1). The history, the physical examination, and x-rays often provide the information needed to understand the character of the fracture.

A complete history is also essential for medicolegal reasons. The history should not say merely that the patient fell on her outstretched wrist: it should include much more detail. The physician should try to get a complete history of how the fall occurred, using the patient's words. If the events are unclear, such a statement should be included in the documentation.

The physician should also consider whether the energy of the injury explains the findings. For instance, if a trivial amount of trauma causes an arm to break, a pathologic process may have weakened the bone.

PHYSICAL EXAMINATION AND CLINICAL FINDINGS

The injured part should be evaluated before ordering x-rays. A neurovascular examination, as complete as possible, must be done. In a cooperative patient, the physician can start by doing a sensory examination of the limb distal to the injury. The sensory distribution of all of the major nerves must be evaluated and any deficiencies recorded. Light touch or pin prick is the most useful test. Any deficiencies in sensation must be noted before the patient goes to the x-ray department for an hour and before the fracture is reduced, in case changes are ongoing.

The motor examination may be difficult due to pain, but intact motor function and nerve supply can be verified. In the upper extremity, median, ulnar, and radial nerve function is easily verified. This is quickly done by asking the patient to make a circle with the index and thumb (median nerve), to separate the fingers (ulnar nerve), and to extend the index finger (radial nerve). In the lower extremity, peroneal and posterior tibial nerve function is also easily verified. Resisted extension of the great toe confirms peroneal function, and flexion confirms posterior tibial nerve function. These tests can be done even in the presence of a shattered tibia. Knowing the status of nerves early is essential to diagnosing compartment syndrome in evolution.

This is a good time to check for compartment syndrome as well. Pain on passive stretch of the deep compartment muscles is the first sign of compartment syndrome. Extreme pain with passive extension of the index finger is an early warning sign if there is forearm swelling. In the lower extremity, pain on passive plantar-flexion of the great toe, with a tense swollen anterior leg compartment, is a red flag for compartment syndrome. An immediate consultation is required.

After completing the preliminary neurosensory examination, the physician should carefully palpate the injured part, evaluating the areas of maximal swelling and ecchymosis and paying close attention to the skin status.

A superficial abrasion or laceration must be distinguished from skin penetration that communicates with the fracture site. In a com-

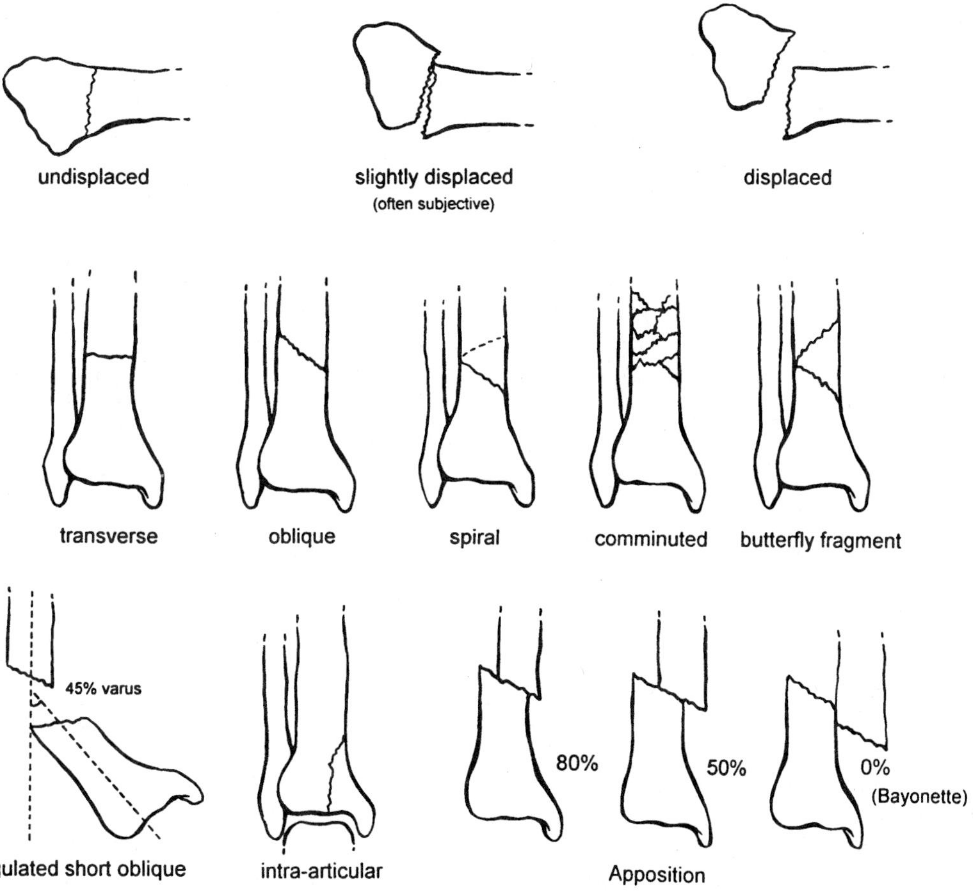

Figure 103-2. Vocabulary of fracture terms.

pound (open) fracture, the fracture communicates with the outside environment through a break in the skin. Often a grade 1 puncture exists where a sharp fragment of bone has punctured the skin from inside out. No matter how small the opening, there is the potential for bacterial contamination. These wounds often have a characteristic appearance, with bloody, fat-filled drainage due to their communication with the marrow cavity. Open fractures should be referred to the orthopedist. It is helpful to culture these wounds and provide tetanus prophylaxis. A distal phalanx fracture with bleeding around the nail bed is probably also a compound fracture.

Pain and tenderness are always present in neurologically intact patients. The physician should palpate and identify the points of maximal tenderness. Bony crepitus, the sound and feel of broken bone edges rubbing together, can sometimes be felt. Often deformity is noted and fracture bleeding leads to swelling.

After this examination, appropriate x-rays should be ordered. The best way to get better at ordering x-rays and diagnosing the appearance of the fracture is to try to guess what the x-ray will show based on the examination. Before the days of radiography, physicians treated fractures correctly by feel and familiarity with a fracture type. The Colles fracture was described well before the first roentgen ray passed through bone.

LABORATORY AND IMAGING STUDIES

The injured patient sent for imaging studies must be well protected in a temporary supportive splint that immobilizes the injured part. This provides comfort and protection for the soft-tissue structures as the patient is positioned for x-rays.

Communication can be a problem when ordering and interpreting x-rays. Proper use of the following terms can help guarantee effective communication with radiologists and orthopedists (Figs. 103-2 and 103-3):

- *Diaphysis:* the shaft of a long bone; made up primarily of compact cortical bone
- *Metaphysis:* the portion of a long bone that widens at both ends; made up of a high percentage of spongy trabecular bone
- *Epiphysis:* the ends of a long bone, from which growth occurs
- *Torus* or *greenstick fractures:* fractures in which one cortex breaks and the opposite bends (like a "green stick"). These occur in children, whose bones have higher elasticity.
- *Undisplaced:* a visible crack in the bone with no displacement of the component parts
- *Slightly displaced:* Because this means different things to different people, it is better to say "displaced" and quantify it by measurement in millimeters.
- *Displaced:* The component parts of the fracture are displaced. Measurement in distance or angular displacement should be given.
- *Transverse:* The fracture crosses the bone perpendicular to its long axis.
- *Oblique:* The fracture line crosses the bone at an angle. This can be modified to short or long oblique.
- *Spiral:* The fracture line winds around the long axis of the bone.
- *Extraarticular:* The fracture line does not enter a joint.
- *Intraarticular:* The fracture line enters a joint.
- *Comminuted:* There are multiple fragments and fracture lines.
- *Butterfly fragment:* A large third fragment is separate from the proximal and distal fragments. It is more or less triangular on the x-ray.

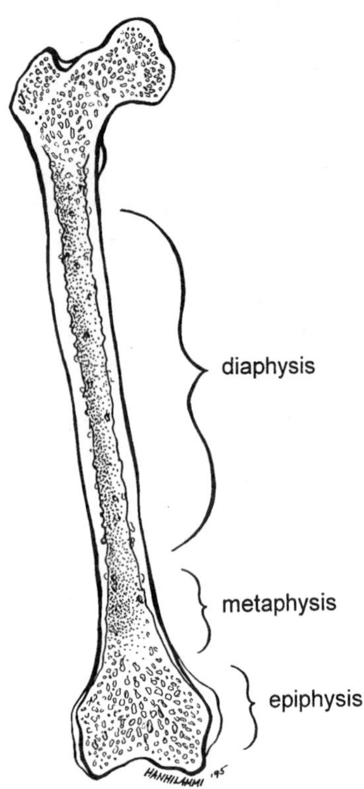

Figure 103-3. Parts of a "typical" bone.

- *Segmental fracture:* There are two distinct areas of fracture in one bone, creating three major fragments.
- *Apposition:* percentage of the cross section of the shaft of the bone in contact
- *Angulated:* A line through the proximal fragment of a long bone is displaced from a line through the distal fragment.
- *Varus angulation:* apex away from the midline
- *Valgus angulation:* apex toward the midline.

It is important to describe the appearance in two planes because they often differ. An anteroposterior view of a short oblique tibia may appear to have 90% apposition and 5° of varus, but on the lateral view there is 10% apposition and 40° of angulation apex anterior.

TREATMENT

Once the initial evaluation of the limb is completed, the patient should be made as comfortable as possible while restoring alignment and protecting the fracture to maintain it safely (usually a splint or cast). The fracture pain is due to swelling and motion, neither of which can be eliminated. However, a well-applied cast helps reduce swelling and pain by means of circumferential pressure. With molding by three-point fixation, it helps reduce fracture motion. Many patients with fractures feel motion of the bone ends for several weeks, even in a well-fitting cast.

Many fractures have several equally correct means of management. A transverse tibial fracture can be treated in a long-leg cast, a short-leg cast, or a plastic orthosis. Different types of surgical intermedullary rodding may be equally correct. The correct treatment depends on the patient's age and occupation, bone quality, other injuries, and other medical problems. It also depends on the physician's experience and comfort with various treatment techniques. Treatment must be individualized, as each fracture has a unique personality.

CONSIDERATIONS IN PREGNANCY

Fractures heal at the same rate in pregnant women as they do in nonpregnant ones. However, fracture healing may be impaired by deficiencies of vitamin D or calcium.

Fractures that are best treated operatively in the nonpregnant patient should be treated the same way in the pregnant patient. Treatment with prolonged bed rest and immobilization can have complications. The goal of early mobilization often realized by early surgical treatment can be valuable in the pregnant patient. Anesthesia can be delivered effectively for both mother and fetus with minimal disturbance of physiology.

Motor vehicle accidents are the leading cause of death of pregnant women. Seatbelts should be fastened properly low across the anterior superior iliac spines to protect the mother and fetus.

BIBLIOGRAPHY

Chapman MW. Operative orthopaedics. Philadelphia: JB Lippincott, 1988.

Charnley J. The closed treatment of common fractures. In: Green DP, ed. Operative hand surgery, 3d ed. New York: Churchill-Livingstone, 1993.

Fildes J, Reed L, Jones N, Martin M, Barrett J. Trauma: the leading cause of maternal death. J Trauma 1992;32:643.

Heckman JD. Managing musculoskeletal problems in pregnant patients. J Musculoskel Med 1984;1(7):35.

Heckman JD, Sassard R. Musculoskeletal considerations in pregnancy. J Bone Jt Surg [Am] 1994;76:1720.

Rockwood CA, Green DP, Heckman JD, Bucholz RW, eds. Rockwood & Green's fractures in adults, 4th ed. Philadelphia: Lippincott-Raven, 1996.

Wolf ME, Alexander BH, Rivara FP, Hickok DE, Maier RV, Starzyk PM. A retrospective cohort study of seatbelt use and pregnancy outcome after a motor vehicle crash. J Trauma 1993;34:116.

Primary Care for Women, edited by Phyllis C. Leppert and Fred M. Howard. Lippincott-Raven Publishers, Philadelphia © 1997.

104
Injuries of the Wrist and Hand

RICHARD A. LEWIS

The hand and wrist facilitate most of our interaction with the world. They are unique in their ability to feel and manipulate the environment and are also subject to varied injuries. A brief review of common hand and wrist injuries will provide the primary care practitioner with an understanding and a basis for approaching the care of these common maladies.

FINGERTIP INJURY

Fingertip injuries come in great variety, and most of us know from experience how painful a blow to the distal finger is. These tactile surfaces have an extraordinary high density of pain, touch, and pressure receptors, so anything that causes bleeding and swelling in the pulp space of the finger is acutely painful. Many blunt traumatic injuries to the pulp space cause subungual bleeding. This subungual blood under pressure causes severe pain, and decompression relieves it. However, if there is an underlying closed fracture of the distal phalanx, decompressing a subungual hematoma must be done in a sterile manner. Some emergency departments use a small sterile hand drill to place a small hole at the base of the nail, allowing the hematoma to drain. A sterile dressing is then applied. A paper clip heated to red-hot can be gently held against the nail; it quickly melts through the nail, making a small hole for drainage. The trick in either case is not to press too hard, because the pressure hurts. If one goes through too fast, the underlying tissue is sensitive. Very light pressure does the job with no need for anesthesia. However, the pulp cannot be drained by this method, as it is divided into compartments. Therefore, when dealing with an infection of the pulp space, the incision must cross all the septae to provide effective drainage.

TUFT FRACTURES

Fractures of the distal phalanx that involve the tuft and not the joint are usually easy to treat. A lightweight aluminum splint or cage that keeps pressure off the tip of the finger is all that is necessary. It can be taped on in a way that does not obstruct circulation to the digit. These heal to comfort in 3 or 4 weeks and do well with just protection. One of these fractures that is associated with a nail bed avulsion should probably be considered an open fracture. These require fastidious irrigation and sterile dressings and prophylactic antibiotics for a few days.

MALLET FINGER

The mallet or baseball finger is an avulsion of the distal extensor mechanism. Sometimes there is a characteristic "chip" fracture off the proximal dorsal aspect of the distal phalanx. This is known as a bony mallet finger. A mallet finger deformity can be of soft-tissue origin if the extensor insertion is avulsed without a bone fragment. This is known as a soft-tissue mallet finger. The treatment is to support the finger in extension until it heals. One needs only to extend the distal interphalangeal joint with a small dorsal splint. It should be worn continuously and should remain in place for 6 weeks. Severe hyperextension can cause a skin slough, but slight hyperextension is desirable. The skin must be checked periodically, and the patient must be taught to hold the tip in extension when changing or cleaning the splint. After 6 weeks, with a soft-tissue mallet finger, night splinting only for an additional 6 weeks is recommended. With a bone avulsion, the physician must carefully check the films to ensure that the fragment is not too large, especially as it relates to the joint surface. Very large dorsal chips that approach a third of the joint surface probably are better treated by pinning the fragment or temporarily pinning the joint. A large neglected fragment can allow the entire distal phalanx to sublux volarly.

FRACTURES OF THE MIDDLE AND PROXIMAL PHALANX

Fractures of the middle and proximal phalanx can be some of the simplest and some of the hardest to treat. Treatment requires an understanding of the anatomy of the flexor and extensor mechanism. Chip fractures from the dorsal proximal middle phalanx are injuries of the central insertion of the extensor mechanism. If left untreated, the lateral bands of the extensor mechanism sublux forward and a difficult boutonnière deformity ensues. This can be a bony or a soft-tissue injury. The physician should check for local tenderness over the middorsal proximal interphalangeal joint and just proximal to it and also should check for a chip fracture in the same spot. The boutonnière deformity of a flexed proximal interphalangeal joint and an extended distal interphalangeal joint is usually a late problem. Acutely, these avulsions, if small, are treated with the proximal interphalangeal joint in full extension.

A volar chip fracture is usually a result of hyperextension of the proximal interphalangeal joint and avulsion of a piece of bone by the volar plate. If small, it can be treated in about 30° of flexion with a small splint, switching to buddy tapping for a few weeks after that. Large volar fragments can make the joint unstable in extension. Large ones must be referred for open reduction or extension block splinting, a technique best handled by a specialist.

In all these injuries, the patient must be advised that some fusiform swelling will persist for a long time and might even be permanent.

Condylar fractures of both the proximal and middle phalanx must be carefully evaluated radiologically for any rotation. If these intraarticular fractures show any displacement, a consultation should be requested. If it is undisplaced and treated with an immobilizing splint, it should be monitored carefully at 5 to 7 days and again at 8 to 14 days to ensure it did not go on to displace. Displacement causes joint malfunction, rotation, and deformity. Most of these cases must be pinned surgically.

Shaft fractures of the phalanges must be in good alignment, with special attention to rotary alignment. X-rays do not give much information about axial rotation. The way to check rotary alignment is to look at the hand. As you flex your own fingers, they overlap a bit, and they all tend to point to the tuberosity of the navicular at the wrist. If the patient's injured finger points differently, it is malaligned in rotation and must be reduced (Fig. 104-1). The nail beds offer another clue about malrotation: if the injured digit's nail bed looks tilted when viewed on end, it is malaligned.

The proximal phalanx has a great deal of tight anatomy adjacent to it. It is easy for this apparatus to get stuck to the healing fracture, so early range of motion is essential. The finger should never be immobilized longer than necessary, as it becomes harder to regain motion as structures become adherent.

In summary, with finger fractures the physician should be familiar with the anatomy; should follow the injury closely, watching for displacement or angulation; and should mobilize as early as possible.

DISLOCATIONS OF THE PROXIMAL AND DISTAL INTERPHALANGEAL JOINTS

Dislocations of the proximal and distal interphalangeal joints are usually easy to reduce. The trick is not to pull too hard or too quickly. The deformity must be increased only slightly to slip it gently back in place. The common dorsal dislocation has torn volar structures and needs hyperextension to slip it back in place. After it is reduced and an x-ray confirms the absence of fracture, it can be immobilized with a splint in mild flexion. It may be unstable if allowed to return to extension. Early motion is again important.

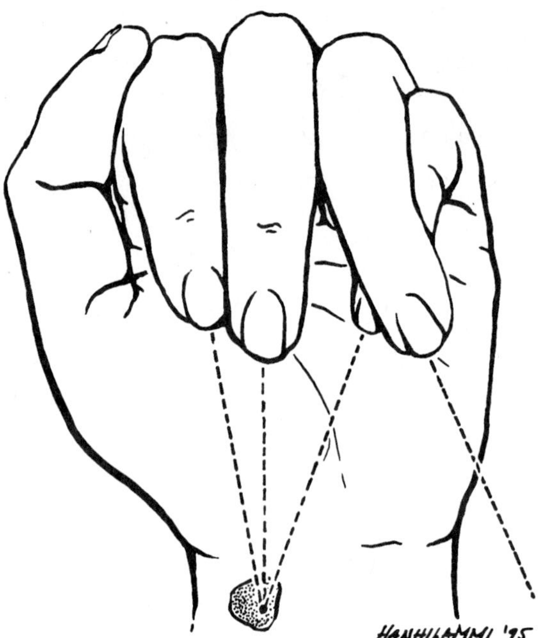

Figure 104-1. Rotary malunion, fourth ray.

DISLOCATIONS OF THE METACARPOPHALANGEAL JOINTS

Dislocations of the metacarpophalangeal joints, in contrast, are not always easy to reduce; the thumb in particular can be a problem. The problem is that the head of the metacarpal can get trapped by the flexor tendons in such a way that it locks like a button in a buttonhole. This can be recognized by a dimple in the skin over the palmar aspect of the metacarpal. The primary care physician who sees this should not even consider attempting the reduction but should seek help. This type usually cannot be done closed.

Some metacarpophalangeal joint dislocations are easy to reduce and to treat closed, if they do not get trapped by soft tissues. If reducible, they are usually stable and require only 3 to 4 weeks of immobilization to heal.

METACARPAL FRACTURES

Metacarpal fractures are among the most common hand injuries. The striking of an immovable object with a clenched fist is the usual mechanism of injury. This is also a typical injury after a fist fight, when the unwary aggressor strikes a part of the opponent's anatomy that is much harder than his or her own hand. The physician should look carefully for a small laceration over the hand and ask where the patient struck his or her opponent. In one minor fifth metacarpal fracture I saw, a small puncture wound over the metacarpal head was not initially appreciated. An x-ray confirmed a small radiodense foreign object in the tissues that turned out to be a tooth. An aggressive infection developed that resulted in the amputation of the fourth and fifth rays of the hand. Early treatment and recognition might have avoided this disaster.

Closed metacarpal fractures are easy to treat as long as the basic rules of fractures are respected. Alignment and correct rotary alignment must be achieved in the anteroposterior and lateral views (see Fig. 104-1). The ring and fifth fingers are much more forgiving on apex dorsal angulation than the index and long fingers. The reason for this is clear: on the normal hand, the fourth and fifth rays can easily be wiggled by grasping the metacarpal heads and moving them from dorsal to volar. The same maneuver on the index and long fingers illustrates the stability of their bases. Thus, if a metacarpal fracture heals with 30° of angulation on the fifth ray, the metacarpal merely moves dorsally when the patient grasps a broad-based tool such as the handle of a hammer. However, the same degree of angulation in a long finger metacarpal is perceived as a painful prominent lump in the palm that irritates the patient when a hammer is grasped. Therefore, the index and long fingers, with their stable bases, must be reduced more exactly than does a similar-looking fracture in the fourth or fifth ray.

The physician must also keep in mind the effects of shortening. A long oblique fracture may yield a successful result with good function. However, shortening of a metacarpal is seen when looking at the knuckles, or metaphalangeal joints, of the closed fist. It is nice to tell the patient about this before she reports it.

A fracture that enters the proximal or distal joint has a worse prognosis due to the joint injury and may develop posttraumatic arthritis. Fracture lines extending into the mobile carpometacarpal joints of the fourth and fifth fingers have a particularly poor prognosis. Fracture into these joints should always be looked for. Posttraumatic changes are difficult to treat because of the need to preserve mobility in this part of the hand to allow cupping of the palm.

CARPOMETACARPAL JOINT DISLOCATION

The key to making the diagnosis of carpometacarpal joint dislocation is to look carefully at the lateral x-ray and to make sure that the x-ray technician provides a true lateral view. If there is tenderness at the carpometacarpal level, the dorsal prominence of the metacarpal can sometimes be felt. The skin in this area quickly swells with fluid in the dorsal space, making it impossible to palpate. If the diagnosis of dislocation is made, it may be reducible, but it is often so unstable that a percutaneous pinning is necessary. This also must be done if the reduction is unstable or if, on close follow-up, it is noted to displace on the lateral x-ray.

THUMB METAPHALANGEAL JOINT

The importance of the thumb to hand function and the unique way it opposes the other digits create special considerations regarding injury to its function. The ulnar and radial collateral ligaments allow power grip and accurate key pinch. They are essential to power and delicate activity. A fall on the thumb, often from a ski injury, is the common mechanism of injury. The x-ray is negative in these collateral ligament injuries. However, an unrecognized complete rupture of the ulnar collateral ligament can create a painful unstable thumb. The avulsed collateral ligament can pull out of its normal placement and come to rest above the thumb extensor mechanism, where healing is impossible. A complete rupture of a collateral can be recognized by gentle manual testing in extension and in 30° of flexion. This is compared to the uninjured opposite side. If there is more than 30° difference between the sides, the patient should be referred for surgical evaluation and possible acute repair. If there is less instability, a well-fitting thumb spica cast is satisfactory treatment for 6 weeks. Late reconstruction of a collateral ligament is more difficult than early recognition and treatment. The ulnar ligament is a greater problem than the radial ligament because of how it is used in grasp and pinch grip.

THUMB METACARPAL FRACTURES

Thumb metacarpal fractures are straightforward until the joints are involved. The universal joint at the base of the thumb can compensate for fracture-induced malalignment in the metacarpal shaft. The physician should attempt to reduce angular deformity, but if it recurs and cannot be reduced, the thumb is most forgiving in tolerating healing with angulation.

Fractures near the base of the metacarpal require special consideration. A transverse proximal metacarpal fracture or a comminuted proximal metacarpal fracture must be differentiated from one that enters the joint. The fracture that enters the joint, a Bennett fracture (Fig. 104-2), is intrinsically unstable. The fracture line enters the joint in such a way that the pull of the abductor pollicis longus can separate the metacarpal shaft from the variable-sized volar lip fragment. It is really a fracture–dislocation of the thumb carpometacarpal joint. Accurate x-rays are mandatory. If a fracture line into the joint is visualized, this injury should be referred to a specialist. However, if the fracture lines do not enter the joint, the primary care physician can easily manage a closed extraarticular fracture without a specialist's involvement.

WRIST INJURY

With new knowledge of the anatomy and pathomechanics of wrist function, the "wrist sprain" has become a myriad of specific diagnoses related to soft-tissue injury in and about the wrist. Instability patterns have been described, explaining patterns of dynamic and static carpal position changes on the loss or attenuation of specific ligamentous structures. These are beyond the purview of primary care physicians (and in fact many general orthopedists); they need the attention of the hand subspecialist. Chronic wrist pain with x-rays showing any of the instability wrist pattern signs should be referred. One that can be easily recognized is the widening of the space between the lunate and the navicular. Arthrography, magnetic resonance imaging, and arthroscopy are playing a part in better understanding and treatment of the wrist.

WRIST FRACTURES

A fall on the outstretched wrist is one of the most common mechanisms by which wrist fractures occur. So many easy, undisplaced,

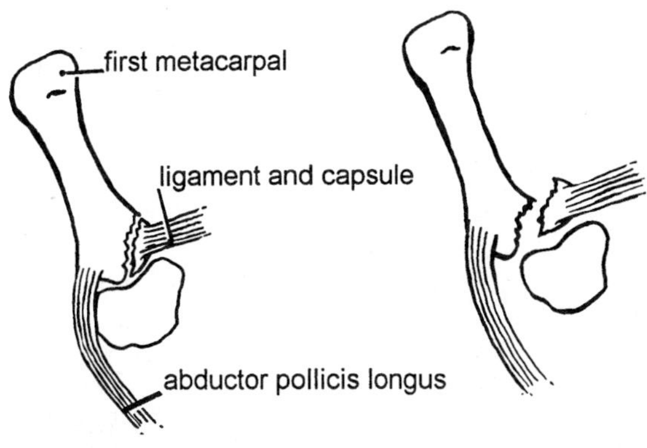

Figure 104-2. Bennett's fracture and how it displaces.

extraarticular fractures occur with this mechanism that the primary care physician can enjoy evaluating and treating with a good outcome. There are a few pitfalls, however. A slightly displaced or undisplaced fracture can displace further in the first few weeks if not immobilized properly with three-point fixation. Fractures into the radioulnar joint may impair pronation and supination.

The physician should always look for the fracture line in the navicular on every film seen, late and early. An occult fracture in this area can occur along with other fractures. The physician should always palpate for tenderness in the "anatomic snuff box." This is a sign of occult navicular fracture, and tenderness alone requires a thumb spica splint or cast, with x-ray reevaluation in 2 or 3 weeks to ensure that a fracture has not occurred. With a fracture of the navicular, the primary care physician should make the diagnosis and send the patient to a hand specialist.

When evaluating wrist injuries, the physician should consider the lunate and should look at it on every film to recognize its proper appearance. This permits recognition of the rare lunate or perilunate dislocation. The physician can also note the early signs of Kienböck disease (avascular necrosis of the navicular), when treatment can improve the outcome.

TENDINITIS

Tendinitis is a common, often vague form of hand pain that is difficult to treat and diagnose. Stenosing tenosynovitis of the first dorsal compartment (de Quervain disease) is probably an exception, in that it is specific and easy to treat. Tenderness over the first dorsal compartment and pain on passive stretch of the thumb (the Finklestein test) are classic signs of de Quervain disease. Active extension against resistance also causes pain. The tendon (or too many slips of tendon) gets inflamed as it enters the first dorsal compartment, where a groove in the radius is roofed over by a rigid ligament. The treatment is to reduce this inflammation. Antiinflammatory drugs can be given orally, or a local well-placed antiinflammatory steroid injection can be administered. Immobilization may help, but the wrist should not be immobilized without including the thumb; this worsens the situation. The injection alone resolves many of these cases without much fuss. If conservative treatment fails, then a surgical release of the roof of the tunnel can be done in a few minutes.

It would be nice if the generalized vague dorsal extensor tendinitis were as easy to understand and resolve as is de Quervain disease. Rest, immobilization, and nonsteroidal antiinflammatories are used with mixed results for these tendinitis conditions. Trying to reduce the repetitive activity that induces the pain is essential. The physician must rule out connective tissue diseases, collagen vascular diseases, neurologic diseases, and psychological disorders, as well as malingering.

BIBLIOGRAPHY

Blount WP. Fractures in children. Baltimore: Williams & Wilkins, 1955.

Charnley J. The closed treatment of common fractures. In: Green DP. Operative hand surgery, 2d ed. New York: Churchill-Livingstone, 1991.

Rockwood CA, Green DP, Heckman JD, Bucholz RW, eds. Rockwood & Green's fractures in adults, 4th ed. Philadelphia: Lippincott-Raven, 1996.

Sandzen SC. Atlas of wrist and hand fractures, 2d ed. Boston: PSG Publishing Co., 1978.

Weeks PM, Wray RC. Management of acute hand injuries: a biological approach, 2d ed. St. Louis: CV Mosby Co., 1978.

105

Injuries of the Ankle and Foot

RICHARD A. LEWIS

Primary Care for Women, edited by Phyllis C. Leppert and Fred M. Howard. Lippincott-Raven Publishers, Philadelphia © 1997.

We are so accustomed to our feet working well that when they fail, we are surprised how much disability is incurred. We take for granted the magnificent design and mechanical accomplishments of this masterpiece of bioengineering called the human foot. Great endurance is required for the hours we spend on our feet. The ability to bear the loads and stresses of standing is remarkable. It is amazing to think of the foot's ability to tolerate the stresses of running or sprinting or rapid changes of direction, not to mention the added stresses of carrying a 60-lb bag, or the demands of excess loads in the morbidly obese. In pregnancy, the gradual physiologic changes add weight across the foot at the same time that there is an increase in the level of hormones that relax the connective tissues, the tissues that hold the architecture of the foot together. This is why foot pain can occur in the third trimester.

Fashionable footwear does not help the situation. It is hard to see the logic in placing the foot into a pointed-toe, high-heeled shoe that compresses the forefoot and wedges the weightbearing area onto the anterior aspect of the longitudinal arch. Early in pregnancy is a good time to advise a patient about wearing sensible supportive and comfortable shoes that will prevent foot problems and falls as her weight increases and as the ligaments become more lax. This is an opportunity to practice preventive medicine, as a good shoe may prevent a fall or a twisted ankle.

TOE FRACTURES

Most toe fractures respond well to general fracture care. The physician must be sure that the fracture is a closed injury and that it does not enter a joint. The fracture is then reduced and aligned as anatomically as possible and then taped to adjacent toes. A cast is rarely needed. A good shoe can often be a part of treatment by allowing weightbearing on the rest of the foot. One trick to decrease motion in a distal foot fracture is to ask the shoemaker to place a second stiff, thick sole on the outside of the shoe to stiffen it and to decrease motion at the metaphalangeal level and beyond.

Intraarticular fractures are often no great problem either, but there may be future problems. The great toe needs careful attention to intraarticular problems and is less forgiving of small amounts of displacement than the lesser toes. The rule of anatomic reduction of all intraarticular fractures should be obeyed. Any deviation from this rule should be by the specialist, not the primary care physician.

FRACTURES OF THE SESAMOID BONES

The sesamoids are weightbearing bones that lie beneath the first metatarsal head. They can sustain trauma, and a fracture may be suspected. However, the sesamoids may be congenital bipartite structures that just look fractured. The foot should be examined carefully for tenderness and the radiograph scrutinized with a magnifying glass in search of cortical disruption. If there is a fracture, it needs protection from weightbearing.

METATARSAL FRACTURES

Weightbearing is the foot's primary function. The forefoot takes 50% of the weight and the hindfoot the other 50% in static loading. Each metacarpal head bears weight. The forefoot's weight is distributed so that the great toe, with its two underlying sesamoid bones, takes one third, and each of the lesser four toes takes one sixth. With a fracture of a metacarpal, the physician must bear in mind the weightbearing function. As soon as the initial fracture pain and swelling is over (usually within 2 to 3 weeks), some weightbearing can usually begin. With single metacarpal fractures, the adjacent metacarpals can splint and support the fractured one. The weightbearing force can actually allow the fractured metacarpal head to rise or fall into the correct alignment.

A fracture in the proximal diaphysis of the fifth metacarpal can often be slow to heal and requires a cast or open reduction. The adjacent common avulsion fracture of the base of the fifth metacarpal is quick to heal, and a stiff shoe is often adequate treatment (Fig. 105-1).

TARSOMETATARSAL FRACTURE AND FRACTURE-DISLOCATION

The proximal end of the metacarpals forms the roof of the longitudinal arch of the foot. Disruption of these joints often is hard to treat and results in chronic foot pain. These Lisfranc joint injuries are easily missed on x-rays unless the physician is careful to look at the alignment between the metatarsal shafts and the tarsal bones. Comparing the injured foot with the uninjured one gives a clue to the patient's normal anatomy. There is often subtle widening between the base of the first and second rays, indicating a large soft-tissue injury to the tarsometatarsal joints. A fracture in this location may have the same consequence. The alignment of the medial aspect of the cuboid on the oblique view should project along the medial border of the fourth ray. If it does not, the larger injury should be suspected. These fracture-dislocations are often unstable and require pin fixation or open reduction. Tarsometatarsal fracture-dislocations deserve an evaluation by a consultant. It is difficult to regain a normal foot after a Lisfranc tarsometatarsal fracture-dislocation.

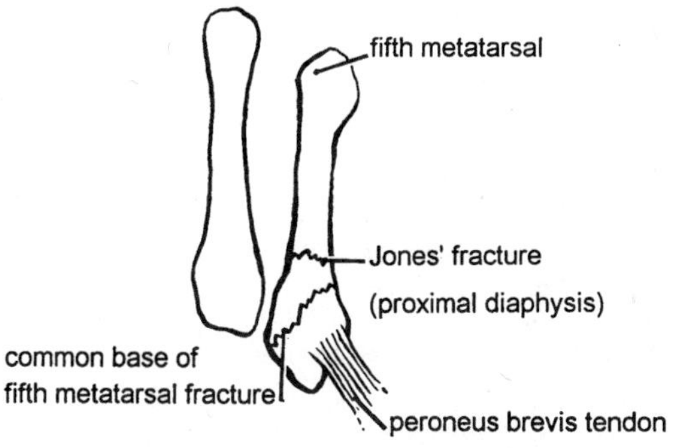

Figure 105-1. Different types of fifth metatarsal fractures.

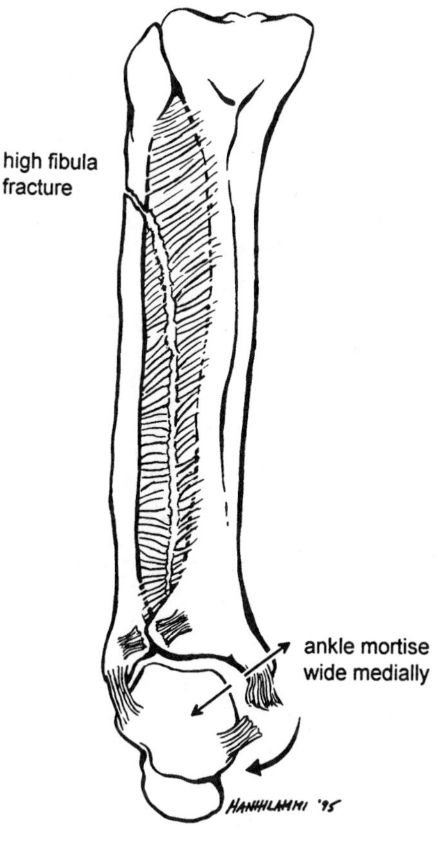

Figure 105-2. The swollen ankle with severe ligamentous injury and the high fibular fracture.

TARSAL INJURY

The small bones of the foot, like those of the hand, often sustain small avulsion fractures. Rest, immobilization, and elevation often improve comfort and produce good outcomes. The anterior avulsion chip off the anterior talus is a common sprain-equivalent fracture. Fractures of the body or neck of the talus are not of the same ilk, however. The talus has an easily compromised blood supply that is at risk even in undisplaced fractures. The dome of the talus is the surface of the ankle joint and must be reduced perfectly. The distal surface of the talus is the bulk of the subtalar joint, which also must be reduced well, and all injury to the surface must be recognized for optimal treatment. The calcaneus makes up the other side of the subtalar joint and has a complex surface anatomy. All calcaneal fractures must be seen by a specialist. The axial loading that produces a fractured heel often simultaneously produces vertebral fractures, so the physician should check for back tenderness in the patient with a broken heel who fell from a height.

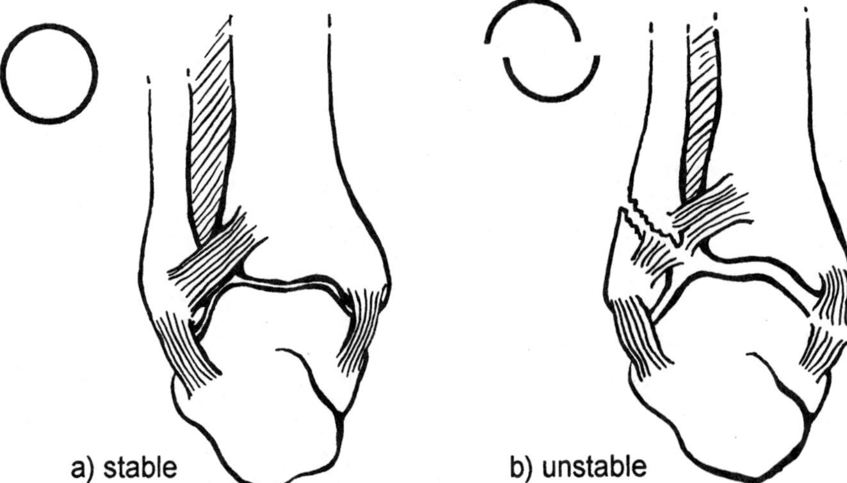

Figure 105-3. The stable ring analogy for stable versus unstable ankle fractures.

The tarsal navicular often has a small accessory ossicle at its medial aspect, called an accessory navicular or a pro-hallux. This is often confused with an acute avulsion fracture, but a fracture is usually more locally tender. The x-ray on careful study shows a round shell of cortical bone with an accessory navicular; in contrast, a fracture shows a sharp disruption of the cortex. This is the attachment site of the posterior tibial tendon. A fracture of the tarsal navicular can result in avascular necrosis, nonunion, and chronic foot pain.

RUPTURED ACHILLES TENDON

Patients with a ruptured Achilles tendon describe being struck or feeling a pop in the leg at the moment of a rapid change in direction. This history is that of a heel cord tear or the less serious gastrocnemius muscle tear. The examiner must confirm whether the Achilles tendon is intact. The patient can plantar-flex the foot even with a complete rupture of the Achilles tendon. This is possible because of the pull of the toe flexors and the peroneal and posterior tibial tendon, whose course behind the axis of rotation of the ankle allows plantar-flexion. Also, the power of the gastrocsoleus group is missing. To test the heel cord, the patient should lie prone on the examining table with the foot off the end of the table. The physician should observe and palpate the area of swelling. Usually the defect in the Achilles tendon can be felt above the calcaneus up to the level of the musculotendinous junction. A gastrocnemius tear is higher, from halfway between the ankle and knee toward the knee. A positive Thompson test also suggests a ruptured Achilles tendon: gentle compression of the gastrocnemius from medial to lateral should make the foot plantar-flex a small amount. If there is no foot motion, the Thompson test is positive and the Achilles tendon is ruptured.

There is debate in orthopedic circles about whether to treat these injuries by open or closed means. In general, more active athletic patients have surgical repairs, and older, nonathletic patients are treated with equinus casting.

ANKLE FRACTURES

Over the last decade we have become more demanding about what is considered acceptable in ankle fractures. Only simple, closed, undisplaced fractures should be treated by the primary care practitioner. This includes small avulsions. Any fracture pattern that shows a wide mortise or even slight displacement must go to the specialist.

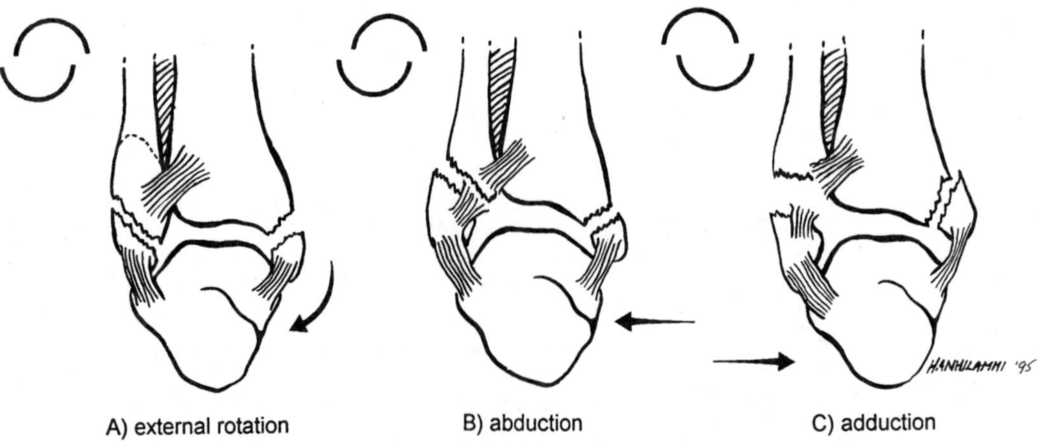

Figure 105-4. Mechanisms of ankle injury disrupting the ankle mortise.

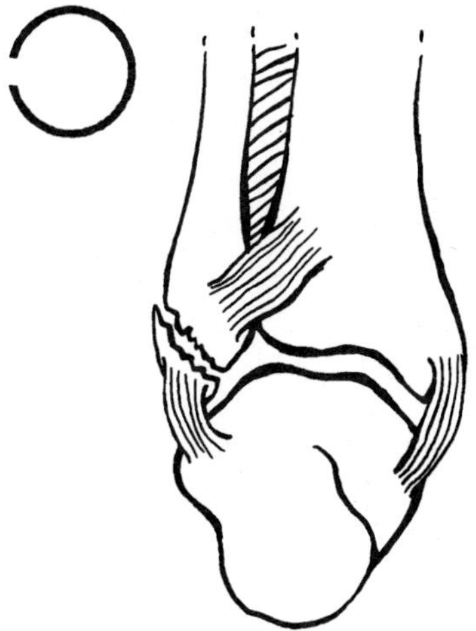

Figure 105-5. The stable ankle fracture with unilateral ring disruption.

One patient to watch for is one who has a negative x-ray and is sent home from the emergency department with the diagnosis of sprain. If there is more swelling and ecchymosis than one would expect, the patient may have a grade 3 ligament injury, which is better treated in a cast. Also, a pronation eversion injury of the ankle may involve a complete tear of the deltoid ligament and the tibiofibular syndesmosis with a high fibula fracture that is not even visible on the routine ankle film. If this is suspected, the physician should palpate the entire length of the fibula and x-ray the entire fibula. The high fracture is presumptive evidence that the other structures are torn. A screw across the syndesmosis is often recommended while it heals. It is hard to hold this injury to reduce the mortise in a cast. The fracture of the fibula is not a problem; the restoration of ankle anatomy to perfection is the problem (Fig. 105-2).

The ankle joint's components can be thought of as a closed ring—that is, the talus, the lateral ligaments, the distal fibula, the tibia, and the syndesmosis between the tibia and fibula make a stable ring-like structure, and this ring makes the mortise stable. If the ring is disrupted in one spot, it is still quite stable, but if it is broken in two places, it becomes quite unstable (Fig. 105-3). Figure 105-4 shows three basic fracture patterns. All three are unstable because the ring has broken in two places, one medial and one lateral. A ligament can tear without a fracture and produces the same kind of instability. The best way to ensure that the ring is broken in one place only is by careful examination. In an undisplaced fibula fracture with lateral tenderness and swelling, the physician should carefully examine the medial side. If the medial side is not tender, it is good evidence that the deltoid ligament is intact (Fig. 105-5). If the medial deltoid is intact and the lateral fibula is fractured, then the ring is broken in one spot and the pattern is stable. It is unlikely that the mortise will widen in this situation, but it should still be monitored for change.

BIBLIOGRAPHY

Crenshaw AH. Campbell's operative orthopedics, 8th ed. St. Louis: Mosby Year Book, 1992.

Dee R, Mango E, Hurst LL. Principles of orthopedic practice, New York: McGraw-Hill, 1988.

Rockwood CA, Green DP Heckman JD, Bucholz RW, eds. Fractures in adults, 4th ed. Philadelphia: Lippincott-Raven, 1996.

Jahss MH. Disorders of the foot and ankle. Philadelphia: WB Saunders, 1982.

Yablon IG, Segal D, Leach RE. Ankle injuries. New York: Churchill-Livingstone, 1983.

Primary Care for Women, edited by Phyllis C. Leppert and Fred M. Howard. Lippincott-Raven Publishers, Philadelphia © 1997.

XII
Neurologic Problems

106
Headache

JOSHUA HOLLANDER

Headache is a problem encountered at some time by most people. It is generally infrequent and not excessively severe. Most patients deal with occasional headaches with over-the-counter (OTC) drugs and without consulting a physician. About a third of the population suffers more severe or frequent headaches. Some even suffer disabling symptoms without troubling their physician because of the common belief that physicians can do little for a headache anyway. The patient complaining to a physician constitutes a minor portion of the affected population who has reached the point of being unable to cope. This, combined with the major advances in management that have taken place, means that the complaint of headache should be dealt with in a serious and sustained fashion. When the patient does resort to medical help, careful attention to the symptoms and proper diagnosis require the physician's time and interest more than technology. The problem requires a clear explanation of the cause of the problem as well as pain relief. Infrequent headaches can respond to abortives, but frequent occurrences require an attempt at prophylaxis. Chronicity implies a benign origin but also necessitates more care and support by the physician. Multiple agents may be tried, and the patient's understanding and cooperation are required. Because the problem is not life-threatening it is too often dismissed all too casually by the treating physician.

ETIOLOGY AND DIFFERENTIAL DIAGNOSIS

Although brain tissue per se is not pain-sensitive, there are numerous intracranial structures that are nociceptive. The scalp, dural sinuses, falx, and proximal larger arteries are innervated by the trigeminal nerve in the anterior and middle fossa and the upper cervical roots and glossopharyngeal and vagus nerves in the posterior fossa. Pain is elicited by traction and distortion of nociceptive structures. It is generally referred frontotemporally when arising in anterior and middle fossa and posterior cervically or to the ear or throat when posterior fossa structures are involved. Sinus headache occurs but should manifest itself by frank purulent material. This is the term popularized on television for migraine without aura. The eyes may be a source of headache primarily when glaucoma or injection is present.

The overwhelming majority of headache sufferers have benign conditions, but many insist that there must be a structural reason for headache. The misconception that brain tumors commonly present with severe headaches contributes to the anxiety provoked by recurrent and resistant severe headaches. The first consideration for the caregiver is to distinguish those common benign headaches from the infrequent ominous headache presentation. The physician must always balance the need to recognize these life-threatening conditions against the cost of imaging studies. The differential is quite different in a first acute headache and in a chronic, recurrent one. A headache that stands out against a background of infrequent, deep aching or is described as the "worst headache of my life" is probably only a migraine but is worrisome, especially when sudden in onset. A change in the pattern of a chronic headache is also disturbing and requires careful reevaluation. A first severe, explosive headache, especially if associated with a stiff neck, draws attention to the possibility of meningeal irritation. It is important to remember that full expression of meningeal signs may await blood breakdown or progression of meningitis. Explosive onset of headache and stiff neck without fever suggests subarachnoid hemorrhage, and a more gradual development of headache and stiff neck with fever suggests meningitis. Consideration of either pus or blood will require lumbar puncture. The presence of history or physical findings suggestive of lateralized masses, posterior fossa masses, or increased intracranial pressure may require a computed tomography (CT) scan prior to lumbar puncture.

The headache of increased intracranial pressure occurs in the morning or after naps and remits after arising. It occurs during more than 50% of mornings and displays a crescendo time profile over weeks to months. Intensity is variable. The headache associated with a local lesion is constant and nonpulsating and is maximal in a small area determined by the lesion.

The International Headache Society has developed a new classification of headache; Table 106-1 reflects a simplified version of this classification. Only some classes of headache are reviewed here.

Table 106-1. Headache Classification (International Headache Society)

- Migraine
  - Migraine without aura
  - Migraine with aura
    - Migraine with typical aura
    - Migraine with prolonged aura
    - Isolated migrainous aura
    - Familial hemiplegic migraine
    - Basilar migraine
  - Ophthalmoplegic migraine
  - Retinal migraine
  - Complications of migraine
    - Status migrainosus
    - Migrainous infarction
- Tension-type headache
  - Episodic tension-type headache
  - Chronic tension-type headache
- Cluster headache and chronic paroxysmal hemicrania
  - Cluster headache
    - Episodic cluster headache
    - Chronic cluster headache
  - Chronic paroxysmal hemicrania
- Miscellaneous headaches unassociated with structural lesion
  - Idiopathic stabbing headache
  - External compression headache
  - Cold stimulus headache
  - Benign cough headache
  - Benign exertional headache
  - Headache associated with sexual activity
- Headache associated with head trauma
- Headache associated with vascular disorders
- Headache associated with nonvascular intracranial disorder
- Headache associated with substances or their withdrawal
- Headache associated with noncephalic infection
- Headache associated with metabolic disorder
- Headache or facial pain associated with disorder of cranium, neck, eyes, nose, sinuses, teeth, mouth, or other facial or cranial structures

Migraine

Migraine is the most common headache type, affecting almost half of significant headache sufferers. It is a complex blend of head pain and neurologic and vegetative symptoms. Diagnosis is based on history. All headache sufferers have headaches of varying severity. Mild migraine without aura may blend into tension-type headache, but a severe headache tends to be of a type usually associated with migraine. It most typically is unilateral, throbbing, aggravated by routine activity, of a severity interfering with daily activities, and associated with photophobia and phonophobia. The sufferer prefers to lie down in a quiet, dark place. Headache will last 4 to 72 hours but may be terminated by sleep. Ice-pick pains and ice cream headache increase in frequency in migraine.

Prevalence is significantly higher in women, peaking at age 40, abating some to age 55, with a significant decrease later in life. Incidence peaks somewhat earlier in teens in migraine with aura. Female-to-male prevelence ratio diverges at puberty and peaks at 3.5 to 1 at age 40. Genetic factors are noted in twin studies. An individual has a 40% chance of migraine if one parent is affected, rising to 70% when both parents have migraine. The migraine personality has not stood up to scrutiny, but psychogenic factors as triggers remain important. Depression is almost universal in people with daily headaches, but it is less clear which is primary. It may well be that each feeds on the other.

Some migraineurs can identify no clear precipitants for headache, but the majority can identify some stimulus likely to provoke an attack. Psychosocial factors may manifest as a slump headache on days off rather than at times of peak stress. Emotional stress, too much or too little sleep, bright light, loud, blaring music, and olfactory stimulants all probably act on central mechanisms. Missed meals, foodstuffs, food additives, medications, and altered barometric pressure presumably act systemically. Many potentially precipitating agents such as sharp cheddar, chocolate, or nuts contain vasoactive agents such as tyramine or phenylethyl amine. Vasodilators such as nitrates or nitrites may precipitate migraine in susceptible individuals. Red wine and alterations in barometric pressure are of uncertain mechanism. Excitatory amino acid transmitters, such as monosodium glutamate and aspartame, may be precipitants. Foodstuffs are important triggers for a small number of individuals, and it is not generally helpful to embark on massive dietary restrictions unless it is clearly relevant to the individual patient. Medications said to cause headache include antihypertensives, vasodilators, calcium channel blockers, H_2 blockers, hormones, and antibiotics. Agents such as ergotamine and caffeine are associated with rebound headache. A factor in conversion of migraine to chronic daily headache is the analgesic rebound headache. The effects of menses and pregnancy are discussed later in this chapter.

Premonitory symptoms or prodromes are warnings of impending headache but may precede the attack by hours or days. These include changes in mood, behavior, energy level, and appetite, or vague cervical and cephalic sensations. These may not always occur but may be sufficiently striking to alert family and friends to an impending attack.

The aura is a transient attack of neurologic dysfunction gradually developing over 5 to 20 minutes and lasting less than 60 minutes. This usually precedes the head pain. It is most commonly a sensory disturbance, either visual or somatosensory. The most characteristic is a C-shaped, shimmering, prismatic, jagged scotoma best seen with the eyes closed. It is usually in one hemifield and slowly moves across the field to the periphery. As it moves off it may be replaced by either visual loss or a new scintillation. A large variety of visual phenomena may occur, including hemianopia, blindness, and photopsias. Monocular phenomena raise the specter of retinal or nerve disease, but may be a retinal migraine with a bright-colored light progressing to visual loss and clearing with headache onset. Cheiro-oral dysesthesias are the most common somatosensory phenomenon. Other phenomena include motor abnormalities, vertiginous states, aphasia, and behavioral and perceptual states. The metamorphopsias and perceptual alterations have been referred to as the "Alice in Wonderland" syndrome.

Although migraine with aura is easy to recognize in its most typical form, it must be recognized that the patients with prolonged aura or with aphasia and hemiplegia will provoke greater concern and need for evaluation. Patients with migraine with aura may have some headaches without aura and may also experience aura without headache. Patients whose headaches stopped earlier in life may later develop transient neurologic dysfunction, to be differentiated from transient ischemic attacks. Transient migrainous attacks spread slowly across the cortex, and the visual, motor, or sensory loss may take 5 to 20 minutes to fully spread, whereas transient ischemia is manifest in its full distribution almost immediately.

Despite great advances in clarifying the pathophysiology of migraine, major gaps remain. For many years a vascular mechanism was hypothesized that suggested intracranial vasospasm as the cause of the migrainous aura, with subsequent vasodilatation and vessel stretching as the cause of the pain. This could not be confirmed experimentally and failed to reconcile major clinical findings in migraine. Modern experimental studies have led to the neurogenic inflammation theory. The trigeminal vascular system innervates the proximal portions of the large intracranial vessels and can transmit nociceptive stimuli centrally, but at branch points can also conduct antidromically with release of algesic substances promoting vascular inflammation and increasing pain. Vomiting might then occur because of the trigeminal activation of brainstem centers involved in vomiting. The migrainous aura is now believed to relate to spreading cortical depression of Leao rather than vasospasm. Potassium is released in spreading depression and a leading wave of depolarization, commencing in calcarine cortex (aura of "classical migraine"), which reaches trigeminal fibers, and can initiate the nociceptive trigeminal vascular circuit. This fails to explain the initiation of the spreading cortical depression in migraine with aura, the initiation of nociception in migraine without aura, or the role of precipitating perceptual or psychic factors. Important roles have been postulated for the mesencephalic periaqueductal gray matter and the medullary raphe nuclei. These are pain-modulating centers and a failure of these negative feedback loops because of either hereditary instability or neural inputs could then allow the trigeminal vascular system to spiral out of control. There are a host of observations of altered serotonin function in migraine at many levels, but no certain role. Regrettably a unified theory of migraine capable of explaining all of the complex phenomenology characterizing this common disorder is lacking.

Tension-Type Headache

Recurrent episodic bilateral headaches of mild-to-moderate intensity, not worsened by activity and unaccompanied by nausea, may last 30 minutes to 7 days. The pain is of a pressing, tightening quality. These headaches do not occur on a daily basis (<15 per month); when they do occur more frequently on a sustained basis, they are referred to as chronic tension-type headaches. Both intermittent episodic and chronic tension headaches show a higher incidence in women. Tension-type headache has a significant component of psychosocial stress. Analgesic abuse and withdrawal are important considerations in the chronic form, especially when it blends into chronic daily headache. Oromandibular dysfunction is also more prominent in chronic forms.

This disorder was formerly called muscle contraction headache when it was thought that it developed due to cervical or fronto-occipital muscle spasm. Electromyography has failed to confirm this mechanism. It is now postulated that an acute attack might occur in an otherwise normal individual as a result of a complex interaction of pericranial muscle strain, myofascial pain sensitivity, and descending limbic effect on brainstem nociception. Chronicity may manifest with predominant central mechanisms.

Cluster Headache and Chronic Paroxysmal Hemicrania

Cluster headache is a dramatic disorder (0.1% of population) with a host of synonyms. Strictly unilateral, abrupt in onset, and severe orbital, supraorbital, and temporal pain may occur in periods of weeks to months at a frequency of several times a week to multiple (up to 8) per day. Individual attacks affect the same side and last 15 to 180 minutes. One or more of the following associated signs are seen on the painful side: conjunctival injection, lacrimation, nasal congestion, rhinorrhea, forehead and facial sweating, miosis, ptosis, and eyelid edema. The pain may be described as boring, burning, or throbbing. It elicits a local sensitivity and a tendency to perform short, intense physical activity unlike the rest sought by migraine sufferers. This type of headache is unusual in that it is more common in men and, unlike migraine, has little family history. Headaches usually occur in periodic clusters with many months between. During the cluster small amounts of alcohol can have a precipitating effect. Most commonly these headaches will awaken the subject from sleep. Chronic cluster headache lacks the periodicity but is of minor frequency.

An uncommon (only 1% as frequent as cluster headache) related disorder that primarily affects women with onset in adulthood is chronic paroxysmal hemicrania, which differs from cluster primarily in brevity and frequency of attacks. Attacks are excruciating and usually last only 2 to 24 minutes, but may recur 2 to 30 times a day. These patients are usually still during attacks, which may be mechanically triggered. An absolute responsiveness to indomethacin is a diagnostic feature.

Miscellaneous Headaches Without Associated Structural Lesion

Idiopathic Stabbing Headache

Idiopathic stabbing headache (jabs and jolts, icepick-like pains) manifests itself by fleeting stabs or a series of stabs confined to the head and most specifically the distribution of the first division of the trigeminal nerve. These occur at irregular intervals and are a common feature in migraineurs, usually on the side habitually affected by migraine. Structural disease must be excluded.

External Compression Headache

External compression headache is a constant pain, resulting from the application of external pressure to the head (eg, swim goggles, tight hat, tight wig). It is felt in the area of pressure and relieved by removal of the compression.

Cold Stimulus Headache

Cold stimulus headache can be elicited by external cold or, more commonly, ingestion of a cold substance (ice cream headache). After rapid ingestion of the cold stimulus, pain rises to the middle of the forehead. It may be intense but subsides within 5 minutes. It is benign but is associated with migraine.

Benign Cough Headache

Benign cough headache is a brief bilateral headache of sudden onset precipitated by coughing. This is identical in presentation to that seen in posterior fossa masses and imaging is required. Straining or heavy lifting will induce a similar phenomenon in intracranial masses and should be distinguished from a benign exertional headache, which is a bilateral throbbing headache brought on by exercise that lasts 5 minutes to 24 hours.

Headache Associated With Sexual Activity

Headache associated with sexual activity (benign coital cephalgia), precipitated by the sexual excitement of masturbation or coitus, is a bilateral headache that occurs in three varieties: a dull ache increasing to orgasm, an explosive orgasmic headache to be distinguished from subarachnoid hemorrhage, and a postural headache like that of low cerebrospinal fluid (CSF) pressure.

Specific Considerations With Regard to Menses

Menstrual migraine is a category that has not been specifically defined in the new headache classification. Migraine is worsened around menses, but this term refers specifically to migraine without aura which occurs primarily during or just prior to menses. The headache seems to be precipitated by a fall in plasma estradiol and manifested by a severe, 2- to 3-day attack with nausea and vomiting. Recurrent menstrual migraine can be delayed by estrogen but not progesterone. Headache still is seen when estradiol level is allowed to fall. There do not seem to be estrogen levels distinctive to this population of women. Although altered hypothalamic control systems have been said to occur, this would still not explain estradiol-withdrawal headache. Numerous hormonal manipulations have been tried with dubious benefit.

The track record of oral contraceptive pills has been colored by the viewpoint of neurology or gynecology. All series tend to be weak, but neurologists claim a significant increase in frequency and duration of headache, while gynecologists seem unconcerned. Both worsening of headache and onset of menstrual migraine with oral contraceptives are probably problems for some women. Headaches that worsened may return to their former severity 1 to 12 months after cessation of oral contraceptives. Stroke risk is probably increased by oral contraceptives, especially in association with smoking and hypertension.

Pregnancy has a beneficial effect on migraine in most women, particularly in the last two trimesters and in women with menstrual exacerbation. A few patients may have their first attack in pregnancy. Relapse is not uncommon in the first week postpartum.

Menopause is said to cause a transient worsening followed by improvement, but large numbers of women have no change or a worsening of their headaches. Because of considerations of arterial disease and osteoporosis, hormone replacement is common. Daily administration of estrogens may lessen headache. Cyclic therapy reduces the risk of endometrial carcinoma, but worsens headache.

HISTORY

The patient will often have difficulty describing in detail all the headaches experienced, so it is simpler to focus on the current headache, the typical headache, and the worst headache. Frequency, duration, location, quality, and severity are determined. Is there more than one variety? Has the pattern changed? When did headaches first appear? Are there typical times or modes of onset?

After exploration of the pain itself, associated symptoms such as prodromal symptoms, aura, autonomic features, and residua are sought. Precipitating, exacerbating, and ameliorating factors may shed light. A careful history of previous workups is necessary. What treatments have been employed, at what dose, and for how long? Many useful agents are discarded prematurely. Toxicity should be clarified. OTC agents are frequently omitted by patients who do not consider them real medicine. Recent imaging studies need not be repeated. Is there a family history of headache? What is the occupational or home life like? Does the patient have an exposure to precipitating foods, medicines, recreational drugs, or occupational agents? Marital discord may make management impossible. Does the patient already know what brings them on or relieves these headaches? The interview frequently establishes a relationship, which is then built upon to ensure patient trust and compliance with maneuvers needed to deal with a chronic illness.

PHYSICAL EXAMINATION

The physical examination is primarily of value in the elicitation of findings signaling structural causes of headache. Blood pressure is freely blamed for headache but should not be invoked unless there has been an acute rise of over 25% in diastolic pressure. Careful examination of the head should include visual fields, funduscopic examination, conjunctival injection, tympanic membranes, temporomandibular joints, occipital nerve tenderness, carotid or superficial artery tenderness, or meningeal signs. In addition to nuchal rigidity (present on flexion and sparing rotation), one should test for Kernig sign (with the hip and knee at 90°, the leg is extended on the thigh and pain is elicited), the more specific leg Brudzinski (on testing Kernig sign, the contralateral hip and knee flex), and the neck Brudzinski (neck flexion elicits flexion of hips and knees). During headache, migraine patients look ill and may well have difficulty complying with a detailed physical and neurologic examination. The neurologic examination may be dismissed as nonfocal, with no attention to visual fields, cortical sensory examination, or higher cortical function.

LABORATORY AND IMAGING STUDIES

Lumbar puncture may be required in subarachnoid hemorrhage, central nervous system inflammation, and benign intracranial hypertension. The erythrocyte sedimentation rate may alert the physician to temporal arteritis in older patients. Lupus anticoagulant or antiphospholipid antibodies are useful in atypical migraine, especially if there is a history of spontaneous abortion or venous thrombosis. The usual headache sufferer learns more from the laboratory about toxicity to chronic medication use than about the headache.

Although some physicians have advocated obtaining imaging studies on all headache sufferers to avoid later problems of a medicolegal sort, the cost to the health care system of ordering 20,000,000 CT or magnetic resonance imaging (MRI) studies for the 10% of the U.S. population who have migraine is prohibitive. The decision to order a study is based on a sense of disquiet about the headache or associated symptom history. A typical history without abnormalities on a physical or neurologic examination should not necessitate imaging. A neurologic consultation is generally cheaper and more helpful. Computed tomography is usually more readily available in emergency situations to rule out intracranial hemorrhage (not subarachnoid hemorrhage), hydrocephalus, or a large mass lesion. MRI is generally a more definitive study in less acute situations, especially to exclude posterior fossa lesions or Arnold-Chiari lesions. Magnetic resonance angiography is the procedure of choice to exclude dural venous sinus thrombosis.

TREATMENT

Management of any patient with recurrent headache requires establishing a relationship and the ability to address the major concerns of the patient as to possible brain tumor and the need for a definable cause for pain. This requires some discussion of the nature of the headache syndrome as well as reassurance that others are experiencing similar phenomena. This may improve the outlook for some patients. A "headache log" is necessary to establish a baseline; then pharmacotherapy may be undertaken.

Migraine

Two major approaches to migraine therapy are available: abortive and prophylactic. Abortive therapy attempts to terminate an already established headache. Abortive therapy is preferable when headaches are infrequent. This should be optimized and care should be taken to include all medications in the assessment. Patients frequently do not regard over-the-counter nonsteroidal antiinflammatory drugs (NSAIDs), aspirin, acetaminophen, or mixtures as true medications and may be ingesting large quantities without volunteering the information. Consideration of analgesic rebound headache as well as analgesic hepatic or renal toxicity must be considered when headache frequency is weekly or more frequent. Specific problems associated with migraine include nausea and vomiting with gastric stasis, which may eliminate oral therapy. Migraine may respond to aspirin or NSAIDs, but the patients will usually have tried acetaminophen, aspirin, ibuprofen, or naproxen in OTC preparations before consulting a physician. A variety of OTC headache mixtures are also available. Caffeine appears to provide an added benefit. Many patients will have tried a variety of medications in suboptimal dosage or time. After a careful history to assess headache type and medication history, a trial of naproxen (500 to 1000 mg) or ibuprofen (600 mg) may be tried. For patients unable to tolerate NSAIDs, acetaminophen (1000 mg) or isometheptene (Midrin) may be tried. Caffeine is a useful adjutant, as is rest in a quiet, dark place. For more severe headaches or for patients with poor NSAID response, a trial of rectal ergotamine may be made in younger patients without arterial disease. This should be administered early in the headache. Unfortunately nausea from the headache may blend into nausea from the ergotamine. It is helpful to cut the suppository and test 0.5, 1, and 2 mg doses when the patient is in the interictal phase to assess the maximum tolerated dose. Cafergot should not be repeated on a daily basis to avoid ergotism or ergot-withdrawal headache. Much more costly preparations include 6 mg sumatriptan SC or 1 mg D.H.E 45 IM or IV. Sumatriptan is an arterial constrictor and must be avoided in patients with angina. It causes a peculiar sensation in the chest, and it is often useful to administer the first dose in the physician's office. It comes in a fixed dose injector. The attack recurs in about 40% and a repeat dose may be needed. It should not be repeated for lack of efficacy. No more than 12 mg is given in 24 hours. A less effective oral preparation is now available. D.H.E. 45 is an older agent that can be very effective. It is a venoconstrictor rather than an arterial constrictor. Dosage can be varied, but nausea may be a common accompaniment and 10 mg metaclopramide IM or IV is usually given first. In the emergency department one can also use a small dose of intravenous prochlorperazine (10 mg) or, less optimally, chlorpromazine (1 mg/kg). Hypotension may result and intravenous fluids and careful observation are in order.

Prophylactic therapies are warranted to avoid analgesic toxicity or rebound headache. This approach may fail if serious interpersonal problems exist (eg, if the patient is having serious marital problems, prophylactic therapy is probably doomed to failure) or the patient is suffering a chronic daily headache, perhaps from analgesic rebound or depression. Considerable time seems needed to achieve efficacy and to avoid confusing minor fluctuations in headache frequency or intensity from true headache reduction. It is probably best to not worry about how each agent may be reducing headache while so much of headache mechanisms remain controversial. Each agent may not be acting in the manner implied by its classification in the therapeutic armamentarium. Effective dosage varies with the individual and may require titration. Dosages are frequently assumed to be very low and potentially valuable agents are abandoned because of the lack of efficacy at inadequate dosage. Major prophylactic agents include β-adrenoreceptor blocking agents, antidepressants, calcium channel blocking agents, methyl ergonovine, valproate. Less popular because of toxicity is methysergide, and of low efficacy is cyproheptadine.

β-adrenoreceptor blocking agents show variable efficacy in migraine. Effective agents include propranolol, nadolol, timolol, atenolol, and metoprolol. Ineffective β-blockers include alprenolol, oxprenolol, pindolol, and acebutolol. Lack of efficacy does not relate to cardioselectivity, penetration into the central nervous system, membrane-stabilizing activity, or affinity for serotonin-binding sites. Partial agonist activity has a negative correlation to efficacy. The main effect is to reduce headache frequency. Side effects include fatigue, sleep disturbances, depression, dizziness, and hypotension. Equipotent doses for hypotension and bradycardia are probably equipotent in migraine prophylaxis.

Calcium channel blocking agents also have a variable role with poor response to nifedipine and nimodipine. The best documented efficacy studies show a strong benefit to flunarizine, an agent not available in the United States. Verapamil in doses of 240 to 320+ mg/day has less rigorous documentation of efficacy, but when maintained for 6 to 8 weeks is probably quite effective. Side effects include constipation, nausea, edema, hypotension, and atrioventricular block. It should not be used with a β-blocker, bradycardia, sick sinus syndrome, or atrioventricular block.

Antidepressant medications have been known to have benefits comparable to propranolol. The cyclic compounds documented in control trials were amitriptyline and doxepin. These drugs are tolerated relatively poorly by migraine patients and must be titrated up from 10 to 25 mg to 75 to 100 mg. The disturbing sedation usually wears off, but dry mouth, constipation, aggravation of glaucoma, and urinary retention can all be problems. Excess sweating and altered myocardial depolarization can also occur. The other tricyclic antidepressants, as well as the heterocyclic trazodone, may be better tolerated but lack as clear documentation of efficacy. Imipramine appears ineffective. Of the serotonin reuptake inhibitors, fluoxetene has been proven effective. This is one of the few migraine prophylactic agents not causing weight gain. Sertraline has less stimulant effect and has been thought effective. Monamine oxidase inhibitors such as phenelzine have been shown to be helpful, but concern about food-precipitated hypertension, as well as other toxicities, have caused most physicians to hold this as a last resort.

The α-agonist clonidine showed some early promise but is ineffective.

The anticonvulsant valproate has clear antimigraine effect, but phenytoin and carbamazepine do not. Valproate can be titrated by blood level. Care must be taken over possible teratogenic neural tube defects. Other toxicities include hyperammonemia, hair loss, and weight gain. Serious hepatic toxicity is only reported in children.

The antiserotonin methysergide is an effective agent in migraine prophylaxis but causes significant gastrointestinal and mood disturbances even when the dose is titrated slowly, and must be stopped for 2 to 3 months after taking it for 5 to 6 months because of risk of retroperitoneal fibrosis. Interaction with ergotamine is also a problem. Methysergide should only be used in severely affected individuals by an experienced physician. The antihistamine cyproheptadine is also a weak antiserotonin agent, but gives only minimal benefit.

Tension Headaches

Tension headaches are not easily managed if they have passed from an episodic event responding to OTC preparations to chronic intractable headache. Finding a suitable explanation for the pain is something that most physicians have difficulty with in view of our lack of understanding of this process. The process can be explained as one in which spiraling headache and depression or anxiety feed on each other. After a strong dose of reassurance, aspirin, acetaminophen, or nonsteroidal antiinflammatory agents may be used. For chronic tension-type headaches, amitriptyline seems highly beneficial. For some patients nonpharmacologic therapy such as relaxation exercises or biofeedback may prove helpful. Possible oromandibular dysfunction should be explored.

Cluster Headaches

Cluster headaches are relatively intense and brief. One hundred percent oxygen at 7 L/min by tight mask can abort a headache in 5 to 10 minutes, even though no increase in cerebral oxygen consumption occurs. Oxygen availability may be a problem. Sumatriptan has been very effective, but the patient may suffer relapses. It retains efficacy despite prolonged use. Less popular now is ergotamine and dihydroergotamine. Prophylactic therapy is obviously in order in patients whose cluster is prolonged or in whom the problem is chronic. Rectal ergotamine-caffeine is effective for nocturnal attacks. Verapamil is usually used before lithium or methysergide is tried. Steroids have been widely used but efficacy has never been clearly demonstrated. Methysergide has been quite effective and in patients with the intermittent variety can be stopped before concerns about retroperitoneal fibrosis become a major factor. Valproate is claimed to be effective but further study is in order.

There is a group of indomethacin-responsive headaches which include chronic paroxysmal hemicrania, idiopathic stabbing headache, and benign exertional headache. Headache associated with sexual activity is indomethacin-responsive when associated with benign exertional headache. Propranolol may be helpful because exertional headaches may be associated with hypertensive surges. Diltiazem has been claimed to be effective. The main consideration here is concern about possible subarachnoid hemorrhage.

CONSIDERATIONS DURING PREGNANCY

Although many women experience some headache early in pregnancy, this is usually a minor problem and responds to acetaminophen. Migraine, especially menstrually exacerbated migraine, remits in approximately 70% of pregnant women. This is most striking during the last trimester. Unfortunately, there are some individuals who experience migraine throughout pregnancy, and the small number who experience the onset of migraine with pregnancy. Tension-type headaches continue through pregnancy.

Pharmacologic management of the headache combines concern about possible teratogenicity early in pregnancy and possible labor-related problems later in pregnancy. Abortive therapy tends to evolve about acetaminophen. The teratogenicity of NSAIDs has not been adequately studied; aspirin is probably the best-studied, without much known about its teratogenicity. Concern about acetylsalicylic acid (aspirin) relates primarily to labor-related problems, but some other NSAIDs are teratogenic. While ibuprofen is relatively safe, it is probably best to avoid all prostaglandin synthesis inhibitors. β-blockers such as propranolol and atenolol are thought safe but may cause neonatal bradycardia. All ergot derivatives are probably inappropriate because of their potential uterine involvement. Acetaminophen for abortive therapy and amitriptyline for prophylaxis are the best options. Biofeedback, meditation, and other nonpharmacologic means can also be used.

BIBLIOGRAPHY

Davidoff RA. Migraine: manifestations, pathogenesis, and management. Philadelphia: FA Davis, 1995.

Headache Classification Committee. Classification and diagnostic criteria for headache disorders, cranial neuralgia and facial pain. Cephalalgia, an international journal of headache. Trondheim, Norway: Norwegian University Press, 1988;8(7):1.

Olesen J, Tfelt-Hansen P, Welch KMA. The headaches. New York: Raven Press, 1993.

Raskin NH. Headache, 2nd ed. New York: Churchill Livingstone, 1988.

107
Dizziness

JOSHUA HOLLANDER

Primary Care for Women, edited by Phyllis C. Leppert and Fred M. Howard. Lippincott-Raven Publishers, Philadelphia © 1997.

Sensations of heat or cold are consistently learned experiences of childhood. No such uniformity exists for dizziness, and the physician must first understand what the patient means by it. Most patients are relating a loss of spatial orientation. Correct sensory input, proper central integration, and appropriate motor response are all needed. Vision, vestibular input, proprioception, touch and pressure, and hearing all serve as orienting sensations. Attention and alertness are required for full spatial orientation. Vision contributes horizontal and vertical meridians and is a primary orienting sensation in humans. The labyrinth provides angular acceleration in three perpendicular axes through the semicircular canals and the otoliths measure linear acceleration in the vertical (gravity) and horizontal (fore-and-aft) planes.

Problems causing dizziness include spontaneous false sensations, such as acute vestibular dysfunction; sensory mismatch, as in reading a book in a rocking boat cabin; sensory distortion, as seen with new cataract lenses; poor central integration, seen in multiple sclerosis; impaired motor execution with cerebellar dysfunction; and servoloop failure, as in Parkinson disease. Most patients with true rotational vertigo have vestibular disease, but the range of problems referred to as dizziness is quite broad.

The vestibuloocular reflex (VOR) is more important in humans than the vestibulospinal reflex and requires some clarification of eye movement systems. Vergence systems (convergence and divergence) permit independent eye movements to allow binocular fusion at varying target distances. Saccadic eye movements are quick flicks that change the line of sight and include nystagmus fast phases. These bring the target to the high-acuity fovea. The moving image is stabilized on the retina by optokinetic and pursuit systems. The VOR allows for ocular stabilization despite head movements.

Voluntary saccades are ballistic eye movements initiated by the frontal eye field's signals to the paramedian pontine reticular formation, with the superior colliculus reorienting gaze to novel stimuli. A complex process produces signals via the median longitudinal fasciculus to the oculomotor and abducens nuclei, allowing both yoked eye movements and reciprocal inhibition. Smooth pursuit is triggered by retinal slip with low target speed.

The vestibular end organ has two interconnected subsystems, the three perpendicularly oriented semicircular canals and the otolith. The canals detect angular acceleration by endolymph motion, bending a group of hair cells with nonmotile stereocilia. This is bidirectional and results in conjugate deviation of the eyes through the yoked medial and lateral recti. The eye movements should be equal in amplitude and opposite in direction to the head movement; this is the VOR and is much faster than the smooth pursuit system. The resultant slow deviation of the eyes may result in a corrective saccade. The resultant alternating fast and slow eye movements in the plane of the stimulated semicircular canal is called vestibular nystagmus. The utricle and saccule have otoliths (calcium carbonate crystals) attached to hair cells oriented to provide responses to linear acceleration in the vertical or horizontal plane. The vestibular system then adjusts the position of the eyes in the orbit to compensate for the head position in space.

Vestibulospinal reflexes contribute to posture and tone. Unilateral labyrinthectomy decreases ipsilateral extensor tone and increases contralateral tone. Bilateral lesions abolish decerebrate rigidity.

ETIOLOGY AND DIFFERENTIAL DIAGNOSIS

In a large number of unselected patients presenting to Northwestern University with the complaint of dizziness, many actually suffered low-level hyperventilation or multisensory impairments (Fig. 107-1) Symptoms of vertigo syndromes include the illusion of movement caused by impaired perception of a stationary environment by CNS space-constancy mechanisms.

Multisensory impairments provide the added loss of an outside stationary reference system required for orientation and postural regulation, contributing to a sense that oneself or one's surroundings are moving. These impairments might include large-fiber peripheral neuropathy with diminished position sense; visual disturbances such as cataract removal without implant, major refractive change, or macular degeneration; cervical osteoarthritis with limited neck movement; or impaired auditory or vestibular sensitivity.

Otolithic lesions produce static head tilts or ocular skew or torsion. Unilateral labyrinthine lesions produce an imbalance in the tonic vestibular firing rate as the ipsilateral vestibular nucleus loses its spontaneous activity and becomes unresponsive to ipsilateral rotational signals. The symptoms usually reflect the horizontal semicircular canals, as the vertical canals cancel each other out. Such a patient attempting fixation experiences visual blurring as an object appears to move away from the side of the lesion toward the fast phase of the vestibular nystagmus. Eye proprioception is lacking, and target displacement on the retina is perceived as motion. Eye closure eliminates visual correction, and the vestibular input imbalance is perceived as subjective rotation toward the affected labyrinth.

Dizziness reflects cortical spatial disorientation. Nystagmus is due to direction-specific VOR imbalance. Ataxia or imbalance is due to impaired vestibulospinal signals. Nausea and vomiting are due to activation of the adjacent medullary vomiting center. Compensation occurs as the normal vestibular nuclei reduce their firing rate and the commissural fibers induce a new tonic firing. Compensation probably requires cerebellum and reticular formation; this is why central vertigo is less easily compensated. The "double-hit" problem occurs in the face of central and peripheral lesions with poor compensation. Compensation is poor for otolithic lesions, and chronic mild imbalance may be perceived. Compensation occurs most rapidly if vestibular exercises and stimulation begin as soon as possible after injury. Patients with bilateral vestibular dysfunction experience visual blurring when walking or driving because they are left with only a slow smooth pursuit system and without the VOR cannot maintain fixation.

Symptoms are thus influenced by laterality, chronicity, and severity. The clinical axioms are:

- Acute unilateral vestibular dysfunction causes vertigo.
- Compensated unilateral vestibular dysfunction does not cause vertigo.
- Uncompensated intermittent unilateral vestibular dysfunction causes vertigo.
- Recurrent dysfunction of the same or opposite labyrinth may cause vertigo.
- Bilateral absent vestibular function may cause lifelong symptoms but not vertigo.

Physiologic vertigo occurs when a sense of vertigo is produced by external stimuli acting on a normally functioning sensory system. Motion sickness, the most common, is elicited by unfamiliar body accelerations or intersensory mismatch, accentuated by fear or insecurity. Visuovestibular conflict is important and is reduced with ample peripheral vision. Provocative activities might include reading a book in the back of a car on a winding road. Symptoms include apathy, salivation, nausea and vomiting, pallor, perspiration, and prostration.

Height vertigo is a visually induced subjective instability in postural balance and locomotion, with fear of falling and vegetative symptoms. The response is subject to adaptation, but a phobic reaction may supervene.

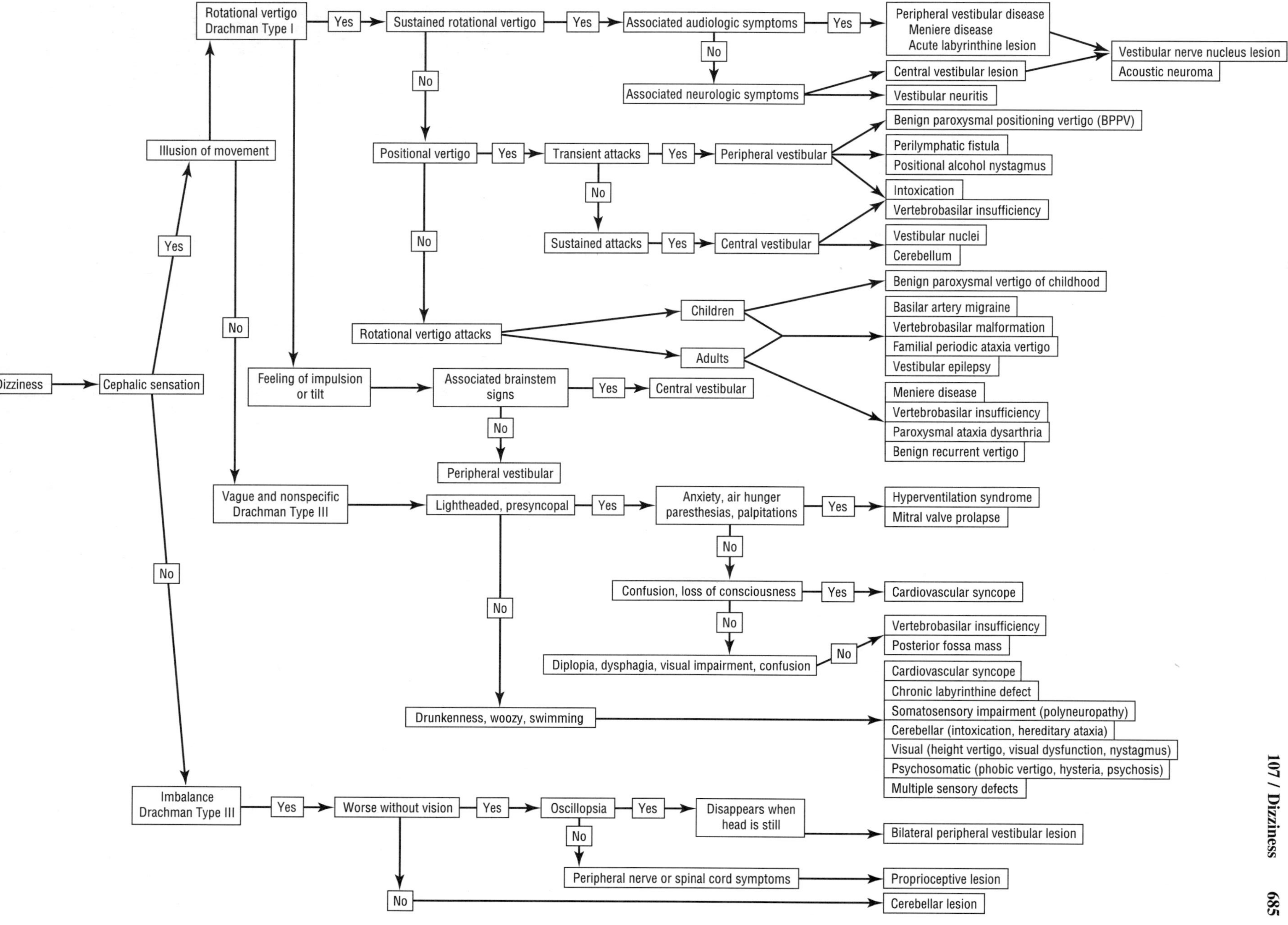

Dizziness
Cephalic sensation
Yes
Illusion of movement
Yes
Rotational vertigo
Drachman Type I
Yes
Sustained rotational vertigo
Yes
Associated audiologic symptoms
Yes
Peripheral vestibular disease
Meniere disease
Acute labyrinthine lesion
Vestibular nerve nucleus lesion
Acoustic neuroma
No
Associated neurologic symptoms
Central vestibular lesion
Vestibular neuritis
No
Positional vertigo
Yes
Transient attacks
Yes
Peripheral vestibular
Benign paroxysmal positioning vertigo (BPPV)
Perilymphatic fistula
Positional alcohol nystagmus
Intoxication
Vertebrobasilar insufficiency
No
Sustained attacks
Yes
Central vestibular
Vestibular nuclei
Cerebellum
No
Rotational vertigo attacks
Children
Adults
Benign paroxysmal vertigo of childhood
Basilar artery migraine
Vertebrobasilar malformation
Familial periodic ataxia vertigo
Vestibular epilepsy
Meniere disease
Vertebrobasilar insufficiency
Paroxysmal ataxia dysarthria
Benign recurrent vertigo
Feeling of impulsion or tilt
Associated brainstem signs
Yes
Central vestibular
No
Peripheral vestibular
No
Vague and nonspecific
Drachman Type III
Lightheaded, presyncopal
Yes
Anxiety, air hunger
paresthesias, palpitations
Yes
Hyperventilation syndrome
Mitral valve prolapse
No
Confusion, loss of consciousness
Yes
Cardiovascular syncope
No
Diplopia, dysphagia, visual impairment, confusion
No
Vertebrobasilar insufficiency
Posterior fossa mass
No
Drunkenness, woozy, swimming
Cardiovascular syncope
Chronic labyrinthine defect
Somatosensory impairment (polyneuropathy)
Cerebellar (intoxication, hereditary ataxia)
Visual (height vertigo, visual dysfunction, nystagmus)
Psychosomatic (phobic vertigo, hysteria, psychosis)
Multiple sensory defects
No
Imbalance
Drachman Type III
Yes
Worse without vision
Yes
Oscillopsia
Yes
Disappears when
head is still
Bilateral peripheral vestibular lesion
No
Peripheral nerve or spinal cord symptoms
Proprioceptive lesion
No
Cerebellar lesion

Head extension vertigo is important because it is often confused with vertebrobasilar insufficiency. The otoliths are nonfunctional in head extension and flexion. Flexion is a more common position, and we accommodate. When we look up with no visual cues (darkness) or conflicting cues (moving clouds without a horizon line), we may fall when we lift a foot.

Space sickness, visual vertigo, somatosensory vertigo, auditory vertigo, alternobaric vertigo, and pilot's vertigo (spatial disorientation) are all manifestations of physiologic vertigo. They are important but are not discussed further here.

As previously discussed, visual and somatosensory problems may cause pathologic vertigo. More detailed discussion follows on vestibularly mediated vertigo.

Peripheral Vestibular Vertigo

Acute unilateral peripheral vestibulopathy or vestibular dysfunction has been suggested in patients with poorly understood pathogenetic mechanisms. These patients are acutely vertiginous and experience vegetative distress. They lie with the affected ear up and avoid looking toward the good ear. Vestibular neuritis describes a single episode of acute vertigo, nausea, and vomiting. These patients tend to be younger. Hearing is unaffected. Vertigo is severe, with commensurate spontaneous nystagmus.

Antecedent infection has been described, but the cause is unknown. It may be related to epidemic vertigo seen in the spring and summer. Viral labyrinthitis is a similar disorder that follows a childhood exanthem and is usually associated with hearing loss. Ramsay Hunt syndrome (herpes zoster oticus) may be associated with facial paresis as well as vertigo, hearing loss, and canalicular vesicles.

Patients with Meniere disease experience the classic tetrad of aural fullness, fluctuating sensorineural hearing loss, low-pitched tinnitus, and decrescendo nystagmus-vertigo attacks. Recovery is over hours or days, with remissions of a month or longer. Most patients experience remission in 5 years. Electronystagmography may be normal but usually displays positional nystagmus or canal paresis. It is usually unilateral. It is thought that problems with endolymphatic duct drainage result in endolymphatic hydrops. Periodic rupture decompresses the membranous labyrinth but releases high-potassium endolymph into the perilymph, causing vestibular nerve discharge and then paresis. This may present at end stage with otolithic catastrophes of Tumarkin, abrupt alterations of postural tilt until the patient crashes to the floor.

Posttraumatic vertigo is a mixed group of disorders ranging from postconcussive syndrome to benign paroxysmal positional vertigo, labyrinthine concussion, perilymph fistula, and temporal bone fracture. Syphilis may present with labyrinthitis or hydrops. Vascular problems include internal auditory artery occlusions, small vessel infarcts from diabetes, or hemorrhage from bleeding diatheses. Acoustic neurinoma is slow growing, and vestibular compensation usually causes hearing loss without much vertigo.

Recurrent Unilateral Vestibular Dysfunction

Recurrent unilateral vestibular dysfunction may be caused by Meniere syndrome. Otosclerosis, a familial disorder due to abnormal bone growth and resorption, results in hearing loss in the second or third decade. Some of these patients experience gait disturbances and episodic vertigo.

Paroxysmal Positional Vertigo

Benign paroxysmal positional vertigo is common and is usually seen in women age 50 to 60. Rotational vertigo begins 10 to 15 seconds after head tilt toward the affected ear and subsides after 10 to 60 seconds, and the response fatigues. Vertigo is usually worse in the morning but is triggered by lying down, rolling over in bed, or extending the head when upright. It is confirmed on examination by a classical Hallpike response. The mechanism is presumed to be disruption of otoconia from the utricular macule, with lodgment in the ampulla of the posterior semicircular canal. This converts the canal to a gravity receptor rather than an angular acceleration receptor.

Other types of positional nystagmus have been divided into central and peripheral types, but this classification may not have merit. Failure of fixation suppression and direction-changing nystagmus may be the best indicators of central pathology.

Bilateral Vestibular Dysfunction

Positional alcohol nystagmus is the most common and results from overindulgence. Alcohol enters and leaves the cupula at a different rate than the endolymph, inducing a specific gravity differential that causes movement-induced vertigo during intoxication and 5 to 10 hours later, when recovering. A similar mechanism may relate to the vertigo of macroglobulinemia.

Ototoxicity is a symptom complex without vertigo. It is associated with impaired balance in darkness as well as impaired VOR. The patient has visual difficulty when the head is in motion and unsteadiness with head turns. The patient presents as an outpatient or when mobilized after a major illness or surgery. Aminoglycosides are concentrated in endolymph and are common offenders. Diagnosis depends on the electronystagmographic demonstration of bilateral canal paresis and a history of ingestion of a potentially ototoxic drug or of major illness or surgery. Prophylactic or therapeutic use in any patient, but especially in one with impaired renal function, may be all the history obtained. Other ototoxic drugs include nonsteroidal anti-inflammatories, loop diuretics, antiprotozoal agents, anticancer agents, and a host of less common offenders. This must be distinguished from the long list of agents causing nonvestibular dizziness, which clears on drug withdrawal.

Disequilibrium of aging is a complex of disorders. Degenerative cupulolithiasis causes benign paroxysmal positional vertigo. Loss of end organ function (depressed VOR) may cause the vestibular ataxia of aging. These patients are asymptomatic when still but have trouble controlling the center of gravity when walking and trying to maintain a fixed head position for visual reference. Loss of central inhibition (hypersensitive VOR) may result in vertigo with angular head movements. Vertigo ensues with changing head position relative to gravity. The patient sits on the edge of the bed before walking. Orthostatic hypotension must be excluded.

Multiple sensory defects may also contribute to disequilibrium of aging. Age-associated changes occur in the vestibular system and in proprioception. These changes may combine with hearing loss and visual loss due to cataract or senile macular degeneration to result in disequilibrium, even though no single system is sufficiently involved by itself.

Bilateral Meniere syndrome may occur, but the symptoms are no different from those of the unilateral form. Autoimmune sensorineural hearing loss manifests as progressive hearing loss, tinnitus, pressure, and reduced vestibular function. Bilateral relentless hydrops or an associated autoimmune disorder may suggest this rare entity.

Central Vestibular Vertigo

Central vestibular vertigo may be caused by lesions of the vestibular nuclei, the vestibular cerebellum, or their connections. Pure nystagmus vectors tend to be central in origin, and a neurologic examination usually elicits associated findings.

Vascular disease tends to be invoked in older patients quite freely, disregarding other possibilities. Although vertebrobasilar insufficiency is commonly associated with vertigo (reduced supply to the vestibular nuclei and cerebellum), associated brain stem or cerebellar symptoms or signs may occur, including vegetative signs, dysarthria, postural imbalance, visual loss, diplopia, paresis, or paresthesias of one or both sides. Occipital headache is common. Onset is abrupt, tapering over 30 minutes or less. Vertebrobasilar insufficiency may be hemodynamic in origin, and Stokes-Adams attacks and subclavian steal must be considered. Vertebral artery occlusion may produce the lateral medullary syndrome (posterior inferior cerebellar artery syndrome) of ipsilateral ataxia, loss of ipsilateral facial pain and temperature sensibility, loss of contralateral pain and temperature sensibility, and Horner syndrome. The vestibular nuclear lesion causes vertigo and fall to the affected side; utricular involvement produces skew deviation. Anterior inferior cerebellar artery syndrome produces a lateral pontomedullary syndrome often associated with labyrinthine infarction and deafness. Cerebellar hemorrhage is a potentially lethal disorder easily seen on computed tomography in a patient with sudden onset of headache, nausea, vomiting, vertigo, and ataxia.

Multiple sclerosis with brain stem or cerebellar involvement may cause dizziness, but associated brain stem signs should be present unless only the vestibular nerve root entry zone is affected.

Basilar artery migraine is an uncommon disorder seen primarily in adolescent girls or young women. The aura is of vertigo, ataxia, and bilateral visual changes. This is followed by an occipital throbbing headache. Benign paroxysmal vertigo of childhood is thought to be a migraine variant. Various foramen magnum lesions and eye-movement disorders may induce dizziness, usually through the development of oscillopsia (conscious perception of visual movement in nystagmus).

Psychogenic Vertigo

Psychogenic vertigo is common in anxiety neurosis, hysteria, depression, and schizophrenia. Low-grade hyperventilation is common. Panic attacks with vertigo as a major complaint may occur with or without agoraphobia.

HISTORY

There are four areas to explore in the neurotologic history: time course, precipitating factors, predisposing factors, and associated symptoms.

Time Course

Dizziness of sudden onset and offset may suggest a cardiac or vascular etiology. Psychogenic vertigo builds gradually with an abrupt offset. A single bout tapering over days to weeks suggests acute peripheral vestibulopathy. Brief episodes of minutes to hours occur in Meniere disease. Brief paroxysms elicited by changing head position suggest benign paroxysmal positional vertigo. New-onset nystagmus may cause an illusory environmental movement (oscillopsia).

Precipitating Factors

Orthostatic dizziness may also be seen in orthostatic hypotension, but dizziness elicited when lying down or rolling over in bed is characteristic of benign paroxysmal positional vertigo. Other movements are nonspecific. Carotid kinking can occur and is as common as vertebral kinking. The Tullio phenomenon of vertigo induced by loud noise is seen in perilymph fistula or Meniere disease.

Predisposing Factors

Alcohol may affect the relative specific gravity of endolymph and macula. Phenytoin is a cerebellar toxin, and aminoglycosides are ototoxic. Anticoagulants may induce bleeding. Sedatives may cause extravestibular dizziness.

Associated Symptoms

- Aural: hearing loss, tinnitus, fullness, otalgia, otorrhea
- Autonomic: nausea, vomiting, sweating
- Neurologic: facial motor or sensory loss, dysarthria, dysphagia, loss of coordination, visual problems, altered consciousness, weakness, paresthesias
- Psychogenic: Phobias (particularly agoraphobia) are suggested if fear of dizziness confines the patient to home.
- Visual: Oscillopsia from nystagmus and the inability to focus on the macula while in motion, reflecting bilateral vestibular impairment, must be distinguished on history and explored on the physical examination.

PHYSICAL EXAMINATION

When performing the general neurologic examination, the physician must pay particular attention to the cranial nerves, proprioception, and the cerebellum. The general physical examination must include otoscopic inspection of the drum for vesicles (Ramsay Hunt), drainage, and inflammation. A blue drum suggests glomus tympanicum. Hearing can be grossly checked with a watch tick or 512 tuning fork. Rubbing fingers may mask the other ear and whispered words may reveal the impaired verbal discrimination of nerve deafness.

Vestibular imbalance may be manifest as nystagmus that is fixation-suppressed. It may be detected on ophthalmoscopy and accentuated by covering the viewing eye to block fixation suppression. The head may be shaken while the subject reads, and visual blur or corrective saccades imply abnormal vestibular gain. A minimal caloric test can be performed using 1 cc of ice water in the ear with the erect head tipped back 60° or the supine head elevated 30°. Normally, the ensuing nystagmus is named for the fast component and is cold opposite. A secretarial swivel chair may be used to perform an approximate Barany rotation; ten rotations with the head tipped back 60° usually suffices. Nystagmus and dizziness can be elicited. The patient should be able to suppress the nystagmus by fixing on an outstretched finger. Failure to do so (failure of fixation suppression) is a central sign. The otolithic system may manifest by head tilt or visual skew deviation.

The vestibulospinal system is tested by gait and station. The Romberg maneuver requires intact cerebellar function to allow the patient to stand in place with her feet together. The eyes are then closed. Without visual cues, position sense and vestibular sense are required to maintain stance. If position sense is significantly impaired, the patient falls in a random manner. If unilateral vestibular impairment is present, the fall is to the paretic side or the direction of the nystagmus slow phases. The patient is asked to march in place and slowly rotates in the direction of Romberg fall. Past pointing is tested by having the outstretched arm come down on the examiner's finger with the eyes closed. The patient's finger deviates to the direction of Romberg fall.

Saccades may be dysmetric in cerebellar dysfunction and are best tested by having the patient look from lateral gaze to a medial target. Smooth pursuit may be tested by having the patient follow a slowly moving target. The eye movement should not break up into multiple jerky saccades. The patient is examined for nystagmus. Nystagmus may be pendular (symmetric in both directions) or jerk (rapid in one direction and slow in reverse). The fast component of jerk nystagmus is a corrective saccade. Optokinetic nystagmus is elicited by moving a series of targets across the visual field; a nystagmus ensues that is fast component in the direction from which the target is coming (as though the eye followed the target until it passed by and then moved to find a new one at the edge of the field). Asymmetric optokinetic responses are seen in parietal lobe disease. Endpoint nystagmus is also a physiologic nystagmus occurring in the direction of gaze. It should not be asymmetric and is not seen at less than 20° lateral gaze (when the limbus crosses the lachrymal puncta). Gaze-evoked nystagmus is the pathologic form and is seen in association with drugs, myasthenia, multiple sclerosis, and so forth. When the adducting eye is limited and there is dissociated nystagmus in the abducting eye, this reflects a median longitudinal fasciculus lesion commonly seen in multiple sclerosis. Positional nystagmus is not seen in the primary position (head and eyes facing forward) but is manifest in any other position. Vestibular nystagmus is always conjugate and is more evident in the direction of gaze of the fast component (away from the nonfunctioning vestibular system). Peripheral vestibular nystagmus is common, is always conjugate, is never vertical and is not usually pure horizontal, is reduced by visual fixation (fixation suppression), may be marked, and is often associated with tinnitus or deafness. Romberg fall, past pointing, and compass turn are in the direction of the slow phase, but subjective environmental spin is to the fast phase.

Provocative maneuvers are useful if a sensation is elicited that is comparable to the patient's subjective sensation. Both physician and patient are reassured that there is a mutual understanding of the patient's complaint. Orthostatic hypotension is sought by measuring pulse and blood pressure supine and after 3 minutes of standing. A potentiated Valsalva maneuver can be performed by having the patient squat, stand, and blow forcefully for 15 seconds. A limited Barany rotation in a swivel chair was described earlier, as was the limited ice water caloric test. The Nylan-Barany maneuver (also called the Dix-Hallpike) can be performed before the patient is placed supine for examinations. The patient's head is turned to one side 45° and the patient is brought down to a 45° hanging head position and observed for 1 minute. Typical nystagmus may appear after 15 to 20 seconds, associated with vertigo and fatigue in about 1 minute. The patient is then returned to the sitting position; vertigo and reversed nystagmus then appear after a similar delay. Fixation suppression may eliminate the nystagmus. The patient should avoid fixation, and Frenzel lenses should be used if available.

LABORATORY AND IMAGING STUDIES

Routine laboratory studies are not often helpful but should include a complete blood count and measurement of T4, TSH, GTT, SPEP, ANA, FTA-ABS, and lipids.

Audiometry is used if a vestibular mechanism is suspected. Routine pure-tone audiometry with air conduction, bone conduction, and masking is supplemented with impedance audiometry and tympanometry. The diagnostic audiologist should know that site-of-lesion testing is desired.

Short latency brain stem auditory evoked potentials (auditory evoked responses) play a major role in site-of-lesion testing. Electrodes are placed on the head and the far-field potentials are recorded. A repetitive click is the auditory stimulus, and time-locked signal averaging allows the resolution of the potentials elicited by the auditory stimulus from the more random electrical activity. The first five waves occur within less than 10 msec and are little affected by drugs or level of awareness. Despite lack of certainty about the specific generators, prolonged interwave latencies or loss of later waves can localize the pathology. An increase in wave 1 to 3 interwave latency is a sensitive test for acoustic neuroma; a wave 3 to 5 prolongation indicates intrinsic brain stem pathology.

Electronystagmography allows observation of nystagmus behind closed lids and recording of eye movements, and a more leisurely and quantitative analysis becomes possible. This is because a corneal-retinal potential difference makes the eye a dipole and allows electrical tracking of eye movements. Variability is present, and this is really only a semiquantitative test. The tests usually performed include a search for pathologic nystagmus with changes in gaze position, head position, and fixation. Saccades, smooth pursuit, and optokinetic nystagmus are usually tested to assess central oculomotor control systems. The VOR is studied by a bithermal caloric test. Major findings include unilateral canal paresis in unilateral vestibular dysfunction, as in vestibular neuritis or acoustic neuroma; bilateral canal paresis of ototoxicity; failure of fixation suppression of central pathology; or the classical Hallpike response of benign paroxysmal positional vertigo.

Rotational or sinusoidal testing is better tolerated than caloric stimulation and is good at detecting bilateral canal paresis and failure of fixation suppression. It does poorly with unilateral vestibular dysfunction, is expensive, and has limited clinical use.

Posturography is a test of the vestibulospinal reflex. The patient stands on a force platform and undergoes a computer analysis of Romberg sway. Linear acceleration stimuli and shifts in platform angle and visual surround provoke compensatory force shifts that can be analyzed. The use of this test is increasing, but its utility has not been fully defined.

Thin-cut computed tomography through the internal auditory canal allows visualization of small intracanalicular acoustic neuromas but has been surpassed by magnetic resonance imaging, which does not suffer from bone artifact. The cochlea and semicircular canals, as well as the eighth nerve, can be seen on imaging studies, but these have little relevance to most patients with dizziness.

TREATMENT

Spatial disorientation and postural instability are frightening by themselves but are accompanied by dread of a more ominous cause. Despite the distressing lack of therapeutic accompaniment to the growing sophistication of research in vestibular and oculomotor physiology, the physician can provide a careful explanation of the basis of the patient's complaint. There is a powerful therapeutic effect to the explanation of what the patient is experiencing and what is not happening. Learning about vestibular compensation may sustain a patient through a trying time.

The acutely vertiginous patient must lie still with sedation and antiemetics and fluids as needed. As soon as the nausea and vomiting have subsided enough, the patient should be mobilized to promote early vestibular compensation. Excessive sedation or maintenance therapy should be avoided with recurrent attacks in favor of standby therapy. Medication is often given inappropriately for positional vertigo, even though the symptoms usually subside before the medication takes effect, and the medication may delay vestibular compensation. Physical therapy is probably preferable.

Pharmacologic Measures

There is a balanced spontaneous firing rate of the vestibular primary afferent neurons and transmission of this through the vestibular nuclei. Transmission from primary to secondary vestibular neurons is thought to be cholinergic. A cholinergic facilitatory reticulovestibular system is balanced by a monoaminergic inhibitory reticulospinal system. An imbalance in the spontaneous firing rate could be corrected by suppressing both sides' spontaneous firing. Anticholinergic drugs can do this but are limited by mental status changes as well as the more common dry mouth, constipation, prostatism, and glaucoma. Transdermal scopolamine (0.5 mg three times daily) is effective for motion sickness when instituted several hours before anticipated exposure. Inadvertent ophthalmic contamination because of lack of sufficient care in handling the disc can cause mydriasis, visual impairment, and anxiety.

Antihistamines are the most commonly prescribed agents, but their mode of action is unknown. Meclizine is usually given for vertigo and dimenhydrinate for motion sickness. Trimethobenzamide has antiemetic properties and may be more useful in acute vertigo. Adrenergic agents such as ephedrine may be adjunctive.

Phenothiazines have been used for their antiemetic properties. Chlorpromazine is a classic dopaminergic blocking agent with some antihistaminic and anticholinergic properties. It suppresses both the spontaneous vestibular and stimulation-induced firing rates and offers sedative and antiemetic effects. The use of prochlorperazine should be avoided because it can induce severe dystonic reactions as well as antiemetic effects. Butyrophenones are potent agents and can be used when others fail, bearing in mind the risk of extrapyramidal side effects. Benzodiazepines depress the spontaneous vestibular firing rate and interact with central pathways.

Vestibular compensation requires exposure to the vertiginous stimulus, and suppressant medication should be discontinued as soon as possible after the most severe symptoms have subsided.

Meniere disease is usually treated by salt restriction and the use of thiazides. Topical gentamicin may be used transtympanically in patients with bilateral disease over several weeks in a fashion designed to reduce vestibular function without ablation.

Patients with central vertigo are difficult to treat. If they fail to respond to benzodiazepines, a trial of acetazolamide may be used. Carbamazepine may be useful in patients with quick spins who fail to respond to other approaches.

Vestibular Physical Therapy

Since it became clear that vestibular compensation was facilitated by early exercise, Cooksey-Cawthorne exercises and the later Brandt modification have been used. Exposure to mismatch by eye, head, and body movements somehow leads to a restoration in the fragile balance in vestibular firing, presumably by restoration of the depressed spontaneous firing rate. It is not surprising that centrally mediated vertigo is helped less by vestibular compensation, which requires a central recalibration of sensory mismatch. This compensation requires cerebellar function and can be lost if a later cerebellar stroke occurs ("double hit"). Sedatives and alcohol can induce transient loss.

Positional vertigo can be managed by having the patient assume the appropriate ear-down supine position, hold it until the response fatigues, and then sit up to reelicit the responses. This is repeated until the response does not occur. This is done several times a day until symptoms improve. Patients are often so terrified of the symptoms that they will not hold the position, so sometimes a family member must assist. Whether this helps by shaking an otoconia loose or by vestibular compensation is unknown.

Surgical Therapies

Meniere disease may undergo spontaneous remission or respond to salt restriction or diuretics. When this fails, various procedures have been undertaken. The efficacy of endolymphatic sac shunting is questionable. Vestibular nerve section may preserve hearing, but this may be involved, and separation of vestibular from auditory nerves is not always feasible. When little or no residual hearing exists in unilateral disease, destructive labyrinthectomy may be undertaken. Medical ablation with streptomycin may also be used. When cupulolithiasis is unremitting, the posterior semicircular canal may be deafferented by singular nerve section, allowing preservation of hearing. "Disabling positional vertigo" is reportedly due to microvascular loops that compress the vestibular nerve; surgery has been done to correct this.

CONSIDERATIONS DURING PREGNANCY

Considerations relate primarily to possible orthostasis and hypoglycemia associated with pregnancy. Vascular tumors and arteriovenous malformations enlarge during pregnancy. Posterior fossa meningiomas and acoustic schwannomas might be involved in this enlargement, but this is unlikely.

BIBLIOGRAPHY

Baloh RW, Honrubia V. Clinical neurophysiology of the vestibular system, 2d ed. Philadelphia: FA Davis Co., 1990.

Brandt T. Vertigo: its multisensory syndromes. Great Britain: Springer-Verlag, 1991.

Hollander J. Dizziness. Sem Neurol 1987;7:317.

Jackler RK, Brachmann DE. Neurotology. St. Louis: Mosby, 1994.

Primary Care for Women, edited by Phyllis C. Leppert and Fred M. Howard. Lippincott-Raven Publishers, Philadelphia © 1997.

108
Seizures

GERALD W. HONCH

Epilepsy is a chronic heterogeneous neurologic condition characterized by abnormal electrical discharges in the brain, manifested clinically as two or more unprovoked seizures. It is clinically important to separate the observation of seizures from the diagnosis of epilepsy. Seizures arise from abnormal, paroxysmal electrical discharges of cerebral neurons. They are symptomatic of an underlying process affecting cortical electrical excitability. Seizures are the manifestation of this electrical excitability. Many conditions, such as infections, metabolic changes, or toxic states, may temporarily produce seizures. These are potentially treatable or reversible and once corrected will free the patient of the risk of further seizures. Epilepsy is characterized by recurrent seizures that are not provoked by a metabolic or toxic disturbance. The causes of epilepsy are diverse, and many types of epilepsy have been described. These are treatable conditions with an enlarging group of drugs at the clinician's disposal.

It is difficult to accurately examine the scope of this medical problem because of inability to identify all individuals with the disease. Reporting biases limit these data. The social stigma of these disorders causes individuals to be reluctant to report the condition. Those patients whose seizures are controlled with medication or who have not had a recent seizure may not report epilepsy as a medical problem in a survey. In data from the National Health Interview Survey (NHIS) of 1986 to 1990, approximately 1.1 million persons in the United States annually report having epilepsy. The overall prevalence of epilepsy is 4.7 cases per 1000 persons. The prevalence is lowest (3.1) for persons aged 65 years or older and highest (5.2) for persons aged 15 to 64 years. The age-adjusted prevalence is similar for women and men (5.1 and 4.2, respectively), and the age-specific pattern is consistent for both sexes. The age- and race-adjusted prevalence of epilepsy is similar among the regions of the country. The age-adjusted prevalence of epilepsy is higher for blacks (6.7) than whites (4.5). This pattern is similar for both black males and black females.

TERMS

The terms or language of epilepsy and epileptologists are confusing and require some definition:

- *Absence*—a brief lapse of consciousness
- *Antiepileptic*—drug or mechanism to prevent seizures
- *Aura*—the warning that precedes an epileptic seizure. Regarded as part of the seizure itself.
- *Clonic*—rhythmic motor activity alternating with motor relaxation
- *Cure*—a term not freely used by epileptologists. There is a certain reluctance to declare with absolute confidence that seizures will not recur. The clinical test lasts a lifetime.
- *Epileptogenic lesion*—a structural disturbance (such as a tumor or a scar) which gives rise to seizures.
- *Focal*—a single epileptic focus. May be bilateral or multifocal and independent. Contrast with diffuse or generalized (nonfocal).
- *Generalized seizures*—bilateral involvement of the brain
- *Grand mal*—an unfortunate and outdated term. Usually taken to mean seizures with loss of both consciousness and postural tone, both tonic and clonic components, tongue biting, incontinence. It is what most witnesses mean when they refer to a seizure. This is a "usual" or "regular" seizure.
- *Ictus*—the epileptic seizure itself
- *Major motor seizure*—this is the term that has replaced grand mal seizures
- *Partial seizures*—seizures that begin in a part of the brain or are limited to one hemisphere. *Simple* partial seizures do not impair consciousness. *Complex* partial seizures impair consciousness.
- *Petit mal*—an unfortunate and outdated term. Refers to a specific well-defined clinical event in children (absences) with characteristic EEG (electroencephalogram) features (3-per-second spike and wave). Does not mean "small" events.
- *Postictal*—transient clinical or electrophysiologic abnormalities in brain function that appear when the ictal event has ended. May last minutes to a day or two.
- *Pseudoseizure*—any nonepileptic event that resembles an epileptic seizure. Often a difficult and meddlesome task to clarify and treat. Also known as psychogenic seizures.
- *Secondary epileptogenesis*—when focal epileptogenic abnormalities give rise to distant epileptogenic zones. Also may be referred to as "kindling".
- *Seizure free*—when the patient is no longer having seizures. Not considered "cured" but is used to denote a clinical state without detectable epileptic events.
- *Temporal lobe seizures*—also known as psychomotor seizures. Another unfortunate and outdated set of terms. Modern terminology uses partial complex seizures with focal identification or limbic descriptors.
- *Tonic*—sustained motor activity without rhythmic phenomena. May produce a slow or sustained motor manifestation such as a posture or position.

CLASSIFICATION

A classification of the various seizure types serves many purposes. The most important purpose is an effort to define by type for ease of understanding of the patient's symptoms. Proper identification improves the clarity of communication regarding a specific seizure type. The treatment choices may be directed by the type of seizure experienced. The success of treatment is closely linked to the appropriate choice of anticonvulsant for the seizure type encountered.

The International League Against Epilepsy published the first International Classification of Epileptic Seizures in 1970. This was revised in 1981 (Table 108-1). It is based on distinctive behavioral

Table 108-1. International Classification of Epileptic Seizures

Partial (focal, local) Seizures

A. Simple partial seizures
 1. With motor signs
 2. With somatosensory or special sensory symptoms
 3. With autonomic symptoms or signs
 4. With psychic symptoms

B. Complex partial seizures
 1. Simple partial onset followed by impairment of consciousness
 2. With impairment of consciousness at onset

C. Partial seizures evolving to secondarily generalized seizures
 1. Simple partial seizures evolving to generalized seizures
 2. Complex partial seizures evolving to generalized seizures
 3. Simple partial seizures evolving to complex partial seizures evolving to generalized seizures

Generalized Seizures (convulsive or non-convulsive)

A. Absence seizures
 1. Typical absences
 2. Atypical absences

B. Myoclonic seizures

C. Clonic seizures

D. Tonic seizures

E. Tonic–clonic seizures

F. Atonic seizures (astatic seizures)

Unclassified Epileptic Seizures

(From Commission on Classification and Terminology of the International League Against Epilepsy. Epilepsia 1981;22:489. Reproduced with permission of the publishers.)

and electrophysiologic features of the epileptic ictal events. This classification does not specify pathophysiologic mechanisms or anatomical substrates. It uses impairment of consciousness as the sole means of distinguishing between simple and complex partial seizures. In addition, it takes into account the symptom progressions that characterize most epileptic seizures. Alternative classifications may be more useful clinically for those working in the field.

ETIOLOGY

Epilepsy can be classified by etiology or by clinical manifestation. Epilepsy with a cause is referred to as symptomatic or secondary epilepsy. Epilepsy without an identifiable cause is referred to as idiopathic epilepsy. This distinction may be clinically important because treatment or relief of the cause of the seizures may improve or favorably affect the ultimate treatment with anticonvulsants.

A seizure may be provoked in any normal individual given the right combination of circumstances. There are individual differences in the threshold for seizures, however. One might think of this threshold as a level which might be raised or lowered depending on various circumstances. The resting state of neuronal excitability and synchronization plus the rapidity of change in the basal state determine the point at which a seizure occurs. In addition, one can consider a number of inhibiting mechanisms which may exert a protective effect. This threshold is not a static phenomenon and changes with maturation and biochemical factors. The incidence of seizures is higher in the very young and the aged.

In some patients there is a genetic susceptibility for seizures. This is a nonspecific susceptibility (aside from inherited metabolic disorders). There is an increased susceptibility to epileptiform EEG patterns and epileptic seizures among first degree relatives of individuals with epilepsy. A genetic basis for nonspecific seizure susceptibility is now generally accepted. A precise genetic model has not been found, hence the manifestation of epileptiform EEG abnormalities or seizures requires the interplay of both genetic and environmental factors. Genetic traits may underlie specific epileptogenic disturbances (eg, the 3-cycle-per-second spike-and-wave EEG discharge or photosensitivity).

Fluctuations in the threshold for seizures occur with normal biological rhythms. Circadian rhythms are related to diurnal cycles in hormone levels or to alterations in neuronal activity accompanying sleep and wakefulness. Some patients may have seizures predominantly in wakefulness and others predominantly during sleep. A particularly vulnerable time for seizures is in the transition or twilight period as one is going to sleep or awakening. Longer cyclical fluctuations in threshold can also occur. A common example of this is catamenial epilepsy. There is an increase in seizure occurrence in women around the time of menses due largely to changes in estrogen and progesterone levels. There is a premenstrual and an ovulatory exacerbation of seizures. Estrogen appears to lower seizure threshold and progesterone raises seizure threshold. Epilepsy also has an effect on hormone levels and function. There may be an interplay between antiepileptic drugs, hepatic enzyme systems, and birth control medication, which may lead to birth control failure and the need for a higher dose of hormone replacement. There are potentially persistent interictal effects of seizures leading to reproductive endocrine disorders. Menstrual disorders occur in more than 50% of women with epilepsy. Amenorrhea occurs in 14% to 20% of women with epilepsy (oligomenorrhea in 20%). Prolonged or shortened menstrual cycles occur in 20%.

Environmental factors may alter the capacity of cerebral neurons to be excited or synchronized. Seizure threshold may be raised or lowered by various means. Nonspecific factors such as systemic illness, psychologic stress, sleep deprivation, alcohol or sedative drug withdrawal, and fever may all lower seizure threshold and precipitate an event. Certain drugs, such as the neuroleptics and antidepressants, are not likely to cause seizures in nonepileptic persons, but can increase the risk of seizures in those in whom specific epileptogenic factors exist. Other drugs, such as cocaine or amphetamines, may produce a seizure at the time of use in an otherwise healthy individual who is not predisposed to epilepsy.

Acquired brain lesions may lower or raise seizure threshold in certain cerebral areas. Often, focal seizures are the result of focal injuries to the cerebral cortex. The cortical scarring and cortical irritation from traumatic injury is the most common example. Other focal cortical injuries, such as those of cerebral infarction, 10% to 15% of stroke patients, regions affected by arteriovenous malformation (berry aneurysms, Sturge-Weber syndrome), multiple sclerosis, and other disorders, are associated with an increased risk of epilepsy. Hypertensive encephalopathy is considered the cause of seizures in toxemia of pregnancy. The residual pathological changes in the cerebral cortex can act as a focus for chronic epilepsy. Seizures can also occur with blood dyscrasias (sickle cell anemia and coagulopathies) and the perivascular infiltrates due to leukemia and cerebral disturbances induced by collagen vascular diseases.

Seizures occur in 20% to 70% of patients with various types of intracranial tumors. It is possible that small, unrecognized tumors account for a higher percentage of focal epileptic disorders. Magnetic resonance imaging (MRI) has been particularly valuable in demonstrating small lesions in difficult to evaluate areas such as the mesial temporal lobes. Meningiomas and arachnoid cysts produce seizures by irritation rather than by destruction. Malignant tumors are more aggressive and are associated with areas of high vascularity and tumor necrosis, which may contribute to cortical irritability. Hamartomas and nonneoplastic masses consist of abnormal mixtures of vascular, glial, and neuronal tissue that may give rise to seizures. Hamartomas are occasionally encountered in temporal lobe tissue removed from patients with complex partial seizures. Tubers are disorganized collections of large pleomorphic astrocytes, often with calcification; these are also occasionally encountered in temporal lobe tissue removed from patients with partial complex seizures. The acute infections associated with meningitis, encephalitis, or abscess commonly precipitate seizures. Cortical irritation, local metabolic changes, reduced glucose levels, and cellular changes all contribute to this production. Chronic infections or more indolent infections can cause seizures. The most common cause of focal seizures in Latin America is cysticercosis. Syphilis is returning as an important cause of seizures. Today, acquired immunodeficiency syndrome (AIDS) is an important cause of neurologic symptoms in adults and children. Opportunistic infections, lymphomas, and AIDS encephalopathy can manifest with epileptic seizures.

Acquired degenerative diseases are occasionally associated with epileptic seizures. Two percent of patients with multiple sclerosis have seizures. Patients with presenile and senile dementia of the Alzheimer's type have a 10-fold increase in the incidence of seizures. Local degenerative changes may cause seizures.

Hippocampal sclerosis is the most common lesion encountered in patients with complex partial seizures. The cause of this change is debated. These changes alone may cause seizures. It has been postulated that hippocampal sclerosis results from epileptic activity. It has been suggested that prolonged febrile convulsions (commonly reported in the history of patients with complex partial seizures) may produce hippocampal damage. Later in life, this structural abnormality itself becomes an epileptogenic lesion.

HISTORY

The clinical story or history is absolutely essential in establishing a diagnosis of a seizure disorder. The history is usually obtained from an observer and even retold through multiple well-meaning sources. There is no substitute for questioning the primary observer. Seizures are dramatic and frightening to witnesses. The records are often incomplete and mixed with the emotional contributions of the observer. The patient may be able to provide valuable information regarding the prodrome or period of time before the event. In addition, the patient may be able to give statements documenting the period of time in recovery from the postictal state. An eyewitness account is usually more reliable than the patient account.

The course of events during a seizure must be recorded logically and concisely. It is never reasonable to accept a diagnosis of a seizure disorder without sifting through the events that took place, no matter how well-qualified or well-intentioned the historian is. A video recording done by family members is particularly valuable and may be analyzed repeatedly by multiple persons. It is very easy to be misled by a wrong diagnosis. The obvious consequences of this are multiple: the correct treatment is not given, various social and financial problems are invited, and the true diagnosis is missed.

It is best to start with the circumstances under which the event occurred: the time of day, the activity of the patient, the general health and condition of the patient, and any contributing circumstances. What was the effect of the episode on consciousness? How long did the event last? Has there been more than one type of event? Stress, sleep deprivation, fatigue, alcohol, drugs, hunger, or bizarre dietary changes may be important.

Was there an aura (warning) or prodrome to the event? Is this warning a recognizable phenomenon that might be useful to predicting or recognizing another event? The usual questions asked relate to olfactory sensations (usually unpleasant), odd tastes, abdominal discomfort, or a rising sensation (in the genital areas). Some visual disturbances occur such as visual distortions of size, shape, color, or form. Were there formed or unformed hallucinations? Was there "forced thinking" (the patient may experience repeated or stereotyped thinking patterns or memories)? Some of these are quite unusual such as a fragment of music, a voice, or a familiar dialogue. Visual or auditory experiences are not usually volunteered by patients out of embarrassment or fear. Feelings of familiarity (such as déjà vu, déjà entendu, and déjà vécu) or strangeness (jamais vu, jamais entendu, jamais vécu) occur in partial complex seizures. Fear is the most common affective symptom.

The observer must record the duration of the event and note the evolution of activity within an event. Focal clonic or tonic movements or forced versive deviations of the limbs or eyes may give an important clue to the origin of the epileptiform activity. Attention should be paid to the number and variety of seizure types. Is there some cycling or clustering of seizures?

The past history needs careful scrutiny. Birth history with gestational risks and the delivery should be explored. A history of past head trauma or surgical procedures on the central nervous system (CNS) may be relevant. Is there a relationship to other CNS disorders? Are there known medical disorders (eg, systemic lupus erythematosus) that might be the genesis for seizures? Is there a family history of a seizure disorder?

PHYSICAL EXAMINATION

The general physical examination may give clues to systemic illnesses which might predispose the patient to seizures. In both the acute and nonacute settings the general physical examination may yield useful signs of such disorders as infection, hypertension, drug intoxication, metabolic disturbances. In addition, signs of trauma must be noted. The skin may give an indication of a phakomatosis (eg, the port-wine stain of Sturge-Weber Syndrome, the café-au-lait spots of neurofibromatosis, or the ash leaf spots and shagreen patches of tuberous sclerosis). Inspection of the scalp and palpation of the skull may reveal evidence of trauma or prior surgical procedures.

The neurologic examination is often normal in the patient with idiopathic epilepsy. Focal or lateralized features can help distinguish partial from generalized epileptic disorders. Careful examination during the immediate postictal period may reveal diagnostically useful fleeting focal or lateralized dysfunction that would not be apparent later. Findings of minimal brain dysfunction such as clumsiness, synkinesis, abnormal posturing of the hands, hyperreflexia, and mild mental retardation or dementia may support a diagnosis of secondary rather than primary epilepsy. Memory disturbances can result from the epileptogenic lesion itself and are often exacerbated by antiepileptic drug effects. It is important to remember that a postictal Todd paralysis or phenomenon (focal paralysis following a seizure) usually does not last longer than 24 to 48 hours.

LABORATORY AND IMAGING STUDIES

The laboratory studies should be tailored to the needs and presentation of the patient. In an acute setting with a first convulsive episode, the laboratory workup is generally more extensive. In the patient with an established seizure disorder, the laboratory workup is more specific.

In the acute setting, the following studies are helpful: complete blood count, electrolytes, glucose, liver and renal screen, urinalysis, and calcium. A serum magnesium is generally not considered useful. A lumbar puncture is done if the history and physical examination suggest that the cerebrospinal fluid might be helpful in establishing another diagnosis. A toxic screen of blood and urine is helpful in selected patients. The serum prolactin is elevated after complex partial and generalized seizures (should be drawn within 20 minutes of the episode). Serum levels of anticonvulsant drugs are very helpful in providing guidance for treating the patient with an established seizure disorder.

The EEG is the single most informative laboratory test for the diagnosis of epilepsy. This is a noninvasive, benign, and relatively inexpensive test. An EEG should be performed in every patient with suspected epilepsy. There is no reason to decrease antiepileptic medication before obtaining an EEG. There is no justification for routinely repeated EEGs at specific intervals without asking specific questions. The EEG can be useful to help establish the following:

- Does the patient have epilepsy? The EEG will help distinguish seizures from other conditions.
- What kind of epilepsy does the patient have? Certain EEG patterns may be very helpful in establishing characteristic types of epilepsy and this knowledge will guide the selection of specific drugs.
- The EEG can help establish signs of drug toxicity. In some instances the EEG is useful as a guide to therapy. For instance, the EEG is indispensable in following the treatment of the patient with status epilepticus.
- The EEG is useful for establishing the location of the interictal EEG spike discharges. This is helpful for locating the focal nature of the electrical activity.

A variety of EEG protocols exist. In a routine study the electrode placement, the duration of the examination, and the use of activation procedures such as hyperventilation and photic stimulation are well-established. Sleep studies are useful to help activate interictal EEG spike activity. Special monitoring facilities for all-night recording or long-term monitoring are available in certain laboratories. Special monitoring facilities are equipped with video facilities in conjunction with simultaneous EEG recording. Additional recording electrodes may be used (eg, nasopharyngeal, sphenoidal). CT (computed tomography) and MRI are useful in demonstrating focal structural lesions of the CNS. A CT scan is cheaper, more often available on an emergency basis, and is generally superior to a MRI in demonstrating hemorrhage or a meningioma. A MRI scan is vastly superior for demonstrating subtle lesions of the mesial temporal lobe as well as vascular lesions (such as an arteriovenous malformation).

TREATMENT

Once the diagnosis of epilepsy is made, long-term treatment with antiepileptic drugs needs to be designed. The goal is to achieve complete seizure control with a minimum of adverse side effects. The cost of medication is also an important consideration in the current era of cost containment. It is well to remember that these medications range from relatively inexpensive to amounts that are enormous when considered over a lifetime of anticonvulsant use. The primary antiepileptic drugs in use today include phenytoin, carbamazepine, valproate, ethosuximide, phenobarbital, and primidone. Newer agents available today include felbamate, gabapentin and lamotrigine. No drug is able to control all seizure types and there is not a drug free of the potential for adverse side effects. Careful selection of the initial antiepileptic drug is based on the identification of the seizure type and the epilepsy syndrome as discussed earlier. Monitoring symptoms as well as drug levels is necessary in a patient with epilepsy. Any anticonvulsant used in subtherapeutic amounts cannot be expected to be effective. The fewer the number of agents being used, the simpler the management scheme.

A thorough appreciation of the medication being used is mandatory in these patients. Anticipation of the problems that may be encountered and the idiosyncrasies of each anticonvulsant being used cannot be emphasized strongly enough. Uncontrolled seizures and disabling side effects will contribute to a compromised quality of life. The patient as well as the physician need to be well informed.

Compliance is a major problem in the treatment of these patients. Poor compliance is often linked to psychological issues. Loss of control over one's health, resentment over the need to take medication, and dependence on medication to lead a normal life are all very real issues to the patient. Denial of illness is very common initially. Lack of understanding of the nature of epilepsy and the proper use of medication are educational issues that the physician must return to over and over again. The social stigmata associated with epilepsy alter the way these patients live and relate to the world in diverse ways, including school, job and career selection, marriage, sports, driving, and living independently. Discrimination is still commonplace.

The vast majority of patients (50% to 80%) will achieve adequate control of their seizures with a minimum of side effects, using only a single drug effectively. There is a role for polypharmacy, but this should be the exceptional case, not the rule. Proper selection of the most effective agent for the correct seizure type is the first step. Table 108-2 lists the major antiepileptic drugs in use today along with their major indications. This list includes some of the newer agents currently in use.

Knowledge of the pharmacokinetics of each drug is necessary to prescribe both the dose and the timing of each dose. Table 108-3 lists these same drugs with notation of the half-life of each one. Drugs with a long half-life may be given once or twice per day. Drugs with a relatively short half-life will need dosing multiple times per day to avoid wide peak and trough variability. The same concept applies to obtaining drug levels; it is generally best to obtain drug levels at the estimated trough time (in the morning). In this way a consistent pattern of analysis is accomplished.

Table 108-2. Drugs for Treatment of Epilepsy

DRUG	PRIMARY AGENT	ADJUNCTIVE AGENT	USED FOR PARTIAL SEIZURES	SECONDARY GENERALIZED	COMMENTS
Carbamazepine	Yes	—	Yes	Yes	—
Clonazepam	Yes	—	—	—	Useful for myoclonic seizures
Ethosuximide	Yes	—	—	—	Useful for petit mal epilepsy
Phenobarbital	Yes	—	Yes	Yes	
Phenytoin	Yes	—	Yes	Yes	
Primidone	Yes	—	Yes	Yes	
Valproic acid	Yes	—	±	Yes	
Felbamate	Yes	Yes	Yes	—	
Gabapentin	No	Yes	Yes	Yes	
Lamotrigine	No	Yes	Yes	—	

Protein binding is more important for some drugs than others. Those drugs with a high degree of protein binding will be affected in those states that affect serum protein (eg, renal failure, pregnancy). It may be necessary to obtain free levels in these special circumstances.

The therapeutic range is meant as a guide, not an absolutely rigid set of numbers. Fixation on achieving these numbers is often difficult to overcome in both the physician and the patient. The pharmacokinetics of these drugs is not a straight line function (first order kinetics). With the majority of antiepileptic drugs zero order kinetics prevail. In zero order kinetics saturation of the enzyme necessary for drug metabolism occurs. The serum drug level then increases exponentially with the increasing dose. After a certain point, very small changes in dose result in very large changes in serum drug levels. It is the physician's mission to control the seizures with the least number of side effects; it is very easy to slip from the therapeutic to toxic range with only a minor increase in medication. Levels are most useful in sorting out questions of toxicity and compliance, as well as planning and monitoring the effects of changes in dose. Steady state levels are reached roughly after a period of five half-lives of the drug in question. This is a very useful guide for monitoring drug levels after a dosage adjustment.

In the acute situation the question of "loading" the patient needs to be considered. Certainly in the patient with status epilepticus or frequent seizures, loading the patient with anticonvulsants is a practical and necessary step. In most patients with a single seizure, loading is unnecessary. Loading with antiepileptic drugs is done generally only with those agents with a relatively long half-life (phenytoin and phenobarbital). The other antiepileptic drugs with short half-lives do not lend themselves to this use (carbamazepine). With short half-lives, the threshold to toxicity is reached quickly. It is also important to remember that certain agents (such as carbamazepine) gradually induce hepatic enzyme systems to higher levels over days to weeks. Hence, the early doses of these agents need to be smaller with titration to higher dose regimens gradually.

Drug interactions are complex both within the family of drugs used to control epilepsy as well as drugs which may be used along with antiepileptic drugs. The effect may be to enhance or retard the metabolism of the drugs being used. Hence, the addition of another agent may render the levels of anticonvulsant subtherapeutic or toxic, depending on the drugs in question. In other situations there is no apparent interaction. Careful selection of antiepileptic drugs, and their interactions with other antiepileptic drugs as well as other drugs, is essential. A safe practice should always include a referral to a source to address these possibilities.

The case of the single seizure is an important and difficult area. With a single unprovoked seizure, the patient does not have epilepsy by definition and does not warrant treatment with anticonvulsant drugs. These patients with isolated seizures have a 16%

Table 108-3. Drugs for Epilepsy: Pharmacokinetics

DRUG	HALF LIFE (H)	PERCENTAGE OF DRUG PROTEIN BOUND	THERAPEUTIC RANGE (mg/mL)	RELATIVE COST PER MONTH (DOLLARS)
Carbamazepine	6–12	72–76	6–12	60
Clonazepam	24–36	50–80	0.025–0.075	90
Ethosuximide	30–70	0	40–100	90
Phenobarbital	70–100	60	15–30	5
Phenytoin	15–24	90	10–20	20
Primidone	12	0	5–15	40
Valproic acid	8–10	95	50–100	90
Felbamate	20–23	22–25	Not established	120
Gabapentin	5–7	<3	Not established	150
Lamotrigine	12–48	55	Not established	160

to 61% chance for recurrent seizures. The likelihood of recurrence is increased in the following situations:

- Patients with remote symptomatic neurologic disease
- A family history of epilepsy
- Partial complex seizures
- Abnormal findings on a neurological examination
- An abnormal EEG.

If seizures are going to recur, they will do so within 1 year. The longer the patient remains seizure free (measured in years), the lower the tendency for recurrence. After a patient has had a second unprovoked seizure, the risk of recurrence is high (79% to 90%).

The question of when and how to discontinue antiepileptic drugs is never easily answered. There are no absolutes to address this question and the "test" or trial off antiepileptics lasts for the lifetime of the patient. However, some general guidelines are quite helpful. The longer the duration of seizure control with antiepileptic drugs, the better the prognosis. The greatest chance for successful drug withdrawal is associated with:

- No seizures for 2 to 5 years on antiepileptic drugs
- A single type of seizure (either partial or generalized)
- Normal neurological examination
- Normal IQ
- EEG that is normalized with treatment.

The question of generic substitution for antiepileptic medication is a frequently asked question of the patient and the third-party payment system. Cost containment is the issue. This cost spread over the lifetime of the patient can be enormous. Table 108-3 provides a list of the relative range of costs for the various antiepileptic agents in use.

Current Federal Drug Administration guidelines assume that bioavailability can vary safely by 20%. There is no scientific evidence that this, or any other range of variability, can be tolerated safely by patients with epilepsy. There are three pharmacologic risk factors to consider: low water solubility, a narrow therapeutic range, and nonlinear pharmacokinetics. With generic preparations there may be variations in time to maximum blood level after each dose. Variability in shelf life may be questioned.

With generic substitution neither the patient nor the physician is kept informed about which manufacturer's generic formulation is actually dispensed at a particular time. There may be multiple manufacturers for a single agent, each with differing binding or coloring agents, differing dissolution and absorption times, differing bioavailability, and differing time to maximum serum concentration. Generic substitution can only be approved if safety and efficacy are not compromised.

The special case of convulsive status epilepticus has been a subject of controversy and special study. The outcome is often linked to the etiology. The setting in which this occurs is important. In patients with life-threatening illnesses such as anoxia or CNS infection, the outcome is less favorable. In patients with status epilepticus as their first manifestation of a seizure disorder or in patients who have suffered an abrupt reduction in their antiepileptic drugs, the outcome is more favorable. Over half of the patients with status epilepticus will respond to therapy with a single agent. Status associated with an acute or progressive neurological disorder is more likely to be refractory.

As with any unresponsive patient, the initial management of status epilepticus includes the ABCs of life support: supporting respiration (**a**irway), maintaining **b**lood pressure, gaining access to **c**irculation, and when possible, identifying and treating the probable cause. Fluid management, electrolyte and glucose levels, and temperature all need to be addressed. Simply correcting a fever may be helpful in stopping the seizure activity.

The goal of therapy is the rapid termination of the clinical and electrical seizure activity. The longer an episode of status epilepticus goes untreated, the more difficult it is to control with medication. There is no substitute for a clear plan of treatment, prompt administration of effective drugs in adequate doses, and attention to the possibility of apnea or hypoventilation. Neuromuscular paralysis without administration of antiepileptic drugs is inappropriate because sustained brain electrical discharges can cause irreversible brain injury. Intramuscular therapy has no place in treating status epilepticus or seizures in general. Drugs should be administered by the IV route only.

Table 108-4 provides a simple comparison of available agents for the treatment of status epilepticus. These should only be given under conditions of close monitoring such as in an intensive care

Table 108-4. Drugs for Status Epilepticus

	DIAZEPAM	LORAZEPAM	PHENYTOIN	PHENOBARBITAL	MIDAZOLAM
Adult IV dose, mg/kg	0.15–0.25	0.1	15–20	20	Bolus of 200 μg/kg followed by continuous infusion of 0.75–10 μg/kg/min
Max. admin. rate mg/min	5	2.0	50	100	
Time to stop status (minutes)	1–3	6–10	10–30	20–30	>5
Effective duration of action (hours)	0.25–0.5	>12–24	24	>48	Titrate
Elimination half-life (hours)	30	14	24	100	1.5–3.5
Side effects					
Depression of consciousness	10–30 min.	Hours	None	Days	Yes
Respiratory depression	Yes	Yes	Rare	Yes	Yes
Hypotension	Rare	Rare	Yes	Rare	Rare
Cardiac arrhythmias	No	No	With history of heart disease	No	No

Table 108-5. Special Effects of Antiepileptic Agents

DRUG	TERATOGENICITY	EXCRETED IN BREAST MILK
Carbamazepine	Spina bifida	Yes
Clonazepam	Unclear	Yes
Ethosuximide	High prevalence of severe birth defects, physical anomalies, growth and mental retardation	Yes
Phenobarbital	Cleft lip and palate; congenital heart and urogenital defects	Yes
Phenytoin	Cleft lip and palate; congenital heart and urogenital defects	Yes
Primidone	Adds to phenobarbital risk	Yes
Valproic Acid	Spina bifida, cardiovascular and urogenital malformations	Yes
Gabapentin	Unknown	Unknown
Lamotrigine	Unknown	Yes
Felbamate	Unknown	Yes

unit or emergency department where ventilatory support is immediately available. Diazepam is probably the most popular agent available and is extremely rapid in its onset. Diazepam suffers in that it is no longer effective to prevent seizures in 15 to 30 minutes. Hence, the seizure activity tends to recur. Lorazepam does not have as rapid an affect as does diazepam, but is very fast. The major advantage of lorazepam is the duration of action. Several hours of anticonvulsant effect can be achieved. As the seizure activity comes under control, a longer acting agent such as phenytoin should be added promptly.

Recently, midazolam has been suggested for cases of refractory generalized status epilepticus. This is reserved for very special circumstances where the patient has had prolonged convulsive status epilepticus unresponsive to standard doses of intravenous benzodiazepines, phenytoin, and phenobarbital. Midazolam is given as a slow bolus followed by a continuous infusion for several hours. EEG monitoring is recommended to follow the seizure activity. An adjustment of the maintenance dose to stop electrographic seizures is based on EEG monitoring. Phenytoin and phenobarbital are continued as maintenance medications. The midazolam is discontinued after about 12 hours while clinically monitoring the patient and the EEG for further clinical or electrographic seizure activity.

CONSIDERATIONS IN PREGNANCY

Concern for the teratogenic potential of antiepileptic drugs has reached the awareness of both the medical and the lay community. It is estimated that one in 250 newborns is exposed to antiepileptic drugs in utero. The risks include major malformations, minor anomalies intrauterine, or postnatal growth failure and psychomotor retardation. The absolute risk is that 7% to 10% of these children exposed to antiepileptic drugs will have these defects. This risk is two or three times higher than the general population. The more serious effects include congenital heart malformations (with phenytoin and phenobarbital) and neural tube defects (with valproate and carbamazepine).

There is concern that there may be a genetic predisposition for some of these defects in certain families. The children of mothers with epilepsy (treated or untreated with antiepileptic drugs) tend to have slightly more minor anomalies than do children of fathers with epilepsy or control subjects. The effects of tonic–clonic seizures on the fetus during pregnancy are not well established. Physical injury to the mother, hypoxia, and hypotension, as well as antiepileptic drugs, may all make significant contributions to that risk. No information is available as to which of the four major antiepileptic drugs (phenytoin, carbamazepine, valproate, or phenobarbital) is the most teratogenic or which causes the most major malformations. Table 108-5 lists the major antiepileptic drugs in use today and their associated potential teratogenic effects. The risk to the fetus is greatest in the first trimester.

Controversy exists over the contribution of folic acid to the birth defect equation. Some have suggested that antiepileptic drugs cause neural tube defects by interfering with folic acid metabolism. After one child has been born with a neural tube defect, supplementation with folic acid (4 mg per day at least 1 month before conception) can reduce the risk of recurrence of neural tube defects in subsequent children from 3.5% to 0.7%. It is safer to recommend that the diets of all women who might bear children contain adequate amounts of folic acid, that all women with epilepsy who are under treatment with antiepileptic drugs receive folic acid daily, and that pregnant women with epilepsy receiving antiepileptic drugs have normal folic acid concentrations determined in serum and red blood cells.

The risk of teratogenicity increases with:

- High daily dose of an antiepileptic drug
- High serum antiepileptic drug levels
- Polypharmacy
- Low folate levels (neural tube defects).

It is important that adequate preconception as well as prenatal counseling be given. More than 90% of women with epilepsy who receive antiepileptic drugs during pregnancy will deliver a normal child free of birth defects. Some simple measures are suggested:

- Discussion and knowledge of potential risk *before* conception
- A realistic and accurate risk potential weighed against alternatives to antiepileptic drugs
- A discussion of diet and assurance of adequate folate
- Seizure control with monotherapy if possible
- If seizure free for at least 2 years, consider withdrawal of antiepileptic drugs
- Lowest antiepileptic drug dose and plasma level that protects against seizures.

During pregnancy the serum antiepileptic drug levels may vary. Altering the dose should be done after consideration of clinical issues, not simply a serum level of antiepileptic drugs. The reasons for fluctuation of serum levels are increased hepatic and renal clearance rates, reduced albumin levels, plasma protein binding of increased levels of unbound drug, and increased plasma volume by the third trimester.

During labor and delivery, a tonic–clonic seizure occurs in 1% to 2% of women with epilepsy. Maintenance of adequate levels of antiepileptic drugs is important during this time when doses may be missed. Attention to the half-life of these drugs (see Table 108-3) will provide a guide to dosing frequency. After delivery, the antiepileptic drug dosages must be returned to prepregnancy levels during the first few weeks of the puerperium to avoid toxicity.

All antiepileptic drugs are present in breast milk (see Table 108-5). The concentration depends on the degree of protein binding in the serum of the mother (the higher the protein binding the less the drug is available for secretion into breast milk (see Table 108-3). Sedation of the infant may be a problem with agents that have sedative potential. Breast-feeding is not recommended with clonazepam or the newer agents (felbamate, gabapentin and lamotrigine). Reported concentrations of antiepileptic drugs in breast milk range from 10% to 80% of the maternal serum levels.

Antiepileptic drugs may induce hepatic microsomal enzymes enough to alter the metabolism of oral contraceptive agents. Breakthrough bleeding may be an early sign of this interference. The effectiveness of the oral contraceptive may be threatened; hence, a higher hormone dose in the oral contraceptive may be necessary. In addition, a similar mechanism of enzyme induction by oral contraceptives may reduce the serum levels of antiepileptic drugs and cause an increased frequency of seizures. Adjustments of antiepileptic drug levels may need to be made when oral contraceptives are started or adjusted.

BIBLIOGRAPHY

Abramowicz M. Drugs for epilepsy. The Medical Letter 1995;37(947):37.

Cascino GD. Epilepsy: contemporary perspectives on evaluation and treatment. Mayo Clin Proc 1994;69:1199.

Commission on Classification and Terminology of the International League Against Epilepsy. Revised clinical and electroencephalographic classification of epileptic seizures. Epilepsia 1981;22:489.

Delgado-Escueta AV, Janz D. Consensus guidelines: preconception counseling, management and care of the pregnant woman with epilepsy. Neurology 1992;42(suppl 5):149.

Devinsky O, Yerby M, eds. Women with epilepsy: reproduction and effects of pregnancy on epilepsy. Philadelphia: WB Saunders, 1994.

Dodson WE, Lorenzo RJ, Pedley TA, Shinnar S, Treiman DM, Wannamaker BB. Treatment of convulsive status epilepticus. JAMA 1993;270(7):854.

Donaldson JO. Epilepsy. In: Donaldson JO, ed. Neurology of pregnancy. Philadelphia: WB Saunders, 1989:229.

Engle J. Seizures and epilepsy. Philadelphia: FA Davis, 1989.

Prevalence of self-reported epilepsy—United States, 1986-1990. JAMA 1994:272(24):1993.

Krumholz A. Epilepsy in pregnancy. In: Goldstein PJ, Stern BJ, eds. Neurological disorders of pregnancy. Mount Kisco, NY: Futura Publishing Co, 1992:25.

Kumar A, Bleck TP. Intravenous midazolam for the treatment of refractory status epilepticus. Crit Care Med 1992;20:483.

Leis AA, Ross MA, Summers AK. Psychogenic seizures: ictal characteristics and diagnostic pitfalls. Neurology 1992;42:95.

Lindhout D, Omtzigt JGC. Pregnancy and the risk of teratogenicity. Epilepsia 1992;33(suppl 4):S41.

Morrell MJ. Hormones and epilepsy through the lifetime. Epilepsia 1992;33(suppl 4):S49.

Noort SVD. Assessment: generic substitution for antiepileptic medication. Neurology 1990;40:1641.

Parent JM, Lowenstein DH. Treatment of refractory generalized status epilepticus with continuous infusion of midazolam. Neurology 1994;44:1837.

Theodore WH, Porter RJ. Epilepsy: 100 elementary principles. Philadelphia: WB Saunders, 1995.

Treiman DM. Epileptic emergencies and status epilepticus. In: Grotta JC, ed. Management of the acutely ill neurological patient. New York: Churchill Livingstone, 1993:111.

Primary Care for Women, edited by Phyllis C. Leppert and Fred M. Howard. Lippincott-Raven Publishers, Philadelphia © 1997.

109

Parkinson's Disease and Other Movement Disorders

JOSHUA HOLLANDER

This group of disorders includes disturbances manifested by difficulty in both initiating and sustaining movements and is therefore divided into *hypokinetic* (akinetic-rigid syndromes) and *hyperkinetic* (dyskinetic) disorders. Despite a rich terminology of words to describe movement disorders, a major advance in this field has been the use of videotaping to allow for analysis and consultation of uncertain movements and the documentation of therapeutic interventions. Because these problems are best visualized on videotape, such tapes have been made available for educational purposes. Some of the specific terms used to describe the phenomenology include rigidity, bradykinesia, tremor, chorea, athetosis, ballism, dystonia, myoclonus, tics, and stereotypies. *Rigidity* refers to a stiffness or resistance throughout the range of passive movement. It is the same in both extensors and flexors, and relatively independent of velocity. It is reinforced by contralateral movement, anxiety, and stress. When interrupted by tremor it is called cogwheel rigidity; without tremor it is lead pipe or plastic rigidity. *Bradykinesia* refers to a complex of delayed motor initiation, slow performance, inability to execute simultaneous or sequential movements, difficulty in reaching a target with a single movement, rapid fatigue with repetition, and defective kinetic automatisms (loss of associated movements, eg, armswing when walking). Akinesia may be a synonym but implies greater severity.

The description of adventitious movements uses potentially overlapping terms. *Dyskinesia* refers to excessive or abnormal involuntary movements. *Tremor* is a rhythmic oscillation of varying frequencies about a point of varying frequencies and varying in relation to motion. *Chorea*, after a word meaning dance, is a quick, irregular, and predominantly distal, semipurposive movement. *Ballism* is a proximal, high amplitude, wild, uncontrollable, and sustained flinging (ballistic) movement which evolves to chorea as it recovers. *Athetosis* refers to continuous, slow, writhing (Balinese dancer) movement. There is a recent tendency to lump all of these movements into the category of chorea. *Myoclonus* is a sudden movement due to contractions of single muscles or groups which may be single or repetitive in the same part of the body. It may be spontaneous or precipitated by movement. Negative myoclonus is induced by inhibition of contraction of agonist and antagonist muscle groups and is called *asterixis* (flap). *Dystonia* is an involuntary, often twisting, movement ending in a sustained contraction. Muscle tone is normal between spasms. Dystonia may only be manifest with action. *Akathisia* is a restlessness resulting in an inability to sit or stand still. *Tics* are sudden, transient, complex, coordinated movements. These tend to be repetitive and are subject to brief voluntary suppression. *Stereotypies* are involuntary coordinated, repetitive, patterned, purposeless, ritualistic appearing movements, postures, or utterances. With the exception of sleep myoclonus and seizures, abnormal involuntary movements cease during sleep.

Parkinson's disease, essential tremor, and the drug-induced movement disorders are the most common problems encountered and will be stressed in this discussion.

ETIOLOGY AND DIFFERENTIAL DIAGNOSIS

The complex connections of the basal ganglia can be reviewed only briefly here. The pars compacta of the substantia nigra contains dopaminergic cells that project to the putamen (striatonigral pathway). It is these cells that are depleted in Parkinson's disease. Striatopallidal pathways are both direct and indirect. The direct gamma-aminobutyric acid (GABAergic) inhibitory path to the internal pallidum reduces GABAergic inhibition of the ventrolateral thalamic nucleus, which results in the release of stimulation of the supplementary motor cortex. The cortex has direct stimulatory connections to the striatum. A similar GABAergic inhibitory path to the external pallidum (GPe) inhibits a GABAergic output to the subthalamic nucleus which has glutamatergic facilitatory output to the internal pallidum (GPi). Omitted are numerous other neurotransmitters, multiple receptor types, and loop pathways. In Parkinson's disease loss of nigral cells results in loss of GPi inhibition and hence loss of thalamic activation of the supplementary motor cortex. This results in bradykinesia and rigidity. In Huntington's chorea there is loss of the striatal inhibition of the GPe and resultant inhibition of the subthalamic nucleus. In hemiballismus, an infarct or tumor of the subthalamic nucleus reduces GPi activation and hence lack of movement suppression.

Parkinson's disease is a progressive neurodegenerative disorder usually beginning in the sixth and seventh decade of life with a prevalence of about 1 per 1000 people. Life expectancy is about 15 years. Cardinal features of the disease are bradykinesia, rigidity, tremor, and impaired postural reflexes. Bradykinesia contributes to the masklike facies, diminished arm swing and other associated movements, slow movements, small step gait, difficulty in initiating movements, hypophonia, and micrographia. The characteristic tremor is a resting tremor of low (4 to 5 Hz) frequency and coarse amplitude, but a low amplitude action tremor may also be seen. The patient sitting at repose, with tremor clearing with movement, is striking. Cogwheel rigidity is seen (primarily upper limbs), reflecting the tremor detected in motion. Loss of postural reflexes results in loss of balance and an inability to invoke righting reflexes. Autonomic dysfunctions include impotence, seborrhea, constipation, and orthostatic hypotension. Eye movements tend to be hypometric. Blepharospasm may be seen. Depression and its associated psychomotor retardation may be erroneously diagnosed in the patient with Parkinson's disease. It is not unusual in Parkinson's disease to see depression. Therapy, as in other depression, is appropriate. Subcortical dementia may be seen in 20% of patients and may confound therapy. A wide variety of psychiatric disorders can be seen with either Parkinson's disease or its treatment.

Parkinson's disease is due to loss of dopaminergic cells of the striatonigral path, but the reason for this is still uncertain. Studies based on the Parkinsonism induced by the designer drug MPTP led to the thesis that chronic exposure to environmental oxidative toxins led to the cell loss. Some cell loss occurs merely as a result of aging, but the cell loss in Parkinson's disease is compounded by oxidative toxicity. Symptoms develop after a critical threshold of cell loss has taken place. Some cases are familial but most are sporadic. A cohort of postencephalitic Parkinsonism related to the world pandemic of von Economo encephalitis of 1919 has aged and is passing from the scene. There are a group of other causes of atypical Parkinsonism, which may share similar pathogenesis.

There is a group of diseases sometimes referred to as Parkinson's plus. Lewy bodies are eosinophilic, hyaline, cytoplasmic inclusions seen in the nerve cells (diffuse Lewy body disease with extensive cortical involvement is discussed in Chap. 111). In Parkinson's disease Lewy bodies tend to be seen preferentially in the basal ganglia, but some cases of Parkinson's disease do not have Lewy bodies at all. Multiple system atrophy refers to a group of disorders making up about 10% of Parkinsonism and include *Shy-Drager syndrome*, *olivopontocerebellar atrophy*, and *striatonigral degeneration*. Oligodendroglial tubular inclusions characterize these disorders. The presence of severe autonomic dysfunction, absence of resting tremor, early postural instability and falls, early dementia, and poor response to levodopa should alert the clinician to this possibility. Corticobasal ganglionic degeneration is an akinetic-rigid syndrome with severe cortical sensory impairments, apraxia, myoclonus, tremors, and other abnormal involuntary movements. Cognitive impairment and oculomotor impairments (gaze apraxia) are also seen. Disordered voluntary gaze characterizes *progressive supranuclear palsy (PSP)*. Decreased upgaze is seen in normal aging and is worse in Parkinson's disease. Progressive supranuclear palsy shows a striking early impairment of downgaze. This results in an inability to use bifocals and a tendency to fall on descending steps. The diagnostic tetrad for PSP is supranuclear oculomotor palsy axial rigidity, pseudobulbar palsy, and subcortical dementia.

The major disorder confused with Parkinson's disease after the akinetic-rigid syndromes is essential tremor. *Essential tremor* is the most common of the movement disorders. When a positive family history (50%) is elicited, it is called familial tremor. When onset is after age 65 it is called senile tremor. Subtetanic motor unit stimulation with intact stretch reflexes results in a low amplitude oscillation whose frequency is proportional to muscle stiffness and inversely to the mass. This physiologic tremor is enhanced to visible levels with adrenergic excess due to anxiety, stage fright, hypoglycemia, hyperthyroidism, caffeine, levodopa, or adrenergic medication. This is an action tremor not present at rest. Quite similar is essential-familial tremor. Quiet at rest, movement such as attempting to drink a glass of water or sign a check produces a distressing and embarrassing tremor. It should be easily distinguished from Parkinsonism because of the absence of rest tremor, rigidity, bradykinesia, and postural instability. It continues to be confused, perhaps because there is an increased incidence of essential tremor in Parkinsonism.

Drug-induced Parkinsonism is usually seen within months of institution of drug therapy. Although it may mimic Parkinson's disease, it occurs at any age, usually resolves within days to months of drug withdrawal, is symmetric, and displays both a relatively rapid resting and an action-postural tremor. Bradykinesia is a major feature. Drugs with the highest affinity for dopaminergic blockade in the nigrostriatal system, such as piperazine phenothiazines and butyrophenones, cause denervation hypersensitivity. These are also associated with a high incidence of both drug-induced Parkinsonism and tardive dyskinesia. The dopamine receptor (D2) antagonist metoclopramide can cause both Parkinsonism and tardive dyskinesia. Dopaminergic blockade causing drug-induced Parkinsonism and subsequent denervation hypersensitivity causing tardive dyskinesia may be an oversimplification, but is conceptually useful in considering these problems.

The *choreiform disorders* fall into hereditary and sporadic types, but the clinician often suffers from inadequate history due to adoptions and unrecognized paternity, as well as lost or suppressed family data. *Huntington's disease* has a United States prevalence of 5 to 10 per 100,000 people and is the best known of the disorders. Mean onset is at age 40, with chorea or disordered motor control the usual presentation, but bradykinetic and psychotic forms occur. Chorea may resemble abnormally quick voluntary movements, especially if the patient incorporates them into seemingly purposeful movements or parakinesias. These are increased with stress and walking and, in Huntington's disease, are frequently associated with slower athetoid or later dystonic movements. There are more generalized motor disorders associated with impairment of eye and tongue movements as well as repetitive movements. This ultimately makes driving or even holding a knife unsafe. Dysarthria and dysphagia become endstage problems. An emotional change near onset is common. Cognitive problems tend to involve attention, concentration, and executive planning. Visual memory is more involved than verbal memory. It is an autosomal dominant disorder carried on chromosome 4 with an excessive number of trinucleotide CAG repeats (coding for glutamine). A direct correlation between the number of repeats and the age of onset has been found. The normal unidentified protein produced in excess has been called Huntington. Other diseases have been found with abnormal CAG repeats and much is yet to be clarified in the pathogenesis. Pathological studies have shown extensive loss of caudate head and striatal GABAergic cells of the indirect path to the external globus pallidus. Senile or essential chorea patients may well be late life forms of Huntington's disease.

Neuroacanthocytosis can have either dominant or recessive inheritance. Less severe chorea may be manifest as myoclonic jerks, tics, vocalizations, dystonia, and self-mutilation. Over 15% of the red blood cells on smear are acanthocytes. Less common hereditary choreas include *benign hereditary chorea* and *paroxysmal dystonic choreoathetosis.*

The most common *sporadic chorea* is *Sydenham's chorea,* which is seen in poststreptococcal infection as part of the rheumatic fever complex. It is decreasing in frequency due to aggressive antibiotic therapy of streptococcal infections. The movements are swifter than in Huntington's disease and the patients are younger. In addition to the risk of cardiac problems, some residual chorea and increased susceptibility to recurrent chorea from medications, birth control pills, and pregnancy may occur. *Chorea gravidarum* is chorea with pregnancy. As noted, there are many patients with a prior history of Sydenham's chorea, but there is a possible hormonal factor as well. Although vasculitis must be excluded, the pregnancy can proceed to term. Chorea associated with birth control pills is quite similar and ceases with withdrawal of these hormonal preparations. Other causes of sporadic chorea include hyperthyroidism, polycythemia vera, and vasculitis such as lupus, dopa, and stroke. Neuroleptics may cause tardive dyskinesia (orobuccolingual dyskinesia), which may be mistaken for chorea but tends to be more repetitive and stereotypic.

Hemiballismus most commonly occurs as a result of a small penetrating artery stroke in the subthalamic nucleus of Luys. Movements are continuous and more violent than chorea and may result in injury. This tends to subside spontaneously and will evolve into a hemichorea phase.

Athetosis is most commonly associated with perinatal injury such as prematurity or kernicterus. There may be a later progression. When this is seen in response to movements in other parts of the body, it is referred to as overflow.

There is a large group of disorders referred to as dystonias, which are the subject of multiple overlapping classifications. *Idiopathic torsion dystonia* has its onset in childhood and is more common among Ashkenazi Jews with a dominant inheritance pattern and chromosome identification. It is not known if this is true in non-Jewish individuals. Idiopathic torsion dystonia is a generalized process beginning as a localized phenomenon and displaying overflow. It can be a seriously disabling disorder. Individuals frequently learn sensory tricks to suppress abnormal movement. While there is a tendency to think of dystonia as a sustained posture, it has associated movements of varying speeds and types. The sporadic and localized dystonias are 10 times more common, occurring at a prevalence of 30 per 100,000. *Spasmodic torticollis* is the most common form of cervical dystonia; it is often interrupted by placing a finger on the chin. When combined with cranial dystonias such as blepharospasm, it is referred to as *Meige syndrome.* Other common dystonias include spastic dysphonia and hand dystonias *(writer's and occupational cramps).* Blepharospasm may be sufficiently severe to cause functional blindness.

Wilson's disease is a rare autosomal recessive disorder (chromosome 13) that presents in childhood with rigidity, bradykinesia, dystonia, and liver dysfunction. Adults may have psychiatric presentations with a tremor (may be coarse) and dysarthria. A Kayser-Fleischer ring in the cornea may be detected as a brown deposition, but often requires an ophthalmologist to perform a slit-lamp examination. This disorder is associated with excessive copper deposition in affected organs due to impaired biliary excretion. The myoclonic disorders are not discussed in this text. However, the presence of myoclonus should prompt consultation of more detailed sources.

HISTORY

The patient's history must include a careful exploration of birth history. Neurologic disease in the family, as well as possible psychiatric illness, must be reviewed, with input from older members of the family to include information about individuals who may have slipped out of family gatherings because of their chronic illness. It may prove necessary to see some family members directly. A history of carbon monoxide exposure must be specifically sought, as must use of street or designer drugs.

The wide range of movement disorders seen after neuroleptic use, as well as their use for nonpsychiatric purposes (eg, nausea and vomiting), may require careful questioning and a high index of suspicion. It is important to remember that tardive movement disorders occur after reduction or withdrawal of neuroleptic medications, and the patient may be diffident about discussing nervous breakdowns.

The disturbance in posture or movement itself must be dissected as to sudden versus insidiously progressive, sensory tricks, ameliorating factors such as alcohol, and exacerbating factors such as stress. Although there is a rich spectrum of psychogenic movement disorders, it is important to remember that many tremors and hyperkinetic disorders are increased by stress. A spouse will bitterly complain that the patient with Parkinson's disease will be more mobile and perform better for the physician than at home. Inquiries about time required to dress in the morning and difficulty adjusting clothing after toileting may be helpful.

Autonomic dysfunction should be sought, including orthostatic symptoms, urinary, bowel, and sweating disturbances, and constipation.

With cognitive impairments seen in many of these disorders, questions about job performance or home responsibilities should be explored.

PHYSICAL EXAMINATION

It may be faster to have an assistant put the patient in a room, but watching the patient walk to the examining room, struggle with clothing, and get on and off the examining table may be more useful than all the rest of the examination. The stooped, small-stepped, shuffling gait of a Parkinson's patient immediately raises the diagnostic possibility. Is there loss or reduction of associated movements? Can the patient rise freely from a sitting posture without needing several attempts or help from arms? Are there overflow movements elicited by walking or contralateral limb movements? Can the patient hold still or maintain a posture? Is the patient merely fidgety or is this abnormal involuntary movement? Unfortunately, this group of disorders requires looking at the patient and making a diagnostic conclusion both when the patient is aware that an examination is underway and when this is not suspected.

Tremor may be present at rest, with posture holding, and with action. What is the speed and amplitude of tremor? Associated cerebellar ataxia should be sought. Warm sweaty palms, tachycardia, or proptosis in a patient with tremor may direct attention to the thyroid. Resting tremor should always be present in Parkinson's disease but can be fairly inconspicuous and asymmetric. Complete absence suggests Parkinson's plus. Although postural tremor may be seen in Parkinson's disease, it is critical to avoid making a diagnosis on tremor alone in the absence of rigidity and bradykinesia.

Tone should be checked in distal and proximal muscles as well as axial musculature such as the neck. This may be brought out by asking the patient to make an alternating movement with the other hand. Cogwheel rigidity may be the only way to detect a subtle tremor when bradykinesia and rigidity are present. Diminished blinking, a bland masked facies, micrographia, and a hypophonic voice fading during a sentence may be seen in akinetic-rigid syndromes. Rigidity is an increase in tone throughout the range of movement unrelated to speed. Spasticity is velocity-dependent and is best characterized by the spastic catch. Spasticity is associated with corticospinal dysfunction. Increasing paratonia is seen with age. This is manifest by gegenhalten (involuntary intermittent resistance to passive movement) and mittgehen (a seeming effort to cooperate with the examiner), and is associated with dementia when marked.

The Babinski reflex is absent in Parkinson's disease, but present in some other disorders. It must be distinguished from the "striatal toe," which is really a dystonic dorsiflexion and is more prolonged and not related to the stimulus.

Eye movements must be examined for ocular dysmetria and hypometric or hypermetric saccades, as well as impairments in vertical or horizontal gaze. The lack of voluntary eye movements in progressive supranuclear palsy are surprisingly full with head turning (eliciting the oculocephalic reflex).

Orthostatic hypotension as well as sweating should be checked. Early orthostasis, anhidrosis, bladder dysfunction, and impotence may reflect multiple system atrophy rather than Parkinson's disease.

Retropulsion and postural instability can be checked by standing behind the patient and giving a quick backward pull. Parkinson's disease may progress to the stage where postural reflexes are lost and the patient falls backward in the direction of the pull with no attempt to compensate. Falls occur in Parkinson's disease, but when they occur early in the course one should suggest progressive supranuclear palsy.

Some interesting phenomena include the retained ability of Parkinson's patients to catch a ball of paper thrown to them despite considerable bradykinesia. Rocking the patient will facilitate walking, as will stripes on the floor.

Normal movements should be smooth and not interrupted by unexplained movements. Motor impersistence may characterize choreic patients and parakinesias should be watched for. The patient who holds a finger or hand to the chin may have either torticollis or myasthenia gravis.

The patient with involuntary movements should be observed long enough to decide whether the movements fall into a recurrent pattern and whether they are generalized or segmental. Videotaping may allow an analysis of the patient's movements outside the office setting.

The neurologic examination must be complete enough to determine whether the problem is really a multisystem atrophy. The mental status examination must determine the presence of either dementia or depression.

LABORATORY AND IMAGING STUDIES

For many of the movement disorders, the diagnosis is made completely on clinical evidence and is therefore based on history and the analysis of the patient's motor function. Imaging studies may be needed to explain an unexpected finding such as an extensor plantar response with the finding of an old stroke or myelopathy. The neurologic workup of all of these disorders follows the neurologic examination. Exceptions would include visualization of the ventricles when hydrocephalus is being considered, atrophy of the caudate head in possible Huntington's disease, and genetic analysis in olivopontocerebellar atrophy (OPCA) and Huntington's disease. Serum ceruloplasmin, urinary copper, or liver biopsy for the effects of copper may help with the diagnosis of Wilson's disease.

TREATMENT

Treatment of Parkinson's disease is evolving as new agents develop and our understanding of the pathogenesis improves. Early disease does not require treatment. Management generally involves slow initiation of medications, preferably at low dosage. When polypharmacy proves necessary, change only one medication at a time. Selegiline is a monoamine oxidase (MAO) B inhibitor that prolongs the efficacy of levodopa. It could thus be used to treat wearing-off. It has a minimal effect on untreated patients, but there is evidence that it slows the progression of the disease. There is no problem of inducing hypertensive crises unless doses above the recommended 10 mg/day are used, when MAO A activity can develop. Problems include interactions with meperidine and fluoxitene, activation of peptic ulcers, orthostatic hypotension, and an increase in levodopa-induced confusion. Insomnia can be avoided by administering the drug early in the day.

The antiviral agent amantadine (100 mg bid) has an effect on rigidity and bradykinesia that is better than anticholinergics and less than levodopa. It may act at pre- and postsynaptic dopaminergic terminals, as well as having an anticholinergic effect. The effect declines with time but some effect can be sustained. Problems include livedo reticularis, edema, dry mouth, and blurred vision. Confusional states may require dosage reduction or elimination, especially in demented patients. Excretion is renal.

Anticholinergic drugs were the old standards. These caused a reduction in symptoms to a modest degree. They are used only minimally now for tremor and rigidity. Slow titration of trihexyphenidyl to 2 mg tid or benztropine to doses of 0.5 mg qid can be used. Side effects of anticholinergics include aggravation of glaucoma, urinary retention, and constipation. Sialorrhea may be decreased by anticholinergics. The most significant problem is a relatively poor tolerance of these agents in the elderly, with delirium, hallucinations, memory loss, and sedation.

The most significant advance in the pharmacotherapy of Parkinson's disease was the discovery of levodopa. Levodopa is able to pass the blood-brain barrier (unlike dopamine) and is decarboxylated there to dopamine. Aromatic amino acid decarboxylase is diminished in Parkinson's disease, but not as severely as the rate-limiting tyrosine hydroxylase. Extensive peripheral decarboxylation was a problem until the concurrent use of a peripherally active decarboxylase inhibitor that does not cross the blood-brain barrier (carbidopa-Sinemet). An unresolved issue is the possibility that the use of dopamine causes increased production of oxidative toxicity and a more rapid progression of the disease. Some physicians would start with dopamine agonists and delay levodopa therapy for this reason. Most neurologists begin Sinemet therapy when the bradykinesia and rigidity begin to impede job performance or interfere with activities of daily living. The medication is usually introduced as half of a 25/100 mg pill tid, gradually working up to 25/100 tid. Early side effects, which tend to subside, include anorexia, nausea and vomiting, orthostatic hypotension, and cardiac rhythm disturbances. When lower doses of Sinemet are used for a protracted period, it may be necessary to add supplemental carbidopa, which is not available in pharmacies but may be obtained from the manufacturer. Initially, gastrointestinal intolerance is avoided by giving with meals. The use of supplemental carbidopa may be helpful, as may be the use of domperidone. (Domperidone is not approved in the United States and must be obtained from Canada at significant patient expense.) Because other aromatic amino acids interfere with absorption of levodopa, the dosage is timed to avoid high concurrent protein meals after initial therapy seems satisfactory. The effect is gradual, and weeks must be allowed to assess maximum therapeutic benefit. The bulk of patients with Parkinson's disease show sustained improvement with therapy, and the absence of such improvement calls the diagnosis into question. Reasons for levodopa failure include inadequate dosage or concurrent administration of a dopaminergic blocking agent such as metaclopromide, phenothiazines, or butyrophenones. Patients and referring physicians are often disturbed by lack of control of tremor or even an increase of tremor. This reflects a lack of use of the correct index of rigidity or bradykinesia. Levodopa is a poor agent for control of tremor and reduction of rigidity and bradykinesia may allow tremor to be manifest. Patients can clearly benefit by increased dosage (25/250 tid or qid) to titrate against side effects. A large minority of neurologists try to minimize the levodopa dosage by the early use of dopamine agonists when moderate doses of levodopa prove inadequate.

Levodopa therapy is complicated by a variety of intercurrent problems. Although Parkinson's disease has always shown fluctuations in severity associated with stress (jumping up from the porch rocker and running away when someone shouts "Fire" only to subsequently freeze), there is a return to the bradykinetic state when safe. These fluctuations increase with the severity of disease and duration of therapy. Freezing may occur on turns or when reaching a doorway. Freezing is the term used when the patient who had been ambulating successfully suddenly stops. This is most distressing to both the patient and caregivers who may think this is a voluntary effort of the patient to be ornery. Initially these tend to be simple wearing-off phenomena that benefit from more frequent dosage, use of the sustained release form, selegiline, or longer-acting dopamine agonists. When these fluctuations occur, the patient must keep a log indicating the time of "off" periods. The patient may not distinguish between tremor and chorea unless this log is reviewed. Although the sustained release preparation would seem an easy solution (substituting Sinemet CR 50/200 for Sinemet 25/100), this is not the case. There is a need to retitrate the patient. There may be an inordinate delay in response in the morning. As the central storage capability decreases, frequent small doses are helpful, but it may be difficult for patients to comply with this suggestion. Supplemental agonists may be helpful because of their lesser tendency to induce dyskinesias. These will be discussed later. There is a rich variety of abnormal movements induced by levodopa. High- and low-dose dopa dyskinesias occur and are being clarified by dopamine receptor subtype analysis. Foot dystonia is often a low-dose phenomenon. High-dose chorea and low-dose dystonia often respond to lowering the levodopa dose at the price of decreased mobility. Levodopa holidays fail to produce lasting effects and can be life threatening.

The dopamine agonists are semisynthetic ergot derivatives that readily enter the brain and require no metabolic conversion. The ones in current use have long half-lives and high potency. Because, unlike Levodopa, they are not generators of free radicals, they have the theoretical advantage of not causing an increase in the rate of progression of the disease. The main ones currently in use are bromocriptine (D2 receptor) and pergolide (D1 and D2 receptor). These drugs are familiar to gynecologists because of their use to block galactorrhea. They have a long blood half-life, but their anti-Parkinson's effect is significantly shorter. When used as initial monotherapy they require levodopa supplementation within a year. As a supplementation of levodopa, they may allow dose reduction, and their greater duration of action may reduce nocturnal or early morning immobility or dystonia. Some reduction in wearing off can be anticipated. Agonist side effects resemble levodopa side effects. Except for dyskinesias they tend to be more severe and last longer. The dosage varies from bromocriptine (15 to 60 mg/day) to pergolide (2 to 4 mg/day). Pergolide is titratable in smaller increments.

Depression is seen in almost half of Parkinson's patients and can be treated with a serotonin reuptake inhibitor or a tricyclic agent, but MAO A inhibitors must be avoided because of possible hypertensive crises when combined with Sinemet.

All of the anti-Parkinsonian medications have mental side effects, and too frequently these limit therapy. Dementia occurs in about 15% of Parkinson's patients and is higher in the Parkinson's plus group. The caregiver should be alert to possible delirium because this is probably a reversible process. Although this may be a sign of systemic illness, it may also be drug-induced. An early feature in levodopa therapy is visual hallucinosis. This may manifest as a hallucination that there are soft, fuzzy non-frightening critters in the patient's bed or figures standing in the room at night. This benign hallucinosis may progress to a state where these things are perceived as real and paranoid ideation may appear. Reduction in medications may allow resolution of this but at a loss of therapeutic benefit. Overt psychosis is more commonly seen in patients with incipient dementia and generally includes florid visual hallucinations and paranoia as features. There has been the suggestion that clozapine in very low doses may be effective and allow continuation of anti-Parkinson's medications, and studies are in progress. Clozapine is associated with agranulocytosis.

Sleep disturbances are common in the elderly and are increased by nocturia, sleep fragmentation by alcohol and other sedative drugs, pain from arthritis, and many other factors. This chapter is concerned only with the Parkinson's-related factors. Sleep apnea is increased in Parkinson's disease. Restless legs and nocturnal myoclonus may benefit from clonazepam or propoxyphene. Depression should be treated if present. Rigidity makes rolling over in bed a problem, and tremor may retard sleep. A trapeze will help the patient roll over and will facilitate arising for toileting.

Pain may occur primarily in the shoulder girdle and may respond to anti-Parkinson's medications. Dystonia may be painful and akathesia may be described as pain.

Constipation is almost the rule. High-fiber diets, bulk-forming agents, and stool softeners should be tried early. Cisapride seems well tolerated and is effective. Lactulose and other osmotic agents may induce a watery diarrhea that is difficult for a patient with reduced mobility. Mineral oil predisposes to aspiration in this population.

Swallowing problems and aspiration are not unusual.

Urinary problems are multifactorial in this population. Nocturia may be reduced by oxybutinin or propantheline. Detrussor hyperreflexia may be suppressed by anticholinergics which may also cause retention. Risk of retention is less problematic in women who are free of prostatism. One can not assume that this problem is either disease- or drug-related without evaluation. Sexual dysfunction is common and relates to chronic illness, immobility, mental status changes, and autonomic dysfunction.

Falling is complex and does not respond to levodopa.

Surgical procedures include ventrolateral thalamotomy, which reduces tremor and rigidity but not bradykinesia. Posteroventral pallidotomy has relieved tremor, rigidity, and bradykinesia. Surgical procedures decreased markedly with the advent of levodopa but are making some recovery. Fetal cell transplantation is now only experimental.

Neuroleptic malignant syndrome is a potentially lethal condition characterized by fever, muscle rigidity, autonomic instability, and altered consciousness that can be precipitated by dopaminergic withdrawal, lithium, and neuroleptics. Prompt dopaminergic restitution is in order.

Essential tremor is reduced by alcohol, but this therapy is problematic because of abuse. Primidone in low dosage has proven the most effective agent for management, but problems with nausea, unsteadiness, vertigo, and clouding of consciousness require very slow initiation of therapy. Use of more than 250 mg seems to add little to effectiveness. Blood levels are not helpful. Propranolol in a range of 240 to 360 mg/day if tolerated seems optimal. This may be tried if primidone is not tolerated.

Wilson's disease is managed with copper chelators. A wide range of agents is used for Huntington's disease, including dopamine receptor antagonists, dopamine depleting agents, benzodiazepines, and anticonvulsants. Therapy for Huntington's disease must be considered unsatisfactory.

Dystonias may be managed by local injections of botulinum toxin when symptoms are sufficiently discrete, such as blepharospasm, spastic dysphonia, and cervical dystonia. The generalized dystonias have been variously treated with anticholinergics, dopaminergics, antidopaminergics, benzodiazepines, and baclofen. Surgical therapy includes thalamotomy, selective nerve root section, and myotomy. Myoclonus may be reduced by clonazepam. Therapy of dystonia, myoclonus, and tic disorders including Tourette's syndrome is complex and best referred to experienced physicians. Tardive dyskinesias can be managed by titrating the neuroleptic to the lowest possible dose in unstable patients and then considering specific therapy with dopamine depletors or benzodiazepines. Stable patients may be slowly tapered and observed off drug for the degree of disability. Management is complex and fraught with medicolegal problems. Referral to experienced physicians is urged.

CONSIDERATIONS DURING PREGNANCY

Major issues for consideration in pregnancy include specific issues of teratogenicity of the specific agents employed and risk of drug withdrawal. For essential tremor medication withdrawal seems best. Parkinson's disease rarely affects childbearing ages. Patients with the other movement disorders should be managed in concert with experts. Many of these disorders have hereditary factors and these should be explored with the prospective mother prior to pregnancy.

A specific issue is chorea gravidarum or the development of chorea during pregnancy. A third of these patients have a history of Sydenham chorea. While they should be checked for activation of streptococcal infection, this is infrequent. Thyrotoxicosis and connective tissue disease must be ruled out. There is no reason to terminate pregnancy.

BIBLIOGRAPHY

Beal MF. Aging, energy and oxidative stress in neurodegenerative diseases. Ann Neurol 1995;38:357.

Jankovic J, Tolosa E, eds. Parkinson's disease and movement disorders. Baltimore: Williams & Wilkins, 1993.

Joseph AB, Young RR, eds. Movement disorders. Boston: Blackwell, 1992.

Kurlan R. Treatment of movement disorder. Philadelphia: JB Lippincott, 1995.

Marsden CD, Fahn S, eds. Movement disorders 3. Oxford: Butterworth-Heinemann, 1994.

Nutt JG, Hammerstad JP, Gancher ST. Parkinson's disease: 100 maxims. CV Mosby, 1992.

Thompson PD. Movement disorders. Current Opinion Neurol 1995; 8:303.

Rubin W, Brookler KH. Dizziness: etiologic approach to management. New York: Thieme, 1991.

Sharpe JA, Barber HO, eds. The vestibulo-ocular reflex and vertigo. New York: Raven Press, 1993.

Primary Care for Women, edited by Phyllis C. Leppert and Fred M. Howard. Lippincott-Raven Publishers, Philadelphia © 1997.

110

Transient Cerebral Ischemia and Stroke

JOSHUA HOLLANDER

Stroke remains the third leading cause of death in the United States and is a major cause of disability. Management of stroke is far less effective than prevention, so it is gratifying that major inroads have been made in identifying stroke risk factors and interventions. Research into acute stroke mechanisms and management has dramatically advanced, and the large number of promising treatment trials in progress suggests that we will soon have an array of acute therapeutic options.

In an ischemic stroke, a core area of the cerebrum suffers profound ischemia, and necrosis is a consequence. An area of sublethal ischemia (ischemic penumbra) could be preserved if flow could be restored promptly. The therapeutic window is not well defined but probably is measured in hours, not minutes. The tissue in the ischemic penumbra may recover or may progress to delayed programmed cell death through a series of complex changes not yet fully identified; changes related to increased intracellular calcium levels, calcium-activated cytotoxic enzymes, free radicals, excitatory amino acid toxicity, cytokines, intercellular adhesion molecules, and programmed cell death have all been explored. We are at the stage of excellent management of experimental stroke in rodents, but in humans successful treatments are as yet unproved.

The older classification of stroke by temporal profile has fallen into disfavor because of the realization that transient ischemic attacks (TIA) last no more than 1 hour and the finding on neuroimaging studies of frequent areas of minor infarction in TIA patients, as well as the absence of clear areas of infarction in many patients with clearly persistent deficits. Temporal classification and the TIA concept was of considerable early value but later served to retard stroke research. Treatment was withheld for 24 hours in trials to prevent confusing stroke with TIA. This allowed the therapeutic window (3 to 8 hours) to pass and almost guaranteed failure for any treatment under consideration. Rational stroke therapy requires the treating physician to analyze the probable stroke mechanism and select appropriate measures for treatment and prevention.

Many stroke treatment trials will produce results within the next few years. We are faced with a need to enroll patients into hyperacute (90 to 180 minutes) or acute (3 to 8 hours) trials because we must fall within the therapeutic window. However, the public and many health care professionals have not yet accepted the concept of a stroke as a "brain attack" worthy of care as serious and urgent as that of a heart attack. Time may be muscle, but it is also brain. The more we delay in getting stroke patients into the system, the fewer patients will be available for trials and the more years will elapse before a meaningful therapeutic intervention is discovered.

Predictors of stroke include factors that we do not control such as age and male sex. Race is a complex factor: blacks are excessively prone to hypertension, hemorrhagic and ischemic stroke, and intracranial vascular disease. The Japanese experience different stroke profiles in Japan, Hawaii, and the mainland United States, presumably due to dietary factors. Hispanics (a mixed population) occupy an intermediate position. Genetic factors are not fully defined. Modifiable risk factors include hypertension for all stroke types and heart disease for ischemic stroke. Nonvalvular atrial fibrillation becomes a progressively more important risk with increasing age. Coronary heart disease, left ventricular hypertrophy on electrocardiogram, and congestive failure all increase the risk of stroke. Prior major stroke, minor stroke, transient hemispheric ischemia, transient monocular blindness, and asymptomatic carotid stenosis increase stroke risk, in declining order of importance. Diabetes increases the risk of all ischemic stroke types, and cigarette smoking is associated with a lower increase in all stroke types. Hypercholesterolemia is a minor risk factor independent of heart disease. Alcohol is more of a risk factor for hemorrhagic stroke, and hypocholesterolemia increases the risk of intracerebral hemorrhagic stroke.

There has been a gradual decline in deaths due to stroke for many years. This trend accelerated with the availability of effective, well-tolerated therapy for hypertension. Effective treatment of streptococcal infections reduced the rate of rheumatic heart disease, and attention to lifestyle and serum lipid levels reduced or delayed ischemic heart disease. Carotid endarterectomy markedly reduces the risk in patients with symptomatic stenosis greater than 70%. The beneficial effect is much lower in asymptomatic patients and occurs primarily in men. Warfarin therapy markedly reduces cardioembolic events, including those due to nonvalvular atrial fibrillation.

ETIOLOGY AND DIFFERENTIAL DIAGNOSIS

The older temporal profile classification of stroke is being replaced by one that emphasizes mechanism (Table 110-1). When assessing etiologic stroke mechanisms, a large percentage fall into cryptogenic stroke, but newer diagnostic techniques are reducing the size of this group. This group is thought to contain many embolic cases in which the source has not been identified.

Large vessel thrombosis is usually associated with atherosclerosis. Extracranial vascular disease is more common among whites, but blacks have a higher incidence of intracranial stenosis. Atherosclerosis of the coronary arteries tends to occur 10 years earlier than carotid disease. The risk of carotid stenosis is higher in

Table 110-1. Classification of Stroke by Mechanism

Ischemic
Thrombosis
Large vessel extracranial occlusion
Large vessel intracranial occlusion
Small vessel intracranial occlusion
Embolism
Cardiogenic
Paradoxic
Arterioarterial
Impaired systemic perfusion
Other known cause
Coagulopathies
Vasculitis
Cryptogenic
Hemorrhagic
Subarachnoid hemorrhage
Intracerebral hemorrhage

patients with peripheral vascular disease. This may present with major vascular territory symptoms or with tandem branch occlusions. Anterior cerebral territory strokes show major involvement of the lower limb; the far more common middle cerebral territory stroke tends to have greater face and hand involvement. Dysphasia, acalculia, and apraxias tend to favor left perisylvian lesions (especially in right-handed patients); dysprosodies and spatial perceptual problems favor the right parietal area. Carotid occlusions may be asymptomatic or present with partial or complete middle cerebral territory infarcts, or even combined massive anterior and middle cerebral combined infarcts. Partial infarcts may be arterioarterial emboli or distal field ischemia. Distal field ischemia tends to favor watershed involvement; this displays more proximal weakness, rather than the typical distal weakness. Posterior cerebral infarcts are more commonly embolic and cause visual field loss and memory loss if bilateral. Basilar territory stroke presents with crossed cranial nerve and long tract signs. The "top of the basilar" is the first narrow point in the posterior circulation, and various syndromes occur from these saddle emboli, based on whether the embolus fragments and occludes the mesencephalic or thalamoperforate vessels or the superior cerebellar or posterior cerebral arteries. Posterior circulation strokes may affect consciousness.

Small vessel intracranial disease is primarily associated with hypertension, but the rate is also increased among diabetics. Lacunar strokes, infarcts of about 5 mm, are due to occlusion of small deep penetrating arteries (primarily from hypertension). Multiple clinical syndromes have been defined such as pure motor hemiplegia, pure sensory stroke, ataxic hemiparesis, sensory-motor stroke, or clumsy hand–dysarthria syndrome.

Embolic stroke may be cardiogenic, paradoxic, or arterioarterial. Some cardiogenic mechanisms are listed in Table 110-2. The risk of recurrent embolization varies with the source: it is high in transmural anterior wall myocardial infarction and low in mitral valve prolapse. Some cardiac lesions, such as mitral annulus calcification, are associated with an increased stroke risk but may be associated with intracranial pathology rather than embolization. Paradoxic emboli require a connection between the pulmonary and systemic circulations such as an atrial septal defect or an intrapulmonary shunt. Valsalva maneuver or pulmonary embolus may shift pressures and open a foramen ovale or induce right-to-left shunting. Older patients are also prone to aortic arch plaque and clot with secondary embolization. Ulcerated carotid plaque with stenosis may also be a source of arterioarterial embolization. Embolic lesions may cause branch occlusions and present with isolated hand weakness and numbness, isolated aphasia, or isolated hemianopia.

Impaired systemic perfusion results from prolonged hypotension below the limits of autoregulation. Inadequate cerebral blood flow is most marked in the watershed territory between the distribution areas of the major cerebral vessels. This produces the previously described characteristic pattern of deficits.

Generally, thrombosis does not occur in small cortical branches because atherosclerosis does not usually occur there. Vasculitis and hypercoagulable states are exceptions, as is distal field ischemia from a proximal occlusion and inadequate perfusion (with or without overenthusiastic antihypertensive therapy).

Venous sinus thrombosis or cortical vein thrombosis occurs primarily in the context of hypercoagulable states and presents a less familiar pattern. When venous sinuses are involved, hemorrhagic infarction is not unusual, and intracranial pressure may be increased because of impaired venous drainage.

Intracerebral hemorrhage is usually associated with vascular malformations in the young. This continues to be a problem later in life, but other factors, such as hypertensive ganglionic hemorrhage, increase. This was the most common type of intracerebral hemorrhage, but more effective antihypertensive therapy has resulted in its decline. Cerebral amyloid angiopathy has taken over its paramount place and is seen as lobar hemorrhage in elderly patients.

Subarachnoid hemorrhage has not decreased in frequency, and we have done poorly in decreasing its mortality. Many patients with aneurysmal subarachnoid hemorrhage die from the first bleed before we even know aneurysm is present. Spontaneous subarachnoid bleeding occurs in children primarily from vascular malformation, but in teenaged patients and older ones, the primary consideration is aneurysm.

Table 110-2. Cardiac Diseases Causing Cerebral Embolism

Cardiac Dysrhythmias and Cerebral Embolism
Nonvalvular atrial fibrillation
Chronic sinoatrial disorder
Ischemic Heart Disease
Acute myocardial infarction
Left ventricular aneurysm
Rheumatic Valvular Disease
Mitral stenosis
Mitral incompetence
Aortic valve disease
Prosthetic Heart Valves
Less Common Sources
Mitral annulus calcification
Mitral valve prolapse
Idiopathic hypertrophic subaortic stenosis
Cardiomyopathies
Nonbacterial thrombotic endocarditis
Infective endocarditis
Cardiac myxoma
Paradoxic embolism

The full definition of stroke requires attention to both the vascular and functional anatomy of the brain. The physician should be able to make a reasonable estimate of the stroke's location and mechanism by combining information from the history, neurologic and vascular examinations, laboratory and imaging studies, and pattern recognition. No single test defines this, but experienced physicians can classify most patients. The stroke's mechanism may remain obscure, either because no mechanism is evident or because multiple factors are possible (eg, atrial fibrillation, hypertension, diabetes, and carotid stenosis are all present). Not every neurologic event or deficit is vascular in origin.

HISTORY

Typically, the stroke syndrome has an abrupt apoplectic onset, but thrombotic strokes may present with a stuttering onset. Carotid strokes may evolve over a day; basilar occlusions may progress over several days. Newer therapies require precise definition of the time of onset of ischemic strokes, and careful probing may be necessary to elicit subtle behavioral changes or mild degrees of unsteadiness or weakness. Patients who awaken with a deficit are more likely to have a thrombotic stroke; abrupt onset in the awake, active patient favors embolic mechanisms. The onset of stroke is dated from the last time the patient was well—for instance, a patient who awakens at 8 a.m. is considered to have stroke onset at bedtime. A history of recurrent stereotypical events such as transient visual loss or hemiparesis favors large vessel extracranial disease. Recurrent pure motor hemiparesis or pure hemisensory syndromes may be signs of lacunar stroke. The nervous system has a limited repertory of responses to injury, and once the lesion is localized, the tempo of the lesion leads to the diagnosis.

The presence of previous TIA favors thrombotic stroke and, depending on the clinical profile, suggests either large vessel or lacunar syndrome. Recurrent symptoms brought on by arm use may suggest subclavian steal, which is due to proximal subclavian occlusion with secondary reversal of flow in the vertebral artery to deliver blood to the involved arm.

There may be multiple potential etiologies for transient neurologic dysfunction. Nocturnal hand numbness and tingling, as well as finger weakness, may reflect carpal tunnel syndrome or cervical radiculopathy from cervical osteoarthritis. The deficit of vascular-origin TIA is abrupt and shows little change during the attack. The hand may drop limply to the bed and have diminished sensation. When the deficit begins in the fingertips and slowly moves up the hand and arm over a 15-minute period, it is more likely a transient migrainous attack. Migraine subsides later in life, and if an isolated migrainous aura develops many years later, the patient may not recall the similarity to her old migrainous aura unless specifically questioned. Such questioning may obviate the need for an expensive work-up.

The "worst headache of my life" suggests subarachnoid hemorrhage. Headache, nausea and vomiting, and a rapidly progressing stroke imply intracranial hemorrhage. Ischemic stroke cannot be fully distinguished from hemorrhagic stroke on history alone.

PHYSICAL EXAMINATION

Evaluation of a stroke patient requires a careful neurologic examination to attempt to localize the lesion and its vascular pattern. The screening neurologic examination should include mental status (level of consciousness, attention, language, memory, gnosis, and praxis), cranial nerves, motor, sensory (including at least one cortical sensory modality), coordination, and reflexes. The examination must include an evaluation of stance and gait. The general examination should include the vital signs. The peripheral pulses should be examined, including the carotid and vertebral pulses and bruits, as well as the timing of radial pulses to exclude subclavian steal. The possibility of aortic dissection should be considered with pulse examination. The heart is checked for murmurs or rhythm disturbances and signs of congestive failure. Funduscopic examination may provide insight into the severity and duration of diabetes mellitus and hypertension. Subhyaloid hemorrhages are characteristic of subarachnoid hemorrhage. The skin, mucous membranes, and conjunctivae should be surveyed for embolic lesions. Fever may occur with time in subarachnoid or pontine hemorrhage but is otherwise unusual with stroke; if present, it suggests endocarditis as an etiology for embolic stroke or intercurrent pulmonary or urinary tract infection.

Loss of consciousness is uncommon in stroke and should alert the examiner to the possibility of subdural hematoma or other intracranial mass lesion. Brain stem or large hemispheric strokes or bleeds may cause altered consciousness, but the "sleepy stroke" warrants prompt imaging studies.

Patients with small sentinel bleeds of subarachnoid hemorrhage may not have focal neurologic findings; if this is suspected because of a thunderclap headache, they should be examined for meningeal signs (photophobia, nuchal rigidity [resistance to neck flexion, not rotation], and Kernig and Brudzinski signs). The Kernig sign is relatively nonspecific and is merely pain in the back of the thigh in response to knee extension when the hip, knee, and ankle are at 90°. The leg Brudzinski sign is seen as contralateral hip flexion elicited when performing the Kernig maneuver. The neck Brudzinski sign is seen when the neck is passively flexed and both hips flex. Meningeal signs may take time to develop, as they are most striking when blood breakdown has already occurred.

Forced eye deviation away from the hemiplegic side is seen in supratentorial lesions; the reverse may be seen in brain stem stroke. Eyes beating to the side of the hemiparesis should alert the examiner to the likelihood of status epilepticus as the cause of the problem. The presence of a Horner syndrome, with or without neck and orbital pain, may suggest carotid dissection. Intracerebral hemorrhage may cause characteristic disturbances in eye movement. Putaminal hemorrhage may cause early transtentorial herniation, with development of a nearly blown pupil on the side of the lesion due to third nerve compromise. Thalamic hemorrhage may cause downward pressure on the superior colliculi, with impairment of upgaze and the so-called "sunset sign," with one or both eyes looking to the nose. Cerebellar hemorrhage may display nystagmus and gaze palsy without hemiparesis early in the bleed. Pontine hemorrhage is associated with pinpoint pupils due to loss of descending sympathetics.

LABORATORY AND IMAGING STUDIES

Routine laboratory studies should include a complete blood count, platelet count, prothrombin time, and partial thromboplastin time to screen for sepsis, blood dyscrasias, and coagulopathies as potential causes. Urinalysis and Westergren sedimentation rate may provide clues to concurrent vasculitis. Hyperglycemia is a poor prognostic sign. Screening chemistries should also be done. A chest film and an electrocardiogram are done and may be followed by a Holter examination if intermittent atrial fibrillation is suspected but not seen on the initial cardiogram.

Patients younger than 60 should have a more detailed battery of studies to exclude a procoagulant state before the use of anticoagulants. Such a screen might include protein C, protein S, antithrombin III, resistance to activated protein C (factor V Leiden), lupus anticoagulant, serologic test for syphilis, and anticardiolipin antibodies. This is important mainly in cryptogenic stroke or in patients with a history of recurrent thrombotic episodes.

Cerebral computed tomography (CT) takes time to show a stroke, and the National Stroke Data Bank studies indicate that up to 40% of strokes never show on CT. A CT is usually done early in the stroke because it is exquisitely sensitive to intracranial hemorrhage and can exclude mass lesions. Early changes may include subtle effacement of the sulci or a white vessel suggestive of an occlusion. CT is less sensitive to subarachnoid hemorrhage but detects more than 90% of cases on day 1, decreasing in sensitivity with time from ictus. The thickness of the clot on CT is a good predictor of the development of delayed ischemic neurologic deficit.

When the stroke mechanism remains obscure despite studies, it sometimes helps to do a repeat imaging study after 3 to 5 days. Magnetic resonance imaging (MRI) can be used for this purpose. MRI is more sensitive than CT and can detect lesions in the posterior fossa and significantly smaller lesions than can be seen on CT. It is less specific for acute hemorrhage than CT.

Selective angiography from a femoral route is the definitive method of visualizing the cerebral circulation. Digital subtraction techniques allow more rapid studies with less catheter time and a lower contrast dose. This minimizes risk, but about 1% of patients still experience transient or permanent neurologic deficit. Arch aortography has a comparable risk, gives overlapping shadows, and lacks intracranial images. MRI can be combined with magnetic resonance angiography. This technique takes advantage of the lack of signal of blood moving rapidly perpendicular to the plane of examination to show vessels without contrast. Magnetic resonance angiography tends to overestimate stenoses and has other limitations that do not allow it to serve as a gold standard, but nevertheless it often provides adequate information to obviate the need for more invasive studies.

Spiral CT combines a slipped conduction ring (allows the radiation source and detectors to make continuous circular movements) and a steadily moving table (thrusting the head through the gantry). This allows for ultrarapid filming of the CT. With a contrast injection, a reliable image of the carotid bifurcation can be obtained.

Carotid duplex examinations (B-mode image of vessel combined with pulsed-wave Doppler velocity measurement) have a sensitivity and specificity of more than 90% for high-grade carotid stenoses and should be performed especially on patients with anterior circulation strokes. Transcranial Doppler sonography offers a picture of the collateral circulation, the cerebrovascular reserve, and the intracranial posterior circulation. A pattern of microembolic signals may provide evidence for cardiogenic or arterioarterial sources. Transcranial Doppler sonography requires a temporal bone thinning (window) and planar arrangement of the circle of Willis. Distal branches cannot be examined. Two-dimensional imaging has not added much to the usual blind technique.

Transthoracic echocardiography is performed when the patient does not have atrial fibrillation or other known source of embolic stroke. The presence of left ventricular wall dysfunction or ventricular aneurysm may indicate a potential embolic source. A 3- to 4-mm clot is sufficient to obstruct the middle cerebral artery, and performing transthoracic echocardiography to see clot is unrewarding.

When the stroke mechanism remains cryptogenic, especially when the patient is young, transesophageal echocardiography may be helpful. This tends to be avoided because the patient must swallow the probe catheter and often requires sedation. The view displays the left atrium and appendage as well as the interatrial septum; part of the thoracic aorta can also be seen. This is the best study for cardioembolic disease, showing the mitral valve, interatrial septal aneurysm, interatrial septal defect, spontaneous echo contrast (smoke), and aortic wall clot. Injection of agitated saline provides microbubble contrast, which clarifies the presence of a right-to-left shunt. A Valsalva maneuver may be needed to open the flap of a patent foramen ovale. Transcranial Doppler sonography can also be used to demonstrate right-to-left shunt. It provides no direct evidence of the intracardiac defect but may detect intrapulmonary shunts. Almost 15% of normal patients have a patent foramen ovale, but young patients with cryptogenic stroke tend to have larger shunts at three times the frequency.

Lumbar puncture has become less important in stroke patients with the advent of new technology but remains the definitive test for subarachnoid hemorrhage. If this is clinically suspected but the CT is negative, a careful lumbar puncture should be performed. The opening pressure should be recorded and three or four tubes collected. If the fluid is bloody, the first and fourth tube counts should be compared to assess clearing. The spun supernatant fluid should be examined for xanthochromia. There are usually 700 red cells to each white cell and 1 mg extra protein. When the tap is done several days after subarachnoid hemorrhage, there is usually an excess of white cells, and only a culture can definitively confirm infection.

TREATMENT

Prevention of stroke is far more effective than treatment. Control of hypertension, cessation of smoking, and reduction in cardiac disease by risk-factor reduction are all in order. Prophylactic aspirin is ineffective in healthy persons but offers a 20% relative risk reduction in patients at risk. Ticlopidine shows a 30% relative risk reduction compared to aspirin but is associated with infrequent neutropenia and frequent diarrhea. Valvular atrial fibrillation is anticoagulated with warfarin (INR 2 to 3). Nonvalvular atrial fibrillation, especially in older patients with left ventricular dysfunction, is also treated with warfarin. Aspirin offers a 20% relative risk reduction in patients at risk but does not prevent cardioembolic stroke in patients with atrial fibrillation.

TIA is followed fairly soon by stroke in patients with high-grade stenosis (> 70% NASCET index). These patients should be worked up promptly and sent for carotid surgery before stroke ensues.

When stroke occurs, the patient should be admitted promptly to a hospital. Controlled studies have demonstrated better results when admission is to a dedicated stroke unit.

Airway support and ventilatory assistance are in order when consciousness is depressed. Oxygen is appropriate when hypoxia is present. Rapid drops in blood pressure are to be avoided, and hypertension is generally treated orally unless the mean arterial pressure exceeds 130 mm Hg. Treatment is cautious. Fever should be controlled to reduce cerebral metabolic demands. Blood sugar should be normalized, but there are no data indicating a better outcome with this therapy.

Cerebral edema peaks at 3 to 5 days. Corticosteroids are ineffective, but osmotherapy may be used. Shunting or ventricular drainage for hydrocephalus may be helpful, but patients with large cerebellar infarctions or hematomas may need posterior fossa decompression. Anticonvulsants are used to control seizures.

Swallowing is assessed by observing swallowing from a cup of 50 mL of water. If this is followed by coughing or wet speech, a speech pathologist should be asked to help evaluate the safety of deglutition and the quest for a reduced-risk program.

Deep vein thrombosis is common in plegic legs. Prophylactic heparin (5000 U twice daily) is given to patients with thrombotic stroke. Patients with intracranial bleeding should have pneumatic compression stockings.

Aspirin has never been shown to be of acute benefit and can be anticipated to be of marginal benefit. Heparin has never been properly studied. Hemorrhagic transformation of embolic stroke is common in embolic stroke at postmortem examination. Good data do not exist, but it seems likely that patients with large embolic strokes are at higher risk for symptomatic hemorrhagic transformation. Early anticoagulation of embolic strokes is in order to prevent reembolization. The physician can wait 2 to 3 days and repeat the CT scan before heparinizing the patient. If hemorrhagic transformation has occurred, anticoagulation is delayed an additional week. However, this may be unduly cautious.

Secondary stroke prevention measures include carotid endarterectomy for stenoses greater than 70% using the NASCET index, in patients whose life expectancy is a year or more, and in patients whose deficit leaves them with more function to lose. Cardioembolic patients who can be safely anticoagulated with warfarin should be so treated. The relative merit of aspirin versus warfarin in patients with cryptogenic stroke is under study, as is the acute use of aspirin, heparin, heparinoids, and low-molecular-weight heparin. Retrospective data suggest that warfarin may be more effective than aspirin.

Many agents are in clinical trials as cerebral protective agents. Properly selected patients with middle cerebral occlusions seen within 180 minutes of ictus can be safely treated with tissue plasminogen activator and has been approved by the Food and Drug Administration. However, this is a potentially dangerous treatment, and its safe use requires careful understanding.

Medical complications experienced by stroke patients include aspiration, pneumonia, malnutrition, deep vein thrombosis, pulmonary embolism, myocardial infarction, urinary tract infections, decubitus ulcers, contractures, and frozen shoulder.

Experienced physicians should manage patients with subarachnoid hemorrhage. Subarachnoid hemorrhage causes death by direct bleeding, rebleeding, and vasospasm. Little can be done about direct bleeding, but we must do better in recognizing small bleeds. Early angiography and surgery can be done in patients in good condition (low Hunt-Hess grade) with clipping of the aneurysm and elimination of rebleeding. The use of endovascular procedures is growing and may prove effective in many vascular malformations. All patients should be treated with prophylactic nimodipine, which reduces death and disability from the delayed disability that occurs after day 4 in patients with subarachnoid hemorrhage and thick clot. Nicardipine reduces vasospasm but fails to improve either death or disability. Presumably, nimodipine acts as a cerebral protective agent. Blood pressure is controlled but perfusion maintained. Hyposmolar agents should be avoided, and hyponatremia should not be treated with fluid restriction. The intravascular volume must be maintained because of the risk of vasospasm; this may require the use of hypertonic agents.

The management of intracerebral hemorrhage is unsatisfactory and remains controversial. A large cerebellar hemorrhage should be decompressed before the patient becomes comatose.

CONSIDERATIONS DURING PREGNANCY

Pregnancy and the puerperium represent a special risk for stroke because of the procoagulant state. It was once thought that these strokes were usually venous, but recent data have shown that strokes in pregnancy and the first week postpartum are arterial. Venous infarction occurs in the succeeding month. The incidence of strokes is about ten times greater in pregnancy and the puerperium. Equal numbers occur during pregnancy and the puerperium. Careful work-up is necessary and anticoagulation is given when appropriate. Warfarin crosses the placenta, so heparin is usually used. Caution about heparin-induced thrombocytopenia is needed. The anticardiolipin antibody syndrome is associated with increased spontaneous abortion, but patients have carried to term with steroids and aspirin. These strokes are usually in the carotid territory.

Venous thrombosis may be suspected when the patient presents with headache, seizures, and obtundation later in the puerperium. Specific syndromes may point to specific dural venous sinuses. Cranial nerves III, IV, V, and VI suggest the cavernous sinus, aphasia the lateral sinus, and leg weakness the sagittal sinus. Although these lesions often are quite hemorrhagic, heparin therapy seems to be helpful.

Vascular lesions may grow during pregnancy. When a patient experiences subarachnoid hemorrhage during pregnancy, the abdomen should be shielded and prompt angiography performed. The risk of bleeding seems greatest during the second trimester, but rupture may occur during parturition. If the lesion cannot be readily dealt with, careful vaginal delivery can be allowed if the Valsalva maneuver can be avoided, as Valsalva increases the venous pressure and the likelihood of rupture. Cesarean section may be needed to protect the mother. The risk drops after delivery but is still high enough to warrant prophylactic surgery, if feasible.

The risk of aneurysmal bleeding increases with each month of pregnancy. Aneurysmal bleeding is more likely to recur severely and soon. Labor may be triggered by aneurysmal rupture. The risk of rebleeding during vaginal delivery is not prohibitive if the patient is multiparous or in good control. If the patient is late in pregnancy, delivery and aneurysmal surgery should be done. If the patient is early in pregnancy, the aneurysm must be dealt with.

Stroke in pregnancy may create problems for the mother's ability to care for her offspring. The problem of subarachnoid hemorrhage is highly complex even without the pregnancy, and a careful multispecialty effort is critical to a successful outcome. Death of patients treated conservatively is in the range of 60% to 70%, and delay should be avoided.

The increased risk of stroke with oral contraceptives seems associated with risk factors such as hypertension and smoking.

BIBLIOGRAPHY

Barnett HJM, Mohr JP, Stein BM, Yatsu FM, eds. Stroke: pathophysiology, diagnosis, and management, 2d ed. New York: Churchill-Livingstone, 1992.

Bogousslavsky J, Caplan L, eds. Stroke syndromes. New York: Cambridge University Press, 1995.

Caplan LR. Stroke: a clinical approach, 2d ed. Boston: Butterworth-Heinemann, 1993.

Fisher M, ed. Stroke therapy. Boston: Butterworth-Heinemann, 1995.

Fisher M, ed. Clinical atlas of cerebrovascular disorders. London: Mosby-Year Book Europe, Ltd., 1994.

Fisher M, Bogousslavsky J, eds. Current review of cerebrovascular disease, 1st ed. Philadelphia: Current Medicine, 1993.

Fisher M, Bogousslavsky J, eds. Current review of cerebrovascular disease, 2d ed. Philadelphia: Current Medicine, 1996.

Hachinski V, Norris JW. The acute stroke. Philadelphia: FA Davis Co., 1985.

Hankey GJ, Warlow CP, eds. Transient ischaemic attacks of the brain and eye. London: WB Saunders Co. Ltd., 1994.

Norris JW, Hachinski VC, eds. Prevention of stroke. New York: Springer-Verlag, 1991.

Yatsu FM, Grotta JC, Pettigrew LC. Stroke: 100 maxims. St. Louis: Mosby, 1995.

111

Dementia (Alzheimer's Disease and Other Types)

JOSHUA HOLLANDER

Primary Care for Women, edited by Phyllis C. Leppert and Fred M. Howard. Lippincott-Raven Publishers, Philadelphia © 1997.

Dementia is a persistent decline in previous intellectual functioning. Cummings has defined dementia as an acquired persistent impairment of intellectual function with compromise in at least three of the following spheres of mental activity: language, memory, visuospatial skills, emotion or personality, and cognition (eg, abstraction, calculation, judgment, executive functioning). The American Psychiatric Association's Diagnostic and Statistical Manual (DSM-IV) continues to require memory loss as a basic requirement while abandoning the need for demonstration of progression. This allows inclusion of those individuals who have suffered a severe but not progressive brain insult (cardiac arrest). The requirement for memory impairment excludes some early dementing disorders. The decline in memory or other cognitive functions can be determined by history of performance decline, clinical examination, or neuropsychologic testing. The diagnosis can not be made when consciousness is impaired by delirium, drowsiness, stupor, or coma, or when the mental status cannot be adequately evaluated because of other clinical problems (National Institute of Neurologic Diseases and Stroke—Alzheimer's Disease and Related Disorders Association [NINDS-ADRDA]).

Dementia is a growing societal and health care problem due to its increasing frequency with aging and the increasing longevity of our population. Most forms of dementia progress insidiously, and the physician or family members may not be aware of even serious deterioration if the patient is not challenged to provide an orderly detailed history. It is the presence of major gaps or inconsistencies that may alert the physician to a cognitive problem. New difficulty at work may bring these deficiencies to attention. Families tend to cover up problems and may gradually assume responsibility for household finances or cooking. Women make up a greater share of the elderly and have a higher incidence of this problem. Significant dementia may reach a prevalence rate of 20% in the over-80 age group and almost 50% over 85 years. There are multiple causes of dementia, with only a small fraction amenable to therapy. Alzheimer's disease is by far the most common form, affecting almost 50% of all demented people. The dementing illnesses are not homogeneous and it is the discrepancies between different cognitive tasks that characterize these disorders.

ETIOLOGY AND DIFFERENTIAL DIAGNOSIS

Etiologic classifications exist but are not as useful as one might wish because of the large number that fall in the unknown category. As research continues to evolve, the group of degenerative dementias will continue to shrink. There is a vast array of neurologic disorders that can cause dementia because of the limited repertoire of responses the nervous system has to injury. Attention will be paid to the more common as well as the potentially treatable disorders. No attempt at more than a few general categorizations about most of these disorders is possible in this context (Tables 111-1 through 111-3).

Degenerative Dementias

Clinically differentiated forms may allow division into cortical, subcortical and mixed types. Not all dementias fit into this classification, but it allows the clinician to make some useful clinical distinctions at the bedside. While the concept of "axial dementia" has been favored to cover pure impairments of new memory formation (Korsakoff psychosis), this has not acquired general acceptance.

Cortical Dementias

Cortical dementias are characterized by a sparing of motor function until quite late in the course of the illness when the patient finally may be reduced to lying curled in hypertonic flexion. The major features are the early involvement of mental status with impairment of language, calculation, visuospatial perception, memory, judgment, and abstraction. The patient may become disinhibited or apathetic.

A prototype disorder is *Alzheimer's disease*. This disorder alone is the most common form of dementia affecting almost half of demented individuals and has a duration of 10 to 20 years. Incidence increases with age from 10% of those over 65 to reach 35% of individuals over 85. It has been estimated to affect as many as 4 million Americans at an annual cost of $90 billion.

Initial features include memory deficits, which are more severe for new memories. Visuospatial skills decline and mild language

Table 111-1. Dementia—A Brief Etiologic Classification

Degenerative dementias
Cortical dementias
Subcortical dementias
Vascular dementias
Infectious dementias
Metabolic dementias
Inherited disorders with dementia
Hydrocephalic dementias
Pseudodementias
Miscellaneous dementias

dysfunction is present. Indifference or irritability may be present and the patient may be sad. Later the memory defects become more global (recent and remote). Visuospatial skills further deteriorate so that even simple constructions can not be done. A fluent aphasia, acalculia, and apraxia are manifest. Restlessness and possibly delusions occur. Finally, severely deteriorated intellect is combined with rigid, flexed posture and incontinence. Seizures may occur late. This may unfold over 10 years, but the rate of progression is somewhat variable.

Alzheimer's disease primarily damages association areas in the parietal, temporal, and frontal regions. The brain is atrophic and there is neuronal loss and astrocytic gliosis. There are intraneuronal neurofibrillary tangles, neuritic plaques, granuolovacuolar degeneration, and amyloid angiopathy. Dendritic arborization is diminished. Each of these histologic findings is nonspecific.

Risk factors include age, female sex, genetic predisposition, lack of education, and head trauma. Less clear is a potential role for late maternal age. Aluminum toxicity was touted but has not born up to further study. Protective benefits to higher education and intellectual pursuits as well as estrogen therapy and nonsteroidal antiinflammatory agents have been suggested.

The etiology of Alzheimer's disease is unclear as yet, but some important clues are emerging. It is possible that multiple etiologic factors and pathogenetic mechanisms may result in a converging pattern of neuronal dysfunction, synaptic impoverishment, and ultimate neuronal loss. Loss of synaptic function adversely affects signal transmission and correlates with intellectual decline. The involvement of the nucleus basalis results in a major loss in frontal subcortical to cortical cholinergic tone which correlates with memory impairment. This system has nerve growth factor receptors. Other neurotransmitters are also involved, predominantly in younger patients. Excitatory amino acids have been implicated in excessive intracellular calcium influx and have been thought to possibly be a mechanism for cell death. While the role of glutamate transmission in ischemic cell death seems more clearly established, it is possible that injured neurons might be more sensitive to excitatory amino acid toxicity. The role (or lack of it) of the amyloid angiopathy is not clear in the pathogenesis of neuronal loss.

Two abnormal proteins have been identified. Microtubule associated tau protein of normal brain is found in large amounts in an abnormally phosphorylated form in paired helical filaments, which are an important constituent of neurofibrillary tangles. β-amyloid is found in the neuritic plaques and degenerating nerve terminals. Amyloid precursor protein is also a normal constituent of brain across many species with many minor amino acid variants. It is a large protein with high turnover and a coiled glycoprotein with straightened ends, one of which is imbedded in the neuronal membrane. It has serine protease properties and may be involved in cell growth. Degradation of the amyloid precursor protein at the wrong site results in β-amyloid, an insoluble protein resistant to deg tion. Genetic mutations in the amyloid precursor protein are ciated with familial Alzheimer's disease.

The amyloid precursor protein gene is located on chromosome 21, and it is interesting that long-lived Down syndrome individuals (21 trisomy) show Alzheimer's changes. The apoE gene codes for a serum lipoprotein and occurs in three forms. It is located on chromosome 19, and whereas apoE4 is seen in 14% of controls, it occurs in 30% to 40% of late onset sporadic cases and 80% of late onset familial cases. Individuals homozygous for apoE may have a 90% chance of developing Alzheimer's disease by age 85. Estimates are that 25% to 40% of cases are attributable to apoE4. ApoE4 has a high affinity for β-amyloid, and patients with the gene have larger plaques. The continued rapid evolution of understanding of the neurobiology and genetics of this disorder may lead to useful therapeutic manipulations in this common tragic disorder.

Pick's disease is a much less common disorder. Unlike Alzheimer's disease, personality is affected early, with amnesia and visuospatial problems, and acalculia late. Linguistic disturbances also occur but these tend to anomia and stereotypic speech. Because of the selective atrophy of frontal and temporal lobes, Klüver-Bucy syndrome with hypersexuality, gluttony, hyperorality, and emotional blunting may be seen. The pathology includes the presence of argyrophilic intracytoplasmic Pick bodies or inflated cells with argyrophilic cytoplasm. Dendritic spines are lost and white matter gliosis is seen. Other focal cortical degenerations occur including: frontal-lobe degeneration of the non-Alzheimer's type, neuronal intranuclear hyaline inclusion disease, progressive subcortical gliosis, primary progressive aphasia, and posterior cerebral atrophy.

Subcortical Dementias

Unlike the cortical dementias, these disorders manifest by early abnormalities of gait, stance, movement, and tone. Speech is more impaired than language, and speech as well as cognition seem slowed. Mood is apathetic and memory suffers retrieval problems. These patients may really be suffering from loss of frontal-subcortical connections with resultant difficulty in switching sets, and the term may be somewhat of a misnomer. An example might be Huntington's disease or the lacunar state.

Huntington's disease is an autosomal dominant disorder with complete penetrance. Atrophy of the caudate head and loss of cortical neurons occurs. It is localized genetically to the short arm of chromosome 4. The defect is known to be a polymorphic trinucleotide CAG repeat. A potential role for excitotoxic amino acids and depleted γ-amino butyric acid (GABA) have been presented. Onset is usually between 30 to 50 years of age, with duration about 15 years. Prevalence is about 5 per 100,000 people. Features include motor, cognitive, and emotional impairments. The motor disorder is not just chorea but includes athetosis, dystonia, and other movements. Rigidity occurs in juvenile onset and late disease. The cognitive disorder may be preceded by impairment of frontal lobe "executive" functions such as organization and judgment. The cortical features tend to be spared, with memory deficit, cognitive slowing, and apathy the rule. Loss of perception of shapes, impaired comprehension of prosody, and dysarthria are other features. Psychiatric problems include depression, impulsive behavior, intermittent explosive disorder, and, less common, schizophrenia and antisocial behavior. Suicide is excessive as befits a population with a third having major depression.

Table 111-2. Etiologic Classification of Dementias

Degenerative Dementias

- Cortical dementias
  - Dementia of the Alzheimer type
  - Pick disease
  - Focal cortical atrophies
    - Primary progressive aphasia
      - Nonfluent aphasia (anterior perisylvian)
      - Fluent aphasia (temporal and posterior perisylvian)
      - Anomic aphasia (anterior temporal)
      - Mixed aphasia (temporal and perisylvian)
    - Perceptual-motor syndromes
    - Progressive visual syndromes (parieto-occipital/parieto-temporal, posterior cerebral atrophy)
      - Progressive motor syndromes (parietofrontal)
    - Progressive frontal lobe syndromes (frontal lobe dementia)
      - Neuropsychiatric
      - Progressive spasticity/primary lateral sclerosis
      - Mixed
    - Bitemporal syndromes
      - Progressive amnesia
      - Progressive prosopagnosia
      - Progressive neuropsychiatric syndrome with anomia and amnesia
      - Posterior cerebral atrophy
- Subcortical dementias with basal ganglia involvement
  - Huntington disease
  - Parkinson disease
  - Diffuse Lewy body disease
  - Progressive supranuclear palsy
  - Wilson disease
  - Hallervorden-Spatz syndrome
  - Spinocerebellar degenerations
  - Idiopathic calcification of the basal ganglia (Fahr disease)
  - Thalamic degeneration
  - Corticobasal degeneration
  - Progressive subcortical gliosis
  - Motor neuron disease with dementia

Vascular Dementias

- Superficial infarctions
  - Multiple emboli, vasculitis, etc.
- Deep infarctions
  - Lacunar state
  - Binswanger disease
- Combined superficial and deep infarctions
  - Multi-infarct dementia
- Hypoperfusion syndromes

Viral Dementias

- Postencephalitic dementias
  - Arbovirus
  - Herpes simplex
- Postinfectious encephalomyelitis
  - Exanthematous
  - Nonexanthematous
  - Postvaccination
- Progressive dementia due to conventional viruses
  - Human immunodeficiency virus type 1
  - Progressive multifocal leukoencephalopathy
  - Subacute sclerosing panencephalitis
  - Progressive rubella panencephalitis
- Prion diseases
  - Creutzfeldt-Jakob disease
  - Kuru
  - Gerstmann-Straussler-Scheinker disease
  - Alper disease
  - Thalamic dementia

Bacterial, Fungal, and Parasitic Dementias

- Chronic meningitis
  - Fungal
    - Cryptococcus, coccidioides, histoplasmosis, candida, blastomyces, aspergillosis, paracoccidioides, dermatomycosis, clodosporium, allescheria, cephalosporium, sporotrix, actinomyces, nocardia
  - Parasitic
    - Malaria
    - Cysticercosis
    - Coenurosis
    - Toxoplasmosis
    - Amebiasis
  - Chronic bacterial
    - *Mycobacterium tuberculosis*
    - Syphilis
      - General paresis
      - Meningovascular
      - Syphilitic meningitis
    - Neurobrucellosis
    - Lyme borreliosis
    - Whipple disease
    - African trypanosomiasis

Metabolic Dementias

- Medications
- Heavy metals
  - Lead
  - Mercury
  - Manganese
  - Arsenic
  - Thallium
  - Others: aluminum, gold, tin, bismuth, nickel
  - Industrial toxins
- Endocrinopathies
  - Thyroid (myxedema, thyrotoxicosis)
  - Adrenal (Addison, myxedema)
  - Parathyroid (hyper with hypercalcemia, hypo)
  - Hypopituitarism
- Nutritional deficiencies
  - Hypoglycemia
  - Thiamine
  - Niacin
  - Cyancobalamin
- Anoxias
  - Transient severe anoxia with postanoxic dementia
  - Carbon monoxide
  - Chronic hypercapnic encephalopathy
  - Hyperviscosity syndromes
- Chronic renal failure
  - Uremic encephalopathy
  - Dialysis dementia
- Hepatic dysfunction
  - Portosystemic encephalopathy
  - Chronic non-Wilsonian hepatocerebral degeneration
- Pancreatic disorders

Inherited Disorders With Dementia

- Leukodystrophies
  - Metachromatic leukodystrophy
  - Adrenoleukodystrophy
  - Cerebrotendinous xanthomatosis
- Poliodystrophies
  - Adult GM_1 gangliosidosis
  - Adult GM_2 gangliosidosis
  - Adult Gaucher disease
  - Membranous lipodystrophy
  - Neuronal ceroid lipofuscinosis (Kuft disease)
  - Niemann-Pick disease, Type C

(continues)

Table 111-2. *(Continued)*

Inherited Disorders With Dementia *(continued)*	Hydrocephalic Dementia
Corencephalopathies	Spontaneously arrested hydrocephalus
Subacute necrotizing encephalomyelitis (Leigh disease)	Obstructive, noncommunicating hydrocephalus
Hepatolenticular degeneration (Wilson disease)	Obstructive, communicating hydrocephalus (normal pressure)
Hallervorden-Spatz	Subarachnoid hemorrhage
Neuroacanthocytosis	Superficial hemosiderosis of the CNS
Diffuse encephalopathies	Hydrocephalus ex vacuo
Acute intermittent porphyria	**Pseudodementias**
Adult polyglycosan body disease / Fabry disease (multiinfarct dementia)	Dementia syndrome of depression
Mitochondrial encephalomyelopathies	Ganser syndrome
Kearns-Sayre syndrome	Malingering
Myoclonus epilepsy with ragged red fibers (MERRF)	Miscellaneous psychiatric disorders
Mitochondrial myopathy, encephalopathy, lactic acidosis, and stroke-like episodes (MELAS)	Miscellaneous dementias
Progressive myoclonus epilepsy (Unverricht-Lundborg)	Trauma
With Lafora bodies	Dementia pugilistica
Without Lafora bodies	Closed head injury
Spinocerebellar degenerations	Chronic subdural hematoma
Friedreich syndrome	Multiple sclerosis
Olivopontocerebellar atrophies	Tumors
Dentatorubral-pallidoluysian atrophy	Direct
MAST syndrome	Mass
Sensory radicular neuropathy	Local
Myotonic dystrophy	Neoplastic meningitis
Homocystinuria	Paraneoplastic limbic encephalitis

Parkinson's disease is a common (1 per 1000 people prevalence) disorder with the four cardinal features of rigidity, bradykinesia, tremor, and postural instability. Onset is at about 60 years and duration is about 10 years. There is a loss of pigmented neurons most severe in the pars compacta of the substantia nigra. Neuronal loss and gliosis are associated with the more specific finding of cytoplasmic round eosinophilic hyaline bodies with halos called Lewy bodies. The movement disorder is related to the loss of nigral dopaminergic input to the striatum. Some mental impairment occurs in 20% to 30% of patients, especially at late stages of the disorder. The dementia in most is of only mild to moderate type with bradyphrenia, impaired problem solving, slowed and impaired recall, decreased spontaneity, impaired visuospatial perception, impaired set shift, and depression. There exists a strong association of limbic cortex Lewy bodies and large numbers in the mesencephalon. This limbic Lewy body concentration is strongly associated with dementia. When severe cognitive deficits occur, there may be associated Alzheimer's changes. There is a group of patients with moderate cortical Lewy body involvement and dementia without Parkinson's disease. These patients are referred to as having *diffuse Lewy body disease* and present with a primarily cortical dementia. An additional complexity is the ability of the anti-Parkinson's medications to induce delirium.

Progressive supranuclear palsy is only 1/100th as common as Parkinson's disease; it may be confused with Parkinson's disease early in the illness. It presents with axial rigidity, pseudobulbar palsy, dysarthria, and supranuclear ophthalmoplegia. Posture tends to be in extension rather than flexion as in Parkinson's disease. Parkinson's patients develop an impairment of upgaze, but these patients characteristically have a striking impairment of downgaze. The eye movement problem is supranuclear as evidenced by the ability to induce reflex eye movements in response to head turning (oculocephalic reflex). This impaired downgaze produces severe reading problems for patients requiring bifocals. Combined with instability of posture, falls are frequent. The dementia occurs late and is typically frontal subcortical in type.

Other causes of subcortical dementia include Wilson hepatolenticular degeneration, Hallevorden-Spatz Syndrome, ALS-Parkinsonism-dementia complex of Guam, and spinocerebellar degenerations.

Mixed cortical and subcortical dementias also exist and include some forms of vascular dementia and neurosyphilis.

Vascular Dementia

Vascular dementia presents special problems because it harkens back to the days when cerebral arteriosclerosis was accepted by general physicians as *the* cause of dementia. While the term is used more cautiously, a clear definition and an understanding of the relationship between the vascular lesion and the dementia is still lacking. It is recognized that some 25% of stroke patients from the Stroke Data Bank have dementia. Of those with dementia, 56% are thought it is because of the stroke and an additional 36% are thought to have mixed vascular and Alzheimer's disease. The extent of the vascular disease, location, bilaterality, and total volume seem determinants of the development of dementia, rather than the nature of the vascular disease itself. For each of the factors cited, no clear criteria exist. Evidence for a slow strangulation of nerve cells rather than multiple infarctions has not been pre-

Table 111-3. An Abbreviated Classification

D	drug
E	emotional
M	metabolic
E	eyes and ears
N	nutritional
T	tumor
I	infection
A	atherosclerosis

sented. Controversy exists over whether this diagnosis is over or underused.

The classic clinical points to imply vascular etiology are: male sex, sudden onset, stepwise course, focal signs, relative preservation of personality, history of vascular disease, vascular risk factors, and hypertension. They are quantified into an ischemic scale by Hachinski, then evolved and simplified by Rosen. This does serve to divide patients into those with high probability of stroke from those with low probability (Table 111-4)

Patients with large areas of infarction are not controversial because they also present with obvious neurologic findings and are therefore not easily confused with other patients with dementia. Elderly individuals with chronic nonvalvular atrial fibrillation experience an excessive embolic stroke burden. They are therefore subject to possible granular cerebral atrophy which can cause a cortical dementia, but the frequency of this in the elderly is unclear.

Lacunes are small deep infarcts of gray and white matter due to hypertensive fibrinoid changes in the small penetrating arteries at the base of the brain. They also result from atherosclerosis of the mouth of these vessels. Less commonly, they may be caused by emboli or small bleeds. When these lesions are bilateral and multiple it is called the *lacunar state.* The subcortical dementia which ensues shows apathetic behavior, memory disturbances, emotional lability, and preservation of insight. This is superimposed on a background of incontinence, pseudobulbar palsy, and pyramidal and extrapyramidal signs.

The hemispheric white matter is supplied by long fine penetrating vessels that arise from major cortical branches, but are themselves end vessels subject to similar hypertension-induced changes as cause lacunar infarction. This may result in subcortical infarcts or incomplete lesions where the tissue integrity is preserved but axons and myelin are lost, and can cause disconnection of overlying cortex. This has been referred to as Binswanger disease. In addition, these areas are also in the watershed between major blood vessels and may suffer if hypotension or overzealous antihypertensive regimens are used, especially if large vessel disease is also present. These patients share many of the features of lacunar state, but may show more cortical features. Large vessel involvement may result in the *angular gyrus syndrome*, which may be confused with Alzheimer's disease, but which spares topographic skills and memory when nonverbal testing is used.

Leukoaraiosis was a name coined to refer to changes seen in white matter on computed tomography, to distinguish a radiographic appearance of uncertain nature from Binswanger disease. Magnetic resonance imaging offers finer resolution of these changes, which are very common. Leukoaraiosis correlates with age, stroke, and hypertension. Mild changes seen as ventricular caps are common, and some change merely reflects the cribriform state, which is an increase in perivascular spaces in atrophic brains of hypertensive patients. Some patients show large confluent areas which are associated with white matter pathology as described in Binswanger disease. It bears some relation to cognitive decline and focal neurologic findings. Increased leukoaraiosis in Alzheimer's disease has been attributed to Wallerian degeneration or hypotension and hypoperfusion. Leukoaraiosis has a strong correlation with multiinfarct dementia and, when severe, has been said to be itself a cause of dementia. A too common error has been to attempt to define the presence of dementia or its etiology in radiographic terms.

Table 111-4. Rosen Modification of Hachinski Ischemic Scale

Abrupt onset	2
Stepwise deterioration	1
Somatic complaints	1
Emotional incontinence	1
History of hypertension	1
History of strokes	2
Focal neurologic symptoms	2
Focal neurologic signs	2

Degenerative dementia suggested by score < 3, vascular if > 3.

It is not possible to cover all of the dementing illnesses, but several infectious causes are worthy of mention. Creutzfeld-Jakob disease is a rare, rapidly progressive dementia with myoclonic jerks. Several clinical varieties have been described. Of great importance was the discovery that the etiology of this disorder is a transmissible agent. This and other spongiform encephalopathies have been shown to be transmitted by prions—small proteinacious infectious particles that resist inactivation by procedures which modify nucleic acids. This can occur in sporadic, inherited, and iatrogenic forms. This has been the subject of human transmission through organ transplantation, and therefore dementia must be regarded as an absolute contraindication to such grafts.

A growing cause of dementia, especially among the young, is the acquired immunodeficiency syndrome (AIDS) dementia complex (human immunodeficiency virus [HIV] encephalopathy). Patients may present with dementia before they have full-blown AIDS. The disorder usually presents as a subcortical dementia, but ultimately expresses itself as a more generalized process. It is not amenable to therapy thus far and leads to an early demise. A critical consideration for the physician is ruling out such opportunistic infections as toxoplasmosis, cryptococcal meningitis, cytomegalovirus, progressive multifocal leukoencephalopathy, or primary central nervous system (CNS) lymphoma.

Neurosyphilis is a major cause of dementia, but it has undergone a profound decline, with new cases now rare. Despite reemergence of syphilis as a problem, it will be some years before new cases of tertiary syphilis are seen again.

A rare, but much discussed, syndrome is normal pressure hydrocephalus. This is most readily diagnosed after subarachnoid hemorrhage or meningitis and manifests itself in a dementia with slowed mental processing deteriorating to apathetic forgetfulness, suggestive of a subcortical type, but it may display admixtures of cortical dysfunction. There is always an associated gait disturbance and it is commonly more of an ataxic type rather than a spastic gait (more common in high pressure hydrocephalus). Urinary incontinence is a later feature of the diagnostic triad. This is due to a communicating hydrocephalus (no blockage in spinal fluid flow from ventricles to subarachnoid space) associated with an impairment in spinal fluid absorption into the pacchionian granulations and the sagittal sinus. Difficulty in distinguishing enlarged ventricles from atrophy (hydrocephalus ex vacuo) leads to its frequent consideration. Diagnosis is somewhat problematic, as less than a third of patients seem to improve with ventriculoperitoneal shunting. Improvement is more common when the syndrome is new and may be least effective for the mental changes.

Early in the course of the dementing illness, distinction from the normal cognitive changes of aging must be made. As individuals age, they experience a normal increase in problems of immediate recall and may assume that this is a manifestation of impending dementia. Physician reassurance is essential to their sense of well-being. Early in the illness, when the complaints may reflect a high achiever's loss of a subtle edge, the standard interview may prove quite inadequate. Patients may be brought back in follow-up when the distinction between normal aging and excess responsibilities, as opposed to incipient dementia, may not be evident to the examiner. The family benefits not only from knowledge of the presence of an illness but also from projection of its possible course. Diagnosis currently is based primarily on clinical judgment and knowledge of the possibilities. Unfortunately, there are no simple blood or imaging tests available and a careful cognitive examination takes time. Detailed neuropsychologic testing is available and often quite helpful, but many insurance plans are reluctant to pay for this testing. The physician should be reluctant to accept a diagnosis as gloomy as this without serious consideration of possible alternatives. Specific diagnosis will be more imperative as more specific treatments become available.

HISTORY

A general medical history must include a history directed at endocrine, hematologic, or infectious (including HIV) factors. Inquiries about neurologic dysfunction, such as head injury, stroke, or seizure, should be made. Family history of dementing illness may not be volunteered and must be elicited. Early features such as forgetting names must be distinguished from the normal age-associated memory impairment. Mismanaging work or financial affairs is seen and may require independent history from family or coworkers. It is important to remember that the organ that gives the history is the one that is ill. It is said that when the physician feels more and more frustrated or provoked by the patient's inability to provide a consistent reasonable history, dementia should be considered as a possible diagnosis. Many families will cover for patients, and indirect questions about who handles the checkbook and if the cooking has changed may give clues. Difficulty with appointments or scheduled medications may follow. Loss of creativity or inability to learn new skills or retain topographic orientation usually precedes any loss of linguistic or perceptuomotor skills. The pattern of developing disorder will vary both by individual and by dementia type. Apathy must be distinguished from depression. Depression may also follow loss of intellect. It is not usually a key etiologic factor unless the patient has a prior history of mood disturbance. The use of prescription, over-the-counter, or recreational drugs or alcohol should be queried. This may require a family check on the medication cabinet for such things as a dead spouse's medication, multiple out-dated prescriptions, prescriptions by multiple physicians.

The family or friends may contribute information about changes in the patient's personality and routines. Appetite, weight, sleep, dress, and toilet must all be assessed. The office situation can usually be manipulated to allow private conversation with the caregiver except in very paranoid patients. Failure to do so will necessitate a specific arrangement to get a history from family or coworkers in the patient's absence.

PHYSICAL EXAMINATION

A general physical examination is necessary because intercurrent illness can seriously compromise mental status testing, particularly in the elderly. The so-called frontal signs are more reflective of diffuse disease. These include the glabellar response (inability to suppress forced eye closure in response to tapping the forehead), suck reflex, forced grasp response, impaired visual smooth pursuit, impaired upgaze, and paratonia (resistance to passive movements intermingled with facilitation of such).

The patient's level of consciousness, as well as attention, must be assessed. An *alert* person with the ability to attend to the task is needed before a reliable mental status test can be performed. *Attention* is gauged by spelling "world" backward or performing serial subtractions. Delirium with clouding of consciousness may be present in a demented patient, but one should not rush to diagnose dementia when delirium is present. The mental status examination should take cognizance of general behavior and mood. Language function must be evaluated early because the ability to comprehend the cognitive testing may be compromised by aphasia. Aphasia with severe neologisms and paraphasias may be confused with the sudden onset of schizophrenia, an unlikely event in the elderly. Delusions, illusions, and hallucinations may have a paranoid flavor but tend to be more commonly visual and simpler than in primary psychotic disorders. Insight may be lacking.

Cognition is tested by a series of questions that are directed at different aspects of higher function. The patient's prior level of intellect and education will have a major impact on performance. Most physicians do not have available a set of testing materials and make do with pencil and paper. The Folstein Mini-Mental Status test is quite well known to many physicians and medical students. This 5-minute test can be quite helpful when it is recognized that results are affected by illness and medication and also may be inadequate to evaluate early and late disease. For example, mild deficits fail to distinguish between age-associated memory impairment and Alzheimer's disease. Many areas are covered in this scale, but finding of deficits should lead to further exploration.

Orientation to time, place, and person is assessed. A patient with a long hospitalization is frequently fuzzy on the day of the month.

Memory is frequently tested by immediate recall, but this is primarily a function of attention. *Fund of information* (old learning) may be measured by questions directed at age of children and schooling, occupational history, geography, politics, sports, or hobbies. The ability to retain new information as well as retrieve old information may be tested. A memory task, usually three objects, is given and the examination continues after the examiner is assured that the objects have indeed been learned. Other parts of the mental status are pursued and later the examiner returns to this task. Aged patients may have better recognition than recall.

Comprehension, judgment, and abstractions may be tested by proverbs ("Rome wasn't built in a day"), similarities ("What do an orange and an apple have in common?"), and problems ("Why do we pay taxes?"; "What would you do if you found a sealed stamped addressed envelope?").

Apraxia has been defined as an inability to carry out purposeful movements on oral command, in the absence of comprehension or motor deficits. *Constructional tasks* may ask for a drawing of a daisy or a clock face, copying a design, or building with blocks or matches. Other *apraxias* may be tested by asking the subject to show how to use a comb or scissors. The patient should be observed dressing.

Motor aspects of *speech* are tested, but dysarthria is not usually seen early in cortical dementias, as opposed to the more symbolic processing of language. *Language* is evident during the history through *comprehension* of the questions and the *spontaneous speech*. Abnormal language may be either nonfluent with sparse, slow, effortful, telegraphic speech, or fluent but devoid of nouns, verbs, and content. Letter or word substitutions (paraphasias) or nonwords (neologisms) may be interspersed or the sentence be directed around a word that will not be found. *Naming* is tested, as are reading, writing, and repetition.

Other cognitive functions that may be affected include topographic disorientation, right–left confusion, finger agnosia, unilateral neglect, impaired motor sequences (rock, paper, scissors), and calculation.

Formal neuropsychologic evaluation is quite helpful, but much useful information may be obtained by a physician with sufficient time to spend with a patient. The references should be consulted for more details of the technique of the mental status examination, if this is desired.

LABORATORY AND IMAGING STUDIES

The laboratory is usually not of great help in evaluating dementias because the most frequent causes lack diagnostic tests. The importance of the laboratory lies both in excluding potentially treatable disorders and in the ability to make specific diagnoses in many of the rarer cases. This type of bleak outlook deserves some effort at the more treatable possibilities. Routine blood counts and serum chemistries, including glucose, renal, hepatic, and protein studies, are done. B_{12} determinations are necessary, even if the blood picture is unremarkable, to exclude combined degeneration. Thyroid studies including TSH are indicated, as well as calcium and perhaps cortisol. Sedimentation rate and perhaps antinuclear antibodies may help exclude inflammatory diseases. A serum VDRL or similar test may be negative in 40% to 50% of tertiary syphilis and an FTA-ABS is needed. When anything raises the clinical suspicion a toxic drug screen or heavy metal analysis may be in order. A lumbar puncture is not part of the routine diagnostic workup but is needed when chronic fungal meningitis is considered. Specific tests may be ordered to rule out some of the more exotic causes.

An imaging study is usually obtained to exclude chronic subdural hematoma, which may present with more behavioral than motor signs. This will also be helpful in the chronic meningitides and other intracranial masses and will exclude normal pressure hydrocephalus (NPH). Magnetic resonance imaging (MRI) will provide more information and is usually done in preference to a computed tomographic (CT) scan. In NPH, an acute angle between the frontal horns and a depressed third ventricular floor with ventriculomegaly and minimal sulcal enlargement are most easily seen in MRI, as is transependymal absorption of spinal fluid. In suspicious cases assessment of the spinal fluid flow pattern by Indium cisternography may be helpful. The isotope is injected into the lumbar cerebral spinal fluid and should flow over the convexities and be absorbed normally. In NPH the isotope enters the ventricle and stays for days without passing to the sagittal sinus. Plain x-rays are seldom helpful.

Electroencephalography (EEG) is generally unrewarding but can show characteristic suppression bursts (sharp waves on a low-voltage slow background), which may be seen in Creutzfeld-Jakob disease, and triphasic slow waves in some metabolic encephalopathies. Cerebral evoked potentials are specific EEG activity seen in response to a stimulus. A signal averager or computer averages out the background variable EEG activity as background noise after hundreds of stimuli, leaving only EEG activity that is stimulus-linked. Event-related potentials with long latency, in response to distinguishing a novel stimulus, have been claimed to distinguish depression from true dementia. This is not fully established and is not done routinely.

Positron emission tomography (PET) and single photon emission tomography (SPECT) can provide functional brain imaging which can be most useful in supplementing clinical and neuropsychologic data. These, combined with a CT or MRI, may yield only equivocal results. While SPECT is more likely to be clearly positive in a more advanced disease, it is also less likely to be needed. While SPECT may display a pattern of cerebral blood flow more suggestive of Alzheimer's disease than other types of dementia, no pattern is completely diagnostic.

TREATMENT

The first step in management of dementia is deciding that a cognitive deficit is present; the second is deciding whether progression is present and to determine its rate. Once treatable causes have been excluded, treatment is primarily supportive. The patient and family will require considerable information about the process and expectations for the future. Considerable repetition and review is needed. The physician or nurse can be a significant source of support, but most families can derive much benefit from linkage with the Alzheimer's Association. This is especially true if a local support group is available.

Little specific therapy exists for Alzheimer's disease. There is a cholinergic deficit in this disorder due to involvement of the nucleus basalis of Meynert. Tacrine is a cholinergic agent (a reversible cholinesterase inhibitor) that has been shown to improve cognitive scores and global assessments in 10% to 26% of patients treated with a high dose (160 mg/day) of tacrine daily. Fifty percent of patients experience transaminase elevations to 3 times the upper limit of normal. The transaminase must be monitored every 2 to 4 weeks and the drug discontinued if enzyme changes occur. Seventy-five percent tolerate rechallenge, and most problems occur in the first 18 weeks. The treatment is begun at 40 mg and increased by 40 mg every 6 weeks to 160 mg/day. Most common side effects are nausea, vomiting, anorexia, and diarrhea. Only 27% of patients could be titrated to the effective dose. Probably no more than 10% of mild-to-moderate patients can be expected to benefit. Because the effect is not expected to be sustained, some formal assessment of cognitive function should be made, and if efficacy cannot be sustained, the drug should be slowly withdrawn. This should only be used in mild-to-moderately effected patients with well-motivated caregivers and little general illness. This is an expensive drug requiring repeated blood testing and marginal benefit.

In my experience most families and patients will consider entry into clinical trials, and the physician should be aware of local trials. The efficacy of tacrine is limited and one should make every effort to facilitate development of better-tolerated, more effective agents.

Mild-to-moderate disease may still manifest disturbing behavior. Restless agitation may benefit from a calm routine, food, familiar surroundings, and quiet. Catastrophic reactions may have common triggers, which should be avoided. Feeding problems may be reduced with favorite foods that require little effort to eat and may be left out if the patient likes to eat but cannot handle the structure of regular infrequent meals. Bathing may cause conflict, especially if incontinence is present. The caregiver may execute a strategic withdrawal and try again another time. Urinary incontinence is not uncommon with moderate-to-severe disease, but can also reflect problems of the prostate or pelvic floor. A workup is in order when this occurs inappropriate to the mental status. Evening fluids and diuretics should be minimized. Lights left on at night and scheduled toileting may be helpful. Protective garments are a last resort, but may be needed to avoid decisions for institutional care. Sundowning refers to an evening exacerbation of deficits. This may be severe. It is alleviated by adequate light and reorienting. Lower activity levels and a companion may help.

Even more disruptive for the caregiver, who may have a day job, is an exaggeration of the patient's normal increased nocturnal awakening and loss of deep sleep. This may lead to caregiver burnout and must be addressed. Long restful naps in the day should be avoided, and bedtime snacks and afternoon activity help. Avoidance of nocturnal diuretics, pain, and disorientation is desirable. Sleep medications are avoided, but they may be necessary briefly. Benadryl may cause confusion because of its anticholinergic properties. A sedating antidepressant in small doses may be more beneficial over time than the more direct intermediate-acting benzodiazepines.

Wandering may occur at any time but is more of a problem if the caregiver is asleep or if it takes the patient out of the house inappropriately attired and unable to find the way home. A double lock may restrict departure, and the patient should have an identification bracelet with a phone number. A well-lighted path to the toilet may reduce the problem. The ability to pace in an enclosed space such as a yard or garden may also be helpful.

An additional stress on the caregiver is the need of the patient to shadow the caregiver, preventing any rest and personal time. If possible, a friend or relative can spend some time with the patient to allow the caregiver a chance for shopping or relaxation. An audiotape of the caregiver's voice may also be helpful. Agitation may be relieved by thioridazine or, if this fails, low doses of haloperidol can be used. However, haloperidol has a high propensity for extrapyramidal effects.

Fecal soiling may be reduced by avoiding cathartics and using bulk, exercise, bran, fluids, and planned evacuations or enemas. If this is due to the inability to remove clothing, simpler attire with elastic or Velcro straps may help. Feeding problems and refusal of food are usually an endstage phenomenon.

It is important to remind the caregiver that the patient is not trying to be difficult. Instructions should be given simply and one step at a time. It is useful to capitalize on the patient's strengths and perhaps assign a simple repetitive task. The Alzheimer's Association has patient information sheets with clues on communication and guidelines for caregivers. A major problem can be taking away the car keys. A face-saving excuse may be better accepted unless the patient has had many accidents or has repeatedly been lost. This is a serious issue in communities where the automobile is the major means of transportation. With the widespread availability of guns, this, too, can be a problem.

As the disease becomes worse, institutionalization must be considered. Legal and financial questions should be explored well in advance. Early in the disease, while the patient retains insight, consideration of living wills or health-care proxies should be made. Unless the patient is abusive or caregiver burnout has occurred, institutionalization should be delayed, as deterioration frequently occurs afterward.

CONSIDERATIONS DURING PREGNANCY

Dementia is not a common problem in pregnancy but is of great concern when it occurs because possible etiologic factors are disorders such as HIV dementia and neurosyphilis, which could be transmitted to the fetus. The physician should be alert to possible dementia and thoroughly explore treatable disorders or transmittable disorders.

BIBLIOGRAPHY

American Psychiatric Association, eds. Diagnostic and statistical manual of mental disorders, 4th ed. Washington, DC, 1994.

Appel SH, ed. Current Neurology, vol 15. St. Louis, Mosby-Year Book Inc, 1995.

Burns A, Levy R, eds. Dementia. London: Chapman & Hall, 1994.

Cummings JL. Dementia: the failing brain. Ann Neurol 1993;33:568.

Cummings JL, Benson DF, eds. Dementia: a clinical approach, 2nd ed. Boston: Butterworth-Heinemann, 1992.

Cummings JL, ed. Subcortical dementia. New York: Oxford University Press Inc, 1990.

Gruetzner HM, ed. Alzheimer's: a caregiver's guide and sourcebook. New York: John Wiley & Sons Inc, 1988.

Heilman KM, Valenstein E, eds. Clinical neuropsychology. New York: Oxford University Press, 1993.

Meyer JS, Lechner H, Marshall J, Toole JF, eds. Vascular and multi-infarct dementia. New York: Futura Publishing Co Inc, 1988.

Patient care. Montvale, New Jersey: Medical Economics Publishing, 1991.

Shuaib A. Stroke clinical updates. National Stroke Association 1995; 1:3.

Tatemichi TK, Desmond DW, Paik M. Clinical determinants of dementia related to stroke. Lancet 1993;33:568.

Waldemar G. Functional brain imaging with SPECT in normal aging and dementia: methodological, pathophysiological, and diagnostic aspects. Cerebrovasc Brain Metab Rev 1995;7:89.

Whitehouse PJ, ed. Dementia. Philadelphia: FA Davis, 1993.

Primary Care for Women, edited by Phyllis C. Leppert and Fred M. Howard. Lippincott-Raven Publishers, Philadelphia © 1997.

112
Brain Tumors

GERALD W. HONCH

Brain tumors are relatively common in both children and adults. In adults, about 17,000 new primary brain tumors occur each year in the United States. About half of these are relatively benign and can be successfully treated with an excellent prognosis. The others are more aggressive, are less successfully treated, and carry a limited survival rate. The more common primary brain tumors are listed in Table 112-1. The mean age (in years) at diagnosis is included.

Although neurons are the most common cells in the brain, they cannot reproduce. The glial cells are the supporting cells of the brain. They are numerous and perform many structural and metabolic functions. Glial cells do reproduce and are the source of most of the primary tumors of the CNS. Cancer arises in association with the accumulation of specific structural molecular genetic alterations (mutations) within cells. These cells proliferate inap-

Table 112-1. Primary Brain Tumors—Distribution by Tumor Type

TUMOR	PERCENT OF CASES	MEAN AGE AT DIAGNOSIS
Glioblastoma	40	54
Astrocytoma	16	37
Meningioma	18	55
Schwannoma	2	57
Pituitary adenoma	12	39
Lymphoma	2	46
Other	10	—

propriately, lose the differentiated characteristics of the cells of origin, acquire the ability to invade surrounding normal tissues, and gain the ability to resist antineoplastic therapies.

Two types of molecular alterations cause these changes. There is loss of or a decrease in cellular activities that operate physiologically to restrain growth (tumor suppressor genes). There is also an inappropriate activation of genes that enhance cellular proliferation (protooncogenes). Many malignant tumors induce the formation of new blood vessels, thereby increasing their own nutrient supply and enhancing their own growth. Both benign and malignant tumors may cause edema in the surrounding brain; some secrete factors that increase vascular permeability.

SYMPTOMS AND DIAGNOSIS

Brain tumors present with a variety of clinical signs and symptoms, largely dependent on the type of tumor and its location. Commonly seizures (partial or generalized), visual loss, hearing loss, focal motor or sensory phenomena, ataxia, double vision, and headache occur. Increased intracranial pressure may cause nonspecific complaints of headache, nausea, and vomiting. Personality changes may be seen with increased intracranial pressure as well as masses in the frontal region or posterior fossa. Changes in libido or menstrual cycles may occur. This mixture of protean and specific complaints is the reason medical attention is sought.

On physical examination, the focal signs may help direct the work-up. The fundi may reveal papilledema. With slow-growing tumors, the findings are generally more subtle, as the CNS may be more accommodating. A rapid evolution of signs and symptoms is generally cause for alarm.

In the past, lumbar puncture with CSF analysis, electroencephalography, nuclear scanning, pneumoencephalography, ventriculography, and angiography were the mainstays of the work-up for brain tumors. These studies have been supplanted by computed tomography (CT) and magnetic resonance imaging (MRI). The MRI may offer a better evaluation of the anatomy of the CNS, as well as better definition of edema versus tumor mass. Angiography remains a useful modality, especially for vascular tumors.

CLASSIFICATION

Neuropathology has played a major part in the improved understanding of tumor pathogenesis. Tissue by biopsy or resection is the only method of exact diagnosis. Although the location and behavior of the mass and its character on CT or MRI scanning may give important clues to the diagnosis, there is no substitute for the microscopic examination with differential staining and other advanced pathologic techniques.

There are several different scales or classification protocols that are followed. The Karnofsky performance score is an important clinical grading scale commonly used to evaluate the patient across various stages of treatment and follow-up. Other scales used are the WHO, the Bailey and Cushing, the Kernohan, and the Dauma-Duport classification. Patients are assigned a score of 10 to 100 according to their ability to perform daily tasks. Thus, simple survival scores have been expanded to include the quality of that survival.

BENIGN TUMORS

The benign tumors of the nervous system (Table 112-2) are generally characterized by slow growth and lack of invasion of surrounding structures. They are often subtle in their presentation. A benign tumor is benign on the basis of its cellular character and behavior. However, benign tumors may not be resectable because of their adherence to adjacent tissues or their tendency to surround essential structures.

Meningioma

Meningiomas occur twice as often in women as in men and tend to occur in later life. They are more common after previous cranial radiation and in persons with neurofibromatosis. There is an increased incidence in patients with breast carcinoma. Meningiomas have receptors for sex hormones and other ligands that include progesterone, estrogen, androgen, dopamine, and the β-receptor for platelet-derived growth factor; of these, the progesterone receptor is the most robust. These may have important implications for pathophysiology and future therapies. The characteristic histologic features are whorls formed around central hyaline material. This eventually calcifies and forms psammoma bodies or interlacing bundles of elongated fibroblasts with narrow nuclei. Several pathologic classifications have been developed.

The classic primary treatment has been surgical, but size, location, and relation to neighboring structures may preclude total resection. Radiation therapy has been shown to be of potential benefit in selected patients with inoperable, partially resected, or recurrent meningiomas. Hormonal therapy has been tried. Tamoxifen (antiestrogen) has been ineffective; RU486 (an antiprogesterone) has shown some promise.

Pituitary Adenoma

Pituitary adenomas have four common presentations: a hypersecretory endocrine syndrome, visual symptoms, symptoms of mass effect such as headache, or as an incidental finding on MRI or CT.

There are four hypersecretory adenomas. The most common hypersecretory syndrome is hyperprolactinemia from a prolactin-secreting tumor (40%). Women develop galactorrhea and amenorrhea. Serum prolactin levels can be monitored. Growth hormone-secreting adenomas (15%) produce acromegaly in adults. Major changes in other organs (eg, hypertension, cardiomyopathy, hepatosplenomegaly, arthritis) may occur. The third hypersecretion syndrome is Cushing syndrome, caused by excess cortisol or adrenocorticotropic hormone (10%). The clinical signs include moon facies, truncal obesity, abdominal striae, buffalo hump, facial hirsutism, diabetes mellitus, and hypertension. Follicle-stimulating

Table 112-2. Benign Tumors of the CNS

TUMOR	CLINICAL PRESENTATION	LOCATION	CT FEATURES	MRI FEATURES	TREATMENT ISSUES
Meningioma	Subtle. Slow growth and lack of invasion. Seizures, headache, focal deficits	Arachnoid origin. Along dural planes	Well defined. Enhanced well with contrast	Similar to brain on T1 and T2. Enhance with contrast	Not always curable. Site, accessibility, and biologic aggressiveness. Hormone relation
Pituitary adenoma	Endocrine Visual symptoms. Mass effect Incidental	Sella turcica and suprasellar region	Use contrast; transaxial and coronal views (bone and tissue)	Best on T1 Contrast Sagittal, coronal, and transaxial	Observation Hormone (bromocriptine) Surgery
Acoustic neuroma	Sensorineural hearing loss, tinnitus, dizziness	Vestibular nerve in internal auditory meatus	Bony changes and mass	Best seen with MRI and contrast	Observation, surgery, radiation
Craniopharyngioma	Growth failure in children. Sexual dysfunction/ visual loss in adults	Suprasellar	Low density with calcification	Low density with calcification	Observation, radiation, stereotactic and surgical resection. Combination
Epidermoid	Seizures, cranial nerve abnormalities, and hydrocephalus	Cisterns at base of brain	Low density. Irregular rim that enhances	Low density. Irregular rim that enhances	Surgical only
Colloid cyst	Headache or obtundation due to obstruction of foramen of Monro	Third ventricle	Low, isodense or enhancing. Location is key.	Low, isodense or enhancing. Location is key.	Surgery; may need shunting. Stereotactic aspiration
Hemangioblastoma	Posterior fossa obstruction and hydrocephalus	Cerebellum	Vascular nodule with surrounding cyst	Vascular nodule with surrounding cyst	Surgical resection

hormone, luteinizing hormone, and thyroid-stimulating hormone may all be affected.

Pituitary adenomas typically produce a bitemporal hemianopia as the tumor compresses the fibers within the optic chiasm. Symptoms of a mass effect with headache are often nonspecific. Pituitary apoplexy with hemorrhage or infarction into the pituitary gland can cause collapse and symptoms similar to those of subarachnoid hemorrhage. Several other problems can mimic a pituitary adenoma by occupying the sellar and suprasellar regions. These include meningiomas, craniopharyngiomas, and rare primary and metastatic tumors.

MRI is the modality of choice for imaging pituitary structures. Excellent definition of the suprasellar extent of the tumor, as well as retrosellar and parasellar extension, can be accomplished. CT scanning is an excellent second choice. Both MRI and CT scanning should be done with contrast.

The management of these tumors depends on their size and type and the clinical syndrome. Often neurology, neurosurgery, ophthalmology, and endocrine consultants are necessary. With prolactin-secreting tumors, a dopamine agonist (eg, bromocriptine) lowers prolactin levels and shrinks the tumor mass. The other pituitary tumors are best treated by surgery. Transsphenoidal surgery is the procedure of choice, with a morbidity rate of 5% to 10% and a mortality rate of near zero. CSF leak is the most common postsurgical problem. Radiation therapy is used adjunctively.

Acoustic Neuroma

Acoustic neuromas are more correctly called vestibular schwannomas, as they are composed of Schwann cells and arise from the vestibular nerve. They have an incidence of about one per 100,000. Ninety-five percent are unilateral and are not associated with other entities. Five percent are bilateral and are associated with neurofibromatosis type II (von Recklinghausen disease), an autosomal dominant disorder. There is no sexual predilection.

The most common presenting complaint is sensorineural hearing loss. Other complaints include tinnitus, dizziness, and disequilibrium. As the tumor expands, it fills the internal auditory meatus, compressing the cochlear and facial nerves. Late signs include brain stem compression, ataxia, and hydrocephalus. Audiometry shows a sensorineural hearing loss, usually for high frequencies. Brain stem auditory evoked potentials testing demonstrates prolongation of waves I–III. MRI with gadolinium is the imaging modality of choice. Other lesions of the cerebellopontine angle include meningiomas, gliomas, cholesteatomas, arachnoid cysts, metastatic tumors, lipomas, hemangiomas, and aneurysms.

The therapeutic options include observation, surgery, and radiation therapy. Acoustic neuromas tend to be slow-growing tumors; hence, an incidental finding of a small tumor in an elderly patient may warrant observation for an extended period. A young patient with progressive neurologic deficits or evidence of tumor growth requires definitive treatment. Surgery is the treatment of choice. CSF leakage is a potential postoperative problem. Preserving hearing and avoiding facial nerve damage is enhanced with newer microsurgical techniques. Large tumors and those that have enveloped cranial nerves or distorted the brain stem render the patient at higher risk. Radiation therapy has had limited success.

Craniopharyngioma

Craniopharyngiomas are suprasellar tumors arising from epithelial remnants of the Rathke pouch. They present in children with growth failure and in adults with sexual dysfunction. MRI and CT scanning may be diagnostic because of location and the variable contents, ranging from low density to calcification. Treatment options include observation, various surgical approaches, and radiation. Postoperative problems include memory deficits, appetite and behavioral disturbances, and endocrine dysfunction.

Epidermoid

Epidermoids are collections of misplaced ectoderm (by implantation or sequestration). They generally occur at the cerebellopontine angle and the base of the skull. They generally present with headache, signs of obstruction, or cranial nerve abnormalities. On CT scanning, they are of low attenuation and lobulated in the expected location. On MRI, they have prolonged T1 and T2 values. The treatment is surgical, although their tendency to insinuate along cranial nerves may preclude removal. Cyst contents are notorious for inciting an aseptic meningitis (responsive to steroids).

Colloid Cyst

Colloid cysts are spherical cysts in the roof of the third ventricle. They present with headache and other signs of obstructive hydrocephalus. Sometimes they are found incidentally on a scan done for other reasons. They are low or isodense spheres on CT and MRI scanning; some enhance. The treatment is surgical, but their location can make removal difficult.

Hemangioblastoma

Hemangioblastomas are most commonly found in the cerebellum. About 10% of these patients have polycythemia from tumor production of erythropoietin. They occur sporadically or as the autosomal dominant von Hippel-Lindau disease. They are associated with retinal angiomatosis, renal cell carcinoma, visceral cysts, and adrenal pheochromocytomas. A cystic lesion with a nodule is seen on CT and MRI scanning. Surgical resection is the preferred treatment.

MALIGNANT TUMORS

The term *malignant* generally refers to the ability of a tumor to metastasize. This has no relevance in the CNS, but seeding or spreading of tumor along surfaces does occur. Malignant CNS tumors infiltrate the parenchyma and are poorly circumscribed (Table 112-3). Metaplasia (a nonneoplastic conversion of one adult cell type to another) and anaplasia (change from a more differentiated to a less differentiated state) occurs. Tumor necrosis occurs by outpacing blood supply. Other important signs of malignancy include grading by histologic differentiation, palisading and pseudopalisading, rosette formation, desmoplasia (proliferation of mesenchymal tissue), and endothelial proliferation (capillaries).

Astroglial Neoplasms

The astrocytic series is the largest and most heterogeneous group of neuroepithelial tumors. Astrocytoma, anaplastic astrocytoma, and glioblastoma form a continuum of the same process. Malignant changes may transform a well-differentiated astrocytoma over time. The astrocytoma is considered a mildly hypercellular tumor with pleomorphism but no vascular proliferation or necrosis. The anaplastic astrocytoma has vascular proliferation, moderate pleomorphism, and moderate hypercellularity. The glioblastoma has these characteristics plus necrosis. The absence of necrosis is the principal criterion separating anaplastic astrocytoma from glioblastoma.

The astroglial tumors are also described on the basis of their location: optic nerve glioma, hypothalamic glioma, brain stem (tectal, pontine, or medullary) glioma, cerebellar astrocytoma, corpus callosum glioma, cerebral hemisphere astrocytoma, and so forth. The location of the tumor may have important implications for treatment. Brain stem gliomas occur primarily in children. Widespread infiltration of the brain parenchyma is rare; when it occurs, it is termed gliomatosis cerebri.

Anaplastic astrocytomas have a mean age of onset of 46 years. They are usually located in the cerebral hemispheres. The average survival time from diagnosis is 2 years.

Glioblastoma multiforme is the most common primary brain tumor in adults and comprises about 50% of all gliomas. It is the most aggressive, malignant, and lethal primary tumor of the CNS parenchyma. The peak age at onset is 40 to 60 years; the average survival time from diagnosis is 10 months. It occurs in the deep white matter, basal ganglia, or thalamus; rarely it is found in the cerebellum or spinal cord. The affected portion of the brain is usually replaced by a single well-circumscribed lesion that infiltrates the cerebral cortex and spreads to the opposite hemisphere via the corpus callosum.

Most patients with an astrocytoma present with headaches, a progressive neurologic deficit, or seizures. A seizure occurring for the first time in an adult (without evident cause) should alert the clinician to the possibility of a brain tumor. This should be investigated by CT or MRI scanning. Their appearance is quite varied. Low-grade tumors are seen on CT scanning as low-density areas (containing either tumor cells or fluid due to edema). MRI scanning is more sensitive than CT scanning in separating tumor from edema. Glioblastoma multiforme has a border that enhances with contrast medium.

Surgical resection is the mainstay of treatment. The width of the resection should be as vigorous as possible with guidance and limitation by location. Radiation to the whole brain plus the tumor itself prolongs survival. Brachytherapy (stereotactic implantation of radiation) may be useful for recurrence. Various chemotherapeutic agents have been used; some have small but definite advantages over surgical resection and radiation therapy.

Oligodendroglioma

Oligodendroglial tumors comprise only 1% of brain tumors in children and less than 5% of brain tumors in all ages. The frontal lobes are often the site of these tumors. Almost 25% are hemorrhagic. On occasion they bleed sufficiently to manifest a strokelike presentation, but headache and seizures are the usual presenting features.

These tumors do not enhance with contrast on CT or MRI scanning. They characteristically are of low density and contain areas of calcification. Histologically, the cells have uniform nuclei surrounded by clear cytoplasm, producing a "fried egg" appearance.

Table 112-3. Malignant Tumors of the CNS

TUMOR	CLINICAL PRESENTATION	LOCATION	T1 FEATURES	MRI FEATURES	TREATMENT ISSUES
Astroglial neoplasm	Headache, progressive neurologic deficit, seizures	Range from optic nerve to brain stem	Range from low density to contrast-enhancing rim with variable edema	More sensitive than CT. Better demarcation of tumor vs. edema	Surgical resection with radiation. Chemotherapy options
Oligodendroglioma	Seizures and headache, rarely hemorrhage	Variable	Hypodense, often with calcification. No enhancement	Hypodense, often with calcification. No enhancement	Surgical resection. Radiation is questionable. Chemotherapy is option.
Ependymoma	Headache, obstructive hydrocephalus, seizures	Posterior fossa masses in children; supratentorial in adults	Isodense or hyperintense lesions that enhance with contrast	Variably enhancing, heterogeneous tumors lining the ventricles	Surgical resection with radiation
Ganglioglioma	Seizures	Temporal or frontal lobe	Hyperdense; no enhancement. Ca^+	Hyperdense; no enhancement. Ca^+	Surgical resection. Radiation is option.
Medulloblastoma	Headache, gait disturbance, diplopia, increased intracranial pressure	Cerebellar vermis in children; cerebellar hemisphere in adults	Nonspecific posterior fossa mass with hydrocephalus	Nonspecific posterior fossa mass with hydrocephalus	Surgical resection when possible. Radiation therapy
Pineal region	Headache, gait disturbance, Parinaud syndrome	In region of the pineal gland with obstruction and compression of adjacent structures	Variable: isodense, hyperdense, heterogeneous. Contrast enhancing	Best study. Variable: isodense, hyperdense, heterogeneous. Contrast enhancing	Variable depending on type, size, and extension. Surgery and radiation
Lymphoma	Focal symptoms and signs, headache, increased intracranial pressure. Immune compromised	Mass in periventricular region of deep white matter	Isodense or hyperdense in supratentorial periventricular regions. Enhances. Ring enhancing at times	Isodense or hyperdense in supratentorial periventricular regions. Enhances. Ring enhancing at times. Little edema	Steroids are oncolytic. Surgery for biopsy only. Radiation therapy is treatment of choice. Chemotherapy in selected cases
Cerebral metastases	Occur in 30% with systemic cancer. Melanoma, breast, small cell lung	Distal arterial fields. Progressive deficit, seizure, hemorrhage	Enhancing lesions with edema	More sensitive than CT. Enhancing lesions with edema	Biopsy if primary is not known. Surgical excision for single accessible lesion. Radiation

The accepted treatment is surgical. Radiation treatment is optional, with several studies demonstrating benefit; controversy exists regarding timing, dose, and response. Chemotherapy has been shown to benefit some of these patients.

Ependymoma

Ependymomas arise from the cells that line the ventricles, and the tumors project from the ependymal surface to occupy the ventricle. Obstructive hydrocephalus is the common mode of presentation. They comprise 4% of all brain tumors and are the third most common CNS tumor in children. They are most common below age 10. Ninety percent are in the brain; the rest are in the spinal cord. Most are infratentorial.

Radiographically, they appear on CT scans as isodense or hyperintense lesions that enhance with contrast. Forty percent are calcified. MRI demonstrates the anatomic location well and may demonstrate spread. These may seed the subarachnoid space and the spinal canal. Histologically, they are characterized by sheets of cells interrupted by perivascular rosettes and canals (gland-like structures lined by cells resembling those that line the ventricles).

The treatment is surgical resection with radiation. If seeding is evident, full craniospinal radiation is done. Chemotherapy for these tumors is not well established.

Ganglioglioma

Gangliogliomas occur in children and young adults; 80% of the patients are under age 30. They may occur anywhere in the brain, but the temporal lobe is the most common site. These patients present with longstanding epilepsy. CT and MRI scans are often nonspecific. They are nonenhancing hyperdense lesions, but occasionally a nodule enhances. Calcifications may occur.

Pathologically, they resemble low-grade astrocytomas with sheets or bundles of spindle cells. A dysplastic appearance of some neurons may occur.

The treatment is surgical resection. Radiation therapy is added for unresectable recurrent tumors and for subtotally resected gangliogliomas with an anaplastic component.

Medulloblastoma

Medulloblastoma is the most common malignant brain tumor of childhood. Twenty-five percent occur in adults, but most of these patients are under 20. These are rare after the fourth decade. Patients present with posterior fossa signs or signs of obstruction (headache, nausea, vomiting, diplopia, gait disturbance ataxia, nystagmus, papilledema). In children, these tumors arise in the cerebellar vermis; in adults, they arise in the cerebellar hemisphere.

Histologically, these are highly cellular tumors with abundant dark-staining round or oval nuclei, scant cytoplasm, and frequent mitoses. Pseudorosettes, characterized by carrot-shaped nuclei arranged radially around amorphous, eosinophilic centers, are present in 40% of the cases.

The CT and MRI appearance of medulloblastoma is nonspecific. They appear as isodense or hyperdense masses arising either from the cerebellar vermis or cerebellar hemisphere. There is variable contrast enhancement. Hydrocephalus is common.

These tumors tent to spread locally within the ventricles or seed the subarachnoid space and spine. Staging is helpful for planning treatment and establishing prognosis.

The first line of treatment is surgical. The goal is to remove as much tumor as possible without neurologic compromise. Shunting for hydrocephalus may be necessary. Craniospinal radiation is the mainstay of postoperative treatment. Chemotherapy has had limited interest.

Pineal Region

Tumors in this area account for only 1% of adult brain tumors; they are more common in children. Various tumors occur in this area, more than half of them of germ cell origin. Germinomas (accounting for two thirds of the germ cell tumors), teratomas, dermoids, malignant choriocarcinomas, endodermal sinus tumors, and embryonal tumors form the germ cell list, in descending order of frequency. Twenty percent are of pineal cell origin (pinealocytoma and pineoblastoma).

These tumors produce symptoms by obstruction of CSF flow at the aqueduct or posterior third ventricle and by compression of adjacent brain stem structures. Hydrocephalus is common. Presenting symptoms include headache, lethargy, nausea, vomiting, and gait disturbance. Tectal compression produces Parinaud syndrome (impairment of upgaze, loss of convergence, pupillary abnormalities, and retraction nystagmus).

These tumors are of variable cell type and are also variable in their appearance on CT and MRI. They vary from isodense to hyperdense to heterogeneous. Some are calcified. Contrast may enhance them.

Surgical treatment with attention to the hydrocephalus is the usual approach. Seeding along CSF pathways may be a concern. Radiation may be helpful.

Lymphoma

Primary CNS lymphomas occur in both immunocompetent and immunosuppressed populations, but the highest incidence is in patients with AIDS. They are also associated with other immunodeficiency states, both congenital (eg, Wiskott-Aldrich syndrome) and acquired (eg, organ transplant recipients). The origin is unknown, as there are no lymph nodes or lymphatics in the CNS. These are not likely to be a metastasis from an occult systemic lymphoma.

These tumors typically occur as a mass lesion in the periventricular region of the deep white matter. Seventy-five percent are supratentorial. Primary CNS lymphoma is multifocal in about 50% of immunocompetent patients but is multifocal in all AIDS patients (often with leptomeningeal spread). Hemorrhage into the tumor is uncommon in primary CNS lymphoma, but it occurs often in patients with AIDS (especially after surgery). Tumor necrosis is characteristic of AIDS-related lymphomas. Lesions in identical locations in the two hemispheres (mirror images) are commonly encountered in AIDS patients.

Most tumors are of B-cell origin. The tumor cells are usually large, of high grade, pleomorphic, discohesive, and infiltrative. The tumor is often infiltrated by reactive T lymphocytes.

Primary CNS lymphoma occurs in all age groups. The peak incidence is in the sixth and seventh decades in immunocompetent patients, earlier in the immunosuppressed population. These patients present with focal symptoms and those of increased intracranial pressure. Personality and cognitive changes are common. Seizures are uncommon. Symptoms progress over weeks to months.

Contrast-enhanced CT or MRI scanning reveals periventricular masses with indistinct borders, homogeneous enhancement, and little surrounding edema. Before enhancement, the tumors are isodense or hyperdense. Multiple lesions are seen in 50% of patients.

CSF analysis may be helpful. The CSF protein level is elevated in 85% of patients. The CSF glucose level may be low with leptomeningeal spread. Lymphocytic pleocytosis is present in 50% of the patients. Immunohistochemical staining may establish the malignant nature of the pleocytosis.

Corticosteroids are oncolytic agents in primary CNS lymphoma and should not be given until the disease is established by biopsy. Steroid responsiveness should not be used as a diagnostic test. Surgery is limited to biopsy only.

The radiographic appearance in patients with AIDS may mimic that of toxoplasmosis. In patients with AIDS and a CNS mass lesion, empiric antitoxoplasmosis therapy is usually given first. If the patient has primary CNS lymphoma, neurologic deterioration usually occurs during antibiotic treatment.

Whole brain radiation therapy must be used because of lymphoma's widespread distribution within the brain. Primary CNS lymphoma can recur within the brain, but distant from the original tumor. Radiation therapy provides a complete response in 90% of patients. The median survival is 12 to 18 months, with a 3% to 4% 5-year survival rate. Chemotherapy together with radiation has been shown to be of some benefit.

CEREBRAL METASTASIS

Neurologic symptoms occur in about 20% of patients with cancer. Metabolic encephalopathy is the most common neurologic sequela in the patient with cancer, but it is usually a terminal complication representing organ failure. Parenchymal brain metastatic lesions are the most common nonterminal neurologic event in patients with cancer. Almost 25% of patients with cancer have brain metastases at autopsy, and about 10% have metastases confined to the brain parenchyma.

More than 25% of all autopsy-proven brain metastases have a pulmonary source; those from breast cancer and melanoma are second and third most common, respectively. Malignant melanoma (which represents only 1% of all cancers) has the highest propensity of all systemic malignant tumors to metastasize to the brain. Most brain metastases are spread hematogenously, arising from circulating tumor cells or from frank tumor emboli. They occur at the gray/white matter junction, characteristic of an embolic event. Metastases are multiple in about 50% of patients and typically are well demarcated and solid. Occasionally, they are cystic, necrotic, or hemorrhagic. Tumors arising from the kidney, colon, breast, and thyroid and adenocarcinoma of the lung are most often associated with a single metastasis; metastases from melanoma, small cell carcinoma of the lung, and tumor of unknown origin tend to be multiple. Melanoma, renal cell carcinoma, and germ cell malignant tumors (especially choriocarcinoma) tend to be hemorrhagic. Brain metastases of lung origin are often identified early in the course of the disease; metastases from breast cancer typically develop late, usually after the disease has spread systemically.

Most brain metastases present with a combination of focal and generalized symptoms and signs in a subacute progressive time frame. Hemorrhage or seizures present acutely in a dramatic fashion. CT scanning usually provides sufficient information. Contrast enhancement and the presence of white matter edema and multiple lesions are the compelling features of metastases. MRI scanning can detect CT-occult metastases, identify associated leptomeningeal disease, and disclose early therapeutic complications.

Treatment options are tempered by the patient's neurologic condition, functional and overall performance status, the extent of the primary tumor and other sites of systemic disease, the number and sites of the brain metastases, and the radiosensitivity of the tumor type. The goal of treatment is to control the neurologic symptoms; cure is rarely possible. Corticosteroids produce a prompt improvement in most patients with brain metastases. This improvement may be seen in just a few hours, and 70% of patients experience substantial improvement within 48 hours. Corticosteroids may have a specific oncolytic effect in lymphomas and breast cancer. The long-term use of corticosteroid medication is associated with substantial side effects and risks. Whole brain radiation and other radiation techniques may extend the duration and the quality of life. Chemotherapy of cerebral metastases remains uncertain.

Surgical options include the resection of solitary lesions, treatment of increased intracranial pressure, biopsy of tumors from an unknown primary cancer, and administration of stereotactic radiosurgical therapy. A solitary metastasis occurs in up to 50% of patients. About half of these are not surgical candidates because of tumor inaccessibility, extensive systemic metastases, or other medical problems. In patients who qualify, resection of an isolated metastasis followed by radiation therapy offers better survival than does radiation therapy alone.

CONSIDERATIONS DURING PREGNANCY

Intracranial tumors (except pituitary tumors) do not have an increased incidence during pregnancy. Intracranial neoplasms may manifest initially during pregnancy because of three factors. First, tumors may enlarge during pregnancy as a result of retention of salt and water by the systemic vasculature. Vascular tumors such as meningiomas are most likely to manifest in this way. Second, mild immunologic suppression during pregnancy may decrease the patient's ability to tolerate a tumor. Third, some tumors may be hormonally dependent.

The pituitary gland may enlarge up to 70% during pregnancy because of a proliferation of prolactin-secreting cells. When a woman with an unknown adenoma or other pituitary tumor becomes pregnant, the tumor may rapidly enlarge and rapidly become symptomatic. The most common symptoms include headache and a bitemporal hemianopic visual field defect. As stated earlier, adenomas may be hypersecretory or hyposecretory for prolactin, growth hormone, or adrenocorticotropic hormone.

Management depends on the degree of symptoms. If vision is threatened, surgical management is unavoidable. In most instances, however, surgery may be delayed if the tumor can be controlled with steroids and bromocriptine (for prolactin-secreting tumors). These agents are safe to use during pregnancy. Bromocriptine suppresses lactation in the postpartum period. Abrupt blindness due to pituitary apoplexy mandates urgent surgical intervention.

Meningiomas and vascular tumors have been frequently reported to present during pregnancy. These tumors have been reported to show rapid progression of symptoms during the course of pregnancy, followed by a decrease of symptoms after parturition. Progesterone and estrogen receptors are frequently detected in meningioma cells and are thought to have a direct hormonal effect on the tumor's growth rate. Indeed, the symptoms of a meningioma may fluctuate with the menstrual cycle. Tamoxifen (a potent antiestrogen agent useful in breast cancer) does not clinically affect tumor size or symptoms in patients with inoperable meningiomas.

Choriocarcinoma is a malignant tumor that arises from fetal trophoblastic tissue. This trophoblastic tumor invades maternal uterine blood vessels and metastasizes. There is a high rate (up to 28%) of cerebral metastases. These may manifest as an embolic stroke, subarachnoid hemorrhage, or intracerebral hematoma. These are highly vascular tumors that bleed at the site of metastatic involvement. There is a strong relation between cerebral metastatic lesions and mortality due to choriocarcinoma. Chemotherapy and radiation therapy are the initial treatment modalities for these cerebral metastatic tumors. Surgery is reserved for acute hemorrhagic complications.

In the management of brain tumors diagnosed during pregnancy, several important considerations must be weighed: the suspected nature of the tumor, the stage of pregnancy during which the tumor is detected, the patient's neurologic stability, the maternal and fetal outcomes with medical versus surgical management, the efficacy of vaginal versus cesarean delivery, and fetal viability.

BIBLIOGRAPHY

Black PM. Brain tumors. N Engl J Med 1991;324:1471.

Donaldson JO. Neurology of pregnancy. In: Walton J, ed. Major problems in neurology. Philadelphia: WB Saunders, 1989.

Fox MW, Harms RW, Davis DH. Selected neurologic complications of pregnancy. Mayo Clin Proc 1990;65:1595.

Heffner RR. Pathology of nervous system tumors. In: Bradley WG, Daroff RB, Fenichel GM, Marsden CD, eds. Neurology in clinical practice. Boston: Butterworth-Heinimann, 1996.

Jaeckle KA, Cohen ME, Duffner PK. Clinical presentation and therapy of nervous system tumors. In: Bradley WG, Daroff RB, Fenichel GM,

Marsden CD, eds. Neurology in clinical practice. Boston: Butterworth-Heinimann, 1996.
Laws ER, Thapar K. Brain tumors. CA 1993;43:263.
Olivi A, Brem RF, McPherson R, Brem H. Brain tumors in pregnancy. In: Goldstein PJ, Stern BJ, eds. Neurological disorders of pregnancy. New York: Futura, 1992.
O'Neill BP, Buckner JC, Coffey RJ, Dinapoli RP, Shaw EG. Brain metastatic lesions. Mayo Clin Proc 1994;69:1062.
Weinreb HJ. Demyelinating and neoplastic diseases in pregnancy. In: Yerby M, Devinsky O, eds. Neurologic complications of pregnancy. Philadelphia: WB Saunders, 1994.
Wen PY, Black PM. Brain tumors in adults. Neurol Clin 1995;13:4.

113A
Spinal Cord Syndromes

JOSHUA HOLLANDER

Primary Care for Women, edited by Phyllis C. Leppert and Fred M. Howard. Lippincott-Raven Publishers, Philadelphia © 1997.

Spinal cord diseases can be confusing if the clinician is not familiar with the anatomy of the cord and its circulation and the cord's relation to the spinal canal and its bony levels. The cord does not match the growth of the spinal column and slowly recedes in a rostral direction. In adulthood, the cord ends at the L1-2 vertebral level. In the cervical region, there are seven vertebrae and eight roots. C1 through C7 emerge above the vertebral level; the C8 root emerges below the vertebra in the manner characteristic of the rest of the vertebral column. The clinician must remember the discrepancy between the cord and column levels in planning investigations. The dermatomal distribution is discussed in the section on radiculopathy.

In cross section, the cord is seen to have white matter columns surrounding the interior gray. Posterior columns are involved with ipsilateral discriminative touch and limb proprioception crossing in the brain stem. The ventrolateral spinothalamic and spinoreticular columns conduct pain, temperature, touch, and pressure. Sensory neurons have their cell bodies in the dorsal root ganglia and may synapse in the dorsal horn of the cord. Most spinothalamic fibers cross through the central cord. The lateral columns contain descending motor fibers. The anterior horns of the central gray contain the lower motor neurons, which exit through the anterior root. Many complex interneurons and multiple transmitters exist in the cord but are not dealt with here.

The circulation of the cord is complex. Two posterior spinal arteries course downward near the dorsal root entry zones with multiple radicular collaterals (Fig. 113-1). The anterior cord is less well endowed, with an anterior spinal artery arising from branches from each vertebral artery. Anterior collaterals are less frequent and may include small ones at about C6 and some in the thoracic cord. A major lateralized collateral is the great radicular artery of Adamkiewicz in the lumbar area. This is somewhat variable but is usually at T11 on the left. Blood flow is such that the major watershed area is around T4, but there may be another at T12.

ETIOLOGY AND DIFFERENTIAL DIAGNOSIS

Woolsey and Young's format (1995) for approaching these diseases is followed here, and their work can be consulted for a more complete discussion. They divided these disorders into five neurologic abnormalities and nine cord syndromes; this allows clinical classification before performing any expensive studies.

Low back pain and sciatica are covered in the continuation of Chapter 113, beginning on page 755.

The five neurologic abnormalities are pain, motor, sensory, reflex and motor tone, and bladder symptoms.

Pain includes local, radicular, or central pain. Local pain relates to ligamentous and bony structures involved at the level of the lesion; the time course of its evolution can indicate the type of process. Radicular pain in intrinsic disease usually occurs at the level of the lesion and tends to radiate only short distances. It is less useful in localization than paresthesias. Central pain has a diffuse burning, aching quality associated with sensory loss in the appropriate area.

The most significant motor abnormality is weakness, which requires loss of 50% of descending motor neurons or a similar loss of anterior horn cells. This is most striking in abrupt-onset lesions. Slowly progressive lesions may be reflected more by fatigability, clumsiness, and unsteadiness. Spasticity of the upper motor neuron type may be prominent but is usually less of a problem. Involvement of anterior horn cells may be associated with atrophy and fasciculations. Hand problems are more readily detected.

Sensory abnormalities include positive and negative features. Positive features, or paresthesias, are manifest in damaged sensory pathways. Presentation is either posterior column type ("pins and needles" or tingling) or spinothalamic pathway (thermal or itching). The Lhermitte sign is an electric shock-like sensation down the back or limbs produced by cervical flexion in association with cervical myelopathy. Negative symptoms of numbness or "deadness" reflect posterior column involvement. Spinothalamic loss may be noted only by loss of ability to recognize shower temperature with one side. Characteristic patterns include loss of position and vibratory sense in the feet with spared reflexes (dorsal cord syndrome), loss of position and vibratory sense in the feet with a clear sensory level to pinprick on the trunk (thoracic cord lesion), bilateral segmental upper limb sensory loss sparing the lower limbs (central cord syndrome), loss of pinprick and contralateral position and vibration (Brown-Séquard syndrome), loss of pinprick on the trunk and lower limbs with a level but preserved perianal sensation (sacral sparing; intramedullary or anterior extramedullary cord lesion), loss of perianal and posterior thigh sensation (conus medullaris or high cauda lesion), and loss of pinprick on the trunk and lower limbs with a level (anterior cord syndrome).

Reflex changes include spinal shock (when acute lesions result in paralysis) and areflexia (from loss of descending facilitative impulses). More slowly developing lesions manifest hyperactive reflexes below the level of the lesion and may show absent or hypoactive reflexes at the level of the lesion. Hyperactive limb

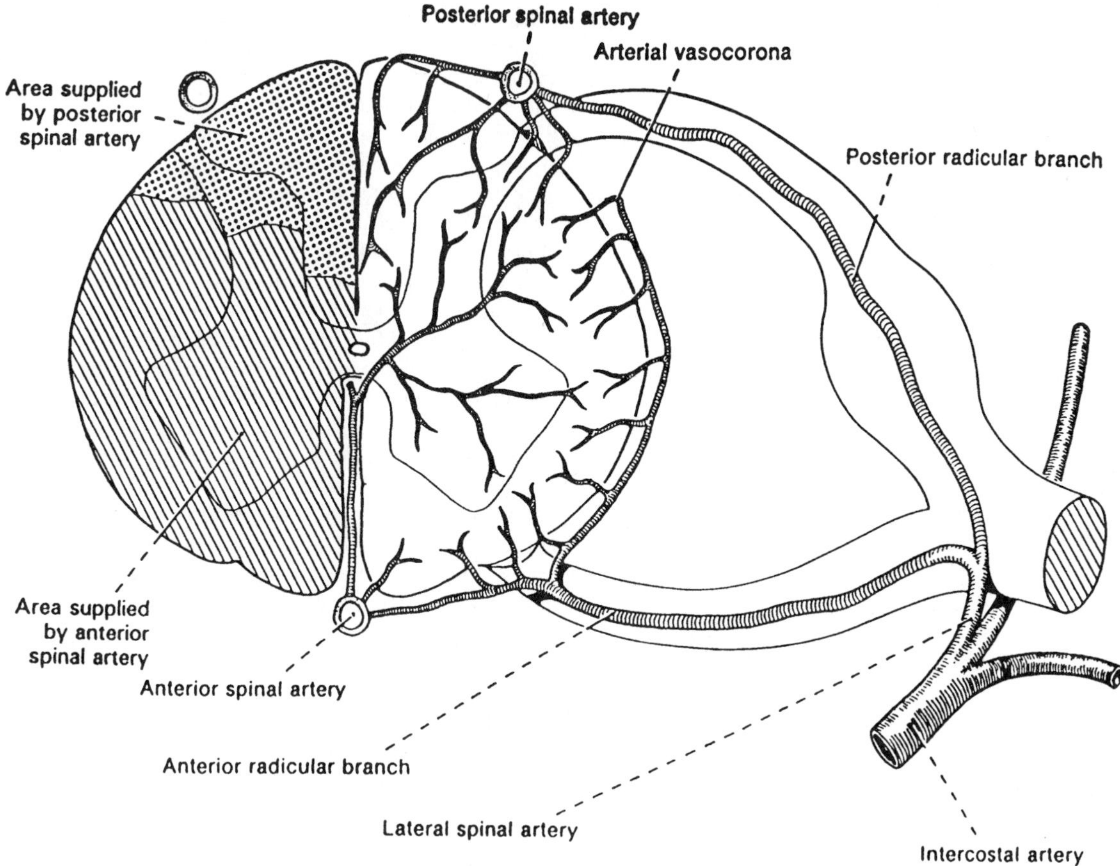

Figure 113-1. Circulation of the spinal cord.

reflexes with a hyperactive jaw jerk suggest an intracranial localization; a hypoactive jaw jerk suggests a high cervical localization. The extensor plantar response is a polysynaptic reflex that may be seen early in cord disease.

Bladder dysfunction varies with the level of the lesion and the rate of development. Urinary retention with overflow incontinence is seen with acute cord lesions and lesions of the conus medullaris and cauda equina. More slowly progressive myelopathies result in hyperactive detrusor reflexes that present as urgency, frequency, and incontinence. A more confusing problem is detrusor/sphincter dyssynergia seen with disorders causing multiple-level lesions.

The nine cord syndromes of Woolsey and Young are as follows.

The complete cord syndromes (paraplegia or quadriplegia with local pain, altered reflexes, nonselective sensory loss, and loss of bladder function) occur as acute or subacute disorders. *Acute complete cord syndromes* occur primarily through vascular or traumatic mechanisms. Trauma is usually associated with a history of injury and local pain. Infarction tends to occur in the more vulnerable anterior cord, sparing posterior columns. Spontaneous epidural hemorrhage and acute cord compression from herniated disk are rare. These conditions are associated with spinal shock. *Subacute complete cord syndromes* may evolve over hours or weeks. More rapid syndromes such as transverse myelitis may display areflexia; more slowly evolving syndromes show hyperreflexia and extensor plantar responses. A spinal epidural tumor or abscess shows early radicular pain. The bladder is involved acutely and late in subacute processes.

Chronic spastic paraplegia with gait ataxia evolving over months or years has three syndromes. *Pure motor syndromes* include motor neuron diseases, familial spastic paraplegia, and the myelopathy of cervical spondylosis. Bladder involvement is minor. The *dorsal cord syndromes* (paraplegia or quadriplegia with loss of position and vibratory sense) include multiple sclerosis, subacute combined degeneration of the spinal cord (B_{12} deficiency), myelopathy of cervical spondylosis, arteriovenous malformations, axial or extraaxial cord tumors, spinocerebellar degeneration, arachnoiditis, and spinal cord trauma. Bladder involvement is a late event. *Disorders with loss of pain sensation* include bilateral (anterior cord syndrome) and unilateral (Brown-Séquard syndrome) variants. Etiologies include extrinsic cord tumors, spondylotic myelopathy, radiation myelopathy, cord trauma, and myelitis.

Chronic atrophic paralysis of the hands evolving over months or years can be grouped by the presence or absence of sensory loss. These disorders include segmental loss of pain sensation (*central cord syndrome*) and multiple modalities. It begins as a cape or glove distribution. Problems include syringomyelia, intrinsic cord tumors, and trauma. *Pure motor syndromes* include motor neuron disease, cervical spondylosis, and extrinsic high cervical tumors.

Cauda equina syndromes (paraplegia with low back pain, areflexia, saddle anesthesia, and loss of bladder function) can be grouped by time course. *Acute syndromes* can be precipitated by lumbar spine trauma with fracture, a central lumbar disk herniation, or AIDS lumbosacral polyradiculopathy. *Subacute or chronic*

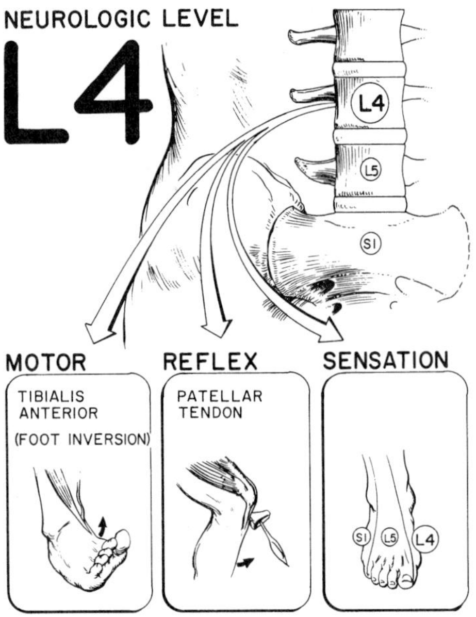

Figure 113-2. Fourth lumbar root. (Hoppenfeld S. Orthopadedic Neurology. Philadelphia: JB Lippincott, 1977:52.)

syndromes may be caused by lumbar disk protrusion, lumbar spinal stenosis, arachnoiditis, and tumor.

Acute transverse myelitis is a rare monophasic demyelinative disorder; although its name implies a segmental lesion, the pathology may extend more broadly. The typical scenario is that of an antecedent viral illness followed by back pain, weakness, sensory loss and paresthesias, and urinary retention. Predilection is for the lower thoracic cord. More acute onset is associated with more severe necrosis and residua. There is an association with multiple sclerosis, but the frequency is controversial (perhaps 5% to 10%). Specific infectious agents have rarely been associated with acute transverse myelitis, but they more commonly present with a necrotizing myelopathy or more subacute involvement. These include herpes viruses, toxoplasmosis, schistosomiasis, and Lyme borreliosis. Toxic myelopathy is seen with intrathecal methotrexate and cytosine arabinoside. Enthusiasm for chymopapain treatment for herniated disk waned when transverse myelitis became associated with this therapy. Acute transverse myelitis is seen in systemic lupus erythematosus similar to other types but with a rapid onset, clear sensory level, and back pain. Lupus is also associated with a subacute multiple sclerosis-like fluctuating course. There is no clear association with anticardiolipin antibodies.

Spinal cord ischemia is rare, possibly due to the rich collateral supply and relative resistance to ischemia (compared to the brain). The most vulnerable areas are the central gray matter and the watershed area in the thoracic cord. Most cases occur from loss of segmental radicular arteries of the aorta. Loss of the great radicular artery (Adamkiewicz) may occur in spontaneous dissection of the aorta involving the descending thoracic or abdominal aorta or during surgery on this section of the aorta. This usually presents with sudden tearing chest or abdominal pain and paraplegia and a sensory level.

The cord is usually spared by atheromatous (aorta), myxomatous (heart), or fibrinocartilaginous (disk) emboli, but these have been reported. Spinal cord claudication (exercise-induced painless paraparesis and sphincter disturbance) has been implicated in some patients with aortic atherosclerosis, but again vascular disease of the cord is rare. Iatrogenic vascular lesions of the cord are more common than spontaneous ones and include aortic surgery, intraaortic counterpulse balloons, radiographic catheters, and possibly spinal or epidural continuous anesthesia with vasoconstrictive potentiators. Systemic hypotension has also been implicated.

Spinal cord vascular malformations include true arteriovenous malformations of both intramedullary and intrathecal, extramedullary types and dural arteriovenous fistulas. The true malformations tend to be thoracic and dorsal to the cord. They may have multiple feeders but frequently have a large one in the lumbar area. Onset may be from subarachnoid hemorrhage associated with stabbing pain in the back (coup de poignard) and perhaps paraparesis. Exertional or postprandial paraparesis has also been noted. The dural lesions may manifest as a progressive myelopathy later in life due to increased venous pressure.

Progressive necrotic myelitis (syndrome of Foix and Alajouanine) usually presents with sensory, motor, and sphincter loss, progressing to higher cord levels over years, associated with abnormal hypertrophied vessels and spastic paraparesis with ascending amyotrophy.

Radiation myelopathy presents as a gradual symmetric loss of long tracts due to vascular changes. It is related to the dose and fractionation and may occur 6 to 48 months after exposure. A transient cord syndrome has been described, but this syndrome usually develops over weeks and is permanent.

The perivenous demyelinative diseases include acute disseminated encephalomyelitis and multiple sclerosis (see Chap. 114). The nervous system is affected more widely in these disorders and diagnosis is not made by the spinal findings alone, as these are nonspecific. An uncommon variety of multiple sclerosis presents late in life as a chronic progressive or relapsing/progressive spinal degeneration, with or without a remote spinal or optic event. Asymmetric onset and asynchrony in posterior column and motor signs may help distinguish this from vitamin B_{12} deficiency. Because B_{12} deficiency tends to occur later in life, the concurrent presence of some cervical spine degeneration with osteophytic ridges may cause confusion.

Degeneration of the cervical spine is associated with osteophyte formation and subluxation of joints; disk herniation may occur in association. Spinal canal or neural foramina, or both, may be compromised. The usual presentation of cervical spondylosis is of a painful stiff neck, pain and numbness in the arms and hands, and spastic (?ataxic) paraparesis. Evolution is over months or years, with some intermittent painful exacerbations. Bladder problems may include urgency incontinence. Purely radicular syndromes are more suggestive of herniated disk. The most common vertebral spaces involved are C4-5 (C5), C5-6(C6), and C6-7(C8). The severity does not always correlate with the size of the osteophyte. Other determinants are the size of the cervical canal (cervical stenosis) and the presence of redundant ligaments, which could contribute to a myelopathy by repeated cord trauma from flexion and extension. Diagnosis requires good correlation of location and severity of signs and radiographic findings.

Motor neuron or motor system diseases include progressive muscular atrophy, progressive bulbar palsy, primary lateral sclerosis, and amyotrophic lateral sclerosis. The latter disorder is the most common form. The combination of upper and lower motor neuron features in the same muscle groups is important for the diagnosis. Lower motor neuron features are atrophy, weakness, and fasciculations at rest; upper motor neuron features are spasticity, hyperreflexia, and extensor plantar responses. The affected limb shows atrophy and weakness, but reflexes are preserved. Cervical spondylosis may cause atrophy in the hands, but the only hyperreflexia is in the legs. Onset may be asymmetric, and bulbar muscles may be involved. Intellect and sensation are spared. Either lower motor neuron or upper motor neuron signs may be prominent early. The predominantly lower motor neuron variant, progressive muscular atrophy, tends to pursue a more indolent course rather than death at 4 to 7 years. Hereditary spinal muscular atrophies have their onset in infancy or childhood.

Familial spastic paraplegia is a progressive syndrome of childhood or adult onset presenting with progressive weakness and spasticity of the legs. It probably represents a mixture of disorders.

Spinocerebellar degenerations present with ataxia as a prominent sign. The best known is Friedreich ataxia. Onset is in childhood or adolescence, progressing slowly over decades. This autosomal recessive disorder affects the dorsal root ganglia, posterior columns, and spinocerebellar and corticospinal tracts. Progressive ataxia and loss of touch, vibration, and position sense are combined with areflexia. Dysarthric speech, swallowing impairment, and nystagmus are present. Skeletal deformities such as pes cavus and kyphoscoliosis are secondary. Death is usually from the associated cardiomyopathy.

Syringomyelia refers to a cavitation of the central cord, usually in the cervical region, presenting with a central cord syndrome. There is usually loss of pain and temperature sensation in a glove or shawl distribution; painless injuries to the fingers are not unusual. Other sensory modalities are usually spared, but they may be involved below the lesion. There is segmental muscle atrophy and weakness. The differential diagnosis includes intramedullary tumor, which may also be associated with a syrinx. The cavity may extend to involve the medulla, with resultant cranial nerve dysfunction. The medulla is also affected in the half of these patients who have an associated Chiari type 1 malformation (plugging of the foramen magnum and downward protrusion of a medullary tongue and cerebellum). A syrinx may also develop in response to trauma and arachnoiditis.

Subacute combined degeneration of the spinal cord (B_{12} deficiency) is becoming less common. Paresthesias and sensory ataxia are followed by spastic paraparesis. Neuropathy is seen as well. Presentation is usually symmetric, progressing from paresthesias to sensory ataxia and then an ataxic paraparesis. The reflexes vary, depending on the stage of the disease. A spongiform appearance is seen in the involved tracts. Primary nutritional deficiency of B_{12} is rare, and the classic syndromes result from malabsorption of B_{12} due to lack of intrinsic factor (addisonian pernicious anemia) or problems of gastrectomy, blind loops of bowel, or extensive bowel resection. Rarer forms are due to metabolic defects in cobalamin or methyl group metabolism. A macrocytic anemia with hypersegmented polymorphs and a marrow picture of megaloblasts may provide the needed clues. Administration of folate may obscure this, and this is important to remember in women of childbearing age who must have folate supplementation.

Infectious causes of myelopathy include tropical spastic paraparesis, which has been found to be due to human T-cell lymphotropic virus (HTLV-1). A chronic meningoencephalitis produces a spastic leg weakness with variable sensory and sphincter problems. It is usually seen in middle-aged persons who lived

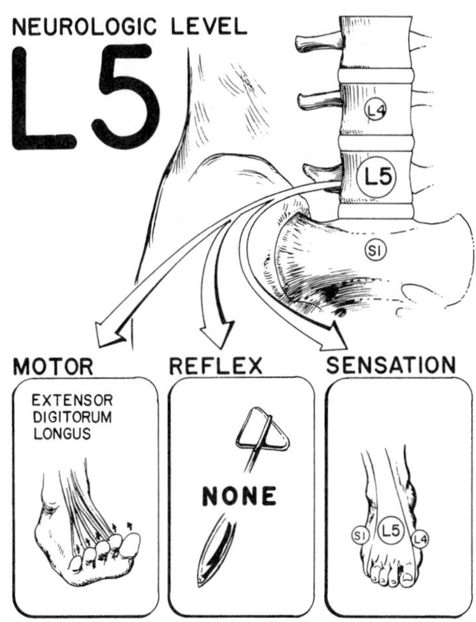

Figure 113-3. Fifth lumbar root. (Hoppenfeld S. Orthopadedic Neurology. Philadelphia: JB Lippincott, 1977:54.)

in North Africa or the West Indies. It may be transmitted by transfusion. Infection with HTLV-1 is usually asymptomatic.

AIDS is associated with various infections such as the herpes group, but a vacuolar myelopathy occurs in 10% to 30% of patients. It resembles subacute combined degeneration, but no B_{12} deficiency is present. The variable clinical picture tends to include spastic ataxic gait, proprioceptive sensory loss, and sphincter disturbance. The etiology is unclear.

Adhesive arachnoiditis is decreasing in frequency as greater care is taken as to what is placed in the spinal fluid. This progressive fibrosis of the pia/arachnoid can manifest as chronic low back, thigh, and leg pain, with adhesions seen on myelography. Another picture is that of a progressive spastic ataxia.

Spinal tumors are only 25% as common as intracranial tumors. The most common spinal tumors are meningiomas and neurofibromas, which represent over half. Ependymas and metastases represent an additional quarter, with ependymomas and a miscellaneous group completing the list. Meningiomas are more common in women, ependymomas in men—this means that spinal cord tumor is more common in women overall. Peak incidence is in the fifth decade. Tumors are classified as intramedullary, intradural extramedullary, or extradural. Neurofibromas may present as dumbbell lesions projecting through the neural foramen.

Intramedullary tumors include both primary and metastatic lesions. Intramedullary metastases usually occur in advanced disease and there are lesions elsewhere as well. Primary intramedullary tumors resemble extramedullary tumor if localized to a segment. If the root entry zone is affected, pain is prominent. Most commonly, multiple segments are involved and the patient presents with a central cord syndrome resembling syringomyelia. If the lesion is thoracic and the expanding tumor affects spinothalamic tracts, the sacral fibers are affected last, resulting in sacral sparing.

Extramedullary tumors tend to involve few segments and present with local and radicular pain and paresthesias. Radicular

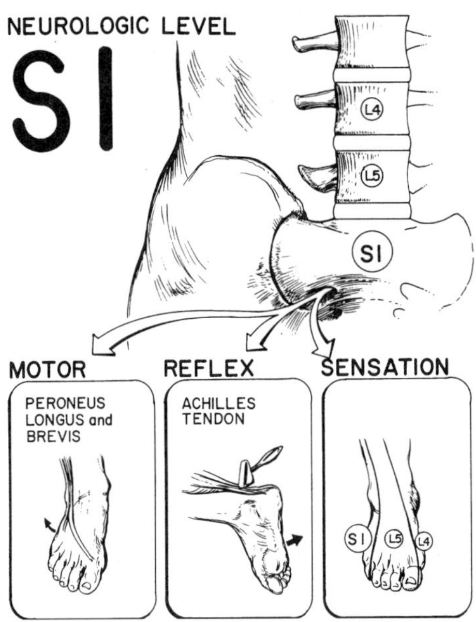

Figure 113-4. First sacral root. (Hoppenfeld S. Orthopadedic Neurology. Philadelphia: JB Lippincott, 1977:58.)

weakness and wasting follows with ultimate cord compression. Cord compression affects the outer pathways first. The clinical syndrome of spinal cord compression is a neurologic emergency. Clinical features include spastic weakness below the lesion, a sensory level at the level of the lesion, reflex hyperactivity, loss of superficial reflexes and extensor plantar responses, and impaired bladder (ultimately rectal) control. If effective treatment is not promptly instituted, progression to complete cord transection follows. When epidural cord compression occurs in the context of advanced cancer, symptoms may be overlooked. Unsteady gait may be sensory ataxia; limb weakness or paresthesia or unrelenting pain may be bony metastases with incipient cord compression. Primaries include lung, breast, or gastrointestinal tumors, melanoma, or lymphoma. Intradural tumors are more likely to be neurofibromas, meningiomas, or schwannomas.

Foramen magnum tumors may involve posterior column sensation as well as a spastic paraparesis. Lower cranial nerves (C9–12) may be involved if the tumor extends rostrally. The C2 dermatome is on the occiput and may be missed. Cervical tumors present with features related to the specific level. Upper cervical lesions produce spastic tetraplegia, but lower lesions produce a level at which there is flaccid atrophic muscle; below the level there is spastic paresis. The C4 dermatome involves sensation to the epaulet area and innervation of the diaphragm. The C5 dermatome provides sensation to the outer upper arm and motor innervation to the deltoid, biceps, supinator, and spinati muscles. The upper arm hangs limply and the biceps reflex is lost. The C6 dermatome provides sensation to the radial forearm and the first two digits. Motor supply is to the triceps and wrist extensors. The triceps reflex is lost and the partly flexed forearm has a partial wrist drop. The C7 dermatome provides sensation to the middle finger and motor supply to the wrist flexors and finger flexors and extensors; attempted hand closure produces mild wrist extension and slight finger flexion ("preacher's hand"). The C8 dermatome provides sensation to the ulnar forearm and the fourth and fifth digits and motor supply to the intrinsic muscles of the hand. A claw hand (main-en-griffe) is seen. Horner syndrome (ptosis, miosis, hypohidrosis, and relative enophthalmos) can be subtle. Although it is caused by involvement of the C8 root, descending sympathetic fibers can be caught anywhere along their descent by intramedullary tumors.

Thoracic tumors depend primarily on the sensory level. Lumbar tumors of L3-4 sparing the cauda equina leave weak quadriceps with loss of reflex and preservation of ankle jerk. The cauda is usually involved with lower limb flaccid areflexic paralysis or some combination of findings. Conus or cauda tumors give pain in the low back, perirectal area, and both lower legs, with sensory loss in the saddle area and the remaining lumbosacral dermatomes. Bladder function is lost early. Flaccid lower limbs with atrophy and areflexia develop later.

HISTORY

Spinal cord trauma has an estimated incidence of 900 per 1 million persons; almost 80% of patients are male. The etiologies include motor vehicle accidents, falls, recreational activities (diving), and assaults. Major sites of injury are cervical (especially C5, C6) and the thoracolumbar junction. These patients should be stabilized and transported to a suitable facility for specialized care after ensuring that no further cord injury occurs.

The history is of paramount importance. The temporal sequence and rate of progression are defined. Attention is directed toward the five features previously described. Pain (or its absence) is localized, radicular, or diffuse. Weakness may be manifest by fatigability or clumsiness. Gait may be unsteady. The patient may describe specific functions she cannot perform; this suggests a direction for the muscle examination. Paresthesias may define root involvement more specifically than associated pain or sensory loss. The Lhermitte sign is a specific sensation indicative of cervical cord pathology. It indicates posterior column involvement and is nonspecific for multiple sclerosis. Flexion of the neck releases an fleeting electric shock down the spine and perhaps the limbs.

Some patients are reluctant to discuss bladder or bowel function, but this must be specifically inquired about, as must sexual function. An atonic bladder may present as urinary retention with overflow incontinence. Urgency, frequency, and incontinence reflect a spastic neurogenic bladder. Detrusor/sphincter dyssynergia has more variable symptoms. Urinary tract infection may manifest as retention, urgency, or frequency and must be ruled out. Incontinence should suggest neurologic involvement.

The history should also explore features suggestive of other levels of nervous system involvement. Cerebral hemisphere involvement is more likely to produce position sense loss than pinprick. Dementia may favor frontal lobe dysfunction. Cough or exertional headache may favor a concurrent Chiari malformation. Exposure to toxic or infectious agents should be explored. Antecedent optic neuritis can be overlooked if remote. The family history should not be overlooked.

PHYSICAL EXAMINATION

The physical examination should include the spine curvature and mobility. Tenderness is elicited. Skin lesions may suggest neurofibromatosis, and axillary freckles should be sought. Pulses may indicate aortic involvement. The bladder can be palpated and percussed. A cutaneous angioma may be present in patients with arteriovenous malformations.

The cranial nerves are checked with funduscopic examination and fields, as well as the lower cranial nerves. Horner syndrome is subtle because the bright lights usually used for examination cause pupillary constriction in the normal eye, obscuring the pathology. A faint light from the side allows estimation of pupillary size in relative darkness.

Sensory examination is most quickly done with a pin to ascertain the presence of a sensory level, proceeding from the area of decreased sensation to more normal areas. Sacral areas must be checked for clues to conus or cauda syndromes, as well as the presence of sacral sparing. It is useful to elicit clues from the history as to possible radicular sensory loss. A mental dermatome map is needed to allow fluid sensory testing. The sensory examination is the most difficult for both the patient and the examiner and is best done briskly to avoid excessive fatigue. Posterior column sensation is less readily defined in terms of a sensory level, although vibratory sense on the spine may provide useful information of level. The evaluation of both spinothalamic tracts and posterior columns is necessary to define the nature of the syndrome.

Motor strength and tone are evaluated. Atrophy is carefully assessed in weak muscles and the presence of fasciculations is evaluated by examining exposed limbs at rest. These small subcutaneous ripples represent spontaneous firing of large motor units. They should be present in weak muscles and should not be restricted to a single muscle group. The tongue can be examined in the floor of the mouth and the "bag of worms" effect seen.

Reflexes are checked for a level above which reflexes are normal and below which they are increased. Landry-Guillain-Barré syndrome may involve areflexic weakness, but it does not usually show diminished pinprick. The presence of weakness and atrophy associated with preserved or increased reflexes suggests amyotrophic lateral sclerosis.

LABORATORY AND IMAGING STUDIES

New technology has made evaluation of the spinal cord safer and more accurate; however, it cannot be used efficiently if the region and question are not adequately defined.

Evoked potentials are obtained by providing a repetitive stimulus and recording electrical activity from the skin overlying the spine or skull. This activity is then averaged when time-yoked to the stimulus. Somatosensory potentials are elicited by providing repetitive electrical stimuli to the area of the median, ulnar, posterior tibial, and peroneal nerves. Potentials can be elicited from the back, cervical spine, thalamus, and sensory cortex. This allows a central conduction time to be obtained. Because the large myelinated fibers of the posterior columns conduct most rapidly, this test reflects primarily posterior column function. Transcranial or transspinal magnetic stimulation allows painless activation of corticospinal tracts with recording of complex polyphasic electromyographic waveforms, thereby providing a central motor conduction time. These electrophysiologic tests allow noninvasive measurement of cord function.

Filming the spinal canal with the CSF rendered radiodense with a water-soluble contrast medium is called myelography. The contrast medium is introduced by lumbar arachnoid puncture and is excreted by the kidneys. The use of contrast allows visualization of the cord shadow and anything impinging on it. Carcinomatous meningitis may reveal multiple nodules on nerves. Because a full-spine study requires intrathecal contrast and high doses may be toxic, the technique of combining lumbar myelography with cervical or thoracic computed tomography has been used to image the cord.

Magnetic resonance imaging has replaced most other imaging modalities. T1-weighted images show great anatomic detail, with black CSF and a gray-white cord. Sagittal images permit visualization of syringes and vascular malformations. T2-weighted images are less crisp but tend to highlight pathology. Intravenous injection of gadolinium allows enhancement of many pathologic lesions.

Lumbar puncture allows the cells to be examined for inflammation and malignancy. An elevated protein level may suggest tumor or other neoplasia. A low sugar level is consistent with infection or neoplasia. Cytology may be helpful. The need for and use of lumbar puncture is decreasing.

TREATMENT

Treatment must be directed at the primary disease process. Meningiomas and schwannomas are benign tumors that may be removed without definite neurologic injury. Neurofibromas are benign but are intermingled with nerve fibers, so removal of the tumor requires loss of the nerve root. Ependymomas may exist as a string of beads that may be shelled out of the central cord, but there may be recurrence. Astrocytomas require radiation, with potential cord injury. Epidural metastatic lesions are best managed by radiation without surgery. The tumor may have destroyed the anterior elements, and decompression by posterior laminectomy may render the spine unstable. Anterior procedures are more complex. The lesion must be approached surgically when a prior diagnosis of cancer has not been made.

Spinal cord trauma patients may be helped by high-dose steroids, and surgery is indicated in some to decompress the cord and stabilize the vertebrae. As for all too many of these conditions, there are no therapeutic options for spinal cord ischemia.

Cervical spondylosis may benefit from anterior fusion or posterior laminectomy. Foraminotomy is less successful but may be needed for intense pain. The problem is susceptibility of the root to traumatic injury. Many patients are relieved by short courses of steroids or nonsteroidal antiinflammatory agents. Controversy exists about the utility of collar and traction, but some patients seem to benefit.

Syringomyelia may have periods of stabilization, making it difficult to evaluate the many surgical procedures available. Posterior fossa decompression is useful in patients with concurrent Chiari malformations. Drainage of the cyst itself may be necessary in others. The goal is to arrest the process, but some patients do improve.

Subacute combined degeneration of the spinal cord is the most optimistic of all. All but the most severely affected patients show some response to intramuscular administration of vitamin B_{12}.

Advances in our understanding of amyotrophic lateral sclerosis have led to a new treatment, Riluzole. It offers limited benefit, but there is the promise of more meaningful therapy in the future.

CONSIDERATIONS DURING PREGNANCY

Meningiomas are vascular tumors that increase in size during pregnancy. Arteriovenous malformations also increase in size during pregnancy because of the estrogen and perhaps because of enhanced perfusion.

Diagnostic problems related to the high radiation to the fetus in myelography can be avoided with magnetic resonance imaging, which may well be safe in pregnancy.

Because of the lower frequency and less readily measurable responses, female sexual dysfunction has been far less completely studied in spinal cord injury. Traumatic injury has been the best studied, and problems may include loss of psychogenic or reflex stimulation of vaginal lubrication, clitoral enlargement, and labial swelling. Bowel and bladder soiling, as well as pelvic muscle spasticity, may be avoided by elimination before intercourse and muscle relaxants to reduce the spasticity. Once a seriously embarrassing event has occurred, sexual contact may be avoided. Pregnancy can occur and contraception may be indicated. Women with higher cord lesions may have problems with autonomic stability and ineffectual contractions. Blood-pressure control may be a problem, as may recurrent urinary tract infections. Before delivery, careful planning should be done to allay the mother's anxiety about caring for her child.

BIBLIOGRAPHY

Barnett HJM, Foster JB, Hudgson P. Syringomyelia. London: WB Saunders, 1973.

Byrne TN, Waxman SG. Spinal cord compression: diagnosis and principles of management. Philadelphia: FA Davis, 1990.

Chiles III BW, Cooper PR. Current concepts: acute spinal injury. N Engl J Med 1996;334:514.

Hoppenfeld S. Orthopaedic neurology; a diagnostic guide to neurologic levels. Philadelphia: JB Lippincott, 1977.

Ropper AH, Wijdicks EFM, Truax BT. Guillain-Barré syndrome. Philadelphia: FA Davis, 1991.

Young RR, Woolsey RM. Diagnosis and management of disorders of the spinal cord. Philadelphia: WB Saunders, 1995.

Primary Care for Women, edited by Phyllis C. Leppert and Fred M. Howard. Lippincott-Raven Publishers, Philadelphia © 1997.

114

Multiple Sclerosis

JOSHUA HOLLANDER

Multiple sclerosis (MS) is the most common serious neurologic disease of young adults. It may have its onset in childhood and later years. It shows a sharp rise in incidence in the late teens, peaking early and falling briskly in later years. The median age of incidence is 30 years. The actual incidence shows a geographic gradient, increasing with latitude from the equator. Exceptions exist, and there are pockets of high and low incidence not otherwise explained. The female:male ratio is about 1.5 : 1.

Acute disseminated encephalomyelitis is a perivenous inflammatory demyelinating disease that may follow a number of viral illnesses and vaccinia virus inoculation. A similarity of this monophasic illness and the illness following rabies immunization with rabbit brain–derived antigen to the pathology of experimental allergic encephalomyelitis led to extensive studies of this experimental disorder. This illness seems to be attributable to induction of an immune response to myelin basic protein, proteolipid protein, and myelin-associated oligodendrocyte glycoprotein. This monophasic illness has been a model for the polyphasic demyelinating disease MS.

MS is a demyelinating disease, by which it is meant that the myelin sheaths are more severely affected than the axis cylinders. It is one of a group of perivenous inflammatory demyelinative diseases. When tiny foci of perivenous demyelination become confluent, a true plaque is formed. When the myelin loss is incomplete, a shadow plaque is formed; this represents an area of increased vulnerability to future attacks. There are multiple areas of inflammation, demyelination, and glial scarring (sclerosis)—hence the name. Remyelination by oligodendroglia may occur, but the internodal gap tends to be shorter.

MS may attack CNS myelin anywhere along the neuraxis but spares peripheral myelin. Because the symptoms correlate with areas of demyelination, a bewildering array of symptoms is theoretically possible, although certain characteristic patterns do emerge.

ETIOLOGY AND DIFFERENTIAL DIAGNOSIS

The pathogenesis of MS is presumably immunologic, but certain features suggest environmental factors. Population migrations from areas of high to low incidence have indicated that if a person lives for 15 years in a high-incidence area, he or she continues to be at high risk, even if he or she moves to a low-risk area. Despite this evidence, which might suggest a viral or other infectious factor, none has been identified. It is thought that the illness may be triggered by various viral infections, perhaps multiple.

Studies of the major histocompatibility complex (MHC—chromosome 6) class II alleles (DR and DQ regions—DR15, DQ6, Dw2) have suggested increased susceptibility in these populations without consistent correlations. There may also be an overrepresentation of a variant of a portion of the T-cell receptor. The search for a specific MS antigen has failed, perhaps because there may be no single antigen. There is no systemic evidence of immune dysfunction in MS.

The disease is rare among Japanese, Chinese, and Africans but is higher among African-Americans than Africans. Siblings have an increased prevalence of six to eight times, parents and offspring only two to four times. Concordance of twin studies shows a 10-fold greater concordance among identical twins. Hereditary factors in MS may reflect multifactorial genetic immunologic capabilities rather than disease-specific inheritance.

The following is a hypothetical pathogenesis. An initiation phase occurs when a person with an appropriate genetic immune system is exposed to an environmental factor. Over the next decade or more (latent phase), a population of myelin-specific T lymphocytes is established. The initial neurologic event (provocative phase) occurs when a provocative event such as a mild febrile illness (eg, an upper respiratory viral illness), an enhanced level of γ-interferon, pregnancy, or other unidentified event (80%) occurs. This triggers the transmigration phase, in which the previously myelin-specific, activated, autoaggressive T lymphocytes (CD4, Th-1) enter the CNS. These persist and release the inflammatory cytokines interleukin-2, interleukin-3, γ-interferon, and tumor necrosis factor-α, initiating the inflammatory phase. Recruitment of further T lymphocytes, B lymphocytes, and macrophages into the CNS ensues. Reactive astrocytes develop and oligodendrocytes are injured, leading to demyelination. The subsequent two- to three-week demyelinative phase involves macrophages stripping injured myelin from axons. Oligodendrocytes are not abolished from the lesion area unless multiple attacks have occurred. The recovery phase may include improved transmission, with subsidence of the inflammatory response, remyelination, and perhaps axonal sprouting. The residual phase may be a stable phase with or without residual neurologic deficit (benign, relapsing/remitting, relapsing/progressive). When a gradual loss of function continues, this is termed chronic progressive disease. The residual neurologic disability relates to the volume and location of MS plaques and the potential for axon destruction and wallerian degeneration.

As recurrent attacks increase the tissue burden and decrease the reserve, each subsequent attack may result in further loss of neurologic function. Why relapses occur is unknown. Decreases in suppressor cells and increases in helper cells occur with attacks, but the trigger is unknown. Studies using magnetic resonance imaging (MRI) have shown that patients thought to be in remission experience asymptomatic attacks of demyelination.

The course of MS is highly variable and cannot be predicted. About 10% of patients have a benign course; a similar number begin with a progressive course. Early relapses occur at intervals of 1 to 4 years. The prognosis is adversely correlated with the frequency, duration, and severity of relapse. Patterns of deficit include cerebral, brain stem/cerebellar, and spinal. Patients with a later onset tend to experience a spinal type of disease that displays a chronic progressive course. A prolonged remission may be terminated by a disabling course. About 70% of patients have some interference with employment. Half will require a cane for ambulation in 15 years; 30% will ultimately require a wheelchair. Life expectancy is shortened by only 2 years, and death is rarely from MS itself.

An acute or subacute monosymptomatic onset is more common than a polysymptomatic or apoplectic onset. Weakness in one or more limbs is most common, followed by optic neuritis and paresthesias. Diplopia is twice as common as vertigo, ataxia, or micturition problems. Other problems are found to be initial symptoms in less than 5% of patients.

Various symptoms and signs occur throughout the course of the disease (Tables 114-1 and 114-2) and are discussed in more detail in the section on history and physical examination. The diagnosis of MS has been notoriously difficult because it has been primarily clinical and has required evolution of the disease to demonstrate two attacks and involvement of two discrete areas of the nervous system. However, newer CSF, electrophysiologic, and MRI studies may allow the clinician to make a confident diagnosis earlier in the course.

An attack is defined as neurologic dysfunction lasting more than 48 hours. It is synonymous with bout, episode, and exacerbation. The classification divides patients into clinically definite, laboratory-supported definite, clinically probable, and possible MS. A patient with clinically definite MS has two attacks and clinical or paraclinical evidence of two separate lesions. The findings are preferably confirmed by the physician. Laboratory-supported definite MS substitutes CSF and paraclinical evidence for one of the requirements of clinically definite MS. In other words, two attacks with only or lesion but CSF findings; one attack with two lesions and CSF findings; and one attack with one clinical and one paraclinical lesion and CSF changes may all qualify if syphilis, connective tissue disease, sarcoid, and subacute sclerosing panencephalitis have been ruled out. Clinically probable MS requires two attacks and evidence of only one lesion; one attack and clinical evidence of two lesions; or one attack, clinical evidence of one lesion, and paraclinical evidence of another discrete lesion. Laboratory-supported probable MS requires two attacks in different parts of the nervous system with abnormal CSF.

Major diagnoses to exclude are collagen vascular diseases such as systemic lupus erythematosus, polyarteritis nodosa, Sjögren syndrome; infections such as syphilis, Lyme disease, HIV myelopathy, HTLV-1 myelopathy, and progressive multifocal leukoencephalopathy; disorders of unclear etiology such as sarcoidosis and Behçet syndrome; toxic metabolic disorders such as subacute combined degeneration of the spinal cord, adrenomyeloneuropathy, subacute myelooptic neuropathy; degenerative disorders such as spinocerebellar degenerations and hereditary spastic paraplegias; and demyelinating diseases such as acute disseminated encephalomyelitis. The time factor between attacks may eliminate the monophasic acute disseminated encephalomyelitis. The varied presentation of syphilis requires a serology in any patient with suspected MS. Hereditary spastic paraplegia may be confused with the chronic spinal progressive form but does not show sensory findings. Adrenomyeloneuropathy has elevated levels of plasma very-long-chain fatty acids. It is sex-linked, but obligatory heterozygous females may have an MS-like state. Vitamin B_{12} levels may be needed to exclude subacute combined degeneration of the spinal cord. Subacute myelo-optic neuropathy is most common in Japanese with a high intake of chlorhydroxyquinolin. Lyme borreliosis may present in endemic areas with cranial neuropathies, spastic paraparesis, and cerebellar deficits; CSF and serum antibodies should be tested. The presence of oral and genital ulcers may suggest Behçet syndrome. Appropriate antibodies may alert the clinician to collagen vascular disease, as might systemic signs. Bony deformities may suggest spinocerebellar degeneration.

Optic neuritis and transverse myelitis may present as the initial attack of MS or may never recur. Optic neuritis most commonly presents as retrobulbar neuritis, in which the patient loses central vision and may experience pain on movement of the eye. It usually affects only one eye at a time. When the lesion is in the region of the nerve head, it is called papillitis. This is a common presenting manifestation of MS but is not always due to MS. The exact percentage of cases of optic neuritis later found to be MS is controversial but may be 25% to 50%. Transverse myelitis, a disorder that infrequently is a premonitory sign of MS, presents with a sensory and motor level suggesting that the lesion is at a specific cord level. It is usually much less well localized. Because subacute progression of spinal cord disease is common in MS, it is all too often assumed that this and MS are synonymous. Actually, the incidence is quite low, with only 5% of MS patients presenting with transverse myelitis and only 1% of cases of transverse myelitis developing into MS. Neuromyelitis optica (Devic disease), a condition restricted to optic nerve and spinal cord involvement, is most common in Asia.

Brain stem/cerebellar dysfunction is another pattern of disease, with tremor, ataxia, and dysarthria (Charcot triad) frequently asso-

Table 114-1. Common Symptoms and Signs of Multiple Sclerosis

FUNCTIONAL SYSTEM	FREQUENCY (%)
Motor	
Muscle weakness	65–100
Spasticity	73–100
Reflexes (hyperreflexia, Babinski, absent)	62–98
Sensory	
Impairment of vibratory/position sense	48–82
Impairment of pain, temperature, or touch	16–72
Pain (moderate to severe)	11–37
Lhermitte sign	1–42
Cerebellar	
Ataxia (limb/gait/truncal)	37–78
Tremor	36–81
Nystagmus (brain stem or cerebellar)	54–73
Dysarthria (brain stem or cerebellar)	29–62
Cranial Nerve/Brain Stem	
Vision affected	27–55
Ocular disturbances (including nystagmus)	18–39
Cranial nerves V, VII, VIII	5–52
Bulbar signs	9–49
Vertigo	7–27
Autonomic	
Bladder dysfunction	49–93
Bowel dysfunction	39–64
Sexual dysfunction	33–59
Others (sweating and vascular abnormalities)	38–43
Psychiatric	
Depression	8–55
Euphoria	4–18
Cognitive abnormalities	11–59
Miscellaneous	
Fatigue	59–85

ciated. Nystagmus, oculomotor disturbances, and other cranial neuropathies may be seen. A characteristic problem is internuclear ophthalmoplegia. In the paramedian pontine reticular formation near the abducens nucleus is a center for ipsilateral lateral gaze. Lateral gaze requires yoked action of the contralateral medial rectus, innervated by the contralateral oculomotor nucleus. The two nuclei are linked by the median longitudinal fasciculus. Lesions in this tract dissociate these movements, with impaired adduction on the side of the lesion and contralateral nystagmus. This tract lies near the midline, and the vascular supply respects the midline. Thus, ischemic lesions may cause unilateral internuclear ophthalmoplegia, but bilateral internuclear ophthalmoplegia is most common with MS or brain stem tumors or bleeds. Vertigo may be seen. Hearing loss is rare.

Cognitive abnormalities occur, as do mood changes. Euphoria is frequently commented on, but depression is more common.

Table 114-2. Infrequent Symptoms and Signs Associated With Multiple Sclerosis

WELL-RECOGNIZED ASSOCIATIONS	RARE ASSOCIATIONS
Generalized seizures	Aphasia
Tonic seizure	Anosmia
Headache	Hiccoughs
Trigeminal neuralgia	Deafness
Paroxysmal dysarthria/ataxia	Horner syndrome
Chorea/athetosis	Paroxysmal itching
Myoclonus	Cardiac arrhythmias
Facial hemispasm	Acute pulmonary edema
Myokymia	Hypothalamic dysfunction
Spasmodic torticollis/focal dystonia	Narcolepsy
Lower motor neuron signs—wasting, decreased tone, areflexia	
Restless legs	
Hysteria	

Aphasia and similar disturbances are unusual except as late end-stage phenomena in severe cerebral MS.

MS is usually thought not to be a painful disorder, but back pain is not unusual in spinal MS. Trigeminal neuralgia is disproportionately frequent in MS and may be associated with sensory loss. Multiple uncommon localized painful syndromes occur, such as the band paresthesias, burning pains, and painful spasms.

Seizures are usually ascribed to gray matter disease but may also occur in MS. Unusual in the general population are brief painful tonic seizures. Another paroxysmal problem is a peculiar fleeting paroxysmal dysarthria and ataxia.

Diagnostic confidence is enhanced by the findings on neurologic examination, although no specific features allow a definitive diagnosis. The diagnosis in patients with only sensory findings is tenuous: only the history, corroborated by examination, allows a confident diagnosis. Diagnosis should not be made on the basis of imaging studies alone, as despite major improvements in the laboratory diagnosis, it remains supplemental to the clinical evaluation. The uncertainty about the initial diagnosis and confusion about the natural history in a given patient cause great anxiety. Patients find the uncertainty unbearable, and the stress may exceed that seen in a progressive disorder. The ability to resolve this issue is extremely important, but the physician should be accurate.

HISTORY

The history is burdened by the need to explore the possibility of past nervous system involvement. Mild optic neuritis in the remote past may be the only clue in an older patient with chronic progressive spinal MS. A complete system review is needed to exclude other diagnostic considerations that involve non-CNS problems. A review of possible motor, sensory, cerebellar, brain stem, cranial nerve, autonomic, and psychiatric symptoms, as well as excessive fatigue, must be done. The physician must try to define the symptoms precisely. Records must be sought from other physicians to establish the presence of corroboratory physical findings. Many of the historical items may be reported in a convincing way by knowledgeable patients who have a need for this diagnosis. Reports of diplopia should be explored to separate horizontal, diagonal, and pure vertical diplopia. Diplopia may be thought of as visual blurring and confused with optic neuritis. Patients with optic neuritis often experience pain on eye movement. The perceptive patient may report color desaturation or loss of central vision. The Lhermitte sign must usually be specifically sought. Paresthesias may include a feeling of a tight band around a limb or trunk. Numbness may be a sensory loss but is commonly a motor phenomenon. Gait disturbances may be difficult for the patient to define in terms of ataxia versus weakness.

As the diagnosis requires multiple (relapses or exacerbations) attacks, it is essential that an attack last longer than 48 hours and not be associated with an intercurrent febrile illness. Patients may experience a transient exacerbation in their symptoms when exposed to heat. The Uhthoff phenomenon is a transient return of central field loss with exertion. This process can be seen with other previous MS lesions. Long days at work may also result in decreased strength or dysarthria late in the day. These are merely transient problems of CNS function, not true attacks of demyelination.

PHYSICAL EXAMINATION

A careful general physical examination is in order to explore possible embolic sources and signs of infection or connective tissue dysfunction. Patients with MS usually have more findings than symptoms, and the physician should be alerted when the history is suggestive but the examination is unproductive.

The cranial nerves are examined, with particular attention to the eyes. It is important to assess visual acuity (near card in the office) and visual field. Formal visual field testing is desirable but impractical in the office. Central fields can be defined simply by asking the patient to cover one eye and look at the examiner's nose. Missing parts of the face can usually be described by the patient. Moving fingers is a relatively crude way to examine peripheral fields, but counting briefly displayed fingers can be more precise in a cooperative patient. Patients with optic neuritis (papillitis or retrobulbar neuritis) have a central or cecocentral scotoma. Examination of the optic disc is normal in retrobulbar neuritis (neither patient nor physician sees anything) and shows papilledema in papillitis. True papilledema can be distinguished from papillitis by the acuity, which is preserved in papilledema and lost in papillitis. The Marcus Gunn pupil (afferent pupillary defect—swinging flashlight test) may be seen in both present and remote optic neuritis. In this phenomenon, the pupil responds poorly ipsilaterally and normally on consensual stimulation. The pupil thus appears to dilate when the light shines in the affected eye after shining the light in the normal eye. The optic nerve head may appear pale (temporal or full) after resolution of the process—thus, the afferent pupillary defect and optic atrophy may provide a clue to remote optic neuritis.

The presence of bilateral internuclear ophthalmoplegia can be seen on lateral gaze by impaired adduction and dissociated jerk nystagmus of the abducting eye. Nystagmus is common and can be horizontal, vertical, or rotatory. Eye signs of cerebellar disease include nystagmus, ocular dysmetria, loss of smooth pursuit, and macro-square wave jerks. Gaze paresis and oculomotor palsies may be present.

Dysarthria has multiple etiologies that may be hard to sort out because of multiple possible concurrent mechanisms. Facial asymmetry may be seen.

Muscle strength problems are most common in the lower limbs as an asymmetric paraparesis. Hemiparesis and tetraparesis or -plegia may occur. Spasticity may be severe enough to interfere with positioning the limb. Ataxia is not unusual. An action tremor may be minimal or severely disabling. A spastic ataxic gait is not unusual. Movements may be of adequate strength but merely slowed.

Sensory disturbances affect position and vibratory sense more readily, but any modality may be involved. Sensory ataxia may be a problem. It is best elicited by observing the limb with the eyes closed. A typist who has a position sense deficit may be unable to work. Loss of sensation may lead to Charcot joints, but usually concurrent motor loss protects the limb.

Muscle stretch reflexes are commonly hyperactive with extensor plantar responses. Lesions at the root entry zone may cause lost reflexes; those in the exit zone may cause lower motor weakness and atrophy. The polysynaptic cutaneous reflexes are commonly lost. The abdominals are elicited in each quadrant by drawing a pin over the skin in the direction of the dermatome. However, postpartum or postoperative abdomens often fail to display abdominal responses.

Stance, Romberg, and gait are all evaluated, perhaps by watching the patient walk to the examining room. An inner corridor sheltered from the waiting room may be necessary for this evaluation.

LABORATORY AND IMAGING STUDIES

Laboratory studies may serve as screening studies to rule out other systemic etiologies. First attacks limited to one location in the nervous system may require other studies to exclude other CNS possibilities such as tumor. Testing may be done in an effort to find evidence for an unrecognized lesion elsewhere in the nervous system, which would allow an earlier diagnosis to be made. Laboratory studies such as urinalysis, serologic test for syphilis, Westergren sedimentation rate, antinuclear antibody (ANA), vitamin B_{12}, angiotensin-converting enzyme, Lyme titers (in endemic areas), HIV, and HTLV-1 (spastic paraparesis) may be done.

MRI is the most useful imaging study and has replaced most other studies in the evaluation of MS. White matter lesions are seen in 90% of T2-weighted images. They are most readily detected as hyperintense signal in the periventricular area and can be located in centrum semiovale white matter, but are particularly notable in the white matter just posterior to the occipital horn in proton-density and T2-weighted images. Activity may be reflected by enhancement with gadolinium in T1-weighted images. The lesions in benign MS may require delayed scanning with high-dose gadolinium. MRI findings must be interpreted carefully: they may be falsely interpreted as positive in older patients and those in whom lesions are small or few in number.

The CSF is abnormal in over 90% of patients. Cell counts may show five to 20 lymphocytes but are usually normal. Cells are mostly CD4 cells. Glucose is normal and mild protein elevation may be seen. IgG is abnormal in most patients. Sensitivity can exceed 90% when the IgG is examined for oligoclonal bands not present in serum. There is increased IgG synthesis and a high IgG index. κ-Chains tend to be increased. Myelin basic protein is elevated in the face of active demyelination. Other inflammatory diseases may raise the IgG and the myelin basic protein, however, so neither test is truly specific.

Evoked potentials can be elicited by providing a stimulus and then signal-averaging the brain electrical activity time yoked to the stimulus. Typically, these are visual, auditory, and somatosensory. Visual responses are usually performed by pattern shift. The patient is asked to fix on a black-on-white checkerboard that alternates with a white-on-black checkerboard. This is very sensitive, with prolongation in the latency of the P100 wave in one or both eyes and an interocular difference in many patients. It is positive in 85% of cases of definite MS. It is most useful when findings indicate optic nerve conduction delay in previously unrecognized optic dysfunction or in patients with complaints referable to the eyes but lacking other objective confirmation. Less sensitive in MS are the brain stem auditory evoked responses; although positive in many patients with brain stem dysfunction, they are less likely to define new lesions in MS. Somatosensory evoked potentials can be elicited by electrical stimulation of median, peroneal, or posterior tibial nerves. These are also less sensitive than visual evoked potentials.

Although primary care providers may need to refer patients with suspected MS for these tests, they must understand their role in the diagnosis of this disease.

TREATMENT

Treatment of patients with MS is directed at managing symptoms and altering the immune process thought causative of disease progression. Good nutrition is always in order, but no dietary additive or supplement has ever been demonstrated to be of benefit. Any chronic disease of unpredictable course subject to frequent remission lends itself to large numbers of dubious claims of successful treatment, and this is clearly true for MS. Some dietary manipulations have included fish oil and megavitamins. Patients should be encouraged to discuss these claims before embarking on a protracted trial of unproven therapies.

Symptomatic therapy is inherently poor, as the intensity of the problem is decreased but not removed. Fatigue may be relieved in some patients by modifying activities to minimize effort or by scheduling a formal rest period. The patient should understand that this problem is not the same as one of strengthening a weak muscle; aggressive physical therapy is not in order. Some patients benefit from amantadine 100 mg twice or three times daily.

Spasticity can become severe but is never alone because weakness is always present. Complete relief of the spasticity may render a lower limb incapable of supporting the patient. Physical therapy with stretching exercises can be helpful. Titration of baclofen against weakness and lethargy is common; the use of dantrolene and diazepam is less common. With nonambulatory patients, destructive procedures cutting nerves or tendons may be needed to facilitate toileting and hygiene.

The problems of a spastic neurogenic bladder may be helped by anticholinergic agents, which may lengthen the time between voidings and decrease urgency. Poor bladder emptying may benefit from the Credé technique of pressing down on the abdomen while bearing down. If this is inadequate, intermittent self-catheterization is useful. If the problem is dyssynergia or does not respond, referral to a urologist and urodynamics are in order. Foley catheters may be the only solution for some patients. Urinary acidification may reduce the incidence of urinary tract infections.

Two thirds of women with MS have sexual difficulties. Problems arise from impaired self-image, impaired bowel and bladder control, the presence of a catheter, and flexor spasms. Men and women report decreased genital sensation, loss of sexual interest, and decreased orgasm. Women may complain of vaginal itching and dryness; lubrication may help. Timing of voiding, taping catheters out of the way, timing spasmolytic drugs, and adjusting intercourse positions may be of benefit. Some couples are helped by mechanical stimulators or oral sex.

Constipation is more frequent than fecal incontinence and may be helped by fluids and bulk. Laxatives or suppositories may be needed to induce regularity.

Problems of decreased mobility include decubitus ulcers and swollen feet. Decubitus ulcers may be helped by the use of doughnuts, cushions, or other ways of reducing pressure. Swollen feet can be reduced by the use of elastic stockings and elevation.

Painful tonic seizures may be reduced by the use of carbamazepine, which is also effective in trigeminal neuralgia. Tricyclic antidepressants may relieve the inappropriate forced laughter or crying seen in pseudobulbar palsy.

Increased neurologic deficits associated with fever should be managed with fluids and antipyretics.

Specific therapies may be divided into those for relapsing/remitting disease and those for progressive disease. Antigen-nonselective immunomodulating therapies include steroids and interferon-α and -β. Acute therapy of an exacerbation (as previously defined) means steroid therapy. High-dose therapy is usually used because of the results of the optic neuritis trial and evidence that it seems to work faster. The dose is not established, but 1000 mg/day methylprednisolone IV for 5 days is used at Rochester General Hospital. Admission to the hospital makes this simpler and permits physical therapy. However, managed care systems generally demand outpatient infusions or home infusions unless the disability demands hospitalization. Use of H_2 blockers is not established but may be safer. Whether it is best to follow the intravenous therapy with a short- or long-taper regimen, or no tapering, is unknown. The no-taper plan attempts to reduce steroid complications. High-dose steroids are lympholytic in a nonspecific way and also restore the integrity of the blood–brain barrier. Furthermore, cytokine production and other aspects of the immune and inflammatory response are reduced. It remains to be proven whether this therapy affects the long-term course of the disease. Toxicity of chronic use precludes long-term therapy.

The interferons are a family of proteins of four groups. They are involved in the response to viral and other infections as well as tumor resistance. Interferon-α and -β activate a cell surface receptor and are antagonistic to interferon-γ, which is a proinflammatory agent increasing the relapse rate in MS. There are multiple areas of antagonistic effect on the immune system. Interferon-β1B (Betaseron) has been approved for therapy of chronic relapsing/remitting MS. In the pivotal study, it reduced the relapse rate by 35% and the incidence of severe exacerbations by 50% and reduced the area and activity of MRI involvement. The study was not designed to allow evaluation of long-term change in disability. Interferon-β1B is made by transfected *Escherichia coli* and is nonglycosylated. It is injected subcutaneously every other day and causes flu-like symptoms, fevers, myalgias, headache, local skin reaction, marrow suppression, and elevation of hepatic enzymes. Patients who have one or more attacks per year and do not have unacceptable side effects should be treated with interferon. The cost (about $10,000/year) make selective use an issue for payers. Interferon-β1A (Avonex), a new drug, is made from a transfected mammalian cell and is said to be better tolerated. It is injected intramuscularly weekly. However, the high price might make this treatment less desirable.

Other nonselective immunomodulating agents are being investigated. An antigen-selective immunomodulatory agent nearing approval by the FDA is Cop1 (Copolymer1, Copaxone). It is a basic amino acid copolymer partially cross-reactive with myelin basic protein. In experimental allergic encephalomyelitis, it is protective, but the mechanism is controversial. It is given subcutaneously daily. It seems to be better tolerated but has comparable efficacy. The notion of combining several agents—with enormous expense and poorly understood mechanisms—will probably preclude combining Cop1 with interferon. Oral myelin basic protein is said to have potential benefit and is in trial.

These agents have not yet been demonstrated to be of benefit in chronic progressive disease. Cytotoxic immunosuppressants have been used in chronic progressive disease. These have included azathioprine, cyclophosphamide, cyclosporine, methotrexate, and cladrabine, with little efficacy demonstrated. Plasma exchange and total lymphoid radiation have also been used.

Snake venom, bee stings, hyperbaric oxygen, and many other therapies have been announced as cures. Unfortunately, the matter requires more than unsubstantiated claims.

CONSIDERATIONS DURING PREGNANCY

It was formerly held, on the basis of no data, that pregnancy presented a severe risk to patients with MS; there was even a famous surrogate mother case involving a woman with MS. Studies have failed to show any negative impact of MS on pregnancy. There is no difference in the relapse rate between married and single women. The risk of relapse during pregnancy is equal to that during the 3 months postpartum. There is probably an increase in the relapse rate in the 6 months after delivery. The relapse rate is probably only 0.25 relapses per person per pregnancy year. Termination of pregnancy does not reduce this, nor does postpartum steroid therapy. Oral contraceptives have not been shown to have any effect on MS.

Women contemplating pregnancy should arrange for additional help with night feedings and should avoid undue exhaustion. They should consider their current degree of disability and the burden of caring for the child. If analysis of these considerations and the defined risk are known and the woman wishes to have a child, there are no clear medical contraindications.

BIBLIOGRAPHY

Bauer HJ, Hanefeld FA. Multiple sclerosis: its impact from childhood to old age. London: WB Saunders, 1993.

Donaldson OJ. Neurology of pregnancy, 2d ed. London: WB Saunders, 1989.

Herndon RM, Seil FJ. Multiple sclerosis: current status of research and treatment. New York: Demos Publications, 1994.

Lisak RP. Rational approach to drug therapy in multiple sclerosis. American Academy of Neurology, Annual Courses, 1996;5:346.

McDonald WI, Silverberg DH. Multiple sclerosis. London: Butterworths & Co., 1986.

Matthews WB, Acheson ED, Batchelor JR, Weller RO. McAlpine's multiple sclerosis. New York: Churchill Livingstone, 1985.

Paty DW, Scheinberg L, McDonald WI, Ebers GC. The diagnosis of multiple sclerosis. New York: Thieme-Stratton Inc., 1984.

Saud AS, Miller JR. Demyelinating diseases. In: Rowland LP, ed. Merritt's textbook of neurology, 9th ed. Philadelphia: Williams & Wilkins, 1995.

Schapiro RT. Symptom management in multiple sclerosis. New York: Demos Publications, 1987.

Vollmer TL. Multiple sclerosis: new approaches to immunotherapy. Neuroscientist 1996;2:127.

Primary Care for Women, edited by Phyllis C. Leppert and Fred M. Howard. Lippincott-Raven Publishers, Philadelphia

115
Mononeuropathies

HAROLD LESSER

Isolated injuries to peripheral nerves frequently are seen in the primary care setting. The most common are injuries to the median nerve at the wrist, ulnar nerve at the elbow, and peroneal nerve at the fibular head. Whereas many mononeuropathies are isolated events, others develop in patients with underlying systemic illnesses or significant risk factors for nerve injury. Identifying underlying risk factors may help to limit recurrent trauma to an affected nerve, prevent future nerve injury, and predict prognosis.

The clinical course and management of nerve injuries depend on the severity of the injury. Injuries that affect only the myelin sheath carry a better prognosis than those affecting the integrity of axons themselves. In neurapraxia, the mildest of nerve injures, there is temporary focal disruption of nerve function without disruption of the anatomic integrity of the nerve or its sustaining structures. The limb that "falls asleep" and recovers over minutes is a common example. Repeated or more severe neurapraxia injuries can produce symptoms lasting for days. When the myelin sheath surrounding the nerve sustains a significant injury, conduction block (focal nerve conduction failure) can develop at the site of injury. The acute functional consequences of severe conduction block are identical to nerve transection: loss of sensorimotor function distal to the site of injury.

Axonotmesis describes a more severe form of nerve injury in which there is some degree of axon loss but the integrity of the supporting structures of the nerve is preserved. Weakness, sensory loss, and loss of reflexes develop acutely. Over time, wallerian degeneration develops in the axons disconnected from their sustaining cell bodies. The most distal portions of the axons and their myelin coating degenerate first, then degeneration spreads proximally. When axonotmesis is mild by both clinical and electrodiagnostic measures, functional recovery is more likely because regenerating axons can regrow along intact nerve infrastructure.

Neurotmesis or transection is the most severe form of nerve injury. Immediate and potentially permanent loss of sensorimotor and autonomic function is seen distal to the transection site. Severe muscle atrophy develops during subsequent months. Surgical exploration should be attempted when neurotmesis is suspected because surgical reanastomosis provides the only hope for functional recovery. Unfortunately, despite surgical intervention, scarring and neuroma formation at the transection site often inhibit regeneration and may lead to chronic nerve irritation and pain.

Nerve conduction studies provide an accurate estimate of the degree of axonal loss if they are performed after Wallerian degeneration has had time to develop. If performed too early (ie, within the first few weeks after injury), they underestimate the ultimate degree of axon injury. Needle electromyography is exquisitely sensitive to axon loss, but again, timing is critical. When motor axons are injured and die, there is a loss of trophic (nutritional) support to the muscle fibers that they previously innervated. Denervated muscle fibers undergo degeneration, causing membrane instability, which leads to abnormal spontaneous discharges known as p-waves and fibrillations. Abnormal spontaneous activity (also known as denervation) can be detected after injury to as few as 3% of motor axons.

In cases of severe axonotmesis, the question often arises whether *any* axons remain intact. When only a few motor axons survive, they often activate so few muscle fibers that no muscle contraction is visible. Electromyographic demonstration of volitional motor unit activation implies a better prognosis for recovery than when no volitional motor units can be activated. Electromyographic evidence of ongoing axonal sprouting and reinnervation, when present, also is a hopeful sign.

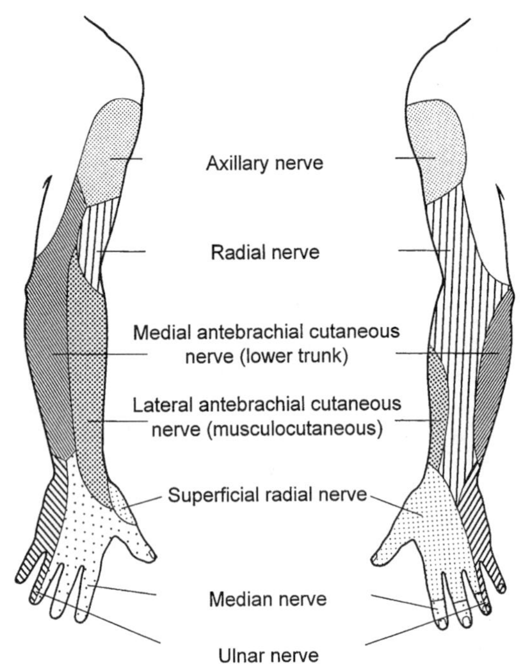

Figure 115-1. Cutaneous innervation of the left arm. (Modified from Binney CD, Cooper R, Fowler CJ, Mauguière F, Prior PF. Clinical neurophysiology: EMG, nerve conduction and evoked potentials. Oxford: Butterworth-Heinemann, 1995:114.)

ETIOLOGY AND DIFFERENTIAL DIAGNOSIS

The common compressive mononeuropathies (median at the wrist, ulnar at the elbow, and peroneal at the fibular head) often are associated with underlying disorders or risk factors that increase the probability of developing mononeuropathies. A mild, diffuse polyneuropathy (eg, diabetes, hypothyroidism, uremia) predisposes to compressive injury of individual nerves. Prolonged unconsciousness or immobility and severe weight loss are risk factors for compressive injuries to the ulnar nerve at the elbow, the radial nerve at the spiral groove, and the peroneal nerve at the fibular head. Carpal tunnel syndrome (CTS) or lateral femoral cutaneous neuropathy (meralgia paresthetica) often develop during pregnancy.

HISTORY

When evaluating mononeuropathies, a patient's handedness, occupation, and hobbies should be ascertained. A history of trauma to the symptomatic limb, even in the distant past, may be relevant. Recent use of casts, orthotic devices, or crutches should be considered. If the patient has been hospitalized recently, inquire about periods of immobility or unconsciousness and intravenous or phlebotomy sites.

A detailed medical history should be obtained, and family history should be probed for diabetes, hypothyroidism, connective tissue disorders, and neuropathy. A family history of high arched feet, hammer toes, gait disorders late in life or simply "funny feet" should suggest the possibility of an inherited neuropathy.

PHYSICAL EXAMINATION

Identifying a mononeuropathy requires a fairly detailed knowledge of peripheral nerve anatomy. Figures 115-1 through 115-3 show the cutaneous distribution of the peripheral nerves in the limbs. This information needs to be compared and contrasted with the dermatomal patterns of Figures 115-4 and 115-5 because the differential diagnosis of peripheral nerve lesions often includes nerve root compression (eg, ulnar neuropathy versus C8-T1 radiculopathy).

CLINICAL FINDINGS

Upper Extremity Mononeuropathies

Median Mononeuropathies

Compression of the median nerve at the wrist, or CTS, is the most common mononeuropathy. The carpal tunnel is a fibrous channel bound by the transverse carpal ligament through which the median nerve and nine finger flexor tendons enter the wrist. Overuse of the hands, particularly by repetitive motions performed under stress, produces focal nerve injury. Other predisposing factors for CTS include weight gain, pregnancy, hypothyroidism, and rheumatoid arthritis. Women are more likely to get CTS than are men.

Classically, patients complain of numbness and tingling involving their thumb and index and middle fingers. Difficulty holding a newspaper or a steering wheel and clumsiness of the hand often are reported, and nocturnal awakening with paresthesia is usually present. The discomfort of CTS may be poorly localized, involving the whole hand, forearm, shoulder, or even neck. Alternate diagnoses such as a proximal median mononeuropathy at the elbow, brachial plexopathy, or cervical radiculopathy must be considered when evaluating such complaints.

With mild CTS, there may be a paucity of findings on examination. The presence of Tinel's sign—paresthesias (abnormal sensation of pins and needles) provoked by percussion over the median nerve at the wrist—indicates local axonal injury and regeneration at the site of percussion. Phalen's sign—the reproduction of symptoms by forcible hyperflexion of the wrist for 30 to 60 seconds—also suggests local nerve injury. Decreased sensation on the median (lateral) half of the fourth digit with sparing of sensation on the ulnar half is characteristic. Sensory loss and thenar atrophy are

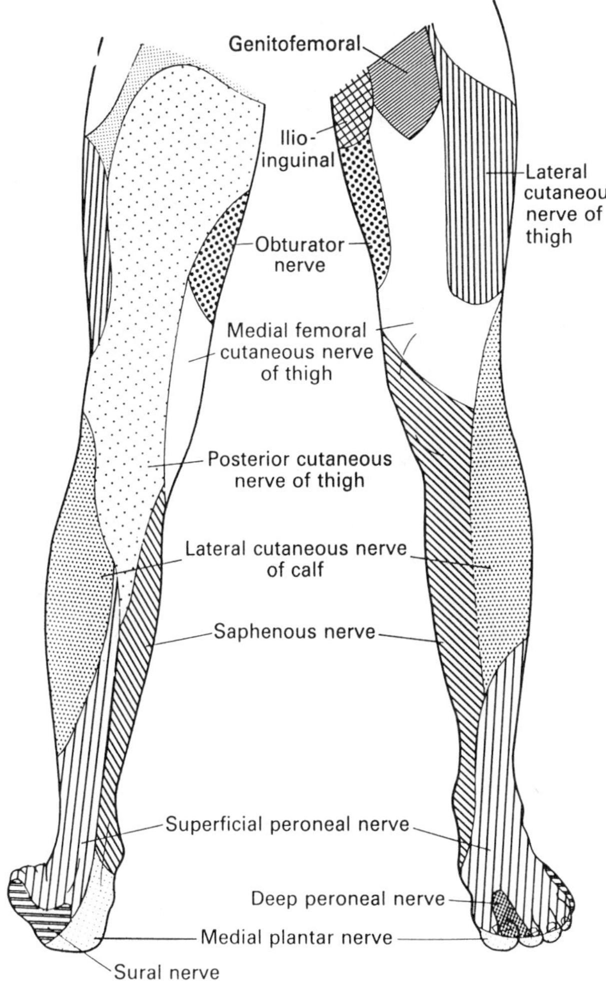

Figure 115-2. Cutaneous innervation of the left leg. (Modified from Binney CD, Cooper R, Fowler CJ, Mauguière F, Prior PF. Clinical neurophysiology: EMG, nerve conduction and evoked potentials. Oxford: Butterworth-Heinemann, 1995:127.)

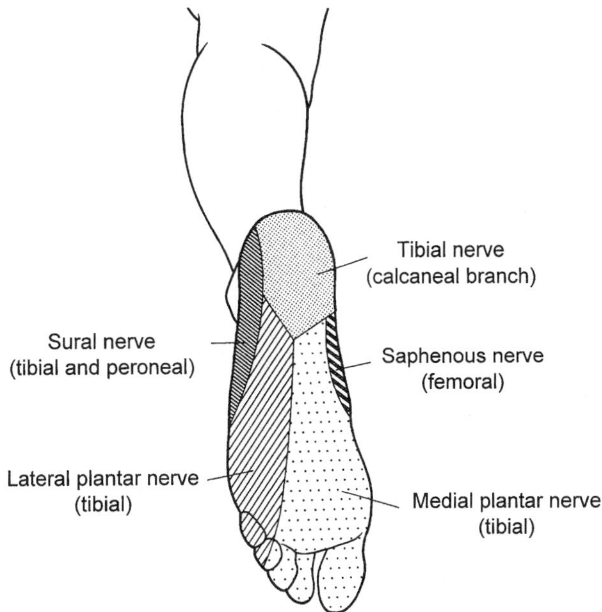

Figure 115-3. Cutaneous innervation of the sole of the left foot. (Modified from Binney CD, Cooper R, Fowler CJ, Mauguière F, Prior PF. Clinical neurophysiology: EMG, nerve conduction and evoked potentials. Oxford: Butterworth-Heinemann, 1995:135.)

seen in more advanced cases. Both hands always should be evaluated for signs and symptoms because the syndrome is commonly bilateral. The differential diagnosis of CTS should include DeQuervain syndrome (tenosynovitis of the thumb extensor tendon), C_6 radiculopathy, and proximal median mononeuropathy.

Mild CTS can be managed with nocturnal wrist splinting to prevent passive flexion of the wrist during sleep. Splints reduce both nocturnal awakening and the associated ongoing nerve injury that is associated with daytime symptoms. Reducing repetitive movements and strain at work and home also can be helpful. Symptoms often progress despite these interventions. Local injections of long-acting steroids into the carpal tunnel may be of use in patients without evidence of axonal injury. Injections can provide temporary or occasionally sustained relief in some patients; however, no controlled trial supports the efficacy of this treatment.

Electrodiagnostic testing can be used to confirm the diagnosis of CTS, assess the need for surgical management, and rule out alternate etiologies. Surgical intervention generally is warranted for axon-loss injuries. Once significant atrophy develops, the recovery of function after surgery may be incomplete. A more conservative approach should be taken when symptoms arise during pregnancy.

Ulnar Mononeuropathy

Ulnar mononeuropathy at the elbow is the second most common compressive mononeuropathy. Leaning on the elbows is the most frequent cause. It also occurs commonly in unconscious and immobilized patients. Antecedent trauma can predispose some patients to developing ulnar mononeuropathy years or even decades later: the so-called "tardy ulnar palsy." Bony overgrowth from the original injury renders the nerve more susceptible to injury. Specific inquiry about previous trauma is important because patients rarely associate their past injury with current difficulties. Because all ulnar-innervated muscles share common C8-T1 root supply via the lower trunk of the brachial plexus, both cervicothoracic radiculopathy and lower trunk plexopathy must be considered in the differential diagnosis.

When clinical examination, electrodiagnostic testing, or both indicate significant axon loss at the elbow, surgical ulnar transposition should be considered. The nerve is typically relocated anterior to the cubital tunnel, although alternative approaches exist. Surgical intervention should be considered cautiously in those with an underlying polyneuropathy (eg, diabetes).

Radial Mononeuropathy

The radial nerve is vulnerable to injury in the axilla (crutch injury) and as it wraps behind the distal third of the humerus at the spiral groove. "Saturday-night palsy" is radial neuropathy resulting from prolonged pressure on the nerve in the spiral groove, frequently after alcoholic stupor. Humeral fracture is a common cause of injury as well. Lead toxicity characteristically produces radial mononeuropathies.

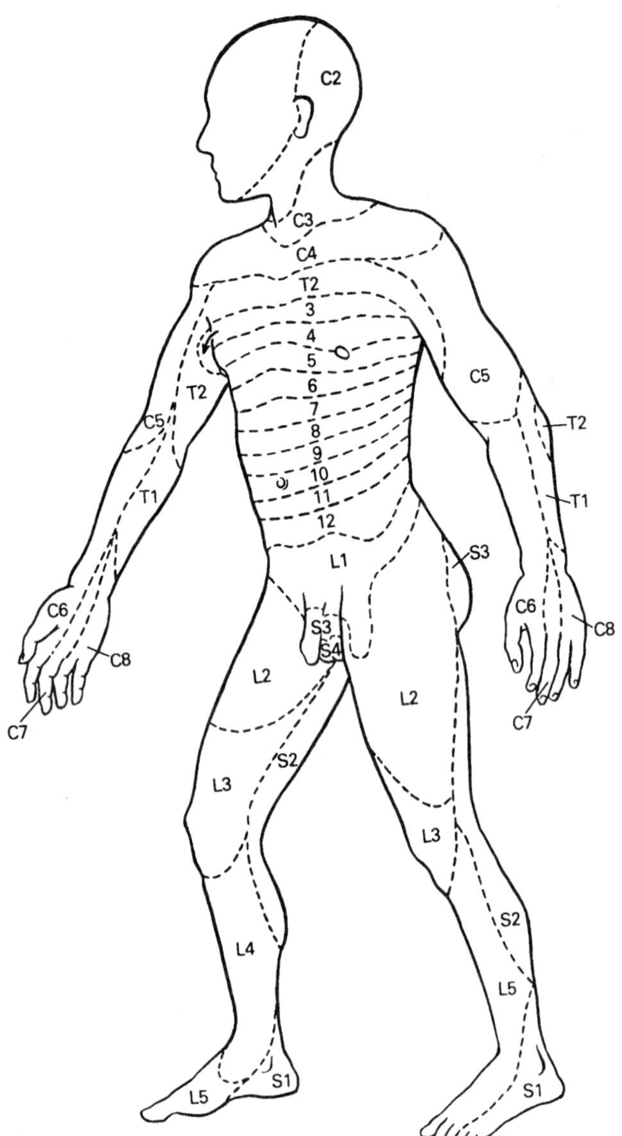

Figure 115-4. Dermatomes in anterior oblique view. The arm is supplied by C5–T2, the leg by L2–S2. Common landmarks include the T4 dermatome at the level of the nipples and the T10 dermatome at the level of the umbilicus. (Devinsky O, Feldmann E. Examination of the cranial and peripheral nerves. Oxford: Churchill Livingstone, 1988:37.)

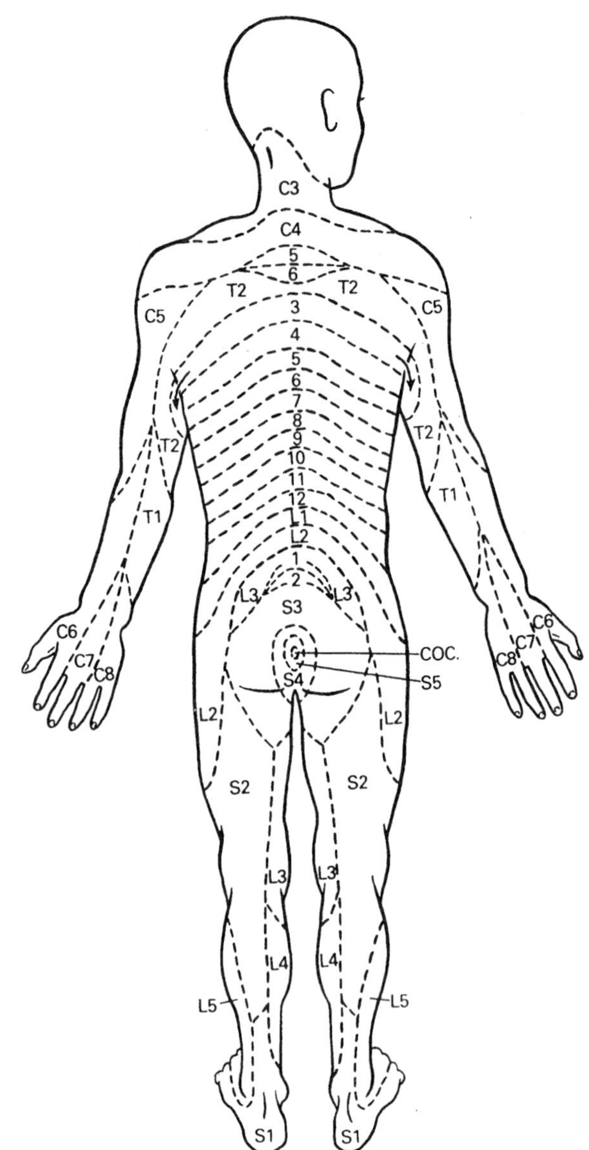

Figure 115-5. Dermatomes in the posterior view. (Devinsky O, Feldmann E. Examination of the cranial and peripheral nerves. Oxford: Churchill Livingstone, 1988:37.)

A finding of wrist drop, finger drop, or both is the hallmark of most radial mononeuropathies, but triceps weakness is seen only with the most proximal of radial injuries. Weakness of the brachioradialis suggests a lesion at or proximal to the spiral groove. To test this muscle, place the patient's forearm midway between pronation and supination (as if ready to pound the fist on the table) and have the patient flex the arm at the elbow.

Weakness from radial mononeuropathy is often mistaken either for a stroke, which causes extensor greater than flexor weakness in the upper extremity, or for an ulnar mononeuropathy, which causes weakness of hand intrinsic muscles. The hand intrinsics help to spread the fingers apart and work to mechanical advantage only when the fingers are fully extended. Without radial-mediated finger extension, the fingers assume a flexed position in which they do not generate full power. Placing the hand placed flat on the examination table before testing hand intrinsics restores the optimal mechanical advantage and permits the demonstration of normal strength.

Other Upper Extremity Mononeuropathies

The long thoracic nerve supplies the serratus anterior, which helps to stabilize the scapula against the chest wall. Traction or blunt injuries lead to scapular winging with medial translocation of the scapula. Stretch injury or direct trauma to the nerve is an infrequent complication of mastectomy or thoracotomy. The suprascapular nerve can be compressed as it passes under the suprascapular notch on its way to supply the infraspinatus. A suprascapular mononeuropathy results in weakness of external rotation of the arm. The axillary nerve supplies the teres minor and deltoid muscles and provides sensory supply to a small patch of skin overlying the deltoid muscle. Humeral neck injuries, blunt trauma, and injection injuries account for most axillary mononeuropathies. The cutaneous territory of the axillary nerve is shown in Figure 115-1.

Lower Extremity Mononeuropathies

Pelvic masses, pregnancy, vaginal delivery, and certain pelvic procedures commonly are complicated by focal nerve compression, placing women at special risk for developing mononeuropathies of the lower extremity. Evaluation of lower extremity abnormalities is complicated by the close anatomic interrelationships among its peripheral nerves. The sciatic nerve gives rise to both the peroneal and tibial nerves, and all three share a similar root supply. To further complicate matters, the sheer strength of the leg muscles makes it difficult to detect mild muscle weakness. Sensory findings often are most helpful in localizing a problem to a particular root level.

Sciatic Mononeuropathy

The sciatic nerve innervates the hamstrings, and its branches supply all of the muscles below the knee. It is composed of both peroneal and tibial fascicles, which remain anatomically distinct along the entire course of the nerve. The peroneal and tibial fascicles finally separate to form the common peroneal and tibial nerves in the distal third of the thigh. The sensory territory of the sciatic includes portions of the lateral leg and the lower leg and foot. Injuries to the sciatic nerve are often partial, which is a testament to its size and deep location.

Sciatica is a common presenting complaint in outpatients. The term *sciatica* is used loosely by patients and physicians to cover a wide range of symptoms referable to the low back and lower extremity. The history and physical should narrow the differential diagnosis of sciatica. The differential diagnosis includes spinal cord pathology (typically in the low thoracic cord or the conus medullaris), lumbosacral radiculopathy (particularly at the L5-S1 level), mononeuropathies (sciatic, posterior femoral cutaneous, peroneal or tibial), lumbosacral plexopathy, or simply nonspecific low back pain. Electrodiagnostic testing may be required to distinguish among these possibilities.

Trauma to the proximal sciatic occurs with pelvic fractures and dislocations, fractures of the acetabula, and penetrating wounds. Misplaced buttock injections (inferomedially instead of superolaterally near the ischial rim) are the most common iatrogenic cause, followed by hip arthroplasty and malpositioning during surgery. Hematomas can arise after trauma or surgery, or can develop spontaneously in patients on anticoagulant therapy. More unusual causes include prolonged sitting in the yoga position or sitting on a large wallet in the hip pocket. Pelvic tumors can produce direct sciatic compression. Endometriosis can produce *catamenial sciatic,* symptoms of sciatic compression which vary with the menstrual cycle, by compression of the nerve either at the sciatic notch or as it passes under the piriformis muscle.

In the piriformis syndrome, patients experience groin discomfort when internally rotating their flexed and adducted hip (ie, sitting on the floor with legs crossed) and often complain of dyspareunia. The syndrome is said to result from compression of the sciatic or its peroneal division as it passes under the piriformis muscle toward the greater sciatic foramen. Despite the anatomic plausibility of this syndrome, little firm electrodiagnostic evidence supports its existence.

Peroneal Mononeuropathy

The common peroneal nerve separates from the sciatic nerve in the distal third of the thigh. It winds around the fibula relatively unprotected from external compression, making common peroneal mononeuropathy at the fibular head one of the most frequently seen compressive mononeuropathies. The common peroneal gives off superficial and deep branches, each with their respective motor and sensory supplies. The deep peroneal nerve supplies the "anterior compartment" of the ankle and leg, including the ankle and toe dorsiflexors, and provides sensation to the web space between the great toe and the second toe. The superficial peroneal nerve supplies the ankle evertors and provides sensation to the dorsum of the foot, except for the most lateral portions, which are supplied by the sural nerve (see Figs. 115-2 and 115-3). The lateral (external) hamstring jerk is mediated by the peroneal nerve; the medial (internal) hamstring jerk is tibial nerve mediated.

Compression at the fibular head produces painless footdrop, toe drop, or both, often with little sensory loss. Eversion of the foot is also weak. The most common etiology in healthy patients is habitual or prolonged leg crossing or squatting. Thin individuals, patients with significant recent weight loss (either intentional or in the setting of cachexia), and diabetics all are at increased risk. Patients who deliver in the lithotomy position may compress their peroneal nerves by improper use of stirrups, or even by exerting pressure from their own hands as they attempt to forcefully flex and externally rotate their hips.

Patients with footdrop have a characteristic gait. The inability to dorsiflex the foot makes it impossible to advance the affected leg without external (lateral) rotation or unnatural elevation of the hip. Patients report tripping over their toes, catching the edge of carpeting, or scuffing the tops of their shoes. An ankle-foot orthosis (AFO) "cures" footdrop and permits a nearly normal gait, even when the ankle dorsiflexors are flaccid. When footdrop is mild, high-top sneakers may substitute for an AFO.

Chronic footdrop places patients at risk for developing Achilles tendon shortening and contractures. Once contractures develop, dorsiflexion of the foot becomes impossible, even with normal ankle dorsiflexor strength. Use of a foot board at night, appropriate supports (AFO or high-top shoes) during the day, and passive lengthening exercises can help to preserve normal heel cord length.

The differential diagnosis of peroneal mononeuropathy includes L5 radiculopathy, sciatic mononeuropathy, lumbosacral plexopathy, and other conditions. Upper motor neuron injuries (ie, stroke, spinal cord injury) also can produce footdrop. L5 radiculopathies typically are associated with back pain and weakness of both foot inversion *and* eversion, whereas peroneal mononeuropathies produce greater eversion weakness. The peroneal fascicles in the sciatic nerve are selectively vulnerable to compression and often mimic more distal injuries to the common or deep peroneal nerve. Electromyographic evaluation should be sufficiently detailed to exclude this possibility.

Tibial Mononeuropathy

The tibial nerve arises from the medial portion of the sciatic nerve. It supplies the posterior calf muscles and foot intrinsics. Tibial mononeuropathies produce weakness of ankle plantar flexion ("stepping on the gas") and inversion. The ankle jerk and medial hamstring jerk are both tibial nerve mediated. The sensory territory of the nerve includes the posterior leg, the lateral border of the foot, and the sole via the medial and lateral plantar nerves (see Figs. 115-2 and 115-3).

The tibial nerve and the medial sciatic nerve from which it arises are relatively immune to injury. Proximal injuries are rare, occurring with total knee replacement, severe knee trauma, Baker's cysts, and aneurysms of the popliteal artery. Distal compressive injuries at or below the ankle are more common but still unusual. Tarsal tunnel syndrome is the most common of the tibial mononeuropathies. The syndrome results from entrapment of the tibial nerve under the flexor retinaculum (just behind the medial malleolus). Sensory loss is prominent on the plantar surface of the foot in the distribution of the median and lateral plantar nerves (see Fig. 115-3). Sensation in the heel is spared as the calcaneal branch of the tibial arises just proximal to the tarsal tunnel and is not compressed. Weakness of the lateral toe flexors develops. Tinel's sign may be elicited below the medial malleolus. As with other entrapments, diabetic and hypothyroid patients are at increased risk.

Femoral Mononeuropathies

The femoral nerve supplies the quadriceps (knee extensors), the iliopsoas (hip flexor), and the sartorius (external rotator of the knee) and provides sensory supply to the anteromedial thigh, knee, and medial calf via the saphenous nerve. The patellar jerk is mediated by fibers of the femoral nerve. Placing a patient in the lithotomy position, either for surgical procedures or delivery, can compress the femoral nerve under the inguinal ligament, and cephalopelvic disproportion can lead to direct compression of either the femoral nerve or the lumbosacral plexus from which it arises. Retroperitoneal hemorrhage can produce devastating proximal femoral mononeuropathies. Spontaneous retroperitoneal bleeding often develops in patients on anticoagulation therapy. Inguinal pain followed by weakness of both the proximally innervated iliopsoas and the quadriceps muscles strongly suggest the diagnosis, which can be confirmed by a pelvic computed tomography scan. Timely surgical intervention may spare femoral nerve function.

Diabetic amyotrophy, a severe subacute thigh pain followed by pronounced quadriceps atrophy, is discussed in Chapter 117. Whereas the distribution of signs and symptoms are reminiscent of an ischemic femoral mononeuropathy, a more proximal injury at the level of the lumbosacral plexus is more likely.

Obturator Mononeuropathy

The obturator nerve supplies the hip adductors. Mononeuropathies are uncommon but can occur in the setting of difficult vaginal deliveries or gynecologic surgery because it lies in close approximation to the uterus. Endometriosis can produce nerve compression in rare instances. Weakness of hip adduction and flexion (a secondary action of the adductor muscles) is seen. An L2-3 radiculopathy can produce a similar picture, although hip flexion, mediated by the femoral-innervated iliopsoas muscle, is more severely affected and back pain is likely.

Gluteal Mononeuropathies

The gluteal nerves supply the gluteal muscles (gluteus maximus, minimus, and medius) and the tensor fascia lata, the fibrous band of a muscle on the lateral thigh. Both nerves exit the sciatic foramen with the sciatic nerve and can be injured by misplaced injections into the buttock. The inferior gluteal nerve supplies the gluteus maximus, which primarily extends but also abducts and laterally rotates the thigh. The superior gluteal nerve supplies the gluteus medius and minimus and the tensor fascia lata.

Pudendal Mononeuropathies

The pudendal nerve exits the greater sciatic foramen along with the sciatic and both gluteal nerves. It reaches the perineum via the pudendal canal. Injury to the nerve can occur because of misplaced injections, bicycle riding, or trauma during vaginal delivery or surgery. Branches of the nerve subserve sexual function and bowel and bladder control, making mononeuropathies particularly devastating. More proximal injuries to either the lumbosacral plexus or the sacral roots in the cauda equina can produce a clinical and electrodiagnostic picture similar to a pudendal mononeuropathy and must be considered in the differential diagnosis.

The first branch of the pudendal nerve within the pudendal canal is the inferior rectal nerve, which provides motor supply to the levator ani and external anal sphincter and perirectal cutaneous sensation. The perineal nerve arises from the pudendal shortly after the inferior rectal branch and supplies both the posterior labia and the external urethral sphincters. The dorsal nerve of the clitoris is the final pudendal branch.

Electrodiagnostic studies are useful in the evaluation of urinary and fecal incontinence. Pudendal motor conduction studies can be performed using a flexible St. Mark's electrode attached to an examination glove. Needle electromyography of the urethral and anal sphincters also can be performed.

Sensory Mononeuropathies of the Lower Extremity

Several of the proximal mononeuropathies of the lower extremities produce sensory-only symptoms. Figure 115-2 shows the cutaneous distribution of these nerves. The most common of these is the lateral femoral cutaneous neuropathy—the syndrome known as meralgia paresthetica ("painful thigh"). The lateral femoral cutaneous nerve of the thigh is typically injured by tight pants, seat belts, leaning against the edge of a table, or during pregnancy. Diabetics and obese patients also are particularly prone to this condition. Patients report sensory loss or dysesthesia over the anterolateral thigh. Symptoms typically resolve spontaneously, so conservative management generally is appropriate. Nonsteroidal antiinflammatory agents may provide sufficient relief in some, but others may require local steroid injection or nerve block for adequate pain relief. The presence of motor signs or symptoms, back pain, or an atypical pattern of sensory loss should raise suspicion of an alternate diagnosis. The differential should include a high lumbar radiculopathy (L2-3 level) as well as lumbosacral plexopathy. Nerve conduction studies may be helpful, although they are often most difficult to perform in the very patients who are at risk: the obese and diabetic.

The saphenous nerve is the terminal branch of the femoral nerve. It is a purely sensory nerve that supplies the medial calf and medial dorsum of the foot. Inadvertent injury during saphenous vein grafting, knee surgery, and varicose vein surgery are most common causes of mononeuropathy. Improper stirrup use can result in isolated injury. Both a proximal femoral mononeuropathy and an L4 radiculopathy produce a similar pattern of sensory loss.

Cutaneous sensation in the perineum is mediated by nerves arising from the lumbar plexus, as shown in Figure 115-6. Most mononeuropathies result from abdominal or pelvic surgery, although retroperitoneal malignancy must be considered. When

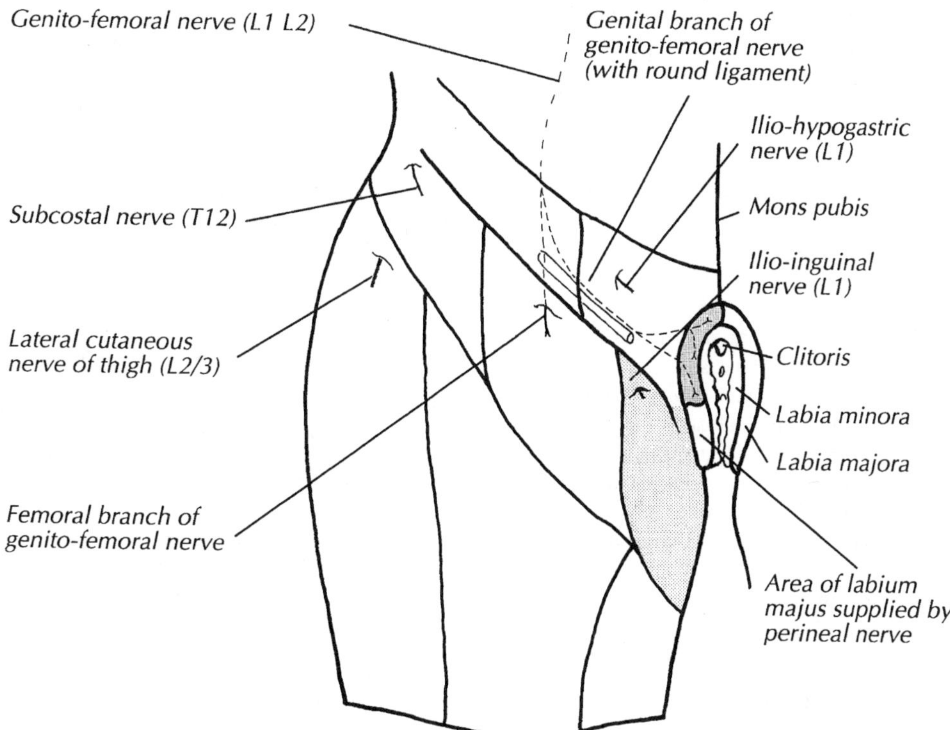

Figure 115-6. Cutaneous nerve supply to the female perineum. The superior portion of the labia majora is supplied by both the ilioinguinal nerve and the genital branch of the genitofermoral nerve. The inferior portion of the labia majorum is supplied by the perineal nerve. The ilioinguinal nerve supplies the superomedial thigh adjacent to the perineum. (Modified from Patten J. Neurological differential diagnosis, 2nd ed. Berlin: Springer-Verlag, 1996:313.)

bilateral abnormalities are present, spinal cord disease must be ruled out. The iliohypogastric nerve supplies the skin overlying the medial portion of the inguinal ligament. It is most commonly injured during procedures requiring transverse low abdominal or suprapubic incisions. The ilioinguinal and genitofemoral nerves traverse the inguinal canal and are therefore more at risk during herniorrhaphy, appendectomy, and pregnancy. Ilioinguinal nerve injuries produce sensory loss or pain overlying the extreme medial portion of the thigh and the upper half of the labia majora. Thus sensation to the labia majora is subserved by two anatomically distinct pathways; the upper half of the labia majora by the ilioinguinal nerve and L1 nerve roots and the lower half by the pudendal nerve and S2-3 nerve roots. Iatrogenic causes of genitofemoral neuropathy predominate. Sensory loss involves the femoral triangle: the anterior thigh below the inguinal ligament in the region of the femoral nerve, artery, and vein. The sensory supply of the clitoris is supplied by the dorsal nerve of the clitoris, a terminal branch of the pudendal nerve. The lower half of the labia majora and the labial minora share this root supply. The posterior femoral cutaneous nerve (S1-3) arises from the sacral plexus and traverses the greater sciatic foramen beside the sciatic nerve. It courses under the piriformis to supply the medial aspect of the buttock, the posterior inner thigh, and the upper portion of the posterior calf. Hip or upper femur fractures or misplaced buttock injections can

Table 115-1. Common Pregnancy-Associated Mononeuropathies

	PREGNANCY	VAGINAL DELIVERY	CESAREAN DELIVERY	SURGICAL POSITIONING
Sensorimotor	Median (CTS)	Lumbosacral plexus	Lumbosacral plexus	Ulnar
	Sciatic	Pudendal	Pudendal	Sciatic
	Obturator	Obturator	Femoral	Obturator
		Peroneal		Femoral
		Femoral		Peroneal
Sensory only	Median (CTS)	Saphenous	Genitofemoral	Saphenous
	Meralgia paresthetica		Ilioinguinal	
			Iliohypogastric	
			Saphenous	

CTS, carpal tunnel syndrome.

injure the nerve. The inferior rectal nerves, discussed under "Pudendal Mononeuropathies," subserve perirectal sensation.

The sural nerve receives contributions from both the tibial and common peroneal nerves. It supplies the medial third of the posterior calf and portions of the lateral calf and foot. Sural injury can develop when the posterior calf is pressed against a hard edge or from wearing improperly fitting ski boots. The sural nerve is commonly harvested for nerve biopsy because of its accessibility and the inconsequential nature of the postbiopsy sensory deficit. Unfortunately, a small percentage of patients develop chronic pain from neuroma formation at the distal stump of the transected nerve.

Injury to the tibial-derived interdigital nerves under the metatarsal heads of the lateral toes produces Morton's metatarsalgia. Patients complain of chronic toe pain exacerbated by weight bearing and walking. Deep interdigital palpation may reveal local tenderness or local nerve enlargement. Tight shoes and high heels are major risk factors for local nerve injury, hence the most patients with this condition are women. Conservative measures such as changing footwear should be attempted before surgical exploration is considered. At surgery, some patients have local nerve enlargement (neuromas). Resection of the neuroma or nerve transection more proximally can lead to symptomatic relief.

CONSIDERATIONS IN PREGNANCY

Table 115-1 lists the most common mononeuropathies seen in pregnancy, vaginal or cesarean delivery, and as iatrogenic complications of surgical positioning. Most are self-limiting conditions that can be managed conservatively. The most common, CTS, occurs in up to 2% of patients and often is bilateral. Vaginal delivery can result in mononeuropathies because of direct compression of the lumbosacral plexus or peripheral nerves by the descending fetal head. Surgical instruments used to assist in delivery also can result in injury. Cesarean sections and other surgeries can produce local injuries to the nerves of the lower abdominal wall and inguinal region or compressive injuries caused by improper patient positioning.

BIBLIOGRAPHY

The Editorial Committee for the guarantors of Brain. Aids to the examination of the nervous system. East Sussex, UK: Balliere Tindall, 1986.

Asbury AK, Thomas PK. Peripheral nerve disorders. II. Blue books of practical neurology, no 15. Oxford: Butterworth-Heinemann, 1995.

Cohen BS, Felsenthal G. Peripheral nervous system disorders and pregnancy. In: Goldstein PJ ed. Neurological disorders of pregnancy. Mt Kisco, NY: Futura, 1986:153.

Devinsky O, Feldmann E. Examination of the cranial and peripheral nerves. Oxford: Churchill Livingstone, 1988.

Donaldson JO. Neurology of pregnancy. In: Walton J, ed. Major problems in neurology, 2nd ed, vol 19. London: WB Saunders, 1989.

Patten J. Neurological differential diagnosis, 2nd ed. Berlin: Springer-Verlag, 1996:282.

Stewart JD. Focal peripheral neuropathies, 2nd ed. New York: Raven Press, 1993.

116
Cranial Neuropathies

GERALD W. HONCH

Primary Care for Women, edited by Phyllis C. Leppert and Fred M. Howard. Lippincott-Raven Publishers, Philadelphia © 1997.

The cranial nerves are 12 paired sets of nerves named for their functional innervation. The first two cranial nerves do not originate in the brain stem, but the rest do. Knowledge of brain stem anatomy is essential for localizing a lesion at that level. Understanding the anatomic relations within the brain stem and appreciating space within the brain stem and functional relations at the brain stem level will provide a framework for localization. As the cranial nerves leave the brain stem and course toward an end organ or structure, they may be vulnerable to injury. Knowledge of this course and the anatomic pitfalls of entrapment or injury will help diagnostically.

DIFFERENTIAL DIAGNOSIS

If the clinician can discern where the insult occurred from the clinical clues at presentation, more than half the diagnostic challenge has been met. Diagnostic tools can be selected only after the insult has been localized by clinical examination. The judicious investigation is both logical and economical. X-rays are useful for evaluating bony structures. Computed tomography (CT) scanning is ideal for bony structures and the sinuses, but its utility is limited for the brain stem parenchyma. Magnetic resonance imaging (MRI) is ideal for brain stem structures but not very helpful for bone. Angiography is useful for vascular anatomy and its anomalies but is invasive. Functional electrical testing (electromyography and nerve conduction studies) requires experienced neurophysiologic personnel and knowledge of the specific questions to be answered. Evoked response testing of vision and the brain stem can be helpful but again require specific questions to be answered.

CLINICAL FINDINGS, IMAGING STUDIES, AND TREATMENT

An exhaustive review of neuroanatomy and functional anatomy within the skull is not intended here. Table 116-1 provides a quick guide to the 12 cranial nerves and their relations within and outside the brain stem. Landmarks are given to help the clinician recognize valuable clues to localization. Only cranial nerves II through VIII are discussed in detail here; these have been chosen because of their importance and frequency of involvement.

Cranial Nerve II—-Optic

The optic nerve receives neural input from the rods and cones in the retina. The optic nerves extend from the posterior orbit to the optic chiasm just in front of the pituitary stalk. The course of this

Table 116-1. Summary of Cranial Nerves

NERVE		FUNCTION	BRAIN STEM ANATOMY	LANDMARKS	RELATED NERVES	ISSUES/ PROBLEMS
Number	*Name*					
I	Olfactory	Sensory	Not applicable	Upper nose, cribriform plate, olfactory bulb, olfactory tract	None	Odors to supplant basic taste. Diseases within the nose or trauma.
II	Optic	Sensory	Not applicable	Orbit, carotid artery, pituitary, chiasm	None	Vision. Field defects. Unilateral vs bilateral. Optic neuritis.
III	Oculomotor	Motor	Midbrain near midline. Relates to medial longitudinal fasciculus.	MLF, tentorial edge, cavernous sinus, orbit	IV, V, VI	All extraocular muscles except superior oblique and lateral rectus. Pupillary constrictor muscle.
IV	Trochlear	Motor	Medial tegmentum of midbrain at inferior colliculus	Exits brain stem ventrally; petrous bone, cavernous sinus, orbit	III, V, VI	Motor to superior oblique
V	Trigeminal	Motor/sensory	Pons to the gasserian ganglion. Three sensory divisions to face.	Meckel cave in petrous part of temporal bone. Exits skull via foramen ovale.	III, IV, VI	Motor to muscles of mastication. Sensory from surface of head and neck, sinuses, meninges and tympanic membrane.
VI	Abducens	Motor	Dorsal medial pons near 4th ventricle	Petrous bone, cavernous sinus, orbit	III, IV, V	Motor to lateral rectus muscle
VII	Facial	Motor/sensory	Pontine tegmentum. Winds around the 6th nerve nucleus.	Enters the interval auditory canal via cerebellopontine angle. Travels in facial canal. Exits skull at stylomastoid foramen.	Special relation to 6th nerve nucleus in brain stem. Travels with 8th nerve in facial canal.	Muscles of facial expression and stapedius. Sensation from tympanic membrane. Taste on anterior 2/3 of tongue.
VIII	Vestibulocochlear	Sensory	Enters medulla at junction with pons. Lateral to 7th nerve	Travels with the 7th nerve in the internal auditory canal	VII	Balance and hearing
IX	Glossopharyngeal	Motor/sensory	Series of rootlets between inferior olive and restiform body of lateral medulla	Travels the jugular fossa. Exits skull via jugular foramen.	X, XI	Motor to stylopharyngeal m. Parotid gland. Sensation around ext. ear and tympanic membrane. Taste posterior third of tongue.
X	Vagus	Motor/sensory	Dorsal motor nerve of vagus and nucleus ambiguus	Wanders from brain stem to splenic flexure. Exits skull via jugular foramen. Travels in carotid sheath. Laryngeal, recurrent laryngeal, and cardiac branches.	IX, XI	Motor/sensory to pharynx and larynx. Parasympathetic to thoracic and abdominal viscera.
XI	Accessory	Motor	Lower motor neuron cell bodies in spinal cord	Exits cranium via jugular foramen	IX, X	Motor to sternomastoid and trapezius muscle
XII	Hypoglossal	Motor	Medullary tegmentum near midline	Exit brain stem as rootlets between pyramid and inferior olive. Exits skull via hypoglossal canal near foramen mag.	None	Motor to intrinsic and extrinsic muscles of the tongue

nerve as it leaves the globe is extremely complex. Its relations with the extraocular nerves, the bones of the orbit, the carotid artery, and the pituitary gland may provide anatomic clues of great localizing value. The appearance of the retina and optic disc must be assessed. The size, shape, and extent of a visual field defect must be recorded. Whether the field defect and changes on funduscopic examination are unilateral or bilateral is of great localizing significance (to define whether the problem is within the eye, in the supporting structures, or in the brain). Papilledema (swelling of the optic nerve head) may be difficult to appreciate in mild cases but is dramatic in others. Optic atrophy as a residua from prior papilledema or optic neuritis appears as a pale disc color, a reduction in the fine retinal vasculature, and a reduction in the disc size.

Optic neuritis is more common in women (77%) and is associated with ocular pain and visual loss of varying severity. Optic disc edema may occur. Color vision is impaired in 90% of patients. Most patients recover visual acuity with time alone; treatment with high-dose steroids is controversial. Many patients with a history of optic neuritis are subject to future attacks. Some patients who have suffered an episode of optic neuritis later develop multiple sclerosis. An MRI is not warranted in an episode of optic neuritis. It is unclear how to interpret an MRI that demonstrates white matter lesions in the absence of other symptoms. Most neurologists would be reluctant to diagnose multiple sclerosis on the basis of an episode of optic neuritis and an abnormal MRI without other supportive historical, laboratory, or physical changes.

Anterior ischemic optic neuropathy is caused by impairment of perfusion in the anterior portion of the optic nerve (supplied by the posterior ciliary arteries). Clinically, the patient experiences sudden painless visual loss in one eye. The cause may be systemic or local hypotension, glaucoma, vasculitides such as giant cell arteritis, hypertension, diabetes mellitus, or atherosclerosis. Recovery is poor.

Tumors may develop in the optic nerve, chiasm, or tract. Children tend to have more aggressive tumors. Neurofibromas may also occur in this region. Many other neoplastic lesions occur in the optic nerve pathway, such as metastases, germinomas, dermoids, craniopharyngiomas, meningiomas, pituitary adenomas, hamartomas, and epidermoids. Mass effects from aneurysms, arachnoid cysts, sarcoidosis, or a craniopharyngioma may be a cause of symptoms referable to the optic nerve pathways.

Cranial Nerves III, IV, and VI—-Oculomotor, Trochlear, and Abducens

These three motor nerves move the eye within the orbit. Six extraocular muscles in each eye rotate the eye about three mutually orthogonal axes. The patient presents with double vision (diplopia). An understanding of the function of these three nerves and their relation to the muscles they serve will help the clinician describe the diplopia and decide whether referral to a neurologist or ophthalmologist is appropriate.

The lateral and medial rectus muscles abduct and adduct the eye, respectively. The superior rectus and inferior oblique muscles elevate the eye. The inferior rectus and superior oblique muscles depress the eye. The superior and inferior oblique muscles and the superior and inferior recti act in concert to provide torsion movements to the eye.

The central control of eye movement must be divided between the supranuclear, internuclear, and nuclear areas. In supranuclear and internuclear lesions, damage occurs to the premotor input to the nerve nucleus; certain types of eye movements may be affected, but others are spared. The classic example is with internuclear ophthalmoplegias in which conjugate horizontal eye movements are affected but vergence eye movements are spared. In nuclear lesions or beyond the nucleus into the nerve itself, there is disruption of all types of eye movements that use the involved nerve.

Oculomotor Nerve

The oculomotor nucleus is located in the medial tegmentum of the midbrain near the periaqueductal gray matter at the level of the superior colliculus. This oculomotor complex of subnuclei innervates the ipsilateral medial rectus, inferior rectus, superior rectus, and inferior oblique muscles of each eye, as well as the levator palpebrae muscles of the eyelid. Control of pupillary function also is mediated by related nuclear structures. The medial longitudinal fasciculus relates components of the third and sixth nerve nuclei on the opposite sides of the brain stem to coordinate horizontal eye movements.

The course of the third nerve, after exiting the brain stem, is complex. It passes between the posterior cerebral and superior cerebellar arteries and runs parallel to the posterior communicating artery (relations to vascular structures may give clues to localization of berry aneurysms that occur in this area). It passes on the edge of the tentorium (providing localizing clues in uncal herniation). The third nerve passes along the superior region of the cavernous sinus and relates to other cranial nerves (IV, V, and VI) in this intimate crossroads. Finally, it enters the orbit through the superior orbital fissure (a bony landmark).

A complete oculomotor nerve palsy causes ptosis and a fixed, dilated pupil. The eye is abducted at rest as a result of unopposed tonic activity in the lateral rectus. Adduction, elevation, and depression of the eye are lost. With less severe palsies, all the features are less severe or even incomplete. If the pupil is spared, the physician must consider myasthenia gravis, hypertension, diabetes mellitus, restrictive orbit disease, or rarely an aneurysm. A tonic (Adie) pupil or a dorsal midbrain lesion (Parinaud syndrome) may produce light near dissociation. Local instillation of drugs that affect the pupil should be considered when a patient has a dilated pupil and no other findings. Anatomic localization of lesions damaging the oculomotor nerve depends on associated neurologic and orbital signs. These clues may place the lesion at various locations within the brain stem, along the course of the third nerve and adjacent structures, or within the orbit. An accurate assessment of these findings simplifies and directs the work-up.

Trochlear Nerve

The trochlear nucleus is located in the medial tegmentum of the midbrain, ventral to the periaqueductal gray matter and at the level of the inferior colliculus. It decussates before exiting the brain stem. This is the only cranial nerve to exit the brain stem dorsally. The trochlear nerve passes ventrally around the cerebral peduncle and then enters the cavernous sinus (lateral). The nerve enters the orbit through the superior orbital fissure to innervate the superior oblique muscle (contralateral to the trochlear nerve nucleus of origin).

The superior oblique muscle depresses the eye when the eye is adducted and intorts the eye when the eye is abducted. Hence, trochlear nerve palsies cause vertical and torsional diplopia. The diplopia is most severe with gaze downward and with the head tilted toward the side of the paretic muscle. These patients often maintain a typical head posture to minimize the diplopia (chin down and head tilted toward the normal eye). A trochlear nerve lesion is easy to identify when an oculomotor nerve lesion coexists (when the abnormal eye is examined on attempted downward gaze, subtle rotatory movement can be seen in the conjunctival vessels if the trochlear nerve is intact).

The trochlear nerve can be damaged by lesions in the brain stem, subarachnoid space, cavernous sinus, or orbit. Trauma is the most common cause of acquired trochlear nerve palsy.

Abducens Nerve

The abducens nerve nucleus is located in the dorsal medial pons, under the floor of the fourth ventricle. The nerve exits the brain stem ventrally at the pontomedullary junction and then ascends in the prepontine cistern. It travels along the apex of the petrous bone, passes through the cavernous sinus, and enters the orbit through the superior orbital fissure. It innervates the lateral rectus muscle. This nerve has a tortuous course, making it vulnerable to various injuries in multiple anatomic locations.

Abducens nerve palsies present with horizontal diplopia. The distance between the images becomes more pronounced as the patient looks toward the paretic lateral rectus muscle. The diplopia worsens with distance vision and is less severe with near vision. On examination, there is often a grossly apparent reduced abduction of the involved eye. In primary position, there may be esodeviation of the involved eye, as the medial rectus is unopposed. Restrictive orbital problems (as in Graves disease) and ocular myasthenia gravis may need to be considered.

Lesions that damage the abducens nucleus or nerve often involve adjacent neural structures. With a brain stem lesion that affects the abducens nucleus, an ipsilateral nuclear facial palsy and a contralateral hemiparesis are common. Involvement of the medial longitudinal fasciculus may produce a contralateral medial rectus dysfunction. The combination of an abducens nucleus lesion and involvement of the ipsilateral medial longitudinal fasciculus is referred to as the "one-and-one-half syndrome" (the only remaining horizontal eye movement is abduction of the contralateral eye). Pontine lesions involving the abducens nucleus or nerve can result from ischemic infarction, hemorrhage, abscess, neoplasm, Wernicke encephalopathy, and demyelination. Many disorders that involve the subarachnoid space (eg, meningioma, carcinomatous meningitis, infection) can affect the abducens nerve. Lesions at the bony petrous apex (usually from complicated otitis media) can cause an abducens nerve palsy associated with ipsilateral facial (retroorbital) pain and decreased facial and corneal sensation (Gradenigo syndrome). Neoplastic processes may also invade the petrous apex. Increased intracranial pressure may produce an abducens palsy solely on the basis of pressure on the nerve with its very long subarachnoid course (as a false localizing sign). In the cavernous sinus and the orbit, abducens nerve palsies occur in conjunction with losses in adjacent cranial nerves (III, IV, and V). Isolated abducens palsies can occur as the result of occlusion of the vasa nervorum secondary to hypertension or diabetes mellitus.

Cranial Nerve V—Trigeminal

The trigeminal nerve has three sensory divisions: ophthalmic (V_1), maxillary (V_2), and mandibular (V_3). These three divisions cover the facial territory extending from the vertex of the scalp (but not the scalp posterior to the ear) to the lower margin of the mandible. The outer canthus of the eye separates V_1 from V_2, and the corner of the mouth separates V_2 from V_3. The three sensory divisions merge at the gasserian ganglion (in a depression of the petrous part of the temporal bone called Meckel's cave). The trigeminal nerve extends proximally from the gasserian ganglion and merges with the ventrolateral aspect of the pons. Within the pons, some sensory fibers remain in the main trigeminal nucleus; others extend caudally to the level of the second cervical segment, and still other sensory fibers terminate in the mesencephalic nuclei at the edge of the periaqueductal gray matter. The motor nucleus of the trigeminal nerve is in the lateral pontine tegmentum. Motor fibers pass forward along the inferior surface of the gasserian ganglion to become incorporated into the mandibular division. The motor component of the mandibular division leaves the skull through the foramen ovale and enters the anterior trunk of the mandibular division to innervate the muscles of mastication (masseter, temporalis, and medial and lateral pterygoid). Branches are sent to the tensor tympani, tensor veli palatini, mylohyoid, and anterior belly of the digastric muscles.

Primary vascular afferents contain neuropeptides that modulate pain. This trigeminovascular system is central to the pathogenesis of migraine headaches.

Injury to one or all of the divisions or branches of the trigeminal nerve results in loss of sensibility in the corresponding cutaneous area. The range of sensory losses include loss of light touch, pain, and temperature. Dysesthesia or hyperpathia can occur. Interruption of the ophthalmic division can cause diminution or loss of the corneal reflex. Lesions of the mandibular nerve lead to loss of the masseter or jaw reflex. Paralysis of the masseter or temporalis muscle may be seen.

Trigeminal neuralgia (tic douloureux) is intense lightning-like pain that occurs in one or more divisions of the trigeminal nerve. The pathophysiology is unclear but relates to increased afferent activity and diminished inhibitory control, with paroxysmal discharges in the trigeminal nucleus in response to sensory input. The neurologic examination is usually normal. Trigeminal neuralgia is more common in women than men (1.74 : 1) with an incidence of 4.7 per 100,000. It is rarely familial. The patient experiences brief episodes of severe, focal pain described as electric, jabbing, or lancinating. The pain is usually within a single dermatome (usually V_2 or V_3). The painful paroxysms can occur repeatedly around the clock, often with a characteristic trigger point. The trigger point may be so sensitive that the patient avoids washing an affected area, brushing certain teeth, or even eating or talking in an effort to avoid pain. These episodes have an extremely rapid onset and a slightly slower offset. Each paroxysm of pain lasts only a few seconds but is so intense that the patient may distort the length. Between attacks, the patient is free of pain and can carry on usual activities with caution to the trigger areas. Some patients have a prodromal pain syndrome that consists of a continuous dull, achy discomfort. After a paroxysm of pain, there can be a refractory period during which stimulation of the trigger zone does not precipitate pain. Hence, immediately after suffering a painful episode, the patient may be able to eat or wash her face without triggering another episode. The episodes of pain may remit spontaneously for months or years. The patient lives in dread of the next episode of pain.

The precise pathophysiology of trigeminal neuralgia is unclear, but vascular compression of the trigeminal nerve root entry zone is favored. Several studies have demonstrated compression of the nerve by an artery (less commonly by a vein). Trigeminal neuralgia is more common in patients with multiple sclerosis. Trigeminal neuralgia is also seen in other causes of stretching of the nerve, as in mass lesions, syringobulbia, brain stem infarctions, aneurysms, and vascular malformations.

Most patients (90%) respond to carbamazepine. Other medical therapies include phenytoin, baclofen, and pimozide, alone or in combination. Once the patient has obtained relief, the dosage should be tapered slowly to define a maintenance level. Once the patient has experienced remission of symptoms, the medication should be tapered and discontinued. Surgical procedures are best used when conservative approaches have failed. These include percutaneous radiofrequency neurolysis, glycerol or alcohol block, microvascular decompression, and peripheral neurectomy. Some neurosurgical procedures (radiofrequency) attempt to destroy pain-transmitting fibers and spare touch sensation. Complete anesthesia may cause loss of the corneal reflex or could lead to a painful anesthesia of the face (anesthesia dolorosa). Some recommend microvascular decompression of the trigeminal nerve with a retromastoid craniectomy. The success rate is improved if vascular distortion of the nerve can be demonstrated.

Sensory trigeminal neuropathy is a sensory loss in the trigeminal nerve distribution. It may occur as an isolated complaint or as part of a more widespread neurologic constellation. The symptoms may be acute or subacute, unilateral or bilateral, and may involve parts of or the entire trigeminal nerve distribution. It may be painless or associated with constant pain or even paroxysmal trigeminal neuralgia symptoms. Headache may occur also. Motor findings are absent. The causes or associated diseases cover a wide spectrum: idiopathic, inflammatory diseases, multiple sclerosis, neoplastic disease (primary or metastatic), trauma, infections, and so forth.

Mental neuropathy (numb chin syndrome) may be caused by a lesion of the mandibular division of the trigeminal nerve or the inferior alveolar nerve and its terminal branch, the mental nerve. There are various causes, but the most common etiology is cancer.

Cranial Nerve VII—Facial

Voluntary motor control of the face, including eyelid closure, originates in the cortex (lower third of the precentral gyrus). The fibers course downward in the genu of the internal capsule and decussate in the basis pontis to terminate in the facial nucleus. The nuclear component of the forehead receives cortical contributions bilaterally. The innervation of the lower facial muscles is predominately contralateral. Hence, in an upper motor lesion (above the facial nucleus), sparing of the forehead is an important finding. In a lower motor lesion (at the facial nucleus or in the facial nerve), the forehead is involved.

The facial nerve originates from the facial nucleus at the level of the pontine tegmentum. Fibers from the nucleus wind around the sixth nerve nucleus and then exit the pons in the region of the cerebellopontine angle medial to the acoustic nerve. The nerve enters the internal auditory meatus (in the facial canal) accompanying the eighth nerve. The facial canal is 1 cm long and contains the geniculate ganglion. Within the facial canal, branches are given off to the stapedius muscle and chorda tympani. After leaving the skull via the stylomastoid foramen, the facial nerve passes through the parotid gland, where it divides into a number of branches to supply the muscles of facial expression.

The parasympathetic component of the facial nerve originates from the lacrimal and superior salivatory nuclei. The fibers from these nuclei emerge from the pons as the nervus intermedius. It merges with the motor root of the facial nerve in the internal auditory canal, although it may run a separate course from the seventh and eighth nerves. The parasympathetic fibers pass through the geniculate ganglion on their way to the lacrimal and nasopalatine glands as well as the sphenopalatine ganglion. The parasympathetic fibers destined for the submaxillary and sublingual glands also pass through the geniculate ganglion and proceed with the seventh nerve to the chorda tympani.

The taste chemoreceptor cells of the tongue reside in the anterior two thirds of the tongue. This sensory information travels through the lingual nerve to the chorda tympani and hence to the facial nerve. Stimuli are conveyed centrally via the nervous intermedius to the nucleus solitarius. Second-order fibers go to the thalamus through the medial lemniscus on their way to the sensory cortex.

Supranuclear lesions cause predominant weakness of the lower half of the contralateral face. The greatest weakness is around the mouth, with drooping of the corner of the mouth and flattening of the nasolabial fold. Any weakness of the forehead is usually slight and transient. Closure of the eyelid may be compromised slightly. Emotional and associated movements of the face may be retained, but voluntary movement is compromised.

Most pontine lesions do not affect the facial function without affecting neighboring structures such as the abducens nucleus. A proximal pontine facial nerve lesion can spare the parasympathetic and taste components of the facial nerve.

With complete peripheral facial nerve palsies, all movements of the affected side of the face are lost, both voluntary as well as associated and emotional. The weakness extends from the mouth and nasolabial fold to eyelid closure and the forehead. On attempting eye closure, the eye rotates up and out (Bell's phenomenon). Blinking is lost, and tears collect and overflow. Food tends to collect between the gum and cheek. Corneal sensation is intact, but the blink reflex is lost. If the nerve to the stapedius muscle is affected, there may be increased auditory acuity (hyperacusis). Loss or distortion of taste occurs over the anterior two thirds of the tongue with compromise of the chorda tympani nerve. Most patients who report loss of taste actually have loss of smell: taste on the tongue is limited to sweet, sour, bitter, and salty.

Peripheral facial nerve palsy can occur secondary to many causes. It can occur as part of a constellation of other neurologic findings, or it can occur in isolation. The onset may be acute or slowly progressive. It can be unilateral or bilateral. It can be recurrent. It can be congenital.

Idiopathic facial nerve palsy or Bell palsy is an inflammatory demyelinating neuropathy. It is rare in childhood, and the incidence increases with age. There is no sexual preference, although it is more common during pregnancy by a factor of three. It is more common during the third trimester and in the first 2 weeks postpartum. In some series, toxemia appears to be a risk factor, but in other series this is not significant. It may be recurrent. Sixty percent of patients have periauricular pain, 57% have dysgeusia, 30% have hyperacusis, and 17% have diminished tearing. A mild mononuclear pleocytosis and mild elevation of the protein may be found in the CSF. The facial nerve and muscles can be examined with nerve stimulation studies and electromyography. Within the first few days of paralysis, there is minimal distal nerve degeneration, so nerve conduction studies are normal distal to the stylomastoid foramen. If recovery has not spontaneously occurred in days to weeks, repeat studies may demonstrate abnormalities. These findings may be useful prognostically. About 85% of the patients recover completely in 3 months. If the patient does not recover fully within 3 months, complete remission is unlikely. Older patients have a poorer recovery rate than younger ones. The more severe the facial weakness, the poorer the rate of recovery.

Protection of the eye from drying and foreign material cannot be overemphasized. Closure of the eyelid with paper tape or ophthalmologic consultation to stitch the eyelid closed (tarsorrhaphy) may be necessary. Artificial tears are often prescribed but are useful only briefly because they dry out. Protecting the eye during sleep must not be overlooked. Steroid treatment remains controversial because of the large portion of patients who recover spontaneously. Those who advocate steroids use prednisone 1 mg/kg/day as soon as possible after onset and continue it for 1 to 2 weeks. There is no evidence that surgical intervention to treat typical patients with idiopathic facial nerve palsy is helpful.

Ramsay Hunt syndrome is peripheral facial nerve palsy with herpes zoster oticus. The varicella zoster represents activation of the virus residing in the geniculate ganglion. Recovery is less certain than with idiopathic or Bell palsy. Treatment with acyclovir alone or in combination with corticosteroids may lead to a better outcome.

Melkersson-Rosenthal syndrome is characterized by recurrent facial paralysis, fissured tongue, and unilateral, recurrent, nonpitting facial and lip edema. Only part of the triad may be present. This may be a spectrum of orofacial granulomatous disorders.

Facial palsies may be caused by various infectious and inflammatory diseases, including Lyme disease, sarcoidosis, tuberculosis, syphilis, HIV, infectious mononucleosis, rubella, mumps, Guillain-Barré, Behçet syndrome, and Wegener granulomatosis. Various neoplasms, as well as carcinomatous meningitis, may produce facial palsies. Facial palsies are more common in metabolic disorders such as diabetes mellitus, uremia, hypothyroidism, and porphyria.

Surgical techniques to reinnervate facial muscles are considered within the context of serious traumatic injury to the facial nerve, surgical resection causing discontinuity of the facial nerve, and the rare patient with a poor recovery 1 year after the onset of facial neuropathy. In traumatic injury, efforts are directed at reapproximating the nerve and stump. Nerve grafts are sometimes used. A hypoglossal—-facial nerve or spinal accessory—-facial nerve anastomosis can be created.

Hemifacial spasm is characterized by paroxysmal involuntary tonic and clonic contractions of muscles innervated by the facial nerve on one side. Women are affected twice as often as men. The orbicularis oculi is usually the first muscle affected. The orbicularis oris is the other most commonly affected muscle, but all the facial muscles can be involved. The spasms may continue during sleep and are worsened by stress, chewing, speaking, light, and cold. The most common cause is microvascular compression of the facial nerve at its root exit zone, although many other causes have been cited. Carbamazepine or clonazepam may be helpful. Botulinum toxin injections can be tried. Decompressive surgery may be helpful.

Facial myokymia is characterized by continuous involuntary mild facial muscle contractions (usually unilateral). It is associated with many causes.

Möbius syndrome is characterized by the sporadic occurrence of congenital sixth and seventh nerve palsies and associated skeletal deformities (syndactyly, brachydactyly, and oligodactyly). There is hypoplasia or absence of brain stem nuclei.

The facial nerve can be imaged with CT and MRI. High-resolution CT scanning provides excellent bone detail of the internal auditory canal, facial canal, and adjacent vestibular and auditory structures. MRI scanning with contrast provides visualization of the brain stem, proximal facial nerve, and facial nerve within the facial canal. These two modalities should be used to complement each other, not as exclusive studies.

Cranial Nerve VIII—-Vestibulocochlear

The vestibulocochlear nerve carries two kinds of sensation, vestibular (balance) and audition (hearing), from special sensory receptors in the inner ear. The central processes of these neurons form the eighth nerve, which travels through the internal auditory meatus in the company of the seventh nerve. This complex enters the medulla at its junction with the pons, just lateral to the seventh nerve.

The end organ of the vestibular system is the vestibular labyrinth, which is divided into two components: the semicircular canals and the otolith organs. In each ear, there are three semicircular canals arranged at right angles to each other in the three planes of the body. The semicircular canals sense head rotation. The otolith organs (utricle and saccule) sense linear acceleration, including that caused by gravity. These structures are constantly active, firing at a basal rate even when the subject is stationary. With movement, the baseline firing increases. The structures are physiologically paired with the opposite side such that rotation or movement that activates a semicircular canal on one side inhibits the paired semicircular canal on the other side. There is a relation between head rotation and eye movements. With the vestibuloocular reflex, there is an opposite response of the eyes to rotational movement of the head (ie, head turning to the right results in eye turning to the left). Both the saccule and utricle have a patch of sensory receptors (macula) that consist of ciliated hair cells covered by a gelatinous mass. Tiny crystals of calcium carbonate (otoliths) are embedded in the gel. When the head changes position relative to gravity or accelerates linearly, the otoliths stimulate the hair cells by bending the cilia in different directions.

The vestibular ganglion in the periphery collects this sensory information regarding motion. Central processes of the ganglion cells form the vestibular portion of the eighth nerve. These axons run with the cochlear division and with the seventh cranial nerve through the internal auditory meatus to terminate in the vestibular nuclear complex in the floor of the fourth ventricle. Secondary neurons go to the cerebellum and to lower motor neurons in the brain stem and spinal cord (to maintain balance). All nuclei in the vestibular complex contribute fibers to the medial longitudinal fasciculus. This complex arrangement allows the eyes to maintain fixation on an object while the head is moving.

Damage to or dysfunction of the vestibular apparatus results in dizziness, falling, and abnormal eye movements. Nausea and vomiting may accompany these symptoms because of connections between the vestibular nucleus and the vagal nucleus. The clinical clues to localization relate to onset of symptoms (acute versus chronic), constant versus intermittent, presence or absence of hearing changes, positional relations, contribution of motion, disorders of eye movement (including nystagmus), and findings within other cranial nerves. Chapter 107 provides more information.

The cochlear component of eighth nerve function serves to convert sound waves (which distort and move structures within the external ear) to mechanical vibrations of the middle ear. Essentially, the sound waves cause the tympanic membrane to vibrate. The vibrations are transmitted via the round window to move three small ossicles (the malleus, incus, and stapes). Vibrations of the stapes set up waves in the fluid within the cochlea. The cochlea contains a complex array of organized structures that receive, sort, and convert these mechanical changes. The mechanical changes are converted into an electrical signal that is transmitted along the acoustic portion of the eighth nerve. The cochlear nuclei at the junction of the pons and the medulla receive these primary sensory neurons. The pathway to the auditory cortex is complex and not well understood.

Damage to the auditory apparatus (tympanic membrane, ossicles, cochlea) or nerve is commonly the result of skull fractures or infections. These cause a loss of hearing in the affected ear. Mass lesions within the internal auditory meatus (meningioma or acoustic neuroma) may damage components of the eighth nerve as well as the accompanying seventh nerve.

BIBLIOGRAPHY

Albers JW, Bromberg MB. Bell's palsy. In: Johnson RT, ed. Current therapy in neurologic disease. New York: BC Decker, 1990.

Bromberg MB. Bell's palsy and idiopathic cranial neuritis. In: Feldmann E, ed. Current diagnosis in neurology. St. Louis: Mosby, 1994.

Donaldson JO. Neurology of pregnancy. Philadelphia: WB Saunders, 1989.

Goldstein PJ, Stern BJ. Neurologic disorders of pregnancy. Mt. Kisco, NY: Futura, 1992.

Rosenbaum RB, Donaldson JO, eds. Neurologic complications of pregnancy. Neurol Clin North Am 1994;12.

Stern BJ, Wityk RJ, Lewis RF. Disorders of the cranial Nerves and brain stem. In: Joynt RJ, ed. Clinical neurology. Philadelphia: JB Lippincott, 1993.

Wilson-Pauwels L, Akesson EJ, Stewart PA. Cranial nerves: anatomy and clinical comments. New York: BC Decker, 1988.

Primary Care for Women, edited by Phyllis C. Leppert and Fred M. Howard. Lippincott-Raven Publishers, Philadelphia © 1997.

117
Polyneuropathies

HAROLD LESSER

Unlike mononeuropathies, which affect individual nerves, polyneuropathies affect all of the peripheral nerves in varying degrees. They produce a wide range of pathology and symptomatology and are often associated with underlying systemic disorders. The differential diagnosis of neuropathy is so extensive as to be both daunting and confusing. The history and physical examination can determine the relative involvement of sensory, motor, and autonomic function and the temporal course of the illness. Once classified in this manner, the differential diagnosis becomes more focused and can help guide further work-up. The distinction between axonal and demyelinating neuropathies can be difficult to make without electrodiagnostic testing or nerve biopsy and thus is less helpful in directing the early investigation of a neuropathy.

ETIOLOGY AND DIFFERENTIAL DIAGNOSIS

Sensorimotor polyneuropathies are the most common polyneuropathies; conditions affecting predominantly sensory, motor, or autonomic function are less common. The differential diagnosis for each of these neuropathies is shown in Table 117-1. For simplicity, many rarer inherited disorders and less common drug toxicities have been omitted.

Sensorimotor Polyneuropathy

Sensorimotor polyneuropathy is the most common pattern of polyneuropathy. Diabetes, alcohol abuse, and hypothyroidism account for a large percentage of cases, making these neuropathies common in the primary care setting.

Diabetic Polyneuropathy

The neuropathy of diabetes is prototypical of the sensorimotor polyneuropathies. Symptomatic neuropathy occurs in 15% to 20% of diabetics, and neuropathy can be detected in twice that many patients. Neuropathic symptoms commonly lead to a previously unsuspected diagnosis of diabetes. Like many other neuropathies, the neuropathy of diabetes is characterized by length-dependent axonal injury. The longest axons, those subserving sensation to the toes, are affected earliest; the shorter axons supplying the fingers are not typically affected until lower extremity symptoms reach the knees. As the neuropathy progresses, a glove-and-stocking pattern of sensory loss (ie, distal and symmetric) emerges. The deep tendon reflexes are reduced or absent, and vibratory sensation and position sense are impaired. Motor signs appear somewhat later and are manifested by symmetric distal weakness (eg, footdrop or, somewhat later, wrist drop). Loss of trophic (nutritional) support may produce chronic skin and nail changes. Profound sensory loss can lead patients to traumatize their extremities repeatedly, producing bony destruction of digits in the hand or foot (Charcot joints). Nerve conduction studies show low-amplitude sensory and motor compound action potentials, reflecting the axonal nature of the neuropathy. Conduction velocities may be mildly decreased due to secondary demyelination accompanying the axonal loss.

Other Diabetes-Associated Conditions

Diabetics are at increased risk for developing compressive mononeuropathies at the common sites of compression (median at the wrist, ulnar at the elbow, peroneal at the fibular head). Patients presenting with multiple mononeuropathies, such as bilateral carpal tunnel syndrome, or cranial mononeuropathies, such as Bell palsy, should undergo screening for diabetes.

Diabetic autonomic neuropathy can develop when significant small-fiber injury occurs. Its effects on orthostasis, gastrointestinal and bladder function, thermoregulation, sexual function, and the ability to detect hypoglycemia can be disabling.

Diabetic amyotrophy presents with the sudden onset of severe pain in one or both lower extremities, followed days to weeks later by atrophy. The condition may be due either to an ischemic injury to the femoral nerve or, more likely, to a proximal process within the lumbosacral plexus. The pain of diabetic amyotrophy is intense, requiring narcotics acutely and tricyclic antidepressants for chronic discomfort. Recovery of motor function can be pro-

Table 117-1 Polyneuropathy

	SENSORIMOTOR	SENSORY OR SENSORY > MOTOR	MOTOR OR MOTOR > SENSORY	AUTONOMIC
Common	Diabetes[M], alcohol, hypothyroidism[M], uremia[M]	Diabetes[M], alcohol, uremia, hypothyroidism[M]	*AIDP*[D] Diabetic amyotrophy, ALS[N]	Diabetes[M], amyloid, alcohol, renal & hepatic failure
AIDS-associated	HIV infection[AD] *Meds:* ddI/ddC	Distal symmetric polyneuropathy of AIDS *Meds:* ddI/ddC, thalidomide	*AIDP/CIDP*[D] Cytomegalovirus-associated polyradiculoneuropathy, distal symmetric polyneuropathy, motor neuron disease	
Chemotherapy	Chlorambucil, vincristine, Suramin[M]	Cisplatinum, docetaxel, paclitaxel, vincristine		Paclitaxel, vincristine
Connective tissue disorders	*Rheumatoid arthritis*[D] Periarteritis nodosa, systemic lupus erythematosus[M]	Sjögren[N]	Systemic lupus erythematosus[M]	Rheumatoid arthritis[D]
Endocrine	*Acromegaly*[D] Diabetes[M], hypothyroidism[M]	Diabetes[M], hypothyroidism[M]	Diabetic amyotrophy	Diabetes[M]
Idiopathic	Critical-illness polyneuropathy	Dorsal root ganglionitis[N]	ALS[N]	Shy-Drager, primary idiopathic orthostatic hypotension
Immune	*CIDP*[D] Amyloid, cryoglobulinemia, multiple myeloma, osteosclerotic myeloma[M], sarcoid, Waldenström macroglobulinemia	*anti-MAG*[D] Amyloid, Crohn, cryoglobulinemia, hepatitis C, paraproteinemia, primary biliary cirrhosis, Sjögren	*AIDP*[D], *MMN/CB with anti-GM$_1$ antibodies*[D] Axonal AIDP, brachial neuritis	AIDP[D] Amyloid
Infectious	*Diptheria*[D] Lyme	AIDS, Lyme, leprosy[M], syphilis (tabes dorsalis)	*Diphtheria*[D] AIDS, botulism, leprosy[M], polio[N], tick paralysis	AIDS, leprosy[M], botulism
Inherited	*HMSN I*[D], HMSN II, *hereditary neuropathy with tendency to pressure palsy (HNPP)*[D] Myotonic dystrophy	Friedreich ataxia, amyloid, rare hereditary sensory neuropathies	*Porphyria*[D] Hereditary ALS[N], Werdnig-Hoffman syndrome[N]	Amyloid, porphyria
Medications (nonchemo)	*Amiodarone*[D] Chlorpropamide, colchicine, ddI, ddC, disulfiram, ergots, gold, indomethacin, isoniazid, lithium, metronidazole, phenytoin tolbutamide, tricyclic antidepressants	ddI, ddC, isoniazid (slow acetylators),metronidazole, phenytoin thalidomide, vitamin B_6 overdose[N]	Dapsone, tricyclic antidepressants	
Metals	Arsenic, gold[M], mercury, thallium	Arsenic, gold[M], thallium, methyl mercury	Gold[M], lead	Arsenic, inorganic mercury
Neuronopathy		anti-Hu[N] (see paraneoplastic) dorsal root ganglionitis[N], Sjögren[N]	See paraneoplastic	
Nutritional	B_{12}, folate, thiamine deficiencies, gestational	B_{12} deficiency, vitamin E deficiency		B_{12} deficiency
Paraneoplastic	Mild distal neuropathy of cancer	anti-Hu (lung > breast > ovary > lymphoma)	Lymphoma, Hodgkin motor neuron disease	Adenocarcinoma, anti-Hu, Lambert-Eaton syndrome
Toxic	Ethylene oxide, nitrous oxide, hexacarbons (glue sniffing)	Ethylene oxide, nitrous oxide	Acrylamide, hexacarbons, organophosphate poisoning	Acrylamide

Unless noted, all neuropathies are axonal. Exceptions are indicated by superscript as in demyelinating[D], mixed[M], neuronopathy[N], axonal[A].

AIDP, acute inflammatory demyelinating polyradiculoneuropathy; *ALS*, amyotrophic lateral sclerosis, *Anti-GM*, anti-GM$_1$ gangliosides; Anti-Hu, aka: anti-ANNwA (antineuronal nuclear antibody); *CIDP*, chronic inflammatory demyelinating polyradiculoneuropathy; *ddC*, 2′,3′-dideoxycytidine (zalcitabine); *ddI*, 2′,3′-dideoxyinosine (didanosine); *HMSN I*, hereditary motor sensory neuropathy type I (Charcot-Marie-Tooth disease); *MMN/CB*, multifocal motor neuropathy with conduction block.

longed when severe atrophy develops. The association between amyotrophy and diabetes is strong enough to warrant a careful screen for diabetes in all patients with this clinical picture.

Diabetic neuropathic cachexia is a frightening complication of diabetes often associated with attempts to bring severe diabetes under better control. Patients experience months of profoundly decreased appetite, severe weight loss, and depression, leading most to undergo an unrevealing work-up for occult malignancy. The pathophysiology of the disorder is unknown. Treatment is supportive, with antidepressants and analgesics. The end of the illness is often heralded by the return of an appetite sufficient to permit the patient to gain weight. Many patients ultimately make a good recovery after a year or more of debilitating illness.

Alcoholic Polyneuropathy

Chronic alcohol abuse, even heavy social drinking, can lead to alcoholic polyneuropathy. A symmetric, axonal sensorimotor polyneuropathy affecting distal more than proximal fibers results. Most patients with an alcoholic neuropathy have other physical, neuropsychological, and social stigmata of alcohol abuse. Direct ethanol toxicity and nutritional depletion (especially of thiamine, vitamin B_{12}, and folate), the result of substituting alcohol for normal caloric intake, have been implicated as potential causes of neuropathy. A clinically indistinguishable polyneuropathy can develop secondary to B_{12} and folate deficiencies in strict vegetarians and in AIDS patients with intestinal malabsorption.

Lancinating foot pain is often the first sign of an alcoholic polyneuropathy. With continued alcohol use, the upper extremities ultimately develop similar symptoms. A gait disorder often develops later. The cause of gait difficulties in alcoholics is multifactorial, including impaired sensory inflow to the cerebellum due to neuropathy and direct ethanol toxicity to the cerebellum itself.

Other Acquired Sensorimotor Polyneuropathies

As shown in Table 117-1, there are numerous other causes of acquired sensorimotor polyneuropathy. Specific inquiry should be made about exposure to the medications and chemotherapeutic agents listed, possible toxic exposures, unusual dietary practices, recreational drug use, and other active illnesses. Critical-illness polyneuropathy and chronic inflammatory demyelinating polyradiculoneuropathy and its related disorders are discussed later in this chapter.

Inherited Sensorimotor Neuropathies

There are dozens of inherited neuropathies, including sensorimotor, sensory, motor, and autonomic types. Almost all are rare and are the province of the neuromuscular specialist. Two fairly common sensorimotor neuropathies deserve mention, as they are likely to be encountered frequently in the primary care setting.

Charcot-Marie-Tooth disease (hereditary motor sensory neuropathy type I [HMSN I] or peroneal muscular atrophy) is the most common inherited neuropathy. This autosomal dominant disorder has an extremely indolent course, beginning in the first or second decade. It often goes unrecognized even in families with many affected members. Pathologically, the neuropathy has a predilection for the largest myelinated fibers, where it causes repeated bouts of demyelination and remyelination, leading to a microscopic appearance reminiscent of onion bulbs and to palpable nerve hypertrophy. Patients usually present with motor complaints. On examination, they often have high-arched feet (pes cavus), hammertoes, and "stork legs" (peroneal muscle atrophy). The deep tendon reflexes are diminished or lost, vibratory sensation is reduced, and nerve hypertrophy may be appreciated. Footdrop may be present. Despite these abnormalities, many patients with HMSN I have minimal disability. Nerve conduction studies reveal conduction velocities reduced far below the lower limits of normal. The diagnosis can also be established by DNA testing, which is available pre- and postnatally.

A similar clinical picture can arise from the axonal form of Charcot-Marie-Tooth (HMSN II), although the underlying pathology and electrophysiology are dominated by axon loss. Inheritance is also typically autosomal dominant. Symptoms begin somewhat later, in the second decade. Nerve enlargement is absent and arm involvement is less common. Electrodiagnostic studies show essentially normal conduction velocities and evidence of axon loss. No genetic test is available for HMSN II. In rare cases, the distinction between HMSN I and II is made only after nerve biopsy.

Sensory-Predominant Polyneuropathies

The differential diagnosis of the sensory neuropathies differs from that of the more common sensorimotor polyneuropathies, although several conditions can lead to either. The presence of a purely sensory neuropathy is often unsuspected early in the course, as most patients with the more common sensorimotor polyneuropathy develop sensory symptoms first. The diagnosis is often first suggested when electrodiagnostic tests reveal the near-absence of motor involvement. The most common sensory neuropathies are due to diabetes, alcohol abuse, and uremia. Of the nearly two dozen other causes listed in Table 117-1, a few deserve special mention.

Nutritional deficiency states, especially B_{12} and folate deficiencies, produce selective injury to sensory fibers. B_{12} and folate deficiencies are most common in alcoholics and less common in strict vegetarians, as noted above. A macrocytic anemia is anticipated. Spasticity and extensor plantar responses, which indicate upper motor neuron damage, coexist with lower motor findings such as areflexia. Vitamin E deficiency, typically associated with fat malabsorption syndromes, can produce both a sensory neuropathy and spinocerebellar degeneration.

Several chemotherapeutic agents commonly used in the treatment of malignancies of the reproductive organs—vincristine, cisplatin, paclitaxel, and docetaxel—produce fairly predictable dose-dependent sensory neuropathies. Progressive loss of deep tendon reflexes is followed by distal-predominant sensory loss. Vincristine can also produce significant autonomic problems, including orthostatic hypotension, impotence, and abdominal pain. Paclitaxel doses above 200 mg/m^2 are likely to result in an acute distal sensory-predominant neuropathy. With doses of cisplatin below 500 mg/m^2, the neuropathy may be reversible.

Leprosy (Hansen disease) is the most common cause of peripheral neuropathy worldwide, although it is uncommon in the United States (except for a few southern states). In the lepromatous form, local bacterial invasion and sensory loss are seen in cooler areas of the body, with sparing of the palms and soles. The tuberculoid form produces hypopigmented skin lesions with reduced pain and temperature sensation. Isolated or multiple mononeuropathies may develop. Chronic joint injury, leading to autoamputation, is common. Dapsone, a common drug used treat leprosy, can can produce a motor-predominant neuropathy.

Sensory Neuropathies

The most disabling sensory neuropathies occur when the cell bodies, which reside in the dorsal root ganglia, are damaged. The term neuronopathy is used to indicate a process which damages the cell body or neuron as a whole, in contrast to a neuropathy where damage is limited to the axon. Sensory neuronopathies are caused by toxic agents. Selective and severe damage to the sensory fibers mediating joint position sense leads to profound functional disability with little weakness and few sensory complaints. The inability to detect either movement or static position of the limbs may lead to apparent weakness that often resolves if the patient is retested while watching the limb being evaluated. Patients often cannot sit or stand unsupported.

When a sensory neuronopathy develops over days, the cause is probably idiopathic. Subacute and chronic sensory neuropathies are more likely to be due to carcinoma or Sjögren syndrome, although idiopathic cases can occur as well. Among the carcinomas, small cell lung tumors are the most common, followed by breast, esophagus, kidney, and liver cancer. A careful history can help exclude prior toxic exposures to heavy metals, drugs, or toxins.

Friedreich Ataxia

Friedreich ataxia is an autosomal recessive disorder in which sensory abnormalities are prominent. Patients present in the preteen years with gait difficulties due to lower extremity ataxia. Over time, there is involvement of the arms and dysarthria. High-arched feet (pes cavus) and scoliosis are common. Like B_{12}-deficient patients, the curious combination of areflexia and bilateral Babinski signs is seen. Large-fiber sensory loss results in the loss of vibratory sensation and position sense. Motor weakness is often seen later in the illness. Cardiomyopathy is common, and many patients develop diabetes mellitus. Pathologic findings are present in the dorsal root ganglia and posterior columns, accounting for the prominent large-fiber sensory loss. Abnormalities in the corticospinal tracts explain the spasticity and extensor plantar responses.

Motor-Predominant Polyneuropathies

Several polyneuropathies affect motor fibers nearly exclusively. Acute causes include acute inflammatory demyelinating polyradiculoneuropathy (Guillain-Barré syndrome) and critical-illness polyneuropathy; chronic disorders include chronic inflammatory demyelinating polyradiculoneuropathy. The remaining illnesses in Table 117-1 are uncommon.

Acute Inflammatory Demyelinating Polyradiculoneuropathy

Acute inflammatory demyelinating polyradiculoneuropathy (AIDP) is treatable but dangerous. In two thirds of patients, the disorder is preceded by a viral respiratory illness, diarrhea, vaccination, or surgery. Distal-predominant weakness develops over hours or days. At initial presentation, patients may have vague complaints of distal paresthesias and back pain and subtle weakness. Many are initially diagnosed with viral syndrome, anxiety, or hysteria. Subtle bilateral facial weakness or complaints consistent with autonomic instability (tachycardia, excessive sweating, orthostasis) are easily overlooked. The persistence of reflexes, which are classically absent or depressed, can falsely reassure the unwary physician early in the clinical course. Ultimately, the constellation of symptoms becomes clearer, making the proper diagnosis more likely.

AIDP typically progresses over days to at most a month. Symptoms often stabilize during a plateau phase of 1 or 2 weeks; this is followed by recovery over many months. The vast majority of AIDP patients make a substantial and often complete recovery, but up to 20% have residual motor deficits at 1 year. Progressive weakness over more than a month or exacerbations and remissions should suggest an alternate diagnosis.

As many as 10% to 20% of AIDP patients require mechanical ventilation during the early phase of the illness. Failure to recognize impending respiratory distress can be a fatal mistake. When called about a patient with possible AIDP, the first question should be, "Can she cough?" Patients who can cough have a vital capacity well over 1 L and are unlikely to suffer immediate respiratory failure. If the cough is weak or absent, the patient should be transferred to an intensive care unit, regardless of how well she otherwise appears. Blood gas measurements are often falsely reassuring; elective intubation should be performed in patients who show signs of respiratory fatigue, including but not limited to a forced vital capacity below 12 to 15 mL/kg or a negative inspiratory force below −30 mm H_20. When respiratory failure is properly managed, the mortality in AIDP drops to 2% to 4%, with most deaths from cardiac arrhythmias and hospital-acquired infections.

A particularly severe form of AIDP often follows a bout of bloody diarrhea secondary to infection with *Campylobacter jejuni*. Unlike typical AIDP, in which the primary pathology is demyelinating, axonal injury predominates. The illness is often explosive, with profound weakness developing over hours to a day. Early electrodiagnostic testing reveals absent responses from both motor and sensory fibers. The prognosis for recovery is guarded, as axonal regeneration is often incomplete.

Chronic Inflammatory Demyelinating Polyradiculoneuropathy

Chronic inflammatory demyelinating polyradiculoneuropathy (CIDP) is the chronic cousin of AIDP. It shares many of the same clinical features, but its management is much different. CIDP presents as a progressive, symmetric sensorimotor polyneuropathy. Unlike AIDP, CIDP progresses over months to years, and exacerbations and remissions are common. CIDP accounts for nearly 20% of cases of chronic neuropathy. It often presages the development of another disorder: up to a third of patients later develop a paraproteinemia, lymphoma, granulomatous disease, an autoimmune disease (eg, lupus, rheumatoid arthritis, Sjögren), or HIV infection. Plasma cell dyscrasias from multiple myeloma are especially common. A few patients demonstrate antibodies directed against myelin (anti-MAG [myelin-associated glycoprotein]).

Symptoms are often more prominent in the legs, and sensory symptoms are often more prominent than in AIDP. Tremor and nerve hypertrophy are fairly common in CIDP but not in AIDP. As in AIDP, there is a cytoalbuminologic dissociation in the CSF. Electrodiagnostic criteria have been established for CIDP, although some patients may require nerve biopsy to establish the diagnosis. Onion bulb pathology, the residua of bouts of demyelination and remyelination, strongly supports the diagnosis.

Multifocal Motor Neuropathy With Conduction Block

Multifocal motor neuropathy with conduction block is a recently described, treatable disorder. Its presentation can mimic that of amyotrophic lateral sclerosis. Patients present with asymmetric, progressive weakness that is often worse in the arms. Anti-GM_1 antibodies are present in the serum in most patients. Electrodiagnostic studies play a crucial role, as they demonstrate evidence of conduction block in affected limbs. Treatment with intravenous immunoglobulin or immunosuppression with cyclophosphamide is effective.

Critical-Illness Polyneuropathy

Critical-illness polyneuropathy often develops in the setting of sepsis but has also been associated with the concomitant use of neuromuscular blocking agents and high-dose steroids. A generalized neuropathy ensues, producing diffuse weakness and diaphragmatic weakness or paralysis. This diagnosis should be considered in the acutely ill patient with unexplained ventilatory dependence or weakness. AIDP can also develop in this setting and must be considered as well.

Autonomic Neuropathies

Autonomic involvement is characteristic of a few neuropathies, many with concurrent involvement of sensorimotor fibers. The most common associated neuropathies are diabetes, alcoholism, and amyloidosis. Autonomic instability is common in patients with AIDP; some suffer bouts of severe hypotension and hypertension within minutes of each other. Autonomic instability and its associated cardiac rhythm disturbances account for a large percentage of AIDP-associated deaths. Severe autonomic involvement is also seen in the Shy-Drager syndrome, a parkinsonian syndrome characterized by rigidity, gait disturbances, impotence, and relative unresponsiveness to L-DOPA.

Mononeuritis Multiplex

Mononeuritis multiplex is the term applied to conditions that injure multiple peripheral nerves in a haphazard pattern. At onset, the condition often appears to be a simple mononeuropathy, but as additional nerves are affected the process declares itself to be multifocal. The inability to classify the neuropathy under one of the common schemas (ie, distal, axonal, sensorimotor) should suggest this diagnosis. Mononeuritis multiplex follows no simple rules. In some cases, there is preferential injury to distal nerve fibers. Multiple nerve injuries may produce confluent sensory loss that replicates the glove-and-stocking pattern of distal symmetric polyneuropathies. Clues to the correct diagnosis are often obtained from a careful history revealing either abrupt, stepwise changes in sensorimotor function or events in the distant past that the patient thought insignificant (eg, old carpal tunnel syndrome). A detailed physical or electrodiagnostic examination may uncover evidence of unsuspected neuropathies.

The most common conditions causing mononeuritis multiplex are diabetes, rheumatoid arthritis, sarcoid, polyarteritis nodosa, HIV infection, and leprosy. Although routine laboratory studies (fasting blood glucose, rheumatoid factor, serum angiotensin-converting enzyme (ACE) level, HIV titer) may be useful, a definitive diagnosis often requires nerve biopsy.

HISTORY

Sensory complaints are usually the first symptom in sensorimotor polyneuropathy. Patients experience paresthesias or burning discomfort or state they feel like they are "walking on cardboard" or "wearing too many socks." They rarely complain of sensory loss itself. Gait instability, particularly in the dark, can be seen due to the loss of joint position sense that accompanies the loss of large sensory axons. Distal hand numbness may produce clumsiness or trouble identifying objects deep in one's pockets. Injuries to the feet such as blisters, puncture wounds, and infections may go unnoticed. The motor component of neuropathy leads to distal-predominant weakness and only much later to atrophy. Footdrop or toe drop develops first. Patients may report catching their toes on the edge of carpeting, scuffing the tops of their shoes, or slapping their feet as they walk. Autonomic complaints such as feeling faint on standing, nausea, vomiting, diarrhea, and impotence are often prominent but may be mistakenly attributed to nonneuropathic causes.

The clinical course of the neuropathies varies from acute (progressing over hours or days) to very indolent (over decades). Ischemic neuropathies result in symptoms of immediate onset. Chronic demyelinating neuropathies, both acquired and inherited, have a slow, relentless course.

PHYSICAL EXAMINATION AND CLINICAL FINDINGS

Early in the course of a neuropathy, symptoms may be unaccompanied by signs of nerve dysfunction on examination. Later in the illness, the physical examination is more revealing. The goal of the peripheral nervous system examination is to describe the findings concisely—for example, "a distal, symmetric sensory greater than motor polyneuropathy with evidence of axonal features." While taking the history and examining the patient, the physician should consider several questions: When did symptoms begin? What type of clinical course did this process have (eg, acute, subacute, chronic, relapsing, progressive)? Where did symptoms start? Is it symmetric? Is there a glove-and-stocking pattern of abnormalities (suggestive of a distal-to-proximal dying-back neuropathy), or does the sensory loss suggest a radicular (dermatomal) pattern or that of an individual mononeuropathy? Are small or large nerve fibers preferentially affected? Sometimes these questions can be answered by a careful history; in other cases, even a detailed physical examination leaves many questions unanswered. An electrodiagnostic evaluation often helps clarify the nature and degree of pathology, but sometimes only nerve biopsy can reveal the specific diagnosis.

The sensory examination is particularly helpful in assessing patients with polyneuropathy because distal sensory signs occur so early in the clinical course. When large sensory fibers are involved, there is progressive loss of distal vibratory sensation and decreased joint position sense (the ability to detect passive movement of a joint or its position in space), and the deep tendon reflexes are diminished. Small sensory fibers, which mediate pain and temperature sensation, can be spared in some neuropathies and preferentially involved in others. Small-fiber diseases, such as amyloidosis, may also produce significant autonomic dysfunction, with decreased sweating and orthostasis.

The motor examination assesses large motor axon function. Muscle weakness and atrophy occur only after fairly significant axonal loss has occurred; thus, the physical examination often misses signs of early motor neuropathy. Needle electromyography, however, is exquisitely sensitive to axonal loss: the loss of just 3% of motor axons within a nerve produces increased membrane instability in muscle detectable as p-waves and fibrillations (denervation). Denervation can be found when strength, bulk, and reflexes are all normal.

LABORATORY EVALUATION

Polyneuropathy is not a diagnosis unto itself. The physician must establish a probable cause for the polyneuropathy, excluding the treatable (predominantly demyelinating) neuropathies and reducing or eliminating ongoing risks to the peripheral nervous system (eg, medications, alcohol, toxins). The laboratory evaluation should begin by focusing on the most common conditions associated with each subtype of polyneuropathy. If screening laboratory studies for the relevant conditions fail to establish a diagnosis, the patient should be referred to a neuromuscular specialist for further evaluation. The cost of screening neuropathy panels, touted by some laboratories as a one-size-fits-all work-up, far exceeds that of a neurologic consultation; furthermore, these panels are often unrevealing. Unfortunately, even exhaustive work-ups at major referral centers fail to identify the etiology of a neuropathy in up to 30% of patients.

Nerve conduction studies are crucial in some patients to help classify the neuropathy and to serve as a possible prelude to nerve biopsy. Biopsies of clinically and electrically normal nerves are rarely abnormal. When severely affected nerves are biopsied, end stage pathologic changes may obscure the primary pathologic process. Nerve conduction studies can help determine whether a biopsy should be performed and which nerve should be selected.

In patients with a sensorimotor polyneuropathy, screening laboratory tests should include a random glucose study, hemoglobin A_1C level, thyroid function tests, and levels of blood urea nitrogen, creatinine, B_{12}, folate, serum and urine protein electrophoreses (SPEP and UPEP), and serum immunofixation. If the history suggests heavy metal exposure, a 24-hour urine sample should be done.

In sensory neuronopathy, laboratory studies should include a B_{12} level, a vitamin E level in patients at risk for fat malabsorption, and a serum and urine protein electrophoresis and immunofixation. A chest x-ray should be obtained in all patients and an anti-Hu in those at risk for lung malignancy by history or chest x-ray. CSF should be obtained, looking for abnormal cytology or the anti-Hu antibody (although the latter can often be detected in serum). An AIDS test should be considered in patients with risk factors or an unrevealing laboratory work-up. Laboratory screening for Sjögren syndrome should include anti-Ro (SS-A) and anti-La (SS-B) tests. An ophthalmologic evaluation, including a Schirmer test for tear production and Rose-Bengal staining of the cornea, can establish the diagnosis. The gold standard for diagnosing Sjögren syndrome is a minor salivary gland biopsy.

Laboratory tests play a central role in diagnosing the acquired demyelinating polyneuropathies. In AIDP, the most useful confirmatory tests are CSF analysis and electrodiagnostic testing. Additional tests should be performed to exclude the most common AIDP look-alikes and to look for possible causes. CSF analysis should be performed, looking for the characteristic cytoalbuminologic dissociation (protein elevation without elevation in white cells in the CSF). The CSF may remain normal during the early days of the illness, and up to 10% of patients never develop CSF protein elevation. A significant leukocytosis in the CSF should raise concern about the polyradiculopathies associated with carcinoma, AIDS, Lyme disease, or cytomegalovirus. Nerve conduction studies can demonstrate evidence of distal conduction block or temporal dispersion due to early demyelinating changes. Electromyography can detect denervation secondary to motor axon injury after 1 to 2 weeks. Ancillary testing should probably include an HIV test, a porphyria screen, *C jejuni* titers, a hepatitis screen, and a mononucleosis spot. If clinically indicated, a urinary heavy metal screen or diphtheria titers should be done.

In CIDP, the CSF should be evaluated as in AIDP. It is critical to look for evidence of plasma cell dyscrasia. Screening tests should include a serum and urine protein electrophoresis and immunofixation. A bone marrow analysis may be necessary to exclude an underlying hematologic malignancy. A skeletal survey should be performed to look for evidence of lytic lesions, which would suggest multiple myeloma. Lifelong surveillance for myeloma is required. Worsening CIDP or the appearance of a new protein spike on serum protein electrophoresis warrants a repeat skeletal survey. Radiation or resection of a new lytic lesion results in improvement in the neuropathy in some patients. AIDP and CIDP are more common in HIV-positive patients and can be the initial manifestation of HIV infection.

TREATMENT

Many of the polyneuropathies have no specific therapy, although there are interventions that may be of benefit. When the neuropathy accompanies a systemic disorder such as diabetes or hypothyroidism, treatment of the underlying condition may slow the progress of the neuropathy. Uremic patients may do especially well as their condition improves. The toxic effects of drugs, alcohol, heavy metals, or industrial solvents must be considered (see Table 117-1) and all potential offending agents eliminated.

A few polyneuropathies require specific interventions. Diabetic neuropathy requires preventive and symptomatic treatment. Prevention consists of redoubling efforts to control blood sugar levels and, when necessary, symptomatic treatment of the positive symptoms. The Diabetic Control and Complications Trial, completed in 1994, demonstrated that long-term tight control of blood sugar levels slows the progression of diabetic neuropathy in insulin-dependent patients. Symptomatic treatments can help reduce the chronic burning dysesthesias that bother many patients. The tricyclic antidepressants in low nocturnal doses (eg, amitriptyline 10 to 50 mg orally at bedtime) are often helpful; carbamazepine and phenytoin are also effective. Some patients benefit from the local application of capsaicin cream (derived from pepper plants), although a 30-day trial of four-times-daily application may be necessary to establish efficacy.

Effective treatments are available for the acquired demyelinating polyneuropathies (AIDP and CIDP). Therapy for AIDP uses total plasma exchange or infusions of intravenous immunoglobulin. Steroids, once the standard of care, are ineffective. Plasma exchange is most effective when begun during the first 2 weeks of the illness, but treatment during the first month is probably warranted if the patient is sufficiently weak. Typically, five or six plasma exchanges are performed on an alternate-day schedule. If the final exchange is completed during the second or third week of the illness, the patient may require one or two weekly "clean-up" exchanges to prevent relapse during the first month of the illness. Intravenous immunoglobulin is also effective treatment for AIDP, but the relapse rate may be higher than with plasma exchange. Intravenous immunoglobulin is particularly useful in children and in patients with limited intravenous access or vascular instability.

In CIDP, unlike AIDP, there is a therapeutic role for steroids. Many patients require chronic immunosuppression with steroids or steroid-sparing agents such as azathioprine (Imuran), although some can be managed with intermittent plasma exchange or intravenous immunoglobulin. CIDP patients with gammopathy require lifelong screening for worsening gammopathy or lytic bony lesions. The detection and treatment of a previously occult malignancy can result in improvement in the neuropathy.

CONSIDERATIONS DURING PREGNANCY

Few of the polyneuropathies are specifically exacerbated in pregnancy; the two exceptions are the inflammatory demyelinating polyneuropathies (AIDP and CIDP). AIDP appears to be no more common in pregnancy than at other times. The primary treatment modalities, plasma exchanges and intravenous immunoglobulin therapy, can both be used safely during pregnancy. CIDP may present or relapse at higher rates during pregnancy. Normally, CIDP is treated with prednisone, but this should be avoided during pregnancy if possible; plasma exchange is a safe alternative. Chronic immunosuppressive therapy is commonly used in CIDP patients. Women of childbearing age must be counseled about the considerable teratogenicity of these therapies, and a highly effective form of birth control should be used.

A gestational distal-predominant sensorimotor polyneuropathy can develop in women with significant nutritional deficiency, but it is uncommon in developed countries. In rare families predisposed to brachial plexopathy or mononeuritis multiplex, pregnancy may provoke a new attack.

BIBLIOGRAPHY

Aminoff MJ, ed. Neurology and general medicine. London: Churchill-Livingstone, 1995.

Asbury AK, Thomas PK, eds. Peripheral nerve disorders: blue books of practical neurology. Oxford: Butterworth-Heinemann, 1995.

Bosch EP, Mitsumoto H. Disorders of peripheral nerves. In: Bradley WG, Daroff RB, Fenichel GM, Marsden CD, eds. Neurology in clinical practice, 2d ed. Oxford: Butterworth-Heinemann, 1996:1881.

Donaldson JO. Neurology of pregnancy. In: Walton J, ed. Major problems in neurology, 2d ed. Philadelphia: WB Saunders, 1989.

Dyck PJ, Thomas PK, Griffin JW, Low PA, Poduslo JF. Peripheral neuropathy. Philadelphia: WB Saunders, 1993.

Cohen BS, Felsenthal G. Peripheral nervous system disorders and pregnancy. In: Goldstein PJ, ed. Neurological disorders of pregnancy. Mt. Kisco, NY:

Primary Care for Women, edited by Phyllis C. Leppert and Fred M. Howard. Lippincott-Raven Publishers, Philadelphia

118
Myasthenia Gravis

HAROLD LESSER

Myasthenia gravis (MG) is the most common disorder of neuromuscular junction transmission and probably the best understood autoimmune disease. Patients with MG experience fatigable weakness that can be restricted to the ocular muscles (ocular MG), the oculopharyngeal muscles (bulbar MG), or the skeletal and respiratory muscles (generalized MG). MG was recognized over 300 years ago, but effective treatments were not discovered until the early 1900s. As recently as the late 1950s, MG was a disabling disorder with a 30% mortality rate. Today, MG is manageable, most patients lead full lives, and fatalities are unusual. The disorder is sporadic, with an incidence of two to five cases per year per million persons, and a prevalence of five to 12 cases per 100,000. There are 35,000 cases in the United States. Women tend to get MG in their 20s and 30s, men in their 60s and 70s.

ETIOLOGY AND DIFFERENTIAL DIAGNOSIS

Weakness, the primary symptom in MG, results from disturbed transmission across the synapse that bridges the motor axon and the muscle membrane. Neurotransmission is mediated by acetylcholine (ACh), which is released from synaptic vesicles in the axon terminal and crosses the synaptic cleft, where it binds to acetylcholine receptors (AChR) embedded in the muscle endplate. ACh binding leads to action potential production in the postsynaptic muscle membrane. Autoantibodies to the AChR reduce the number of available receptors, thereby decreasing the ability of ACh to generate an action potential. At rest or with minimal effort, there is sufficient physiologic reserve to make action potential generation likely; with exertion, the probability of successful neurotransmission is reduced, and weakness results. In addition to decreasing the number of available postsynaptic receptors, autoantibody binding and complement activation result in structural simplification of the muscle membrane and shorten the life of the AChR; both of these impair neuromuscular transmission.

The autoimmune basis of MG is well established. Passive transfer of patient sera to experimental animals produces disease, IgG autoantibodies to the AChR have been isolated from sera, and the AChR and its autoantibodies have been characterized at the molecular level. The autoimmune nature of the disease is further supported by the increased risk of autoimmune disorders such as lupus, rheumatoid arthritis, and thyroiditis in patients and their first-degree relatives. As with most autoimmune diseases, the primary trigger for the disorder is not well understood; however, evidence suggests a pathophysiologic link to the thymus.

The differential diagnosis of MG is limited in patients who present with marked clear diurnal variation. The differential is broader in patients with symptoms limited to the ocular or oculopharyngeal muscles, particularly when there is some degree of fixed weakness. Disorders to consider include thyroid eye disease, intracranial mass lesions in the region of the superior orbital fissure, multiple sclerosis, brain stem masses, multiple cranial mononeuropathies, and myopathy (oculopharyngeal dystrophy, progressive external ophthalmoplegia). In cases without definite laboratory evidence of MG, a brain imaging study may be necessary to exclude other conditions.

Weakness that involves both the bulbar and limb musculature suggests several other disorders, including amyotrophic lateral sclerosis (ALS), polio, botulism, and some myopathies. Patients with ALS usually have both upper motor neuron signs (spasticity, diffuse hyperreflexia, and extensor plantar responses) and lower motor neuron signs (weakness, fasciculations, and atrophy). Polio and botulism have fairly acute clinical courses, and pupillary abnormalities are typical in botulism. Proximal muscle weakness is common in many myopathies, including polymyositis. Except for a few rare metabolic myopathies, the characteristic pattern of myopathy is fixed rather than variable weakness. Many myopathies are associated with an elevated creatine kinase (CK) level, particularly in the acute phase. The CK level is not elevated in MG.

The Lambert-Eaton myasthenic syndrome is another disorder of neuromuscular transmission that is occasionally confused with MG. The unfortunate choice of "myasthenic syndrome" to refer to Lambert-Eaton syndrome makes confusion with "myasthenia" all too easy. Fortunately the differential diagnosis is usually straightforward. Like patients with MG, those with Lambert-Eaton syndrome complain of variable weakness; however, their strength may improve with repeated effort. They often complain of dry mouth, and they are frequently areflexic. The antibodies that cause Lambert-Eaton syndrome attack the voltage-gated calcium channels of the presynaptic axon terminal, thereby reducing ACh release. Antibody testing for Lambert-Eaton syndrome is not generally available at this time.

Drug-induced MG can occur in patients who receive D-penicillamine for rheumatoid arthritis. These patients have otherwise typical MG with positive antibodies and abnormal repetitive stimulation studies. The myasthenic symptoms typically disappear after the medication is discontinued.

HISTORY

The symptoms of MG develop insidiously. Patients with ocular MG may notice blurring of vision after prolonged reading or driving. Ptosis can develop in this setting as well. Questions about new ptosis or facial weakness can often be settled by reviewing old photographs; a driver's license photo is often readily available. Patients with bulbar MG may report nasal speech, decreased speech volume, nasal regurgitation of fluids, and trouble swallowing. Weakness of facial muscles can make it difficult to drink from a straw. When a "myasthenic snarl" replaces a normal smile, family and friends often mistakenly believe the patient to be depressed or angry. In generalized MG, patients may have difficulty accomplishing activities of daily living. They have often subconsciously adjusted their activities to accommodate their symptoms. The ability to accomplish activities of daily living requiring good proximal muscle strength should be assessed (eg, washing one's hair, lifting heavy objects out of cupboards, climbing stairs, getting in and out of a car, arising from a low couch, and standing from a squat). A good history may reveal a significant worsening in strength either as the day goes on (ie, diurnal variation) or following exertion.

PHYSICAL EXAMINATION AND CLINICAL FINDINGS

The physical examination should be directed at demonstrating either fatigable or fixed weakness. Fatigable weakness of extraocular or limb muscles is the hallmark of MG. Ptosis or diplopia may be elicited by having the patient stare at the ceiling for 1 or 2 minutes. The palpebral fissures should be measured both before and after testing. The pattern of diplopia may be confusing, as multiple muscles in both eyes are often affected. Limb weakness can be provoked by repetitive exertion of specific muscle groups. The patient is asked to exert a maximal effort five to ten times against the examiner's resistance. Patients with significant MG may demonstrate decreasing strength with repeated efforts. After a few minutes of rest, strength returns to normal. Tests of upper extremity fatigability are usually performed on the deltoid; lower extremity strength can be evaluated by having the patient repeatedly stand from a squat.

Fixed weakness often develops in the neck extensors and facial muscles. In a normal person, the examiner should not be able to overcome forcefully closed eyes or lips or forcefully extended necks. When profound neck extensor weakness develops, the patient may have her chin on her chest or resort to propping her head up with her hands. This symptom can also be seen in polymyositis and ALS. MG is not associated with sensory deficits or reflex abnormalities.

LABORATORY EVALUATION

The laboratory evaluation of MG is important to confirm the diagnosis and to help with treatment decisions. The major categories of testing are serologic testing, electrodiagnostic studies, supplementary laboratory evaluation, and imaging studies.

Antibody testing should be performed whenever the diagnosis of MG is seriously considered. AChR antibodies are present in 85% of those with generalized MG and 50% of those with ocular or bulbar MG. The absolute titer of AChR antibodies does not predict disease severity between patients, but a rising titer in an individual patient may indicate disease progression. Seronegative patients are clinically indistinguishable from seropositive ones and respond to similar treatments. False-positive antibody tests are rare. False-negative results are occasionally obtained during the first year of the disease, so repeating the AChR antibody test 1 year after an initially negative work-up may be revealing.

Electrodiagnostic testing is helpful in evaluating MG. Repetitive motor conduction studies can demonstrate neuromuscular junction fatigue. At a normal neuromuscular junction, repetitive nerve stimulation at low rates of two to five/second evokes motor responses of equal amplitude. In MG, neuromuscular fatigue causes the amplitude of the response to decline. The effect is most pronounced in proximal muscles (eg, trapezius, facial muscles) and is absent in some patients. In contrast, Lambert-Eaton patients have low-amplitude motor responses at rest and a marked increase in response amplitudes after exercise or repetitive stimulation at high rates (50/second).

In patients with a normal repetitive stimulation test, single-fiber electromyography may be helpful. This test looks for abnormally increased variability ("jitter") in the timing of activation of adjacent muscle fibers. The degree of jitter correlates well with the severity of the neuromuscular transmission defects. Abnormalities are often seen even in clinically normal muscles. Single-fiber electromyography has a sensitivity well over 95% and may be the only abnormal laboratory test in some myasthenics.

Supplementary laboratory testing is critical to rule out underlying conditions that could be confused with MG or could complicate its management. Given the association of MG with autoimmune disorders, it is rational to order thyroid function tests, an anti-nuclear antibody (ANA), and a rheumatoid factor assay. If the diagnosis is in question, it is reasonable to obtain thyroid function tests, a CK measurement, and vitamin B_{12} and folate levels. If the diagnosis is established, baseline laboratory studies may be appropriate before embarking on steroid treatment or immunosuppression. Tuberculosis should be excluded in any patient in whom chronic immunosuppression is anticipated. In patients with newly diagnosed MG, a chest computed tomography scan should be performed to look for an enlarged thymus in the mediastinum; a chest x-ray detects only the largest of masses and is therefore an inadequate screening test.

Malignant thymoma should be suspected in all patients with newly diagnosed MG. A chest x-ray will detect only the largest of thymomas; therefore, computed tomography scan of the chest should be performed instead. If an anti-striated muscle antibody titer is positive, malignant thymoma is highly probable. Patients with suspected thymoma require more aggressive therapy as discussed below.

In some centers, the Tensilon (edrophonium) test is routinely used to evaluate patients with possible MG, however, modern electrodiagnostic and serologic techniques have led to decreased use of the test. Patients must have a definite abnormality on examination, such as objective ptosis or diplopia, dysphonia, or weakness. The test should be done by experienced practitioners in a facility where atropine and resuscitation equipment are available, as anticholinergic agents can precipitate profound bradycardia or respiratory arrest. In a positive test, muscle strength improves for up to 5 minutes after the injection. Some physicians perform the test in a blinded fashion to avoid observer bias. False-positive tests can occur in other diseases that produce weakness.

TREATMENT

MG should be managed by a specialist. All the treatments have serious potential side effects, and mismanagement can lead to unnecessary morbidity and mortality. Treatment consists of both symptomatic and immunosuppressive arms.

Symptomatic treatment is accomplished with anticholinesterase agents such as pyridostigmine (Mestinon). By inhibiting the action of acetylcholinesterase, pyridostigmine increases the availability of ACh in the neuromuscular junction, thereby facilitating neuromuscular transmission. Side effects of pyridostigmine include cramps, nausea, vomiting, or diarrhea. Excessive doses may lead to a cholinergic crisis, severe weakness that is clinically indistinguishable from MG itself. In addition to the oral form of pyridostigmine, there are parenteral and sustained-release (Mestinon Timespan) formulations.

Immunosuppressive treatments help by reducing the production of AChR antibodies. Prednisone and prednisone-sparing agents, as well as immunomodulating therapies such as plasma exchange and immunoglobulin infusions, are used. Prednisone is the mainstay of therapy for many patients. The initiation of therapy with this drug should be done on an inpatient basis, as nearly half of patients develop increased weakness during the first week of treatment. A rare patient may even develop respiratory failure during this time. Initial prednisone doses of 60 mg/day are often required to bring symptoms under control, but ultimately many patients can be managed on alternate-day therapy in doses as low as 2.5 to 5 mg.

Some patients fail to respond to prednisone or require such large doses that chronic side effects are inevitable. Prednisone-sparing agents are particularly helpful to these patients. Azathioprine (Imuran) is commonly used. Because it may take up to 6 months to work, it is often started concurrently with oral steroids. At least 10% of patients treated with azathioprine develop an intolerable flu-like syndrome and must be taken off it. Others develop severe neutropenia. Patients of childbearing age must be cautioned about the significant risk of this and other immunosuppressive agents to the fetus and should be offered highly effective contraceptives.

Cyclosporine is an alternate immunosuppressant that is effective in MG. Its primary side effects are nephrotoxicity and hypertension. It acts sooner than azathioprine, beginning 1 to 2 months after treatment is initiated.

Plasma exchange is a highly effective, rapidly acting immunotherapy for MG. It is particularly useful in acute crises. A series of four to six exchanges given every other day removes circulating autoantibodies and improves neuromuscular transmission. It may also exert modulatory effects on antibody production by mechanisms that are not well understood. Intravenous immunoglobulin is also effective in MG and may be suitable for children and patients with difficult vascular access. It is less reliable than plasma exchange but is useful in some patients.

Thymectomy may be the most powerful immunomodulatory therapy. Unlike any of the treatments mentioned above, it can increase the remission rate up to 40%. The value of thymectomy was first recognized in the 1930s, when malignant thymomas were first resected. Although patients with thymoma had more severe MG, a surprising number went into remission postoperatively. The observation that the remission rate improved even among patients whose preoperative "thymoma" was pathologically benign led to trials of thymectomy in patients without thymoma. Surgery is nonelective in those with thymoma, and radiation therapy is usually employed postoperatively. In patients without thymoma, series have demonstrated increased remission rates during the 3 to 5 years after surgery. Surgery benefits even very young children, but the benefit is uncertain in patients over 60. Before surgery, symptomatic patients should undergo a course of plasma exchange to maximize their ventilatory capacity and strength. Transsternal thymectomy should be performed, as it affords better exposure of the mediastinum and permits more complete resection of both the thymus and scattered ectopic rests of thymic tissue.

When the symptoms of MG worsen, several possibilities must be considered. Medication compliance is always a consideration, but in its absence an underlying infection is the most likely culprit. Patients can develop severe respiratory compromise in the setting of a "simple" urinary tract infection or pneumonia—the myasthenic crisis. Increased body temperature increases the rate at which acetylcholinesterase degrades ACh, thereby compromising neuromuscular transmission. Patients experiencing frank dysphagia or coughing after eating or drinking are at high risk for aspiration and respiratory failure and require close attention, often in an intensive care setting. Vital capacities below 15 mL/kg or negative inspiratory forces below −20 cm H_2O are indications for intubation, even if blood gas measurements are normal. A brief course of plasma exchange is often the best way to improve neuromuscular junction function rapidly in this setting.

Cholinergic crisis, the result of excessive use of pyridostigmine, can produce progressive weakness as well. Often patients have signs of cholinergic excess. Salivation can be misleading, as it could just as easily reflect difficulty handling secretions from bulbar weakness. Profound bradycardia and diarrhea may be more helpful signs. Management involves the discontinuation of medications, respiratory support, and slow reintroduction of low doses of anticholinesterases at a later time.

Concurrent medications are a potential concern, as several different drugs can compromise the function of the neuromuscular junction. However, few, if any, are absolutely contraindicated. The aminoglycoside antibiotics such as gentamicin are commonly cited as a potential risk, but they should not be withheld in the setting of significant gram-negative infection.

Thymic hyperplasia and thymoma can also lead to worsening MG. Patients who have undergone thymectomy should have a repeat chest computed tomography scan to look for residual thymic rests that may have hypertrophied after surgery. "Second-look" surgery may lead to substantial improvement in such cases.

CONSIDERATIONS IN PREGNANCY

Myasthenics require special attention in all phases of pregnancy, beginning before conception and continuing through the postpartum period. Women of childbearing age should use highly effective contraceptives if they are treated with azathioprine or cyclosporine. Prednisone should be avoided but can be used in pregnancy if it is essential. Plasma exchange is safe throughout pregnancy and may be used in patients whose condition deteriorates. Treatment with pyridostigmine can be continued, but the parenteral form should be avoided, as it can induce uterine contractions.

MG is not an indication for cesarean section. Spinal anesthesia should be used whenever possible. Nondepolarizing neuromuscular blocking agents should be avoided, as myasthenics may have a prolonged response to these medications.

If preeclampsia develops in a myasthenic patient (a chance occurrence, as the two conditions are not related), caution should be used with the administration of magnesium sulfate. Magnesium is a neuromuscular depressant, and the effect may be more pronounced in a patient with preexisting neuromuscular transmission difficulties.

During the first few postpartum days, neonates born thenic mothers must be monitored for signs of weakne 15% of infants have evidence of transitory neonatal MG; feeding or breathing or a weak cry is a common sign. Passi fer of AChR antibodies from mother to fetus during gestation underlies this condition. Neonatal weakness can persist for weeks to months until maternal antibodies are cleared. Although breast milk contains measurable amounts of maternal antibodies to AChR, there is no evidence that it poses a significant threat, even to infants with transitory neonatal MG. Symptomatic treatment of infants with pyridostigmine is usually adequate, although intravenous immunoglobulin or plasma exchange is needed in some. Affected infants are not at increased risk of developing MG later in life, although like all first-degree relatives they are at increased risk for developing other autoimmune disorders.

BIBLIOGRAPHY

Drachman DB. Medical progress: myasthenia gravis. N Engl J Med 1994;330:1797.

Drug-induced myasthenia gravis. Micromedex 1996;87.

Gilchrist JM. Myasthenia gravis. In: Feldmann E, ed. Current diagnosis in neurology. St. Louis: CV Mosby, 1994:350.

Lopate G, Pestronk A. Autoimmune myasthenia gravis. Hospital Practice 1993;28:55.

Sanders DB, Howard JF Jr. Disorders of neuromuscular transmission. In: Bradley WG, Daroff RB, Fenichel GM, Marsden CD, eds. Neurology in clinical practice, 2nd ed. Oxford: Butterworth-Heinemann, 1996.

Toyka KV. Myasthenia gravis. In: Johnson RT, ed. Current therapy in neurologic disease. Philadelphia: BC Decker, 1990:85.

113B

Low Back Pain and Sciatica

JOSHUA HOLLANDER

Primary Care for Women, edited by Phyllis C. Leppert and Fred M. Howard. Lippincott-Raven Publishers, Philadelphia © 1997.

Affecting the area between the rib cage and the gluteal folds, low back pain is the most common patient complaint heard by primary care physicians and the most common cause of disability among persons less than 45 years of age. About 75% of the population experiences low back pain (lumbago). The annual prevalence is 15% to 20% in the United States. About 25% of patients with low back pain have back-related leg pain that radiates along the course of the sciatic nerve to one or both legs, distal to the knee (sciatica). Although there is no gender difference with regard to low back pain, men more often undergo surgery. Physically fit people recover more readily from back pain. Related physical factors include heavy work, lifting, static posture, bending, and twisting, and muscle fatigue and reconditioning predispose to injury. Job dissatisfaction and monotony increase the likelihood of complaint.

The lumbar spine is a series of vertebrae linked by anterior discs and posterior facet joints. The vertebral discs are fibrocartilaginous remnants of the notochord. They have an ovoid gelatinous nucleus pulposus within the firm concentric collagenous fibrous rings of the annulus fibrosus. Discs have minimal blood supply and are innervated by a branch of the posterior primary ramus. Their water content drops from 88% at birth to 66% at age 70. A normally functioning disc allows for an incompressible cushion to distribute forces. An isolated vertebra compresses before a disc does, but the in situ spine withstands forces far in excess of that tolerated ex vivo. The abdomen, its muscle wall, and the paraspinal muscles disseminate forces widely, protecting the spinal column. The typical weight lifter's trochanter belt serves a similar function.

The aging (early) spine loses both water and proteoglycans and its collagen content increases, resulting in a loss of gel behavior. Tears may develop in the annulus and cause lumbago. Disc herniation and fragment compression of a root cause sciatica. There are thus three stages of disc degeneration: a dysfunctional stage manifested by nuclear degeneration with traumatic tears of the annulus that lead to nuclear prolapse, an unstable stage with disc and facet degeneration and capsular laxity, and a restabilization stage of disc collapse and fibrosis and osteophyte formation, producing a stiff joint. Goldthwait related lumbago and sciatica to the lumbar disc. Mister and Barr demonstrated a clear relationship between herniated lumbar discs and lumbago and sciatica as well as therapy by lumbar disc excision. The role of muscle spasm and injury is controversial and may be only an epiphenomenon.

The clinical symptoms that signal a need for caution and early workup include sciatica with an evolving neurologic deficit, unrelenting rest pain suggesting cancer or infection, and writhing pain of intra-abdominal or vascular processes.

Mechanical disorders of the lower back are covered in Chapter 100.

NEURAL COMPRESSION SYNDROMES

A herniated lumbar disc may cause an easily recognized acute onset of lumbago and sciatica. It may also present in a patient with chronic lumbago and segmental (hip and thigh) pain who is experiencing less back and proximal pain but rather primarily distal radicular discomfort. Specific symptoms relate to the root affected and whether the lesion is lateral and compressing a single root or central and compressing the conus. *Lumbar spinal stenosis* may present in a manner similar to a herniated disc. Central stenosis presents with neurogenic claudication and neurogenic bowel and bladder. Confusion with vascular claudication arises when a patient has leg pain with walking that is relieved by rest. Patients can comfortably ride a stationary bike, however, because the legs are flexed. Lateral stenosis may be vague, with only segmental leg pain. The syndrome of neurogenic claudication with pain on walking that is relieved by rest may possibly be related to nerve root ischemia induced by the compression of the roots. Mechanical (instability) syndromes may be manifested by low back or segmental pain aggravated by weight bearing, bending, or twisting and relieved by recumbency.

HISTORY

Only infrequently associated with a specific diagnosis, acute low back pain is pain of less than 6 weeks' duration. Subacute back pain is of 7 to 12 weeks' duration, and chronic low back pain is of longer duration. Sciatica is pain radiating along the course of the sciatic nerve to one or both legs, distal to the knee. A damaged lumbar disc may cause pain to the knee, as may hip disease, but pain does not radiate below. Patient history should include pain onset, duration, distribution, course, and quality. Factors that aggravate or alleviate symptoms should be explored. Radiation in a radicular pattern, paresthesias, motor loss, and bowel or bladder dysfunction should alert the physician to potentially more serious problems. Other potentially serious problems can be signaled by fever (especially in drugs users, diabetics, or immunocompromised patients), abdominal symptoms, known cancer, unexplained weight loss, or osteoporosis. Lack of fitness, psychosocial problems, and marked scoliosis are risk factors. Patients must be asked about traumatic causes. Inflammatory spondylopathies may worsen pain after bed rest and cause morning stiffness. Tumor pain is usually increased by recumbency. Patients with disc disease have difficulty sitting, and those with lumbar spinal stenosis may suffer neurogenic claudication and require rest after walking modest distances. Patients who are unable to be at rest may have abdominal pathology with colic.

PHYSICAL EXAMINATION

The physical examination should include the general physical examination, especially that of the abdomen. Motor and sensory skills, coordination, and reflexes are checked. Sphincter tone and anal wink assessment may be needed. The spine should be evaluated for normal curvature, tenderness, mobility (flexion, extension, later flexion), and paravertebral spasm. A shelf suggests spondylolisthesis. Tenderness should be sought 2 or 3 cm lateral to the spine for facet joint disease. A sciatic list is away from the irritated nerve root when the herniation is lateral to the root and toward the side of the irritated root when the herniation is medial. Sciatic notch tenderness is checked with the Valsalva maneuver. The jugular compression test reproduces the pain in the radicular distribution, as does coughing and straining. Gait testing includes toe and heel walking. The usual upper limb muscle is weaker than a lower limb muscle, and patients with questionable weakness on formal strength testing may have obvious weakness when tested functionally. The knee and ankle reflexes are most easily elicited with the hip, knee, and ankle flexed at 90 degrees and the foot pressing lightly down on a supporting hand. The straight leg raising (Lasègue) test stretches a trapped nerve root at less than 50 degrees of hip flexion. This test can also be performed with the patient in the sitting position by extending the knee in such a manner as to disguise one's purpose if the examiner is suspicious of the patient's symptoms. Sensitivity is increased by Bragard's test, which involves lowering the leg after a positive straight-leg-raising test and then dorsiflexing the foot, reproducing the patient's pain. The well leg straight-leg-raising test has high specificity but low sensitivity. Hoover's sign is elicited by placing the examiner's hand under the heel of the good leg in a supine patient. The patient attempts to raise the weak leg, exerting a downward force on the examiner's hand with the good leg. If this force is not present, the patient is not really trying.

Simplified schemas of dermatome features are presented in Figures 113-2 to 113-4 on pages 724 to 726.

LABORATORY AND IMAGING STUDIES

Investigation of uncomplicated acute low back pain requires only the taking of a history and performance of a physical examination unless the examiner's impression after this evaluation suggests that the patient falls into a group at risk that requires early workup.

Acute low back pain with sciatica is more worrisome. If a cauda equina syndrome is suggested or neurologic deficit progresses, workup must be considered. Multiple imaging techniques are available. Plain spine films are inexpensive, and they are useful in the less common causes of back pain, such as tumor, congenital anomalies, and spondylolisthesis. They also have the advantage of being low in radiation. These films provide little information about the disc itself or the spinal canal, however. Magnetic resonance imaging (MRI) is expensive but provides visualization of the spine, the disc spaces, and the contents of the spinal canal. It has replaced most other lumbar imaging studies. It provides information about far lateral disc protrusion that does not disturb the canal. Computed tomography (CT) may be sufficient for straightforward disc disease but does not give any information about the contents of the spinal canal. It does, however, show the details of cortical bone and is preferred over MRI for visualization of bony disorders, because MRI sees marrow but not dense bone. Myelography may be performed with water-soluble contrast material and used in concert with CT to evaluate the contents of the spinal canal. In most cases adequate images can be obtained using only one modality. If the findings are equivocal, however, or if there are inconsistencies between the clinical and imaging findings, multiple investigations are in order. Isotope bone scan is helpful in inflammatory disease of bone or joint, as well as tumor. The use of discograms had a recent minor resurgence, but they have generally been abandoned. Epidural venography is no longer held in high esteem. EMG is, unfortunately, overly sensitive and less specific and, therefore, less useful than it might be. It is valuable for (1) excluding a more distal lesion; (2) confirming evidence of root compression; and (3) localizing the compression to one or more roots.

In evaluating the results of any of these studies, it is important to remember that in one third of patients disc herniation may not be accompanied by sciatica. Weakness and paresthesias may occur without pain. Disc herniation may cause back pain without sciatica.

TREATMENT

Many patients' acute low back pain may be relieved by 2 days of bed rest (supine in modified Fowler's position) or by back mobilization exercises. Acute low back pain with sciatica is of greater concern, but more than 50% of patients recover without surgery. Some clinicians have greater reservations about manipulation in the face of sciatica.

Subacute low back pain (a residual 10% of acute low back pain sufferers) requires more extensive treatment. A limited workup is in order. Limited bed rest may help. Lumbar traction probably exerts its benefit by confining the patient to bed. Heat and cold may be used, with variable effect. Injections of facet joints, epidural steroids, and peripheral nerve blocks are of questionable benefit. Many patients seem to benefit from the use of a lightweight flexible support with a molded plastic insert, which restricts lumbosacral motion and provides abdominal support and postural correction.

Subacute low back pain with sciatica requires an attempt at more specific diagnosis, with therapy then directed at the presumed etiology. In most case this kind of pain is caused by a herniated nucleus pulposus. Surgical removal of a disc fragment visualized and correlated with symptoms and signs promotes recovery in the 10% of patients who seem to require surgery. Chymopapain injections have become less favored because of a high incidence of anaphylaxis and reports of transverse myelopathy. Lumbar fusion is performed infrequently. Newer procedures for disc removal are far less extensive and do not seem to lead to an unstable back.

Many patients with severe neurogenic claudication from lumbar spinal stenosis are elderly. They nevertheless tend to benefit from large-scale decompressive laminectomy. This procedure should not be withheld purely on the basis of age.

Chronic back pain, despite conservative measures and a serious effort at finding a treatable cause, may require referral to a pain specialist. These patients may have to learn to live with some pain. Concurrent depression should be treated.

CONSIDERATIONS DURING PREGNANCY

Although only half of pregnant women complain of back pain, it is almost certainly more common. The need to maintain an erect posture while the enlarging uterus protrudes anterior to the center of gravity forces an increasingly lordotic posture. Periodic bed rest and avoidance of high-heeled shoes are in order. Alternating the feet on a step while standing may help. When, infrequently, sudden severe pain with sciatica and features of herniated disc occurs, bed rest is in order. The presence of cauda equina syndrome requires surgical intervention even during Pregnancy, but other deficits should be managed conservatively, if possible. MRI may be undertaken if either cauda equina syndrome or progressing neurologic disability indicate that surgery may be appropriate.

BIBLIOGRAPHY

Acute low back problems in adults. Clinical Practice Guidelines. U.S. Dept. of Health and Human Services Pub. No. 14, 1994.

Barnett HJM, Foster JB, Hudgson P. Syringomyelia. London: WB Saunders, 1973.

Borenstein DG, Wiesel SW, Boden SD. Low back pain: medical diagnosis and comprehensive management. 2nd ed. Philadelphia: WB Saunders, 1995.

Byrne TN, Waxman SG. Spinal cord compression: diagnosis and principles of management. Philadelphia: FA Davis, 1990.

Chiles III BW, Cooper PR. Current concepts: Acute spinal injury. N Engl J Med 1996;334:514.

Devereaux M. Acute low back pain. Am Acad Neurol Annual Courses. San Francisco, 1996; 7:423.

Empting LD. Ten questions about lower back pain. Neurologist 1996;2:2.

Frymoyer JW. Back pain and sciatica. N Engl J Med 1988;318:291.

Hoppenfeld S. Orthopaedic neurology: a diagnostic guide to neurologic levels. Philadelphia: JB Lippincott, 1977.

Malmivaara A, Hakkinen U, Aro T, et al. The treatment of acute low back pain—bed rest, exercises, or ordinary activity? N Engl J Med 1995;332:351.

Ropper AH, Wijdicks EFM, Truax BT. Gullain-Barré syndrome. Philadelphia: FA Davis, 1991

Young RR, Woolsey RM. Diagnosis and management of disorders of the spinal cord. Philadelphia: WB Saunders, 1995.

XIII

Ophthalmologic Problems

Primary Care for Women, edited by Phyllis C. Leppert and Fred M. Howard. Lippincott-Raven Publishers, Philadelphia © 1997.

119

Examination of the Eye

GWEN K. STERNS
JAMES FRANK

Taking a systematic approach to the examination of the eye helps the primary physician uncover pathology that threatens vision. A properly conducted, organized examination ensures appropriate intervention and timely referral.

OCULAR HISTORY

The basic eye examination begins with a thorough patient history of current symptoms and complaints, including their onset, duration, and severity. Loss of vision should be noted and defined as monocular, binocular, episodic, complete, or partial. Other symptoms, including glare, photosensitivity, spontaneous pain, pain with motion, discharge, and crusting (especially in the morning on awakening), should also be included. A detailed past ocular history and medical history, including current medications, allergies to medications, social history, and family history, should be elicited.

The patient's age is an important part of the history and should be considered strongly in the differential diagnosis. For example, a 40-year-old patient complaining of gradual onset of blurred vision for near tasks may lead the clinician to a presumptive diagnosis of presbyopia. An 80-year-old patient with the same complaints is more likely to have a cataract.

Past history can reveal important information to aid in the diagnosis. A young woman with a long history of cold sores on her lip who now presents with a red, painful eye may have a herpes simplex keratitis. A contact lens wearer with similar complaints may have a vision-threatening corneal ulcer from her contact lenses. Sudden loss of vision in an eye of a woman who has a prosthetic heart valve may suggest an embolus. Severe headaches in a woman with fluctuating vision should suggest the possibility of an intracranial process such as pseudotumor cerebri or a pituitary mass.

ASSESSING VISUAL FUNCTION

Visual Acuity

Every eye examination should include visual acuity testing, regardless of presenting complaints. A vision testing chart such as a Snellen chart for distance acuity is placed 20 feet from the patient under adequate diffuse illumination. Each eye is tested independently with and without the patient's most recent distance spectacle correction. Acuity is noted as cc (with correction) or sc (without correction). If the patient can see all letters on the 20/20 line at a distance of 20 feet from the chart, this is recorded as 20/20. If the patient missed two letters on the 20/20 line, then the vision should be recorded as 20/20–2. A patient who reads all the letters on the 20/40 line and two additional letters on the 20/30 line would have an acuity of 20/30+2. Ophthalmologists use the Latin designation of OD for right eye and OS for left eye.

Acuity is recorded as a ratio of the distance at which the patient can see an object divided by the distance at which the object can be seen by someone with normal vision. For most patients, the test objects are letters or numbers. For example, an acuity of 20/50 means the patient can read at 20 feet an object that a person with normal vision can read at 50 feet. Alternatively, the testing distance can be moved closer to the patient, with the numerator adjusted accordingly. This can be helpful in evaluating patients with severely reduced vision who require standardized testing to monitor their progress. For example, a patient with a retrobulbar neuritis might have an acuity reduced to 3/100. This means that the patient could read a test object at 3 feet that a person with normal vision could read at 100 feet.

If the patient cannot read the largest letter on the Snellen chart at any distance, then the distance at which the patient can perceive hand motion is noted and is recorded as HM at stated distance. If no hand motion is detected by the patient, then the presence of light perception or no light perception is recorded as LP or NLP. If only light perception is seen by the patient, the light should be shined from each of the four field quadrants and the patient asked to identify the direction from which the light is shining. If the answers are consistently correct, the vision may be recorded as light perception with projection in four quadrants. Each eye must be tested independently.

The pinhole visual acuity test helps identify patients with uncorrected refractive errors and corneal irregularity. The test should be performed on patients with a visual acuity less than 20/30 in either eye. The pinhole aperture is placed in front of each eye independently and the patient is asked to read the Snellen chart through one of the pinholes. The pinhole compensates for any uncorrected refractive error down to the 20/25 line. Therefore, a patient with a refractive error as the sole reason for diminished visual acuity should see the 20/25 Snellen acuity line. A patient who has 20/40 vision in the right eye without correction who pinholes to 20/25 should be recorded as OD VA sc 20/40, PH 20/25. If there is no improvement in vision with the pinhole aperture, the examiner should suspect a cause other than refractive error or corneal irregularity. Such causes may include media opacity (eg, vitreous hemorrhage), cataract, diabetic retinopathy, or optic nerve disease. These patients should be referred to an ophthalmologist for further evaluation.

Near vision should be tested with the patient wearing reading glasses or bifocals. Near vision is tested using the Rosenbaum Pocket Vision Screener or other equivalent near card. The patient should hold the card about 14 inches away, and the smallest line discernible should be read. The vision may be recorded in the Jaeger notation as J1, specifying the testing distance and whether the test was done with or without correction. Again, each eye is tested separately.

Confrontation Visual Fields

Many conditions are associated with loss of the peripheral visual field. Specialized visual field equipment is usually available only in a specialist's office. Confrontation visual field testing can be performed to screen for gross visual field defects and often is as accurate as formal perimetry testing. Often it is the only method available for patients with physical disabilities that prevent them from sitting at a field analyzer.

In one technique of confrontation field testing, the examiner and the patient face each other about an arm's length apart. The patient is instructed to occlude the left eye with an occluder or hand and to look at the examiner's left eye with her right eye. The field of the examiner's left eye is used as a standard for measuring the field in the patient's right eye and vice versa. The examiner asks the patient to count the number of fingers on the hand that the examiner presents to each of the four quadrants. Next, the examiner uses both hands and simultaneously presents fingers to both the nasal and temporal field of the eye. The patient's responses are recorded and visual field loss is noted. This examination can reveal visual field loss and help direct further examination and referral for more formalized testing.

Color Testing

Color defects in women are rare and may be associated with other vision problems. Color testing can be performed by use of standardized color test charts such as the pseudoisochromatic plates of Ishihara. Color perception may be diminished in conditions such as optic neuritis, and this may help in the diagnosis. The patient with optic neuritis may perceive a red target as a dull brown in the affected eye.

INTRAOCULAR PRESSURE

Tonometry, the determination of intraocular pressure, is easy to obtain in the typical office setting and can be performed by the primary care physician as part of a general physical examination. Tonometry should always be part of the formal eye examination. It should also be performed in patients who give a positive family history for glaucoma.

Intraocular pressure can be measured with the readily ava[illegible] Schiotz tonometer. A topical anesthetic is required. The patient [illegible] lay her head back or be supine. The eyelids are held open and [illegible] tonometer is held gently over the cornea. The amount of indentation of the cornea by a specific weight determines the intraocular pressure.

EXTERNAL EXAMINATION

The examination of the ocular adnexa should proceed in an orderly fashion. Using a penlight, the lids can be examined for evidence of infection such as crusting, swelling, and erythema. Lid position should be noted, checking for ptosis, proptosis, and lid lag. Lesions on the lid margin should be noted. An entropion—a lid that turns in—may produce tearing and irritation; an ectropion—eversion of the lid margin—suggests a lid neoplasm in a young patient and lid laxity causing excessive tearing in an older patient.

PUPILS

The pupils should be inspected for size, shape, reaction to light and near stimuli, and the presence or absence of the consensual light response. An irregularly shaped iris may suggest synechiae (adhesions) between the iris and lens due to an iritis, trauma, or acute glaucoma. An afferent pupillary defect can alert the examiner to an optic neuritis or retrobulbar neuritis.

MOTILITY

Eye movement is assessed in the cardinal positions of gaze: up and right, right, down and right, left and up, left, and left and down. The primary position of gaze should also be evaluated by having the patient fixate on a distant target, observing the position of the corneal light reflex. Any gross asymmetry of the light reflex in one or both eyes indicates a deviation of that eye.

OPHTHALMOSCOPY

The technique of direct ophthalmoscopy should be a part of all ophthalmic and general physical examinations. The first step in ophthalmoscopy is to look for the red fundus reflection, which can easily be seen without magnification at a distance of 20 to 40 cm. A full red reflex quickly rules out gross corneal lesions, dense media opacities, and complete retinal detachments. Any opacities present appear as black forms against the red background of the reflex. Next, the cornea is inspected with a strong plus lens of about +10.00 to +15.00 diopters. From a distance of 2 cm, one may easily see corneal scars, ulcers, and foreign bodies. In ocular herpes simplex keratitis, dendritic corneal lesions may also be seen using this technique.

Abnormalities of the anterior chamber aqueous such as hyphema or hypopyon may be seen. Adequate detail of the iris architecture using a +15.00 diopter lens may be used to rule out tumor, nodules, or synechiae. With a slightly lower power of +4.00 to +8.00 diopters, the lens may be examined, looking for cataract formation.

Extending the focus into the vitreous cavity using +4.00 to +8.00 power, opacities in the vitreous can be seen. Blood in the vitreous appears as bright-red blood if there has been a recent hemorrhage or as dark-brown clumping if the hemorrhage is more chronic.

The funduscopic examination should include inspection of the optic nerve, vessels, macula, and mid-periphery. The disc is normally round or oval, with the nasal edge less distinct than the temporal edge. The sclera may be seen surrounding the optic nerve in myopic patients. The disc, with a central white depression (cup), may be seen. Cup-to-disc ratios should be recorded; larger than normal ratios suggest glaucoma.

The macula is temporal to the disc. It may appear darker than the surrounding retina. The central reflex in the macula is the foveal reflex. Clumping or loss of pigment in this region, with resultant loss of central vision, suggests macular degeneration.

The retinal vessels should be examined for caliber, course, and crossing appearance. The ratio of the normal venous diameter to the arteriole diameter is 3:2. Changes in this ratio, defects in the crossings, and increases in the light reflex of the arteriolar color suggest arteriolar sclerotic or hypertensive retinopathy.

SUMMARY

If the examination described yields an abnormal finding that requires additional evaluation, the patient should be referred to an ophthalmologist. Supplemental diagnostic testing such as indirect ophthalmoscopy, neuroimaging, gonioscopy, perimetry, ultrasonography, or fluorescein angiography may be performed.

BIBLIOGRAPHY

Berson FG, ed. Ophthalmology study guide. American Academy of Ophthalmology, 1987.

Tasman W, Jaeger EA, eds. Duane's clinical ophthalmology. Philadelphia: JB Lippincott, 1994.

120
Red Eye

RONALD D. PLOTNIK
GWEN K. STERNS

Primary Care for Women, edited by Phyllis C. Leppert and Fred M. Howard. Lippincott-Raven Publishers, Philadelphia © 1997.

Conjunctivitis refers to any disorder causing inflammation of the conjunctiva, usually manifested as a "red eye" or "pink eye." These conditions range from inconsequential to severe. Etiologies include infection, trauma, allergy, and toxins. Further, a variety of conditions are unique to the eye (eg, glaucoma, dry eye) that may result in redness.

In these conditions, the eye appears red because of inflammation of the conjunctiva. The conjunctiva is the outermost layer adjacent to the white sclera and normally is clear. Injection or dilation of the blood vessels results in the redness seen. The conjunctiva can be affected primarily, such as in cases of infection, or can become red as a generalized reaction to other ocular conditions. In the primary care setting, the history often gives a clue as to the etiology, and the associated symptoms often are helpful in delineating a cause.

Most primary care settings do not provide the physician with a biomicroscope or "slit lamp," which is the device ophthalmologists use to examine the eye. This allows a magnified detailed inspection of the eye and often gives a definitive answer as to the cause of the red eye. It becomes imperative, then, to be able to decide who can be treated empirically and who needs urgent referral. Further, the range of treatment in a primary care setting should be broad enough to allow treatment of the most common conditions but narrow enough to prevent inappropriate treatment. In a practical sense, common bacterial and viral conjunctivitis can be treated by the primary care physician whereas most other causes need referral. Warning signs exist as to which patients need referral—"red flags" that topical antibiotics for conjunctivitis are not the appropriate treatment.

ETIOLOGY AND DIFFERENTIAL DIAGNOSIS

The following provides a partial list of some of the more common causes of a red eye. Each has characteristic signs and symptoms, as well as specific treatment. The most common cause of a red eye is bacterial or viral conjunctivitis (Table 120-1).

HISTORY

In the ophthalmologist's office, the history may be important, depending on what signs are present on the slit-lamp examination. In the primary care setting, however, the history is imperative in that the only other information available are the signs seen by the primary care provider's naked eye.

The history can be divided into two parts. The first includes onset, exposure history, past medical history, course, and symptoms. The second includes specific exclusion of all symptoms that require urgent referral.

The course of onset can be an important differentiating historical point. More severe conditions tend to come on more quickly. History of exposure to other individuals with a red eye is important. Bacterial and viral forms of conjunctivitis often are antedated by close contact with another person with a red eye, especially contact with children. Certain sexually transmitted diseases are transmittable to the eye. "Cold sore" exposure may be important. A previous upper respiratory infection or fever may give additional information. A history of connective tissue disease, shingles, chicken pox, atopy, rosacea, herpes simplex labialis, or previous red eye provides clues to the etiology. A history of trauma, contact lens wear, eye drop usage, chemical exposure, occupational history, or previous ocular surgery or conditions also is helpful.

Ocular symptoms include tearing, light sensitivity (photophobia), reactive eye lid closure (blepharospasm), discharge, decreased vision, eye pain or irritation, foreign body sensation, itching, double vision, pain on eye movement, periocular swelling, unequal pupil size, decreased or restricted eye movement, headache, proptosis (eye projecting somewhat out of the socket), or associated nausea and vomiting. The warning signs and symptoms that the condition is more than a simple case of conjunctivitis and needs urgent referral are listed here:

- Decreased vision
- Unequal pupils
- Significant ocular or periocular swelling

- Significant photophobia
- Associated nausea or vomiting
- Significant ocular pain
- Double vision
- Proptosis
- History of contact lens wear

Often, these symptoms indicate cornea involvement, significant ocular inflammation, infection, or an elevated eye pressure (glaucoma). Treatment of these conditions requires an ophthalmologist's attention.

PHYSICAL EXAMINATION AND CLINICAL FINDINGS

In the primary care setting, the ocular examination should be directed to diagnose conjunctivitis and to exclude other ocular diseases. Certain signs can be evaluated, even without the use of specialized equipment. The examination should begin with a determination of visual acuity. A wall or hand-held chart is optimal. If the patient wears corrective glasses, they should be worn for this test. Conjunctivitis usually does not decrease visual acuity.

The penlight can be a very useful instrument. Pupil size and reactivity should be determined. The pupils should be equal, round, and reactive to the light. The cornea surface can be evaluated by shining the penlight directly on the eye. The cornea light reflection or "reflex" is usually smooth and bright. Irregularities of the cornea surface may dull or distort the reflex. A whitish opacity or spot, graying, or a foreign body on the cornea may be visualized in some conditions.

The periorbital skin should be inspected for signs such as vesicles, redness, thickening, swelling, purulence, scaling, or excoriation. The conjunctiva should be grossly inspected for injection (redness) and chemosis (swelling). Gross purulence usually is present with bacterial and sometimes with viral conjunctivitis.

The nature of the ocular redness also may be important. Redness primarily in a circle around the cornea, redness with a purple hue, redness that affects only one portion of the eye, intense redness, or marked enlargement of vessels should prompt referral.

Fluorescein dye can be instilled in the eye and viewed with a cobalt blue light filter. This blue filter is built into most direct ophthalmoscopes, or it may be available as a penlight attachment. Defects in the corneal surface cell layer (epithelium) show up as bright green in ordinary light and as bright yellow in the cobalt blue light. Any dye uptake by the cornea suggests corneal disease (as opposed to primary conjunctivitis) and requires referral. If a slit-lamp biomicroscope is available (such as in some offices and emergency rooms), the eye should be examined to rule out other disease.

LABORATORY STUDIES

In the ophthalmologist's office, cultures often are helpful. This is especially so if the symptoms and signs are nonspecific and infection is suspected. Certain bacteria are considered to be normal flora on the eye (such as coagulase-negative *Staphylococcus*), but even these can cause infection in certain situations. In suspected bacterial conjunctivitis, cultures are obtained only if there is a poor clinical response to treatment. Most topical antibiotics are effective for bacterial conjunctivitis and, therefore, cultures usually are not helpful. Cultures must be obtained with antibiotic sensitivities for any corneal ulcer because this is a much more serious condition.

Table 120-1. Common Causes of Conjuntivitis

Infectious
Bacterial conjunctivitis
Viral conjunctivitis
Bacterial keratitis
Herpes simplex
Herpes zoster
Fungal keratitis
Orbital/preseptal cellulitis
Chlamydia
Traumatic
Subconjunctival hemorrhage
Traumatic iritis
Corneal abrasion
Conjunctival lacerations
Foreign bodies
Chemical injury
Ocular Conditions
Contact lens overwear
Blepharoconjunctivitis
Acute glaucoma
Dry eye (Sjögren syndrome)
Iritis (intraocular inflammation)
Scleritis (inflammation of the sclera)
Allergy/Toxic
Contact
Hayfever
Contact lens reactions
Atopy
Chemicals

Typical herpes simplex or herpes zoster lesions do not require cultures because the clinical picture often is sufficiently clear without cultures. Probable viral conjunctivitis, likewise, is usually not worth culturing if the clinical suspicion is high enough. Herpes lesions and adenovirus may affect the cornea in the form of an immune reaction, but cultures during this phase usually give negative results. With certain slit-lamp findings, testing for infection with *Chlamydia* can be helpful.

In the primary care setting, cultures usually are not warranted. If the clinician is sufficiently concerned—either in terms of the diagnosis or in terms of antibiotic sensitivity—to obtain a culture, the patient should be referred to an ophthalmologist so that a slit-lamp examination can be performed.

CLINICAL FINDINGS AND TREATMENT CONSIDERATIONS

The following discussion covers many of the more common causes of red eye. It is by no means exhaustive, and the patient's broader clinical situation must be taken into consideration.

Infectious Conjunctivitis

Bacterial Conjunctivitis

Bacterial conjunctivitis is common and may have been preceded by exposure to a child or adult with "pink eye." The infection causes tearing, occasional mild blurring of vision because of the purulence on the eye (which can be "blinked away"), and redness. The discharge ranges from mucoid to frank yellow or green purulence. Usual organisms isolated include *Staphylococcus aureus*, coagulase-negative *Staphylococcus*, *Streptococcus*, and, in children, *Haemophilus influenzae*. Although uncommon, gonococcal conjunctivitis produces copious purulent discharge and requires systemic treatment. Other organisms usually require only 7 days of topical antibiotic treatment. Most organisms are overwhelmed by the antibiotic, and specific sensitivity tests usually are not needed unless the patient does not respond to treatment.

Never use an antibiotic–steroid combination or steroids alone because this may lead to significant complications, including the potentiation of herpes simplex virus as well as worsened bacterial and viral infections. As a general rule, primary care physicians should not use steroids at all before a detailed slit-lamp examination, which usually requires a referral. Contagious precautions should be taken because patients may be infectious for several days. Additionally, topical anesthetics should never be dispensed because they are toxic to the ocular surface and prevent healing.

Viral Conjunctivitis

Viral conjunctivitis usually is caused by adenovirus. The incubation period can be as long as 2 weeks, and often there is a history of exposure. There may have been an antecedent upper respiratory tract infection, and an associated fever may be present. It is typically bilateral, although one side usually is more severely affected. The eyes are red, and the discharge is watery to mucoid. The vision may be decreased later in the course of the disease. Mild photophobia may be present, and often there is an enlarged tender preauricular node. Viral conjunctivitis usually runs its course without major aftereffects but may lead to corneal findings with decreased vision. Treatment consists of keeping the eye clear of accumulating discharge, using cool compresses, and employing contagious precautions. Viral conjunctivitis is extremely contagious and can be transmissible for approximately 2 weeks from the onset of symptoms. Patients should be advised to use prudent hand washing and to avoid sharing towels or pillows. Because of the infectious and often epidemic nature of viral adenovirus conjunctivitis, health care providers and others, including day-care workers, often must be secluded for 2 weeks. The virus can live on dry surfaces for many hours.

Bacterial Keratitis

Bacterial keratitis is an ophthalmic emergency requiring frequent fortified antibiotic drops. It is significant for the primary care provider to exclude this diagnosis. The vision usually is markedly decreased, but not always. The eye is typically extremely red, and there may be copious discharge. Contact lens wear, especially extended-wear lens use, is a risk factor. Sometimes a white opacity can be seen on the cornea, or the cornea luster may be decreased. If there is doubt as to whether this entity is present, urgent referral is needed.

Chlamydia

Infection with *Chlamydia* is sexually transmitted and usually is spread to the eyes by way of the fingers. A history of urethral or vaginal discharge may be elicited. Infection with *Chlamydia* causes a red eye minimally responsive to topical antibiotics. The vision may be decreased slightly. Treatment should consist of systemic doxycycline or similar medication for 2 to 3 weeks. It is important to additionally treat the sexual partners of these patients. Coinfection with *Chlamydia* also should be considered when treating other sexually transmitted eye infections, such as infection with gonococcus.

Herpes Simplex

Herpes simplex may affect the eye as the primary infection, but more often it represents a reactivation of latent infection in the trigeminal ganglion. Herpes simplex virus travels out the nerve axons and causes infectious herpes simplex conjunctivitis or keratitis. Precipitating factors may include a fever, "flu," or a history of trauma. Although used for the sequelae of the virus, treatment with topical steroids during acute infection may cause marked worsening with permanent visual loss. This is the most cogent reason that the "red eye" should not be treated by primary care physicians with steroid or antibiotic–steroid combinations. Acute infection often takes the form of a "dendrite" or branch-like lesion on the cornea that stains with fluorescein dye. Treatment consists of topical antiviral agents tapered over the course of 3 weeks. Oral antiviral agents may be of additional benefit.

Herpes Zoster

Herpes zoster may affect the eye in the form of "shingles" or, less often, after a case of chicken pox. In the more common form, an adult presents after having had chicken pox as a child, with right- or left-sided dermatomal skin involvement that may involve the scalp, forehead, eye, nose, and cheek. Eye findings range from minimal conjunctivitis to severe ischemic ocular disease. The corneal sequelae of herpes zoster can last for many years and may require topical steroids to control inflammation. Topical antiviral agents usually are not given, but oral antiviral agents have been shown to significantly decrease ocular complications of the disease. Postherpetic neuralgia often can be controlled with topical capsaicin, a substance P inhibitor.

Fungal Keratitis

Fungal keratitis or corneal infection is more common in tropical climates and may be associated with contact lens wear. Treatment consists of topical and oral antifungal agents. The corneal surface usually displays a defect that stains with fluorescein dye, and an underlying white spot usually is present.

Orbital and Preseptal Cellulitis

The orbital septum divides the outer periorbital skin from the eye orbit or socket itself. Infection of the preseptal or skin region requires oral antibiotics. Gram-positive organisms usually are etiologic. Deeper infection of the orbit itself is an ocular emergency, requiring intravenous antibiotics. Urgent computed tomography or magnetic resonance scanning also is indicated to rule out orbital abscess, which require incision and drainage. Although preseptal cellulitis may give a mild red eye, no other signs are present in the eye or orbit. With orbital cellulitis, the clinician can see proptosis, restriction of eye movement, abnormal pupil responses, marked swelling, decreased vision, copious discharge, and abnormalities of the fifth cranial nerve (ie, paresthesia).

Traumatic Causes of Conjunctivitis

Subconjunctival Hemorrhage

With subconjunctival hemorrhage, mild bleeding can occur in the space beneath the conjunctiva, over the white sclera. The blood appears vibrant red and is homogenous. Blood vessels are not engorged. Subconjunctival hemorrhage usually is sectoral; it is inconsequential and needs no treatment. Resolution may take as long as 2 weeks. Subconjunctival hemorrhage may be caused by minor trauma, significant coughing, systemic anticoagulation, daily aspirin use, or as an isolated event.

Traumatic Iritis

Any blunt trauma to the eye can cause intraocular inflammation. At the slit-lamp examination, this is evidenced by white blood cells floating free in the anterior chamber of the eye. There is often associated photophobia, decreased vision, tearing, and pain. Topical steroids and a dilating drops usually are prescribed. A slit lamp is needed to make the diagnosis.

Corneal Abrasion

The surface layer of cells of the cornea or epithelium can be abraded by a variety of means. Patients may report having been hit in the eye by a baby's finger, tree branch, or piece of paper. Topical antibiotic ointment, either with or without patching, is usually indicated. One type of abrasion deserves special mention. Contact lens wearers may present with what is believed by the patient to be an abrasion. Clinical examination also can be consistent with this, but corneal infection must be ruled out. It is safer not to patch contact lens "abrasions" and to treat with topical antibiotic ointment. Patching may make infection worse, but this is not of concern for most abrasions of other etiologies.

Conjunctival Lacerations

Trauma may cause a laceration of the conjunctiva, which may involve the underlying sclera. Referral is indicated if this is suspected.

Foreign Bodies

Conjunctival and corneal foreign bodies are relatively common. Many are metallic and are occupationally related. Conjunctival and corneal foreign bodies can be removed easily with a needle or burr at the slit lamp. Sometimes the foreign body can be seen with the naked eye, and a moistened cotton swab can be used for removal. Conjunctival foreign bodies are more amenable to removal than corneal by this method. Antibiotic ointments usually are prescribed for several days as prophylaxis.

Chemical Injury

Chemical injuries vary from mild to catastrophic. Mild injuries cause a red eye with no decreased vision. Topical antibiotic–steroid combinations may be used if other causes of red eye have been ruled out. Referral usually is indicated if symptoms are severe or persistent. More severe injuries are caused by alkali or acid. Alkali injuries are worse and may cause significant and permanent ocular damage. Immediate treatment for chemical injury consists of copious irrigation at the site of injury, which is continued into the emergency room. The pH level must be checked periodically to assess progress and then again after irrigation to make sure no residual alkali or acidic particles remain. Urgent referral is indicated for most chemical injuries. Patients with minor injuries, a mild red eye, no fluorescein staining, and no other symptoms may be observed carefully.

Ocular Conditions Causing Red Eye

Contact Lens Overwear

Contact lens overwear may cause a severe red eye. There is often tearing, photophobia, and decreased vision. The history often includes sleeping in daily wear lenses. Temporary cessation of lens wear is necessary. The frequency of infectious keratitis is significantly increased in these patients, and referral is needed for slit-lamp examination to rule out signs of infection. Cultures may be taken. Patching is not indicated, nor is topical steroid use. Contact lens solution toxicity may be an additional factor. Often, topical antibiotics are used empirically.

Blepharitis and Dry Eye Syndrome

The tear film is composed of water from the lacrimal glands and oil from the meibomianum glands. Aging causes decreased water production from the lacrimal glands, which gives rise to dry eye syndrome. Sjögren syndrome is a form of this. Blepharitis, or plugging of the oil glands in the eye lids, results in decreased lubricating oil in the tears. These conditions give rise to chronic irritation and redness from poor quantity and quality of the tear film. The history of gradual onset and long-lasting symptoms in an adult, especially in women, can be characteristic. Slit-lamp examination and special testing can confirm the diagnosis.

Acute Glaucoma

In predisposed individuals, pupil dilation in low light conditions can cause acute angle closure glaucoma. "Angle closure" refers to the anatomic changes that occur to cause this type of glaucoma. The eye pressure is extremely high, causing severe pain, a red eye, a hazy cornea, and often nausea and vomiting. Urgent referral is needed to prevent visual loss. Treatment consists of lowering the pressure with drops and oral medications and then performing a laser procedure as the definitive treatment. The low light conditions of a movie theater in an older adult is the classic setting. Pupil dilation as part of the eye examination also can precipitate this in certain individuals.

Iritis (Intraocular Inflammation)

Although mentioned previously as precipitated by trauma, iritis can be seen as an intrinsic entity with intraocular inflammation without precipitating factors. Iritis often is seen in the setting of connective tissue diseases, which are associated with significantly increased incidence. Treatment includes topical steroids and a dilating drop, which can prevent intraocular scarring. In an otherwise healthy individual, a systemic workup may be indicated if the iritis is bilateral, recurrent, or severe. Visual loss, photophobia, tearing, and pain are usual accompanying symptoms.

Scleritis (Inflammation of the Sclera)

Inflammation of sclera presents as a red eye. It can be severe and may be associated with visual loss, a small nodule on the eye, sectoral redness, corneal inflammation, and iritis. Although scleritis is not necessarily associated with systemic connective tissue disease, it often is, and a systemic workup usually is indicated. Although topical steroid and nonsteroidal antiinflammatory drugs may be helpful, systemic treatment usually is needed. This consists of indomethacin (Indocin) or another nonsteroidal antiinflammatory agent, with prednisone or systemic immunosuppressants used for more severe cases.

Allergic Reactions

Hay Fever

Seasonal allergies may give rise to a red eye accompanied by prominent itching. Tearing and conjunctival swelling may be present. Allergic conjunctivitis can be treated with cool compresses and systemic antihistamines. Several topical products exist that may help, including antihistamines, mast cell stabilizers, and nonsteroidal antiinflammatory drugs.

CONSIDERATIONS IN PREGNANCY

A primary consideration in pregnancy is the use of diagnostic and therapeutic drops. The small amount of each drop instilled is absorbed systemically. Two techniques diminish this significantly. Normally the excess drop is removed from the eye surface through the lacrimal drainage system. This consists of two small openings (puncta) in the medial lids (one upper and one lower) that connect to a lumen, which empties into the nose. This is why crying results in clear rhinorrhea. The blinking action helps propel the excess drop into this system. Five minutes of lid closure, without blinking, after drop instillation decreases systemic absorption. As a second technique, pinching the bridge of the nose, including the medial corner of each eye, effectively closes the openings to the system. Combined lid closure and punctal occlusion may be even more effective.

The usual course of antibiotic treatment is dosing four times daily for 1 week. Treatment for 5 days may be effective. Eye drops, as opposed to ointments, usually are preferred. Antiviral drops may need to be used and are often continued, at a tapering dose, for 3 weeks. The use of fluorescein dye and dilating drops, especially phenylephrine, should be avoided. Topical steroids should be used at the lowest needed dose. Antihistamines and other drops should be avoided unless symptoms necessitate their use. Lid closure and punctal occlusion after dosing should always be performed. Obstetric consultation should be obtained before using any drops.

BIBLIOGRAPHY

Arffa RC. Grayson's diseases of the cornea, 3rd ed. St Louis: Mosby Year Book, 1991.

Fraunfelder FT, Roy FH. Current ocular therapy, 4th ed. Philadelphi: WB Saunders, 1995.

Smolin G, Thoft RA. The cornea: scientific foundations and clinical practice, 2nd ed. Boston: Little, Brown, 1987.

Primary Care for Women, edited by Phyllis C. Leppert and Fred M. Howard. Lippincott-Raven Publishers, Philadelphia © 1997.

121
Eye Trauma

HENRY S. METZ

Eye trauma is common among both men and women. However, certain types of trauma may be seen more frequently in one sex than in the other. For example, workplace forms of injury, specifically those involved with activities such as hammering, chiseling, and grinding, are found more often in men. Ocular trauma secondary to spousal abuse, facial cosmetics and their applicators, or an infant's fingernail scratch of the cornea are noted more frequently in women.

Although most forms of eye injury are not specific to either males or females, emphasis in this chapter will be placed on trauma found more commonly among women.

DIFFERENTIAL DIAGNOSIS

In most cases there is little question about the etiology of the ocular trauma or its differential diagnosis. The history should contain the information necessary to explain the cause of the eye problem. Examination findings are used to verify the history and to evaluate the extent of the damage to the globe and lids. If these findings are not consistent, the history should be questioned. Imaging studies in certain types of trauma may also assist in making the correct diagnosis. These types include, for example, orbital floor or medial wall fracture, or a suspected intraocular foreign body.

HISTORY

The details of the mechanism of eye injury are most important. For example, what were the size and speed of the object that struck the eye? Was it sharp or blunt? In the case of a chemical injury, what type of material was involved? Was it acidic or alkaline? It is often useful if the patient can bring in the label from the box or bottle of the offending agent. What immediate treatment has been given, either ocular irrigation or medication? Is the eye painful? Has there been a change in visual acuity? If there has been solar injury or ultraviolet light exposure, how long did the exposure last?

Usually, the history will reveal a great deal about the nature and severity of the injury. However, it may be difficult to get sufficient or accurate information from a patient who has been unconscious, or from a young child who was out of the view of an adult at the time of the ocular trauma.

PHYSICAL EXAMINATION AND CLINICAL FINDINGS

The eye examination after trauma must be done carefully, so as not to increase the damage. When the injury has not been penetrating, a topical anesthetic will often provide increased comfort and improved cooperation from the patient. While holding the lids apart to inspect the globe, pressure on the eye should be avoided. If possible, visual acuity should be measured with the patient's own corrective lenses or through a pinhole aperture.

Corneal Abrasion and Foreign Body on the Eye or Eyelid

Patients generally complain of a foreign body sensation and often give a history of something blowing into their eye or of getting scratched with a foreign object. This could be from such diverse sources as a tree branch, a baby's fingernail, or a mascara brush while applying makeup. Fluorescein instillation in the cul-de-sac will show the abrasion or foreign particle very well with a cobalt blue light illuminator. The fluorescein collects in the defect in the cornea and is seen as a bright green fluorescent color. Contact lens overwear, especially with older hard plastic, polymethylmethacrylate (PMMA) lenses, will result in a foreign body sensation and a punctate staining pattern centrally on the cornea. Eversion of the upper lid may be needed to locate a foreign particle on the conjunctival surface of the lid.

Blunt Injury

Blunt injuries may be caused by a fist, elbow, or knee, and often occur in an altercation or during a sporting event. They may also be caused by a ball, such as a baseball or soccer ball. Ecchymoses (black eye) and lid swelling are often noted first. The lids may be swollen shut so that the globe is not easily seen. When examining the eye, the lids should be separated gently and carefully to avoid causing additional injury. In severe cases, it may be necessary to instill a topical anesthetic and cautiously use lid retractors to gain exposure.

Injury to the globe may include a hyphema, which is blood in the anterior chamber (Fig. 121-1), dialysis of the root of the iris, lens subluxation, cataract (Fig. 121-2), vitreous bleeding, retinal detachment, and macula edema. Even when a sharp object was not involved, the globe may be ruptured, with protrusion of the iris, uveal tissue, and vitreous.

Trauma from spousal abuse has produced many of the problems just mentioned. In addition, orbital damage may be found with fracture of the floor or medial wall of the orbit (Fig. 121-3). With floor fractures, up gaze is restricted and down gaze may also be limited. Often, there is vertical strabismus with diplopia. Exophthalmos, secondary to orbital edema, may be noted initially, but enophthalmos may be found later due to orbital tissue sunken into the maxillary antrum. With fracture of the medial wall, there is esotropia and limited abduction.

Perforating Injury

Perforating injuries are caused by sharp objects, such as knives and glass. The globe can be lacerated, with lid, cornea, or scleral involvement. This may be accompanied by cataract formation, vitreous hemorrhage, and retinal damage. Occasionally, one or more of the extraocular muscles and the optic nerve may be lacerated. Vision may be extremely poor, and the eyeball may be soft to palpation or on intraocular pressure measurement. Trauma of this type may have surprisingly little associated pain.

Small perforations may be caused by metallic foreign bodies entering the eye with great speed in a heated state. This occurs most often when hammering against a chisel. Glass foreign particles may also enter the globe. This injury can occur as a result of a motor vehicle accident or from an object striking a patient's non–shatterproof spectacles, causing pieces of glass to enter the eye. Particles may remain wedged in the cornea, or enter the anterior chamber, lens, vitreous, or retina. Retinal tear and hemorrhage are usually seen with a foreign body in the posterior segment of the eye (Fig. 121-4). Occasionally, the foreign body will enter with sufficient velocity to perforate the posterior sclera also, causing a double perforation. The prognosis in these injuries is very poor.

Chemical Injury

Almost any chemical agent can accidentally get in the eye. Soap, in the form of shampoo, is the most common agent to irritate the globe. Fortunately, this usually results in only mild-to-moderate conjunctival injection and temporary burning of the eyes without any permanent damage.

More serious ocular injury can be caused by acidic or alkaline substances. Acids produce damage that is somewhat less severe, because alkaline agents penetrate the tissues more rapidly. Findings include not only redness, which is often marked, but loss of corneal epithelium, coagulation of the vessels around the limbus, corneal opacities in the more severe cases, and a great deal of pain. Substances around the home that contain concentrated alkalis include oven and drain cleaners. Accidental splashes causing eye injury can be prevented, or minimized, by using protective goggles or glasses.

Photosensitized Radiation Injury

Ultraviolet radiation may be the most common form of radiation producing damage to the eye. A diffuse, punctate keratitis usu-

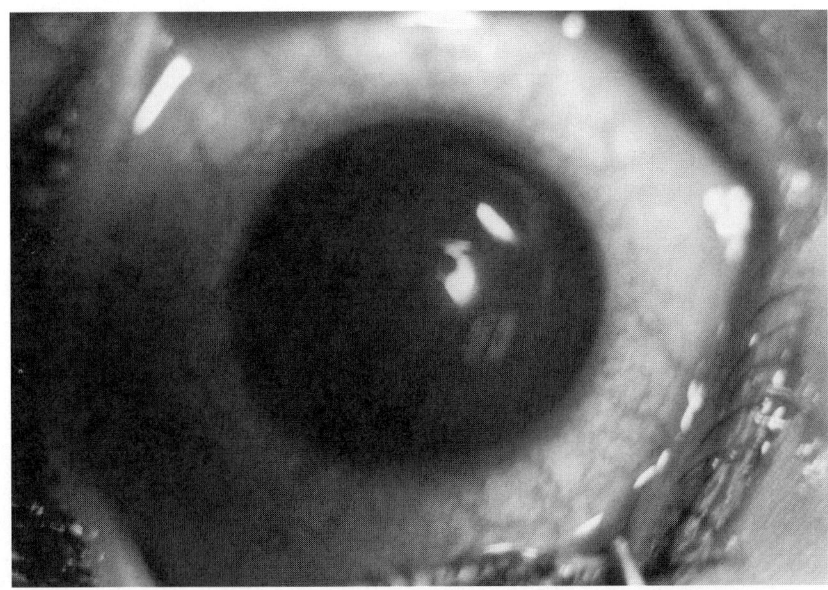

Figure 121-1. Traumatic hyphema. The anterior chamber is completely filled with dark red blood (eight-ball hemorrhage), obscuring all iris details.

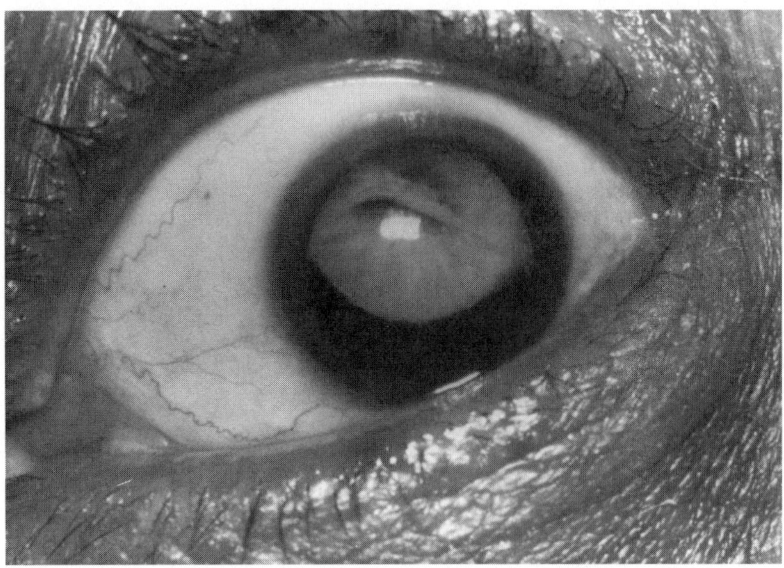

Figure 121-2. Traumatic cataract with lens subluxation (partial dislocation).

ally results, with marked pain, blurred vision, redness, and tearing, often waking the patient in the middle of the night. This damage may be caused by exposure to a welder's arc or to ultraviolet light from lamps at a tanning parlor. The use of protective goggles can prevent corneal trauma in these cases.

X-irradiation and gamma irradiation, usually given in the course of treatment of a lesion near the eye, also can cause severe ocular damage. Cataracts are seen commonly, and radiation retinopathy may appear later. Decreased or absent tear formation, with drying of the ocular surface, has been described following irradiation. Proper shielding during therapy may be helpful but does not always avoid the problem.

Solar retinopathy can occur following prolonged, direct gazing at the sun. Looking directly at an eclipse can produce this effect. Foveal depigmentation is frequently noted, with a surrounding ring of pigmentation in the perifoveal area. Central vision is reduced, with a central scotoma found on visual field testing.

Thermal Injury

Burns can affect the eye in two ways: a direct corneal burn, as from a cigarette ash, or more severely, a burn injury to the face, with resultant lid involvement. Tears usually cool hot ashes as they touch the eye, and an epithelial defect, such as an abrasion, may be the only result. With marked facial and lid burns, the eyes can lose their protective lid covering and the problem of drying caused by corneal exposure becomes paramount. Less marked involvement may cause lid ectropion, also resulting in corneal exposure, or entropion, with the difficulty of the lashes turning inwards, rubbing against the cornea.

Freezing injury to the cornea is more unusual. Localized edema may be noted, which often resolves spontaneously.

LABORATORY AND IMAGING STUDIES

Generally, laboratory studies are not especially useful in assessing ocular injuries. The one instance where they may be of help is in cases of penetrating eye trauma or an intraocular foreign body. These injuries may result in secondary intraocular infection, and cultures taken from the area of the wound, from aqueous fluid in the anterior chamber, or from the vitreous may be helpful in diagnosing the responsible organism. With this knowledge, drug therapy can be more precisely targeted.

Imaging studies can be useful in several situations. Orbital floor and medial wall fractures can often be demonstrated radiologically (Fig. 121-5).The location of an intraocular foreign particle, if radiopaque, can be determined with the appropriate x-rays. In some cases, the foreign material may be found to lie outside the globe, thus obviating the need for a surgical extraction from the eye.

Another type of imaging study can be of value when the media (cornea, lens, vitreous) are cloudy. An ultrasound examination can locate a foreign body that is not radiopaque, as well as reveal the presence of vitreous hemorrhage and a trauma-induced retinal detachment (Fig. 121-6).

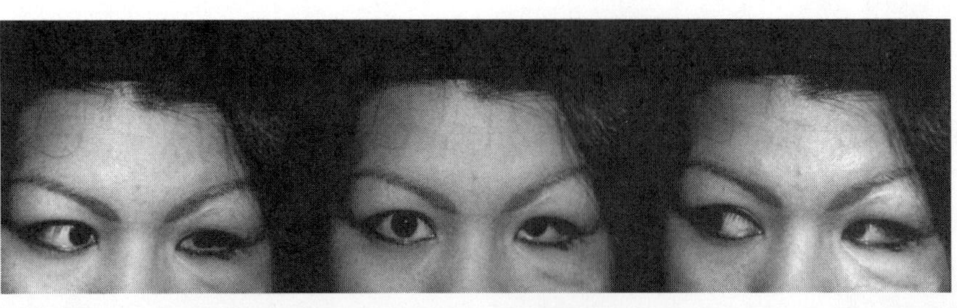

Figure 121-3. Traumatic fracture of the medial wall of the orbit. Left gaze (*left*), shows a decreased range of abduction of the left eye; central gaze, demonstrating a left esotropia (*middle*), and right gaze (*right*).

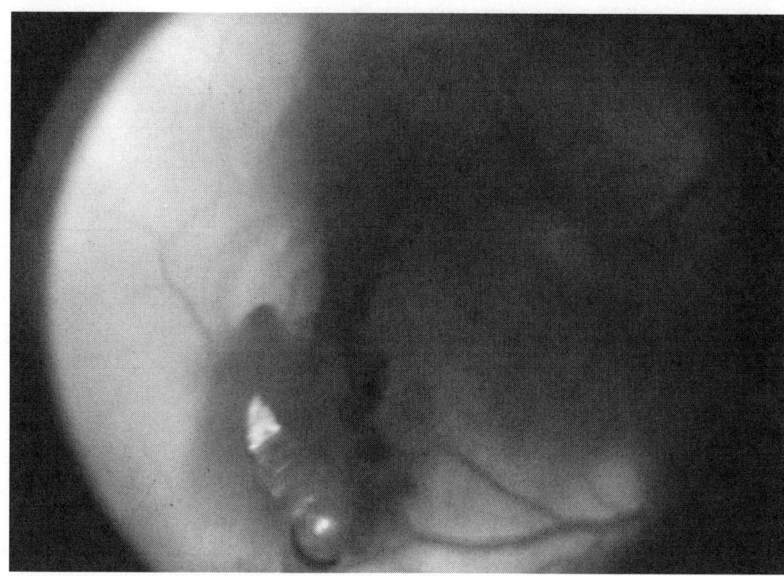

Figure 121-4. Metallic intraocular foreign body with vitreous hemorrhage partially obscuring some of the retinal details.

TREATMENT

Corneal Abrasion and Foreign Body of the Eye or Eye Lid

Foreign bodies on the cornea or under the eyelid should be wiped away with a cotton-tipped applicator after instilling a topical anesthetic into the cul-de-sac. If the particle is adherent, a corneal spud can be used to remove the foreign body. An abrasion is usually found after the particle has been removed.

Abrasions are treated by instilling a topical, broad-spectrum antibiotic drop or ointment, and then applying a pressure dressing for 1 to 2 days until the epithelial defect is covered and no longer picks up fluorescein stain. The pressure patch usually improves the patient's comfort and speeds up corneal healing. An intact epithelium provides a barrier to corneal infection. The aim of treatment is to prevent the occurrence of corneal ulceration.

Blunt Injury

The lid edema and ecchymosis often found following blunt injury may require little treatment other than the application of an ice pack.

Hyphema must be considered a serious injury and the patient placed at rest for 5 days. Bilateral eye patching, formerly a common treatment, is no longer the standard form of therapy. The hyphema will usually clear in 4 to 5 days. Rebleeding can be more severe than the original episode of hemorrhage, and is most common in the first 5 days following trauma. For this reason, the patient should be advised to rest for 5 days after the injury. Aminocaproic acid, an antifibrinolytic agent, has been recommended by some clinicians to prevent breakup of the blood clot in the anterior chamber and reduce the incidence of secondary hemorrhage. If the hemorrhage does not resorb, or if there is a rebleeding episode, glaucoma may ensue with subsequent damage to the optic nerve and blood staining of the cornea. Diamox, taken orally to reduce aqueous production, and topical glaucoma eye medication to both increase aqueous outflow and decrease fluid production, can be helpful. If adequate control is not obtained, the blood must be surgically irrigated from the anterior chamber.

Lens subluxation, persistent vitreous hemorrhage, retinal detachment, or glaucoma, should be referred to the appropriate ophthalmologic specialist for definitive therapy.

Orbital floor fractures can be left alone if diplopia is absent in primary gaze and down gaze, and if there is no evidence of enophthalmos. In the presence of these complications, surgery is usually required to remove the entrapped orbital tissue from the fracture site and to repair the orbital floor. The same general principles apply to treatment of fractures of the medial orbital wall.

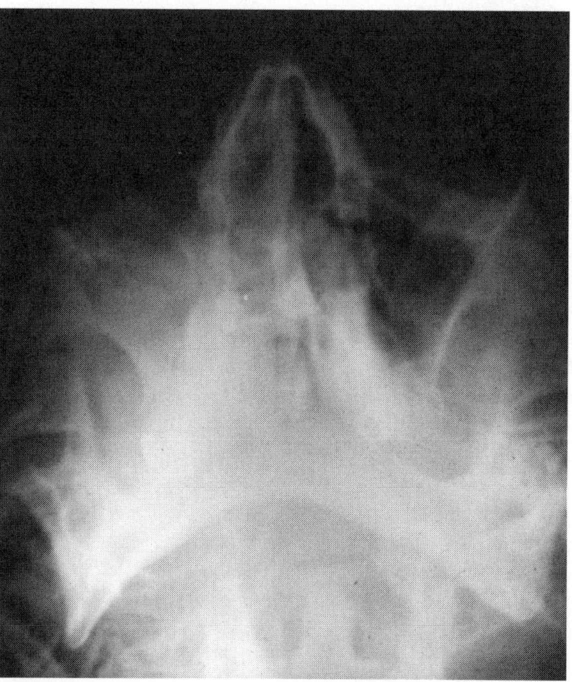

Figure 121-5. X-ray of the face, in the chin up position, demonstrating a fracture of the floor of the orbit on the right side, with clouding of the maxillary antrum secondary to fluid in the sinus cavity.

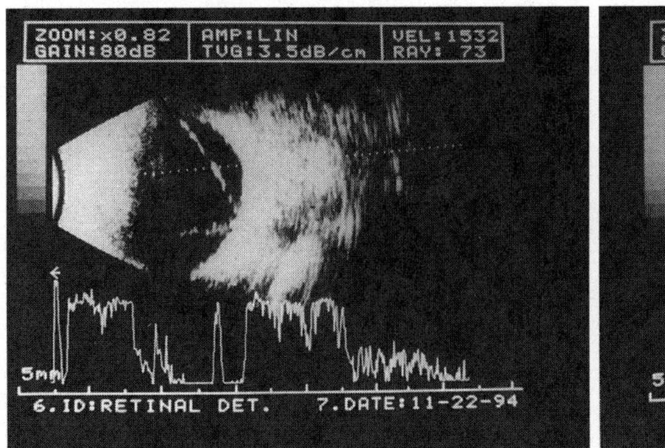

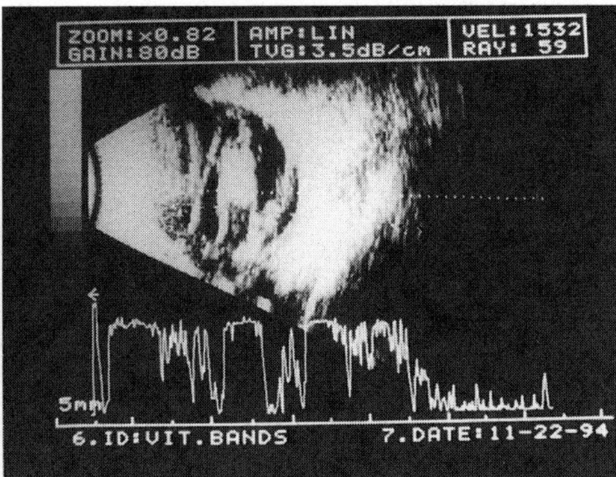

Figure 121-6. Ultrasound (B scan) of the eye showing a retinal detachment (*left*) and vitreous hemorrhage and band (*right*).

Perforating Injury

Perforating injuries require surgical repair as soon as possible. This is usually done using general anesthesia, because the injection of a local anesthetic around the eye may cause increased pressure on the globe and extrusion of intraocular contents. Both intravenous and topical antibiotics are used to try to prevent endophthalmitis.

Penetrating intraocular foreign bodies require surgical removal. If the foreign particle is metallic, a powerful magnet may be used in the extraction. With nonmagnetic objects, direct removal, using vitreoretinal instrumentation, can be successful. If the injury is complicated by retinal detachment, repair can usually be performed later, after the original injury has been operated on and the globe has had a short time to heal.

Chemical Injury

The most important treatment for chemical injuries of the eye is immediate irrigation with tap water, usually the most available solution. Especially with acid or alkali accidents, time is of the essence, and seconds and minutes count. Any attempt, for example, to locate a solution to neutralize the offending chemical agent is a waste of valuable time.

Milder types of chemical injury, such as soap or shampoo in the eye, will usually respond well to treatment with topical steroids. More severe damage to the anterior segment of the globe may be treated with topical antibiotics, steroids, and, in some cases, anticollagenase medication. Corneal transplant surgery is sometimes indicated when the cornea has become severely scarred, but the rate of success may not be very high.

Photosensitized Radiation Injury

The punctate keratitis seen secondary to ultraviolet exposure may be uncomfortable, but is not serious. The short term use of topical steroids is usually helpful. Cataracts from x-ray exposure can be removed surgically, but there is no successful treatment for radiation retinopathy. Dry eye problems can benefit from the use of artificial tears or, in more severe cases, punctal occlusion. Solar or eclipse retinopathy also does not respond well to therapy.

Thermal Injury

Most thermal injuries will be ameliorated by the presence of tears, which cool heat trauma or warm a frozen area. If there is residual loss of corneal epithelium, treatment similar to that described for an abrasion can be useful. When the injury is severe enough to cause an iritis, topical steroids and cycloplegic agents are indicated.

If the lids have been burned, causing the lashes to turn inwards, a protective contact lens can prevent corneal irritation and erosion. Subsequently, corrective surgery can be used to reposition the lid into a more normal position.

CONSIDERATIONS IN PREGNANCY

For the most part, there are no significant considerations in the treatment of eye trauma during pregnancy. When surgical treatment is required, it is best if general anesthesia can be avoided in the pregnant patient. In some perforating injuries or ruptures of the globe, local anesthesia may produce pressure on the eye and result in extrusion of intraocular contents. Therefore, general anesthesia may be necessary for the success of surgery, even during pregnancy.

The use of aminocaproic acid to reduce the incidence of rebleeding in patients with hyphema is not recommended in pregnancy.

BIBLIOGRAPHY

Fraunfelder FT Roy FH, eds. Current ocular therapy, 4th ed. Philadelphia: WB Saunders, 1995:362.

Gombos GM. Handbook of ophthalmic emergencies, 2nd ed. Garden City, NY: Medical Examination Publishing Co, 1973.

Hicks E. Ocular trauma. In: Metz HS, Rosenbaum AL, eds. Pediatric Ophthalmology. Garden City, NY: Medical Examination Publishing Co, 1982:25.

Keeney AH. Trauma of the globe, adnexa and orbital walls: prophylaxis and immediate therapy. In: Harley RD, ed. Pediatric Ophthalmology. Philadelphia: WB Saunders, 1975.

Paton D, Goldberg MF. Management of ocular injuries. Philadelphia: WB Saunders, 1976.

Primary Care for Women, edited by Phyllis C. Leppert and Fred M. Howard. Lippincott-Raven Publishers, Philadelphia © 1997.

122 Corneal Diseases and Contact Lenses

RONALD D. PLOTNIK

CORNEA

Eye Anatomy

The eye is roughly spherical and averages about 24 mm in diameter. The posterior 80% of the eye surface consists of sclera, which is composed of connective tissue with collagen fibrils. It is opaque, white, and about 1 mm thick. The muscles that move the eye attach to the sclera, and the nerves and vessels must penetrate the sclera to reach the deeper layers of the eye wall.

The anterior fifth of the eye is composed of the cornea. The cornea, due to its unique collagen structure, is clear. It is 12 mm in diameter, varies from 0.5 to 1 mm thick, and meets the sclera at a transition zone called the limbus. The cornea is composed of five layers.

Layers

The outermost layer of the cornea is called the epithelium. It is five to seven cells thick. This is the layer damaged when the cornea suffers an abrasion. The cell layer rejuvenates itself and there is progression of cells from the basal layer to the surface. Fluorescein dye can be added to the eye to help evaluate the corneal surface. The orange dye is taken up and stains the surface only in areas where the cells are damaged or missing. Corneal abrasions and herpes simplex infections classically produce fluorescein dye uptake.

The next two layers are composed of collagen lamellae and connective tissue. Directly beneath the epithelium is Bowman's membrane. This thin, compact, homogeneous layer of connective tissue supports the overlying cells. Beneath this is the stroma. This makes up the bulk of the corneal thickness and is the region that becomes swollen when there is corneal edema. The stroma is made of an orderly array of collagen fibrils. Fine cells are scattered throughout.

Beneath the stroma is a layer called Descemet's membrane. This layer is the basement membrane for the fifth and deepest layer, the endothelium. The endothelium is a single layer of cells that do not divide. They actively pump fluid out of the cornea into the eye. This pumping action is crucial to maintain a relatively dehydrated, thin, and clear cornea. Nerves are scattered throughout the superficial cornea, but there are no blood vessels: the blood vessels of the sclera stop at the limbus.

Functions

The cornea serves several functions. As a clear layer, it allows the light from images to reach the retina unimpeded, much like the lens in a camera. The retina gathers the light in the back of the eye; it is analogous to the film in a camera. The surface cells keep fluid from the tear film from entering the cornea by tight junctions that form a watertight seal. The cornea acts as the anterior eye wall and as such maintains the integrity of the eyeball.

The cornea also provides the bulk of the eye's refracting power. It is responsible for bending the light rays so they form a clear image on the retina. The crystalline lens in the interior of the eye also contributes. Most eyes have similar refracting power. The difference in image focus, with its concomitant need to wear glasses, is primarily determined by the eye's length: images may fall short of the retina or be focused behind the retina. Glasses and contact lenses bend the light so the image falls directly on the retina.

The refractive condition of the cornea may be altered by various modalities. Glasses can correct most refractive errors by either diverging or converging the light rays. Nearsightedness is caused by the eye being too long; farsightedness, too short. Astigmatism is due to differences in power of the cornea at different places on the cornea. It requires additional spectacle correction only at one axis to bend the light. Contact lenses also work by bending the light. The power of the lens is specified by the eye care provider. Soft lenses sit directly on the eye; hard lenses float more on the tear film.

Surgical procedures of the cornea may alter corneal shape to achieve better uncorrected visual acuity. These include but are not limited to radial keratotomy (RK) and photorefractive keratectomy (PRK). The former involves making radial partial-thickness deep cuts into the cornea to flatten the central refractive area. The latter involves a laser that essentially grinds a lens from the corneal surface, effectively flattening it.

Clinical Conditions

The cornea may be affected by a wide variety of conditions. Traumatic abrasions may leave a defect in the surface epithelial layer. Deeper lacerations may involve all the layers of the cornea. Foreign bodies may become embedded in the cornea. Viral, bacterial, and fungal infections may involve the cornea. Numerous dystrophic conditions primarily affect one layer of the cornea. Congenital conditions may affect any of the layers and may manifest clinically at varying times of life. Corneal warpage disorders may involve corneal bulging or thinning. The cornea may be damaged by ocular surgery, either in the immediate or more delayed postoperative period. Abnormalities of the corneal endothelium may allow fluid to accumulate in the cornea, resulting in corneal swelling or edema. The cornea may be damaged by ocular dryness or Sjögren syndrome. Contact lens complications of the cornea have various causes.

Evaluation

Evaluation of the cornea involves unique diagnostic modalities. The most commonly used instrument is the biomicroscope or slit lamp. The slit lamp passes a slit of light through the cornea, providing a magnified view of the illuminated cornea. It allows the production of an optical cross section, as the beam can be viewed from the side. This permits an evaluation of the depth, extent, and morphologic characteristics of corneal lesions. It is one of the few areas of medicine in which the disease process can be visualized directly, sometimes down to the cellular level. The examination can be photographed or videotaped.

The second most common modality is keratometry, which allows subjective and objective evaluation of the corneal surface curvature. It allows a quantification of corneal power, refractive ability, and astigmatism. A more powerful tool is the cornea videotopography system. Light rings are projected onto the cornea; a video capture system retrieves the reflected image and a computer digitizes it and produces a color-coded "topographic" map of the cornea. Each area of the cornea can be evaluated for irregularity, steepness, curvature, symmetry, power, and astigmatism. This is especially useful in the diagnosis of corneal warpage disorders.

In the posterior cornea, the monolayer of endothelial cells can be photographed with a special camera, and a calibrated grid can be used to determine the number and density of cells in the photographs. Certain disorders cause a loss of cells and may result in corneal edema. Corneal thickness can be determined, as can corneal nerve sensitivity.

The cornea can be cultured if infection is suspected. Adenovirus, herpes simplex, fungus, chlamydia, and bacterial cultures can yield diagnostic information and often provide antibiotic sensitivities. Culture techniques include direct inoculation of agar plates. A spatula is used to scrape the corneal surface or conjunctiva after a topical anesthetic is instilled. The spatula is used to inoculate the plates, slants, broths, slides, or transport media directly; this significantly increases the yield. If cultures are taken in the primary care setting, standard bacterial swabs can be obtained. Chlamydia and viral testing are also available in some settings, such as the gynecologist's office. Wetting the swab with unpreserved saline can further increase the yield significantly. Respiratory saline vials or certain unpreserved artificial tears are also effective as wetting agents.

Other tests are occasionally performed, such as biopsy, immunofluorescent antibody techniques, polymerase chain reaction, and impression cytology.

Other techniques can be used to diagnose the dry eye. Dry eye syndrome is more common among women and can harm the cornea. Symptoms include a dry feeling of the eyes, a foreign body or gritty sensation, light sensitivity, and, paradoxically, tearing. The cornea shows signs of dryness, with abnormalities of the surface epithelial cells. The accessory lacrimal glands are small glands that produce tears. With age, and more frequently in women, tear production is markedly diminished. The main lacrimal gland, which is responsible for reflex tearing with crying or ocular irritation, may actually produce intermittent gushes of tears due to the chronic underlying dryness. Dry eye is increased in patients with connective tissue diseases and can increase in severity after menopause. Testing includes the use of Schirmer test strips. These short strips of filter paper are tucked in the lower lid and can be used to estimate the amount of tears produced.

In Sjögren syndrome, patients develop dryness of other mucous membranes as well, primarily the mouth. Sjögren syndrome can be primary or secondary to connective tissue diseases. Antibody tests for Sjögren syndrome can be useful. The mainstay of treatment involves the use of artificial tears as well as cautery occlusion of the lacrimal puncta, the openings that drain tears from the eye into the lacrimal drainage system.

Corneal Transplantation

Cornea transplantation involves replacing an abnormal cornea with that of a recently deceased person. Corneas were the first successfully transplanted solid tissue. Since that time, technique, suture materials, indications, and postoperative care have advanced significantly. All living cellular elements are transplanted as part of the cornea transplant graft. About 40,000 cornea transplants are performed each year in the United States.

Immunology

The low rejection rate of cornea transplants, despite disparate antigens between donor and recipient, is primarily due to the lack of blood vessels and lymph channels in nonvascularized corneas. Routine systemic immunosuppressives are not needed after a corneal transplant. Topical steroid drops are used to help prevent rejection. Rejection can be directed at any level of the cornea, but the most serious type of rejection is against the deepest layer, the endothelium. Patients may present after transplantation with pain, decreased vision, or a red eye. Thickening of the cornea and inflammatory debris on the back of the cornea can be diagnosed at the slit lamp examination. Treatment of rejection consists of intensive topical steroids and occasionally systemic steroids as well. Although about 30% of all transplant patients experience a transplant rejection episode, most of these can be reversed by treatment. Close clinical supervision is required to diagnose subclinical rejection episodes. The average time for rejection is 8 months after surgery; the frequency of rejection declines after that point. Most patients can be tapered down to topical steroid drops ranging in frequency from once a week to twice a day.

Technique

The donor cornea is retrieved from the cadaver by either removing the eye and then preparing the cornea or by retrieving the cornea directly. Trained eye bank technicians harvest tissue from those who elect to donate their corneas at death. The cornea is placed in a special culture media that is enriched to keep the corneal cells viable and healthy. In the operating room, most patients receive local anesthesia by injecting an anesthetic mixture behind the eye. This numbs the eye, blocks vision for the duration of the case, and prevents the eye or lid from moving. Corneal transplantation consists of cutting a round corneal "button" of about 8 mm from the recipient's abnormal cornea and replacing it with the normal donor cornea. A round trephine, resembling a cookie cutter, is used to cut the corneas. The donor cornea is usually oversized at the time of surgery by 0.25 mm to ensure a tight fit and good seal. The new cornea is sewed into the hole created by trephination with 10-0 nylon suture; this is done under an operating microscope. The suture effectively seals the eye, making tight, close contact between the graft button and the recipient. Other procedures, such as cataract extraction or exchange of faulty plastic lens implants, can be performed when the abnormal cornea is removed. The eye is patched and shielded at the end of the operation and the patient is seen in follow-up the following day.

In the past, restrictions included a week of bed rest with sandbags around the head. Today, restrictions are normally limited to lifting, bending, and some sporting activities. Most surgeons lift all restrictions by 3 months after surgery.

Indications

Corneal Trauma

Corneal transplantation in traumatic injuries either restores the integrity of the globe or clears the visual axis of scarring. Traumatic lacerations and perforations of the cornea must be repaired urgently. Examples include tree branch injuries, high-speed metallic foreign bodies, broken glass injuries, and injuries due to such objects as fish hooks and screwdrivers. Trauma can result in infection of the cornea or even the entire eye. The prognosis with ocular infection (endophthalmitis) is poor. Injuries are repaired using 10-0 nylon suture. Intensive topical fortified antibiotic drops are often used for prophylaxis.

Alkali and acid injuries to the cornea range from minor to catastrophic. If severely burned, the cornea may need to be transplanted due to melting of corneal tissue or due to severe scarring. It is often advisable to wait until the inflammation has subsided if transplantation is indicated. Alkali injuries tend to be worse. Initial first aid for such injuries includes copious irrigation. Many complications may ensue, and the prognosis can be grim.

Less serious but common injuries may be caused by such objects as a hot curling iron, pieces of paper (paper cuts), or Superglue (mistaken for eyedrops). Corneal scarring of any cause may necessitate corneal transplantation for visual rehabilitation.

Rheumatoid Diseases

Rheumatoid arthritis and other connective tissue diseases may adversely affect the eye. In their most severe form, immunologically mediated corneal melting may occur. This may progress to a corneal perforation requiring repair. Ulcers close to the sclera and limbus are often due to immune complex deposition. Collagenase and other collagenolytic agents are activated with thinning of the corneal tissue. More centrally, the mechanism is less clear, but inflammatory cells can be found in surgical pathology specimens. The corneal graft is usually a full-thickness or, in some cases a partial-thickness "patch graft" that may be performed of partial-thickness donor corneal material that can be frozen and stored.

Other ocular diseases associated with rheumatoid arthritis include severe dry eye, inflammation within the eye (iritis), and scleritis. Scleritis involves immune-mediated inflammation of the scleral tissue. This ranges from mild to severe and may even progress to full-thickness scleral melting. Scleromalacia perforans, an ischemic destructive scleritis, can cause widespread thinning of the sclera with associated complications. Often the sclera and cornea are affected, giving rise to a sclerokeratitis. Both tissues show evidence of ongoing immune-mediated inflammation. Treatment includes systemic nonsteroidal antiinflammatory drugs, systemic prednisone, and even systemic immunosuppressives. Severe forms of scleritis often indicate systemic immune process, and long-term survival, as well as the localized scleritis, may be significantly improved by systemic immunosuppression.

Corneal Warpage Diseases

Although the cornea may have natural astigmatism, extreme degrees are abnormal. An analogy is that the normal cornea is to a basketball as the astigmatic cornea is to a football. The curvature and refracting power are not equal for the entire 360° of the cornea. In keratoconus, the cornea, usually inferiorly, bulges outward, with corneal thinning and eventual scarring. The severity ranges from mild (glasses for optical correction) to moderate (gas-permeable contact lenses for optical correction) to severe (corneal transplantation). Gas-permeable contact lenses may be effective in that they sit above the eye on the tear film and may provide a relatively smooth refracting surface. There may be genetic factors, and both corneas are usually affected, although asymmetrically. The prognosis for corneal transplantation in these patients is excellent. The success rate is over 95%, and most patients achieve 20/40 or better visual acuity. Many of these patients are young, and corneal transplantation allows them to resume an active lifestyle.

Other warpage diseases include keratoglobus (the entire cornea bulges with thinning at the periphery for 360°) and pellucid degeneration (inferior thinning near the inferior limbus). Trauma, previous infections, and scarring due to other causes may also cause significant astigmatism requiring either a gas-permeable hard contact lens or corneal transplantation.

Corneal Endothelial Abnormality

The endothelial cells must be able to dehydrate the cornea for the cornea to stay thin and clear. These cells actively pump fluid out of the cornea and into the anterior chamber, the fluid reservoir immediately behind the cornea. Several conditions may decrease the number of cells on the posterior corneal surface. As these cells do not divide, they may reach a critically small number, resulting in corneal edema or swelling. Although a topical ointment with a high salt concentration can be used to try to draw some fluid out the front of the cornea (by osmosis), this usually helps only temporarily once corneal edema has ensued.

In some conditions, the cellular number falls. Fuchs corneal dystrophy, an autosomal dominant condition, causes excrescences to form on the back of the cornea, giving a peau d'orange appearance on the slit lamp examination. It is associated with a precipitous and progressive premature cellular loss, sometimes to the point of corneal edema. This usually worsens with age. Surgical procedures on the eye such as cataract extraction can reduce the cell number still further, and corneal edema often ensues after cataract surgery.

Corneal transplantation replaces the main bulk of the cornea and also the living endothelial layer. These cells then pump fluid out of the recipient eye as they did when the donor was living. Unstable lens implants, as were often placed in the past, also contribute to premature cellular loss. Modern cataract extraction, outside the setting of Fuchs corneal dystrophy, rarely results in corneal decompensation.

Complications

Rejection of the corneal transplant is the most common complication. Patients are advised to call the office for urgent evaluation if they develop pain, a red eye, or decreased vision. Most rejection episodes can be treated successfully. A major bleed in the eye or severe infection at or about the time of surgery can result in poor or no vision in the eye. These complications are rare, and all precautions are taken to avoid them. Glaucoma (elevated pressure in the eye requiring drops for normalization), retinal detachment (requiring surgical intervention to replace the retina on the posterior eye wall), cataract formation, ocular inflammation, and corneal bacterial infection are all increased in frequency but still remain uncommon.

Postoperatively, astigmatism may be a problem. Sutures are selectively removed to make the transplant rounder. At the location on the cornea where the sutures are relatively tight, there is more astigmatism. Tight sutures are removed first, looser ones later or not at all. Glasses are given for visual rehabilitation as soon as possible. Some patients see better soon after surgery if a gas-permeable hard contact lens is used. If areas of the transplant remain "tight" even after suture removal, partial-thickness cuts are sometimes made in the interface between the corneal transplant button and the recipient's cornea. This loosens the area of healing and scar formation between the donor and recipient corneas. The procedure is done in the office using the slit lamp, and healing is rapid.

CONTACT LENSES

Contact lenses place a plus (convex, for hyperopia or farsightedness) or minus (concave, for myopia or nearsightedness) refracting lens on the eye, precluding the need for spectacles. Many patients appreciate the freedom from glasses, given the lenses' convenience, light weight, and increased peripheral vision.

Types

Lenses may be soft or hard. Soft or hydrogel lenses consist of two components: a stable cross-linked polymer matrix and a less stable aqueous component that exchanges with the tear film. The water conveys a high degree of oxygen flow through the lens. Lenses then must have a very high water content or be very thin to provide adequate oxygen flow. Soft lenses conform to the eye and therefore do not correct astigmatism; astigmatism on the corneal surface is conveyed to the lens. For small degrees of astigmatism, some clinicians prescribe toric soft contacts, which put additional correction in one axis of the lens. The lens must stay oriented in a specific direction, and there are ways to prevent significant lens rotation on the eye. For the most part, the ideal soft lens candidate has little astigmatism and does not have an especially dry eye. Soft lenses stay on the eye more securely than hard ones and are better for athletes. Lenses must be removed each day and for such activities as swimming and sleeping.

Hard lenses have changed over the years. Previous hard lenses had little oxygen permeability, and oxygen from the tear film got through to the ocular surface around the lens as the patient blinked. Today, gas-permeable lenses have extremely high oxygen flow through the lens itself. Advantages of gas-permeable lenses include astigmatism correction and easier handling. Disadvantages include a longer adjustment period for the patient and a tendency for the lenses to fall out during sports and similar activities.

Fitting

Careful attention to such parameters as lens composition, design, fit, and care can help minimize adverse effects. To fit a lens appropriately, the clinician must know the curvature of the cornea. This is determined easily by the keratometer, which gives a precise measurement of central corneal curvature. Contact lens curvature and diameter are specified by the eye care professional to provide an appropriate fit. If the lens is too tight, ischemia results, and complications are much more frequent. If the lens is too loose, it moves excessively on the eye, with discomfort and even pain. Once the lenses are dispensed, it is important to see the patient again, as fit can change over time.

Care

Contact lenses must be cleaned, disinfected, and enzymatically treated. Various care regimens exist, and some solutions are "all in one." Lens cleaning involves placing the lens in the hand and rubbing it with cleaning solution. Disinfecting usually involves leaving the lens overnight in the disinfecting solution. Once a week or so, enzymatic cleaning helps remove stubborn deposits from the lenses.

Complications

The patient must be able to insert and remove the lenses each day and provide appropriate lens hygiene and care. Failure to perform the care regimen properly may predispose to corneal infection. Contact lens wear presents a potential risk for infection due to microtrauma of the cornea, relative hypoxia of the surface epithelial cells, and repeated inoculum of bacteria if allowed to grow on the contact lenses or lens cases or in contaminated solutions. Overnight extended wear of soft lenses may present an additional risk of infection. Lenses may become a problem in older women, as dry eye may make lens wear difficult.

Toxic or allergic reactions to contact lenses or solutions may also occur. Some solutions are worse than others in terms of potential toxic reactions. These reactions, although very symptomatic, usually do not present long-term complications. In giant papillary conjunctivitis, papilla larger than 1 mm in diameter form on the undersurface of the upper lid. This is usually accompanied by mucous discharge, itching, irritation, and an inability to keep the lenses clean. Medications can be used to decrease the signs and symptoms. A change of contact lens type or solutions often helps.

BIBLIOGRAPHY

Arffa RC. Grayson's diseases of the cornea, 3d ed. St. Louis: Mosby Year Book, 1991.

Kaufman HE, Barron BA, McDonald MB, Waltman SR, et al. The cornea. New York: Churchill-Livingstone, 1988.

Smolin G, Thoft RA. The cornea—scientific foundations and clinical practice, 2d ed. Boston: Little, Brown & Co., 1987.

Primary Care for Women, edited by Phyllis C. Leppert and Fred M. Howard. Lippincott-Raven Publishers, Philadelphia © 1997.

123
Retinal Diseases

STEVEN J. ROSE

The retina is the specialized tissue that lines the back of the eye and is most commonly associated with the transformation of light energy into perceived visual images. The anatomic arrangement of the nine layers of the retina (Fig. 123-1). clearly identifies this tissue as one of the most highly organized tissues of the body. Light energy is received at the level of the photoreceptors and is modified and reorganized as it travels through the retina to the optic nerve and then onto the occipital cortex of the brain, where visual imaging actually takes place.

The vitreous body, which constitutes most of the volume of the eye, is essentially an optically empty chamber. In normal healthy individuals, the vitreous body has various structural and physiologic roles that maintain optical integrity. Abnormal vitreoretinal relationships can, however, lead to a number of disease states that ultimately affect vision.

This chapter presents the most common retinal diseases encountered in a primary care setting. Recognition of these disease states and the need for referral to the appropriate ophthalmologist is stressed.

The retinal diseases covered in this chapter include retinal vascular diseases, diabetic retinopathy, age-related macular degeneration, inflammatory and infectious diseases, retinal tears, and retinal detachment.

EXAMINATION OF THE FUNDUS

Before proceeding with the clinical description of the retinal diseases likely to be encountered in practice, the practical aspects of the retinal examination are presented.

A thorough examination of the fundus requires excellent powers of observation, and clinical experience with ophthalmoscopy is necessary. Most clinicians have been introduced to the direct ophthalmoscope at the beginning of their clinical training in medical school. The emphasis was placed on observation of the optic nerve head and, secondarily, the blood vessels. Unfortunately, the most helpful adjunct to examining the retina, pupillary dilatation, has never been stressed consistently. Examination of the fundus, and especially the retinal periphery, is greatly facilitated by a well-dilated pupil. Suggested dilating medications include 1% tropicamide (Mydriacyl) and 2.5% phenylephrine drops (Mydfrin), one drop of each in both eyes. Most patients' eyes dilate adequately after 20 to 30 minutes; however, darkly pigmented irises dilate more slowly. The reluctance to dilate eyes originated from the concern that narrow angle glaucoma attacks would be precipitated. Although this is a concern for only a few patients, the amount of disease missed through an undilated pupil is, according to my opinion, potentially more harmful to the patient thαn the glaucoma, which can be safely treated.

To examine the ocular fundus, specialized instruments are necessary. The simplest and most familiar to primary care practitioners is the direct ophthalmoscope, which is, in essence, a miniature flashlight held close to the examiner's and patient's eyes and shined through the pupil (Fig. 123-2). The fundus is viewed monocularly through a small aperture just above the illumination source, producing an upright, virtual image that magnifies the area being examined about 15 times. The ophthalmoscope has a set of neutralizing lenses built in that can be dialed to achieve the sharpest image for the examiner.

Although magnification and resolution are good with the direct ophthalmoscope, it has disadvantages that limit its effectiveness. The lack of stereopsis (depth perception), inadequate illumination in the presence of media opacities (corneal scars), a retinal image covering only about 8% of the total retinal area, and significant degradation of the image with significant lens opacities all contribute to a suboptimal screening examination. Furthermore, the direct ophthalmoscope does not allow an undistorted view of the peripheral retina, limiting its use to the posterior retina only. The use of other ophthalmoscopes such as the binocular indirect ophthalmoscope is beyond the scope of practice for the primary care provider and is not covered here.

In summary, the direct ophthalmoscope, in conjunction with pupillary dilation, serves the primary care practitioner well as a useful screening device for evaluating papilledema, macular degeneration, and diabetic and hypertensive retinopathy.

RETINAL VASCULAR DISEASES

Diabetic Retinopathy

Diabetic retinopathy is one of the four most frequent causes of new blindness in the United States and the leading cause in the 20- to 64-year-old age group. An estimated 14 million Americans have diabetes mellitus. Ten percent to 15% of the diabetic population has insulin-dependent diabetes mellitus (type I), which usually is diagnosed before 40 years of age. Most patients, however, have non—-insulin-dependent diabetes mellitus (type II), which is usually diagnosed in patients older than 40 years of age. Although those with type I diabetes mellitus experience a higher incidence of severe ocular complications, those with type II diabetes mellitus make up the majority of clinical cases because of their larger overall numbers.

The prevalence of all types of retinopathy in the diabetic population increases with the duration of diabetes and patient age. The prevalence of any degree of retinopathy reaches 50% by 7 years' duration of disease and approaches 90% after a duration of 17 to 25 years. Systemic hormonal changes occurring at puberty result in an increased prevalence of retinopathy after 13 years of age. Furthermore, associated health and medical problems present a significant risk for the development and progression of diabetic retinopathy. These factors include pregnancy, hypertension, chronic hyperglycemia, renal disease, and hyperlipidemia.

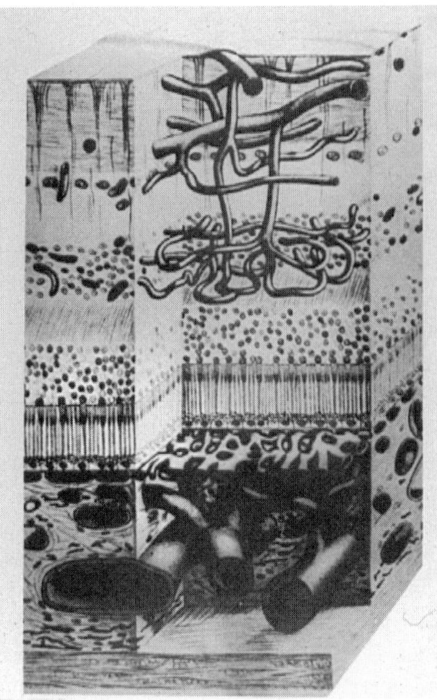

Figure 123-1. Anatomic arrangement of the retina. The top of the figure represents the vitreous side; the bottom is choroidal.

The cause of diabetic microvascular disease is not known. It has been suggested that exposure to hyperglycemia over an extended period of time results in glycosylation of tissue proteins and ultimate damage. Certain physiologic abnormalities have been identified to occur early in the course of diabetic retinopathy. These include impaired autoregulation of retinal blood vessels, alterations in blood flow, and breakdown of the blood-—retinal barrier, a normally impermeable vascular entity.

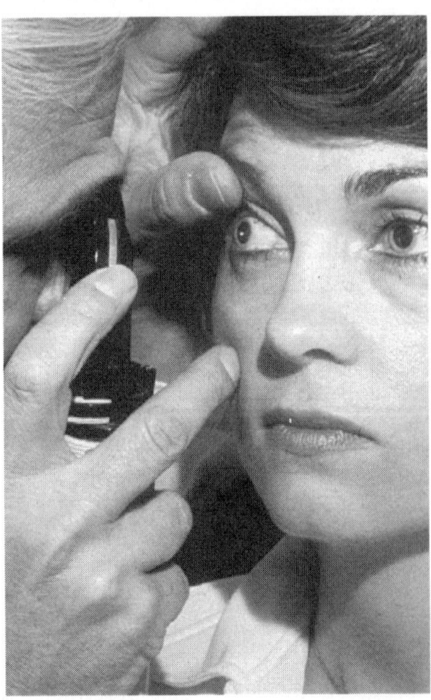

Figure 123-2. Examination of the fundus using direct ophthalmoscope.

Studies suggest that the speed of retinal blood flow in large vessels increases with progressive disease. Capillary closure results, causing retinal ischemia, which at some critical point, causes the release of a vasoproliferative factor, stimulating new blood vessel growth from the retina, optic nerve, or iris.

The clinical findings of diabetic retinopathy most likely are present before any visual symptoms occur; therefore, it is critical to screen for this disease in the yearly examinations performed in the primary practitioner's office. Various retinal lesions identify the risk of progression of retinopathy and visual loss.

The first clinical signs of diabetic retinopathy are microaneurysms, which are saccular outpouchings of retinal capillaries (Fig. 123-3). Ruptured microaneurysms and decompensated capillaries result in intraretinal hemorrhages. The clinical appearance of these hemorrhages reflects the retinal level at which the hemorrhage occurs. Hemorrhages at the nerve fiber layer are more flame shaped, whereas hemorrhages deeper in the retina assume a pinpoint or dot shape. Venous caliber abnormalities are indicators of severe retinal hypoxia. These changes can be venous dilatation, venous beading, or loop formation (Fig. 123-4).

Proliferative diabetic retinopathy (Fig. 123-5) is marked by proliferating endothelial cell tubules. They grow either at or near the optic disc (neovascularization of the disc) or elsewhere in the retina (neovascularization elsewhere). Fibrous tissue can appear to grow with these new vessels.

Diabetic retinopathy is classified into two main stages: nonproliferative and proliferative. The nonproliferative stage is characterized by focal intraretinal capillary closure and increased retinal vascular permeability. The hemorrhagic changes described earlier are the clinical manifestations of this stage. In addition, exudation of serum proteins, including lipoproteins, is seen as hard exudates (Fig. 123-6).

Retinal thickening is an important consequence of abnormal retinal vascular permeability. Edema involving the macula is probably the most common cause of decreased vision in diabetic retinopathy. Diabetic maculopathy may present as focal or diffuse retinal thickening with or without deposits of intraretinal lipoprotein exudates.

The diagnosis of diabetic retinopathy, although mainly a clinical diagnosis, is aided by an imaging technique known as fluorescein angiography. Sodium fluorescein is a dye injected into a peripheral vein. Up to 70% of the injected dye molecules are bound to serum

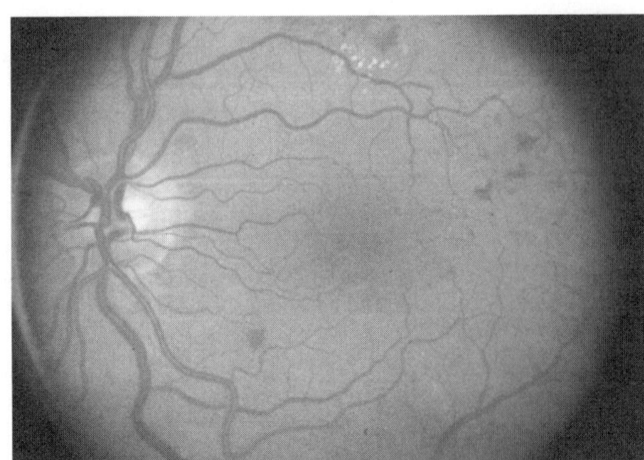

Figure 123-3. Macular area of a diabetic with small hemorrhages from microaneurysms.

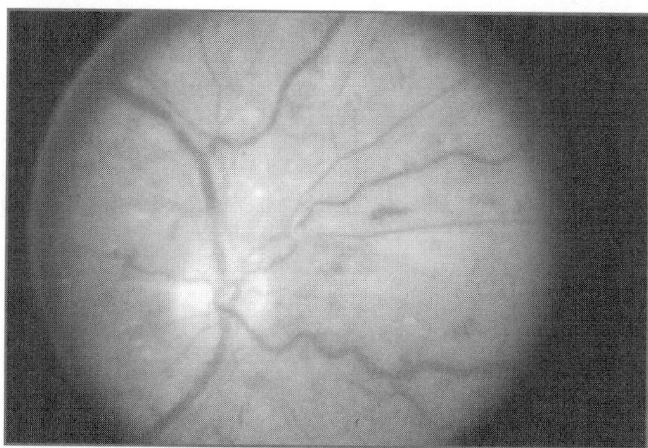

Figure 123-4. Venous abnormalities in a patient with diabetic retinopathy. Note the sausage shape to the vasculature.

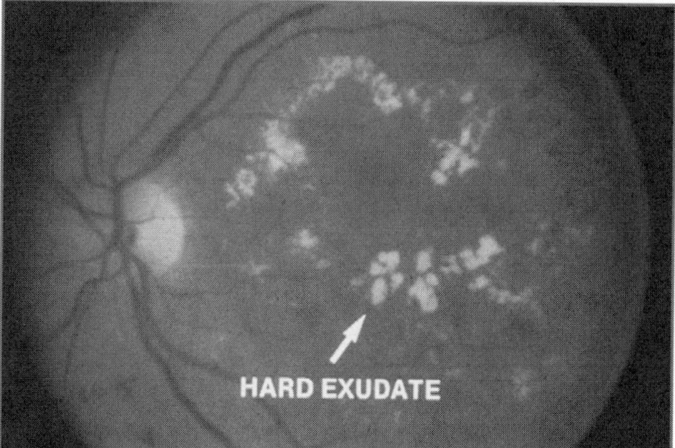

Figure 123-6. Macular edema with significant hard exudates.

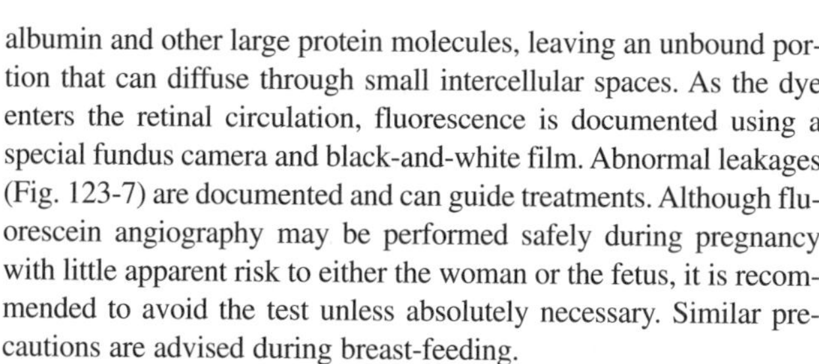

albumin and other large protein molecules, leaving an unbound portion that can diffuse through small intercellular spaces. As the dye enters the retinal circulation, fluorescence is documented using a special fundus camera and black-and-white film. Abnormal leakages (Fig. 123-7) are documented and can guide treatments. Although fluorescein angiography may be performed safely during pregnancy with little apparent risk to either the woman or the fetus, it is recommended to avoid the test unless absolutely necessary. Similar precautions are advised during breast-feeding.

The treatment of diabetic retinopathy can be divided into three categories: medical control of retinopathy, laser therapy, and surgical treatment.

The medical control of diabetic retinopathy has been a long-sought but elusive ideal. The recent Diabetes Control and Complications Trial, a nationwide clinical trial testing tight control of blood glucose levels versus standard control of blood glucose levels, has been completed and shows that tight control significantly reduces the rate of progression and severity of diabetic retinopathy.

The association of hypertension with the development of diabetic retinopathy is well documented, but the degree to which it causes exacerbation of retinopathy is uncertain. One study shows systolic blood pressure to be a predictor of the incidence of diabetic retinopathy, and diastolic blood pressure to be a predictor of the progression of retinopathy.

Laser photocoagulation remains the cornerstone of treatment for both nonproliferative and proliferative diabetic retinopathy. Laser photocoagulation uses a collimated beam of light energy at certain wavelengths to create focal burns at the level of the retina. Focal macular edema is treated by focal closure of the leaking blood vessels directly, whereas diffuse macular edema is treated with an indirect grid laser pattern (Fig. 123-8). In contrast, scatter photocoagulation (Fig. 123-9) is used for treating proliferative diabetic retinopathy. It involves placing multiple laser burns in the midperipheral retina over the course of two or more sessions, consisting of 1500 to 2500 total burns.

The response to laser treatment varies, but its introduction in the latter half of this century has saved millions of diabetics from certain blindness.

If a patient fails to respond to laser treatment, surgical intervention using removal of the vitreous (vitrectomy) and abnormal fibroproliferative tissues also can save many eyes from severe visual loss. These techniques require specialized training and experience and are performed by ophthalmologists who subspecialize in vitreoretinal diseases and surgery.

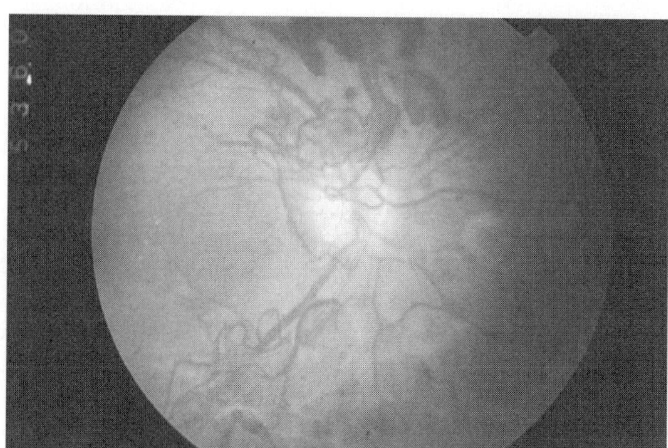

Figure 123-5. Proliferative diabetic retinopathy with florid neovascularization of the optic nerve.

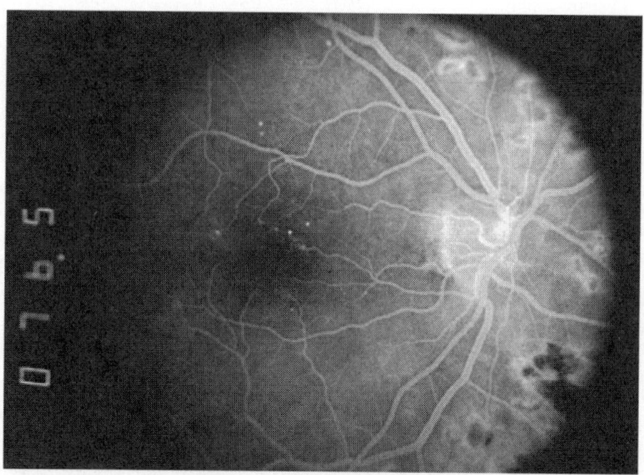

Figure 123-7. Fluorescein angiogram of macula with pinpoint leaks near the fovea from diabetic microaneurysms.

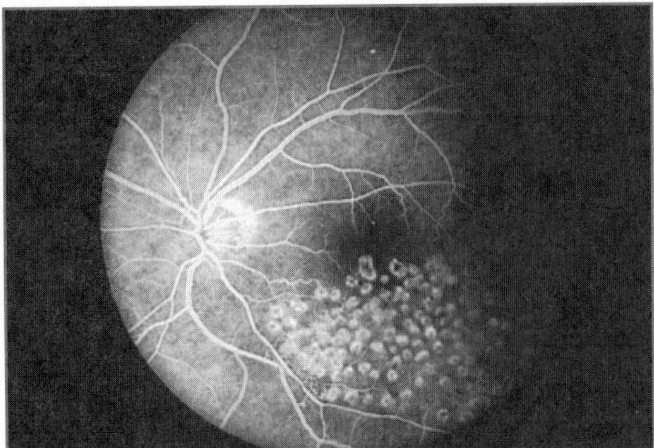

Figure 123-8. Fluorescein angiogram depicting grid laser treatment pattern.

Pregnancy presents a unique situation with regard to diabetic retinopathy. The acceleration of proliferative retinopathy and the poor control of hyperglycemia is a well-known clinical phenomenon in pregnant diabetics. Glucose metabolism is disturbed by the anabolic needs of the developing fetus and by the hormonal state of pregnancy. Patients with advanced retinopathy formerly were cautioned against pregnancy because of retinopathy and maternal and neonatal complications. Currently, the efficacy of laser photocoagulation has eliminated retinopathy as a contraindication to pregnancy.

The effect of pregnancy on the progression of retinopathy is controversial. Few randomized prospective studies compare pregnant and nonpregnant diabetic women. Among diabetic women, those with either no or minimal nonproliferative retinopathy have minimal risk of developing vision-threatening complications during pregnancy. Macular edema can be marked during pregnancy, especially in those with hypertension or nephropathy, but is unlikely to lead to permanent visual loss.

Pregnant women with more severe nonproliferative retinopathy have a higher risk of progressing to proliferative retinopathy. More than half will progress to proliferative retinopathy during pregnancy without laser treatment. Increased intravascular volume and

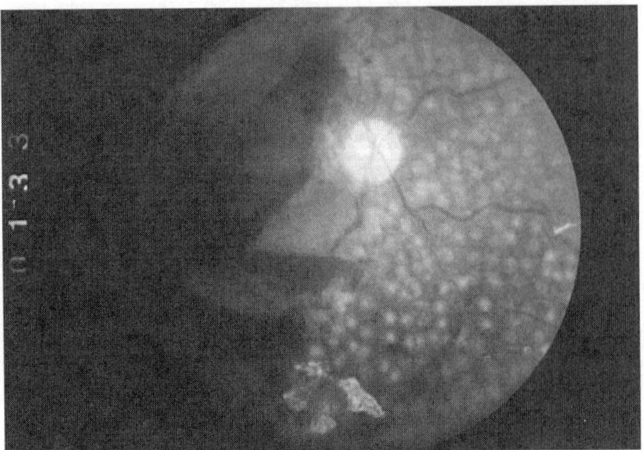

Figure 123-9. Scatter laser photocoagulation for proliferatire diabetic retinopathy.

Valsalva maneuvers during delivery may increase the risk of vitreous hemorrhage. Pregnant women with severe nonproliferative diabetic retinopathy (NPDR) or early proliferative retinopathy should be considered for prompt laser photocoagulation. Macular edema can be treated at the same time. Notice that patients who have had laser treatment for proliferative retinopathy with complete regression have been shown to experience progression with a subsequent pregnancy.

Until a cure for diabetes is found, the emphasis must be on identification, careful follow-up, and timely laser intervention. Proper care results in reduction of personal suffering as well as a substantial cost savings for all involved. Table 123-1 provides guidelines regarding an eye examination schedule.

Hypertensive Retinopathy

Systemic hypertension initially causes local or generalized vasoconstriction of the retinal arterioles. Prolonged acute systemic hypertension may cause disruption of the blood—retinal barrier, resulting in leakage of plasma and formed blood elements into the retina, similar to the diabetic changes mentioned earlier.

Prolonged systemic hypertension results in thickening of the walls of the retinal arterioles. Clinically, the thickened arterioles have a broader and brighter reflex. Because the arteries and veins have a common adventitial sheath where they cross, arteriovenous (AV) crossing changes can be seen. Characteristic changes include AV nicking (Fig. 123-10). If arteriolar sclerosis advances significantly, several complications may occur, including macroaneurysm formation and central retinal artery or vein occlusion.

During pregnancy, hypertensive retinal changes may occur because of preeclampsia or toxemia of pregnancy. Visual loss ranging from mild to total blindness can occur. The pathologic changes are seen at the level of the choroid or blood supply under the retina. The acute hypertensive crisis causes reversible damage to the smallest blood vessels (choriocapillaris), which in turn cause damage to the overlying retinal pigment epithelium. The resultant breakdown in the pigment epithelial barrier allows fluid to collect under the retina. In extreme cases, a total exudative retinal detachment occurs with total loss of vision.

Toxemia also can cause optic nerve swelling with or without concomitant retinal damage.

Treatment is directed at the underlying cause, and rarely is any direct treatment of the retina required. In most cases, vision returns to normal. The primary care provider and the ophthalmologist should work closely together during these periods.

Arterial Occlusive Disease

The blood supply to the inner layers of the retina is entirely from the central retinal artery, a branch of the ophthalmic artery, which is a branch of the internal carotid. Retinal ischemia results from disease affecting the afferent vessels, anywhere from the common carotid artery to the intraretinal arterioles. The signs and symptoms of arteriole obstruction are dependent on the vessel involved. Ophthalmic artery disease can cause total blindness, whereas occlusion of an extramacular arteriole may be asymptomatic. The loss of vision usually is abrupt, although symptoms of intermittent loss of vision or amaurosis fugax may precede the final event.

The two major kinds of arterial occlusion are branch retinal artery occlusion (BRAO) and central retinal artery occlusion

Table 123-1. Eye Examination Schedule

TYPE OF DIABETES	RECOMMENDED TIME OF FIRST EXAMINATION	ROUTINE MINIMAL FOLLOW-UP INTERVAL
Type I; IDDM	5 y after onset or at time of diagnosis	Yearly
Type II; NIDDM		Yearly
During pregnancy	Prior to pregnancy for counseling	3–6 months postpartum
	Early in first trimester	
	Each trimester or more frequently as indicated	

(CRAO). In BRAO, the patient usually notices a partial blind spot or scotoma near their central visual field. Clinically, acute BRAO causes an edematous, white retina caused by infarction of the affected vessel (Fig. 123-11). With time, the edema resolves and the vessel reopens or recanalizes. A permanent field defect results. Three main varieties of emboli are recognized: cholesterol emboli arising from the carotid artery, platelet—fibrin emboli associated with large vessel arteriosclerosis, and calcific emboli resulting from diseased cardiac valves. Rare causes of emboli include fat emboli from long bone fractures, cardiac myxoma, septic emboli from infective endocarditis, and talc emboli in intravenous drug abusers.

Management is directed toward determination of the systemic etiologic factors. No specific, proven ocular therapy is possible.

CRAO is characterized by sudden, painless loss of vision in one eye. The retina becomes opaque and edematous, particularly in the posterior pole where the nerve fiber and ganglion cell layers are the thickest. This permits an orange reflex, from the intact choroidal vasculature beneath the intact foveola, to stand out in contrast to the surrounding opaque retina, producing a "cherry red" spot (Fig. 123-12). With time, the central retinal artery reopens and the retinal edema clears.

The effect on visual acuity usually is devastating, with most eyes ending up with a vision of hand motions or less than 20/400 vision. Loss of vision to no light perception usually results from concomitant choroidal vascular obstruction.

CRAO usually is caused by arteriosclerosis-related thrombosis, occurring at the level of the optic nerve. Emboli may be important in some cases. Any patient in 60- to 80-year-old age range presenting with CRAO or BRAO should have temporal arteritis high on the differential diagnosis list, and a sedimentation rate should be obtained as a screening test.

Therapy for CRAO is an ophthalmic emergency, and patients must be referred immediately. Steps include reduction of the intraocular pressure by paracentesis, ocular massage, inhalation therapy with carbogyn (95% oxygen–5% carbon dioxide), and the use of aspirin. A recent study shows the prognosis to be poor with or without treatment; however, anecdotal cases of visual recovery are common.

Venous Occlusive Disease

The venous supply from the retina also is at risk for blockage, causing disease with mild to severe visual loss. Similar to arterial disease, the venous diseases can be divided into branch retinal vein occlusion (BRVO) and central retinal vein occlusion (CRVO).

The ophthalmoscopic findings of acute BRVO include superficial hemorrhages, retinal edema, and often cotton-wool spots in a sector of the retina affected (Fig. 123-13). The obstructed vein is dilated and tortuous, and the corresponding artery may become narrowed and sheathed. The superotemporal quadrant is most commonly affected, and the site of occlusion is usually at an AV crossing point. Histologic studies suggest that the common adventitia at these points bind the artery and vein together and that disease of the arterial wall impinges on the vein, resulting in turbulent flow, endothelial cell damage, and thrombotic occlusion. Arterial disease related to systemic hypertension, diabetes, or arteriosclerosis may predispose to BRVO.

The visual prognosis is related to the extent of capillary damage, retinal ischemia, and the presence of macular edema. Fluorescein angiography is used to assess the extent and location of capillary damage. Acutely, vision may be reduced from macular edema, hemorrhage, or capillary occlusion. With time, capillary

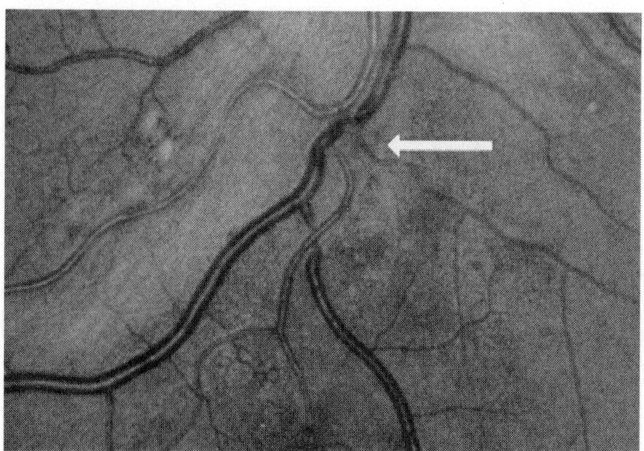

Figure 123-10. Hypertensive retinal vascular changes illustrating arteriovenous nicking.

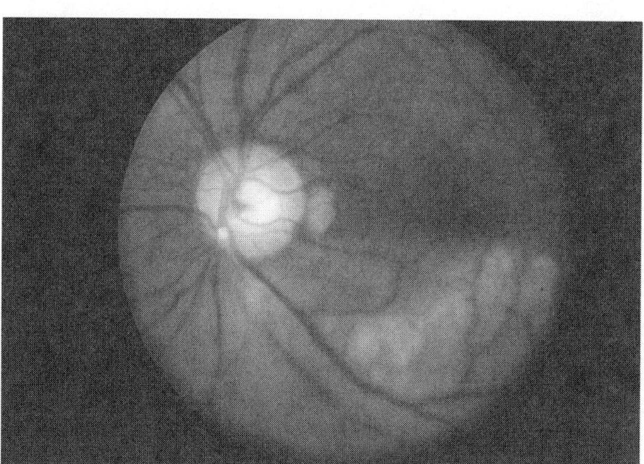

Figure 123-11. Occlusion of the inferior macular branch artery. Note white, edematous retinal tissue.

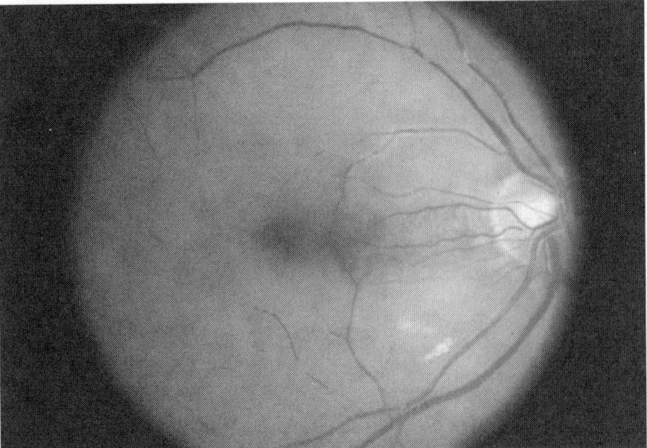

Figure 123-12. Central retinal artery occlusion with cherry-red spot.

compensation and reperfusion may allow recovery of flow with resolution of edema and improvement in visual acuity. In other eyes, progressive capillary occlusion may occur. Extensive retinal ischemia can result in the growth of new blood vessels on the retina or optic nerve, similar to neovascularization from diabetes. This can cause visual loss from vitreous hemorrhage.

Laser photocoagulation therapy in BRVO is considered for the two major complications: chronic macular edema and neovascularization. For eye with macular edema, delaying treatment for 4 months is important to allow maximum spontaneous resolution. Therapy has been shown to enhance resolution of the edema.

For eyes with neovascularization, scatter photocoagulation in the diseased quadrant of the retina is effective in causing regression of the new vessels. For eyes that develop nonclearing vitreous hemorrhage, vitrectomy surgery may be indicated.

CRVO usually is a much more dangerous and devastating disease. Several forms of the disease are recognized. A milder form, called partial or venous stasis retinopathy, has early findings of a full CRVO, yet visual acuity usually is good. This type of fundus picture commonly is seen in younger women with no significant medical history. Histologic studies suggest that all forms of CRVO have a common mechanism, which is thrombosis of the central retinal vein at the level of the optic nerve. The completeness of the thrombosis seems to determine the severity of retinal findings and the variable course.

Partial CRVO is characterized by mild optic disc swelling with mild dilatation and tortuosity of all branches of the central retinal vein. Dot and flame hemorrhages are present in all quadrants of the retina. Macular edema with loss of visual acuity may be present. Complete resolution can occur in a significant percentage of patients. Partial resolution can be seen in about one third of patients, and progression to complete CRVO occurs in about one third to one half of patients.

Complete CRVO is characterized by extensive four-quadrant retinal edema and hemorrhage. Marked venous dilatation and a variable number of cotton-wool spots are found (Fig. 123-14). The visual prognosis is extremely poor for this group as a whole: only 10% of this group will achieve vision better than 20/400. In addition, there is a high incidence rate (20% to 60%) of abnormal blood vessel growth in the front of the eye (iris neovascularization), which can result in a painful type of glaucoma that is difficult to treat.

Both types of CRVO are similar in age of onset, associated local and systemic findings, and laboratory studies. Ninety percent of patients are older than 50 years of age at onset. CRVO can occur at younger ages and is not always benign. Frequent systemic associations include cardiovascular disease, hypertension, and diabetes. Unusual diseases that affect the blood vessel wall or cause clotting abnormalities or changes in blood viscosity may be associated with a CRVO, including blood dyscrasia, dysproteinemia, and causes of vasculitis (eg, syphilis, sarcoidosis, lupus). Oral contraceptive use also has been implicated in CRVO.

Commonly, abnormal laboratory studies in patients with CRVO include glucose tolerance, serum cholesterol, lipoproteins, triglycerides, and γ-globulins. All patients presenting with CRVO should undergo a complete systemic evaluation with the appropriate laboratory studies to identify factors that may promote thrombus formation.

In eyes with partial CRVO, no treatment is useful unless an underlying systemic cause is found. In eyes with ischemic CRVO, full-scatter laser photocoagulation is effective therapy for preventing glaucoma.

MACULAR DISEASES

The macula, or central area of the retina, is a highly specialized structure that is made up of pure cones. This area allows normal indi-

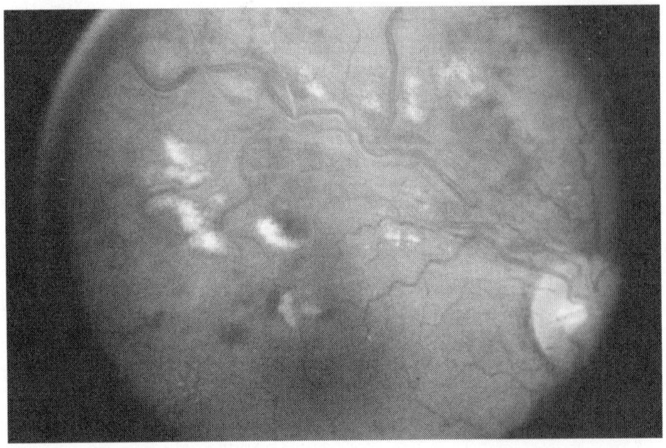

Figure 123-13. Superotemporal branch vein occlusion with hemorrhages and cotton-wool spots.

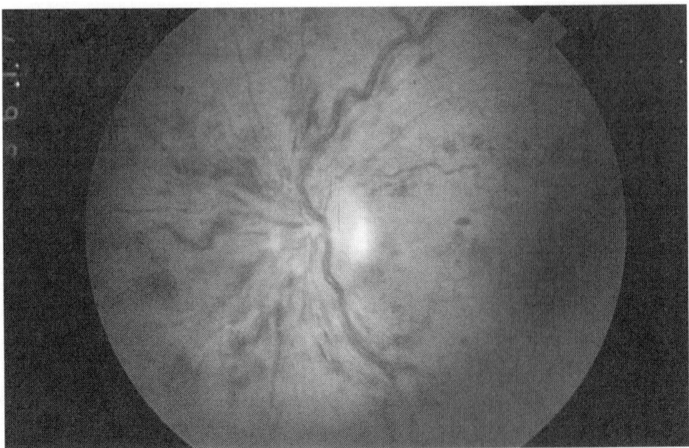

Figure 123-14. Occlusion of the central retinal vein.

viduals to achieve 20/20 vision or better in the healthy state. A variety of retinal diseases affect the macula preferentially, and the more common ones to be encountered in primary care are reviewed.

Age-Related Macular Degeneration

Age-related macular degeneration is extremely prevalent in the United States, affecting over 20 million individuals. Although it is most common in the group of individuals older than 65 years of age, younger patients also may be affected, and early signs of the disease can be seen in the third and fourth decades. This is a disease that primarily affects central vision, which is the vision relied on for close work such as reading and writing. It can also affect the ability to drive if severe enough. Normal senescence results in a spectrum of clinical and histologic changes in the macula, affecting all layers. The principle cell affected seems to be the retinal pigment epithelial cell (RPE).

This cell layer lies beneath the retina and has an important role in maintaining macular health. The anatomy of the RPE is unique, and the RPE promotes normal macular function in three ways: (1) formation of a blood-—retinal barrier between the blood supply to the retina and the sensory retina, (2) phagocytosis of rod and cone segments, and (3) vitamin A metabolism.

Changes in the RPE with age and disease include a loss of pigment granules and the formation of hyaline deposits on the supporting structure of the RPE, called Bruch's membrane. These deposits are called *drusen* and are the hallmark for this disease (Fig. 123-15). Bruch's membrane may thicken and then weaken, allowing vascular ingrowth from the blood vessel layer beneath the retina (choriocapillaris).

As a result of the processes associated with drusen formation, complications may ensue that cause visual loss. The most frequent complication is loss of the RPE leading to atrophy. Visual loss occurs because of the attendant loss of photoreceptors. This is more commonly known as *dry macular degeneration.* A second complication of drusen, accounting for almost 90% of severe visual loss from macular degeneration, is subretinal neovascularization. This is more commonly called *wet macular degeneration* and is caused by neovascular membranes entering through Bruch's membrane into the subretinal space, where they leak fluid, blood, or both, causing severe visual loss. The hemorrhage stimulates proliferation of scar tissue with loss of cone function.

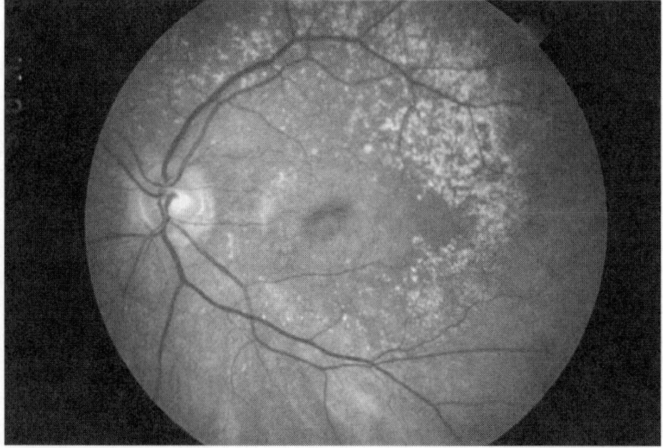

Figure 123-15. Macular drusen are the hallmark of age-related macular degeneration.

The pathogenesis of macular degeneration is unclear. The primary abnormality seems to be degeneration or a metabolic disturbance of the RPE and its biochemical relationship with the photoreceptor cells, resulting in a thickening of Bruch's membrane and the formation of drusen. Hereditary factors will most likely prove to be the most important determinant for the development of this disease.

No effective medical treatment is known for the dry form of macular degeneration. Patients with drusen, particularly when the fellow eye has a macular scar, should be instructed to monitor the central acuity. The standard is called an Amsler grid and is essentially a graph paper pattern with a central fixation point. Patients monitor each eye independently and look for any blind spots or distortion in the lines. Any abnormal symptom should be reported to their ophthalmologist. Fluorescein angiography can be performed to look for any evidence of treatable subretinal neovascular complexes.

Recent reports of the efficacy of zinc in the diet has spawned a host of dietary "eye vitamins," none of which have been proven to delay the onset or cure the damage of macular degeneration. Other studies have, however, shown some stabilization of the disease in which patients consumed a diet high in green leafy vegetables such as spinach and collard greens.

The efficacy of laser treatment for the wet or exudative form of macular degeneration has been demonstrated by a national randomized double-blind study called the Macular Photocoagulation Study. In this study, patients had angiographic evidence of a choroidal neovascular membrane at least 200 μm from the center of the fovea. After 18 months, 65% of untreated eyes, compared with 25% of treated eyes, had experienced severe visual loss.

Many eyes cannot be treated effectively, and a patient can progress to legal blindness in each eye in a short period of time. For an otherwise healthy independent adult, this can result in a dramatic change in lifestyle. An individual may no longer be able to drive or live by themselves. A joint effort by the ophthalmologist and primary care provider is essential to watch for signs of depression during this period. Low vision aids and support groups can be useful. Referral for evaluation by the local state services for the visually handicapped may be appropriate.

Central Serous Choroidopathy

Central serous choroidopathy (CSR) is characterized by the development of a serous detachment of the sensory retina caused by a focal leakage in the RPE. It occurs preferentially in young men who present with symptoms of sudden onset of blurred vision and distortion. Women are affected, although rarely.

The sensory retina is elevated, and the leakage point sometimes is identified as a small area of RPE clumping or atrophy. Occasionally, an extensive serous detachment of the retina may develop from one or more leak points outside of the macula and clinically can resemble a large retinal detachment.

Most eyes with CSR (80% to 90%) undergo spontaneous resorption of the subretinal fluid and recovery of vision within 1 to 6 months of the onset of symptoms, although the patient may continue to complain that the vision is not right. Some eyes develop permanent visual loss, and many experience recurrent episodes.

Although CSR is less common in women, there have been some studies on the effects of pregnancy on this disease. There presence of subretinal fibrinous exudates in this particular population of women was common. There seemed to be no race predilection, and all patients studied showed that the resolution phase of CSR occurred during the term of the pregnancy. One patient had a subsequent pregnancy without involvement.

Laser treatment of the site of leakage has been shown to shorten the duration of this disease, but does not affect the final visual acuity when compared with eyes that are not undergoing treatment. Most ophthalmologists elect to observe the first episode of CSR and treat only if it persists beyond 6 months. Recurrences are more likely to be treated, and eyes with visual loss in the fellow eye from CSR also should be treated.

Macular Hole

Macular hole is a condition occurring primarily in women in the sixth through eighth decades of life. A hole forms in the central macula, causing loss of reading vision (Fig. 123-16). The symptoms usually worsen over a period of time; however, some patients report a sudden visual loss. Visual acuity can drop to the 20/400 level with preservation of peripheral visual field. Developing macular holes can present with much better vision.

The pathogenesis of macular hole formation is not known; however, the relationship between the macula and its overlying vitreous is implicated. Tractional or pulling forces exerted by a thin layer of vitreous seem to cause hole development in patients who are susceptible.

Previously, there was no successful treatment for this condition, but within the last decade surgery has allowed recovery of most of the visual loss. Removal of the vitreous gel using microsurgical techniques, in addition to peeling the thin layer of adherent vitreous over the macula, is the mainstay of treatment. The vitreous is replaced with a premeasured concentration of a long-acting gas bubble, and the patient is instructed to maintain a face-down position for 12 to 14 hours per day for up to 2 weeks postoperatively. The success rate of this procedure approaches 90%.

The incidence rate of bilateral disease has been reported to be up to 10%, so an effective treatment has had a considerable impact on this group of patients. Patient selection remains crucial in the success of this procedure.

Epiretinal Membrane

Epiretinal membranes are extraretinal tissues that have a propensity to form at or near the macula and cause blurring and distortion of vision (Fig. 123-17). These membranes occur in patients in the sixth through eighth decades, and, if they develop enough pulling properties, can cause a marked reduction in visual acuity associated with macular edema. The pathogenesis of these membranes is unclear; however, histologic studies show some of the cells that make up the membranes to both RPE and retinal glial cells.

The treatment of these membranes is surgery if vision drops to a level that makes reading or driving difficult. Whereas most of these membranes are idiopathic, some can be secondary to a variety of conditions, including retinal vascular occlusions, uveitis, trauma, and intraocular surgery.

INFLAMMATORY AND INFECTIOUS DISEASES

A variety of inflammatory and infectious diseases can affect the retina and vitreous. The degree of inflammation varies, and visual loss ranges from mild to severe. The importance of accurate diagnosis cannot be overemphasized because appropriate and timely treatment makes a considerable difference in outcome. The major diseases to be reviewed are toxoplasmosis and AIDS-related diseases found in the eye.

Toxoplasmosis

Patients with ocular toxoplasmosis usually present with symptoms of floaters and blurred vision. The floaters are caused by inflammatory cells in the vitreous. The source of the cells is a focus of inflammation in the retina that usually can be seen ophthalmoscopically as a white, raised retinal lesion with indistinct borders. The causative organism is *Toxoplasma gondii*, which multiplies preferentially in the inner retinal layers.

The acute retinal lesions heal spontaneously within 6 months and leave a chorioretinal scar with variable pigmentation (Fig. 123-18). Usually the vitreous clears, and vision returns as long as the retinitis has not involved the macula.

Repeated attacks are caused by recurrent foci of retinitis, most often at the edge of old atrophic lesions, thought to be caused by the breakdown of *Toxoplasma* cysts in the retina and subsequent release of viable organisms. The encysted organism may remain latent in the retina for many years.

The congenital form of toxoplasmosis is transmitted in an infected pregnant woman across the placenta to the fetus and

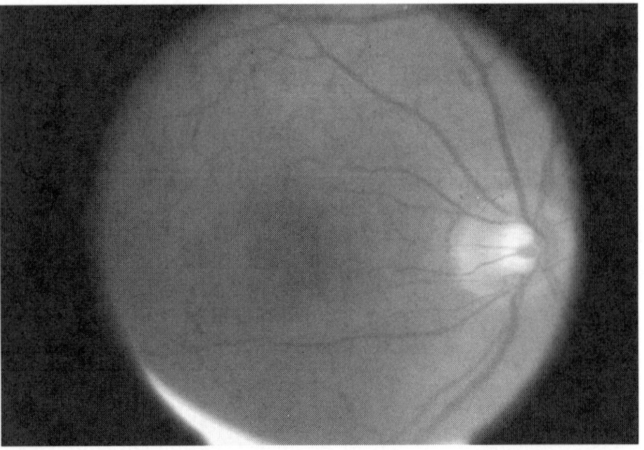

Figure 123-16. Macular hole measuring approximately 300 μm.

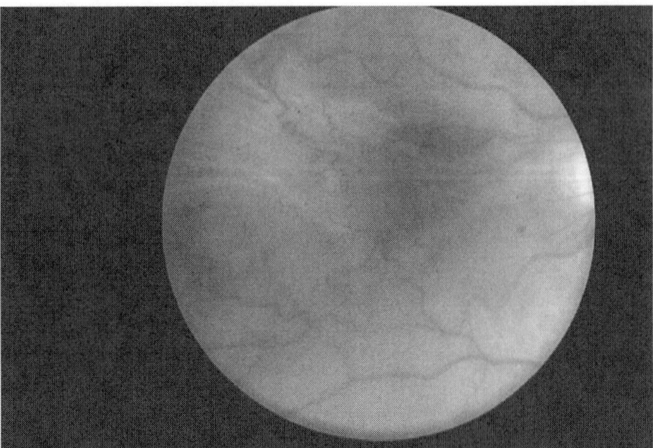

Figure 123-17. Epiretinal membrane over the macula causing distortion of the underlying retina.

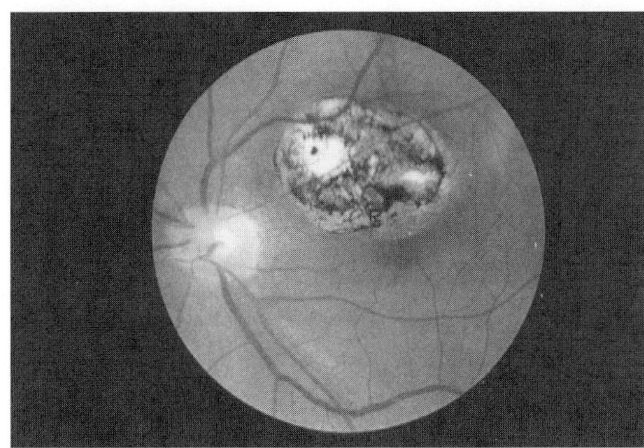

Figure 123-18. Typical toxoplasmosis scar with heavy pigment present.

affects multiple organs. The eye and brain are especially susceptible, particularly if the fetus acquires the infection during the first trimester. Infants born with congenital toxoplasmosis often are born with large macular scars and may show recurrences over the rest of their lives.

Cats are the natural host of the organism and shed the cysts in their feces. This can contaminate foods or infect animals eaten by humans. Raw or undercooked meat is a major and avoidable source of infection.

The diagnosis of ocular toxoplasmosis is made by observing a focal, necrotizing retinitis in association with an old chorioretinal scar and by detecting any levels of anti-*Toxoplasma* antibodies in the sera. The enzyme-linked immunosorbent assay is most useful for this purpose.

Treatment of active ocular toxoplasmosis generally is recommended in patients with extensive involvement and when the lesions threaten the macula. Treatment consists of orally administered pyrimethamine and sulfonamide along with prednisone for 6 weeks. Clindamycin also has been found to be effective in place of sulfonamides.

AIDS: Retinal and Choroidal Infections

At least a dozen infectious agents have been identified in the retina or choroid of patients with AIDS. They vary in prevalence, but all can lead to loss of vision or blindness. Because of the difficulty involved with retinal biopsy and vitreous culture and the inaccuracy of serologic testing for ocular pathogens, clinical diagnosis remains the major method of differentiating the cause of an AIDS-related retinopathy.

The most common retinal manifestation of AIDS is a microangiopathy clinically manifested by the presence of single or multiple cotton-wool spots. The lesions usually are found in the macular area. Retinal hemorrhages, microaneurysms, or other microvascular changes also can be found.

No specific treatment is required; however, the presence of these changes is probably a marker for an advanced stage of the illness. Human immunodeficiency virus retinopathy has been shown to be related to a decreasing CD4–CD8 ratio.

Cytomegalovirus (CMV) retinitis is the most common retinal infection seen in AIDS. The exact prevalence is not known, but most investigators believe that at least 20% of patients with AIDS will develop CMV retinitis during the course of their disease. Cytomegalovirus retinopathy is usually a late manifestation of the AIDS syndrome, its presence alone is sufficient for making a diagnosis of AIDS.

The diagnosis of CMV retinopathy is based on clinical findings. The presence of anti-CMV antibodies or the presence of CMV from other body sites cannot be used to confirm the diagnosis of CMV retinopathy because most patients with AIDS have been infected with CMV.

CMV retinitis can be bilateral or unilateral. Clinically, there are two presentations of CMV retinitis described. The first is the classically described form usually seen in or near the macula. This presentation may be referred to as the hemorrhagic type and has a "crumbled cheese and ketchup" appearance. Large areas of retinal hemorrhage associated with areas of thick, whitish retinal necrosis are seen along blood vessels (Fig. 123-19). The second form, most often seen in the peripheral retina, is the granular type. In this form, the lesions spread out from a central focus. The advancing border has a yellow-—white granular appearance with little or no hemorrhage. The location of these changes is mostly impossible to see with the direct ophthalmoscope, so it is important for the ophthalmologist to screen these patients at risk for the development of CMV retinitis every 90 days.

CMV retinitis is an indolent infection, spreading slowly over the course of many weeks to eventually involve the entire retina. Without treatment, vision usually is lost because of optic nerve involvement. Spontaneous remission is rare. Treatment was successfully undertaken in 1985 using ganciclovir, an analogue of the antiviral acyclovir. Ganciclovir stabilizes the retinitis, halting or delaying progression and visual loss, and decreasing viral shedding. The drug is used intravenously for a 2- to 3-week induction period at a dose of 5 mg/kg twice daily. After induction, patients continue on maintenance of 5 to 6 mg/kg/day given 5 to 7 days during the week. Renal function and the development of neutropenia need to be monitored while on this therapy. Therapy continues indefinitely unless the patient develops a resistant CMV infection or experiences life-threatening side effects.

Initially, 70% to 80% of patients with CMV retinitis respond to ganciclovir; however, recurrent CMV can occur in up to 40% of patients on maintenance therapy. Patients need to be followed closely every 2 to 3 weeks while undergoing treatment.

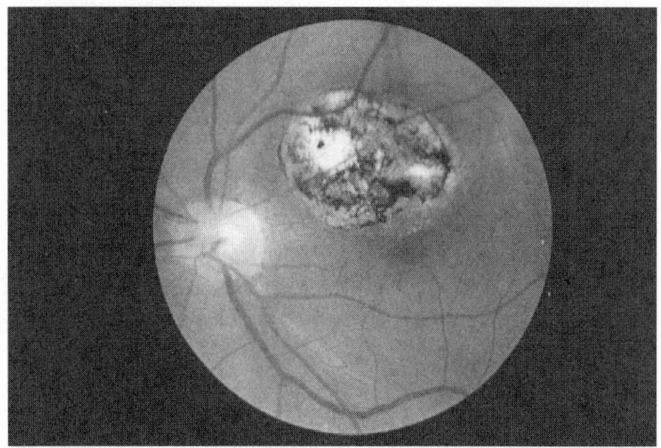

Figure 123-19. CMV retinitis with hemorrhages and retinal necrosis.

The primary alternative to ganciclovir is foscarnet, which is a potent inhibitor of herpes simplex virus DNA polymerase as well as retrovirus reverse transcriptase. Foscarnet also is virustatic for CMV and requires continuous therapy. The most problematic side effect is nephrotoxicity.

Other treatment modalities include direct injection of ganciclovir into the vitreous cavity in patients unable to tolerate the systemic side effects. A long-acting ganciclovir pellet, which can be surgically inserted into the vitreous, recently has been approved by the Food and Drug Administration. The pellet lasts about 5 months and obviates the need for systemic treatment. This will probably become the standard of care shortly.

The presence of CMV retinitis used to be associated with a mean survival of 4 to 6 months. With improved treatments of AIDS in general, this survival has been lengthened to years. The ability to preserve vision becomes more important with increased survival time.

Several other opportunistic infections affect the retina and underlying choroid. These are only mentioned here, and the interested reader is referred to sources cited at the end of this chapter for more detailed information. Infection with *Pneumocystis carinii* usually is seen in advanced cases of AIDS. Syphilis, herpes zoster infection, toxoplasmosis, and infections with *Mycobacterium* and *Cryptococcus* all have been described.

RETINAL TEARS AND RETINAL DETACHMENT

The development of retinal tears or retinal detachment can occur at any time during a person's lifetime. A retinal break is a full-thickness discontinuity of the retinal tissue, usually located in the peripheral retina. Its clinical significance lies in the fact that it provides an access route for vitreous fluid to enter the subretinal space, causing a retinal detachment. Normally, the retina is kept in place by a variety of mechanical, physical, and metabolic forces. The RPE has a strong pumping mechanism that keeps the subretinal space relatively dry. When forces of fluid movement are strong enough to overcome that pump mechanism, the retina detaches.

The precursor of a retinal tear is the condition known as posterior vitreous detachment (PVD). The vitreous in young individuals uniformly fills the vitreous cavity. With senescence, the vitreous gel liquefies and can pull away from its adhesion at the back of the eye (Fig. 123-20). The adhesion in the peripheral retina is strongest near the insertion of the vitreous, here called the vitreous base. This is the location where tears usually occur. Symptomatic PVD causes patients to complain of the sudden onset of floaters or flashing lights. These flashing lights, or photopsias, are an indication of persistent pulling or traction on the retina and can be present with or without a retinal tear. Symptomatic PVD requires immediate referral to an ophthalmologist and a careful retinal examination. If the collapsing vitreous pulls on the retinal blood vessels, a vitreous hemorrhage can occur with a dramatic loss of vision.

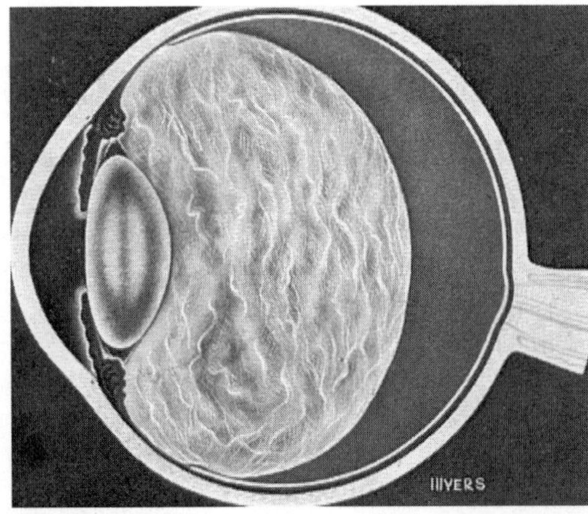

Figure 123-20. Posterior vitreous detachment. Note the adhesions remaining anteriorly.

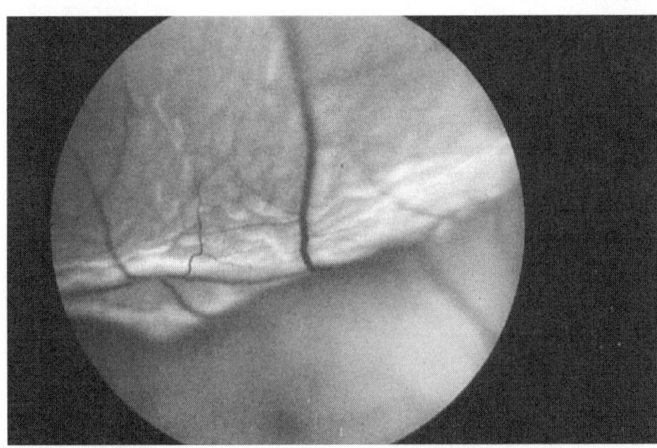

Figure 123-21. Typical appearance of a retinal detachment.

If a retinal tear is identified, it is usually treated the same day. As long as the tear is not associated with the development of large amounts of subretinal fluid, laser or freezing (cryopexy) can be performed. These are office-based procedures and are associated with minimal morbidity and high success rates.

If too much fluid has accumulated under the retina, then a retinal detachment has occurred (Fig. 123-21) and major eye surgery usually is indicated. Retinal detachments usually are an ophthalmic emergency, and surgery is performed within 12 to 24 hours. If the detachment is limited to a peripheral part of the retina not involving the macula, then the surgery takes on added urgency. If the detached retina can be repaired before fluid accumulates under the macula, the chances of preserving 20/20 vision are much greater. Patient with detachments threatening the macula usually undergo surgery within hours.

Surgery usually involves outpatient or inpatient hospital services. The standard procedure is called a scleral buckle. The tears all are identified under controlled conditions in the operating room suite

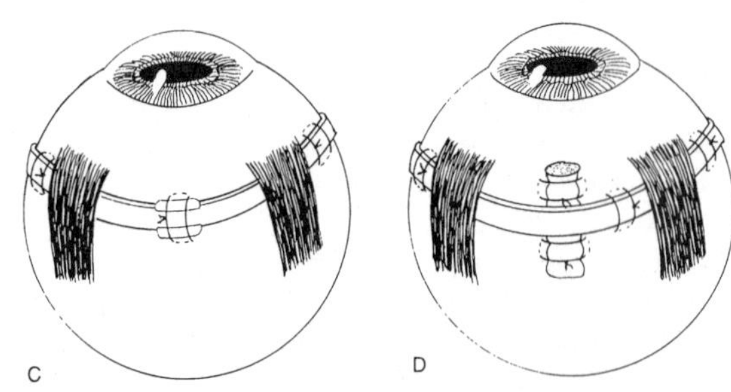

Figure 123-22. Location of scleral buckle surgery.

and treated with cryopexy to induce RPE adhesion. A silicone or sponge material is then sutured onto the wall of the eye under the tears to support the weakened areas of tear. The eye wall is indented effectively, relieving the pulling on the retinal tear (Fig. 123-22). Some retinal detachments require more involved surgery such as vitrectomy. An office-based procedure for certain selected retinal detachments is called pneumatic retinopexy. This technique involves instillation of a long-acting gas (2 to 4 weeks) into the vitreous cavity and after treatment of the tears with laser or cryopexy. The patient then is positioned so that the intraocular gas bubble remains in contact with the tear for 12 to 16 hours per day. Obviously, this procedure is tolerable for superior detachments primarily.

Retinal detachment surgery is successful greater than 90% of the time. Failure of the retina to reattach results from a variety of reasons, and reoperation may be necessary.

BIBLIOGRAPHY

Diabetes Control and Complications Trial Research Group. retinopathy with intensive versus conventional treatmen Control and Complications Trial. *Ophthalmology* 1995;10

Duane T, ed. Clinical ophthalmology, vol 3. Philadelphia: Harper & Row, 19

Gass JDM. Stereoscopic atlas of macular diseases. St Louis: CV Mosby, 1987.

Lewis H, Ryan SJ, eds. Medical and surgical retina: advances, controversies and management. St Louis: CV Mosby, 1994.

Macular Photocoagulation Study Group. Argon laser photocoagulation for senile macular degeneration: results of a randomized clinical trial. *Arch Ophthalmol* 1982;100:912.

Ryan SJ, ed. Retina. St Louis: CV Mosby, 1989.

Schepens C. Retinal detachment and allied diseases, vols 1 & 2. Philadelphia: WB Saunders, 1983.

Stenson S, Friedberg D. AIDS and the eye. Contact Lens Association of America, 1995.

Primary Care for Women, edited by Phyllis C. Leppert and Fred M. Howard. Lippincott-Raven Publishers, Philadelphia © 1997.

124

Neuro-Ophthalmologic Disorders

ERIC L. BERMAN

In the field of neuro-ophthalmology a number of conditions are encountered that occur more commonly, although not exclusively, in women. Some of these disorders are well-known; others are more obscure. This chapter discusses several of these conditions. Demyelinating and inflammatory conditions, autoimmune disorders, conditions causing papilledema associated with elevated cerebrospinal fluid pressures, tumors involving the anterior visual pathways, and changes seen in pregnancy will be reviewed.

DEMYELINATING AND INFLAMMATORY CONDITIONS

Etiology

Optic neuritis is one of the most common conditions seen by the neuro-ophthalmologist. In children it is often bilateral, symmetric, and of viral etiology. The prognosis for recovery is excellent without treatment. In adults, optic neuritis is one of the classic events seen in multiple sclerosis. Patients presenting with this condition may be found to have multiple sclerosis after workup, or may have a known diagnosis of demyelinating disease. All patients with optic neuritis do not have multiple sclerosis; all patients with multiple sclerosis do not develop optic neuritis.

History

The clinical course of optic neuritis is often classic. Patients describe a subacute loss of vision, occurring over hours to days. The vision stabilizes and begins to improve over the next few weeks to months. The loss of vision is often associated with a dull pain behind the eye that increases on ocular movement. High temperatures or exercise may exacerbate the visual difficulty (Uhtoff phenomenon). Careful history should be undertaken to look for previous neurologic events that may represent other evidence of multiple sclerosis. Syphilis, lupus, Lyme disease, and other inflammatory, infectious, and autoimmune conditions may also cause optic neuritis.

Physical Examination

Clinical examination shows decreased vision in the involved eye ranging from 20/20 to no light perception, along with a relative afferent pupillary defect (RAPD). This latter finding is the sine qua non of optic nerve injury. Unless both nerves have been involved, the diagnosis of optic neuritis requires the presence of an RAPD. To look for an RAPD, shine a bright halogen handlight into one pupil and then rapidly swing it to the other. When the light strikes the contralateral pupil it should constrict. If one pupil constricts and the other dilates or remains the same size, an RAPD is present. The remainder of the clinical examination is usually normal. In one third of cases the inflammation can be observed directly as swelling of the optic nerve, or papillitis. The remaining two thirds of patients have retrobulbar optic neuritis, with normal-appearing optic nerveheads on direct ophthalmoscopy. Further evidence of optic nerve insult can be confirmed by having the patient compare the brightness of a light, or a red test object between the two eyes. The loss of brightness or color saturation is further evidence of optic neuritis. All patients with evidence of optic neuritis should undergo a careful neurologic examination to look for other signs consistent with multiple sclerosis.

Differential Diagnosis

The differential diagnosis of optic nerve disease includes optic neuritis, papilledema (where the optic nerve is swollen due to increased intracranial pressure), ischemic optic neuropathy, and compressive optic neuropathy. Papilledema, as discussed below, is usually bilateral and does not cause acute loss of vision. Ischemic optic neuropathy is an infarction of the optic nerve, causing an acute loss of vision with little chance for recovery. Compressive optic neuropathy usually is a more chronic process, occurring over weeks and continuing as a progressive loss of vision without stabilization or improvement.

Treatment

Until recently, treatment of optic neuritis was anecdotal with no good, controlled studies looking at the optimal treatment. The Optic Neuritis Treatment Trial (ONTT), a multicenter, randomized prospective study, was designed to look at risk factors, appropriate workup, and treatment of this disorder. Three groups of patients suffering from an initial attack of optic neuritis in one eye were randomized to receive a placebo, oral prednisone, or intravenous solumedrol. Each group was compared for visual function, including visual acuity, color vision, contrast sensitivity, and visual field testing. One year after randomization all groups recovered to the same level in all tests. On average all groups recovered to 20/16 vision in the involved eye. A difference between groups was that those receiving intravenous solumedrol recovered more rapidly than the other two groups. An unexpected finding was that the oral prednisone group had a statistically higher rate of developing additional neurologic events. As a result, the conclusion of the study was that oral prednisone is contraindicated in acute optic neuritis.

Imaging Studies

In later publications the ONTT has shed light on other factors involved in optic neuritis. If there is no evidence in the history or physical examination for other pertinent medical conditions, there is no yield in obtaining routine blood work. Most recently a publication has documented that those patients with MRI scans showing specific changes consistent with multiple sclerosis have suffered fewer subsequent demyelinating attacks over the following two years if treated with intravenous steroids. Thus, at this time, any patient with routine optic neuritis should have a magnetic resonance (MR) imaging scan of the head and, if changes consistent with multiple sclerosis are seen, intravenous steroids are recommended.

ANTERIOR ISCHEMIC OPTIC NEURITIS

After the age of 45 acute loss of vision caused by optic nerve disease is more often ischemic than demyelinating. This condition is referred to as anterior ischemic optic neuropathy (AION) because optic disc swelling is almost always seen. The typical complaint is unilateral, instantaneous, and painless loss of vision, which is often severe and may be total. Etiology is divided into arteritic and nonarteritic types. The arteritic form of AION is caused by giant cell arteritis and is diagnosed with an erythrocyte sedimentation rate and temporal artery biopsy. Careful history should be directed toward symptoms of temporal arteritis, including scalp tenderness, headache, jaw claudication, unexplained fevers, weight loss, anorexia, or aches and pains consistent with polymyalgia rheumatica. Acute loss of vision in the setting of temporal arteritis is not always due to AION. Thirty percent of central retinal artery occlusions are caused by giant cell arteritis.

The nonarteritic form of AION is not associated with temporal arteritis and is the more common form. It is usually seen in conjunction with hypertension or diabetes.

Findings on physical examination are similar to optic neuritis, with decreased vision and a relative afferent pupillary defect. In contradistinction to the majority of optic neuritis patients, the optic nervehead is swollen and often pale. There may be a segmental swelling of the disc and adjacent hemorrhages. Other fundus changes may point to hypertension or diabetes as an underlying risk factor. These include arteriolar narrowing, venous tortuosity, flame or dot hemorrhages, and soft and hard exudates. Some patients may have a small cup-to-disc ratio of 0.1 or less in the contralateral eye.

Workup of AION requires an immediate erythrocyte sedimentation rate to rule out giant cell arteritis. If there is any question about this diagnosis, a biopsy of the superficial temporal artery is mandatory. If the biopsy is positive, the patient should be started on steroids in an attempt to decrease the risk of stroke or AION in the contralateral eye. If the suspicion is strong enough, oral or intravenous steroids should be initiated prior to biopsy. Most neuro-ophthalmologists start treatment with 1 g/day of intravenous solumedrol for 2 to 3 days before switching over to oral therapy. Left untreated, temporal arteritis will cause AION on the other side in greater that 50% of cases. If temporal arteritis can be excluded, treatment mandates aggressive control of underlying factors, including blood pressure and blood glucose. No study has documented a positive effect for steroids in the nonarteritic form of this disease.

AUTOIMMUNE DISORDERS

The two major autoimmune disorders encountered by the neuro-ophthalmologist are myasthenia gravis and thyroid eye disease. Although systemic disease may be seen in both conditions, it is not unusual for ocular disease to be the sole manifestation of the entity or to precede the systemic findings and allow the diagnosis to be made.

Myasthenia Gravis

Etiology

Myasthenia gravis is a disease in which antibodies to the neuromuscular junction cause muscular weakness. The weakness may be due to blockage or destruction of acetylcholine receptors by antibodies. There is a 2-to-1 female preponderance. The disease may begin at any age of life, but is most common in the third decade. Patients or family members may have other autoimmune diseases, such as Graves disease, lupus, ulcerative colitis, or rheumatoid arthritis.

Clinical Findings

The classic complaint is of fatigue of the involved muscles that increases over the course of the day or when extremely tired. In the most serious form of the disease, involvement of the diaphragm may be life-threatening. The weakness recovers after rest or introduction of anticholinesterase medication. Approximately 75% of all cases of myasthenia gravis begin with ocular complaints. Over 90% of generalized myasthenia patients have ocular findings. Thus it is essential to pick up early clues to allow diagnosis and treatment before more serious effects have occurred.

Myasthenia gravis may involve any or all extraocular and facial muscles. The most commonly seen manifestations are ptosis, drooping of one or both eyelids, and paretic strabismus. Ptosis is characterized by an inability to keep the eyes open by the end of the day. Characteristically, patients report that the eyes open normally on awakening or after a nap. By late morning or early afternoon the problem develops and worsens steadily until evening. Often patients describe taping the eyelids open or using their fingers to allow them to drive. Fatigability can be documented by observing increased drooping of the eyelid after having the patient fixate in upgaze for 20 to 30 seconds. In addition, there may be weakness of the orbicularis muscle. On attempted forced closure the eye may be seen through the weakened lids, a "peek sign."

Virtually any oculomotor paresis may be seen in myasthenia. The only muscles that are not involved are those innervated by the autonomic nervous system. Thus, pupillary abnormalities suggest another diagnosis. Diplopia is binocular and may be vertical, horizontal, or torsional in nature. One classic pattern is "pseudointernuclear ophthalmoplegia." The paresis resembles that seen in damage to the medial longitudinal fasciculus with weakness of adduction in one eye and abducting nystagmus of the contralateral eye. Any diplopia which does not fit a classic cranial nerve palsy pattern or is variable should raise the possibility of myasthenia gravis.

Diagnosis

The diagnosis of myasthenia gravis is made by observing improvement or normalization of muscular function after intravenous administration of edrophonium chloride (Tensilon), an acetylcholinesterase inhibitor. False positive results are rare, but false negatives may occur. If clinical suspicion is high the test should be repeated. The test should not be considered negative unless fasciculation of the eyelid or other systemic signs of therapeutic levels of the medication are noted. In some cases this test is negative in clinically classic myasthenia gravis. In these cases anti-acetylcholine receptor antibodies should be assayed. There are three subtypes of antibody, receptor, modulating, and sensitizing, all of which need to be tested. In purely ocular myasthenia the receptor antibody is positive in slightly greater than 50% of cases, while the modulating antibody is positive in close to 75%. Studies have shown that ocular myasthenia becomes systemic within 2 years of diagnosis if generalized myasthenia is to develop.

Treatment

Treatment of myasthenia gravis is with systemic anticholinergic medications, steroids, or a combination of the two. Often the ptosis and diplopia are only partially improved. If the condition stabilizes for more than 1 year, conservative surgical repair of ptosis or strabismus can be considered.

Thyroid Eye Disease

Etiology

Thyroid eye disease is an autoimmune disease that can affect all aspects of the ophthalmologic examination. Changes may include proptosis, eyelid retraction or swelling, corneal exposure, extraocular motility problems, conjunctival injection, and optic neuropathy. Common to all these conditions is an underlying autoimmune disorder. The exact nature of the problem has not been identified; research has suggested common antigens expressed on the thyroid gland and orbital tissues. Patients with thyroid eye disease may clinically be hyperthyroid, euthyroid, or hypothyroid. Some patients may not develop Graves disease until many years later; other cases may remain purely ocular in nature. Thus, systemic assays to look for abnormal thyroid hormones may be negative, even in classic thyroid eye disease. Nonetheless, most cases of ocular disease are associated with Graves disease.

A mnemonic to help remember the spectrum of thyroid eye signs is NO SPECS (Fig. 124-1).

Clinical Findings

There is no typical progression of changes. Patients may have only motility difficulty or sight loss, or may have multiple changes. The most common changes seen are proptosis, lid retraction, and diplopia. The corneal changes are due to lagophthalmos, the inability to close the eyes, which is caused by lid changes or severe proptosis. Frequent lubrication is important in reducing the likelihood of permanent damage or perforation. Sight loss is the most feared complication, caused by compression of the optic nerve by enlarged extraocular muscles in the posterior orbit. This requires emergent treatment by oral steroids, radiation, or bony decompression of the orbit.

The duration of active inflammation on each side is typically less than 3 years. Each orbit may be involved over different periods of time. The goal of treatment is to be as conservative as possible during the period of acute inflammation and perform any surgical repairs later, after fibrosis has occurred. Surgery in an inflamed orbit may actually increase the inflammatory response and make the situation worse. After the changes have been noted to be stable for more than 6 months surgical repair may be considered.

PSEUDOTUMOR CEREBRI

The term *papilledema* refers to swollen optic nerveheads associated with increased cerebrospinal fluid pressure. There are many other causes of optic nerve swelling, as discussed earlier, which should be described as a swollen optic nerve, not papilledema. Only when a lumbar puncture is performed or neuroimaging documents obstruction to cerebrospinal fluid flow should the term papilledema be used. Unfortunately, the appearance of the swelling does not always allow one to make this distinction. The clinical picture should allow papilledema to be differentiated from inflammation, infarction, or compression of the optic nerve.

Etiology and Differential Diagnosis

Pseudotumor cerebri, or idiopathic intracranial hypertension (IIH), is a clinical syndrome in which signs and symptoms of papilledema are associated with normal neuroimaging studies and elevated opening pressure on lumbar puncture. By definition, this condition requires exclusion of other infectious or mass lesions that may produce a similar picture. IIH may occur before puberty

N No signs or symptoms
O Only signs (increased stare)
S Signs and symptoms (tearing)
P Proptosis
E Extraocular motility problems
C Corneal changes
S Sight loss

Figure 124-1. A mnemonic to help remember the spectrum of eye signs in thyroid disease.

or after menopause, but is most common during the early adult years. Approximately 85% of patients are obese women of child-bearing age. Before puberty and after menopause the male to female ratio is equal. There is not a strong relationship between IIH and obesity in men.

In a minority of patients an underlying factor is identified. One cause of IIH is venous sinus thrombosis. While the most common sinus involved is the superior sagittal sinus, any sinus may be involved. This diagnosis requires careful magnetic resonance angiography (MRA), with flow rates set to look at venous flow. The usual MRA sequences, designed to look at the arterial system, may miss this finding. Suggestions of thrombosis should be seen on high quality MRI scans, and often on computed tomography (CT) scanning of the head. Another potential cause of IIH is medications. The most commonly identified agents are listed in Table 124-1.

Of these agents the most commonly used clinically are tetracycline and vitamin A. Despite common opinion, no controlled study has documented a relationship between IIH and birth control pills. If there is a question of relationship, it is prudent to discontinue any potential causes.

The majority of cases have no predisposing conditions. The most common complaint is headache. This is usually a bilateral, nonlocalized headache, not relieved with over-the-counter analgesic medications. The second most common complaint is transient obscurations of vision. These are short-lived "gray-outs" of vision, often induced by rapid standing or bending over. The symptoms may be described as white, gray, or black, but do not typically last longer than 4 or 5 seconds and should not be confused with amaurosis fugax, which typically is not shorter than 5 minutes. Papilledema does not cause loss of vision unless chronic. Most patients with IIH report normal vision between obscurations, differentiating this state from acute inflammatory or ischemic conditions. A third complaint is pulsatile tinnitus. While present in up to 60% of IIH patients, this is not generally volunteered by the patient and should be specifically sought out. The patient hears a pulsation in one or both ears which is synchronous with the arterial pulse. Patients may also have diplopia, secondary to sixth nerve palsy. This is the only neurologic sign seen in IIH. The sixth nerve is tethered under the petroclinoid ligament while coursing over the petrous ridge of the temporal bone and is the only cranial nerve affected by increased intracranial pressure.

Physical Examination and Clinical Findings

Findings on physical examination are usually minimal. Abduction deficit may be seen in the setting of sixth nerve palsy, but usually the only finding is swollen optic nerves. While unilateral disc swelling is possible, bilateral swelling is the rule. The margin between the optic nervehead and the adjacent retina is blurred and no spontaneous venous pulsations are seen. With the direct ophthalmoscope, elevation of the disc can be documented by starting at a +7 setting, putting the focus on the ocular lens. By dialing in additional minus, one can appreciate that the swollen, elevated part of the optic nervehead comes into focus earlier than the central, cup, or retina. Numerous soft exudates and hemorrhage are often seen around the optic nervehead.

Table 124-1. Medications and Other Agents That May Cause Idiopathic Intracranial Hypertension

Definite Relationship
Tetracycline
Nalidixic acid
Vitamin A
Lithium
Withdrawal from steroids
Possible Relationship
Birth control pills

Laboratory and Imaging Studies

The workup of IIH includes visual field testing. Usually the only findings are the enlargement of the blind spot and constriction of the inferonasal periphery. Additional changes may be seen in chronic cases. If the enlarged blind spot approaches within 5° of fixation, aggressive care is mandated.

All cases of suspected IIH require neuroimaging. At this time high quality MRI scanning with MRA is the procedure of choice. If not available, CT scanning is an acceptable alternative. If these studies do not reveal pathology, lumbar puncture is the next step. These are often difficult procedures due to obesity, and referral to an experienced practitioner may be indicated. The opening pressure is measured in a relaxed, lateral position and fluid is then sent for routine chemistries, cell count, and culture. Often the pressure is at or above 400 mm and may be above the scale of the usual manometer. In such cases patients often note immediate relief of headaches after the procedure. While the upper range of normal cerebrospinal pressures are directly related to body weight, any opening pressure above 250 in a relaxed patient is elevated.

Treatment

Treatment of IIH is based on the severity of symptoms and signs. Some patients have papilledema noted on routine examination. If there is no evidence of visual dysfunction these patients may be safely observed at close intervals. All obese patients should be advised to lose weight. Practitioners who see many pseudotumor patients have witnessed complete disappearance of symptoms with weight loss. Years later, if patients regain the weight they may witness the return of symptoms. If there is only mild headache patients may choose not to receive any treatment. If treatment is indicated, medical therapy is the initial regimen. Oral furosemide is the medication with the lowest rate of side effects, and works by decreasing total body water, including that in the cerebrospinal fluid. If this is not sufficient, or if the initial symptoms are severe, acetazolamide therapy is the next agent. This medication decreases cerebrospinal fluid production by about 50%. If patients are quite obese doses of 2 g/day may be needed. For patients who cannot tolerate acetazolamide or who are allergic to sulfa medications, digoxin is another alternative. Digoxin also decreases cerebrospinal fluid production and has few side effects in patients without cardiac disease or electrolyte abnormalities. Because of the relationship between IIH and withdrawal from steroids, most experts do not recommend steroid therapy for this entity.

If medical therapy is not sufficient to relieve symptoms or reverse visual dysfunction, surgical therapy is indicated. The two major procedures performed are lumboperitoneal shunt and optic nerve sheath decompression (ONSD). Shunting of the cerebrospinal fluid effectively reduces the pressure and reverses symptoms. Unfortunately, shunting procedures often need revision and permanent visual loss may develop at the time of failure. For visual dysfunction ONSD is now the procedure of choice. This procedure entails creating an opening in the dural sheath surrounding the optic nerve and allowing escape of cerebrospinal fluid through the subarachnoid space. Whether a permanent fistula or removal of the elevated pressure from a critical portion of the optic nerve is responsible for the results is not known. Whatever the explanation, the procedure is effective in reversing some of the visual loss and in decreasing headache in some patients.

ADIE'S PUPIL

A fixed, dilated pupil elicits fear in most patients and physicians. When seen in the emergency room a presumptive diagnosis of impending third nerve palsy is usually made and the patient is rushed to the radiology suite for CT scanning and cerebral angiography to rule out an aneurysm. A number of these patients do not have a pending third nerve palsy, but rather a benign condition often called Adie's pupil. It is important to differentiate this from third nerve palsy to save the patient the expense and invasiveness of angiography.

Etiology

Adie's pupil represents denervation hypersensitivity of the ciliary ganglion. This ganglion contains nuclei that control the parasympathetic innervation to the pupillary sphincter and ciliary body. Loss of function of these cells produces pupillary dilation secondary to unopposed sympathetic tone and inability to accommodate (change focus to view near objects). These symptoms are part of a third nerve palsy, but in the absence of pain and other oculomotor signs of third nerve palsy other causes should be considered. One other cause of a fixed, dilated pupil is accidental or purposeful instillation of medication into the eye causing dilation. This would include parasympatholytic agents such as atropine and scopolamine that can accidentally reach the eye after application of a patch for motion sickness.

Physical Examination and Clinical Findings

The workup of a fixed, dilated pupil in the absence of pain and other signs of third nerve palsy includes careful examination of the reaction of the pupil to near stimuli. The patient must intently fixate on a near target, preferably her own finger, for at least 25 or 30 seconds. Often after a prolonged period the pupil will begin to constrict in an irregular, tonic manner. Once attention is again directed to the distance, redilation may also be tonic. If this pattern is seen, Adie's pupil is the likely diagnosis. This can be confirmed by instilling a dilute solution ($^1/_8$%) of pilocarpine into both eyes. The normal pupil will not react, but the hypersensitive Adie's pupil will. If the pupil does not react to dilute solutions, 1% or 4 % pilocarpine should be instilled. If the pupil still does not react, there is blockage of the receptors and pharmacologic dilation is the diagnosis. Caution must be observed when using these guidelines. Acute Adie's pupils may not react to dilute pilocarpine for days to weeks after the initial insult. If there is a question, immediate neuro-ophthalmologic consultation should be requested.

Treatment

In young women Adie's pupil is often associated with decreased deep tendon reflexes in the lower extremities. This is called Adie's syndrome, a benign condition. The management of Adie's pupil is based on symptoms. If the patient is having no problems, no therapy is indicated. Over time the pupil will reduce to a more normal size and may become smaller than the contralateral pupil. If the patient complains of light sensitivity, dilute pilocarpine or a cosmetic contact lens with a colored area simulating the contralateral iris may be tried. Often patients require reading lenses due to the inability to accommodate.

PITUITARY TUMORS

The pituitary-hypothalamic axis controls the majority of the body's hormone production. Tumors of the pituitary traditionally were described based on their light microscopic characteristics (eg, basophilic, acidophilic). Now they are described based on their hormonal activity. From 20% to 40% are nonsecreting, and the remainder may affect various parts of the body through changes in the levels of adrenocorticotropic hormone, prolactin, growth hormone, thyroid stimulating hormone, follicle stimulating hormone, luteinizing hormone, melanocyte stimulating hormone, oxytocin, and vasopressin. These tumors are often diagnosed earlier in women than men due to changes in menstruation.

Neuro-ophthalmologic disease in the context of pituitary disease is not due to hormonal changes, with the exception of hyperthyroidism. In general, changes are related to direct mechanical mass effect on adjacent structures and thus are not related to the type of adenoma and its resulting oversecretion. Pituitary tumors must be fairly large to involve the visual pathways. The optic chiasm lies 1 cm superior to the top of the sella on average. Anatomically the chiasm may be "pre-fixed", with the optic tracts directly over the sella, or "post-fixed", with the optic nerves directly over the sella. Depending on this anatomy, various visual field defects will be seen. The classic defect is a bitemporal hemianopia, due to involvement of the chiasm. If the chiasm is prefixed a homonymous defect may be seen; if the chiasm is post-fixed a unilateral defect may be seen. In addition, combinations of the above may be seen if the chiasm is involved on one side and the optic nerve or tract on the other. RAPDs are not characteristically seen unless one optic nerve or tract is mainly involved.

Pituitary tumors may also cause diplopia due to involvement of the oculomotor nerves in the cavernous sinus or superior orbital fissure. Cranial nerves 3, 4, and 6 all may be involved. This is often due to pituitary apoplexy, a rapid expansion of the mass due to infarction or hemorrhage. This may cause hemiparesis, loss of vision, ocular motor palsy, disturbance of consciousness, sudden and severe headache, and double vision. The diagnosis of this condition is made by changes seen on MRI. Treatment is with high-dose steroids. Some cases may need urgent transsphenoidal decompression of the anterior visual pathways.

A separate class of pituitary adenoma is prolactinoma, due to its medical management. Prolactinoma makes up 35% of all pituitary adenomas. The diagnosis is made on the basis of symptoms of amenorrhea-galactorrhea, and assays reveal serum levels of prolactin over 1000. These masses may increase in size during pregnancy. As opposed to other tumors where the primary mode of treatment is transsphenoidal resection, bromocriptine may shrink the size of prolactinomas without surgery. Unfortunately, this requires prolonged therapy and regrowth occurs after cessation of medication.

MENINGIOMA

Sphenoid ridge meningiomas are slow-growing lesions arising from the tuberculum sellae and planum sphenoidale, which grow in the parasellar region. They may cause a slow progressive visual loss due to involvement of the optic chiasm, intracranial optic nerves, or growth into the optic canal. These lesions may progress in pregnancy. The Foster-Kennedy syndrome is described as optic disc swelling on one side, with optic atrophy on the other. The classic etiology for this is an olfactory groove meningioma that grew initially on one side, producing optic nerve damage and crossing the midline to cause an optic neuropathy on the other. At present the most common cause of this syndrome is AION.

The diagnosis of meningioma is made by the presence of hyperostosis of bone on CT scanning. Other tumors in the region rarely cause similar bony changes. Unfortunately, meningiomas commonly involve adjacent tissue extensively, and complete excision is often not possible. Partial excision is undertaken in an effort to protect vision. Radiation therapy is often given later due the difficulty of repeat attempts at excision.

CONSIDERATIONS IN PREGNANCY

Many of the disorders mentioned heretofore are affected by pregnancy. Fortunately, pregnancy does not seem to have any effect on the optic nerve or chiasm. The nerves and chiasm may be compressed by growth of adjacent tumors during pregnancy. Hormonal changes may cause pituitary adenomas to grow and may accelerate involvement of the optic chiasm. With the introduction of bromocriptine, many of these tumors can be controlled without surgery before delivery. If necessary, transsphenoidal decompression of the sella has been performed without deleterious effects. Meningiomas may contain estrogen or progesterone receptors on their surface and can grow rapidly during pregnancy with the normal rise in blood estrogen levels. Pseudotumor cerebri may be seen during pregnancy. This is not surprising, because it is normally seen in overweight women of child-bearing age. No studies have documented a higher rate of IIH in pregnancy than in age-matched controls. Many investigators have postulated a hormonal basis for IIH, which makes an association with pregnancy more likely. In addition, there may be a relationship between IIH and acute decreases in some endogenous steroid levels in pregnancy. Patients can usually be controlled conservatively, but if necessary optic nerve sheath decompression can be performed under local anesthesia to prevent permanent loss of vision. Pseudotumor cerebri can also be seen in the setting of disseminated intravascular coagulopathy (DIC). DIC may occur in complicated pregnancies or preeclampsia, and may cause thrombotic events, including venous sinus thrombosis.

The most serious neuro-ophthalmologic disease seen in pregnancy is in patients suffering from severe preeclampsia or eclampsia. A number of cases have been reported of visual disturbances ranging from retinal ischemia anteriorly to cortical ischemia posteriorly. In some cases, edema of the occipital lobe has been documented on CT scanning, causing cortical blindness. Vision usually recovers, although rare patients may have permanent visual loss. Elevated blood pressure before or during delivery has also been reported to cause retinal artery occlusion, optic neuritis, ischemic optic neuropathy, and psychogenic disturbances with functional visual loss. These conditions may be caused by the elevated pressures or by overly aggressive reduction of pressure, causing ischemia.

BIBLIOGRAPHY

Beck RW, Cleary P. Optic neuritis treatment trial. One year follow-up results. Arch Ophthalmol 1993;111:773.

Boghen DA, Glaser JS. Ischemic optic neuropathy: the clinical profile and natural history. Brain 1975;98:689.

Corbett JJ. Problems in the diagnosis and treatment of pseudotumor cerebri. Can J Neurol Sci 1983;10:225.

Duane TD, ed. Clinical ophthalmology, volume 2. Philadelphia: JB Lippincott, 1986:7.

Ehlers N, Malmros R. The suprasellar meningioma: a review of the literature and presentation of a series of 31 cases. Acta Ophthalmol 1973; (suppl 121):1.

Jacobson DH, Gorman CA. Endocrine ophthalmopathy: current ideas concerning etiology, pathogenesis and treatment. Endocr Rev 1984;5:200.

Seybold ME. Myasthenia gravis. A clinical and basic science review. JAMA 1983;250:2516.

Sunness JS. The pregnant woman's eye. Surv Ophthalmol 1988;32:219.

Thompson HS, Bell RA, Bourgon P. The natural history of Adie's syndrome. In: Thompson HS, Daroff RB, Frisen L, et al, eds. Topics in neuro-ophthalmology. Baltimore: Williams and Wilkins, 1979:96.

125

Cataracts

STEVEN S.T. CHING

Primary Care for Women, edited by Phyllis C. Leppert and Fred M. Howard. Lippincott-Raven Publishers, Philadelphia © 1997.

A cataract is the result of a change in clarity of the crystalline lens. About 1.3 million cataract surgeries are done yearly in the United States. Ninety-five percent of people over age 65 have some form of lens change; therefore, the definition of the term "cataract" should include a change in visual function with the noted anatomic change. Fifty percent of people between ages 65 and 74 and 70% of those over age 75 have visual impairment due to cataract.

CATARACT FORMATION

The eye captures images of the world and transmits them to the brain. As in any camera, a lens system refracts or focuses light. The eye has an external lens, the cornea, and an internal lens, the crystalline lens. A cataract occurs when the internal lens loses its clarity or focuses light abnormally.

The crystalline lens grows throughout life. Growth occurs by the proliferation and differentiation of lens cells in layers. Like the growth rings of a tree, the external layers are the newest. The cells in the new layers have nuclei but lose them with age. On slit-lamp examination, the center of the lens is the nucleus and the periphery is the cortex.

Cataract formation due to aging presents in three forms: nuclear sclerosis, peripheral cortical opacification, and posterior subcapsular opacification (Fig. 125-1). After age 65, the nucleus

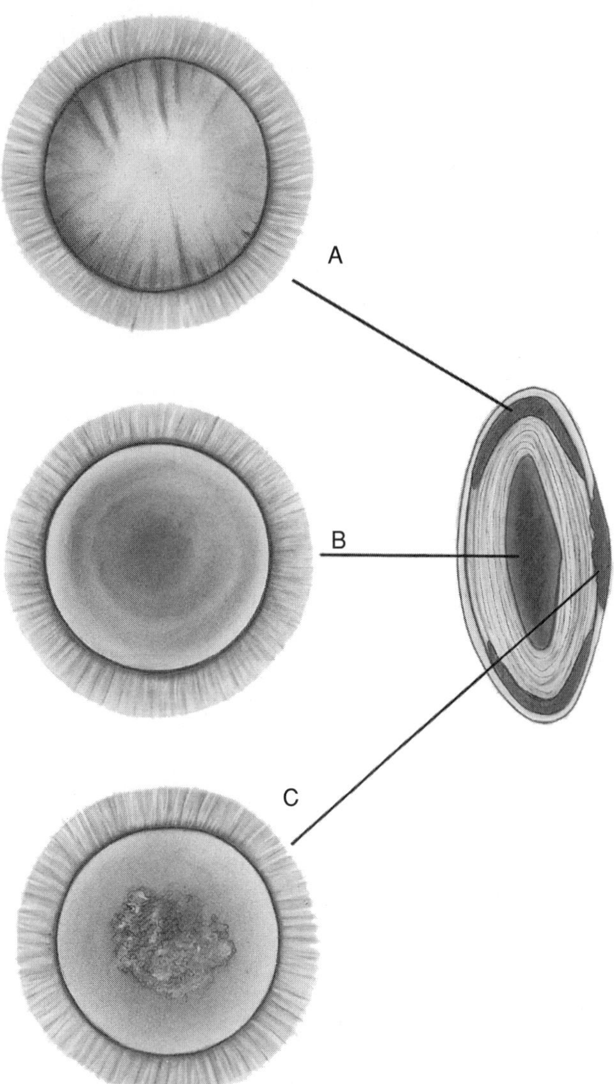

Figure 125-1. (***A***) Cortical cataract. Peripheral lens fiber abnormalities give the clinical appearance of spokes of a wheel, "cortical spokes" or cuneiform cataract. (***B***) Nuclear cataract. The nucleus of the lens is denser than the periphery. This causes a "bull's eye" appearance. (***C***) Posterior subcapsular cataract. Posterior axial abnormal lens fibers cause focal opacification. The axial location of the opacity causes early visual symptoms.

begins to increase in density and change in color from clear crystalline to yellow brown. This change is termed *nuclear sclerosis*. Nuclear sclerosis results from the formation of insoluble protein aggregates. This changes the refractive index, scatters light rays, and reduces transparency. Initially, the increased index of refraction tends to make the lens have greater refracting power. This may induce myopia or nearsightedness, and the person may be able to see near objects without glasses. This phenomenon of regaining near vision with advancing age is termed "second sight." As the nuclear sclerosis progresses, vision eventually becomes distorted, with loss of visual clarity.

If the growth of the cortical lens fibers is disturbed, a focal opacity of the lens results. This phenomenon occurs with age with the formation of peripheral lens opacities. It appears, on slit-lamp examination and ophthalmoscopy, to be similar to spokes wheel and is termed *cortical spokes*. Because of its peripheral tion, this form of cataract causes symptoms of glare, with a mild decrease in visual acuity.

In the third form of cataract, lens fibers migrate posteriorly near the posterior capsule and fail to differentiate. This results in an opacity in the posterior lens and is termed a *posterior subcapsular cataract*. Due to its axial and posterior location, this form of cataract causes the most visual disability. Patients usually complain of light sensitivity and decreased vision in bright light.

ETIOLOGY

In the normal aging process, a photooxidative stress is thought to be induced by UVA and UVB radiation on lens proteins and lens cells. The radiation effects may be mediated by a loss of intralenticular antioxidant activity or photosensitization of lens proteins. This eventually causes protein aggregation, areas of varying indices of refraction, and light scattering.

Ultraviolet light, alcohol, and smoking increase the risk of cataract. Two important causes of cataract are the use of systemic steroids and diabetes mellitus. The use of systemic steroids is associated with an increased incidence of cataract, as can be seen with rheumatoid arthritis patients. Thirty percent to 40% of rheumatoid arthritis patients develop cataract if they are maintained on prednisone at doses of 10 mg/day for 2 years; this increases to 100% of those treated for 4 years. Diabetes mellitus is thought to accelerate the rate of cataract formation by 20 to 30 years because of damage by sorbitol to the lens cells. Hyperglycemia also decreases the antioxidative activity of the lens and thereby potentiates other lens damage.

DIAGNOSIS

Patients complain of decreased visual acuity, light sensitivity, monocular multiple images, halos, loss of stereopsis, and the appearance of flaring around point sources of lights. They may regain reading vision and have an increased frequency of eyeglass changes.

The examiner may notice a discoloration of the pupil. The direct and indirect pupillary response to light should be normal—cataracts, even if severe, do not alter the pupillary light response. An abnormal pupillary response indicates optic nerve dysfunction, retinal disease, or CNS disease. To view the lens and retina, the pupil should be dilated with phenylephrine 2.5% (Neo-Synephrine) and tropicamide 1% (Mydriacyl). Before dilation, the examiner should estimate the anterior chamber depth to ensure that the patient is not at risk for an angle closure glaucoma attack. The examiner should view the lens with a direct ophthalmoscope with a +10 diopter setting at 10 cm or a +3 diopter setting at 33 cm. The red reflex in nuclear sclerosis appears as a bull's-eye with a central dark reflex and peripheral lucency. As a consequence of nuclear sclerosis, there are varying indices of refraction of the central lens. When the fundus is viewed through the ophthalmoscope, there may be optical distortion of the retinal structures. Cortical spokes appear as peripheral linear opacities and the posterior subcapsular cataract appears as a central axial dark spot.

DIFFERENTIAL DIAGNOSIS

Cataract is the most common cause of visual disability in the elderly. However, because it may coexist with other ocular diseases such as glaucoma and macular degeneration, other causes of visual loss should be ruled out.

Optical aberrations viewed by the direct ophthalmoscope can be localized by parallax. By varying the observer's position, the location of the opacity can be determined in relation to the lens. Anterior visual aberrations arise from the cornea; posterior opacities are in the vitreous.

A late stage of cataract formation gives the appearance of a white pupil or leukocoria. In the adult, leukocoria can be secondary to cataract, retinal detachment, intraocular tumor, or vitreous membranes.

MEDICAL MANAGEMENT

There is no effective chemical agent to reduce the incidence or progression of cataract. Clinical trials of aspirin, aldose reductase inhibitors to lower sorbitol, and antioxidants are underway. Damage of the lens secondary to UV radiation comes from a lifetime of exposure, and short-term measures to reduce this exposure probably would have little effect.

Colored lenses, usually amber to brown, limit the spectra of incoming light and may limit glare and increase contrast. Optimizing lighting and using magnifiers may be beneficial. If the cataract is axial and of limited area, pupillary dilatation is sometimes helpful.

Referral to an ophthalmologist is advised with a diagnosis, or suspected diagnosis, of cataract.

INDICATIONS FOR SURGERY

The decision to pursue surgical intervention is based on the patient's visual disability induced by the cataract, the patient's visual needs, the surgical risks, and the medical risks of the ocular disease. Cataracts can cause symptoms of glare and monocular diplopia. The blurred vision caused by a monocular cataract can interfere with the functioning of the opposite eye. If these symptoms are bothersome and interfere with the patient's life, cataract surgery could be considered.

The visual needs of patients vary considerably. For example, a machinist or pilot may need stereopsis and fine binocular acuity. Other persons may not need stereo vision and may not need to undertake the risks of surgery. Persons with nuclear sclerotic cataracts usually have limited distance vision but may have excellent near vision. If perfect distance vision is not crucial to the patient, surgery may not be necessary. Usually a critical level of vision in the elderly is the vision necessary to maintain a driver's license. In most states, 20/40 vision from either eye is required to maintain an unrestricted driver's license; the requirements for a limited day license vary from 20/50 to 20/70, depending on the state. Patients may need to maintain other minimum visual standards as mandated by government or industry.

In some instances, cataracts need removal for medical reasons. For example, in patients with diabetic retinopathy or glaucoma, visualization of the retina and optic nerve is necessary to monitor and treat the underlying ocular disease. If the cataract is significantly advanced, inflammatory or angle closure glaucomas can be precipitated.

The surgical risk of an ocular complication from cataract varies from 1% to 3%. The patient must be able to lie flat and tolerate local anesthesia.

SURGICAL TECHNIQUES

There are three major surgical methods for cataract removal: intracapsular, extracapsular with a standard incision, and extracapsular by phacoemulsification with a small incision. Intracapsular surgery, which involves removing the entire lens, was popular through the 1970s but is used infrequently in the United States today because it limits intraocular lens choices. This procedure is relatively simple—in fact, it is still used in Third World countries because of its simplicity—and does not require extensive surgical instrumentation.

Extracapsular cataract surgery involves removing the lens contents, leaving the external lens capsule. The capsular remnant serves to hold or anchor an artificial intraocular lens. Both the standard technique and the small-incision phacoemulsification technique appear to have the same visual results and complications when measured 4 months postoperatively. The small-incision phacoemulsification technique allows quicker rehabilitation but may not be suitable for all types of cataract.

VISUAL CORRECTION AFTER SURGERY

The internal crystalline lens accounts for 35% of the eye's refracting power, so this must be compensated for after cataract surgery. This can be done by high power-plus lenses (cataract spectacles), a contact lens, or an intraocular artificial lens. Cataract spectacles are safe but have significant optical disadvantages. They magnify the image by about 30%, causing significant perceptual problems. In

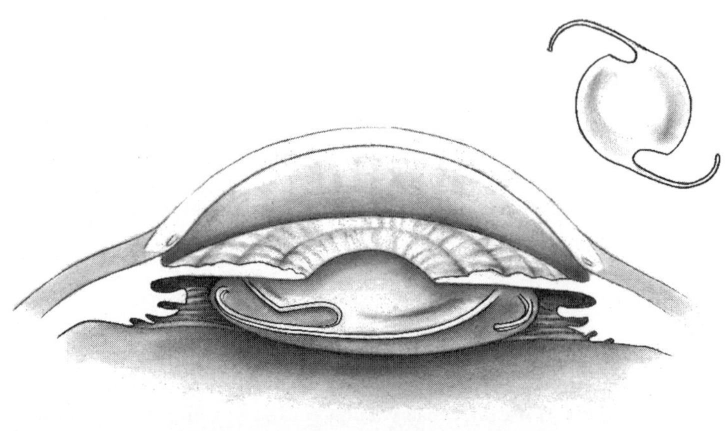

Figure 125-2. The intraocular lens is a plastic prosthetic lens. This schematic shows a lens situated in the capsule of the original crystalline lens in the posterior chamber. The arms of the lens act as springs to stabilize the lens against the peripheral capsule.

addition, high-plus lenses significantly limit peripheral vision and have peripheral distortion. Contact lenses are difficult for most patients to manage. Elderly persons have an increased incidence of dry eyes and may not be candidates for contact lenses.

Intraocular lenses have been used since 1949 and are considered the standard of care in the United States. Ninety-eight percent of all cataract surgeries are performed using intraocular lens implants. Some types of intraocular lenses in the 1970s and early 1980s had significant complications of intraocular inflammation, bleeding, glaucoma, and corneal edema. Today's implants are placed either in the posterior chamber (Fig. 125-2) or the anterior chamber and have a low risk of complications. The use of intraocular lenses in patients younger than age 18 is investigational.

OCULAR COMPLICATIONS AFTER CATARACT SURGERY

The risk of cataract surgery is usually low. Severe early complications include severe hemorrhage (choroidal hemorrhage, 0.3%) and intraocular infection (endophthalmitis, 0.08% to 0.13%). Significant late complications include corneal edema (0.3%), clinically significant macular edema (1.4%), and retinal detachment (0.8%). There rarely may be persistent intraocular inflammation (uveitis) and long-term raised intraocular pressure.

LASER AFTER CATARACT SURGERY

After extracapsular cataract surgery, the capsular remnants undergo opacification in about 20% of patients in the first year after surgery. A neodymium:YAG laser is used to create a pupil in the posterior capsule. This procedure is sometimes mistakenly interpreted by patients as having a cataract removed by laser.

BIBLIOGRAPHY

American Academy of Ophthalmology. Cataract symposium, 1994.

Andley U. Photooxidative stress. In: Albert DM, Jakobiec FA, Robinson NL, eds. Principles and practice of ophthalmology. Philadelphia: WB Saunders, 1994:575.

Berson FG, ed. Ophthalmology study guide for students and practitioners of medicine, 6th ed. American Academy of Ophthalmology, 1993.

Floyd RP. History of cataract surgery. In: Albert DM, Jakobiec FA, Robinson NL, eds. Principles and practice of ophthalmology. Philadelphia: WB Saunders, 1994:606.

Gans LA, Cobo LM, Johns KJ, Roussel TJ, Schanzlin DJ, Van Meter WS. Basic and clinical science course, section 11: lens and cataract. San Francisco: American Academy of Ophthalmology, 1994.

Javitt JC, Street DA, Tielsch JM, Wang Q, et al. National outcomes of cataract extraction: retinal detachment and endophthalmitis after outpatient cataract surgery. Ophthalmology 1994;101:100.

Newell FW. Ophthalmology, principles and concepts, 7th ed. St. Louis: Mosby, 1992.

Powe NR, Schein OD, Gieser SC, Tielsch JM, et al. Synthesis of the literature on visual acuity and complications following cataract extraction with intraocular lens implantation. Arch Ophthalmol 1994;112:239.

Schein OD, Steinberg EP, Javitt JC, Cassard SD, et al. Variation in cataract surgery practice and clinical outcomes. Ophthalmology 1994;101:1142.

Streeten BW. Pathology of the lens. In: Albert DM, Jakobiec FA, Robinson NL, eds. Principles and practice of ophthalmology. Philadelphia: WB Saunders, 1994:2180.

West SK, Valmadrid CT. Epidemiology of risk factors for age-related cataract. Surv Ophthalmol 1995;39:323.

Primary Care for Women, edited by Phyllis C. Leppert and Fred M. Howard. Lippincott-Raven Publishers, Philadelphia © 1997.

126

Glaucoma

STEVEN S.T. CHING

Glaucoma refers to a group of ocular disorders that are associated with raised intraocular pressure (IOP), optic atrophy, and visual field changes. Anatomically, the glaucomas can be classified according to the anatomy of the anterior chamber angle. In angle closure glaucoma, the peripheral iris apposes and occludes the trabecular meshwork of the anterior chamber angle. In open angle glaucoma, the iris is not in apposition to the trabecular meshwork. Glaucomas are termed primary if no secondary causes (eg, inflammation, abnormal neovascularization, congenital anatomic abnormalities) can be ascribed.

Glaucoma causes 12% to 15% of cases of blindness in the United States. Two million Americans have glaucoma. It is the leading cause of blindness in American blacks and the second leading cause of blindness in American whites, after macular degeneration.

INTRAOCULAR PRESSURE AND AQUEOUS HUMOR PRODUCTION

Eyes with raised IOP have a characteristic form of optic atrophy and visual field loss. The level of IOP at which damage to the optic nerve occurs varies with individuals. The mean IOP, as judged by pooled epidemiologic studies, is 15.5 mm Hg (standard deviation, 2.5 mm Hg). Any IOP above 21 mm Hg is considered suspicious. However, there is no level of IOP that is clearly safe. Some eyes undergo damage with an IOP of 18 mm Hg; others tolerate an IOP above 30 mm Hg without damage. Major risk factors for glaucomatous damage include diabetes mellitus, cardiovascular disease, a history of central retinal vein occlusion in either eye, age, and race (blacks have a greater incidence of glaucoma). For a patient at greater risk who has borderline raised IOP, treatment would be more likely to be undertaken. The ophthalmologist must weigh the benefits of treatment against the side effects and cost. Eyes with a higher IOP have a greater incidence of optic nerve damage; therefore, most ophthalmologists institute treatment if the IOP exceeds 30 mm Hg.

IOP measurements are subject to considerable variability. Normal eyes have a diurnal variation of 6.5 mm Hg. In patients with primary open angle glaucoma, the average diurnal variation is 10 mm Hg. Other causes of transient alteration in IOP include exercise, postural position, and drugs such as alcohol and tobacco.

These fluctuations make it difficult to judge when the IOP is well controlled. Sometimes it is necessary to take multiple readings through the day and night to ensure that peak levels of IOP are not excessive.

The level of IOP is the result of aqueous humor production and the rate of aqueous outflow from the eye (Fig. 126-1). Most glaucomas result from some form of obstruction or increased resistance to aqueous outflow. Aqueous humor maintains IOP, provides metabolic substrates, and helps remove metabolic products. It is formed in an area posterior to the iris, the ciliary body. It is secreted into the posterior chamber and then passes forward to the anterior chamber through the pupil. The major drainage of aqueous occurs through the trabecular meshwork at the juncture of the cornea and the iris; 5% to 15% of aqueous drains from the eye via an alternate pathway, the uveoscleral pathway, which involves the ciliary muscle, supraciliary space, and suprachoroidal space.

There are several methods for measuring IOP. The Schiotz tonometer is inexpensive, durable, and relatively easy to use. It is well suited for use by primary care providers for glaucoma screening. It gives an indirect assessment of pressure by measuring the amount of indentation of the globe produced by standardized weights. Errors in measurement can occur if the tonometer is not perpendicular to the globe, if the patient squeezes her eyelids or performs the Valsalva maneuver, or if the examiner unknowingly presses on the globe through the eyelids. The instrument may not be accurate in patients with thyroid disease and high myopia.

For Schiotz tonometry to be performed, the patient lies in a supine position. The tonometer should be tested on the test block; the scale reading should read 0 regardless of the standardized weight being used. Both eyes are anesthetized with topical proparacaine. A right-handed observer should stand on the patient's right side; the converse is true for the left-handed observer. The patient is asked to look down toward her feet. The examiner gently retracts the upper and lower lids with the left hand. Care should be taken to retract the lids against the rims of the orbits and not against the globe. The Schiotz tonometer is placed just above the globe. The patient is asked to fixate with her contralateral eye on a point on the ceiling such that the visual axis of the globe is oriented per-

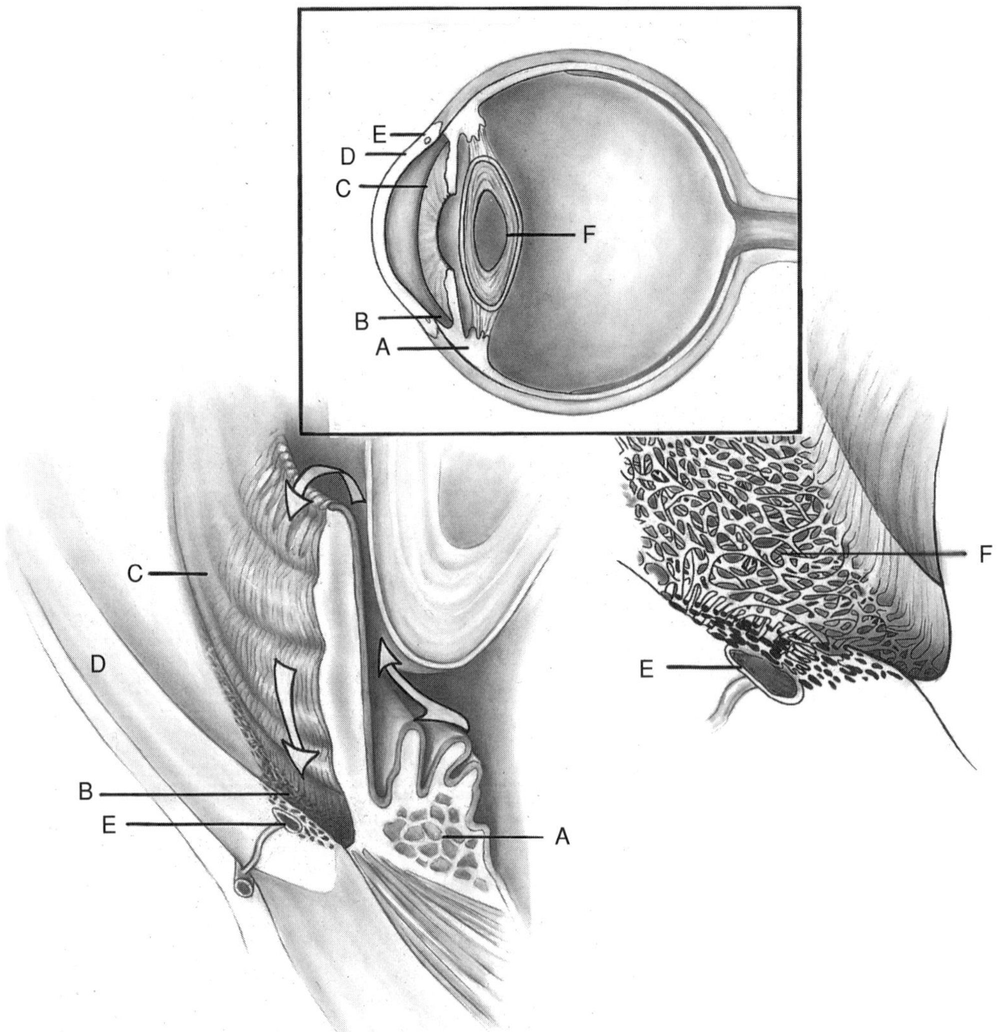

Figure 126-1. (***A***) Ciliary body. (***B***) Trabecular meshwork. (***C***) Iris. (***D***) Cornea. (***E***) Schlemm's canal. (***F***) Crystalline lens. Aqueous is formed in the ciliary body, flows through the pupil, exits the anterior chamber through the trabecular meshwork to Schlemm's canal, and subsequently drains to an episcleral venous network.

pendicular to the floor. The tonometer may then be lowered to contact the center of the cornea. Again, the tonometer must be oriented perpendicularly to the globe along the visual axis. The scale reading is noted and the procedure is repeated on the opposite eye.

The scale reading of the tonometer is most accurate in the range of 3.0 to 8.5. The standard weights are 5.5, 7.5, 10.0, and 15.0 g. The reading is correlated to the IOP and may be read off the conversion tables that accompany the tonometer. For example, a scale reading of 4.0 with a 5.5-g weight corresponds to an IOP of 21 mm Hg.

OPTIC NERVE HEAD

The optic nerve contains 1.2 million nerve fibers. The intraocular portion of the optic nerve has an average area of 1.5 mm. The intraocular normal nerve may be divided into three areas: the neural rim, a central depression termed the optic cup, and an area of central pallor. The optic cup is delineated by retinal vessels and usually corresponds to the area of pallor. The area of the optic cup (C) compared to the total area of the nerve (D) is termed the cup/disc ratio (C/D). Similarly, a pallor/disc ratio can be defined. Most eyes have a C/D ratio below 0.5; it exceeds 0.7 in only 5% of the population (Fig. 126-2) The average C/D ratio may be greater for blacks than for whites because blacks have a larger optic nerve. The areas of the optic cup and pallor are significant because their enlargement over time indicates optic nerve damage due to glaucoma.

The direct ophthalmoscope is an important tool to screen for and follow the progress of glaucoma. When using the direct ophthalmoscope, the observer should use his or her right eye to observe the patient's right eye, and his or her left to observe the patient's left; this prevents noses from colliding and allows the patient to maintain fixation. The observer should keep his or her contralateral eye open to minimize observer accommodation. The clinician should view the nasal retina first to identify a retinal vessel and then should follow this vessel back to the optic nerve head. The nasal retina causes less photophobia for the patient than the temporal retina, thereby facilitating a better view.

The following should be observed:

- Optic nerve margins and course of the nerve vessels
- Optic cup as delineated by the optic nerve vessels
- Area of central pallor
- Symmetry of the cup in relation to the neural rim
- Presence of peripapillary hemorrhages
- Symmetry of the C/D ratio with respect to the other eye.

The optic cup and pallor are usually best seen with lower levels of light intensity of the direct ophthalmoscope. Also, directing the light to an area just adjacent to the cup may retroilluminate the cup and allow better study of subtle variations in color and vessel topography of the optic nerve head.

The optic cup and pallor are the key indicators of glaucomatous damage. Any C/D ratio above 0.5 should be considered suspicious. In glaucoma, the cup and pallor seem to enlarge as the neural rim diminishes. This elongation is often asymmetric in a vertical direction or in a specific sector. The observer must note the relation of the optic cup and the area of pallor. The cup enlargement, as demarcated by optic nerve vessels, may precede pallor enlargement in glaucoma. The reverse, in which pallor extends beyond the circumlinear cup vessel, may also indicate optic nerve damage. Glaucoma is frequently asymmetric between the right and left eyes. A disparity of 0.2 or greater between the C/D ratios of the two

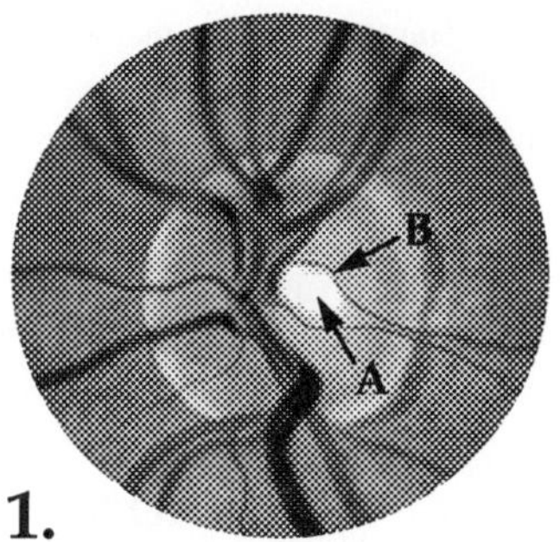

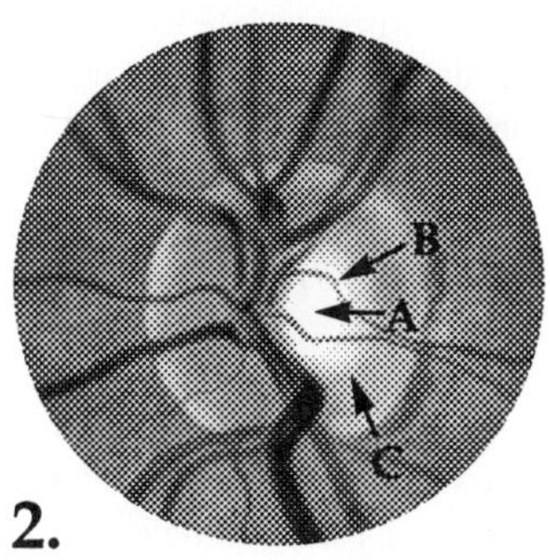

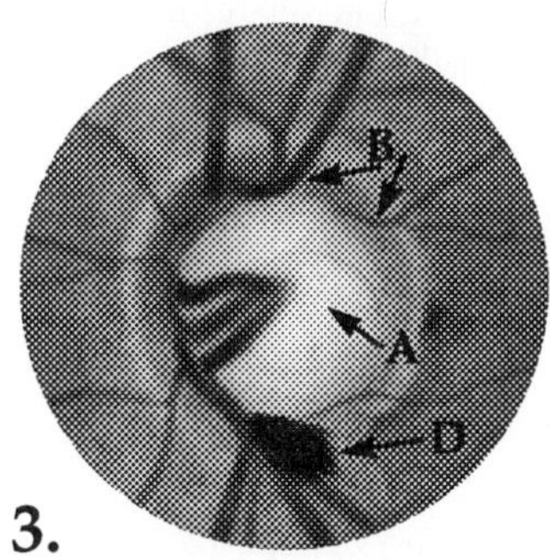

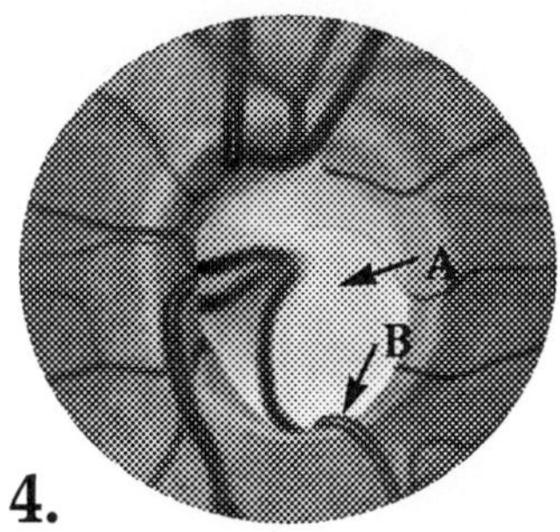

Figure 126-2. 1. Normal optic nerve head. Note the circumlinear blood vessel (***B***) that outlines the optic cup. The central pallor (***A***) usually occupies the same area as the optic cup. 2. The area of pallor (***C***) is beginning to exceed the optic cup. 3. The optic cup and area of pallor are markedly increased. There is a hemorrhage (***D***) inferiorly on the neural rim. The borders of the cup are shown by the circumlinear vessel. 4. Note the extensive cupping and pallor of this glaucomatous optic nerve head. The cup is asymmetric in a vertical direction. Very little neural rim remains at the inferior pole of the nerve head.

eyes is significant. Hemorrhages on the neural rim are frequently seen in glaucoma; subsequent sectoral atrophy at the hemorrhage site on the neural rim occurs.

Optic nerve damage in glaucoma is thought to occur in two ways. Raised IOP causes compression of the optic nerve fibers and decreased axoplasmic flow with the resultant optic atrophy. Abnormal IOP can also cause damage by decreasing the vascular perfusion of the optic nerve.

VISUAL FIELDS

Visual fields aid in the identification of glaucomatous damage in initial screening and allow the practitioner to judge the effectiveness of therapy over time. The visual field defects noted in glaucoma follow the distribution of the retinal nerve fiber layer. These fibers do not cross the horizontal midline. Usually, damage to the inferior and superior retinal fibers is not concurrent; glaucomatous visual field defects, therefore, do not cross the horizontal midline unless there is simultaneous damage to each hemifield. The site of nerve fiber damage determines the resultant visual field defect (Fig. 126-3).

The classic defect is the arcuate scotoma, and other defects may be thought of as partial arcuate defects. The nasal visual field (corresponding to the axons that enter the optic nerve temporally from the temporal retina) is the most susceptible to damage and causes the classic nasal step visual defect. The retinal fibers from the fovea are the most resistant to glaucomatous damage. Thus, the central visual field is often the last area to be lost from glaucoma.

Visual field defects that respect the horizontal midline indicate pathology of the optic nerve and retinal nerve fibers. Typically, defects of this nature are caused by glaucoma or vascular insults to the retina. Visual field defects that honor the vertical midline typically arise from the optic tracts or further posteriorly in the optic radiations and visual cortex and therefore indicate neurologic disease.

PRIMARY OPEN ANGLE GLAUCOMA

Primary open angle glaucoma affects more than 60% to 70% of the patients with glaucoma in the United States. As many as 1% of Americans over age 40 have this disease; the incidence increases to 3% for those over age 70. The disease is more severe and prevalent in the Caribbean and African populations. In the United States, 4% of the patients are blind; in Nigeria, 34% of patients with the disease are blind bilaterally and 91% are monocularly blind.

The prevalence of the disease is higher in relatives of glaucoma patients. In relatives of affected persons, the risk of developing glaucoma is five to six times the rate of the general population. Genetically, it is thought to be polygenic.

Clinical Features

Glaucoma is insidious, slowly progressive, and painless. Because the central vision is affected last, the disease may go unnoticed until severe damage has occurred. Raised IOP is the primary risk factor, but 50% of patients have normal IOP at the initial screening. Not all patients with an IOP above 21 mm Hg have glaucoma. Primary open angle glaucoma may be diagnosed if there is a combination of raised IOP, optic nerve changes, visual field deficits, an open anterior chamber angle by gonioscopy, and no other factors causing raised IOP. The percentage of the population with raised IOP increases with age. Table 126-1 shows the prevalence of raised IOP and glaucoma as a function of age.

One of the greatest challenges for the ophthalmologist is to decide when raised IOP poses a threat and consequently requires therapy. Practitioners have three choices. The first option is to treat all patients with an IOP above 21 mm Hg, but this treats many patients who might not need therapy. The second option is to treat only patients with accompanying disc and visual field deficits.

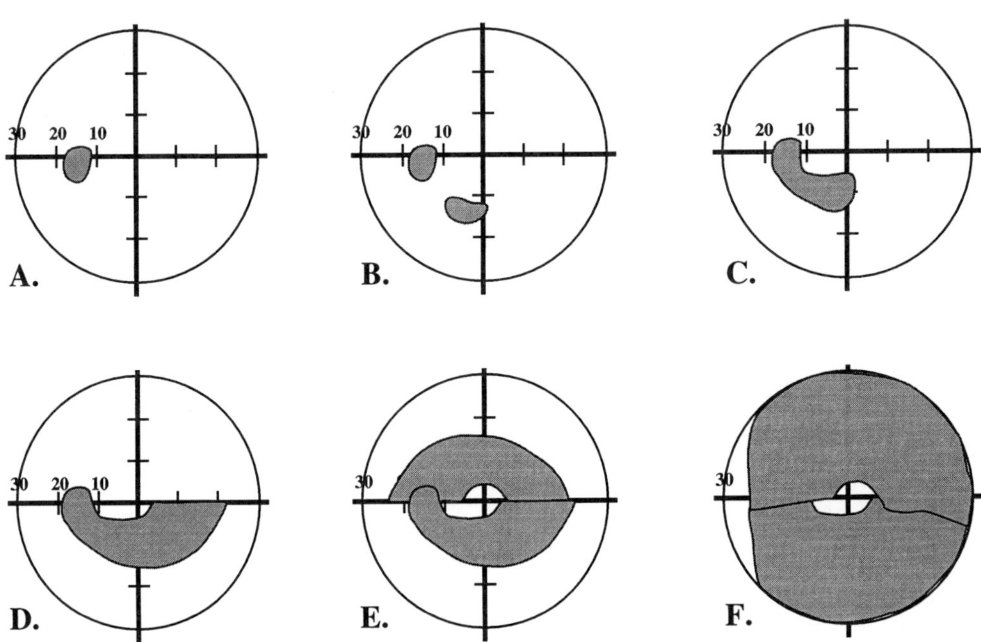

Figure 126-3. (***A***) The normal visual field. (***B, C***) Partial lesions. (***D***) The arcuate nerve fiber defect. (***E***) An arcuate defect in the upper and lower hemifields. (***F***) A late stage of glaucoma with sparing only of a central and temporal island of vision.

Table 126-1. Prevalence of Raised Intraocular Pressure and Glaucoma as a Function of Age

AGE	PERCENTAGE OF POPULATION WITH IOP > 21 mm Hg	PERCENTAGE OF POPULATION WITH PRIMARY OPEN ANGLE GLAUCOMA
Total population	4%	0.5%
Under 30 y	2%	—
30–39 y	6%	—
50–55 y	—	1.5%
70 y and older	10%	3%

However, significant loss of nerve fibers may occur before the first detectable visual field loss. The third option is to treat patients who have risk factors (eg, diabetes mellitus, cardiovascular disease, a strong family history), an excessively high IOP, or suspicious optic nerve changes. Most clinicians choose the third option. The primary care physician must refer patients in this category to an ophthalmologist for evaluation and possible treatment.

Medical Therapy

Topical agents used in ophthalmology can have systemic side effects. This tendency can be lessened by applying digital pressure to the medial canthal area for 5 minutes after application of the agent to the eye. This maneuver limits drainage through the lacrimal ducts and nasal mucosa, thereby minimizing systemic absorption.

β-Adrenergic Antagonists

β-Adrenergic antagonists lower IOP by decreasing aqueous humor production. Five topical β-adrenergic antagonists are available: betaxolol, carteolol, levobunolol, metipranolol, and timolol. Betaxolol is a relatively selective β1 blocking agent; the other agents have both β1 and β2 effects. Systemic side effects are infrequent but include bradycardia, heart block, bronchospasm, decreased libido, and mood changes. β-blockade in the neonate has been described when timolol was used during delivery. Timolol is excreted in breast milk, but studies thus far indicate the daily dose would be below that expected to produce cardiac effects in infants.

Adrenergic Agonists

Topical epinephrine was used before the introduction of dipivefrin. Dipivefrin is a prodrug of epinephrine that increases therapeutic effectiveness locally in the eye while minimizing systemic side effects. This class of glaucoma agent is thought to enhance the outflow of aqueous through the uveoscleral pathway. Systemic side effects include hypertension, extrasystoles, and headache.

Cholinergic Agonists

Cholinergic agonists cause pupillary miosis and ciliary muscle contraction; this increases fluid outflow through the trabecular meshwork. Pilocarpine works directly on the motor endplates as a cholinergic agonist. Echothiophate and demecarium bromide act indirectly by inhibiting the effect of acetylcholinesterase and thus increase the duration of action of acetylcholine. Carbachol has direct and indirect actions on the cholinergic system. The systemic side effects of this family of drugs (diarrhea, abdominal cramps, increased salivation, and enuresis) usually arise from the indirect agents. The indirect agents inhibit systemic anticholinesterase levels; therefore, agents used in general surgery such as succinylcholine should not be used for at least 6 weeks after discontinuing the topical medication.

Carbonic Anhydrase Inhibitors

These agents decrease aqueous production. Acetazolamide and methazolamide are commonly used; dichlorphenamide and ethoxzolamide used less frequently. These agents are often associated with systemic side effects. Patients may experience paresthesias of the fingers, toes, and lips and may complain of weight loss, abdominal cramping, diarrhea, fatigue, and depression. Acetazolamide causes congenital defects in rats, rabbits, and mice, but despite widespread use, no reports link the use of acetazolamide with human congenital defects. Acetazolamide is secreted in breast milk, but there are no reported effects in infants or on lactation. The American Academy of Pediatrics notes that this drug is compatible with breast-feeding.

Hyperosmotic Agents

Hyperosmotic agents dehydrate the vitreous humor and thereby lower IOP. They are usually used for a short treatment course, as they cause significant systemic effects and lose their efficacy as osmotic gradients equalize in the body. Reported side effects are headache, backache, and confusion. Glycerin can cause hyperglycemia in diabetics. Because of the increased intravascular volume, these agents can aggravate congestive heart failure. The most common agents used are oral glycerin, isosorbide, and intravenous mannitol.

Surgical Therapy

In argon laser trabeculoplasty, laser burns are delivered to the trabecular meshwork. This therapy increases aqueous outflow through the trabecular meshwork and is indicated if medical therapy is inadequate. If medical and laser therapy does not control IOP sufficiently to prevent progressive optic nerve damage, surgical filtration surgery can be performed. An internal fistula can be created to allow aqueous to drain to the episcleral space. The complications of these procedures are cataract formation as well as all those noted in cataract surgery.

PRIMARY ANGLE CLOSURE GLAUCOMA

The most common cause of angle closure glaucoma is primary angle closure glaucoma with pupillary block. Other causes include neovascular glaucoma secondary to inflammation or diabetes mellitus, intraocular tumors, or other ocular diseases.

Pathophysiology

The precipitating event may be mild pupillary dilation (iatrogenic or in normal situations, as with a darkened room or sympathetic stimulation). In angle closure glaucoma, the peripupillary iris maintains contact with the crystalline lens; fluid formed by the ciliary body in the posterior chamber cannot travel forward through the pupil to the anterior chamber and is trapped. The peripheral iris bulges forward to appose the trabecular meshwork. The egress of aqueous fluid is blocked. Aqueous continues to be formed, and the IOP builds.

Epidemiology

Angle closure glaucoma with pupillary block has a hereditary component. The prevalence is much lower than primary open angle glaucoma in the United States. However, in Eskimos, Japanese, and Southeast Asians, it is a significant form of glaucoma. Hyperopic eyes, because they tend to have shallower anterior chambers, are more susceptible to this problem. With age, the lens continues to grow and displaces the iris anteriorly. Also with age, the pupil becomes more miotic. Therefore, angle closure glaucoma tends to occur in people over age 60.

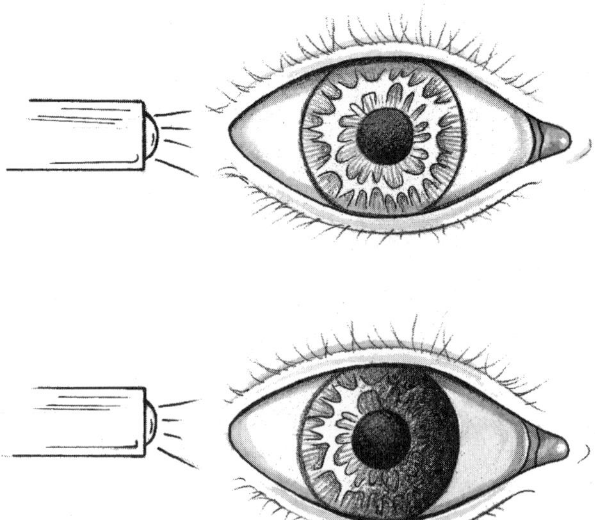

Figure 126-4. Shine a penlight across the anterior chamber from temporal to nasal. A shallow anterior chamber can be demonstrated by the shadow cast by the temporal iris.

Significance

This glaucoma occurs precipitously and is an ocular emergency. Because pressures rise precipitously and to high levels, vision can be lost in a relatively short period of time. Patients may have severe pain with nausea, vomiting, and dehydration. The patient may present in an obtunded fashion secondary to dehydration. This form of glaucoma may be precipitated by pupillary dilatation from the use of systemic drugs with atropinic effects.

Symptoms and Signs

Patients may experience mild to severe eye pain. The pain may be severe enough to cause severe nausea and vomiting. Patients may complain of seeing halos around light, blurred vision, or severe loss of vision. Engorgement of the limbal blood vessels, decreased visual acuity, corneal edema as manifested by an irregular corneal luster and light reflex, decreased corneal clarity, an irregular pupil, a nonreactive, midposition pupil, raised IOP, and poor view of the retina with ophthalmoscopy may be found.

Diagnosis

The examiner should use a hand light and examine the conjunctiva. The injection and distribution of the redness are noted. In angle closure glaucoma, the circumcorneal blood vessels are engorged: there appears to be a red halo surrounding the cornea. By projecting the hand light across the anterior chamber from temporal to nasal, the anterior displacement of the iris can be estimated. In shallow anterior chambers, the iris bows forward and blocks the light pathway; consequently, a shadow is seen on the nasal iris (Fig. 126-4).

With a hand light, the clinician should examine the reflection of the light off the cornea. Normally, the corneal light reflection is uniform and smooth. With corneal edema, the light reflex is pebbly and irregular. The reflection may appear as multiple light reflexes rather than one. The clarity of the cornea should be compared to that of the contralateral eye. Through a normal cornea, the clinician should be able to visualize iris, lens, and retinal detail. If the cornea is edematous, it appears hazy and provides a poor view of the iris, lens, and retina. The pupil may be misshapen and react poorly to light compared to the contralateral eye.

The IOP is usually elevated. However, angle closure attacks may abate spontaneously and occur episodically (subacute angle closure glaucoma). Therefore, the IOP may be normal if the patient is seen in the recovery phase of the episode. In the subacute phase, the cornea may be clear. Varying degrees of optic atrophy or optic nerve pallor may be observed.

Treatment

Laser iridectomy is the treatment of choice. By creating a hole in the iris, an alternate pathway is created from the posterior chamber to the anterior chamber. This decreases the entrapment of aqueous and the resultant iris anterior displacement.

If laser iridotomy is impossible, the attack can be treated medically with the use of topical and systemic agents (see the earlier section on the medical treatment of primary open angle glaucoma).

Surgical iridectomy can be performed if the previous therapies are unsuccessful.

SUMMARY

Glaucoma affects more than 2 million Americans. The disease is often silent, but if it is treated early, visual loss can be prevented. The primary care physician may recognize early signs of the disease primarily by optic disc changes (a C/D ratio > 0.5, an asymmetry of C/D ratios between eyes, and an asymmetric optic cup relative to the neural rim). Other indications for referral include an IOP above 21 mm Hg, risk factors for glaucoma (family history of glaucoma, diabetes mellitus, or severe cardiovascular disease), or signs of acute angle closure glaucoma.

BIBLIOGRAPHY

Berson FG, ed. Ophthalmology study guide, 5th ed. San Francisco: American Academy of Ophthalmology, 1993.

Briggs GG, Freeman RK, Yaffe SJ, et al. Drugs in pregnancy and lactation, 4th ed. Baltimore: Williams & Wilkins, 1994.

Committee on Drugs for the American Academy of Pediatrics. The transfer of drugs and other chemicals into human milk. Pediatrics 1994; 93:137.

Haley MJ, ed. The field analyzer primer. San Leandro, Calif.: Allergan Humphrey, 1987.

Hart WM. The epidemiology of primary open angle glaucoma and ocular hypertension. In: Ritch R, Shields MB, Krupin T, eds. The glaucomas. St. Louis: Mosby, 1989.

Newell FW. Ophthalmology, principles and concepts. St. Louis: Mosby, 1992.

Shields MB. Textbook of glaucoma, 3d ed. Baltimore: Williams & Wilkins, 1992.

Shingleton BJ, Berson FG, Cantor L, Hodapp EA, Lee DA, Anderson LS. Basic science course section 10, Glaucoma. San Francisco: American Academy of Ophthalmology, 1994.

Thomas JV. Primary open-angle glaucoma. In: Albert DM, Jakobiec FA, Robinson NL, eds. Principles and practice of ophthalmology, vol. 3. Philadelphia: WB Saunders, 1994:1342.

Primary Care for Women, edited by Phyllis C. Leppert and Fred M. Howard. Lippincott-Raven Publishers, Philadelphia © 1997.

XIV

Ear, Nose and Throat Problems

127

Acute and Chronic Rhinosinusitis

JAMES A. HADLEY

HISTORY

Acute infectious rhinosinusitis is an extremely common medical problem, affecting more than 20% of the U.S. population each year and accounting for nearly 25 million office visits per year. It is an inflammatory and usually infectious process of the linings of the paranasal sinuses and the nasal cavity. The disease is responsible for the expenditure of millions of dollars for medications and antibiotics to alleviate the symptoms of pain, nasal congestion, and lethargy characteristic of the process. Some experts feel that acute and chronic rhinosinusitis is becoming more prevalent, perhaps due to air pollution damage to the respiratory linings and increased exposure to upper respiratory infections in day-care settings and "tight" buildings.

The symptoms of acute rhinosinusitis (nasal congestion, post-nasal discharge, facial discomfort, and cough) are often confused with the common head cold, and this misunderstanding leads to prolonged inflammation due to lack of early treatment. Primary care physicians must be aware of the symptoms to render early effective treatment and to differentiate between other causes of sinonasal disorders. For example, pregnancy often renders the nose stuffy, primarily due to the estrogenic effects on the nasal mucosa; allergic rhinitis may affect up to 20% of the population and may be seasonal or perennial.

Treatment of infectious rhinosinusitis is necessary to prevent possible serious complications and is based on appropriate antibiotic therapy. The recent emergence of antibiotic-resistant bacteria, especially *Streptococcus pneumoniae*, has made selection of appropriate antibiotic regimens crucial.

In the past decade, technical advances in paranasal imaging and endoscopic examination have led to a new understanding of the physiology of the paranasal sinuses. The concepts that have developed have led to a better overall management of this common problem. Medical therapy should be effective for most patients with persistent rhinosinusitis, but surgery may be recommended for recalcitrant cases and specifically for patients with complications of acute or chronic rhinosinusitis.

ANATOMY AND PHYSIOLOGY

The paranasal sinuses, paired air-containing cavities in the anterior skull, include the maxillary, ethmoid, frontal, and sphenoid sinuses. Phylogenetically presumed to lighten the otherwise heavy skull, they are lined by the same respiratory pseudostratified ciliated squamous epithelium characteristic of the bronchial tree. They develop as outpouchings of respiratory epithelium within the facial bones, and their primary role is to provide aeration, humidification, and warming of inhaled air, as well as protection from foreign objects inhaled through the nose. Ventilation and transport of mucus occurs through the small ostia from the sinuses into the nose. These important mechanisms depend on the ability of the ciliated respiratory epithelium to move mucus through the narrow ostia.

Maxillary Sinus

The maxillary sinuses are the largest and develop first from pea-sized pouches extending into the cheeks from the nose. They begin to develop around the third month of gestation and change shape during the child's growth to a triangular cavity. The maxillary sinus ultimately develops into a pyramidal cavity occupying most of the maxilla. The maxillary antrum communicates with the middle meatus via the infundibulum of the middle meatus through a natural ostium. The natural ostium drains into the hiatus semilunaris, a slit-like ostium between the ethmoid cells, the uncinate process, and the orbit. Accessory ostia may develop as a result of chronic infection.

Ethmoid Sinus

The ethmoid sinuses develop during the third trimester into a labyrinth of small sinus cells medial and superior to the maxillary sinuses. They enlarge by pneumatization over the person's growth. The ethmoid cells vary in number (from four to 50 individual cells) and location. The most anterior cells are the frontal cells; next to them, the infundibular cells are anterior to the ethmoid bulla. These cells drain the frontal sinuses into the nose. The bullar cells may form a large cell and drain into the middle meatus just posterior to the agger nasi cells. Conchal cells of the ethmoids involve the anterior aspect of the middle turbinate and may cause obstruction of the middle meatus or give rise to pressure points. The posterior ethmoid cells lie behind the basal lamella of the middle turbinate and drain into the sphenoethmoidal recess.

Frontal Sinus

The frontal sinuses become pneumatized from the ethmoids directly into the frontal bone after about the third year of life. This pneumatization of the frontal bones is often asymmetric, and the sinuses are sometimes hypoplastic or nonexistent, or large with several compartments. They drain into the nasofrontal recess directly into the middle meatus alongside the anterior ethmoid cells.

Sphenoid Sinus

The sphenoid sinus does not appear until about the third year of life, growing as an outpouching of the sphenoethmoidal recess. Pneumatization enlarges the sinus to the sella turcica, attaining maximal growth in midadolescence. It drains usually through a small ostium in the sphenoethmoidal recess that is superior to the floor of the sphenoid sinus.

Physiology of the Paranasal Sinuses

The sinuses are lined by a respiratory epithelium composed of a pseudostratified columnar layer of cells lying on a supporting layer of fibroelastic tissue associated with goblet cells. The function of this layer of respiratory epithelium is to provide the sinuses with a supporting blanket of mucus.

The nose is designed to protect the respiratory tract from a hostile environment, and the sinuses play a major role in this defense through the elaboration of a mucous blanket. This blanket functions to warm and humidify ambient air and clears debris and pathogens from the body.

A mucous lining consisting of a biphase inner sol layer and an outer thick layer coats the respiratory epithelium. It is made from seromucinous glands within the epithelium and provides both protective and barrier functions. Respiratory mucus, found in the nose, sinuses, and eustachian tube, can insulate, lubricate, waterproof, humidify, and provide a medium for ciliary action. The outer gel layer traps foreign material, which is then transported to the natural drainage ostia by means of the ciliary action of the cells beating in the inner, thinner layer of mucus. Enzymatic proteins including lysozyme, lactoferrin, and secretory IgA are contained in the inner serous layer. These digest foreign bacteria and viruses and are the first line of defense. In the healthy state, the cilia propel the mucus to the natural ostia of the nose, from which it is eventually expelled.

Mucociliary clearance through the natural ostia may become impaired after a viral infection. Stasis of secretions occurs, and a secondary bacterial infection may result from this stagnation. The small size of the natural drainage pathways predisposes to obstruction of the natural ostia from even minor swelling of the mucous membranes after an upper respiratory inflammation, allergic inflammatory response, or infection (Fig. 127-1). These events set the stage for sinus infection.

The ventilation and drainage portals of the sinuses are small ostia that vary in size and position. The natural ostium of the maxillary sinus is located behind a lamella of bone termed the uncinate process. The frontal sinus drains and ventilates through a recess superior to the ethmoid bullar cell (the largest of the many ethmoid cells) directly into the middle meatus, along with the ethmoid cells (Fig. 127-2). The sphenoid sinuses have their own ostia, which drain into the sphenoethmoidal recess posterior and medial to the middle turbinate (Fig. 127-3).

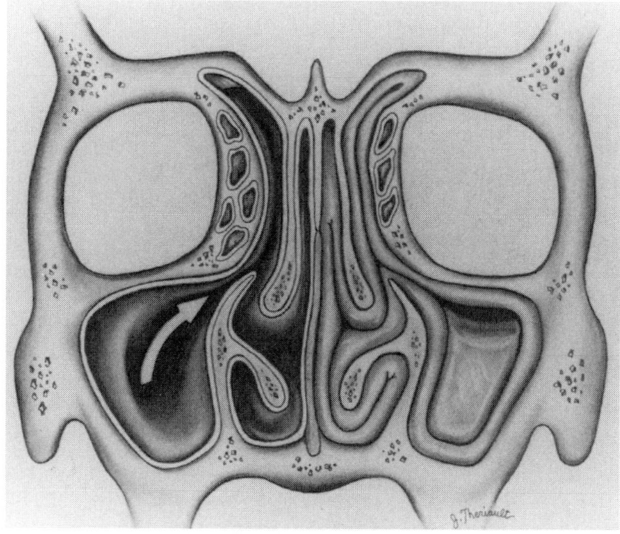

Figure 127-1. Coronal view of the paranasal sinuses showing natural drainage of the maxillary sinus through the ostium and chronic inflammation with obstruction and air–fluid level on the opposite side.

After a viral upper respiratory infection, the seromucinous glands secrete an increased amount of plasma proteins to help fight the infectious process. The increased vascular permeability that results creates the symptoms of nasal congestion and engorgement with increased rhinorrhea. These secretions thicken as the infection progresses, resulting in the symptoms of thick postnasal discharge.

Allergic reactions play a role in the development of inflammations within the paranasal sinuses. Type I hypersensitivity reactions involve the release of inflammatory mediators from the mast cell after sensitization. During the early stage of this reaction, histamine and other preformed kinins are released, causing increased capillary permeability, edema formation, and increased mucous production. This is followed by a late phase several hours later, characterized by the influx of cells into the inflammatory site. These cells include neutrophils, eosinophils, and lymphocytes that elaborate lymphokines and other mediators, prolonging the inflammation within the mucosa. This inflammatory state within the sinus mucous membranes may predispose the patient to secondary invasion of bacterial pathogens, giving rise to an episode of rhinosinusitis.

Histopathologic examination of paranasal sinus tissue from patients with chronic rhinosinusitis reveals an infiltration of the mucosa by eosinophils. These cells liberate major basic protein, eosinophil cationic protein, and other chemical mediators that affect the mucosa, stimulating the generation of polypoid mucous membranes.

Cytokines released by the late phase of the inflammatory reaction attract eosinophils and other inflammatory cells to prolong the inflammatory state. These cytokines include histamine and the

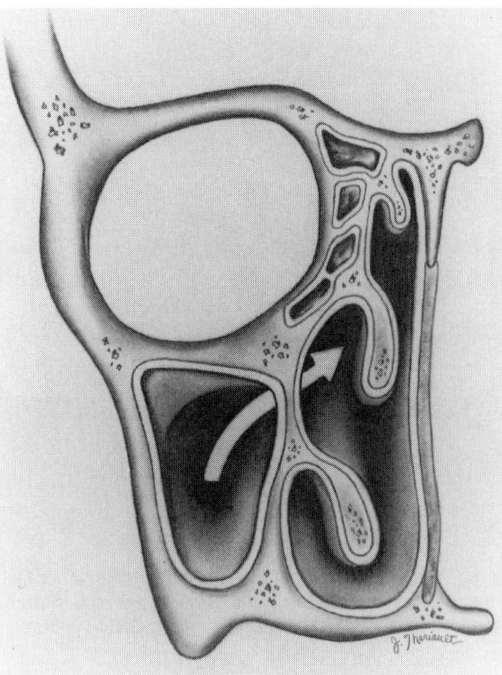

Figure 127-2. Drainage pathway through the natural ostium located at the osteomeatal complex.

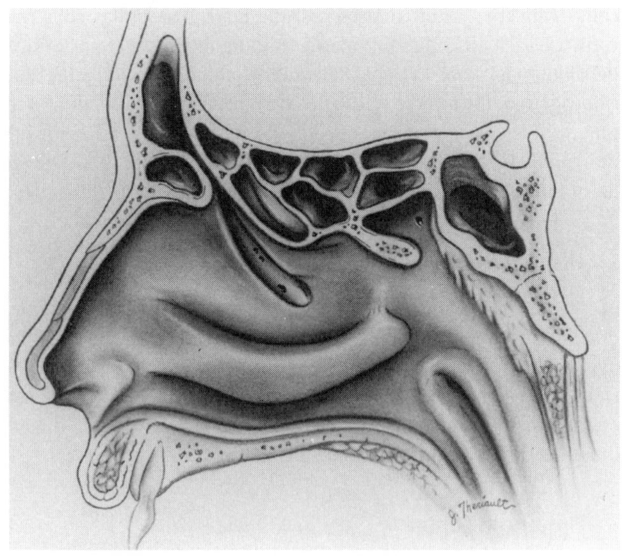

Figure 127-3. Lateral view of the paranasal sinuses with the ethmoid labyrinth and frontal sinus recess draining into the hiatus semilunaris. The sphenoid sinus ostium is clearly seen in the sphenoethmoidal recess. The middle turbinate has been removed for clarification.

leukotrienes LTB4, LTC4, LTD4, and LTE4, which are potent bronchoconstrictors inducing symptoms of asthma with cough in many patients with inflammations of the paranasal sinuses. We now begin to comprehend the association of asthma and acute or chronic sinusitis due to the release of these inflammatory mediators during the late-phase reaction.

PREDISPOSING FACTORS FOR RHINOSINUSITIS

Certain patients have a predisposition to the development of acute or chronic rhinosinusitis. For example, this predisposition occurs in 15% to 20% of patients with allergic rhinitis. Other factors predisposing to infection include structural abnormalities (nasal septal deviations, concha bullosa formation of the middle turbinates, paradoxic middle turbinates) and nasal polyps or tumors that block the outflow tract of the osteomeatal complex (Table 127-1). Metabolic abnormalities include cystic fibrosis, ciliary dyskinesia, immune deficiencies, AIDS, and hyperreactive respiratory lining, especially in patients with asthma.

ETIOLOGY OF SINUS INFECTIONS

A primary respiratory event (either viral or allergic) leads to an inflammatory reaction and consequent edema of the respiratory epithelium. The inflammation of the mucosa at the narrow ostia eventually shuts down the ventilation and drainage of the sinus cavity. With the change in aeration, a vicious cycle develops that leads to continued inflammation and poor drainage (Fig. 127-4). A change in the pH occurs and the mucosal gas metabolism is altered, with resultant damage to the cilia of the epithelium. Secretions stagnate, creating a culture medium for bacterial overgrowth within a closed cavity. Sneezing, nose blowing, or sniffling may allow bacteria to enter the sinus. A secondary infection, usually bacterial, decreases the mucociliary clearance and continues the inflammatory process (Fig. 127-5).

The source of the inflammation is usually at the osteomeatal complex, the narrowest channel between the maxillary and the ethmoid sinuses. Experience with computed tomography (CT) and diagnostic nasal endoscopy has proved that the pathogenesis of sinus infections is within this narrow region.

CLINICAL MANIFESTATIONS

The symptoms of rhinosinusitis are often confused with those of allergic disease or a common upper respiratory infection. The practitioner must be able to differentiate among these disorders to manage the acute manifestations before they become chronic.

Acute Rhinosinusitis

Acute rhinosinusitis presents with symptoms of thick, purulent nasal discharge, facial pain, and severe nasal congestion, often

Table 127-1. Predisposing Factors in Rhinosinusitis

Local Problems	Systemic Problems
Nasal septal abnormalities	Cystic fibrosis
Turbinate abnormalities	Allergic rhinitis
Rhinitis medicamentosa	Ciliary dyskinesia
Environmental aberrations	Immunodepression (AIDS)
Choanal atresia	Immunoglobulin deficiencies
Barotrauma	
Nasal polyps or tumors	
Foreign bodies	

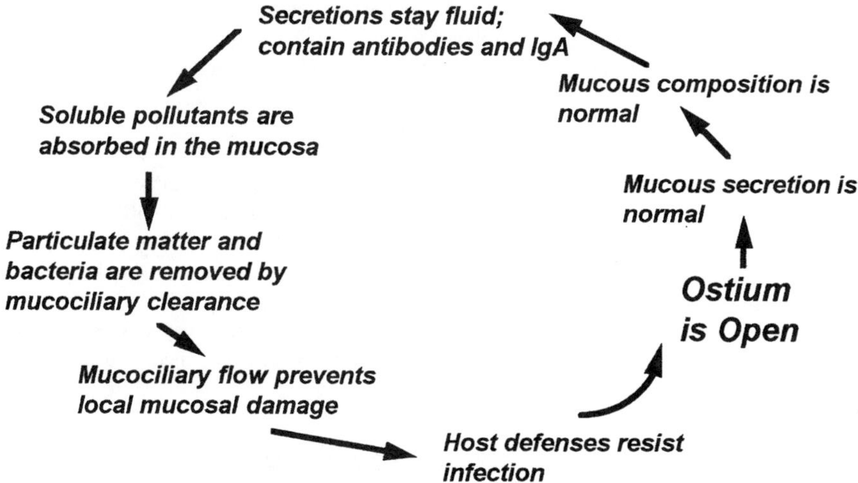

Figure 127-4. Vicious cycle of sinusitis.

accompanied by cough and fever. The facial pain may localize to the maxillary region, with associated dental pain, or to the periorbital and forehead regions, with associated severe headache. These acute headaches may be confused with migraine or temporal arteritis. Younger patients may not have as much pain, but they have purulent rhinorrhea and bad breath. Younger patients often present with cough, which may be confused with an asthma-like picture. Rhinosinusitis is considered acute if the symptoms persist no longer than 6 to 8 weeks or if there are fewer than four episodes per year of acute symptoms lasting 10 days or less, and no mucosal damage remains.

Acute ethmoid sinusitis presents with symptoms of nasal congestion, purulent rhinorrhea, and pain localized to the inner canthal area or periorbital pain and pressure. The infection is often accompanied by infection in the maxillary sinus as well. Patients feel worse when supine or coughing and when wearing glasses. Minimal disease within this small cavity often leads to maximal symptoms.

Acute maxillary sinusitis tends to localize over the cheekbone or on one side of the face. The pain may resemble a toothache, and consequently the patient may present to the dentist. Thick purulent discharge comes primarily from the middle meatus on the involved side. The pain becomes more intense while walking or in an upright position and may improve when supine.

Acute frontal sinusitis presents with severe forehead discomfort. This may rapidly progress to an intracranial complication, especially in younger patients. The headache is usually the worst the patient has experienced and may be confused with meningitis. Patients need early referral to an otolaryngologist to avoid the complications of intracranial spread, epidural abscess, subdural empyema, and brain abscess.

Acute sphenoid sinusitis is relatively rare and is a medical emergency for surgical drainage. Patients complain of a deep occipital-type headache with referral to the top of the head.

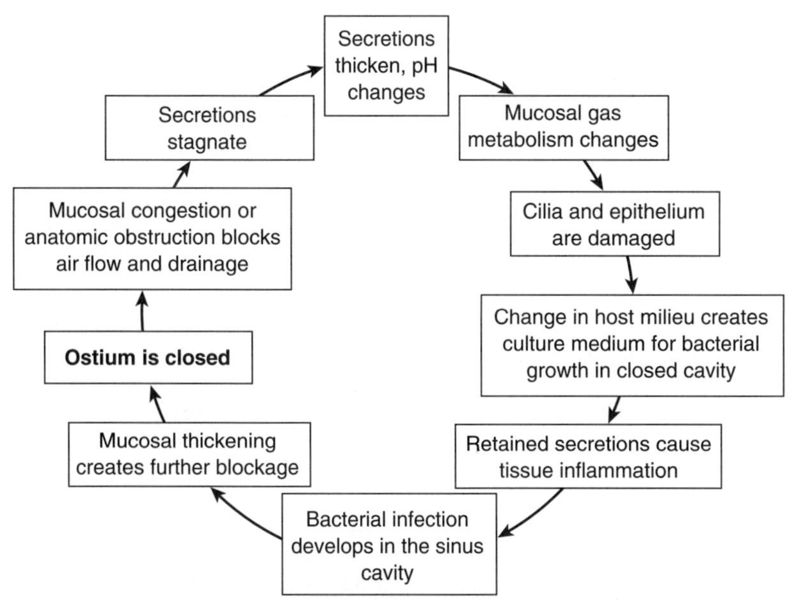

Figure 127-5. Vicious cycle leading to chronic rhinosinusitis.

Impending CNS complications include visual loss and cavernous sinus thrombosis.

Chronic Rhinosinusitis

The clinical manifestations of chronic rhinosinusitis present a diagnostic challenge because they are poorly localized to any one area and are usually more subtle and mild than those of acute rhinosinusitis.

After a period of persistent inflammation, the ostia of the sinuses become blocked with an inflammatory reaction. This leads to stasis and thickened secretions, predisposing to an anaerobic environment. Symptoms include all the common complaints seen in the acute phase of the infection, including purulent yellow or green postnasal discharge and facial discomfort (not typically pain, but a constant feeling of pressure). Fever may coexist but may be low-grade or subclinical. Other symptoms include decreased sense of smell, chronic sore throat with or without hoarseness, and lethargy or generalized fatigue.

Chronic rhinosinusitis may precipitate a worsening of an underlying asthmatic condition. Patients who have asthma frequently have associated chronic rhinosinusitis, and the asthmatic inflammatory state is not resolved until the infection is cleared. Between 30% and 50% of patients with asthma have radiologic evidence of mucous membrane abnormalities of the paranasal sinuses. The lower respiratory tract inflammation may be due to several factors, including reflex increase of vagal tone from trigeminal stimulation within the sinuses and liberation of inflammatory mediators (leukotrienes), which are strong bronchoconstrictors.

COMPLICATIONS

Sinus infections, unless treated early and with proper antibiotics, can lead to severe complications, including blindness and intracranial abscess. Physicians must become familiar with the symptoms of acute sinus infection so they can prevent the spread of the disease into the orbit or brain.

Orbital Complications

Infection within the sinus can easily transgress the thin lamella of bone that separates the ethmoid and maxillary sinuses. Inflammation of the sinus mucosa creates a thrombophlebitis within the veins draining the ethmoid sinuses, and infection can spread easily through the valveless veins of the diploic bone of the skull. The development of vasculitis and early inflammation with cellulitis around the orbit can eventually lead to subperiosteal abscess, then orbital abscess, and finally cavernous sinus thrombosis.

The symptoms of periorbital cellulitis include edema and erythema of the ipsilateral eyelid. This may be confused with an eye infection, but the underlying cause is directly related to the ethmoid sinus infection. Severe headache and fever are common. If not treated aggressively, this process may progress to orbital subperiosteal abscess formation. At this stage, the patient may have decreased motion of the involved eye, chemosis of the eyelid, and proptosis. The CT scan shows a subperiosteal collection of purulence that requires immediate surgical drainage.

Progression of orbital involvement may lead to thrombophlebitis of the veins of the paranasal sinuses, which may progress to the development of cavernous sinus thrombosis. Signs of this potentially fatal infection include severe deep orbital pain, complete ophthalmoplegia, and spiking fevers. This is a medical and surgical emergency requiring intravenous antibiotics and surgical drainage.

Intracranial Complications

The spread of the infection from the paranasal sinus into the brain is rare with the use of broad-spectrum antibiotics. Usually this infection occurs as a direct result of frontal sinus infection. The signs of intracranial infection include prostration, severe headache with nausea and vomiting, photophobia, and papilledema. The CT scan confirms the diagnosis. Lumbar puncture may show infection but may be contraindicated in the presence of increased intracranial pressure.

DIAGNOSIS AND EVALUATION

Historically, physicians relied on the chief complaints and physical examination to diagnose rhinosinusitis. Modern diagnostic techniques involve direct examination of the nasal cavity and sinus ostia, which permits direct culture, and radiographic studies, including CT scanning.

History

A comprehensive history is important to evaluate the patient's complaints and to rule out other causes of nasal complaints, including an evaluation for allergy. The history should include the type, consistency, and duration of nasal discharge, the location of facial pain (to determine the involved sinus cavity), and associated symptoms (eg, loss of sense of smell, presence of cough or fever).

The past medical history should be reviewed with reference to asthma, allergies, chronic bronchitis, or possible immunologic disorders. A thorough review of prior medications, including OTC medications and drug reactions, is necessary.

Physical Examination

Face

The face is observed for evidence of swelling or erythema over an involved sinus. In frontal sinusitis, the physician may note significant edema and tenderness to palpation. Percussion over the cheeks or forehead may elicit tenderness.

Nose

The nose is inspected using ample light via headlamp and nasal speculum (an otoscope may be used for a child), looking for mucosal edema and swelling within the middle meatal region between the middle and inferior turbinates. Direct cultures can be obtained from this region. Otolaryngologists may use a nasal endoscope, which provides superior illumination and visualization of the drainage pathways. The nose is inspected for obvious anatomic abnormalities, including nasal septal deformities and nasal polyps or tumors. The color, texture, and quality of any nasal discharge are assessed.

Sinuses

Transillumination of the paranasal sinuses is performed in a darkened room using a bright light source applied against the patient's cheek, looking into the open mouth, and applied under the eyebrow, looking at the forehead. Swollen, infected sinuses block the transillumination of the light.

Head and Neck

The examiner should evaluate the throat for discharge, swollen membranes, and foul breath. The ears may present with serous middle ear effusions or symptoms of eustachian tube dysfunction, with a retracted or reddened ear drum.

Laboratory Tests

Direct culture of sinus fluid is the best way to diagnose sinusitis. Maxillary sinus puncture is an invasive procedure that represents the gold standard. Direct nasal cultures have not correlated well with the results of the fluid within the involved sinus cavity and should not necessarily be relied on to direct antibiotic coverage (Table 127-2).

Radiography

X-ray evaluation of the paranasal sinuses has evolved with CT scanning, and more precise images can be obtained that make plain views of the sinuses almost obsolete. Plain sinus radiography gives limited information but may be sufficient for the practitioner to justify therapy or referral. It is useful to document maxillary or frontal sinus disease and may have a role in following the progress of infection, but it cannot evaluate the ethmoid sinuses properly. CT is preferred because it provides the best images of the relation of the mucous membranes to the surrounding bony structures.

When nasal endoscopy fails to document the source of presumed infection, CT scanning is indicated to search for inflammation or obstruction, primarily within the anterior ethmoid sinuses. This evaluation is also needed by the otolaryngologist when a patient is a candidate for surgery. CT scanning may also confirm the presence of chronic sinusitis and the need for referral for definitive therapy.

Magnetic resonance imaging is generally not indicated: it does not address the bony confines but shows primarily mucosal disease or possible fungal invasion. This technique is helpful, however, for the differential diagnosis of tumors or the possibility of intracranial complications of acute or chronic sinusitis.

Ultrasonography, using either a-mode or b-mode scanning, reportedly has had some success in diagnosis, but the technique is not well established and requires considerable experience. For now, ultrasonography provides little diagnostic or therapeutic information.

Table 127-2. Common Pathogens in Acute Rhinosinusitis

Species	Positive Cultures (%)*
Streptococcus pneumoniae	41
Haemophilus influenzae	35
Anaerobes	7
Streptococcal spp.	7
Moraxella catarrhalis	3.5
Staphylococcus aureus	3
Others	3.5

*In 383 pretreatment sinus aspirates.
(Gwaltney JM Jr, Scheld WM, Sande MA, Syndor A. The microbiology, etiology and antimicrobial therapy of adults with community-acquired sinusitis: a 15-year experience at the University of Virginia and review of other selected sites. J Allergy Clin Immunol 1992;90:457.)

DIFFERENTIAL DIAGNOSIS

Allergic Rhinitis

Allergic rhinitis presents with very similar symptoms of nasal congestion, facial pressure, and rhinorrhea, but the nasal discharge is primarily clear (Table 127-3). The patient also has a history of seasonal or year-round symptoms of an itchy and runny nose associated with sneezing. Other allergic symptoms may coexist, including red, itchy eyes and dark circles under the eyes ("allergic shiners") due to vascular blush from nasal congestion. Usually these and other symptoms of the allergic state tip the practitioner to this diagnosis. However, allergic patients may become acutely infected; treatment relies on reduction of infection first, with subsequent allergy control.

Nasal Polyposis

Nasal polyps are benign, frequently large sac-like appendages of nasal and sinus mucosa that arise primarily from the lateral wall of the nose, from the ethmoid sinuses and middle turbinate. They develop as a result of an inflammatory process that occurs after an infection or allergic process. Patients complain of constant nasal congestion, anosmia, and chronic nasal discharge. Secondary infection of the sinuses can occur as well. The inflammatory reactions that result from nasal polyps can progress to involve all the paranasal sinuses with a hyperplastic mucosa that fills all the sinuses. Earlier surgical treatments of nasal polypectomy led to recurrence, but current techniques usually avoid this problem.

Fungal Infection of the Sinuses

Fungal infections of the sinuses may occur after ineffective treatment of a sinusitis or de novo. These infections may be asymptomatic or present with symptoms of facial pressure or an infection that persists despite adequate antibiotic therapy. The discharge associated with allergic fungal sinusitis is characteristically thick, tenacious, and dark green or brown; patients may also present with nasal polyposis. CT scans reveal an opacified sinus and areas of hyperdensity but usually no invasion into the bone. The most common fungus is *Aspergillus*, although other species are beginning to appear in case reports. Diagnosis is based on review of the CT scan and identification of allergic mucin by rhinoscopy or at the time of surgery. Treatment is primarily surgical debridement or removal of

Table 127-3. Sinus Infection versus Allergy

Infection	Allergy
Nasal obstruction/congestion	Nasal obstruction/congestion
Pressure with pain	Itchy, runny nose
Thick nasal discharge	Paroxysmal sneezing
Toothache	Thin, watery nasal discharge
Fever	History of sinusitis during allergy season
Cough or irritability	Other allergic symptoms

the fungus ball. Invasive fungal infections of the sinuses present as surgical emergencies.

Sampter Triad

These patients present with symptoms of recurrent rhinosinusitis, usually with nasal polyposis, asthma, and sensitivity to aspirin. Their asthma symptoms worsen after ingestion of aspirin products or other nonsteroidal antiinflammatory agents, due to a blockade of the cyclooxygenase pathway of arachidonic acid metabolism, favoring the production of leukotrienes. These mediators stimulate bronchial smooth muscle contraction. Patients depend on the combination of medical management and surgical removal of nasal polyps with sinus ventilation to improve their quality of life.

Cystic Fibrosis

This disease is due to an autosomal recessive gene affecting the exocrine glands, resulting in the combination of pancreatic insufficiency, pulmonary dysfunction due to excessive mucus, and abnormal sweat. These children present with rhinosinusitis due to nasal polyposis, an otherwise rare finding in children.

Cysts and Tumors

Mucous retention cysts, benign lesions within the maxillary sinuses, develop in patients with inflammation of the sinuses due to allergy or infection. They are found incidentally on radiographic evaluation. Mucoceles are more symptomatic and can cause expansile masses within the frontal sinus.

TREATMENT

The treatment of paranasal sinusitis centers around proper medical management in the acute stages and consideration of surgical drainage and ventilation in chronic sinusitis or refractory cases.

Acute Rhinosinusitis

The management goals in the treatment of acute rhinosinusitis include control of infection, reduction of mucosal edema, improvement of sinus drainage, restoration and maintenance of sinus ostia patency, and breakup of the vicious cycle leading to chronic rhinosinusitis (Table 127-4).

Antibiotics are the mainstay of management of acute rhinosinusitis. Once the diagnosis has been established, the decision to place the patient on appropriate antibacterial medications should be made. Antibiotic therapy should be directed against the primary pathogens in acute sinusitis (see Table 127-2). The recent emergence of resistant bacteria has presented a problem in the choice of appropriate antibiotics. Strains of *S pneumoniae* and especially *Haemophilus influenzae* have become resistant to ampicillin-like agents due to the production of β-lactamase. Current antibiotics recommended for the treatment of acute rhinosinusitis are listed in Table 127-5.

The clinician must consider the efficacy of the medication, the side effect profile, the convenience of administration, and the cost. Erythromycin and tetracycline are ineffective in acute rhinosinusitis. Certain second-generation cephalosporin antibiotics may not have activity against *H influenzae* and should be avoided.

Adjunctive medical therapy is helpful to reduce tissue edema and promote drainage of the sinus cavity. Topical and systemic decongestants may be used to provide relief of tissue edema and subjective improvement of nasal congestion. Topical decongestants (oxymetazoline) act on adrenergic receptors in the nasal mucosa, shrink the swollen inflamed tissue, and promote oxygenation of the sinus. They should be used for no longer than 3 days to avoid rebound effects. Systemic decongestants (pseudoephedrine, phenylpropanolamine) also stimulate α-adrenergic receptors in the nose to provide subjective relief, and they may improve ostial patency by reducing nasal blood flow. Their use in the first trimester of pregnancy is contraindicated, and the use of OTC medications should be discouraged.

Antihistamines are indicated solely for allergic rhinitis and are not useful in acute rhinosinusitis. They control type I hypersensitivity reactions by reducing the release of histamine and other chemical mediators, and thus should be used only when allergy is a predisposing factor for infection. They are effective for reducing the symptoms of rhinorrhea, sneezing, and nasal itching, but the older classic antihistamines may cause too much drying, inhibiting clearance of nasal secretions.

Other adjunctive measures are important. The patient frequently complains of significant pain, so analgesics are important. Humidification of the nasal membranes is important and may be delivered by nasal saline spray, steam inhalation, or cool vapor humidifiers. Mucolytic agents have potential benefit, especially in patients with thick nasal secretions. Guaifenesin is the mucolytic of choice and may be combined with a systemic decongestant.

Maxillary sinus irrigation is occasionally indicated in acute rhinosinusitis. This office procedure is relatively benign and allows direct culture of the involved sinus cavity with the removal of the infected sinus material. Irrigation of the sinus cavity may help restore sinus ostial patency. It should be considered in patients who are immunocompromised, especially in AIDS patients.

The role of topical nasal steroids in acute rhinosinusitis has not been established. These medications are indicated for the treatment of chronic sinusitis. Topical nasal steroids reduce the inflammation

Table 127-4. Medical Therapy for Rhinosinusitis

Adequate medical therapy is the key to successful treatment.
Antibiotics help control the infection in the closed sinus cavity.
Decongestants may help to maintain ostial patency.
Mucoevacuants may also help to maintain patency and thin secretions.
Topical or oral corticosteroids help in chronic rhinosinusitis but are not indicated in acute rhinosinusitis.

Table 127-5. Antibiotics for Acute and Recurrent Acute Rhinosinusitis

Trimethoprim–sulfisoxazole DS (bid)
Loracarbef (400 mg bid)
Amoxicillin–clavulanate (500/125 mg tid)
Cefuroxime axetil (250 mg bid)
Cefprozil (250 mg bid)
Duration of therapy, 10–14 days

Table 127-6. Topical Steroids in Rhinosinusitis*

Beclomethasone dipropionate
Triamcinolone acetonide
Flunisolide
Budesonide
Fluticasone
Dexamethasone

*Topical corticosteroids reduce edema, inflammation, and mucus secretion in chronic rhinosinusitis but are not indicated in acute rhinosinusitis.

within the nasal mucosa but require several days before subjective improvement is obtained.

In summary, therapy for acute rhinosinusitis includes antibiotics, analgesics, decongestants (topical or systemic), mucolytic therapy (saline or systemic mucolytics), adjunctive therapy (topical saline or humidification), and sinus irrigation in refractory or immunocompromised cases.

Chronic Rhinosinusitis

Chronic rhinosinusitis is a direct result of persistent inflammation within the mucous membranes of the paranasal sinuses. This problem occurs after recurrent acute episodes or persistent infection lasting more than 3 months. At this stage, the sinus ostia are more or less irreversibly blocked by fibrous tissue or hyperplastic mucosa that prevents adequate ventilation and drainage of the involved sinus cavities. As the sinus cavity becomes depleted of oxygen, the bacterial species change and become anaerobic; treatment regimens must change accordingly.

Chronic rhinosinusitis in adults should be managed using the same therapies as for acute disease: antibiotics, analgesics if necessary, decongestants, mucolytics, and the addition of topical nasal and sometimes systemic steroids.

Antibiotics directed against anaerobic bacteria should be prescribed (eg, amoxicillin/clavulanate, clindamycin, or the association of penicillin and metronidazole [Flagyl]). They should be prescribed for at least 3 weeks to achieve maximal effect. However, even intensive and prolonged antibiotic therapy may not effect a cure.

Medical therapy to reduce tissue edema is important. Topical nasal steroids are the primary medications used to help reduce tissue edema around the sinus ostia. Used appropriately, the risk of systemic side effects is very low; however, their use in pregnancy is controversial. Five topical steroids are available: dexamethasone, beclomethasone, budesonide, flunisolide, and triamcinolone acetonide. Dexamethasone is prescribed as a short-term, high-potency topical nasal steroid. It is recommended when a rapid onset of action is desired and for cases of hyperplastic nasal polyposis. The other second-generation topical nasal steroids have a slower onset of action but are effective in the management of inflammation. Patients should be cautioned to use the topical corticosteroids at their recommended dosage; the risk of systemic absorption is small at appropriate dosages. Dosages should be adjusted according to the response and reduced to the lowest possible maintenance level. Side effects with the use of topical nasal steroids include nasal irritation, epistaxis, and minor headache (Table 127-6)

Consultation with an otolaryngologist should be considered when the patient does not respond to this regimen. Surgical procedures may afford greater success when the patient has had symptoms for more than 6 months or three or more episodes of acute sinusitis each year for 3 years in a row.

CONSIDERATIONS IN PREGNANCY

Rhinosinusitis may be confused with the symptoms of nasal congestion induced by estrogens during pregnancy. Patients often complain of a stuffy nose, which can be ameliorated with the use of a topical nasal steroid during the second trimester. Topical decongestants may also give relief, and they have less risk to the fetus than systemic medications.

Patients with infections of the sinuses require antibiotics. Penicillins (ampicillin, ampicillin/clavulanate) are the antibiotics of choice. Their risk to the fetus is small. Cephalosporins also have a low risk of teratogenicity, although they cross the placenta and are excreted into the amniotic fluid like the penicillins.

Sulfonamides and combinations with trimethoprim cause no risk to the fetus during the first trimester. They may be combined synergistically with erythromycin.

Antibiotics for chronic rhinosinusitis include clindamycin, which has not been associated with any congenital defects. It crosses the placenta and achieves serum cord levels 50% of those in maternal serum.

BIBLIOGRAPHY

Gwaltney JM, Scheld WM, Sande MA, Syndor A. The microbiology, etiology and antimicrobial therapy of adults with community-acquired sinusitis: a 15-year experience at the University of Virginia and review of other selected sites. J Allergy Clin Immunol 1992;90:457.

Hadley JA, Bakos R, Regenbogen V. Middle cranial fossa epidural abscess, an unusual complication of acute sinusitis: etiology, Evaluation and Treatment. Am J Rhinol 1991;5:181.

Kaliner MA. Human nasal host defense. In: Shapiro G, Rachelefsky G, eds. Mechanism, diagnosis and treatment of sinusitis in children and adults. J Allergy Clin Immunol 1992;90(suppl):424.

Kennedy DW, Zinreich SJ, Rosenbaum AE. Functional endoscopic sinus surgery: theory and diagnostic evaluation. Arch Otolaryngol Head Neck Surg 1985;111:576.

Kennedy DW, Zinreich SJ, Rosenbaum AE. Functional endoscopic sinus surgery: technique. Arch Otolaryngol Head Neck Surg 1985;111:643.

Mabry RL. Corticosteroids in rhinology. Otolaryngol Head Neck Surg 1993;108:768.

Raphael GD, Baraniuk JN, Kaliner MA. How and why the nose runs. J Allergy Clin Immunol 1991;87:457.

Stammberger H. Endoscopic endonasal surgery—concepts in treatment of recurring rhinosinusitis. Otolaryngol Head Neck Surg 1986;94:143.

128
Otitis

PETER MULBURY

Primary Care for Women, edited by Phyllis C. Leppert and Fred M. Howard. Lippincott-Raven Publishers, Philadelphia © 1997.

Otitis is divided into external otitis, otitis media, and labyrinthitis. Each type represents a distinctly separate entity in terms of cause, treatment, and potential sequelae.

EXTERNAL OTITIS

The ear canal inclusive of the tympanic membrane is covered with desquamating squamous epithelium. The epithelium in the cartilaginous lateral portion of the canal is relatively thick, containing a subcutaneous layer that is absent in the bony canal. Within this subcutaneous tissue are the hair follicles and apocrine glands, including the cerumen glands. Cerumen provides lubrication to the epithelium as well as a protective coating.

Etiology

Cerumen accumulation poses a problem for many individuals. Most people, however, are overly concerned about the potential reflection on our hygienic appearance, and cleaning with cotton-tipped applicators often affects the cerumen. If such cleaning is done excessively,the epithelium is stripped of its protective coating, resulting in irritation or a dermatitis. Because the character of cerumen varies dramatically from one individual to another, the easiest removal technique will therefore also vary from curettage to suction to irrigation. Softeners are available, but they may cause the cerumen to swell and occasionally can result in a dermatitis if left in the canal for too long. A simple solution of soap and water or mineral oil used on several subsequent nights at bedtime followed by a gentle irrigation with warm water (to avoid caloric stimulation) is usually an effective home remedy. Care should be taken to avoid any substantial pressure when irrigating, and perforation of the tympanic membrane contraindicates irrigation.

Inflammation of the ear canal is best considered a dermatitis. Because of its relatively narrow diameter, any significant inflammation with the attendant edema or induration may rapidly lead to obstruction. This causes discomfort and interferes with drainage and also with access for topical agents.

Physical Examination and Clinical Findings

Typically, the patient presents with a 2- to 3-day history of unilateral otalgia not associated with an upper respiratory infection or temperature elevation. There often is a history of water exposure, from either swimming or showering. Examination reveals an acutely inflamed canal tender to the touch. Drainage and crusting are usually present in the canal and about the meatus. Because of the otalgia, examination of the tympanic membrane is often not possible. Impacted cerumen may be present; this requires removal. Attendant hearing loss depends on the degree of obstruction and is conductive in character. Often there is significant pre- and postauricular lymphadenitis with variable cellulitis of the adjacent skin.

Cultures are usually positive for *Staphylococcus* and *Pseudomonas* species. Occasionally, cotton-like debris representing the mycelia and the attached spores of a fungal infection are obvious in the canal. The most common of these is aspergillosis nigrans. An underlying history of a dermatitis and recurrences is typical with these patients.

Treatment

Treatment of external otitis must include local therapy. Debris or cerumen should be removed from the canal. Often, the insertion of a wick is necessary to allow penetration of a topical medication medially beyond the swollen outer canal. This may be a strip of gauze or a compressed sponge available commercially. It must be emphasized that the principal therapy is topical, not systemic. Most commonly the preparation is a combination of neomycin, polymixin, and hydrocortisone administered for a period of 1 week.

Fungal infections are also treated topically after cleansing of the canal. Specific examples of antifungal agents include clotrimazole, germicidin, or tolnaftate. Bacterial and fungal infections may often be treated more simply with an acidifying solution such as Burow's solution. These solutions are particularly useful for extending therapy after a specific agent or when used as prophylaxis after water exposure in the patient with a recurrent history. A preparation of a 50 : 50 solution of alcohol and white vinegar used in this manner is an excellent preventative.

Occasionally, a significant cellulitis or periauricular lymphadenitis requires the addition of a systemic antibiotic directed at coverage of *Staphylococcus* or *Streptococcus* species. This should be in addition to the topical medication. Especially in patients with underlying dermatitis and recurrences, a sensitivity to neomycin may exist. A progression of the erythema or the development of a rash of the pinna should serve as a warning of this allergic reaction.

Other Forms of External Otitis

Malignant external otitis is an unusual form of external otitis that occurs almost exclusively in the diabetic patient. Granulation tissue is classically found in the canal. A boring pain is described, and cultures reveal the presence of *Pseudomonas*. The granulation tissue and infection are erosive and may travel medially, eventually into the CNS. Multiple cranial nerves may become involved; the mortality rate is as high as 50% when cranial nerves are involved. Treatment must be aggressive, both topically and with parenteral anti-*Pseudomonas* therapy. With currently available agents, surgical debridement is only rarely necessary. Prophylaxis with an acidifying solution is beneficial in preventing recurrences.

Bullous myringitis is another unusual form of external otitis. Patients present with a characteristic history of a brief (< 24 hours) duration of severe, increasing otalgia, not associated with an upper respiratory infection. The pain is reported to culminate with drainage that may be serous or bloody, but brings relief. Examination reveals multiple bullae within the canal and often on the tympanic membrane. These may be distended or ruptured with discharge present. The tympanic membrane is intact, as is the hearing, although the maceration and inflammation may obscure the drum. These are not the bullae that may be seen on the tympanic membrane associated with the typical otitis media. It is generally held that bullous myringitis has a viral etiology, but *Mycoplasma* has been implicated. Therefore, many practitioners use either a tetracycline or erythromycin in their treatment regimen.

Furuncles are not uncommon in the lateral aspect of the ear canal. These are infections of the glands or hair follicles with staphylococcal organisms. Incision and drainage may occasionally be required, but avoidance of manipulation is usually all that is necessary.

Herpes zoster can cause a shingles-like rash periauricularly. This is a very painful disorder that is most typically associated with a facial paralysis. However, multiple cranial nerves may be involved. Treatment is symptomatic and expectant, similar to Bell's palsy but with a poorer rate of complete resolution. Steroidal and anti-viral therapy may be added, particularly in the debilitated or immunosuppressed patient. Care of the cornea to prevent abrasion is provided.

OTITIS MEDIA

The middle ear, connected to the nasopharynx by the eustachian tube, may be considered an extension of the nasal cavity, and is lined by essentially the same upper respiratory epithelium. Otitis media (OM) and the potential sequelae of otitis media with effusion (OME) and chronic otitis media (COM) are best considered secondary to eustachian tube dysfunction. The eustachian tube is responsible for ventilation of the middle ear. The air within the middle ear space is slowly absorbed, resulting in a relative negative pressure. This negative pressure is relieved by opening the eustachian tube, equilibrating the pressure with that of ambient air. This maximizes the efficiency of the system.

When the eustachian tube does not function properly, a negative pressure persists. This may draw secretions up from the nasopharynx, causing an infection, or result in chronic negative middle ear pressure. In turn there is a thickening of the middle ear mucosa and hyperplasia of the goblet cells that produce a mucoid effusion. Over time the chronic negative pressure may cause atrophic changes in the tympanic membrane, retraction pockets, ossicular problems, or cholesteatomas.

Etiology

Eustachian tube dysfunction is most often a result of whatever is occurring in the nose and nasopharynx. In children this is usually a reflection on the shape of the skull or the status of the adenoids. In adults, upper respiratory infection (URI), allergies, sinusitis, neoplasm, or a general rhinitis are the most frequent causes. The adult patient with an isolated OM or SOM is an unusual occurrence.

Clinical Findings

Similarly, the changes associated with COM are seen only in a patient with a history of previous or ongoing difficulties with otitis. The changes may be tympanosclerosis (scarring), atrophic portions of the tympanic membrane, retraction pockets, perforations, or cholesteatomas. Perforations are classified by size, location (marginal or central), and active or inactive (draining or dry) status. Desquamating squamous epithelium belongs only on the surface of the tympanic membrane. If this epithelium becomes trapped medial to the drum, the desquamated material collects, similar to a sebaceous cyst. The slowly enlarging cyst or collection causes erosion and drainage. A cholesteatoma may be acquired through a perforation or retraction pocket, or, in the rare case, may be congenital.

In the adult patient acute otitis media is usually associated with a URI, the "flu," acute bronchitis, or sinusitis. The patient presents with inflammatory signs and symptoms: fever, dolor, and rubor developing over several days. The tympanic membrane is inflamed, opaque (because of the middle ear purulence), and bulging with the frequent attendant symptoms of rhinorrhea, cough, and generalized malaise. A small number of patients present with more serious symptomatology including a perforation (providing relief), vertigo, or a facial paresis.

Streptococcus pneumoniae, *Haemophilus influenzae*, and type B *Streptococcus* account for the vast majority of infections. A small number are caused by anaerobes, gram-negative bacteria, or *Mycoplasma*. Amoxicillin or sulfamethoxazole-trimethoprim remains the antibiotic of choice; a third-generation cephalosporin or erythromycin is the alternative. Decongestants and antihistamines provide little benefit except in specific circumstances, and topical

Table 128-1. Diagnosis and Treatment for Otitis

DIAGNOSIS	SYMPTOMS	PHYSICAL EXAMINATION	TREATMENT	CAUSE	CONSIDER
External otitis	Painful canal, pain on chewing, no associated URI	Tender canal, no T nodes, with or without hearing, loss, conduct, otorrhea	Topical agents, cleaning, wick	Staphylococcus, Pseudomonas, fungal	Malignant external otitis, mastoiditis, perforated tympanic membrane, dermatitis
Otitis media	Otalgia, hearing loss, associated URI	Fever, URI symptoms, bulging inflamed tympanic membrane, conductive loss, otorrhea with perforation	Systemic antibiotics, with or without topical decongestants. ?Myringotomy	S. pneumoniae, Haemophilus influenzae, Streptococcus	Mastoiditis, facial paralysis
Labyrinthine or vestibular neuronitis	Vertigo, vegetative symptoms, with or without hearing loss	Nystagmus, with or without sensorineural hearing loss, no T	Meclizine, diazepam	Viral	Meniere disease, syphilis

T, temperature.

decongestants offer limited adjuvant aid, limited to 3 days. Unfortunately, the incidence of *S. pneumoniae* resistance to penicillin is now reported as high as 10% to 20%. Beta-lactamase production by *H. influenzae* providing resistance to ampicillin is 20% to 40%. Injudicious use of antibiotics, including inappropriate prophylaxis, is thought to lead to the development of new resistance.

Treatment

The unusual patients listed above, those with abnormal pain, or those intolerant of the pressure and hearing loss are candidates for a myringotomy.

Following the acute episode, a middle ear effusion is the norm, persisting for days to weeks. The tympanic membrane is now visualized as dull and retracted. The patient complains of inability to "pop" the ear, hearing loss, and variable fleeting discomfort. During the phase of resolution, these symptoms gradually improve, with complete resolution anticipated. Persistence with no improvement for weeks, bilaterality, significant hearing loss, and vertigo are again indications for a myringotomy and possible ventilation tube insertion. As in AOM, topical decongestants, steroid nasal sprays, or systemic decongestant/antihistamines are of little benefit except in the allergic or severely congested patient. Pregnancy usually restricts the patient to the limited use of topical agents.

The patient who experiences discomfort while flying can benefit from the use of systemic and topical decongestants on the day of the flight. The difficulty arises on descent only, as one passes from a lower to a higher pressure system. Maintaining a decongested eustachian tube aids in allowing equilibration. The topical agent is used 30 minutes before each descent and repeated once after 5 minutes.

Differential Diagnosis

Temporomandibular joint dysfunction must be discussed because of the frequency with which it is misdiagnosed as otitis. Because the joint occupies a position that is anatomically immediately anterior to the canal and separated from it by only a thin bony wall, irritation in the joint is perceived to originate in the ear. Bruxism, anxiety, ill-fitting dentures, and dental disease may all result in this irritation. The discomfort radiates to the muscles of mastication (temporalis, pterygoids, and masseter) and is associated with a fullness or pressure in the ear, but a normal ear exam. The examiner can often appreciate this by palpation joint asymmetry or crepitus.

LABYRINTHITIS

Labyrinthitis is an inflammation of the inner ear. The vast majority of these illnesses are viral, preceded by a URI. Because the fluid within the cochlea and vestibular portions of the labyrinth communicates, an inflammatory process should involve both. The patient should experience a sensorineural hearing loss with associated tinnitus and true rotary vertigo with the associated vegetative symptoms of nausea, vomiting, pallor, and diaphoresis. More commonly, however, the patient presents with vertigo without the cochlear symptoms. The viral lesion is felt to be in the vestibular portion of the eighth cranial nerve before reaching the labyrinth, thereby sparing the cochlea. This is similar to the seventh cranial nerve paresis in Bell's palsy.

Occasionally, sudden hearing loss does accompany the vertigo, representing a true labyrinthitis. In either situation the acute viral illness lasts for 1 to 3 days. Treatment is symptomatic, directed at the vegetative symptoms with antivagal and antivertiginous medications such as diazepam and meclizine. This period is often followed by a more minor vestibular dysfunction manifested as benign positioning paroxysmal vertigo. Patients experience very brief, repeatable, fatigable, true rotary vertigo on assuming certain head positions, usually extension and rotation of the head to one side or a head hanging position. Ninety percent of these patients have resolution over a variable time period of weeks to months. Unfortunately, recovery of the sensorineural hearing loss is as low as 50%.

The differential diagnosis includes a purulent labyrinthitis (from meningitis or mastoiditis), syphilis (which may present with sensorineural hearing loss and vertigo), and Meniere's disease. Patients with Meniere's disease experience recurrent episodes of true rotary vertigo associated with fluctuating sensorineural hearing loss, tinnitus, and extreme pressure in one ear.

129
Pharyngitis

HOWARD A. FARRELL

Primary Care for Women, edited by Phyllis C. Leppert and Fred M. Howard. Lippincott-Raven Publishers, Philadelphia © 1997.

Pharyngitis is defined as an inflammation of the mucosal and submucosal structures of the throat.

This inflammation can be infectious or noninfectious. Tissues involved include the nasopharynx, oropharynx, and the hypopharynx and are rich in lymphoid tissue. This lymphoid tissue is defined as the Waldyer's ring consisting of the palatine tonsils, the adenoids, and the lingual tonsils. These tissues are prone to reactive change in response to both viral and bacterial infection. They also are potential sites of both solid and hematologic neoplasms. The most commonly recognized form of pharyngitis is tonsillitis.

ETIOLOGY

Inflammation in the pharynx can be of various etiologies. Bacterial causes primarily consist of gram-positive organisms, including alpha- and gamma-hemolytic *Streptococcus*, along with anaerobic bacteria such as *Fusobacterium*, *Peptostreptococcus*, and *Bacteroides*. Other important pathogens include *Staphylococcus aureus*, *Haemophilus influenzae*, *Diplococcus pneumoniae*, and *Streptococcus pyogenes*. Less common organisms include *Corynebacterium diphtheriae*, *Bordetella pertussis*, *Treponema pallidum*, and *Neisseria gonorrhoeae*.

Viral causes of pharyngitis also are common. In the immunocompetent individual, these infections are self-limited.

Common organisms causing these infections include coxsackievirus, rhinovirus, parainfluenza, adenovirus, herpes simplex, Epstein-Barr virus (EBV), cytomegalovirus, and echovirus. Viral infections can be problematic and difficult to eradicate in the immunosuppressed host.

Fungal infections also can be present, especially in the immunosuppressed and the debilitated patient.

The most common fungal pathogen is *Candida albicans*. Other potential fungal organisms include *Cryptococcus neoformans*, *Rhinosporidium seeberi*, and *Blastomyces dermatitidis*.

Granulomatous diseases such as tuberculosis and leprosy can involve the pharynx. Noninfectious causes of pharyngeal inflammation include disorders such as Wegner granulomatosis, Crohn disease, Stevens-Johnson syndrome, pemphigus, pemphigoid, and lupus erythematosus.

HISTORY

In evaluating the patient with pharyngitis, determining the acuity of the infection is important. Bacterial and viral processes tend to have a more rapid onset. Acute infections are accompanied by odynophagia (painful swallow), cervical tenderness, and fever. Viral processes tend to be associated with a low-grade fever, malaise, and rhinorrhea. Bacterial processes such as streptococcal tonsillitis are associated with high fever, chills, and intense pharyngeal pain. A history of more prolonged generalized fatigue along with pharyngeal pain can be associated with infectious mononucleosis. This should be considered in pharyngitis in all young adults aged 10 to 30 years. A history of oral sexual contact along with diffuse erythema can be the hallmarks of gonococcal pharyngitis or syphilis. A history of an inability to open the mouth along with a recent bacterial pharyngitis may indicate a peritonsillar abscess. Investigating a patient's medial history also is important: a history of systemic illness or immunodeficiency can be essential in diagnosing fungal and chronic viral disorders, or can alert the clinician as to the added virulence of an acute infection.

CLINICAL FINDINGS

Physical examination of the head and neck should be thorough and consistent. The lips and facial skin are observed. Mobility of the mandible is noted. Trismus, an impaired opening of the mouth, can indicate a peritonsillar or parapharyngeal abscess. Tongue mobility is noted. Examination of all mucosal surfaces is performed. This must be done after removal of all dental appliances. The floor of mouth and buccal mucosa is observed. The tonsils are observed for symmetry, inflammation, and exudate. The posterior pharyngeal wall also should be observed for swelling and palpated for fluctuation to rule out a retropharyngeal abscess. Mirror examination is performed to observe normal laryngeal structures in the presence of pharyngitis. This should not be done when epiglottis is suspected for fear of inducing laryngeal spasm. Signs of epiglottis are progressive stridor, drooling, odynophagia, and anterior laryngeal tenderness. If epiglottis is suspected, rapid otolaryngologic consultation should be obtained. Careful palpation of the neck also is done, noting adenopathy and fluctuation. Deep neck infection is indicated by cervical erythema, tenderness, firmness, and fluctuation. This can be confirmed by computed tomography scan or radiologic imaging of the neck.

SPECIFIC INFECTIONS

Patients with streptococcal pharyngitis and tonsillitis have a history of sore throat and fever. On physical examination, the pharynx is inflamed and commonly there is tonsilar enlargement with exudate; the oral pharynx must be carefully examined. Physical signs indicating a peritonsillar abscess such as trismus (difficulty with mouth opening), peritonsillar swelling, and deviation of the uvula should be noted. Cervical adenopathy is present in as many as 60% of patients. The neck must be palpated to verify adenopathy and to evaluate for a deep neck infection.

Scarlet fever is an acute streptococcal pharyngotonsillitis accompanied by rash and the production of an erythrogenic toxin. The rash appears on the trunk and chest; it commonly spares the face, soles, and palms. A "strawberry tongue" that is red and swollen also occurs with this disorder. Other potential complications of streptococcal infection include rheumatic fever, rheumatic heart disease, and glomerulonephritis.

Diagnosis is verified with culture. Patients strongly believed to have a streptococcal infection should be started on an antibiotic before culture results are obtained. Treatment for streptococcal pharyngitis is antibiotics. Initial treatment in nonallergic adults consists of penicillin, 500 mg orally four times daily. Patients who fail to improve after penicillin treatment should be given clindamycin, 300 mg orally three times daily. Occasionally, when a patient is unable to take medications orally, hospital admission is required for intravenous hydration and parenteral antibiotics.

Pharyngitis associated with Staphylococcus and *Haemophilus* infection may be associated with purulent drainage, mucosal erythema, and localized pustules, especially in the tonsils. Culture is indicated. Treatment with penicillinase and beta-lactamase–resistant antibiotics is indicated when treatment with amoxicillin fails.

Diphtheria caused by infection with *Corynebacterium diphtheria* was common in the past but, because of routine vaccination, is rare. These gram-positive nonfilamentous rods infest the upper respiratory tract, producing a localized necrosis and inflammation, along with a gray–black membrane that adheres to underlying tissues. Exotoxins also are produced that have cardiac and neurologic effects. Respiratory difficulty arises with an inability to clear secretions and subsequent respiratory obstruction. Indicated treatments include giving antitoxin along with antibiotics such as penicillin and erythromycin.

Pertussis, or "whooping cough" caused by *B pertussis*, is a contagious childhood disease characterized by a violent cough with inspiratory sounds. *B pertussis* is a nonmotile, pleomorphic gram-negative coccobacillus that multiplies only when infecting ciliated epithelium. The disease has three stages characterized by an early upper respiratory infection with a low-grade temperature, progressing to a loud cough with a mucopurulent exudate. Infection primarily effects the tracheobronchial tree but also may involve the pharynx and larynx. The disease is self-limited and rarely is fatal. It has been nearly eradicated in the United States as a result of immunization.

Venereal diseases of the pharynx are also possible. Syphilis, gonorrhea, herpes, and venereal warts all can involve the pharynx. Syphilis caused by *T pallidum* has three clinical stages. The primary stage occurs 3 days to 3 months after initial inoculation. A raised indurated papule, the chancre, presents initially in the infected throat at the site of inoculation. The chancre heals within approximately 6 weeks. The secondary stage occurs with in 8 weeks of chancre formation. This stage is characterized by a disseminated infection; skin lesions and lymphadenopathy are present. Pharyngeal involvement also occurs with patches consisting of gray erosions surrounded by red, raised peripheral edges. Untreated syphilis then becomes latent, with the possibility of developing tertiary manifestations. Serologic tests for syphilis include the venereal disease research laboratory test and the rapid plasma reagin test. These tests are less reliable in tertiary syphilis. The fluorescein treponema antibody absorption test (FTA-ABS) is a sensitive and reliable, albeit expensive, test. This test is reserved for screening test confirmation and to diagnose tertiary infection. Penicillin is used to treat syphilis, with erythromycin being given in the penicillin-allergic patient.

N gonorrhoeae infection is a cause of pharyngitis related to sexual contact. Infection with this gram-negative diplococcus can be asymptotic in the throat, or the organism may cause tonsilar inflammation and cervical adenopathy. Treatment is with penicillin or tetracycline. There are penicillin-resistant strains that are sensitive to trimethoprim sulfate and other antibiotics. Culture in chocolate agar media is required for diagnosis.

Viral infections in the immunocompetent host tend to be self-limited. Viral pharyngitis tends to occur with inflammation in the absence of purulent exudate. Infectious mononucleosis is a common cause of pharyngitis in adolescents and young adults. EBV is the underlying pathogen in "mono." In this disorder, patients present with a sore throat, fever, and malaise. Other systemic effects may include generalized lymphadenopathy and hepatosplenomegaly. Rupture of the spleen can occur with even minor trauma when splenomegaly is present. Patients must be warned to avoid contact sports when infected. Infection with EBV also can result in hepatitis; therefore, alcohol consumption should be restricted in infected patients. Posterior cervical adenopathy is common. Diagnosis often is made with a positive monospot test result. This test involves the demonstration of serum antibodies to horse red cells. The lymphocyte count also is abnormal: the absolute lymphocyte count is increased, and often greater than 10% of these are atypical lymphocytes. Antibody serodiagnosis with viral capsid antigen, IgM, and IgG identification can be useful in establishing the diagnosis in the case of a patient with clinically suspicious but monospot-negative infection. Treatment of infectious mononucleosis is rest and avoidance of alcohol and contact sports. If antibiotics are required for treatment of bacterial superinfection, amoxicillin should be avoided because of an increased incidence of drug-induced rash.

Fungal infections generally are not a source of acute pharyngitis unless they occur in the immunocompromised host. *C albicans* is the most frequent pathogen. Invasion is possible in the immunocompromised host. Symptoms are pain and dysphagia, with a cheesy mucosal plaque being present. Treatment is with topical antifungal agents such as nystatin; if systemic involvement is notable, intravenous amphotericin is given. Oral candidiasis is discussed in more detail in Chapter 130.

CONSIDERATIONS IN PREGNANCY

Bacterial pharyngitis in pregnancy occurs with the same symptoms as in the nonpregnant patient. Symptoms include odynophagia with tonsilar exudate. A throat culture should be performed and appropriate antibiotics started. Antibiotics thought to be safe in pregnancy include the following: penicillins, cephalosporins, erythromycin (except erythromycin estolate), nitrofurantoin, isoniazid, and ethambutol. Antibiotics that may be used with caution but do present some risk include sulfonamides, nalidixic acid, metronidazole, clindamycin, rifampin, and amphotericin B. Antibiotics not recommended for pregnancy include tetracycline, chloramphenicol, trimethoprim–sulfamethoxazole, aminoglycosides, flucytosine, and griseofulvin.

Viral pharyngeal infections should be treated with supportive therapy. EBV infection occurs infrequently during pregnancy. Diagnosis is made via monospot testing or by specific antibody testing. Early EBV infection has been associated loosely with congenital abnormalities of the heart and eyes; it also may be associated with increased spontaneous abortion and stillbirth. The influence of infection with EBV during pregnancy, however, is still inconclusive.

BIBLIOGRAPHY

Andereoli T, Carpenter C, Plum F, Smith L. Infections in the head and neck. In: Cecil R, Andreoli T, Carpenter C, Plum F, Smith C, eds. Essentials of medicine. Philadelphia: WB Saunders, 1986:557.

Davidson T. Clinical manual of otolaryngology, 2nd ed. New York: McGraw-Hill, 1992:372.

Saltsmen R, Jordan M. Viral infections. In: Burrow G, Ferris T, eds. Medical complications during pregnancy. Philadelphia: WB Saunders, 1988.

Simpson M, Gaziano E. Bacterial infections during pregnancy. In: Burrow G, Ferris T, eds. Medical complications during pregnancy. Philadelphia: WB Saunders, 1988:345.

Sobol S, Guida R. Throat pain. In: Lucente F, Sobol S, eds. Essentials of otolaryngology, 2nd ed. New York: Raven Press, 1988:242.

Wenig B, Kornblut A. Pharyngitis. In: Bailey B, ed. Head and neck surgery: otolaryngology. Philadelphia: JB Lippincott, 1993:551.

130

Common Oral Lesions

HOWARD A. FARRELL

Primary Care for Women, edited by Phyllis C. Leppert and Fred M. Howard. Lippincott-Raven Publishers, Philadelphia © 1997.

Multiple lesions can occur in the oral cavity and oral pharynx. Lesions can be inflammatory or neoplastic. Inflammatory lesions in the oral cavity are commonly referred to as stomatitis, or inflammation of the oral cavity. Inflammation can be secondary to infection, trauma, systemic disease, or autoimmune mechanisms. Neoplasms occurring in the oral cavity are numerous, ranging from benign papillomas to oral cavity malignancies such as squamous cell carcinoma. Neoplasms are discussed in greater detail in Chapter 132. Inflammatory lesions of the oral cavity are numerous. Stomatitis frequently is a cause for a primary care visit. Oral cavity inflammation sometimes is associated with systemic disease. A simplified way of categorizing lesions is to consider them as vesiculobullous, ulcerative, red, or white lesions.

VESICULOBULLOUS LESIONS

Vesiculobullous lesions result from pemphigoid, pemphigus vulgaris, and erythema multiforme, and from infection with herpes simplex and herpes zoster viruses. Herpes simplex virus 1 involves the lips and oral mucosa. The virus also may involve the skin, eyes, and rarely the CNS. Herpes simplex virus has an incubation period of approximately 7 days. The route of infection is by direct contact with infected fluids. Primary herpetic gingivostomatitis is rare in adults and usually is seen in children aged 1 to 3 years. The clinical presentation consists of vesicles on any mucosal surface and may be associated with fever, malaise, headache, and cervical adenopathy. Common sites of involvement include the palate, buccal mucosa, and gingiva. The most common area of involvement is the mucocutaneous junction of the lips and the gingiva. Healing without scarring occurs within 2 weeks. The virus migrates along the axonal sheath of the involved nerve and lies dormant until reactivation. Reactivation of latent virus can be induced by ultraviolet light, stress, fever, or immunosuppression. There is typically a prodrome of tingling or burning that is followed by rapid progression to vesicle formation. The vesicle then ruptures and crusts, healing within 7 to 10 days. Histopathologically, a ballooning of the lesion and degeneration of the basal layer with intraepithelial vesicles is seen. The vesicles are formed by the degeneration of the epithelial cells. Virally infected cells may be multinucleated. The nucleus is homogeneous or glassy, with nuclear material being on the perimeter of the cell. Vesicle formation is the key point for diagnosis. Clinical suspicion can be confirmed by viral culture. Treatment is supportive with hydration, analgesics, and antipyretics. Antiviral agents are primarily used in the immunocompromised host. Acyclovir, a acyclic guanosine derivative, is highly selective for viral DNA polymerase and has no effect on the host epithelium. Best results occur if it is used early in the course of the disease. Recurrent herpes labialis may be treated with acyclovir cream, which, if used during the prodromal period, may prevent or greatly shorten the duration of the lesions. Primary herpetic gingivostomatitis in the nonimmunocompromised patient is treated with systemic acyclovir, 100 to 200 mg orally per day, with a high or intravenous dose being given in the immunocompromised host. Prophylactic acyclovir is used in immunocompromised patients to reduce the incidence of recurrence.

Infection with varicella-zoster and herpes zoster viruses also produce vesiculobullous lesions that can occur in the oral cavity. Varicella (chickenpox) is the primary disease caused by the varicella-zoster virus. Herpes zoster (shingles) is the secondary disease caused by reactivation of the latent virus. Varicella is contracted by direct contact or exposure to aerosolized droplets. Clinical features include a rash involving the trunk, head, and neck. This rash progresses to formation of vesicles that ulcerate and crust. Oral mucosal involvement occurs most commonly on the buccal mucosa palate and the pharynx. Treatment is supportive in the nonimmunocompromised patient. Immunocompromised patients may require antiviral drugs such as acyclovir and vidarabine. Herpes zoster is the reactivation of latent virus that traveled along sensory nerves to sensory ganglia during primary infection. Reactivation then occurs during immunocompromised states such as malignancy, trauma, radiation therapy, or high-dose steroid treatment. This commonly occurs in adults. The clinical features are fever and malaise, with pain and tenderness occurring along the course of the involved nerve. Vesicular lesions then develop, with subsequent ulceration and crusting. Involvement along the mucous membranes usually occurs with skin involvement; however, it may occur with oral involvement only. Ramsay Hunt syndrome is facial nerve involvement with facial nerve paralysis, tinnitus, vertigo, and external auditory canal involvement. Treatment is supportive. In the immunosuppressed patient, antiviral therapy—topical, systemic, or both—is employed.

Herpangina is another vesiculobullous lesion of the oral cavity. Herpangina is a coxsackievirus-induced febrile illness of children and young adults. The illness is characterized by fever, malaise, sore throat, and gastrointestinal symptoms. In several days, these symptoms are followed by the formation of vesicles in the oropharynx, which resolve without complication.

Pemphigoid is a disorder that also causes vesiculobullous lesions. The disorder is an autoimmune disease with antibody formation to the basement membrane zone of epithelium. The result is a separation of the basement membrane and formation of subepithelial blisters. This disorder is more common in women in the 40- to 50-year-old age group. Oral mucosa is commonly involved and can be the only site of involvement. Ocular involvement can result in scarring and blindness. Lesions start as bulla and then form ulcers, which can resolve with residual scaring. Gentle rubbing of the uninvolved mucosa denudes the surface epithelium, producing a vesicle or ulcer. This is referred to as a positive Nikolsky's sign. Histopathologically, these lesions reveal subepithelial clefting from the dissolution of basement membrane. There is a relative lack of inflammatory cell infiltration. Direct immunofluorescence reveals a linear pattern of IgG fluorescence at the basement membrane in both the lesion and the uninvolved mucosa. Indirect immunofluorescence usually gives negative results. Treatment for mild involvement is topical steroids. Intralesional steroid use sometimes is effective in oral or conjunctival involvement. Systemic steroids are used in severe oral cases or cases with ocular involvement. A daily dose of 20 to 60 mg of prednisone is given daily, which is then tapered to maintain control. Tetracycline and niacin, 500 mg four times daily, also can be used for treatment. In advanced cases, immunosuppressants such as azathioprine, cyclophosphamide, or methotrexate are given. Dapsone and sulfapyridine also have been used with steroids.

Pemphigus vulgaris is an autoimmune disease caused by the formation of antibodies against intercellular bridges between squamous cells' desmosome–tonofilament complexes. This results in loss of epithelial cohesiveness and acantholysis, with the formation of intraepithelial blisters. The antibodies producing this effect are IgG class antibodies. This disorder is most common in male patients of Mediterranean descent. In its worst form it can be fatal. The most common sites of involvement are the buccal mucosa, palate, and gingiva. Lesions are painful vesicles that rapidly rupture, producing an ulcer with a gray membrane. A positive Nikolsky's sign is seen; gentle rubbing or scraping of the adjacent mucosa strips the mucosa. Pemphigus vulgaris may be associated with other autoimmune diseases such as rheumatoid arthritis, Sjögren syndrome, lupus erythematosus, and Hashimoto thyroiditis. Microscopically, lesions show intracellular edema and loss of intercellular bridges. Basal cells remain attached to the lamina propria, creating a "row of tombstones" effect. Free acantholytic squamous cells assume a spherical form called the *Tzanck cell.* Tzanck cell formation is pathognomonic for this disorder. Direct immunofluorescence shows antibodies against intercellular bridges. Serum levels of intercellular antibody correlate with severity of disease. This disorder can be difficult to control. High-dose steroids are used in initial control. Prolonged use sometimes is required. Immunosuppressants and intramuscular gold also have been used.

Erythema multiforme is a rapidly progressive vesiculobullous lesion of unknown etiology, most commonly affecting young adults. A reaction to drugs, infection, food, or alcohol is thought to result in an antigen–antibody complex that is deposited in the vessels of the subdermis. This forms a ring-like target lesion on the skin. This lesion is not seen in the oral mucosa. Diffuse ulceration and crusting of the lips, tongue, and buccal mucosa are the common oral manifestations. Key to the diagnosis is the history of exposure. Treatment is supportive. Stevens-Johnson syndrome is a severe form of this disorder with systemic involvement; it affects vision and is life-threatening. Treatment requires systemic steroids.

Any patient with a persistent vesiculobullous lesion should be referred to an otolaryngologist or oral surgeon for evaluation and biopsy.

ULCERATIVE LESIONS

Aphthous stomatitis is a relatively common oral cavity lesion (Fig. 130-1). The etiology of aphthous stomatitis is unknown. Potential contributing factors include infection, nutrition, trauma, stress, and hormonal factors. Suspected infectious factors are both viral (herpes) and bacterial (*Streptococcus sanguis*) infestations. Nutritional factors such as vitamin B_{12}, folic acid, and iron deficiencies have been hypothesized. Food allergies to nuts, chocolate, and gluten also have been suspected. The current theory is that the most likely etiology is immunologic. Autoantibodies to oral mucosal membranes have been found. An autoimmune response also has been found to tissues coated with mucopolysaccharides of alpha-hemolytic *Streptococcus*. The ratio of T-helper to T-suppressor cells in the analysis of peripheral T-lymphocytes in patients with aphthae has been noted to be decreased, implying an immunologic influence. The true etiology, however, remains unknown.

Certain general characteristics are seen in patients with aphthous stomatitis. Patients often have other family members affected with the disorder. The painful area of the lesion often exceeds the size of the lesion. Outbreaks can be associated with prolonged stress or systemic illness. The lesions often evolve through a vesicular stage and are most often noted on the mobile keratinized mucosa of the mouth. The lesions appear as well-defined white ulcers with an erythematous halo. Histopathologic features consist of a mixed infiltrate containing mononuclear cells, neutrophils, macrophages, and extravasated red cells. There are, however, no diagnostic histologic features to aphthous ulcers.

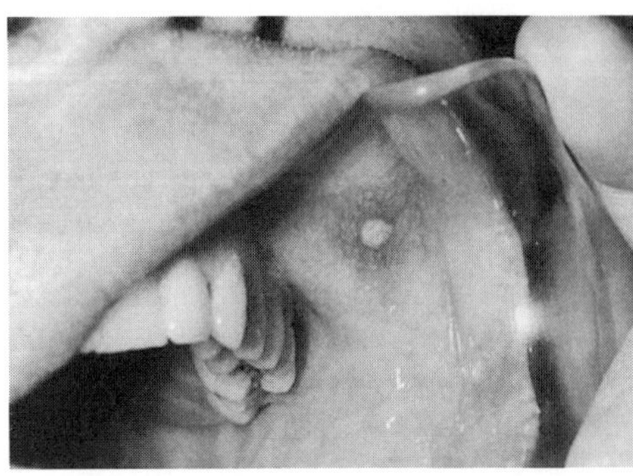

Figure 130-1. Recurrent aphthous stomatitis. A minor aphthous ulcer with a central white ulceration is surrounded by an erythematous halo on the buccal mucosa. (Bailey BJ, ed. Head and neck surgery: otolaryngology. Philadelphia: JB Lippincott, 1993.)

Types of ulcers include simple recurrent aphthae, clusterform aphthae, or recurrent scarring aphthae. Simple recurrent aphthae (or canker sores) affect approximately 60% of the population. Lesions often are multiple. Eruption typically lasts 3 to 10 days. The treatment may involve cautery or steroid cream application. Improvement typically occurs rapidly.

Clusterform lesions (herpetiform aphthae) occur in multiples. The lesions are small ulcerations that can coalesce into larger zones of ulceration. Often the ulcers are chronic. A fever may be related to these lesions. Treatment consists of topical steroids and antibiotics. Tetracycline syrup swish and swallow is given at a dosage of 250 mg four times daily. Dexamethasone elixir (0.5 mg/5.0 mL) also is given as a 2-minute swish and spit two to three times per day. Immediate steroid treatment is given if lesions recur.

Recurring scarring aphthae also are described. These ulcers persist from weeks to months. Deep necrosis results from these lesions, which is associated with scarring. Treatment for the lesions includes systemic steroids and topical tetracycline. Sometimes no complete resolution is obtained, with steroids being used for lesion control. Other treatments include antiinflammatory agents such as sulfones and sulfonamides. Immunosuppressants such as azathioprine also have been used for recurring scaring aphthae.

Acute necrotizing ulcerative gingivitis is another example of an ulcerative lesion of the oral cavity. This disorder also is known as trench mouth or Vincent's stomatitis. Its incidence is increased with the increased prevalence of acquired immunodeficiency syndrome (AIDS). Ulceration of the interdental papillae with bleeding and pseudomembrane formation occurs with a fetid odor. Systemic symptoms of fever, malaise, and lymphadenopathy also occur. Culture of these lesions reveals fusiform bacilli and spirochetes. Treatment consists of superficial debridement and antibiotics. Any patient with a persistent lesion should be referred to an otolaryngologist or oral surgeon for evaluation and biopsy.

Lupus erythematosus may have oral involvement occurring as an erythematous plaque that develops a painful ulceration. It occurs most often in chronic discoid lupus, but any form may have oral involvement. Diagnosis requires biopsy. Histologically, degeneration of the basal cell layer is observed with lymphocytic infiltration. Immunofluorescence most often reveals IgG deposition in the basement membrane.

Treatment is with nonsteroidal antiinflammatory drugs. Steroids are used in severe cases.

WHITE LESIONS

Lichen planus is a chronic disease of the skin and mucous membranes. It is believed to be caused by basal cell layer destruction by activated lymphocytes. The lesions in this disorder are painful, fine, raised white or violaceous lesions in a ring-like pattern called "Wickham's striae." Lesions look much like leukoplakia with a homogenous white plaques. The lesions also can be erosive with erythematous shallow ulcers. Histopathologically, lichen planus shows hyperkeratosis with saw-tooth rete ridges and liquefactive degeneration of the basal cell layer with a band-like subepithelial inflammatory infiltrate. Civatte bodies, or discrete eosinophilic ovoid bodies, also can be seen in the basal cell layer. Treatment is symptomatic. Mild cases do not require therapy. Topical steroids and retinoids can be used. Dapsone in severe forms can yield success.

Candidiasis is another source of white lesions in the mouth. *Candida albicans* is found as an oral commensal organism in 40% to 60%

of normal individuals. Infection usually happens in immunocompromised hosts. Local factors such as decreased salivation or irritants (dentures) can increase the likelihood of infection. Systemic factors such as diabetes, antibiotic use, steroid use, or an immunocompromised state can predispose to infection. Clinical forms of candidiasis have been described including pseudomembranous, hyperplastic, and denture stomatitis. Pseudomembranous candidiasis, or thrush, is the most common form (Fig. 130-2). The lesions are soft yellow plaques that consist of fungi, bacteria, desquamated cells, and food debris. The epithelial surface can be wiped free of lesions with a cotton-tipped applicator, leaving a tender, eroded epithelial surface beneath. Most common sites of involvement are the oral cavity, buccal mucosa, mucobuccal folds, and the lateral tongue. The hyperplastic variant, *Candida* leukoplakia, consists of white firm plaques that involve the buccal mucosa, tongue, or lips. The lesions are leukoplakic and do not wipe away easily. Denture stomatitis occurs in older patients and is most commonly associated with a maxillary denture. It is associated with prolonged denture use and poor oral hygiene. The lesions involve the site of denture mucosal coverage. The lesions are red flat plaques having a pebbly to velvety surface. Histologically, a cytologic smear stained with 20% potassium hydroxide shows hyphae. Culture is of limited use because *Candida* is a normal oral flora in 40% of the population. Diagnosis usually is made on clinical grounds. Medical therapy with antifungal agents is the primary mode of treatment. Four commonly used antifungal agents are nystatin, clotrimazole, ketoconazole, and fluconazole. Nystatin swish and expectorate has the advantage of being effective and safe for long-term use. Clotrimazole is given as a lozenge; it is metabolized in the liver. Ketoconazole is given in oral tablet form and also is metabolized in the liver. Both are used to treat all forms of candidiasis and are useful in immunocompromised hosts. Fluconazole is a synthetic antifungal used for oral pharyngeal, esophageal, or systemic candidiasis. It has no liver effects and is excreted unchanged by the kidneys. Dosage is adjusted for renal patients.

Leukoplakia is defined as white mucosal patches or plaques. This is a descriptive term rather than a disease entity. Most leukoplakic lesions are histologically benign. Some lesions, however, are cancerous or precancerous. A history of cigarette smoking, alcohol use, or both in any patient with an oral lesion should raise concern and should be a motivating factor for referral for biopsy.

Papillomavirus can result in white lesions in the upper aerodigestive tract. They are the result of human papillomavirus infection. Raised pedunculated or flat growths occur. They are common in larynx and oral cavity. Treatment for oral lesions is excision.

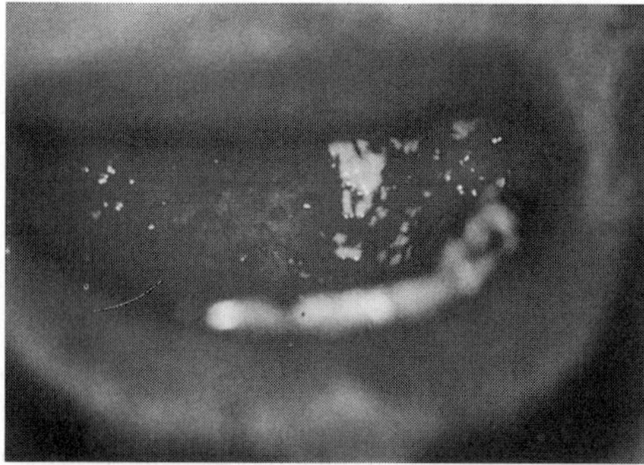

Figure 130-2. Soft white plaques of pseudomembranous candidiasis (thrush). (Courtesy of Dr. Robert O. Greer.) (Bailey BJ, ed. Head and neck surgery: otolaryngology. Philadelphia: JB Lippincott, 1993.)

Laryngeal papilloma can be difficult to eradicate, often requiring frequent treatment.

RED LESIONS

Erythroplakia is a red lesion or plaque of the mucosa. This, like leukoplakia, is a description of a lesion rather than a true disease process. In contrast to leukoplakia, most erythroplakic lesions are worrisome, with 80% to 90% of lesions ranging from severely dysplastic to squamous cell carcinoma. These lesions often are asymptomatic, homogeneous, velvety red plaques. Biopsy is mandatory.

Radiation mucositis is a painful inflammatory reaction of the oral mucosa to radiation therapy. The degree of injury varies with dose, portal of the beam, age, and general health. Radiation mucositis does not occur until at least the second week of a 6-week treatment. The lesions initially occur with diffuse erythema and then are followed by desquamation and ulceration. Pain is associated with this process. Alteration in taste precedes the mucosal reaction. Therapy is primarily supportive. Hydrogen peroxide, water, and bicarbonate rinse may help the symptoms. Benadryl, viscous lidocaine, and dicyclone combinations can be used for mucosal coverage and anesthesia. Severe radiation mucositis can result in notable pain and an inability to maintain oral intake. On these occasions, nutritional support with nasogastric enteral tube feedings is required until the mucositis resolves.

ORAL LESIONS AND THE AIDS PATIENT

The incidence of AIDS is increasing in the female population. AIDS-related diseases have a variety of oral manifestations. Most of these are the result of opportunistic infections. Oral candidiasis occurs in 45% to 75% of AIDS patients. Pseudomembranous candidiasis is the most common form. Erythematous fissures and cracks also can be the precursor of more advanced fungal disease. Treatment of oral candidiasis is mandatory to prevent spread to the pharynx or esophagus.

Herpes simplex infection is the most common viral infection seen in the patient with human immunodeficiency virus (HIV). Painful vesicles occur on the palate or gingiva, which then rupture into a painful ulcer. The prolonged presence of herpes simplex lesions in the HIV-infected patient can herald the advancement to full-blown AIDS. Antiviral therapy is required.

Herpes zoster and varicella also can be problematic in the HIV-infected patient. Oral facial vesicles can involve one or more trigeminal branches. Facial nerve involvement with Ramsay Hunt syndrome also can occur. Treatment with acyclovir orally or intravenously is required.

Hairy leukoplakia also is reported in HIV-infected patients. The lesion is a white thickening with vertical folds resembling a hairy surface. The lesions most often involve the lateral border of the tongue but also may involve other areas of the mouth. Histologically, the lesions show epithelial projections in a hair-like configuration with epithelial hyperparakeratosis and hyperplasia. Little to no inflammatory infiltrate is associated with these lesions. Epstein-Barr virus is considered to be the causative agent. These lesions may respond to high-dose acyclovir. The onset of hairy leukoplakia in the HIV-infected patient is associated with an increased probability of developing AIDS within 30 months.

Non-Hodgkin's lymphoma has an increased prevalence in AIDS patients. Oral lesions are characterized as a swelling or mass that exhibits rapid growth. Lesions most commonly occur along vestibular and buccal mucosa, palate, or alveolar ridges. Biopsy reveals infiltration of B-lineage cells with large round irregular nucleoli. Lesions are responsive to radiation therapy, with control being obtained but with a low cure rate.

CONSIDERATIONS IN PREGNANCY

Oral lesions can be a source of difficulty during pregnancy. Patients with a history of aphthous stomatitis may manifest the disease during pregnancy. Hypothesis have been made attempting to link the occurrence of aphthous stomatitis with hormonal changes of pregnancy or the menstrual cycle. Currently, however, no link has been made between the variations in hormone levels and the lesions. Treatment should be similar to that in the nonpregnant state; however, steroids should be limited and given under the supervision of the obstetrician. Tetracycline use is prohibited because of the effects on fetal teeth and bones.

Herpes simplex stomatitis also can occur during pregnancy. Antiviral agents should be avoided in pregnancy, particularly in the first trimester. The major exception is life-threatening infection. Acyclovir has no known teratogenicity, but little is known about the extent of placental transfer of this drug. Supervision of the obstetrician is required in management of herpes simplex stomatitis during pregnancy.

Both in the pregnant and nonpregnant state, any persistent lesions of unknown etiology should be referred to the otolaryngologist or oral surgeon for evaluation and possible biopsy.

BIBLIOGRAPHY

Aragon S, Jafek B. Stomatitis. In: Bailey B, ed. Head and neck surgery: otolaryngology. Philadelphia: JB Lippincott, 1993:531.

Lee KW. Color atlas of oral pathology. Philadelphia: Lea & Febiger, 1885.

Pindborg J. Atlas of diseases of the oral mucosa. Munksgaard, Copenhagen: WB Saunders, 1993.

Rogers R. Common lesions of the oral mucosa. Postgrad Med 1992;141:53.

Rondu B, Mattingly B. Oral mucosal ulcers: diagnosis and management. J Am Diet Assoc 1992;123:883.

Saltsmen R, Jordan M. Viral infections. In: Burrow G, Ferris T, eds. Medical complications during pregnancy. Philadelphia: WB Saunders, 1988:372.

Simpson M, Gaziano E. Bacterial infections during pregnancy. In: Burrow G, Ferris T, eds. Medical complications during pregnancy. Philadelphia: WB Saunders, 1988:342.

Smith RM, et al. Atlas of oral pathology. Toronto: CV Mosby, 1981.

Zigarreli D. Fungal infections of the oral cavity. Otolaryngol Clin North Am 1993;26:1069.

Primary Care for Women, edited by Phyllis C. Leppert and Fred M. Howard. Lippincott-Raven Publishers, Philadelphia © 1997.

131
Epistaxis

PETER MULBURY

Epistaxis is a common disorder that is usually a minor event and is easily controlled. However, it may present a more significant challenge, requiring the consideration of other causes.

ANATOMY

The blood supply of the nose is derived from both the external and internal carotid systems. The external carotid artery terminates in the sphenopalatine and the descending palatine arteries. The sphenopalatine enters the lateral wall of the nose just at or behind the posterior tip of the inferior turbinate, distributing to the lateral wall and the posterior septum. The descending palatine passes inferiorly from the pterygomaxillary space, entering the oral cavity through the greater palatine foramen. Advancing anteriorly, a branch passes back into the nasal cavity via the incisive canal. This nasopalatine branch supplies the anterior septum and anterior lateral wall of the nose in association with a septal branch of the superior labial artery. This area of the anterior septum with multiple arterial sources is known as Little's or Kiesselbach's area; it is easily the most common site of nose bleeds.

The anterior and posterior ethmoidal arteries represent the branches of the internal carotid system via the opthalmic artery. These enter the superior lateral nasal vault through their respective foramina found in the frontoethmoidal suture line. These vessels supply the superior lateral wall of the nose and the superior septum.

ETIOLOGY

As noted, most nose bleeds occur in Little's area of the septum, approximately 2 cm posterior to the mucocutaneous junction. This area is the site of crusting secondary to air and irritant exposure as well as accessibility to digital manipulation. Deviation of the septum frequently causes turbulent air flow with subsequent drying and crusting. Surgery, cocaine abuse, and excessive crusting all may lead to a perforation of the septum. Perforations collect secretions and crust; in turn, the irritation results in frequent episodes of bleeding.

Congestion secondary to rhinitis is associated with hyperemia. The rhinitis may be vasomotor, allergic, irritative, or the rhinitis of pregnancy. The subsequent nose blowing can be the source of epistaxis.

Differential Diagnosis

For obvious reasons, bleeding disorders such as hemophilia, von Willebrand disease, and Osler-Weber-Rendu disease are not usually a consideration in women but should be mentioned for completeness. Acquired bleeding disorders create problems clinically. Most clinicians are aware of the inhibitory effect on platelet adhesiveness caused by aspirin or the nonsteroidal antiinflammatory drugs. More patients seem to be placed on warfarin (Coumadin) for therapeutic reasons with the frequent results of epistaxis. Finally, more patients currently are receiving chemotherapy or are hemo- or immune-suppressed, with depressed platelet counts or other coagulopathies.

Only rarely is a tumor the cause of epistaxis. Benign tumors include granulomas, polyps (usually infected), and hemangiomas. Particularly noteworthy is the granuloma graviderium; these granulomas generally appear in the last trimester of pregnancy. Histologically, there are no differences from other inflammatory or pyogenic granulomas. These may occur anywhere in the nasal or oral cavities but typically are found on the anterior septum or interdental papillae. The lesion recurs rapidly despite biopsy and cauterization until the termination of the pregnancy when they spontaneously resolve. Malignant tumors include squamous cell carcinoma, melanoma, lymphoma, tumors of olfactory derivation, and the rare sarcoma.

Epistaxis after trauma, such as the nasal fracture, is common; intervention usually is unnecessary. Occasionally, the fracture extends posteriorly to include the lamina papyracea portion of the ethmoid bone. Here the anterior ethmoidal artery may be severed, requiring clipping.

TREATMENT

The patient presenting to the office with epistaxis should require minimal intervention with the appropriate equipment available. A headlight, nasal speculum, bayonet forceps, suction, cotton, silver nitrate applicator sticks, and a topical anesthetic all are readily available and inexpensive. Initially—and frequently over the telephone—therapy may be instituted with the use of topical ephedrine on cotton inserted into the anterior nasal cavity plus pinching the cartilaginous portion of the nose for 5 minutes. This may then be followed by judicious suctioning, leading to the identification of the bleeding site. This is often a linear vessel at the mucocutaneous junction of the septum or a small excrescence of the caudal septum. The appropriate area is topically anesthetized with benzocaine or cocaine and then cauterized with the silver nitrate applicator, typically holding this in place for 30 to 60 seconds. Because of the expected crusting, a topical antibiotic ointment is applied digitally twice daily for 5 days.

Failure to control the site or recurrence of the epistaxis requires more aggressive electrocautery or packing. A simple anterior nasal pack can be achieved by layering strips of antibiotic coated gauze or Vaseline gauze in the anterior nasal cavity from top to bottom. Alternatives are the expansile nasal sponges or absorbable hemostatic agents such as Gelfoam or Surgicel, the latter agents being of special benefit in the patient with a bleeding diathesis.

If this fails, particularly if there has not been a site identified, or if the bleeding is brisk and is associated with spitting and hematemesis, a posterior epistaxis should be considered. These are arterial bleeds either from a high ethmoidal source or a posterior sphenopalatine source. Control requires a nasopharyngeal pack of either gauze or a balloon in conjunction with a tight anterior pack. Alternatives that are less effective but more easily used are the double- or triple-balloon nasal devices. These usually are used to temporize until a more effective pack is inserted. Patients with a posterior nasal pack require hospitalization and close monitoring. Failure of control leads to surgical intervention, involving the ligation or clipping of the appropriate vessels.

Primary Care for Women, edited by Phyllis C. Leppert and Fred M. Howard. Lippincott-Raven Publishers, Philadelphia © 1997.

132

Oral Tumors and Cancers

JAY K. ROBERTS

The oral cavity and oropharynx are the sites of many different mass lesions. There are tumors that occur in one location exclusively, but most occur commonly in either location, so both regions will be discussed together. Brief mention will be made of tumors of the parapharyngeal space as well as of odontogenic tumors, and fissural and odontogenic cysts. Except where specifically noted, when surgical intervention is suggested it should most often be accomplished by an otolaryngologist–head and neck surgeon.

ANATOMY

The oral cavity extends from the mucocutaneous junction of the lips anteriorly. Posteriorly, the limits are the posterior edge of the hard palate superiorly and the line of circumvallate papillae inferiorly. This space contains the lips, buccal mucosa, maxillary and mandibular alveolar ridges, retromolar trigone, floor of mouth, oral tongue (anterior ⅔), and hard palate.

The oropharynx is bounded by the oral cavity anteriorly, and extends to the plane of the hard palate superiorly and to the plane of the hyoid bone inferiorly. This space includes both surfaces of the entire soft palate, the tonsils, including their pillars, the tongue base from the circumvallate papillae to the base of the epiglottis, and the posterior and lateral oropharyngeal walls.

The parapharyngeal space lies lateral to the oropharynx and medial to the mandible and muscles of mastication. Structures of interest in this area include the deep lobe of the parotid, cranial nerves 9 through 12, the jugular vein, and the carotid artery.

BENIGN LESIONS OF THE ORAL CAVITY AND OROPHARYNX

Oral tori are exostoses rather than true neoplasms of the palate (torus palatinus) or mandible (torus mandibularis). They are bony hard protuberances that are located in the midline of the hard palate or along the lingual surface of the mandible in the region of the bicuspid. Tori occur in about 20% of the population, and the palatal location is more common. They are asymptomatic and do not require imaging. Surgery is required only rarely when they interfere with the fitting of dental prostheses.

A granular cell tumor occurs in two forms and is currently felt to be a benign proliferation of Schwann cell origin, rather than a true neoplasm. Epulis of the newborn is the congenital form and occurs on the gingiva (Fig. 132-1). It predominates 8 to 1 in females, occurs three times more commonly on the maxilla than the mandible, does not recur, and has been reported to regress spontaneously. The other form is a lesion of young adults, seen

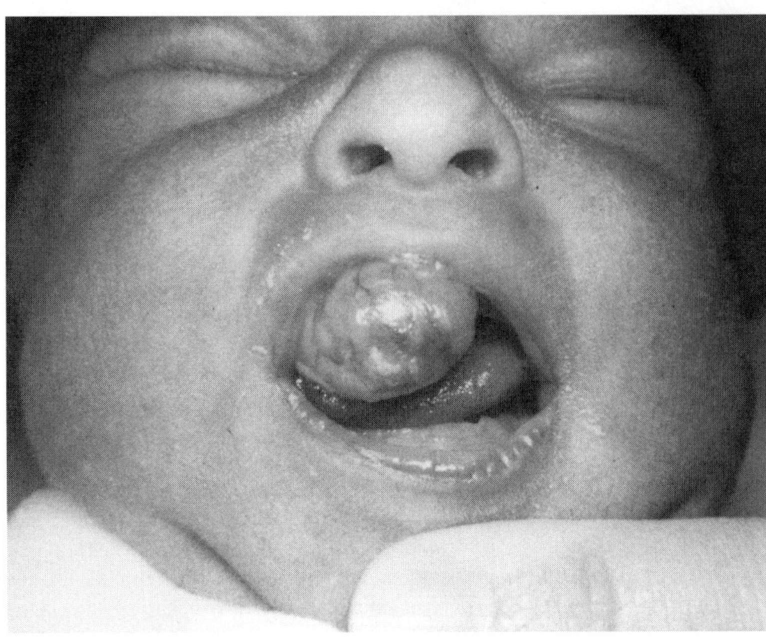

Figure 132-1. Epulis of the newborn. Granular cell tumor of the anterior maxillary alveolus in a 1-day-old girl. Removed under local anesthesia in the nursery.

slightly more often in women and blacks. The mass appears as a firm submucosal nodule most often in the tongue. Treatment of either form is conservative surgical excision.

A number of vascular lesions are seen in the oral cavity. Hereditary hemorrhagic telangiectasia (Osler-Weber-Rendu) is manifested by small bright red vascular lesions of the tongue and other oral mucous membranes. They are generally asymptomatic, but patients often require treatment due to bleeding from lesions elsewhere in the body. Varicosities of the ventral tongue and lateral tongue base are quite common in older individuals. They never require treatment. Lymphangioma and hemangioma are benign proliferations of blood and lymphatic vessels. Tongue and floor of mouth are the most common sites for these lesions in the oral cavity. They are often present at birth or shortly after. Most hemangiomas regress during the first few years of life. Management of large hemangiomas is especially challenging, although a conservative approach is advocated. Temporary tracheotomy is sometimes required for airway compromise. When intervention is required, steroids or percutaneous embolization have been found to be more efficacious than cryosurgery, laser surgery, sclerotherapy, or radiation. Lymphangiomas are managed with antibiotics and steroids when infected, and may be treated with surgical excision if extensive or markedly symptomatic.

Several other lingual lesions are commonly noted, including geographic tongue, median rhomboid glossitis, hairy tongue, and lingual thyroid. Geographic tongue is a condition in which certain areas of the tongue are denuded of papillae and the epithelium appears very thin. The remainder of the tongue appears normal. The surface configuration of the tongue changes over time as areas alternately desquamate and regenerate. Patients are asymptomatic, and no treatment is required. Median rhomboid glossitis is due to an embryologic abnormality. When development proceeds as expected, the tuberculum impar becomes depressed as the lateral halves of the tongue medialize. If this does not occur, the tuberculum impar is left as a surface structure. The absence of papillae in the central portion of the anterior tongue allows the underlying vessels to be very apparent, leading to the typical appearance of median rhomboid glossitis. Hairy tongue is a condition in which the filiform papillae of the dorsal surface of the tongue are markedly elongated. They are usually black or brown in color. The condition is harmless. Lingual thyroid is a condition in which the thyroid gland failed to make its descent into the neck from the foramen cecum during embryologic development. This condition becomes manifest almost exclusively in women. It is most often diagnosed in the teen years. It appears as a mass in the area of the foramen cecum, and the patient frequently complains of dysphagia, a sense of fullness, or dysphonia. The differential includes lingual tonsil, thyroglossal duct tissue, or neoplasms seen in this location such as squamous cell carcinoma, lymphoma, or minor salivary gland tumors. A thyroid scan is mandatory, since if it is the lingual thyroid it usually is the patient's only functioning thyroid, and therefore excisional biopsy should certainly be avoided.

A fibroma is a very common benign lesion composed of proliferating fibroblasts and is not a neoplasm. It is a fibrous overgrowth caused by chronic irritation. Some authors refer to this as fibrous hyperplasia or as fibroepithelial polyp. They occur most commonly on the tongue or buccal mucosa and appear as smooth round masses. Most often they are sessile, although they may be pedunculated. Their size ranges between several millimeters and a few centimeters, although most are less than 1 cm in size. A fibroma is not encapsulated and has a variable amount of vascularity. Conservative excision is suggested when the lesion is symptomatic, but any obvious irritating cause should also be addressed.

There are a number of white lesions that involve the mucosa of the oral cavity and oropharynx. Lichen planus is a dermatological disease which may manifest itself in the mouth with or without cutaneous lesions. It typically occurs in middle-aged adults and in most series, females predominate. The raised striae of reticular lichen planus seen in the buccal mucosa is characteristic, and biopsy is usually unnecessary to make the diagnosis. Erosive lichen planus is usually painful, and may involve buccal mucosa, gingiva, or lateral tongue. This will sometimes be confused with discoid lupus erythematosus or squamous cell carcinoma, so biopsy is often indicated. This should be taken at the periphery of the lesion, as the central portion will often not be diagnostic. Reticular lichen planus does not require treatment; however, erosive lichen planus is best managed by steroid therapy. Focal disease may be treated topically, while more diffuse lesions may require topical and oral steroids.

The term *leukoplakia* is used clinically to indicate a lesion which appears white, cannot be scraped off, and which cannot be diagnosed as another lesion (Fig. 132-2). These lesions occur more commonly in elderly people, and less often in women. Histologically, the majority of these show hyperkeratosis without atypia. However, approximately one fifth reveal atypia, carcinoma in situ, or invasive squamous cell carcinoma. Biopsy should be undertaken to establish a diagnosis. Further aspects of this will be discussed later in this chapter under the heading Malignant Neoplasms of the Oral Cavity and Oropharynx.

A pyogenic granuloma is a benign, raised, capillary-rich lesion, which, when it occurs in the oral cavity, tends to involve the gingiva. The term "pregnancy tumor" may be used for this lesion when it occurs at the gingiva of pregnant women. It is thought to be the result of overreaction to minor trauma, although hormonal changes may also be an etiologic factor. Lesions are usually sessile and friable, often between 0.5 and 2 cm in greatest dimension. They sometimes grow rapidly, suggesting malignancy. The differential diagnosis includes Kaposi sarcoma. Histologically, the pyogenic granuloma has many dilated endothelial-lined vascular spaces, budding endothelial cells, and a marked proliferation of fibroblasts. Surgical removal is the treatment of choice, although some have suggested that the pregnancy tumor not be removed until after pregnancy because of the likelihood of recurrence.

Necrotizing sialometaplasia is a benign lesion of the salivary tissue of minor salivary glands in the oral cavity occurring spontaneously or as a reaction to injury. There can be startling mucosal ulceration of the palate, which certainly could suggest squamous cell carcinoma. Because of marked squamous metaplasia of the ductal epithelium seen histopathologically, a general surgical pathologist might mistake this for squamous cell or mucoepidermoid carcinoma. Confirming the diagnosis is important to prevent unnecessary surgery. Patients heal spontaneously whether treated with biopsy, partial excision, or complete excision.

CYSTS

The mucocele is believed to occur because of traumatic injury to the duct of a minor salivary gland, allowing saliva to escape into surrounding tissues. It typically appears on the inner surface of the lower lip as a soft, compressible, slightly bluish swelling. A mucocele may also be seen in the floor of the mouth. In this location the lesion is called a ranula. The swelling generally occurs rapidly, and the lesion frequently ruptures and exudes a mucoid saliva. The lesion usually recurs quickly after each episode of spontaneous (or patient-induced) rupture. When the mucocele is recurrent or persistent, it should be excised.

Odontogenic cysts typically appear in the alveolus–gingiva, as submucosal swelling. They also may be apparent in x-rays that include dentoalveolar structures. They include the dentigerous cyst, radicular cysts, keratocysts, eruption cysts, and gingival cysts. The dentigerous cyst is most often seen in the mandible associated with the crown of an unerupted molar. It is thought to come from accumulation of fluid between the tooth crown and the reduced-enamel epithelium. A radicular cyst is asymptomatic and arises within a periodontal granuloma in the periapical area of a nonvital tooth. A keratocyst is a locally aggressive form of any of the above. The diagnosis is made on histopathology. When keratinization is seen within one of the above cysts, it is called a keratocyst. An eruption cyst is the accumulation of blood around the crown of an erupting tooth. Gingival cysts occur due to the entrapment of epithelium during palatal closure. When one discovers an asymptomatic swelling of the upper or lower jaw seen as a radiolucency on x-rays taken to include these areas, it should be evaluated by the patient's dentist or oral surgeon.

Fissural cysts occur in embryonic fusion planes and may not be apparent until young adulthood. They include the globulomaxillary cyst, which occurs in the maxilla between the canine and incisor teeth; the nasopalatine cyst, which occurs in the area of the incisive foramen and causes a mass in the midline of the hard palate anteriorly; and the nasoalveolar cyst, which may manifest as a swelling in the canine fossa beneath the base of the nostril. These may be excised surgically using an intraoral approach.

Dermoid cysts are uncommon in the oral cavity, and rare in the oropharynx. They are felt to be due to entrapment of epithelial cells during embryonic development. They appear simply as a cystic

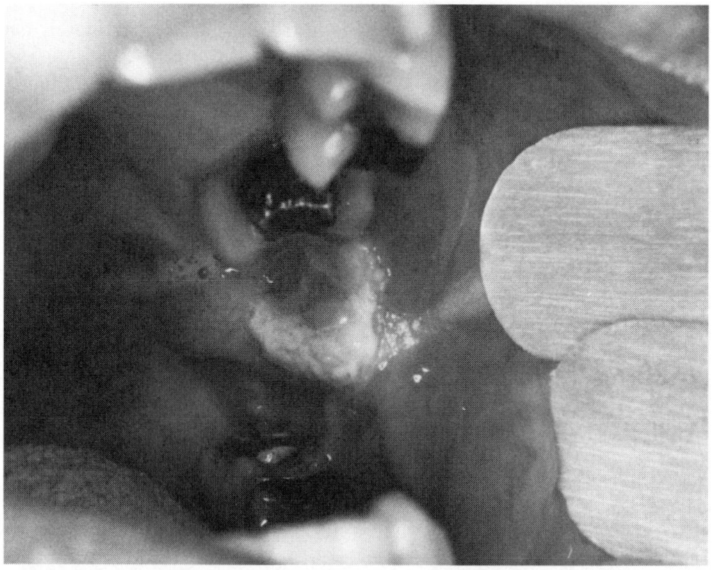

Figure 132-2. Leukoplakia. Keratosis with marked atypia was revealed on a biopsy of this lesion appearing in the posterior aspect of the left buccal mucosa in an 84-year-old woman with no history of tobacco use.

swelling. Stratified squamous epithelium lines the cyst. In most instances surgical excision is recommended.

BENIGN NEOPLASMS

Squamous papilloma is a benign neoplasm seen frequently in the oral cavity and oropharynx, most commonly attached to the free edge of the soft palate or uvula. There can be multiple papillomas, usually appearing as pedunculated wart-like masses. The papilloma is rarely more than a few millimeters in greatest dimension. It is composed of finger-like projections of squamous epithelium, and it is felt to be of viral etiology. Dysplasia is distinctly unusual. The differential diagnosis includes condyloma acuminatum, focal epithelial hyperplasia, and verruciform xanthoma. If symptomatic, it may easily be excised in the office under topical or local anesthesia. Recurrence is rare.

An important category of benign neoplasms that occurs in the oral cavity and oropharynx is that of the minor salivary gland tumors. There are approximately 500 minor salivary glands in the oral cavity and oropharynx. The ratio of neoplasms of the major salivary glands (parotid, submandibular, and sublingual) to those of the minor salivary glands is 5 to 1. Over half of the minor salivary gland neoplasms occur on the palate. The distribution of minor salivary gland neoplasms parallels the distribution of the glands themselves. In the palate, minor salivary glands are not found anterior to the first molars, nor are they found in the midline. Approximately 20% of minor salivary gland tumors are benign. Benign minor salivary gland tumors appear as asymptomatic masses which have been present typically for months before diagnosis. Pain is uncommon, as is ulceration. Pleomorphic and monomorphic adenoma are the most common histologic benignities. Lack of a capsule is a common histologic feature. Despite this, surgical removal is rarely followed by recurrence.

A number of other neoplasms occur rarely in the oral cavity and oropharynx, and their characteristics are similar to those which they manifest elsewhere in the body. The primary symptoms are due to mass effect. Examples include lipoma, leiomyoma, rhabdomyoma, neurogenic tumors (eg, schwannoma, neurofibroma), mesenchymoma, and plasmacytoma.

MALIGNANT NEOPLASMS OF THE ORAL CAVITY AND OROPHARYNX

Malignant tumors of the oral cavity and oropharynx account for only about 2% of all cancers occurring in women in the United States, and account for only about 1% of cancer deaths in this group. The relatively low death rate is offset by the fact that successful elimination of the tumor often comes with significant functional compromise and cosmetic disability. Patients often present to the treating head and neck surgeon with advanced disease, despite the fact that the oral cavity is easy to inspect and palpate. Dentists often discover intraoral cancers before either the patient or the primary care physician becomes aware of the problem. Signs and symptoms of particular concern are otalgia, hemoptysis, voice change, dysphagia, odynophagia, ulceration or mass in the mouth that fails to resolve, or a neck mass. By far the most common histopathology is squamous cell carcinoma, which may arise anywhere in the oral cavity or oropharynx. Lymphoma is not uncommon in Waldeyer's ring (pharyngeal and lingual tonsils). Malignant minor salivary gland tumors are seen with some frequency, and mucosal melanoma is encountered rarely. Other tumors, such as sarcomas, are quite unusual.

SQUAMOUS CELL CARCINOMA

The incidence of oral carcinoma varies greatly around the world as well as in different parts of the United States. Whereas in the United States it constitutes less than 5% of the new cancers to be diagnosed each year, in certain parts of Asia it approaches 50%. This reflects different habits. As tobacco use in women has increased to approach that of men in the United States, a corresponding increase (although, of course, delayed) in the incidence of squamous cell cancer has been noted in women. In 1995, it is expected that one third of all oral and oropharyngeal carcinomas diagnosed in the United States will occur in women. This is a markedly higher proportion than noted even 5 or 10 years ago. In certain parts of the United States, the use of smokeless tobacco has been common in women for many decades. When one examines series published from these areas concerning oral cancers, one is struck by the fact that up to 93% of the tumors reported in these series occur in women.

Several etiologic factors are associated with oral cancer. The disease is most closely associated with the use of tobacco in any form. More than 90% of the patients in published series were tobacco users. Tobacco exposure causes progressive change in the exposed mucosa over time. This is demonstrated in the relatively high incidence of second synchronous or metachronous primary tumors in about 15% of the patients with squamous cell carcinoma of the upper aero–digestive tract. The extremes are a 40% to 50% incidence of second primaries in those patients who continue to smoke after presumed curative treatment of their first cancer, to about 5% in those who quit tobacco use at the time of diagnosis and treatment of their first cancers. Pipe smokers have a higher incidence of cancer of the lip. It is felt that the high temperature of the pipe stem may cause irritation that leads to dysplastic change. Alcohol consumption has been shown to be correlated with oral cancers. About 75% of the patients in published series have a history of significant alcohol consumption. Tobacco and alcohol seem to work synergistically, as patients who use both seem to have a higher risk of developing oral or oropharyngeal cancer than they would with the sum of the risks of each. Solar exposure (ultraviolet light) is a risk factor for carcinoma of the lip especially. It occurs much more often in individuals who work outdoors, and much more commonly in the lower lip, which is exposed more directly to sunlight. Poor dental and oral hygiene seem also to be associated with oral cancers, but this is often compounded by the use of tobacco, alcohol, or both. Poor dentition, ill-fitting dentures, and restorative dental work in poor repair may cause irritation leading to dysplastic changes. When two different metals come in contact, an electromotive force is set up, allowing for the flow of an electric current. This occurs, for instance, when a gold crown is placed in contact with a silver amalgam. This has been associated with recurrent dysplasia and even carcinoma in situ in the tongue on its lateral border where it contacts the interface of the two metals. Iron and riboflavin deficiencies have been associated with oral cancers. Plummer-Vinson syndrome is observed most frequently in women and is associated with achlorhydric iron deficiency, pharyngoesophageal strictures, and oral–oropharyngeal dysplasia. There are suggestions that certain occupational exposures are associated, and one sees more oral malignancy than expected in the immunocompromised, particularly those with acquired immunodeficiency syndrome (AIDS), and those who have received organ transplants.

A persistent sore in the mouth is the most common symptom of oral cavity cancer. Dysphagia is the most common complaint when the primary site is in the oropharynx. Pain tends to occur rather late, and, unfortunately, many patients do not seek attention until they note pain. Often patients consult dentists because of loosening of the teeth, or tooth or jaw pain. Approximately one third of the patients present with a neck mass, most often representing regional metastasis, but occasionally an ulcerated tumor will be markedly inflamed, leading to adenopathy on that basis. Weight loss is seen if the tumor has caused significant dysphagia or odynophagia. As noted earlier, the vast majority of patients have a history of tobacco abuse and substantial alcohol consumption.

The physical examination is the key to diagnosing and evaluating oral cavity and oropharyngeal carcinoma. Bimanual palpation is an important part of the physical examination, as it allows one to get a better sense of the volume of tumor present. With ulcerative and endophytic tumors especially, the observable portion of the tumor may be quite unimpressive (Figs. 132-3 and 132-4). If one is examining a patient who has a heavy smoking history, it is not uncommon to see several areas of suspicious mucosa. An excellent, simple aid to the diagnosis of mucosal dysplasia is the toluidine blue test. This is a painless test that allows the physician to distinguish between malignancy and other lesions that may be of concern, such as lichen planus, trauma, leukoplakia, and various benign tumors. Carcinoma in situ and invasive cancer stain bluish, whereas other lesions do not. The test helps delineate the best site for biopsy as well. False positives can occur. The procedure is as follows:

1. Rinse the mouth thoroughly with water.
2. Apply 1% acetic acid to the areas of concern with a cotton swab.
3. Remove any necrotic debris.
4. Apply 1% toluidine blue to suspicious areas.
5. Rinse the mouth with water.
6. Areas stained blue are sites for biopsy.

A careful examination of the neck is carried out to assess the patient for possible regional metastases.

Radiologic evaluation is often a useful adjunct in assessing the extent of local disease. CT scanning is particularly helpful in assessing mandibular involvement if the tumor encroaches upon it grossly. The same is true for the bone of the hard palate and pterygoid plates. Magnetic resonance imaging (MRI) can be more beneficial in assessing parapharyngeal space involvement. Other studies such as sialography, barium swallow, bone scan, and arteriography may be indicated in certain circumstances.

The most important step in evaluation of a patient with a squamous cell carcinoma of the oral cavity or oropharynx is panendoscopy with biopsy of the primary tumor, usually carried out by the otolaryngologist–head and neck surgeon. Under general anesthesia, the lesion is carefully examined and mapped, and a biopsy is obtained. Because of the significant number of patients with second primary tumors in the upper aerodigestive tract, laryngoscopy, bronchoscopy, and esophagoscopy are carried out at the same time. Any lesion found in this portion of the examination is of course mapped and biopsied as well. Some surgeons tattoo the mucosa at the margins of the tumor to assist with surgical resection should planned preoperative radiation be given, or in case salvage surgery is required after failure of radiation for cure. At this point all information is available to allow appropriate staging, which is mandatory for proper treatment planning. Staging is carried out with reference to data from the American Joint Committee on Cancer (Tables 132-1 through 132-4).

A number of modalities are used in the treatment of oral and oropharyngeal squamous cell carcinomas. Surgery, radiotherapy, chemotherapy, and combinations of these are all used with some frequency. In general, radiation and surgery are equally efficacious in Stage I and II disease, and often the two are used together in Stage III and IV lesions. Most would choose to use radiation for Stage I and II lesions because the functional results tend to be superior with regard to speech and swallowing. Radiation, however, is likely to lead to permanent xerostomia, which patients find quite distressing. It also often leads to extraction of all dentition prior to treatment if the teeth are not in excellent shape.

Stage III and IV lesions, in general, benefit from treatment with both surgery and radiation. There is still some argument about whether planned preoperative irradiation followed by surgery is preferred over surgery with postoperative radiation. The advantages of planned preoperative radiation are several:

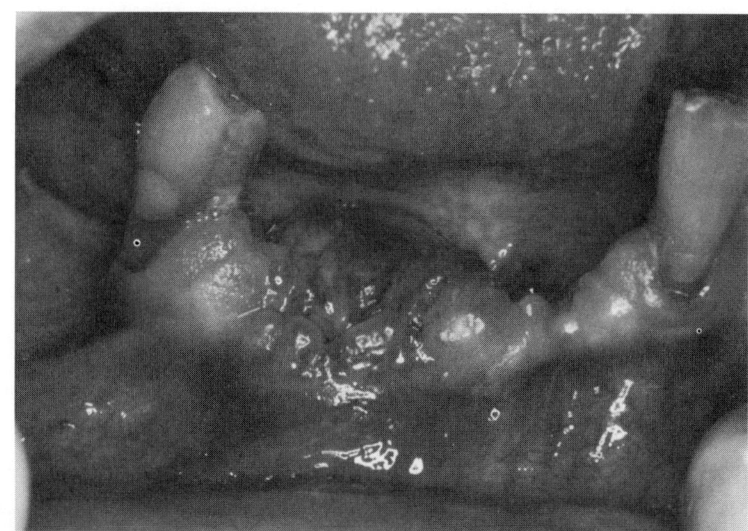

Figure 132-3. Squamous cell carcinoma. Epidermoid carcinoma of the anterior aspect of the mandibular alveolus in an 83-year-old woman with no history of tobacco use. This was removed transorally and the resection included a marginal mandibulectomy. The patient received excellent rehabilitation through the use of a denture.

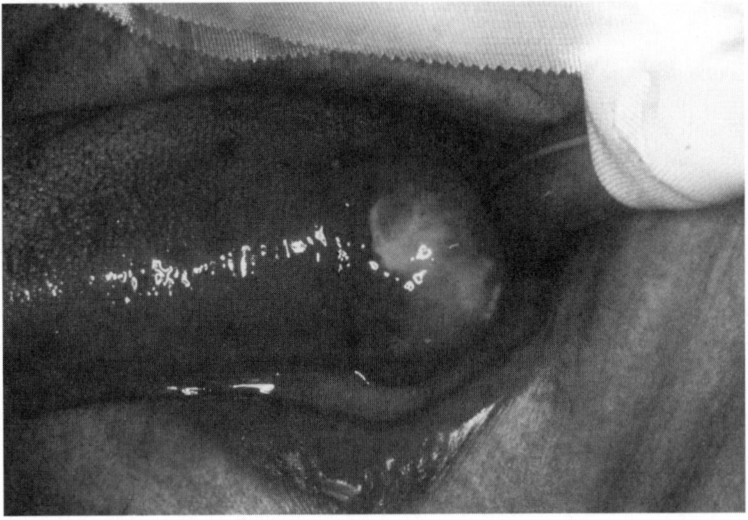

Figure 132-4. Squamous cell carcinoma. This left lateral tongue tumor appears in a 78-year-old woman with a history of heavy tobacco and alcohol abuse. At presentation, she was staged as T1N1M0. Despite control of her local and regional disease with surgery and radiation therapy, she died of distant metastases about 18 months after treatment.

- The occasional patient has a complete response to the radiation (preoperative levels are normally about 5500 cGy) and is taken to curative levels (usually about 7000 cGy), thus avoiding the morbidity of surgery altogether.
- There is a theoretical advantage to irradiating tissue upon which there has been no operation. Irradiation works best in well oxygenated tissue, and there is often significant scar tissue in the area of a major head and neck surgery. With postoperative radiation, persistent tumor is most likely to exist at the margins of resection, the area of greatest scarring, and the area of lowest oxygen tension.
- Preoperative radiation will be given. Occasionally, when postoperative radiation is planned, there is a major wound complication after the surgery, such as an orocutaneous or a pharyngocutaneous fistula, requiring many weeks of hospitalization and sometimes several reconstructive procedures. Many radiation oncologists will not irradiate an unhealed wound, and since radiation should be begun within 6 weeks of operation, a postoperative wound complication sometimes means that the radiation is not given at all. In this instance one tends to observe for recurrence, and if it occurs, salvage surgery is performed with postoperative radiotherapy, assuming there is adequate wound healing.
- There is a significant reduction in recurrent disease in the cervical lymphatics when preoperative radiotherapy is given.

There are also advantages to surgery followed by radiation:

- There are fewer wound complications when surgery precedes radiation.
- Some surgeons find it easier to operate on tissue that has not been irradiated.
- In general, higher levels of radiation may be given postoperatively than preoperatively.

Table 132-1. Primary Tumor Classification, Oral Cavity Cancer

T1: tumor ≤ 2 cm in greatest dimension
T2: tumor > 2 cm, but ≤ 4 cm in greatest dimension
T3: tumor > 4 cm in greatest dimension
T4: tumor invades bone, deep musculature of tongue, sinus, or skin

(Beahrs OH, Henson DE, Hutter RVP, Kennedy BJ [eds]. Manual for staging of cancer. 4th ed. Philadelphia: JB Lippincott, 1992.)

It is noted that when radiation is given, the ports include the cervical lymph nodes which drain the area of the primary tumor. If low cervical metastases are noted, the mediastinum is often included as well.

Surgery for squamous cell carcinoma of the oral cavity or oropharynx involves a number of considerations. Among the surgeon's concerns are whether to use a transoral, mandibulotomy, or mandibulectomy approach. Neck dissection is carried out in the presence of clinical disease, but prophylactic neck dissection is often indicated even in the apparent absence of regional disease. The reconstructive options are constantly increasing in number. Primary closure may be used for some defects, as can placement of a dermal graft. Local and regional pedicled flaps are useful in many circumstances. Consideration should be given to the use of osteomyocutaneous free vascularized flaps, particularly when there is an anterior mandibular defect. The procedure often requires several hours in the operating room. Consideration should be given to measures to prevent deep vein thrombosis. A heating blanket should be employed, and blood should be available. The patient will often need to be cared for in an intensive care unit setting for the first postoperative day or two. A tracheotomy is often required for airway management postoperatively. There may be difficulties with aspiration due to postoperative swelling or the presence of an asensate regional flap or free flap placed for reconstruction. Usually the tracheotomy tube may be removed within a week or two of surgery. The patient will most often require nasogastric feeding for 5 to 10 days following surgery. Speech pathologists often are required to provide the patient with extensive retraining with regard to speech and swallowing.

Table 132-2. Primary Tumor Classification Oropharyngeal Cancer

T1: tumor ≤ 2 cm in greatest dimension
T2: tumor > 2 cm, but < 4 cm in greatest dimension
T3: tumor > 4 cm in greatest dimension
T4: tumor invades cortical bone, soft tissue of neck, or deep tongue musculature

(Beahrs OH, Henson DE, Hutter RVP, Kennedy BJ [eds]. Manual for staging of cancer. 4th ed. Philadelphia: JB Lippincott, 1992.)

Table 132-3. Classification of Cervical Metastatic Disease of Oral or Oropharyngeal Cancer

N0: No clinically positive node

N1: Single ipsilateral node ≤ 3 cm in diameter

N2: Single ipsilateral node > 3 cm but < 6 cm in diameter, or multiple ipsilateral nodes ≤ 6 cm in diameter, or bilateral or contralateral nodes ≤ 6 cm

N2a: Single ipsilateral node > 3 cm, but < 6 cm in diameter

N2b: Multiple ipsilateral nodes ≤ 6 cm

N2c: Bilateral or contralateral nodes ≤ 6 cm

N3: Nodes > 6 cm

(Beahrs OH, Henson DE, Hutter RVP, Kennedy BJ [eds]. Manual for staging of cancer. 4th ed. Philadelphia: JB Lippincott, 1992.)

Table 132-4. Stage Groupings of Oral and Oropharyngeal Cancer, TNM Classification

Stage I	T1N0M0
Stage II	T2N0M0
Stage III	T3N0M0, T1, T2, or T3N1M0
Stage IV	T4N0 or N1M0
	Any TN2 or N3M0
	Any T or NM1

(Beahrs OH, Henson DE, Hutter RVP, Kennedy BJ [eds]. Manual for staging of cancer. 4th ed. Philadelphia: JB Lippincott, 1992.)

Chemotherapy has been used extensively in the treatment of head and neck squamous cell carcinoma. Many controlled trials have demonstrated various complete and partial response rates to numerous combinations of agents. At present, there is very little to suggest that the use of chemotherapy provides a significant advantage to the patient suffering from head and neck squamous cell carcinoma. Although several combinations of agents have demonstrated impressive response rates (up to 65%), none has documented an increase in survival. Adjuvant, induction, and maintenance chemotherapy have all been used, but none has yet demonstrated prolonged disease-free intervals or an increase in survival. Currently, if chemotherapy is considered in a patient with oral cavity or oropharyngeal squamous cell carcinoma, they should be enrolled in a protocol within the environment of a clinical trial.

When one considers the entire population of patients currently being treated for oral cavity cancer, including all stages and all combinations of treatment modalities, one can expect a 5-year disease-free survival of about 70%. For oropharyngeal cancer, the figure is about 55%.

NONEPIDERMOID MALIGNANCIES OF THE ORAL CAVITY AND OROPHARYNX

Lymphoma in the oral cavity and oropharynx arises from the structures in Waldeyer's ring and appears as masses in the oropharynx. Treatment depends on cell type and extent of disease. This is within the purview of the hematologist–oncologist.

Oral cavity–oropharyngeal melanoma is rare, representing only about 1% of all melanomas (Fig. 132-5). About one third of all mucosal melanomas occur in the oral cavity. This must be differentiated from the amalgam tattoo, which is a very common iatrogenic phenomenon. Mucosal melanoma most often appears as a darkly pigmented soft mass that is smooth and painless in a patient in the sixth to eighth decade of life. Amelanotic melanoma is very rare. The treatment is wide surgical excision including neck dissection if clinical disease is apparent there. Survival is extremely poor, with most patients progressing to develop multiple metastases within a year or two. Five-year survival is only about 5% to 10%.

Minor salivary gland malignancies are seen with the same general distribution as that of the benign minor salivary gland tumors. Approximately 80% of minor salivary gland tumors are malignancies. These tumors are seen much more often in atomic bomb survivors than in other groups. There also appears to be a somewhat increased risk of salivary gland tumors of all types in women who have had breast tumors. Minor salivary gland cancers appear as painless submucosal masses which enlarge slowly over time. Imaging often reveals that these lesions have extended into the maxillary sinus, parapharyngeal space, or pterygopalatine fossa. It is uncommon for patients to present with cervical metastases. Forty percent of these malignancies are adenoid cystic carcinoma. Perineural invasion is common with this particular tumor, so local recurrence is common. There is a high incidence of distant metastasis, particularly to the lung. This distant disease may show up 20

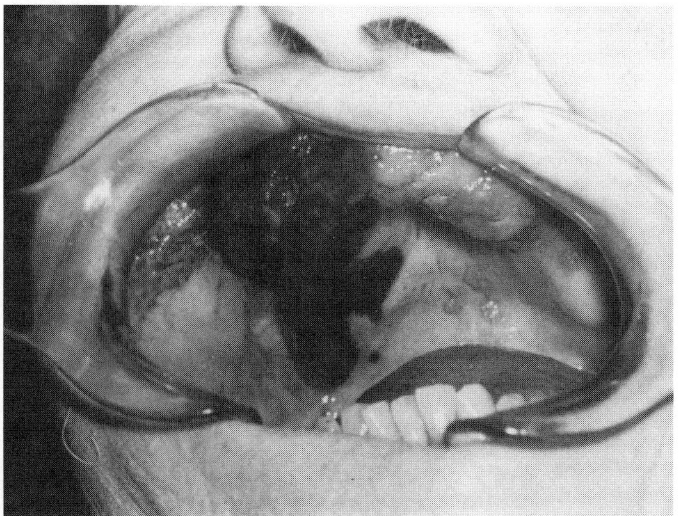

Figure 132-5. Mucosal melanoma. This large melanoma involves the right maxillary alveolus, hard palate, and gingivobuccal sulcus in a 91-year-old woman. She also had clinical cervical adenopathy and brain metastases at the time of presentation.

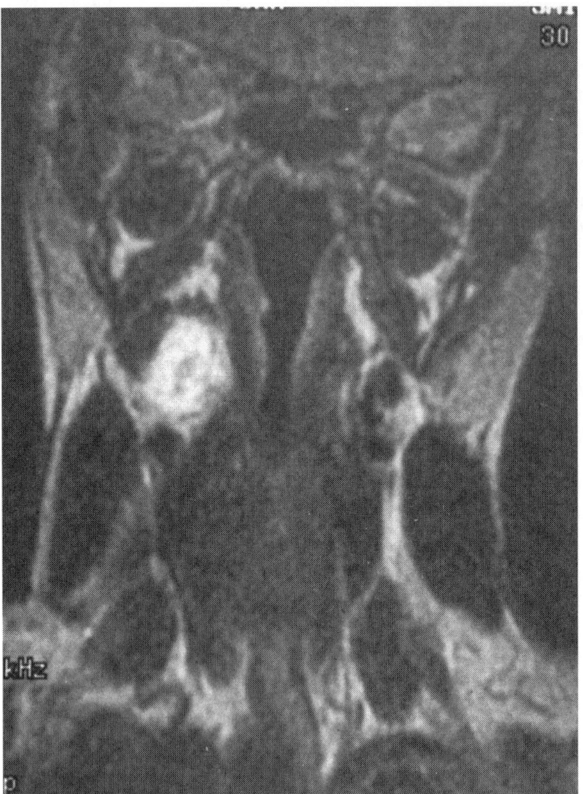

Figure 132-6. Parapharyngeal space neoplasm. Asymptomatic ganglioneuroma of the right cervical sympathetic chain demonstrated on an MRI of a 34-year-old woman.

years or more after initial diagnosis and treatment. Adenocarcinoma is the histopathology identified in about 30% of minor salivary gland malignancies. They are locally aggressive and occur in older patients. Mucoepidermoid carcinoma represents about 20% of minor salivary gland cancers. This tumor is distinctly more common in women, and tends to present between age 40 and 50. The majority of mucoepidermoid cancers are classified as low-grade and have a very favorable prognosis. Minor salivary gland malignancies are treated with wide surgical excision and neck dissection when nodes are present clinically. Prophylactic neck dissection is not indicated because of the low incidence of cervical disease. Most would advocate radiation therapy to the primary site when dealing with a high grade malignancy such as adenoid cystic, high grade mucoepidermoid, or adenocarcinoma. Because a relatively large percentage of minor salivary gland malignancies demonstrate recurrences at 10 or even 20 years after treatment, discussing five-year survival does not necessarily give an accurate picture of the behavior of these tumors. Five, ten, and fifteen-year survivals are in the range of 50%, 33%, and 20%, respectively.

Sarcomas may arise from numerous tissues in the oral cavity and oropharynx, including angiosarcoma, fibrosarcoma, leiomyosarcoma, liposarcoma, osteogenic sarcoma, and rhabdomyosarcoma. The latter two occur with greater frequency than the others listed. Osteogenic sarcoma is treated most often with chemotherapy and surgery. With rhabdomyosarcoma, the most favorable results are when complete surgical excision is possible. Because significant functional compromise is usual when dealing with a patient who has had a large resection, radiation and chemotherapy after conservative surgical treatment, or even biopsy only, is the frequent mode of treatment when it occurs in the head and neck area.

PARAPHARYNGEAL SPACE

Tumors of the parapharyngeal space impinge upon the oropharynx and therefore may mimic primary tumors of that area (Fig. 132-6). The structures found in this area include the deep lobe of the parotid gland, the major vessels, and several cranial nerves, as well as the cervical sympathetic chain and occasionally lymph nodes. It is not a surprise, therefore, to find that the largest numbers of tumors of this region derive from these tissues. The most common tumor found in this region is a benign mixed tumor of the deep lobe of the parotid, although all salivary gland histopathologies are seen here. Vascular lesions such as carotid body paragangliomas (chemodectoma) and aneurysms may be encountered. Schwanno-

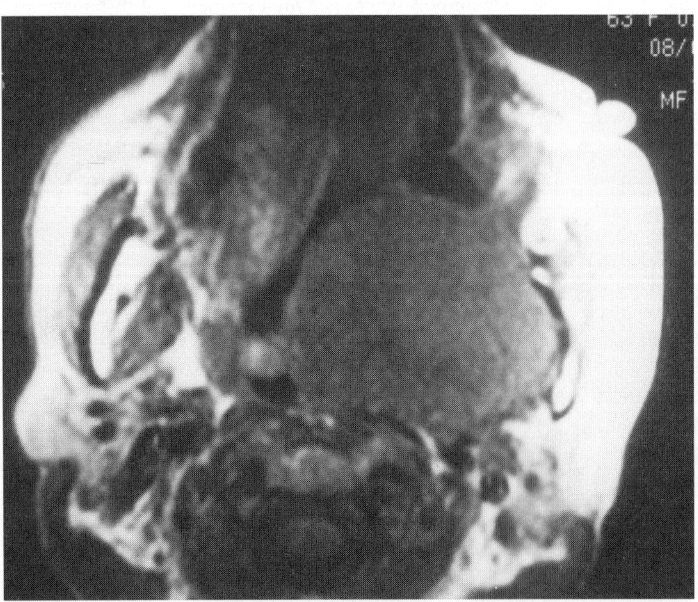

Figure 132-7. Parapharyngeal space neoplasm. This 63-year-old woman presented with a short history of trismus. Tumor was known to have been present at least 6 years at the time of this MRI. Resection required a lateral skull base approach. The final pathology demonstrated malignant granular cell tumor.

mas, ganglioneuromas, and others may arise from the neural structures in this region. Lesions occurring within the parapharyngeal space are most often benign and often asymptomatic until impressively large (Fig. 132-7). Rarely one may find malignancy within a lymph node in this region, either a lymphoma or metastatic disease as from a squamous cell carcinoma or from a thyroid malignancy. The majority are detected by the primary physician on routine physical exam of the oropharynx, where asymmetry is noted. Occasionally the patient may present with complaints of dysphagia, voice change, sensation of a lump in the throat, or sleep apnea due to the impingement of the mass on the oropharyngeal airway at night. The best imaging of this region is obtained by an MRI scan. Depending on the size and histopathology of the tumor, it may be approached best transcervically or transorally, or a mandibular osteotomy may be required.

CONSIDERATIONS IN PREGNANCY

The majority of the aforementioned lesions are benign or occur in older individuals. Nonetheless, occasionally one sees an oral or oropharyngeal lesion of concern in a pregnant woman. Fortunately, the vast majority of these lesions may be biopsied in the office under local anesthesia. Those that lie deep to the surface may be biopsied under ultrasound guidance at no risk to the developing fetus. If further imaging is required, MRI may be safely accomplished during pregnancy. Once the histopathology of the lesion is known, decisions may be made as to how to manage best the pregnancy, the lesion, and the two individuals involved. Benign lesions requiring surgery may be dealt with at some point after the delivery. The difficult question comes with those pregnant patients who have a malignancy. When head and neck surgery is carried out on the mother, the major risk to the fetus is during the first trimester. Major resections have been carried out during the second and third trimesters without adverse outcome to either the fetus or the mother. If a major resection cannot be delayed until after the first trimester, consideration may be given to ending the pregnancy. Radiation therapy should also be deferred until after pregnancy.

SUMMARY

Evaluation and management of oral and oropharyngeal lesions is the life-work of many otolaryngologist–head and neck surgeons, as well as some oral surgeons, general surgeons, and plastic surgeons. Because most tumors in this region are easily recognized or easily identified by appropriate biopsy, timely treatment may be effected, and most often the patient may expect a very satisfactory outcome.

BIBLIOGRAPHY

Batsakis JG. Tumors of the head and neck. Baltimore: Williams and Wilkins, 1979.

Cummings CW, Fredrickson JM, Harker LA, et al. Otolaryngology-head and neck surgery. St. Louis: CV Mosby, 1993.

Tran LM, Mark R, Meier R, et al. Sarcomas of the head and neck. Cancer 1992;70(1):169.

Wingo PA, Tong T, Bolden S. Cancer statistics, 1995. Ca Cancer J Clin 1995;45:8.

Wray A, McGuirt WF. Smokeless tobacco usage associated with oral carcinoma. Arch Otolaryngol Head Neck Surg 1993;119:929.

133
Laryngeal Neoplasms

PAUL TOPF

Primary Care for Women, edited by Phyllis C. Leppert and Fred M. Howard. Lippincott-Raven Publishers, Philadelphia © 1997.

The larynx is a structure in the neck that is involved in respiration, phonation, and deglutition. A woman presenting to her primary care physician with a tumor of the larynx may experience changes in voice, breathing ability, or swallowing. Most laryngeal neoplasms are one of numerous benign tumors, but a malignancy also may be seen. This chapter discusses the various laryngeal neoplasms, beginning with the usual presenting history, methods of evaluation of the larynx, and treatment options for specific tumors.

HISTORY

A patient with a laryngeal tumor usually presents with a disorder of voice. This is most notable if the tumor is present on the vocal cords rather than elsewhere in the larynx. Symptoms related to respiration such as dyspnea or stridor are rare with laryngeal tumors and are seen only in larger, more advanced lesions. Disorders of swallowing produce more vague, less noticeable symptoms and are not as common on presentation.

The most common presenting voice disorder in a patient with a laryngeal tumor is hoarseness or a raspy quality to the voice. This results from the mass effect of a neoplasm inhibiting the proper closure of the vocal cords on phonation. A less common voice disorder is a breathy voice, which occurs when a vocal cord is paralyzed. A paralyzed vocal cord usually occurs from hindrance of vocal cord motion by a malignant tumor present elsewhere in the larynx.

The two most important aspects in the medical history of a patient with vocal dysfunction and a possible laryngeal tumor are a history of cigarette smoking and the duration of the patient's symptoms. Malignant neoplasms of the larynx are extremely rare in nonsmokers. Vocal dysfunction of a few days' duration is most commonly associated with infections or an inflammatory process. If vocal problems have been present for several weeks or months, the likelihood of a benign or malignant neoplasm is higher.

Apart from the two initial points of the history just mentioned, other contributory information needs to be elicited. Respiratory disturbances can occur with large, usually malignant neoplasms. Dysphagia or odynophagia also may be seen with a neoplasm of the larynx.

A background of vocal abuse and misuse is another point that should be obtained in the history. Singers and other vocal abusers such as teachers have a higher incidence of benign laryngeal lesions such as vocal nodules, polyps, or cysts. Throat pain with associated referred otalgia, hemoptysis, or weight loss are worrisome symptoms and raise the possibility of malignancy, especially in cigarette smokers.

PHYSICAL EXAMINATION

After obtaining a history, the assessment of the patient begins with a subjective evaluation of the voice quality. A rough or raspy quality to the voice is consistent with a mass lesion on the vocal cords such as a neoplasm. A breathy voice most commonly occurs with a paralysis of the vocal cord. A tremulous or spasmodic quality to the voice may be a sign of a neurologic problem such as spasmodic dysphonia (laryngeal dystonia).

The following is a list of the different ways to perform a physical examination of the larynx:

- Mirror direct laryngoscopy
- Flexible fiberoptic laryngoscopy
- Direct laryngoscopy (with or without microscope)
- Videostroboscopic laryngoscopy.

Indirect laryngoscopy involves the use of a mirror to examine the larynx through the mouth. This is sufficient in many patients. If a more detailed evaluation is necessary or if the patient's anatomy makes the mirror examination impossible, flexible fiberoptic nasopharyngolaryngoscopy can be performed. After administration of topical anesthesia to the nose and throat, a flexible scope is passed through the nasal cavity into the throat to evaluate the larynx.

Indirect mirror laryngoscopy and flexible fiberoptic laryngoscopy are routine office evaluations. If a tumor of the larynx is observed, the next step usually is direct laryngoscopy in the operating room. This is usually performed under general anesthesia with endotracheal intubation. Biopsy or complete excision of laryngeal neoplasms is performed during the procedure. For greater magnification and visualization, a microscope can be used. Carbon dioxide laser is readily available to remove certain lesions when indicated.

Some patients, such as professional singers, may benefit from videostroboscopy of the larynx. Videostroboscopy is performed in the office using either a rigid scope transorally or a flexible nasopharyngolaryngoscope. The scope is attached to a camera, and the image appears on a monitor. The entire evaluation can be recorded on videotape.

The stroboscopic light source allows slow-motion evaluation of the functioning vocal cord. For vocal cord tumors, it helps to differentiate between the following benign lesions:

- Nodules
- Polyps
- Papillomas
- Cysts
- Granulomas.

BENIGN LARYNGEAL NEOPLASMS

Vocal Cord Nodules

Patients with vocal cord nodules usually present with a previous history of vocal abuse and misuse. This lesion commonly is seen in singers and often causes deep concern for the patient. Vocal cord nodules also are the most common cause for hoarseness in children and teenagers.

The pathologic features of a vocal cord nodule include a thickened epithelium with acanthosis and superficial keratinization. These are seen bilaterally on the vocal cords at the junction of the anterior and middle thirds.

Conservative treatment is the usual approach for vocal nodules. Most resolve with limited voice rest and speech therapy. Microsurgical techniques can be used at the time of microlaryngoscopy to remove the nodules if the nodules have not resolved after 6 months of speech therapy.

Vocal Cord Polyps

Vocal cord polyps differ from nodules in that they usually are unilateral and require surgical excision. Vocal cord polyps do not usually resolve spontaneously or with speech therapy. Most polyps are edematous, but some are found with many red blood cells and resemble angiomatous polyps. Polyps are more erythematous than nodules. Microsurgical removal during microlaryngoscopy is the treatment of choice. Postoperative speech therapy should follow to prevent recurrence of the polyps.

Papillomas

Laryngeal papillomas are tumor-like proliferations of stratified squamous epithelium most commonly seen on the vocal cords. An association is believed to exist between laryngeal papillomas and the human papillomavirus. Juvenile laryngeal papillomatosis is a much more aggressive entity than the laryngeal papillomas seen in adults. The treatment of choice is endoscopic removal with the carbon dioxide laser.

Cysts

Benign mucus retention cysts commonly are seen in various locations in the supraglottic larynx. Treatment is indicated if symptoms such as dysphagia are present. Treatment usually involves endoscopic marsupialization.

Granulomas

Granulomas occur most commonly over the medial edge of the posterior portion of the vocal cords. The presence of vocal cord granulomas is associated with a history of recent endotracheal intubation and gastroesophageal reflux disease. The most common presenting symptom is vocal dysfunction, but referred otalgia also can be seen.

Most granulomas resolve with antireflux measures. If laser excision is indicated, intraoperative steroid injection and postoperative treatment of reflux is important to prevent recurrence.

MALIGNANT TUMORS OF THE LARYNX

Over 90% of malignant tumors of the larynx are squamous cell carcinoma. Cancer of the larynx represents 0.4% of all malignant tumors in women, with a higher incidence in men. Approximately 11,000 cases of laryngeal malignancy are diagnosed per year in the United States.

The most important risk factor for squamous cell carcinoma of the larynx is smoking. Alcohol intake also is an important factor, and there is a synergistic effect with cigarette smoking. Carcinoma of the larynx most commonly originates on the vocal cords. When occurring elsewhere in the larynx, because of the inherent difficulty in diagnosis and the aggressiveness of the tumor, cure rates are not as high as with vocal cord carcinoma.

Treatment of early carcinomas of the larynx either involves endoscopic excision or radiation therapy. Moderately advanced lesions are treated either with partial laryngeal resection or radiation therapy. Advanced tumors frequently require dual-modality treatment such as total laryngectomy and postoperative radiation therapy. Except for early vocal cord carcinomas, the cervical lymphatics require treatment either with radiation therapy or surgical lymph node dissection.

CONSIDERATIONS IN PREGNANCY

Previously described squamous papillomas of the larynx occur with a higher incidence in children whose mothers had genital warts during pregnancy. Papillomavirus infection of the female genital tract is common; however, laryngeal papillomatosis is rare. The risk of developing the disease for a child born to an infected mother was calculated to be one in several hundred exposures. Because these lesions may be hormonally dependent, there have been occasional remissions or significant worsening during pregnancy in patients with laryngeal papillomas.

Overall, the incidence of laryngeal tumors during pregnancy is extremely low. The effect of these tumors on the upper airway must be considered during the course of the pregnancy and the delivery. Paragangliomas and supraglottic hemangiomas are two extremely rare tumors of the larynx that are suspected of increased growth potential during pregnancy. Squamous cell carcinoma of the larynx during pregnancy was first reported in 1973, and there does not appear to be a significant association.

BIBLIOGRAPHY

Ford CN, Bless DM. Phonosurgery. New York: Raven Press, 1991.

Gould WJ, Sataloff RT, Spiegel JR. Voice surgery. St Louis: CV Mosby, 1993.

Paparella M, Shumrick D, Gluckman J, Meyerhoff W. Otolaryngology. Philadelphia: WB Saunders, 1991.

XV
Dermatologic Problems

Primary Care for Women, edited by Phyllis C. Leppert and Fred M. Howard. Lippincott-Raven Publishers, Philadelphia © 1997.

134
Everyday Skin, Hair, and Nail Care

SOPHIE M. WOROBEC

Healthy skin requires little maintenance. Its main needs are proper cleansing, maintenance of an optimal moisture level, and protection from excessive sun exposure or exposure to excessive heat, cold, and wind. Nevertheless, women in our society are pressured by advertisements to spend time and money on products that will "repair," "revitalize," and "reveal newer, more youthful skin." Some of these products are good in that they cleanse, moisturize, and help protect the skin, but simpler, less expensive products usually suffice. Physical fitness, cheerfulness, and a sense of self-esteem, even in the face of disabilities and advancing age, do more for beauty than any "rejuvenating" cream.

SKIN CLEANSING

Skin cleansing removes dead skin cells, sweat, body secretions, microorganisms, and dirt. A person's daily activities, her environment, and her skin characteristics determine how frequently she wishes or needs to wash. Water removes most dirt; other cleansers, such as liquid soaps, soap bars, and detergent bars, help remove lipid-soluble materials. In cold climates in the winter and with advancing age, less frequent bathing (sometimes only once or twice a week) is necessary, and soap needs to be used only in body folds such as the axillae and groin. Some cleansing products have incorporated moisturizers; some are fragrance free. The use of sponges and loofahs is appropriate if they are not excessively abrasive. Newer plastic cleansing poufs are soft and help decrease the amount of product needed to work up a lather. Astringents, fresheners, toners, or refining lotions consist of water and alcohol solutions and can be used to remove sebum or makeup.

BODY ODOR, FOOT ODOR, AND SWEATING

Personal cleanliness and the wearing of clean clothes are the most important aspects of controlling body odor. Deodorants are products that may have some antibacterial agents and contain fragrances to mask body odor. Antiperspirants contain aluminum salts that block the eccrine sweat ducts and obstruct delivery of sweat to the skin. They can cause a 20% to 40% reduction in armpit sweating. In some women, they may be irritating and should not be used soon after shaving. Obese women may find it helpful to use talcum powder dusted in the axillae and groin to help prevent chafing; professional bicyclists use talcum powder for the same purpose.

Heavy footwear made of synthetic materials may create a damp environment that promotes the growth of the fungi that cause athlete's foot. Dusting the feet with drying powders such as Zeasorb (or, in the presence of fungal infection, Zeasorb-AF, which contains the antifungal agent miconazole) is helpful.

MOISTURIZATION

Optimal water content for the top layer of the skin, the stratum corneum, is at least 10%. At this level, a nice, smooth skin surface is maintained. In dry weather or during the winter in heated rooms, the ambient humidity is often insufficient to maintain this level of moisture in our skin. The skin begins to feel rough and may become itchy. Use of moisturizers is recommended to prevent and treat this common problem. Moisturizers are emulsions that help prevent water loss from the skin. They are best applied immediately after bathing and patting oneself dry, but while the skin is still hydrated from bathing. The least expensive moisturizers are Crisco and Vaseline, but many people consider them too greasy. Many of the moisturizers on the market contain water and glycerin (eg, Curel lotion, Aveeno moisturizing cream). Thicker preparations include Absorbase, Aquaphor, and Eucerin. Agents such as lactic acid and urea also have water-binding properties. A prescription lotion, Lac-Hydrin, contains 12% lactic acid and is very helpful, especially on dry intact skin and for smoothing out dry cracked skin over the heels and plantar foot surfaces. Women with a tendency to acne should choose a noncomedogenic moisturizer such as Moisturel.

PREVENTION OF SUN DAMAGE

In the past 30 years, there has been increasing recognition that there is a intrinsic skin aging process and an extrinsic aging process that affects predominantly sun-exposed areas (photodamage). The skin can be protected from the sun by minimizing midday (10 a.m. to 4 p.m.) sun exposure, wearing hats and protective clothing, and using sunblock skin care products. It is important to use a product offering both UV-B and UV-A wavelength protection. Some are marketed for adolescents with oily, acne-prone skin; others are marketed for persons with sensitive skin. Clothing manufactured under the trademark Solumbra has been approved by the FDA as a sun protectant. In general, colored synthetics protect better than white cotton fabrics; however, heavy cotton denim protects quite well.

Sunblock products are regulated as OTC drugs, and women should try different products to see which they prefer. The use of sunblock products helps reduce the risk of skin cancer and photodamage only if the person does not extend the amount of time she spends in the sun. The Sun Protection Factor (SPF) associated with these products is a laboratory-derived figure produced under strictly defined conditions. An SPF 2 figure means that 50% of incipient UV-B radiation is blocked. At SPF 8, it is 87.5%; at SPF 16, 93.75%. However, there is no way of calculating a person's "burn time" on a day-to-day basis using SPF figures as a way to promote increased "safe" sun exposure.

Tretinoin or retinoic acid has been prescribed widely for use on sun-damaged skin for reducing fine wrinkles, roughness, and brown spots. However, it alters the skin's barrier properties and may make the skin more vulnerable to ultraviolet damage.

Renova (tretinoin emollient cream) has been granted marketing approval as an adjunctive agent for the palliation of fine wrinkles, mottled hyperpigmentation, and tactile roughness of facial skin in patients who do not achieve these results using a program of comprehensive skin care and sun avoidance alone. Renova does not eliminate wrinkles or repair sun-damaged skin, nor does it reverse photoaging or restore a more youthful or younger dermal histologic pattern, according to its package insert. The 1996 package insert also contains a "black box" warning stating that it is a dermal irritant and that there is evidence of atypical changes in melanocytes and keratinocytes and of increased dermal elastosis in some patients treated with Renova for longer than 48 weeks; the significance of these findings is unknown. The second bullet in the black box warning states that the "safety and effectiveness of Renova in individuals with moderately or heavily pigmented skin have not been established."

HAIR CARE

Shampoos remove hair oils, cellular debris, microorganisms, and other soils. Depending on the woman and other hair treatments (eg, tinting and permanents) she uses, different shampoos appeal to different women. Women with less dense hair may prefer one that gives "extra body." Women who swim daily may find that a swimmer's shampoo and conditioner leaves their hair softer and more manageable. Additional shampoo information is given in Chapter 140. Conditioners are added to shampoos or used separately to enhance the combability of the hair and to prevent damage from traction after washing. The frequency of shampooing varies from daily to twice a week or less, depending on personal grooming practices.

The amount of facial and body hair depends on a woman's genetic background. However, a sudden change or increase in facial or body hair warrants a hormonal evaluation.

NAIL CARE

Fingernails vary in thickness and flexibility from person to person. As we age, the fingernails grow more slowly, become thinner, and may develop longitudinal ridges. Ingestion of gelatin or calcium does not strengthen a normal fingernail. Protection of the hands prevents nail injuries. Hands exposed to dry, cold weather or frequent washing should be protected with gloves and emollients. An intact eponychium (cuticle) prevents infection of the posterior nail fold and should not be removed. Hangnails are partially detached, dried pieces of skin at the lateral nail fold. They should be cut close to the base and covered with a bandage; they should not be picked or torn because this may lead to secondary infection.

Carefully applied and maintained manicures are aesthetically beneficial. However, the use of methacrylates as glues for wrapping nails can result in onycholysis, paronychia, and permanent damage to the nail.

Care of the toenails means wearing well-fitting footwear, as the most common cause for ingrown toenails is ill-fitting shoes. Toenails should be clipped straight across. Cutting them down in the corners causes the sharp ends to dig into the lateral nail folds, and ultimately granulation tissue or "proud flesh" may form. If this happens, the patient should be shown how to put a little piece of cotton between the sharp corner of the nail and the skin. The cotton should be replaced daily after a shower or bath until the nail has grown out enough to allow it to be trimmed properly.

"NATURAL" INGREDIENTS

Natural does not mean better: poison ivy is "all natural," yet it is the most common cause of severe contact dermatitis in North America. Skin care products may be labeled as "natural" because they contain ingredients found in nature, such as alpha-hydroxy acids; however, these ingredients may be synthesized or manufactured when they are used in these products. Natural substances such as vitamin E, lanolin, and aloe occasionally cause contact dermatitis. In other words, "natural" materials can cause skin problems as well as being useful products. For example, lanolin can be a good moisturizer in persons who are not allergic to it, and aloe can be very soothing. Allantoin, glycerin, and oatmeal at designated concentrations are described as safe and effective in the FDA's "Tentative Final Monograph of Over-the-Counter Skin Protectant Drugs." As for AHA-containing products, it is the responsibility of the company or person recommending them to have the proof backing any therapeutic claims.

In short, if a woman has a skin or hair care product that she is pleased with, it does not make sense to switch to a more expensive product simply because it is labeled as being "natural."

BIBLIOGRAPHY

Bech-Thomsen N, Wulf HC, Ullman S. Xeroderma pigmentosum lesions related to ultraviolet transmittance by clothes. J Am Acad Dermatol 1991;24:365.

Engasser PG. Care of normal skin, hair and nails. In: Orkin M, Maibach HI, Dahl MV, eds. Dermatology. Norwalk, Conn.: Appleton & Lange, 1991.

Jackson EM. An overview of natural cosmetic ingredient use. Cosmetic Dermatology 1994;7:42.

Marks R. Summer in Australia: skin cancer and the great SPF debate. Arch Dermatol 1995;131:462.

Renova (tretinoin emollient cream) 0.05% Package Insert, January 1996. Dermatological Division, Ortho Pharmaceutical Corp., Raritan, NJ.

Sayre RM, Hughes SNG. Sun protective apparel: advancements in sun protection. Skin Cancer J 1993;8:41.

Steinem G. Revolution from within: a book of self-esteem. Boston: Little, Brown & Co., 1991.

Stern RS. Sunscreens for cancer protection. Arch Dermatol 1995;131:220.

Wolf N. The beauty myth: how images of beauty are used against women. New York: William Morrow & Co., Inc., 1991.

Primary Care for Women, edited by Phyllis C. Leppert and Fred M. Howard. Lippincott-Raven Publishers, Philadelphia © 1997.

135
Rashes

SOPHIE M. WOROBEC

Every day, the physician in practice is asked about skin findings. Sometimes the question is about checking a mole or "growth," but the statement that may produce the most disquiet is, "Doc, I've got a rash." The approach to a rash is the same as that applied to any illness: obtaining a history, performing a physical examination, and formulating a differential diagnosis and a treatment plan.

The dermatologic history includes onset (when and where it first appeared), course (how it progressed, any remissions, exacerbation), change in appearance since onset, any systemic symptoms (eg, fever, joint pain), local symptoms (eg, itching), menstrual history, and whether anyone close to the patient has had a skin disease. Most patients will already have used something for their rash, and this should be ascertained. Any exacerbating factors (eg, sun exposure, cold, medications) should be discussed. The patient profile should cover occupational history, lifestyle and hobbies, and travel history.

The past medical history includes chronic and recent illnesses, any past skin problems, known allergies and what they were like, and any manifestation of atopy such as asthma, hay fever, or eczema. The family history should include questions regarding skin diseases such as psoriasis or eczema, cancer, hair or nail problems, and infectious diseases such as impetigo, scabies, or herpes simplex.

The medication history includes not only prescription medications but also over-the-counter preparations, home remedies, and personal care products.

The diagnosis is facilitated by dividing the physical examination findings into two groups: primary and secondary lesions. Primary lesions are the original skin changes; secondary lesions develop with the passage of time. Pustules can be primary lesions, as in folliculitis, or secondary lesions (eg, the clear umbilicated vesicles of herpes simplex infection becoming pustular).

Dermatology is unique in that direct visual recognition often establishes the diagnosis. Many diagnoses consist of identifying the unique diagnostic primary lesions, such as the comedones of acne or the "black dots in callus" of a wart, and recognizing secondary lesions, such as crusting in impetigo or lichenification of neurodermatitis.

The morphologic terms used to describe primary and secondary lesions are listed in Table 135-1. Rashes can be further characterized by their configurations (Table 135-2) and their regional distributions (Table 135-3).

Annular lesions, by their configuration, alert the physician to the consideration of tinea corporis, urticaria, syphilis, granuloma annulare, psoriasis, and pityriasis rosea. In examining the patient with a rash, the more systematic or global examination yields the greatest yield. The physician should look at more than the immediate rash pointed out by the patient; the patient should be examined thoroughly, looking at the scalp, face, eyelids, behind the ears, the mouth, and so on. This examination may yield clues to patterns of psoriasis, eczema, or contact dermatitis. Commonly, a tinea pedis

Table 135-1. Morphology of Skin Lesions

Primary Skin Lesions	
Macule	Flat discoloration < 1 cm in diameter
Patch	Flat discoloration > 1 cm in diameter
Papule	Elevated lesion < 1 cm in diameter
Plaque	Flat, elevated lesion > 1.5 cm in diameter
Nodule	Elevated lesion > 1 cm in diameter
Tumor	Rounded elevated lesion > 2–3 cm in diameter
Vesicle	Fluid-filled elevated lesion < 1 cm in diameter
Bulla	Fluid-filled elevated lesion > 1 cm in diameter
Pustule	Elevated lesion filled with pus
Wheal	Elevated pink to red pruritic lesion
Secondary Skin Lesions	
Crust	Dried exudate attached to skin surface
Scale	Accumulation of skin "flakes"
Pustule	Elevated lesion filled with pus
Purpura	Hemorrhage into the skin. Doesn't blanch with pressure from glass slide. Small lesions are petechiae; larger ones are ecchymoses.
Erosion	Surface denudation limited to the skin's top layer
Fissure	Linear break in the skin going down to the dermis
Ulcer	Skin defect involving at least part of the dermis
Excoriation	Area of erosion or ulceration produced by the patient
Atrophy	Decrease in the thickness of the skin caused by partial loss of dermis or subcutaneous fat
Pigmentation	Increase of color—hyperpigmentation; decrease—hypopigmentation
Papilloma	Elevated cauliflower-like lesion
Cyst	Fluid- or solid material-filled cavity surrounded by a sac
Lichenification	Thick, leathery skin

Table 135-2. Configurations of Skin Lesions

Annular	Ring-like
Arciform	Incompletely formed ring; like an arc
Serpiginous	Winding, like a snake
Linear	In a straight line (eg, poison ivy dermatitis)
Guttate	Drop-like individual lesions, like spots in a field
Dermatomal	Following a dermatome distribution
Target-like or iris-like	Ring around a central lesion
Reticulate	Net-like
Grouped	Clustering of lesions in a well-demarcated area

may help explain a hand rash, which may itself be a tinea manuum or an id reaction to the dermatophytic infection of the feet.

The spectrum of skin problems can be broadly divided into the groupings shown in Table 135-4.

Once diagnosed, a skin problem can then be treated. Individual chapters in this text address the therapy of specific diseases.

If after seeing and interviewing the patient and consulting reference books, no specific diagnoses can be made, it is best to refer the patient to another physician. A dermatologist's experience allows more prompt recognition of a dermatosis or the need for a biopsy. Although a skin biopsy is relatively easy to perform, a dermatologist is well versed in choosing the most appropriate lesion or lesions (in the case of cutaneous T-cell lymphoma) for a biopsy. In difficult cases, a dermatopathologist can be asked to read the skin biopsy. His or her expertise, gained by reading of thousands of skin slides, can help guide the patient's care. The dermatologist can help communicate clinical findings and the differential diagnosis to the dermatopathologist. Sometimes additional laboratory work, not a biopsy, is in order (an RPR and FTA-Abs for the diagnosis of syphilis, positive hepatitis serology in the patient with itching, or a positive mononucleosis test in the patient with an ampicillin rash).

Some rashes, such as a well-developed herpes zoster, are instantly recognizable; others stump even experienced and astute dermatologists. However, careful observation, a thorough history, testing, and consultation with other physicians and the literature usually narrow the diagnostic possibilities.

Table 135-3. Distributions of Skin Lesions

TYPE	EXAMPLES
Generalized	Viral eruption
Photosensitive	Systemic lupus erythematosus
Intertriginous	Intertrigo candidiasis
Symmetric	Psoriasis
Asymmetric	Poison ivy
Along cleavage lines	Pityriasis rosea

Table 135-4. Skin Disease Groupings by Clinical Presentation

TYPE	EXAMPLES
Eczematous	Contact dermatitis, infestations, infections, drugs. Atopic dermatitis dyshidrosis, nummular eczema, stasis dermatitis, xerotic eczema
Papulosquamous	Psoriasis, seborrhea, pityriasis rosea, secondary syphilis, tinea, lichen planus, discoid lupus, lichen simplex chronicus, cutaneous T-cell lymphoma
Vascular reactivity	Urticaria, erythema multiforme, annular erythemas, toxic erythema, viral exanthems
Inflammatory	Erythema nodosum, bacterial infections, insect bites, infestations, panniculitis and nodules papules
Vesiculobullous	Eczematous dermatoses, viral eruptions, insect bites, scabies, bullous impetigo. Stevens-Johnson syndrome, pemphigoid, porphyria cutanea tarda, fixed drug eruption, diabetic bullae, bullae with coma, pemphigus vulgaris, dermatitis herpetiformis
Pustular	Acne vulgaris, acne rosacea, folliculitis, steroid acne, gonococcemia, pustular psoriasis candidiasis
Purpuric	Leukocytoclastic vasculitis, senile purpura, corticosteroid excess, vascular defects, platelet disorders, clotting factor disorders
Pruritus	Various causes: xerosis; drug-induced; dermatologic diseases (eg, eczema, scabies); systemic disease (eg, renal failure, polycythemia vera, iron-deficiency anemia, hepatobiliary problems); HIV infection; psychological
Psychocutaneous	Neurotic excoriations, lip biting, hair pulling, factitial dermatitis, delusions of skin disease
Life-threatening	Staphylococcal scalded skin syndrome, toxic epidermal necrolysis, toxic shock syndrome, Kawasaki disease, Rocky Mountain spotted fever

BIBLIOGRAPHY

Fitzpatrick TB, Eisen AZ, Wolff K, Freedberg IM, Austen KF, eds. Dermatology in general medicine, 4th ed. New York: McGraw-Hill, 1993.

Flowers FP, Krusinski PA, eds. Dermatology in ambulatory and emergency medicine: a clinical guide with algorithms. Chicago: Year Book Medical Publishers, 1984.

Lynch PJ, Edwards L. Genital dermatology. New York: Churchill-Livingstone, 1994.

McKee PH. Pathology of the skin. Philadelphia: JB Lippincott, 1989.

Orkin M, Maibach HI, Dahl MV, eds. Dermatology, 1st ed. Norwalk, CT: Appleton & Lange, 1991.

Sams WM, Lynch PJ, eds. Principles and practice of dermatology. New York: Churchill-Livingstone, 1990.

136
Pigmentation Disorders

SOPHIE M. WOROBEC

Primary Care for Women, edited by Phyllis C. Leppert and Fred M. Howard. Lippincott-Raven Publishers, Philadelphia © 1997.

Patients are often concerned about any increase (hyperpigmentation) or decrease (hypopigmentation) in their normal skin color. The most common reason for changes in pigmentation is an alteration in the formation of melanin within melanosomes and the subsequent dispersal of melanin to keratinocytes. Pigmentary demarcation lines are a normal finding in up to 26% of African-American patients, most commonly on the dorsal and ventral surfaces of the arms, extending onto the chest.

ETIOLOGY AND DIFFERENTIAL DIAGNOSIS

Skin color can be altered by heat exposure, solar radiation, ionizing radiation, drugs, trauma, and heavy metals. Local trauma due to disease or therapeutic measures (eg, dermabrasion, liquid nitrogen, curettage, chemical peels) can destroy melanocytes, causing temporary or permanent hypo- or hyperpigmentation.

Hyperpigmentation

Hyperpigmentation can be circumscribed or diffuse. Common nevi, freckles, and lentigines are the most common circumscribed hyperpigmented lesions.

Mongolian spots (dermal melanocytosis) occur as aggregates of melanocytes in the dermis; due to the Tyndall effect, they appear blue-gray to blue-black because of the deep location of the melanin pigment. Most Mongolian spots regress by adolescence, but some persist into adulthood. They are most common on the lumbosacral area but can also occur on the shoulders, upper back, arms, and legs.

Nevus of Ota is a localized hyperpigmented blue-gray or blue-black macular lesion caused by an upper dermal nevoid aggregate of dendritic melanocytes over the distribution of the ophthalmic and maxillary divisions of the trigeminal nerve. It can extend to involve eye structures, especially the sclera; rarely, ocular malignant melanoma develops. It is most common in Asian, Hispanic, and African-American persons.

Melasma or chloasma occurs as a blotchy hyperpigmentation on the forehead, cheeks, nose, upper lip, and chin. It is more common in women and is sometimes related to pregnancy or the use of oral contraceptives. Sunlight exposure aggravates and perpetuates this condition.

Lentigines are circumscribed hyperpigmented macular lesions, slightly larger and darker than freckles. Senile lentigines (liver spots) are caused by chronic sun exposure of lighter-pigmented persons and occur in most elderly Caucasians and many Asians. Generalized lentigines in a young person may be part of a clinical syndrome such as Peutz-Jeghers or leopard syndrome. With the use of long-term chemophototherapy, PUVA-induced lentigines, some with cellular atypia, have been reported in up to 4% of patients.

Café-au-lait spots are light to dark brown, well-circumscribed macules ranging from 1 to 20 cm in size. They can be round or oval or have an irregular border. They can be present at birth or appear later in childhood. Up to 20% of all people have them, but the presence of multiple lesions suggests the possibility of an associated clinical syndrome such as neurofibromatosis or Albright syndrome. Café-au-lait spots, even with associated axillary freckles, are not in themselves diagnostic of neurofibromatosis. Lisch nodules (melanocytic hematomas of the iris) are present in over 97% of adult women with neurofibromatosis. Albright syndrome consists of polyostotic fibrous dysplasia, precocious puberty in females, endocrine dysfunction, and large café-au-lait spots with jagged margins resembling the coast of Maine.

Diffuse hyperpigmentation can be seen in Addison disease due to increased pituitary secretion of melanocyte stimulating hormone (MSH) and ACTH. Other metabolic diseases associated with diffuse hyperpigmentation include Wilson disease (also with sky-blue nail lunulae), alkaptonuria, hemochromatosis, biliary cirrhosis, and porphyria cutanea tarda.

Drugs responsible for hyperpigmentation include amiodarone, busulphan, cyclophosphamide, clofazimine, zidovudine (AZT), topical nitrogen mustard, chlorpromazine, gold, and minocycline. Silver, bismuth, mercury, and arsenic can produce hyperpigmentation. Topical use of benzoyl peroxide, tretinoin, and fluorouracil can result in hyperpigmentation. Fixed drug eruptions, caused most commonly by phenolphthalein in laxatives, barbiturates, and sometimes tetracycline, can result in one or several hyperpigmented macular lesions. Bleomycin can produce a linear, flagellate pattern of hyperpigmentation. Berloque dermatitis is caused by bercapten (5-methoxy psoralen), which is present in oil of bergamot, a component of many perfumes and some hair-care products. It occurs on areas of skin application as a photosensitization reaction and leaves a streaky, long-lasting hyperpigmentation.

Many dermatoses, even the inflamed papules and pustules of common acne, can leave postinflammatory hyperpigmentation. Even tanning is triggered by the activation of DNA-repair enzymes following DNA damage induced by ultraviolet radiation.

Yellow discoloration of the skin is seen in jaundice. Jaundice often includes the sclerae. The yellow color of carotenemia does not involve the sclerae and is accentuated on the palms and soles. Quinacrine, an antimalarial agent sometimes used to treat lupus, can also cause yellowish skin discoloration. Other drugs imparting a yellow color include cathaxanthin and phenazopyridine.

Hypopigmentation

Intrinsic hypopigmentation disorders include vitiligo, albinism, and piebaldism.

Vitiligo affects 1% to 2% of the population. Women are affected more frequently than men, and the peak incidence is in the second and third decades. Lesions of vitiligo are asymptomatic and show hypopigmentation or complete depigmentation. Early lesions may show areas of perifollicular hypopigmentation, which progress to depigmentation and extend to coalesce, with resulting larger macular lesions. Lesions tend to occur over bony prominences such as the knuckles, elbows, knees, and ankles; in photoexposed facial, neck, and chest areas; and around orifices such as the mouth, eyes, and genital areas. Halo nevi, white patches of hair (poliosis), and premature hair graying are common associated problems. In African-Americans in particular, vitiligo can show trichrome coloration of complete depigmentation (white), partial depigmentation (light brown), and a deeper normal brown. In vitiligo, there is local destruction of melanocytes. The cause is unknown, but there is an association with hyperthyroidism, hypothyroidism, pernicious anemia, diabetes mellitus, Addison disease, and rarely internal malignancy. Most cases are idiopathic, with formation of antibodies to melanocytes. Often there is a history of stress, although given the amount of stress in most people's lives it is difficult to créate a causal relation.

Oculocutaneous albinism may affect the eye, hair, and skin color or the eyes alone (ocular albinism). Oculocutaneous albinism has been classified into nine forms, depending on the type of defect present—in other words, whether there is missing or aberrant tyrosinase activity or still unclassified alterations in melanin formation. In all forms, there is a reduction or absence of normal melanin in the skin. Albinism is congenital and best diagnosed by comparing the patient's coloration with that of her family members. Photophobia and nystagmus are common but not essential for diagnosis.

Piebaldism is rare and occurs as an autosomal dominant trait. It is characterized by a congenital white forelock (> 90% of cases) and vitiligo-like depigmented macules, which often contain isolated normally pigmented or hyperpigmented macules. Hyperpigmented macules are usually less than 1 cm in diameter (although larger ones have occurred) and are characteristically present within the depigmented areas and on normal skin.

Hypopigmented macules that are polygonal and range from 2 to 9 mm in diameter are seen in idiopathic guttate hypomelanosis. In this common condition, lesions appear on sun-exposed areas of the upper and lower extremities, and more rarely on the face, neck, and trunk. Lesions start in early adulthood and increase in number. They are often of cosmetic concern. The cause is unknown, although aging, sun exposure, and genetic background all play a role.

Skin diseases (eg, tinea versicolor, pityriasis alba, chronic erythema ab igne, sarcoidosis, mycosis fungoides, and scleroderma) may be associated with hypopigmentation. Hypopigmented oval to lance-ovate macules are seen in tuberous sclerosis. Hereditary metabolic diseases such as phenylketonuria can result in hypopigmentation; it is subtle and best appreciated by comparison with family members.

Chemical exposure to phenolic compounds that interfere with tyrosinase activity may cause chemical leukoderma. The use of liquid nitrogen on brown to brown-black skin can cause areas of hypopigmentation or depigmentation. Intralesional injection or long-term topical use of corticosteroids can cause hypopigmentation.

HISTORY AND PHYSICAL EXAMINATION

In both hyperpigmentation and hypopigmentation disorders, a careful history (date of onset, any progression, general health status, diet, prior or concomitant therapy, and family history of pigmentary lesions) and a careful visual inspection help the clinician reach a diagnosis. Other dermatologic conditions can cause postinflammatory hyperpigmentation. Increased sun exposure with the use of oral contraceptives, residence in the southern United States, or pregnancy is often associated with melasma or chloasma. Certain drugs can cause hyperpigmentation. Increasing tiredness with hyperpigmentation, especially of skin crease lines and scars, points to Addison disease. The use of tanning parlors may be associated with increased freckles and lentigines. Exposure to antioxidants (eg, monobenzyl ether of hydroquinone) in rubber goods such as gloves or rubber pads can cause hypopigmentation.

In the evaluation of any pigmented lesion, if there is suspicion of malignant melanoma, an excisional biopsy is in order. Skin punch biopsies may also be needed to confirm or exclude other diagnoses such as scleroderma, Hansen disease (leprosy), heavy metal exposure, and hemosiderosis.

LABORATORY AND IMAGING STUDIES

Well-defined macular lesions that are hyperpigmented on sun-protected areas and hypopigmented on sun-exposed areas should be scraped with a #15 blade and the skin scale scrapings examined with potassium hydroxide (KOH) to check for pityriasis versicolor. A Wood's light examination can be helpful in determining the true extent of hypopigmented lesions, especially in very fair-skinned persons. An ophthalmoscopic examination can help detect retinal pigment changes. If tuberous sclerosis, neurofibromatosis, Albright syndrome, or one of the syndromes with generalized lentigines is suspected, special imaging studies and further work-up may be indicated. Tyrosinase studies can be performed when albinism is a diagnostic possibility. In persons with vitiligo, consideration should be given to testing levels of vitamin B_{12}, thyroid-stimulating hormone, and antimicrosomal antibodies and performing a random glucose test. These and other tests (eg, gastric endoscopy) should be done as indicated by the history and physical examination.

TREATMENT

Hyperpigmentation

The sine qua non of reducing the occurrence or intensity of melasma, freckles, and solar lentigines is protection from sun exposure by the use of broad-spectrum sunblocks, hats, and protective clothing such as Solumbra. These lesions and some cases of postinflammatory hyperpigmentation respond variably to treatment with bleaching creams and solutions containing hydroquinone (eg, Solaquin, Eldoquin, Melanex). Tretinoin cream or gel 0.025% to 0.05% may be added at bedtime to increase bleaching. Topical corticosteroids also can lighten pigment. However, all these agents have the potential to produce untoward side effects such as irritation, undesired hypopigmentation, or hyperpigmentation. Treatment can take months and must be combined with scrupulous avoidance of ultraviolet light, either in natural sunlight or tanning parlors. Some lentigines and the nevus of Ota respond to laser treatment. If part of a syndrome or systemic disease, treatment is tailored to ameliorate or correct the signs and symptoms of the more serious disorder.

Hypopigmentation

Persons with vitiligo and albinism are at increased risk for the development of actinic keratoses, basal cell epitheliomas, squamous cell epitheliomas, and melanomas. Photoprotection with broad-spectrum sunblocks, hats, and clothing is essential.

Albinism is stable. Vitiligo, because it is usually idiopathic, rarely repigments, and many persons go through cycles of improvement and worsening. If an associated finding, such as hypothyroidism, is found in a patient with vitiligo and treated, the vitiligo may disappear. Secondary hypopigmentation, as in pityriasis versicolor and even Hansen disease, improves as the underlying cause is treated. Camouflage cosmetics such as Covermark and Dermablend are helpful in concealing vitiligo. Treatment of vitiligo with topical or systemic photochemotherapy with psoralens and UVA light (PUVA) requires a large time commitment, with visits at least weekly; burns may occur. Side effects of oral PUVA therapy include nausea and vomiting, hyperpigmentation of normally pigmented skin, itching, photoaging, increased risk of skin cancer, and increased risk of cataracts. Ultraviolet-protective sunglasses and sunblocks must be used for 24 hours after oral dosing. Grafting of uninvolved pigmented skin into the vitiliginous area, together with PUVA therapy, has been successful in a few centers.

Patients over age 12 who have vitiligo over 50% or more of their body surface can try to depigment the remaining skin with topical 20% monobenzyl ether of hydroquinone. Side effects include irritation and contact sensitization. The resultant depigmentation is permanent, and lifetime protection against excessive sun exposure is necessary.

CONSIDERATIONS IN PREGNANCY

Melasma in pregnancy is best treated by avoiding excessive sun exposure. Other common changes during pregnancy are darkening of the nipples, areolae, external genitalia, and sometimes the axillae and inner thighs. The linea alba becomes darkened and is then termed the linea nigra. Existing moles and freckles may darken. These changes partially or completely regress once pregnancy is completed. Hormonal changes such as increases in estrogen, progesterone, MSH, and ACTH levels are probably responsible for the changes.

The histology of moles during pregnancy is similar to that of those removed from nonpregnant patients. If there is doubt as to whether an existing mole is undergoing expected physiologic changes or is undergoing a malignant change, it is best to excise the lesion.

BIBLIOGRAPHY

Bolognia JL, Pawelek JM. Biology of hypopigmentation. J Am Acad Dermatol 1988;19:217.

Falabella R. Idiopathic guttate hypomelanosis. Dermatol Clin 1988;6:241.

Fulk CS. Primary disorders of hyperpigmentation. J Am Acad Dermatol 1984;10:1.

Grimes PE. Diseases of hyperpigmentation and Diseases of hypopigmentation. In: Sams WM, Lynch PJ, eds. Principles and practice of dermatology. New York: Churchill-Livingstone, 1990:807.

Hendrix JD Jr, Greer KE. Cutaneous hyperpigmentation caused by systemic drugs. Int J Dermatol 1992;31:458.

Khalid M, Mujtaba G, Haroon TS. Comparison of 0.05% clobetasol propionate cream and topical Puvasol in childhood vitiligo. Int J Dermatol 1995;34:203.

Ortonne J-P, Mosher DB, Fitzpatrick TB, eds. Vitiligo and other hypomelanoses of hair and skin. New York: Plenum, 1983.

Porter JR, Beuf AH, Lerner AB, Nordlund JJ. The effect of vitiligo on sexual relationships. J Am Acad Dermatol 1990;22:221.

Tal A, Gagel RF. The diagnostic dilemma of hyperpigmentation in patients with acquired immunodeficiency syndrome. Cutis 1991;48:153.

Wildfang IL, Jacobsen FK, Thestrup-Pedersen K. PUVA treatment of vitiligo: a retrospective study of 59 patients. Acta Derm-Venereol 1992;72:305.

137
Acne

ANITA S. PAKULA

Primary Care for Women, edited by Phyllis C. Leppert and Fred M. Howard. Lippincott-Raven Publishers, Philadelphia © 1997.

Acne is the most common skin disease treated by physicians. Although it is most prevalent in adolescents, it may either persist into or initially present in adulthood. The pathogenesis of acne is multifactorial and involves hormonally induced excessive sebum production, abnormal follicular keratinization, proliferation of *Propionibacterium acnes*, and inflammation, which is modulated by the host immune system. The clinical presentation may range from noninflammatory comedones to inflammatory papules, pustules, nodules, and cysts that may result in permanent scarring. With as many as 30% of women in their 30s, 20% of women in their 40s, and 8% of women in their 50s having acne to some degree, the chronic nature of this disease and its psychosocial impact on the patient must not be ignored. The goals of treatment are to limit the duration and degree of disease and to prevent scarring—hence, to minimize the psychosocial consequences. There are various therapeutic modalities that are directed toward specific pathogenic factors. A successful treatment regimen can be devised based on an understanding of the polygenic and multifactorial nature of this disease and good communication with the patient.

PATHOGENESIS

Acne vulgaris is a disorder of the sebaceous follicles, which consist of large sebaceous glands and miniature hairs. The sebaceous follicles are present in highest concentration on the face, back, and chest. The four key pathogenic factors of acne vulgaris are androgen-induced production of sebum, abnormal keratinization and desquamation of the sebaceous follicle epithelium (comedogenesis), proliferation of *P acnes*, and inflammation.

Sebum Production

The sebaceous glands are androgen-dependent appendages of hair follicles that secrete lipids to lubricate the skin and hair and contain enzymes for the peripheral metabolism of androgens. Increased production of androgenic hormones in puberty appears to stimulate enlargement of the sebaceous gland and increase production of sebum. The serum dehydroepiandrosterone sulfate (DHEA-S) level increases in adrenarche and appears to be the earliest marker for the development of acne. Androgens may also decrease the linoleic acid concentration in the sebum of acne patients, contributing to retention hyperkeratosis and obstruction of the pilosebaceous ducts.

Comedogenesis

Abnormal keratinization of the sebaceous and follicular ducts causes the epithelial cells lining the ducts to become more cohesive, forming a plug that blocks the follicular orifice. This process is also referred to as retention hyperkeratosis and comedogenesis. The result is formation of a microcomedo, the precursor lesion of acne.

Propionibacterium acnes and Inflammation

The combination of excessive sebum and the anaerobic environment created by the plugged follicles results in the proliferation of the anaerobic diphtheroid *P acnes*. These bacteria trigger immune and nonimmune inflammatory reactions that cause further damage to the follicular epithelium. *P acnes* produce lipases that hydrolyze the triglycerides of sebum into irritating free fatty acids. These bacteria also release chemotactic factors that attract neutrophils, which in turn release hydrolytic enzymes that damage the follicular wall, allowing leakage into the dermis. This results in further inflammation and irritation.

HISTORY AND PHYSICAL EXAMINATION

A complete history should include inquiry into menstrual irregularities, medication and cosmetic use, pregnancy status, and a family history of acne and endocrine disorders. Physical examination should address the location, type, severity, and complications, such as scarring, of the acne. In addition, signs of androgen excess, such as hirsutism, androgenic alopecia, and obesity, should be noted. If an underlying androgenic disorder, such as polycystic ovarian syndrome, Cushing syndrome, or late-onset congenital adrenal hyperplasia, is suspected, then appropriate laboratory studies should be obtained.

There is no uniformly accepted method for grading the severity of acne, but the classification should take into account the morphology, distribution, complications, response to therapy, and the impact of the disease on the patient. Acne should be classified by the predominant type of lesion, such as comedonal, papulopustular, or nodular, and then should be graded as mild, moderate, or severe.

CLINICAL MANIFESTATIONS

Acne lesions can be divided into two categories, noninflammatory and inflammatory. Noninflammatory lesions consist of open and closed comedones. The accumulation of sebum results in the closed comedo or whitehead. The open comedo or blackhead results from continued distention of the follicular orifice, resulting in dilatation and protrusion of the keratinous plug. The dark color of a blackhead is due to melanin, not dirt. Usually, this keratinous material is sloughed without inflammation unless the lesion is traumatized.

The inflammatory lesions consist of papules, pustules, and nodules. When the follicular wall ruptures superficially, an inflamed pustule develops. Pustules have a visible central core of purulent material. Deeper rupture of the follicular wall results in a papule or nodule. Papules are inflammatory lesions measuring less than 5 mm; nodules are inflammatory lesions measuring greater than 5 mm. True cysts are lined by epithelium and are the rare residua of healed pustules or nodules.

DIFFERENTIAL DIAGNOSIS

Acne rosacea is a chronic disorder of vascular hyperreactivity that more commonly affects adults between 30 and 60 years of age. A history of recurrent facial flushing is usually obtained. Comedones are usually absent, but pustules, papules, and nodules with a predilection for the nose, cheeks, and chin are common. Persistent erythema, telangiectase, and, less commonly in women, rhinophyma may result. Perioral dermatitis often occurs in younger patients and is characterized by erythema, slight scaling, and papulopustules in a perioral, perinasal, and at times periorbital distribution. Topical corticosteroids may aggravate or uncover this condition in predisposed persons. Oral antibiotics, particularly the tetracyclines and topical metronidazole (MetroGel and MetroCream), are effective. Avoidance of stimuli that provoke flushing, such as alcohol, hot or spicy foods, and ultraviolet light, is important.

Acne cosmetica results from the frequent use of cosmetics containing lanolin, petrolatum, lauryl alcohol, butyl-stearate, vegetable oils, and oleic acid. The acne is usually of the closed comedonal type. Pomade acne is a form of acne cosmetica that occurs most frequently in African-American patients who use pomades or oils on their scalp and face that result in numerous comedones.

Occupational acne may occur in workers exposed to chlorinated hydrocarbons, cutting oils, coal tar derivatives, and animal and vegetable oils.

Acne mechanica occurs at sites of repeated trauma or friction. Acne lesions occurring under helmets, chin straps, bra straps, football shoulder pads, and headbands are examples.

Drug-induced acne may result from injury to the follicular epithelium, causing the follicular contents to spill into the dermis and resulting in an inflammatory response. Many drugs have been reported to cause or exacerbate acne; these are listed in Table 137-1. Acne may be caused by oral contraceptives and implants containing androgenic progestins. Systemic corticosteroids may cause a folliculitis consisting of monomorphous papules on the upper trunk, arms, neck, and face.

Pyoderma faciale is an uncommon form of acne, possibly related to rosacea, that typically occurs in women between ages 20 and 40 years, with the rapid onset of numerous tender papules, pustules, and nodules localized to the face. Abscess formation and a reddish discoloration of the involved areas are common, as is extensive scarring.

Acne excoriée des jeunes filles is the term used to describe patients who excoriate or manipulate their acne lesions. It is most common in adolescent girls and may be a manifestation of underlying emotional stress or obsessive-compulsive disorder.

Hidradenitis suppurativa is a chronic disease involving deep inflammatory nodules, cysts, and sinus tracts in the axilla, groin, and perianal area. Women are more frequently affected than men.

TREATMENT

Selection of therapy should take into account the type and severity of the acne lesions. The patient must be reminded that it takes several weeks for improvement to be noted, and maximal efficacy of treatment may not be apparent for at least 2 to 3 months. Topical treatment should be applied to acne-prone areas, not just individual

Table 137-1. Drugs That Cause or Exacerbate Acne or an Acneiform Eruption

ACTH	Lithium
Anabolic steroids	Phenytoin
Azathioprine	Progestins (oral and implanted)
Chloral hydrate	Quinine
Corticosteroids	Rifampin
Cyclosporine	Stanazolol
Dantrolene	Testosterone
Disulfiram	Thiouracil
Halides	Thiourea
Halothane	Vitamin B_1, B_6, B_{12} (high dose)
Isoniazid	

lesions. A list of the topical agents used in the treatment of acne is given in Table 137-2.

Noninflammatory Acne

Mild comedonal acne may respond to over-the-counter products, which generally contain 1% to 2% salicylic acid or benzoyl peroxide in concentrations of 2.5%, 5%, or 10%. Benzoyl peroxide shows bactericidal activity against *P acnes* and is mildly comedolytic. The aqueous gels are generally better tolerated than compounds prepared in an alcohol and acetone vehicle. The gel form is usually more effective than soaps, washes, and lotions but tends to be more irritating. An irritant dermatitis manifested by erythema and peeling is common and can often be circumvented by starting at a lower concentration. Contact sensitivity develops in about 1% of patients. Use of benzoyl peroxide during pregnancy has not been fully evaluated, and it is classified as a category C drug.

Moderate to severe comedonal acne may benefit from the addition of the keratolytic agent Retin-A (tretinoin) at bedtime.

Table 137-2. Topical Therapy for Acne

Azelaic acid 20% (Azelex)
Benzoyl peroxide (2.5%, 4%, 5%, 8%, 10%)
5% Benzoyl peroxide–3% erythromycin (Benzamycin gel)
Benzoyl peroxide–sulfur (Sulfoxyl lotion, regular and strong)
Tretinoin (Retin-A)
Salicylic acid
Alpha-hydroxy acids
Resorcinol
Resorcinol–sulfur
Sulfacetamide–sulfur (Novacet, Sulfacet-R)
Topical Antibiotics
Clindamycin (Cleocin T)
Erythromycin
Erythromycin–zinc (Theramycin Z)
Metronidazole (MetroGel and MetroCream)
Tetracycline (Topicycline solution)

Tretinoin is available in a cream base at concentrations of 0.025%, 0.05%, and 0.1%; the liquid is available in a 0.05% concentration. Therapy should be started with the 0.025% cream, and the concentration is gradually increased as tolerated. For the patient with very oily skin, gel formulations at a 0.01% or 0.025% concentration are available. The patient should be instructed to apply a small amount to the acne-prone areas at bedtime, 20 to 30 minutes after washing the face. Potential side effects include photosensitivity, irritation, and, rarely, a contact dermatitis. The patient should be warned that a transient pustular flare is common in the first few weeks of therapy. The combination of benzoyl peroxide in the morning and tretinoin at bedtime seems to have a synergistic effect; however, the potential for irritation is increased. Tretinoin may also allow topical antibiotics to penetrate more readily.

Open comedones can be easily removed with a comedo extractor. Closed comedones require puncture with a small needle or lancet first. Manipulation of inflamed lesions should be avoided.

Inflammatory Acne

Mild inflammatory papular acne benefits from the addition of a topical antibiotic. Choices include erythromycin in a solution, gel, or pad; clindamycin phosphate in a solution, lotion, gel, or pledget; and tetracycline in a solution (Topicycline). Topical tetracycline is rarely used because of its fluorescence under black light. A combination of 5% benzoyl peroxide and 3% erythromycin gel (Benzamycin) appears to result in less bacterial resistance than using a topical antibiotic alone. Resistance should be considered if improvement diminishes. Side effects of topical antibiotics are rare but may include local irritation and pseudomembranous colitis, which has been reported to occur with topical clindamycin.

Azelaic acid cream (Azelex) is a new topical agent for the treatment of mild to moderate inflammatory acne. The mechanism of action is unknown, but it appears to normalize keratinization and to have antimicrobial activity against *P acnes.* It is applied twice daily, and although interactions with other topical agents have not been reported, it may cause irritation or allergic contact dermatitis and hypopigmentation, which requires vigilance in darkly complected patients. Azelaic acid is classified as a pregnancy category B drug.

Unresponsive or moderate to severe inflammatory acne requires the addition of a systemic antibiotic. Systemic antibiotics decrease bacterial colonization and free fatty acid concentration in the sebum, and inflammation is decreased by inhibiting neutrophil chemotaxis. Tetracycline, erythromycin, sulfonamides, and clindamycin are effective in the treatment of inflammatory acne, and their use is summarized in Table 137-3. Systemic antibiotics must be continued for at least 6 to 8 weeks to establish whether the patient will respond. Routine laboratory testing is generally unnecessary during long-term oral antibiotic therapy in the healthy patient. Systemic antibiotics may decrease the efficacy of oral contraceptives and cause *Candida* vaginitis.

Treatment with tetracycline or erythromycin should be initiated at a dose of 500 mg twice daily. Tetracycline must be given 1 hour before or 2 hours after meals. Calcium-containing foods or supplements decrease its absorption. The estolate form of erythromycin if used during pregnancy has been associated with maternal hepatotoxicity. Tetracyclines are contraindicated during pregnancy and in children less than 12 years of age. Doxycycline hyclate or monohydrate can be substituted in doses of 50 to 100 mg twice daily, but these drugs are more photosensitizing. The monohydrate form has a decreased incidence of esophageal ulcerations. Minocycline in a dose of 50 to 100 mg twice daily is less photosensitizing and results in less resistance but may cause ototoxicity, pigmentation of the teeth and skin, hepatotoxicity, and a drug-induced systemic lupus erythematosus-like syndrome.

Gram-negative folliculitis should be suspected in the acne patient on oral antibiotics who develops multiple pustules and nodules emanating from the nasal area. A bacterial culture reveals secondary colonization with *Escherichia coli, Klebsiella*, *Pseudomonas*, or *Proteus* spp.

Severe scarring or inflammatory or nodulocystic acne that fails oral antibiotics may require referral to a dermatologist for treatment with isotretinoin (Accutane). Isotretinoin is a synthetic vitamin A derivative that affects keratinization by suppressing sebum production and diminishing the growth of *P acnes*. Its use is limited by the fact that it is a potent teratogen and has numerous side effects. The usual dose is 1 mg/kg/day in two divided doses. The range can be up to 2 mg/kg/day, with these higher doses used for back and chest involvement or for patients who failed an initial course of isotretinoin. The length of therapy is usually 15 to 20 weeks, with clinical improvement continuing after stopping the medication. Relapse is less likely to occur if a dose of at least 1 mg/kg/day is used or a total cumulative dose of 120 mg/kg is reached. However, there appears to be no additional benefit of cumulative doses of greater than 150 mg/kg.

Because of the teratogenic effect of the drug, it should be prescribed only in females who are on two forms of contraception for at least 1 month before beginning therapy and for 1 month after completing therapy. The potential side effects should be discussed both verbally and in writing with the patient. Written forms are available in a packet supplied by the manufacturer. Baseline laboratory tests, including a complete blood count, liver function tests, measurement of cholesterol and triglycerides, urinalysis, and serum or urinary pregnancy test with a sensitivity of at least 50 mIU/mL should be obtained within 1 week of starting therapy. The patient should be instructed to start therapy on the second or third day of her next normal menstrual period. A transient flare of the acne is common in the first few weeks of therapy; if severe, it may require the administration of systemic corticosteroids. Laboratory tests are then repeated after 2 weeks and at monthly intervals.

The potential side effects of this drug are numerous. Cheilitis and hypertriglyceridemia are common and may be dose-dependent. Depression, photosensitivity, elevated liver function tests, pyoderma, hair loss, proteinuria, hematuria, leukopenia, pseudotumor cerebri, headaches, and decreased night vision are some of the possible complications that should be monitored. Patients should be advised not to wear contact lenses during the course of therapy.

Individual papulonodular or nodulocystic lesions can be treated with intralesional corticosteroids. Injection of 0.05 to 0.1 mL of 1.0 to 2.5 mg of triamcinolone acetonide diluted in normal saline is performed with a 30-gauge needle. Local atrophy and hypopigmentation are potential side effects.

Hormonal Therapy

Female acne patients with abnormal hormone studies or recalcitrant acne, or those who are not candidates for isotretinoin, may respond to hormonal therapy with estrogens, glucocorticoids, or systemic antiandrogens.

Low-dose glucocorticoids, such as dexamethasone 0.125 to 0.5 mg/day or prednisone 2.5 to 5 mg/day, suppress adrenal androgen production in women with persistent acne and elevated DHEA-S levels. Treatment is often combined with an oral contraceptive.

Estrogens in a dose of 50 mg or more of ethinyl estradiol or mestranol suppress sebaceous gland activity, but the potential side effects preclude its use in most females. Low-dose estrogens in the form of oral contraceptive pills may lessen acne, particularly the newer ones that contain less androgenic progestins, such as deso-

Table 137-3. Summary of Systemic Antibiotic Therapy

DRUG	DOSE	ADVANTAGES	DISADVANTAGES
Tetracycline	250–1500 mg/day	Inexpensive	Poor compliance, GI upset
Doxycycline hyclate	50–200 mg/day	Inexpensive, improved compliance	Increased photosensitivity, esophageal ulceration
Doxycycline monohydrate	50–200 mg/day	Less esophageal irritation	Relatively expensive
Minocycline	50–200 mg/day	Low resistance, low photo-sensitivity	Expensive, vertigo-like symptoms, rare tooth and skin discoloration, Löffler-like syndrome, drug-induced lupus
Erythromycin	500–1000 mg/day	Inexpensive	30% GI upset, frequent resistance
Trimethoprim–sulfamethoxazole	1–2 double-strength tablets/day	Lipophilic, effective in gram-negative folliculitis	Bone marrow suppression, drug eruptions
Clindamycin	300–450 mg/day	Effective	Limited to short-term use, psuedomembranous colitis

gestrel (DesOgen, Ortho-Cept) or norgestimate (Ortho-Cyclen, Ortho Tri-cyclen). Recent reports, however, suggest an increased incidence of deep vein thrombosis associated with desogestrel use.

Spironolactone is an aldosterone antagonist with potent antiandrogen effects. It is effective in the treatment of acne at doses of 50 to 200 mg/day but is not labeled for this indication. Side effects include menstrual irregularities, breast tenderness, decreased blood pressure, headaches, and hyperkalemia. Spironolactone is contraindicated in pregnancy. The problem of menstrual irregularities can be ameliorated by the concomitant use of an oral contraceptive pill. Cyproterone acetate is a competitive inhibitor of the androgen receptor and is effective for acne at low doses in combination with estrogens, but it is not approved for use in the United States. Flutamide is a nonsteroidal antiandrogen with potential hepatotoxic effects and is not recommended for routine use. Finasteride is a 5α-reductase inhibitor used in the treatment of benign prostatic hyperplasia and may have a future use in the treatment of acne.

CONSIDERATIONS IN PREGNANCY

Acne can either be exacerbated or ameliorated during pregnancy. It may affect the patient's self-image differently during this time, when other bodily changes are occurring. If the patient requests treatment and if there is the potential for scarring, treatment should be offered.

Topical erythromycin for mild acne and systemic erythromycin for severe acne are acceptable therapies during pregnancy; however, the estolate form of erythromycin must be avoided during pregnancy. Gastrointestinal upset and candidal vulvovaginitis may occur and may be especially difficult to deal with during pregnancy.

Physicians treating acne in women of childbearing age, as well as during pregnancy, should be aware of the FDA pregnancy categories of prescribed medications.

BIBLIOGRAPHY

Bigby M, Stern RS. Adverse reactions to isotretinoin. A report from the Adverse Drug Reactions Reporting System. J Am Acad Dermatol 1988;18:543.

Burkman RT Jr. The role of oral contraceptives in the treatment of hyperandrogenic disorders. Am J Med 1995;98 (suppl 1A):130S.

Lucky AW, Biro FM, Huster GA, Leach AD, Morrison JA, Ratterman J. Acne vulgaris in premenarchal girls: an early sign of puberty associated with rising levels of dehydroepiandrosterone. Arch Dermatol 1994;130:308.

Nguyen QH, Kim AY, Schwartz RA. Management of acne vulgaris. Am Fam Physician 1994;50:89.

Pochi PE. The pathogenesis and treatment of acne. Ann Rev Med 1990;41:187.

Report of the Consensus of Acne Classification. J Am Acad Dermatol 1991;24:495.

Rothman, KF, Lucky AW. Acne vulgaris. Adv Dermatol 1993;8:347.

Thiboutot DM. Acne rosacea. Am Fam Physician 1994;50:1691.

Primary Care for Women, edited by Phyllis C. Leppert and Fred M. Howard. Lippincott-Raven Publishers, Philadelphia © 1997.

138

Hair Loss

MARIA K. HORDINSKY

This chapter focuses on the history, etiology, differential diagnosis, physical examination, laboratory and imaging studies, and treatment of hair diseases. Androgenetic alopecia, hirsutism, telogen effluvium hair loss, alopecia areata, structural abnormalities, and the scarring alopecias are discussed.

Hair diseases of the scalp affect both men and women, but the presentation may differ. For example, in contrast to men, women with androgenetic alopecia tend to retain their frontal hair line, presumably because of increased aromatase activity. In frontal scalp skin, aromatase aromatizes testosterone to estradiol, thereby decreasing the amount of dihydrotestosterone, the hormone implicated in the pathogenesis of androgenetic alopecia.

Women, like men, may also experience telogen effluvium hair loss, alopecia areata, or structural changes in their hair because of acquired structural hair abnormalities related to the use of hair cosmetics or grooming procedures. The development of hair loss or hair thinning related to poor nutrition or abnormal thyroid function is also common to both men and women. Permanent loss of hair follicles occurs in both men and women when there is significant inflammation or infiltration of hair follicles with tumor cells or a granulomatous process. Some examples of inflammatory diseases associated with a scarring alopecia include lichen planopilaris, pseudopelade, and discoid lupus erythematosus.

In contrast to men, women may experience changes in hair growth and structure related to excess androgen production from the ovaries. Changes in hair have also been reported during and after pregnancy. More recently, a fibrosing alopecia has been described in the frontal recession common in postmenopausal women.

Inherited hair diseases affect men and women differently depending on the mode of inheritance. For example, in one of the most common X-linked ectodermal dysplasia syndromes, Christ-Siemens-Touraine syndrome, affected males have sparse or absent body hair whereas heterozygous females exhibit less obvious hair abnormalities.

Hair loss in women, as in men, is occasionally associated with psychological changes. Sometimes the patient becomes so preoccupied with the hair loss that she becomes incapacitated; such patients may be given the diagnosis of dysmorphic syndrome.

HAIR CYCLE

Patients with hair problems often use the term "hair loss" to describe many things, including hair thinning, change in hair texture, hair breakage, a decrease in hair growth, and hair falling out by the roots. To understand this complaint, the physician must understand the hair cycle and the multitude of factors that can affect normal hair differentiation.

Hair follicles proceed through three major cycles: anagen, catagen, and telogen. Anagen is the stage of active growth and on the scalp is estimated to last up to 3 years. Catagen is the transitional stage and heralds the end of the anagen stage. During telogen, the hair follicle releases the hair fiber. These shed hairs have a club-shaped appearance, and patients frequently describe such hairs as "falling out by the roots." The duration of anagen is important to hair length and is under genetic control. Some of the factors that influence the anagen stage include age, sex, and body site.

There are an estimated 100,000 hairs on the scalp, and because 10% to 15% of these hairs may be in telogen at one time, an average daily loss of 100 telogen hairs can be expected. This number can be used as a guide when patients present with the chief complaint of hair loss. In some situations, the complaint of hair loss may reflect that hairs are breaking and not falling out by the roots. These patients may have either an inherited or acquired structural hair abnormality.

HISTORY

All patients who present with the chief complaint of hair loss should be asked routine questions to ascertain whether there is a genetic, medical, dietary, or physical explanation for the hair disorder or whether there could be more than one etiology.

Information about the onset of the hair disorder and whether it is associated with too much or too little hair elsewhere may help differentiate a genetic from an acquired hair disease. Medication use must be carefully reviewed, as many medications can affect hair growth and differentiation. The patient's past medical history may provide useful information. The physician should also ask whether there is a family history of hair diseases. Hair-care procedures and products need to be reviewed, as they can cause or aggravate hair loss.

ANDROGENETIC ALOPECIA

History

For a woman presenting with androgenetic alopecia, the clinician must ascertain whether the hair problem is related to pituitary, adrenal, or ovarian disease or the use of specific hormones such as those found in birth-control pills, anabolic steroids, and replacement therapy (or lack thereof) in the postmenopausal period. The patient should be questioned about her menstrual cycle, pregnancy history, use of oral contraceptives or hormone replacement therapy, and history of infertility, galactorrhea, hirsutism, virilization, or severe cystic acne. Another clue to the diagnosis is the complaint that the patient's hair is less dense and that her hair style has become shorter to compensate for this. Some patients report that their androgenetic alopecia became noticeable after an episode of telogen effluvium, as often occurs after childbirth.

Etiology and Differential Diagnosis

Androgenetic alopecia is an inherited, androgen-dependent condition. The male pattern of androgenetic alopecia does occur in women, but more commonly the part width widens and there is a diffuse decrease in hair density on the crown. Androgenetic alopecia is related to increased reduction of testosterone to dihydrotestosterone by the enzyme 5α-reductase. Androgenetic alopecia not associated with underlying endocrinologic problems is considered idiopathic and is the main presentation of androgen excess in most women. However, 30% to 40% of patients have underlying adrenal or ovarian disease associated with the androgenetic alopecia. If the underlying disease is addressed, the hair disease may also improve.

Androgens are thought to regulate hair growth by acting on the dermal papilla cells, which in turn influence other follicular components. In addition to skin, the major sources of androgens in women are the ovaries and adrenal glands. The same enzymatic pathways are used by the ovaries and adrenal glands for the production of androgens. However, the ovaries do not produce cortisol or aldosterone, and the adrenal gland does not produce estrogen or progesterone. When androgens are released, only a small fraction exists as free steroid. About 80% of circulating testosterone is bound to sex hormone binding globulin (SHBG) and 19% to albumin; about 1% remains unbound. This implies that whenever SHBG levels are decreased, levels of free testosterone increase and androgenetic alopecia may worsen.

An inflammatory infiltrate is typically present in androgenetic alopecia at the bulge region, the site of hair follicle stem cells. The role of this inflammation is not well understood.

Physical Examination

Women experience diffuse thinning, most pronounced over the frontal/temporal scalp. This is often preceded by a telogen effluvium type of hair loss. The density is typically greater over the occipital scalp and the hair along the frontal hairline, which may be straight or M-shaped. The central part appears widened because of increased spacing between the hairs. The hairs here become miniaturized and vary in diameter and length. In general, women follow the pattern described by Ludwig:

- Ludwig grade I: perceptible thinning of the hair on the crown with no loss of the frontal hair line and a relatively normal part width
- Ludwig grade II: pronounced thinning of the hair on the crown and an increase in the part width
- Ludwig grade III: extreme baldness on the crown and further widening of the part width (Fig. 138-1).

Male androgenetic alopecia is usually described using the Hamilton classification system, later modified by Norwood. In this system, the balding process begins with bitemporal recession, followed by midfrontal and vertex recession to the point where there is increased loss from the vertex and frontotemporal region, with the areas of baldness eventually becoming confluent. An estimated 80% of women develop type II androgenetic alopecia (bitemporal recession) after puberty, and about 25% develop type IV androgenetic alopecia by age 50. In uncomplicated androgenetic alopecia, there is no evidence of hair breakage, patchy loss, or scarring, but the distal hair fiber ends are thinner.

Laboratory and Imaging Studies

Usually the diagnosis of androgenetic alopecia is made from the history and clinical findings. An extensive hormonal evaluation is usually unnecessary if the patient has no menstrual irregularities, hirsutism, severe cystic acne, infertility, galactorrhea, or history of infertility. However, if any of these are present, levels of free and total testosterone, dehydroepiandrosterone sulfate (DHEA-S), and prolactin should be measured. Subtle abnormalities may also exist in the adrenal steroidogenic pathway; these can be detected only by adrenocorticotropic hormone (ACTH) stimulation tests. Patients with virilization

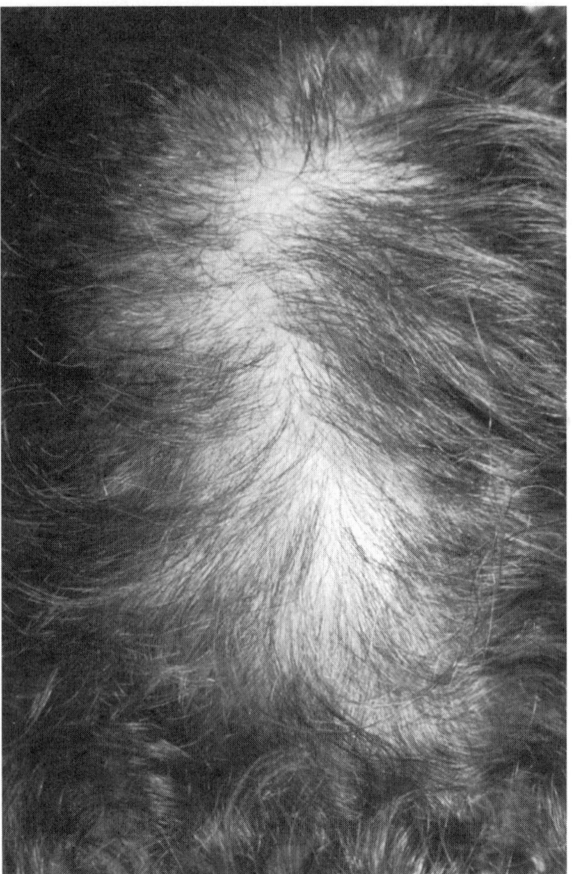

Figure 138-1. Grade II female androgenetic alopecia.

and androgenetic alopecia probably have a significant abnormality in androgen metabolism; an underlying tumor must be ruled out.

Additional laboratory studies can be ordered to exclude other common causes of diffuse hair loss and thinning, as concurrent diseases could be present. Tests measuring the levels of thyroid-stimulating hormone, serum iron, and ferritin and the total iron-binding capacity and a complete white blood count can be ordered to rule out anemia or thyroid disease.

Analysis of vertical and horizontal scalp biopsy samples (4 mm in diameter) may be useful. Such an analysis may establish the diagnosis of androgenetic alopecia and can provide information about the number of follicular units, the number of hairs in anagen and in telogen, and the degree of hair differentiation, which be helpful in predicting responsiveness to therapy. For example, a patient with significant follicular dropout will probably not respond well to therapy; instead, she may benefit most from a surgical procedure to correct the balding process.

Treatment

The goals of treatment are to decrease further hair thinning and to promote hair regrowth. Minoxidil is the only drug approved by the FDA for female androgenetic alopecia; application of 2% minoxidil topically promotes hair growth in women with androgenetic alopecia. The recommended daily application is 1 cc twice daily. Hair growth typically peaks at 1 year. When therapy is discontinued, the hair gained is usually lost within 4 to 6 months after stopping drug application.

Antiandrogens have been used topically, orally, or intralesionally to retard hair loss and to try to regrow hair. Antiandrogens may inhibit either the conversion of testosterone to dihydrotestosterone by 5-α reductase (finasteride) or dihydrotestosterone binding to the steroid receptor. Estrogens decrease ovarian and adrenal androgen production and stimulate SHBG from the liver. Spironolactone decreases testosterone production by the adrenal gland. It affects the cytochrome P-450 enzyme system, a system needed for the 17-hydroxylase and desmolase enzymes to synthesize androgens. Spironolactone is also a mild competitive inhibitor of dihydrotestosterone binding to the androgen receptor, thereby interfering with the translocation of the receptor complex to the nucleus. Progesterone and 17-α progesterone are competitive inhibitors. However, these agents themselves have an androgenic potential that can potentially aggravate the hair loss problem.

Other therapies that have been tried include penetration enhancers such as SEPA or topical tretinoin in conjunction with topical minoxidil. The nonsteroidal drugs flutamide and cimetidine have also been tried, with limited success. Cyproterone acetate is a potent antiandrogen that is used in Europe but is unavailable in the United States.

Hair dyes, permanent waving, sprays, and mousses can be recommended to the woman with androgenetic alopecia. Camouflage techniques may also be used to hide the extent of disease. The use of creams, crayons, and sprays may be helpful. Some patients find integration pieces, hair swatches, hair weaving, and scalp prostheses (full or partial) to be beneficial. Surgical removal of the involved area is another alternative.

Considerations in Pregnancy

No unnecessary drugs should be used during pregnancy, and this includes the use of agents that promote hair growth. Antiandrogens can affect the fetus, and feminization of the male fetus may occur.

HIRSUTISM

History

The patient with hirsutism should be asked the same questions as the patient with androgenetic alopecia. In both cases, the clinician must try to determine whether there is evidence for pituitary, adrenal, or ovarian disease.

Etiology and Differential Diagnosis

The main causes of androgen dysfunction in females include abnormalities in the pituitary/adrenal and pituitary/ovarian axes or abnormal target cell hormone metabolism and use. Many drugs may also cause hirsutism, including progestational agents, steroids, and testosterone. Hyperprolactinemia may be associated with hirsutism and may be the result of a pituitary adenoma, hypothalamic disease, or hypothyroidism. The exact mechanism by which hyperprolactinemia leads to hyperandrogenism is unclear but is thought to involve a direct effect on adrenal or ovarian steroidogenesis or decreased SHBG.

Physical Examination

The degree of hirsutism may be assessed using the Ferriman and Gallwey scoring system (Fig. 138-2). In this system, 11 body areas are assessed, with a maximum grade of 4 points for each area. This scale was later modified to include only the following nine body areas with sex hormone-sensitive hair follicles: upper lip, chin, chest, upper abdomen, lower abdomen, arm, thigh, upper back, and lower back. The degree of hair growth in each area is then graded from 1 (minimal terminal hair) to 4 (frank virilization). The scores are summed, and a total score of 8 or more indicates hirsutism. In women with hirsutism and amenorrhea, or those with signs of virilization, a pelvic examination and radiographic tests may be indicated.

Laboratory and Imaging Studies

Screening studies for women with hirsutism, like those for women with androgenetic alopecia, include measurement of serum testosterone, DHEA-S, 17-hydroxyprogesterone, follicle-stimulating hormone (FSH), luteinizing hormone (LH), and prolactin levels. If the serum testosterone level is normal and the menses are regular, the patient probably has idiopathic hirsutism. A serum testosterone level above 200 ng/dL with a mildly elevated serum DHEA-S level suggests an ovarian tumor. An elevated DHEA-S level is very suggestive of an adrenal tumor. If Cushing syndrome is suspected, an ACTH stimulation test is recommended. 17-hydroxyprogesterone has been used as a screening test for late-onset congenital adrenal hyperplasia, but it is now recommended that this be done (if at all) with an ACTH stimulation test. A high-dose dexamethasone test may help distinguish Cushing disease from Cushing syndrome from ectopic ACTH production or an adrenal tumor. If a tumor is suspected, sonography, computed tomography, and magnetic resonance imaging may be indicated. Patients with polycystic ovarian disease have elevated serum concentrations of testosterone, and their LH/FSH ratio often exceeds 3 : 1.

Treatment

Whenever possible, the underlying cause of the hirsutism should be treated. The antiandrogens used to treat hirsutism include oral contraceptives, spironolactone, glucocorticoids, cimetidine, and flutamide. The use of oral contraceptives is considered if the elevated level of androgens can be attributed to the ovary. The estrogen component of oral contraceptives decreases ovarian and adrenal androgen production and stimulates production of SHBG from the liver. Typically, oral contraceptives with an estrogen and progestin of low androgen activity are prescribed.

Spironolactone has been used for years to treat hirsutism, with about 25% of patients noting improvement after 6 months of use. Doses used range from 100 to 200 mg/day.

Glucocorticoids suppress adrenal androgen production. Dexamethasone is prescribed in doses of 0.25 to 0.75 mg at night to reduce ACTH secretion, with 30% to 50% of patients demonstrating improvement. The treatment of Cushing syndrome depends on the cause. Bromocriptine may be used in the treatment of hyper-

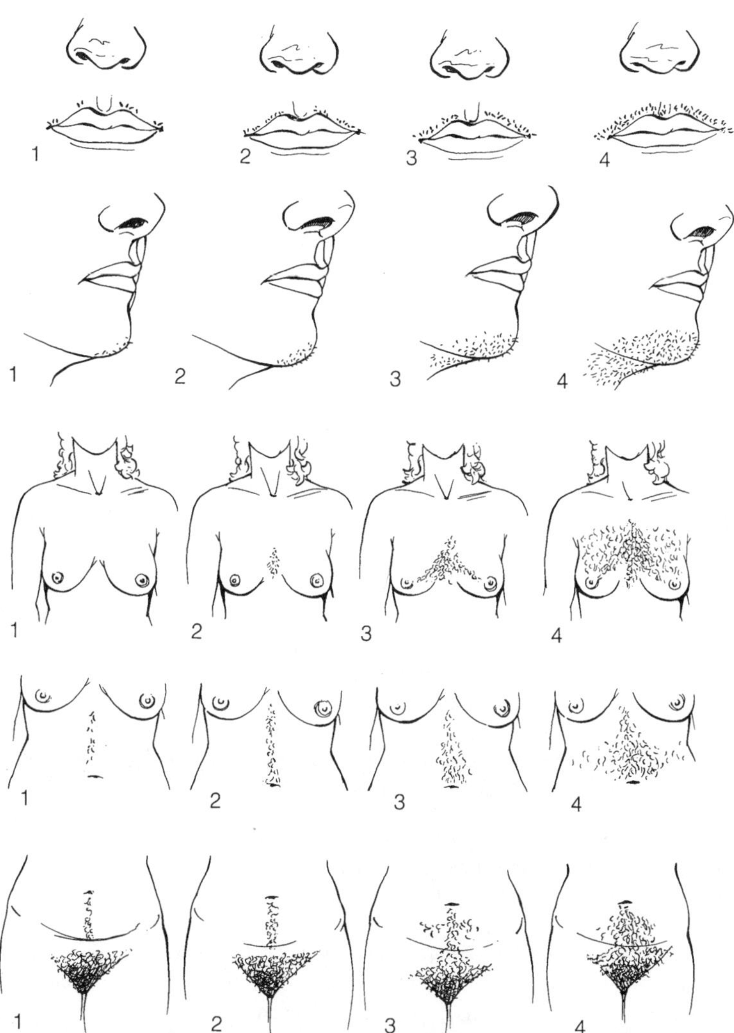

Figure 138-2. Hirsutism scoring standards, showing the spectrum from minimal hirsutism (grade 1) to frank virilization (grade 4) in several body regions. The scores in each of these areas are summed: a total score of 8 or more indicates hirsutism. (Redrawn from Hatch R, Rosenfield RL, Kim MH, Tredway D. Hirsutism: implications, etiology, and management. Am J Obstet Gynecol, 1981;140:815. Used by permission. Adapted from Ferriman D, Gallwey JD. Clinical assessment of body hair growth in women. J Clin Endocrinol Metab 1961;21:1440, and Lorenzo EM. Familial study of hirsutism. J Clin Endocrinol Metab 1970;31:556. *(continues)*.

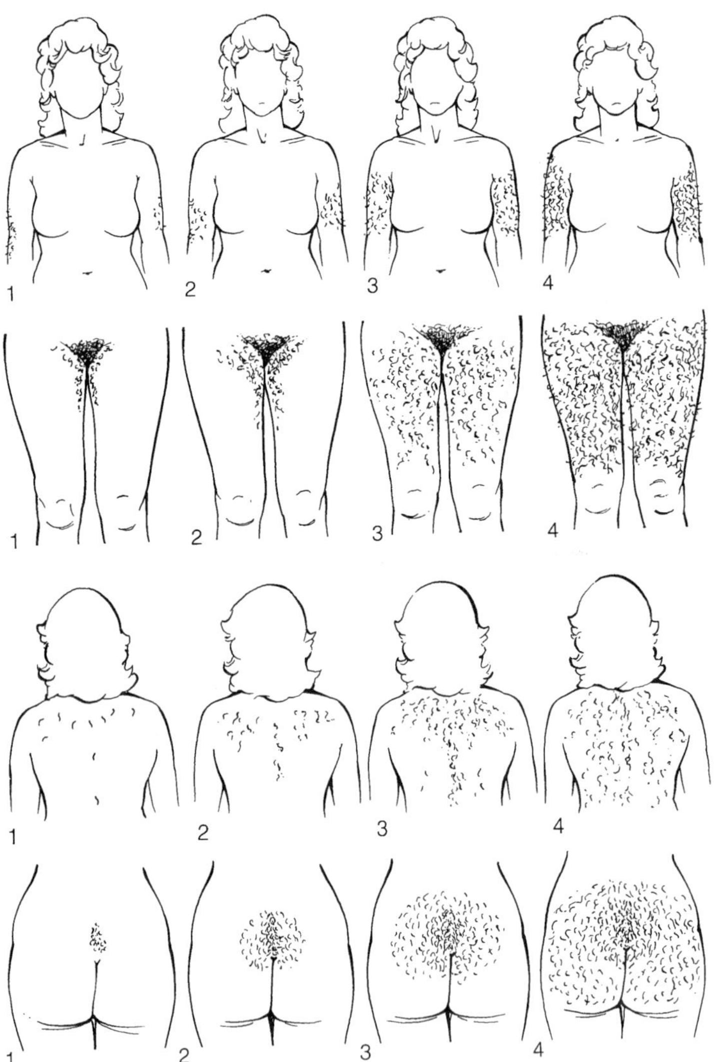

Figure 138-2. (*Continued.*)

prolactinemia. Virilizing ovarian or adrenal tumors usually must be surgically removed.

Cosmetic procedures can also be helpful. Depending on the body region, plucking, shaving, waxing, and bleaching can be recommended.

Considerations in Pregnancy

Antiandrogens can be associated with feminization of the male fetus.

TELOGEN EFFLUVIUM

History

Immediate, short, and delayed anagen and immediate and delayed telogen release have been implicated in telogen effluvium hair loss. Patients who experience a telogen effluvium hair loss characterized by immediate anagen release often report an association with a drug or a history of physiologic stress (including episodes of high fever). Delayed anagen release is most commonly associated with postpartum hair loss, whereas short anagen telogen effluvium hair loss appears to characterize patients who experience increased shedding associated with decreased hair length. One factor in the history that may be relevant to identifying delayed telogen release is discovering increased hair loss occurring with travel from areas of low daylight to those of high daylight, suggesting that in some women, light affects the hair cycle.

Etiology and Differential Diagnosis

The diffuse hair loss seen with telogen effluvium typically affects the entire scalp, but bitemporal recession may become prominent. Typically, a normal hair cycle is resumed after the telogen effluvium process has resolved. Five types of telogen effluvium hair loss have been proposed:

- Immediate anagen release is very common and affects follicles by having them prematurely leave anagen and enter telogen. It may be related to the use of drugs, a high fever, or another physiologic stress.
- Delayed anagen release is associated with postpartum hair loss.
- Short anagen characterizes patients with persistent hair loss. These patients cannot grow long hair.

- Immediate telogen release is characterized by a shortened normal telogen and initiation of anagen and is thought to occur with drugs such as minoxidil.
- In delayed telogen release, hair shedding occurs after a period of decreased shedding. In some cases, it may be seen at predictable times.

Physical Examination

The physical examination may be relatively unremarkable. However, the patient with an active telogen effluvium has positive light hair pull tests, demonstrating primarily telogen hairs (Fig. 138-3).

Laboratory and Imaging Studies

The patient typically presents after the most active hair shedding has occurred. Therefore, most of the tests that can be easily done may not exclude the diagnosis of telogen effluvium, as the hair disease may be resolving.

Clip and pull tests may be helpful. A clip test is done by grasping 25 to 30 hairs between the thumb and forefinger at the scalp. The hair sample is cut with scissors, and hair 1 cm or so above the fingers is cut and discarded. The remaining sample is transferred to a glass slide, held in place with a mounting medium, and then covered with a coverslip. Hair shaft diameters are evaluated under the microscope. In a negative test, the hair shafts are of nearly uniform diameter; fewer than 10% of the shafts are of small diameter. In patients with a resolving telogen effluvium, typically more than 10% of the hairs are of small diameter.

Pull tests are done by grasping 25 to 30 hairs and extracting them from the scalp by hand or with an instrument. In the normal scalp, fewer than five or six telogen hairs are detected.

If the patient presents with diffuse, active hair loss and a positive light hair pull test, a scalp biopsy (two 4-mm punch biopsies

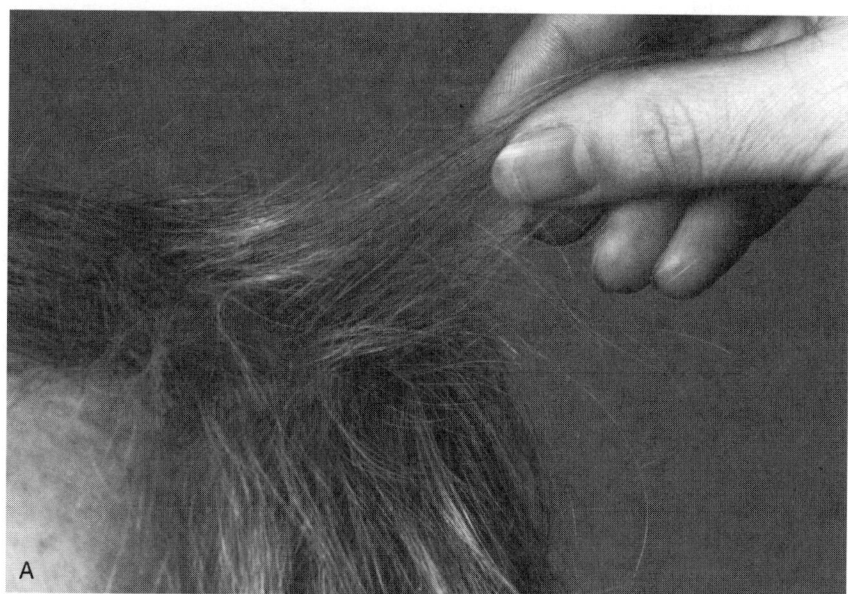

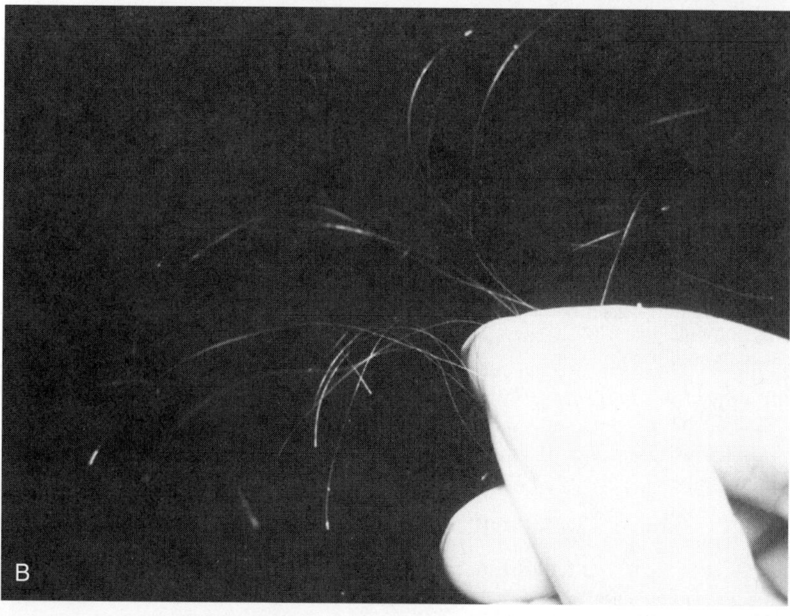

Figure 138-3. (***A***) Patient with telogen effluvium hair loss. (***B***) Positive light hair pull test from the same patient. A similar finding is seen in patients with diffuse, active alopecia areata.

for vertical and horizontal sectioning) is helpful to differentiate telogen effluvium hair loss from active alopecia areata. Establishing the correct diagnosis ensures that the patient is properly counseled.

Women who are anemic or nutritionally deficient or who have thyroid disease may present with a telogen effluvium hair loss. Therefore, it may be helpful to measure levels of thyroid-stimulating hormone, serum iron, transferrin, and ferritin, to check the iron-binding capacity, and to perform a hematologic screen. Copper and zinc levels could be checked in women thought to have a poor diet.

Treatment

In general, the prognosis is good with most cases of telogen effluvium, particularly cases of seasonal telogen effluvium and immediate anagen release effluvium due to drugs or acute-onset physiologic events. Hair growth after delayed anagen release postpartum is usually reversible, but the hair density may not return to that before pregnancy.

Once the diagnosis has been established, patients must be taught about the hair cycle and advised that hair growth will occur. Hair grows at about 0.25 mm/day, so some time will pass before the patient sees significant growth. Patients with short anagen syndrome may be responsive to a drug such as 2% topical minoxidil; this drug may prolong the anagen stage, allowing the opportunity to grow long hair. Correcting an underlying abnormality such as iron deficiency may also be associated with a decrease in hair shedding and hair regrowth, but this cannot be guaranteed.

Considerations in Pregnancy

During pregnancy, many women report that their hair appears thicker. It has been suggested that estrogens prolong the anagen stage or that there is a delayed telogen release because of the need to conserve metabolic resources. Pregnant women and women in the postpartum period who complain of diffuse hair loss should have their iron metabolism, hematologic profile, and thyroid status examined. If they are found to be hypothyroid or anemic, replacement therapy can be initiated; hair loss may decrease and regrowth may be seen.

ALOPECIA AREATA

History

The etiology of alopecia areata remains unknown, but most investigators agree that it is mediated by the immune system and probably is an autoimmune disease. In most epidemiologic studies, alopecia areata has generally been grouped with atopic diseases such as asthma, atopic dermatitis, and allergic rhinitis, or with other autoimmune diseases such as pernicious anemia, ulcerative colitis, or thyroiditis. In addition to the general questions asked of all patients presenting with hair loss, patients with alopecia areata should be questioned about autoimmune diseases and stressful life events, as many patients report a significant event around the time the alopecia areata developed. In most studies, alopecia areata patients with atopy have been found to have a more severe form of the disease. These patients may also have a longer disease duration. Obtaining this history is therefore important.

Etiology and Differential Diagnosis

Alopecia areata is thought to be an immunologically mediated disease. Other theories are that it is an inherited disease, is mediated by the nervous system, or is related to exposure to chemicals or infectious agents. Alopecia areata is characterized in its limited form by circumscribed patches of alopecia with well-demarcated borders between normal and affected scalp. There typically is no prior history of inflammation. Disease extent may progress from this limited form to complete loss of all scalp and body hair (alopecia totalis and alopecia universalis). Alopecia areata typically recurs and is sometimes refractory to treatment.

Alopecia areata is usually easy to diagnose, but patients with less common variants may be misdiagnosed. For example, the patient with the diffuse variant may be diagnosed as having trichotillomania, a hair-pulling disorder.

Physical Examination

The most common presentation is a round or oval patch of hair loss. This type of nonscarring alopecia may progress to total scalp hair loss or to total body hair loss (Fig. 138-4). Variants from this pattern include the reticular and diffuse variants. Patients with the reticular variant experience loss of hair in one site, concurrent with spontaneous hair regrowth in another site. Those with the diffuse variant cannot grow long anagen hairs in involved areas.

In early active alopecia areata, most hair follicles convert to telogen. The light hair pull test, done by lightly pulling on several hairs, reveals telogen hairs. Fractured hairs, which appear as black dots on the scalp, may also be seen; these reflect the distal segment of a hair that fractured as it exited the scalp. Patients who do not regrow normal terminal hair may appear totally bald or may show short, white, vellus, or indeterminate hair regrowth that may come and go.

Laboratory and Imaging Studies

Alopecia areata is commonly associated with the atopic conditions asthma, allergic rhinitis, and atopic dermatitis, as well as diseases of the thyroid gland. It has also been associated with several autoimmune diseases. Children with alopecia areata often have circulating antibodies to thyroid microsome and thyroglobulin. Therefore, assessment of thyroid function may be indicated, including the presence of antibodies to thyroid microsome or thyroglobulin. Other laboratory tests may be ordered, depending on the history and physical examination.

Scalp biopsies may be useful for diagnostic purposes and possibly for predicting responsiveness to therapy. When the patient presents with diffuse active hair loss, it may be difficult to differentiate active alopecia areata from telogen effluvium hair loss. Establishing an accurate diagnosis with an evaluation of a scalp biopsy specimen then becomes important, as the outcome for each hair disease is so different. In contrast, when a patient presents with extensive hair loss and seeks a treatment to induce hair growth, it becomes important to document follicular dropout or loss, the presence or absence of inflammation, and the predominant stage of the hair cycle, as all these factors can influence the choice of therapy and outcome.

Treatment

Many treatments may help stimulate hair growth in alopecia areata, but at best they only suppress the underlying process. The

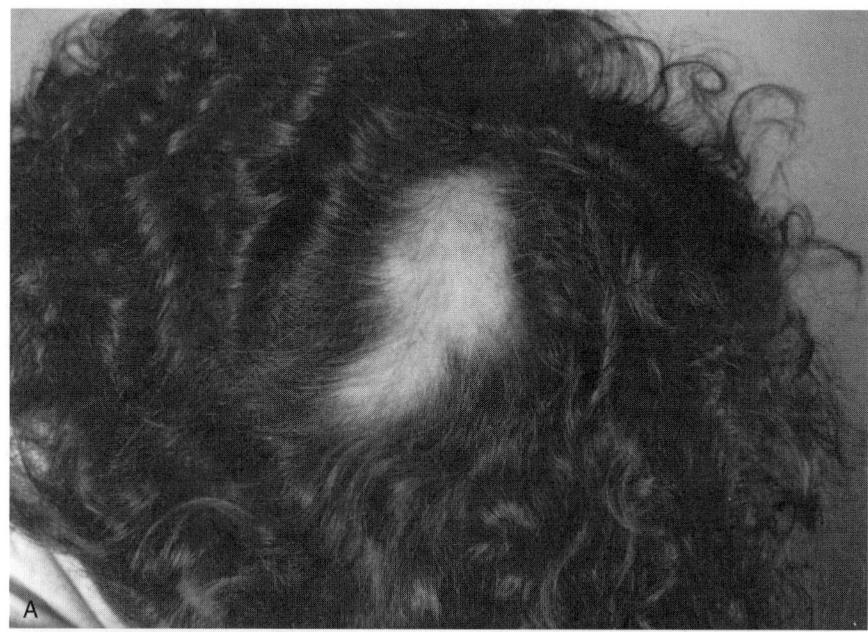

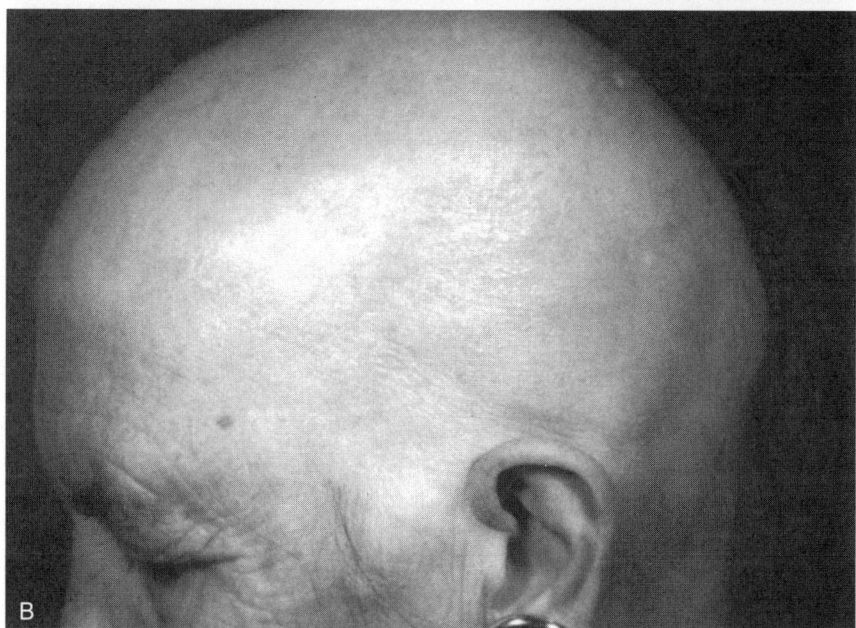

Figure 138-4. (***A***) Patchy alopecia areata. (***B***) Extensive alopecia areata.

most commonly used treatments are immunomodulating agents and the irritant anthralin. Of the many immunomodulating agents, topical and intralesional corticosteroids are the most commonly prescribed. These can be used successfully in patchy, limited alopecia areata, but their efficacy is diminished when more than 50% of the scalp is involved. The minimum strength or class of topical steroid to use to manage alopecia areata has not been determined, although it appears as if 1% hydrocortisone is too weak. The maximum effective strength remains to be determined. Different intralesional steroid preparations are also available. The most commonly used are triamcinolone acetonide or triamcinolone hexacetonide, in a dosage of 10 mg/mL for scalp lesions and 3 to 5 mg/mL for eyebrow areas. Complications include atrophy, telangiectasias, folliculitis, hypertrichosis, and acneiform eruptions. In addition, the administration of intralesional injections can be painful. Intralesional injections are typically administered every 6 to 8 weeks. Topical therapy can be continued for several months, as long as the patient is responsive and there are no complications.

The mechanism by which anthralin regrows hair is unknown. The use of anthralin cream (Dritho-Creme) can be initiated at low concentrations, and as tolerated the concentration can be raised up to 1% to maintain a clinical response. Specific scalp preparations of anthralin are available and can be used in place of the cream formulations.

Considerations in Pregnancy

All unnecessary drugs, including those prescribed for the therapy of alopecia areata, should be discontinued during pregnancy. Exacerbation and remission of the disease can be seen during pregnancy. Patients with alopecia areata who experience a postpartum thyroiditis may also experience a flare of alopecia areata.

STRUCTURAL HAIR ABNORMALITIES

History

Structural hair abnormalities may be acquired or inherited, so it is important to ask whether the abnormality has been present from birth. A thorough review of hair-care habits is recommended: in either case, some hair-care habits may injure the hair fiber, particularly fibers that are already abnormal. Questions about sun exposure, hair styling, the frequency of shampooing, the use of hair-care products, and activities such as swimming may help the clinician discern the etiology of a structural hair abnormality.

Etiology and Differential Diagnosis

The normal hair shaft consists of three major parts: the cortex, cuticle, and medulla. Structural abnormalities have been divided into four main categories: fractures, irregularities, twisting, and extraneous matter. Fractures may be related to a genetic disease such as monilethrix or physical or chemical trauma. Irregularities can be seen in congenital or acquired hair diseases, as can coiling and twisting of the hair fiber. Extraneous matter on the hair shaft includes fungi, bacteria, or lice. A unique acquired abnormality is "bubble hair," characterized by bubble-like areas in the hair shaft caused by heat, as from a hair dryer.

Physical Examination

Patients may present with short hair and the chief complaint that their hair does not grow. This typically occurs in patients with structural hair abnormalities that result in fractures when the hair is manipulated, as with combing or brushing. Other patients may present with unruly hair related to knotting of the hair, the presence of longitudinal grooves, or pili bifurcati (Fig. 138-5). Patients with short, fine, brittle, dry hair from birth probably have a type of ectodermal dysplasia.

Laboratory and Imaging Studies

To be significant, hair shaft abnormalities should be seen consistently on hairs from different areas of the scalp. Hair samples

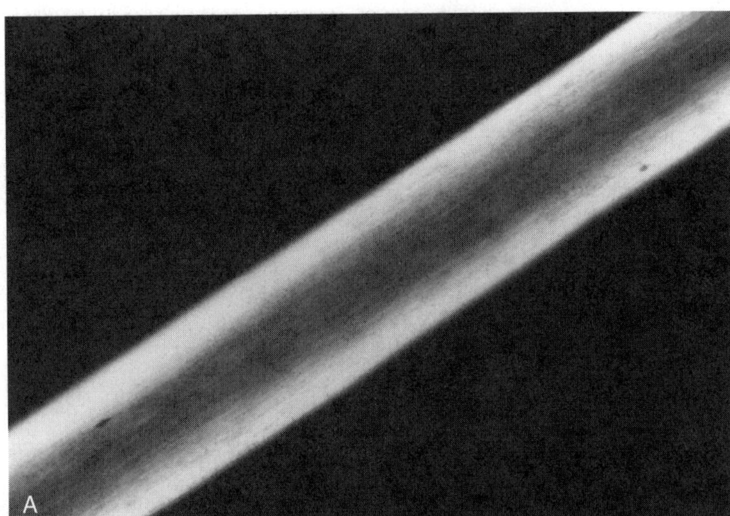

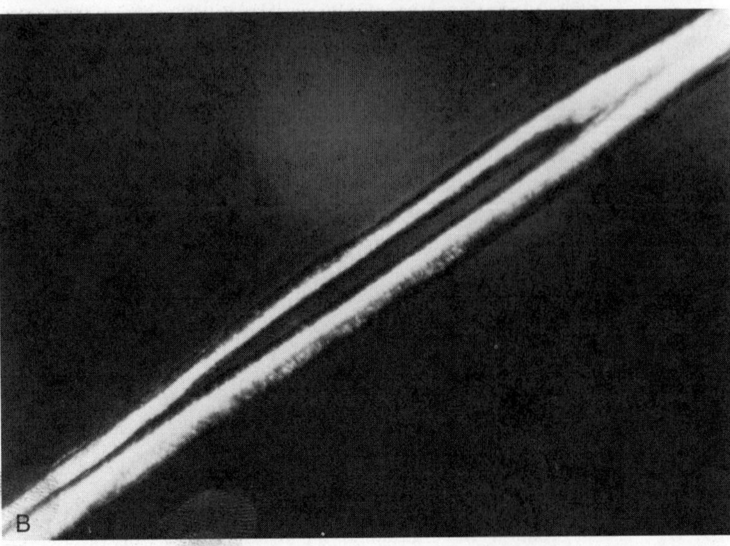

Figure 138-5. Light microscopic examination of hair mounts from (***A***) a normal person and (***B***) a patient with uncombable hair syndrome.

should be cut at the base of the scalp and mounted in parallel on glass slides previously coated with double-faced clear tape or a mounting medium. The latter provides a permanent preparation that is free of optical distortion when examined microscopically. Scanning electron microscopy may be helpful in further identifying the structural abnormality. Polarization of mounted hairs may demonstrate alternating light and dark bands characteristic of trichothiodystrophy.

Treatment

When a structural hair abnormality is present, the hair fiber is more prone to breakage and weathering. Therefore, simple measures such as using conditioners and avoiding the use of hair dryers may help avoid additional damage. For patients with woolly hair or uncombable hair syndrome, hair straightening methods may be tried. These can minimize the unruly appearance.

Considerations in Pregnancy

Structural hair abnormalities are usually not affected during pregnancy.

SCARRING ALOPECIAS

History

Patients with a scarring alopecia who do not have an antecedent history of scalp symptoms, trauma, or infections may have pseudopelade. Others, as is the case with patients with lichen planopilaris, may have an antecedent history of lichen planus. Patients should be questioned about the presence of other dermatologic diseases that could manifest themselves on the scalp as a scarring alopecia. Recession of the frontal hairline commonly occurs in postmenopausal women. Typically, this is a nonscarring alopecia, but in some cases a perifollicular erythema develops that may be associated with a frontal fibrosing alopecia.

Etiology and Differential Diagnosis

Permanent loss of a hair follicle occurs if the follicle is destroyed by inflammation, related either to an infectious process or to a primary skin disease of the scalp such as lichen planopilaris. Similarly, permanent scarring occurs if the hair-bearing area becomes infiltrated with a granulomatous process such as sarcoidosis or tumor cells, as can be seen with metastatic disease to the scalp. Postmenopausal frontal fibrosing alopecia, a newly described variant, may be a variant of lichen planopilaris or may be a unique entity.

Physical Examination

Pseudopelade presents with small, glistening white patches of alopecia that resemble footprints in the snow. There is usually no associated erythema or scale. Patients with lichen planus show atrophic, circumscribed patches with hyperkeratotic follicular areas and surrounding scale. in some cases, follicular spinous keratotic papules are present. If the scarring process is chronic, white areas of scalp are apparent. The scarring alopecia called "tufted hair folliculitis" presents with areas of scarring and tufts of hairs emerging from single openings. There is often an associated superficial staphylococcal infection. Women with postmenopausal frontal fibrosing alopecia of the scalp show prominent frontal and frontoparietal recession associated with pale, smooth skin.

Patients with infiltrative processes or primary dermatologic diseases associated with scarring require a biopsy to make the correct diagnosis and formulate a treatment plan. Patients with infectious processes involving the scalp may develop a scarring alopecia if the underlying infectious disease is not treated.

Laboratory and Imaging Studies

Hair follicles can be destroyed for many reasons. Infiltrative and infectious processes can destroy the hair follicle, as can primary diseases of the scalp and hair follicle. Therefore, a scalp biopsy can help establish the etiology. If the entire scalp is not scarred and the disease is still active in some hair-bearing areas, it may be useful to take biopsies of both areas. A 4-mm biopsy taken from a scarred area provides information about the degree of scarring. If no or few follicles are present, the patient may elect to have a surgical procedure to remove the scarred areas. In contrast, a biopsy taken from an area of active hair loss may provide information about the diagnosis. If an immunobullous disease is suspected, another biopsy can be obtained for immunofluorescence examination. If purulent drainage is present, the material should be cultured for bacteria and fungi.

Treatment

When *Staphylococcus aureus* is cultured from the skin of patients with inflammatory scalp diseases, antibiotic treatment may need to be prescribed for many weeks to eradicate the organism. If the scarring alopecia is related to an infiltrative process identified on biopsy, treatment should be directed toward the underlying process, whether a malignancy or a granulomatous process. Similarly, if a connective tissue disease or blistering disease is identified, treatment should be directed toward the primary disease. If the primary cause of the scarring alopecia is physical and the result of an injury such as a burn, the affected area can be removed surgically.

Considerations in Pregnancy

Unnecessary treatments should be avoided during pregnancy.

BIBLIOGRAPHY

Fanti PA, Tosti A, Bardazzi F, Guerra L, Morelli R, Cameli N. Alopecia areata. A pathologic study of nonresponder patients. Am J Dermatol 1994;16:167.

Ferriman D, Gallwey JD. Clinical assessment of body hair growth in women. J Clin Endocrinol Metab 1961;21:1440.

Hatch R, Rosenfield RL, Kim MH, Tredway D. Hirsutism: implications, etiology, and management. Am J Obstet Gynecol 1981;1140:815.

Headington JT. Telogen effluvium. Arch Dermatol 1993;129:356.

Hordinsky M. Alopecia areata. In: Olsen ED, ed. Disorders of hair growth. New York: McGraw-Hill, 1994:195.

Leung AKC. Hirsutism. Int J Dermatol 1993;32:773.

Kossard S. Postmenopausal frontal fibrosing alopecia. Arch Dermatol 1994;130:770.

Maffei C, Fossati A, Rinaldi F, Riva E. Personality disorders and psychopathologic symptoms in patients with androgenetic alopecia. Arch Dermatol 1994;130:868.

Moyes AL, Hordinsky MK, Holland E. Ectodermal dysplasias. In: Diseases of the eye and skin. New York: Raven Press (in press).

Nayar M, Schomberg K, Dawber RPR, Millard PR. A clinicopathological study of scarring alopecia. Br J Dermatol 1993;128:533.

Olsen E. Androgenetic alopecia. In: Olsen ED, ed. Disorders of hair growth. New York: McGraw-Hill, 1994:257.

Rushton DH, Ramsay ID, James KC, Norris MJ, Gilkes JJH. Biochemical and trichological characterization of diffuse alopecia in women. Br J Dermatol 1990;123:187.

Sawaya ME, Hordinsky MK. The antiandrogens. Dermatol Clin 1993;11:65.

Siegel SF, Finegold DN, Lanes R, Lee PA. ACTH stimulation tests and plasma dehydroepiandrosterone sulfate levels in women with hirsutism. N Engl J Med 1990;323:849.

Whiting DA. Structural abnormalities of the hair shaft. J Am Acad Dermatol 1987;16:1.

139
Eczema

SOPHIE M. WOROBEC

Primary Care for Women, edited by Phyllis C. Leppert and Fred M. Howard. Lippincott-Raven Publishers, Philadelphia © 1997.

Eczema or atopic dermatitis is characterized by skin inflammation and itching. It usually occurs in persons with a personal or family history of at least one manifestation of the atopic triad of asthma, allergic rhinitis, and eczema. Eczema usually starts before age 5 years. The appearance of lesions varies with their duration: acute lesions present with erythema, edema, and vesicles, and lesions of longer standing or chronic eczematous lesions are characterized by skin thickening or lichenification and scaling. The distribution is predominantly facial and on extensor surfaces in infants, but in later childhood the areas of involvement become flexural, involving the wrists and the antecubital and popliteal fossae. Adults may continue to have pruritic erythematous or lichenified lesions or may simply have "sensitive skin," with itching brought on by mechanical friction (as from wool fabrics), temperature changes, or excessive bathing with hot water. Variants of eczema include nummular eczema, lichen simplex chronicus or neurodermatitis, hand dermatitis, and dyshidrotic eczema.

The prevalence of eczema is believed to have increased in the past decade to over 10%. The cause of this increase is not well understood, but theories include urbanization, with exposure to multiple allergens, and increased washing and bathing, with increased skin dryness. Studies of immigrant populations have demonstrated an increased incidence of eczema among Chinese immigrants to Hawaii and among the London-born children of African-Caribbean parents.

ETIOLOGY AND DIFFERENTIAL DIAGNOSIS

Primary care physicians are often asked what causes eczema and must be able to answer questions about the role of allergens and how to avoid various trigger factors of itching. The etiology of eczema is unknown. Studies suggest that in some patients, ingested foods or inhaled allergens may aggravate or cause a flare of dermatitis. IgE elevations are found in 40% to 80% of patients, and those who have concomitant asthma or allergic rhinitis have the highest IgE levels. However, these high IgE levels may not be causal, as many patients with classic atopic dermatitis do not have IgE elevations. In some patients, a challenge with certain foods (eg, eggs, peanuts, milk, soy, wheat, fish) causes itching, followed by an erythematous rash within 2 hours. The frequency of a food-aggravated pathogenesis is unknown and may be related to a subset of patients with a food-induced urticaria that on subsequent scratching becomes eczematous. There is no shortcut alternative to detecting these patients with a challenge and controlled observation, because the food allergens correlate poorly with positive immediate skin tests or radioallergosorbent (RAST) food tests. Other allergens suspected of playing a role in eczema include house dust mites, pollens, and animal dander. One theory is that the chronic exposure to and introduction of these allergens into traumatized skin keeps the eczematous reaction going rather than an IgE-mediated reaction.

The skin of atopic patients is often colonized by *Staphylococcus aureus*, but fewer than 5% of nonatopics carry *S aureus*. This bacterial pathogen may be another source of antigenic stimulation in the atopic patient, as elevated levels of serum IgE directed against *S aureus* have been found in atopics with high (75,000 IU/mL) IgE levels.

Defective cell-mediated immunity is estimated to occur in up to 80% of atopics, with decreased resistance to infections with bacteria, viruses, and dermatophytes. This may be related to differences in functional subsets of $CD4^+$ T-helper cells. These subsets consist of TH1, TH2, and TH0 cells. The predominant subset of CD4 cells in atopics is the TH2 subset, which produces the cytokines interleukin 4 (IL-4) and interleukin 5 (IL-5), but not gamma-interferon (IFN-γ). IFN-γ, produced by TH1 cells in vitro, inhibits IL-4–induced IgE synthesis and is itself inhibited by IL-4. The predominance of these cytokines (IL-4 and IL-5) may promote IgE synthesis and the formation of eosinophils, which, along with other mediators, may promote the sensation of itch. This hallmark of eczema, itch, in turn leads to scratching, which in turn leads to keratinocyte activation, with further cytokine release and an expansion of the inflammatory cascade.

Other differences of atopic skin include:

- Alteration of vascular reactivity, as demonstrated by white dermatographism (formation of a white line instead of a red one when the skin surface is stroked)
- Greater sweating response to acetylcholine than in normal controls
- Deficiency of lipids derived from sebaceous glands on the surface of the skin
- Lower threshold for histamine release from basophils
- Increased histamine levels in plasma and skin.

Analogous to the classification of asthma as being either allergic extrinsic or intrinsic, eczema can be considered to have two components: that of allergen interaction with IgE, causing increased inflammation, and that of an intrinsic hyperirritability of the skin.

Differential diagnoses include seborrheic dermatitis, superficial fungal infections, contact dermatitis, pityriasis rosea, pityriasis versicolor, stasis dermatitis, hyperimmunoglobulin-E syndrome, necrolytic migratory erythema, drug eruptions, parapsoriasis, psoriasis, and early-stage mycosis fungoides. In children, rare diseases presenting with eczematous lesions include Wiskott-Aldrich syndrome, Shwachman syndrome, histiocytosis X, acrodermatitis enteropathica, and chronic granulomatous disease. An abrupt onset of eczema in adulthood may be a sign of internal malignancy and warrants an appropriate work-up.

HISTORY

Eczema usually is not seen before age 4 weeks. The infantile phase extends to 2 years of age and is manifested by acute eczema with erythema, edema, vesiculation, scratching, oozing, and possible secondary infection. Sites of involvement include the scalp, face, neck, trunk, forearms, knees, and legs. By age 2 months, infants have sufficient coordination to scratch. Scratching, a family history of atopy (asthma, eczema, or hay fever), and the characteristic areas of involvement help distinguish eczema from seborrheic dermatitis in this age group. Food intolerance may also be present. At age 2, some children may heal. From ages 3 to 11, skin thickening or lichenification starts, predominantly on flexural areas such as the antecubital and popliteal fossae, the hands and wrists, and the soles. African-American children may have a more papular presentation, follicular eczema, instead of dry, scaly patches. In later childhood and adolescence, the lesions become more flexural. Only a few patients continue to have full-blown eczema throughout life, although most continue to have "sensitive skin" and are prone to ill-defined hand eczema, dyshidrotic eczema, nummular eczema, or neurodermatitis.

PHYSICAL FINDINGS

The physical appearance of eczema varies with the patient's age and race and the duration of disease. Early lesions are erythematous and edematous, with varying vesiculation and oozing. More chronic lesions become drier and more scaly and show skin thickening. In more deeply pigmented persons, the chronic eczema areas may look ashy and show a tendency to follicular papules or follicular lichenification. Dry skin or xerosis is common, and there is an increased incidence of ichthyosis vulgaris in atopics. Hyperlinearity of palmar skin markings may be present. Facial pallor with infraorbital darkening or "allergic shiners" is common. A redundant fold of the lower eyelids, the Dennie-Morgan fold, may be present. There is a higher incidence of cataracts among adults with severe eczema. Pityriasis alba, or dry hypopigmented patches on the face, arms, and trunk, is common in children and young adults. In African-American patients with severe, longstanding eczema, affected skin areas may develop hyperpigmentation, with smaller areas of depigmentation where the inflammation has been so severe as to destroy melanocytes.

Dyshidrotic eczema or pompholyx is characterized by a vesicular eruption on the palms, soles, and digits. This type of eczema is occasionally precipitated by emotional stress such as bereavement or a favorite child's impending marriage. Nickel allergy and the ingestion of nickel-rich foods have also been proposed as aggravating factors for dyshidrotic eczema.

Nummular eczema is common among adults, especially during the winter, when heating is used and the ambient air humidity decreases. It is manifested by nummular or coin-shaped patches 1 to 2.5 cm in diameter, predominantly seen on the shoulders, hips, arms, thighs, and legs.

Neurodermatitis or lichen simplex chronicus is common in adults and is occasionally seen in adolescents. It presents as an ill-defined, intensely pruritic area that on intense rubbing and scratching becomes lichenified.

LABORATORY STUDIES

Laboratory studies, including scratch and intradermal tests, do not correlate with disease exacerbation. The same is true for RAST tests. Elevated IgE levels and eosinophils may be present, but there is no need to test these parameters routinely for diagnosis. If secondary infection is suspected, appropriate confirmatory tests (eg, KOH, fungal, viral, or bacterial cultures) should be done. A sudden flare of eczema with intense itching and scratching, especially if burrows are present, indicates that scabies may have infested the patient, and appropriate diagnostic scraping and treatment should be done.

TREATMENT

Atopic dermatitis patients need to avoid drying or irritating the skin. General measures include not bathing more than once daily, avoiding very hot baths or showers, using mild soaps, restricting soap use to the armpits, groin, and feet, patting the skin dry instead of rubbing, and using emollients such as Plastibase, Eutra, Eucerin, Vaseline, Aquaphor, and Albolene. Summertime emollients should be lighter in consistency than winter ones and include creams such as Unibase, Nivea, Aveeno, and Moisturel and lotions such as Curel, Moisturel, Aveeno, and Oil of Olay. Fabrics that feel stiff, rough, and itchy (eg, certain woolens and mohair) should be avoided. If a food allergy is thought to cause flares, the best test is to eliminate one food at a time. A problem food should cause a flare within minutes to hours, although in one study even 3 days was suggested as a time to flare after food challenge. Airborne allergens are more difficult to uncover. If the patient also has asthma or hay fever, referral for testing by an allergist for dust mite or other environmental allergens is reasonable.

Local treatment of eczema lesions is done with corticosteroid creams and ointments of varying potency, depending on the severity of the eczema. Antibiotics are used as necessary for secondary infection. The use of topical corticosteroids may reduce *S aureus* colonization, along with reducing itch and dermatitis. Application within 3 minutes after bathing on hydrated skin increases the efficacy of these topical corticosteroids. In general, creams are more comfortable in the summer, ointments in the winter. Their use should be tapered to once or twice a week as soon as significant improvement is noted. Every effort should be made to substitute plain emollients (also best applied soon after bathing for maximum efficiency) as the mainstay of treatment. This avoids the side effects of long-term topical corticosteroid use, as well as tolerance or tachyphylaxis. Corticosteroids should be avoided on the face and in body folds and genital areas. Weeping lesions should be treated with compresses two to four times daily. Infections should be treated as appropriate. Coal tar preparations are useful as a steroid-sparing alternative therapy. Antihistamines, especially taken at bedtime, may be useful in combating pruritus.

Even the agents used for therapy may be responsible for irritant or allergic contact dermatitis. There is increasing recognition of corticosteroid contact allergic dermatitis, and this should be considered when a patient does not improve. Referral to a dermatologist is appropriate in such cases. Selected patients may benefit from phototherapy, either with UVB light without or with coal tar products, or with PUVA (psoralen and UVA light).

Rarely, systemic agents such as prednisone, IFN-γ1B, cyclosporine, or azathioprine are used to bring severe eczema under control. Hospitalization with intense topical care, removal from everyday stress, and parenteral antibiotics if necessary helps bring severe eczema under control and often results in better long-term control once patients see that the disease can be controlled.

CONSIDERATIONS IN PREGNANCY

Treatment should be as conservative as possible, focusing on emollients and mild soaps and cleansing agents and as little use of topical corticosteroids as possible. There is no consistent pattern of improvement or worsening of eczema with the hormonal changes associated with menstruation, pregnancy, parturition, and menopause.

BIBLIOGRAPHY

Hanifin JM. Atopic dermatitis: new therapeutic considerations. J Am Acad Dermatol 1991;24:1097.

Kemmett D. Tidman MJ. The influence of the menstrual cycle and pregnancy on atopic dermatitis. Br J Dermatol 1991;125:59.

Lepoittevin JP, Drieghe J, Dooms-Goosens A. Studies in patients with corticosteroid contact allergy. Arch Dermatol 1995;131:31.

Leung DYM, Rhodes AS, Geha RS, et al. Atopic dermatitis (atopic eczema). In: Fitzpatrick TB, Eisen AZ, Wolff K, et al, eds. Dermatology in general medicine, 4th ed. New York: McGraw-Hill, 1993:1543.

Reitschel RL. Patch testing for corticosteroid allergy in the United States. Arch Dermatol 1995;131:91.

Sehgal VN, Jain S. Atopic dermatitis: ocular changes. Int J Dermatol 1994;33:11.

Sheehan MP, Atherton DJ, Norris P, Hawk J. Oral psoralen photochemotherapy in severe childhood atopic eczema: an update. Br J Dermatol 1993;129:431.

Stalder JF, Fleury M, Sourisse M, Rostin M, Pheline F, Litoux P. Local steroid therapy and bacterial skin flora in atopic dermatitis. Br J Dermatol 1994;131:536.

Williams HC, Pembroke AC, Forsdyke H, et al. London-born black Caribbean children are at increased risk of atopic dermatitis. J Am Acad Dermatol 1995;32:212.

140
Seborrheic Dermatitis

DOUGLAS L. POWELL

Primary Care for Women, edited by Phyllis C. Leppert and Fred M. Howard. Lippincott-Raven Publishers, Philadelphia © 1997.

Although seborrheic dermatitis was described over 100 years ago, debate still exists over the cause of this common skin condition, which affects 2% to 5% of the population. Its name may also be a misnomer, as the inflammation does not appear to be tied to increased sebaceous output or changes in sebum. Nevertheless, diagnosis of the condition is usually easy, and various treatments are often effective in controlling this chronic condition.

The disease has a wide clinical range. Many investigators think that common dandruff is the mildest expression of seborrheic dermatitis. Documentation of flares causing total body erythroderma, or complete cutaneous involvement, demonstrates the other end of the spectrum. Most patients have milder disease, however, and treatment can give satisfying results both symptomatically and cosmetically.

ETIOLOGY

Debate exists as to whether seborrheic dermatitis and dandruff are primarily inflammatory disorders or hyperproliferative disorders, or whether a small lipophilic yeast, *Pityrosporum ovale* (also known as *Malassezia furfur*), is the etiologic agent. In 1874, Malassez described a yeast-like cell in the stratum corneum of patients and considered the organism to be an etiologic agent in scalp scaling. In 1904, Sabouraud associated yeast (*P ovale*) with seborrheic dermatitis; however, due to inability to culture the yeast, this was only speculative. In the 1950s, after the introduction of corticosteroids, the inflammatory theories gained ground due to disease response to topical steroids. Favor for the yeast theory once again surfaced in the 1980s, when new antifungal therapies were marketed that also controlled the condition.

Those who think that *P ovale* is the primary etiologic agent point to studies that demonstrate higher *P ovale* concentrations in areas of seborrheic dermatitis in HIV-positive patients when compared to nonaffected skin. Response to antifungals, particularly topical ketoconazole, favors yeast as the etiology. Various immunologic studies tying low antibody titers specific to *P ovale*, decreased T-cell function in affected patients, and complement-activating capabilities of *P ovale* could account for the inflammation associated with the disease.

Others question how *P ovale* could be the primary etiologic agent, as it is part of normal skin flora and does not cause disease in most people. Likewise, topical steroids, which are not fungicidal or fungistatic, clear seborrheic dermatitis without directly treating the yeast. Many who believe that seborrheic dermatitis is a primary inflammatory disease argue that yeast proliferation exacerbates the disease through an increased inflammatory response to yeast antigens. Thus, treatment of the inflammation or treatment directed against *P ovale* results in clinical improvement. Quite possibly, seborrheic dermatitis may be similar to atopic dermatitis in that it is an inflammatory condition in patients who are genetically predisposed, but it is frequently triggered or aggravated by a microscopic organism (*P ovale*).

Some studies have demonstrated a decreased transit time of cells from the basal layer in the epidermis to the cornified layer, similar to psoriasis. This is the basis for the hyperproliferative theory.

HISTORY

Although seborrheic dermatitis is more common in males, it is common enough that it is often seen in females. It is a chronic condition with periodic flares. It is most prevalent in the fourth and fifth decades but can occur early during puberty, and there is a peak of transient disease in infancy. Onset is insidious. Seborrheic dermatitis flares in the summer for some, but does not seem to have seasonal variations in others. Pruritus of the scalp is common. Burning or stinging in other locations occurs, but often the lesions are asymptomatic and are more of a cosmetic concern, as the face is frequently involved.

Some cases occur after the onset of neurologic conditions such as Parkinson disease or peripheral neuropathies. It is also seen frequently and extensively in patients who are HIV-positive.

PHYSICAL EXAMINATION

The face and scalp appear to have greasy scales with underlying erythema in well-demarcated plaques. The scales sometimes appear yellow. Affected areas usually include the scalp, eyebrows, nasolabial folds, ear canals, and retroauricular regions. The eruption is symmetric. Less common locations are the presternal and interscapular regions, the axilla, and the groin. In the flexural regions, the erythema and scaliness is often accompanied by crusting and fissuring. Secondary infection with *Staphylococcus aureus* is common. All these areas of involvement are regions of high sebaceous gland concentration, thus the disease's name. The affected areas are often sharply demarcated on the scalp and trunk, but they are not always well demarcated on the face. Occasionally, seborrheic dermatitis is manifested solely by erythema and crusting of the eyelid margins, also known as blepharitis.

Clues to the diagnosis include asking the patient about dandruff, looking carefully in and around the ears, and observing for central facial redness, which often spares the bulbous part of the nose.

DIFFERENTIAL DIAGNOSIS

Psoriasis of the scalp is often difficult to distinguish from seborrheic dermatitis; frequent overlap of the two conditions occurs and is termed sebopsoriasis. Plaques with dry silvery scale are more typical of psoriasis. The scale in seborrheic dermatitis is often greasy. The distribution and appearance of lesions at other locations on the body give clues to the correct diagnosis.

Contact dermatitis can be another look-alike on the face but is often asymmetric and does not often affect the ears. A thorough history often elicits the cause of contact dermatitis.

Individual lesions of pityriasis rosea on the trunk can look seborrheic, but they are smaller oval plaques, occur in a Christmas tree pattern, and are not commonly found in seborrheic areas.

Candidiasis can mimic or complicate seborrheic dermatitis in the inguinal folds, thus warranting a potassium hydroxide preparation of some scales.

Tinea capitis must be considered when usual treatments fail, particularly if scaling is accompanied by hair breakage or alopecia.

No specific laboratory or imaging tests are needed.

TREATMENT

Seborrheic dermatitis responds well to both antifungal and antiinflammatory agents. Low-potency, nonfluorinated topical steroids applied twice daily work well for flares of seborrhea. Many different shampoos are effective long-term treatments when used twice a week; the suds should be rubbed over affected facial areas before rinsing. Some of the shampoos are selenium sulfide 2.5%, zinc pyrithione 1%, and others that contain sulfur or coal tar. Patients with markedly thickened scalp scales can be treated with salicylic acid shampoos to remove the scales so that other medications can penetrate more effectively. Of the antifungal agents, ketoconazole 2% shampoo and ketoconazole cream have been particularly effective in treating seborrheic dermatitis. Combination treatment, such as a topical steroid cream combined with antifungal shampoo, often is the treatment of choice.

Nightly cleansing of the eyelid margins with baby shampoo on a cotton swab is used to treat blepharitis.

If the condition does not improve with basic treatment or if the diagnosis is uncertain, the patient should be referred to a dermatologist.

CONSIDERATIONS IN PREGNANCY

Little is mentioned in the literature regarding seborrheic dermatitis in pregnancy; however, because cell-mediated immunity is lessened during pregnancy and corticosteroid levels are raised, changes in the intensity of seborrheic dermatitis would not be surprising. It could vary during pregnancy, as does atopic dermatitis, which can undergo flares or resolution. Because many women wish to minimize the use of any medication during pregnancy, frequent shampooing and washing with nonmedicated products may be sufficient treatment.

BIBLIOGRAPHY

Berbrant IM, Faergemann J. The role of *Pityrosporum ovale* in seborrheic dermatitis. Semin Dermatol 1990;9:262.

Faergemann J. *Pityrosporum* infections. J Am Acad Dermatology 1994;31(3 pt 2):S18.

Ive FA. An overview of experience with ketoconazole shampoo. Br J Clin Pract 1991;45(4):279.

Kligman AM, Leyden JJ. Seborrheic dermatitis. Semin Dermatol 1983;2:57.

McGrath J, Murphy GM. The control of seborrheic dermatitis and dandruff by antipityrosporal drugs. Drugs 1991;41(2):178.

Sabouraud R. Les maladies desquamitives: maladies du cuir chevelu. Paris: Masson, 1904.

Stratigos JD, Antoniou C, Katsambas A, et al. Ketoconazole 2% cream vs. hydrocortisone 1% cream in the treatment of seborrheic dermatitis. J Am Acad Dermatol 1988;19(5 pt 1):850.

Webster G. Seborrheic dermatitis. Int J Dermatol 1991;30(12):843.

141
Psoriasis

SOPHIE M. WOROBEC

Primary Care for Women, edited by Phyllis C. Leppert and Fred M. Howard. Lippincott-Raven Publishers, Philadelphia © 1997.

Psoriasis is a common skin disease with no sex predilection. It is believed to affect some 4 million Americans, or 2% of the population, at an annual cost of $1.6 billion. Most patients first develop the disease before age 30, and some 10,000 new cases annually occur in children below age 10. The disease is troublesome, with itching and scaliness being everyday difficulties. In the United States, some 400 people die annually of psoriasis complications, and 5% of psoriatics eventually develop severe disabling arthritis.

Primary care physicians should feel comfortable treating localized psoriasis, with referral to dermatologists and collaborative follow-up of severe disease.

ETIOLOGY

The cutaneous lesions of psoriasis can consist of plaques, guttate (drop-like) lesions, localized pustules, widespread pustules, and erythrodermic involvement. Psoriasis is a skin disease of genetic predisposition with a wide range of trigger factors (eg, drugs, skin injury, infection) that cause inflammatory, hyperproliferative lesions. Among monozygotic twins, if one twin is affected, there is a 65% concordance for psoriasis in the second twin. This would indicate that both a hereditary genetic factor and an environmental triggering event are necessary for disease development; therefore, many people who have a genetic tendency for psoriasis may never develop it.

Linkage to HLA-Cw6 and HLA-DR7 antigens is strong for people who develop psoriasis before age 40. About one third of affected patients have relatives with psoriasis. It is unknown whether a genetic model fits all patients with psoriasis, or whether there should be a division of psoriasis into early-onset disease (before age 40) and late-onset disease (after age 40), with a differing disease pathogenesis resulting in similar cutaneous expression in both groups.

On histopathologic examination, psoriatic lesions show abnormal cellular proliferation with a thickened epidermis and retention of epidermal cell nuclei in the stratum corneum. Often, sterile subcorneal pustules containing polymorphonuclear leukocytes (PMNLs) are present. Labeling studies have revealed that psoriatic epidermis is hyperproliferative: the normal epidermal transit time from the basal layer to the granular cell layer is reduced from 14 days to 2 days. The mechanism responsible for this increased cell proliferation is unknown. The finding of PMNLs within the epidermis has led to theories that they play an important role in stimulating this proliferation. Psoriatic scale, in which are found bacteria, immune complexes, denatured proteins, prostaglandins and their precursors, and even PMNLs, is chemotactic for PMNLs.

The subepidermal capillaries are dilated and present in increased numbers, with an activated T-cell mononuclear cell infiltrate often surrounding them. The dilated and tortuous capillaries, found in uninvolved as well as involved skin of psoriatic patients, show a marked attenuation of their walls, with gaps between the endothelial cells. This may result in an easier route of exit of both inflammatory mediators and PMNLs and their subsequent entry into the epidermis.

DIFFERENTIAL DIAGNOSIS

The differential diagnosis of psoriasis includes lichen planus, nummular eczema, the lichen simplex chronicus type of eczema, seborrheic dermatitis, parapsoriasis, pityriasis rubra pilaris, pityriasis rosea, drug eruptions, mycosis fungoides, psoriasiform tertiary syphilis, Reiter syndrome, and congenital ichthyosiform erythroderma. Localized acral pustular psoriasis must be distinguished from Bazex syndrome, in which a pustular and scaly acral eruption is an external sign of internal malignancy.

HISTORY

Psoriasis can occur at any age, from infancy until well into old age, but most patients develop the disease as young adults. Onset can be slow and insidious, with a few red, scaly papules that coalesce into a plaque. In most patients the disease waxes and wanes, requiring rotation of available therapies.

Triggering factors can include infections, skin injury, stress (eg, grief over a spouse's death), and drugs. Drug therapies associated with new onset or exacerbation of psoriasis include lithium, antimalarials, interferons, gemfibrozil, nonsteroidal antiinflammatory agents (phenylbutazone and meclofenamate), and angiotensin-converting enzyme inhibitors (captopril and lisinopril). Fluoxetine (Prozac) has been associated with the development of psoriasis after 6 and 12 months of use, a time frame similar to that observed with lithium-induced psoriasis. Both lithium and fluoxetine modulate serotonergic function; therefore, a common mechanism may contribute to the induction of psoriatic lesions.

CLINICAL FINDINGS

Psoriasis can occur at any age. Plaque psoriasis, the most common presentation, presents with sharply marginated erythematous plaques and papules with a tenacious silvery-white scale that if picked off reveals pinpoint bleeding spots (known as the Auspitz sign). Plaque psoriasis may become confluent and cover large areas of skin. Plaques may also appear annular or arcuate due to central clearing. The extensor surfaces of the arms and legs, especially the knees and elbows, and the lumbar area are the most common sites of involvement. The thickness of these lesions varies with location, usually being thicker on nonfold body areas (arms, legs, knees, elbows, lumbar area, sacral/lower back area) and thinner on flexural areas (axillae and groin). Psoriasis appearing on flexural areas also tends to lack scale and often has secondary *Can-*

dida colonization. The presence of scalp and nail involvement helps establish a diagnosis of inverse psoriasis. Characteristic nail changes include nail pitting (punctate), ridging, onycholysis, subungual hyperkeratosis, and nail plate "oil spots" or "salmon patches," which are oval to round areas of pink to reddish-brown discoloration.

The incidence of psoriatic arthritis is difficult to ascertain, but it occurs in as many as 21% of severely affected patients. This seronegative arthritis usually is polyarticular and asymmetric but can be monoarticular. Five basic patterns of psoriatic arthritis have been defined:

- Asymmetric oligoarthropathy involving both the proximal and distal interphalangeal joints, giving the appearance of "sausage digits." Only one digit may be involved.
- Predominant distal interphalangeal joint involvement
- Rheumatoid pattern. This is symmetric and involves the metacarpophalangeal and proximal interphalangeal joints, as in rheumatoid arthritis; however, it is seronegative and less destructive and has a different radiologic picture than rheumatoid arthritis. Also, unlike rheumatoid arthritis, distal interphalangeal joint involvement is common.
- Psoriatic arthritis mutilans. This disabling form is manifested by foreshortened digits due to osteolysis.
- Predominant spondylitis or sacroiliitis. This occurs alone or in conjunction with the other manifestations of psoriatic arthritis. Even asymptomatic persons may have radiologic evidence of spondylitis.

Guttate psoriasis is characterized by the rapid onset of multiple, small (0.5 to 1.5 cm), finely scaly, pink to erythematous papules over the trunk and extremities. It may present as the original manifestation of psoriasis, especially with a current or recent upper respiratory infection (either viral or β-hemolytic streptococcal), or it may be a sign of worsening disease in patients with established plaque psoriasis.

Localized pustular psoriasis occurs as either a sterile pustular eruption of the palms and soles or a pustular eruption of the fingers and toes with nail involvement. There may be loss of the nail plate, with pustules persisting in the nail bed and paronychial area. The pustules are a cloudy yellow, then turn brown and develop a hard keratinaceous surface.

Generalized pustular psoriasis (von Zumbusch type) is marked by a sudden onset of sterile pustules that may come in successive waves, with accompanying fever, malaise, weakness, peripheral leukocytosis, raised erythrocyte sedimentation rate, and sometimes hypocalcemia. Pustules can coalesce into lakes of pus or pus-laden annular lesions. This can occur as an initial manifestation of psoriasis or in patients with a prior history of psoriatic lesions. A common precipitating factor for generalized pustular psoriasis is the withdrawal of systemic corticosteroid therapy. Therefore, such therapy must be avoided in the treatment of known stable long-term plaque psoriasis, or used with great caution for disabling psoriatic arthritis.

An exfoliative or erythrodermic form of psoriasis shows generalized erythema. This rare explosive form usually develops in patients who previously had plaque-type psoriasis. Exfoliative erythroderma occurs also in T-cell lymphoma, ichthyosis, drug reactions, pityriasis rubra pilaris, contact dermatitis, and eczematous disease. Associated findings can include chills, rigors, and fever due to poor temperature regulation, protein loss, fluid and electrolyte imbalances, and high-output cardiac failure.

LABORATORY AND IMAGING STUDIES

The diagnosis of psoriasis is established by the history and clinical examination and a skin biopsy (especially in uncertain cases). Additional skin tissue for direct immunofluorescence studies should be obtained when lupus is in the differential diagnosis. Syphilis serology may be indicated, as luetic lesions can be psoriasiform. Wood's light examination, potassium hydroxide preparation, fungal cultures, Gram stain, and bacterial cultures should be done as appropriate to diagnose secondary yeast, fungal, or bacterial infections. Because acral pustulosis and Bazex syndrome are clinically difficult to differentiate, a complete history and physical examination with age-appropriate malignancy screening should be done. There is a fourfold incidence of psoriasis in patients with Crohn disease (regional enteritis); therefore, if the history is compatible with this affliction, an appropriate work-up is indicated.

TREATMENT

All treatment approaches are directed at lessening inflammation and epidermal hyperproliferation. Topical treatments include corticosteroids, the vitamin D analog calcipotriene, coal tar and its derivatives, and anthralin. Sun exposure in summertime, with care to avoid a sunburn (as burns can trigger a Koebner reaction), is helpful for about 85% of psoriatic patients. However, this should not be recommended for those who are at increased risk of skin cancer (eg, past history of skin cancer, personal or family history of melanoma or atypical moles, fair-skinned with light eye color, easily burned, past exposure to arsenicals or ionizing radiation).

Avoiding skin dryness by the use of emollients and lubricants is useful adjunctive therapy. Prompt treatment of any concurrent infections is essential, as they may act as trigger factors for psoriatic flares.

Major shortcomings of topical corticosteroids include cutaneous atrophy, folliculitis, and tachyphylaxis; however, they are useful in controlling localized disease. Many dermatologists start therapy with high-potency topical steroids (Ultravate, Temovate, Diprolene, Psorcon) until a lesion is suppressed, then switch to maintenance therapy with emollients and once- or twice-weekly "pulsing" with a topical corticosteroid. Many patients prefer a cream to an ointment base, as there is less greasiness to soil clothes. However, if thick scale is present, an ointment applied at bedtime may be more effective. Salves should be applied shortly after bathing and the skin should be patted dry, because percutaneous absorption is best on hydrated skin. Solutions, gels, and lotions can be used for scalp treatment. Long-term use of high-potency corticosteroids on the scalp or on extensive body areas can result in adrenal suppression and a cushingoid habitus. Therefore, every attempt should be made to wean patients off superpotent corticosteroids or decrease the frequency of their usage.

Tar gels and shampoos are available over the counter and help most patients; however, an irritant folliculitis that can koebnerize precludes their use in sensitive patients. Anthralin products can produce long-term remissions of plaque psoriasis, but irritation and staining of skin and clothing limit their acceptability.

Calcipotriene ointment or cream applied twice a day is effective in reducing thick psoriatic plaques. It can be used as a first-line alternative to topical steroids or in rotation with topical steroids. The face and intertriginous areas may become irritated and should not be treated with calcipotriene. Irritation develops in 10% to 17% of users, and patients should apply it sparingly for maximum benefit.

Mild to moderate disease affecting 10% or less of the total surface area can be treated by the primary care physician. Patients with more serious or refractory disease should be referred to a dermatologist. The primary care physician should attempt to avoid or reduce the use of medications that are potential exacerbants (lithium, β-blockers, nonsteroidal antiinflammatory drugs).

Severe psoriasis is treated with phototherapy (UVB or UVA), the Goeckerman regime (UVB and topical coal tar preparations), chemophototherapy with either oral or topical psoralens and UVA, retinoids, and methotrexate. Resistant cases have been treated with cyclosporine in investigational use, with significant improvement. However, relapse and even generalized pustular flares have occurred within several weeks of discontinuing therapy. Climatotherapy (eg, vacationing at the Dead Sea) is helpful and is an approved therapy accepted by several European health care systems.

Erythrodermic psoriasis and generalized pustular psoriasis can be life-threatening, and most affected patients need inpatient management. Major complications include sepsis, electrolyte imbalance, and negative nitrogen balance. The retinoid etretinate at 1 mg/kg/day is highly effective in controlling generalized pustular psoriasis.

CONSIDERATIONS IN PREGNANCY

There are anecdotal reports of improvement of psoriasis during pregnancy. In Dunna and Findlay's survey of 65 women who experienced at least a single pregnancy after the onset of psoriasis, this observation held true. Psoriases tended to improve gradually during pregnancy, but worsened again within 3 months after delivery. The same observation has held true for the course of psoriatic arthritis. These improvements during pregnancy are probably due to higher levels of circulating corticosteroids.

Generalized pustular psoriasis occurs rarely during pregnancy and may be life-threatening. In the past, it was given the misnomer "impetigo herpetiformis." It usually occurs in the second half of pregnancy, and only one third of affected patients have a prior clinical history of psoriasis. The cutaneous eruption consists of expanding symmetric red patches, starting usually in the flexures (groin, axillae, and neck). Grouped pustules occur at the margins; old pustules interior to the margin form crusts or become impetiginized. It is associated with fever, chills, asthenia, nausea, vomiting, and diarrhea. Neurologic disturbances such as confusion and convulsions were more common in the past and were probably due to untreated hypocalcemia. Fetal death occurs in half of cases. The disease disappears in the postpartum period, but there is increased risk for recurrence with subsequent pregnancies.

The histopathology of the cutaneous lesions is that of pustular psoriasis. High white cell counts and sedimentation rates are common. Infection must be ruled out in the presence of fever. The intact pustules are sterile, but broken skin may become secondarily infected. Serum calcium and albumin levels may be low, and therapeutic replacement is indicated.

Prednisone in doses up to 60 mg/day has been used to control the eruption, but it must be tapered slowly, as a too-sudden lowering may result in a flare-up. There is some doubt in the European literature as to whether corticosteroids produce a consistent response to this disease. It is necessary to monitor and treat any secondary cutaneous or systemic infection.

BIBLIOGRAPHY

Abel EA. Diagnosis of drug-induced psoriasis. Semin Dermatol 1992;11:269.

Baker H, Ryan TJ. Generalized pustular psoriasis: a clinical and epidemiological study of 104 cases. Br J Dermatol 1968;80:771.

Beveridge GW, Harkness RA, Livingstone JR. Impetigo herpetiformis in two successive pregnancies. Br J Dermatol 1966;78:106.

Dunna SF, Finlay AY. Psoriasis: improvement during and worsening after pregnancy. Br J Dermatol 1989;120:584.

Elder JT, Nair RP, Voorhees JJ. Epidemiology and the genetics of psoriasis. J Invest Dermatol 1994;102:245.

Hemlock C, Rosenthal JS, Winston A. Fluoxetine-induced psoriasis. Ann Pharmacother 1992;26:211.

Lotem M, Katzenelson V, Rotem A, Hod M, Sandbank M. Impetigo herpetiformis: a variant of pustular psoriasis or a separate entity? J Am Acad Dermatol 1989;20:338.

Oosterling RJ, Nobrega RE, DuBoeuff JA, et al. Impetigo herpetiformis or generalized pustular psoriasis? Arch Dermatol 1978;114:1527.

Oumeish OY, Farraj SE, Bataineh AS. Some aspects of impetigo herpetiformis. Arch Dermatol 1982;118:103.

Sauer G. Impetigo herpetiformis. Arch Dermatol 1961;83:119.

142
Stasis Skin Changes and Disorders

SOPHIE M. WOROBEC

Primary Care for Women, edited by Phyllis C. Leppert and Fred M. Howard. Lippincott-Raven Publishers, Philadelphia © 1997.

Chronic venous insufficiency usually occurs as a result of incompetent valvular function in the deep venous channels of the lower limbs and in the perforating veins connecting the superficial to the deep venous systems. Stasis dermatitis, ulcers, and other changes are the consequences of chronic venous insufficiency. The incidence of leg and foot ulcers increases greatly with age, with venous ulceration occurring in 1% to 4% of people over age 70.

ETIOLOGY AND DIFFERENTIAL DIAGNOSIS

The venous vasculature of the lower extremities consists of two major vein groups: the deep venous system within the muscular system and the superficial system, which lies above the muscle groups. About 90% of the venous return is by the deep venous system, which is subject to muscular compression. Ideally, the deep veins draw blood from the superficial system, which drains the skin venules. The contraction of calf muscles can generate a pressure of 200 to 300 mm Hg, which normally is transmitted to the deep venous system. The superficial venous system of the lower extremities is a lower-pressure system than the deep venous system. Valves within the deep veins and perforator veins (connecting the deep and superficial venous systems) prevent the transmission of the higher pressure to the superficial veins. In venous insufficiency, valvular dysfunction allows retrograde blood flow (up to 25% of total femoral flow) and the transmission of high pressure into the superficial veins. This pressure is then transmitted to the capillary beds of the skin and subcutaneous tissue. This widens the endothelial pores, allowing fibrinogen molecules to exude into the extracellular fluid and form fibrin complexes around the capillaries. This, in turn, forms a diffusion barrier for oxygen and other nutrients necessary for the healthy function of the skin and subcutaneous tissue. Decreased fibrinolytic activity and increased collagen synthesis have also been demonstrated in sclerotic areas of long-term stasis changes.

Venous insufficiency can be secondary to deep vein thrombosis (DVT) that blocks the proximal flow of blood in the deep venous system, but most patients do not have a definite clinical history of DVT or phlebitis. The incidence rises with advancing age and with an increasing number of pregnancies. Edema of the lower legs is common. Other causes of such edema can include neoplastic obstruction of the pelvic veins, congenital or acquired vascular malformations of the venous or lymphatic systems, cardiac failure, or renal disease.

HISTORY

Chronic venous insufficiency is first characterized by edema of the lower legs, then by secondary changes of the skin and subcutaneous tissue. There may be a history of one or more episodes of phlebitis, associated with pregnancy or prolonged bed rest or after trauma. Symptoms include a persistent dull ache that worsens at the end of a long period of standing or sitting with the legs in a dependent position. Stasis dermatitis consists of pruritic eczematous changes. Leg trauma can cause bleeding of superficial varicosities.

PHYSICAL EXAMINATION AND CLINICAL FINDINGS

The earliest change of venous insufficiency, edema, is at first mild and present only at the end of the day. Gradually, it worsens and is accompanied by a mild erythema, pinpoint petechiae, and brownish pigmentation due to hemosiderin deposits left by extravasated red blood cells. The skin may become thin and shiny as the edema progresses. The sites involved include the medial ankle area, the dorsa of the feet (where shoe compression stops), and gradually the entire lower legs and ankles. As stasis dermatitis develops, the erythema becomes more extensive, and scaling, weeping, and crusting occur. Superficial secondary infection may occur and develop into cellulitis. Applied remedies can result in contact dermatitis of the irritant or allergic type; a new onset of vesicular lesions should alert the clinician to this possibility.

Lipodermatosclerosis (LDS) is a scleroderma-like induration and fibrosis of the skin and subcutaneous tissue. It occurs in up to 30% of affected patients and often precedes venous ulceration. In the acute stage of LDS, the skin is bright red, scaly, very tender, and warm. It often starts above the medial malleolus. There is no preceding trauma or illness, and the lesion is not well demarcated from adjacent normal skin. In this acute stage, it is often misdiagnosed as morphea, cellulitis, erythema nodosum, or another panniculitis. In the chronic stage, there is less erythema, scaling, pain, and discomfort, and the involved sclerotic area is sharply demarcated from the surrounding normal skin. Eventually, the entire lower third of the leg may become hard and woody, and the legs resemble inverted champagne bottles.

Venous ulcers usually develop first over the medial malleoli or the anterior aspect of the leg. They usually have an irregular erythematous border and a moist, granulating base. Healing often results in a thin scar that can break down with trauma. Repeated episodes of ulceration and secondary infection can result in loss of ankle mobility. Rarely, carcinoma (squamous cell or basal cell) develops in a longstanding ulcer.

LABORATORY AND IMAGING STUDIES

Doppler examination or duplex scanning can help confirm the existence of venous insufficiency. More than 20% of patients with leg ulceration have evidence of arterial insufficiency on Doppler studies. Feeling pulses may be inaccurate; arterial studies are needed to exclude arterial insufficiency in any patient before compression therapy is used.

Skin biopsy is rarely necessary. The histology of stasis dermatitis is nonspecific. Occasionally, if acute LDS is suspected, a biopsy must be performed to rule out other diseases. The biopsy should be performed at the edge of an erythematous and indurated area and closed primarily after a longitudinal thin excision to prevent dehiscence and the creation of an ulcer. A nonhealing ulcer may necessitate referral to a dermatologist for work-up and biopsy to rule out a carcinoma, unusual infection, vasoocclusive disease, or granulomatous disease. Biopsy for this purpose should be large enough to include both an ulcer edge and part of the ulcer base. An exophytic component to the edge, if present, should be chosen as the biopsy site.

TREATMENT

Coexistent arterial disease, if present, must be treated before effective treatment is possible for venous disease. Graded compression stockings with 30 to 40 mm Hg of pressure at the ankle are essential. These should be individualized for the patient. Several brands are available. These stockings should be put on immediately on arising in the morning, before edema develops, and removed in the evening. Ill-fitting stockings should not be used. Ace wraps can be used temporarily. Sclerotherapy, skin grafting, venous ligation, and venous reconstruction are therapeutic options. All of these are palliative measures and must be part of a comprehensive management program that includes compression therapy.

Stasis dermatitis responds to low- or mid-potency corticosteroids. Tap water compresses can be used for weeping, crusted, or scaly dermatitis, followed by a very thin layer of a corticosteroid. Both should be discontinued or tapered once the dermatitis resolves. Infections are treated as appropriate. Topical neomycin and garamycin should be avoided, as their use in stasis areas is associated with an increased incidence of allergic sensitization. If secondary allergic or irritant dermatitis is suspected, referral to a dermatologist is appropriate to help determine its etiology.

Stanozolol 5 mg twice a day has been used successfully to treat acute LDS. Its fibrinolytic activity is thought to be the mechanism by which it exerts a beneficial effect. Taking short walks, elevating the leg during the day, and avoiding constricting garments are advisable.

Stasis ulcers should be monitored for signs of infection, and the infections should be treated. Deep ulcers do well with Sorbsan dressings. Duoderm dressings with an overlying Unna boot are helpful for multiple ulcers. Large ulcers with an adequate vascular supply to support a graft may need to be grafted to heal, as they may worsen without grafting.

CONSIDERATIONS IN PREGNANCY

Venous disease is more common in women with a family history of it. The relative risk of venous disease in women increases with an increasing number of full-term pregnancies. The risk of developing venous disease during pregnancy increases with age: it is four times higher for women over age 35 than it is for women age 24 or less. During late pregnancy, significant improvement of venous function and a subjective decrease of swelling, tiredness, and pain can be achieved with graduated compression hosiery.

BIBLIOGRAPHY

Callam MJ, Harper DR, Dale JJ, Ruckley CV. Arterial disease in chronic leg ulceration: an underestimated hazard? Lothian and Forth Valley leg ulcer study. Br Med J 1987;294:929.

Dindelli M, Parazzini F, Basellini A, et al. Risk factors for varicose disease before and during pregnancy. Angiology 1993;44:361.

Goldman MP, Weiss RA, Bergan JJ. Diagnosis and treatment of varicose veins: a review. J Am Acad Dermatol 1994;31:393.

Kirsner RS, Pardes JB, Eglestein WH, Falanga V. The clinical spectrum of lipodermatosclerosis. J Am Acad Dermatol 1993;28:623.

Korstanje MJ. Venous stasis ulcers: diagnostic and surgical considerations. Dermatol Surg 1995;21:635.

McCarthy WJ, Dann C, Pearce WH, Yao JS. Management of sudden profuse bleeding from varicose veins. Surgery 1993;113:178.

Nilsson L, Austrell C, Norgren L. Venous function during late pregnancy: the effect of elastic compression hosiery. Vasa 1992;21:203.

Phillips TJ, Dover JS. Leg ulcers. J Am Acad Dermatol 1991;25:965.

White JW. Localized eczematous disease: stasis dermatitis. In: Sams WM Jr., Lynch PJ, eds. Principles and practice of dermatology. New York: Churchill-Livingstone, 1990:413.

143

Superficial Fungal Infections

WILLIAM V.R. SHELLOW

Primary Care for Women, edited by Phyllis C. Leppert and Fred M. Howard. Lippincott-Raven Publishers, Philadelphia © 1997.

Superficial fungal infections of the skin are much less common in women than in men. The reasons for this are unclear, but may result from factors such as differences in clothing and footwear as well as intrinsic differences such as less profuse sweating in women and less body hair. In general, many nonfungal infections are incorrectly diagnosed as being fungal in origin, whereas many true fungal infections are not diagnosed as such. The primary care physician must be familiar with definitive methods of diagnosing cutaneous fungal infections and also should be able to prescribe cost-effective therapy. Correct diagnosis is the key to successful therapy. Cutaneous fungal infections usually are not serious but they can create significant discomfort and a great deal of unhappiness in patients. Because of the tendency to recur, patient education by the physician is an important adjunct to proper therapy.

ETIOLOGY AND DIFFERENTIAL DIAGNOSIS

Fungal infections of the skin can be divided into three types: (1) ultrasuperficial infections caused by *Malassezia furfur*; (2) infections of the skin, hair, and nails caused by the dermatophytes; and (3) diseases of the skin, nails, and mucous membranes caused by the yeasts. Tinea versicolor, which is characterized by hyperpigmented macules, hypopigmented macules, or both together can be confused with vitiligo or postinflammatory hyperpigmentation. Dermatophyte infections of the skin can resemble psoriasis, erythema multiforme, gyrate erythemas, and drug eruptions, to name just a few. Psoriasis and various nail dystrophies look similar to fungal infections of nails. Hair loss caused by tinea capitis may look like alopecia areata or trichotillomania.

HISTORY

The presence of pets in the house is important when the diagnosis of tinea corporis is made. Most acute infections in women are acquired from the cat or dog. Of course, the presence of other family members with acute or chronic fungal infections is a significant factor. The presence of diabetes mellitus is a significant contributor to the development of candidiasis. Recent dental work often precedes the onset of perlèche. Recent antibiotic therapy also can contribute to the development of candidiasis in the perianal and submammary areas. Occupations that involve wet work contribute to candidal nail and web space infections. A recent manicure, perhaps by a new manicurist, often precedes an acute paronychia. Manicuring technique, such as forceful pushing back of the cuticle, may prompt the continuation of a chronic paronychia.

PHYSICAL EXAMINATION AND CLINICAL FINDINGS

Tinea versicolor (Pityriasis versicolor) is characterized by brown, pink, red, or white scaly patches. These occur primarily on the chest, back, and shoulders but may also involve the neck and proximal extremities. During the summer, the infection may be noticed by the patient as small hypopigmented areas. The etiologic agent prevents transfer of melanin from melanocytes to epidermal cells; therefore, infected patches of skin do not tan like the uninfected skin. If this diagnosis is suspected, some scale should be present in addition to the color change. This can be demonstrated by scratching one of the macular areas with the finger nail. This will raise a small amount of fine scale. Examination of the skin with a Wood's light may reveal a weak gold or orange-brown fluorescence. Tinea versicolor is diagnosed with certainty by scraping a scaly lesion with a No. 15 scalpel blade, placing the scale obtained on a microscope slide, and adding a drop of 20% potassium hydroxide (KOH). Examination under the microscope reveals the characteristic short hyphae and spores, sometimes referred to as "spaghetti and meatballs."

Dermatophytic and candidal infections are scaly and erythematous lesions with well-defined margins, occurring in characteristic areas of the body that promote the growth of fungi. Lesions on the nonhairy skin often show clearing in the center, leaving an annular, erythematous lesion with scaly borders. This type of lesion has been called a "ringworm." Dermatophyte infections are defined by the area of the body they affect. Tinea pedis, when acute, may be characterized by small blisters and inflammation on the edges of the soles and in the interdigital areas of the feet. Chronic tinea pedis is characterized by erythema, scaling, and sometimes hyperkeratosis of the soles. Tinea corporis affects other areas of the body, including the trunk, buttocks, and extremities. When there is involvement of the face, it may be called tinea faciei. Tinea cruris, or infection of the inguinal folds, is extremely uncommon in women.

Onychomycosis, or tinea unguium, is characterized by the accumulation of subungual keratin and invasion of the nail plate by fungus, resulting in a thickened, distorted, discolored, and crumbly nail. Tinea capitis, or scalp ringworm, occurs almost exclusively in children, although there are rare reports of tinea capitis in adults.

Confirmatory diagnosis of a dermatophyte infection requires microscopic examination of the lesion for hyphae, using a KOH wet-mount. The border of the lesion is scraped lightly using a No. 15 scalpel blade. A clean microscope slide is placed so that the scale obtained falls on top of the slide. A coverslip can be used to push all of the scale into a small mound. One, or at most two, drops of 20% KOH solution or KOH with dimethylsulfoxide (DMSO) is dropped in the center of the collected scale, and a coverslip is placed over the drop. If the KOH solution does not contain DMSO, the slide must be heated lightly over an alcohol lamp to improve "clearing" of the epithelial cells. If DMSO is present, heating is not required. Under low power (40×) with reduced light, thread-like hyphae can be seen. Branched, septate hyphae are confirmed under higher power (100×).This second step is necessary to make sure that artifacts are not being mistaken for hyphae. In candidal infections, small thin-walled spores are seen. These actually may be budding but usually are not. Pseudohyphae, which are elongated budding spores that have failed to detach, are pathognomonic for *Candida albicans*.

In women, *Candida* infections of the skin occur principally in intertriginous locations such as the axillae, groin, intergluteal folds, inframammary area, and perianal areas. Physical examination of involved skin reveals bright red erythema, oozing, and superficial erosions with the subjective symptoms of burning, itching, or both. Another presentation is as acute, but more commonly, chronic infections of the posterior nail folds of the fingers. Chronic paronychia is characterized by loss of the cuticle and retraction of the proximal nail fold with erythema. Gentle pressure on the affected area may express a small amount of yellow pus or cheesy material. This material is excellent for examination by KOH preparation and for culturing. Crusted involvement of the labial commissures, known as perlèche, is another form of candidiasis. Lesions are pustular and thin walled on a red base, often producing burning and itching. In general, candidiasis may be clinically suspected as a result of the presence of characteristic satellite pustules outside of the margin of the primary lesion.

Onychomycosis of the fingernails, toenails, or both usually results from a dermatophyte infection elsewhere, especially on the feet. Candidal onychomycosis of the fingernails may result if there is a chronic candidal paronychia. *Candida* then invade the nail plate itself rather than just the soft tissues of the nail fold.

LABORATORY STUDIES

Before systemic therapy is considered, a positive culture result should be obtained. It is more than reasonable to begin topical antifungal therapy based on a positive finding from the KOH preparation. It is convenient to use dermatophyte test medium, which is an agar-containing phenolphthalein, as a color indicator. If planted scale or pus turns to medium red within 14 days, the presence of a pathogen can be assumed. Clinical Laboratory Improvement Act of 1988 (CLIA) regulations allow the physician to perform fungal cultures in an office laboratory, as long as their findings are read as "positive" or "negative." Attempting to speciate the organism brings with it more onerous regulations. Many outside laboratories provide a fungal culture that reports the exact organisms growing. This may be important when choosing a drug for systemic therapy.

TREATMENT

Tinea versicolor can be treated effectively with selenium sulfide, zinc pyrithione, sulfur—salicylic acid combinations, or with one of the antifungal agents such as miconazole, clotrimazole, econazole, ketoconazole, or ciclopirox. Over-the-counter shampoos such as 1% selenium sulfide (Head and Shoulders Intensive Treatment) or a zinc pyrithione shampoo (Zincon, Head and Shoulders) can be applied with a rough washcloth. It should be allowed to remain on the affected areas for 10 minutes and then rinsed off. Daily application for 1 week is recommended. The prescription shampoos like a 2.5% suspension of selenium sulfide (Selsun), or ketoconazole shampoo (Nizoral) usually are effective for treating tinea versicolor. In refractory cases, selenium sulfide suspension can be left on the skin overnight. The topical antifungal agents are much more expensive but useful in recalcitrant involvement of small areas. When the infection is too widespread for topical therapy, systemic ketoconazole (Nizoral), 200 mg daily, for 7 to 10 days is effective for extensive involvement. Ketoconazole should be taken with an acidic fruit juice. An alternative method is two tablets followed by exercise-induced sweating. The patient is advised not to shower until the next day. This regimen is repeated 1 week later and also can be repeated monthly to prevent recurrences. There is no evidence that a course of ketoconazole of less than 14 days' duration is associated with the idiosyncratic hepatotoxicity that is seen in 1:15,000 patients taking the drug for longer periods of time. After successful treatment, the hypopigmented areas remain lighter than the rest of the skin until the patient has a chance to tan those areas. The absence of fine scaling on the lighter areas is a good indication that no active infection is present.

In tineas other than versicolor, *Trichophyton rubrum*, *Trichophyton mentagrophytes*, and *Microsporum canis* are the most common infecting organisms. Unless systemic therapy is being considered, the actual etiologic agent may be less important than the firm establishment of a fungal etiology by KOH preparation. Regardless of location, the lesion should be kept dry, and an effective topical agent applied. The patient should dry oozing lesions by applying compresses soaked in Burow's solution from 30 to 60 minutes one to three times daily. In intertriginous areas, either a nonmedicated or an antifungal powder may be used to absorb moisture. Topical treatment usually suffices for involvement of glabrous skin, but systemic antifungal agents may be required in hairy areas, where there is widespread involvement of the skin, or when there is an associated folliculitis.

New topical antifungal agents are constantly being approved by the Food and Drug Administration (FDA). Many claims of efficacy are made by drug representatives. Most topical antifungal agents provide a cure in approximately 85% of acute infections, but the cure rate is much less when used for chronic infections.

Four distinct classes of topical antifungal agents currently are available. The largest is the azoles, which contains the first-approved imidiazoles and some variations on the basic molecule. The older agents, miconazole and clotrimazole, are available both over-the-counter and by prescription. The following is a list of available azoles:

- Clotrimazole (Mycelex, Lotrimin AF, Lotrimin)
- Econazole (Spectazole)
- Ketoconazole (Nizoral)
- Miconazole (Micatin, Monistat)
- Oxiconazole (Oxistat)
- Sulconazole (Exelderm).

The second class is the ethanolamines, which contains only ciclopirox olamine (Loprox).

The third class is the allylamines, which contains naftifine (Naftin) and terbinafine (Lamisil).

The fourth class is the polyene antibiotics, amphotericin and nystatin, which are anticandidal.

Costs to patients are similar for most of these agents. Some are promoted as being effective when used only once a day, and these would then be relatively less expensive to the patient.

Clotrimazole, miconazole (MicaTin), and tolnaftate (Tinactin, Aftate) can be purchased without a prescription, so the patient may have already tried a topical antifungal before visiting her physician. (It is more likely that the patient would have tried an over-the-counter hydrocortisone or topical antibiotic). It is important to learn what the patient has already used, so that the physician is not embarrassed by giving the patient a prescription version of an agent she has already tried. When choosing a prescription antifungal agent for such a patient, it is especially helpful to choose one from a different class such as naftifine or terbinafine, the two members of the allylamine class. These agents are unique in being fungicidal rather than fungistatic. Similarly, ciclopirox olamine is from a different class of drugs that is completely unrelated chemically to the azoles.

General principles to be considered when choosing a topical antifungal are the following:

For intertriginous involvement, lotions are more drying and can be applied in the morning and on return from work; a cream can be used at night but should be applied sparingly. In erythematous pruritic lesions, therapy may be initiated with an antifungal agent in combination with steroids such as clotrimazole and betamethasone (Lotrisone). Refractory cases may respond to a combination of agents, employing a topical from one class during the day and a topical from another class at night. For onychomycosis, ciclopirox may penetrate the nail plate better than some of the other agents.

If marked improvement of clinical lesions and symptoms is not seen within 3 weeks, it probably is necessary to use systemic antifungal agents. Griseofulvin is the first choice and usually is effective for superficial infections. A regimen for treatment with ultramicrosize griseofulvin is as follows: 5 to 7 mg/kg/day for skin infections for 2 to 4 weeks. Ketoconazole, 200 mg per day, also can be used. If therapy is planned for more than 2 weeks, it makes sense to get a baseline chemistry 18 panel and a complete blood cell count. Itraconazole (Sporanox) has a much better safety profile than ketoconazole and can be prescribed at doses of 100 mg twice daily for several weeks.

For infections shown to be caused by *M canis*, itraconazole is a better choice than ketoconazole because the organism is more sensitive to the former than to the latter.

Tinea pedis is much less prevalent in women than in men, but nonetheless requires some additional instruction. For maceration between the toes, wearing sandals may be helpful. If nylon stockings or panty hose are worn, the toes can be separated with lamb's wool, which absorbs moisture better than cotton. After bathing or showering, it is helpful to dry between the toes using a hair dryer set on a cool setting. Topical antifungal agents alone often suffice, but when widespread scaling with hyperkeratosis occurs (the so-called "moccasin" type of tinea pedis), keratolytic agents are required. The nightly application of 10% to 20% salicylic acid in petrolatum with antifungal creams used two or three times daily may successfully treat this difficult problem.

Onychomycosis of the toenails is extremely refractory to treatment, but fingernail infections may respond to griseofulvin; a polyethylene glycol vehicle preparation may facilitate absorption. A dosage of 250 mg two to four times daily, depending on the response, must be taken until the infected portion of the nail has grown out to the end of the nail. Periodic blood counts are advised because leukopenia has been observed. It may be necessary to remove the affected nail surgically or chemically using a 40% urea paste. Even if a cure is obtained, reinfection is common. Ketoconazole has been used in patients who do not respond to griseofulvin or who cannot tolerate it. Baseline liver function tests should be documented, and then laboratory studies should be repeated at least monthly. Itraconazole is very effective and recently was approved by the FDA for continuous therapy for this indication. A 54% mycologic cure rate was seen in the American studies used to support the claim for approval. Studies are currently evaluating pulse dosing of itraconazole (200 mg twice daily for 1 week a month for 4 months). Based on similar regimens in Europe, including one result with a 93% clinical cure, this is a safe, effective, and less expensive way to treat onychomycosis. Studies also are ongoing with pulsed fluconazole therapy.

Women with onychomycosis of the fingernails or toenails have the advantage over men with this problem in that they can cover the onychomyctoic nails with nail polish, which camouflages the unsightliness. Reducing the hyperkeratotic nail with filing or by using an emery board helps the appearance of the nails. Fingernail infections usually respond better than toenail infections. Topical ciclopirox may penetrate the nail plate and might be tried with nightly applications under occlusion.

Treatment of candidiasis requires meticulous drying of the area, adequate exposure to air, and specific anticandidal therapy. Gentian violet or Castellani's paint are more effective than the old-fashioned methods of drying intertriginous areas, but they have the disadvantage of coloring the skin purple. Topical antifungal creams or lotions should be used two or three times daily. The use of powder in body folds as well as the wearing of loose clothing and cotton underwear and brassieres is a useful adjunct. In highly inflamed infections, initiating therapy with a topical corticosteroid cream in combination with clotrimazole (Lotrisone), which is lightly applied to the affected areas, proves to be beneficial. For resistant candidal infections, oral nystatin, 500,000-U tablets taken orally three times daily, can be prescribed. This is a safe and inexpensive drug, which reportedly is not absorbed from the gastrointestinal tract, but on a pragmatic basis is helpful for perianal, crural, and inframammary infections. Fluconazole (Diflucan) is an expensive oral agent that is effective against *Candida* infections. A dose of 100 or 150 mg per day for 7 to 10 days is the usual regimen. Itraconazole also is effective against *Candida* infections and can be prescribed as 100 mg twice daily. The clinician should ask the patient about predisposing factors to candidiasis, such as use of systemic corticosteroids, birth control pills, or oral antibiotics. Pregnancy, diabetes, Cushing syndrome, and acquired immunodeficiency also predispose the patient to candidiasis.

Candidal paronychial infections are difficult to treat. Therapy consists of avoiding exposure to water, and rubber gloves with cotton lining should be worn whenever contact is unavoidable. Nystatin or amphotericin B (Fungizone) lotion should be applied two to four times daily to the affected area. In highly inflamed conditions, clotrimazole with steroids may be used for short periods. Chronic paronychia may cause rippling or other deformation of the nails, but eventually the nails grow out normally after the paronychia has been cured. Ketoconazole, itraconazole, or fluconazole may be required if local therapy fails.

CONSIDERATIONS IN PREGNANCY

Fluconazole is teratogenic and must not be prescribed during pregnancy. It is also believed that pregnant women should not be treated with oral ketoconazole or itraconazole. Nystatin is safe to use during pregnancy because no adverse effects or complications have been seen in infants born to women treated with oral nystatin.

BIBLIOGRAPHY

Borelli D, Jacobs PH, Nall L. Tinea versicolor: epidemiologic, clinical and therapeutic aspects. J Am Acad Dermatol 1991;25:300.

Chren M-M. Costs of therapy for dermatophyte infections. J Am Acad Dermatol 1994;31:S103.

Cohn MS. Superficial fungal infections: topical and oral treatment of common types. Postgrad Med 1992;91:239, 249.

Cohen PR, Scher RK. Topical and surgical treatment of onychomycosis. J Am Acad Dermatol 1994:31:S74.

Degreef HJ, DeDoncker PRG. Current therapy of dermatophytosis. J Am Acad Dermatol 1994;31:S25.

Hay RJ. Antifungal therapy of yeast infections. J Am Acad Dermatol 1994;31:S6.

Korting HC, Schäfer-Korting M. Is tinea unguium still widely incurable? Arch Dermatol 1992;128:243.

Leyden JL. Tinea pedis pathophysiology and treatment. J Am Acad Dermatol 1994;31:S31.

Odds FC. Pathogenesis of *Candida* infections. J Am Acad Dermatol 1994;31:S2.

Roberts DT. Oral therapeutic agents in fungal nail disease. J Am Acad Dermatol 1994;31:S78.

Sanchez JL, Torres VM. Double-blind efficacy study of selenium sulfide in tinea versicolor. J Am Acad Dermatol 1984;11:235.

Vidimos AT, Camisa C, Tomecki KJ. Tinea capitis in three adults. Intl J Dermatol 1991;30:206.

Primary Care for Women, edited by Phyllis C. Leppert and Fred M. Howard. Lippincott-Raven Publishers, Philadelphia © 1997.

144

Herpes Simplex Virus Infections

DAVID L. CROSBY

Herpes simplex viruses (HSVs) are near-perfect human parasites. The organisms infect a significant percentage of the population: 95% of urban adults are serologically positive for HSV 1, and almost half of patients at STD clinics and 20% of U.S. females are serologically positive for HSV 2. HSVs cause an initial mild (in 80% to 90% of cases clinically silent) primary infection, followed by lifelong latent carriage of the virus in the dorsal sensory root ganglia. Periodic infectious clinical and subclinical recurrences of the infection aid in transmission of the virus through the population. Rarely is the human host seriously injured by the virus by such untoward sequelae as encephalitis, neonatal herpes, or disseminated herpes. Although herpesviruses rarely cause significant physical harm to their hosts, severe emotional distress and disruption of interpersonal relationships can accompany the diagnosis of herpes.

ETIOLOGY

The family *Herpesviridae* includes the group of viruses with the characteristics of double-stranded, linear DNA in the viral cord; icosadeltahedral (20-sided) capsid containing 162 protein capsomeres assembled in the host cellular nucleus; and a lipid bilayer envelope surrounding the capsid, derived from the nuclear membrane of the infected cell (Table 144-1). The subfamily *alpha Herpesviridae,* characterized by a short reproductive cycle, rapid spread in culture, efficient destruction of infected cells, and capacity to establish latent infection in sensory nerve ganglia, includes HSV 1 and 2 and varicella zoster virus (VZV). HSV 1 and 2 are the most closely related of the six human herpesviruses, sharing 50% DNA homology and common surface antigens that are neutralized by antisera from heterologous types.

Numerous herpesviruses infect animal species, but they are highly specific for their target hosts. Occasionally, the B virus (*Herpesvirus simiae*), a primate herpesvirus unique to Asian monkeys of the *Macaca* genus, infects laboratory workers by a bite from an infected monkey. This rare cross-species transmission may lead to severe infection with a high mortality.

Estimates of the incidence of genital HSV infection in the United States are as high as 500,000 new cases per year. The incidence doubled in the United Kingdom between 1979 and 1985. Serologic evidence of prior HSV 2 infection rose to 21.7% of the U.S. population by 1993, a 31% increase in the past decade alone.

After initial HSV infection, there is lifelong carriage of latent virus in the dorsal sensory root ganglia. There may be no further eruption of the virus after the initial clinical manifestation of HSV. Reactivation of the latent virus with recurrent clinical lesions occurs more commonly in genital than orolabial sites (in 50% and 30% of cases, respectively). Recurrence is much more common in genital herpes with HSV 2 than HSV 1 (95% and 50% of cases, respectively). The fact that fewer surface antigens are found on the envelope of HSV 2 than HSV 1 may account for this difference in reactivation by less effective immune surveillance. Women are less likely than men to develop a recurrence or frequent recurrences (more than ten recurrences in the first year of infection) after primary genital herpes: recurrence occurs in 74% of women and frequent recurrences occur in 14%. The risk of developing subsequent recurrences is associated with the severity of the primary infection, the patient's age, and the HSV type. Patients with HSV 2 averaged four recurrences in the first year after primary infection; those with HSV 1 had only one. Reactivation may be associated with menses, stress, sunburn, fever, or immunosuppression, but most reactivations are idiopathic.

Table 144-1. The Human Herpesviruses

VIRUS	PRIMARY DISEASE MANIFESTATION
Herpes simplex virus 1	Orolabial herpes (cold sores)
Herpes simplex virus 2	Genital herpes
Varicella zoster virus	Varicella (chickenpox) and herpes zoster (shingles)
Cytomegalovirus	CMV mononucleosis and CMV inclusion disease
Epstein-Barr virus	Mononucleosis
Human herpes virus 6	Roseola infantum (exanthem subitum)

HSV 1 generally infects orolabial regions, HSV 2 genital regions. However, either virus can infect any mucocutaneous site. Oral–genital contact can facilitate the spread of the HSV 2 to the mouth or HSV 1 to the genitals. Other sites of viral infection are usually associated with traumatic breaks in the skin and can be exogenous or autoinoculations (eg, fingers of thumb-suckers, nipples of women nursing babies with orolabial HSV, and fingers of health care workers).

The clinical subtypes of HSV infection include primary infection of an immunologically naive host, nonprimary first episode (the first clinical appearance of infection in a patient with serologic evidence of previous herpesvirus infection), and recurrent disease (a reactivation of clinical lesions in a patient with a history of previous herpesvirus infection). Primary infections are usually asymptomatic, but when clinically evident they tend to be more severe.

HISTORY

Most cases of primary infection of the orolabial mucosa by HSV 1 are asymptomatic during childhood between 6 months and 5 years of age. Maternal antibodies prevent primary infection before age 6 months. However, any person not previously infected with HSV is at risk. Women raised in rural areas may remain immunologically naive well into adulthood. Most clinically silent infections occur between age 6 months and 2 years. Symptomatic cases are most common between ages 2 and 5 years, arising after a 3- to 5-day incubation period. Severe erosive stomatitis with drooling, foul breath, and resistance to eating and drinking then erupts in association with fever, malaise, and tender cervical adenopathy. The febrile period lasts 3 to 5 days, followed by complete recovery within 2 weeks. Primary genital herpes infection arises 3 to 5 days after sexual activity. Many cases of primary genital herpes are asymptomatic or mild and are not recognized by the patient. Most symptomatic women present with painful genital lesions, dysuria, or a mucopurulent discharge. They may have noted lesions on the genitals of their sexual partners. Associated systemic symptoms of primary HSV infection include headache, dysuria, fever, malaise, and tender inguinal adenopathy.

Recurrent herpetic lesions may be preceded by 12 to 24 hours of tingling paresthesias or mild burning pain. Recurrent orolabial lesions (cold sores) are usually located on the vermilion border of the lip. Genital recurrent lesions may be present on any part of the genitalia, although cervical involvement is noted in only 10% of cases. Lesions that recur tend to reactivate in the same area again and again and may leave scarring. Any cutaneous eruption that recurs repeatedly in the same location should raise the suspicion of a recurrent herpesvirus lesion.

PHYSICAL EXAMINATION

The sine qua non lesion of herpesvirus infections consists of grouped vesicles or pustules on an erythematous base (Fig. 144-1). The primary herpesvirus infection tends to be more severe and to last longer than recurrent lesions. Primary orolabial HSV presents with tender mucositis, drooling, and decreased oral intake, primarily in toddlers. Blisters are rare; rather, erythematous macules with ragged white centers progress over a period of 1 to 2 days to superficial erosions covered by adherent yellow exudate. Primary genital HSV in women presents with an extensive painful eruption of vesicles and papules on erythematous plaques distributed over the external genitalia, introitus, vagina, and occasionally the cervix. Erosive cervicitis is a rare complication. The blisters progress to shallow ulcerations, then crusts, over a period of 5 to 7 days. Complete healing of primary HSV progresses over a 10- to 14-day period.

Pharyngitis is noted in some patients with primary genital HSV, and HSV can be cultured from the pharynx in 11% of patients. Aseptic meningitis with photophobia, headache, stiff neck, and CSF pleocytosis is noted in 35% of women with primary HSV.

Clinical variants of HSV infection include Kaposi varicelliform eruption, a secondary infection of another primary dermatosis such as atopic dermatitis, Darier disease, ichthyosis, or cutaneous T-cell lymphoma with HSV (Fig. 144-2). The multiple breaks in the skin provided by the primary dermatosis allows widespread dissemination of the virus; rarely, systemic infection occurs. Large necrotic ulcers that grow over a period of months may develop in patients with profound, longstanding immunosuppression such as AIDS (Fig. 144-3). Herpes encephalitis, which occurs in one in 250,000 to 500,000 persons per year, is usually due to HSV 1. It is the most common form of sporadic encephalitis in the Western world. Herpes keratoconjunctivitis is the leading cause of infectious blindness in the United States. Epithelial infection of the cornea develops during the initial episode. Recurrent HSV infection of the eye can lead to deeper stromal involvement and corneal destruction.

LABORATORY STUDIES

The most direct way to diagnose HSV infection is via the Tzanck smear, performed by unroofing a vesicle and scraping the undersurface of the roof and floor of the resulting erosion with a scalpel blade. The material obtained is gently smeared onto a glass slide

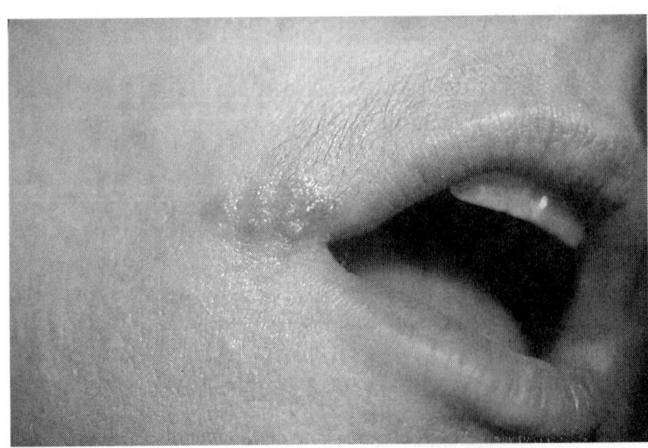

Figure 144-1. Orolabial herpes simplex infection (a cold sore), demonstrating the primary lesion of HSV 1 and 2 and VZV, grouped vesicles, pustules, or papules on an erythematous base.

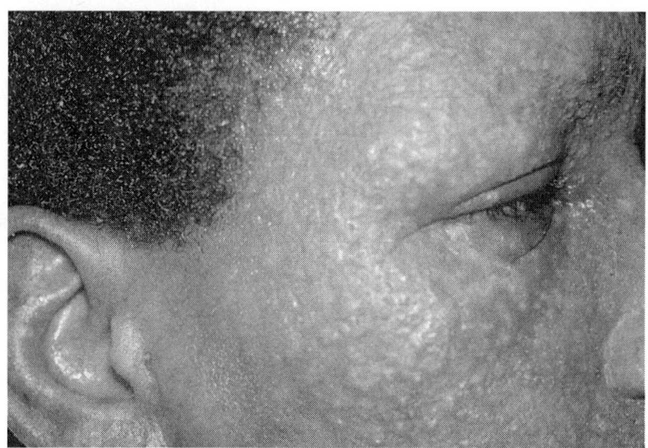

Figure 144-2. Kaposi varicelliform eruption in a patient with atopic dermatitis. The cribriform superficial vesicles and ulcerations arose over a 2-day period. This patient had had two similar episodes within the past 18 months.

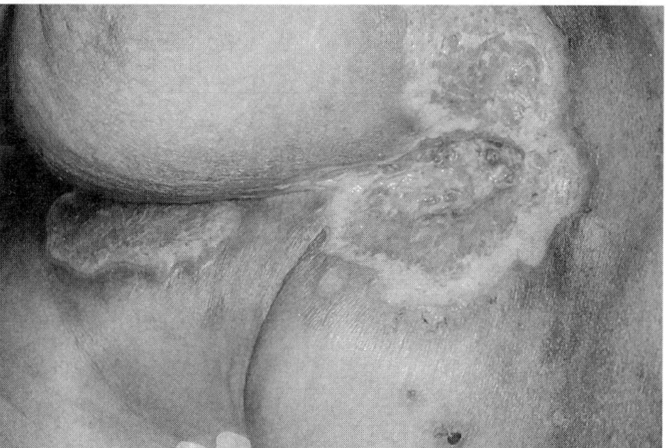

Figure 144-3. This painful, necrotic ulceration arose over a 3-month period in this woman with AIDS. Biopsy demonstrated the cytopathologic changes of herpes infection, and culture grew HSV 2. This healed over a five-week period on acyclovir.

and stained with Wright, Giemsa, or Papanicolaou stain. The presence of multinucleate, giant epithelial cells with characteristic large nuclei and rather scant cytoplasm seen on Tzanck smears and biopsy specimens of herpetic lesions is diagnostic of a herpesvirus infection (Fig. 144-4). HSV 1 and 2 and VZV infections produce indistinguishable cytopathic changes.

The cytologic diagnosis and specific viral etiology of the eruption can be confirmed by viral culture. HSV grows readily from 95% of swab specimens from vesicular lesions in 2 to 3 days. As lesions age, the yield on viral culture drops appreciably (87% of pustules, 70% of ulcers, and 29% of crusted lesions). Differentiation of HSV 1 from HSV 2 in culture requires the use of immunofluorescence techniques. The use of immunofluorescence techniques to search for the expression of viral antigens in HSV cultures can also reduce the time to a positive result to 24 hours from the 3 to 5 days required for cytopathic changes to occur.

TREATMENT

Attempts at vaccination against HSV have been disappointing. Various antigens have been used, including HSV glycoproteins D and B and HSV immune stimulating complexes. Adjuvants used with these antigens to stimulate the immune response include muramyl tetrapeptide and alum. These vaccines have shown efficacy in guinea pig models of HSV infection, but human studies have failed to show efficacy.

Herpesviruses, like all viruses, are obligate intracellular parasites. Steps in viral reproduction include receptor-mediated absorption and penetration of the cellular membrane, uncoating and disassembly of the virion in the cytoplasm, translocation of the viral DNA to the nucleus, viral protein synthesis and DNA replication, reassembly of the virion, and release of the infectious viral particle via host cell cytolysis. Each step is a potential target for antiviral therapy.

The most effective antiviral therapies for herpesvirus infections have been directed at viral-encoded thymidine kinase, an enzyme produced by the virally infected cells to allow viral replication and latency in nondividing cells, which do not usually express thymidine kinase (eg, neurons) (Fig. 144-5). The first nucleoside analog to exploit thymidine kinase as an antiherpetic target was acyclovir. Topical acyclovir is effective in the treatment of herpetic keratoconjunctivitis, primary HSV, and recurrent HSV in immunocompromised hosts. Parenteral acyclovir is indicated for primary HSV, recurrent HSV in immunocompromised hosts, and chronic prophylaxis in frequently recurring HSV. The widespread practice of episodic treatment of recurrent HSV in immunocompetent patients with parenteral acyclovir at the onset of prodrome symptoms has shown limited efficacy in a few patients.

The dosage of acyclovir for primary and nonprimary first-episode HSV is 200 mg five times daily for 7 to 10 days. It may be given intravenously at 5 to 10 mg every 8 hours. Acyclovir ointment should be applied every 3 hours, six times daily for 7 days. Downward dosage adjustment is necessary in cases of renal compromise. For chronic prophylaxis of frequently recurrent HSV, acyclovir 400 mg can be given twice or three times daily without the risk of inducing antiviral resistance or other untoward sequelae. However, this expensive and inconvenient treatment is usually reserved for patients with more than six symptomatic recurrences per year or severe emotional distress due to the recurrent disease. Suppressive acyclovir also may reduce asymptomatic viral shedding in women with frequently recurrent genital herpes.

Famciclovir at a dosage of 125 mg three times per day for 5 days and valacyclovir, a prodrug of acyclovir with better oral bioavailability, at a dosage of 500 mg three times per day for 5 days will both decrease the duration and severity of recurrent herpes eruptions. Both drugs must be started as soon as possible after the onset of the eruption, during the prodrome if present, to have an effect. Acyclovir-resistant HSV has been found in HSV 2 infections. Resistance is a clinical problem in immunocompromised patients, primarily AIDS patients, treated previously with suppressive or, especially, frequent short courses of acyclovir. The mechanisms of acyclovir resistance includes deletion of the viral-encoded thymidine kinase, an altered viral-encoded thymidine kinase with greater substrate specificity, and alterations in DNA polymerase. DNA polymerase mutations are rare, as this is a highly conserved enzyme with a specific, unalterable function in cellular and viral propagation. Thymidine kinase-deficient clones have significantly reduced virulence because the virus lacking this enzyme cannot infect and establish latent infection in neurons effectively.

Patients with genital HSV often feel stigmatized and express feelings of reduced self-worth. This emotional turmoil may be

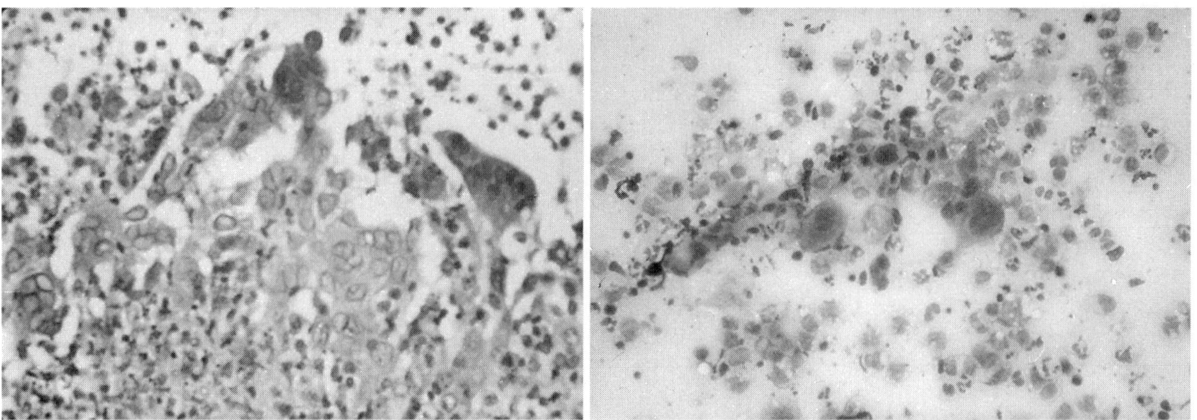

Figure 144-4. Cytopathologic changes of herpesvirus infection. The multinucleate giant epithelial cells are diagnostic of herpesvirus infection, due to HSV 1 or 2 or VZV. *Left*, hematoxylin and eosin stain of a biopsy specimen (original magnification x400). *Right*, rapid Wright stain of a smear from a vesicle (original magnification x100).

compounded by concerns over present and future interpersonal relationships, the source of the infection, and fidelity. It is important to stress to the patient that is impossible to tell when she or her partner may have first been infected with HSV, as the primary, asymptomatic infection may have occurred years before the present outbreak. Counseling regarding spread of the herpetic infection to others, both when lesions are present and during times of asymptomatic viral shedding, is imperative. Although condoms are not completely effective at preventing the spread of the infection, their use should be encouraged. As with all STDs, careful examination for any other venereal disease is warranted. Patients interested in further information and local support groups can contact the Herpes Hotline, staffed by personnel from the American Social Health Association, at (919) 361-8488.

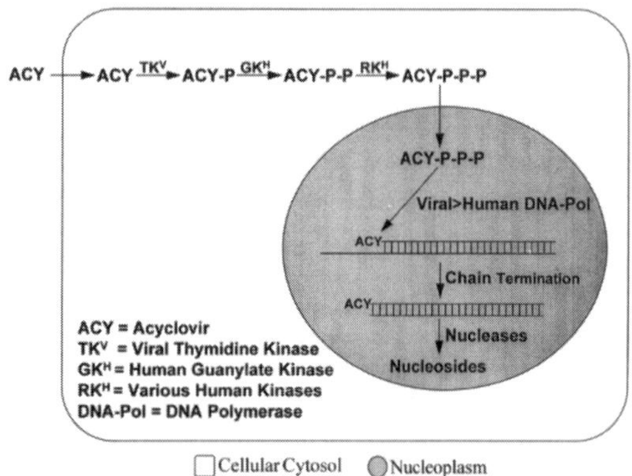

Figure 144-5. Acyclovir enters cells via passive diffusion. Viral thymidine kinase selectivity phosphorylates acyclovir to acyclovir monophosphate at a rate 3000 times that of human thymidine kinase. Guanylate kinase then places a second phosphate onto the acyclovir monophosphate, with the third phosphate added by a variety of kinases. Acyclovir triphosphate is incorporated into the growing DNA chain via DNA polymerase. Viral DNA polymerase is also selective in picking up acyclovir triphosphate at a rate three to four times greater than guanidine triphosphate. Acyclovir is an obligate chain terminator, ending the replication of the growing DNA chain. The terminated DNA chain is broken down by nucleases, and the cell cannot produce the viral DNA. The infection is therefore inhibited.

CONSIDERATIONS IN PREGNANCY

Neonatal HSV infection is a serious problem because of the possibility of severe untoward effects on the infected neonate. Neonatal HSV is due to HSV 2 in 70% of cases and occurs once in every 3500 to 5000 deliveries per year in the United States. Only the skin and mucosa are affected in 42% of cases, but 35% of patients have CNS involvement, and in 22% of cases the infection disseminates. Significant morbidity and mortality can arise despite adequate antiviral therapy. Viral shedding has been reported at delivery in 0.09% to 0.8% of mothers. Thus, at most, one in every 280 babies delivered through an infected birth canal develops neonatal HSV. Factors that influence transmission include the type of maternal infection (primary infection of the mother is the most dangerous), maternal antibody status (children of seronegative mothers are at highest risk), the duration of ruptured membranes greater than 24 hours, and the presence of a fetal scalp monitor.

There is no consensus on the appropriate management of expectant mothers with genital HSV infection. The most prudent approach would seem to be that mothers with clinical lesions of HSV at the time of parturition should be delivered via cesarean section if the membranes have not ruptured. After rupture of membranes, cesarean section might still be appropriate in mothers with true primary infection. Cesarean section, however, does not prevent all cases of neonatal infection. Antepartum cultures weekly from week 32 would predict only 25% of neonatal cases. Therefore, herpesvirus cultures should be obtained only when a woman is symptomatic, and cultures should be obtained at delivery only if there is a history of HSV infection in the mother or active lesions in her partner. Pediatricians should be alerted when active lesions are noted at the time of labor, even if a cesarean section is performed. Babies born to mothers with genital HSV should be monitored closely for any signs of infection and treated at the earliest opportunity with acyclovir if the disease develops.

Acyclovir is a pregnancy category C drug. A database of pregnancy outcomes in acyclovir-exposed fetuses has been enrolling patients for over 10 years now. In 811 exposures with 601 known outcomes, 70% of these during the first trimester, no consistent pattern of defects have been associated with acyclovir use during pregnancy. Combining these safety data with the risk of neonatal herpes suggests that prophylactic acyclovir may reduce the risk of maternal–fetal transmission of the virus in mothers with frequent recurrences or, especially, primary infections. Studies supporting this hypothesis are lacking. Limited trials in small numbers of patients have shown reduced viral shedding at the time of delivery and lower rates of cesarean section in acyclovir-treated mothers with frequent recurrences.

BIBLIOGRAPHY

Benedetti J, Corey L, Ashley R. Recurrence rates in genital herpes after symptomatic first-episode infection. Ann Intern Med 1994;121:847.

Benson PM, Malane SL, Banks R, Hicks CB, Hilliard J. B virus (*Herpesvirus simiae*) and human infection. Arch Dermatol 1989;125:1247.

Blank H, Haines HG. Viral diseases of the skin, 1975: a 25-year perspective. J Invest Dermatol 1976;67:169.

Bryson YJ, Dillon M, Lovett M, et al. Treatment of first episodes of genital herpes simplex virus infection with oral acyclovir. N Engl J Med 1983;308:916.

Communicable Disease Surveillance Centre. Sexually transmitted disease in Britain, 1985. Communicable Dis Rep 1987;45:3.

Corey L. First-episode, recurrent, and asymptomatic herpes simplex infections. J Am Acad Dermatol 1988;18:169.

Corey L, Adams HG, Brown ZA, Holmes KK. Genital herpes simplex virus infections: clinical manifestations, course, and complications. Ann Intern Med 1983;98:958.

Corey L, Nahmias AJ, Guinan ME, et al. A trial of topical acyclovir in genital herpes simplex virus infections. N Engl J Med 1982;306:1313.

Crumpacker CS 2d. Molecular targets of antiviral therapy. N Engl J Med 1989;321:163.

Fife KH, Crumpacker CS, Mertz GJ, et al. Recurrence and resistance patterns of herpes simplex virus following cessation of ≥6 years of chronic suppression with acyclovir. J Infect Dis 1994;169:1338.

Goldberg LH, Kaufman R, Kurtz TO, et al. Long-term suppression of recurrent genital herpes with acyclovir. Arch Dermatol 1993;129:582.

Johnson RE, Nahmias AJ, Magder LS, et al. A seroepidemiological survey of the prevalence of herpes simplex virus type 2 infection in the United States. N Engl J Med 1989;321:7.

Liesegang TJ. Ocular herpes simplex infection: pathogenesis and current therapy. Mayo Clin Proc 1988;63:1092.

Moseley RC, Corey L, Benjamin D, Winter C, Remington ML. Comparison of viral isolation, direct immunofluorescence, and indirect immunoperoxidase techniques for detection of genital herpes simplex virus infection. J Clin Microbiol 1981;13:913.

Nugier F, Colin JN, Aymard N, et al. Occurrence and characterization of acyclovir-resistant herpes simplex virus isolates: report on a two-year sensitivity screening survey. J Med Virol 1992;36:1.

Olson LC, Buescher EL, Artenstein MS, Parkman PD. Herpesvirus infections of the human central nervous system. N Engl J Med 1967;277:1271.

Pregnancy outcomes following systemic prenatal acyclovir exposure. MMWR 1993;42:806.

Stray-Pedersen B. Acyclovir in late pregnancy to prevent neonatal herpes simplex [letter]. Lancet 1990;336:756.

Wald A, Barnum G, Selke S, et al. Acyclovir suppresses asymptomatic shedding of HSV 2 in the genital tract. 34th Interscience conference on antimicrobial agents and chemotherapy, Orlando, October 1994.

Whatley JD, Thin RN. Episodic acyclovir therapy to abort recurrent attacks of genital herpes simplex infection. J Antimicrobial Chemother 1991;27:677.

Whitley RJ. Neonatal herpes simplex virus infections. J Med Virol 1993;Suppl 1:13.

Primary Care for Women, edited by Phyllis C. Leppert and Fred M. Howard. Lippincott-Raven Publishers, Philadelphia © 1997.

145

Varicella Zoster Virus Infections

DAVID L. CROSBY

The varicella zoster virus (VZV) is the most ubiquitous of human infections. Almost all humans are infected with the virus by the time they reach adulthood. VZV has two distinct clinical presentations, varicella (chickenpox) in the previously uninfected host and herpes zoster (shingles) due to reactivation of the virus in previously infected persons (Table 145-1). Varicella tends to be a minor (asymptomatic in one third of cases) infection of early childhood. Only rarely are there untoward sequelae of varicella, with fewer than 1000 deaths nationwide each year. During the primary infection, VZV establishes latent infection in the dorsal sensory root ganglia that persists throughout the patient's entire life. Waning of the host immune response to the virus due to drug- or disease-induced immune suppression or, more commonly, advanced age can lead to a reactivation of the virus in a single nerve root, leading to the dermatomal eruption of herpes zoster.

Although there is limited morbidity and mortality from acute varicella and herpes zoster, the severe, chronic pain of postherpetic neuralgia is a significant complication of herpes zoster, especially in people over age 50. Vaccination against VZV is possible, but at a potential cost to society in terms of dollars and indeterminate long-term morbidity and mortality. Treatments for VZV have a limited impact on the acute course of both varicella and herpes zoster, but some marginal improvement in postherpetic pain has been realized with the nucleoside analog famciclovir. Newer products might increase this benefit even further.

ETIOLOGY

VZV is a member of the subfamily *alpha Herpesviridae*. Its virology is similar to that of herpes simplex virus (HSV). More than 95% of people are infected with VZV by the time they are adults. One third of these infections are asymptomatic; therefore, in patients without a history of chickenpox in childhood, more than 90% are VZV serologically positive. The virus is carried in the sensory ganglia neurons for life after primary varicella infection. Reactivation of VZV as herpes zoster in a single nerve distribution is associated with stress (both physical and emotional) and immunosuppression. Thirty percent of bone marrow transplant patients develop herpes zoster within the first year after the transplant. However, most cases of herpes zoster are idiopathic.

Varicella is a disease of childhood. The disease is much less severe in younger children than in older children and is highly infectious. Most subsequent cases in a family are more severe than the index case, possibly due to exposure to a higher viral load

Table 145-1. Distinguishing Features of Varicella and Herpes Zoster

	VARICELLA	HERPES ZOSTER
Type of infection	Primary	Recurrent
Varicella zoster immune globulin (VZIG) status of patient	Seronegative	Seropositive
Mode of transmission	Exogenous infection from a person with varicella or, rarely, herpes zoster	Endogenous from reactivation of latent viral infection in dorsal sensory root ganglia neurons
Primary lesion	Solitary vesicle on an erythematous base	Grouped vesicles on an erythematous base
Distribution	Disseminated	Solitary dermatome
Duration of eruption	7–14 days	7–14 d
Infectivity	High, via direct contact with the eruption and respiratory route	Low, only via direct contact with the eruption (immunologically naive persons develop varicella, not herpes zoster)
Complications	Pneumonitis is rare, encephalitis and disseminated infection are very rare	Postherapetic neuralgia, especially in the elderly, and rare dissemination

through extensive household contact. In severe cases, defined as patients with more than 500 lesions, leukopenia is seen in 20%, thrombocytopenia in 5%, and hepatitis in 25%. Severe dissemination with pneumonitis and encephalitis is rare and usually seen only in adult cases.

The reactivation of VZV as herpes zoster (shingles) is directly related to the patient's age. The annual incidence climbs from 25 cases per 100,000 in people less than age 14 to more than 400 cases per 100,000 in patients over age 75. This increased incidence is proportional to the declining immune response to VZV as people age. Both the skin test reactivity and cell-mediated immune response to VZV antigens decrease dramatically with age, especially after age 50.

HISTORY

After an incubation period of 14 to 17 days, fevers, chills, and malaise are the herald of varicella. The fever may be absent or mild in young children; older children and adults tend to be more ill, with higher temperatures. A fleeting scarlatiniform eruption starts on day 2 to 4 of the fever, followed rapidly by the eruption of numerous small papules. These papules turn into clear, tense vesicles over a period of hours. The individual lesions become turbid and umbilicate in the center and crust over a period of 3 to 7 days. Three to five new crops of vesicles generally erupt over a 2- to 4-day period.

Herpes zoster may be preceded by 1 to 2 weeks of dermatomal pain. The degree of pain does not correlate well with the extent of the eruption. The pain is frequently described as burning or like an electric shock. The dermatomes involved with herpes zoster are thoracic in 53%, cervical in 20%, trigeminal in 15%, and lumbosacral in 11% of cases. This distribution does not parallel the number of nerve roots or the percentage of body surface area innervated by these dermatomes.

Postherpetic neuralgia is pain persisting beyond 4 weeks after the onset of the acute eruption of herpes zoster. This pain syndrome of unknown etiology arises in a third of patients with herpes zoster. This frequency increases with age; over two thirds of patients over age 70 are affected. This burning neuralgia pain, with occasional knife-like jabs or sensations akin to electric shocks, is unusual in patients who do not have acute pain. The intensity of the pain usually peaks within the first month and then gradually resolves over 3 to 6 months. Ten percent to 15% of patients with postherpetic neuralgia have pain beyond 6 months after the acute eruption; this unfortunate group may suffer for months or even years without respite.

PHYSICAL EXAMINATION

The primary lesions of herpes zoster are identical to those of HSV: grouped papules, vesicles, or pustules on an erythematous base. In varicella, these lesions are distributed singly and have been described as "dew drops on a rose petal" (Fig. 145-1). Clustered lesions in a dermatomal array are seen in herpes zoster (Fig. 145-2). Dermatomal maps prepared to assist in describing the distribution of nerve roots are of limited utility and should be considered only a rough approximation of nature, as much interindividual variation exists. Care should be taken to ensure that the patient is not misdiagnosed with multidermatomal herpes zoster, which is rare. Usually contiguous or bilateral dermatomes are involved; only rarely are disparate dermatomes involved at the same time.

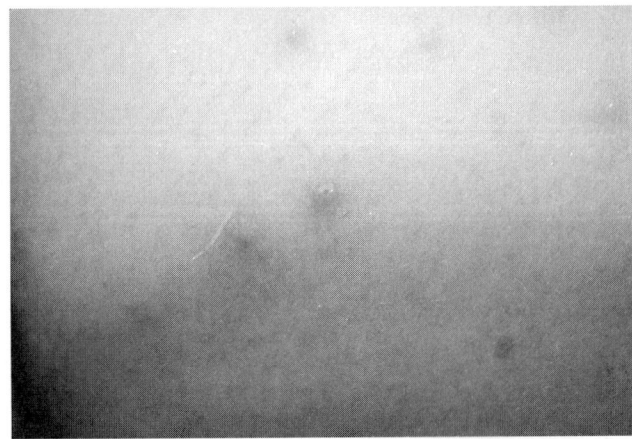

Figure 145-1. Small (1- to 3-mm) vesicles surmounting an erythematous macule in varicella. The vesicles develop central umbilication, as in the lesion in the center of the figure, then crust over a period of 3 to 7 days.

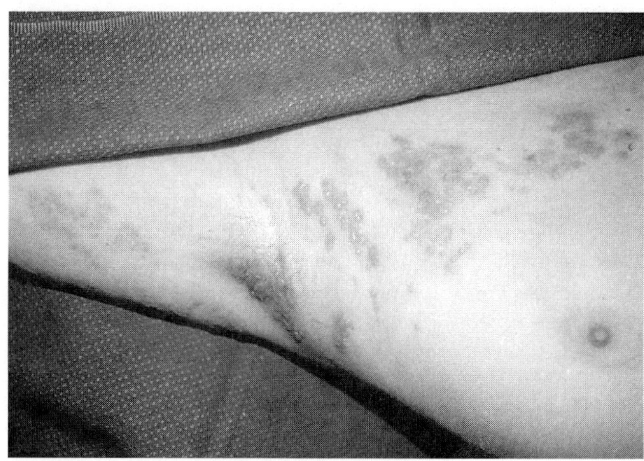

Figure 145-2. Herpes zoster (shingles) in the left T1 dermatome. This painful eruption was preceded by 2 weeks of hyperesthesia and severe burning pain in the dermatome.

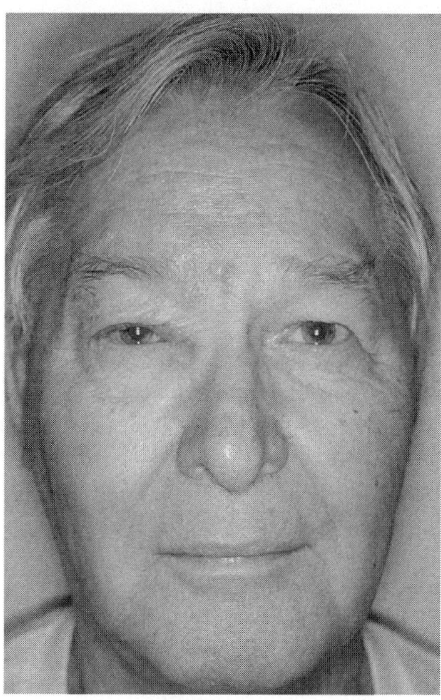

Figure 145-3. This eruption arose 36 hours previously, after 5 days of tingling paresthesias. The patient complained of right eye tearing and photophobia. Slit-lamp examination revealed a dendritic corneal erosion. There was slight erythema and a small vesicle on the tip of the nose, the area innervated by the nasociliary branch of the ophthalmic division of the trigeminal nerve.

Extradermatomal lesions of herpes zoster occur in up to a third of patients. These lesions, akin to the "dew drops on a rose petal" of varicella, are randomly distributed outside the involved dermatome. The presence of fewer than ten of these common lesions does not indicate dissemination. Disseminated herpes zoster is rare, even in severely immunocompromised patients. The widespread dissemination of herpetic lesions usually occurs in the second week of the outbreak. Dissemination of VZV from herpes zoster is a severe disease with the potential for untoward sequelae, including viral pneumonitis, encephalitis, and hepatitis. Herpes zoster in the ophthalmic division of the trigeminal nerve is of special concern because of the possibility of corneal damage (Fig. 145-3). The nasal tip is innervated by the nasociliary branch of the ophthalmic nerve, which also innervates the cornea. When the lesions of ophthalmic herpes zoster are found on the nasal tip, corneal involvement is common. Therefore, patients with ophthalmic herpes zoster should be evaluated by an ophthalmologist to exclude corneal involvement.

Occasional motor nerve syndromes occur in concurrence with the sensory nerve spread of the VZV to the skin in herpes zoster. The Ramsay Hunt syndrome is seen in facial nerve herpes zoster. Distal facial nerve palsy causing face drop develops in conjunction with vesicles on the upper half of the ear, uvula, anterior soft palate, and hard palate. Glossopharyngeal herpes zoster presents with vesicles on the earlobe and severe palatal pain. Vagal nerve herpes zoster is an unusual syndrome of lesions on the base of the tongue, epiglottis, and arytenoids in association with hoarseness, from involvement of the recurrent laryngeal nerve, and gastrointestinal and cardiac distress, which can mimic an acute abdomen and myocardial infarction. Herpes zoster involvement of the C2-C4 nerve roots has been associated with temporary diaphragmatic paralysis from phrenic nerve involvement.

Herpes zoster has several unique features in immunocompromised patients. The eruption may involve more than one dermatome. Recurrent herpes zoster may occur in patients with profound and longstanding immunosuppression because their damaged immune system does not respond with the usual boost in immunity to VZV antigens on rechallenge. Chronic, crusted herpes zoster is a unique form of the disease seen in patients with profound immunosuppression (Fig. 145-4). After acute herpes zoster, crusted papules, plaques, or erosions persist for months in the distribution of the previous herpes zoster. Biopsy reveals the cytopathic changes of viral infection, and VZV can be grown in culture from these atypical lesions.

The most severe and longstanding complication of herpes zoster is postherpetic neuralgia. Postherpetic neuralgia is not affected by acute treatment with acyclovir with or without steroids, although famciclovir may reduce its incidence.

LABORATORY STUDIES

The findings on histologic examination and Tzanck preparation of VZV lesions are identical to those of HSV infection. VZV is much more fastidious and difficult to grow in viral cultures than HSV. A culture yield of 50% from vesicular lesions is the most that can be expected of excellent virology laboratories; average laboratories fare much worse. The viral cultures must be held much longer when VZV is suspected, as the virus may take 10 to 14 days to grow. The use of immunofluorescence techniques to search the culture for the expression of viral antigens may reduce this time to 3 to 5 days.

Although most cases of HSV and VZV infections can be separated on clinical grounds, occasional cases of herpes zoster with a limited number of lesions may be confused with HSV infection. When evaluating an eruption with the clinical appearance of a herpesvirus infection (grouped vesicles on an erythematous base) and a positive Tzanck preparation, viral culture can help distinguish HSV from VZV. If the culture grows HSV 1 or 2, the diagnosis is established. If the culture grows VZV or no viral pathogens from a vesicular lesion, then VZV is the most likely etiology.

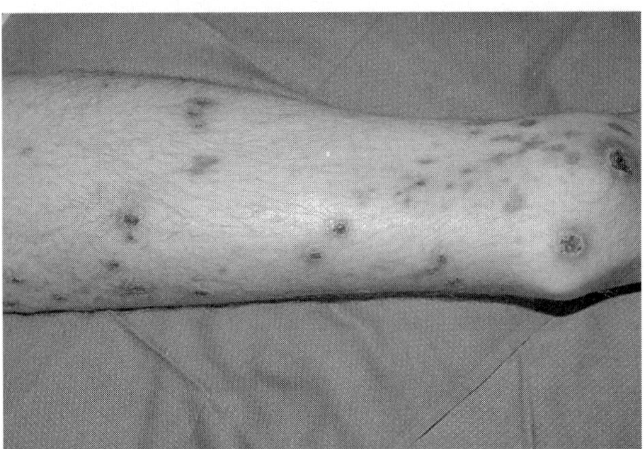

Figure 145-4. This patient with a CD4 count of 64/μL had developed OL3 zoster 3 months previously. The vesicles resolved over a 3-week period, leaving the tender, 2- to 4-cm, keratotic plaques of chronic, crusted herpes zoster as a residua.

TREATMENT

The varicella vaccine is a live attenuated vaccine produced by passing VZV through a series of culture systems. The original viral strain for the vaccine was obtained from a healthy Japanese boy with varicella named Oka; thus, the vaccine's name (Oka/Merck). This vaccine has been used in Japan and Korea under the Oka/Biken label for almost a decade. It has also been available in Europe. The vaccine induces partial immunity in immunized normal and immunocompromised children without significant side effects. After asymptomatic immunization (in 5% of normal and 50% of leukemic children, there is a mild eruption of varicella), there is lifelong carriage of the attenuated Oka VZV in sensory ganglia.

Vaccinated healthy children develop protection that is 95% effective at preventing varicella for 5 years, with antibody persistence for at least 6 years. Vaccinated healthy adults are protected only 70% of the time for 5 years, and 75% maintain their seropositivity at 6 years. Varicella that breaks through the vaccine protection is not uncommon, seen in 58 of 4171 vaccinated children in one study. A much more mild disease, with fewer lesions and fewer systemic signs of infection, is seen in vaccinated children than in children who acquire the natural infection.

Although the indication and effectiveness of the varicella vaccine in preventing untoward sequelae of varicella in previously uninfected, immunocompromised hosts (eg, leukemic children, transplant patients) are indisputable, there are grave concerns regarding routine vaccination of all American children. The immunity induced by vaccination may not be lifelong and boosters may be required in adulthood, making compliance difficult. Without the repeated exposure to VZV in the community, the "herd" immunity could dwindle over time after mass vaccination. Thus, the varicella vaccine could lead to an increased incidence of adult varicella, with its more serious complications. It is also uncertain what the clinical presentation or incidence of herpes zoster will be later in life in immunized children.

Cost analyses have shown that vaccination of children would reduce the cost to society as a whole; this benefit is due almost wholly to allowing parents of an infected child to avoid work loss while caring for the ill child. A simple maneuver that would reduce this cost benefit back toward nil would be to allow children with varicella to return to school once they are afebrile, despite the presence of lesions on their skin. Such a public health policy has been shown to be appropriate by various studies demonstrating that most varicella infections occur during the varicella prodrome, before the rash arises. Such a policy could be widely accepted if only society were to acknowledge that all children must be infected with VZV at some point during their life.

Acyclovir 20 mg/kg four times/day (maximum dose, 800 mg four times/day) is efficacious for the treatment of varicella within 24 hours of eruption onset, decreasing the number of lesions and the severity of infection. The treatment of herpes zoster is more controversial. Acyclovir shortens the acute course of herpes zoster by 1 to 2 days at a dosage of 800 mg five times/day or 10 to 15 mg intravenously every 8 hours for 7 to 10 days. Acyclovir must be started within the first 48 hours after the onset of the eruption to have any impact on the course of the disease. Acyclovir is ineffective in preventing postherpetic neuralgia. Adding steroids to the regimen or extending the duration of acyclovir therapy to 21 days is also ineffective in reducing postherpetic neuralgia.

Famciclovir, an antiviral agent for the treatment of herpes zoster, is given at 500 mg three times/day for 7 days. Famciclovir is a prodrug that is rapidly and completely absorbed by the bowel and converted to penciclovir, the active nucleoside analog. Penciclovir follows the same intracellular activation steps as acyclovir; however, penciclovir is more rapidly and completely converted to penciclovir triphosphate, due to higher avidity of binding to viral-encoded thymidine kinase. Famciclovir has a similar limited impact on the acute course of herpes zoster as acyclovir. However, famciclovir has shown efficacy in reducing the duration of postherpetic neuralgia in patients treated within 72 hours of eruption onset.

Valacyclovir, a prodrug of acyclovir that increases its oral bioavailability, is given at 100 mg three times per day for 7 days. Valacyclovir also reduces the duration of posttherpetic neuralgia, although not quite as profoundly as famciclovir.

CONSIDERATIONS IN PREGNANCY

The congenital varicella syndrome presents in newborns with fetal exposure to VZV as limb hypoplasia, dermatomal skin scarring, and CNS and eye damage. The highest risk of developing the syndrome (2% of exposed fetuses) occurs in mothers who have varicella between weeks 13 and 20 of gestation. Fetuses born to mothers with herpes zoster during pregnancy do not appear to be at risk of this developmental damage. If the mother develops varicella within 4 days before and 2 days after delivery, the neonate is at risk of developing severe congenital varicella with a mortality approaching 30%, because he or she is unprotected by maternal antibodies. The effect of acyclovir treatment of mothers with varicella on the development of fetal infection and subsequent birth defects is unknown. Considering the encouraging safety data of acyclovir exposure during pregnancy, antiviral intervention with acyclovir early in the course of varicella during pregnancy may be warranted.

BIBLIOGRAPHY

Bernstein HH, Rothstein EP, Watson BM, et al. Clinical survey of natural varicella compared with breakthrough varicella after immunization with live attenuated Oka/Merck varicella vaccine. Pediatrics 1993;92:833.

Degreef H, Andrejevic L, Aoki F, et al. Famciclovir, a new oral antiherpes drug: results of the first controlled clinical study demonstrating its efficacy and safety in the treatment of uncomplicated herpes zoster in immunocompetent patients. Internatl J Antimicrobial Agents 1994;4:241.

de Moragas JM, Kierland RR. The outcome of patients with herpes zoster. Arch Dermatol 1957;75:193.

Dunkle LM, Arvin AM, Whitley RJ, et al. A controlled trial of acyclovir for chickenpox in normal children. N Engl J Med 1991;325:1539.

Enders G, Miller E, Cradock-Watson J, Bolly I, Ridehalgh M. Consequences of varicella and herpes zoster in pregnancy: prospective study of 1739 cases. Lancet 1994;343:1548.

Gershon AA, LaRussa P, Hardy I, Sternberg S, Silverstein S. Varicella vaccine: the American experience. J Infect Dis 1992;166(Suppl 1):S63.

Lieu TA, Cochi SL, Black SB, et al. Cost-effectiveness of a routine varicella vaccination program for U.S. children. JAMA 1994;271:375.

McKendrick MW, McGill JI, White JE, Wood MJ. Oral acyclovir in acute herpes zoster. Br Med J 1986;293:1529.

McKendrick MW, McGill JI, Wood MJ. Lack of effect of acyclovir on postherpetic neuralgia. Br Med J 1989;298:431.

Meyers JD. Congenital varicella in term infants: risk reconsidered. J Infect Dis 1974:129:215.

Moore DA, Hopkins RS. Assessment of a school exclusion policy during a chickenpox outbreak. Am J Epidemiol 1991;133:1161.

Pregnancy outcomes following systemic prenatal acyclovir exposure. MMWR 1993;42:806.

Ragozzino MW, Melton LJ 3d, Kurland LT, Chu CP, Perry HO. Population-based study of herpes zoster and its sequelae. Medicine 1982; 61:310.

Watson B, Gupta R, Randall T, Starr S. Persistence of cell-mediated and humoral immune responses in healthy children immunized with live attenuated varicella vaccine. J Infect Dis 1994;169:197.

Wood MJ, Johnson RW, McKendrick MW, et al. A randomized trial of acyclovir for 7 days or 21 days with and without prednisolone for treatment of acute herpes zoster. N Engl J Med 1994;330:896.

Primary Care for Women, edited by Phyllis C. Leppert and Fred M. Howard. Lippincott-Raven Publishers, Philadelphia © 1997.

146

HPV Infection (Warts)

KARL R. BEUTNER

Infection of cutaneous surfaces with human papillomavirus (HPV) is ubiquitous. The major clinical manifestations of this infection, warts, are common. Although the diagnosis usually is simple and is based on physical findings, there can be some pitfalls in the diagnosis. Once the diagnosis has been established, treatment often is challenging and a source of frustration to both the patient and the clinician. Understanding the nature of the infection and its natural history provides the clinician with information necessary to not only counsel the patient but also to make proper decisions regarding therapy. As with other viral infections, before it is possible to effectively treat or educate, it is necessary to understand the natural history.

ETIOLOGY AND EPIDEMIOLOGY

Warts are the most commonly recognized clinical manifestation of cutaneous infection with the HPV. Based on differences in their DNA, there are multiple genotypes of HPV, perhaps 80 or more. The important concept regarding HPV types is that different types tend to infect different anatomic areas and cause different types of warts. For example, a few types cause common warts and other types cause flat warts; another large group of HPVs—often referred to as genital HPVs—are, in reality, the HPVs found on moist surfaces of the conjunctiva, nasal cavity, oral cavity, larynx, and the genital area. The virus replicates only in the epidermis; it does not spread inward, nor is it spread by the blood stream.

When the skin is infected with the wart virus, the skin cells grow in an abnormal fashion, clinically producing warts. Warts are classified in several ways, depending either on how they look (morphology) or on their anatomic location (Table 146-1). Warts often are referred to according to their anatomic location—for example, as hand warts, or periungual warts (warts around the fingernail), or plantar warts (warts on the plantar aspect [soles] of the feet).

Morphologically, nongenital warts are essentially of two varieties: (1) the keratotic verruca vulgaris; or (2) flat warts, which are small, flat, often tan to flesh-colored, slightly raised, 1- to 2-mm papules. In the genital area, there are four morphologic types of warts: (1) the cauliflower or hypertrophic type—condyloma acuminatum; (2) smooth papular warts, which consist of small, 1- to 5-mm, sometimes dome-shaped, flesh-colored papules; (3) keratotic genital warts, which can mimic seborrheic keratoses; and (4) flat warts.

In the genital area, the major differential diagnosis includes molluscum contagiosum, squamous cell carcinoma in situ, lichen planus, seborrheic keratoses, pearly penile papules, sebaceous (Tyson's) glands, condyloma lata, and skin tags. Squamous cell carcinoma in situ of the genitalia (or bowenoid papulosis) is a clinical manifestation of high-risk genital HPV infection. This is the cutaneous manifestation of the oncogenic HPVs. If the diagnosis is in doubt, simple biopsy helps to clarify the issue. In general, if a patient is failing frequent treatments or is getting worse with treatment, a biopsy should be considered. The progression of squamous cell carcinoma in situ on the external genitalia to invasive cancer in immunocompetent patients is extremely rare. However, women with vulvar squamous cell carcinoma in situ and female partners of men with this condition are at significant risk for developing abnormalities of their cervix. Women with any form of genital HPV infection or whose male sexual partners have genital HPV infection should have a pap smear and be retained in the pap smear system, because HPV—if not the cause—is a major risk factor for developing cervical cancer.

The epidemiology of nongenital warts has not been well-characterized other than to say they are common. In terms of genital HPV infection, it has been estimated that 25% to 50% of all sexually active adults have genital HPV infection. Approximately 1% have visible genital warts at any given time. The predominant mode of transmission of genital warts in sexually active adults is through sexual contact. Nonsexual transmission can occur, but it is relatively rare in the sexually active population. In children with genital warts,

Table 146-1. Wart Classification

Location
Nongenital warts
Hand warts
Periungual warts
Plantar warts
Genital warts
Morphology
Nongenital warts
Verruca vulgaris
Flat warts
Genital warts
Hypertrophic, cauliflower, or condyloma acuminata
Smooth papular
Keratotic
Flat

sexual abuse needs to be considered. Although most (perhaps 75% to 90%) of genital warts in children have been transmitted by other than sexual routes, child sexual abuse needs to be excluded.

Both the clinicians treating warts and the patients being treated for warts need to have reasonable expectations of therapy. Considerable evidence suggests that once a patient is infected with the wart virus they may be infected for life. This is analogous to the situation with herpes simplex infection in that once infection is established the clinician is left with treating symptoms, but currently the infection is untreatable. Therefore, the goal of treatment is the induction of wart-free periods. Optimally, this should be achieved with a treatment that is no worse than the disease. Often, when patients do not respond well to treatment, the treatment gets increasingly aggressive. More aggressive therapies often are not met with better clinical outcomes.

Nongenital warts are thought to be transmitted by casual contact with others who are infected or through fomites. HPVs do not have a lipid envelope and, thus, are inherently relatively resistant to physical and chemical destruction. This resistance facilitates transmission by fomites. Currently, the incubation period (the time from infection with HPV until warts develop) is believed to be weeks to months. There is also reason to believe that many, if not most, people infected may never express the infection in terms of a recognized wart.

Some factors increase susceptibility to the development of warts. These include age, immunologic status, and chronic exposure to moisture. Whereas nongenital warts can occur at all ages, they are clearly more common in children than adults. Patients who are immunosuppressed because of medications, other illnesses, or infections are particularly susceptible to developing warts, which are often multiple and difficult to treat. In the immunocompromised host, particularly on sun-exposed areas, warts may evolve into squamous cell carcinomata.

Individuals who have either hands or feet that are chronically wet either because of hyperhidrosis from avocational or vocational activities are more prone to develop warts. It has been speculated that the chronic exposure to moisture facilitates the entrance of the wart virus into the skin. Periungual warts, for example, are associated with improper sterilization technique on the part of manicurists as a vector for transmitting the infection.

Differential diagnoses of nongenital warts includes seborrheic keratoses, Gottron's papules (a manifestation of dermatomyositis), granuloma annulare, lichen planus, molluscum contagiosum, skin tags, lichen nitidus, seborrheic keratosis, actinic keratosis and squamous cell carcinoma. On the feet, it is often difficult to distinguish between a plantar wart and a clavus or corn, or acquired digital fibrokeratoma, or foreign body. In general, the plantar warts have small, blue-black stippling representing thrombosed capillaries and, in general, warts do not have dermatoglyphics. Corns and calluses often are found over bony prominences, but they lack the blue-black stippling and, although dense and keratinous, they do maintain normal dermatoglyphics.

The main reason for treating nongenital warts is that they present a mechanical problem in that they can be tender or traumatized and often are cosmetically bothersome. One option with warts is simple observation. It has been estimated that about two thirds of warts go away in 2 years without treatment. For the patient who does not desire treatment, it is not unreasonable to simply observe. Genital warts need to be treated because they may facilitate transmission or acquisition of blood-borne infections such as hepatitis and human immunodeficiency virus. When selecting treatment, the patient's preference, anatomic location of the wart, and the availability of different treatment modalities often are the major determining factors.

COMMON WARTS

Common warts occur anywhere on the cutaneous surface and can be traumatized, resulting in pain and discomfort. They are most common, however, on the hands and feet. Cryotherapy with liquid nitrogen is a common treatment modality. When done properly, this results in a good response with minimal, if any, scarring. When using cryotherapy, remember that a wart is a benign tumor of the top layer of the skin. Contrary to popular belief, warts do not have "roots." A wart is never any thicker than the top layer of skin (epidermis). However, the top layer of skin (epidermis) can vary considerably in thickness in different anatomic sites, and is particularly thick on the palms and soles and thinner on the face and genitalia. Liquid nitrogen can be applied either with spray technique, loosely wound cotton on a wooden stick, or a cryoprobe. It is difficult, if not impossible, to absolutely freeze a wart using a tightly wound cotton swab. Liquid nitrogen should be applied long enough so that the wart is completely frozen and so that it forms a 1- to 2-mm halo around the wart. For mid- to larger warts, repeated freeze–thaw cycle may improve efficacy. Cryotherapy for warts essentially induces frostbite, with a resulting necrosis of the tissue and slough, leaving an erosion that needs to be treated.

Inadequate freezing of the wart results in poor therapeutic response. Overly aggressive therapy, in addition to unnecessary pain, results in scarring and, on the digits, potential nerve damage. In some patients, more than a simple necrosis results: a blister or bulla, which may be hemorrhagic, can form. The patient should be told ahead of time that this may develop and be given appropriate wound care instructions.

Other than cryotherapy, surgery also can be applied to common warts; modalities often employed include curettage, electrodesiccation, hot cautery, and laser surgery. These require special training and proctoring to be effectively performed, and in inexperienced hands can result in a variety of surgical complications. Caustic agents in the form of nitric acid as well as monochloracetic, bichloracetic, and trichloracetic acids are alternatives.

FLAT WARTS

Flat warts occur on the face, hands, and arms but are a particular problem on the legs of women. Shaving of the legs can spread the warts up and down the legs. Because the patient often is aware of these but they are visible only with bright lighting or side illumination, deciding to observe rather than to treat flat warts is reasonable. If the patient insists on treatment, cryotherapy is effective but should be done gently so as to avoid hypopigmented and hyperpigmented scars. Other therapies that have been used include topical 5-fluorouracil cream, which should be used cautiously because it is a teratogen; tretinoin acid, which has anecdotally been reported to have some efficacy; and keratolytic agents containing salicylic acid.

PLANTAR WARTS

Care should be taken in the treatment of plantar warts because a scar on the plantar aspect of the foot can result in a great deal of discomfort, essentially for the lifetime of the patient. Because the epidermis is thick on the plantar aspect of the foot, plantar warts are thick. An inexpensive but labor-intensive treatment for plantar warts is the use of 40% salicylic acid plasters. The patient should be instructed to apply the plaster to the wart and a small area of surrounding tissue and to hold the plaster in place with a cloth-type adhesive tape. The plaster should be left in place for 2 to 3 days. After removing the plaster, the area should be soaked in warm water and then pared by the patient. Paring can be achieved with sandpaper or an emery board. The patient should be instructed to continue this until the wart is gone, which often is signified by the return of normal dermatoglyphics. The patient should be instructed that pain or bleeding should not occur at any time during this treatment. The major shortcoming of this therapy is that it takes several weeks and a conscientious patient.

If the patient has hyperhidrosis or if occupationally or avocationally the feet are frequently wet, attempts should be made to keep the feet drier, which may facilitate treatment. If salicylic acid fails, other modalities can be used with caution, including surgery, cryotherapy, formalin, and glutaraldehyde.

GENITAL WARTS

The current treatment for genital warts includes cryotherapy, interferon, podophyllin resin, podofilox (Condylox), surgery, and trichloroacetic acid. Not all therapies are equally effective for all patients with genital warts. The factors to be considered when selecting treatment for genital warts include the morphologic type of the wart, wart size, anatomic site, wart area, wart count, the clinician's experience, and the patient's preference. When undertaking therapy of genital warts, having a plan is important. After three to four treatments, if a significant clinical response has not occurred, the modality should be changed or the patient should be referred to a dermatologist or gynecologist.

Cryotherapy works well for genital warts. Other than the patient who has just a few small warts, patients should be offered a local anesthetic, either injectable lidocaine or topical Emla (midocaine 2.5% and prilocaine 2.5%). Using local anesthesia allows the patient a greater degree of comfort and the clinician greater ease at achieving adequate cryotherapy.

Interferon was the first drug shown to be effective in the treatment of genital warts, and it is administered by injections into the dermis at the base of the wart. It is administered three times a week for 3 weeks or twice a week for 8 weeks. However, the large number of visits, the expense of the drug, and the fact that it offers no greater efficacy than other modalities clearly has made this the second line of therapy.

Surgery for genital warts has a major advantage in that it rapidly renders the patients wart-free, and the only question remaining is recurrence. Modalities that have been used include simple tangential scissors excision, curettage, electrocautery, hot cautery, and laser surgery.

Trichloroacetic acid is a caustic agent that chemically coagulates the wart and adjacent tissue. It seems to have the greatest efficacy on small to average-sized warts on moist surfaces. Larger warts on nonmoist surfaces may be made smaller with this modality but are rarely cleared completely in an expedient fashion.

Podophyllin resin is the extract from a plant *Podophyllin emodii* or *Podophyllin peltatum*. It is not a caustic agent but rather contains biologically active compounds that interfere with mitoses and other cell functions that need intact microtubles. The major shortcoming of the podophyllin resin is a lack of a readily available standardized preparation with a known shelf-life. Podophyllin resin should be avoided during pregnancy. It is most commonly used as a 25% podophyllin in tincture of benzoin. A small amount should be applied to the wart and allowed to air-dry before the patient assumes a normal anatomic position. Whereas it is often recommended to wash off the podophyllin in 2 to 4 hours, in reality, because benzoin is not water soluble, it is difficult to wash off with water. If only a small amount is applied initially and allowed to dry, the patient can safely leave it on overnight.

Podofilox as a 0.5% solution (Condylox) is available for patients' self-treatment of external genital warts. It is limited to the treatment of warts that the patients can visualize themselves. Like podophyllin resin, it should be avoid during pregnancy.

When treating genital warts, in addition to treating the warts and, thus, alleviating the patient's symptoms, the patient should be provided with education regarding the natural history and implications of having this sexually transmitted disease. Whereas some HPV types are associated with cervical cancer, the major impact of this infection on patients is the emotional impact. By educating patients regarding the natural history and the normal emotional response to this infection, the most common complication can be prevented, that is, psychological stigma. Patients should be given both verbal and written educational material in this regard. (Patient educational material is available from the American Social Health Association at 1-919-361-8422.) Although treating warts removes the symptoms, it is not clear whether it alters the patient's infectivity. Patients should be told to tell their partners, both present and future, that they have this infection and may be infectious even after the warts are gone.

CONSIDERATIONS IN PREGNANCY

Genital HPV is rarely spread perinatally to the neonate. When this occurs, it takes the clinical form of juvenile laryngeal papillomatosis. In this condition, the infant develops multiple laryngeal warts caused by acquisition of an HPV infection while transiting the birth canal. This is a devastating but rare condition. In general, the presence of genital warts at the time of delivery is not an indication for cesarean section.

BIBLIOGRAPHY

Androphy EJ, Beutner, KR, Olbricht S. Human papillomavirus infection. In: Arndt KA, LeBoit PE, Robinson JK, Wintroub BU, eds. Cutaneous medicine and surgery: an integrated program in dermatology. Philadelphia, WB Saunders, 1996.

Beutner KR, Becker TM, Stone KM. Epidemiology of human papillomavirus infections. Dermatol Clin 1991;9:211.

Bunney MH, Benton C, Cubix HA. Viral warts: biology and treatment. New York: Oxford University Press, 1992.

Gross G, Jablonska S, Pfister H, Stequer HE, eds. Genital papillomavirus infections: modern diagnosis and treatment. Berlin, Heidelberg: Springer-Verlag, 1990.

Kautsky LA, Galloway DA, Holmes KK. Epidemiology of genital human papillomavirus infection. Epidemiol Rev 1983;10:122.

Kling AR. Genital warts. Ther Semin Dermatol 1992;11:247.

Patient educational material. Park, NC: American Social Health Associates.

147
Scabies and Pediculosis

ALLISON HOLM

Primary Care for Women, edited by Phyllis C. Leppert and Fred M. Howard. Lippincott-Raven Publishers, Philadelphia © 1997.

SCABIES

Scabies is a common disorder caused by infestation with the mite *Sarcoptes scabiei.* The adult female mite is 300 to 500 μm long, has four pairs of legs, and produces two or three eggs daily as she burrows into the stratum corneum. The eggs hatch within 3 to 4 days, producing larvae with only three pairs of legs. The larvae undergo two nymphal stages before maturing into adult mites at about 2 weeks. The female mite has a life span of 30 days.

Scabies is contracted by close personal contact, usually in situations such as families with school-aged children or persons in close living quarters (including institutionalized patients), or via sexual contact. Less frequently, scabies is spread from contaminated linens or clothing, but the mite survives only 2 to 3 days off the human host. If sexual transmission is suspected, patients should be evaluated for other sexually transmitted diseases.

The clinical features of scabies infestation include pruritic papules and burrows around the hands, especially finger webs, wrists, axillae, areolae, lower abdomen, genitals, and buttocks. In adults, the scalp and face are usually spared, but young children and infants may be affected on the entire skin surface, including the scalp, palms, and soles. Other primary lesions that may be present include pustules, vesicles, bullae, and nodules. Secondary lesions include excoriations, crusts, scars, and bacterial infections. Common causes of pyoderma are *Streptococcus pyogenes* and *Staphylococcus aureus.*

Crusted (Norwegian) scabies, a variant that manifests as severe hyperkeratosis, occurs in patients with AIDS and those receiving immunosuppressive agents. These patients have thick, extensive crusts and mites numbering in the thousands to millions.

Patients with primary scabies infestations often have no symptoms for 2 to 4 weeks, during which time sensitization to the mite occurs. Thereafter, the host remains truly sensitized to scabies but does not develop absolute immunity, so that recurrent infestations are common. When they do occur, symptoms appear immediately and are often more intense.

Positive diagnosis is based on microscopic identification of scabies mites, eggs, or fecal pellets. Mineral oil is applied to several suspicious papules and burrows, especially around the hands and wrists, and the epidermis is gently scraped with a scalpel blade. The scraping is then placed on a slide and examined microscopically under low power. Another helpful technique is the burrow ink test, in which black ink is applied to suspicious areas and the excess ink is wiped away with alcohol. This technique highlights burrows and may help the clinician determine the best areas for scraping. If scabies is not confirmed by scraping or skin biopsy, a therapeutic trial of antiscabetic treatment may be necessary.

Lindane 1% lotion (gamma benzene hexachloride [Kwell]) has for many years been the standard treatment for scabies. It is applied at bedtime to the entire skin surface below the head, including the neck, umbilicus, and subungual and intertriginous areas. The scalp of infants and young children should also be treated. The medication is washed off after 8 to 12 hours and the treatment is repeated in 4 to 7 days to treat any newly hatched mites and to ensure that all body surfaces have been treated. The estimated cure rate is 65% to 95%, but most failures result from inadequate application.

Permethrin 5% cream (Elimite), available since 1989, is a safe and effective treatment for scabies. Application is the same as with topical lindane, and the estimated cure rate exceeds 90%. Toxicity is lower than that of lindane because only 2% of the applied dose is absorbed. Permethrin is currently the treatment of choice for scabies infestations, especially in patients with neurologic disorders, infants and young children, and those who have failed lindane therapy.

Other treatments include crotamiton (Eurax), which is applied once or twice daily for 3 to 5 days in a row. It is safe in young infants but has only a 50% to 70% cure rate. Five percent to 10% precipitated sulfur in petrolatum can be applied nightly for 2 or 3 nights, but its cure rate has not been established and it is a messy and malodorous treatment.

Successful treatment necessitates careful explanation of the proper use of antiscabetic therapy and thorough inquiry into the patient's living situation. All clothing, towels, and bedding in contact with the patient require treatment, which can be done by laundering at 120°F or by dry cleaning. Alternatively, items may be placed in a sealed environment (eg, a plastic bag) for several days to prevent live mites from reinfesting a human host. All family members and close contacts, including sexual contacts, should be treated simultaneously to prevent reinfection of the patient.

Although itching often decreases within 48 hours of treatment, many patients experience postscabetic pruritus that may persist for days to weeks until mites, eggs, and feces are shed from the stratum corneum. The pruritus can be treated with oral antihistamines, lubricants, and topical steroids. As a result of numerous excoriations, pyodermas such as impetigo, ecthyma, furunculosis, and cellulitis can occur, necessitating appropriate antimicrobial therapy. A more serious complication is poststreptococcal glomerulonephritis.

LICE

Lice are 2- to 4-mm-long, flattened wingless insects that can infect the scalp (*Pediculus humanus capitis*), body (*Pediculus humanus corporis*), and pubic area (*Phthirus pubis*). They commonly attack humans, and although each variety prefers certain parts of the body, they occasionally migrate to other areas. Lice live by attaching themselves to the skin and taking a blood meal, thereby releasing a salivary secretion that produces a pruritic dermatitis.

Pediculosis Capitis

Head lice infestation occurs most frequently in children, but it may also occur in adults. It is more common in urban communities than in rural areas and affects females more frequently than males. African-Americans are affected less frequently than Caucasians, most likely because lice have adapted to gripping the cylindric hair of Caucasians.

Because head lice can survive for 2 to 3 days off the host, pediculosis capitis can be transmitted by infested clothing, hats, hairbrushes, combs, towels, bedding, and upholstery. Head lice infestations are characterized by nits (white, hatched eggs) attached to hairs about ¼ inch from the scalp. The nits are firmly fixed to the scalp hair; scale and hair casts are distinguished by their nonfixed nature and ability to slide up and down the hair shaft. Once the eggs hatch, the nymph goes through three larval stages before becoming a mature louse 10 days later. The female survives about 40 days, during which time she lays 100 to 300 eggs.

Head lice infestations produce few symptoms other than mild itching. Excoriations and secondary bacterial infections from chronic scratching can occur.

The treatment of choice for head lice infestation is synthetic pyrethrin, 1% permethrin creme rinse (Nix), which is applied to the hair and scalp for 10 minutes and then rinsed. Permethrin is both pediculicidal and ovicidal; therefore, one treatment is generally adequate. A second treatment 7 to 14 days later ensures the cure and has a 95% success rate for head lice. Natural pyrethrins (eg, Rid shampoo) are also efficacious, but they have an increased risk of allergic contact dermatitis. Moreover, they are not ovicidal, so treatment must be repeated in 1 week to ensure treatment of any newly hatched eggs. A 1% lindane preparation (Kwell) may be applied as a shampoo or left on overnight as a lotion. Lindane has been used for many years as an effective treatment for head lice.

After treatment, the remaining nits can be removed with a fine-toothed comb. In addition, all personal hair items such as combs and brushes should be treated with pediculicides or soaked in alcohol. Bedding and clothing should be treated as outlined for scabies treatment.

Family members of patients should be examined and the school contacted to detect any additional affected persons. No uniform recommendation exists for treating all household members of close contacts who have not been examined; each case must be evaluated individually. The determination regarding treatment is based on the degree of crowding and the likelihood of widespread infection.

Pediculosis Corporis

The body louse lives primarily in the seams of clothing adjacent to the skin rather than on the skin itself. This infestation occurs most commonly in indigents and those with poor hygiene who do not change clothes frequently.

The bite of the louse produces a papule or wheal with a central hemorrhagic punctum. The clinical presentation is usually one of generalized pruritus with excoriations, secondary impetiginization, and bloody crusts. The diagnosis is confirmed by identifying lice or eggs on clothing.

Pediculosis Pubis

The pubic louse differs from body and head lice in that it has a short, crab-like body and three pairs of large legs. It prefers to infest areas of the body where the hairs are shorter and less dense than those on the scalp, such as pubic hair, axillary hair, eyebrows, eyelashes, beards, and body hair. Pubic lice are spread primarily through sexual contact and fomites such as clothing and bedding. Because pediculosis pubis is a sexually transmitted disease, patients should be evaluated for other sexually transmitted disorders such as syphilis, gonorrhea, and HIV. Pubic lice in the eyelashes of children is a sign of possible sexual abuse.

The diagnosis is confirmed by finding live lice among the pubic hairs. Some lice may be attached to two hairs, and as with head lice, nits are seen fixed to hairs. Treatment is similar to that for pediculosis capitis. Natural and synthetic pyrethrins, as well as lindane, can be applied as shampoos for 10 minutes or as lotions for several hours. Treatment should be repeated in 1 week to treat any newly hatched lice. Lice and nits of the eyelashes can be treated by manual removal or simple occlusion using agents such as petrolatum several times daily to asphyxiate the lice. Sexual partners should be treated simultaneously.

CONSIDERATIONS IN PREGNANCY

Lindane treatment for scabies has not been shown to be safe in pregnant women or nursing mothers. There have been reports of neurotoxicity in infants and young children. Neurotoxicity has almost always been associated with misuse or accidental ingestion of the drug.

Elimite (permethrin) 5% cream is classified as a pregnancy category B drug. However, because no adequate and well-controlled studies exist in pregnant women, permethrin should be used in pregnancy only if clearly needed. The same is true for permethrin products for the treatment of pediculosis.

Eurax (crotamiton USP) lotion/cream is in pregnancy category C and should be used in pregnancy only if clearly needed (eg, allergy to permethrin).

BIBLIOGRAPHY

Cabrera R, Agar A, Dahl MV. The immunology of scabies. Semin Dermatol 1993;12(1):15.

Clore ER, Longyear LA. A comparative study of seven pediculicides and their packaged nit removal combs. J Pediatr Health Care 1993;7:55.

Elgart ML. Pediculosis. Dermatol Clin 1990;8:219.
Elgart ML. Scabies. Dermatol Clin 1990;8:253.
Jucowics P, Ramon ME, Don PC, Stone RK, Bamji M. Norwegian scabies in an infant with acquired immunodeficiency syndrome. Arch Dermatol 1989;125:1670.
Orkin M, Maibach HI. Scabies therapy 1993. Semin Dermatol 1993; 12(1):22.
Paller AS. Scabies in infants and small children. Semin Dermatol 1993; 12(1):3.
Purvis RS, Tyring SK. An outbreak of lindane-resistant scabies treated successfully with permethrin 5% cream. J Am Acad Dermatol 1991; 25:1015.
Schultz MW, Gomez M, Hansen RC, et al. Comparative study of 5% permethrin cream and 1% lindane lotion for the treatment of scabies. Arch Dermatol 1990;126:167.
Taplin D, Meinking TL, Chen JA, Sanchez R. Comparison of crotamiton 10% cream (Eurax) and permethrin 5% cream (Elimite) for the treatment of scabies in children. Pediatr Dermatol 1990;7(1):67.
Taplin D, Meinking TL, Porcelain SL, Castellero PM, Chen JA. Permethrin 5% dermal cream: a new treatment for scabies. J Am Acad Dermatol 1986;15:995.

148
Cellulitis

SOPHIE M. WOROBEC

Primary Care for Women, edited by Phyllis C. Leppert and Fred M. Howard. Lippincott-Raven Publishers, Philadelphia © 1997.

Cellulitis is an acute spreading bacterial infection of the skin and subcutaneous tissue. A superficial infection of the skin is termed impetigo. More invasive forms of infection include streptococcal gangrene (necrotizing fasciitis) and myositis.

ETIOLOGY

The causative agents are almost always group A β-hemolytic streptococci or *Staphylococcus aureus*. Group G, B, and C streptococci can also be causative, especially at sites of saphenous vein harvesting for coronary artery bypass surgery. Diabetic patients are at risk for polymicrobial cellulitis, including both gram-positive and gram-negative bacteria and anaerobic organisms. Other causes include: *Haemophilus influenzae* type b, a gram-negative organism, especially as a cause of facial cellulitis in young children; and *Pasteurella multocida*, a gram-negative rod, particularly after animal bites or scratches.

The body's foremost defense against skin and soft tissue infections is an intact cutaneous barrier. A skin disease such as eczema or psoriasis, unrecognized minor skin trauma, or even preexisting tinea pedis (after saphenous vein harvesting and resultant lymphatic stasis) may provide a portal of entry for various bacteria. The normal skin flora includes various aerobic and anaerobic organisms, including coagulase-negative staphylococci (eg, *Staphylococcus epidermidis*), micrococci, diphtheroids, and Propionibacteria. Transient colonizers of the skin include various streptococci, *S aureus*, and gram-negative enteric bacteria such as *Escherichia coli* and *Proteus mirabilis*. Any organism can become an opportunistic pathogen in an immunocompromised host.

Conditions commonly predisposing to cellulitis include diabetes, neoplastic disease, chronic obstructive pulmonary disease, alcoholism, malnutrition, immunosuppression, nephrotic syndrome, preexisting skin disease, and lymphatic or venous obstruction, atherosclerotic vascular diseases, and intravenous drug abuse.

HISTORY AND PHYSICAL EXAMINATION

The diagnosis of cellulitis is based on the abrupt development, usually over 1 to 2 days, of a rapidly progressing area of redness, warmth, swelling, and tenderness. Lymphadenitis and lymphadenopathy as well as malaise, fever, chills, and other systemic symptoms of infection may be present. Cellulitis most often affects the lower extremities, but any part of the body may be affected.

Erysipelas is a characteristic superficial type of cellulitis that affects dermal tissue, primarily without involvement of subcutaneous tissue. Erysipelas is characterized by a hot, bright-red lesion with a sharply demarcated border; cellulitis has an indistinct border. The areas involved may develop blisters, purpura, erosions, small areas of necrosis, and scaliness.

Blistering distal dactylitis is a superficial infection of the anterior fat pad of the distal portion of the finger or toe. Most cases occur in children. Both hemolytic streptococci and hemolytic staphylococci have been isolated from these lesions. Blistering distal dactylitis is characterized by large tense blisters on a tender erythematous base.

DIFFERENTIAL DIAGNOSIS

Impetigo is a superficial bacterial skin infection consisting of pustular or bullous skin lesions; on breaking, they develop crusts. Ecthyma is a variant of impetigo, manifested by punched-out, ulcerated, and often painful lesions that usually occur on the lower extremities.

The differential diagnosis of cellulitis includes acute contact dermatitis (lacks systemic symptoms of malaise, fever, chills), venous thrombosis (may occur with cellulitis), recurrent breast cancer (ie, erysipeloid carcinoma on the chest wall), and lymphatic obstruction by other tumors.

On the hand, the finding of a dorsal, purple, red, or violet, warm, and tender plaque should alert one to the diagnosis of erysipeloid. Erysipeloid, a cutaneous infection caused by *Erysipelothrix rhusiopathiae*, is acquired via skin trauma while handling contaminated fish, shellfish, or meat.

Cellulitis should be differentiated from necrotizing soft-tissue infections: necrotizing fasciitis, Fournier gangrene, streptococcal gangrene, and clostridial myonecrosis (gas gangrene). These severe deep infections require hospitalization, antibiotic coverage, and surgical and infectious disease consultation.

LABORATORY AND IMAGING STUDIES

In cellulitis, the presenting clinical picture is the basis of the diagnosis. Cultures of aspirates or lesional biopsies are frequently (in

70% or more of cases) negative. Blood cultures should be done if sepsis is suspected and always in immunocompromised or debilitated patients. White blood counts show a leukocytosis and bandemia. Skin biopsy is usually unnecessary, but if done it shows edema, a mixed lymphocytic and polymorphonuclear infiltrate, and sometimes bacteria with special stains. In postoperative wound streptococcal cellulitis, the discharge may show chains of gram-positive cocci on Gram staining.

Special imaging is usually unnecessary unless gangrene or osteomyelitis is suspected. Rarely, bacterial skin infections may originate in a contiguous deeper focus (eg, perforated viscus or osteomyelitis) or with hematogenous dissemination of systemic disease. Soft-tissue infections of the hands should be carefully evaluated by a hand specialist to determine if deep structures such as tendon sheaths, joints, and muscular spaces are involved. Orbital cellulitis requires urgent consultation with an ophthalmologist or a head and neck surgeon for evaluation.

TREATMENT

Most uncomplicated cases of cellulitis can be treated on an outpatient basis with a penicillinase-resistant penicillin or cefazolin. Erythromycin is a next-line agent but requires careful monitoring for response because of increasing resistance. It is not indicated for erysipelas. In erysipelas, the treatment of choice is penicillin orally or intravenously; the alternatives are oral amoxicillin, intravenous ampicillin, intravenous cefazolin, or vancomycin.

Because new antibiotics are constantly being introduced, and because patterns of resistance may change, consultation with an infectious disease service or a local microbiology laboratory may be indicated to choose the best antibiotic coverage. Hospitalization may be necessary for a compromised host at risk for sepsis; a patient who cannot reliably care for herself at home; a patient who is progressing despite the use of oral antibiotics; or a patient who presents with high fever, rigors, severe and rapid progression, or involvement of the face, orbit, or perineum.

Abscesses must be drained, and devitalized tissue must be debrided, necessitating surgical intervention.

If an open wound is present and no tetanus toxoid booster has been received in the last 5 years, it should be administered. If no initial tetanus series was ever received, both tetanus toxoid and tetanus immune globulin should be given.

Diabetic patients in whom gram-negative organisms are a concern have been treated with amoxicillin-clavulanate potassium. However, this drug is expensive and side effects include diarrhea and rash. Various quinolones are also indicated for soft-tissue infections; however, cost is also an issue with them. Cefoxitin is another option. If there are signs of sepsis in a diabetic patient, she should be given parenteral therapy with imipenem or a penicillinase-resistant penicillin plus an aminoglycoside antibiotic.

Outpatient parenteral antibiotic therapy of cellulitis has been used to complete treatment after hospitalization or to initiate outpatient oral therapy. A single daily parenteral dose of ceftriaxone can effectively treat most cases, except some diabetic foot infections, possibly because of poor coverage of anaerobic bacteria or associated peripheral vascular disease. Teicoplanin, a glycopeptide related to vancomycin, has pharmacokinetics supporting once-daily intravenous use. However, it cannot treat gram-negative organisms; thus, a second drug is necessary when gram-negative organisms may be involved.

Nonpharmacologic therapy should be used together with antibiotics: the affected area should be rested and moist compresses applied.

CONSIDERATIONS IN PREGNANCY

Although cellulitis is not uncommon during pregnancy, little has been written specifically about cellulitis and pregnancy.

Two severe infections due to *Pasteurella multocida* have been reported in pregnant women who had contact with animals (licked by a dog and a cat) but no history of an animal bite. One patient developed meningitis; the other developed cellulitis with a deep abscess. Both were successfully treated with parenteral penicillin and cephalosporin after failing to respond to oral phenoxymethylpenicillin. One affected woman had a slightly decreased IgG level, but no other immunologic defects were detected in these women. Partial suppression of cell-mediated immunity during pregnancy may have interfered with their resistance to this infection. However, most infectious diseases do not have an increased risk of acquisition and severity during pregnancy. In contrast, infectious diseases caused by intracellular bacterial pathogens such as tuberculosis, viral infections, and systemic fungal, protozoal, and helminthic infections are significantly more severe during pregnancy.

In pregnancy, higher doses of antibiotics may be needed for pharmacokinetic reasons. Changes in renal function and also in the composition and amount of body fluids occur as pregnancy progresses. However, little has been published about pharmacokinetics in pregnancy. Lower antibiotic levels in serum or plasma have been documented during pregnancy for ampicillin and are suspected for other antibiotics. In severe infections, the magnitude and duration of peak serum levels are crucial for obtaining optimal drug levels at the site of infection, which rarely is located in the bloodstream. Treatment in pregnancy may fail because lower antibiotic levels are reached at the site of infection, where the antibiotic is needed. The one exception is the treatment of lower urinary tract infections, as antibiotic levels in urine seem to be unchanged in pregnancy.

BIBLIOGRAPHY

Kahn RM, Goldstein EJ. Common bacterial skin infections: diagnostic clues and therapeutic options. Postgrad Med 1993;93:175.

Lindbeck G, Powers R. Cellulitis. Hosp Prac (Office Edition) 1993;28(suppl 2):10.

Morantes MC, Lipsky BA. "Flesh-eating bacteria": return of an old nemesis. Intl J Dermatol 1995;34:461.

Philipson A. Pharmacokinetics of antibiotics in pregnancy and labour. Clin Pharmacokinet 1979;4:297.

Rollof J, Johansson PT, Host E. Severe *Pasteurella multocida* infections in pregnant women. Scand J Infect Dis 1992;24:453.

Weinberg ED. Pregnancy-associated depression of cell-mediated immunity. Rev Infect Dis 1984;6:814.

Zemstov A, Veitschegger M. *Staphylococcus aureus*-induced blistering distal dactylitis in an adult immunosuppressed patient. J Am Acad Dermatol 1992;26:784.

Primary Care for Women, edited by Phyllis C. Leppert and Fred M. Howard. Lippincott-Raven Publishers, Philadelphia © 1997.

149
Corns and Calluses

DOUGLAS L. POWELL

Nature's method of protecting skin from the trauma of constant rubbing is through the development of calluses. Someone who is exposed to frequent friction in localized skin areas, such as a gymnast, can appreciate the protective effects of calluses. However, when calluses form in areas of constant pressure such as the foot, pain ensues and the lesions become more bothersome than helpful. Corns and calluses can cause sufficient morbidity to make ambulation difficult. Because the lesions are so common, particularly in older women, primary care physicians often have the opportunity to evaluate and treat them. Often simple measures give significant results.

ETIOLOGY

On both the histologic and clinical level, the skin thickens and calluses form from the stresses of friction, compression, tension, shear, and torsion. These stresses on the feet are exaggerated and distorted by ill- or tight-fitting shoes, gait abnormalities, atypical foot architecture, osteoarthritis, or impaired sensory nerve input. Corns (clavi) apparently develop from increased pressure by a shoe on a previously formed callus. Increased pressure on the soft tissues created by calluses, or pressure on the central core of the corn, creates the pain associated with these lesions.

Ill-fitting shoes that create the above-mentioned stresses are the most common etiologic agent. The increased pressure and friction is often so subtle that it is not noticed until after the development of the callus or corn. The chronicity of the stress creates the lesions. A simple visual comparison of the shape and size of a foot with that of a person's shoe reinforces the realization that some parts of the foot receive greater trauma than others. According to a 1990 U.S. National Health Interview study, women are $2\frac{1}{2}$ times more likely to be bothered by corns and calluses than men. This difference is probably not due to musculoskeletal differences between men and women but, rather, to wearing shoes that cause foot problems.

Diabetic patients with peripheral neuropathy are even less likely to sense increased friction on the foot and have a greater propensity to develop calluses. Also, the neuropathy of diabetes frequently leads to a "claw foot" position that places more pressure on the metatarsal heads during ambulation. Calluses develop at these locations, and their formation can increase localized pressure by as much as 30%. Studies have documented the predictive value of calluses in creating ulcers in diabetic patients. These calluses develop into ulcers greater than 70% of the time, according to some studies. The difficulty of treating these ulcers and the morbidity they cause emphasize the need to treat and prevent calluses in diabetic patients.

HISTORY

Often the patient visits the doctor for other medical reasons but then mentions the calluses or corns during the examination. Pain while walking is the most common complaint. Some patients realize that their tight shoes worsen the situation but persist in wearing them. Sometimes the lesions are not mentioned by the patient but are found on a careful foot examination. Although the patient may not have any complaints about shoes, friction is occurring if calluses are present.

PHYSICAL EXAMINATION

Calluses are skin-colored or yellow elevated, thickened plaques in which regular dermatoglyphics (fine skin ridges) are continuous over the top. They occur anywhere friction is occurring.

Two types of corns are common: hard and soft corns. Hard corns are thick calluses with small, central, cone-shaped cores that point into the foot. The dermatoglyphics of corns are interrupted at the core. Hard corns commonly occur under the metatarsal heads on the plantar surface of the foot or on the lateral aspect of the small toe (Fig. 149-1), but they can occur anywhere there is pressure. Soft corns occur in interdigital spaces, particularly the fourth web space. They are not hard but still are quite tender and worsen with pressure. Soft corns present as soft white or gray papules. Occasionally they are associated with underlying bony exostoses.

DIFFERENTIAL DIAGNOSIS

Corns and simple calluses look most like plantar warts, which also can be associated with a fair amount of callosity. By paring the lesions down with a scalpel blade, the three can be differentiated. Warts demonstrate small dark-brown or black dots that correlate with thrombosed capillaries extending up into elongated dermal papillae histologically. Warts are often less painful in patients with intact sensation. Hard corns reveal the solid central core, which when removed carefully with a scalpel blade reveals a central pit. Simple calluses show no interruption of the dermatoglyphics.

IMAGING STUDIES

If underlying bony abnormalities are suspected, x-rays of the foot should be taken. Referral to an orthopedic surgeon is appropriate if bony changes are found.

TREATMENT

Treatment comes in two categories: preventive and therapeutic. Patients should select shoes with lower heels and cushiony soles or wider shoes that lace up. A half-inch of space should be allowed in the front of the shoes. Other preventive measures are the use of circular pads around corns or a molded shoe insert device, which can be obtained from a podiatrist; both of these help remove pressure from corns and calluses. These simple measures must be empha-

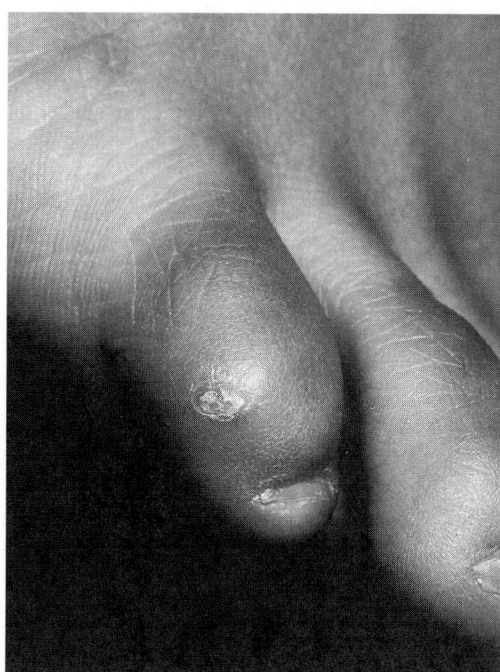

Figure 149-1. A hard corn on the lateral toe.

sized, as the lesions will recur after treatment if prevention is not used. To prevent further formation of soft corns, cotton should be inserted between the toes and the patient should wear wider shoes.

The simplest therapeutic treatment consists of paring the corns and calluses down with a scalpel blade. Caution should be used in treating diabetics or others with peripheral neuropathies, as any aberrant injury to the skin can act as a nidus for infection or an ulcer. The patient can help with treatment by applying OTC salicylic acid preparations (used for warts) daily, soaking the foot daily, and removing excess skin after soaking with a pumice stone. Forty percent salicylic acid in a plaster, available OTC, can be taped to the callus or corn 1 day to 1 week at a time; this is followed by rubbing with a pumice stone.

If abnormalities of foot structure or walking gait are suspected, the patient should be referred to an orthopedic surgeon. Diabetic patients with persistent lesions or calluses should be referred to a podiatrist or dermatologist.

CONSIDERATIONS IN PREGNANCY

No specific changes to corns during pregnancy have been noted in the literature; however, some women's feet widen late in pregnancy, so wider shoes should be worn.

BIBLIOGRAPHY

Baker B. Presence of plantar callus raised risk of diabetic foot ulcers. Skin Allergy News 1995;26(3):15.

Caputo M, Cavanagh PR, Ulbrecht JS, Gibbons GW, Karchmer AW. Assessment and management of foot disease in patients with diabetes. N Engl J Med 1994;331:854.

Collier JH, Brodbeck CA. Assessing the diabetic foot: plantar callus and pressure sensation. Diabet Educ 1993;19:503.

Kennedy CTC. Callosities and corns. In: Rook AJ, ed. Textbook of dermatology, 5th ed. Oxford: Blackwell, 1992:783.

Levy LA. Prevalence of chronic podiatric conditions in the U.S.: National Health Survery 1990. J Am Podiatr Med Assoc 1992;82:221.

Richards RN. Calluses, corns, and shoes. Semin Dermatol 1991;10(2):112.

Sheard C. Simple management of plantar clavi. Cutis 1992;50(2):138.

Primary Care for Women, edited by Phyllis C. Leppert and Fred M. Howard. Lippincott-Raven Publishers, Philadelphia © 1997.

150

Skin Cancer

MARC D. BROWN

Skin cancer continues to be the most common form of cancer, with an estimated 1 million cases per year in the United States. Fortunately, the vast majority of these skin neoplasms are easily diagnosed, can be treated with a high cure rate with several therapeutic modalities, and are usually not a cause of significant morbidity or mortality. The exceptions are melanoma and certain high-risk squamous cell carcinomas. Skin cancers do kill over 10,000 persons annually in the United States, however, and many of these deaths may have been preventable.

The three most common types of skin cancers are basal cell carcinoma (BCC), squamous cell carcinoma (SCC), and melanoma, of which there are various histologic and clinical subtypes. The most common etiologic factor of these skin cancers is acute and chronic exposure to ultraviolet radiation (sun exposure). BCC and SCC are more common in middle-aged to elderly patients; melanoma is often seen in a younger population. The biologic behavior of these skin cancers ranges from slow-growing tumors that invade only locally, to rapidly growing and metastasizing malignant carcinomas.

BASAL CELL CARCINOMA

Etiology

Basal cell carcinoma is the most common cancer, with an estimated 600,000 to 700,000 new cases annually in the United States. Despite the high incidence, very few people die from BCC. This cancer is typically slow-growing, with a very low risk of metastasis. BCC affects males slightly more than females, but this gap is narrowing as women increasingly expose their skin to the sun. The incidence of BCC increases as a person ages; however, younger persons (in their 20s and 30s) are being seen more frequently with an initial BCC tumor.

The most common etiologic factor is ultraviolet exposure. BCC is more common on sun-exposed areas such as the central face (especially the nose), ears, forehead, cheek, and neck, as well as upper back and chest. About 90% of all BCCs are on the head and neck. BCC is more common in fair-skinned persons who sunburn

Table 150-1. Etiology of Basal Cell Carcinoma

Sun exposure
Previous radiation treatment
Arsenic exposure
Trauma
Genodermatoses

easily. It is also more common in those with outdoor occupations and those who live in sunny climates. BCC is rare in blacks. Other factors are listed in Table 150-1.

BCCs that develop at a site of previous irradiation can be very aggressive in their growth. The tumor appears 15 to 30 years after the x-ray treatment. Unfortunately, x-ray treatment was used in the past for dermatologic conditions such as acne and tinea capitis. Arsenic exposure is now rare, but in the past arsenic was used in medications (Fowler solution) and fertilizer. Patients with arsenic exposure have an associated clinical finding of small pits in the palmar surface of the hands.

Trauma as an etiologic factor is difficult to prove, but historically some patients note that the BCC started after a traumatic event to the skin.

With albinism, patients lack protective melanin. With xeroderma pigmentosum, an autosomal recessive disease, there is abnormal DNA repair after normal sun exposure and patients develop skin cancers at an early age. There are associated ocular and neurologic abnormalities. Basal cell nevus syndrome is a rare autosomal dominant disorder characterized by frequent and multiple BCCs that begin to develop early in life. Patients may develop hundreds of BCCs. Associated clinical findings include jaw cysts, frontal bossing, hypertelorism, bifid ribs, palmar pits, and internal neoplasms.

Clinical Findings

There are several clinical types of BCC (Table 150-2). The most common type is the nodular BCC, which appears as a pink to flesh-colored papule or nodule with a translucent (pearly) surface, telangiectasias, and rolled borders (Fig. 150-1). Patients describe a pimple that waxes and wanes in clinical appearance, but slowly gets larger. As the nodular BCC grows, there may be central erosion or ulceration; failure to heal, crusting, and bleeding typically bring the patient to see the doctor. Pain is usually absent unless there is perineural invasion or invasion of deeper structures such as cartilage, which may result in tenderness. Although the BCC can be clinically recognized and diagnosed when quite small, the typical size at diagnosis is about 1 cm. If ignored or misdiagnosed, the BCC can reach an impressive size and may result in destruction and loss of important structures such as an ear, nose, or eyelid.

Variants of the nodular BCC include the pigmented and cystic BCC. The pigmented BCC is brown to black due to melanin deposition in the tumor. The pigmented BCC resembles a nodular melanoma, but close inspection reveals an elevated, rolled, translucent border. The cystic BCC appears as a smooth, round cystic lesion. If near the eyelid, it can resemble a benign hidrocystoma.

Table 150-2. Types of Basal Cell Carcinoma

Nodular
Superficial
Morpheaform
Pigmented
Cystic
Basosquamous

The morpheaform BCC is the most aggressive BCC. Synonyms include sclerosing, infiltrative, or micronodular BCC. Clinically, this BCC is poorly defined, with a scar-like appearance: it is white to yellow, flat, indurated, and firm. The infiltrative BCC has the greatest potential for deep and insidious subclinical growth and extension. A nodular BCC has a soft, mushy quality and feel that is easily distinguished, and it can be removed with a sharp curet; in contrast, the infiltrative BCC is difficult or impossible to curet. The infiltrative BCC has the highest risk of local recurrence after treatment. The basosquamous BCC is a variant of the aggressive growth BCC and histologically shows areas of squamous differentiation within the basaloid neoplasm.

The superficial BCC appears as an ill-defined, red, scaly patch or plaque, frequently on the upper back or chest but also on the face. The superficial BCC grows and spreads peripherally and rarely invades deeper subdermal structures. Due to its appearance, the superficial BCC may be misdiagnosed as a dermatitis or fungal infection and may slowly enlarge over several years before a skin biopsy confirms the correct diagnosis.

Laboratory Studies

The definitive diagnosis of a BCC is made with a skin biopsy. In most cases, histologic confirmation should be obtained before treatment, as the histologic subtype may determine the best treatment option. A biopsy can be performed by shave or punch excision. A punch biopsy provides a deeper tissue sample and should be used for a probable morpheaform BCC. The classic histologic picture of a BCC is that of basaloid tumor islands extending from the epidermis into the dermis or subcutaneous tissue. The tumor islands stain a deep blue with hematoxylin and eosin. There is an orderly line of cells around the periphery of dermal tumor nests (peripheral palisading), as well as stromal retraction. The infiltrative BCC shows numerous small nests and finger-like tumor islands with a background fibrous stroma.

Treatment

Despite the pattern of slow growth, the BCC tumor is characterized by relentless, often extensive subclinical local invasion through soft tissue, cartilage, muscle, and even bone. Thus, treatment is imperative but not necessarily urgent. The best treatment method for a BCC depends on several factors, including tumor size, histology, location, and previous treatment. These criteria help to define and distinguish low-risk from high-risk BCCs. Tumors greater than 1 cm on the face and 2 to 3 cm on the trunk are considered to be high risk. Superficial and nodular BCCs are lower risk than the infiltrative, aggressive BCCs. Histologic evidence of perineural invasion also defines a high-risk BCC. Location is particularly important; difficult-to-treat areas include the nose and ear and the periocular, perioral, and pre- and postauricular facial regions. Previously treated BCCs (especially those treated with radiation) that are locally recurrent are also more difficult to treat.

A clear understanding of the indications, advantages, and disadvantages of the treatment modalities will help the physician adopt a uniform approach to the treatment of BCCs. Most BCCs are low-risk

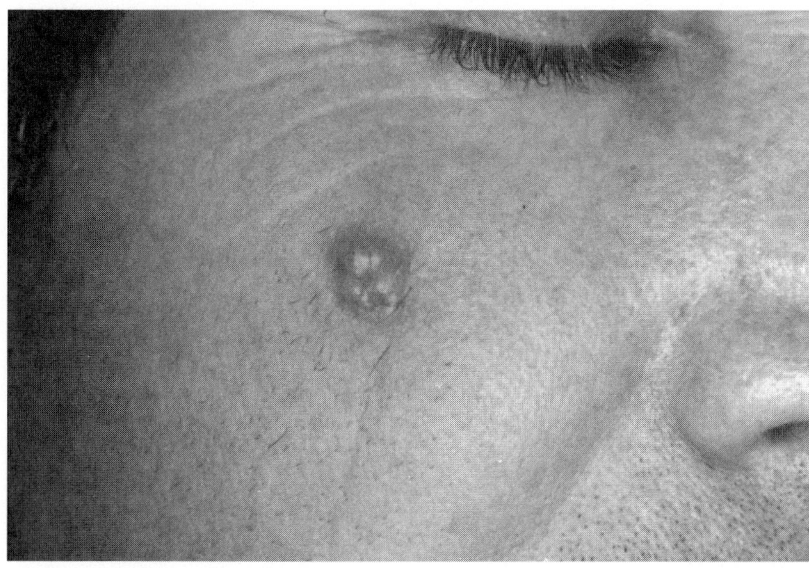

Figure 150-1. Basal cell cancer (nodular type).

tumors and can be treated with a high cure rate via curettage, excision, cryosurgery, radiation, or laser (Table 150-3).

Electrodesiccation and Curettage

Electrodesiccation and curettage (ED&C) is probably the most frequently used method of tumor ablation by dermatologists for a small nodular or superficial BCC. The tumor is removed with a sharp curet, followed by electrodesiccation to the base and periphery. This process is then repeated two more times. Curettage should not be used on an infiltrative BCC, a recurrent BCC with scar tissue, or a nodular BCC that extends deeply into the subcutaneous tissue. Small tumors treated with ED&C typically heal in 2 to 4 weeks with a whitish scar; large BCC tumors treated with ED&C may leave cosmetically unacceptable scars. The disadvantage of ED&C is a lack of clear histologic margin control.

Excision

Excision and layered closure is best used for larger tumors, or where cosmesis is more critical and there is looser skin, such as the neck, cheek, and forehead. Curettage of the tumor before excision allows clearer delineation of margins. A surgical margin of 4 to 6 mm is recommended. Excision allows for permanent-section margin control. Excision followed by local flap reconstruction is best done with frozen-section margin control before suturing the flap in place.

Cryosurgery

Freezing with liquid nitrogen is excellent for premalignant lesions and superficial skin cancers. Treating deeper tumors with cryosurgery requires the use of a thermocouple to measure the depth and degree of freezing adequately. Healing may require 4 to 6 weeks.

Table 150-3. Skin Cancer Treatment

Electrodesiccation and curettage
Excision
Radiation
Cryosurgery
Laser
Mohs

Radiation

Because radiation can induce skin cancers, it is best used in older patients. For patients reluctant to undergo surgery, radiation is an excellent alternative, with good cure rates and acceptable cosmesis. Disadvantages include multiple treatments, possible radiation dermatitis, and lack of margin control.

Lasers

The CO_2 laser is destructive and can adequately remove smaller and superficial skin cancers. Wounds heal slowly. Bleeding is minimal, so this may be a good choice for patients who are anticoagulated.

Investigations are underway using lasers and photosensitizing agents taken up by the tumor (photodynamic therapy). This may hold promise for the nonsurgical treatment of multiple, smaller skin cancers.

Mohs Surgery

In Mohs surgery, serial layers of skin and soft tissue are removed systematically, with precise frozen-section margin control. Mohs surgery offers the highest cure rates and is indicated for high-risk tumors (eg, large, recurrent, location on the eyes, ears, nose, or lips, infiltrative histology, and perineural invasion). Mohs surgery requires precise layered excision and tumor mapping, along with horizontal histologic frozen-section and microscopic examination of all tissue removed. The procedure allows the dermatologic surgeon to track out subclinical extensions of skin cancers while minimizing removal of normal tissue. Mohs surgery is performed in an outpatient setting under local anesthesia and allows for immediate reconstruction of the defect after ascertaining clear margins.

Appropriate follow-up of patients with BCC is important, as up to 35% of patients subsequently develop another skin cancer. Most patients should be seen twice a year for a full skin examination. Use of sunscreens and sun avoidance should be stressed at each visit. Preventive steps are outlined in Table 150-4.

Table 150-4. Prevention of Skin Cancer

Use sunscreens SPF ≥ 15.
Begin sunscreen use in childhood.
Avoid most intense sun (10 a.m.–2 p.m.).
Wear protective clothing (hat, long-sleeved shirt).
Avoid tanning parlors.
Perform self-skin examination on a regular basis.

SQUAMOUS CELL CARCINOMA

Etiology

SCC is the second most common skin malignancy. There are over 100,000 new cases in the United States each year, resulting in about 2500 deaths. SCC originates from the epidermal squamous cell and invades the dermis. If confined to the epidermis, it is referred to as SCC in situ or Bowen disease. Like BCC, SCC is most common in sun-exposed areas, as ultraviolet light exposure is the primary etiologic factor. Common sites of involvement include the lower lip, ear, dorsal hand, and scalp. Bowen disease can be seen on the lower legs of females. SCC commonly afflicts persons in their 60s or 70s.

Beside sun exposure, other etiologic factors for the development of SCC include previous radiation treatment or exposure, chronic scarring processes (eg, burn scars, chronic skin ulcers, chronic osteomyelitis), genodermatoses, and chronic exposure to polycyclic hydrocarbons. Of interest is the association of some SCC with human papilloma virus infection. These SCC, resembling a warty growth, can be seen on the digits or genitalia. Immunosuppressed patients are also at increased risk for SCC, especially renal transplant patients.

Clinical Findings

SCCs that develop in actinically damaged skin typically begin as a hyperkeratotic pink to red papule, plaque, or nodule (Fig. 150-2). The SCC can grow rapidly and ulcerate centrally; when aggressive, it can double in size within weeks to months. SCC also can metastasize, especially to the regional lymph nodes or lungs. Thus, treatment is more urgent than for the slow-growing BCC.

The common precursor lesion for SCC is the actinic keratosis (AK). The AK is a solar-induced premalignant lesion seen most commonly in fair-skinned persons on the face, hands, arms, and scalp. The AK appears as a flat to slightly raised, pink, scaling lesion, usually less than 1 cm in size. A hypertrophic AK is difficult to distinguish from an early SCC, and a skin biopsy is necessary to confirm the diagnosis. Many patients with both BCC and SCC have a background of diffuse AK. Bowen disease appears as an erythematous, scaling patch and clinically resembles a superficial BCC (Fig. 150-3).

An SCC that arises in an AK was thought to have minimal potential for metastatic disease. However, more recent studies indicate that these SCCs can be very aggressive. Metastatic rates for SCC range from 2% to 40%. SCCs that develop in old scars or ulcers have a greater metastatic potential. Other risk factors for aggressive biologic behavior include size (> 2 cm), depth of invasion, location on the lower lip or ear, underlying immunosuppression, perineural invasion, poorly differentiated histology, and previous treatment (Table 150-5).

Laboratory Studies

As with BCC, a skin biopsy is necessary to confirm the diagnosis of SCC. A punch biopsy is preferred to obtain a deeper specimen and thus to avoid missing evidence of invasion. The pathologist should report if the invasive SCC is well differentiated, moderately differentiated, or poorly differentiated.

The classic histology of SCC is that of a neoplastic proliferation of keratinocytes that arise from the epidermis with extension through the dermis and potentially into deeper subcutaneous tissue. The well-differentiated SCC shows keratin formation with horn pearls. Mitotic figures range from few with fairly normal keratinocyte architecture to frequent and atypical (poorly differentiated). Less common subtypes include lobular, acantholytic, and spindle cell variants.

Treatment

Smaller, low-risk lesions can be treated by standard methods, similar to BCC, with cure rates exceeding 90%. For in situ SCC, topical 5-fluorouracil, cryosurgery, and curettage offer quick and simple treatment. For more invasive SCC, excision and margin

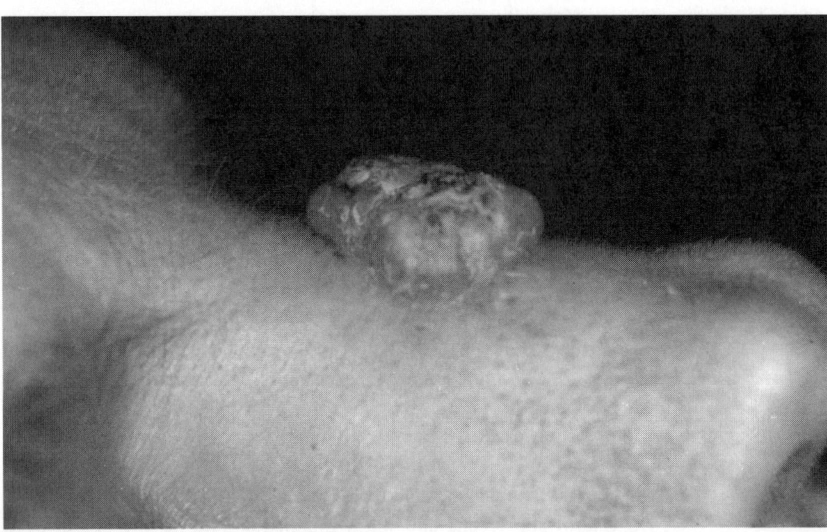

Figure 150-2. Well-differentiated squamous cell carcinoma.

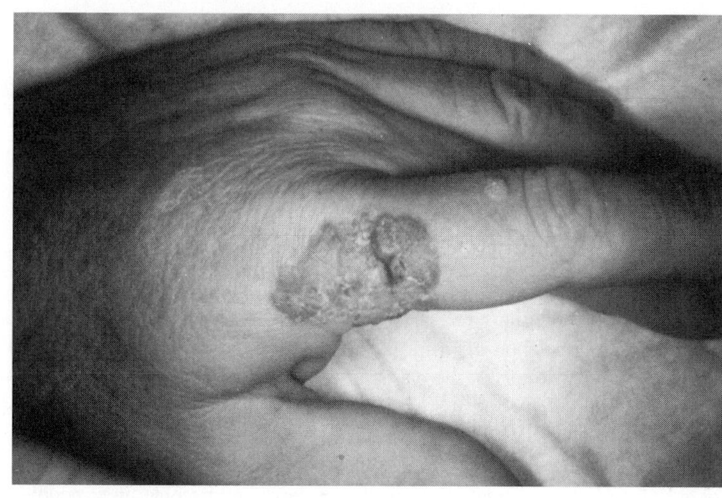

Figure 150-3. Bowen disease (squamous cell in situ).

control becomes more important. For high-risk SCC, Mohs surgery or wide local excision is necessary; even then, the cure rate may only be 90% to 95%. Careful palpation of regional nodes is important, as is a screening chest x-ray. Sometimes, high-risk tumors that are deeply invasive on the head and neck may require elective lymph node dissection or postoperative radiation therapy. For high-risk SCC, follow-up is recommended every 3 to 4 months for the first 2 to 3 years, and then every 6 months thereafter. Patients with extensive AK may need to be seen on a regular basis.

MELANOMA

Etiology

The incidence of melanoma continues to rise at a rapid and predictable rate: over the past 50 years, the incidence has increased almost 1000-fold. Currently, the estimated lifetime risk is about 1:100. An estimated 32,000 new cases develop annually in the United States, resulting in about 6500 deaths. Melanoma is the most common cancer in women ages 25 and 29 and is second only to breast cancer in women ages 30 to 35. The good news is that the overall 5-year survival rate has improved, probably due to earlier detection, diagnosis, and treatment.

Ultraviolet radiation has been consistently implicated as a major etiologic factor in the development of melanoma. Patients at high risk are those with fair skin, a tendency to freckle, light-colored hair and eyes, and a history of severe sunburns. A family history of melanoma places the patient at increased risk. Patients with atypical moles or a large number of moles are at increased risk, as are patients with large congenital nevi. Intermittent, limited but intense sun exposure appears to be the major element in the development of melanoma. Melanoma is more prevalent among those who have indoor occupations and are of a higher socioeconomic class and tend to spend weekends and vacations outdoors. Ozone depletion may also have an effect on the increased incidence of melanoma, with an estimated 5% to 8% increase in incidence expected from a 5% depletion of the ozone layer by the year 2000.

Table 150-5. High-Risk Squamous Cell Carcinoma

Size > 2 cm
Poorly differentiated histology
Depth of invasion
Perineural invasion
Etiology (burn scar)
Location (ear, lip)

The three major precursor lesions to the development of melanoma are dysplastic nevi (atypical moles), congenital nevi, and lentigo maligna.

A dysplastic nevus is an acquired pigmented lesion of the skin whose clinical and histologic appearance differs from that of the typical common mole. The dysplastic nevus serves as both a precursor and a marker lesion for the development of malignant melanoma. The dysplastic nevus is often larger than a common mole and has a variegated color, ranging from tan to dark brown. The margins are irregular and ill defined, and there is often a raised center. The exact incidence of dysplastic nevi in the general population is unknown, with estimates ranging from 2% to 50%. Any dysplastic nevus can develop into a melanoma, although the vast majority do not. Malignant melanoma can also occur de novo on normal skin. Thus, removing all dysplastic nevi from a patient does not ensure that a melanoma will not develop. Changing moles and atypical moles should be evaluated for surgical excision.

Congenital nevi are moles that are present at birth or shortly thereafter. Most are small; only 1:20,000 newborns has a large congenital nevus. A large ("giant") congenital nevus is usually defined as larger than 10 cm. The lifetime risk of a large congenital nevus developing into a malignant melanoma is estimated to be 6% to 8%. Excision is recommended as early as possible, although removal frequently requires extensive multistaged surgical procedures. Small congenital nevi, which are present in 1% of newborns, are far easier to treat, but there is no agreement about the need for surgical excision. The risk of melanoma associated with a small congenital nevus is unknown: they may be responsible for 3% to 15% of all melanomas, but clear data are lacking. Prompt excision is advised for small congenital nevi that show evidence of change other than the normal enlargement that occurs in proportion to the child's growth. Small congenital nevi may be excised prophylactically sometime around puberty, when the child can more easily tolerate excision under local anesthesia in an outpatient setting.

Table 150-6. Risk Factors for Melanoma

Precursor lesions
  Lentigo maligna
  Congenital nevus
  Dysplastic nevi

Large number of moles
Fair skin, light-colored hair, tendency to freckle
Poor tanning, history of sunburns, sun exposure
Family history of melanoma

A lentigo maligna is a flat, macular pigmented lesion that appears on sun-exposed areas in older persons. Sunlight is thought to have a causative role. The lentigo maligna begins as a tan, irregular, freckle-like lesion; it subsequently enlarges and may develop a highly irregular pigment pattern and border. Its growth is typically slow, but it can get quite large. Lentigo maligna is best thought of as a melanoma in situ that has the potential to evolve into an invasive melanoma. Surgical excision is the treatment of choice. Superficial treatment methods such as cryosurgery are less reliable because the atypical melanocytes may extend along hair follicles and dermal appendages. Nonexcisional treatment modalities include radiation, cryotherapy, laser ablation, and dermabrasion, but these treatments are associated with higher recurrence rates.

Melanoma risk factors are outlined in Table 150-6.

Clinical Findings

The key to successful treatment of malignant melanoma is early recognition. The characteristic clinical features of early melanoma can best be remembered as the ABCDs of melanoma (Table 150-7): *A* is asymmetry, *B* is border irregularity, *C* is color variegation, and *D* is diameter of more than 6 mm. Whereas most moles are round, oval, and uniform, one half of a typical melanoma is asymmetric compared to the other half. Margins are typically irregular. The color ranges from hues of tan and brown to black, sometimes mixed with red and pink.

Melanoma is classically divided into four subtypes. Superficial spreading melanoma, the most common, occurs on any anatomic site but is most common on the trunk and extremities. Nodular melanomas present as elevated or polypoid tumors that grow rapidly and sometimes show ulceration with more advanced growth.

Table 150-7. ABCDs of Melanoma Diagnosis

A—Asymmetry
B—Border irregularity
C—Color variegation
D—Diameter > 6 mm

Lentigo maligna melanomas (Fig. 150-4) develop from the precursor lentigo maligna, as described earlier; they are brown to black macular lesions on the sun-exposed neck areas of older persons. Acral melanoma (Fig. 150-5) presents as a darkly pigmented flat to nodular lesion on the palms or soles or under the nails and is more common in African-Americans and Asians.

Any change in a preexisting mole may signal an evolving melanoma. Although most melanomas are asymptomatic, pruritus and bleeding may occur as they enlarge and become more nodular. Any mole that is symptomatic should be removed for histologic examination.

Laboratory Studies

One of the most important steps in the diagnosis and proper management of melanoma is a timely and appropriate biopsy. The best biopsy procedure is the total excisional removal of the pigmented lesion, usually with a narrow resection margin. Dissection should be carried to the level of the subcutaneous tissue to achieve an accurate measure of tumor infiltration for prognostication and formulation of a treatment plan. Sometimes an incisional or punch biopsy may be necessary due to the larger size or location of a melanoma (eg, a large lentigo maligna melanoma on the face). In this case, a punch biopsy should be taken from the most deeply pigmented or nodular area of the suspected melanoma. There is no evidence that the melanoma will spread from a biopsy procedure. Removal of a suspicious pigmented lesion by shave excision or curettage is not recommended.

An important element of the histologic diagnosis is the Breslow depth, the vertical thickness (in mm) from the stratum granulosum to the deepest portion of the melanoma. The Breslow depth most accurately determines the prognosis of the melanoma, its likelihood of metastasis, and treatment recommendations. Other helpful information contained in the pathology report includes evidence of

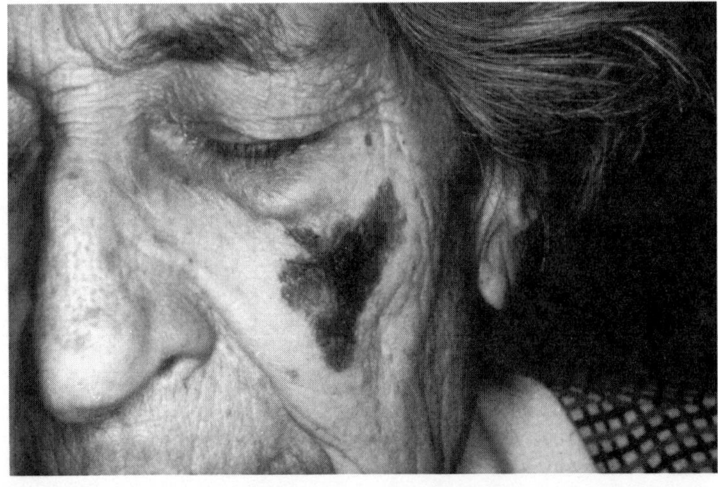

Figure 150-4. Lentigo maligna melanoma.

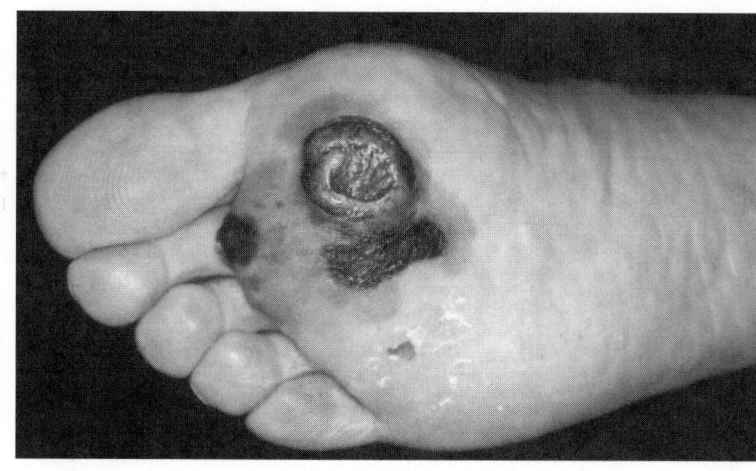

Figure 150-5. Acral melanoma.

ulceration, regression, angiolymphatic invasion, the degree of mitotic activity, and the presence or absence of precursor lesions.

The value of routine laboratory tests in patients with early melanoma is controversial. There are no data that clearly support the value of routine chest x-rays, a complete blood count, or chemistry profiles. Nonetheless, many physicians think they are warranted as baseline studies. More extensive diagnostic investigations, such as computed tomography (CT), magnetic resonance imaging, and nuclear scans clearly are not indicated in staging asymptomatic patients with thin melanomas unless suggested by a specific finding on physical examination. Lymph node biopsy or aspiration is indicated if the lymph nodes are clinically enlarged. If clinical palpation reveals grossly involved lymph nodes, nodal dissection without a prior biopsy is reasonable. If nodal biopsy or dissection shows metastatic melanoma, then full-body CT scans should be performed to determine evidence of distant or visceral involvement of the melanoma. More complete diagnostic radiologic studies may also be indicated for deep melanomas (> 4 mm), which have a greater than 50% risk for metastatic spread.

A complete physical examination is important in all patients with melanoma. This begins with careful inspection and palpation around the area of the melanoma, looking for cutaneous metastatic lesions. Regional and distant lymph nodes are carefully palpated to determine any clinical presence of metastatic disease. A thorough cutaneous evaluation includes examination of the scalp, conjunctiva, oral mucosa, genitalia, perianal area, nails, palms, and soles. Note should be made of possible liver or spleen enlargement.

Treatment

Treatment options for melanoma are based on the Breslow depth of invasion and the clinical staging (Table 150-8). A major trend has been the decreasing margin size needed for reexcision after the diagnosis of melanoma is made. Previously, the approach for melanoma was to excise lesions with up to a 5-cm margin of normal skin. This often resulted in a cosmetically unacceptable skin-grafting procedure for reconstruction. More recent clinical trials indicate that thin melanomas can be excised with much narrower margins. The optimal margin of resection is uncertain, but data suggest that resection margins greater than 3 cm do not improve survival. The dissection should be carried to the level of the deep subcutaneous tissue, but muscle fascia does not need to be removed. In most cases, the resulting defect can be closed in a side-to-side fashion or with a local flap. For melanoma in situ, where there is no evidence of invasive disease, excision with a 5-mm border of clinically normal skin is sufficient. Theoretically, this should result in a 100% cure rate. For invasive melanomas with a Breslow thickness of less than 1 mm, a 1-cm margin of clinically normal skin is required. This results in a 5-year survival rate exceeding 95%. Thicker melanomas have a higher risk of microscopic satellitosis and therefore require a wider margin of resection (usually 1 to 3 cm, depending on the Breslow depth of invasion).

Long-term follow-up is important for patients with melanoma. Late recurrences are possible even in patients who have had thin melanomas. Of greater concern is the development of a second primary melanoma. It is estimated that 3% of those who have had a melanoma develop a second melanoma within 3 years. Up to one third of patients with the familial atypical mole and melanoma syndrome develop a secondary primary melanoma. In addition, immunocompromised patients tend to be at high risk for multiple primary melanomas. Although somewhat arbitrary, 6 months appears to be an appropriate interval between examinations for thin melanomas. For thicker, high-risk melanomas, return visits three or four times a year are recommended.

Table 150-8 Surgical Margin for Melanoma

BRESLOW THICKNESS (mm)	SURGICAL MARGIN (cm)	FIVE-YEAR SURVIVAL (%)
In situ	0.5–1	100
>1	1	95–99
1.1–1.49	1–2	80–90
1.5–4.0	2	60–75
>4	2–3	<50

Considerations in Pregnancy

Controversy has surrounded the issue of whether pregnancy before, during, or after the melanoma diagnosis affects the prognosis and outcome. There are no unequivocal data suggesting that pregnancy worsens the prognosis. However, melanoma can cross the placental barrier and affect the fetus. If a melanoma is diagnosed during pregnancy, it should be removed immediately. Some physicians advise women with melanoma to avoid pregnancy for several years after the diagnosis and thus avoid the possibility of becoming pregnant if they develop metastatic disease. Obviously, this is a highly individual decision on the part of the patient.

BIBLIOGRAPHY

Guidelines of care for basal cell carcinoma. American Academy of Dermatology Bulletin 1990;8(suppl):9.

Johnson TM, Smith JW 2d, Nelson BR, Chang A. Current therapy for cutaneous melanoma. J Am Acad Dermatol 1995;32:689.

Koh HK. Cutaneous melanoma. N Engl J Med 1991;325:171.

Kwa RE, Campana K, May R. Biology of cutaneous squamous cell carcinoma. J Am Acad Dermatol 1992;26:1.

Miller SJ. Biology of basal cell carcinoma. J Am Acad Dermatol 1991;24:1.

Schwartz RA. Skin cancer: recognition and management. New York, Springer-Verlag, 1988.

Swanson NA. Basal cell carcinoma: treatment modalities and recommendations. Primary Care 1983;10:443.

151
Diagnostic Techniques in Dermatology

SOPHIE M. WOROBEC

Primary Care for Women, edited by Phyllis C. Leppert and Fred M. Howard. Lippincott-Raven Publishers, Philadelphia © 1997.

Dermatologists use several procedures to diagnose skin diseases. The most frequently used procedures are skin biopsy, potassium hydroxide (KOH) preparation for the demonstration of fungi or yeast, Wood's light examination, cytodiagnosis (Tzanck smear), diascopy, testing for dermatographism, phototesting, patch testing, fungal cultures, and microscopic examination of scabies preparations.

SKIN BIOPSY

A simple procedure, skin biopsy provides relevant diagnostic information to the physician who properly considers when to do one, the type of lesion on which biopsy should be performed, and the appropriate size of the biopsy specimen. The recently developed Episcope deserves mention here because of its potential usefulness in distinguishing benign from malignant lesions. An Episcope is a hand-held instrument similar in size to an ophthalmoscope that magnifies skin surface characteristics by 10×. It is not a replacement for biopsy but helps to determine the lesions on which to perform biopsy.

Choice of Biopsy Site

The choice of biopsy site depends on the nature of the skin disease being studied. When possible, a dermatologist should evaluate the patient and make this decision. Similarly, skin biopsy material is best sent to a dermatopathologist for interpretation.

If the eruption is widespread, then an early typical lesion on the site that most easily hides a small scar is the optimal site for biopsy. For blistering diseases, an entire early, small lesion should be removed.

For large, chronic lesions such as patches or plaques suggestive of cutaneous T-cell lymphoma or mycosis fungoides, the most indurated lesions should be chosen, and multiple biopsy specimens often are needed. Ideally, no corticosteroids should have been used for at least 4 weeks before biopsy.

When malignant melanoma is strongly suspected, it is best to refer the patient to a physician who will be responsible for the removal of the entire lesion and subsequent follow-up. If a punch or other type of incisional biopsy is chosen, it is important that it be adequate so as not to miss the crucial pathology. For example, areas of regression that clinically can be white or pink may reveal deeper foci of melanoma extension. A shave biopsy should be avoided on a suspected malignant melanoma because this may completely eliminate the possibility of getting an estimate of the true depth of the lesion.

Size of the Biopsy Specimen

A 3-mm punch biopsy specimen is frequently sufficient to establish the diagnosis. In certain cases of deeper tumors or lesions that are suspected of extending to the subcutaneous tissue, at least a 4-mm punch biopsy or an excisional biopsy should be performed.

Shave biopsies may also be appropriate, especially in cases of benign tumors such as seborrheic keratosis. All of these may leave scars. The size of an excisional biopsy should be dictated by the area where the biopsy is going to be done and by ease of closure.

Skin Biopsy Materials

The following materials are used in skin biopsies. For anesthesia, 1% or 2% lidocaine (Xylocaine) with or without epinephrine, a 3- or 5-mL syringe, and a 27- or 30-gauge needle are used. Epinephrine should not be used on the fingers, toes, or nose tip because skin sloughing may result from excessive vasoconstriction. Skin preparation solutions consist of alcohol and povidone-iodine (Betadine) or chlorhexidine gluconate (Hibiclens). Three or four sterile drapes should be available. Instruments consist of a No. 11 or No. 15 scalpel blade and handle, a sterile skin biopsy punch, Adson forceps, suture scissors, and a needle holder. The following also are needed: nylon or Prolene suture, five or six sterile gauze pads, pathology specimen container, and sterile gloves. Dressing material consists of Gelfoam, Telfa pads, gauze pads, and tape or a Kerlix gauze roll.

Skin Biopsy Technique

Preparation for biopsy includes shaving the hairy areas. The site is then washed gently. The area to undergo biopsy is then infiltrated with a local anesthetic. In a punch biopsy, a sharp punch is firmly pressed against the skin and then gently rotated until a slight give is felt. The punch is then removed, and the skin plug is elevated using gentle pressure with an Adson forceps. The bottom of the plug is then cut with the sterile scissors. The skin tissue should not be squeezed. The specimen is then placed in the pathology specimen container. The bottle should be shaken to make sure that the skin plug is immersed in the preservative formalin. The bottle should be immediately labeled with the patient's name, the date, and the site of the biopsy.

Excisional biopsies are performed by creating an ellipse with a scalpel blade surrounding the lesion in question. Once the ellipse is created, it is gently elevated with forceps by one of the corners, and then underlying subcutaneous tissue is separated from the base with sharp scissors. Hemostasis usually is obtained by gentle pressure for 1 to 2 minutes. Wound closure then follows. After suturing, the wound should then be covered with a dressing held in place securely with tape or gauze. It is desirable to inform the pathologist of the differential diagnosis being considered and to give the pathologist a description of the skin lesion. If tissue is being sent for electron microscopic study, it should be placed in a special buffered glutaraldehyde solution. Tissue being sent for direct immunofluorescence study is put in Michel's transport media or is snap-frozen in liquid nitrogen.

Complications of Skin Biopsy

Possible complications that need to be included in the informed consent include allergic reaction, scarring, bleeding, and infection. Antibiotic prophylaxis should be provided if indicated.

POTASSIUM HYDROXIDE PREPARATION FOR THE DEMONSTRATION OF FUNGI

Material from the affected area is collected on a microscope slide in the following ways. The suspected tinea corporis, or candidiasis, skin lesion is gently scraped at its outer, scaly edge with a no. 15 blade, being careful to collect scale, without drawing any blood. Suspected pityriasis versicolor lesions are gently rubbed with a no. 15 blade, and the fine scale throughout the surface of the lesion is collected. Thick scaly hyperkeratotic palmar and plantar lesions are scraped similarly over areas of greatest scaliness, which may be at the center or periphery. If bullous or vesicular lesions are present, a blister roof is gently held by a forceps and removed by a curved iris scissors. Nail material can be collected with a tiny curette. Hairs from suspected areas of tinea capitis can be gently plucked with an Adson forceps.

A cover slide is applied. A drop of 5% to 20% KOH or other specialized fungal stains, such as chlorazol black E or Swartz Lamkins containing counter stains, dimethylsulfoxide, or both, is then added at the side of the cover slip and allowed to percolate under the cover slip to cover the collected tissue. (These are available from Delasco Dermatologic Lab & Supply, Council Bluffs, Iowa, 1-800-831-6273.)

The slide is briefly heated (to avoid crystallization of the KOH) over an alcohol burner before any bubbling appears. Heating can be omitted, but more time will be required for clarification of the specimen. Thick specimens such as nails, blister tops, or hair may require a 30-minute wait or longer.

The preparation then is examined microscopically with subdued light with the condenser turned to its lowest position. Fungal elements appear as thread-like, birefringent, branching, linear elements that cross the outlines of the fading cell walls. Yeast spores vary in size, and budding is extremely useful in differentiating yeast spores from trapped air bubbles. A typical "spaghetti and meatballs" pattern of hyphae and spores representing *Pityrosporum orbiculare* (*ovale*) is seen in pityriasis (tinea) versicolor lesional scrapings.

CYTODIAGNOSIS (TZANCK SMEAR)

Changes induced by viruses that occur in lesions of herpes simplex, herpes zoster varicella, and molluscum contagiosum can be seen be preparing a smear of cells from the base of a fresh blister or papule. For the smear, an early unruptured blister is chosen. The roof of the blister is gently removed with sharp scissors, and the base is then gently blotted with gauze; the base is then firmly scraped with a blunt scalpel without inducing bleeding. The material on the scalpel is then spread on the glass slide and stained with Giemsa or Sedi-Stain. In lesions of herpes simplex and herpes zoster varicella, a peculiar ballooning degeneration of the keratinocytes and multinucleated giant cells is seen. Microscopic examination of material expressed from a papule of molluscum contagiosum shows large, round, brick-shaped eosinophilic bodies termed *molluscum bodies*.

WOOD'S LIGHT EXAMINATION

A Wood's lamp is an instrument containing a mercury lamp fitted with a filter that limits the emission to 360 nm; it is used to examine skin and hair in a darkened room. In disorders of depigmentation or hypopigmentation, such as vitiligo, a Wood's light examination helps to visualize early developing areas that are not visible to the naked eye. The lesions of vitiligo shine a lighter color than the surrounding normal skin. Hyperpigmented lesions can be seen more intensely with a Wood's lamp than with visible light if the melanin pigmentation is predominantly in the epidermis. Examples of lesions accentuated with a Wood's lamp are melasma, lentigo maligna melanoma, acral lentiginous melanoma, and ephelides (freckles). However, dermal hypermelanosis, as is present in a Mongolian spot, is not accentuated by a Wood's lamp illumination.

A pinkish red fluorescence is seen in urine from patients with porphyria when the urine is exposed to the Wood's lamp. Addition of dilute hydrochloric acid, which converts porphyrinogens to porphyrins, increases the fluorescence. However, urine fluorescence is not always detectable, and laboratory analysis of blood, urine, and stool is necessary to establish a porphyria diagnosis.

Erythrasma is a common bacterial infection caused by *Corynebacterium minutissimum*, which occurs as brownish red patches in body fold areas. These patches emit a coral-pink to orange-red fluorescence on Wood's lamp examination. *Pseudomonas* infection shows a yellow-green fluorescence of affected skin and nails.

When the result is positive, a Wood's lamp examination can delineate the extent of fungal infections. Tinea corporis and capitis lesions caused by small-spored *Microsporum* species fluoresce a bright blue-green when lighted by a Wood's lamp. Some fungal species give off a pale green fluorescence, but not all fungal infections fluoresce. The organism currently responsible for most cases of tinea capitis, *Trichophyton tonsurans*, does not cause a fluorescence and gives a negative finding on Wood's lamp examination.

DIASCOPY

Diascopy is a procedure in which gentle pressure is applied on top of skin lesions with two microscope slides to observe color changes. Erythema from capillary dilatation then blanches. Purpuric lesions from extravasated red blood cells do not blanch, which indicates a diagnosis of vasculitis. A yellow-brown color is revealed in granulomatous lesions such as sarcoidosis, granuloma annulare, and cutaneous tuberculosis, and also in some cases of cutaneous lymphoma.

TESTS FOR DERMATOGRAPHISM

When testing for dermatographism, the skin is gently stroked with a blunt instrument such as a tongue depressor. The usual response is the triple response of Lewis, which consists of a red line within 15 seconds, followed by a red flare extending laterally in 15 to 45 seconds, followed in 1 to 3 minutes by a wheal occurring in the central area of stroking. In white dermatographism, a white line develops instead and no flare or wheal is seen. The mechanism of white dermatographism is not clearly understood, but this finding confirms that a patient has atopic dermatitis (eczema).

PHOTOTESTING

Phototesting is done to determine heightened reactivity to portions (UVA, UVB, and visible light) of the sunlight spectrum. This is done to diagnose certain photosensitivity disorders. It also is done before phototherapy or photopatch testing to determine threshold sensitivities to light.

PATCH TESTING

Patch testing is done to detect delayed hypersensitivity reactions causing allergic contact dermatitis. The indications for patch testing include a persistent eczematous dermatitis or other dermatologic diseases, such as stasis dermatitis that is nonhealing, to determine if a contact hypersensitivity component exists. A screening series, the T.R.U.E. TEST, is available from Glaxo-Dermatology (Glaxo Research, Triangle Park, NC).

Patch testing should *never* be done on inflamed skin. If extensive inflammation is present, false-positive reactions may occur more readily.

In photopatch testing, duplicate patch tests are applied, with one set being exposed to light. It is indicated when a dermatitis is present in a photodistribution and a photo allergen is suspected.

Although simple in principle, the interpretation of patch test reactions and patient counseling on their relevance is complex. When a suspected contact dermatitis cannot be resolved using a screening series, referral to a dermatologist with a special interest in contact dermatitis is indicated for further workup.

BIBLIOGRAPHY

Caplan RM. Medical uses of the Wood's lamp. JAMA 1967;202:1035.

Cram DL. Common diagnostic procedures. In: Solomon LM, Esterly NB, Loeffel ED, eds. Adolescent dermatology. Philadelphia: WB Saunders, 1978:39.

Fitzpatrick TB, Bernhard JD. The structure of skin lesions and fundamentals of diagnosis. In: Fitzpatrick TB, Eisen AL, Wolff K, Freedberg IM, Austen KF, eds. Dermatology in general medicine, 4th ed. New York: McGraw-Hill, 1993:27.

Hoke AW. Scabies scraping. Arch Dermatol 1973;108:424.

Patterson JW, Blaylock WK. Cutaneous diagnostic procedures for the clinician. In: Dermatology: a concise textbook. New York: Medical Examination Publishing, Division of Elsevier Science, 1987:35.

Storrs FJ, Rosenthal LE, Adams RM, et al. Prevalence and relevance of allergic reactions in patients patch tested in North America, 1984–1985. J Am Acad Dermatol 1989;20:1038.

T.R.U.E. TEST Thin-layer rapid use epicutaneous test. Allergen patch test. Product monograph. Triangle Park, NC: Glaxo Research, 1994.

152

Dermatoses of Pregnancy

SOPHIE M. WOROBEC

Primary Care for Women, edited by Phyllis C. Leppert and Fred M. Howard. Lippincott-Raven Publishers, Philadelphia © 1997.

The skin exhibits many changes during pregnancy: the nipples, areolae, and external genitalia become more darkly pigmented; a linea nigra develops on the lower abdomen; existing moles may darken; and a facial blotchy hyperpigmentation termed melasma develops in over 50% of women.

Hair growth resulting in mild to moderate hirsutism is common, and resolves either in the third trimester or after delivery. In 1 to 5 months postpartum, telogen effluvium occurs, with regrowth usually happening within 1 year.

Stretch marks, or striae distensae, occur over the abdomen, hips, buttocks, and breasts, often with the initial presentation of itching. Skin tags may enlarge and proliferate.

Hyperemia results in palmar erythema in up to two thirds of women. Both spider angiomas and new cherry angiomas may appear. Existing angiomas tend to enlarge. Varicosities of the lower extremities may worsen.

Sweet syndrome, which includes a constellation of signs (fever, leukocytosis, tender red plaques, and biopsy findings of a subepidermal edema with a neutrophilic dermal infiltrate) has been reported in six patients during pregnancy. In two women, it recurred during subsequent pregnancies (Fig. 152-1).

The dermatoses of pregnancy can be divided into those that have been best defined and those that are poorly defined. Among the well-defined entities are pemphigoid (herpes) gestationis (PG), pruritic urticarial papules and plaques of pregnancy (PUPPP), recurrent cholestasis of pregnancy, and "impetigo herpetiformis," which is a form of pustular psoriasis. The first three are described in this chapter, and the last in Chapter 141.

PEMPHIGOID (HERPES) GESTATIONIS

Pemphigoid (herpes) gestationis is an immunologically mediated bullous disease of pregnancy and the postpartum period. It is recurrent and is marked by small papulovesicles, which often are grouped and occur on an erythematous background. Urticarial plaques may be present, and bullae may evolve from the vesicles. Excoriations and crusts are common (Figs. 152-2 and 152-3).

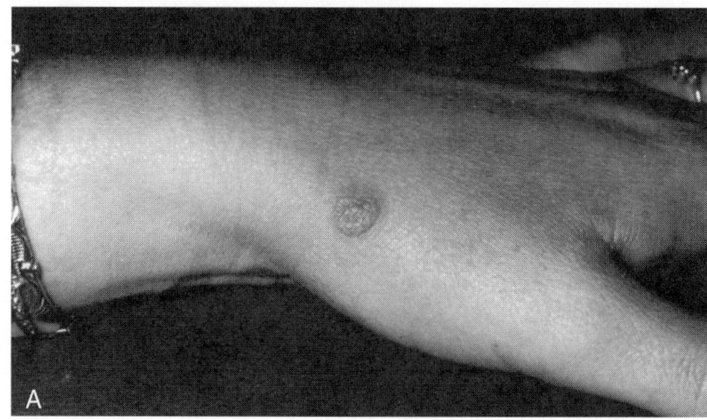

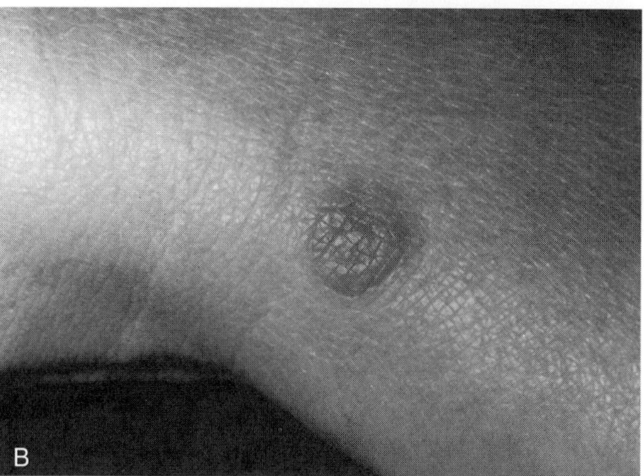

Figure 152-1. (***A***) A pseudovesicular plaque that is seen in Sweet syndrome. (***B***) Close-up of same plaque. These are firm, red, edematous plaques that can be recurrent and have an edematous feel to them with a suggestion of translucency, which has led to the use of the term of *pseudovesicular* in describing them. They occur as multiple lesions of varying sizes and of varying duration, and heal leaving a dusky red or hyperpigmented patch. Diagnosis is by biopsy, which reveals a dense, neutrophilic infiltrate in the upper dermis. This syndrome is associated with malignancy in approximately 30% of cases and should trigger an age-appropriate workup for malignancy. However, six case reports of Sweet syndrome have been associated with pregancy in normal individuals. When associated with pregancy, Sweet syndrome can be recurrent with subsequent pregnancies.

Etiology

In PG, circulating IgG1 autoantibodies have been demonstrated that bind to one of two antigen sites within the epidermal basal membrane zone. One of these sites consists of a 180-kd protein, which has been identified as the bullous pemphigoid antigen (BPA-2); the other antigen is a 230-kd protein known as BPA-1. These antigens are present in extracts of human placenta and amnion, and also are recognized by sera from patients with bullous pemphigoid.

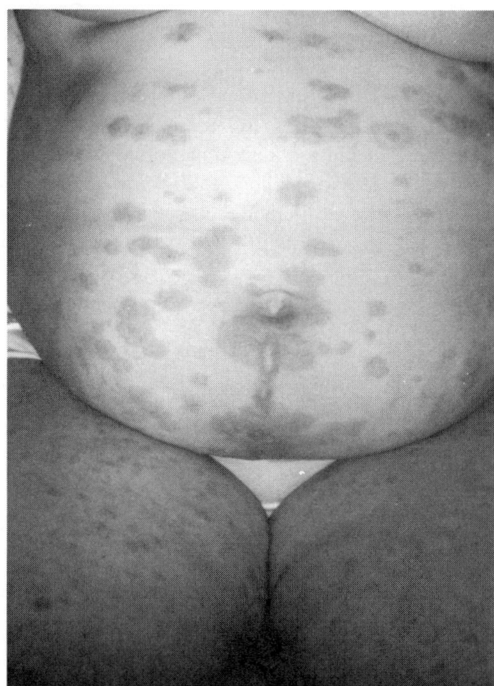

Figure 152-2. Pemphigoid (herpes) gestationis (PG). PG is an immunologically mediated bullous disease of pregnancy in the postpartum period. The eruption is marked by small papulovesicles with an erythematous rim. Urticarial plaques also may be present. The lesions are generalized in distribution. (Courtesy of Dr. Kim B. Yancey.)

History

The eruption can start any time during pregnancy, with flares common at the time of delivery or in the postpartum period. Onset also can occur in the postpartum period. There are recurrences with subsequent pregnancies, with disease starting earlier in the course of the subsequent pregnancy. The use of birth control pills also may cause flare. One study showed an increased fetal mortality and morbidity, but this was not confirmed in a subsequent large study. There may be an increased incidence of small-for-gestational-age infants born to affected mothers. Infants may rarely have a transient eruption.

Physical Examination

The eruption consists of papules, plaques, vesicles, and sometimes tense bullae, occurring anywhere on the body. Target lesions may be present, leading to a differential diagnosis of erythema multiforme or bullous pemphigoid.

Laboratory Studies

Skin biopsy shows edema of the dermal papillae with an infiltrate consisting of eosinophils, lymphocytes, and a few neutrophils. A subepidermal blister with necrosis of basal cells may be found, but routine histopathologic study alone does not distinguish PG from other blistering diseases. The diagnostic test is direct immunofluorescence of a perilesional skin biopsy specimen with the demonstration of C_3 in a linear pattern along the basement membrane (Fig. 152-4). These deposits have persisted for over 1 year after the eruption has cleared, and also have been demon-

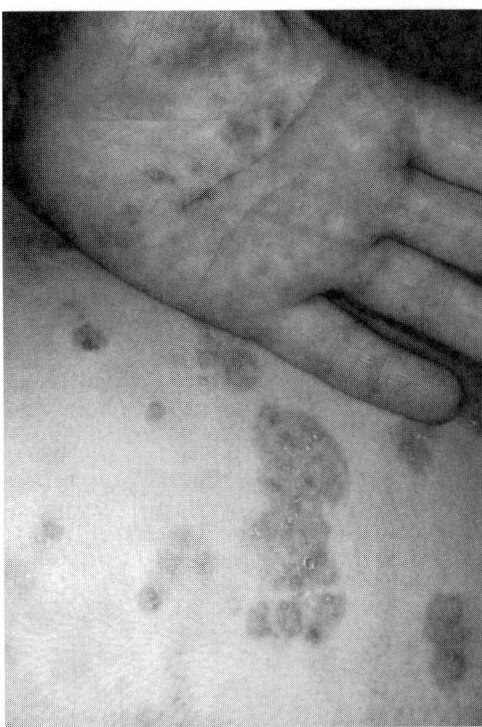

Figure 152-3. This is a close-up of lesions of pemphigoid (herpes) gestationis. Small papules vesicles are grouped and occur on a red background. Excoriations and crusts are common. (Courtesy of Dr. Kim B. Yancey.)

strated in the skin of infants born to affected mothers. Other immunoreactants, most commonly IgG, also have been found along the basement membrane.

Treatment

Systemic glucocorticosteroids and antihistamines with increased doses during delivery and the postpartum period have been used in treatment. Occasionally, topical corticosteroids have controlled milder cases. If the mother is treated with prolonged high-dose corticosteroids, infants should be monitored for adrenal insufficiency. There are no data on the effect of maternal treatment on infant morbidity and mortality. Dapsone also has been used.

PRURITIC URTICARIAL PAPULES AND PLAQUES OF PREGNANCY

Pruritic urticarial papules and plaques of pregnancy (PUPPP) is a common, itchy disorder seen toward the end of the third trimester of pregnancy. It is characterized by red urticarial papules and plaques that usually begin on the abdomen, especially within stretch marks, and then spread onto the thighs and sometimes the buttocks and arms (Fig. 152-5).

Etiology

The etiology of PUPPP is unknown. Increased maternal weight gain, increased neonatal weight gain, and an increased incidence of twinning in 30 patients have led to the hypothesis that increased abdominal distention, or a reaction to it, may be important.

PUPPP is more common in prima gravidae but can be seen in any pregnancy. In half of the patients, lesions first start within periumbilical striae.

Physical Examination

The lesions of PUPPP are those of its name. Rarely, a microvesicle appears within a few papules.

Laboratory Studies

Routine histopathologic findings are nonspecific, showing upper dermal edema, a lymphohistiocytic perivascular infiltrate, and sometimes eosinophils. Direct immunofluorescence of perilesional skin yields negative findings and should be performed if a diagnosis of PG is in the differential diagnosis.

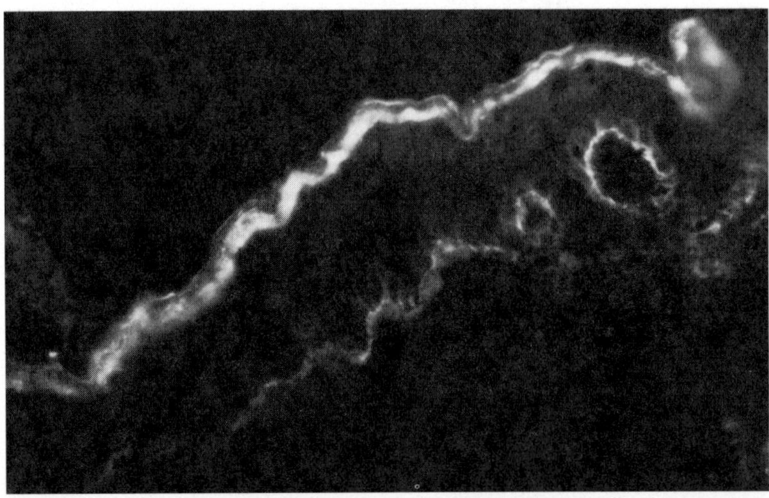

Figure 152-4. Pemphigoid (herpes) gestationis (PG). Direct immunofluorescence of perilesional skin is the diagnostic test that determines whether a patient has PG. Here deposition of C3 in a linear pattern along the basement membrane is demonstrated. Other immunoreactins, most commonly IgG, also can be found along the basement membrane. (Courtesy of Dr. Kim B. Yancey.)

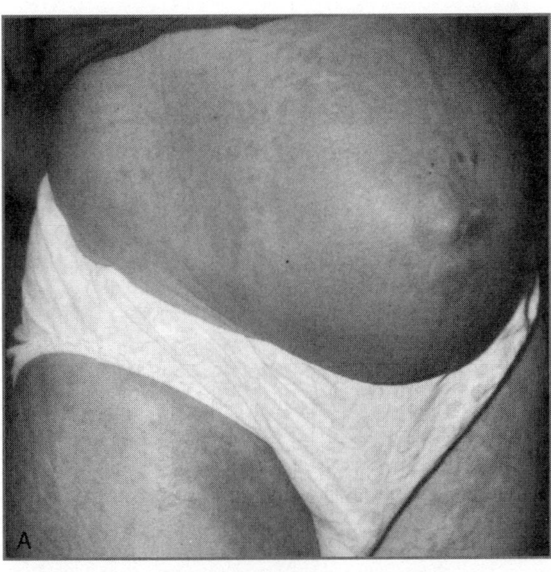

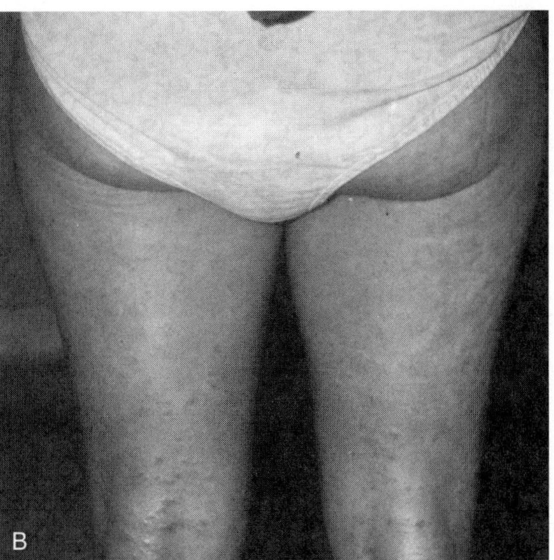

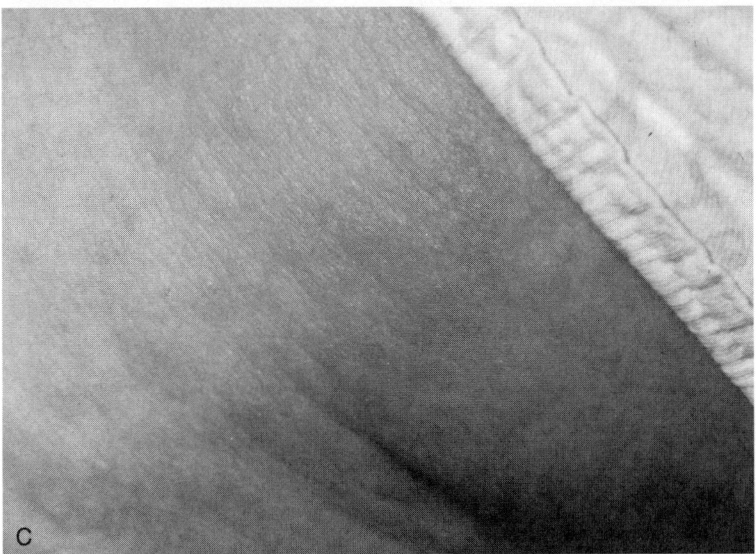

Figure 152-5. Pruritic urticarial papules and plaques of pregnancy (PUPPP). (***A***) PUPPP is characterized by red, urticarial papules as seen here on the thighs and urticarial plaques, which usually begin on the abdomen and (***B***) then spread onto the thighs and sometimes onto the buttocks and arms. (***C***) Close-up of urticarial papules of PUPPP on the lower buttock.

Treatment

Treatment of PUPP consists of emollients, topical corticosteroids, and, rarely, short courses of systemic steroids. Some have advocated the use of potent topical corticosteroids five to six times per day.

RECURRENT CHOLESTASIS OF PREGNANCY (PRURIGO GRAVIDARUM)

Recurrent cholestasis of pregnancy (prurigo gravidarum) is a disorder that is marked by severe itching followed by jaundice. It usually occurs in the late third trimester but also is seen earlier in pregnancy.

Etiology

Agenetic predisposition is suggested by reports of several members of the same family having developed recurrent cholestasis of pregnancy. Whether increased levels of estrogen, progesterone, or both contribute to the cholestasis is unknown.

History

Severe generalized itching, with no other predisposing cause, is the hallmark of the medical history. Fatigue, anorexia, nausea, right-quadrant fullness, light-colored stools, dark urine, and vomiting also may be present. Symptoms may return with subsequent pregnancies or with oral contraceptive use.

Physical Examination

Icterus may not develop until 4 weeks or later after the onset of itching. Secondary excoriations may be widespread. The liver may be enlarged and slightly tender.

Laboratory Studies

Hyperbilirubinemia, elevated serum alkaline phosphatase levels, and impaired bromsulphalein retention all may be found in women with recurrent cholestasis of pregnancy.

Treatment

Bland emollients, topical anti-itch remedies, antihistamines, and cholestyraminebeen all have been used in treatment.

OTHER DERMATOSES OF PREGNANCY

The following sections discuss four of the poorly defined dermatoses of pregnancy.

Prurigo Gestationis of Besnier

Prurigo gestationis of Besnier is described as itchy papules occurring over the upper trunk and extremities. It resolves during the postpartum period, with residual hyperpigmentation. There is no blistering and no associated fetal morbidity or mortality.

Papular Dermatitis of Pregnancy

Papular dermatitis of pregnancy is an entity described as consisting of 3- to 5-mm red papules that quickly become crusted and excoriated, leaving a hyperpigmented scar. It is controversial whether it actually exists as a separate entity.

Pruritic Folliculitis of Pregnancy

Pruritic folliculitis of pregnancy has been reported in six patients. It, too, consists of 3- to 5-mm excoriated red papules, and on skin biopsy, folliculitis was seen in five of the six patients. All offspring were healthy; direct immunofluorescence gave negative findings. The eruption has resolved at delivery, within 1 month after delivery, and within 1 week of onset.

Immune Progesterone Dermatitis of Pregnancy

Immune progesterone dermatitis of pregnancy was reported in 1973 in one patient who had a first-trimester papulopustular eruption over the extremities, buttocks, and thighs. Some lesions were acneiform and some had a psoriasiform scale. Peripheral eosinophilia, pulmonary infiltrates, and polyarteritis were associated findings. The pregnancy ended in a spontaneous abortion, as had a previous one in which the patient reported a similar dermatitis. Skin biopsy of lesional skin revealed intraepidermal eosinophilic abscesses, along with lymphocytes and histiocytes, dense perivascular infiltrates, and a lobular panniculitis with eosinophilic abscesses within the subcutaneous tissue. An intradermal aqueous progesterone injection produced similar histologic results. The dermatitis resolved after the abortion. No premenstrual flare of this dermatitis was reported, although a progesterone-containing contraceptive worsened this patient's symptoms.

CONSIDERATIONS IN PREGNANCY

A recent report demonstrated that 12% of sera from pregnant women versus 2% of sera from nonpregnant women contained IgM, which reacted with the epidermal proteins of 180 kd or 230 to 240 kd (BPA-2 and BPA-1 antigens, respectively) in the basement membrane zone. Yet, these women had no clinical disease; therefore, these anti-basement membrane zone antibodies may be regarded as "natural autoantibodies." The IgM antibodies have low affinity, in contrast to the high affinity of the IgG antibodies that bind to the BPA-2 and BPA-1 in PG. Recent research in immunology indicates that women in general have stronger humoral reactivity than men. A further extension of this finding is that pregnant women have heightened humoral reactivity compared with nonpregnant women. Pregnant women produce several antibodies to both paternal and fetal antigens. The immunologic changes of pregnancy, coupled with the profound physiologic changes occurring during pregnancy, probably are responsible for the skin disorders and changes seen during pregnancy.

BIBLIOGRAPHY

Bierman SM. Autoimmune progesterone dermatitis. Arch Dermatol 1973;107:896.

Borradori L, Didierjean L, Bernard P, et al. IgM autoantibodies to 180- and 230- to 240-kd human epidermal proteins in pregnancy. Arch Dermatol 1995;131:43.

Cohen LM, Capeless EL, Krusinski PA, Maloney ME. Pruritic urticarial papules and plaques of pregnancy and its relationship to maternal-fetal weight gain and twin pregnancy. Arch Dermatol 1989;125:1534.

Diaz LA, Ratrie H III, Saunders WS, et al. Isolation of a human epidermal cDNA corresponding to the 180-kD autoantigen recognized by bullous pemphigoid and herpes gestationis sera: immunolocalization of this protein to the hemides mosome. J Clin Invest 1990;86:1088.

Laatikainen T. Effect of cholestyramine and phenobarbital on pruritus and serum bile acid levels in cholestasis of pregnancy. Am J Obstet Gynecol 1978;132:501.

Lawley TJ, Stingl G, Katz SI. Fetal and maternal risk factors in herpes gestations. Arch Dermatol 1978;114:552.

Lawley TJ, Yancey KB. Skin changes and diseases in pregnancy. In: Fitzpatrick TB, Eisen AZ, Wolff K, Freedberg IM, Austen KF, eds. Dermatology in general medicine. New York: McGraw-Hill, 1993:2105.

Primary Care for Women, edited by Phyllis C. Leppert and Fred M. Howard. Lippincott-Raven Publishers, Philadelphia © 1997.

XVI

Psychologic and Behavioral Problems

153

Depression

ADRIAN LEIBOVICI

Depression, one of the most common mental disorders, is an important source of disability for both men and women. It is associated with emotional and physical distress, with dysfunction at work and in personal relations, and in extreme cases with suicide. About one fourth of all persons in the United States will experience some form of depression in their lifetime, and in about 9% of the population the symptoms will reach clinical proportions.

CLASSIFICATION AND EPIDEMIOLOGY

From a clinical viewpoint, depression can be construed as a symptom (feeling down, blue, sad, with low mood), a sign (affect depressed as observed by an objective examiner), a syndrome, or an illness.

Syndrome of Depression

Depressed mood and inability to experience pleasure (anhedonia) are the most common features of depression. They must be sustained and severe. Appetite is decreased or less frequently increased, and weight loss or gain follows in severe cases. Sleep is disturbed, in the form of insomnia or hypersomnia. Patients complain of fatigue, lack of energy, and difficulty with concentration or decision making. Thinking is dominated by ideas of poverty, worthlessness, and guilt. Thought processes and motor functions can be either slowed or sped up (psychomotor retardation or agitation). In the most extreme cases, patients exhibit delusions and suicidal thinking and behavior.

Depressive Illness

The nosology of depression is complex and evolving due to the phenomenologic and etiologic diversity of this common psychiatric condition. The official psychiatric classification of depression (DSM-IV) recognizes several broad diagnostic categories: major depressive disorder (unipolar), dysthymic disorder, bipolar disorder, cyclothymic disorder, substance-induced mood disorder, and mood disorder due to a general medical condition.

Major depressive disorder is characterized by a rather severe and prolonged depressive syndrome that lasts at least 2 weeks, more often several months. The natural course is usually episodic. The severity, frequency of episodes, extent of interepisodic recovery, and response to treatment vary. Women are twice as likely to develop major depression as men: lifetime prevalence in the community is 10% to 25% for women and only 5% to 12% for men. Ethnicity, education, income, and marital status do not predict depression, but the illness is 1.5 to three times more frequent in first-degree relatives of afflicted persons.

The most severe cases of depression present with extreme psychomotor retardation, nihilistic or paranoid delusions, severe weight loss, early-morning awakening, and a tendency to feel worse in the morning (diurnal mood variation): this clinical picture is called melancholia.

Bipolar disorder or manic-depressive illness typically consists of alternating episodes of depression and mania. The manic state consists of elevated or irritable mood, grandiosity, decreased need for sleep, pressured speech, racing thoughts, distractibility, and increased levels of energy and goal-directed activity (sexual, professional, social). The same syndrome of somewhat lesser intensity is called hypomania. The diagnosis of bipolar disorder is made if at least one manic or hypomanic episode occurs, even in the absence of documented depressive episodes. The interval between episodes often is asymptomatic, especially earlier in the course of illness. Some patients tend to cycle more rapidly with aging. In severe cases, so-called mixed affective states are described: the patient experiences a mixture of depressive and manic symptoms at the same time—for instance, hyperactivity and flight of ideas on one hand and unhappiness and suicidal ideation on the other. When true mania is present, bipolar disorder 1 is diagnosed. It is equally common in both sexes and has a lifetime community prevalence of 0.4% to 1.6%. Bipolar disorder 2 is diagnosed when hypomania but not mania is present. It tends to be more common in women and its prevalence is only 0.5%.

Dysthymic disorder is characterized by a depressive syndrome of somewhat lesser intensity but of longer duration than major depression. The diagnostic time criterion is at least 2 years, although in most cases the illness lasts much longer. The terms chronic depression and depressive personality have also been applied. The disorder is two to three times more frequent in women. The lifetime community prevalence is 6%.

Cyclothymic disorder is a chronic condition characterized by periods of depression and periods of manic-like acceleration. The severity of symptoms and extent of disability are less than with bipolar disorder. As with dysthymia, cyclothymia lasts very long and many times defines a person's behavioral and interacting style: it used to be called cyclothymic personality disorder. The lifetime community prevalence is 0.4% to 1%, and the genders are equally affected.

These four diagnostic categories can be seen as primary, because their etiology is largely unknown. *Secondary depression* (Table 153-1) is also very common. It can be caused by an emotional stressor (adjustment reaction with depressed mood), by a foreign substance taken for medical or recreational reasons (substance-induced mood disorder), or by a concurrent medical condition (mood disorder due to a general medical condition). Depressive syndromes are also quite prevalent as concomitants or complications of other psychiatric conditions such as anxiety disorders, schizophrenia, and certain personality disorders. The clinical picture of secondary depression is quite variable, ranging from brief and mild sadness to the most severe forms of melancholia. Many times the course is atypical, following that of the primary etiologic factor. Prevalence is known for certain conditions (eg, 25% to 40% of patients with Parkinson disease have depression) but less studied for others.

Table 153-1. Some Conditions Associated With Secondary Depression

Infections	AIDS, influenza, mononucleosis, viral hepatitis, tuberculosis, syphilis
Collagen disease	Systemic lupus, rheumatoid arthritis, scleroderma
Malignancy	Carcinomatosis, pancreatic carcinoma
Endocrine disease	Hypothyroidism, hyperthyroidism, hypopituitarism, Cushing disease, Addison disease
Neurologic disease	Stroke, multiinfarct dementia, other dementias, brain tumor, head trauma, epilepsy (temporal lobe), Parkinson disease, multiple sclerosis
Avitaminosis	Pellagra, pernicious anemia
Iatrogenic	Antihypertensives (β-blockers, α-methyldopa), vincristine, vinblastine, cycloserine, steroidal contraceptives, cimetidine
Accidental intoxications	Thallium, mercury
Drugs of addiction	Intoxication and withdrawal (alcohol, anxiolytic, cocaine, amphetamines); intoxication (opioids, inhalants, hallucinogens, PCP)

ETIOLOGY AND PATHOGENESIS

Primary Depression

The exact cause and mechanism are unknown, but a multifactorial paradigm is generally accepted, as it accommodates facts and findings from different and sometimes competing fields. Heredity, neurochemistry and neurophysiology, gender, personality type, early emotional trauma, and life stressors have all been shown to correlate with the occurrence of depressive illness and with its natural course.

Heredity

Adoption and twin studies support the notion that both bipolar and unipolar major depression recurrent subtypes have genetic transmission, although efforts to identify a locus or depressive gene have not been successful. It is unknown if inheritance is based on a single dominant gene or a polygenic continuum, or if the gene or genes are autosomal or X-linked. The phenotypic expression of genetic vulnerability is reflected in the 1.5- to threefold increase in prevalence in first-degree relatives of patients with major depression. First-degree relatives of persons with bipolar depression are also at increased risk of developing mood disorders.

Neurobiology

The discovery more than three decades ago that pharmacologic monoamine oxidase inhibition was associated with an antidepressant effect raised the possibility that metabolic pathways influenced by this group of enzymes could be involved in the pathogenesis of depression. Much research has been done in this area, leading to the identification of neurotransmitters, brain receptors, and specific pathways thought to be connected with mood and mood disorders. Abnormalities in serotonin and norepinephrine systems are thought to occur in mood disorders, as most antidepressants influence predominantly these two systems.

Gender

Women's greater vulnerability to depression is well documented but poorly understood. Research into gender differences has not yielded significant insights into the mechanisms of depression in general, although several theories have been advanced:

- Women have higher concentrations of monoamine oxidase, the very enzyme inhibited by one class of antidepressants.
- Women respond with mood swings to physiologic changes mediated by sexual hormones.
- Clinical and even subclinical abnormalities in thyroid hormone secretion are more common in women and have been linked to certain types of depression
- In a male-dominated society, women are thought to display more passivity, reliance on interpersonal associations, and helplessness, which might make them vulnerable to depression when confronted with adversity and loss.

Emotional Deprivation

Animal studies in primates point to the fact that separation from the mother and the group in the first month of life leads to severe behavioral disturbance, consisting of withdrawal and self-aggression (anaclitic depression). Depression might be more severe and start earlier in life in persons who lose a parent in childhood; child abuse and neglect are considered important elements in the history of some patients with chronic depressive syndromes.

Stress

Adverse life events such as separation and loss (real or anticipated) are linked to depressive syndromes. They may cause depression, as in adjustment reactions, or precipitate a depressive decompensation in patients with preexisting vulnerability. Sometimes the connection between life stressors and depression is obvious, but other times it takes an astute and persistent clinician to reveal it: many women deliberately or unconsciously conceal abandonment, painful anniversaries, sexual problems, or victimization.

Secondary Depression

Virtually any medical condition can cause depression, via some known or presumed neurochemical effect, by means of the psychological trauma of being ill (incapacity, severe prognosis, deformity), or as a combined psychobiologic reaction. For instance, severe depression associated with carcinoma of the pancreas sometimes precedes diagnosis or severe symptoms, but when the patient becomes aware of this most malignant illness, a reactive component is often superimposed.

Mood disorders are described in association with collagen diseases, infections, endocrinopathies, neoplasms, and avitaminosis. Organic processes in the brain are frequently complicated by depression. Degenerative diseases such as multiple sclerosis, Parkinson disease, or temporal lobe epilepsy can cause symptoms that are more severe than what would be expected from a psychological response to illness. Poststroke depression can pose major management problems because it interferes with the victim's effective participation in rehabilitation at a critical time. Left and anterior locations of the stroke predict a high incidence and typical clinical picture of depression; right and posterior localizations lead to less typical brain syndromes, where affect is mostly restricted and flat. Lack of energy and motivation, poor appetite and sleep, and even psychomotor retardation are characteristic to end-stage organ failure (hepatic, renal, cardiac). Depressive thought content and depressed affect and mood are sometimes present.

Steroidal contraceptives have been associated with depression, which can be severe. Other medications causing iatrogenic depression include antihypertensives (eg, β-blockers, α-methyldopa, reserpine), cytostatics (eg, vincristine, vinblastine), and antipsychotic drugs.

Drugs of abuse and addiction can cause mood pathology during or after either intoxication or withdrawal. Cocaine withdrawal and alcohol intoxication, for instance, are often accompanied by intense dysphoria and suicidal tendencies, which are generally short-lived.

DIAGNOSIS

The clinical diagnosis of depression is relatively easy and should be made by any informed clinician. Several simple rules should be observed:

- The clinician should maintain a high level of suspicion in the presence of major life stressors.
- Some patients do not complain unless specific questions are asked.
- When avoided, questions about substance abuse, sexual function, and suicidality reflect the interviewer's rather than the patient's awkwardness.
- The physician's office is not always conducive to the free expression of intimate thoughts and feelings, so the clinician should try to put the patient at ease as much as possible.
- Rushing to comfort and reassure a patient who starts complaining might shut her off, and the full scope of her distress will not become apparent.
- When in doubt, the clinician should obtain psychiatric consultation.

GOALS OF TREATMENT

Symptom reduction is crucial in the acute phase of treatment: not only is the subjective distress associated with this illness extreme (severe psychological pain), but the risks of suicide can be lowered considerably by initiating supervision and effective interventions early. Restoring function and preventing depressive relapse are the other two major objectives of treatment, becoming more relevant as the patient starts to improve.

Psychological autopsy shows that depression is a major factor in most suicides. Each time depression is diagnosed, the practitioner should assess suicide risk immediately and take appropriate action. Direct questions about the presence of death wishes, suicidal thoughts, and concrete plans to commit suicide, and the availability of means to carry out such plans should be asked without hesitation. The myth that such questions might lead the patient into hurting herself is disproved by clinical reality. In fact, many times suicidal patients are reassured when unacceptable, self-destructive fantasies can be shared with a sympathetic, nonjudgmental professional. Certain history and clinical features are known risk factors for suicide and their presence or absence should be determined: prior suicide attempts, family history of suicide, alcoholism in the patient or family, coexistence of severe medical illness (incurable or with intractable pain), psychotic depression, living alone, hopelessness, old age, and white race. When a significant risk of suicide is determined to be present or when in doubt, immediate evaluation by a psychiatrist should be obtained. Procrastination can be fatal: many patients who commit suicide had seen a physician shortly before the act. This underscores the need to protect patients at risk. Mobilizing supportive family members to supervise the patient until she can be seen by a psychiatrist (suicide watch), or even calling an ambulance and forcefully transporting the patient to the hospital for evaluation is sometimes necessary.

A thorough diagnostic effort helps the clinician identify conditions that are directly causal or only contributing factors to the depressive syndrome. Specific treatment, when available, may obviate or minimize the scope of antidepressant treatment. Examples include hormone replacement in hypothyroidism, aggressive treatment of congestive heart failure, finding alternatives to offending drugs such as propranolol, oral contraceptives, and cimetidine, or addressing the patient's cocaine or alcohol addiction.

Symptomatic treatment for depression includes antidepressant medication, electroconvulsant therapy (ECT), and psychotherapy. Severity of illness, affordability, patient preference, type of depression, and previous response to treatment all play a role in the choice.

Research has been conducted in an effort to objectify the relation between the use of medication, standardized psychotherapies, or both and the outcome of antidepressant treatment. It is generally accepted that mild depression, especially so-called reactive depression, can be treated with psychotherapy alone, but severe depression will not respond without antidepressant medication or ECT. In depression of moderate severity, the choice of treatment is less clear. It appears that both psychotherapy and antidepressant medication are more effective than placebo, and that coadministration of medication and psychotherapy is more effective than either one alone.

ANTIDEPRESSANT MEDICATION

With the advent of newer, better tolerated antidepressants, the use of medication in primary practice and in less severe forms of depression has expanded significantly. The generalist who chooses to treat depression should maintain a certain level of familiarity with the use of different therapies. In practice, antidepressant medication is tried rather than psychotherapy, as the latter is time-consuming and requires special training and expertise.

There are several classes of antidepressant medication (Table 153-2). All antidepressants are equally effective in therapeutic doses, although a particular patient might respond to one antidepressant but not to another. The choice of antidepressant is based on the side effect profile, price, and convenience of use. The only predictors of therapeutic response for a particular drug are previous good response in the patient or in another family member. Therapeutic effect can be seen after 10 to 14 days, although in some cases it takes 6 or 8 weeks. It is important to stress with patients the lack of instant response to antidepressant medication: along with side effects, impatience with the lack of quick symptom relief is a major source of noncompliance. Another important circumstance associated with therapeutic failure in depression is the use of antidepressant medication in insufficient dosage or for an insufficient amount of time.

The mechanism of action of antidepressants is not entirely understood, but they all seem to influence neurotransmission by enhancing noradrenergic, serotonergic, and to a lesser extent dopaminergic systems.

Selective Serotonin Reuptake Inhibitors

Selective serotonin reuptake inhibitors (SSRIs) such as fluoxetine, sertraline, paroxetine, and fluvoxamine have become the most popular antidepressants among general practitioners. They are as effective as traditional antidepressants, at least in outpatient settings, and in most cases have a more favorable side effect profile; specifically, they are practically devoid of side effects such as orthostatic hypotension, tachycardia, or heart block. Jitteriness, insomnia, and gastric discomfort are among the most common side effects and with few exceptions are tolerable. Sexual dysfunction, especially anorgasmia, can be a problem for some patients. All SSRIs compete for the cytochrome P450 2D6 enzyme system, which can increase levels of other medications administered concurrently (eg, tricyclic antidepressants, some antipsychotics, coumadin, quinidine, flecainide). The newly approved fluvoxamine inhibits 3A4 isoenzyme and may increase cardiotoxicity when coadministered with antihistaminic drugs such as terfenadine or astemizole. Overall, however, SSRIs are well tolerated and not as dangerous as other antidepressants when taken in overdose, a dis-

Table 153-2. Commonly Used Antidepressants

CLASS	GENERIC NAME	BRAND NAME	DOSE RANGE (MG/DAY)
Heterocyclics			
Tertiary amines	Imipramine	Tofranil	150–300
	Amitriptyline	Elavil	150–300
	Doxepin	Adapin, Sinequan	150–300
	Clomipramine	Anafranil	150–300
Secondary amines	Desipramine	Norpramin	150–300
	Nortriptyline	Aventil, Parlor	75–150
	Amoxapine	Asendin	150–450
	Protriptyline	Vivactil	15–60
	Trimipramine	Surmontil	150–300
	Maprotiline	Ludiomil	150–200
SSRIs	Fluoxetine	Prozac	20–80
	Fluvoxamine	Luvox	100–300
	Sertraline	Zoloft	50–200
	Paroxetine	Paxil	20–60
MAOIs	Phenelzine	Nardil	45–90
	Tranylcypromine	Parnate	30–50
	Isocarboxazid	Marplan	30–50
Other	Trazodone	Desyrel	200–450
	Nefazodone	Serzone	100–600
	Bupropion	Wellbutrin	150–350
	Venlafaxine	Effexor	75–375

tinct possibility in some depressed patients. Other appealing features of this class of antidepressants are easy administration (once a day in most cases), lack of association with undesirable weight gain, and anticompulsive, antianxiety properties. Sensational reports in the media linking fluoxetine (Prozac) to suicidal and homicidal ideation and behavior were based on case reports and to date have been disproved by systematic research. One major drawback of SSRIs is their high price, which should be taken into consideration with women who have limited resources.

Heterocyclic Antidepressants

There are two subgroups of heterocyclics: tertiary amines (eg, imipramine, amitriptyline, doxepin, clomipramine) and secondary amines (eg, desipramine, nortriptyline, protriptyline, maprotiline). Side effects include orthostatic hypotension, tachycardia, quinidine-like delays in atrioventricular conduction, constipation, urinary retention, dry mouth, blurred vision, confusion, sedation, insomnia, and restlessness. Tertiary amines are more anticholinergic and sedative, so they are more useful in agitated depression and when insomnia is prominent. Secondary amines are "activating" and less anticholinergic: they are more suitable when psychomotor retardation is present, or when it is important to avoid sedation, as in patients who work or drive. Among tricyclics, nortriptyline has become popular with psychiatrists because there seems to be a more reliable therapeutic window when blood levels are measured. Amitriptyline, which for a long time was the most popular antidepressant, is avoided now, especially in the elderly, because it is the most anticholinergic and sedative agent. It is as effective as the other antidepressants and is the least expensive agent, which can be relevant in uninsured patients. Clomipramine, the first drug marketed in the United States specifically for obsessive-compulsive disorder, works as a potent antidepressant also.

Treatment with tricyclic antidepressants requires monitoring of physical status. A baseline electrocardiogram should be obtained, especially in at-risk patients such as the very old and the very young. Vital signs, including orthostatic changes, should be checked periodically. A typical trial in a young healthy woman might start with desipramine 50 mg at bedtime. The dose is increased gradually to 150 mg at bedtime over 1 week as tolerated. If no improvement is noted after 4 weeks, further increments in dose are attempted, up to 300 mg a day. Measuring blood levels can be useful; however, a steady state for any given dose is reached in about 5 days. In the elderly, the dosage needed and tolerated can be considerably lower, and increments should be more gradual—in other words, "start low, go slow."

Monoamine Oxidase Inhibitors

The monoamine oxidase inhibitors (MAOIs) phenelzine, tranylcypromine, and isocarboxazid are the most widely used antidepressants in this class. Unlike other antidepressants, they act by inhibiting the metabolism of catecholamine neurotransmitters and do not have direct effects on neuroreceptors. They are as effective as tricyclics or SSRIs, especially in depressions with an important anxiety component. It is said that the so-called atypical or "rejection sensitivity" depression that is most common in young women responds best to MAOIs; tricyclic antidepressants might worsen the situation. The most common side effects include orthostatic hypotension, mild anticholinergic toxicity, and sedation. Rarely, patients might experience a hypertensive crisis resulting from the ingestion of catecholamine precursors because the physiologic defense against such an occurrence, intestinal monoamine oxidases, is suppressed by the drug. Patients taking MAOIs must eliminate tyramine-rich foods from the diet (eg, chocolate, coffee, wine, processed cheese, canned meats) and avoid using medications such as L-dopa or cold remedies containing sympathomimetics. Another severe complication is a serotonin syndrome (extreme, even fatal hyperpyrexia), which was associated with the coadministration of MAOIs and meperidine or other analgesics.

Other Antidepressants

Several antidepressants that do not belong to the main three classes can be very useful. *Trazodone*, which primarily influences the serotonin system, has a separate soporific effect that is dose-related; many patients with insomnia experience better sleep immediately, before the other symptoms of depression abate. *Bupropion* is notable for its lack of negative effect on sexual function. It also has no notable cardiotoxicity, but in high doses it is associated with a higher incidence of seizures. *Venlafaxine* and *nefazodone* have been recently released, and their role remains unclear.

Drug Combinations and Antidepressant Augmentation

In psychotic depression, an antipsychotic agent is added to the antidepressant. When insomnia, agitation, or anxiety accompanying depression are severe, a benzodiazepine can be given for several weeks, until the antidepressant medication takes effect. Lithium carbonate, stimulants, and triiodothyronine are thought to enhance the action of antidepressants and are sometimes added to an established antidepressant regimen. Such associations, as well as combinations of two antidepressants, are used in refractory depression and should best be handled by a psychiatrist.

ELECTROCONVULSANT THERAPY

ECT is the most effective treatment for severe depression. It is especially indicated in patients with high suicidal risk, catatonia, agitated depression, inability to tolerate medication, lack of response to several good trials with antidepressants, and a previous response to ECT, and if it is the patient's preference. There are no absolute contraindications, and it has been given without ill effects to pregnant women. It is administered by a psychiatrist, usually in an inpatient setting, but the primary care physician should remain involved, providing support to the patient and medical consultation as needed to the psychiatrist.

TREATMENT OF BIPOLAR DISORDER

Mania and hypomania are best treated with mood stabilizers such as lithium, carbamazepine, and valproic acid. The same agents can be used when the patient is asymptomatic to prevent future episodes, but alone they are ineffective in treating depression. In acute mania, antipsychotics are necessary for sedation; in extreme cases, ECT may be needed. When a patient with bipolar disorder is being treated with antidepressants, the clinician must monitor her closely for early signs of acceleration, as one of the side effects of antidepressants in this group of patients is reversal to mania.

PSYCHOTHERAPY

Mild and moderate forms of depression may respond to psychotherapy alone; in severe depression, psychotherapy can be used as an adjunct to somatic treatments. Of the more than 200 forms of psychotherapy described, several deserve to be mentioned because they are widely used, consist of better standardized techniques, and have been systematically studied against medication and against each other for efficacy.

Cognitive therapy is based on the assumption that negatively distorted thinking about oneself is crucial to the depressive syndrome and that helping the patient identify such distortions and correct them as they occur can lead to symptom reduction. *Interpersonal therapy* focuses on the patient's social relations, which are almost always disrupted. Whether such difficulties are causal or concomitant to or consequences of depression, the interventions are the same—namely, helping the patient resolve a grief reaction, eliminate social isolation, and negotiate new social roles. *Brief dynamic psychotherapy* decreases symptoms by identifying and resolving a core conflict between unacceptable wishes and social and moral constraints. *Supportive psychotherapy* is patient- and problem-driven rather than based on a particular theory and allows for the flexible application of many techniques, including discussion, advice, reassurance, limit setting, persuasion, confrontation, interpretation, and clarification.

In depressed women, issues such as guilt, loss, dependency, painful memories of abuse and abandonment, and low self-esteem are pertinent regardless of the treatment modality and should be investigated and addressed.

Education about the nature of the depressive illness and the rationale and specifics of different treatments, including medication and ECT, can take a fair amount of time in the self-absorbed, indecisive, distraught patient. Such minimal supportive interventions can and should be attempted by all primary care providers who choose to prescribe antidepressant medication. If the practitioner is too busy for such a time commitment, it is better to refer the patient directly to a mental health professional.

SPECIAL CONSIDERATIONS IN WOMEN

Differences in prevalence notwithstanding, mood disorders have a similar clinical picture regardless of gender. In an eclectic model of illness, gender-specific social, biologic, and psychological factors are taken into account in each case, but in general "female depression" cannot be seen as a separate illness. Nonetheless, several subtypes of depression are associated with women.

Premenstrual Syndrome

Premenstrual syndrome, also known as premenstrual dysphoric disorder or late luteal dysphoric disorder, is a poorly defined, controversial nosologic entity consisting of physical and psychological symptoms of variable severity that have in common a specific temporal correlation with the menstrual cycle. They occur about 1 week before menses and disappear during the follicular phase. Mood lability, irritability, sadness, anxiety, abdominal pain, bloating, and breast tenderness are the most common symptoms. It is unclear if mild symptoms should be defined as pathologic, as most menstruating women or women taking replacement hormones experience some discomfort premenstrually. At the other end of the spectrum, the most severe forms occur as exacerbations of symptoms that persist throughout the cycle. When rigorous research criteria, as defined in the psychiatric literature for late luteal phase dysphoric disorder, were applied, the community prevalence ranged from 3% to 5%. The disability can be severe, extending to occupational functioning and personal relations. Fluoxetine and other SSRIs have been used with anecdotal good response.

Postpartum Mood Disorder

About 10% of women are affected by a depressive syndrome that meets the criteria for major depression and begins in the first 3 to 6 months postpartum. Symptoms include tearfulness, mood lability, irritability, negative thoughts about oneself and one's ability to be a good parent, poor appetite, insomnia, lack of energy, and mild cognitive disturbance due to poor concentration and inattention. The etiology is unknown, but risk factors to consider are a personal or family history of depression and life stressors, especially a poor relationship with the child's father. Attempts to identify biologic determinants for postpartum depression, including estrogen, progesterone, thyroid hormones, or cortisone, have been unsuccessful. Treatment consists of a combination of pharmacotherapy (tricyclics or SSRIs in usual doses have been effective) and supportive psychotherapy (individual or group). The focus of psychotherapy is to explain the nature of symptoms and their relation to the patient's circumstances and to reassure the patient that the prognosis for full remission is quite good.

Psychotic depression, a severe form of postpartum depression, is potentially dangerous, as the patient can engage in violent behavior toward herself or her child in response to delusions or hallucinations. It responds to aggressive treatment with antidepressants and antipsychotics or with ECT and may require psychiatric hospitalization (see Chap. 155).

Postpartum depression must be distinguished from the so-called maternity blues, a period of mild depressive mood and lability starting 3 days after delivery and lasting no more than 2 weeks. It is self-limited, but physician reassurance and support from the family are helpful. Postpartum depression usually starts after an interval of apparent well-being after delivery, but in some cases what seems to have started as maternity blues progresses to a full-blown major depression.

Other Circumstances Specific to Women

For women, depression is a rather common response to gender-specific difficulties in overcoming crises and developmental milestones. The breakup of a romantic relationship, marital oppression by a dominant partner and other conflicts in which the woman feels powerless, becoming a widow, menopause, hysterectomy, and nursing home placement and living are situations in which women become extremely vulnerable to psychopathology in general and to depression in particular. The primary care provider, not the mental health professional, has the opportunity to notice the first manifestations and to take appropriate action.

Considerations in Pregnancy

No link between the use of heterocyclic antidepressants during pregnancy and congenital malformations could be established in several large-scale European retrospective studies of either consecutive random births or consecutive deliveries of malformed babies. Preliminary postmarketing analysis of outcome in women treated with fluoxetine during pregnancy seems to indicate that this drug should be relatively safe as well. Other new drugs, such as bupropion and the rest of the SSRIs, are less well studied from this point of view. There is some indication that MAOIs are associated with teratogenesis in animals and humans, and they should probably be avoided in pregnancy.

The use of heterocyclics late in pregnancy has been associated with toxicity and withdrawal in the neonate. Symptoms include respiratory distress, heart failure, seizures, irritability, and anticholinergic effects such as urinary retention and tachycardia. Until better data become available, women should not breastfeed if they take antidepressants: some studies suggest that tricyclics such as imipramine and desipramine reach milk in concentrations similar to those in plasma, but other studies conclude that the milk concentration of antidepressants is very low.

Mood stabilizers, including lithium, carbamazepine, and valproic acid, have all been shown to be teratogenic in humans. Lithium taken in the first trimester of pregnancy has been associated with a 20-fold increase in congenital malformations compared with the general population. Most frequently noted were Ebstein anomaly and other cardiovascular abnormalities. Even so, many children exposed to lithium in the first trimester have normal development. Therefore, if exposure does occur, the fetus should be monitored echocardiographically rather than automatically prescribing therapeutic abortion. Lithium equilibrates across the placenta and can be toxic to both mother and fetus, especially when given close to delivery. The newborn can present with "floppy baby syndrome" (hypotonia, lethargy, cyanosis), fetal goiter, arrhythmia, and poor sucking response. Blood levels in the mother can show dangerous increments immediately after delivery due to the sudden decrease in glomerular filtration rate. Other factors, such as edema and the use of sodium-depleting diuretics and sodium restriction for hypertension, can affect lithium le[illegible] must be considered. The concentration of lithium in milk [illegible] half of that in plasma, and cases of lithium toxicity i[illegible] breast-fed by women taking lithium have been documented. If treatment with lithium cannot be avoided, the baby should be closely monitored.

Carbamazepine was considered relatively safe until it was associated with craniofacial defects, nail hypoplasia, and developmental delay. There is a well-documented association between the use of valproic acid in the first trimester and spina bifida in the offspring; therefore, this medication is contraindicated in pregnancy.

It is important to counsel women of childbearing age regarding the implications of using psychotropics in pregnancy before starting the medication. Decisions regarding treatment should try to balance the goal of using as little medication as possible to minimize teratogenesis and toxicity to the baby against the risk of decompensation, with its severe consequences to both mother and child.

BIBLIOGRAPHY

American Psychiatric Association. Diagnostic and statistical manual of mental disorders, 4th ed. Washington DC: American Psychiatric Association, 1994.

Elia J, Katz IR, Simpson GM. Teratogenicity of psychotherapeutic medications. Psychopharm Bull 1987;23:531.

Kaplan HI, Sadock BJ, eds. Comprehensive textbook of psychiatry, 4th ed. Baltimore: Williams & Wilkins, 1985.

Novalis PN, Rojcewicz SJ, Peele R. Clinical manual of supportive psychotherapy. Washington DC: American Psychiatric Press, 1993.

Bech P. Acute therapy of depression. J Clin Psychiatry 1993;54:(suppl)18.

Schatzberg AF, Cole JO. Manual of clinical psychopharmacology, 2d ed. Washington DC: American Psychiatric Press, 1991.

Stewart DE, Stotland NL, eds. Psychological aspects of women's health care: the interface between psychiatry and obstetrics and gynecology. Washington DC: American Psychiatric Press, 1993.

Primary Care for Women, edited by Phyllis C. Leppert and Fred M. Howard. Lippincott-Raven Publishers, Philadelphia © 1997.

154
Anxiety

ADRIAN LEIBOVICI

Anxiety disorders are the most common psychiatric problems encountered in the community. They vary in clinical presentation, etiology, prognosis, and treatment, but all have in common an excessive display of concern, fear, and worry. Proper recognition and treatment of anxiety is an important task for the primary care physician, as many cases present with physical symptoms suggestive of medical illness and many medical conditions are accompanied by anxiety. Women are particularly prone to anxiety, and overall the prevalence of anxiety is much higher than in men.

CLASSIFICATION AND PHENOMENOLOGY

Panic Disorder

Panic anxiety is characterized by discrete episodes of very intense fear with a rather sudden onset and many somatic concomitants. The object of the fear varies (eg, death, heart attack, stroke, losing one's mind). At other times, the fear is intense but not defined. Among the most common physical symptoms are sweating, palpitations, racing heart, chest pain, shortness of breath, choking, shaking, numbness or tingling, abdominal distress, dizziness, and a fainting sensation. The frequency and intensity of attacks vary widely: some patients have one or several each day for weeks in a row; others have symptom-free intervals of weeks and even months. Typically, patients become concerned with the meaning of symptoms ("Do I have a severe medical condition?" or "Am I going insane?") and with the possibility of additional attacks in the near future. Many times, untreated cases are complicated by avoidance of situations from which escape might be difficult in the event of a panic attack (agoraphobia). Examples include fear and avoidance of going out alone, being in a crowd, and using public transportation. Agoraphobia occurs most often as a complication of panic, but there are cases of agoraphobia without a history of panic disorder in which avoidance is caused by fear of, for instance, diarrhea or dizziness.

Generalized Anxiety Disorder

In generalized anxiety disorder, patients cannot stop worrying about upcoming events or about possible but not probable negative outcomes. This apprehensive expectation is considered excessive. Other symptoms include fatigue, feeling restless or on edge, irritability, insomnia, difficulty concentrating, and muscle tension. In general, the disorder lasts a long time, often characterizing the person's style or temperament. According to modern diagnostic criteria, symptoms must be present for at least 6 months. Similar symptoms, usually in reaction to a significant psychosocial stressor but lasting less than 6 months, are labeled adjustment reaction with anxious mood.

Obsessive-Compulsive Disorder

Obsessions are recurrent thoughts that are perceived as intrusive and inappropriate. They cause subjective distress and are time-consuming for the patient. Examples include aggressive impulses (to hurt a defenseless person or shout profanity at a funeral), fear of contamination (getting AIDS by shaking hands), preoccupation with remembering names of public figures, concern with having things placed in a certain order (papers on a desk or shirts in a drawer must be symmetrically arranged), repeated doubts (wondering whether one has turned off the oven or locked the door before leaving the house). Some obsessive thoughts are abnormal only because of their repetitive nature, but other have little basis in reality—for instance, the recurrent fear that one has hit someone in traffic. Patients recognize obsessions as unreasonable and try to ignore or suppress them.

Compulsions are behaviors performed repeatedly and with a sense of urgency by patients to alleviate anxiety. Frequently, compulsive behavior alleviates the distress caused by a specific obsession. For instance, a patient concerned with cleanliness will engage in repetitive handwashing; the concern with having completed certain tasks like locking the door will trigger repetitive checking of the knob. Sometimes compulsions take a ritualistic, magical form—for instance, counting up to a certain number or pacing a certain number of steps for each occurrence of an obsessive blasphemous thought. As with obsessions, compulsions are recognized as excessive and irrational by the patient. Attempts to suppress compulsive behavior cause increasing levels of urge and distress. Satisfying a compulsive need relieves the anxiety for a while, but it is not pleasurable and can make the patient feel guilty and inadequate.

Patients with obsessive-compulsive disorder have either both obsessions and compulsions or only one of the symptoms. Typically, the illness starts in childhood in men and in the third decade of life in women. The course is chronic and fluctuating, with exacerbations in response to stress. A few patients deteriorate to the point of not being able to function, even requiring institutionalization.

Specific Phobia

Patients experience severe fear in the presence or mere anticipation of a specific situation or object. Virtually anything can become the stimulus for a phobic response, but some types of exposure are more common: animals such as snakes and insects, receiving injections and seeing blood, heights, water, storms, different situations such as flying or using elevators, or being in closed spaces (claustrophobia). The fear is recognized as unreasonable and excessive by an adult patient but not by a young child. The common reaction to a phobic stimulus is avoidance, which protects the patient against experiencing anxiety. The extent of disability is proportional to the patient's circumstances in terms of the object of her phobia. A fear of heights could be inconsequential for a woman living in a flat rural region but devastating for the urban professional who must use air travel for transportation. When forcefully exposed to the object of her phobia, the patient experiences anxiety of panic proportions. The harder it seems to escape from such a situation, the more severe the symptoms are. In most phobias the patient's heart rate and breathing are accelerated, but in the blood-injection subtype most patients experience a vasovagal reaction, with hypotension and fainting.

Social Phobia

The cardinal symptom of social phobia is marked apprehension of performing in public, anticipating failure and embarrassment. The most common example is public speaking, be it a lecture, an examination, or even a friendly social gathering. Other situations include eating, drinking, or writing in public. The fear is recognized as excessive and unreasonable by adult patients. It leads to avoidance of social exposure, a more restricted life, and a fair amount of emotional suffering. Sometimes the person decides to endure the anxiety associated with exposure. The actual performance can be much better than anticipated, but not uncommonly the patient's nervousness will sabotage her efforts, leading to a poor outcome, confirmation of her fears, and a reinforcement of the phobia. The anxiety experienced by patients with social phobia ranges from anticipatory apprehension to panic. Physical symptoms such as abdominal pain, diarrhea, blushing, sweating, shaking, and palpitation are likely and tend to peak right before the feared event is scheduled to start.

Posttraumatic Stress Disorder and Acute Stress Disorder

In posttraumatic stress disorder and acute stress disorder, symptoms develop in reaction to situations in which a person is confronted with an extremely traumatic event, such as death, serious injury, assault, or credible threats of the same nature. The victim can be the person herself or others around her. The initial response is one of horror and helplessness. The traumatic event is reexperienced many times as nightmares; the imagery includes painfully realistic flashbacks. There is intense emotional distress when an unrelated memory or unintended external cue reminds the subject of the original event. There is numbing of emotional response and a deliberate effort to reject recollections associated with the trauma. For instance, patients tend to avoid people, places, or conversational subjects directly or even tangentially related. Patients have selective amnesia, a feeling of detachment, constriction of affect, and a decrease in goal-directed activities. They show increased overall arousal (insomnia, hypervigilance, irritability, exaggerated startling response, outbursts of anger).

Symptoms that develop soon after exposure and subside in no more than a month make up an acute stress disorder. When the illness lasts more than a month, a diagnosis of posttraumatic stress disorder is warranted. Traditionally, events such as war, terrorist acts, earthquakes, and other catastrophes are considered common causes of posttraumatic disorder. The chronic and severe abuse (physical, sexual, emotional) suffered in childhood by many patients has recently been added to the list. This is significant for women, who tend to be victimized more often (see Chap. 162).

Anxiety Disorder Due to a General Medical Condition and Substance-Induced Anxiety Disorder

Anxiety in all its forms (generalized, panic, obsessions, compulsions) can be the physiologic consequence of a medical illness or of an exogenous chemical introduced into the body (eg, medication, food, recreational drug; Table 154-1). Certain conditions associated with secondary anxiety are more common in women: hyperthyroidism, certain collagen diseases, and the use of stimulants for weight loss or of nonsteroidal antiinflammatory drugs for pain. Other common causes of anxiety include pulmonary embolism, chronic obstructive pulmonary disease and asthma, angina, arrhythmias, mitral valve prolapse, and congestive heart failure. Medications such as steroids, sympathomimetics, and coffee and caffeine-containing foods are also common offenders. Substances of abuse such as alcohol and cocaine can cause anxiety both during intoxication and withdrawal. The diagnosis of substance or illness-induced anxiety is warranted when the onset, course, and resolution of the primary condition are correlated in time with the symptoms of anxiety.

Anxiety can be a sign or symptom in many other psychiatric disorders, including schizophrenia, personality disorders, and depression. The relation between anxiety and depression is a close and important one but remains poorly understood. Especially in women, a syndrome characterized by anxiety attacks and severe dysphoria, meeting the criteria for both panic disorder and major depression, has been described. Both diagnoses can be made, but some advocate a separate nosologic category for mixed depression and anxiety syndromes. Somatic treatments for both depression and anxiety overlap.

A diagnosis of anxiety disorder is justified only when the extent of symptoms causes disability: some measure of anticipatory apprehension or anxiety is a universal and normative psychophysiologic response to perceived danger. When its intensity is commensurate with the originating stimulus, anxiety has an important adaptive value, allowing the person faced with a challenging situation to mobilize her coping and fighting resources.

Table 154-1. Secondary Anxiety

Respiratory
Chronic obstructive lung disease
Emphysema
Pneumonia
Acute respiratory failure
Cardiovascular
Pulmonary embolism
Congestive heart failure
Arrhythmias
Coronary ischemia
Endocrine/metabolic
Cushing disease and syndrome
Hypoglycemia
Hyperthyroidism
Pheochromocytoma
Porphyria
Carcinoid
Neurologic
Encephalitis
Vestibular dysfunction
Tumors
Cerebrovascular events
Recreational drug intoxication
Alcohol, cannabis, phencyclidine, inhalants, hallucinogens, caffeine, cocaine, and amphetamine-related drugs
Recreational drug withdrawal
Alcohol, cocaine, hypnotics, sedatives
Prescription drugs
Analgesics, anesthetics, sympathomimetics, oral contraceptives and other steroids, antihypertensives, anticonvulsants, antiparkinsonians, antipsychotics, lithium, anxiolytics, antidepressants, insulin
Toxic agents
Heavy metals, paint, gasoline, pesticides, carbon monoxide, nerve gas

EPIDEMIOLOGY

Anxiety disorders are the most prevalent psychiatric illnesses in community studies. Women are three times more likely to have an anxiety disorder than men.

The lifetime prevalence of panic disorder in the general population ranges from 1.5% to 3.5%. Panic without agoraphobia is twice as common in women than in men; for panic with agoraphobia, the ratio is three to one. Social phobia is more common in women than in men in community samples, but the sexes are equally represented in clinical settings. The lifetime community prevalence for this disorder is estimated to be as low as 3% and as high as 13%. Simple phobia is considerably more common in women (ratios of up to 9 : 1 for certain subtypes). Its lifetime community prevalence is about 12%. Obsessive-compulsive disorder is equally common in women and men and afflicts about 2.5% of the general population. The epidemiology of stress-induced anxiety disorders is less well defined.

ETIOLOGY

Biological, psychological, and sociologic factors have been shown to play a role in generating, perpetuating, and exacerbating anxiety. A unifying theory is lacking and, at best, one can say that the etiology of anxiety is multifactorial. A genetic factor probably exists, at least in some conditions such as generalized anxiety disorder, obsessive-compulsive disorder, and panic disorder; however, a single locus on the genome was not identified, and they have lower heritability than other major psychiatric illnesses (eg, schizophrenia and bipolar disorder). This opens the door to psychosocial theories, which tend to stress the connection between anxiety and fear as an instinctual response to danger. Behavioralists regard anxiety as a conditioned response to fear.

According to cognitive theory, thought distortions allow the misreading of benign stimuli as signs of real danger, which in turn leads to autonomic hyperactivity. In psychoanalytic theory, anxiety is the price we pay to keep unacceptable archaic wishes out of the realm of our awareness.

The ability to provoke attacks reliably in panic disorder patients with lactate, bicarbonate, or carbon dioxide has lent strong support to biologic theories on the etiology of all anxiety disorders. The locus ceruleus, with its high concentration of noradrenergic neurons, is implicated in the sympathetic response associated with anxiety. Other areas, such as the septohippocampal region, are thought to analyze and compare stimuli from the environment, body, and memory: hypersensitivity of this area might explain some forms of paroxysmal anxiety. Positron emission tomography has shown hypermetabolism in the frontal lobes, especially the orbital gyri of patients with obsessive-compulsive disorder. These areas contain serotonergic neurons consistent with the efficacy of serotonin-enhancing drugs in reducing obsessions and compulsions. The neurochemical theory of anxiety revolves around the role of the gamma-aminobutyric acid (GABA) receptor complex: benzodiazepines link to it, opening calcium ion channels, and the action of GABA, the brain's main inhibitory neurotransmitter, is enhanced.

An extracranial theory for the pathogenesis of panic has been advanced. The carotid body directly stimulates a response in the brain's respiratory and circulatory centers via the ninth and tenth cranial nerves in response to subtle changes in the concentration of blood gases. According to this theory, panic is merely hypersensitivity of such a "suffocation alarm system."

COMPLICATIONS

Anxiety disorders, even when severe, may remain unrecognized and therefore untreated for long periods of time, sometimes even for a lifetime. This was particularly true for women who were cast in social roles consistent with dependency, acceptability of displays of fear and weakness, and lack of pressure to overcome their symptoms. Extreme examples of women who had not left their home for decades because of agoraphobia have been documented in the literature. In general, patients with untreated anxiety disorders have a more restricted life and tend to achieve below their potential.

Many patients discover that, at least initially, drinking alcohol provides symptomatic relief. Slowly, they develop tolerance and increase their consumption. Such self-medication leads to alcoholism in many uninformed patients. Similarly, chemical alleviation of severe anxiety can lead to abuse of and addiction to benzodiazepines, barbiturates, or illicit drugs.

Up to 60% of patients with panic disorder develop major depression sometime in the course of their illness. For some, this is an apparent complication of the unrelenting stress of living with intense anxiety attacks and especially with the fearful anticipation of their occurrence.

Epidemiologic data suggest that extreme anxiety may represent a risk factor for suicide.

GENDER-RELATED CLINICAL ISSUES

Although the epidemiology of anxiety points to a greater vulnerability for women, the phenomenology is no different between the genders. In the absence of definitive genetic data to suggest a sex-linked transmission of anxiety disorders between generations, the psychological and sociologic literature has tried to fill in the gap by identifying the risk factors for developing anxiety that are more common in women. Modern life and the new demands and opportunities for women have received special attention: women with underlying low self-esteem are faced with competitive careers and expectations of success, and this leads them to become apprehensive, fearful, and insecure. Phobic and panic symptoms develop as a result of new conflicts centering around such dichotomies as success versus failure, sensitive versus aggressive, feminine versus macho, and being accepted versus loss of love.

The reproductive cycle is marked by the exacerbation of preexistent anxiety or new-onset anxiety at each of its milestones (menarche, pregnancy, delivery or abortion, menopause). Many times, anxiety is self-limited and commensurate with the situation at hand. For instance, women, especially new mothers, tend to experience high levels of worry and nervousness during the first trimester of pregnancy and again close to delivery. This is in reaction to concerns about their adequacy as mothers, the well-being of the baby, and the way in which relations with their partner and family might be affected. Sympathetic listening to elicit such worries and gentle reassurance is enough in most cases. However, the practitioner must be able to recognize situations where the level of anxiety reaches clinical proportions and specific interventions are required. For instance, postpartum panic disorder and postpartum obsessive-compulsive disorder have been described. There are anecdotes of women who developed obsessional ideas about harm to the baby or compulsive rituals involving some aspect of infant care. It is hypothesized that the rapid decline of estrogen and progesterone after delivery affects serotonergic transmission in the brain, which in turn leads to anxiety symptoms. Indeed, serotonergic agents such as clomipramine or selective serotonergic reuptake inhibitors (eg, fluoxetine, fluvoxamine) are effective in the treatment of perinatal anxiety disorders.

DIAGNOSIS

Anxiety is more difficult to diagnose than other psychiatric conditions such as depression or psychosis. Not infrequently, the clinical picture is confusing due to the vagueness of the patient's complaints, the coexistence of other emotional problems, and the tendency of the anxious patient to report numerous physical symptoms. A patient might be seen many times in the office for chest pain, shortness of breath, intolerance to cold, poor concentration, or tearfulness before mentioning more suggestive symptoms such as discrete periods of paroxysmal fear or intrusive thoughts and ritualistic behavior. The key to the successful identification of an anxiety disorder is the physician's willingness to listen to the patient's account of complaints in her own words. In the opening phase of the interview, the patient should not be interrupted—according to one study, the average primary care physician waits less than half a minute before interrupting the patient with a question that is usually meant to mold the story into a familiar nosologic category. In the second phase of the interview, if a suspicion of anxiety was generated, the physician should elicit additional information methodically, asking specific questions about the presence of other anxiety conditions (many times they coexist); the presence of medical conditions; the use of medications, drugs, alcohol, and caffeine-containing products; exposure to toxic agents implicated in the etiology of anxiety; a family history of anxiety or other psychiatric disorders; and current psychosocial stressors or past exposure to traumatic events. A thorough assessment includes a physical examination and a mental status examination. When in doubt, a formal consultation with a psychiatrist is helpful.

TREATMENT

Starting in the mid-1960s, the treatment for anxiety shifted from psychoanalytic approaches to a balanced combination between biologic and behavioral therapies. The net result is probably quite positive, with better symptom control, reduced disability, and fewer complications.

Pharmacologic Treatment

Many classes of psychotropic drugs have a role in the treatment of anxiety.

Benzodiazepines

Primary care physicians write 80% of all prescriptions for antianxiety medications, psychiatrists only 20%. Of all anxiolytics prescribed, 90% are benzodiazepines. These numbers underscore the need for primary care physicians to be familiar with the proper use of benzodiazepines. Drugs in this class were first developed as muscle relaxants, but their use has extended rapidly to the treatment of insomnia, status epilepticus, and anxiety.

The first to be released was chlordiazepoxide, in 1960. About a dozen drugs in this class are approved for use in the United States. In equivalent doses, they are equally effective (Table 154-2). Benzodiazepines link to a specific receptor, part of a larger macromolecular complex that also contains receptors for the inhibitory neurotransmitter GABA. The action of this neurotransmitter is facilitated when the benzodiazepine receptors are occupied by the drug. The net result is hyperpolarization and therefore decreased firing of GABA-ergic neurons, which in turn could explain seizure and anxiety suppression.

Pharmacokinetic considerations are important when choosing a particular drug. For instance, the rate of onset of the therapeutic effect is very short for diazepam and flurazepam and slow for oxazepam; lorazepam and alprazolam fall somewhere in the middle. The duration of action varies with the distribution half-life when drugs are given acutely (short for diazepam, long for chlordiazepoxide, intermediate for lorazepam) and with the elimination half-life when they are given daily and a steady state is established (short with triazolam, intermediate with lorazepam, long for clonazepam). A few benzodiazepines, such as lorazepam and oxazepam, are metabolized in the liver through conjugation with glucuronic acid only, but most other drugs in this class undergo oxidative degradation. The distinction is important because effective glucuronic conjugation occurs even when liver function is restricted due to illness or age; therefore, oxazepam and lorazepam are preferable in the elderly or in the presence of advanced liver disease.

Compared with other psychotropics, benzodiazepines have a favorable side effect profile. The most common side effects are sedation, anterograde amnesia, dizziness, ataxia, and other forms of motor discoordination. They are relatively safe when taken in overdose, unlike barbiturates, the drugs they have replaced in the treatment of anxiety. Most patients treated continuously with benzodiazepines develop tolerance and a need for ever-increasing doses to sustain the therapeutic effect. Cases of addiction, iatrogenic or illicit, are not rare, and in many states the prescribing of these drugs is highly regulated.

Dosage varies with indication and must be individualized. In generalized anxiety disorder, one starts with diazepam 2 mg three times a day and titrates up as needed. Most patients do not need more than the equivalent of 20 mg of diazepam daily. In panic disorder, alprazolam 0.25 mg four times a day is a good starting dose. If the patient needs more than 1 mg four times a day, a referral to a specialist should be strongly considered. Ideally, benzodiazepines should be used for limited periods only (eg, several weeks) or on an as-needed basis to avoid habituation.

Table 154-2. Benzodiazepines

GENERIC NAME	BRAND NAME	DOSAGE EQUIVALENCY (MG)
Clonazepam	Klonopin	0.25
Alprazolam	Xanax	0.5
Triazolam	Halcion	0.5
Lorazepam	Ativan	1.0
Diazepam	Valium	5.0
Clorazepate	Tranxene	7.5
Prazepam	Centrax	10
Oxazepam	Serax	15
Chlordiazepoxide	Librium	25
Flurazepam	Dalmane	30
Temazepam	Restoril	30

Buspirone

Buspirone, a relatively new nonbenzodiazepine, nonsedating anxiolytic, is relatively well tolerated and nonaddictive. It probably works by inhibiting the firing of serotonergic neurons in the raphe. Its effectiveness in generalized anxiety disorder is at best mild, but some patients find it useful. The usual dose is 5 to 10 mg three times a day, but some patients need considerably more (up to 80 mg/day).

Other Anxiolytics

Barbiturates such as amobarbital, pentobarbital, or phenobarbital were used extensively to control anxiety before the advent of benzodiazepines. They should probably be avoided because they are hepatotoxic and addictive and have no notable advantage over benzodiazepines. Meprobamate and antihistamines such as hydroxyzine have also been used for control of anxiety. Antipsychotic drugs (eg, chlorpromazine, haloperidol), also called major tranquilizers, are strong anxiolytics, but their long-term use in the absence of psychotic symptoms is not indicated, given the risk of tardive dyskinesia and other movement disorders.

β-Blockers

Drugs such as propranolol and atenolol have been advocated for use in social phobia and generalized anxiety disorder and when the peripheric consequences of anxiety (eg, tachycardia, hyperventilation, excessive perspiration) are prominent. One starts with doses as low as 10 mg twice a day of propranolol and titrates up to 120 to 160 mg/day. Heart rate and blood pressure must be monitored for bradycardia and hypotension.

Antidepressants

A major advance in the treatment of anxiety disorders was the recognition that many so-called antidepressant drugs are effective in controlling specific conditions and symptoms such as panic, phobias, and compulsions. Such drugs are discussed in Chapter 153. In general, the same dosages are used as for depression.

Pharmacologic Treatment for Specific Anxiety Disorders

Panic disorder responds to various antidepressants. Phenelzine 45 to 90 mg/day and other monoamine oxidase inhibitors (tranylcypromine, isocarboxazid) are considered by some to provide the most comprehensive pharmacologic treatment, as they seem to diminish social apprehension better than other drugs. Among tricyclic antidepressants, imipramine has been the most widely studied, but other drugs in this class (eg, nortriptyline, doxepine) should be equally effective. The same dosage guidelines and blood levels apply as in the treatment of depression. Some studies suggest that clomipramine is a more powerful antipanic agent than imipramine. Preliminary data indicate that fluoxetine and other selective serotonin reuptake inhibitors (SSRIs) have antipanic properties, but it is unclear how they compare with the other antidepressants. High-potency benzodiazepines such as alprazolam and clonazepam are also being used in the treatment of panic disorder. They work faster but lose their effectiveness in time due to tolerance. One strategy is to start an antidepressant and a benzodiazepine concomitantly and to taper the benzodiazepine after several weeks, when the antidepressant has become effective. Regardless of what drug is chosen, effective treatment translates into a decreased frequency and intensity of panic attacks and a better ability to confront the avoidance that is characteristic of agoraphobia.

Generalized anxiety disorder responds to judicious use of benzodiazepines. Antidepressants such as tricyclics work better than placebo but are less effective than benzodiazepines in this disorder, and β-blocking drugs might have a role in diminishing the consequences of autonomic hyperactivity.

Obsessive-compulsive disorder has been more resistant to therapeutic intervention than other anxiety disorders. Compulsions can be decreased by up to 60% to 80% with the use of clomipramine in usual antidepressant doses. The other tricyclics are not very effective. Sometimes a therapeutic response occurs only after 6 to 8 weeks. Obsessions are less responsive to medication than compulsions. SSRIs are somewhat useful in the treatment of this illness: they are better tolerated but less effective than clomipramine. Benzodiazepines and the other antianxiety drugs do not work in patients with obsessive-compulsive disorder.

Social phobia responds best to MAOIs. Very mild and circumscribed cases of social phobia, such as performance anxiety, respond to β-blocking agents, but this class of drugs does not work when social avoidance is pervasive.

In acute stress disorder, the as-needed use of benzodiazepines controls the most extreme manifestations until patients regain behavioral control. Posttraumatic stress disorder has been treated with tricyclic antidepressants, MAOIs, lithium, carbamazepine, benzodiazepines, and β-blocking agents.

Antianxiety Medication and Pregnancy

Some studies indicate that the use of benzodiazepines during the first trimester of pregnancy is associated with a higher incidence of cleft palate in the newborn. Most of the data refers specifically to diazepam, and it is not unanimous. Other benzodiazepines, such as clonazepam, are thought to have low teratogenic potential. Meprobamate is associated with an assortment of congenital defects when used during pregnancy.

Benzodiazepines cross the placenta easily due to their low molecular weight. This tendency becomes more accentuated toward the end of pregnancy. When benzodiazepines with long half-lives are used chronically, they tend to accumulate in the fetus. The neonate experiences a withdrawal syndrome consisting of hypotonia ("floppy infant"), tremor, hyperreflexia, irritability, intolerance to cold, and respiratory depression. The use of barbiturates during pregnancy can also cause withdrawal in the newborn. Nursing mothers pass benzodiazepines in milk in active form, leading to lethargy in the infant.

When weighing the risks of psychotropic medication in the pregnant or nursing woman with clinical anxiety, one must factor in the extent of her subjective distress and the relative risks to mother and child if severe symptoms are not addressed (see the earlier section on complications). It is often recommended that tricyclic antidepressants should be used as a first choice in such situations, as they are generally better accepted for use in pregnancy (see Chap. 153).

Psychotherapy

Psychoeducation

Much of the "talk" therapy involved in the treatment of anxiety disorders is initiated in the primary care physician's office. Regardless of the specific disorder, the primary care physician is in an excellent position to educate the patient about her illness and its treatment. In conditions such as panic disorder, psychoeducation has great therapeutic value: telling the patient that her symptoms are due to anxiety rather than heart disease, stroke, or insanity and teaching her to relax in such circumstances can bring considerable relief. In fact, in all anxiety disorders, informing patients about the name of their condition and its prevalence has positive effects, as it gives them the needed vocabulary to refer to their illness and a sense that they are not alone experiencing it. Explaining the biologic nature of anxiety is reassuring for some patients; others do better when the role of situational factors is stressed.

Dealing with the somatic concomitants of anxiety can be challenging in patients who feel uncomfortable conceptualizing their distress in emotional terms and hope that a physical condition can be identified and treated. The physician must decide how far to go in ordering diagnostic tests and specialist consultations before exploring the psychological aspects of the problem. An "either/or" (organic versus psychogenic) approach is counterproductive, as it can lead to such iatrogenic outcomes as excessive use of diagnostic tests and consultations, overlooking legitimate coincidental medical problems, and alienating the patient by telling her that she has no medical problem but that she should see a psychiatrist. Referral for consultation or treatment, when necessary, should be discussed openly as a way of obtaining expert advice and care. The physician should reassure the patient that she is not being abandoned as a hopeless "mental case" and that the referring physician will remain involved.

The patient's lifestyle must be explored and anxiety precipitants identified and eliminated if possible. Simple measures such as proper rest and exercise, a predictable sleep/activity schedule, healthy eating, and elimination of coffee and caffeine-containing beverages can go a long way. The association between alcohol and anxiety is a very strong one: many uninformed patients become alcoholics as they try to alleviate a preexisting anxiety disorder by drinking. The chronic drinker who tries to quit may experience various degrees of anxiety, part of a withdrawal syndrome. It is generally very difficult to treat anxiety successfully if the patient continues to drink, and patients must be forcefully confronted with this fact.

Behavioral Therapy

The focus of behavioral therapy is to obtain symptom reduction by increasing the patient's ability to tolerate the very situations likely to make her uncomfortable. Phobias, panic, and compulsive rituals respond best to this approach. Patients are helped to identify anxiety-producing situations and list them hierarchically. A structured program of gradual exposure to these stimuli is then agreed on between therapist and patient. For instance, a woman afraid of riding the bus because that is where she had her first panic attack starts by going to the bus station to watch buses come and go. In the next stage, she gets on the bus and gets off immediately. Then she rides longer and longer distances, starting with off hours when few people are likely to ride and ending with rush hours when the bus is crowded. At each point during treatment, the patient experiences anxiety and is taught to be aware of it and to reflect on its intensity and on her ability to master it. The patient is tempted to interrupt her exposure to the anxiety-producing stimulus (for instance, by getting off the bus sooner than planned) but forces herself not to (response prevention). Gradually, tolerance to even the most dreaded situations develops and the patient becomes able to function without avoidance. The overall level of anxiety decreases, and she now uses buses without difficulty. If panic has been mitigated with medication, behavioral therapy can progress much faster and with more dramatic results.

Cognitive Therapy

Initially developed for depression, cognitive therapy is now being applied in the treatment of selected anxiety conditions such as performance anxiety and social phobia. It is based on the assumption that symptoms are the result of cognitive distortions in which a negative view of oneself plays a central role. Patients are taught to consider alternative explanations to the negative assessment of situations leading to symptoms.

Other therapies used in the treatment of anxiety disorders include biofeedback and relaxation, psychoanalysis or psychodynamic psychotherapy, interpersonal psychotherapy, and supportive psychotherapy. Generally, patients are referred to mental health professionals for formal psychotherapy. It is important, however, for the primary care physician to monitor progress and to be available to coordinate care with the psychotherapist as needed.

BIBLIOGRAPHY

American Psychiatric Association. Diagnostic and statistical manual of mental disorders, 4th ed. Washington DC: American Psychiatric Association, 1994.

Elia J, Katz IR, Simpson GM. Teratogenicity of psychotherapeutic medications. Psychopharmacol Bull 1987;23:531.

Kaplan H, Sadock BJ, ed. Comprehensive textbook of psychiatry, 4th ed. Baltimore: Williams & Wilkins, 1985.

Klein D. Testing the suffocation false alarm theory of panic disorder. Anxiety 1994;1:1.

McGlynn T, Metcalf H, eds. Diagnosis and treatment of anxiety disorders: a physician's handbook. Washington DC: American Psychiatric Press, 1989.

Schatzberg AF, Cole JO. Manual of clinical psychopharmacology, 2d ed. Washington DC: American Psychiatric Press, 1991.

Stewart DE, Stotland NL, eds. Psychological aspects of women's health care: the interface between psychiatry and obstetrics and gynecology. Washington DC: American Psychiatric Press, 1993.

Weissman MM, Klerman GL, Markowitz JS, Ouellette R. Suicidal ideation and suicide attempts in panic disorder and attacks. N Engl J Med 1989;321:1209.

Zerbe JK. Anxiety disorders in women. Bulletin of the Menninger Clinic 1995;59 (suppl A):38.

Primary Care for Women, edited by Phyllis C. Leppert and Fred M. Howard. Lippincott-Raven Publishers, Philadelphia © 1997.

155
Psychosis

ADRIAN LEIBOVICI

None of the current definitions of psychosis has received universal acceptance. In a broad sense, psychosis refers to a psychiatric syndrome characterized by severe impairment in the ability to separate what is real from what is imagined (loss of reality testing). A more technical and narrow definition requires the presence of specific signs and symptoms, such as delusions or hallucinations.

A delusion is a false belief that is so rigid that it does not change, even in the face of compelling and repeated refuting evidence. The content of delusional thoughts is varied but is usually organized around several familiar themes: persecution, reference, religion, somatic symptoms, jealousy, guilt, poverty, grandiosity, and nihilism.

Hallucinations are severe perceptual distortions occurring in any sensory domain (auditory, visual, tactile, olfactory, or gustatory). Unlike illusions, where a real stimulus is perceived erroneously, hallucinations have no basis in reality whatsoever. Examples include hearing noises or voices, seeing persons or animals, feeling bugs crawling on one's skin, and being bothered by an unpleasant and otherwise unexplained smell.

Other features of the psychotic syndrome include disorganization of thinking and bizarre behavior.

EPIDEMIOLOGY AND CLINICAL DESCRIPTION

Psychosis can be secondary to various physical or emotional factors, or the central manifestation of a number of still idiopathic psychiatric illnesses, the most common and disabling of which is schizophrenia.

Schizophrenia

This severe, usually chronic psychiatric illness is characterized by the severe disturbance of many psychological functions, although sensorium is generally preserved. The clinical picture is characterized by the presence of delusions, hallucinations, abnormal behavior and speech, and so-called "negative symptoms." Patients remain oriented and generally intact cognitively. Delusions can be bizarre, such as the belief that one's internal organs have been altered by hostile forces, or that one is monitored by special FBI agents with cosmic weapons. The search for pathognomonic content to schizophrenic delusions has not been fruitful, but in general ideas of reference are very suggestive of a schizophrenic process. Examples include the belief that certain events, such as radio and television broadcasts, convey special messages to the patient, or that someone puts thoughts in the patient's mind (thought insertion), removes thoughts (thought withdrawal), or manipulates the patient's thinking (thought control).

Auditory hallucinations are the most prominent perceptual distortion, although virtually any sensory modality can be affected. Often patients hear voices running a distinct discourse that is perceived as separate from their thoughts. Threats, pejorative statements, or commands that the patient is more or less able to resist are common. A particular type of hallucination is almost exclusively encountered in schizophrenia: it consists of one or several voices continuously commenting on the person's thoughts or behavior.

Thought processes in schizophrenia are profoundly disturbed. This is reflected in disorganized speech, rapid and illogical associations (loose associations), answers that are only marginally connected with the question asked (tangentiality), and in severe cases total loss of comprehensible structure or meaning (incoherence).

Deficits in volition, production of speech, and affective expression are described under the generic term "negative symptoms." Patients display difficulty initiating goal-directed activities, whether related to social interactions or work (avolition). Their speech has little spontaneous flow and their answers are laconic (alogia). The range of emotional response in schizophrenic patients is generally restricted (blunt or flat affect), although exaggerated or incongruent affective states are also described.

The behavior of schizophrenic patients ranges from normal in certain phases of illness to profoundly disorganized in others, paralleling the extent to which thought processes are affected. For instance, a patient may go out into the cold without proper clothing or may wander dangerously in the traffic. At other times, the behavior reflects the content of delusions or hallucinations: the patient becomes hostile or even assaultive when confronted with a "persecutor" or when the voices tell her to defend herself. Negative symptoms also shape behavior, which explains the patient's poor ability to care for herself and the perception that she is morally weak or lazy, contributing to the social and occupational underachievement caused by this illness.

The diagnosis of schizophrenia is justified only if symptoms persist for at least 6 months. In general, the course is chronic, with onset in the late 20s for women and a few years earlier for men. Some patients have exacerbations and remissions; others remain symptomatic all the time. It is not uncommon for patients to have episodes of delusions, hallucinations, and disorganization in response to life stressors and to display only negative symptoms between episodes.

In some patients, the course toward worsening with each new decompensation leads to states of profound deficit and mental disability. Such an outcome was more common before the advent of effective treatment—hence the old term "dementia praecox," which is actually a misnomer.

There are several clinical varieties of schizophrenia. The paranoid type is characterized by the prominence of auditory hallucinations and delusions with persecutory content, although other psychological functions are somewhat better preserved. The disorganized (hebephrenic) type is dominated by disorganized speech or behavior and inappropriate affect: sometimes patients make concrete, cheerful remarks, incongruent with the circumstances. The catatonic type refers to the coexistence of a marked psychomotor disturbance during the acute phase of illness. Mutism, negativism, idiosyncratic complex movements such as immobility and plasticity (waxy flexibility), echolalia and echopraxia (repeating the interviewer's words or movements), stupor, and purposeless hyperactivity can occur in any combination or level of severity. Other types of schizophrenia are residual (predominance of negative symptoms with few if any delusions and hallucinations) and undifferentiated.

The exact prevalence and incidence of schizophrenia are not yet known because different studies have used different definitions of the illness. In general, the illness is equally prevalent throughout the world when the same diagnostic criteria are applied. The lifetime prevalence of schizophrenia is thought to range between 0.5% and 1%. The incidence is one per 10,000/year. Community-based studies show no sex differences in prevalence, although hospital-based studies indicate higher rates for men. This is consistent with the assertion that women have a later onset and a better prognosis, making hospitalization less likely.

Schizophreniform Disorder

Patients presenting with signs and symptoms characteristic of schizophrenia of less than 6 months' duration receive a diagnosis of schizophreniform disorder. About two thirds of such patients progress to develop schizophrenia; the remaining third recover before the 6-month criterion for schizophrenia is met.

Schizoaffective Disorder

When major depression, mania, or a mixed affective state coexists with typical schizophrenic symptoms, a diagnosis of schizoaffective disorder is sometimes warranted, although the relation between psychosis and mood pathology is a more complex one (see the section on differential diagnosis below).

Paranoia

Another major psychotic illness is paranoia or delusional disorder. It is characterized by prominent nonbizarre delusions with better preservation of other psychological functions such as thought processes, volition, and behavior. In the persecutory subtype, patients experience delusions of persecution: one is spied on, poisoned, conspired against, and harassed. The perceived aggressor can be a work supervisor, a government agency, or a relative. The erotomanic type applies to patients with the delusional belief of being loved by another person, usually of a higher social status. The patient tries to contact that person through letters, telephone calls, and gifts. Stalking and even extreme aggression, including murder, can occur as patients are repeatedly rejected and their frustration increases. Although this subtype is equally prevalent in both genders, women are more often seen by clinicians; men are more likely to be handled in the legal system. The grandiose type is characterized by the delusion of having made a discovery or having a special relationship with a prominent public figure, such as the president or the pope. Many such persons apply for patents (eg, perpetual motion devices). In another type of delusional disorder, the somatic type, the psychotic process revolves around one central somatic delusion, such as a foul smell emanating from the mouth or vagina, or the conviction that one is contaminated with germs. Finally, in the jealous type, the central delusion is that the patient's spouse is unfaithful. There is no due cause, and the patient tries to intervene by following her spouse or hiring private detectives. The prevalence and incidence of paranoia does not differ in women and men, but men tend to be afflicted more by the jealous type.

ETIOLOGY AND PATHOPHYSIOLOGY

Most research into the cause and mechanisms by which psychosis develops has focused on patients with schizophrenia, although one favorite method of inquiry is looking at better-understood illnesses with psychotic symptoms and trying to extrapolate findings to schizophrenia. Many theories have been proposed, but no single model can integrate all the important correlative data accumulated. It is said that schizophrenia and related psychiatric conditions are a consequence of a complex interaction between inherited and environmental factors.

Genetic Factors

The risk of schizophrenia is significantly higher in biologic relatives of affected persons than in the general population, and the relative risk increases with the degree of consanguinity, peaking in monozygotic twins. Adoption studies show that biologic but not adoptive relatives are at increased risk, apparently refuting the theories stressing upbringing as an etiologic factor. However, even in monozygotic twins there is a high degree of discordance, which leaves room for an important role to be played by environmental factors.

Current research efforts focus on genetic mapping in hopes of identifying one or several "schizophrenia genes." Another strategy is the study of genetic disorders that may present with a schizophrenic-type psychosis (eg, homocystinuria, porphyria, Huntington chorea, and albinism). The chemical mechanisms of such illnesses might lend insights into the pathophysiology of primary psychotic illnesses such as schizophrenia.

Congenital and Perinatal Disorders

Basic neurodevelopmental processes occurring primarily in the second trimester of pregnancy can be disrupted, resulting in psychotic symptomatology later in life. For instance, corpus callosum agenesis, arachnoid cysts, porencephaly, and other rare conditions have been shown to correlate with psychosis. Brain injury resulting from complicated pregnancy or delivery can also lead to psychotic illness in adulthood. One of the proposed pathways is brain hypoxia of whatever cause, which can disrupt proper neuronal migration in the hippocampus and results in aberrant cytologic architecture of this brain structure, thought to have an important role in cognitive-affective processes and pathology. Some of the obstetric and perinatal factors associated with psychosis later in life are listed in Table 155-1

Table 155-1. Perinatal Factors Associated with Psychosis Later in Life

Viral infections during pregnancy
Maternal age >40
Gestational medical illnesses (eg, diabetes, deep vein thrombosis, hypertension)
Breech presentation
Cesarean section
Forceps application or vacuum extraction
Pathology of the placenta
Hyperbilirubinemia in the newborn
Respiratory distress
Prematurity

Medical Illness

Medical and neurologic illness can cause psychosis. Probably there is more than one mechanism responsible. Here again, it is hoped that by studying the impact on the brain of such conditions, our understanding of the pathogenesis of psychotic phenomena will advance. An example is the association between epilepsy and schizophrenic-like psychosis, which occurs more frequently than would be expected by chance only. Research has shown that this is not a random association but one dependent on certain characteristics of the epileptic process. In particular, foci in the medial aspect of the temporal lobe, especially on the left side, are highly predictive of psychosis. Such observations corroborate with other data supporting notions such as localization and lateralization in schizophrenia. Some of the neurologic, medical, and toxicologic/pharmacologic factors associated with psychotic conditions are listed in Table 155-2.

Structural Brain Abnormalities

Older pneumoencephalographic and newer brain computed tomography (CT) and magnetic resonance imaging (MRI) studies of patients with schizophrenia and other psychotic disorders reveal the presence of subtle structural differences. Ventricles are enlarged and the total cortical mass is reduced. Temporal horns, especially on the left side, are affected more. These changes are less prominent in women than in men. Again, the data seem to point to a special role for the temporal lobes and adjacent structures.

Functional Neuroimaging

The advent of positron emission tomography and single photon emission computed tomography have allowed in vivo studies of the intensity of some neurochemical processes in different regions of the brain. Using these techniques, researchers have shown that patients with schizophrenia have a low level of metabolic activity in the prefrontal cortex. The prefrontal cortex is an area of multimodal association linked to higher cognitive processes such as fluency of thought, volition, attention-shifting, and behavior sequencing, as well as affective expression. Symptoms such as affective blunting, avolition, and alogia are generated via hypofrontality, according to this theory.

Neurochemistry

Based on the fact that all traditional antipsychotic drugs block dopamine (D2) receptor binding, the dopamine hypothesis of psychotic symptom formation was developed. According to this theory, functional overactivity of dopamine in temporolimbic regions leads to "positive" symptoms such as delusions and hallucinations.

Table 155-2. Organic Psychoses

Delirium
Uremic or hepatic encephalopathy
Hyponatremia
Collagen disease
Lupus cerebritis
Infections affecting brain tissue
Meningitis
Encephalitis
Brain abcess
Nutritional deficiency
Megaloblastic anemia (B_{12} or folate deficiency)
Wernicke psychosis (thiamine deficiency)
Pellagra (niacin deficiency)
Porphyria
Endocrinopathies
Hypothyroidism
Addison disease
Hypopituitarism
Cerebrovascular disease (all types of stroke can manifest with psychotic symptoms)
Cerebral tumors (primary or metastatic)
Neurodegenerative disorders
Parkinson disease
Huntington chorea
Wilson disease
Multiple sclerosis
Alzheimer disease
Epilepsy
Intoxication
Alcohol, sedatives, hypnotics, anxiolytics, cocaine, cannabis, phencyclidine, amphetamines and other stimulants
Withdrawal syndromes
Alcohol, sedatives, hypnotics, anxiolytics
Prescription medications
Analgesics, anticholinergics, antihistamines, antiparkinsonians, anticancer agents (cyclosporine), corticosteroids, muscle relaxants, antihypertensives

Dopamine blockade in these regions accounts for the antipsychotic effect of neuroleptics; dopamine blockade in the basal ganglia explains the extrapyramidal side effects of these drugs. Furthermore, based on the fact that dopaminergic fibers originating in the substantia nigra and tegmentum project onto the frontal cortex, a dysfunction of the dopamine neurotransmitter system could explain both the negative symptoms and the dulling effect of antipsychotics.

This formulation is at best simplistic. It does not account for new research identifying a variety of subtypes of dopamine receptors, the absence of D2 receptors in frontal and temporolimbic regions, and the effectiveness of newer antipsychotics such as clozapine and risperidone, which exert potent effects on non-D2 receptors. The role of serotonergic or D1 receptors is being reevaluated, but to date a unifying biochemical theory of psychosis remains elusive.

Psychosocial and Cultural Factors

A complete discussion of the etiology and pathophysiology of psychosis would be incomplete without mentioning nonbiologic theories. Several decades ago such theories prevailed in this country. Severe failure of ego functioning, resulting in a subjective perception of daily tasks as overwhelming and leading to inability to adjust and function, was a common psychoanalytic interpretation of schizophrenia. Developmental failure caused by inappropriate upbringing was another favorite formulation: attention was directed to the "schizophrenogenic" mother, described as anxious, overprotective, and enmeshed. The fact that schizophrenia is more prevalent in lower socioeconomic strata led to theories linking poverty to the etiology of this illness. Other factors, such as urbanization, industrialization, and migration, were similarly interpreted based on prevalence studies.

All these theories fail to analyze the respective connections in both directions, making unproven cause-and-effect presumptions. Does the anxious mother cause her child to develop symptoms, or is the premorbidly aloof and unresponsive child making the sensitive mother overly concerned and protective? Is poverty a cause of schizophrenia, or is schizophrenia, with its disabling functional and occupational failure, throwing the patient at the bottom of the socioeconomic ladder?

Although they do not provide convincing etiologic explanations, psychosociocultural factors are relevant in understanding the context in which psychosis develops, the dynamics of decompensation, and the success or failure of treatment. Their proper consideration allows a more complete definition of the concept of vulnerability. According to this notion, the actual occurrence of symptoms results from the cumulative and coincidental action of diverse predisposing factors, be they genetic predisposition, environmental stress, or noncompliance with treatment.

DIAGNOSIS

It is relatively easy to make a diagnosis of psychosis when the patient presents with bizarre delusions, complains of hearing voices, or displays disorganized speech and behavior. Many times, however, the clinical picture is more subtle. Paranoid patients can be so distrustful that they do not share their delusions with the physician. Indirect clues, such as a guarded attitude in the office or reports by caregivers that the patient makes frequent calls to the police and does not allow people in her house, should be properly interpreted. Depressed patients with psychosis may ruminate about lack of money and difficulty paying bills. The untrained listener may validate such complains as plausible without noticing the fact that they are unusual for that patient or that they are presented in a rigid, exaggerated manner, unresponsive to reassurance. Even more difficult to identify are patients with chronic psychotic illness, presenting only with some measure of affective blunting, poor social functioning, and mild thought process disturbance, such as tangentiality and loose associations. The astute clinician takes note of such signs and obtains a thorough history. The effort could be rewarded by the finding that in the past the patient experienced more florid psychotic symptoms.

When in doubt, referral to a psychiatrist for consultation is appropriate. Rarely, projective psychological testing administered by a certified clinical psychologist can be helpful in unmasking psychotic thinking in patients who cover their thought disorder well and cannot be diagnosed clinically.

DIFFERENTIAL DIAGNOSIS

Two common errors are attributed to primary care providers once the presence of a psychotic syndrome has been established: automatic referral to a mental health professional and instituting treatment immediately, without further diagnostic inquiry. Such actions are justified only in some cases: for instance, a patient with a well-established diagnosis of schizophrenia needs psychiatric follow-up, and an acutely agitated psychotic patient needs sedation right away. In general, however, the clinician's first priority is to rule out a host of medical conditions that can present with psychotic symptoms.

Whenever possible, a thorough physical and neurologic examination should precede any other action. Along with the mental status examination (description of attention, alertness, affect, mood, thought content and processes, perception, memory, and other cognitive functions), the history and a minimum set of laboratory data (blood count and differential, chemistry profile, urinalysis) enable the physician to make a diagnostic presumption that can then be pursued and confirmed.

Delirium

The first entity to consider and rule out should be delirium, a medical emergency. Delirium is a medically induced acute confusional state that can present with high levels of behavioral and thought disorganization, as well as delusions and hallucinations. Unlike other psychotic illnesses, however, it has a rather sudden onset (hours or days). Another distinguishing feature is the fluctuation in level of alertness and orientation (waning and waxing) and the impairment in attention and concentration. Many exogenous substances and acute medical conditions can lead to this transitory insult to brain function, and by definition removal of the cause is followed by resolution of mental symptoms.

The vulnerability of a person to develop delirium and the time necessary to recover from it are increased with age and the preexistence of organic brain pathology. For instance, an elderly woman with mild dementia easily develops delirium in response to moderate dehydration. Her confusion, agitation, and psychosis may linger for weeks and even months after her water and electrolyte balance is restored, much to the frustration of her physician, who might be tempted to label her as insane and in need of psychiatric hospitalization.

Dementia

Loss of memory and other cognitive functions such as speech, praxis, and visual/spatial orientation due to a progressive destruction of brain tissue defines the syndrome of dementia, which is encountered mostly in older persons. Alzheimer disease and cerebrovascular disease, alone or in combination, account for almost 80% of cases. Whatever the cause, patients develop psychopathology during the course of illness, including paranoid delusions, delusions of misidentification, disorganization of thought processes, agitation and aggression, and other psychotic symptoms. Incorrectly attributing these manifestations to a functional psychiatric illness can lead to unrealistic treatment choices and an incorrect prognosis. A history of steady and chronic memory and functional decline; a CT or MRI scan of the head suggestive of atrophy, small infarcts, or both; other associated features (eg, alcoholism, repeated head trauma, hypothyroidism, vitamin B_{12} deficiency); or a family history of dementia should raise the suspicion of dementia.

Substance-Induced Psychosis

Stimulants such as methylphenidate, d-amphetamine, and corresponding drugs of abuse such as cocaine and phencyclidine can cause a psychotic syndrome indistinguishable from acute schizophrenia: auditory command hallucinations, ideas of reference, paranoia, assaultiveness, and intense fear. Psychosis can occur both as a result of intoxication and withdrawal (eg, alcoholic hallucinosis, characterized by visual and tactile hallucinations, begins after alcohol levels have dropped). Many prescription drugs have been reported to cause psychotic symptoms as an untoward effect. Examples include anticholinergic agents, antiparkinsonian drugs, corticosteroids, analgesics, muscle relaxants, antihypertensives, cimetidine, and cytostatics such as cyclosporine or procarbazine.

The physician should remember the role of exogenous substances in generating psychosis and should always obtain a thorough drug history. In cases of suspected abuse, the urine or blood should be checked ("tox screens").

Medical Illness

As mentioned, psychosis can be a nonspecific manifestation of many medical conditions (see Table 155-2). Proper diagnosis avoids traumatic psychiatric labeling and allows institution of specific treatment if available. There are many anecdotes in the literature documenting patients with slow-growing brain tumors, temporal lobe epilepsy, porphyria, or degenerative neurologic conditions who have been diagnosed and treated for many years for "schizophrenia."

Primary Psychosis

In the absence of identifiable medical factors, a functional psychotic illness can be presumed. Given the accumulating evidence that illnesses such as schizophrenia and paranoia have an important biologic substrate, the term "functional" has become something of a misnomer. The term "primary psychosis" seems more appropriate, although such a category must exclude brief reactive psychosis, a nonorganic but secondary illness lasting between 1 day and 1 month that occurs in apparent response to a very stressful event.

The distinctions between schizophrenia, schizoaffective disorder, delusional disorder, and schizophreniform disorder were discussed above. There is an important overlap between affective and psychotic disorders. Sometimes schizophrenic patients experience depressive symptoms, which can be an isolated or combined consequence of three factors: improvement leading to better insight into the devastating consequences of the illness (postpsychotic depression), prominent negative symptoms, and antipsychotic-induced affective blunting. On the other hand, many patients with primary affective illness become psychotic. It is notoriously difficult to distinguish between some forms of mania and florid schizophrenic decompensation.

Several other psychiatric illnesses are sometimes difficult to differentiate from psychosis. Patients with panic anxiety complain of losing their mind. Their perception is genuine and very frightening, but they remain rational throughout the attack. Similarly, patients with obsessive-compulsive disorder have irrational thoughts such as having caused a car accident or being contaminated with germs or dirt. These thoughts are uncontrollably intrusive, but the patients are not psychotic because they know their fears are irrational.

Several personality disorders (borderline, paranoid, schizotypal, schizoid) can present with elements of psychotic thinking, especially when the patient is under increased stress. The diagnosis of personality disorder relies on the presence of a pervasive and stable pattern of behavior and interpersonal relationships that is maladaptive and causes subjective distress and functional disability. Personality disorders can mimic psychosis or coexist with psychotic illness. They are best diagnosed by mental health professionals based on extensive history and ongoing behavioral observations. When suspected, early referral for psychiatric consultation is advised.

TREATMENT

Secondary Psychosis

Good treatment starts with the understanding that psychosis is not an illness but a syndrome cutting across many different entities. A thorough diagnostic effort allows for specific treatment of secondary psychosis, be it correction of hypoxia, dehydration, or infection in a delirious patient, the discontinuation of an offending pharmacologic agent used for another illness, or the surgical removal of a slow-growing meningioma.

Dangerousness

The disturbed behaviors associated with psychosis can, in extreme cases, be dangerous to the patient or others. Suicide is a common complication of both psychotic depression and schizophrenia. Erratic, unsafe acts such as crossing the street without paying attention to traffic or sleeping in the cold can also have life-threatening consequences. Acutely paranoid patients can be aggressive, exhibiting acts ranging from random assaultiveness to thoroughly prepared murderous plots. Caregivers have an ethical and legal duty to protect both patients and their potential victims. Early in the evaluation phase, the clinician must estimate the risks involved and decide if hospitalization, voluntary or not, should be arranged. Factors such as past behavior, command hallucinations, suicidal or homicidal thinking, and availability of social supports must be considered when making such a decision, and psychiatric consultation should be obtained as soon as possible.

Agitation

Acute psychosis is often accompanied by a fair amount of agitation. The patient is distraught and in need of subjective relief. Motor restlessness can be intense and interferes with further diagnostic examination. In such circumstances, sedation and even physical restraints are necessary. Concerns about the patient's civil rights and dignity are legitimately raised only when such measures are applied too late, too early, for excessive periods of time, or without proper clinical justification. Many drugs, including antipsychotics, benzodiazepines, other nonbenzodiazepine anxiolytics, and lithium, are being used for acute sedation. A powerful and safe regimen is the combination of haloperidol 5 mg and lorazepam 2 mg, given together orally or intramuscularly, every 1 to 4 hours as needed. Antipsychotics used for acute sedation act immediately and in a nonspecific way, which is why they are also called major tranquilizers. The more specific antipsychotic effect is delayed for weeks and occurs at different, usually lower, doses.

Pharmacologic Treatment of Psychotic Symptoms

Regardless of etiology, psychotic symptoms (delusions, hallucinations, disorganization) improve with the use of specific pharmacologic and, to a lesser extent, nonpharmacologic interventions.

Antipsychotics

Drugs in this class are also known as neuroleptics or major tranquilizers. Until recently they all had in common the antagonism of dopamine receptors in several areas of the brain, such as the tegmentum, substantia nigra, temporolimbic structures, prefrontal lobes, and basal ganglia. The introduction of nonconventional antipsychotics such as clozapine and risperidone, with mechanisms of action involving other neurotransmitter systems, has changed the thinking on the mechanism of pharmacologic suppression of psychotic phenomena.

Conventional antipsychotics are equally effective in equivalent dosage. They differ in side effects, forming a continuum from high to low potency (Table 155-3). High-potency drugs such as haloperidol or fluphenazine cause extrapyramidal syndromes: parkinsonism, akathisia (a subjective and objective restlessness thought to be one of the major causes of noncompliance with these medications), acute dystonia (a rather frightening, albeit benign, complication that resolves promptly with the administration of diphenhydramine 50 mg intramuscularly). Low-potency drugs such as thioridazine or chlorpromazine cause little movement disorder but are associated with orthostatic hypotension, somnolence, and anticholinergic toxicity (constipation, urinary retention, dry mouth, delirium in the elderly).

All traditional antipsychotics, when used for long periods, can cause tardive dyskinesia, a movement disorder characterized by facial tics and choreoathetoid movements of the tongue, mouth, limbs, or trunk. In some cases it improves with discontinuation of the antipsychotic; in others it is irreversible. In extreme cases it can cause swallowing or breathing problems, although its main impact is aesthetic. Tardive dyskinesia is one of the main sources of malpractice liability in psychiatry, and in some communities written informed consent before starting antipsychotic medication has become standard. Women and the elderly are thought to be at increased risk of developing tardive dyskinesia.

Table 155-3. Antipsychotic Medications

CLASS	GENERIC NAME	BRAND NAME	CPZ EQUIVALENT
Low potency	Chlorpromazine	Thorazine	100
	Thioridazine	Mellaril	95
	Mesoridazine	Serentil	50
Intermediate potency	Molindone	Moban	10
	Loxapine	Loxitan	10
	Perphenazine	Trilafon	8
	Thiothixene	Navane	5
	Trifluoperazine	Stelazine	5
High potency	Fluphenazine	Prolixin	2
	Haloperidol	Haldol	2
Atypical	Risperidone	Risperidal	?
	Clozapine	Clozaril	60

Haloperidol 5 mg twice daily, or any other drug in equivalent dosage, is a usual antipsychotic dose. Higher doses are justified only when sedation is also necessary. Loading a patient with high doses of antipsychotic medication (rapid neuroleptization) does not achieve a faster decrease in delusions or hallucinations. The elderly and patients with coexistent liver disease might need considerably lower doses. For instance, a demented woman with paranoia and agitation might require as little as 0.25 mg of haloperidol once or twice a day. Patients who are noncompliant with oral medication benefit from depot preparations given intramuscularly, such as fluphenazine decanoate every 2 weeks or haloperidol decanoate every 4 weeks. Iatrogenic parkinsonism responds to drugs such as trihexyphenidyl, benztropine, or amantadine. Akathisia responds to small doses of propranolol (eg, 10 mg four times a day).

Although effective in decreasing delusions, hallucinations, acute disorganization, and agitation, most antipsychotics have little effect on negative symptoms. Clozapine, an unconventional antipsychotic drug, has been shown to improve negative symptoms such as avolition, inactivity, and affective blunting. Furthermore, clozapine is effective in about a third of psychotic patients resistant to traditional antipsychotics and does not cause tardive dyskinesia. The high cost, cumbersome dispensing system, and association with severe side effects (eg, agranulocytosis, seizures, tachycardia) limit its wider use. Doses range from 12.5 mg to 900 mg a day, with an average maintenance dose of 300 mg. Weekly blood counts to prevent fatal agranulocytosis are required by the manufacturer. Like clozapine, risperidone is a newer antipsychotic that does not depend only on dopamine inhibition for its action. In doses of up to 3 mg twice a day, it is relatively free of side effects, but at higher doses it behaves like a high-potency antipsychotic.

Other drugs have a more limited role in the treatment of psychosis. Benzodiazepines can be useful in acute sedation, antidepressants in psychotic depression, lithium and carbamazepine in psychotic mania and as prophylaxis in bipolar disorder. Vitamin E is being advocated in the treatment of tardive dyskinesia. Neuroleptic malignant syndrome, a rare but potentially fatal complication of antipsychotics, consists of rigidity, fever, delirium, and myolysis. It responds to dantrolene along with nonspecific intensive medical care. Electroconvulsive therapy is used for affective psychosis and in selected cases of schizophrenia, especially in young patients.

Nonspecific Nonpharmacologic Interventions

Interacting with a psychotic patient can be frightening, frustrating, and perplexing to the caregiver. The myth that only mental health professionals can deal with such patients can be dispelled easily by observing several simple rules. The patient must be treated with respect and the content of her delusional thoughts explored in a nonjudgmental manner. The interviewer must not try to either contradict or pretend to agree with the delusional patient, but rather should focus on areas of agreement, such as the fact that the patient is upset, scared, or in need of help. Many psychotic patients calm down if their "space" is not being violated: for instance, close physical proximity or discussion of sensitive subjects is better avoided. Certain elements of the physical examination, such as the rectal and genital examination, might need to be postponed. Communication with the patient must be kept simple and direct. Too much information presented at once might be overwhelming. Patients with psychosis tend to do better with predictable routines and become anxious and more psychotic when faced with unexpected changes. Even trivial modifications in their medication or appointments should be introduced carefully. Awareness of such basic principles allows the primary care provider to establish the therapeutic relationship necessary for the delivery of nonpsychiatric medical care, for psychiatric management in case this is provided to some extent by the primary care provider, or for successful referral to a psychiatrist. More formal interventions usually require involvement by a psychiatric provider.

Psychosocial Treatments

Several types of nonpharmacologic treatments have proven to be useful in the management of patients with subacute and chronic psychotic illness.

Individual Psychotherapy

Supportive and behavioral therapies are most relevant in the treatment of psychotic patients; psychoanalytic techniques are considered by many to be of limited usefulness, if not outright detrimental. Supportive psychotherapy stresses directive interventions such as clarification, psychoeducation, explanations, encouragement, reassurance, and even advice, in contrast to analytic techniques in which the therapist remains more neutral and detached and the main intervention is interpretation.

Severely regressed patients respond to behavioral techniques such as modeling, reinforcement of desirable behaviors by contingency application of rewards, extinction of psychotic or undesirable behavior, and so forth. Some of the goals of psychotherapy include improving coping ability and social skills, increasing understanding of the illness and its proper treatment, decreasing psychotic thinking and inappropriate behavior, decreasing subjective distress, and avoiding noncompliance and relapse.

Family

Family involvement in the care of psychotic patients is crucial. Family therapy with or without patient participation, multifamily therapeutic groups, and self-help and advocacy groups are all useful modalities. They can achieve important goals such as education about the illness, emotional support, practical tips about dealing with sick relatives, and information about community resources.

Environmental Manipulation

The social management of patients with psychosis centers around creating a protective environment in which exposure to different life stressors is controlled. Group homes, social clubs, day programs, occupational therapy, vocational training, and sheltered workshops are components of such an environment. The goal is to help the patient return to the highest level of socialization tolerable.

CONSIDERATIONS IN PREGNANCY

Puerperal Psychosis

Between one and two per 1000 deliveries are complicated by a psychotic syndrome. The exact definition of puerperal psychosis is controversial. Many believe that most cases reflect either a better-accepted category of postpartum affective disorder or a psychotic episode in an already affected woman who decompensates in response to the psychological stress of pregnancy and delivery. The clinical picture is variable, but there is always a symptom-free interval between delivery and onset of at least 2 to 3 days. Sleep disorder, rapidly changing course, irritability, and mood lability are almost always present. Nihilistic delusions about the infant or pregnancy include the belief that the child is dead or defective, or denial of having a baby altogether. Command hallucinations to harm the baby are of particular concern. In some cases schizophrenic-type symptoms predominate: thought disorganization, bizarre delusions, and hallucinations. The most common presentation is affective psychosis. Symptoms include delusions of guilt and worthlessness, crying, death wishes, and suicidal and infanticidal ideas. Manic and mixed affective states are also described. An infrequent variety of puerperal psychosis is the pseudoorganic type: patients are confused and show memory and other cognitive deficits.

The illness can have an early onset, in which case affective symptoms tend to predominate. Late-onset cases (more than 3 weeks after delivery) present with the schizophreniform syndrome and tend to occur in older women with preexistent psychopathology.

The cause of puerperal psychosis is unknown. In some patients, some form of psychopathology precedes the pregnancy or becomes evident during gestation. Many patients with recurrent psychotic affective illness later in life experience a first episode postpartum. Attempts at finding a correlation between postpartum psychosis and endocrine markers such as progesterone, estrogen, FSH, prolactin, and thyroxin have been unsuccessful.

Treatment includes pharmacotherapy aimed at the most prominent symptoms. Antipsychotics and antidepressants are used in combination for the psychotically depressed patient. Haloperidol 5 mg once to three times daily and nortriptyline 50 to 100 mg once a day exemplifies such a regimen. Lithium or carbamazepine can be used alone or in combination with antipsychotics for manic symptoms. Antipsychotics alone are appropriate for the nonaffective varieties. In all cases, lack of response to medication raises the need for electroconvulsive therapy, which is quite effective.

In the acute phase, the safety of the mother and the baby must be thoroughly evaluated. Suicide, infanticide, and child neglect or abuse are common complications. Hospitalization is almost always necessary; some advocate hospitalizing both patient and child if possible. As the patient improves, she can benefit from supportive psychotherapy. Therapies concentrate on issues such as her relationships with her child, her partner, and her mother. Individual, marital, or group settings can all be useful, and enlisting the support of family, friends, and social services is appropriate. The prognosis for resolution of acute symptoms is good.

Preexistent Psychotic Illness and Pregnancy

Women with already diagnosed psychotic conditions such as schizophrenia pose special management problems when they become pregnant. Even before conception, the practitioner might be faced with the need to provide the would-be mother and her partner with genetic counseling: the offspring of a schizophrenic mother has a tenfold higher risk of developing schizophrenia. The risk of decompensation to the mother during and after pregnancy, her parenting skills, and her suitability to overcome the many challenges of motherhood must be discussed so that an informed decision can be reached. After conception, the mother's mental status should be followed closely and the pregnancy considered high risk. Once the baby has been delivered, social services are always called on to provide support and to assess the safety of the mother and the child.

Use of Somatic Treatments and Pregnancy

Antipsychotic drugs are crucial in the treatment of psychotic illness regardless of etiology, and their use or avoidance during and immediately after pregnancy is associated with several potential problems and risks. When making a prescribing decision, the clinician must consider the risks of structural teratogenicity, behavioral teratogenicity, and maternal and newborn toxicity on the one hand, and danger to the fetus and mother if the untreated patient decompensates on the other.

The few large retrospective and prospective studies of possible correlations between structural congenital malformations and the use of neuroleptics during pregnancy showed conflicting results. There may be a slight increase in malformations, especially if the drugs were used between the 4th and 10th week of pregnancy. This preliminary conclusion is derived primarily from the California Child Health and Development Project, a study of 19,000 births between 1959 and 1966 that originally showed no significant differences between women who had used antipsychotics and women who did not. A reanalysis of the data in 1984 by Edlund and Craig showed that mothers who used neuroleptics between the 4th and 10th week had a 5.4% chance of giving birth to malformed children, as opposed to 3.2% for the rest of the sample. Another large study conducted in France by Rumeau-Rouquette and coworkers found that use of neuroleptics in the first trimester was associated with a 3.5% risk of malformations in the infant, higher than the 1.6% risk for the rest of the sample (chromosomal abnormalities were excluded). On the other hand, a large prospective study of over 50,000 births found no correlation between the use of antipsychotics during pregnancy and congenital malformations. Teratogenicity is somewhat higher in case reports and small retrospective studies. Interpreting the existing data on teratogenicity is made difficult by a number of confounding variables: children of untreated psychotic women may have a higher risk of malformations, many of the women included in the analysis took small doses of phenothiazines as antiemetics only, and no consideration was given to concurrent use of other drugs, diagnosis, age, number of pregnancies, dose, or length of exposure.

Even less is known about the behavioral teratogenicity of antipsychotics. Learning delays, hyperactivity, and other disturbances of motor activity have been blamed on virtually any CNS active medication used by the mother during pregnancy. A critical review of the literature reveals a still undeveloped methodology and a paucity of long enough follow-up studies. None of the antipsychotics available can therefore be considered safe in this regard.

The use of neuroleptics during the third trimester of pregnancy causes an extrapyramidal syndrome in the neonate that lasts up to several months. Symptoms include hypertonia, psychomotor agitation, hyperreflexia, and initial delay in learning tasks. The effect might be dose-related. Exaggerated neonatal jaundice and a syndrome characterized by cyanosis and respiratory distress have been described, especially with the use of high doses of chlorpromazine.

Antipsychotics are excreted in breast milk, haloperidol more than phenothiazines. Several studies showed that except for mild drowsiness, there are no major negative consequences to infants breastfed by mothers taking antipsychotics.

In practice, antipsychotics can be used during and immediately after pregnancy if necessary. Delirium, severe acute psychosis, and the likelihood of psychotic decompensation if medication is withheld are acceptable indications. Treatment of nausea with phenothiazines or the use of antipsychotics for anxiety or nonspecific tranquilization should be avoided. In patients who are well compensated on antipsychotics and want to become pregnant, an attempt to discontinue the medication in the first trimester or in the weeks preceding delivery can be made. During such an effort, the patient must be monitored closely for early signs of decompensation. Some advocate the use of high-potency drugs such as haloperidol during pregnancy, but there are few solid data to support a particular drug over others.

BIBLIOGRAPHY

American Psychiatric Association. Diagnostic and statistical manual of mental disorders, 4th ed. Washington DC: American Psychiatric Press, 1994.

Elia J, Katz IR, Simpson GM. Teratogenicity of psychotherapeutic medications. Psychopharmacol Bull 1987;23:531.

Novalis PN, Rojcewicz SJ, Peele R. Clinical manual of supportive psychotherapy. Washington DC: American Psychiatric Press, 1993.

Schatzberg AF, Cole JO. Manual of clinical psychopharmacology, 2d ed. Washington DC: American Psychiatric Press, 1991.

Stewart D, Stotland NL, eds. Psychological aspects of women's health care: the interface between psychiatry and obstetrics and gynecology. Washington DC: American Psychiatric Press, 1993.

Primary Care for Women, edited by Phyllis C. Leppert and Fred M. Howard. Lippincott-Raven Publishers, Philadelphia

156
Addictive Disorders and Substance Abuse

CESAR BARADA

Epidemiologic surveys of psychiatric disorders in the United States estimate that 13% to 24% of Americans at some time in their lives experience alcohol abuse or dependence, and 6% to 12% experience drug abuse or dependence. The prevalence of substance use disorders varies among different subgroups of the general population and is influenced by age, gender, race, and socioeconomic factors. There is a substantial gender difference in the prevalence of substance abuse and drug dependence disorders. Reiger and colleagues found 1-month prevalence estimates of any substance abuse disorder to be four times higher in men than in women (6.3% versus 1.6%, respectively). Alcohol use disorders were more than five times higher in men than women (5% versus 0.9%, respectively), and drug disorders were 2.6 times more common in men than in women (1.8% versus 0.7%, respectively). Kessler and colleagues found that 32.6% of men and 14.6% of women met lifetime criteria for alcohol abuse or dependence, and 14.6% of men and 4.9% of women met lifetime criteria for drug abuse or dependence. However, as of 1995, about 5.9 million (5%) of American women aged 18 years or older have suffered abuse or dependence within a 12-month period. Approximately 4% of American women admitted to some illicit drug use during the month preceding a 1993 household survey. Rates were highest in women of child-bearing age: 8% among women aged 18 to 25 years, and 6% among those aged 26 to 34 years.

Addictive disorders include a range of disorders related to the use of a substance. These substances are both legal (ie, caffeine, nicotine, and alcohol) and illegal drugs. The latter includes benzodiazepines, barbiturates, marijuana, lysergic acid diethylamide (LSD), phencyclidine (PCP), opiates, cocaine, and amphetamines. The *Diagnostic and Statistical Manual of Mental Disorders* of the American Psychiatric Association classifies these substance-related disorders into two groups: (1) substance use disorders and (2) substance-induced disorders. Substance use disorders include substance abuse and dependence (Tables 156-1 and 156-2).

The term *substance-induced disorders* refers to a group of disorders caused by a substance (ie, substance intoxication or withdrawal). Substance dependence describes a disorder characterized by cognitive, behavioral, and physiological symptoms related to the repeated use of a substance in addition to significant substance-related problems. Substance abuse describes a pattern manifested by recurrent and significant adverse consequences related to repeated use of a substance. Unlike substance dependence, it does not include a pattern of tolerance, withdrawal, or compulsive use (see Table 156-2).

DIAGNOSIS

Substance abuse screening is the first step in identifying a patient who may have a substance-related disorder. Such screening is relatively simple in that it requires no sophisticated tools and only takes a modest amount of time. Primary care physicians need to ask questions aimed at the discovery of substance abuse because few patients spontaneously volunteer this information. In addition, the history, physical examination, and toxicology screening provides information for detecting substance abuse. Several approaches are available to screen for alcohol and other drug problems in women. Two widely used screening tests for alcoholism are the CAGE and T-ACE (Tables 156-3 and 156-4). These clinical interview questions are considered to be effective and useful in helping to make the diagnosis of alcoholism. Primary care providers should be aware that a positive reply is not equivalent to a diagnosis. The physician should use these questionnaires to determine that alcoholism may exist; further evaluation then is necessary.

Although all patients should be asked about substance use, those with a previous history of substance abuse or a family history of such abuse may be at higher risk. A history of infections common among drug abusers such as endocarditis, hepatitis B or C infection, tuberculosis, sexually transmitted diseases, or recurrent pneumonia should alert the physician to the possibility of substance abuse. Certain patient complaints such as insomnia, mood swings, chronic pain, or repetitive trauma may indicate substance abuse. Social and behavioral problems; a history of chaotic relationships, erratic

Table 156-1. Criteria for Substance Abuse

A. A maladaptive pattern of substance use leading to clinically significant impairment or distress, as manifested by one (or more) of the following, occurring within a 12-month period:

(1) Recurrent substance use resulting in a failure to fulfill major role obligations at work, school, or home (eg, repeated absences or poor work performance related to substance use; substance-related absences, suspensions, or expulsions from school; neglect of children or household)

(2) Recurrent substance use in situations in which it is physically hazardous (eg, driving an automobile or operating a machine when impaired by substance use)

(3) Recurrent substance-related legal problems (eg, arrests for substance-related disorderly conduct)

(4) Continued substance use despite having persistent or recurrent social or interpersonal problems caused or exacerbated by the effects of the substance (eg, arguments with spouse about consequences of intoxication; physical fights)

B. The symptoms have never met the criteria for substance dependence for this class of substance.

(American Psychiatric Association. Diagnostic and statistical manual of mental disorders, 4th ed. Washington, DC: APA, 1994:182.)

employment, or both; frequent visits to the emergency room; and criminal incarceration also suggest substance abuse.

During the course of the physical examination, the physician should look for the physical findings associated with substance abuse. These findings often are subtle and may be nonspecific. The woman's vital signs can give a clue to substance overdose or withdrawal. Hypotension and bradycardia can be present in patients with overdoses of central nervous system depressants. In alcohol withdrawal, the patient may have hypertension, tachycardia, and fever.

The patient's general appearance is important and should be noted. Does the patient appear to be her stated age? (Chronic substance abuse and life on the street often have an aging effect.) Is the patient groomed and well dressed, or disheveled and wearing soiled clothes?

A careful examination of the eyes provides clues to several types of substance abuse states (Table 156-5). Chronic use of cocaine by nasal inhalation may result in irritated nasal mucosa, perforated nasal septum, septal necrosis, bleeding, granulation tissue, ulceration, and sinusitis. The skin examination yields clues as well. Needle marks and tracks in the antecubital fossae and forearms, thrombosed veins, bruises, or increased pigmentation over the veins all signal intravenous drug abuse. Skin abscesses also may point to drug injection. Cellulitis is a common finding in drug injectors. Alcoholics often have physical evidence of trauma caused by accidents in the intoxicated state. Typical signs are cigarette burns and multiple bruises at various stages of onset and resolution.

The primary care physician also should be alert to the following clues of substance abuse or dependence: the use of central nervous system depressants or stimulants may decrease or increase the respiratory rate, heart rate, and blood pressure; bronchitis and pneumonia are common in immunosuppressed and debilitated patients; and hemoptysis may indicate pulmonary tuberculosis.

Likewise, the physician needs to be alert to diseases associated with substance abuse. Infective endocarditis should be considered in a patient who presents with fever, chills, chest pain, dyspnea, and a history of intravenous drug use. Atrial fibrillation, myocardial infarction, severe hypertension, and cerebral hemorrhage have been reported in cocaine and crack users. Alcoholics may have an enlarged and tender or small and nonpalpable liver; spider angiomas; and jaundice. Ascites may be present in end-stage liver failure. Ataxic gate may signal acute alcohol intoxication. Decreased peripheral reflexes may indicate use of central nervous system depressants, whereas withdrawal from alcohol, sedatives, or hypnotics may be accompanied by increased peripheral reflexes. Tremors and seizures can be seen in alcohol withdrawal.

Seizures also may be a consequence of cocaine abuse. Transient ischemic attacks and subarachnoid and intraparenchymal hemorrhage also are seen in cocaine abusers.

Table 156-2. Diagnostic Criteria for Substance Dependence

A maladaptive pattern of substance use, leading to clinically significant impairment or distress as manifested by three (or more) of the following, occurring at any time in the same 12-month period:

(1) Tolerance, as defined by either of the following:
  (a) A need for markedly increased amounts of the substance to achieve intoxication or desired effect
  (b) Markedly diminished effect with continued use of the same amount of the substance

(2) Withdrawal, as manifested by either of the following:
  (a) The characteristic withdrawal syndrome for the substance
  (b) The same (or a closely related) substance is taken to relieve or avoid withdrawal symptoms

(3) The substance is often taken in larger amounts or over a longer period than was intended

(4) There is a persistent desire or unsuccessful efforts to cut down or control substance use

(5) A great deal of time is spent in activities necessary to obtain the substance (eg, visiting multiple doctors or driving long distances), use the substance (eg, chain-smoking) or recover from its effects

(6) Important social, occupational, or recreational activities are given up or reduced because of substance use

(7) The substance use is continued despite knowledge of having a persistent or recurrent physical or psychological problem that is likely to have been caused or exacerbated by the substance (eg, current cocaine use despite recognition of cocaine-induced depression, or continued drinking despite recognition that an ulcer was made worse by alcohol consumption)

(American Psychiatric Association. Diagnostic and statistical manual of mental disorders, 4th ed. Washington, DC: APA, 1994:181.)

Table 156-3. CAGE Questions

Have you ever;

Felt the need to **C**ut down drinking?

Felt **A**nnoyed by criticism of drinking?

Had **G**uilty feelings about drinking?

Taken a morning **E**ye-opener?

(Ewing JA. Detecting alcoholism. JAMA 1984;252:1906.)

Table 156-4. The T-ACE Questions Found to Be Significant Identifiers of Risk-Drinking*

T	How many drinks does it take to make you feel high (TOLERANCE)?
A	Have people ANNOYED you by criticizing your drinking?
C	Have you felt you ought to CUT DOWN on your drinking?
E	Have you ever had a drink first thing in the morning to steady your nerves or get rid of a hangover (EYE-OPENER)?

*Risk-drinking is defined as alcohol intake sufficient to potentially damage the embryo/fetus.

(Sokol RJ, Martier SS, Ager JW. The T-ACE questions: practical prenatal detection of risk-drinking. Am J Obstet Gynecol 1989;160:865.)

THE ROLE OF URINE TESTING

Urine testing may be useful in verifying substance abuse suspected by clinical indicators in the history and physical examination. Such testing also is useful in monitoring the progress of drug rehabilitation and in screening for relapse. Obtaining a toxicology screen requires informed consent and the ability to discuss the results in a nonjudgmental manner. Drugs that can be identified in a urine screen include marijuana, cocaine, amphetamines, opiates, PCP, LSD, methaqualone, barbiturates, benzodiazepines, and steroids. However, the urine toxicology test detects only recent use.

Frequent users are more likely to be detected by urine screening than occasional users. Results of urine tests remain positive after the last use of amphetamines for 24 to 72 hours, cocaine for 24 to 72 hours, opiates for 2 to 4 days, marijuana for 7 to 30 days, alcohol for 8 to 16 hours, LSD for 2 to 3 days, phencyclidine for 7 days, and benzodiazepines for several weeks. Once the patient has been screened for substance use, the next step is to assess the extent of this use and the associated adverse effects to determine what treatment, if any, is indicated.

After an initial evaluation, the diagnosis of substance abuse or dependence requires further investigation. The criteria for a clinical diagnosis of substance abuse or dependence, as established in the *Diagnostic and Statistical Manual of Mental Disorders*, is shown in Tables 156-1 and 156-2. In general, substance abuse is a maladaptive pattern of substance use manifested by recurrent and significant adverse consequences related to the repeated use of substances. The substance use may result in failure to fulfill a major role obligation at work, school, or home; the substance is used in situations that are physically hazardous.

Finally, substance abuse may cause legal problems, and there is continued use despite having persistent or recurrent social or interpersonal problems.

Substance dependence is defined by at least three or more of the symptoms listed in Table 156-2.

TREATMENT

The treatment of substance abuse or dependence is aimed at reversing the health and social problems associated with the substance of use. It is also expected to to reduce or eliminate criminal activities associated with the use of illegal drugs. These treatment programs often are expected to produce a permanent state of abstinence in individuals who have been using drugs for a long period of time, in addition to changing behavior related to the multiple psychosocial problems.

Table 156-5. Common Eye Signs With Various Drugs of Abuse

Marijuana
Normal-sized pupil
Slow or no reaction of pupil to light
Nonconvergence
Redness of sclera
Glazing of cornea
Horizontal nystagmus
Swollen eyelids
Watering
Heroin
Constricted pupil
Nonreactive pupil
Ptosis
Glazing of cornea
Decreased corneal reflex
Swollen eyelids
Alcohol/Benzodiazepines
Normal-sized pupil
Slow or no reaction of pupil to light
Nystagmus
Redness of sclera
Glazing of cornea
Nonconvergence
Cocaine/Amphetamine
Dilated pupil; slow or no reaction of pupil to light
Nystagmus
Retracted upper eyelid (walleye or bug-eye)
Decreased corneal reflex
Swollen eyelids

(Tenant F. The rapid eye test to detect drug abuse. Postgrad Med 1988;84:111.)

The first step in treatment is for the individual to accept that substance abuse or dependence is a treatable disease. The provider must have a working knowledge of the treatment resources in the community. Figure 156-1 shows a general approach to the management of substance users. In general, any treatment program is considered successful if safe and comfortable withdrawal has been achieved, whether or not this is followed by a permanent state of abstinence.

Different treatment programs are available, including detoxification, drug-free counseling, outpatient drug-free treatment, self-help groups, inpatient drug-free treatment, drug treatment such as methadone for heroin users, and combinations of these methods.

Detoxification originally was developed for treating alcohol abuse but has been extended to treating abuse of other drugs, including heroin. This treatment involves medical (ie, methadone treatment) and nonmedical or social intervention in a carefully controlled, supportive environment. The staff for detoxification programs is selected, trained, and supervised with great care.

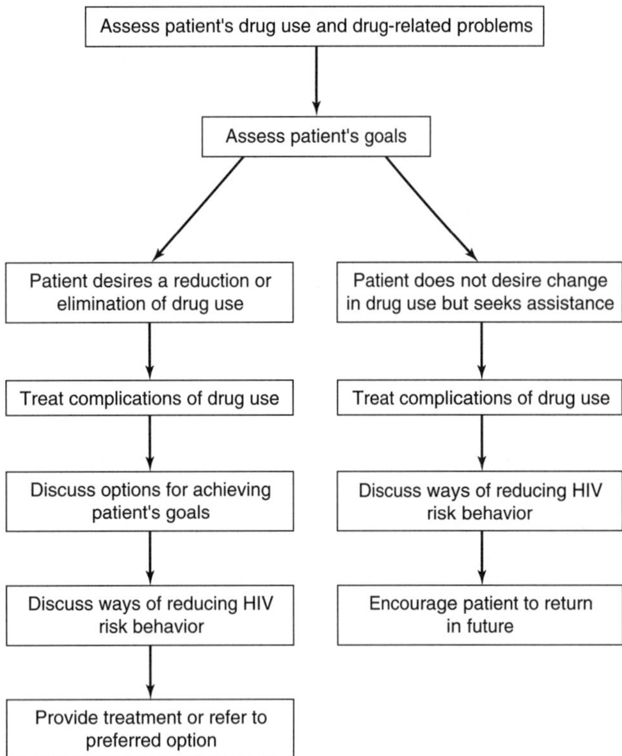

Figure 156-1. Guidelines for the management of substance users. *HIV*, human immunodeficiency virus. (Modified from Wodak A. Managing illicit drug use: a practical guide [review]. Drugs 1994;47:450.)

Drug-free counseling covers a variety of approaches that have in common only the absence of provision of any medication. Outpatient drug-free treatment emphasizes intensive and long-term treatment and involves psychotherapy. This therapy is reserved for individuals who are highly motivated and have better-than-average verbal skills.

Self-help groups (ie, Alcoholics Anonymous) involve a series of meetings in which individuals discuss the experience and problems in a forum. The meetings follow a format and are cost-free, there is no waiting list, no records of the meeting are taken, and a traditional 12-step progression to abstinence and a change in lifestyle is followed.

Inpatient drug-free treatment programs are residential rehabilitation programs that follow the philosophy of personal growth by involvement in a community of individuals who share similar difficulties. Many of these centers admit individuals under court orders who were given the choice of compulsory treatment or a return to incarceration.

The Food and Drug Administration (FDA) has approved three pharmacotherapies for illicit opiate addiction: methadone, L-alpha-acetylmethadol (LAAM), and naltrexone. Clonidine is another agent commonly used for the management of opioid withdrawal in outpatient settings, although it is not approved by the FDA for this purpose.

Methadone is a synthetic potent opioid agonist that is cross-tolerant with heroin.

Methadone is well absorbed orally and has a half-life in plasma of 16 to 48 hours. A single daily dose achieves satisfactory plasma concentrations with only a twofold variation in peak-to-trough concentrations.

Like morphine and heroin, methadone acts mainly on the μ–receptors, which are believed to be important for analgesia, euphoria, respiratory depression, tolerance, and dependence. Methadone can be used both for detoxification of the opioid addict and as maintenance treatment to substitute for heroin and other opioids that are typically injected. The rationale for use of methadone depends on the fact that it can be administered orally and has a long half-life, which prevents withdrawal symptoms from occurring (heroin has a half-life of only 3 to 4 hours). It also can be prescribed legally.

At high doses, usually above 60 mg/dL, methadone attenuates the effects of injected heroin and may decrease the frequency of heroin injection. Doses need to be individually adjusted: most patients can be managed satisfactorily with methadone doses between 60 and 100 mg/dL, but some patients require higher dosages, and a few do well on less. Methadone treatment is the most attractive treatment option for most drug users. It reduces the risk of human immunodeficiency virus (HIV) infection because it decreases the frequency of injection rather than modifying unsafe injections practices. Methadone treatment also retains a higher proportion of illicit drug users on treatment than any other modality.

LAAM is an opiate agonist. It has a half-life of 72 to 92 hours, which is a longer half-life than methadone, but otherwise has similar properties to methadone. LAAM is given orally three times per week.

Naltrexone is an opioid antagonist with no intrinsic agonist properties. It blocks the opiate receptors, thereby preventing the euphoric high produced by opiates. It is well absorbed orally and has a half-life of approximately 72 hours. It is given orally three times per week.

Clonidine is a centrally acting antihypertensive agent that is helpful in managing opiate withdrawal. It works by suppressing the autonomically mediated signs and symptoms of withdrawal.

Desipramine, an antidepressant, has been used both for cocaine detoxification and maintaining abstinence. The rationale for antidepressant treatment in patients with cocaine abuse comes from the clinical observation that depression may precede or follow cocaine use.

Antidepressant treatment seems to be most effective for patients with diagnosed cocaine abuse who have antecedent or consequent symptoms of severe depression.

Dopamimetic agonist has been used to treat cocaine abuse and dependence. It is postulated that these agents block the negative reinforcement of stimulant withdrawal, thereby decreasing the craving for cocaine. Unfortunately, the results of this approach have been mixed.

Disulfiram works as a counter-conditioning agent. It causes acetaldehyde, an alcohol metabolite, to accumulate. This metabolite accumulation causes an adversive syndrome that includes a hot flushed face, headaches, respiratory difficulties, nausea, vomiting, sweating, thirst, chest pain, weakness, vertigo, and blurred vision. This syndrome occurs within 5 to 10 minutes after alcohol ingestion and may last from 30 minutes to several hours.

SUBSTANCE USE AND ABUSE DURING PREGNANCY

Substance abuse by the pregnant woman is a major health problem because of the associated perinatal complications. These include a high incidence of stillbirths, intrauterine growth retardation, meconium-stained amniotic fluid, premature rupture of the membranes,

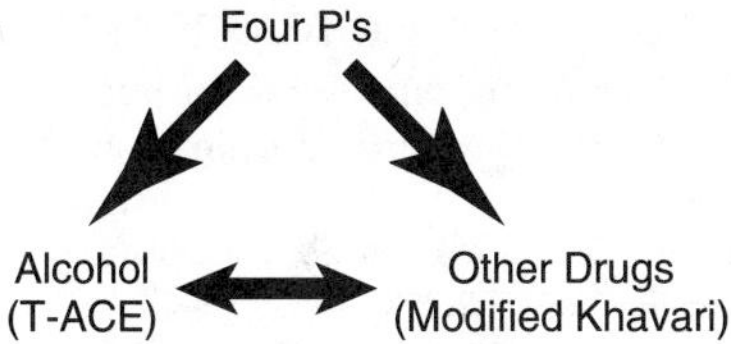

Four P's

1. Does your **P**artner have a problem with (or use) drugs or alcohol?
2. Do you consider one of your **P**arents to be an addict or an alcoholic?
3. Have you used drugs or alcohol during this **P**regnancy?
4. Have you had a problem with drugs or alcohol during the **P**ast?

(Scoring: One positive answer to any question is considered an overall positive screen)

Figure 156-2. The Four P's is a four-point screening instrument designed to assess substance abuse in obstetrical patients in need of further interviewing, referral, education, or monitoring. Any positive answer generates a positive screen result and should lead to further questioning using either the T-ACE (see Table 156-4) or the modified Khavari drug use index shown in Figure 156-3. (Courtesy of Hope Ewing, MD, Director, Born Free Project/Contra Costa County, Martinez, CA.)

maternal hemorrhage (abruptio placenta or placenta previa), and fetal distress. Unfortunately, the true prevalence of substance abuse by the pregnant woman is difficult to establish, partly because of maternal denial of substance abuse; however, it seems to range between 0.4% and 27%.

Identification by the health care worker of substance abuse in pregnant women is not easy. Maternal admission of the substance abuse often is inaccurate because of the fear of medical or social consequences. On the other hand, these patients can be hostile, manipulative, uncooperative, and can create feelings of frustration in the health care provider. The obstetric management of the pregnant patient involves a multidisciplinary team. This team includes nurses, social workers, mental health providers, and substance abuse providers. At the initial visit, a history and physical examination should elicit information relative to substance abuse or dependence. The 4 P's (Fig. 156-2) is a four-question screen designed under the auspices of the Contra Costa County Born Free Project by Hope Ewing, MD, and George Medeiros. It was developed for use in perinatal clinics and for integration within large health care systems. This screening tool is designed to quickly identify obstetric patients in need of further interviewing, referral, education, or monitoring. Any positive answer should lead to further investigation either by T-ACE or a modified Khavari questionnaire (Fig. 156-3). Any sequela of substance abuse (ie, preterm delivery, a low birth weight infant, abruptio placenta, and history of sexually transmitted disease) should be identified in the obstetric history. Those with significant alcohol use should be counseled about the potential risk of fetal alcohol syndrome. In addition to routine laboratory testing, these patients should be screened for hepatitis B and C, syphilis, skin testing for tuberculosis, and cervical cultures for gonorrhea and *Chlamydia* infection. The cervical and blood test for syphilis and hepatitis should be repeated again in the third trimester.

This population of women is prone to multiple sexual encounters and to trading sex for drugs. Thus, education and counseling about HIV infection should be provided and antibody testing offered. Unfortunately, most pregnant substance abusers do not know their last menstrual period. Therefore, a dating ultrasound and an anatomic scan at 18 to 20 weeks' gestation should be ordered to confirm gestational age and identify congenital anomalies. Because of the increased risk of intrauterine growth retardation in this population, frequent examination for fetal growth is indicated. Drug use may be monitored by urine toxicology screening at each prenatal visit. However, some programs have demonstrated that pregnant women may be so afraid of a punitive

Questions for Other Drugs

• Have you ever used marijuana ?	Yes	No
• Have you ever used cocaine ?	Yes	No
• Have you ever used heroin ?	Yes	No
• Have you ever used CAT (cocaine derivative) ?	Yes	No

IF YES TO ANY OF THE ABOVE QUESTIONS

- When was the last time you used any of these drugs ?
- How many days per week ?
- How many times per day ?
- What is the cost per day ?
- What method ? (smoke snort subcutaneous oral inject)

Figure 156-3. Modified Khavari drug use index. These questions are for addressing the use of substances other than tobacco and alcohol by patients. These questions specifically identify frequency and extent of drug use and can be incorporated into the physician's clinical practice. (Adaptation by Susan Martier at Wayne State University.) (Courtesy of K.A. Khavari, Department of Psychology, University of Wisconsin-Milwaukee.)

response from their obstetric providers that they miss prenatal appointments rather than risk identification by a positive finding on urine testing. The prenatal care provider must carefully consider the consequences of routine mandatory screening, realizing that in certain situations flexibility is important. Providing ongoing prenatal care is essential, even if it means that certain pregnant women do not have a urine toxicology screen at every visit. The interval between clinic appointments should be every 1 to 2 weeks to provide careful monitoring of the mother and fetus. At each prenatal visit, substance abuse counseling should be offered to individuals suspected of substance abuse. Antepartum fetal testing is appropriate when there is a reason to expect fetal compromise (ie, with a small-for-date fetus, decreased fetal movement, and intrauterine growth retardation). The labor and delivery management of these patients should be the same as for any other high-risk pregnancy. Fetal well-being should be documented throughout labor. The indications for anesthesia and operative delivery are the same as for most obstetric patients. The health care provider caring for the baby should be informed of the mother's substance abuse. These infants need prolonged observation for signs of withdrawal and for potential future developmental abnormalities. In the postpartum period, the mother should be encouraged to receive treatment for substance abuse. Providing contraception and education to prevent undesired pregnancies is essential. Breast-feeding mothers should be counseled that breast-feeding may expose the infant to substances that the mother is using.

The treatment of opiate abuse during pregnancy does not differ significantly from the nonpregnant state. Typically, the detoxification period is the first step in treating opiate abuse and may take from 3 to 5 days. Women who experience severe agitation because of cocaine withdrawal can be medicated with phenobarbital, 60 mg to 120 mg orally every 4 to 6 hours as needed on days 1 and 2, and 60 mg orally every 6 hours as needed on days 3 and 4; or hydroxyzine (Vistaril) or diphenhydramine (Benadryl) as needed. Pregnant women with heroin abuse can be managed with methadone as an alternative to heroin withdrawal.

Pregnancy and childbirth are times when women can be motivated to change unhealthy behaviors. Health care providers should use this motivating force with counseling and education, realizing that the potential is great for success when child-bearing women are enrolled in a comprehensive multidisciplinary treatment program.

BIBLIOGRAPHY

Ball JC, Ross A. The effectiveness of methadone maintenance treatment: patients, programs, services and outcome. New York: Springer-Verlag, 1991.

Chasnoff IJ: Drug use and women: establishing a standard of care. Ann NY Acad Sci 1989;562:208.

Chasnoff IJ, Burns WJ, Schnoll SH, et al. Cocaine use in pregnancy. N Engl J Med 1985;313:666.

Christie MJ, Harvey AI. Pharmacological options for management of opioid dependence. Drug Alcohol Rev 1993;12:71.

A guide to the detoxification of alcohol and other drug dependent, pregnant women. Cambridge, MA: Coalition on Addiction, Pregnancy and Parenting.

Hawks RL, Chiang CN, eds. Urine testing for drugs of abuse. NIDA Research Monograph 73, 1986.

Isner JM, Chokshi SK. Cardiac complication of cocaine abuse. Annu Rev Med 1991;42:133.

Kessler RC, McGongale KA, Zhao S, et al. Lifetime and 12-month prevalence of DSM-III-R psychiatric disorders in the United States. Arch Gen Psychiatry 1994;51:8.

Kreek MJ. Rationale for maintenance phamacotherapy of opioid dependence. In: O'Brien CP, Jaffe JH, eds. Addictive states. New York: Raven Press, 1992:205

Kuriloff DB, Kimmelman CP. Osteocartilaginous necrosis of the sinonasal tract following cocaine abuse. Laryngoscope 1989;99:918.

Laposata EA. Cocaine-induced heart disease: mechanisms and pathology. J Thorac Imaging 1991;6:68.

Mac Gregor SN, Keith LG, Chasnoff IJ, et al: Cocaine use during pregnancy: adverse perinatal outcome. Am J Obstet Gynecol 1987;157:686.

Mody CK, Miller BL, McIntire HB, et al. Neurologic compliocations of cocaine abuse. Neurology 1988;38:1189.

Oro AS, Dixon SD: Perinatal cocaine and methamphetamine exposure: maternal and neonatal correlates. J Pediatr 1987;111:571.

Ostrea EM, Chavez CS. Perinatal problems (excluding neonatal withdrawal) in maternal drug addiction: a study of 830 cases. J Pediatr 1979;94:292.

Reiger DA, Boyd JH, Burke JD, et al. One-month prevalence of mental disorders in the United States. Arch Gen Psychiatry 1988;45:977.

Reiger DA, Farmer ME, Rae DS, et al. Comorbidity of mental disorders with alcohol and other drug abuse. JAMA 1990;264:2511.

Substance Abuse and Mental Health Services Administration. National Household Survey on Drug Abuse. Population estimates, 1993.

Tennant FS, Rawson RA, Humphrey E, Seecrof R. Clinical experience with 959 opioid dependent patients treated with levo-alpha-acetylmethanol (LAAM). J Subst Abuse Treat 1986;3:195.

Williams GD, Grant BF, Hartford CT, et al. Population projections using DSM 111: criteria, alcohol abuse and dependence 1990–2000. Alcohol Health Res World 1989;13:366.

157

Eating Disorders

MARJORIE A. BOECK

Primary Care for Women, edited by Phyllis C. Leppert and Fred M. Howard. Lippincott-Raven Publishers, Philadelphia © 1997.

The term "eating disorders" usually refers to the conditions anorexia nervosa and bulimia nervosa, which are diagnosed clinically based on criteria set forth by the American Psychiatric Association (DSM-IV). These disorders typically begin during adolescence or young adulthood, and more than 90% of those afflicted are female. Women are much more likely than men to base their perceptions of self-worth on physical appearance. A cultural preoccupation with youth and slimness has resulted in a considerable increase in these disorders over the past several decades. Obesity, however, remains the most common nutritional disorder in the developed world. Ironically, although we have become a nation obsessed with dieting, the percentage of obese women has increased in all age groups and ethnicities.

Obesity does not appear as a clinical diagnosis in the DSM-IV because it has not been established that it is consistently associated with any psychological or behavioral syndrome. It has become apparent that some obese people engage in binging behaviors, but without the compensatory behaviors to maintain weight within a normal range. This new binge eating disorder appears for the first time, as a set of research study criteria, in the appendix of DSM-IV.

Anorexia nervosa, bulimia nervosa, obesity, and binge eating disorder all have in common an incompletely understood, multifactorial etiology with resulting multiple treatments that are less than efficacious.

ANOREXIA NERVOSA

Anorexia nervosa is a disorder in which previously healthy persons lose weight to the point of emaciation while continuing to view themselves as fat. Described by Hilde Bruch as the "relentless pursuit of thinness," the starvation, at least in the initial stages, is self-imposed. The disorder occurs primarily in females (90%) with a mean onset at age 14, or alternatively a bimodal onset at ages 14 and 18. Onset after the third decade is rare. The initial stereotypic patient was a white, intelligent, perfectionistic, upper- or upper-middle-class adolescent, often from an intact, professional family. However, this view is simplistic: the disorder occurs, although less frequently, in males, the elderly, all ethnic backgrounds, and persons in all industrialized countries.

Etiology and Diagnosis

The exact etiology of anorexia nervosa is unknown. It is thought to be a combination of sociocultural, psychological, and organic factors. Although the illness has been traced back as far as the 13th century and described in the medical literature since the 17th century, its incidence and prevalence have increased markedly during the past several decades. Some argue that this increase is due to the current cultural ideal of an extremely thin female body, others attribute it to a glamorized presentation of anorexia nervosa in the mass media, and still others attribute it to the stress on women to succeed as wife, mother, and career professional simultaneously without adequate preparation. The woman who develops this disorder has usually felt helpless and ineffectual for a long time, with her actions always being in response to others. She fears being incompetent and a "nothing," but others have perceived her as being self-assured. She develops a rigid discipline over eating and weight loss, often after experiencing a lifestyle change, to have a feeling of power and control over one aspect of her life. The anorectic person behaves at this point in a way similar to animals and humans starved for other reasons, with a preoccupation with food, high consumption of chewing gum and caffeine-containing beverages, hoarding behavior, and sleep disturbance. One exception is that although most food-deprived persons tend to slow down activity to conserve energy and are aware of their emaciated condition, persons with anorexia nervosa have a high, almost driven energy level and a distorted body image. The family interaction style of many of these patients is one of conflict avoidance.

There appears to be a genetic predisposition that makes some persons susceptible to the disorder after they begin to lose weight. There continues to be controversy over the possible genetic relation between anorexia nervosa and other eating disorders and affective disorders.

The diagnosis of anorexia nervosa is based on clinical criteria developed by the American Psychiatric Association and published in DSM-IV (Table 157-1). They include weight loss or failure to gain weight, leading to a body weight less than 85% of expected; intense fear of fatness; disturbance in body image (not just a feeling of fatness, but an actual exaggeration of their own body measurements but not those of other persons); and amenorrhea of 3 months' duration or failure to menstruate without hormone administration. The new diagnostic criteria divide both anorexia nervosa and bulimia nervosa into purging and nonpurging types. This has eliminated the need to give about 50% of eating disorder patients both diagnoses, simultaneously or sequentially.

Women who have an eating disorder and yet do not fulfill the full criteria for anorexia nervosa or bulimia nervosa, or binge eating may be diagnosed as having "Eating Disorders Not Otherwise Specified" (Table 157-2).

History

The patient with anorexia nervosa may present with a medical complaint such as fatigue, dizziness, weakness, constipation, abdominal pain, or bloating. Many patients present to a gynecologist because of primary or secondary amenorrhea. Alternatively, she may be brought to a physician by concerned parents, teachers, colleagues, or a spouse because of significant weight loss, while she denies any adverse symptomatology and points out her high energy level. Adult patients in therapy may be referred by a therapist and often have not been seen by a physician for years. The patient should be questioned about all the above symptoms.

It is important to get an accurate history of previous weights, both high and low, as well as the degree of weight loss over time. The physician should assess why the patient decided to go on a

Table 157-1. DSM-IV Diagnostic Criterion 307.1: Anorexia Nervosa

A. Refusal to maintain body weight at or above a minimally normal weight for age and height (eg, weight loss leading to maintenance of body weight less than 85% of that expected; or failure to make expected weight gain during period of growth, leading to body weight less than 85% of that expected).

B. Intense fear of gaining weight or becoming fat, even though underweight.

C. Disturbance in the way in which one's body weight or shape is experienced, undue influence of body weight or shape on self-evaluation, or denial of the seriousness of the current low body weight.

D. In postmenarcheal females, amenorrhea (ie, the absence of at least three consecutive menstrual cycles). A woman is considered to have amenorrhea if her periods occur only following hormone (eg, estrogen) administration.

Specify type:

Restricting Type: during the current episode of Anorexia Nervosa, the person has not regularly engaged in binge eating or purging behavior (ie, self-induced vomiting or the misuse of laxatives, diuretics, or enemas)

Binge Eating/Purging Type: during the current episode of Anorexia Nervosa, the person has regularly engaged in binge eating or purging behavior (ie, self-induced vomiting or the misuse of laxative, diuretics, or enemas)

(American Psychiatric Association. Diagnostic and Statistical Manual of Mental Disorders, 4th ed. Washington, DC: American Psychiatric Association, 1994.)

Table 157-2. DSM-IV Diagnostic Criterion 307.50: Eating Disorder Not Otherwise Specified

The Eating Disorder Not Otherwise Specified category is for disorders of eating that do not meet the criteria for any specific eating disorder. Examples include:

1. For females, all of the criteria for Anorexia Nervosa are met except that the individual has regular menses.
2. All of the criteria for Anorexia Nervosa are met except that, despite significant weight loss, the individual's current weight is in the normal range.
3. All of the criteria for Bulimia Nervosa are met except that the binge eating and inappropriate compensatory mechanisms occur at a frequency of less than twice a week or a duration of less than 3 months.
4. The regular use of inappropriate compensatory behavior by an individual of normal body weight after eating small amounts of food (eg, self-induced vomiting after the consumption of two cookies).
5. Repeatedly chewing and spitting out, but not swallowing, large amounts of food.
6. Binge eating disorder: recurrent episodes of binge eating in the absence of the regular use of inappropriate compensatory behaviors characteristic of Bulimia Nervosa.

(American Psychiatric Association. Diagnostic and Statistical Manual of Mental Disorders, 4th ed. Washington, DC: American Psychiatric Association, 1994.)

diet, how she feels about her current appearance, and what weight goal she wishes to attain, if any. Some patients, although not actively suicidal, would like to "shrink away to nothing." As patients have become more sophisticated, most report that they realize their weight is too low. If asked, however, how they feel about their thighs, most readily admit to feeling fat.

It is also important to take a detailed dietary history. The patient with anorexia nervosa does not, at least initially, have a loss of appetite or a decrease in craving for any nutrient. Snacks containing concentrated sweets and any foods with identifiable fats (eg, butter, margarine, salad dressing) are eliminated first. As the disease progresses, intakes frequently reach 300 to 800 calories/day. The patient prefers to eat alone, as the eating process is usually lengthy and highly ritualized, with the food arranged in a specific pattern and eaten in a particular order. Many patients automatically count calories but overestimate the amount of calories they consume. The patient should be questioned about her knowledge of eating disorders, including which television programs or magazine articles and books she has read. This knowledge may prove useful in discussing her own diagnosis.

If the patient admits she has anorexia nervosa, it is important to find out when the diagnosis was made (in contrast to when the patient believes the problem began); past symptoms, especially in comparison with current complaints; and previous treatments, including psychotherapy, pharmacotherapy, and hospitalization.

Physical Examination and Clinical Findings

The most notable finding on physical examination is the degree of loss of subcutaneous fat, which may or may not be accompanied by a degree of muscle wasting. It is crucial to examine these patients without clothing. Because patients with this disorder tend to be cold, they often dress in multiple layers of clothing, which are not perceptible. It is important to measure both height and weight. In the younger teen, there may not be a history of weight loss, but rather failure to gain weight when expected to or, even more serious, growth failure and delayed puberty. Other physical findings are those of any cachectic patient: lower core body temperature, acrocyanosis of extremities, low or low-normal blood pressure, and bradycardia. Indications of extreme starvation requiring emergency intervention include the development of lanugo hair, leg edema, orthostatic hypotension, and a weight loss greater than 40%.

Laboratory and Imaging Studies

Patients may be at considerable medical risk and yet have completely normal laboratory findings. The degree of weight loss, the symptomatology, and the duration of illness do not necessarily correlate with the degree of laboratory abnormalities. The changes that occur in the hypothalamic-pituitary-adrenal axis in patients with anorexia nervosa are closely related to the extent of weight loss and in most instances are consistent with those occurring in other forms of starvation. There is no need to perform these expensive tests, as the findings are unnecessary for diagnosis and require no treatment. Abnormalities related to starvation may include lowered white blood cell count with neutropenia, lowered total red blood cell count, macrocytic anemia, elevated or very low cholesterol, elevated liver function tests, reduced creatinine clearance, and an abnormal creatinine kinase level. A serum creatinine level in the high-normal range should be seen as abnormal, because with reduced muscle mass, the value should be low. A computed tomography scan may show cortical atrophy. An electrocardiogram should be obtained. A prolonged QT interval is an ominous sign. The echocardiogram of the severely anorexic patient reveals small heart size with mitral valve prolapse. The absence of menstrual cycles may result in bone mineral depletion, osteoporosis, and even stress fractures. Therefore, evaluation of bone density with dual photon densitometry is recommended; this finding may not be reversible. Although not yet standard practice, many anorectic females are placed on birth-control pills as a source of estrogen and calcium supplementation.

Treatment

There is no entirely satisfactory treatment approach for anorexia nervosa, and the disorder is associated with a mortality rate of 5% to 18%. Treatment must be individualized and multifaceted. The treatment team, in either an inpatient or outpatient setting, should include at a minimum a physician to monitor weight status and medical condition and a therapist to deal with the underlying psychological issues. If the physician is not dealing with nutritional education and concerns about the eating process, a nutritionist with expertise in eating disorders should be included, as well as additional therapists for group or family therapy. All members of the team must be in close communication to ensure the patient gets a consistent message. A contract signed by the patient and all her providers is recommended.

Initial treatment is directed toward reestablishing a weight compatible with survival and may necessitate an inpatient setting. Behavior modification techniques are often used during this stage. Nutritional supplements may be administered by mouth, by nasogastric or nasoduodenal tube, or rarely by peripheral or central hyperalimentation. The achievement of an appropriate weight and normalized eating habits is a long-term goal. Individual psychotherapy is often augmented by group or family therapy.

Numerous pharmacologic agents, including chlorpromazine, lithium, and tricyclic antidepressants, have been used in the treatment of anorexia nervosa, but with little success. Because severe cachexia results in a flat affect resembling depression, many clinicians reserve the use of antidepressants for patients who meet criteria for depression after the refeeding process. An agent used with some success is the serotonin antagonist cyproheptadine, which in high doses (32 mg/day) may result in appetite increase and mood elevation.

Considerations in Pregnancy

Many patients develop secondary amenorrhea before significant weight loss has occurred. This may reflect psychogenic factors operating on the hypothalamus or some deficit in carbohydrate intake. Starvation ultimately results in prepubertal patterns of luteinizing hormone secretion, but resumption of weight does not necessarily reverse this pattern. Patients meeting full diagnostic criteria for anorexia nervosa have primary or secondary amenorrhea and could not become pregnant under normal circumstances, but there have been anorectic women who have conceived using a fertility agent. Such pregnancies are at very high risk for spontaneous abortion, miscarriage, and prematurity, and there is anecdotal evidence to suggest that the infants may suffer from failure to thrive. There is no evidence that a past history of anorexia nervosa, regardless of length or severity, precludes later normal childbearing.

BULIMIA NERVOSA

Bulimia, from the Greek for "ox-hunger," refers to an eating pattern in which a large quantity of food is consumed over a brief period of time. In bulimia nervosa, patients maintain their weight despite eating binges by engaging in purging behaviors (eg, self-induced vomiting, use of laxatives, diuretics, or diet pills) or periods of starvation or excessive exercise. Although practiced by the ancient Greeks and Romans, bulimia nervosa became a clinical diagnostic entity for the first time in 1980, with the publication of the DSM-III. It affects primarily women (90%) and has its onset most often during mid- to late adolescence. The diagnosis reflects a spectrum of behavior that in its mildest form does not impinge on functioning in aspects of life not connected with food and may be self-limited. At the other end of the spectrum is an extremely severe disorder in which all waking hours are spent eating and purging with significant dysphoric mood, suicide attempts, stealing, and abuse of alcohol and other drugs; the prognosis for this severe form is guarded despite treatment.

Etiology and Differential Diagnosis

The etiology of bulimia nervosa is unknown with biological, psychological, and societal factors all implicated, as with anorexia nervosa. It is hypothesized that patients with bulimia nervosa have a dysregulation of serotonin that results in a loss of normal serotonergic inhibition of carbohydrate intake. Another hypothesis is that bulimic patients may be responding to heightened levels of pancreatic polypeptide Y when they initiate a binge. The endogenous peptide neuropeptide Y has also been implicated, as it stimulates feeding when administered in various hypothalamic areas.

Bulimic persons seem to be at increased genetic risk for the development of affective disorders and alcoholism, as there is often a history of depression or alcoholism in first-degree relatives.

Persons with bulimia usually feel a lack of self-control and manifest poor self-esteem. They are often compulsive, depressed, and anxious and feel a lack of control over their lives. Family interactions are often problematic; the problems vary from parental absence to enmeshment. Despite controversy in the literature, it appears that the incidence, severity, or duration of physical or sexual abuse is not greater among bulimic patients than in the female population as a whole. Such a history, however, may have a negative impact on therapy and perhaps on prognosis. The psychological literature views the binge-and-purge cycle as a mechanism for regulating tension states that may be the result of sexual urges, impulsivity, boredom, anxiety, or aggression. It has been postulated that the binging behavior is maintained because these persons attempt to maintain a weight lower than what is constitutionally comfortable for them by habitually fasting and feeling hungry during parts of the day.

Patients usually report dissatisfaction with their body and a societal pressure to be thin. Obesity may exist in other family members. The patient may also be overweight to some degree and the disorder begins after a period of dietary restriction.

The diagnosis of bulimia nervosa is a clinical one. The current diagnostic criteria from DSM-IV (Table 157-3) include recurrent episodes of rapid consumption of a large amount of food in a discrete period of time (binging), a feeling of lack of control over eating during this binging period, regular engagement in behaviors to prevent weight gain due to the binging, and a fear of being overweight. In addition, patients must engage in an average of at least two binge eating episodes a week for at least 3 months to meet the criteria.

History

The primary care physician, including the family practitioner, pediatrician, internist, or gynecologist, is in a position to make an early diagnosis of an eating disorder. This rarely happens, however, because the patient appears healthy, and it is rare that a teenager or adult voluntarily admits to binging or purging episodes. For this reason, it is recommended that a dietary history aimed at detecting an eating disorder be obtained from all girls, adolescents, and adult women. Psychological treatment is usually not sought for a number of years. Many adult bulimic patients seek medical attention only because it is a prerequisite for their eating disorder treatment program.

The woman with frequent episodes of binging followed by self-induced vomiting often complains of sore throat and hoarseness. Other complaints may include weakness, dizziness, constipation, headache, chest pain, abdominal pain, bloating, muscle cramps, and a general sense of not feeling well. Many patients have episodes of secondary amenorrhea despite appropriate weight for height. The patient should be questioned about the occurrence of any of these symptoms.

In contrast to adult patients who are self-referred, many teenagers are brought to treatment after being discovered by their

Table 157-3. DSM-IV Diagnostic Criterion 307.51: Bulimia Nervosa

A. Recurrent episodes of binge eating. An episode of binge eating is characterized by both of the following:

(1) eating, in a discrete period of time (eg, within any 2-hour period), an amount of food that is definitely larger than most people would eat during a similar period of time and under similar circumstances

(2) a sense of lack of control over eating during the episode (eg, a feeling that one cannot stop eating or control what or how much one is eating)

B. Recurrent inappropriate compensatory behavior in order to prevent weight gain, such as self-induced vomiting; misuse of laxatives, diuretics, enemas, or other medications; fasting; or excessive exercise.

C. The binge eating and inappropriate compensatory behaviors both occur, on average, at least twice a week for 3 months.

D. Self-evaluation is unduly influenced by body shape and weight.

E. The disturbance does not occur exclusively during episodes of Anorexia Nervosa.

Specify type:

Purging Type: during the current episode of Bulimia Nervosa, the person has regularly engaged in self-induced vomiting or the misuse of laxatives, diuretics, or enemas

Nonpurging Type: during the current episode of Bulimia Nervosa, the person has used other inappropriate compensatory behaviors, such as fasting or excessive exercise, but has not regularly engaged in self-induced vomiting or the misuse of laxatives, diuretics, or enemas

(American Psychiatric Association. Diagnostic and Statistical Manual of Mental Disorders, 4th ed. Washington, DC: American Psychiatric Association, 1994.)

parents. They view purging as a weight-control technique and have no desire to change. Unlike the solitary binging of the adult, teenagers may binge and vomit in groups.

Physical Examination and Clinical Findings

The physical examination is usually entirely normal. Benign, painless swelling of the parotid or submandibular glands has been reported and is reversible when the binge-and-purge cycles end. There may also be characteristic superficial ulcerations, hyperpigmented calluses, or scars on the dorsum of the hands of patients who use their fingers to induce vomiting. With repeated emesis, the acid vomitus causes a loss of tooth enamel that affects the palatal side of the upper teeth, beginning with the molars and moving centrally. This ultimately results in dental caries and significant abnormalities of bite.

Other medical complications include reflux esophagitis, esophageal tears, and aspiration pneumonia. Life-threatening complications, such as ventricular fibrillation due to hypokalemia, renal failure, gastric rupture, toxic megacolon after prolonged laxative abuse, seizures, and tetany, have also been reported. The use of syrup of ipecac to induce vomiting has been associated with death in bulimic patients due to cardiotoxic effects.

Laboratory Studies

Laboratory studies are often entirely normal. Many patients are careful not to purge for a day or two before a physician visit. The physician should determine when the last purging episode occurred. The physician must explain the potential medical complications of purging behavior, reminding the patient that normal laboratory studies do not imply that her health may not be placed in danger immediately after purging. The most common electrolyte abnormality is an elevated serum bicarbonate level, indicative of a metabolic alkalosis. Other abnormalities include hypochloremia, hypokalemia, and hypomagnesemia. Occasional patients require oral potassium supplementation on a daily basis. Patients may also have an elevated serum amylase level, which in many cases is a result of an elevation of the salivary (not pancreatic) isoenzyme.

Treatment

Most patients are treated in an outpatient setting. An inpatient or day hospital setting, using a therapeutic approach similar to that used for patients with anorexia nervosa, is occasionally indicated. Treatment of bulimia nervosa with psychotherapy alone is not sufficient. The symptom of binging and purging must be addressed directly through behavioral approaches such as aversion therapy, behavior modification, and most recently cognitive behavioral restructuring. There have been several controlled outpatient psychotherapy trials conducted on bulimic adults with generally good short-term results. Although the details of the programs vary—some use individual therapy, others group therapy or a combination of individual and group therapy—they had several elements in common. Most treatment programs emphasize nutrition counseling; some even prescribe specific dietary intake for patients. There is also a strong emphasis on eliminating binge eating and vomiting, as well as on establishing normal eating patterns. Several programs include assertiveness training or relaxation training. Almost all programs place an emphasis on self-monitoring. Many programs emphasize specific behavioral paradigms, such as stimulus control, response delay, and problem-solving technique.

Pharmacotherapy plays an important adjunctive role in the treatment of bulimia nervosa. Evidence linking bulimia to major affective disorders has led to the hypothesis that antidepressant medications might be an effective treatment. Controlled double-blind placebo trials have been carried out using tricyclic antidepressants with success. A patient who initially has a good response to imipramine may later develop tachyphylaxis and respond well to a different tricyclic.

The mood disturbance of some bulimic patients has been noted to be similar to that of patients with atypical depression. This term is used to describe patients who, when depressed, retain reactivity to environmental events and experience two or more of the following: increased appetite or weight gain, oversleeping, severe fatigue, and extreme sensitivity to personal rejection. Studies suggest that patients with atypical depression respond better to monoamine oxidase inhibitors than to tricyclic antidepressants. The use of monoamine oxidase inhibitors requires strict adherence to a tyramine-free diet and thus calls for careful patient selection and close monitoring.

There has also been interest in and success with use of the specific serotonin agonists, especially fluoxetine. This medication is an antidepressant and also produces a decrease in appetite, particularly for carbohydrates, as a side effect. This drug has a safer and better-tolerated side effect profile (no dry mouth or constipation and little if any cardiotoxicity).

Narcotic antagonists, such as naltrexone, have been reported to reduce the frequency of binging and purging under both double-blind and open label conditions. Such agents remain confined to the research setting.

Because some bulimic women seem to have seasonal fluctuations of binging consistent with seasonal affective disorder, light therapy has been tried with some success.

Considerations in Pregnancy

Obstetricians should take an initial history designed to detect the presence or history of eating disorders in their pregnant patients. The pregnant bulimic patient physically appears normal but represents a high-risk pregnancy. She may be able to eat an adequately balanced diet with vitamin supplementation during the pregnancy and yet continue to binge and purge on a daily basis. Medications such as fluoxetine that may have controlled symptoms in the nonpregnant state are contraindicated. As with other chronic illnesses, the pregnancy should be planned with the patient in remission and off all medications. Normal, full-term infants have been born to actively bulimic women who have received high-risk care throughout their pregnancy. Anecdotally, these women are at higher risk for postpartum depression.

OBESITY

Obesity may be defined as a maladaptive increase in the amount of energy stored as fat. There is no method to determine accurately the optimal amount of body fat stores or the ideal body weight for a given person. Published weight tables, such as those of the Metropolitan Life Insurance Company, are usually used to determine ideal body weight, although they reflect the actual weight of insured adults. A better measure is a body mass index (BMI), which takes into account the relation between height and weight. The most frequently used BMI is the Quetelet index (weight in kilograms divided by height in meters squared [kg/m^2]). The most accurate office measure of body fat is the direct measurement of subcutaneous fat mass at various anatomic sites, usually the triceps and subscapular, using skinfold calipers. Other methods for measuring body fat include hydrostatic weighing, bioelectrical impedance analysis (four-electrode plethysmography used to determine total body water), total body potassium, and total body dual photon densitometry.

Etiology

Obesity is a heterogeneous group of disorders that can result from various pathophysiologic mechanisms. The familial nature of obesity has been noted for generations. When both parents are obese, about 70% of their children will be obese. Studies comparing heights and weights of adult adoptees with those of their adoptive and biologic parents, studies of monozygotic twins reared together and apart, and studies of pairs of monozygotic twins deliberately overfed have indicated a larger role for genetics than previously thought. Although these studies indicate the importance of genetics, they do not tell us what precisely is inherited.

A person may have hypertrophic obesity due to an increase in fat cell size, hyperplastic obesity due to an increase in cell number, or a combination of both. In certain persons, new fat cells may develop during any period of weight gain throughout life. This is probably genetically determined. It is hypothesized that reduction does not decrease the number of fat cells and th individual fat cells reach a normal size, weight reduction stops.

Human studies have lent support to the "set point" theory, which states that each person has a genetically determined biologic weight (the set point). The organism defends its body weight (much like a thermostat) against pressure to change, even if the weight is far above the culture's ideal.

Historically, investigators believed there was a discrete hunger center in the lateral hypothalamus and a satiety center in the ventromedial hypothalamus. It is now recognized that the process of feeding is considerably more complex, and that these "centers" are more like "systems" that regulate feeding behavior via an interplay of central and peripheral pathways, including other brain areas, neurotransmitters, circulating metabolites, and hormones. These include neuropeptide Y, dopamine, norepinephrine and epinephrine, and serotonin.

The high prevalence of obesity in the United States may be due, at least in part, to unlimited access to palatable foods. Sweetness (sugar content) is a weaker determinant of overeating than both fat content and variety. It is thought that some overweight persons may be more prone to eat in response to visual or olfactory cues, regardless of hunger.

Fewer than 1% of obese patients have endogenous obesity as a result of endocrine or hypothalamic abnormalities or defined genetic syndromes. These few patients are usually readily identified in childhood because of growth failure.

Many epidemiologic studies, prospective, cross-sectional, and retrospective, have shown that the risk of developing certain health problems and a shortened life span is higher among overweight persons than among those who are not overweight of the same sex, race, age, and socioeconomic status. The risks increase with the degree of obesity.

There are two patterns of fat distribution. The upper segment obesity pattern (abdominal, apple, or android) is associated with a higher risk of developing physiologic complications than the lower segment pattern (femoral-gluteal, gynoid) pattern. The pattern of fat distribution can be determined visually or by measuring the circumferences of waist and hip. A waist:hip ratio of 0.8 or higher in females is high enough to provide that risk. The body's content of visceral fat, as determined by computed tomography or magnetic resonance imaging, may be a better predictor of risk than the waist:hip ratio.

Physiologic complications include hyperinsulinism, insulin resistance, acanthosis nigricans, noninsulin-dependent diabetes mellitus, cholesterol gallstones, hypertension, atherogenic lipid profile, coronary vascular disease, stroke, gout, exacerbation of arthritis, obstructive sleep apnea, menstrual abnormalities, and complications of anesthesia, surgery, and pregnancy. The types of cancer associated with obesity in women include gallbladder and biliary passages, breast, cervix, endometrium, and ovary. Complications such as acanthosis nigricans, hyperinsulinism, hypertension, atherogenic lipid profile, and obstructive sleep apnea can begin before puberty if the child is sufficiently overweight.

History

The history should include information about the age of onset of excessive weight gain, maximum weight attained, and any identifiable precipitating events or circumstances. Note should be made of the presence of chronic or earlier serious health problems, previous starvation, abdominal surgery, or prolonged bed rest, all of which have been associated with the onset of excessive weight gain. A detailed menstrual history, including any fertility problems or pregnancies, should be elicited. Most obese girls have an early menarche, often by age 10. Soon after, they may develop secondary amenorrhea or dysfunctional uterine bleeding. The clinician should also inquire about the use of pharmacologic agents known to result in obesity (eg, steroids, antipsychotic medications).

The family pattern of weight gain and history of obesity-related conditions such as diabetes, high blood pressure, heart disease, and cancer should be elicited. The clinician should obtain any history of similar disorders in the patient.

Further information about the family's attitude toward obesity and any perceived relation between eating and various moods and life stresses is important in gaining a perspective on which therapeutic strategies have the best probabilities for success. It is important to assess why the patient is seeking medical attention at this time and her motivation to lose weight. Patterns of eating should be investigated, including the number of meals and snacks per day, the rate of eating, food preferences, the degree of hunger and satiety, and the occurrence of binging and nocturnal eating.

The patient should be asked about previous efforts at weight loss, including the type of weight-reduction program, the duration of the effort, the amount of weight lost, the reason for terminating the attempt, and the time and amount of weight regained, if any.

The impact of obesity on social functioning, including peer relationships, leisure activities, and school or work performance, should be assessed. In today's culture, with its emphasis on slimness, the child, adolescent, or adult who is obese may have difficulty with self-image and peer relationships. Several studies have shown that children and adolescents, when offered a choice of friends, prefer a person with a physical handicap rather than one with obesity. Other studies have found a striking similarity between the psychological traits of obese adolescent girls and those of racial minorities who have been victims of prejudice. Discrimination against the obese in education and employment has been well documented. Although most obese adults do not have a poor self-image, a pathologically poor self-image is found in persons who become or remain obese during adolescence. Such persons view themselves as disgusting and avoid looking into a store display window because they will see their own reflection. They divide the world into fat people, who are bad, and thin people, who are good. These severe body image disturbances seem to develop during a critical period of adolescence, when negative views of peers and significant adults are incorporated into the teenager's developing self-concept. Such body image disturbances persist with remarkably little change over long periods of time, even after weight reduction.

Physical Examination and Clinical Findings

The physical examination should include careful measurement of height, weight, and circumferences of waist and hip, with calculation of the BMI and waist:hip ratio. Blood-pressure measurements should be made with an appropriate-size cuff, using a thigh cuff if necessary. Insulin resistance may result in acanthosis nigricans (a velvety darkening of the skin due to melanocyte deposition in the dermis; it is found at the neck and often in the axillary and inguinal regions) and hyperandrogenism, which is manifested as hirsutism. The clinician should note the distribution of body fat, acne, and the color of striae if present. Special attention should be paid to the thyroid gland, the back, and weight-bearing joints. It is often difficult to detect organomegaly or masses on the abdominal examination or to palpate the ovaries on the pelvic examination.

Laboratory Studies

The insulin response to oral glucose is greatly elevated in the obese person, and fasting levels of both glucose and insulin should be obtained. A normal fasting insulin is not sufficient, however, to rule out hyperinsulinism or insulin resistance. Obese females tend to have higher levels of triglycerides, very low-density lipoprotein, low-density lipoprotein, and total cholesterol and lower levels of high-density lipoprotein (HDL) than their lean counterparts. A complete 12-hour fasting lipid profile must be obtained to calculate the ratio of total cholesterol to HDL. A low HDL level responds to weight reduction and exercise.

Obesity may cause infertility due to ovarian dysfunction in the absence of grossly abnormal menses, as may occur in luteal phase insufficiency. Obese females may also develop oligomenorrhea or secondary amenorrhea. The most common cause is polycystic ovary syndrome, which was initially defined as the constellation of hirsutism, obesity, menstrual irregularity, and infertility associated with enlarged sclerocystic ovaries. The extent to which obesity plays a causative role has not been determined. Diagnostic studies include measurement of serum luteinizing hormone, follicle-stimulating hormone, estrone, DHEA, androstenedione, and testosterone. Imaging studies of the ovary, such as pelvic ultrasound, are needed to assess ovarian size and function.

Morbidly obese females are at risk for obstructive sleep apnea, which may develop into hypersomnia and the pickwickian syndrome. Observers may report that the patient snores loudly and sometimes seems to stop breathing. Such patients warrant polysomnography and may benefit from continuous positive airway pressure as an alternative to tonsillectomy, adenoidectomy, and uvulectomy or tracheostomy while losing weight.

Treatment

The basis for the treatment of obesity is to lower energy intake below that of energy expenditure. This might be easier and more effective if we had a classification of human obesity based on etiology and pathogenesis. However, the classification used to determine the type of obesity treatment is that of mild, moderate, and severe or morbid obesity. Mild obesity is characterized as a weight 20% to 40% over ideal body weight, as defined by standard tables of height and weight, or a BMI of 27 to 30 (25 for women); moderate obesity as a weight 41% to 100% over ideal body weight or a BMI of 30.1 to 35; and severe obesity as more than 100% above ideal body weight, with a BMI above 35.

Ninety percent of all obese persons have mild obesity and may not have any physiologic problems for which weight loss would be indicated. Some degree of weight loss may be important for women with upper segment obesity. Mild obesity should be treated with conservative methods, if at all.

Patients with moderate (9.5%) and severe obesity (0.5%) usually require treatment. The amount of weight required to reverse physiologic problems may be in the range of 5% to 10% rather than achieving ideal body weight. Patients who cycle between weight loss and gain might actually be doing themselves more harm than if they just remained obese, but this is not true for the moderately and extremely obese. If conservative treatments fail, these women may be treated with very low calorie diets (VLCD), pharmacotherapy, or surgery.

Conservative Approaches

Most weight-loss programs include a diet, nutrition education, behavior modification, and exercise. Diets are most likely to succeed if they are highly individualized, based on current eating patterns, degree of motivation, intellect, amount of family support, and monetary considerations. Such a diet plan should aim for a loss of 1% of body weight per week. Dozens of weight-loss books are on the market; many make claims that are untrue and a few are actually dangerous. A physician should be consulted before instituting any new diet. The distribution of protein, fat, and carbohydrate is important to lose the maximum amount of adipose tissue with a minimum loss of nitrogen. This is provided by the American Heart Association's step I diet: 20% of calories from protein, 30% of calories from fat (less than one third from saturated, more than one third from monounsaturated, and one third from polyunsaturated), and 50% of calories from carbohydrates, preferably complex carbohydrates that are high in fiber. Vitamin and mineral supplements should be used with diets providing fewer than 1200 calories/day.

Before the diet program begins, the woman must have a realistic expectation about the rate of weight loss. It takes an energy deficit of 3500 to 3600 kcal to lose 1 lb. Compliance with new dietary habits for a prolonged period to attain and maintain weight loss is a major difficulty. Weigh-in and counseling sessions on a weekly or biweekly basis are essential initially, with biweekly or monthly reassessment required for many during both weight loss and maintenance.

Behavioral programs focus on how to eat, on the assumption that eating habits must change to maintain weight loss. Women are asked to keep a diary of all food eaten and the circumstances surrounding its consumption (time, place, activity, mood). This identifies specific behaviors to be targeted for change by the program. Programs may focus on slowing the rate at which food is eaten, using smaller plates, eating mainly in certain areas, and avoiding other activities while eating, such as watching television. This sedentary activity involves exposure to many high-calorie foods, both in commercials and the actual programming. Studies on the effectiveness of behavioral treatment indicate that its advantage is not in the amount of weight lost, but rather in the maintenance of weight once loss has occurred.

Although the role of physical activity in the development of obesity is unclear, an exercise program should be a part of every weight-reduction plan. It is important to recommend kinds of exercise, such as walking and climbing stairs, that do not require elaborate, expensive facilities. As with behavioral change strategies, exercise is more important for weight maintenance than for weight loss. Compliance with exercise programs, however, is poor: studies report a 25% to 75% dropout rate.

Treatment programs for the mildly obese, with their emphasis on lifestyle changes, are conducted primarily within self-help groups and commercial programs. Self-help groups include Overeaters Anonymous and Take Off Pounds Sensibly. The success of such groups parallels that of groups such as Alcoholics Anonymous in the treatment of alcoholism. Commercial diet programs, of which Weight Watchers International is the prototype (the oldest and the largest, claiming a yearly membership of 3 million), include diet, behavior modification, and exercise. Commercial diet programs tend not to collect or release data on attrition and success rates. A recent study of a commercial weight-reduction program in the United States, however, found an attrition rate of 50% at 6 weeks and 70% at 12 weeks. Similar high attrition rates were reported in five other programs on three continents.

Very Low Calorie Diets

There is no universally accepted definition of a VLCD. Most commonly, it provides 400 to 800 calories/day (protein-sparing modified fasts) but is formulated to provide all essential nutrients and to result in a positive nitrogen balance. VLCDs should not be confused with the liquid protein diets of the 1970s, which contained poor-quality protein and resulted in over 60 deaths related to cardiac atrophy. Current diets provide protein from meat, fish, or fowl (served as food) or from egg and milk sources. In the latter case, the protein is powdered, mixed with vitamins and minerals, and hydrated (by the patient) into liquid form. The amount of carbohydrate to be included, if any, is controversial.

These diets should be restricted to persons at least 30% overweight. Contraindications include a recent myocardial infarction; a cardiac conduction disorder; a history of cerebrovascular, renal, or hepatic disease; cancer; type I diabetes; and pregnancy. Attrition rates vary from 15% to 68%. Treatment by VLCD is often delivered by a multidisciplinary team including a physician, a behavioral psychologist, a dietitian, and perhaps an exercise specialist. No studies have been conducted, however, to compare the results of team treatment with those of treatment by a single physician.

Usually, treatment by VLCD involves four phases:

- A 1- to 4-week introductory phase in which the patient is placed on a traditional 1200- to 1500-calorie diet with increased exercise
- The VLCD itself for 8 to 16 weeks
- A 4- to 8-week refeeding period in which conventional foods are gradually reintroduced. The return to eating solid food is often a time of very high anxiety for the patient.
- A maintenance phase, during which the patient is instructed in methods of maintaining weight loss. Less than a third of patients participate in formal weight-maintenance programs.

Patients should be examined by a physician once weekly during the VLCD phase and should have blood studies biweekly. Complications associated with VLCD include gallstones, elevated uric acid level, and anemia. Symptoms are usually confined to the first few days and include fatigue, dizziness, muscle cramping, headache, gastrointestinal distress, cold intolerance, dry skin, and hair loss. Most patients do not report hunger, probably because of ketosis. Although the resting metabolic rate is depressed during the dieting process, it rises to a level appropriate for the patient's new body weight.

The average weight loss on a VLCD for 12 to 16 weeks is 20 kg. The weight loss is usually less for women, especially those who are very short, because they have lower caloric needs. Patients tend to regain most of their weight within 1 to 5 years; it is unknown whether participation in a formal weight-maintenance

Table 157-4. DSM-IV Research Criterion: Binge Eating Disorder

A. Recurrent episodes of binge eating. An episode of binge eating is characterized by both of the following:

(1) eating, in a discrete period of time (eg, within any 2-hour period), an amount of food that is definitely larger than most people would eat in a similar period of time under similar circumstances

(2) a sense of lack of control over eating during the episode (eg, a feeling that one cannot stop eating or control what or how much one is eating)

B. The binge eating episodes are associated with three (or more) of the following:

(1) eating much more rapidly than normal

(2) eating until feeling uncomfortably full

(3) eating large amounts of food when not feeling physically hungry

(4) eating alone because of being embarrassed by how much one is eating

(5) feeling disgusted with oneself, depressed, or very guilty after overeating

C. Marked distress regarding binge eating is present.

D. The binge eating occurs, on average, at least 2 days a week for 6 months.

Note: the method of determining frequency differs from that used for Bulimia Nervosa; future research should address whether the preferred method of setting a frequency threshold is counting the number of days on which binges occur or counting the number of episodes of binge eating.

E. The binge eating is not associated with the regular use of inappropriate compensatory behaviors (eg, purging, fasting, excessive exercise) and does not occur exclusively during the course of Anorexia Nervosa or Bulimia Nervosa.

(American Psychiatric Association. Diagnostic and Statistical Manual of Mental Disorders, 4th ed. Washington, DC: American Psychiatric Association, 1994.)

program would improve these findings. Patients may retain some of the health benefits despite regaining much of the weight.

Pharmacotherapy

Many short-term trials of 4 to 12 weeks have shown that appetite suppressant drugs produce weight losses two to four times that of placebo. These drugs include dexfenfluramine, fluoxetine, and phenylpropanolamine. According to licensing regulations, the pharmacologic treatment of obesity is limited to short periods, usually 12 to 16 weeks. This is based on a belief that obesity can be treated as a short-term disorder, similar to pneumonia, rather than as a chronic disease such as diabetes. The question of longer-term, even lifelong, administration of drugs for the management of obesity has been raised. This is based on the facts that obesity is a major health problem, that the management of severe physiological and psychological disorders depends on weight loss, that only sustained weight loss results in sustained medical benefits, and that current therapy too often ends in failure.

Such an antiobesity agent must have a potent weight-lowering effect in short-term controlled trials, acceptable clinical tolerance, no addictive properties, sustained effects when treatment is continued, absence of major side effects after years of administration, and known mechanism of action. Dexfenfluramine has been studied most extensively, including a 1-year trial known as INDEX (International Dexfenfluramine Study) that involved 822 patients from 24 centers in nine countries. Results from this randomized double-blind trial of dexfenfluramine 15 mg twice daily or placebo indicate that such a drug might aid in extended weight loss over time or would be an aid in maintenance of weight loss after VLCD. In another study, 121 people took part in a 34-week trial of phentermine 15 mg combined with sustained-release fenfluramine 30 mg versus placebo, added to a program of behavior modification, caloric restriction, and exercise. At the end of 34 weeks, only nine subjects had dropped out, the active medication groups had lost significantly more weight, there were no bothersome side effects, and the medication continued to be efficacious. This study, sponsored by the National Institutes of Health, continued for 4 years, studying dose response, intermittent dosing, effects on physiologic parameters, and individual treatment response. Pharmaceutical companies are expanding their efforts to develop new drugs to be used in the long-term treatment of extreme obesity.

Surgery

Surgery is indicated for highly selected patients who are more than 100 lb above ideal body weight and who have a serious illness responsive to weight loss for which no previous treatment has been successful. A woman selected must understand the surgery and the requirement for lifelong postoperative care. She must be emotionally stable, without any tendency toward self-destructive behavior. Perioperative mortality in severely obese patients having a primary operation to control obesity is below 1% in centers specializing in this type of surgery.

Two surgical techniques are reasonably safe and effective: gastric restriction and gastrointestinal bypass. In the former, patients decrease their food intake to avoid the intense discomfort and vomiting that occur when small additional amounts of food are eaten. The greatest flaw with the procedure is that liquids and semisolids of high caloric density can pass through the pouch in excess (eg, potato chips, chocolate) and that overdistention can cause the pouch to distend. Gastric restriction procedures have a higher dropout rate, indicating that conscious modification of eating behavior is more difficult to achieve. Gastrointestinal bypass surgery may result in diarrhea or the dumping syndrome and requires the patient to take vitamin and mineral supplements. These patients also report a change in eating patterns, consuming fewer fats, sweets, and milk and milk products. Studies have shown less depression, anxiety, irritability, and preoccupation with food during weight loss subsequent to the gastric bypass procedure than had occurred during previous nonsurgical attempts at weight reduction. About 50% of severely obese persons maintain a weight loss of greater than 50% of excess weight 5 years after surgery; this exceeds the success of any other treatment.

Considerations During Pregnancy

Among pregnant women, 20% are more than 120% over ideal weight for height and 5% are over 150% of ideal weight for height. Complications of pregnancy such as hypertension, diabetes mellitus, and urinary tract infection, but not anemia, are increased in the obese woman, and the greater the obesity, the higher the risk. The risk of developing gestational diabetes in the severely obese woman is four or more times greater than in the nonobese woman, and the risk of developing all forms of diabetes in pregnancy is more than six times greater. Obese pregnant patients are more likely to have subnormal weight gain, a primary cesarean section, macrosomic infants, and higher morbidity with premature infants.

Maternal obesity had no major effect on neonatal death rates. However, obese mothers with antenatal complications had a neonatal mortality rate three times that of nonobese mothers with antenatal complications. The offspring of obese mothers are more likely to be obese; this has been related to decreased total energy expenditure, not to increased food consumption.

BINGE EATING DISORDER

Estimates of the prevalence of "moderate" binge eating range from 23% to 87%. Some of these obese bingers may be carbohydrate cravers who display a high demand for carbohydrate because of its ultimate action on brain neurotransmitter metabolism. Such persons are described as having more rigid and extreme dieting attitudes and substantial psychological distress. Several studies conducted before the development of the new DSM-IV research criteria (Table 157-4) indicated that obese bingers had less psychopathology and dietary restraint than did patients with bulimia nervosa. Obese binge eaters, as compared to obese nonbingers, had greater lifetime rates of affective disorder and more often had histrionic, borderline, or avoidant personality disorders. This is an active research area.

BIBLIOGRAPHY

American Psychiatric Association. Diagnostic and statistical manual of mental disorders, 4th ed. Washington DC: American Psychiatric Association, 1994:539.

Bachrach LK, Guido D, Katzman D, Litt IF, Marcus R. Decrea density in adolescent girls with anorexia nervosa. P 1990;86:440.

Bjorntorp P, Brodoff BN, eds. Obesity. New York: JB Lippincott, 1992.

Brownell KD, Foreyt JP, eds. Handbook of eating disorders: physiology, psychology, and treatment of obesity, anorexia, and bulimia. New York: Basic Books, 1986.

Brownell KD, Rodin J. Medical, metabolic, and psychological effects of weight cycling. Arch Intern Med 1994;154:1325.

Garbaciak JA, Richter M, Miller S. Maternal weight and pregnancy complications. Am J Obstet Gynecol 1985;152:238.

Garrow JS. Drugs for the treatment of obesity: what do we need? Pharmaceutical Med 1990;4:213.

Guy-Grand B, Apfelbaum M, Crepaldi G, Gries A, Lefebvre P, Turner P. International trial of long-term dexfenfluramine in obesity. Lancet 1989;2:1142.

Hatsukami DK, Mitchell JE, Eckert ED. Eating disorders: a variant of mood disorders? Psychiatr Clin North Am 1984;7:349.

Hudson JL, Pope HG, Jonas JM. Treatment of bulimia with antidepressants: theoretical considerations and clinical findings. In: Stunkard AJ, Stellar E, eds. Eating and its disorders. Research Publications: Association for Research in Nervous and Mental Disease, vol. 62. New York: Raven Press, 1984:259.

Marcus MD, Wing RR, Ewing L, Kern E, Gooding W, McDermott M. Psychiatric disorders among obese binge eaters. Int J Eating Disord 1990;9:69.

Newman MM, Halmi KA. The endocrinology of anorexia nervosa and bulimia nervosa. Endocrinol Metabol Clin North Am 1988;17(1):195.

Schneider LH, Cooper SJ, Halmi KA, eds. The psychobiology of human eating disorders: preclinical and clinical perspectives. Annals of the New York Academy of Sciences, vol. 575. New York: New York Academy of Sciences, 1989.

VanItallie TB, Lew EA. Overweight and underweight. In: Lew EA, Gajewski J, eds. Medical risks: trends in mortality by age and time elapsed. New York: Praeger, 1990.

Primary Care for Women, edited by Phyllis C. Leppert and Fred M. Howard. Lippincott-Raven Publishers, Philadelphia © 1997.

158
Chronic Pain

GILBERT P. PROPER
AJAI K. NEMANI

One in five people suffers from some type of chronic pain. Pain is second only to the common cold as a cause for a visit to the doctor. As the life expectancy of the general population increases, so too does the number of patients with arthritis, osteoporosis, and other painful conditions. Unfortunately, the health care system's ability and desire to treat these persons remain inadequate for several reasons. First, pain is a subjective experience that cannot be assessed by standard means. This is unnerving to health care professionals, who need measurable endpoints to justify their treatment. Second, the belief that pain is an inevitable part of aging inhibits the proper care of the elderly. Third, the fear of addiction, on the part of the physician, nurse, and patient, serves as a major deterrent. The system must get better at initiating and sustaining adequate pain management.

The most common pain problems affect men and women equally, so this chapter concentrates on this non–gender-specific information.

DEFINITIONS

A popular definition of pain is one by the International Association for the Study of Pain: "an unpleasant sensory and emotional experience associated with actual or potential tissue damage, or described in terms of such damage." This definition recognizes both the physiologic and psychological aspects of pain. In other words, pain is not purely a physical experience; rather, it is influenced profoundly by the sufferer's psychological state.

Pain can further be defined based on chronicity. Acute pain (eg, traumatic, postsurgical) usually coincides with new or ongoing tissue injury. It is associated with signs of sympathetic nervous system hyperactivity (eg, tachycardia, hypertension, diaphoresis) and outward signs of distress. It usually resolves within a specific time. If pain from a specific cause lasts longer than expected, then it becomes chronic. Chronic pain is not usually associated with ongoing tissue injury or with signs of sympathetic nervous system hyperactivity. In fact, patients often appear stoic and listless and do not look like they are in pain. In general, the more chronic a pain problem becomes, the harder it is to treat.

Pain can also be classified according to etiology. The three main categories are somatic, visceral, and neuropathic. Somatic pain originates from bone, skin, ligaments, and muscle. It is well localized, aching, gnawing, and throbbing, and responsive to treatment with opioids and nonsteroidal antiinflammatory drugs (NSAIDs). Visceral pain originates from the internal organs and is initiated by stimuli such as distension, traction, and ischemia. It is poorly localized and deep and aching, and it often radiates to the back. Examples include the pain associated with cholecystitis and bowel obstruction. It is usually responsive to treatment with opioids. Neuropathic pain stems from injury to the central or peripheral nervous system. It is burning, shooting, and stabbing. Examples include postherpetic neuralgia and diabetic neuropathy. It may respond to treatment with adjuvant medications (eg, antidepressants, anticonvulsants, sodium-channel blocking drugs) but is much less responsive to treatment with opioids. Most chronic pain problems are a combination of these etiologies.

The evaluation of a patient with chronic pain includes a pain history, physical examination, diagnostic studies, and assessment of psychological issues (eg, quality of life, presence or absence of depression).

HISTORY

The important aspects of a pain history are as follows:

- Primary and secondary pain site or sites
- Duration and evolution
- Pain radiation pattern
- Pattern (constant, intermittent)
- Quality (achy, burning, sharp)
- Exacerbating and relieving factors
- Neurologic abnormalities
- Vasomotor changes
- Analgesic history
- Past treatment history
- Effect on quality of life
- Past medical history.

The duration of pain helps define the chronicity, which helps determine the responsiveness to treatment (longer duration usually means less responsiveness). The site of pain and the presence or absence of radiating symptoms help define its etiology or anatomic origin. The quality of pain allows classification as somatic, visceral, or neuropathic and suggests specific treatment. The pain pattern and exacerbating and relieving factors may suggest an underlying mechanism, as well as treatment options. The presence of neurologic and vasomotor changes helps pinpoint an etiology and may alert the physician to possible emergent situations (eg, spinal cord compression). Analgesic use (past and present), including information on efficacy and side effects, helps form a basis for treatment. The effect the pain has on the patient's quality of life provides information regarding the degree of disability and psychological state.

PHYSICAL EXAMINATION

The physical examination should be tailored to the specific pain problem. The physician should observe the patient's physical appearance (eg, cleanliness, body weight); gait (eg, limp); presence of canes or splints; ease of sitting and standing; presence of scars, bruising, or deformities; skin color and texture changes; and hair and nail growth changes. The physician should also examine the area of pain and surrounding areas, checking for referred pain. This should include a complete musculoskeletal and neurologic examination. It is important to compare the affected side with the unaffected side.

The psychological evaluation often includes the use of specific questionnaires, in addition to a clinical interview. The McGill Pain Questionnaire evaluates the sensory, affective, and evaluative dimensions of pain. The Minnesota Multiphasic Personality Interview assesses personality factors contributing to chronic pain (eg, depression, anxiety, hysteria). The overall evaluation assesses the behavioral response to pain, adjustments to pain and disability, possible secondary gain issues, and personal motivation.

LABORATORY AND IMAGING STUDIES

Laboratory tests are usually nonspecific and of very limited use. Plain radiography is useful in assessing the gross structural integrity of a specific area, but has limited value in evaluating most low back pain conditions (for which it is commonly used). Computed tomography and magnetic resonance imaging demonstrate anatomic and structural abnormalities and are useful in evaluating most chronic pain conditions (eg, low back pain, abdominal pain, headache, cancer pain). Bone scanning is useful in evaluating patients with bone or joint pain (eg, arthritis, metastatic cancer to bone). Myelography is useful in evaluating low back pain, with disc herniation and nerve root compression as possible etiologies. Electrodiagnostic studies (nerve conduction studies, needle electromyographic studies) are useful in assessing pain of possible neuropathic etiology.

TREATMENT

The wide variety of treatment modalities for pain can be divided into pharmacologic, psychological, and physical therapies as the noninvasive techniques, and blocks, regional anesthesia, spinal cord and nerve stimulation, neuroablative procedures, and radiation and chemotherapy as the invasive techniques.

Medication management for pain dates back many centuries and cultures with the use of extracts from the poppy plant, now commonly called opium. Hence, the term *opioids* is given to pharmacologic agents with properties similar to those of opium. Opioids produce their effects by binding to specific opioid receptors in the encephalon and spinal cord. Four receptors are responsible for the effects and side effects: mu, kappa, delta, and sigma. Mu agonism produces supraspinal analgesia, euphoria, respiratory depression, and physical dependence. Kappa agonism mediates spinal analgesia, miosis, and sedation. Delta receptors mediate analgesia and enhance mu analgesia. Sigma receptors are responsible for dysphasia, hallucinations, and stimulation of the respiratory and vasomotor centers.

Opioids are divided into agonists and agonist/antagonists. Some of the common side effects for the opioids may be beneficial or detrimental. There is a great variance from patient to patient and opioid to opioid in the same patient, and this must be considered when prescribing these agents.

Generalized CNS sedation, confusion, unsteadiness, and euphoria are usually seen in the first few days of therapy but then clear. If persistent, amphetamines may help, as well as decreasing the dose and increasing the frequency of administration. Constipation, the most common side effect, should be treated prophylactically because of the serious problem of frank bowel obstruction. Nausea and vomiting are also common but can be treated with antiemetics, prochlorperazine, or haloperidol. Other options are switching to another opioid or another route of administration (rectal, intramuscular, transdermal, intravenous, subcutaneous, or neuraxial) if nausea and vomiting are severe. Pruritus, which is uncommon, can be treated with small doses of naloxone or nalbuphine.

Tolerance and physical and psychological dependence are distinct phenomena and should be discussed with the patient before beginning long-term opioid therapy. Tolerance is a normal pharmacologic response that may be seen to different degrees in patients receiving chronic opioid therapy. Patients usually complain of a decreased degree or duration of pain relief with the same dose of opioid. This is treated by increasing the dose or frequency of the opioid. Cross-tolerance among the opioids is not complete, so switching to an equianalgesic dose of another opioid may provide greater relief. Physical dependence refers to the development of withdrawal symptoms with sudden and complete cessation of the drug. Symptoms usually start about 12 hours after the last dose and peak at 48 to 72 hours. It is rarely life-threatening but can be prevented by decreasing the opioid dose by 15% to 20% daily. Psychological dependence or addiction is characterized by use and drug-seeking behavior for effects other than pain relief. In cancer therapy, this is rarely a problem, and in terminally ill patients who require therapy until death, this should not be considered.

Another large group of pharmacologic agents includes the NSAIDs and acetaminophen. The general mechanism of action both centrally and peripherally is mediated through decreased synthesis and release of prostaglandins. There is an unpredictable variability of response. Therefore, a patient who does not respond to a maximum dose of one agent can be switched to another agent of a different class. Because NSAIDs firmly bind to plasma proteins, care must be taken with concomitant administration of oral anticoagulants, hypoglycemic agents, phenytoin, sulfonamides, and methotrexate. Other considerations are elevated lithium levels; a decrease in the effect of β-blockers, captopril, and thiazides; and a decrease in natriuresis with loop diuretics.

Gastrointestinal disturbances are also mediated through prostaglandin inhibition, but complaints of dyspepsia do not correlate with objective endoscopic findings, which generally are positive in 2% to 5% of patients. Renal side effects, including acute renal insufficiency, are more likely in patients with congestive heart failure, systemic lupus erythematosus, chronic glomerulonephropathy, liver failure with ascites, premature birth, or diuretic use.

The other pharmacologic agents are usually classified as adjuvant analgesics. These include tricyclic antidepressants, anticonvulsants, neuroleptics, sodium channel blocker (mexiletine), γ-aminobutyric acid agonist (baclofen), muscle relaxants, and substance P depleter (capsaicin).

Tricyclic antidepressants have proven useful in neuropathic and myofascial pain. Their effect is probably related to an increased concentration of monoamines in the synapses of descending inhibitory pathways in the CNS. The major side effects are sedative and anticholinergic.

Anticonvulsants are useful for neuropathic pain with a lancinating quality. Carbamazepine and phenytoin have long been used, but valproic acid and clonazepam may also be useful, especially when the other two are not tolerated. Side effects include sedation, confusion, nausea, diplopia, vertigo, liver toxicity, and bone marrow suppression. A complete blood count should be done and liver function tests monitored with carbamazepine use.

Baclofen has been used mainly in the treatment of spasticity. It has been used for pain associated with spasticity but also may help with certain neuropathic pain states such as trigeminal neuralgia. Side effects include drowsiness, confusion, dizziness, nausea, and hypotension.

Mexiletine is an antiarrhythmic that decreases pain associated with diabetic neuropathy. It is also used to treat other neuropathic pain states with lancinating and dysesthetic qualities. Side effects include CNS and gastrointestinal disturbances and arrhythmias.

Capsaicin, applied topically to painful areas, decreases substance P and reduces chemically induced pain as well as pain associated with postherpetic neuralgia. Problems include local burning and the need for frequent applications for at least 3 to 4 weeks before any effect is perceived.

Other agents to consider include benzodiazepines, clonidine, neuroleptics, and combination therapy such as antidepressants and neuroleptics.

Psychological management for pain is directed at patient education and interactions between the patient and the environment. Goals of contingency management include decreasing the use of pain medications, increasing physical activity levels, decreasing pain behaviors, encouraging activities and work, and modifying responses of family members and friends to pain behaviors. Behavioral therapy includes cognitive restructuring, coping skills training, relaxation training, imagery, and biofeedback. Success depends on patient participation and lack of or reduction of secondary gains for the pain behavior.

Physiotherapy is an important tool in the management of chronic pain, including musculoskeletal disorders, myofascial pain, and sympathetically maintained pain (SMP). Activities include exercise, passive joint movement, and application of heat, cold, ultrasound, massage, and transelectrical nerve stimulation (TENS). More invasive therapy ranges from local and regional anesthesia with local anesthetics and steroids to surgery to neurodestructive procedures.

COMMON PAIN PROBLEMS

Low Back Pain

Low back pain (LBP) and sciatica are common complaints: the lifetime prevalence is estimated to be 60% to 80%, with an annual incidence of around 5%. The cost to society depends on many factors, including direct costs (eg, evaluation and treatment) and indirect costs (eg, lost earnings). A conservative estimate would be $25 billion for direct costs and $75 to $100 billion for indirect costs annually. Three quarters of these costs are attributed to the 5% of people who become disabled (either temporarily or permanently) from back pain.

Most patients who present with LBP have an uncomplicated cause for their pain, with resolution of symptoms within 8 weeks with conservative therapy. A few patients have an underlying medical disorder, and others have a life-threatening disease. If patients fail conservative therapy with controlled physical activity and nonnarcotic analgesics, a medical cause should be sought.

A wide variety of rheumatologic diseases, infections, tumors (both primary and metastatic), endocrinologic and metabolic disorders, and hematologic disorders of the lumbosacral spine may cause LBP. There are also referred causes, as from renal colic, cholangitis, and pancreatitis.

The work-up depends on associated symptoms such as fever, weight loss, localized bone pain, viscerogenic pain, or pain with recumbency. Most work-ups start with plain x-rays of the affected area and may progress to bone scans, computed tomography, magnetic resonance imaging, and hematologic tests such as erythrocyte sedimentation rate, chemistry profile, and complete blood count, depending on the symptoms described and associated findings.

Another possibility to consider, especially with a nondiagnostic work-up, is a psychosocial component. This is an important factor when disability (temporary or permanent) is involved.

The approach to a patient with chronic LBP should be conservative and multidisciplinary. Candidates for more invasive therapy must be selected carefully, based on a specific diagnosis.

Treatment goals for chronic LBP, when a definitive diagnosis cannot be made, should be to reduce (as opposed to eliminate) pain, to decrease disability, and to improve function. This requires extensive therapy, with each modality contributing a percentage toward the goals. Improvement requires an active, persistent patient who will comply with a multitude of recommendations.

The goal of medication management is to use the minimum effective dose, especially when the drug in question may be habit-forming. NSAIDs are widely used because of their availability, general safety, and nonaddictive nature. They play a role because inflammation is usually a part of the problem with chronic LBP. They must be given on a time-contingency basis, not on an as-needed basis. Tricyclic antidepressants are also used concurrently or alone. They help decrease pain and may also help return the patient to a normal sleep cycle because of their sedative effect.

The role of nerve blocks in the management of chronic LBP is unclear: there are conflicting reports as to their efficacy. Their role should be only a part of a comprehensive treatment plan, because alone they have little chance of providing long-term pain relief. Most nerve blocks are performed with a corticosteroid deposited at the site of presumed pathology or inflammation, such as the epidural space, sacroiliac joint, or facet joints. The advantages to nerve blocks are ease of administration and a relatively low risk in experienced hands.

Physical therapy plays an important role in management. Many LBP patients are deconditioned, and a structured, active physical therapy program helps increase mobility, range of motion, and endurance. TENS involves the application of controlled low-voltage electrical impulses over painful areas. The effect is probably due to the gate control theory of pain (which states, in short, that pain is transmitted by small-diameter nerves and can be prevented from ascending the dorsal horn to higher centers by stimulating a larger-diameter nerve).

Dorsal column stimulation as a technique for relieving pain is also based on the gate control theory. An electrode is percutaneously placed into the epidural space, and electrical stimulation of the appropriate spinal levels replaces painful sensations in the affected dermatomes with rather pleasant paresthesias. It can be helpful for deafferentation pain, peripheral nerve or radicular injuries, ischemic pain, postherpetic neuralgia, and reflex sympathetic dystrophy. Long-term follow-up shows a success rate of 25% to 40%.

Rehabilitation therapy is designed to return a patient to a functional and productive level. Work hardening programs that have a structured environment and work site simulation and vocational rehabilitation have proven useful in returning patients to employment.

Psychological intervention is exceptionally well suited for these patients. It also gives them an opportunity to play an active role in the management of their pain and promotes independence.

Myofascial Pain Syndrome

Myofascial dysfunction is a common cause of disability and pain. The clinical presentation of myofascial pain (MP) involves regional or diffuse, steady, aching muscle pain and tenderness. It is often associated with reflex muscle spasms, morning stiffness, decreased range of motion, and autonomic dysfunction. The most common cause of MP is trauma to myofascial structures and muscle overload (eg, sprains, strains). Classically, MP is associated with the presence of trigger points, which are well-localized, painful, nodular areas within muscle and surrounding connective tissue. These are exquisitely tender and can be associated with specific referred pain patterns. MP can often mimic the pain of nerve impingement, such as cervical disc disease. The most common areas for MP are the neck, shoulders, hips, and lumbar region. There are usually no radiologic or laboratory abnormalities associated with MP.

Treatment goals include decreasing pain to a tolerable level, improving function, and preventing disability. The most important treatment involves physical therapy and rehabilitation. These modalities are intended to maintain range of motion, reduce muscle spasm, and interrupt the self-perpetuating cycle of pain, spasm, and disuse. Adjuvant treatments, such as medications, nerve blocks, and psychological methods, are often used to facilitate physical therapy. Medications include NSAIDs to decrease inflammation, muscle relaxants to decrease muscle spasms, and antidepressants to improve sleep and to provide an analgesic effect. Trigger point injection involves penetrating the trigger point with a needle and injecting saline or local anesthetic (alone or in combination with steroids). Repeated injections are usually required. Psychological therapy (eg, behavioral modification, biofeedback) may also provide relief.

Neuropathic Pain

Neuropathic pain is perceived after damage to the central or peripheral nervous system. It may persist for months to years, or even permanently. Diseases or injuries associated with small-fiber axonal injury are associated with a higher incidence of pain (eg, diabetic neuropathy). Other examples of neuropathic pain include postherpetic neuralgia, causalgia, reflex sympathetic dystrophy, SMP, central pain, and ischemic neuropathy. Certain chemicals, chemotherapy, and radiation treatment are associated with neuropathic pain.

Patients typically have dysesthesia or an unpleasant abnormal sensation, whether spontaneous or provoked, and complain that the pain has a burning or electrical quality. Pain may be felt in an area that has sensory deficit. Patients may also describe the pain as a shooting sensation or as if a bolt of electricity were traveling through them. They often have allodynia, a painful response to a nonpainful stimulus. It may be painful to wear clothing or have the bedsheets drawn over the painful area.

On physical examination, there may be cutaneous vasomotor changes when compared with the contralateral side. Vasomotor changes of long duration may lead to changes in the nails, skin, and body hair in the affected area. There may be a decrease in or loss of sensory and motor innervation from nerve damage. Electromyography, nerve conduction velocity tests, plain films (demineralization), and bone scans may be helpful.

Neuropathic pain syndromes are difficult to treat: complete relief is the exception rather than the rule. All treatment modalities are usually tried in the hope of finding partial relief. The underlying problem should be removed or corrected if possible. NSAIDs and opioids may be tried but usually do not have a good response. Tricyclic antidepressants and mexiletine are more helpful for the burning pain; anticonvulsants, baclofen, and clonazepam are more helpful for the lancinating pain. Secondary drugs to consider are antipsychotics, clonidine, and capsaicin. Anesthetic interventions range from local and regional blocks to neurolytic procedures. SMP may respond to repeated sympathetic blocks. Physical therapy, TENS, and psychological therapy (eg, biofeedback, relaxation training, behavioral therapy) can be helpful, especially because maintaining function is as much of a goal as pain relief.

Sympathetically Maintained Pain

About 10% of patients seen in pain management centers have SMP, which is characterized by pain and vasomotor and neurologic changes in an extremity. Such changes are mediated by the sympathetic nervous system and usually occur after a traumatic event such as a fracture or surgery. The major subsets of SMP are reflex sympathetic dystrophy, which involves tissue but not specific nerve injury, and causalgia, which involves nerve or nerve trunk injury.

Possible etiologies include sympathetically mediated sensitization of low-threshold mechanoreceptors in the periphery, which sensitize wide-dynamic-range neurons in the dorsal horn, sending abnormally processed pain messages to the CNS. Also, α_1-adrenergic receptors may serve as a link between sympathetic and somatic neurons in the periphery, thereby mediating SMP. Finally, there may be a release of a sympathotrophic factor in the periphery, causing pain.

SMP is characterized by pain out of proportion to the injury and is often described as burning and hyperesthetic (exquisite sensitivity to normal stimulation). It is divided into three stages. The acute phase is characterized by hyperesthesia, burning pain, increased blood flow, warmth, increased hair and nail growth, and rubor. The second stage, the dystrophic phase, is characterized by burning pain, hyperesthesia, decreased blood flow, coolness, sweating, decreased hair and nail growth, edema, and cyanosis. The third stage, the atrophic phase, is characterized by the above changes along with atrophic skin, osteoporosis, muscle wasting, and decreased range of motion. The earlier treatment is started, the better the outcome.

Treatment consists of a combination of sympathetic nerve blocks, which interrupt the SMP cycle, adjuvant medications, physical therapy, and psychological/behavioral therapy. Sympathetic nerve blocks consist of stellate ganglion blocks for upper extremity pain and lumbar sympathetic blocks for lower extremity pain. Usually, a diagnostic block is performed first, followed by a series of blocks. Chemical or surgical sympathectomy can be performed in an attempt to obtain prolonged improvement. Medications consist of NSAIDs, oral steroids, antidepressants, vasodilators (calcium channel blockers, α_1-antagonists), and anticonvulsants. Opioids are an option after more conservative measures have been exhausted. Physical therapy and rehabilitation are important in the overall treatment plan, and psychological therapy (eg, behavioral modification, biofeedback) is also helpful. Some neurostimulation techniques (dorsal column stimulation) and implanted neuraxial opioid pumps are sometimes useful.

Headache

Headache is an almost universal complaint. The International Headache Society has developed a widely accepted classification of headache disorders. Clinically, there is much overlap.

Migraine headaches occur periodically and are separated by pain-free intervals. They affect women more than men and are usually unilateral, localized to the temporal or parietal region. They may occur on a different side with each attack, or switch sides during an attack. They are throbbing and incapacitating, and sometimes are associated with gastrointestinal (nausea and vomiting) and neurologic (photophobia, paresthesias) disturbances.

Cluster headaches primarily affect males, with pain lasting from 15 minutes to 2 hours. They occur daily for 2 weeks to 2 months. If the disorder is episodic, the patient then experiences a remission lasting 6 or more months; if it is chronic, the patient fails to experience a remission of more than 2 weeks during a 6-month period. The pain is intense, burning, and boring in the eye and frontotemporal region, is always unilateral, and always involves the same side of the head. Associated symptoms include tearing, flushing, rhinorrhea, and a partial Horner syndrome.

Tension headaches affect most people at some point. The pain is often described as a tight band around the head, and neck soreness and tightness are often present. This headache is usually worse in the early morning, late afternoon, and evening and is often associated with chronic anxiety and stress. Associated symptoms are usually absent.

Therapy can be divided into abortive (for each attack) and prophylactic. Abortive therapy for migraines includes ergot derivatives (eg, ergotamine), serotonin receptor agonists (eg, sumatriptan), and NSAIDs. Prophylactic migraine therapy includes methysergide, β-blockers, calcium channel blockers, antidepressants, NSAIDs, and valproic acid. For cluster headaches, abortive therapy consists of ergotamine preparations and NSAIDs. Prophylactic therapy includes ergotamine, methysergide, prednisone, lithium carbonate, and calcium channel blockers. For tension headaches, abortive therapy includes using OTC analgesics (eg, aspirin, acetaminophen) and prescription analgesics (eg, NSAIDs, opioids). Prophylactic therapy includes the use of NSAIDs and antidepressants.

Cancer Pain

Overall, about half of patients with cancer have pain, and three fourths of patients with advanced or terminal disease have pain. The pain is usually caused by direct tumor infiltration, either of bone or nerve. Other causes can be secondary to cancer therapy. The leading cause is bone pain from tumor invasion, either primary or metastatic. Therapy must be individualized, depending on the patient's life expectancy, the type of pain, medical feasibility, and the wishes of the patient and family.

Management of cancer pain can be divided into anticancer therapy, medications, neuroablative procedures, and psychological therapy.

Anticancer therapy includes tumor debulking, radiation therapy, and chemotherapy. Radiation therapy is especially useful for bone pain. When anticancer therapy has been exhausted or is not feasible, the next step usually involves trials of medications. Medication management includes nonopioid analgesics, adjuvant drugs, and opioids. NSAIDs are helpful in the management of weak or mild pain and pain associated with bony involvement. Adjuvant analgesics such as tricyclic antidepressants, anticonvulsants, and other membrane stabilizers such as clonazepam and mexiletine, stimulants, and phenothiazines may enhance opioid analgesia or counteract their side effects. They also play a role in pain management on their own, especially with neuropathic pain.

Opioids are especially helpful for moderate to severe pain. A great advantage with opioids is the flexibility as to route of administration. When oral therapy is impossible, rectal, intravenous, intramuscular, and subcutaneous therapy can be instituted. Continuous infusion by a subcutaneous or intravenous route provides constant plasma levels, and newer devices allow the patient to self-administer bolus doses. This can be done in the hospital or at home. Opioids can also be administered epidurally or intrathecally, on a short-term or long-term basis, depending on the delivery system used.

Other conservative therapies to consider include TENS, biofeedback, relaxation training, and hypnosis.

Neurodestructive procedures should be saved for patients who fail conservative therapy. These include injection of alcohol or phenol peripherally, intrathecally, or epidurally to cause chemolysis of nerves. Other procedures include cordotomy and rhizotomy, thermocoagulation, and dorsal root entry zone interruption. Other invasive procedures include hypophysectomy, deep brain stimulation, and dorsal column stimulation.

Pain and Pregnancy

The most common nonobstetric areas of pain associated with pregnancy are LBP and carpal tunnel syndrome. LBP results from mechanical causes such as hyperextension of the lumbar spine, uterine compression on the pelvic wall, relaxation of the pelvic joints, weakening of abdominal muscular support, and discogenic pain with or without nerve root irritation. Due to the possibly deleterious effects of most adjuvant medications (including NSAIDs and antidepressants) on the fetus, treatment of LBP in pregnancy should mainly be supportive. It can usually be helped by abdominal and sacroiliac support (braces), increasing daily rest periods, passive physical therapy (eg, heat, massage, ultrasound, TENS), and mild analgesics (eg, acetaminophen, acetaminophen with codeine). Sometimes epidural steroid injections and trigger point injections are helpful. However, most back pain resolves after delivery.

Carpal tunnel syndrome occurs with increased frequency during pregnancy secondary to fluid retention, which leads to increased pressure on the median nerve within the carpal tunnel. This leads to increased pain in the median nerve distribution, especially at night. Therapy, again conservative, includes the use of wrist splints to immobilize the wrist, minimal use of diuretics on a periodic basis, or injection of a small amount of local steroid directly into the carpal tunnel. Surgical decompression is rarely required, as symptoms usually resolve with delivery.

BIBLIOGRAPHY

Ashburn MA, Lipman AG. Management of pain in the cancer patient. Anesth Analg 1993;76:402.

Bonica J, ed. The management of pain, 2d ed. Philadelphia: Lea & Febiger, 1990.

Diamond S, Freitag F. Treatment of headache. Clin J Pain 1989;5(supp. 2):S7.

Haynes DM. Course and conduct of normal pregnancy. In: Danforth DN, Dignam WJ, et al, eds. Obstetrics and gynecology, 4th ed. Philadelphia: Harper & Row, 1982:355.

Mathew NT, Sabiha A. The pathogenesis and treatment of headache disorders. Hospital Physician 1992:20.

McCowin PR, Borenstein D, Wiesel SW. The current approach to the medical diagnosis of low back pain. Orthop Clin North Am 1991;22:315.

Patt R, Balter K. Posttraumatic reflex sympathetic dystrophy: mechanisms and medical management. J Occup Rehab 1991;1(1):57.

Patt R, Smith JL, Greene D, Flannery M, Millard R. A practical guide to effective cancer pain management. National Cancer Institute, 1993.

Urowitz MB, Gladman BP. Rheumatic diseases. In: Burrow GN, Ferris TF, eds. Medical complications during pregnancy. Philadelphia: WB Saunders, 1982:489.

Wall PD, Melzack R, eds. Textbook of pain, 3d ed. New York: Churchill-Livingstone, 1994.

Walsh NE, Dumiru D, Ramamurthy J, Schoenfeld LS. Treatment of the patient with chronic pain. In: DeLisa JA, ed. Rehabilitation medicine: principles and practice. Philadelphia: JB Lippincott, 1993:973.

Primary Care for Women, edited by Phyllis C. Leppert and Fred M. Howard. Lippincott-Raven Publishers, Philadelphia © 1997.

159

Partner Abuse

ELIZABETH A. DELAHUNTA

Intrafamily violence is becoming acknowledged as a significant, widespread health problem. Family violence can be divided into child abuse, elder abuse, sexual abuse or rape, and spouse or partner abuse. Although lagging behind child abuse, partner abuse is gaining recognition by the medical community. Multiple medical societies are giving a medical perspective to health-related issues resulting from abusive relationships.

Partner abuse occurs between two persons involved in an intimate relationship (dating, cohabitating, or marriage), either heterosexual or homosexual. The violence may be actual or threatened. There is a repetitive pattern of coercive behavior in which one partner's basic rights are unacknowledged. This behavior may include physical, sexual, verbal, or emotional abuse.

HISTORICAL PERSPECTIVE

Children and wives have been regarded as property in many cultures since the beginning of recorded time (Table 159-1). Beatings were condoned as corrective discipline; this abuse was perceived as a necessary form of physical chastisement to maintain family order, as deemed appropriate by the man of the house. The Laws of Hammurabi, written in Babylon in 2000 BC, include the first recorded sanctioning of wife abuse (Table 159-2). Egyptian evidence from paleopathologists revealed that female mummies had more fractures than male mummies, despite the fact that men were the warriors of that society. These fractures of female mummies, primarily skull fractures, were presumed to have been inflicted during domestic disputes. A medieval scholar in the 15th century stated that it was better to damage the body and save the soul than vice versa, thereby condoning partner abuse. British common law placed some limitation on spouse abuse with the "rule of thumb," which allowed a man to beat his wife with a rod no bigger than his thumb. As recently as 1970 in Queens, New York, a woman named Kitty Genovese was murdered by her partner in full view of several neighbors; they failed to intervene on her behalf because they saw the incident as a private matter, not a crime. Until recently, the legal system enforced a "stitch rule" that recognized a complaint as valid only if a woman suffered serious or permanent injury, and only if the abuse was witnessed.

MAGNITUDE OF THE PROBLEM

In the United States, 12 to 15 million women have been physically abused at least once by a male partner. Battering has been declared the most common source of injury to women, more common than auto accidents, muggings, and rapes by a stranger combined. The vast majority of violence against women, including wife battering and sexual assault, is perpetrated by people known to the victim. Partner abuse costs billions of dollars each year. Medical costs include hospitalizations and emergency department and office visits; many of these encounters do not address the underlying abuse, perpetuating the violence. Other costs include absenteeism from work, police responses to incidents, legal interventions, social work involvement, damaged property, and relocation expenses.

ELEMENTS OF DOMESTIC VIOLENCE

The theme of all violent acts is the desire to obtain or retain power and control over another person. Many methods are used by the perpetrator, often without the awareness of anyone but the partner (Fig. 159-1). Psychological torture is often the most injurious over time. Isolation is effective because it alters the victim's perception of reality. With total control over what a woman can do, whom she sees and talks to, and where she goes, the victim soon begins to believe the reality that her partner projects.

Emotional abuse lowers a woman's self-esteem. By putting her down or making her feel bad about herself, calling her names, making her think she is crazy or playing mind games, a man can erode a woman's sense of worth. She is taught repeatedly by her partner that she is incompetent, immoral, unattractive, and unintelligent. She begins to believe that no one else could love her and that she needs her partner to navigate her life.

Economic abuse includes making her ask for money, giving her an allowance, taking her money, making her accountable for every penny spent, not permitting her to have a bank account or credit cards, not permitting her to be employed, and forcing her to sign joint tax returns without reviewing them.

Sexual abuse may involve making her do sexual things against her will, physically attacking the sexual parts of her body, treating her like a sex object, not permitting infection-control measures or birth control, and either not permitting her or forcing her to have an abortion.

Children are also used as an avenue to maintain power. A man may make a woman feel guilty about the children, use the children to give messages, or use visitation as a way to harass her.

Threats psychologically immobilize many women. Often a man makes or carries out threats to hurt a woman, her family, or her possessions: threats to take the children or harm them, to murder or harm the partner, to commit suicide, or to report her to welfare or immigration services are common.

Traditional thinking about male privilege within the home routinely exists. The woman may be treated like a servant, removed from any major decisions, and expected to act as if her partner is the "master of the castle." In the setting of loss of all other means of control and the resulting low self-esteem and fear, intimidation has a large foothold. Looks, actions, gestures, a loud voice, smashing things, and destroying her property readily convey to a woman that she must act as demanded by her partner or deal with the consequences. The threat of physical violence is always present and can lead to severe injury or death.

Table 159-1. Cultural Sayings

China: A bride received into the home is like a horse that you have just bought: you break her in by constantly mounting her and continually beating her.

Great Britain: A woman, an ass, and a walnut tree, bring the more fruit, the more beaten they be.

Italy: As both a good horse and a bad horse heed the spur, so both a good woman and a bad woman need the stick.

Nigeria: A woman is like a horse: he who can drive her is her master.

Poland: He who loves much beats hard.

Russia: A wife is not a pot; she will not break so easily.

United States (Benjamin Franklin): Love well, whip well.

SOCIOPSYCHOLOGICAL INDICATORS

The prototype of an abusive relationship includes previous exposure of both partners to violence in their childhood homes, forced social isolation of the female partner, greater perceived stress (eg, financial concerns, pregnancy), and substance abuse. Traditional views of marriage, family unity, and a commitment for life are common. Societal portrayal of a woman as a nurturer and caretaker with ultimate responsibility for the well-being of the family, even to the sacrifice of herself, is upheld. Marriage is recognized by the couple and their friends and family as the preferred social status for all women. In the event of separation, children are perceived as disadvantaged without both parents, despite previous disharmony within the home and long-term ill effects of exposure to violence.

Characteristics of Battered Women

Battered women cross all racial, religious, socioeconomic, age, and educational boundaries. A battered woman, as a child, was not infrequently portrayed as "Daddy's little girl." The woman often has limited life experience and few job skills, lacks self-esteem, and subscribes to the feminine sex role stereotype. Sex is a means to establish intimacy. She is financially dependent and fearful of rejection by her friends and family. She accepts personal responsibility for the batterer's actions, believing that her inadequacies create conflict. She believes that no one can help her resolve her predicament except herself. She suffers from guilt and may deny the terror and anger she feels. She appears passive to the world but has learned to manipulate her environment so she does not get killed. Severe stress reactions with psychophysiologic complaints develop over time. Unfortunate myths imply that battered women must be masochistic, asking for or provoking repeated batterings, or they would seek outside help and leave the relationship.

Table 159-2. Timeline: Sanctions of Abuse

2000 BC	Babylon, Laws of Hammurabi sanction wife abuse
1000 BC	Egyptian evidence, fracture incidence of female mummies greater than male mummies
15th century	Rules of Marriage
1768	British common law, "Rule of thumb"
1871	Rule of thumb denounced by Massachusetts Supreme Court
1874	Qualifier in North Carolina Supreme Court, "permanent injury ..."
1920	Laws sanctioning spouse abuse are repealed in United States
1960s	First modern reports of wife abuse
1970	Kitty Genovese incident
1971	First shelter for abused women, London

Characteristics of Batterers

Like battered women, batterers come from all racial, religious, socioeconomic, and educational backgrounds. Most are violent only with their partners and may be perceived as congenial in all other aspects of life ("Dr. Jekyll and Mr. Hyde"). The batterer does not necessarily suffer from mental illness. He seeks ultimate control over all components of his family life. The abuser is often an underachiever for his level of education, lacks self-confidence, and has difficulty with intimacy. He uses sex as an act of aggression. He believes in male supremacy and the stereotypic masculine role in the family. He is pathologically jealous without justification and may interrogate his partner until she admits imagined infidelity. He does not accept responsibility for his actions and blames his partner for contrived faults that incite his "justified" response. The batterer poorly controls his aggression. He has severe stress reactions, during which he may use alcohol and other substances along with partner-beating to cope. He does not believe he should suffer negative consequences for his actions and minimizes the extent of the violence. He continues to batter because he has learned that violence, or the threat of violence, maintains his power. Until recently, society has made little effort to end the cycle of violence and has condoned it with silence.

A typical abusive episode occurs in the home, often in the kitchen, during periods of greatest interpersonal interaction. Dinner time, evenings, weekends, and holidays are common. These episodes are rarely witnessed by persons outside the family.

BARRIERS TO IDENTIFICATION

There are significant barriers to the identification of partner abuse. Physicians may distance themselves from the problem to make themselves and their families appear less vulnerable. Some physicians still perceive partner abuse as a private matter in which medical personnel should not meddle. Sadly, some physicians advocate corporal punishment and cannot see partner abuse as a crime. Frustration may be high with a seemingly unchangeable problem and may create a false impression that medical efforts are too time-consuming and ultimately futile. There may be fear of entanglement in legal processes. Psychosocial problems appear complicated, and some physicians may feel powerless outside their area of expertise. Identifying partner abuse can be like opening Pandora's box: numerous, often unforeseen issues arise. To improve the identification of partner abuse, physicians must become knowledgeable about historical, physical, and circumstantial clues that lead to the recognition of a potentially abusive relationship.

PATIENT ASSESSMENT

The role of health care providers who evaluate women is primarily one of identification and acknowledgment of potential abuse. A high level of suspicion is essential. Women should be questioned

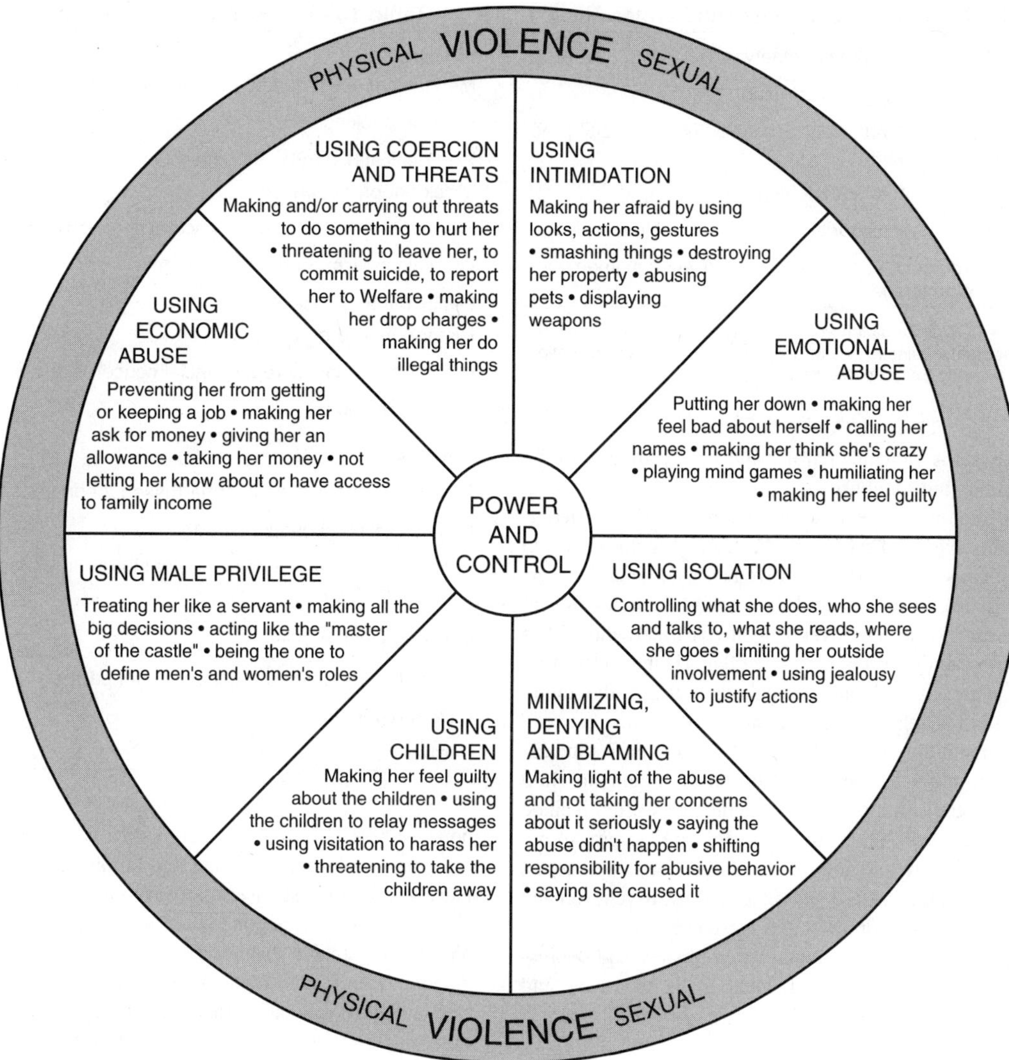

Figure 159-1. Power and control wheel delineates the forms of abuse that may be encountered in an abusive relationship. The central issue is the need for one partner to attain or maintain power and control in the relationship. The rim of the wheel portrays the presence of physical violence or the threat of physical violence as an ever-present element in an abusive relationship. Physicians may use this wheel to help their patients identify abusive aspects of personal relationships.

directly about the potential for domestic violence in their lives as part of any routine or emergency visit. A history must be conducted in a safe environment with a supportive attitude from all health care providers. Confidentiality is paramount.

Table 159-3 lists several misconceptions about partner abuse. One is that an injury is accidental unless proven otherwise. On the contrary, domestic violence must be addressed and excluded to avoid possibly grave consequences if not identified. Other misconceptions include the belief that injuries from abuse are always life-threatening; that alcohol, drugs, depression, or psychological problems cause domestic violence rather than result from domestic violence; and that victims are reluctant to accept help. Unfortunately, lack of acknowledgment of a battered woman's experience can lead to further battering and pathology. If not validated, the victim feels greater isolation and is less likely to pursue efforts to leave the batterer. Psychopathology, including chronic anxiety, and phobias may evolve. Substance abuse, low self-esteem, a sense of hopelessness, and posttraumatic stress disorder often emerge as a consequence (not a precipitant) of domestic violence. Also, the cycle of domestic violence is usually perpetuated and escalates if not interrupted. Therefore, medical providers should ask all women about the existence of domestic violence in their relationships.

In a medical setting, clues to domestic violence can be found in a structured interview. Interviewing should start with general questions that become more direct as needed to allow the patient to reveal her circumstances in a comfortable fashion (Table 159-4). When directly asked, many female trauma patients, across all socioeconomic classes, report domestic violence as the cause of their injuries. The interview must be conducted in a safe, confidential, caring, and nonjudgmental fashion. Victims of domestic violence expect health care providers to initiate discussions sur-

Table 159-3. Misconceptions Regarding Partner Abuse

Injuries are accidental unless proven otherwise.
Abusive injuries are typically life-threatening.
Alcoholism, drug abuse, depression, and other psychosocial problems are the cause of battering.
Abuse victims are reluctant to accept help.
Abuse is a problem of poor, minority, and unemployable people.
Abuse is a family problem that can be prevented when women learn to cope or parent more effectively.

(Flitcraft AH, Stark E. Woman battering, a prevention-oriented approach. In: The physician assistant's guide to health promotion and disease prevention. Atlanta: Emory University School of Medicine, 1986.)

rounding the abuse. A woman's partner and family should not be present when screening for abuse.

Signs and symptoms of the battering syndrome are as varied as the victims themselves. Indicators can be learned to improve the identification of abuse (Table 159-5). A woman who is fearful, nervous, jumpy, hesitant, or embarrassed should raise the index of suspicion for domestic violence. An overly attentive partner who wishes to be present for the entire encounter is a red flag. He may answer all questions for the patient (including personal data such as the timing of her last menses). A delay in presentation, inconsistency between the injury pattern and the explanation provided, and injuries indicative of trauma are clues to abusive relationships, similar to child abuse and elder abuse. Multiple current medications often include sedatives. Repeated presentations to the health care system, sometimes only discovered by a review of substantive medical records, often include recurrent injuries, depression, anxiety, psychosomatic complaints, chronic pain syndromes, and substance abuse.

Constant fear and low self-esteem lead to anxiety and depression. Many women become overwhelmed by helplessness and

Table 159-4. Interviewing Questions and Statements

1. Abuse and violence are epidemics in our society; therefore, we are asking all women about the possibility for abuse in their lives in addition to other health problems.
2. Please be assured that whatever you say will be kept confidential; if you are or have been abused, we would like to give you a chance to talk about it. I will not push you to do anything you do not want to do.
3. Are you (have you ever been) in a relationship with someone who has ever physically hurt or threatened you?
4. We all fight/disagree sometimes with the people we live with. When you disagree at home, are you ever afraid of what your partner might do to you, your children, or your possessions?
5. Has your partner threatened to kill you?
6. Does your partner ever try to control what you do, where you go, your money, or relationships with your family and friends?
7. Does your partner ever force you to engage in unwanted sex or sex that makes you feel uncomfortable?
8. Your injuries concern me. Injuries such as these are often caused by abuse. Could this be happening to you?
9. If you ever are abused, please come back.
10. We see many women who have been abused. Remember, help is available.

Table 159-5. High-Risk History for Partner Abuse

Incident
Mechanism described by patient does not fit injury
Delay in seeking care
Past Medical History
"Accident-prone" patient
Frequent health care visits (review past medical history)
Drug/alcoholism (partner or patient)
Family Circumstances
History of children being abused
High stress in family (eg, financial concerns, pregnancy)
Marital problems
Patient Affect
Patient evasive/guarded, embarrassed, depressed
Patient denies abuse too strongly
Patient minimizes injury or demonstrates inappropriate responses (cries, laughs)
Interaction With Partner
Patient has hypervigilant behavior with partner
Patient defers to partner
Partner hovers

hopelessness and become psychologically immobilized. Repressed rage may evolve into suicidal and homicidal ideation. Hypervigilance and startle responses may develop with stimuli as common as closing a door or someone entering the room. Sleep disturbances, nightmares, eating disturbances, fatigue on awakening, thought disorganization, and mood swings can be presentations of depression and posttraumatic stress disorder. Psychosomatic presentations include phobias, choking sensations, heart palpitations, numbness or tingling of the extremities, dizziness, and nervousness. Complaints of asthma exacerbations and allergies increase. Chronic pain syndromes most often involve headaches, gastrointestinal symptoms, and chest, pelvic, or back pain. A battered woman may complain of abuse directly; however, abusive episodes are sometimes disguised as falls or assaults by a stranger.

PHYSICAL EXAMINATION AND CLINICAL FINDINGS

The physical examination should be conducted with the patient privately. A high suspicion for abuse must exist in the mind of the examiner to avoid missing characteristic signs of abuse (Table 159-6). The pattern of injury may point to domestic violence. The victim may have injuries consistent with using a defensive posture, such as arms raised above the head. Central injuries to the face, head, neck, breasts, abdomen, and genitals are prevalent in domestic violence; accidental injuries, in contrast, normally affect the extremities. Victims of domestic violence are 13 times more likely to sustain injuries to the chest, breast, or abdomen compared with victims of accidents.

Most violence-related injuries are minor, although life-threatening injuries may result after escalating violence. The mechanisms of injury include punching, kicking, slapping, biting, choking, rape or sexual assault, smothering, attempted drowning, scalding, and using

Table 159-6. Typical Findings of Abuse

Central Injuries
Black eyes
Front teeth injuries
Mid-face injury
Neck injury
Breast/abdomen (particularly during pregnancy)
Miscarriage/vague gynecologic complaints (eg, pelvic pain)
Hidden Injuries
Injuries to hidden sites (covered by clothes)
Internal injuries
Defensive Injuries
Mid-arm injuries
Inconsistent Injuries
Injuries to areas not prone to injury by falls
Symmetric injuries
Old as well as new injuries
Injuries to multiple sites
Abusive Mechanism of Injury
Weapon injuries or marks
Strangulation marks
Bites/burns (scald, cigarette)

weapons. Some women report threatening actions and injuries by their partners driving motor vehicles. A pattern of multiple injuries (eg, contusions, lacerations, black eyes, concussions, joint dislocations, fractures, miscarriages) in varying stages of healing is highly suspicious.

LABORATORY AND IMAGING STUDIES

On initial presentation, further assessment of physical injuries should be pursued as with any similar injury from nonabusive circumstances. However, if abuse is identified, evaluation of psychosomatic complaints may be shortened in lieu of psychiatric evaluation and other interventions, as appropriate.

TREATMENT

Treatment must include both physical and emotional care. Referral to subspecialists may be indicated, based on the extent of physical injuries or the degree of psychopathology. However, all primary care physicians or physicians who see women with initial presentations need a basic level of knowledge and understanding of partner abuse to coordinate care, to advise of potential future treatment courses, and to counsel. Unfortunately, the current pattern of medical response often contributes to the battering syndrome. Nonetheless, battered women are most amenable to interventions in the medical setting, especially if they have presented with problems related to abuse. The mnemonic "SCRAPED" can assist health care providers to remember key elements of partner abuse for identification and treatment (Table 159-7).

Table 159-7. Mnemonic to Identify and Treat Partner Abuse

IDENTIFICATION	TREATMENT
S Screen	**S** Safety
C Central injuries	**C** Crime
R Repetitive injuries	**R** Referral
A Abuse (physical + psychological)	**A** Acknowledge abuse
P Possessive partner	**P** Protocols
E Explanation inconsistent	**E** Evidence collection
D Direct questions	**D** Documentation

A team approach is ideal in addressing and intervening in the problem of domestic violence. Prehospital personnel, physicians, nurses, social workers, mental health personnel, clergy, advocacy groups, law enforcement groups, and the legal profession can all contribute.

Mandatory reporting of partner abuse exists in many states. However, as an autonomous and competent adult, a woman can decide if she wishes to file a report with the police or seek legal action. A physician may educate and encourage a particular action but should respect and support the patient's decision. Reporting should be done only with the knowledge of the battered woman. Discussion of restraining orders and how to obtain them would be helpful. The woman is generally acutely aware of her situation and what action will maintain her safety and future options. Patient confidentiality must be observed in all instances.

When domestic violence is suspected, the victim's emotional status must be assessed. A battered woman may experience many sequelae of chronic victimization (eg, substance abuse, hopelessness, posttraumatic stress disorder). She may sense imminent doom and have constant apprehension. The clinician should determine what efforts she has made to cope with the violence and whether she can function at home or work.

The clinician must also assess the future risk to the victim and any children in the home. Without proper identification and intervention, the natural course for domestic violence is chronic battering with escalation over time. At the time of presentation, a woman may be at the greatest risk for serious physical impairment or even death, especially if separation from the partner is pursued. Safety issues must be addressed: 30% of women who were murdered in 1990 were killed by their husbands or boyfriends. Children in the home may also be at risk. Assessing the safety of a woman's environment and her need for alternate lodging is critical to prevent further injuries. Emergency shelters are available across the nation. Factors associated with potential lethality are listed in Table 159-8.

The need for legal assistance, referrals, and follow-up must be determined. Legal assistance and appropriate follow-up should be arranged. The victim may wish to pursue criminal or civil court procedures. A contact person should be identified and a phone

Table 159-8. Risk for Lethality

Escalation of violence
Children in the home
Batterer threatens to kill spouse
Presence of a weapon
Use of drugs and alcohol

(McLeer S. The role of the emergency physician in the prevention of domestic violence. Ann Emerg Med 1987;16:1155.)

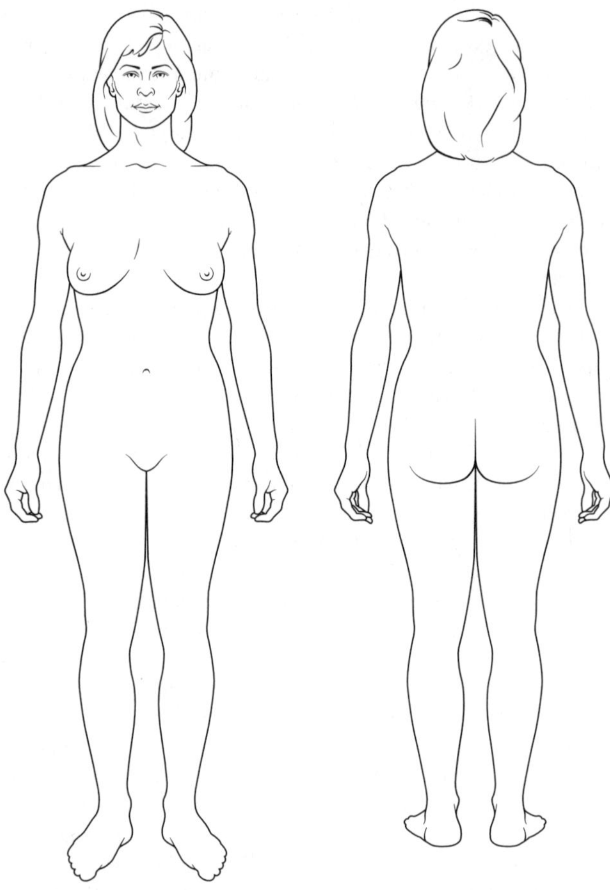

Figure 159-2. Body map. (McFarlane J, Parker B. Abuse during pregnancy: a protocol for prevention and intervention. White Plains, NY: March of Dimes Birth Defects Foundation, 1994.)

number provided. Shelters and other resources should be explained, even if these services are not used.

The physician must avoid blaming the victim and focusing on the woman and her presumed psychopathology. The physician must also avoid the frustration of expecting a single encounter to reverse years of victimization and learned helplessness. Simply recognizing and acknowledging the abuse moves a battered woman immeasurably forward. Options must be presented, but the physician must accept the woman's choice nonjudgmentally. Such acceptance may start to reverse years of low self-esteem and help her make her own informed decisions.

Medical conditions should be diagnosed and managed in the usual fashion. Medications, particularly tranquilizers, are discouraged, as they can erode the woman's ability to solve problems, serve as an advocate for herself, and seek help. Efforts to assist the woman to make substantive changes in her social situation and avoiding blame are integral parts of the health care plan.

Treatment plans that include couple or family counseling are usually unsuccessful and are extremely risky for the woman. Partner abuse is an issue of power and control, not a communication flaw.

Documentation of findings in the medical record establishes the credibility of a battered woman if she seeks legal aid. Repetitive trauma and frequent health-related visits are the usual pattern. Stating the history in the patient's words and using a body map to document injuries are helpful (Fig. 159-2) Photographs should be obtained, when indicated, as part of evidence collection. An objective opinion of any inconsistencies identified during the evaluation should be charted.

BATTERING CYCLE

The cycle of partner abuse includes three phases (Fig. 159-3). The first is a tension-building phase in which small incidents are portrayed as monumental inadequacies of the woman. The male partner becomes more volatile, but the woman accepts this behavior to avoid a more severe outburst. High anxiety in anticipation of imminent abuse causes the woman to "walk on eggshells." The second phase is an acute battering, which may cause serious injury or extreme fear. The third phase involves reconciliation. This "honeymoon" period is filled with remorse and apologies from the batterer and renewed hopefulness on the part of the victim that the abuse will cease. Nurturing attention by the batterer reaffirms the belief that the relationship is stable and enduring.

Why Women Stay

Women stay in abusive relationships for various reasons. There is an ever-present threat of escalating physical violence to herself and her children. The resulting fear is well substantiated by statistics showing that a woman's greatest risk is at the moment she attempts to leave an abusive relationship. There is no guarantee

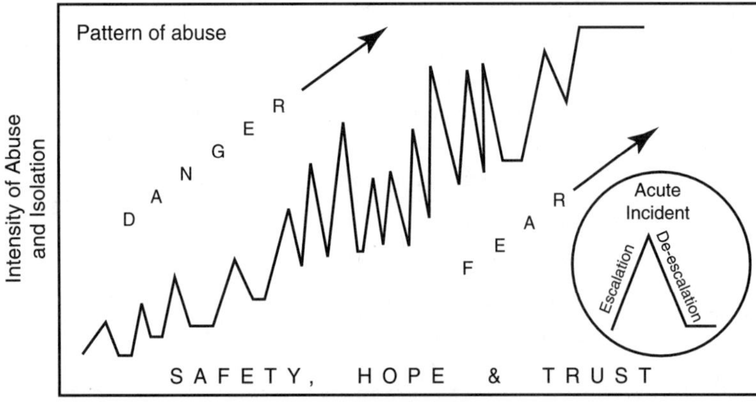

Figure 159-3. Pattern of abuse graph.

that the battering will cease. Any attempt by the woman to assume control over the relationship or life circumstances usually leads to escalation of the violence. She may see no alternative to her circumstances, as she may be without financial resources, alternate housing, or employment. Her dismal situation may still be preferable to the unknown. Immobilization, both physical and psychological, can be a reality. Having learned helplessness, many women cannot avail themselves of new possibilities, even when there are alternatives. Cultural, family, and religious values remind her that she has a duty to her partner and maintaining family unity. Previous experiences with law enforcement agencies may have reinforced the belief that only she can help herself. She accepts partial or complete responsibility for the difficulties in her household. An emotional attachment to the batterer may linger.

Psychological Evolution

A battered woman goes through several psychological stages as she attempts to understand her home situation. Initially, she denies the abuse and refuses to admit that she has been beaten or that there is a problem in the relationship. She offers excuses for her partner's violence and refers to the injuries as accidents. She believes that the violence will never happen again. She feels guilty and accepts the problem as her responsibility. She feels that she deserves to be beaten due to flaws in her character that incite her partner's violent actions. In time, a woman becomes enlightened that she no longer needs to assume responsibility for the battering. She recognizes that no one deserves to be beaten. However, she is still committed to the relationship and hopeful that things will work out. A traumatic bond may have formed in the setting of a power imbalance and the periodic nature of the abuse and nurturing. (Similar bonding has been described between hostages and their captors.) Many women overestimate the benefit of keeping the family unit intact.

Ultimately, the woman realizes and accepts that she cannot stop his violent behavior. She decides that she will no longer submit to his violence and that she can change her attitude about herself and start a new life. This process has a different time frame

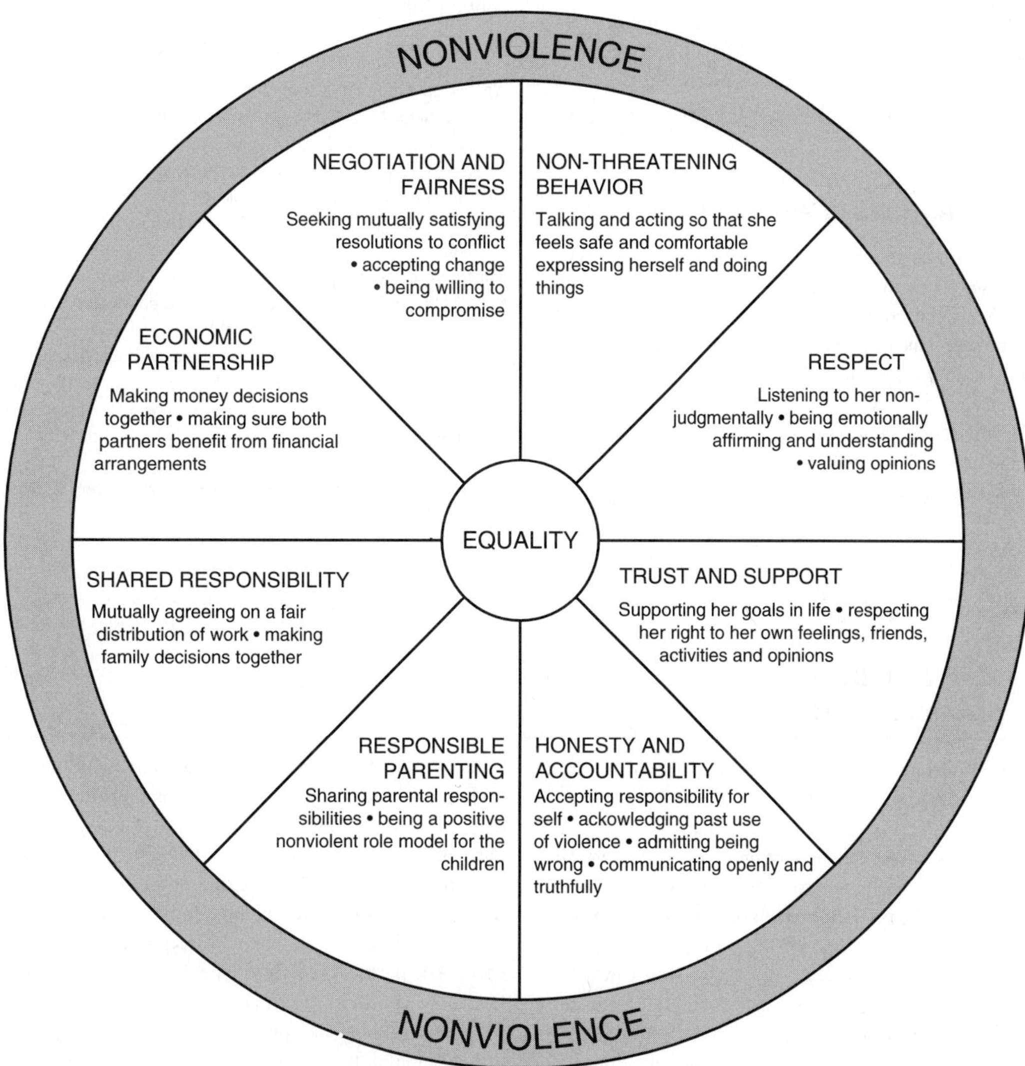

Figure 159-4. The equality wheel shows elements of a mutually supportive relationship. Nonviolent means of interrelating are incorporated into all aspects of the relationship. Physicians may use this wheel to educate their patients about more egalitarian interaction styles.

Table 159-9. Approach to Patients Who Are Victims of Abuse

Screen all women.
Identify abuse.
Validate experience.
Maintain confidentiality.
Report only with patient's knowledge.
Document objectively.
Empower the woman to make her own informed decisions.

for every woman. Most women return to the relationship and the batterer several times before successfully severing all ties. Often an impetus to leave is recognizing the ill effects the violence is having on the children or a recent escalation in the violence. At these moments, the reasons to leave become clearer. A woman sees the potential for safety from mental and physical abuse for herself and her children. She develops increased feelings of control over her life and independence. She can feel self-respect, self-confidence, and a sense of identity. Also, increased peace of mind ensues. Future relationships, ideally, are founded in equality (Fig. 159-4).

CONSIDERATIONS IN PREGNANCY

Partner abuse may occur for the first time or escalate during pregnancy. Physical abuse occurs in 37% of obstetric patients across all class, race, and educational boundaries. In the first 4 months and the last 5 months of pregnancy respectively, 154 per 1000 and 170 per 1000 pregnant women are assaulted by their partners. Morbidity and mortality during pregnancy caused by domestic violence include placental separation, antepartum hemorrhage, fetal fractures, rupture of the uterus, liver, or spleen, preterm labor and miscarriage, and low birthweight.

CONCLUSION

Partner abuse is an epidemic that cannot be ignored. Efforts must be made toward increasing identification of these victims and improving documentation on their behalf. All women must be assessed for possible victimization secondary to partner abuse. A standard approach is listed in Table 159-9. Proper identification and intervention can interrupt the cycle of violence and convey to all victims of domestic violence that:

- The medical profession cares.
- No person deserves to be beaten.
- This is not your fault.
- Battering is a crime.
- Partner abuse is common for all types of women.
- Abuse is usually a repetitive event.
- Help is available.

The most important contribution physicians can make to ending abuse and protecting the health of victims is to identify and acknowledge the abuse. Health care professionals at all levels of training must be taught about identification, assessment, and intervention for survivors of partner abuse.

BIBLIOGRAPHY

American Medical Association. Violence: a compendium from JAMA, American Medical News, and the specialty journals of the American Medical Association. Chicago: AMA, 1992.

Ferrato D. Living with the enemy. New York: Aperture Foundation, 1991.

Hoff L. Battered women as survivors. New York: Routledge, 1990.

Kilgore N. Sourcebook for working with battered women. Volcano, Calif.: Volcano Press, 1992.

Martin D. Battered wives. Volcano, Calif.: Volcano Press, 1981.

Salber PR, Taliaferro E. The physician's guide to domestic violence. Volcano, Calif.: Volcano Press, 1995.

Sonkin DJ, Durphy M. Learning to live without violence: a handbook for men. Volcano, Calif.: Volcano Press, 1989.

Stark E, Flitcraft A. Spouse abuse. In Rosenberg M, Fenley M, eds. Violence in America: a public health approach. New York: Oxford University Press, 1991.

Walker LE. The battered woman. New York: Harper & Row, 1979.

160

Sexuality

PHYLLIS C. LEPPERT

Primary Care for Women, edited by Phyllis C. Leppert and Fred M. Howard. Lippincott-Raven Publishers, Philadelphia © 1997.

Sexual health is an important aspect of life that must be addressed by all primary care providers. Not only is sexual health a part of psychological health, but physical health is affected by sexual behavior as well. A person's sexual behavior can lead to overall satisfaction with life. Conversely, if sexual behavior is allowed to become out of control, adverse health consequences may result (eg, unwanted pregnancies; sexually transmitted diseases, including infection with HIV; acts of violence and aggression toward a sexual partner). It is helpful for primary care providers to present the concept of healthy and safe sex to their patients. Healthy sexuality implies conscious and rational choices, including abstinence.

Althof and Levine have advanced the concept of *sexual equilibrium* to help clinicians understand the intangible, subtle, and powerful forces that occur in the arena of sexuality. In their words, "sexual equilibrium is the delicate changeable balance of psychological forces between partners and is important because the result of this balance is either sexual comfort or sexual anxiety in each partner." They further point out that sexual equilibrium enhances a person's life. In a state of sexual equilibrium, each partner enjoys intimate physical relations and enjoys them frequently. When two people are in a state of sexual disequilibrium, there is disappointment. The partners feel diminished and, therefore, seek sexual contact more and more infrequently.

These authors have proposed that there are three components of sexual identity and three components of sexual function that contribute to sexual equilibrium. The interaction of these components and the regard by a woman that her partner's components are in balance is the state of sexual equilibrium.

COMPONENTS OF SEXUAL IDENTITY

Gender identity is a woman's sense of herself as female and a man's sense of himself as male. This identity is formed in early childhood and evolves throughout life. Life circumstances, such as loss of work, severe illness, or an accident, may make a person feel "less of a woman" or "less of a man." His or her self-worth is decreased. In a subtle, complicated way, a diminished sense of gender identity may cause the person to lose sexual desire. In our society, many able-bodied persons view an ill or injured person as an asexual being.

Sexual orientation refers to the gender of the person with whom one wishes to be sexually intimate. A man who keeps his frequent homosexual liaisons a secret from his wife of many years does not have a state of sexual equilibrium with her.

Intention refers to the degree of aggression in sexual fantasy and behavior. Sexual behavior may be used to dominate others. A girl of 14 will find it difficult to be in a state of equilibrium if her sexual partner is a 40-year-old man.

COMPONENTS OF SEXUAL FUNCTIONING

The three components of sexual functioning are sexual desire, sexual arousal, and orgasm. A lack of sexual desire might be due to hidden sexual identity or orientation. It could also reflect nonsexual problems in the relationship—for instance, the partners may not agree on finances, philosophy, or some other area of life, and may not have been able to discuss them or reconcile their differences. One partner may be clinically depressed. Conversely, some people become hypersexual in response to life's problems. A newly divorced woman may engage in promiscuous sexual behavior to counteract her depression and loss of self-esteem.

Arousal patterns in a relationship may enhance it or may contribute to disequilibrium. A woman may want sexual intercourse four times a week, but her husband may want it only once a week, and then only on weekends. This couple can become chronically frustrated and then asexual. A woman who cannot obtain orgasm except on rare occasions often finds tension occurring with her partner.

When partners have similar sexual drives, their equilibrium is easy to maintain. Couples whose functional components are less compatible must work harder to maintain equilibrium.

Couples must understand, especially as they get older, that sexual intimacy involves more than penile–vaginal intercourse. Americans tends to view this type of intercourse as "the real thing," with anything else being incomplete. Nothing could be further from the truth. A broader range of sexual behavior should be encouraged. Hugging, kissing, petting, and oral–genital contact are all part of sexuality and sharing of love. Humans need warmth, caring, and affection, and a person's sexuality contributes to this.

The primary care physician should be alert to a woman patient's sexuality and sexual health. For instance, adolescents need help with sexual feelings in the form of education and anticipatory guidance. Pregnancy and childbirth often disrupt sexual equilibrium. Many menopausal women have changes in their sex lives due to diminished sexual desire and arousal. Dyspareunia may exist because of vaginal dryness. A male partner may be dysfunctional due to illness. Therapeutic medications can interfere with sexual desire and performance. Many of these changes may be physiologic. Humans are sexual beings throughout life: the elderly have sexual desires and needs as well and can be sexually active.

Many of the problems causing disequilibrium in sexual health can be addressed by the primary provider. Other problems are more serious, and the couple should be referred to a specialist with expertise in sexuality. When to refer a couple is always a difficult decision. In general, a good rule is that the physician should do no harm; thus, when the physician has reached the limit of his or her knowledge and skill, a referral should be made.

Information regarding all aspects of sexuality, including sexually transmitted diseases, contraception, techniques of sexual behavior, sexual battering, and psychological considerations, should be available for patients. Nurses and other professional personnel should be aware of the issues of sexuality and how to intervene or counsel patients. For example, a teenage girl may be more comfortable asking and learning from a nurse strategies to avoid unwanted sexual encounters from aggressive boys and men than from the physician.

Sexual intimacy and intercourse should be encouraged throughout pregnancy. However, it is contraindicated after rupture of membranes and in situations of potential preterm labor. Orgasms cause uterine contractions, which are a problem for women with threatened spontaneous abortion or preterm labor.

Primary care physicians must be alert to the subtle, complex interplay of forces and components of sexuality that contribute to a woman's state of sexual equilibrium. To do so, physicians must understand and accept themselves as sexual beings as well. Physicians who are open to their own sexuality are also open and accepting of their patients' sexuality.

BIBLIOGRAPHY

Althof SE, Levine SB. Clinical approach to the sexuality of patients with spinal cord injury. Urol Clin North Am 1993;20:527.

Bachmann GA, Lieblum SR. Sexuality in sexagenarian women. Maturitas 1991;13:43.

Levine S. Sex is not simple. Columbus, Ohio: Ohio Psychology Publications, 1988.

Masters WH, Johnson VE. Human sexual responses. Boston: Little, Brown & Company, 1966:365.

Sarrel PM. Sexuality in the middle years. Obstet Gynecol Clin North Am 1987;14:49.

Sarrel PM. Sexuality and menopause. Obstet Gynecol 1990;75:265.

Sarrel LJ, Sarrel PM. Sexual unfolding: sexual development and sex therapies in late adolescence. Boston: Little, Brown & Company, 1979:353.

Primary Care for Women, edited by Phyllis C. Leppert and Fred M. Howard. Lippincott-Raven Publishers, Philadelphia © 1997.

161
Sexual Assault

JOSEPH KOZLOWSKI

Sexual assault is a medical emergency and is also one of the fastest-growing violent crimes in this country. In 1990, the Department of Justice reported that the annual incidence of sexual assault was 80 per 100,000 women, compared with 17 per 100,000 in 1960, and that these cases accounted for 7% of all violent crimes. However, experts estimate that only 10% to 33% of all cases of sexual assault are reported to authorities.

The major motive for sexual assault is aggression. Sexual assault is defined as any sexual act performed by one person on another without that person's consent. Rape is defined by the U.S. Justice Department as "carnal knowledge" through the use of force or threat of force. Consent is total agreement and is based on choice. Having sex as a result of being tricked or lied to is not consent.

When a victim is sexually assaulted, she loses control over her life for that period of time. She not only feels fear and pain, but can suffer emotionally. This can affect her sexual, physical, and social functioning. It may take years before a victim can put the experience behind her and function on a somewhat normal level. Victims hesitate to report assault because of humiliation, feelings of guilt, fear of retribution, and disillusionment with the criminal justice system.

There have been many mistaken beliefs about sexual assault. Some of these include the notion that women are asking for sex by smiling at a man or by the way they dress or dance. Other beliefs are that in the absence of physical resistance or injury, sexual assault has not occurred, or that sex is a man's right if he spends money on a date. A similar belief is that if a woman knows a man and invites him into her home or is on a date with him, unwanted sex is not rape. The truth is that being on a date or being alone with someone is not an invitation to have sex. Forced sexual intimacy is a form of violence, not an act of manhood.

Common myths concerning rape stem from society's historical attitudes toward women. Rape is not the result of a spontaneous sexual urge. Rape is much more, because it represents a violent assault, rather than a sexual assault, on a woman's body and psyche that often results in physical injury. Acts of mental brutality, threats, and intimidation are common. Death is a common fear of a woman during rape, and in about 1% of rapes, homicide does occur.

MANAGEMENT OF SEXUAL ASSAULT VICTIMS

An estimated 80,000 victims are treated each year, including infants and the elderly. The staff of each medical facility must determine whether it is prepared to meet the needs of a sexual assault victim. A useful approach is to train a team that can work well together. This limits the number of personnel who come in contact with the victim and provides better security in gathering and storing legal evidence. The team can be composed of nurses, physicians, physician assistants, and nurse practitioners, all of whom should be trained in evaluating a sexual assault victim.

In addition to the team, a well-trained counselor who is available 24 hours a day can counsel victims concerning medical, legal, or social problems. Immediate contact with a counselor may be a way to prevent victims from suppressing memory of the assault. The counselor can also offer emotional support during legal proceedings if the victim wishes to prosecute.

Team members should know state and local laws regarding sexual assault. Informed consent must be obtained before collection of evidence and forensic examination of the victim. Obtaining consent allows the victim to regain a sense of control over the examination. The victim should be placed in a private, secure room where a history can be taken and a physical examination performed. The examiner is responsible for treating injuries and performing appropriate laboratory tests to detect, prevent, and treat sexually transmitted infections. Other tests should be performed to detect pregnancy and to prevent it if the victim desires. The victim should meet a support person, such as a rape crisis counselor, preferably before the examiner sees her. The support person can stay with the victim through the examination.

PHYSICAL EXAMINATION

An initial assessment for unstable vital signs, altered consciousness, peritoneal injury, and pain alerts the examining provider to serious injuries. Rape victims can sustain major nongenital physical injuries, and such injuries should be tended to first. If a weapon such as a knife or gun was involved, treatment should follow appropriate resuscitation maneuvers and diagnostic studies.

A few rape victims have moderate to severe genital injuries. Most of these include upper vaginal lacerations, although intraperitoneal extension of such lacerations is rare. Injuries to the anal canal cause mucosal lacerations. The use of photoscopy to evaluate these injuries is justified. Most mucosal injuries need no intervention, as most minor mucosal bleeding resolves without intervention. For some victims, the impending pelvic and rectal examinations may be their first, and these victims need reassurance. All procedures should be explained and the victims should be involved immediately in all decisions regarding the examination and consent forms. This is done to help restore a victim's feeling of self-respect and dignity. Nothing during the examination should suggest force.

After assessing the acute injuries, a nonjudgmental history should be taken. To spare the victim the distress of having to repeat the narration of the assault unnecessarily, only one member of the team should obtain the history. Basic details about the assault are necessary to ensure that all injuries are detected and to guide the medicolegal examination. The victim's general appearance and demeanor should be noted. Some victims remain calm; others are hysterical or even withdrawn. Most victims feel frightened, humiliated, degraded, and angry. A concise history, not excessively detailed, written in a legible fashion works best. Unnecessary, frivolous information may result in discrepancies with the police report that can adversely affect future criminal proceedings: minute details taken at a time of acute emotional crisis may appear inconsistent or contradictory in court.

The history should include the date, time, and location of the assault; the race, identity, and number of assailants; the nature of the physical contacts; and the use of weapons, restraints, foreign bodies, drugs, and alcohol. The body orifices involved (oral, vaginal, or rectal) should be reported. If digital penetration occurred, or if foreign bodies were used, this should also be reported. Questions should be asked about whether the attacker ejaculated and where this occurred. If ejaculation occurred, the examiner should ask whether it occurred on clothing or on the victim's body. Contraceptive devices, such as condoms, may have been used by the attacker or by the victim. The victim may have bathed, douched, showered, urinated or defecated, washed her mouth, brushed her teeth, used a tampon, or changed her clothing. These activities could alter evidence after the assault and should be documented.

Gynecologic medical history should be recorded, including past infections, contraceptive use, last menstrual period, and last consensual intercourse. Also noted should be the victim's gravidity and parity, whether she is pregnant, and the date of her last Pap smear. The medical history should include allergies, any medications the victim is taking, and tetanus immunization status.

Marks of violence should be documented, including scratches, bruises, rope imprints, bite marks, lacerations, points of tenderness, abrasions, ecchymoses, and linear abrasions. Nongenital injuries occur in 20% to 50% of sexual assaults.

Documentation with photographs is indicated if physical trauma is evident. Police agencies can send a qualified forensic photographer to take the photographs. Documentation on a traumagram or body diagram creates a visual depiction of injuries.

EVIDENCE GATHERING

Saliva

The first step in gathering evidence involves oral swabs and smears. Saliva samples should be obtained and the swabs streaked over clean glass slides and placed in slide folders. The swabs are then air-dried before they are placed in sealed paper box containers marked "oral swabs." An additional saliva sample is obtained on a filter paper the victim places in her mouth. Only the victim may handle the filter paper with bare hands. The filter paper is thoroughly saturated, air-dried, and inserted into the envelope marked "saliva sample."

Trace Evidence

To minimize the loss of evidence, the victim should disrobe over a large piece of examination table paper or a clean sheet. Clothes and the paper or sheet are then placed in a paper (not plastic) bag for forensic testing. Wet or damp clothing should be air-dried before packaging; if wet clothing is wrapped, mold and mildew can damage evidence. The victim's underwear should be collected and placed in the paper bag provided. A Wood's lamp can be used to locate semen stains. Care should be taken not to shake the clothing, as microscopic evidence may be lost. If the victim has changed clothes after the assault, the examiner should ask her to bring the clothing in for the police so evidence may be collected.

Debris Collection

Debris (eg, leaves, fibers, glass, dirt, or hair) is sometimes found on the victim's body. To collect this evidence, the victim is placed on a paper sheet and she brushes off the debris. Any foreign material found on her body is collected, and the folded sheet is placed in the appropriate envelope.

Dried Secretions

Dried secretions from bites or ejaculation deposits are sampled by taking a swab moistened with one or two drops of water or saline. The area of the stain or suspected dry secretion is swabbed carefully, and the swab is allowed to air-dry. These swabs are placed in an envelope marked "dried secretions."

Fingernail Scrapings

Many times women scratch their attackers, although some victims may not realize this. To collect evidence, a paper sheet with a wooden or plastic scraper is provided for each of the victim's hands. Each hand in turn is held over the paper sheet when scraping all fingernails so that any debris falls on the paper. After all the fingers have been scraped, the scraper is placed in the center of the paper, and the paper is folded and placed in an envelope. Each paper is marked "left" or "right" for the respective hands.

Pulled Head Hairs

Pulling hair strands for evidence collection is considered by many to be traumatic to victims of sexual assault. Examiners must use their judgment, based on the victim's physical and emotional well-being and her decision. If the victim agrees to the gathering of head hair, the examiner should use the thumb and forefinger, not forceps or scissors, to pull five hairs from each of five scalp locations for a total of 25 hairs. These hairs are placed in an envelope.

Pubic Hair Combings

A sterile comb and paper sheet should be provided for collecting pubic hair combings. The paper sheet is removed and placed under the victim's genital area. Using the comb provided, pubic hair is combed in downward strokes so that any loose hair or debris falls on the paper sheet. To reduce embarrassment and increase a sense of control for the victim, she may prefer to do the combing. The sheet is carefully removed. The comb is placed in the center of the sheet and the sheet is folded and returned to the envelope marked "pubic hair combings."

Pulled Pubic Hairs

Pulling pubic hair for evidence is another traumatic experience for sexual assault victims. Again, professional judgment regarding whether to complete this step should be based on the victim's physical and emotional well-being and preference. She may feel more comfortable pulling these hairs herself. The thumb and forefingers, not forceps, are used to pull 15 full-length hairs from various locations of the pubic area for sampling. The hairs are placed in the envelope designated "pulled pubic hairs."

PELVIC EXAMINATION

Genital trauma may be a result of sexual assault. The inner thighs, vulva, and vagina are assessed for signs of trauma such as bruises, lacerations, and erythema. Injuries to the genitalia should be characterized and photographs taken. Small abrasions of the fourchette and distal vagina may be evaluated with the aid of a colposcope, if available. Injuries to the labia and clitoris, with evidence of erythema and engorgement, may last for several hours after intercourse. The examination should evaluate the status of the pelvic reproductive organs and should document possible infections. It is generally unnecessary to use a speculum.

When evaluating injuries and collecting specimens in prepubescent or adolescent females, an adult-sized speculum should never be used; even a pediatric speculum may cause further trauma. Specimens for culture and forensic analysis may be obtained by using a glass eyedropper or a cotton-tipped applicator. For prepubescent children, a vaginal, not cervical, specimen is indicated for a culture to test for sexually transmitted disease. If extensive injury or the presence of foreign bodies cannot be ruled out, the examination might cause further trauma to the child. If the child is too distressed to cooperate, an examination under anesthesia is appropriate.

In adults, appropriate specimens include cervical, gonorrhea, and chlamydia cultures. Using two swabs simultaneously, the vaginal vault is carefully swabbed. Both swabs are allowed to air-dry and are placed in boxes marked "vaginal DNA." Using two additional swabs, the same swabbing procedure is repeated and two smears are prepared on slides. These are allowed to air-dry. When the slides are dry, they are placed in slide folders marked "vaginal smears."

ANAL SWABS AND SMEARS

The anal region is examined if anal penetration has occurred. Many victims do not admit that anal penetration has occurred due to embarrassment, so an anal examination should be performed on every victim. Signs of trauma may include laceration, abrasion, or edema. Swabs of the anal region should be moistened with saline or distilled water before the collection process. The anus is carefully swabbed with two swabs, and two smears are prepared on slides. The swabs and smears are allowed to air-dry. Cultures can be taken at this time if appropriate. The swabs and smears are placed in boxes marked "anal."

KNOWN BLOOD SAMPLES

Using the blood tubes provided for collecting serum and plasma, and following normal phlebotomy techniques, blood samples are drawn. The tubes are filled to maximum volume and returned to tube holders. If the victim received a blood transfusion before the examination, "transfusion" should be written on a piece of paper and taped to the blood tubes.

Blood tests to be performed include those for pregnancy, hepatitis B, and HIV, as well as rapid plasma reagin tests (RPR) and the Venereal Disease Research Laboratory (VDRL) test. Basic information about the risk of HIV infection, methods of testing, and confidentiality should be reviewed with the victim. Counseling should also be provided. The patient should be told of the need for HIV retesting in 12 weeks, 6 months, and 1 year. RPR should also be repeated in 12 weeks.

SEXUALLY TRANSMITTED DISEASES

Gonorrhea, syphilis, and *Chlamydia trachomatis* are the three most common STDs transmitted during a sexual assault. Other infections, such as *Trichomonas vaginalis*, genital herpes, genital warts, HIV, and hepatitis B also can be transmitted. Prophylactic antibiotic therapy is routinely prescribed. If the victim is known to be pregnant at the time of the assault, 250 mg erythromycin every 6 hours is given orally for 10 days to prevent chlamydia infection. If the victim is not pregnant, 100 mg doxycycline twice a day is given orally for 10 days. For gonorrhea, one dose of 125 mg ceftriaxone should be given intramuscularly. For trichomonas infection, one dose of 2 g metronidazole is given orally. Hepatitis B vaccine can be offered after confirmation of positive antibody status. Treatment is 0.06 mL/kg hepatitis B immune globulin intramuscularly, to be repeated in 1 month if the victim's serology is negative. Tetanus prophylaxis is appropriate for victims with trauma who are not current with their immunizations.

PREGNANCY PREVENTION

Patients who wish pregnancy prevention can be given two oral contraceptive tablets, each containing 50 mg ethinyl estradiol, taken 12 hours apart, or three contraceptive tablets, each containing 35 mg ethinyl estradiol, taken 12 hours apart. This treatment should be offered regardless of the time of the last menstrual period. An antiemetic (eg, one promethazine [Phenergan] rectal suppository, 25 mg) can prevent nausea and vomiting caused by the oral contraceptives. Statistically, the risk of pregnancy is small: 2% to 4% of women not using contraceptives at the time of assault become pregnant. Hormonal therapy is effective if given within 72 hours of the assault. If pregnancy is diagnosed as a consequence of an assault, the victim can be counseled on her options, including pregnancy termination.

FOLLOW-UP CARE AND REFERRAL

Many sexual assault victims are lost to follow-up care. They also have limited recall about retesting, treatment, and referral. They should receive a sheet that outlines a list of follow-up appointments and treatments received during the evaluation. The outline should list a schedule of follow-up laboratory testing with dates. These tests include STD cultures after antibiotic therapy and repeat blood tests for syphilis and HIV at 3- and 6-month intervals. Information about referral agencies, such as rape crisis groups, and names and telephone numbers of staff members at various medical facilities should also be given.

Some communities have rape crisis centers that provide counseling and support for the victim. Some victims may hesitate to request help because they want to forget the experience. It is desirable to make a referral at the initial visit. Support may include resources for housing, money, child care, notification of significant others, and counseling about future litigation. Talking about the event is helpful. The initial impact of an assault is shock, disorganization, disbelief, and disorientation. Victims do not feel safe even in their own homes. There may be a long period of adjustment. Friends and family may believe that the victim has adjusted to the event, but the victim may be denying the experience and making unrealistic attempts to resume everyday life. Family members may experience the same reactions as the victim. Initially, feelings of hopelessness, disbelief, and shock are common. Victims can experience somatic symptoms, such as headaches, abdominal pain, sleep disturbances, nightmares, eating disorders, nervousness, and irritability. These complaints may actually be signs of posttraumatic stress disorder. Some victims, when exposed to certain stimuli, can undergo flashbacks in which they reexperience the assault. These symptoms can persist for weeks, months, or years.

Recovery is influenced by the victim's personality and by the characteristics of the assault. Date rape victims feel as if they can no longer trust anyone close to them. Victims assaulted by strangers feel as if there is no way to prevent an attack and no environment in which they are completely safe. In the last stages of integration, the victim accepts the reality of the assault and the validity of her emotional response.

Primary care physicians and obstetrician-gynecologists often provide ongoing care for sexual assault victims. Understanding the psychological changes that occur after an assault is paramount in being able to treat these patients. Most victims report fearing death and feeling unsafe. A sense of shame, guilt, helplessness, and lowered self-esteem can affect relationships with boyfriends, spouses, and family. Depression is a common consequence of an assault.

Various sexual dysfunctions can occur, including orgasmic failure. Some victims prefer a prolonged abstinence from sexual activity or experience altered sexual response. Some permanently decrease their sexual activity. The spouse or significant other typically reacts in an overprotective fashion. This may make the victim feel she cannot take care of herself, so such overprotectiveness should be discouraged. Allowing the victim to express herself, particularly with feelings of anger, provides an important step in regaining self-control.

Spouses and significant others of sexual assault victims often feel helpless and vulnerable and may also suffer from depression.

SUMMARY

Sexual assault is one of the fastest-growing violent crimes in the United States. Victims of sexual assault sustain both physical and emotional trauma. Health care professionals caring for these women have a duty to provide sensitive, compassionate treatment. Professional objectivity, in compliance with state statutory requirements, in evaluating sexual assault victims is paramount. This can help ensure that vital information is accessible for criminal proceedings. Follow-up and sustained psychological support are essential to help the victim make the transition from victim to survivor and allow healthy daily activities to resume.

BIBLIOGRAPHY

Beebe DK. Emergency management of the adult female rape victim. Am Fam Physician 1991;43:2041.

Burgess AW, Holmstrom LL. Rape: sexual disruption and recovery. Am J Orthopsychiatry 1979;49:648.

Dupre AR, Hampton HL, Morrison H, Meeks GR. Sexual assault. Obstet Gynecol Survey 1993;48:640.

Dwyer JD. Examination and treatment of the sexual assault victim. Physician Assistant 1987;11:100.

Geist F. Sexually related trauma. Emerg Med Clin North Am 1988;6:439.

Green WM. Rape: the evidential examination and management of the adult female victim. Lexington, Mass.: Lexington Books, 1988.

Hampton HL. Care of the woman who has been raped. N Engl J Med 1995;332:234.

Hick DJ, Minkin MJ, Solola A. Examining the rape victim. Patient Care 1986;20:98.

Jenny C, Hooten TM, Bowers A, et al. Sexually transmitted diseases in victims of rape. N Engl J Med 1990;322:713.

Kirkland K, Mason RE. Victims of crime: the internist's role in treatment. South Med J 1992;85:965.

Kobernick ME, Seifert S, Sanders AB. Emergency department management of the sexual assault victim. J Emerg Med 1985;2:205.

Martin CA, Warfield MC, Braen GR. Physician's management of the psychological aspects of rape. JAMA 1983;249:501.

Silverman D, McCombie SL. Counseling mates and families of rape victims. In: McCombie SL, ed. The rape crisis intervention handbook: a guide to victim care. New York: Plenum Press, 1980:173.

United States Federal Bureau of Investigation. Uniform crime reports for crime in the United States 1988. Washington, DC: U.S. Government Printing Office, 1988:46.

Wertheimer AJ. Examination of the rape victim. Postgrad Med 1982; 71:173.

Woodling BA, Evans JR, Bradbury MD. Sexual assault: rape and molestation. Clin Obstet Gynecol 1977;20:509.

Young WW, Bracken AC, Goddard MA, Mathison S. Sexual assault: review of a national model protocol for forensic and medical evaluation. New Hampshire Sexual Assault Medical Examination Protocol Project Committee. Obstet Gynecol 1992;80:878.

Primary Care for Women, edited by Phyllis C. Leppert and Fred M. Howard. Lippincott-Raven Publishers, Philadelphia © 1997.

162
Posttraumatic Stress Disorder

PHYLLIS C. LEPPERT

In the 19th century, physicians identified a cluster of symptoms associated with trauma and developed treatment methods for this disorder. However, the symptoms of this stress-induced emotional disorder have been known since antiquity. They were well described by Homer and Cicero. What is now known as posttraumatic stress disorder (PTSD) was originally recognized in soldiers exposed to the death and carnage of battle. Pepys described the syndrome in his diary of the Great London Fire of 1666, and physicians described it in the American Civil War. In World War I, it was known as "shell shock." In World War II, the symptoms were correctly identified as both physiologic and psychological. The diagnosis is made only when there is a severe stressor, "outside the range of usual human experience." A modern example is the Oklahoma City bombing in 1995.

The cluster is a triad of symptoms that includes an intrusive, reexperienced event; avoidance responses to evidence of the event and generalized emotional numbing and isolation; and physiologic systemic arousal that does not predate the trauma. Persons experiencing PTSD have witnessed or been confronted with events that involve actual or threatened death, serious injury, or a threat to the physical integrity of others or self. The emotional response in adults is one of intense fear, helplessness, or horror.

Children become disorganized or agitated. The trauma is relived by recurrent and intrusive distressing recollections, including images. In children, this may occur in play. Recurrent dreams occur as well. There is usually a sense that the traumatic event is actually recurring. This is felt as reliving the trauma, with illusions, hallucinations, and dissociative episodes. There is then intense psychological distress from the cues that come to symbolize the trauma. The physiologic symptoms are activated by these internal and external cues, and the victim comes to avoid these disturbing stimuli. The traumatized person avoids thoughts, feelings, or discussions associated with the event, as well as people identified with the trauma. The victim feels detached and estranged, is unable to have loving feelings, and is disinterested in participating in social activities.

To a person with PTSD, the future seems short: "I'll never marry," "I'll die young." Physiologic symptoms include trouble falling asleep or waking up early, outbursts of anger, exaggerated startle, and difficulty in concentration. Many persons affected are hypervigilant. By definition, the symptoms must be of at least 1 month's duration and produce clinically significant distress or social impairment. PTSD is acute if the duration of symptoms is less than 3 months and chronic if it has lasted more than 3 months. In delayed-onset PTSD, the symptoms occur 6 months or more after the stressful event.

In the last decade, the concept of PTSD has been broadened and is used to include symptoms that follow combat trauma, rape, torture, natural disasters, and acute and chronic medical disorders, as well as other categories. This widening of the concept has generated controversy. The current criteria for acute PTSD require that symptoms must follow the trauma, not precede it, and cannot be due to the effect of drug abuse or medication. The symptoms must last at least 2 days and occur within 4 weeks of the event.

Severe trauma, such as torture, rape, or combat, produces PTSD in many persons. The prevalence of PTSD for combat veterans is about 30%; it is over 90% in prisoners of war or victims of torture.

The natural history of PTSD is not always clear, but it seems to be severe for several years and then gradually diminishes. Sleep difficulties and intrusive thoughts persist. Persons so affected carefully avoid anything reminding them of the trauma. Persons who have experienced PTSD usually have a marked decrease in tolerance for serious trauma of any type. However, victims can let go of the memories and the event and lead successful lives. Over time, those who have persistent symptoms have chronic depression and generalized anxiety. The incidence of PTSD after rape or assault in women may exceed 50% during the first months after the occurrence. In several months and up to 1 year, it is 25% to 30%, and after several years it is 5% to 10%.

The differential diagnosis of PTSD must include other disorders with similar symptoms. Other illnesses, such as schizophrenia, could be considered. Depression, anxiety, and substance abuse should also be considered as potential diagnoses. Extreme trauma, such as occurs in concentration camp victims, hostages, or battered women, produces a form of PTSD in which a wide range of symptoms and personality changes occur. In childhood, chronic sexual or physical abuse may lead to a substance abuse disorder, eating disorders, antisocial personality, borderline personality disorder, chronic pain disorder, or hypochondria.

The clinician must be sensitive and allow a person with PTSD to have psychological space. Comments such as, "That must have been very painful" may appear glib. The clinician will have personal emotional reactions to the description of severe trauma as well. PTSD is often missed. The history should be taken gently. The person may be asked, "Have you ever been in a war? a disaster? a severe accident?" "Have you ever been attacked or assaulted?" The clinician could say. "We have learned that physical and sexual abuse is more common than we thought." This statement could be followed by gentle further inquiry. These questions should not be asked initially in the history taking.

PTSD does not involve the normal traumatic stress recovery process: it is more intense and the symptoms are more diverse and more numerous. The primary care provider should be alert to the possibility of PTSD and should refer women to experts for therapy. Therapy may consist of individual psychotherapy, group and family therapy, and pharmacotherapy.

Primary providers, when caring for persons who have sustained acute trauma, can take steps to prevent PTSD. Victims of rape should be offered crisis intervention and counseling. The information given must be honest, adequate, unambiguous, and timely. Victims of a disaster or trauma such as rape need to feel secure. Psychological support, defusing, debriefing, and sometimes psychopharmacologic treatment are needed. Customs and rituals are important in all cultures and assist in the grief and mourning process. They may promote a feeling of safety. Rituals are also carried out within the community, and this helps in expressing feelings and providing a sense of relief.

Emotional first aid involves the following principles:

- Proximity: treat as close as possible to the place where the emotional breakdown occurred
- Immediacy: initiate treatment as quickly as possible
- Expectancy: the patient should be expected to recover quickly
- Simplicity: treatment should be simple.

Emotional first aid also includes acceptance of feelings and symptoms, identification of resources and activities, realization of the psychologically painful situation and acceptance of reality, optimism, not blaming others, acceptance of help and support, and the resumption of daily life.

Persons at high risk for stress-related psychological disorders include survivors with psychiatric problems; close relatives of suddenly or traumatically deceased persons; children, especially if separated from parents; the elderly, mentally retarded, and handicapped; traumatized survivors; and body handlers.

Although primary physicians are not involved in the ongoing therapy of persons with definite PTSD or with the total psychological therapy of persons at risk of developing it, primary physicians should be alert to the existence of PTSD and dedicated to preventing it.

BIBLIOGRAPHY

Allen SN, Bloom SL. Group and family treatment of post-traumatic stress disorder. Psychiatr Clin North Am 1994;17:425.

Blank AS Jr. Clinical detection, diagnosis, and differential diagnosis of post-traumatic stress disorder. Psychiatr Clin North Am 1994;17:351.

Lundin T. The treatment of acute trauma: post-traumatic stress disorder prevention. Psychiatr Clin North Am 1994;17:385.

McFarlane AC. Individual psychotherapy for post-traumatic stress disorder. Psychiatr Clin North Am 1994;17:393.

Sutherland SM, Davidson, JRT. Pharmacotherapy for post-traumatic stress disorder. Psychiatr Clin North Am 1994;17:409.

Tomb DA. The phenomenology of post-traumatic stress disorder. Psychiatr Clin North Am 1994;17:237.

Primary Care for Women, edited by Phyllis C. Leppert and Fred M. Howard. Lippincott-Raven Publishers, Philadelphia © 1997.

163

Cultural Competency

PHYLLIS C. LEPPERT

CULTURE AND HEALTH

The world is made up of numerous groups of peoples, each with different ways of living that have been developed over centuries. These ways of living are transmitted from one generation to another. The sum of the language, ideas, customs, skills, and arts of a given people makes up their culture and tradition. Culture, a people's treasury of information, is reflected in how its members interact with one another. Interactions develop into rules of living aimed at increasing the quality of life of those in the group. Rules of considerate behavior toward others form each society's good manners.

Certain principles of behavior, such as honoring parents and other elders and assuming kinship obligations, as well as taboos against murder and incest, are universal values. All human groups value the arts, music, and education. Group traditions reflect these values. Above all, all human cultures respect and venerate a spiritual life, culminating in deeply held religious and ethical precepts. In all societies, these spiritual values hold the group members to their principles of behavior. Although a culture always includes the group's core values, culture and tradition are ever-changing, so tension can develop between generations.

All cultures have rules of behavior regarding outsiders, intended to protect the society's core values and to provide codes of conduct toward strangers. Most of these rules relate to peaceful methods of conflict resolution. When the deeply held values of one culture are challenged by another culture, dispute ensues. These clashes can escalate into a verbal war or a situation in which all control is lost and force is used to settle the dispute.

Culture and tradition influence the way people look at and respond to health and illness in both spoken and unspoken ways (Table 163-1). Medical and other health professions have cultures with traditional codes of conduct and behavior that have been passed from generation to generation as well. This professional culture is pervasive. When persons of diverse cultures become initiated into the culture of medicine, they become socialized by it and adopt its culture. In the process, to some degree, they do not continue to accept all the values of their culture of birth. Thus, it is not necessarily true that all physicians from one particular cultural group can accept and, therefore, help all nonphysician members of their own culture.

World society includes tremendous cultural diversity. Knowledge of other cultures and contact with persons of other societies have been increasing rapidly in the past 50 years due to the ease of world travel and the ease of communication, first with radio and television and now with computer networks. Language, too, is changing: more societies are incorporating English words into their native tongues (eg, Japanese-English, Spainglish, scientific English, German-English). There is a worldwide youth culture of rock music, Levi's, Coke, fast food, and slang. These youths communicate via the Internet. Often young people have increasingly different cultural values from their parents.

The North American continent, and the United States in particular, is becoming more multiracial and more multicultural than in the past. Our definition of minority is becoming meaningless. There has been an 89.7% increase in the Asian population, a 50% increase in people of Hispanic origin, a 42.8% increase in Native Americans, Eskimos, and Aleuts, and a 14.9% increase in African-Americans from 1981 to 1991, but only a 4.2% increase in whites. In 6% of the states in the U.S., the number of blacks, Hispanics, and Asians combined exceeds that of whites.

As the United States changes, a great challenge to the health care system is to develop ways to welcome newcomers and native-born minority cultures into the mainstream. For people of various cultures to collaborate rather than to develop conflict, most members of a specific culture must accept and understand diversity. Tradition and culture affect in broad ways a person's behavior and attitudes toward illness. Therefore, primary care physicians must develop cultural competency. Such competency reduces the sociocultural barriers to access to health care by improving patient/provider relationships. Sociocultural barriers to health care lead to inefficient use of health care services and negative health outcomes.

The culture of health care is in transition. In the past, and currently, it has emphasized hierarchic attitudes with a paternalism in teaching ("We know what's best for you"). This approach is applied to women in their families and to medical students alike. Progress is measured solely by statistical analysis of outcomes, not by the quality of the interpersonal relationships as well. Patients are expected to conform to physicians' expectations and are not to ask too many or too challenging questions. The health care provider culture assumes that all causes of illness are scientifically based and that spiritual or religious beliefs play no role: technology is supreme. The patient alone is expected to consent to treatment, whereas in many cultures the extended family plays a part in decision making.

The health care system in the United States is designed to offer a diagnosis and a choice of effective methods of treatment to the patient, who in turn is expected to make decisions and comply with all prescribed therapy. Patients, and perhaps one family member, are expected to arrive on time and to understand the course of treatment and the nature of the illness without challenging the physician excessively.

Persons who are ill are dependent, vulnerable, and understandably anxious regarding their disease and its outcome. The need is to trust the physician and other health care providers. In communities, the history and reputation of an institution and the providers have a large role in determining a patient's level of trust. However, many cultures in our country have a profound distrust of the medical establishment. For example, because physicians are required in many states to refer infants of drug-abusing women to child protective agencies, doctors, midwives, and hospitals are thought of as "fetal police," creating a barrier to prenatal care. Native Americans may distrust the Indian Health Service, because in past years Native American women were used as research subjects without their permission. If the customs of individual women are not understood or respected, barriers to health care are created.

The modern, future-thinking health care provider accepts cultural diversity and educates patients for autonomy, personal decision making, and self-care. The emphasis in the new culture of medicine is on personal responsibility for health care. Health care

Table 163-1. Examples of Cross-Cultural Competence

OLD PARADIGM	CROSS-CULTURAL COMPETENCE
A physician addresses a 50-year-old black woman by her first name.	This same patient is addressed by all health care workers as Mrs. Clifford. Using first names for patients, especially for minority patients, shows disrespect.
A nurse insists that a young Hispanic mother sign a consent form for a cesarean section.	The entire staff involves the woman's husband and family in a discussion of the need to undergo a cesarean birth. Among many women of Hispanic heritage, it is customary to have a man give consent for treatment.
A woman misses her appointment for colposcopy. The nurses in the clinic make many attempts to reach her by telephone without success.	The hospital asks a peer health counselor to locate the patient and explain to her the reason why the colposcopy is necessary. When the peer counselor locates the patient, she discovers that the woman's phone has been disconnected because of lack of money to pay the phone bill. The woman's 5-year-old son had a high fever and diarrhea on the day of the colposcopy appointment. She had just enough money and time to get him to a pediatrician. He was hospitalized.
An elderly Chinese woman is asked by her doctor to go to the lab to have blood drawn for tests. She takes the lab slip but does not get the tests as ordered.	The primary care provider notes the woman's hesitation and asks her what she is worried about. She tells him that she believes that blood taken from her body will never be replenished and she is weak already. The provider spends time explaining how blood is replaced.
A woman sees a gynecologist for the first time. He is sensitive to her needs but keeps insisting that she consider using birth control. She had filled in a form saying she was sexually active. She is "not married." The woman is upset and refuses to see this gynecologist again.	The physician takes time in asking the sexual history. In asking about sexual activity, he probes gently. One question asked very openly is, "Do you have sex with men, women, or both?" He then learns that she is a lesbian in a long-term committed relationship.
A couple is newly arrived in the United States from Afghanistan. The wife is obviously in pain. They do not speak English well, so an interpreter is found. The interpreter appears to be having some difficulty interpreting the woman's symptoms. The doctor is rushed. He cannot find any abnormalities on physical examination so he sends the patient home. She returns later with a ruptured ectopic pregnancy and is immediately admitted to the operating room.	The physician notices that the interpreter is not able to communicate well with the couple. He takes the time to discover the problem. The interpreter speaks Farsi; the couple speak Pashto. The couple and the interpreter are attempting to speak to each other in Dari, but much historical information is lost. The physician admits the patient for appropriate tests and an unruptured ectopic is diagnosed.
A civil engineer from Bolivia is visiting a large urban area on business. He becomes ill and seeks care at a hospital. He is talked down to in English and spoken to loudly and very slowly.	The man is greeted courteously by staff. He can relate his circumstances and is given appropriate and concerned care.
A young woman has recently moved to a northern city from a farm in the south. She has four small children and is 4 months pregnant. She is always late for her appointments and is made to wait until everyone else is seen before she can be cared for.	The staff show concern and inquire about her difficulties. She has no one to take care of her children, so she must bring them to the prenatal clinic for her appointments. She needs to take two buses to get to the clinic, and she does not read. A peer counselor arranges for help with learning the bus route and planning her trips. She is also referred to a literacy program for help. One of her first triumphs is learning to recognize the signs on the buses. Over the course of her pregnancy, she learns to read the bus route map and schedules.

is becoming more ambulatory, community-linked, and focused. This transition is more difficult for some members than for others.

SOCIOECONOMIC BARRIERS TO HEALTH CARE ACCESS

Some of the socioeconomic barriers to care are language, cultural traditions, insensitivity of the provider, complexity of the health care system, and an inadequate relation between the hospital and the community.

Despite the widespread use of English worldwide, many persons living in the United States, especially older adults, do not understand English. One person in seven over age 5 grew up or is growing up speaking a language other than English. Millions of persons speaking English as their primary tongue do not read or write it. Most hospitals and health care facilities have taken only limited action in response, posting a few bilingual signs and translating a few brochures into a second language.

Many people also seek traditional healers to remove a hex while under a doctor's care. Others visit spiritual centers or use home herbal remedies. They apply various poultices to reduce fevers, or get massage therapy. When primary care physicians ignore the traditions of various cultures, frustration, miscommunication, and treatment breakdown result.

Health care providers must understand what various cultures believe is appropriate behavior. For instance, some obstetrician-gynecologists tend to call patients by their first names. In many cultures, especially among the elderly and among Asians and African-Americans, this is a sign of disrespect. In some cultures, the man gives permission for health care first before the woman seeking that care.

Many cultures expect physicians and other health care providers to dress formally and wear white coats. When they appear in casual attire, patients distrust them because their clothing is perceived as accompanied by a casual, noncaring attitude.

A geneticist, who is a longtime member of a team of scientists in the forefront of deciphering the human genetic code, was once on vacation and in the neighborhood of a large family who had been the subject of one of his investigations. He had built up over many years a relationship of respect and trust with the elderly patriarch of the family. Because that area of the United States included some interesting and spectacular scenery, the geneticist's family pressed him to take them to the family's neighborhood. The geneticist refused because he had only jeans and sport shirts. "This family has always seen me as a professional in business suit and tie, and I will not belittle them by going to their neighborhood in blue jeans. It will severely jeopardize my relationship with them," he said. In the health care setting, the primary care provider must dress and act in ways those seeking care expect and will accept.

Our system of health care assumes that all persons in need understand how it works and that everyone can comply—and is willing to do so—with its rules and regulations. A hospital's detailed and complex procedures surrounding admission, visiting hours, and meal times are confusing to patients and their families. For instance, dinner is often served at 4:45 to 5:30 p.m., an hour that is not usually considered dinner time. For many people, the incredible size of hospital buildings, the bureaucracy, the voluminous paperwork and documentation, and the constant discussions by staff using professional jargon create a negative ambience.

Our system ignores issues of cultural diversity. Thus, ethnic minorities, newcomers to the United States, and the poor have difficulty negotiating the system's complexities and receiving appropriate and necessary services.

Hospitals and other health care organizations do not adequately assess the needs of the populations they serve. Healthy hospital/community relations mean listening to the women of the community to learn the community's culture and providing services appropriate to them, not in a way that serves the culture of the institution. Therefore, community-based initiatives and partnerships with respected community groups are necessary. Public health issues such as violence and substance abuse must be addressed.

The Opening Doors Project has formulated strategies to identify socioeconomic barriers and to create culturally competent health care organizations. The first step is to discover what local sociocultural barriers exist. The community and providers are asked to define barriers; primary care physicians and other providers often have good insight into culturally based barriers that their patients have identified. Questions are asked through surveys, focus groups, and self-examination. The group should ask what steps need to be taken to attract and keep diverse groups of patients.

The second step is to reach out to the community. Direct services such as education and outreach programs staffed with community members open doors, as do medical services in schools and community settings. Partnerships with churches, social agencies, and other community organizations help establish cultural competency.

Communication obstacles must be removed to increase access for those who do not speak English. Forms, patient education materials, and signs must be translated. Interpreters need to be hired; bilingual staff members are helpful, and language classes can be held for staff members. A phone line for those who do not speak English is helpful. Some communities develop a language book. All staff members must attend cultural sensitivity training to reduce the misunderstandings of nonverbal communication.

The diversity of the Board of Directors and staff should be increased. All levels of workers in the health care institution should represent the racial, cultural, and ethnic diversity of the community. The medical profession must make every effort to recruit members from many racial and cultural groups.

Procedures need to be modified to make the first contact through the last experience less stressful and more responsive. Paperwork needs to be streamlined. Primary care providers must ask if the information obtained is necessary. Communication between various departments of the hospital must be enhanced: for instance, a patient should not need to tell everyone the same facts of her medical history over and over. Important medical historical facts and laboratory information can be put on a form that the patient keeps at home.

The physical setting of the health care facility sends a message, either "welcome" or "this is not a comfortable place." At minimal expense, physical facilities can be made inviting. Meals can be changed to accommodate patients of diverse backgrounds, as food is a vital link to a person's culture.

Finally, others in the profession and in the community should be educated about cultural diversity and acceptance.

STAGES OF CROSS-CULTURAL COMPETENCE

Primary care providers can take the lead in establishing cross-cultural competence in health care institutions. The National Public Health and Hospital Institute identifies five stages of competence in understanding and accepting cultures other than one's own.

Stage 0 is inaction. No activity or organized, conscious approach or planning for cross-cultural competence is demonstrated. Staff and patients navigate the system as best they can.

In stage 1, symbolic action and initial organization, the institution begins to recognize the diversity of its staff and realizes that diversity exists in its patients and neighboring community. Management states that diversity is an important issue and the institution sets aside special days to "celebrate diversity." Staff committees are instructed by management to address issues of cultural diversity. However, funding is minimal and little community involvement is seen. There is relatively little action.

In stage 2, formalized internal action, the institution has consciously recognized the need to formalize cross-cultural competence. Management is to some extent involved in active leadership, and there has been some financial commitment. Cultural sensitivity training or diversity education for staff is initiated. Committees are organized to address staff diversity. However, physicians may still see these activities as too time-consuming and not of concern. Community interaction and community influence remain minimal, and there is little progress in improving patient-related concerns. There is some recognition of and progress in hiring culturally diverse staff.

In stage 3, the institution has made a commitment to diversity of its staff and has begun formally to identify issues within the organization. Institution-wide diversity initiatives are ongoing. There are viable programs in diversity training. Committees exist with both horizontal and vertical reporting and responsibilities on diversity issues. Plans have been developed to recruit a diverse staff. The administration is fully committed to the issue of cross-cultural competency, and there is an adequate commitment of financial resources. Patient-related diversity issues are addressed and are well incorporated into plans and ongoing programs. Community opinions and experience are considered. However, there is no linkage with staff-centered ideas and patient education and information, nor is cross-cultural competency included in quality outcome indicators.

In stage 4, the institution has become cross-culturally competent. The hospital system network has so accepted diversity that it is a seamless piece of the fabric of the health care network. Diversity is considered part of the business and mission of the institution. There are no walls between the institution and the community it serves. Processes and outcome measures to assess the effectiveness of diversity in the institution are linked with community and patient cross-cultural activities. The health network and community are partners, with a common goal of meeting health care objectives.

In summary, a quote from Lee M. Pachter, D.O., in the *Journal of the American Medical Association* is appropriate:

> A culturally sensitive health care system is one that is not only accessible, but also respects the beliefs, attitudes, and cultural lifestyles of its patients. It is a system that is flexible—one that acknowledges that health and illness are in large part molded by variables such as ethnic values, cultural orientation, religious beliefs, and linguistic considerations. It is a system that acknowledges that in addition to the physiological aspects of disease, the culturally constructed meaning of illness is a valid concern of clinical care. And finally, it is a system that is sensitive to intragroup variations in beliefs and behaviors, and avoids labeling and stereotyping.

BIBLIOGRAPHY

Allport GW. The nature of prejudice. Reading, MA: Addison-Wesley, 1979.

Blendon RJ, Scheck AC, Donelan K, et al. How white and African Americans view their health and social problems: different experiences, different expectations. JAMA 1995;273:341.

Kavanagh KH, Kennedy PH. Promoting cultural diversity: strategies for health care professionals. Newbury Park, CA: Sage Publications, 1992.

Kittler PG, Sucher K. Food and culture in America: a nutrition handbook. New York: Van Nostrand Reinhold, 1989.

Kohn S. Dismantling sociocultural barriers to care. Healthcare Forum Journal 1995;38:30.

Pachter LM. Culture and clinical care: folk illness beliefs and behaviors and their implications for health care delivery. JAMA 1994;271:690.

Randall-David E. Strategies for working with culturally diverse communities and clients. Bethesda, MD: The Association for the Care of Children's Health, 1989.

Smith M, Chang P. Race matters: the role of race and ethnicity in health services research. HSR: Health Services Research 1995;30(Pt 2):145.

Sue S, Moore T, eds. The pluralistic society: a community mental health perspective. New York: Human Sciences Press, 1984.

Walker MH. Building bridges: community health outreach worker programs. New York: United Hospital Fund of New York, 1994.

Woloshin S, Bickell N, Schwartz LM, Gany F, Welch HG. Language barriers in medicine in the United States. JAMA 1995;273:724.

Index

Page numbers followed by *f* indicate figures; page numbers followed by *t* indicate tabular material.

A

B

C

D

E

G

I

N

O

P

Q

W

X

Y

Z